PASCH
3/95
P9-CCC-589

OFFICE PRACTICE OF MEDICINE

WILLIAM T. BRANCH, JR., MD
Associate Professor of Medicine
Harvard Medical School;
Associate Director for Clinical and Educational Programs
and Director, Section on Medical Education,
Division of General Medicine and Primary Care,
Brigham and Women's Hospital,
Harvard Medical School,
Boston, Massachusetts

OFFICE PRACTICE OF MEDICINE

THIRD EDITION

W.B. SAUNDERS COMPANY
A Division of Harcourt Brace & Company
Philadelphia London Toronto Montreal Sydney Tokyo

W.B. SAUNDERS COMPANY
A Division of
Harcourt Brace & Company

The Curtis Center
Independence Square West
Philadelphia, Pennsylvania 19106

Library of Congress Cataloging-in-Publication Data

Office practice of medicine / [edited by] William T. Branch, Jr.—
3rd ed.

p. cm.

Includes bibliographical references and index.

ISBN 0-7216-4338-8

1. Internal medicine. 2. Ambulatory medical care.
I. Branch, William T.
[DNLM: 1. Medicine. 2. Ambulatory Care. WB 100 032 1994]

RC48.034 1994 616-dc20

DNLM/DLC 93-20531

Office Practice of Medicine, Third Edition

ISBN 0-7216-4338-8

Copyright © 1994, 1987, 1982 by W.B. Saunders Company

All rights reserved. No part of this publication may be reproduced or transmitted in any form or by any means, electronic or mechanical, including photocopy, recording, or any information storage and retrieval system, without permission in writing from the publisher.

Printed in the United States of America

Last digit is the print number: 9 8 7 6 5 4 3 2

To my wife,
CAROLYN J. BRANCH,

and my daughter,
KATHERINE MARY SEIBELS BRANCH

Contributors

J. BARCLAY ADAMS, MD, PhD

Instructor in Medicine, Harvard Medical School; Active Staff Physician, New England Deaconess Hospital; and Courtesy Staff Physician, Brigham and Women's Hospital and New England Baptist Hospital, Boston, MA

Antibiotic Prophylaxis for Transient Bacteremias

BRUCE H. ALBRECHT, MD

Assistant Clinical Professor, Department of Obstetrics and Gynecology, University of Colorado Health Sciences Center; Associate Director of Videoscopic Surgery Center, Rose Medical Center; and Medical Director, Conceptions: Reproductive Associates, Denver, CO

The Infertile Couple

RONALD J. ANDERSON, MD

Associate Professor of Medicine, Harvard Medical School; and Director of Clinical Training Programs, Department of Rheumatology, Brigham and Women's Hospital, Boston, MA

Chronic Arthritis

MICHAEL D. APSTEIN, MD

Assistant Professor of Medicine, Harvard Medical School, Boston, MA; Chief, Gastroenterology Division, Brockton–West Roxbury Veterans Affairs Medical Center, Brockton, MA; and Associate Physician, Brigham and Women's Hospital, Boston, MA

Gallstones

HENRIETTA N. BARNES, MD

Assistant Professor of Medicine, Harvard Medical School, Boston, MA; and Staff Physician, Department of Medicine, Cambridge Hospital, Cambridge, MA

Substance Abuse and Addiction in Primary Care Medicine

CRAIG D. BARTH, MS

Chief of Audiology, Hebrew Rehabilitation Center for Aged, Roslindale, MA

Basic Assessment of Auditory Function

MONICA BERTAGNOLLI, MD

Instructor in Surgery, Harvard Medical School; Associate Surgeon, Brigham and Women's Hospital, Boston, MA

Lymph Nodes and Subcutaneous Masses

DON C. BIENFANG, MD

Assistant Professor of Ophthalmology, Harvard Medical School; and Surgeon, Brigham and Women's Hospital, Boston, MA

Ophthalmologic Problems

JUDYANN BIGBY, MD

Assistant Professor of Medicine, Harvard Medical School; and Physician, Department of Medicine, Division of General Medicine and Primary Care, Brigham and Women's Hospital, Boston, MA

Substance Abuse and Addiction in Primary Care Medicine

JAMES D. BOWEN, MD

Clinical Associate Professor, Department of Medicine, Division of Neurology, University of Washington School of Medicine; Chief, Division of Neurology, Pacific Medical Center; and Chief, Division of Neurology, Providence Medical Center, Seattle, WA

Dementia

WILLIAM T. BRANCH, Jr., MD

Associate Professor of Medicine, Harvard Medical School; Associate Director for Clinical and Educational Programs and Director, Section on Medical Education, Division of General Medicine and Primary Care, Brigham and Women's Hospital, Harvard Medical School, Boston, MA

The Painful or Discharging Ear;
Dyspepsia and Upper Abdominal Pain;
Abnormal Urinalysis;
Sexually Transmitted Diseases;
Urinary Tract Infections;
Monoarticular Arthritis and Acute Polyarticular Synovitis;
Pain in the Shoulder, Neck, and Arm;
Elbow, Hand, Knee, Hip, and Foot Pain;
Vertigo;
Dermatology in Primary Care;
Periodic Health Assessment of Asymptomatic Adults;
Case Finding for Cancer;
Disorders of Eating

EUGENE BRAUNWALD, MD

Hersey Professor of the Theory and Practice of Medicine, Harvard Medical School; and Chairman, Department of Medicine, Brigham and Women's Hospital, Boston, MA

Congestive Heart Failure

JAMES L. BREELING, MD
Instructor in Medicine, Harvard Medical School; and Physician, Department of Medicine, Infectious Diseases Division, Brigham and Women's Hospital, Boston, MA

Community-Acquired Pneumonia;
Fever of Unknown Origin

EDWARD M. BROWN, MD
Associate Professor of Medicine, Harvard Medical School; and Staff Physician, Endocrine-Hypertension Division, Brigham and Women's Hospital, Boston, MA

Hypercalcemia;
Osteoporosis and Paget's Disease of Bone

T. EDWARD BYNUM, MD
Marlborough Hospital, Marlborough, MA; Brockton–West Roxbury Veterans Affairs Medical Center, Brockton, MA

Dyspepsia and Upper Abdominal Pain

MARTIN C. CAREY, MD, DSc, FRCPI
Professor of Medicine, Harvard Medical School; and Senior Physician, Brigham and Women's Hospital, Boston, MA

Gallstones

ROGER L. CHRISTIAN, MD
Assistant Professor of Surgery, Harvard Medical School; and Associate in Surgery, Brigham and Women's Hospital, Boston, MA

Anorectal Disorders

THOMAS G. COONEY, MD
Professor of Medicine, Residency Program Director, Department of Medicine, Oregon Health Sciences University, Portland, OR

Addressing HIV Infection in Office Practice

MARK A. CREAGER, MD
Associate Professor of Medicine, Harvard Medical School, and Director, Vascular Diagnostic Laboratory, Cardiovascular Division, Brigham and Women's Hospital, Boston, MA

Venous Disease of the Lower Extremities

MITCHELL D. CREININ, MD
Assistant Professor, University of California; and Staff Physician, Department of Obstetrics and Gynecology, San Francisco General Hospital, San Francisco, CA

Contraception

PHILIP D. DARNEY, MD, MSc
Professor in Residence, University of California; and Staff Physician, Department of Obstetrics and Gynecology, San Francisco General Hospital, San Francisco, CA

Contraception

DAVID M. DAWSON, MD
Professor of Neurology, Harvard Medical School; and Chief of Neurology, Brockton–West Roxbury Veterans Administration Medical Center, Brockton, MA

Muscular Weakness

LEWIS DEXTER, MD
Emeritus Professor of Medicine, Brigham and Women's Hospital, Boston, MA

Valvular Heart Disease

RICHARD A. DEYO, MD, MPH
Professor of Medicine, University of Washington School of Medicine; and Staff Physician, Division of General Internal Medicine, Veterans Administration Medical Center, Seattle, WA

Low Back Pain

ROBERT G. DLUHY, MD
Associate Professor of Medicine, Harvard Medical School; and Senior Physician, Brigham and Women's Hospital, Boston, MA

Amenorrhea Syndromes

MAGRUDER C. DONALDSON, MD
Assistant Professor of Surgery, Harvard Medical School, and Surgeon, Brigham and Women's Hospital, Boston, MA

Intermittent Claudication

LAWRENCE M. DU BUSKE, MD
Clinical Instructor of Medicine, Harvard Medical School; and Consultant in Allergy, Brigham and Women's Hospital, Boston, MA

Allergic Rhinitis and Other Diseases of the Nose

BRUCE M. EWENSTEIN, MD, PHD
Assistant Professor of Medicine, Harvard Medical School; and Associate Physician, Brigham and Women's Hospital, Boston, MA

Bleeding and Thrombotic Disorders

CHRISTOPHER H. FANTA, MD
Associate Professor of Medicine, Harvard Medical School; and Clinical Director, Respiratory and Critical Care Division, Brigham and Women's Hospital, Boston, MA

Hemoptysis;
Solitary Pulmonary Nodule

ALISON FIFE, MD
Instructor in Psychiatry, Harvard Medical School; and Associate Director of Consultation–Liaison Psychiatry, Division of Psychiatry, Department of Medicine, Brigham and Women's Hospital, Boston, MA

Anxiety Disorders

PAUL R. FORTIN, MD, MPH
Assistant Professor of Medicine, McGill University; and Assistant Physician, Montreal General Hospital, Montreal, Quebec, Canada

Elbow, Hand, Knee, Hip, and Foot Pain

MARVIN FRIED, MD
Associate Professor of Otology and Laryngology, Harvard Medical School; and Chief, Division of Otolaryngology, Beth Israel Hospital and Brigham and Women's Hospital, Boston, MA

Hoarseness and Diseases of the Larynx

GHADA EL-HAJJ FULEIHAN, MD
Assistant Professor of Medicine, Harvard Medical School; and Associate Physician, Brigham and Women's Hospital, Boston, MA

Osteoporosis and Paget's Disease of Bone

LEE GOLDMAN, MD
Professor of Medicine, Harvard Medical School; Chief Medical Officer, Brigham and Women's Hospital, Boston, MA

Noninvasive Tests in Cardiology

ROBERT C. GOLDSZER, MD
Assistant Professor of Medicine, Harvard Medical School; and Physician, Brigham and Women's Hospital, Boston, MA

Hypertension

LILI A. GOTTFRIED, MD
Instructor in Psychiatry, Harvard Medical School; and Psychiatrist, MIT Medical Department and Brigham and Women's Hospital, Boston, MA

Sexual Problems

THOMAS B. GRABOYS, MD
Associate Clinical Professor of Medicine, Harvard Medical School; and Physician, Brigham and Women's Hospital, Boston, MA

Angina Pectoris

HARRY L. GREENE, MD
Chief of General Medicine, and Associate Chairman of Medicine, University of Arizona Health Sciences Center, Tucson, AZ

Tobacco Use

ROBERT I. HANDIN, MD
Professor of Medicine, Harvard Medical School, and Chief, Hematology–Oncology Division, Brigham and Women's Hospital, Boston, MA

Bleeding and Thrombotic Disorders

L. HOWARD HARTLEY, MD
Associate Professor of Medicine, Harvard Medical School; Physician, and Director, Cardiac Rehabilitation, Brigham and Women's Hospital, Boston, MA

Exercise for Primary Prevention or Rehabilitation in Heart Disease

HARLEY A. HAYNES, MD
Associate Professor of Dermatology, Harvard Medical School; Director, Dermatology Division, Brigham and Women's Hospital; and Chief, Dermatology Service, Brockton–West Roxbury Veterans Affairs Medical Center, Brockton, MA

Dermatology in Primary Care;
Sexually Transmitted Diseases

I. CRAIG HENDERSON, MD
Professor of Medicine, University of California, San Francisco, School of Medicine; Chief, Medical Oncology, University of California San Francisco Medical Center; and Director, Clinical Cancer Programs, Cancer Center, University of California San Francisco, San Francisco, CA

Case Finding for Cancer

PHYLLIS JEN, MD
Assistant Professor of Medicine, Harvard Medical School; and Medical Director, Brigham Internal Medicine Associates, Brigham and Women's Hospital, Boston, MA

Screening, Prophylaxis, and Treatment of Tuberculosis

CRAIG B. KAPLAN, MD, MA
Associate Chairman for Educational Affairs, Department of Internal Medicine, Medical College of Virginia; and Staff Physician, Medical College of Virginia Hospitals, Virginia Commonwealth University, Richmond, VA

Somatization in Primary Care

WISHWA N. KAPOOR, MD, MPH
Professor of Medicine, University of Pittsburgh; and Staff Physician, Presbyterian-University Hospital, Montefiore-University Hospital, and Department of Veterans Affairs Medical Center, Pittsburgh, PA

Syncope

SHAHRAM KHOSHBIN, MD
Associate Professor of Neurology, Harvard Medical School; and Physician, Brigham and Women's Hospital, Boston, MA

Seizure Disorders;
Peripheral Nerve Disorders

ANTHONY L. KOMAROFF, MD
Professor of Medicine, Harvard Medical School; and Director, Division of General Medicine and Primary Care, Department of Medicine, Brigham and Women's Hospital, Boston, MA

Pharyngitis, Coryza, and Related Infections in Adults;
Fatigue and Chronic Fatigue Syndrome

J. THOMAS LAMONT, MD
Chief, Section of Gastroenterology, Boston University Medical Center, and Professor of Medicine, University Hospital, Boston University School of Medicine; and Staff Physician, Boston City Hospital, Veterans Administration Medical Center, and Jewish Memorial Hospital, Boston, MA

Diseases of the Liver

P. REED LARSEN, MD
Professor of Medicine, Harvard Medical School; Chief, Thyroid Division, and Senior Physician, Brigham and Women's Hospital, Boston, MA

Thyroid Diseases

ERIC B. LARSON, MD, MPH
Professor, Department of Medicine, University of Washington; and Medical Director, University of Washington Medical Center, Seattle, WA

Dementia

ROBERT S. LAWRENCE, MD
Adjunct Professor of Medicine, New York University School of Medicine, New York, NY

Periodic Health Assessment of Asymptomatic Adults

MERYL S. LeBOFF, MD
Assistant Professor of Medicine, Harvard Medical School; and Associate Physician, Brigham and Women's Hospital, Boston, MA
Osteoporosis and Paget's Disease of Bone

THOMAS H. LEE Jr., MD
Associate Professor of Medicine, Harvard Medical School; and Director, Clinical Initiatives Development Program, Brigham and Women's Hospital, Boston, MA
Noninvasive Tests in Cardiology

SUSAN M. LETT, MD, MPH
Director, Division of Epidemiology, Massachusetts Department of Public Health; and Staff Physician, Boston City Hospital, Boston, MA
Immunization for Adults

MATTHEW H. LIANG, MD, MPH
Associate Professor of Medicine, Harvard Medical School; and Medical Director, Rehabilitation Services, Brigham and Women's Hospital, Boston, MA
Elbow, Hand, Knee, Hip, and Foot Pain

MACK LIPKIN, Jr., MD
Director, Primary Care Internal Medicine Program, New York University School of Medicine; and President, American Academy on Physician and Patient, New York, NY
The Medical Interview and Related Skills

DON R. LIPSITT, MD
Clinical Professor of Psychiatry, Harvard Medical School, Boston, MA; and Chairman, Department of Psychiatry, Mount Auburn Hospital, Cambridge, MA
The Difficult Doctor-Patient Encounter

KEVIN R. LOUGHLIN, MD
Associate Professor of Surgery, Division of Urology, Brigham and Women's Hospital and Harvard Medical School, Boston, MA
Prostatitis, Epididymitis, and Testicular Enlargement;
Benign and Malignant Enlargement of the Prostate

BERNARD LOWN, MD
Professor of Cardiology Emeritus, Harvard University School of Public Health, Boston, MA; and Senior Physician, Department of Medicine, Brigham and Women's Hospital, Boston, MA
Angina Pectoris

HARVEY J. MAKADON, MD
Assistant Professor of Medicine, Harvard Medical School; and Codirector, Division of General Medicine and Primary Care, Beth Israel Hospital, Boston, MA
Addressing HIV Infection in Office Practice

JOHN A. MANNICK, MD
Mosley Professor of Surgery, Harvard Medical School; and Surgeon-in-Chief, Brigham and Women's Hospital, Boston, MA
Intermittent Claudication

ROBERT C. MAY, MD
Associate Professor of Medicine, Emory University School of Medicine; and Staff Physician, Emory University Hospital, Atlanta, GA
Chronic Renal Failure

WAYNE C. McCORMICK, MD, MPH
Assistant Professor of Medicine, University of Washington; Attending Physician, Division of Gerontology and Geriatric Medicine, and Harborview Medical Center, University of Washington Medical Center, Seattle, WA
Dementia

E. R. McFADDEN, Jr., MD
Argyl J. Beams Professor of Medicine; and Division Director, Airway Disease Center, Department of Medicine, University Hospitals of Cleveland, Cleveland, OH
Obstructive Lung Disease

KENNETH MINAKER, MD
Associate Professor of Medicine, Division on Aging, Harvard Medical School; Director, Brockton/West Roxbury Division of the Boston Area Geriatric Research, Education, and Clinical Center; and Associate Program Director, Clinical Research Center, Beth Israel Hospital, Boston, MA
Clinical Problems in Geriatrics

SARAH L. MINDEN, MD
Assistant Professor of Psychiatry, Harvard Medical School; and Associate in Medicine, Division of Psychiatry, Brigham and Women's Hospital, Boston, MA
Anxiety Disorders

WILLIAM E. MITCH, MD
E. Garland Herndon Professor of Medicine, and Director, Renal Division, Emory University School of Medicine, Atlanta, GA
Chronic Renal Failure

A. JACQUELINE MITUS, MD
Instructor in Medicine, Harvard Medical School; and Associate Physician, Division of Hematology–Oncology, Brigham and Women's Hospital, Boston, MA
Evaluation of an Abnormal Blood Count

THOMAS J. MOORE, MD
Associate Professor of Medicine, Harvard Medical School; and Senior Physician, Endocrine Division, Brigham and Women's Hospital, Boston, MA
Hypercalcemia

JOHN P. MORDES, MD
Professor, Department of Medicine, Associate Professor of Medicine, Diabetes Division, University of Massachusetts Medical School; Physician, University of Massachusetts Medical Center, Worcester, MA
Diabetes Mellitus

MICHAEL J. MUFSON, MD
Instructor in Psychiatry, Harvard Medical School, Boston, MA; Director of Psychiatry, Brockton–West Roxbury Veterans Affairs Medical Center, Brockton, MA; Staff Psychiatrist, and Consultant

to Pain Service, Brigham and Women's Hospital, Boston, MA
Psychotic Disorders;
Chronic Pain Syndrome: Integrating the Medical and Psychiatric Evaluation and Treatment

DAVID NUNES, MB, MRCPI
Assistant Professor of Medicine, Boston University; and Staff Physician, Boston City Hospital, and University Hospital, Boston, MA
Diseases of the Liver

ROBERT OSTEEN, MD
Associate Professor of Surgery, Harvard Medical School; and Co-Chairman, Department of Surgery, Brigham and Women's Hospital, Boston, MA
Lymph Nodes and Subcutaneous Masses

DAVID F. POLAKOFF, MD, MSPH
Instructor in Medicine, Harvard Medical School, Boston, MA; Clinical Director, Geriatric Research, Education, and Clinical Center, Brockton–West Roxbury Veterans Affairs Medical Center, Brockton, MA
Clinical Problems in Geriatrics

DAVID C. PRESTON, MD
Instructor in Neurology, Harvard Medical School; and Director, Neuromuscular Service, Brigham and Women's Hospital, Boston, MA
Peripheral Nerve Disorders

QUENTIN REGESTEIN, MD
Associate Professor of Psychiatry, Harvard Medical School; and Psychiatrist and Director, Sleep Clinic, Brigham and Women's Hospital, Boston, MA
Sleep Disorders

MALCOLM P. ROGERS, MD
Assistant Professor of Psychiatry, Harvard Medical School; and Physician and Attending Psychiatrist, Brigham and Women's Hospital, Boston, MA
Management of Depression

DAVID S. ROSENTHAL, MD
Physician, Brigham and Women's Hospital, Boston, MA
Evaluation of an Abnormal Blood Count

ALDO A. ROSSINI, MD
Professor, Department of Medicine, University of Massachusetts Medical School; and Director, Division of Diabetes, University of Massachusetts Medical Center, Worcester, MA
Diabetes Mellitus

FRANK M. SACKS, MD
Associate Professor of Medicine, Harvard Medical School; Associate Professor in Nutrition, Harvard School of Public Health; and Staff Physician, Brigham and Women's Hospital, Boston, MA
Hyperlipidemia

ISAAC SCHIFF, MD
Joe Vincent Meigs Professor of Gynecology, Harvard Medical School; and Chief, Vincent Memorial Obstetrics and Gynecology Service, Massachusetts General Hospital, Boston, MA
The Infertile Couple

ELLEN E. SHEETS, MD
Assistant Professor of Obstetrics, Gynecology, and Reproductive Biology, and Physician, Division of Gynecologic Oncology, Harvard Medical School; and Director, PAP Smear Evaluation Center, Brigham and Women's Hospital, Boston, MA
Case Finding for Cancer

ALBERT L. SHEFFER, MD
Clinical Professor of Medicine, Harvard Medical School; and Director, Allergy Section, Brigham and Women's Hospital, Boston, MA
Allergic Rhinitis and Other Diseases of the Nose

JANE S. SILLMAN, MD
Instructor in Medicine, Harvard Medical School; and Physician, Brigham and Women's Hospital, Boston, MA
Disorders of Eating

ROBERT P. SMITH, JR., MD, MPH
Clinical Associate Professor of Medicine, University of Vermont College of Medicine, Burlington, VT; and Director, Infectious Disease Fellowship, Maine Medical Center, Portland, ME
Health Advice for Travelers

HAROLD S. SOLOMON, MD
Associate Clinical Professor of Medicine, Harvard Medical School; and Senior Physician, Brigham and Women's Hospital, and Beth Israel Hospital, Boston, MA
Hypertension

STEPHEN T. SONIS, DMD, DMSc
Professor and Chairman, Department of Oral Medicine and Diagnostic Sciences, Harvard School of Dental Medicine; and Chief, Division of Oral Medicine and Dentistry, Brigham and Women's Hospital, Boston, MA
Lesions of the Mouth

EGILIUS L. H. SPIERINGS, MD, PhD
Lecturer in Neurology, Harvard Medical School; Assistant Professor of Neurology, Tufts University School of Medicine; and Director, Headache Section, Division of Neurology, Brigham and Women's Hospital, Boston, MA
Headache

MARSHALL STROME, MD, MS
Chief of Otolaryngology, the Cleveland Clinic, Cleveland, OH
Pain or Congestion of the Paranasal Sinuses;
Hoarseness and Diseases of the Larynx

PHILLIP G. STUBBLEFIELD, MD
Professor of Obstetrics and Gynecology, University of Vermont College of Medicine, Burlington, VT; and Chief of Obstetrics and Gynecology, Maine Medical Center, Portland, ME
Common Gynecologic Problems: Pelvic Mass, Chronic Pelvic Pain, Endometriosis, Premenstrual Syndrome, and Menopause;
Abnormal Uterine Bleeding

LEWIS SUDARSKY, MD
Assistant Professor of Neurology, Harvard Medical School, Boston, MA; Assistant Chief, Neurology Service, Brockton–West Roxbury Veterans Affairs Medical Center, Brockton, MA; and Associate Physician, Brigham and Women's Hospital, Boston, MA

Parkinsonism, Tremors, and Gait Disorders

WILLIAM C. TAYLOR, MD
Assistant Professor of Medicine, Harvard Medical School; and Associate Physician, Beth Israel Hospital, Boston, MA

Immunization for Adults

JERRY S. TRIER, MD
Professor of Medicine, Harvard Medical School; and Senior Physician, Brigham and Women's Hospital, Boston, MA

Chronic Diarrhea

RUTH E. TUOMALA, MD
Assistant Professor of Obstetrics and Gynecology, Harvard Medical School; and Active Staff Physician, Department of Obstetrics and Gynecology, Brigham and Women's Hospital, Boston, MA

Sexually Transmitted Diseases

DAVID M. VERNICK, MD
Assistant Professor of Otology and Laryngology, Harvard Medical School; Associate Surgeon, Brigham and Women's Hospital, and Senior Surgeon in Otolaryngology, Beth Israel Hospital, Boston, MA

The Painful or Discharging Ear

MARTYN A. VICKERS, Jr., MD
Assistant Professor of Urology, Harvard Medical School, Boston, MA; and Staff Physician, Brockton–West Roxbury Veterans Administration Medical Center, Brockton, MA

Sexual Problems

THOMAS M. WALSHE, MD
Assistant Professor of Neurology, Harvard Medical School, Boston, MA; Associate Chief, Neurology Service, Brockton–West Roxbury Veterans Affairs Medical Center, Brockton, MA; and Director, Neurology Clinical Research Unit, Brigham and Women's Hospital, Boston, MA

Transient Ischemic Attacks

LOUIS WEINSTEIN, MD, PhD
Staff Physician, Brigham and Women's Hospital, Boston, MA

Fever of Unknown Origin

WILLET F. WHITMORE, III, MD
Urologic Surgeon, Sarasota Memorial Hospital, Sarasota, FL

Prostatitis, Epididymitis, and Testicular Enlargement

ANTHONY D. WHITTEMORE, MD
Associate Professor of Surgery, Harvard Medical School; and Chief, Division of Vascular Surgery, Brigham and Women's Hospital, Boston, MA

Intermittent Claudication

GORDON H. WILLIAMS, MD
Professor of Medicine, Harvard Medical School; and Chief, Endocrine–Hypertension Division, Brigham and Women's Hospital, Boston, MA

Hirsutism

JOYCE E. WIPF, MD
Assistant Professor of Medicine, University of Washington School of Medicine; Director, Outpatient Resident Training Program, and Staff Physician, Division of General Internal Medicine, Veterans Administration Medical Center, Seattle, WA

Low Back Pain

J. M. WITHERSPOON, MD
Professor of Medicine, Medical College of Virginia, School of Medicine; and Staff Physician, Medical College of Virginia Hospitals, Virginia Commonwealth University, Richmond, VA

Urolithiasis

JACQUELINE L. WOLF, MD
Assistant Professor of Medicine, Harvard Medical School; and Associate Physician, Brigham and Women's Hospital, Boston, MA

Acute Diarrhea

MARSHALL A. WOLF, MD
Associate Professor of Medicine, Harvard Medical School; and Associate Physician-in-Chief, Brigham and Women's Hospital, Boston, MA

Palpitations and Disturbances of Cardiac Rhythm

BEVERLY WOO, MD
Assistant Professor of Medicine, Harvard Medical School; and Physician, Brigham and Women's Hospital, Boston, MA

Vaginitis and Cervicitis

JOSHUA WYNNE, MD
Professor of Medicine and Chief, Division of Cardiology, Wayne State University School of Medicine; and Chief, Section of Cardiology, Harper Hospital, Detroit, MI

Valvular Heart Disease

HOWARD H. ZUBICK, PhD
Instructor in Surgery, Harvard Medical School; and Chief, Speech and Hearing Division, Brigham and Women's Hospital, Boston, MA

Basic Assessment of Auditory Function

Preface to the Third Edition

As primary care becomes the centerpiece of plans for national health care delivery, it is gratifying to offer this third edition of *Office Practice of Medicine*. The book's 86 chapters cover almost all of the clinical problems that generalists and primary care physicians encounter in adults seen in an office or practice setting. Our philosophy has been to present discussions that are both practical and sufficiently in-depth to be of use to the experienced practitioner. I was fortunate in gathering an illustrious group of chapter authors, every one of whom is an experienced clinician with hands-on experience in his or her area of interest, and some of whom are leading investigators in their fields.

As before, the presentation of material in this edition follows a problem-oriented format that corresponds to the approach employed by a clinician when encountering a patient. This format supplements the disease-oriented organization of subjects in standard medical textbooks. Headache, back pain, dizziness, diarrhea, vaginitis, urinary tract infections, vaginal bleeding, painful joints, and many other conditions encountered in office practice receive in-depth coverage.

The expansion of *Office Practice of Medicine* parallels the resurgence of general internal medicine. Our Division of General Medicine and Primary Care at Brigham and Women's Hospital is among the busiest, most productive clinical and research units in our department. The first edition of *Office Practice of Medicine* grew out of the curriculum we devised to train primary care residents at Brigham and Women's Hospital. Today, more than 90% of our medical residents receive at least 3 months of primary care training; and about 25% of our residents are enrolled in the primary care track, which is especially designed for trainees who wish to pursue careers in primary care. I expect that the percentage of residents enrolled in this track will increase in the coming years. *Office Practice of Medicine* represents efforts "to get down on paper" much of what is taught in our program, including the emphasis on health promotion and disease prevention.

Many people contributed generously to this and to the previous two editions of this book. Among those deserving very special mention are my wife, Carolyn Branch, and my daughter, Katherine Branch, who provided the warmth and support that one needs to get through the many hours of editing and writing that go into creating an edition of this book. It has been my special privilege also to be part of the Department of Medicine at Brigham and Women's Hospital, chaired by Eugene Braunwald, MD. Many of the best parts of the book undoubtedly reflect the excellence that Dr. Braunwald has developed and has stressed while building this thriving and intellectually vibrant department. Special thanks also go to Marshall Wolf, MD, my associate in medical practice. Anthony Komaroff, MD, Director of the Division of General Medicine, and others affiliated with this division—including Lee Goldman, MD, Tom Lee, Jr., MD, Phyllis Jen, MD, Beverly Woo, MD, Matthew Liang, MD, and Judyann Bigby, MD—provided encouragement and support in addition to their chapters. My friends, William Mitch, MD, John Witherspoon, MD, and Mack Lipkin, Jr., MD, have continued to contribute their chapters. I wish to say a special word about one person now deceased, Harris Funkenstein, MD, whose three chapters in the previous editions, along with his personal friendship, went a long way to make this book possible. Some new authors, who are colleagues in the Society of General Internal Medicine—Wishwa Kapoor, MD, Rick Deyo, MD, Craig Kaplan, MD, Harry Greene, MD, Bob Lawrence, MD, Harvey Makadon, MD, Bill Taylor, MD, Henrietta Barnes, MD, and Eric Larson, MD—also deserve special thanks for their contributions to this edition. I would also like to mention my mentors and senior colleagues who contributed their efforts to the previous editions as well as to the present one: Louis Weinstein, MD, Lewis Dexter, MD, and Bernard Lown, MD. I wish to acknowledge my secretary, Amy Lowe, for her extra efforts and meticulous work. Finally, several people at the W.B. Saunders Company have helped at every step in preparing this edition: Ray Kersey, David H. Kilmer, Paula Shargel-Green, and Frank Messina.

I want to comment as well on the privilege it has been for me to edit this textbook. It was my hope that the book would be read and not used only as a reference, and comments from many doctors have convinced me that this is the case. To communicate in this way with many thousands of my colleagues has been a special honor for which I am very grateful.

William T. Branch, Jr., MD

Contents

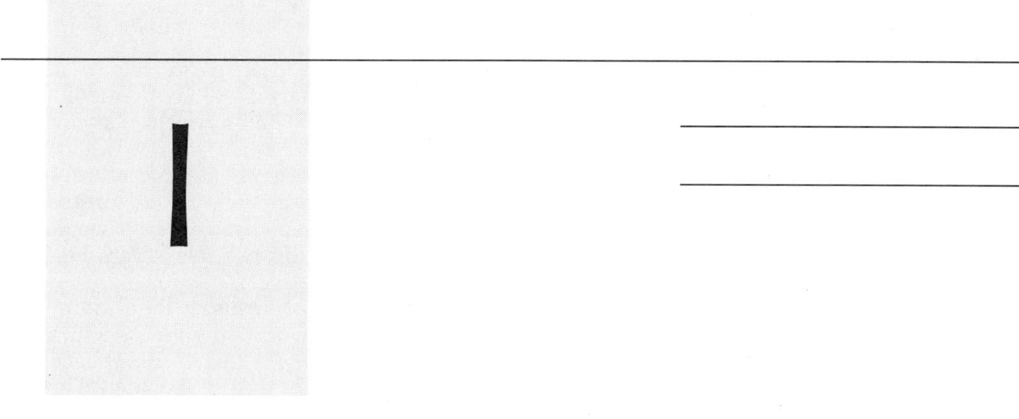

Cardiovascular Disorders

1

Syncope

WISHWA N. KAPOOR, MD, MPH

Syncope is defined as a sudden transient loss of consciousness associated with a loss of postural tone with spontaneous recovery. Syncope must be differentiated from other states of altered consciousness such as dizziness, vertigo, seizures, coma, and narcolepsy. Syncope is a common problem and accounts for 1 to 6% of hospital admissions and 3% of emergency room visits. Loss of consciousness is reported in 12 to 48% of healthy young adults, although most do not seek medical attention. In people older than 75 years of age, residing in a long-term care institution, annual incidence of syncope was reported to be 6%, and 23% had previous lifetime episodes. This chapter reviews the etiologies of syncope and provides a guide to the evaluation of this symptom.

ETIOLOGIES OF SYNCOPE

Table 1–1 shows a list of major causes of syncope reported in recent studies. A brief discussion of these entities is needed for an approach to the evaluation of this symptom.

Vasovagal Syncope

Vasodepressor or vasovagal syncope is characterized by a sudden fall in blood pressure and/or bradycardia in association with increased autonomic activity as manifested by pallor, nausea, sweating, mydriasis, and hyperventilation. Vasovagal syncope often occurs in young individuals and generally in response to fear or injury. Examples of predisposing factors include fatigue, prolonged standing, venipuncture, blood donation, heat, prostatic or pelvic examination, dental surgery, and eye surgery. Vasovagal syncope may also occur without any identifiable predisposing factors and may be provoked if a susceptible individual stands still with an upright posture.

Although it is considered to be a benign entity, sudden death and cardiac arrest have been recorded in association

TABLE 1–1. ETIOLOGIES OF SYNCOPE*

Vasodepressor	Seizure
Situational	Psychogenic
Micturition syncope	Anxiety disorder
Defecation syncope	Panic disorder
Cough syncope	Somatization
Swallow syncope	Depression
Drug-induced syncope	
Orthostatic hypotension	
Cerebrovascular disease	
Carotid sinus syncope	
Glossopharyngeal neuralgia	
Trigeminal neuralgia	
Cardiac Diseases	
Obstruction to flow	
Obstruction to left ventricular outflow: aortic stenosis and hypertrophic cardiomyopathy, left atrial myxoma, mitral stenosis	
Obstruction to pulmonary flow: pulmonic stenosis, pulmonary hypertension, pulmonary embolism, tetralogy of Fallot, right atrial myxomas	
Pump failure: myocardial infarct, unstable angina, coronary spasm	
Cardiac tamponade	
Aortic dissection	
Arrhythmias	
Bradyarrhythmias	
Sinus node disease	
Second- and third-degree atrioventricular block	
Pacemaker malfunction	
Drug-induced bradyarrhythmias	
Tachyarrhythmias	
Ventricular tachycardia	
Torsades de pointes (e.g., associated with congenital long QT syndromes or acquired QT prolongation)	
Supraventricular tachycardia	

*From Kapoor WN: Diagnostic evaluation of syncope. Am J Med 90:91–106, 1991.

with vasovagal syncope.[1] Psychophysiologic processes responsible for vasovagal syncope may also be those leading to sudden death, as sudden collapse and death have occurred after major life crises such as loss of loved ones, humiliation, and other psychological stress.[1]

Situational Syncope

Micturition Syncope. Micturition syncope occurs primarily in healthy young men who, after arising in the early morning, experience sudden loss of consciousness during or immediately after urination. Predisposing factors have included reduced food intake, recent upper respiratory tract infection, fatigue, and ingestion of alcohol. Micturition syncope is also reported in older patients (mean age of 60 years) who have multiple acute and chronic medical problems and orthostatic hypotension.[2] Previous isolated case reports have associated micturition syncope, presyncope or spells with bladder neck obstruction, psychomotor epilepsy, complete atrioventricular (AV) block, and pheochromocytoma of the bladder.

Defecation Syncope. Defecation syncope is defined as a loss of consciousness occurring during or immediately after defecation. In one study a variety of gastrointestinal tract (Meckel's diverticulum, ruptured appendix) and cardiovascular diseases (ventricular arrhythmias), as well as orthostatic hypotension and transient ischemic attacks, were reported to contribute to defecation syncope.[3] No specific predisposing cause for the disorder could be identified in approximately half of the patients. Cases of association with pulmonary embolism have been reported.

Cough Syncope. Syncope after paroxysms of severe cough occurs almost exclusively (>90%) in middle-aged men who drink ethanol, smoke, and have chronic lung disease.

Rare case reports have noted an association of cough syncope with Mobitz II or complete AV block, obstructive cardiomyopathy, hypersensitive carotid sinus syndrome, herniated cerebellar tonsils, and possible severe bilateral carotid artery disease.

Swallow Syncope. Syncope during or immediately following a swallow has been associated with structural abnormalities of the esophagus or the heart.[4] Esophageal disorders have included diverticula, diffuse esophageal spasm, achalasia, and stricture. Cardiac conditions have included acute rheumatic carditis on digitalis, acute myocardial infarction, and a calcified mass over the aortic valve and septum. Bradyarrhythmias have been demonstrated as the cause of swallow syncope and include sinus arrest or asystole, complete AV block, nodal or sinus bradycardia, and sinoatrial block. Vagolytic agents or a pacemaker have abolished symptoms.

Drug-Induced Syncope

Syncope due to drugs may be because of alteration of vascular volume or tone (e.g., antihypertensive agents, nitrates) or arrhythmias (e.g., digoxin toxicity, torsades de pointes associated with prolonged QT interval) or by causing an allergic or anaphylactic reaction. Drugs are responsible for 2 to 9% of symptoms in patients presenting with syncope. The most common drugs causing syncope include nitrates, β-blockers, and vasodilators. Table 1–2 lists various types of drugs that may lead to syncope.

Orthostatic Hypotension

Orthostatic hypotension is generally defined as a decline of 20 mm Hg or more in systolic pressure or 10 mm Hg or more in diastolic pressure after the patient assumes an upright position. Since this finding is common in the elderly and frequently is not associated with symptoms, the clinical diagnosis of orthostatic hypotension should incorporate the presence of symptoms in association with a decrease in systolic blood pressure, and often diastolic blood pressure as well. Symptoms of orthostatic hypotension include dizziness or light-headedness, blurring or loss of vision, weak-

TABLE 1–2. COMMON DRUGS CAUSING SYNCOPE*

Vasodilators
Adrenergic antagonists
Diuretics
Phenothiazines
Antidepressants
Nitrates
Calcium channel blockers
Central nervous system depressants (e.g., barbiturates)
Vincristine and other neuropathic drugs
Quinidine and other drugs that cause prolonged QT interval
Digitalis
Insulin
Marijuana
Alcohol
Cocaine

*From Kapoor WN: Diagnostic evaluation of syncope. Am J Med 90:91–106, 1991.

ness, and syncope. These symptoms are often worse when a person arises in the morning and may be especially prominent after meals or exercise. Table 1–3 shows a list of causes of orthostatic hypotension. Decreased intravascular volume and adverse effects of drugs are the most common causes of symptomatic orthostatic hypotension.[5, 6] Elderly patients are especially vulnerable to symptoms from drugs and volume depletion because of decreased baroreceptor sensitivity, decreased cerebral blood flow, excessive renal sodium wasting, and impaired thirst mechanism with aging.[5]

Cerebrovascular Disease

Syncope is a rare manifestation of cerebrovascular disease. Only about 15% of patients with vertebrobasilar transient ischemic attacks (TIAs) have drop attacks, and syncope is even less common. Loss of consciousness is almost always accompanied by other neurologic symptoms of brain stem ischemia. Syncope is generally not a manifestation of carotid artery ischemia unless accompanied by disease of the vertebrobasilar arteries. TIAs most commonly are caused by atherosclerotic disease but can be caused by inflammatory disorders (e.g., giant cell arteritis, systemic lupus erythematosus), aortic arch syndrome, embolic event from the heart (e.g., rheumatic heart disease, myxoma), sickle cell disease, anomalies of the cervical spine, and others. Subclavian steal syndrome due to subclavian artery stenosis and reversal of blood in the ipsilateral vertebral artery may also lead to brain stem ischemia. A difference in blood pressure (usually >20 mm Hg) and pulse intensity between arms is a helpful clue to this diagnosis.

A "faint sensation" is reported in 12 to 18% of patients with migraine and may often be a vasovagal reaction to pain.[7] Basilar artery migraine is a rare disorder that affects adolescents, and syncope is associated with spasm of the basilar arterial tree. The clinical presentation includes other symptoms of brain stem ischemia.

TABLE 1–3. CAUSES OF ORTHOSTATIC HYPOTENSION*

1. **Primary**
   (a) Pure autonomic failure (idiopathic orthostatic hypotension)
   (b) Autonomic failure with multiple system atrophy (Shy-Drager syndrome)
   (c) Autonomic failure with Parkinson's disease
2. **Secondary**
   (a) General medical disorders: diabetes; amyloid; alcoholism
   (b) Autoimmune disease: acute and subacute dysautonomia; Guillain-Barré syndrome; mixed connective tissue disease; rheumatoid arthritis; Eaton-Lambert syndrome; systemic lupus erythematosus
   (c) Carcinomatous autonomic neuropathy
   (d) Metabolic disease: porphyria; Fabry's disease; Tangier disease; vitamin B_{12} deficiency
   (e) Hereditary sensory neuropathies, dominant or recessive
   (f) Infections of the nervous system: syphilis; Chagas' disease; human immunodeficiency virus infection; botulism; herpes zoster
   (g) Central brain lesions: vascular lesion or tumors involving the hypothalamus and midbrain, for example craniopharyngioma; multiple sclerosis; Wernicke's encephalopathy
   (h) Spinal cord lesions
   (i) Familial dysautonomia
   (j) Familial hyperbradykininism
   (k) Renal failure
   (l) Dopamine β-hydroxylase deficiency
   (m) Aging
3. **Drugs**
   (a) Selective neurotoxic drugs; alcoholism
   (b) Tranquilizers: phenothiazines; barbiturates
   (c) Antidepressants: tricyclics; monoamine oxidase inhibitors
   (d) Vasodilator hypotensive drugs: prazosin; hydralazine
   (e) Centrally acting hypotensive drugs: methyldopa; clonidine
   (f) Adrenergic neuron-blocking drugs: guanethidine
   (g) α-Adrenergic blocking drugs: phenoxybenzamine; labetalol
   (h) Ganglion-blocking drugs: hexamethonium; mecamylamine
   (i) Angiotensin-converting enzyme inhibitors: captopril; enalapril; lisinopril

*Adapted from Bannister SR (ed): Autonomic Failure, 2nd ed. Oxford, Oxford University Press, 1988, p 8. By permission of Oxford University Press.

Carotid Sinus Syncope

Three types of carotid sinus hypersensitivity are described in response to carotid massage done with an electrocardiogram (ECG) and blood pressure monitoring.[8] Cardioinhibitory carotid sinus hypersensitivity is defined as cardiac asystole of 3 seconds or more. A pure vasovagal type is defined as a systolic blood pressure decline of 50 mm Hg or more (in the absence of significant bradycardia). A mixed type consists of a combination of cardioinhibitory and vasovagal responses. Carotid sinus hypersensitivity in an asymptomatic population is reported to be found in 5 to 25%, primarily in older individuals (≥60 years of age) and is found two to four times more commonly in men. The cardioinhibitory variety accounts for 34 to 78% and vasovagal 5 to 10% of cases of carotid sinus hypersensitivity.[8]

Of individuals with carotid hypersensitivity, 5 to 20% suffer spontaneous loss of consciousness, which is called carotid sinus syncope. Attacks may be precipitated by pressure on the carotid sinus (e.g., tight collar, shaving, sudden turning), a history of which is obtained in only a quarter of patients with this syndrome. Syncope occurs predominantly in elderly men, most of whom have coronary artery disease and hypertension. Other predisposing factors include neck pathology such as enlarged lymph nodes, tissue scars, and tumors of the carotid body, parotid, thyroid, and head and neck. A possible association with digitalis, α-methyldopa, and propranolol is also reported.

Neuralgia

Syncope may occur with an attack of glossopharyngeal neuralgia that produces severe unilateral paroxysmal pain in the oropharynx, tonsillar fossa, base of the tongue, or ear precipitated by swallowing, chewing, or coughing. In most cases, syncope is due to asystole or bradycardia and is rarely due to a vasovagal reaction.[9, 10] Neoplasms have been reported in one sixth of the patients with syncope and consist of neck tumors or lymphoma with meningeal involvement. Trigeminal neuralgia has also been associated with syncope and seizures due to bradycardia and asystole or a vasovagal reaction.

Seizure

Seizure and syncope are occasionally difficult to separate clinically for at least three reasons: (1) Convulsion may occur after hypotension leading to cerebral ischemia. For example, 12% of patients with syncope after blood donation develop convulsions, and experimental cerebral ischemia lasting for 15 seconds or more has been associated with seizure-like activity. (2) Akinetic seizures have been described despite a negative interictal electroencephalogram

(EEG). (3) Occasional unwitnessed syncope may actually be a seizure but is difficult to diagnose because the patient may not recall convulsive symptoms. In a study to differentiate seizures from syncope, disorientation after the loss of consciousness was the best distinguishable feature and was correlated with seizure rather than syncope.[11] Other symptoms associated with seizure or syncope are shown in Table 1–4.

Temporal lobe syncope is a term used for complex partial seizures in which loss of consciousness resembles a syncopal episode. Patients have loss of consciousness lasting 2 to 3 minutes followed by partial responsiveness or confusion and may exhibit formed speech or reactive automatisms. Characteristically, an interictal EEG shows temporal lobe epileptic abnormalities.

Psychiatric Illnesses

Psychiatric illnesses may present with syncope.[12] These illnesses should be especially considered in younger patients who are free of organic heart disease and have multiple recurrent episodes. Generalized anxiety may lead to vasovagal reactions, and epidemics of fainting have been described in young individuals that are attributed to transitory anxiety in response to environmental stresses. Syncope is a known symptom of panic disorder, accounting for up to 9% of the presenting somatic complaints in this illness. Patients with somatization disorder have many physical symptoms, and loss of consciousness is reported in 4.5% of patients with this disorder. Depression has also been reported as a cause of syncope.[12]

Drug and alcohol abuse or dependence may result in loss of consciousness. Cocaine use has been reported to lead to syncope; hypnotics, sedatives, and phencyclidine may also cause loss of consciousness by leading to orthostatic hypotension, panic and anxiety attacks, and akinetic seizures. Alcohol ingestion may also cause syncope by leading to reversible autonomic failure as well as to chronic orthostatic hypotension, cardiomyopathy associated with arrhythmias or embolism, and alcohol withdrawal seizures that may mimic syncope.

Cardiac Diseases

Two general types of cardiac problems that lead to syncope include severe obstruction to cardiac output and rhythm disturbance.

Obstruction to Flow. Obstruction to outflow may be due to structural lesions of either the left or right side of the heart that may critically reduce cerebral flow (see Table 1–1). Exertional syncope is a manifestation of all types of heart disease in which cardiac output is fixed and does not rise (or even falls) with exercise. Of patients with severe aortic stenosis, 42% develop syncope that commonly occurs with exercise.[13] Syncope is prognostically important in aortic stenosis, and the average survival rate is 2 to 3 years after the onset of aortic stenosis in the absence of valve replacement.

Syncope is reported in approximately 30% of patients with hypertrophic cardiomyopathy. Left ventricular outflow obstruction is dynamic and worsened by an increase in contractibility, a decrease in chamber size, an afterload, or distending pressure. Thus, states such as Valsalva's maneuver, cough, or drugs (e.g., digitalis) may precipitate hypotension. Ventricular tachycardia is an additional potential cause of syncope in patients with hypertrophic cardiomyopathy. This arrhythmia is reported in approximately 25% of adult patients with hypertrophic cardiomyopathy and is associated with increased risk of sudden death.

Effort syncope commonly occurs in pulmonary hypertension (up to 30% in primary pulmonary hypertension) as well as with severe pulmonic stenosis. Patients with congenital heart disease (e.g., tetralogy of Fallot, patent ductus arteriosus, and interventricular or interatrial septal defects) can experience syncope with effort or crying since a sudden reversal of a left-to-right shunt may occur, leading to a fall in arterial oxygen saturation.

Atrial myxomas may lead to an obstruction of the mitral or tricuspid valve, presenting with symptoms of cardiac failure and rarely syncope. Cardiac murmurs that change with body position are particularly suggestive of myxoma. Mitral stenosis may rarely lead to syncope. The mechanisms include severe obstruction to outflow, atrial fibrillation with rapid ventricular response, pulmonary hypertension, or a cerebral embolic event.

Of elderly patients with acute myocardial infarction, 5 to 12% may present with syncope rather than chest pain. Mechanisms responsible for syncope include sudden pump failure producing a decrease in cardiac output or a rhythm disturbance. Bradycardia secondary to vagal effects is reported in up to 17% of patients with acute myocardial infarction. This occurs usually in patients with inferior or posterior myocardial infarction associated with vascular occlusion of arterial branches that supply the sinus or AV node. Unstable angina and coronary artery spasm also have been rarely associated with syncope.

Syncope is reported in 5% of patients with aortic dissection. Loss of consciousness may be due to a stroke or may be related to rupture into the pericardial space, resulting in sudden cardiac tamponade.[14]

Syncope is reported in 10 to 15% of patients with pulmonary embolism, and it is often associated with massive embolism (>50% obstruction of the pulmonary vascular bed).

Arrhythmias

Bradyarrhythmias. Sinus bradycardia may be caused by excessive vagal tone, decreased sympathetic tone, or sinus node disease. Symptomatic sinus bradycardia also occurs with eye surgery, myxedema, intracranial and mediastinal tumors, and with a large number of parasympathomimetic, sympatholytic, β-blockers, and other drugs including conjunctival instillation of β-blockers.

Syncope occurs in 25 to 70% of patients with sick sinus syndrome. Electrocardiographic manifestations of sick sinus syndrome include sinus bradycardia, pauses, arrest, or exit block. Supraventricular tachycardia or atrial fibril-

TABLE 1–4. SEIZURE VERSUS SYNCOPE*

Symptoms Correlated with Seizure
Blue face or not pale during the event
Frothing at the mouth
Tongue biting
Disoriented
Aching muscles and sleepy after the event
Less than 45 years of age
Unconsciousness for longer than 5 minutes
Symptoms Correlated with Syncope
Sweating or nausea before the event
Oriented after the event according to the eyewitness
45 years of age or over

*Adapted from Hoefnagels WAJ, Padber GW, Overweg J, et al: Transient loss of consciousness: The value of the history for distinguishing seizure from syncope. J Neurol 238:39–43, 1991.

lation may also occur in association with bradycardia or atrial fibrillation with slow ventricular response (tachycardia-bradycardia syndrome).

Tachyarrhythmias. Ventricular tachyarrhythmias are an important cause of syncope and almost always occur in the setting of known organic heart disease. Torsades de pointes or polymorphic ventricular tachycardia occurs in patients with congenital prolongation of QT interval (with or without associated deafness) as well as acquired long QT syndromes that are caused by drugs, electrolyte abnormalities, and central nervous system disorders.[15] Antiarrhythmic drugs are the most common cause of torsades de pointes and are reported with quinidine (quinidine syncope), procainamide, disopyramide, flecainide, encainide, amiodarone, and satolol.[16]

Other tachyarrhythmias that may cause syncope include atrial fibrillation or flutter with rapid ventricular response, AV nodal re-entrant tachycardia, and supraventricular tachycardia in patients with Wolff-Parkinson-White syndrome.

DIAGNOSTIC EVALUATION

As shown in Table 1–5, in patients in whom an etiology could be determined, the history and physical examination identified a potential cause in 49 to 85%.[17–23] Furthermore, many of the cardiac and noncardiac causes (e.g., aortic stenosis, idiopathic hypertrophic subaortic stenosis, pulmonary embolism, subclavian steal) are easily suspected by the history, physical examination, and ECG. These entities often need selective confirmatory tests. Suggestive findings were helpful when assigning the ultimate cause of syncope in 8% of the additional patients.[23]

History

A detailed account of syncope, the events surrounding loss of consciousness, and associated symptoms provide valuable information for diagnosing many of the entities. For example, in vasovagal syncope, precipitating factors, in conjunction with autonomic symptoms, lead to diagnosis. Syncope during or immediately after micturition, cough, defecation, and swallow are easily diagnosed from the patient's history but may require a search for an underlying organic disorder. Syncope associated with symptoms of brain stem ischemia suggest neurologic causes such as TIAs, basilar artery migraines, and subclavian steal syndrome; loss of consciousness with glossopharyngeal or trigeminal neuralgia is due to bradyarrhythmias or a vasovagal response. A detailed drug history is important, and a drug challenge (e.g., with nitroglycerin) in a controlled setting can occasionally provide valuable diagnostic information.

There are specific clinical associations that may suggest various causes of syncope. Examples include syncope with arm exercise suggesting subclavian steal syndrome, loss of consciousness with head rotation or extension suggesting carotid sinus syncope, syncope in a deaf child with effort or emotional distress suggesting prolonged QT syndrome, and fainting with flushing and itching suggesting mastocytosis. Detailed accounts of such associations have been summarized elsewhere.

Physical Examination

The physical examination is important for diagnosis of specific entities and exclusion of others. Orthostatic hypotension and cardiovascular and neurologic findings are particularly important.

Orthostatic blood pressure should be measured after the patient has been supine for 5 minutes; the patient's blood pressure should be measured for at least up to 2 minutes immediately after he or she has been standing. These measurements should be carried out for up to 10 minutes if there is a high suspicion of orthostatic hypotension but a drop in blood pressure has not been found earlier.[24] Blood pressure taken while the patient is sitting is unreliable for detection of orthostatic hypotension. Development of symptoms similar to spontaneous episodes or severe hypotension (systolic blood pressure <90 mm Hg) during standing implicate orthostatic hypotension as a cause of syncope in the absence of another cause.

Several cardiovascular findings serve as clues to specific entities. Differences in the pulse intensity and blood pressure (generally >20 mm Hg) in the arms suggest aortic dissection or subclavian steal syndrome. In all patients with syncope, particular attention should be given to the cardiovascular examination for aortic stenosis, hypertrophic cardiomyopathy, pulmonary hypertension, myxomas, and aortic dissection.

TABLE 1–5. DIAGNOSES BY VARIOUS TESTS IN PATIENTS WITH SYNCOPE*

			No. with Diagnosis		Diagnosis by (n)					
Authors	**Type of Patients**	**No. of Patients**	*n*	*%*	*H&P*	*ECG*	*PEM*	*EPS*	*EEG/CT*	*Other†*
Kapoor et al[17]‡	Admitted SUO	121	13	—	—	—	7	3	—	3
Day et al[22]	ER	198	173	87	147	4	4	—	18	—
Silverstein et al[20]	MICU	108	57	53	42§	—	8	—	—	7‖
Kapoor et al[18]	All	433	254	59	140	30	54	7	2	21
Eagle and Black[19]	Admitted	100	61	61	52§	—	3	—	2	4
Martin et al[21]	ER	170	106	62	90¶	2	5	—	9	—

*From Kapoor WN, et al: Diagnosis and natural history of syncope and the role of invasive electrophysiologic testing. Am J Cardiol 63:730–734, 1989.

†Variety of tests including cardiac catheterization, echocardiogram, cardiac enzymes, stress test, noninvasive cerebrovascular studies, radionuclide brain scan, cerebral angiography, and ventilation/perfusion scan.

‡Excluded patients in whom a diagnosis was made by H&P and ECG.

§On admission examination (may exclude ECG).

‖7 or 8 (data unclear).

¶Calculated; the exact number is not given in the article.

EEG/CT = electroencephalogram/head CT scan; ECG = electrocardiogram; EPS = electrophysiologic studies; ER = emergency room; H&P = history and physical; MICU = medical intensive care unit; PEM = prolonged electrocardiographic monitoring; SUO = syncope of unknown origin.

TABLE 1–6. PROLONGED ELECTROCARDIOGRAPHIC MONITORING IN SYNCOPE*

			Symptoms During Monitoring		No Symptoms During Monitoring	
Study	**No. of Patients**	**Presenting Symptom**	*Arrhythmia (%)*	*No Arrhythmia (%)*	*Arrhythmia (%)*	*No Arrhythmia (%)*
Jonas et al[29]	358†	Dizziness or syncope	4	—	16	80
Boudoulas et al[26]	119	Dizziness or syncope	26	13	27	34
Clark et al[30]	98	Dizziness or syncope	3	39	41	17
Zeldis et al[31]	74‡	Syncope or near-syncope	14	24	—	—
Kala et al[32]	107	Dizziness or syncope	7	7	16	69
Gibson and Heitzman[27]	1512	Dizziness or presyncope	2	15	10	79
Bass et al[28]§	95	Syncope	1	20	26	53
Kapoor[23]‖	249	Syncope	6	22	17	55
TOTAL¶	**2612**		**4**	**17**	**13**	**69**

*From Kapoor WN: Diagnostic evaluation of syncope. Am J Med 90:91–106, 1991.
†12 hours (in 102 patients) or 24 hours (in 256 patients) of monitoring.
‡Total study included 371 with several symptoms (chest pain, palpitations, dizziness, and syncope). Only patients with syncope or near-syncope are included here.
§Prospective study of 72 hours of monitoring.
‖Includes 39 (11%) patients who underwent telemetry only.
¶Total does not add up to 100% because of missing information from two studies.

Laboratory Tests

Routine blood tests rarely yield diagnostically helpful information in patients with syncope. In syncope studies that included patients with seizure, 2 to 3% had hypoglycemia, hyponatremia, hypocalcemia, or renal insufficiency.[18, 22, 23] These tests confirmed clinical suspicion of these problems. In one study only one unexpected finding (hyponatremia) was reported, but that finding was in a patient who had a seizure and did not have syncope.[22] Bleeding was diagnosed clinically rather than on the basis of a complete blood count. The glucose tolerance test did not delineate the cause of syncope in any of the patients undergoing this test.[17]

Carotid Massage

Commonly, carotid massage is done in the supine position and is repeated occasionally in the sitting and standing position if the vasovagal variety of carotid hypersensitivity is suspected and the supine test has a negative result. Electrocardiographic and blood pressure monitoring is necessary. Mixed response (cardioinhibitory and vasovagal) is diagnosed when cardioinhibitory responses are abolished with atropine or AV sequential pacing. The duration of massage should be limited to 5 seconds. At least 15 seconds should be allowed between massage from one side to the other. Simultaneous bilateral massage should never be done. Complication rates are not available but are considered extremely low and include prolonged asystole, ventricular fibrillation, transient or permanent neurologic deficit, and sudden death. In patients with cerebrovascular disease, the test should be done only if all other diagnostic modalities are exhausted and the pretest probability of carotid sinus syncope remains high.

Carotid sinus syncope is diagnosed in patients who have carotid sinus hypersensitivity if they have (1) episodes related to activities that press or stretch the carotid sinus, or (2) recurrent syncope with a negative work-up. Symptom reproduction during carotid sinus massage is generally not necessary.

Diagnosis of Arrhythmias

Assigning arrhythmias as the cause of syncope is often difficult, because in most patients symptoms have already resolved by the time of testing, and thus a causal inference is often made on the basis of arrhythmias detected during asymptomatic periods. This process leads to uncertainty, since at the current time there are no validated criteria for attributing syncope to arrhythmias by the use of electrocardiographic abnormalities during asymptomatic periods. There is no "gold standard" test to determine the performance of ambulatory monitoring or electrophysiologic testing in syncope. A gold standard test is defined as the test used to establish the patient's true disease state. In attributing syncope to arrhythmias, index tests (i.e., tests whose performance is being measured, such as ECG, ambulatory monitoring, or electrophysiologic studies) have been used as elements in the global diagnosis of arrhythmic syncope. Because gold standard tests have not been independent of index tests, it is not possible to estimate the sensitivity and specificity of various tests for arrhythmic syncope.

Electrocardiogram. In recent syncope studies, 2 to 11% of patients had an etiology assigned by an ECG. In our study, 30 of 433 patients had a cause of syncope assigned by an ECG or rhythm strip (20% by paramedics in the field, 20% on rhythm strip in the emergency room or in the hospital with recurrence of syncope, and 60% by 12-lead ECG).[23] This constituted approximately one third of arrhythmias diagnosed in this study. The most common assigned diagnoses included ventricular tachycardia and bradyarrhythmias, but evidence of an acute myocardial infarction was found in five patients with syncope.

Prolonged Electrocardiographic Monitoring. The central problem in attributing syncope to arrhythmias is that the vast majority of detected arrhythmias are brief and result in no symptoms.[25] One method of assessing the yield of ambulatory monitoring in syncope is to determine the presence or absence of arrhythmias in patients who develop symptoms during monitoring.[25] Table 1–6 shows rates of symptomatic arrhythmias in studies on monitoring that met the following criteria: the patient population included those with syncope or presyncope; data on the presence or absence of symptoms during monitoring were reported; and monitoring was for 12 hours or more.[23, 26–32] Only 4% of patients had symptomatic correlation with an arrhythmia. In an additional 17% of patients, symptoms were not associated with arrhythmias, thus potentially excluding arrhythmic syncope. In approximately 80% of patients, no symptoms occurred but arrhythmias were found in 13%.[33] The causal relation between these arrhythmias and syncope is uncertain.

Extending the duration of monitoring to longer than 24 hours does not lead to higher likelihood of detecting symptomatic arrhythmia. In a study of patients undergoing 72 hours of Holter monitoring, arrhythmias by specific criteria were found in 14.7% during the first day, in an additional 11.1% on the second day, and in an additional 4.2% on the third day.[28] However, only one of 95 patients had arrhythmias associated with symptoms, and this occurred during the first 24 hours.

Correlating arrhythmias detected on monitoring to mortality and sudden death in follow-up also does not help to clarify the role of these arrhythmias in causing syncope. Frequent (>10 premature ventricular contractions per hour) or repetitive ventricular ectopy in patients with syncope is an independent predictor of mortality and sudden death (3.7-fold increased risk of mortality and 14.9-fold increased risk of sudden death).[34] Sinus pauses were also associated with a 3.3-fold increased risk of mortality in patients with syncope.[34] The increased mortality is likely to be a manifestation of underlying heart disease, and inferences regarding the cause of syncope are not possible from these data.

Patient-activated intermittent loop recorders can capture the rhythm during syncope after the patient has regained consciousness, since 1 to 4 minutes of retrograde electrocardiographic recording can be obtained. This type of monitor can be worn for weeks at a time. In a study of 57 patients with a history of frequent syncope or presyncope (median number of 10 episodes), only 14 patients were diagnosed by use of the loop recorder of which 7 had arrhythmias and 7 had negative findings, normal sinus rhythm, or sinus tachycardia.[35] This type of a device is more likely to capture an event in patients who have infrequent arrhythmias. Our study of syncope recurrence has shown that only 5% have recurrent syncope at 1 month, 11% by 3 months, and 16% by 6 months.[36] Thus, loop monitoring is likely to be useful for capturing a symptomatic period in a very small subset of patients with a negative initial work-up.

Electrophysiologic Studies. Electrophysiologic studies for evaluation of syncope are more likely to be "positive" or abnormal in patients with known heart disease who have abnormal ventricular function, ECG, or ambulatory monitoring.[37–43] The results of these tests are also more likely to be positive in patients with bundle branch block, providing evidence for isolated conduction disease or ventricular tachyarrhythmia.[44] Predictors of a *negative* electrophysiologic study in patients with syncope include the absence of heart disease; an ejection fraction of more than 40%; normal ECG and Holter monitoring; absence of injury during syncope; and multiple or prolonged (>5 minutes) episodes of syncope.[41]

In studies of syncope patients undergoing electrophysiologic testing, 60% of patients had a positive finding (range of 17 to 75%).[37] Approximately 35% (range of 0 to 80%) had inducible ventricular tachycardia, 20% (range of 0 to 60%) had supraventricular tachycardia, 35% (range of 11 to 60%) had conduction disturbance (abnormal sinus node, AV node, or His-Purkinje function), and 10% (range of 0 to 24%) had other abnormalities (including hypervagotonia and carotid hypersensitivity).

Several issues need to be considered when using electrophysiologic studies in the evaluation of syncope.[37] (1) In most cases, arrhythmias during electrophysiologic evaluation do not produce syncope in the laboratory. Thus, a causal relationship often has to be inferred. (2) The clinical significance of some of the electrophysiologic abnormalities may be difficult to determine. For example, sinus node recovery time is used for diagnosis of sinus node disease. However, this measurement has a low sensitivity for diagnosis of sinus node dysfunction (18 to 69%), although specificity is higher (35 to 100%) when ambulatory monitoring is used as the reference test. The performance of other tests of sinus node function (e.g., sinoatrial conduction time) is also controversial.[42, 43] Tests for AV nodal conduction and refractoriness are also difficult to interpret and vary with autonomic tone.

Similarly, measures of other conduction system diseases (a prolonged HV interval and block between H and V with atrial pacing) are problematic since cutpoints for an abnormal HV interval have widely varied when attributing syncope to conduction system disease (criteria have ranged from >55 msec to >100 msec).

Supraventricular tachycardias and atrial fibrillation or flutter may be occasionally initiated during electrophysiologic studies. The significance of these induced arrhythmias is uncertain unless they reproduce the patient's spontaneous symptoms.[42, 43]

Patients with structural heart disease have higher rates of inducible ventricular tachycardia compared with those without cardiac disease (approximately 55 to 70% versus <20%). The finding of *sustained monomorphic* ventricular tachycardia has a high sensitivity and specificity for presence of spontaneous ventricular tachycardia. However, induction of *polymorphic* or nonsustained ventricular tachycardia may represent a nonspecific response to an aggressive ventricular stimulation protocol.

(3) Regarding patient outcome after therapy, patients with abnormal findings considered to be causally related to syncope are treated with pacemakers, antiarrhythmic agents, or implantable cardioverter defibrillator devices. Recurrence on follow-up is generally used as the endpoint of treatment. In those who have normal studies (i.e., no therapy provided), recurrence rates of 8 to 80% are reported with a mean of 35%, while recurrence rates in those with abnormal testing are 0 to 32% with a mean of 15%.[37] The mean length of follow-up has varied from 11 to 36 months. The interpretation of the rate of recurrence is, however, complicated because it may be caused by many different mechanisms: side effects of drugs, noncompliance, inadequate treatment, or an incorrect initial diagnosis.

The incidence of sudden death in one study was markedly higher in patients with positive studies than in those with negative studies (48% versus 9% at 3 years).[38] Patients with negative electrophysiologic studies have had a low rate of mortality and sudden death, thus defining a low-risk group of patients with syncope.

What is the current role of electrophysiologic studies in syncope? A thorough clinical and noninvasive evaluation using a careful history and physical examination, an ECG, ambulatory monitoring, and other noninvasive or directed tests is generally needed prior to the consideration of electrophysiologic studies. In patients with recurrent syncope who do not have evidence of organic heart disease, the yield of electrophysiologic testing is low and generally should not be performed. In patients with unexplained syncope and organic heart disease (moderate or marked left ventricular dysfunction and/or severe coronary or valvular heart disease), electrophysiologic testing may diagnose potential arrhythmias and guide in empiric therapy.

Upright Tilt Testing

Upright tilt testing refers to maintaining the patient in a head-up position for a brief duration to provoke symptomatic hypotension and bradycardia. The mechanism of syncope with an upright tilt is poorly understood. Upright posture is associated with gravitational pooling of blood, which results in a decline in central venous pressure, stroke volume, and blood pressure. These effects lead to the activation of arterial and cardiopulmonary baroreceptor reflexes as well as activation of the renin-angiotensin system, which lead to vasoconstriction, tachycardia, and fluid retention. However, in individuals susceptible to vasovagal syncope, intense activation of cardiopulmonary mechanoreceptors may occur leading to activation of reflexes that result in bradycardia and hypotension. This type of syncope has been termed vasovagal, vasodepressor, neurally mediated, or neurocardiogenic syncope.

Urinary concentrations of epinephrine and norepinephrine prior to vasovagal syncope are higher than in control subjects, and circulating catecholamine levels measured immediately before loss of consciousness have also occasionally been reported to be high. These findings suggest enhanced adrenergic activity as playing a role in leading to vasovagal syncope. It has been postulated that catecholamine release may enhance susceptibility to bradycardia and hypotension by activation of cardiac mechanoreceptors. These considerations have led to the use of intravenous infusion of catecholamine (e.g., isoproterenol) to provoke syncope. Since upright posture alone is also a provocative stimulus for vasovagal syncope, use of upright tilt testing alone or in conjunction with isoproterenol has been used as a provocative stimulus for vasovagal syncope.

Recent studies of upright tilt testing have primarily investigated patients who have syncope of unknown cause after electrophysiologic testing. In patients with negative electrophysiologic studies, rates of provocation of hypotension on upright tilt testing (without isoproterenol) of 27 to 75% are reported compared with approximately 10% in controls (without syncope).[44–48] Studies using intravenous infusion of isoproterenol during upright tilt testing have reported rates of 50 to 87% in patients who had prior negative electrophysiologic testing compared with 11% in patients who had positive electrophysiologic testing or 11% in control patients (without syncope). False-positive rates of 45% are reported in young healthy control subjects.[48]

Although it is not entirely possible to generalize these results to all patients with syncope of unknown cause, it is likely that a substantial proportion of patients with unexplained syncope have vasovagal reactions that are difficult to diagnose clinically. A wide variety of drugs have been used as treatment in patients with vasovagal syncope. The most common agents are β-blockers, but other drugs include disopyramide, anticholinergic agents, theophylline, fludrocortisone plus salt, and AV sequential pacers. No randomized trials have been done, but treatment is reported to result in decreased recurrence. Intravenous β-blockers have been used in conjunction with repeat tilt testing to show lack of induction of syncope as a test of potential efficacy of therapy with β-blockers. Upright tilt testing may thus be used for potential therapy for patients with recurrent syncope. In patients with isolated or rare episodes of syncope, this test is not likely to have an impact on therapy.

Other Cardiovascular Testing

Echocardiogram, stress testing, ventricular function studies, and cardiac catheterization are generally needed for further evaluation of specific findings on the history and physical examination.[23] These tests can be used in a selective manner to define the type, extent, or severity of cardiac diseases. Similarly, aortogram and cerebrovascular flow studies are used as directed by the clinical presentation. The use of myocardial band isoenzyme of creatine kinase (CK-MB) is based on the clinical and electrocardiographic suspicion of myocardial infarction.

Signal-Averaged Electrocardiogram

Detection of low-amplitude signals (late potentials) has been reported to have a sensitivity of 73 to 89% and specificity of 89 to 100% for prediction of inducible sustained ventricular tachycardia in patients with syncope.[49] Some centers have used signal-averaged ECG as a screening test for ventricular tachycardia in selecting patients for electrophysiologic studies. However, complete electrophysiologic studies are generally needed to evaluate syncope when the decision is made to perform this test since other abnormalities (e.g., sinus node dysfunction, other conduction system disease, supraventricular tachycardia) as well as multiple abnormalities may be of concern.

Electroencephalogram and Computed Tomography Scan of the Head

EEGs and computed tomography (CT) scans have rarely been helpful in determining a cause of syncope (see Table 1–5). These tests have been useful in evaluating patients who have focal neurologic symptoms in association with syncope[22, 23] or when a convulsive disorder is clinically suspected in a patient presenting with syncope. Nonselective use of EEGs and head CT scans has not been rewarding.

PROGNOSIS

The 1-year mortality of patients with a cardiac cause of syncope has been consistently high in all of the recent studies, ranging between 18 and 33%.[18–23] These rates have been higher than those in patients with a noncardiac cause (0 to 12%) or in patients with unknown cause (6%). The incidence of sudden death in patients with a cardiac cause was also markedly higher compared with the other two groups (Fig. 1–1).[23] Even when adjustments for differences in baseline rate of heart and other diseases were made, cardiac syncope was still an independent predictor of mortality and sudden death.

It is not known whether syncope predisposes to increased risk of mortality independent of underlying diseases. In the Framingham study, patients younger than 60 years of age with isolated syncope (i.e., patients with no cardiovascular or neurologic diseases or stigmata) had rates of mortality, sudden death, stroke, and myocardial infarction similar to patients without syncope.[50] However, such information is not available regarding patients with underlying cardiac or noncardiac diseases.

Recurrence of syncope is another clinically important prognostic endpoint. Recurrence rates for syncope of 12 to 15% per year were found in follow-up, and the rates were not significantly different in patients with cardiac causes compared with the other groups.[36] In approximately 5% of patients, new causes were assigned after an evaluation of recurrent syncope. Although recurrences were associated with fractures and soft-tissue injury in 12% of patients, they did not significantly increase the risk of mortality or sudden death.[36]

APPROACH TO DIAGNOSTIC EVALUATION

Using the recent studies on the evaluation of syncope discussed earlier, a diagnostic approach can be suggested (Fig. 1–2):

A careful history and physical examination will identify most causes. In these patients, therapy can be planned based on the diagnosis. The history and physical examination may also reveal findings suggestive of specific entities as possible causes (e.g., findings of aortic stenosis or neurologic signs and symptoms suggestive of a seizure disorder) that may require further noninvasive or invasive directed tests for establishing a diagnosis and initiating treatment.

An ECG is generally needed for the evaluation of patients with syncope, the cause of which is not evident from the history and physical examination. Although the diagnostic yield of an ECG is low (i.e., for arrhythmias or suspicion of myocardial infarction), abnormalities can be acted on quickly if found. Furthermore, patients with a normal ECG have a low likelihood of arrhythmias as a cause of syncope and are at low risk of sudden death.

In patients in whom a cause of syncope is not determined by the history and physical examination and initial ECG, further diagnostic testing can be approached by separating patients into those with and without heart disease.

Patients with coronary artery disease, congestive heart failure, valvular heart disease, obstructive cardiomyopathy, and bundle branch block or bifascicular block have a higher likelihood of arrhythmias. Prolonged ECG monitoring is the first step in the evaluation of these patients. If prolonged monitoring is nondiagnostic, these patients (especially those with recurrent syncope) may be candidates for electrophysiologic studies. The findings of electrophysiologic studies can form the basis for potential therapy.

Patients with negative findings on electrophysiologic studies have a favorable prognosis, and thus empiric therapy with a pacemaker or antiarrhythmics is not justified. Since a large proportion of patients with negative findings on electrophysiologic studies and recurrent unexplained syncope have been reported to have vasovagal syncope by upright tilt testing, this test may help to define a potential cause for syncope in this group of patients. Therapy for this entity can be attempted in patients who have frequent symptoms.

Younger patients (<60 years of age) with syncope and without heart disease have an excellent prognosis.[51] Furthermore, in patients with a normal ECG, the likelihood of arrhythmias is low and prolonged electrocardiographic monitoring rarely leads to a specific diagnosis. The yield of electrophysiologic studies in patients without heart disease is low. Thus, these studies are not justified in the vast majority of these patients. A large proportion of these patients (especially those with recurrent syncope) probably have vasovagal syncope or psychiatric disorders that should be investigated. Similar conclusions probably apply to older patients without heart disease, but further studies are needed in order to better define the role of prolonged electrocardiographic monitoring and other tests in these patients.

Patients with recurrent syncope constitute a difficult group to manage. Patients with multiple episodes (more than five in the last year) are less likely to have arrhythmias and are more likely to have psychiatric illnesses.[41] The extent of initial evaluation of these patients is guided by the presence or absence of heart disease (as noted earlier). In patients with frequent recurrent syncope in whom there is a high suspicion of arrhythmias from the history, patient-activated intermittent electrocardiographic loop recorders are especially attractive if a cause is not established by other means.

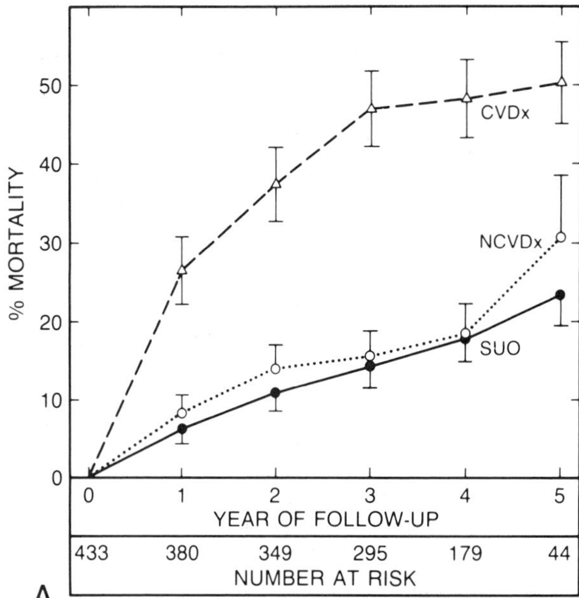

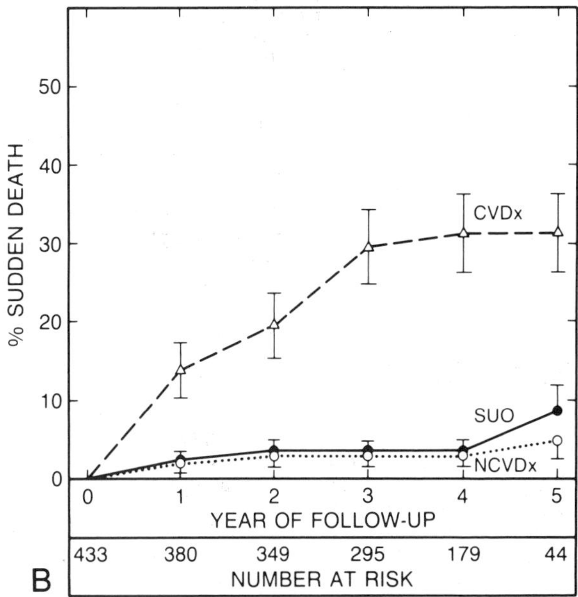

FIGURE 1–1. *A,* Actuarial mortality rates of patients with cardiac cause of syncope (*triangles*); noncardiac cause of syncope (*open circles*); and syncope of unknown cause (*solid circles*). The mortality in patients with a cardiac cause of syncope was significantly higher than in patients with noncardiac cause ($P < .00001$) or in patients with syncope of unknown cause ($P < .00001$). *B,* Actuarial incidence of sudden death of patients with cardiac cause of syncope (*triangles*); noncardiac cause of syncope (*open circles*); and syncope of unknown cause (*solid circles*). The incidence of sudden death in patients with a cardiac cause of syncope was significantly higher than in patients with noncardiac cause ($P < .00001$) or in patients with syncope of unknown cause ($P < .00001$). (From Kapoor WN: Evaluation and outcome of patients with syncope. Medicine 69:160–175, 1990. © 1990, The Williams & Wilkins Company, Baltimore.)

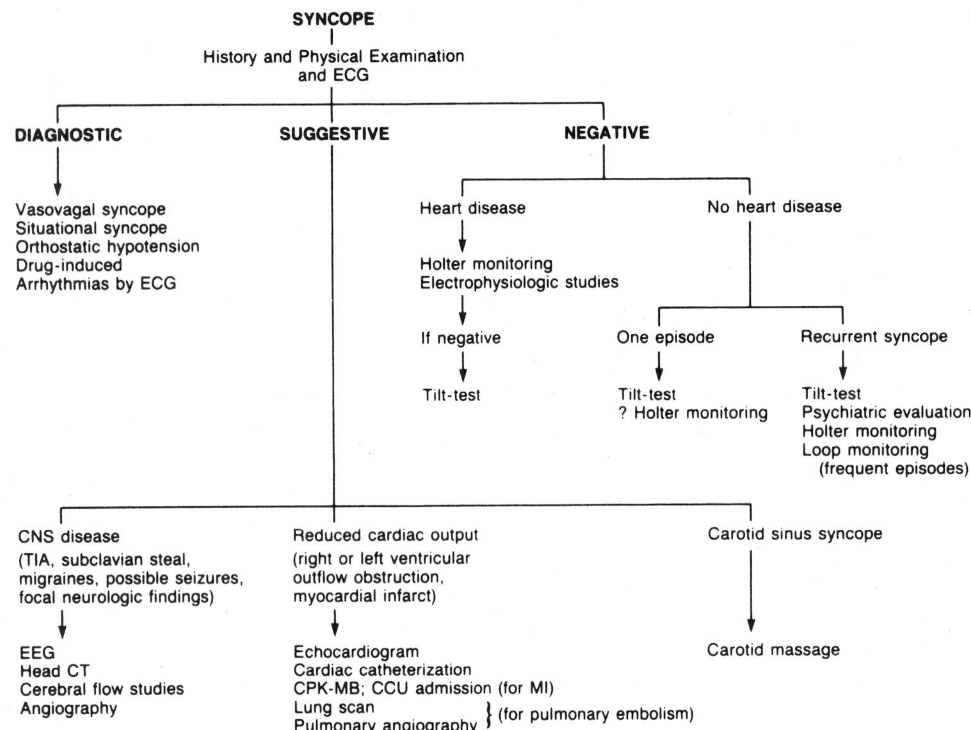

FIGURE 1–2. A flow diagram showing the approach to the evaluation of syncope. (From Kapoor WN: Diagnostic evaluation of syncope. Am J Med 90:93, 1991.)

A cause of syncope is assigned in most patients presenting with this symptom using this approach. Patients without a diagnosis have a favorable prognosis regarding mortality and sudden death, but they must be followed closely and re-evaluated upon recurrence of symptoms, since a potential cause may become apparent in a small proportion of patients after repeated episodes.

REFERENCES

1. Engel GL: Psychologic stress, vasodepressor (vasovagal) syncope, and sudden death. Ann Intern Med 89:403, 1978.
2. Kapoor WN, Peterson JR, and Karpf M: Micturition syncope. JAMA 253:796, 1985.
3. Kapoor W, Peterson J, and Karpf M: Defecation syncope: A symptom with multiple etiologies. Arch Intern Med 146:2377, 1986.
4. Levin B and Posner JB: Swallow syncope: Report of a case and review of the literature. Neurology 22:1086, 1972.
5. Lipsitz L: Orthostatic hypotension in the elderly. N Engl J Med 321:952, 1989.
6. Bannister SR (ed): Autonomic Failure: A Textbook of Clinical Disorders of the Autonomic Nervous System, 2nd ed. Oxford, Oxford Medical Pub, 1988, pp 1–20.
7. Sacquegna T, Cortelli P, Baldrati A, et al: Impairment of consciousness and memory in migraine: A review. Headache 27(1):30, 1987.
8. Strasberg B, Sagie A, Erdman S, et al: Carotid sinus hypersensitivity and the càrotid sinus syndrome. Prog Cardiovasc Dis 5:379, 1989.
9. St. John JN: Glossopharyngeal neuralgia associated with syncope and seizures. Neurosurgery 10:380, 1982.
10. Kapoor WN and Jannetta PJ: Trigeminal neuralgia associated with seizure and syncope. J Neurosurg 61:594, 1984.
11. Hoefnagels WAJ, Padberg GW, Overweg J, et al: Transient loss of consciousness: The value of the history for distinguishing seizure from syncope. J Neurol 238:39, 1991.
12. Linzer M, Felder A, Hackel A, et al: Psychiatric syncope. Psychosomatics 31:181, 1990.
13. Lombard JT and Selzer A: Valvular aortic stenosis: A clinical and hemodynamic profile of patients. Ann Intern Med 106:292, 1987.
14. DeSanctis RW, Doroghazi RM, Austen WG, and Buckley MJ: Aortic dissection. N Engl J Med 317:1060, 1987.
15. Jackman WM, Friday KJ, Anderson JL, et al: The long QT syndromes: A critical review, new clinical observations and a unifying hypothesis. Progr Cardiovasc Dis 31:115, 1988.
16. Laakso M, Aberg A, Savola J, et al: Diseases and drugs causing prolongation of the QT interval. Am J Cardiol 59:862, 1987.
17. Kapoor W, Karpf M, Maher Y, et al: Syncope of unknown origin: The need for a more cost-effective approach to its diagnostic evaluation. JAMA 247:2687, 1982.
18. Kapoor W, Karpf M, Wieand S, et al: A prospective evaluation and follow-up of patients with syncope. N Engl J Med 309:197, 1983.
19. Eagle KA and Black HR: The impact of diagnostic tests in evaluating patients with syncope. Yale J Biol Med 56:1, 1983.
20. Silverstein MD, Singer DE, Mulley A, et al: Patients with syncope admitted to medical intensive care units. JAMA 248:1185, 1982.
21. Martin GJ, Adams SL, Martin HG, et al: Prospective evaluation of syncope. Ann Emerg Med 13:499, 1984.
22. Day SC, Cook EF, Funkenstein H, and Goldman L: Evaluation and outcome of emergency room patients with transient loss of consciousness. Am J Med 73:15, 1982.
23. Kapoor W: Evaluation and outcome of patients with syncope. Medicine 69:160, 1990.
24. Atkins D, Hanusa B, Sefcik T, and Kapoor W: Syncope and orthostatic hypotension. Am J Med 91:179, 1991.
25. DiMarco JP and Philbrick JT: Use of ambulatory electrocardiographic (Holter) monitoring. Ann Intern Med 113:53, 1990.
26. Boudoulas H, Schaael SF, Lewis RP, and Robinson JL: Superiority of 24-hour outpatient monitoring over multi-stage exercise testing for the evaluation of syncope. J Electrocardiol 12:103, 1979.
27. Gibson TC and Heitzman MR: Diagnostic efficacy of 24-hour electrocardiographic monitoring for syncope. Am J Cardiol 53:1013, 1984.
28. Bass EB, Curtiss EI, Arena VC, et al: The duration of Holter monitoring in patients with syncope: Is 24 hours enough? Arch Intern Med 150:1073, 1990.

29. Jonas S, Klein I, and Dimant J: Importance of Holter monitoring in patients with periodic cerebral symptoms. Ann Neurol 1:470, 1977.
30. Clark PI, Glasser SP, and Spoto E: Arrhythmias detected by ambulatory monitoring: Lack of correlation with symptoms of dizziness and syncope. Chest 77:722, 1980.
31. Zeldis SM, Levine BJ, Michelson EL, and Morganroth J: Cardiovascular complaints: Correlation with cardiac arrhythmias on 24-hour electrocardiographic monitoring. Chest 78:456, 1980.
32. Kala R, Viitasalo MT, Tiovenon L, and Eisalo A: Ambulatory ECG recording in patients referred because of syncope or dizziness. Acta Med Scand 668(Suppl):13, 1982.
33. Kapoor WN: Diagnostic evaluation of syncope. Am J Med 90:91, 1991.
34. Kapoor W, Cha R, Peterson J, et al: Prolonged electrocardiographic monitoring in patients with syncope: The importance of frequent or repetitive ventricular ectopy. Am J Med 82:20, 1987.
35. Linzer M, Pritchett ELC, Pontinen M, et al: Incremental diagnostic yield of loop electrocardiographic recorders in unexplained syncope. Am J Cardiol 66:214, 1990.
36. Kapoor W, Peterson J, Wieand HS, and Karpf M: Diagnostic and prognostic implications of recurrences in patients with syncope. Am J Med 83:700, 1987.
37. Kapoor WN, Hammill SC, and Gersh BJ: Diagnosis and natural history of syncope and the role of invasive electrophysiologic testing. Am J Cardiol 63:730, 1989.
38. Bass EB, Elson JJ, Fogoros RN, et al: Long-term prognosis of patients undergoing electrophysiologic studies for syncope of unknown origin. Am J Cardiol 62:1186, 1988.
39. Olshansky B, Mazuz M, and Martins JB: Significance of inducible tachycardia in patients with syncope of unknown origin: A long-term follow-up. J Am Cardiol 5:216, 1985.
40. Doherty JU, Pembrook-Rogers D, Grogan EW, et al: Electrophysiologic evaluation and follow-up characteristics of patients with recurrent unexplained syncope and presyncope. Am J Cardiol 55:703, 1985.
41. Krol RB, Morady F, Flaker GC, et al: Electrophysiologic testing in patients with unexplained syncope: Clinical and noninvasive predictors of outcome. J Am Coll Cardiol 10:358, 1987.
42. DiMarco JP: Electrophysiologic studies in patients with unexplained syncope. Circulation 75(Suppl III):140, 1987.
43. McAnulty JH: Syncope of unknown origin: The role of electrophysiologic studies. Circulation 75(Suppl III):144, 1987.
44. Click RL, Gersh BJ, Sugrue DD, et al: Role of invasive electrophysiologic testing in patients with symptomatic bundle branch block. Am J Cardiol 59(1):817, 1987.
45. Fitzpatrick AP, Theodorakis G, Vardas P, and Sutton R: Methodology of head-up tilt testing in patients with unexplained syncope. J Am Coll Cardiol 17:125, 1991.
46. Almquist A, Goldenberg IF, Milstein S, et al: Provocation of bradycardia and hypotension by isoproterenol and upright posture in patients with unexplained syncope. N Engl J Med 320:346, 1989.
47. Waxman MB, Yao L, Cameron DA, et al: Isoproterenol induction of vasodepressor-type reaction in vasodepressor-prone patients. Am J Cardiol 63(1):58, 1989.
48. Kapoor WN and Brant NL: Evaluation of syncope by upright tilt testing with isoproterenol: A nonspecific test. Ann Intern Med 116:358, 1992.
49. Winters SL, Stewart D, and Gomes JA: Signal averaging of the surface QRS complex predicts inducibility of ventricular tachycardia in patients with syncope of unknown origin: A prospective study. J Am Coll Cardiol 10(4):775, 1987.
50. Savage DD, Corwin L, McGee DL, et al: Epidemiologic features of isolated syncope: The Framingham Study. Stroke 16:626, 1985.
51. Kapoor W, Snustad D, Peterson J, et al: Syncope in the elderly. Am J Med 80:419, 1980.

2

Palpitations and Disturbances of Cardiac Rhythm

MARSHALL A. WOLF, MD

Disturbances of cardiac rhythm may alarm the patient because of sensations that they engender or because of their effects on cardiac output or coronary perfusion. Cardiac function remains relatively stable with changes in heart rate over a fairly wide range; however, if bradycardia or tachycardia is sufficiently extreme even a normal heart will decompensate. In the patient with heart disease, the limits are narrower, and arrhythmias of lesser severity may provoke serious consequences.

In the evaluation of a patient with rhythm disturbance, the actual and potential hazard of the condition should be assessed before initiating extensive diagnostic or therapeutic maneuvers. Occasional extrasystoles are almost ubiquitous; most patients with this problem do not require any intervention except firm reassurance. Similarly, otherwise healthy patients may be well advised to tolerate occasional brief palpitations than to take medications to prevent them. In contrast, some patients with potentially lethal rhythm disturbances minimize their symptoms; the physician must be alert to this possibility. Like most problems in medicine, cardiac arrhythmias require that attention be paid both to the nature of the dysrhythmia as well as to the physical and emotional health of the patient.

PRESENTING MANIFESTATIONS

Some patients are able to sense even minor changes in cardiac activity; other patients, with profound rhythm disturbances, are completely asymptomatic. Although the physician conceives of palpitations as the sensation of rapid or irregular heart beats, patients may describe forceful heart beats as palpitations. It is important, therefore, to ask the patient to define carefully the exact nature of the sensation, especially with regard to rate, regularity, abruptness of onset and termination of the episodes, and associated symptoms.

Patients may present a diagnostic problem if they fail to sense a change in cardiac rhythm and experience only the resultant hemodynamic or physiologic consequences. Some may faint or experience near-syncope. Formerly it was assumed that such spells were usually due to slow heart action, but they are more often the result of tachycardia.[1–4] Occasionally, patients are not aware of arrhythmia prior to their spells, but experience palpitations subsequently.

In addition to spells caused by a precipitous fall in cardiac output, with attendant decreased cerebral perfusion, some patients with arrhythmias experience angina caused by increased myocardial oxygen consumption or decreased coronary perfusion. Others develop congestive heart failure if their hearts are unable to compensate for very slow or fast heart rates or to tolerate the sudden loss of preload caused by atrial dysfunction or atrioventricular (AV) dissociation. The onset of these episodes may be more acute and less predictable than angina or congestive heart failure that occurs in response to exercise or other stresses. Polyuria during or after an arrhythmia is sometimes seen with supraventricular tachycardias.[5, 6]

HISTORY

The history may be sufficient to obviate further diagnostic evaluation. Thus the young patient, who describes infrequent jumping or skipping sensations lasting for only a single beat and who is otherwise in perfect health, probably needs nothing more than the reassurance that this is a common, harmless phenomenon.

When the patient with palpitations is first seen, the clinician should ask whether he or she is experiencing the arrhythmia at that time, since this may provide a unique opportunity to obtain documentation of the nature of the rhythm disturbance. The patient should be asked to describe the symptoms in great detail. It is important to know whether the patient has taken his or her pulse during these episodes and, if so, whether it was regular or irregular or rapid or slow. The abruptness of onset and termination of the arrhythmia may also be useful in distinguishing sinus tachycardia, which begins and ends gradually, from the reentry tachycardias that generally begin and terminate abruptly. Asking the patient to tap out what he or she feels often provides insights into the rate and regularity of arrhythmia.

Some individuals will have learned how to terminate the

arrhythmia, and the maneuvers that they employ may be diagnostically useful. A patient who feels weak and coughs a few times with a prompt return of more normal status is probably experiencing bradycardia; the patient who finds that gagging, bearing down, or moving the bowels terminates the palpitations is more likely to be experiencing a supraventricular re-entry tachycardia.

Possible precipitating circumstances, diseases, and drugs must be carefully evaluated. Weight loss may be the only symptom of thyrotoxicosis in an elderly patient with atrial fibrillation.[7, 8] Sleep apnea syndrome has been associated with supraventricular tachycardia; a history of snoring or daytime somnolence may suggest this diagnosis. Alcoholic beverages and beverages rich in caffeine may be arrhythmogenic.[9, 10] One must also pay attention to the patient's medications (Table 2–1). Diuretics may induce hypokalemia and hypomagnesemia, both of which may predispose to arrhythmia. Arrhythmias have also been attributed to sympathomimetics, theophylline, tricyclic antidepressants, phenothiazines, lithium, pentamidine, and terfenadine. Antiarrhythmic drugs may be arrhythmogenic in some patients.[11] It is important to determine whether the patient's present medications have improved or exacerbated the arrhythmia; concurrence between the onset of an arrhythmia and the administration of a new medication should prompt temporary discontinuation of the medication in an attempt to solve the rhythm problem without more elaborate diagnostic or therapeutic maneuvers.

The pace and intensity of the evaluation are dictated by the effect of the rhythm disturbance on the patient. The patient who has palpitations and finds himself or herself on the floor with a broken pair of glasses and a laceration clearly needs prompt evaluation; a more leisurely evaluation or none at all may be appropriate in a young patient who has brief episodes of otherwise asymptomatic rapid heart action.

Physical examination may provide evidence of congestive heart failure, pulmonary disease, and thyrotoxicosis as well as organic heart disease. If the patient is seen during an episode of arrhythmia, flutter waves or signs of AV dissociation such as variations of the first heart sound or cannon a waves may elucidate the nature of the problem. Laboratory evaluation should include a complete blood count and thyroid function tests as well as serum potassium, calcium, and magnesium determinations.

The physician should always be involved in obtaining the initial electrocardiogram on patients with rhythm disturbances. Leads that permit identification of the P waves should be employed and should be of sufficient length and quality to permit exact measurements of atrial rate and regularity (Fig. 2–1). Although occasionally this requires esophageal or intra-atrial leads, atrial activity can usually be identified by means of double-standard precordial leads recorded from either the high right or left side of the chest. If some or all of the P waves are obscured by QRS complexes or T waves, the rhythm strip should include the results of carotid sinus massage or the Valsalva maneuver or both in an attempt to dissociate the atrial activity from these other complexes and to establish the relationship between atrial and ventricular activity.

Simple maneuvers may elicit arrhythmia that is not present at rest. Isometric exercise, done most conveniently by having the patient squeeze one or two of the physician's fingers, may elicit extrasystoles, a brief episode of tachycardia, or, less often, a significant bradycardia during post-tachycardia recovery. Similar data may be elicited by brief exercise such as sit-ups or running in place (Fig. 2–2). Maneuvers that alter autonomic tone may elicit paroxysmal arrhythmias.

TABLE 2–1. MEDICATIONS THAT MAY BE ARRHYTHMOGENIC

Digitalis preparations
Antiarrhythmic drugs
Diuretics
Antihypertensive drugs
Theophylline
Tricyclic antidepressants
Lithium
Phenothiazines
Thyroid hormone
Sympathomimetics
Terfenadine
Astemizole
Cocaine
Caffeine
Alcohol

Carotid sinus massage plays a central role in the differential diagnosis and occasionally in the treatment of rhythm disorders.[12] The maneuver is contraindicated in patients with carotid artery stenosis or known cerebral vascular insufficiency; it should always be performed with constant electrocardiographic monitoring. Pressure should be applied for only a few seconds and should never be applied bilaterally. An occasional patient may be extremely sensitive to carotid sinus stimulation and may respond with prolonged bradycardia; if the physician asks the patient to cough, this usually produces a prompt return of normal heart action. Some patients will not respond to this maneuver. If the physician stubbornly repeats it for prolonged periods or with greater force, this action will not provide therapeutic or diagnostic data but will only elicit adverse effects. Such patients may respond to the Valsalva maneuver.

Carotid sinus massage can produce several useful responses (Fig. 2–3). Prompt termination of the tachycardia is strong presumptive evidence of a supraventricular re-entry tachycardia; an occasional patient with ventricular tachycardia may also respond in a similar fashion. Slowing of the heart rate with subsequent ventricular irritability is consistent with digitalis toxicity. Gradual atrial slowing and reacceleration is diagnostic of sinus tachycardia. Production of AV block is seen in atrial flutter, ectopic atrial tachycardia with block, and occasionally in sinoatrial re-entry tachycardias. Appearance of ventriculoatrial block is diagnostic of ventricular tachycardia (VT). Occasionally, atrial flutter will convert transiently to atrial fibrillation during carotid stimulation.

Exercise testing is useful in both the diagnosis and treatment of patients with arrhythmias. Some arrhythmias that cannot be documented during prolonged monitoring will be elicited during or immediately after exercise. In addition, for patients whose arrhythmias are consistently elicited by exercise, the efficacy of their antiarrhythmic medications may be assessed by means of exercise testing.

Prolonged electrocardiographic monitoring can be performed with small portable tape recorders that record 12 to 24 hours of continuous data. Comparison of the analysis of such tapes with a log of the patient's activities can provide useful insights regarding the diagnosis, the relationship between the patient's arrhythmia and precipitating or subsequent ischemia, or the relationship of the rhythm disturbance to sleep, meals, activity, and medication. Since multiple tapings may be required before the arrhythmia is detected, monitoring should not be ordered unless the therapeutic implications and the data derived from such studies warrants the expense involved. Usually one or two leads are recorded,[13] and it is essential to place the leads in such

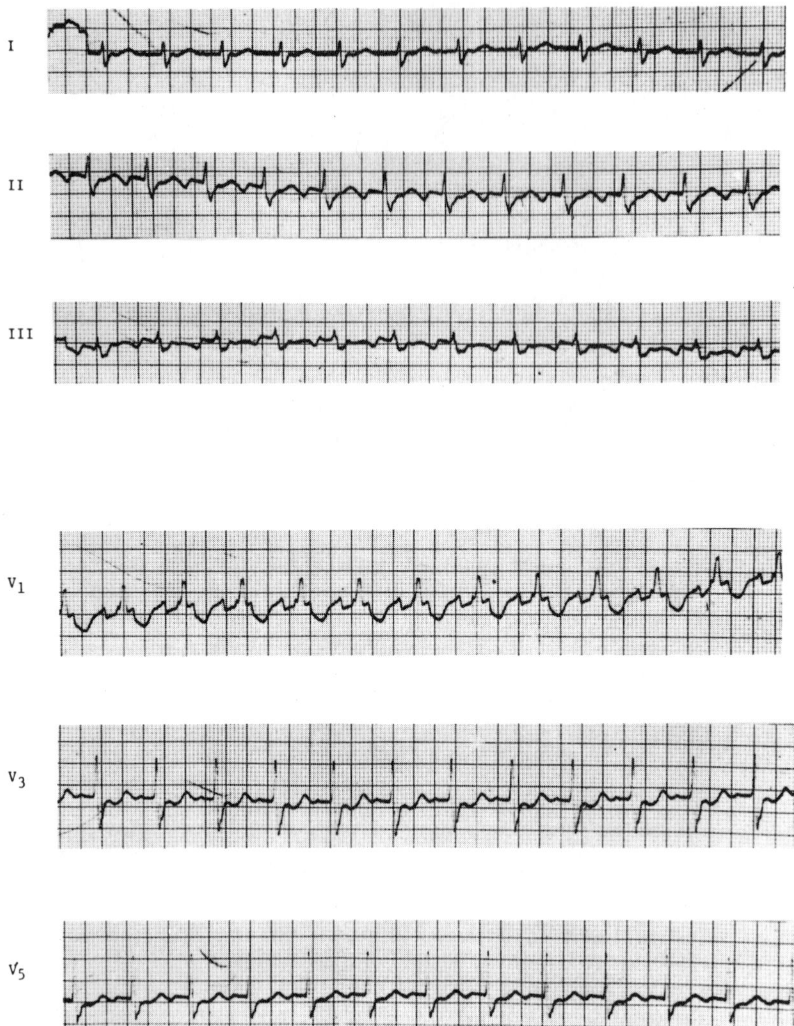

FIGURE 2–1. Slow atrial flutter and 2:1 atrioventricular block in a patient on quinidine. The atrial mechanism is most apparent in V1. The diminutive P waves in ectopic atrial tachycardia with block often can be seen only in the anterior precordial leads (see Fig. 2–11).

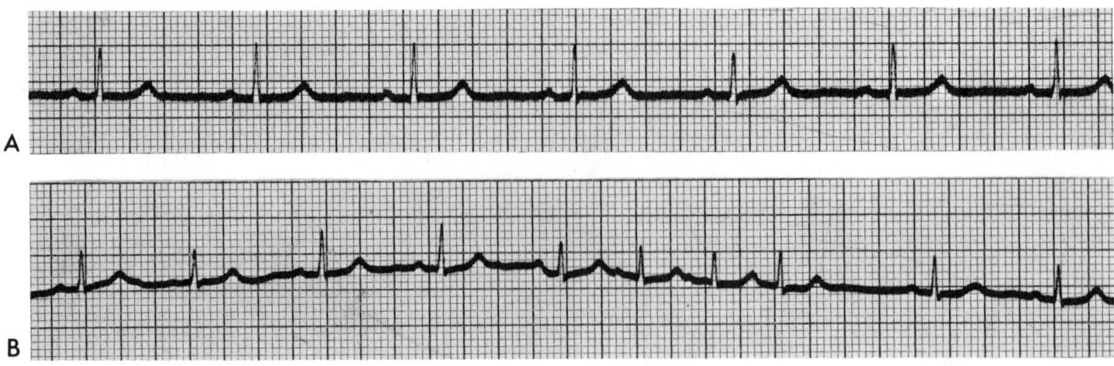

FIGURE 2–2. During rest *(A)*, no abnormalities were noted on the electrocardiogram of a 74-year-old housewife complaining of palpitations. After six sit-ups *(B)*, paroxysmal atrial tachycardia was observed.

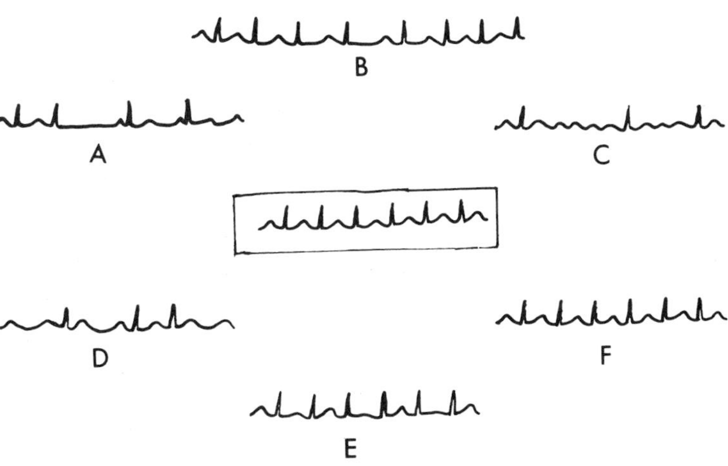

FIGURE 2–3. Carotid sinus massage (CSM) often provides critical information in the differential diagnosis of an arrhythmia. A number of responses may be seen. *A,* Reversion to sinus rhythm. This is considered diagnostic of paroxysmal supraventricular tachycardia; occasionally, ventricular tachycardia may revert with vagal maneuvers. *B,* Gradual slowing and reacceleration. This response may be seen with sinus tachycardia; in critically ill patients, sinus tachycardia often fails to slow with CSM. *C* and *D,* Atrioventricular block. This response is seen with both atrial flutter *(C)* and ectopic atrial tachycardia with block *(D).* The atrial rate is useful in distinguishing between these two arrhythmias. Occasionally atrial flutter may revert to atrial fibrillation with CSM. *E,* Ventriculoatrial block. This rather uncommon response is diagnostic of ventricular tachycardia. *F,* No response. This may be seen with any of the arrhythmias but is distinctly unusual in the patient with digitalis-induced atrial tachycardia with block.

a way as to permit clear identification of the atrial activity, since this may be crucial in identifying the type of arrhythmia recorded. Often the patient fails to have a "spell" during the initial taping. This first tape should be analyzed nonetheless, since many patients with symptomatic arrhythmias will have less prolonged asymptomatic episodes that may suffice for diagnostic purposes. If the initial tapes do not provide a diagnosis, an event recorder may be employed. This device, which provides a constantly updated record of the patient's rhythm, can be worn until an event occurs. Playback of the tape after an event will document the onset and nature of the arrhythmia. This technique is also useful in identifying patients who have palpitations in the absence of arrhythmia.

Electrophysiologic testing (EPT) has greatly increased our understanding of rhythm disturbances. Despite the considerable expense and significant morbidity of the procedure, it is clearly indicated in the evaluation of patients who have survived sudden cardiovascular collapse and in patients with Wolff-Parkinson-White syndrome and atrial fibrillation. EPT is often appropriate for patients with severely symptomatic AV nodal and extranodal pathway reentry tachycardias, since radiofrequency ablation is frequently curative in these disorders. The role of EPT in the evaluation of patients with recurrent syncope is still controversial; it may be appropriate for patients with overt coronary heart disease and unexplained recurrent syncope.

DIFFERENTIAL DIAGNOSIS OF ARRHYTHMIA

The exact nature of most arrhythmias can be clearly established by careful attention to a few important characteristics (Fig. 2–4).

Ventricular Regularity. Completely irregular ventricular activity is usually due to atrial fibrillation; multifocal atrial tachycardia is much less common. Apparently irregular ventricular activity can be seen with varying degrees of AV block or with multiple extrasystoles; in both of these situations, an appreciation of group beating or an underlying regular atrial mechanism should permit ready distinction from atrial fibrillation and multifocal atrial tachycardia, both of which show characteristic irregular or chaotic atrial activity. The ventricular activity in paroxysmal ventricular tachycardia (PVT) is also irregular; the wide QRS complexes and characteristic undulation in QRS voltage permit distinction from the other irregular arrhythmias (see Fig. 2–14). In atrial fibrillation with AV conduction by an accessory pathway, the QRS morphology and the RR intervals are much less variable than in PVT.

QRS Duration. Wide regular QRS complexes (>0.11 second) not due to pre-existent conduction disease are consistent with either VT or supraventricular tachycardia with bundle branch block. AV dissociation and fusion beats are diagnostic of VT. Similarity of the complexes to previously noted premature ventricular contractions or atrial premature beats with aberration is often helpful. Ventricular origin of the arrhythmia is suggested by a QRS duration greater than 0.14 second, a QRS configuration in V1 other than RSR′, the absence of a RS complex in all precordial leads, and an interval greater than 0.10 second between the onset of the R wave and the nadir of the S wave in a precordial lead (see Fig. 2–16).[14, 15] Carotid sinus stimulation may be helpful by provoking ventriculoatrial block, which would be diagnostic of an infranodal origin of the arrhythmia. If carotid sinus stimulation terminates the arrhythmia, it is likely to be supraventricular in origin although an occasional episode of VT will revert with this maneuver. Intravenous adenosine and verapamil have been used to increase AV block as an aid in distinguishing supraventricular tachycardias with aberration from VT. Although neither agent is very effective in this regard, the use of verapamil in this setting is very hazardous. Most patients with VT or atrial fibrillation with an extranodal pathway will suffer life-threatening consequences if they are treated with verapamil.[16]

Atrial Acceleration and Rate. If the atrial rate gradually accelerates over time in a patient with narrow QRS complexes, the arrhythmia is usually sinus tachycardia unless digitalis is being administered; digitalis may accelerate the atrial rate in ectopic atrial tachycardia with block, and in atrial flutter. The atrial rate should be measured carefully; regular atrial activity in excess of 220 beats/min in an adult is suggestive of atrial flutter or re-entry tachycardia in a patient with an AV bypass track.

Relationship Between Atrial and Ventricular Activity. The demonstration of AV dissociation is one of the main criteria for the diagnosis of VT. Similarly, the demonstration of ventriculoatrial conduction, either occurring spontaneously or produced by carotid sinus pressure, establishes this diagnosis. If AV block is present, an effort should be made to distinguish between Wenckebach block and Mobitz type II block, since these two conditions have markedly different prognostic significance.

Response to Carotid Sinus Massage. All arrhythmias may fail to respond to carotid stimulation; this affords no

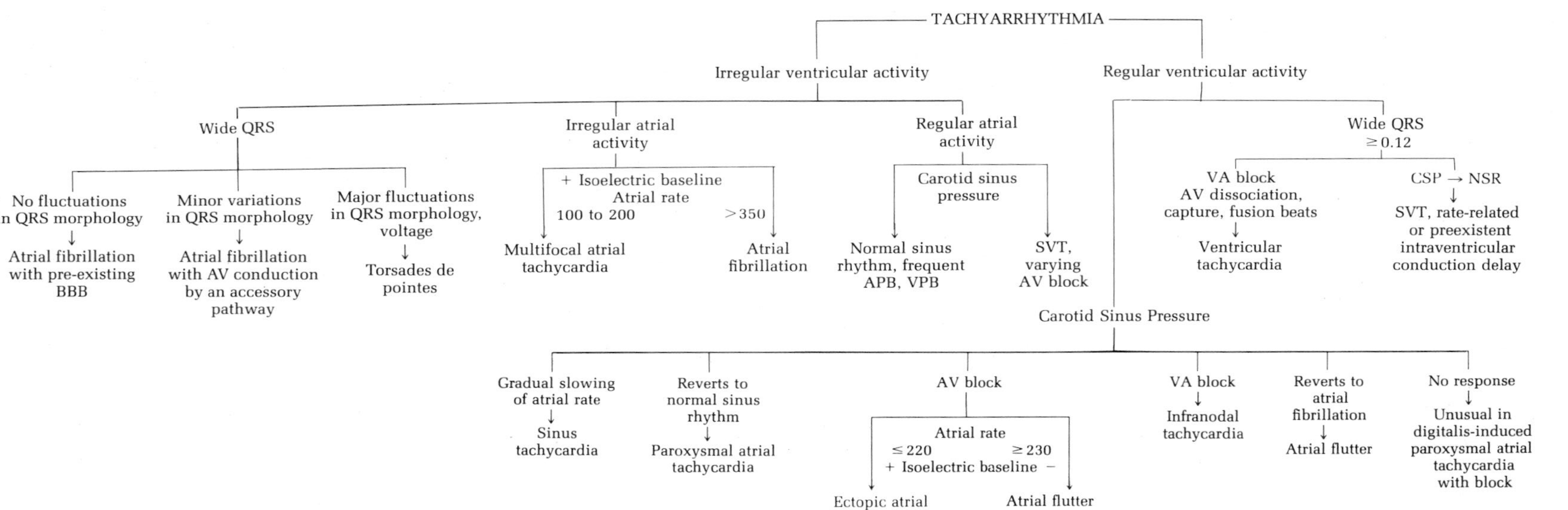

FIGURE 2–4. Differential diagnosis of arrhythmia.

diagnostic information except that it is a highly unusual response with digitalis-induced atrial tachycardia with block. Several other responses are virtually diagnostic: gradual slowing and reacceleration of sinus tachycardia; reversion to sinus rhythm of a re-entry supraventricular tachycardia (or occasionally VT); production of VA block of VT; and development of AV block with unchanged atrial rate of atrial flutter, ectopic atrial tachycardia with block, or less frequently sinoatrial re-entry tachycardia.

GENERAL APPROACH TO THERAPY

Many people assume that any heart trouble is likely to be fatal. The initial therapeutic measure for all individuals with potential or actual rhythm disturbances is reassurance. Although some arrhythmias are truly life-threatening, most arrhythmias are not, and this fact should be emphasized to the patient. In addition, the patient must be ensured that almost all rhythm disturbances eventually respond to therapy even if the initial therapy is unsuccessful. Before prescribing any drug, the physician should identify and modify those factors that might be responsible for the arrhythmia, especially thyroid dysfunction, congestive heart failure, electrolyte disturbances, pulmonary disease, alcohol or caffeine intake, and medications. One must then develop a therapeutic regimen that is both effective and less disagreeable than the complaint being treated.

Clinical circumstances often dictate the choice among several therapeutic alternatives in the patient with acute arrhythmia. For the patient with atrial fibrillation, a rapid ventricular rate, and severe ischemic pain, cardioversion may be the best approach; a patient with a similar arrhythmia who is pain free and may be suffering from digitalis intoxication should not undergo cardioversion but should be treated pharmacologically. In patients with recurrent arrhythmias, several therapeutic alternatives may exist. Patients with only infrequent episodes of a well-tolerated arrhythmia may prefer to take medication only at the time of the episodes; in many cases an effective therapeutic "cocktail" can be developed. Others, whose arrhythmias are more frequent or less well tolerated, clearly require prophylactic therapy. The usual goal of such therapy is to eliminate completely a recurrence of the arrhythmia. Often a less expensive, better tolerated, and equally acceptable program can be designed if the goal is merely to decrease the severity of the arrhythmia, should it recur, or to permit more ready reversion of the arrhythmia. Therapeutic trials are often required to choose the best alternative for the individual patient. In addition, certain noncardiac medical problems may contraindicate some antiarrhythmic medications; for example, the individual with an enlarged prostate is probably not a good candidate for disopyramide therapy, nor a patient with reactive airway disease for propranolol.

Specific Arrhythmias

Tachycardias

Sinus Tachycardia. This arrhythmia is a sign of underlying physiologic or emotional stress. Rather than treat the arrhythmia per se, the physician must identify and treat the various etiologic factors such as emotional stress, pain, fever, anemia, hypoxemia, electrolyte abnormalities, hypovolemia, thyrotoxicosis, or congestive heart failure. Occasional patients may complain of recurrent palpitations, especially at bedtime, due to this arrhythmia. Monitoring will demonstrate sinus tachycardia coincident with their symptoms. Frequently they respond to reassurance or to treatment of their underlying anxiety; sometimes, sedation or a β-blocker is necessary to control the symptoms.

Sinus tachycardia presents as a regular rhythm with a rate greater than 100 and usually less than 180 in the adult. Higher rates are seen in children. The rate often does not change with carotid sinus massage; if it does, the gradual slowing with a gradual return to the original rate aids in differentiating this tachycardia from others.

As mentioned earlier, treatment should be directed toward the etiologic factors rather than toward the tachycardia itself. An infrequent exception to this generalization is the patient with an acute myocardial infarction who does not have congestive heart failure; in this special circumstance, slowing of the rate with a β-blocker may protect the myocardium and decrease infarct size.

Paroxysmal Supraventricular Tachycardia (PSVT). PSVT is one of the commonest of the rhythm disorders; it often occurs in healthy patients with no underlying heart disease. Since little therapeutic benefit results from distinguishing paroxysmal atrial from nodal tachycardias, the two are often grouped under the term PSVT. These supraventricular tachycardias are usually due to re-entry in the AV node; in a significant minority, an accessory AV connection is also involved in the re-entry pathway; a small percentage of these arrhythmias are due to re-entry confined to the SA node and atria. Although occasionally stress or caffeine is implicated in the cause of this disorder, more commonly no etiologic factors can be identified. The rhythm is usually well tolerated in the patient without underlying organic heart disease; patients with organic heart disease, especially mitral stenosis or coronary artery disease, may tolerate this rhythm disturbance poorly. The individual experiencing PSVT is often apprehensive and may describe the heart as "bursting" or beating wildly. Occasionally patients note polyuria during or immediately after the episode. The rhythm begins and ends suddenly, and a clear description of this is useful in distinguishing PSVT from sinus tachycardia. Also many patients have discovered how to achieve reversion of the arrhythmia; a history of palpitations terminated by "bearing down," "straining," gagging, or bowel movements is virtually diagnostic of PSVT.

P waves are useful in distinguishing among the various types of PSVT. In nodal re-entry, the atria and ventricles usually depolarize simultaneously and the P wave is usually buried in the QRS or occurs as a negative deflection just after the QRS. A few patients with nodal re-entry have an inverted P wave just before the QRS. In extranodal pathway re-entry, the ventricular depolarization usually precedes atrial depolarization and an inverted P wave occurs early in the RR interval. In SA re-entry, the P waves are upright (Fig. 2–5). Atrial and ventricular rates in PSVT are usually in the range of 120 to 210; higher rates are seen occasionally in children or in patients with an accessory AV pathway. Extrasystoles rarely occur in paroxysmal atrial tachycardia; when they do, they may interrupt the re-entry cycle and terminate the arrhythmia. Carotid sinus massage either has no effect or terminates the arrhythmia. AV block never occurs with AV nodal or accessory pathway re-entry; an occasional patient with SA re-entry may block down, although more commonly the arrhythmia is unchanged or reverts to sinus rhythm.

Treatment is directed toward terminating the episodes and preventing recurrences. Any maneuver that interrupts the re-entry mechanism responsible for this arrhythmia can terminate it. Altering the autonomic tone is often effective and can be achieved by the Valsalva maneuver or by

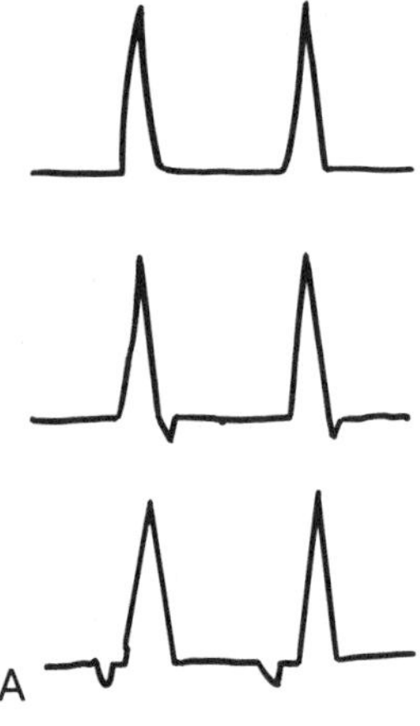

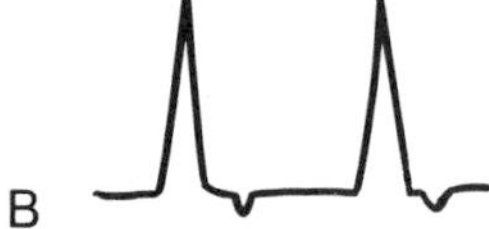

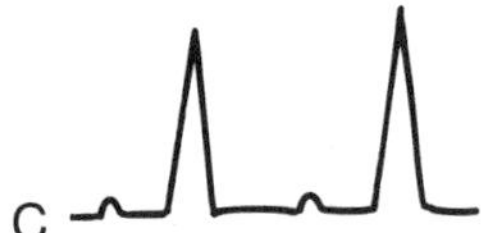

FIGURE 2–5. P wave morphology and paroxysmal supraventricular tachycardia (PSVT). The P wave is often useful in distinguishing the various types of paroxysmal supraventricular re-entry tachycardias. In atrioventricular (AV) nodal re-entry *(A),* the atrial activity most often occurs simultaneously with ventricular activity, and no P wave is seen. Less often in AV nodal re-entry, an inverted P wave occurs during or just after the terminal part of the QRS. Occasionally, when AV nodal re-entry occurs with the antegrade pathway in the faster β fibers, an inverted P wave occurs just before the QRS. In concealed extranodal re-entry *(B),* the atrial activity usually occurs after the ventricular activity, and an inverted P wave is seen after the QRS. In sinoatrial re-entry *(C),* the atria are depolarized antegrade rather than retrograde; the P waves have a normal vector and are upright.

carotid sinus massage as well as by medications. Except in patients with known cerebral insufficiency or carotid artery disease, carotid sinus massage is usually the therapy of choice. Occasionally there is a marked difference in the patient's sensitivity to R and L carotid massage, thus before the maneuver is judged ineffective, each side should be stimulated separately (Fig. 2–6); bilateral compression is hazardous and should never be attempted. Repetition of the maneuver may prove successful after pharmacologic intervention. In some patients the Valsalva maneuver or

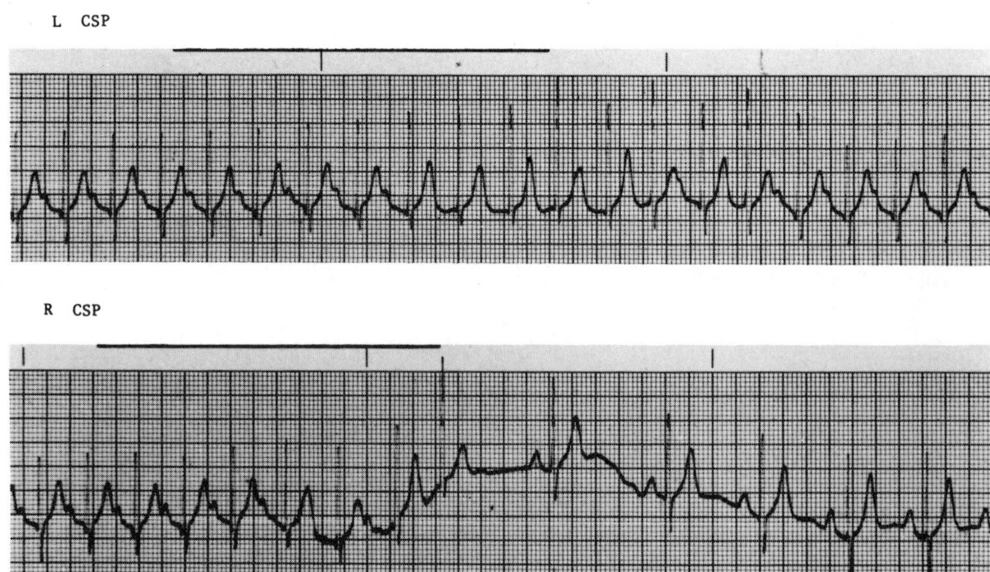

FIGURE 2–6. Left carotid sinus pressure was unsuccessful in terminating paroxysmal supraventricular tachycardia in this 19-year-old student with mitral valve prolapse. The arrhythmia reverted promptly when pressure was applied on the right side.

the induction of gagging may be ineffective when carotid massage has failed.[17]

If vagal maneuvers are contraindicated or unsuccessful, intravenous medications are employed to terminate the arrhythmia. Adenosine, 6 to 12 mg, is successful in more than 95% of patients.[18] It rarely has severe side effects, although prolonged bronchospasm has been seen in patients with asthma, and prolonged AV block may occur in patients taking dipyridamole. Patients taking theophylline may not respond to this agent. Brief chest discomfort and nausea may occur with adenosine. Intravenous verapamil,[18] 0.1 to 0.15 mg/kg, also terminates more than 90% of PSVT. Heart block, digitalis intoxication, a wide QRS complex, and hypotension (unless due solely to the arrhythmia) are contraindications to the use of this agent. The hypotension occasionally produced by this agent can be prevented by pretreating with 1 to 2 g of calcium carbonate. Patients with hypomagnesemia may be refractory to verapamil until the magnesium deficit is corrected.

Cardioversion is usually not required, except in patients with underlying Wolff-Parkinson-White syndrome, acute myocardial infarction, or severe congestive heart failure (Fig. 2–7). Energy levels of 50 to 150 watt-sec usually are effective. If there is any question of digitalis intoxication,

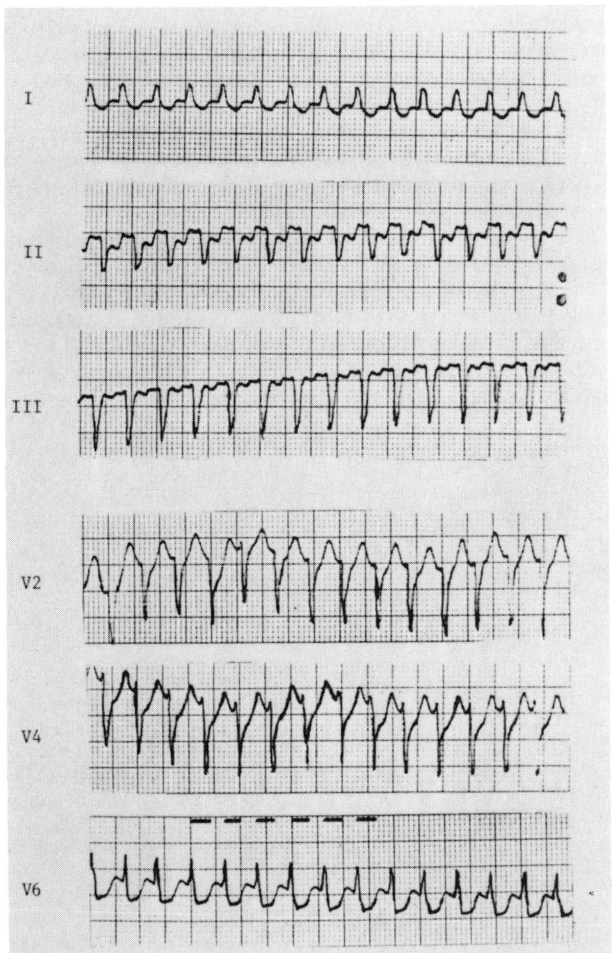

FIGURE 2–7. Rapid supraventricular tachycardia with ischemic changes and chest pain in a patient with Wolff-Parkinson-White syndrome. Such rapid rates are unusual in adults in the absence of an accessory atrioventricular bypass track. The patient did not revert with carotid sinus pressure; cardioversion was successful in terminating the arrhythmia and the discomfort.

test doses of 1 to 2 watt-sec should be given before subjecting the patient to the higher energy levels that are often required for successful reversion.

Once the acute arrhythmia has been terminated, thought must be given to whether or not it is appropriate to institute long-term therapy to prevent recurrences of this arrhythmia. Since many of the patients are otherwise healthy, tolerate the arrhythmia well, and have infrequent episodes, prophylactic medication may not be indicated until there have been several episodes. Patients with infrequent, well-tolerated episodes of PSVT, who cannot terminate their episodes with self-administered vagal maneuvers, may benefit from medications given at the onset of episodes. Verapamil, propranolol, and quinidine as well as some of the newer agents, used in this manner, may terminate the episode or permit termination with vagal maneuvers. The patient who develops syncope, congestive heart failure, or ischemia clearly requires long-term medication. Digoxin, which is often effective, is inexpensive and can be taken once a day. In patients with underlying Wolff-Parkinson-White syndrome or suspected accessory pathway re-entry, digoxin is relatively contraindicated. Verapamil, propanolol, and quinidine are also effective in preventing recurrences; verapamil is also relatively contraindicated in patients with accessory pathway re-entry.

Interruption of one of the limbs of the re-entry pathway prevents further arrhythmia. Initial efforts with surgery or DC shock, although effective, were accompanied by a measurable mortality and considerable morbidity including permanent complete heart block. Radiofrequency ablation is both safer and extremely effective; this is clearly the treatment of choice for patients with significantly symptomatic PSVT who fail to respond to simple medical management.[19]

Atrial Flutter. Atrial flutter is a poorly tolerated arrhythmia that is usually seen in patients with heart or lung disease. In patients without heart or lung disease, the arrhythmia is often a manifestation of multiple pulmonary emboli.[20] The atrial rate is usually 230 to 360, although slower rates may be seen if the patient has received quinidine or another type 1 antiarrhythmic agent or amiodarone. The usual adult patient is unable to sustain 1:1 conduction through the AV node at such rates and presents with 2:1 AV block and a ventricular rate of 115 to 180; occasionally, younger patients may present with 1:1 conduction. The underlying atrial mechanism can often be best appreciated in the inferior leads or in V1 or V2. The atrial activity is usually reflected as a sawtooth pattern rather than as discrete P waves; this may not be apparent in all leads. This arrhythmia is most often confused with sinus tachycardia, PSVT, and ectopic atrial tachycardia with block; carotid sinus pressure or other vagal maneuvers may be useful in establishing the diagnosis (Fig. 2–8). Production of increased AV block, but no change in the underlying atrial rate, distinguishes atrial flutter from sinus tachycardia and PSVT. Distinction between flutter and ectopic atrial tachycardia with block is usually made on the basis of the presence of the sawtooth pattern rather than discrete P waves with an isoelectric baseline and on the basis of atrial rate. Atrial rates in excess of 230 are most consistent with flutter, and atrial rates above 220 are very unusual in ectopic atrial tachycardia with block.[21] Atrial flutter with aberrant intraventricular conduction occasionally may be confused with ventricular tachycardia; production of increased AV block in response to vagal maneuvers will distinguish between the two. Occasional patients fail to respond to vagal maneuvers; a recording from an intra-atrial lead may be necessary to demonstrate the underlying atrial activity.

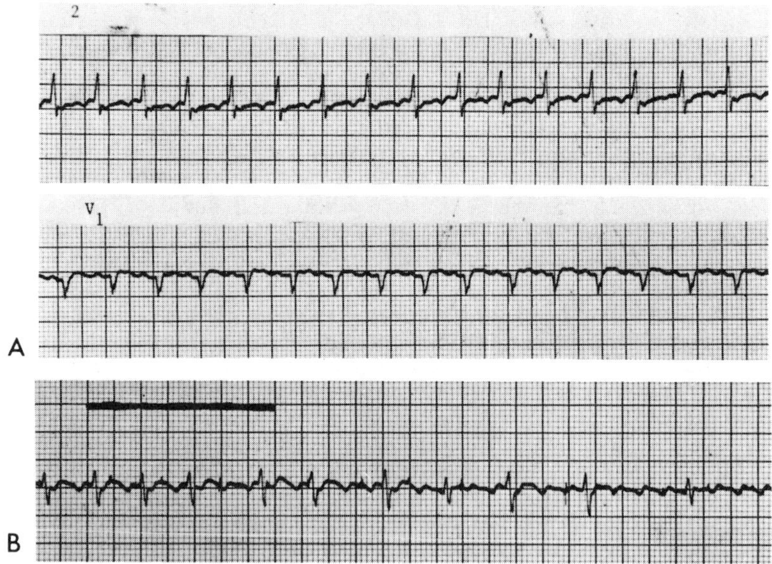

FIGURE 2–8. Palpitations developed in a 47-year-old bookkeeper after cholecystectomy *(A)*. The ventricular rate was 160. Carotid sinus pressure *(B)* increased the atrioventricular block and demonstrated atrial flutter with an atrial rate of 320.

Atrial flutter is often difficult to control pharmacologically, thus cardioversion is probably the treatment of choice. Low energies (5 to 10 watt-sec) usually suffice. Digitalis and quinidine or another type 1 agent are usually employed to prevent recurrences after cardioversion. Atrial flutter can also be managed with drugs. Digitalis increases AV block and, in addition, may convert the patient to atrial fibrillation or sinus rhythm; unfortunately, many patients experience toxicity before such therapeutic effects are achieved. Verapamil increases AV block and slows the ventricular rate; 10% of patients also revert to sinus rhythm. Five to 10 mg is usually given as a bolus or an intravenous infusion; this is contraindicated in the presence of digitalis toxicity, hypotension, a wide QRS complex, or high-grade AV block. β-Blockers also slow the ventricular response and occasionally result in reversion to sinus rhythm. Hypotension and congestive heart failure are relative contraindications to β-blocker therapy unless they are due solely to excessive ventricular rate. Quinidine may revert atrial flutter and also is used to prevent recurrences of this arrhythmia. Since quinidine causes slowing of the flutter rate and enhances AV conduction, some patients may develop 1:1 conduction with ventricular rates of 160 to 220 (Fig. 2–9). Digitalization, which decreases AV conduction, markedly diminishes the risk of this complication. Quinidine increases serum digoxin levels; careful monitoring is required when both agents are employed simultaneously.

Ectopic Atrial Tachycardia with Block. Paroxysmal atrial tachycardia (PAT) with block is a classic misnomer for two arrhythmias that often are not paroxysmal, may occur in the absence of block, and resemble flutter more than PAT.[22] A more accurate name is ectopic atrial tachycardia that blocks. One variant is a manifestation of serious digitalis intoxication; the less common variant is seen in

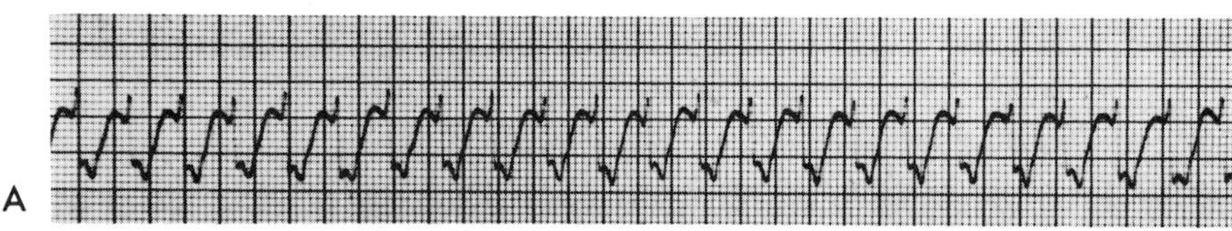

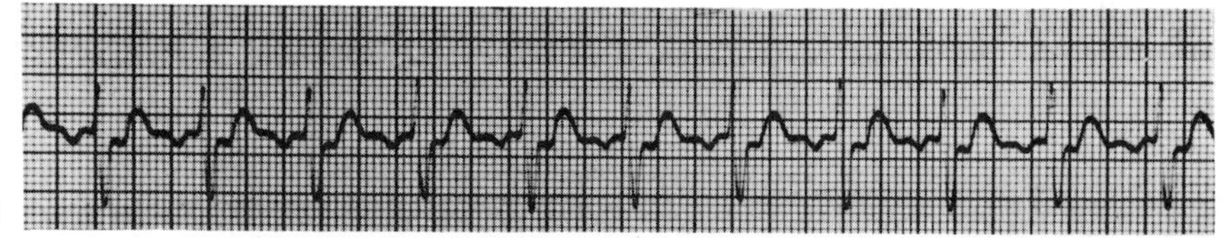

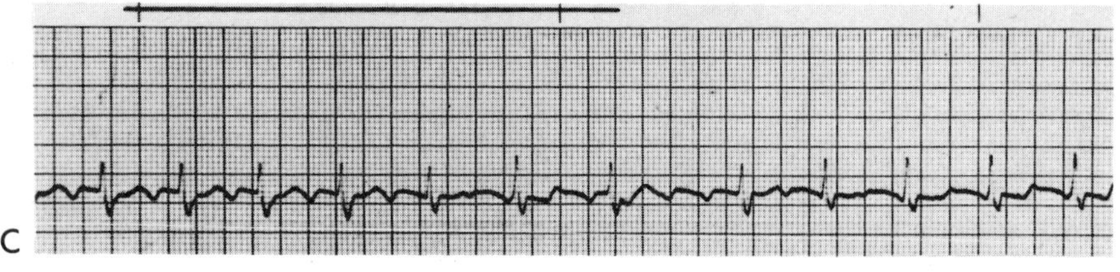

FIGURE 2–9. Atrial flutter, rate 200 with 1:1 conduction *(A)* in a 42-year-old secretary with recurrent atrial flutter and fibrillation who continued to take quinidine but discontinued digoxin. There was spontaneous reversion to 2:1 block *(B)* shortly after the patient arrived in the emergency ward. Carotid sinus pressure *(C)* demonstrates the underlying flutter activity.

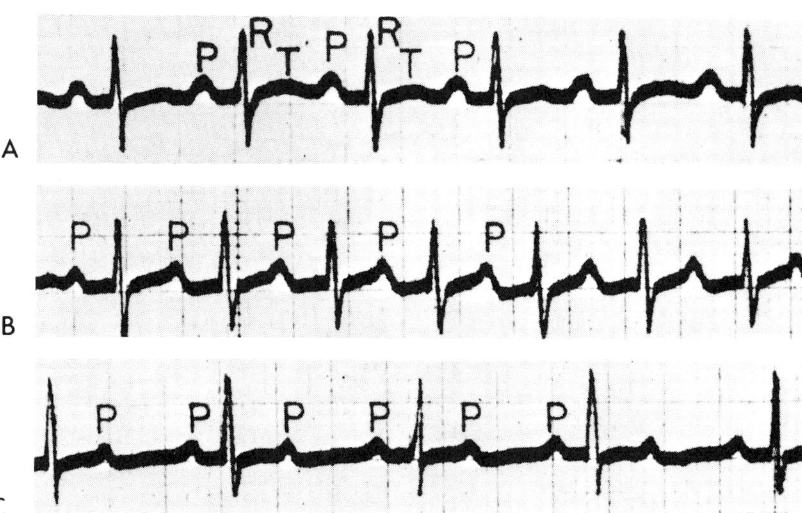

FIGURE 2–10. Development of an ectopic atrial tachycardia with block with progressive digitalization. Sinus rhythm with large, rounded P waves is seen in *A*. An ectopic pacemaker with smaller P waves developed with progressive digitalization *(B)*; carotid sinus pressure would produce atrioventricular block with an unchanged atrial rate. With further digitalization the P voltage decreases, the atrial rate increases, and 2:1 block appears *(C)*. (Adapted from Lown, B, Wyatt, NF, and Levine, HD: Paroxysmal atrial tachycardia with block. Circulation 21:129, 1960. By permission of The American Heart Association, Inc.)

patients with organic heart disease and often responds to digitalis. A rare patient may demonstrate both variants, depending on the degree of digitalization. The arrhythmia induced by digitalis is seen with near-lethal levels of the drug or in mildly intoxicated patients with hypokalemia. Most patients have other manifestations of digitalis intoxication including ventricular premature beats or gastrointestinal, visual, or neurologic/psychiatric symptoms.

The ectopic atrial pacemaker usually develops when the AV node is capable of 1:1 conduction; with continuing digitalization the ectopic pacemaker accelerates, AV conduction deteriorates, and varying degrees of heart block occur (Fig. 2–10). The ectopic P waves are often of low voltage and may be difficult to appreciate (Fig. 2–11). They are usually seen best in leads V1 or V2. Alternate P waves are often obscured by QRS complexes or T waves and appreciated only when more advanced AV block occurs spontaneously or in response to vagal maneuvers (Fig. 2–12). The atrial rate may be as slow as 90 but is usually in the range of 100 to 180 when the arrhythmia is first recognized. Atrial rates in excess of 220 are distinctly unusual and suggest atrial flutter.[21, 22] The P waves are separated by an isoelectric baseline; this, as well as the rate, is useful in distinguishing between this arrhythmia and flutter. Because of the marked vagotonic effect of toxic doses of digitalis, carotid sinus massage is almost always successful in inducing greater degrees of AV block and may be useful in demonstrating this arrhythmia by revealing the P waves hidden in the QRS complexes or T waves. Patients with atrial fibrillation or flutter who have "reverted to sinus rhythm" with digitalis therapy, should always have a rhythm strip with carotid sinus massage to rule out the possibility of their having reverted to ectopic atrial tachycardia with block rather than to sinus rhythm.

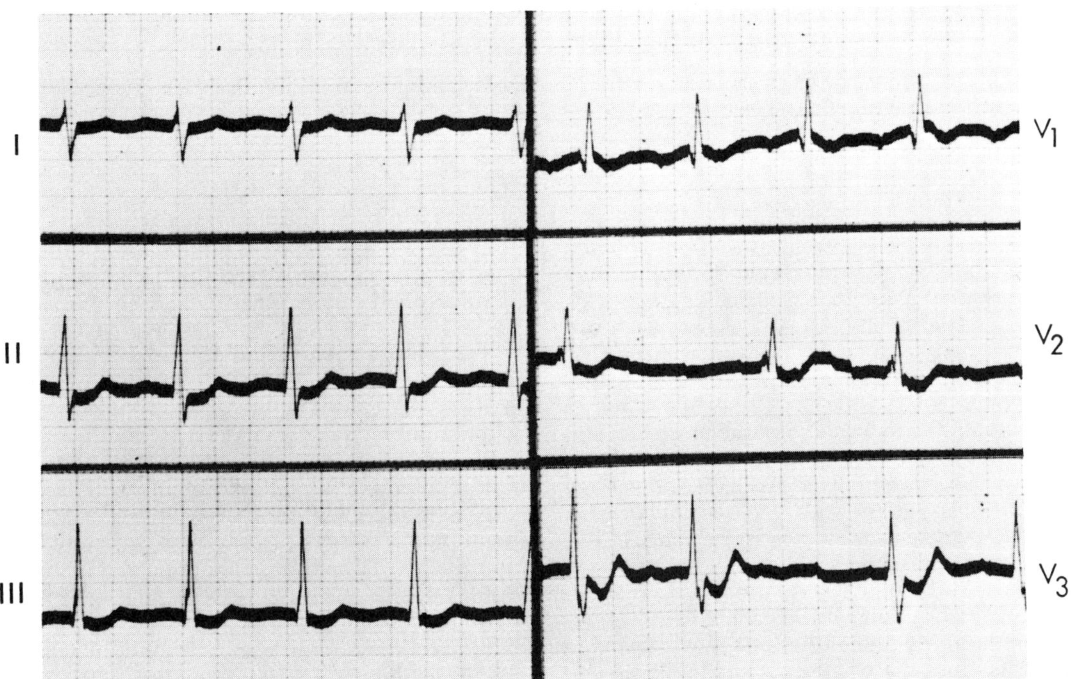

FIGURE 2–11. Diminutive P waves are seen in the anterior precordial leads in this patient with ectopic atrial tachycardia with block. (Courtesy of David Littman, M.D.)

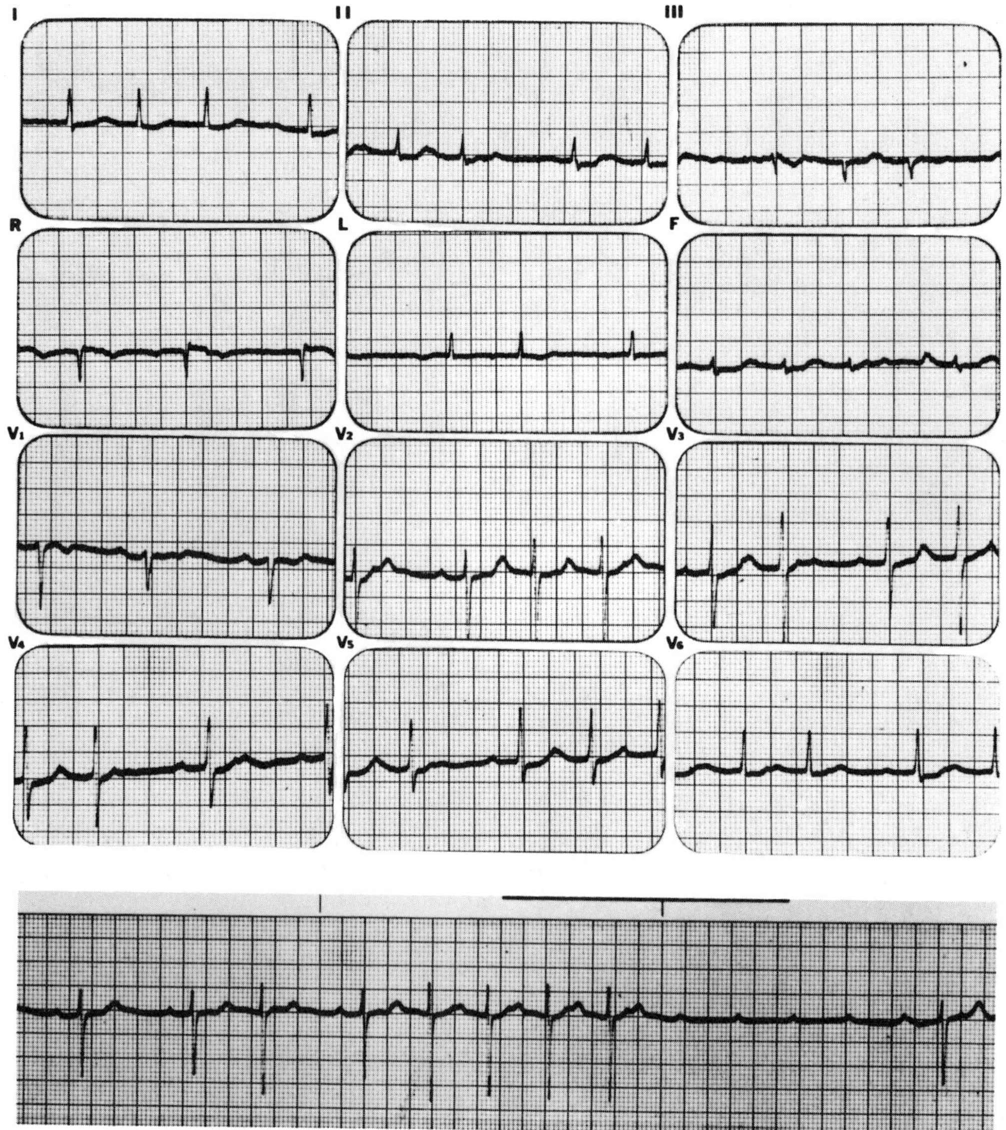

FIGURE 2–12. Digitalis-induced ectopic atrial tachycardia with block in a 64-year-old physician taking digoxin for recurrent atrial fibrillation. The atrial activity is best appreciated in V2. Carotid sinus massage produces transient complete atrioventricular block and makes the atrial mechanism more apparent.

Once the diagnosis is made, the patient should be hospitalized and digitalis should be discontinued. Hypokalemia and hypomagnesemia should be corrected. Lidocaine may be useful in suppressing associated ventricular ectopic activity. Cardioversion is extremely hazardous because it can enhance digitalis toxicity and may elicit ventricular tachycardia or ventricular fibrillation.

Ectopic atrial tachycardia with block that is not due to digitalis usually occurs episodically in patients with valvular heart disease but may be a chronic finding. The ectopic P waves in this variant are usually of much greater voltage than are those seen in patient with digitalis intoxication (Fig. 2–13). The atrial rate is most often in the range of 130 to 220. Carotid sinus pressure usually induces increased degrees of AV block, although some patients may not respond to this maneuver. A diagnosis of ectopic atrial tachycardia with block that is not due to digitalis should be made with great caution, since the treatments employed for this arrhythmia are all potentially lethal in a patient with the digitalis-induced variant. Digoxin and digitoxin levels should be measured before this diagnosis is accepted. Digitalis is effective in increasing AV block in this arrhythmia and in slowing the ventricular rate. Cardioversion often requires high energy levels, and a spontaneous recurrence of the arrhythmia following cardioversion is not uncommon.

Ventricular Tachycardia and Ventricular Extrasystoles. VT usually occurs in patients with acute or chronic heart disease, but it is also seen in some patients as a manifestation of drug toxicity and a few patients with no underlying heart disease. This arrhythmia is often poorly tolerated either because of its tendency to deteriorate to ventricular fibrillation or because of the hemodynamic deterioration that occurs as a result of the rapid rate and the loss of normal atrial preload. Some patients, however, tolerate the rhythm well and may have prolonged episodes with no apparent hemodynamic compromise.

The width of the QRS complex in VT usually exceeds 0.11 second, although narrow complexes are seen occasionally. The ventricular rate is 100 to 250. The ventricular rhythm in established VT is usually very regular, especially at

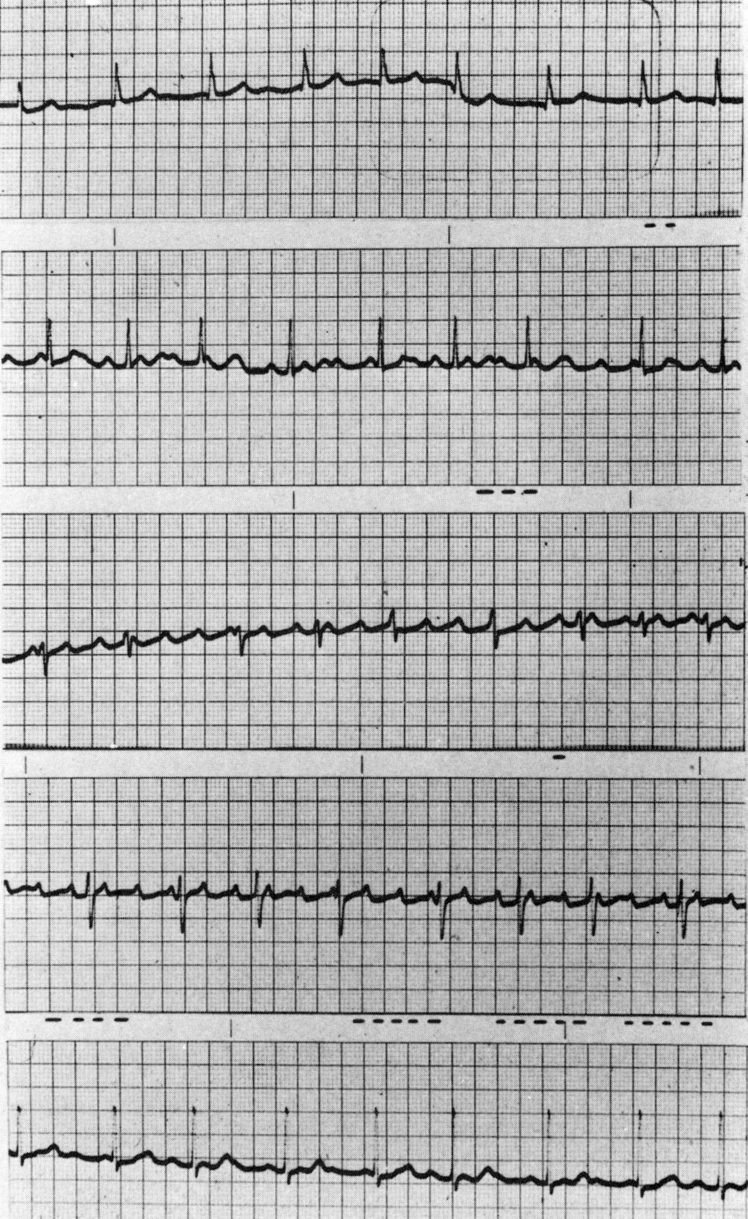

FIGURE 2–13. Ectopic atrial tachycardia with block in a 64-year-old housewife with rheumatic mitral valve disease and no medications. The P voltage is greater than that usually seen in patients with digitalis-induced ectopic atrial tachycardia with block. The atrial rate (200) is too slow for untreated atrial flutter.

faster rates; grossly irregular rapid ventricular activity with a wide QRS is much more likely to be torsades de pointes or atrial fibrillation with pre-existent bundle branch block or with AV conduction via an accessory pathway (Fig. 2–14).

It is often difficult to establish the diagnosis of VT. A physical examination may be useful in patients with AV dissociation, because they may have cannon a waves and their heart sounds may have a characteristic cascading pattern. The electrocardiogram confirms the diagnosis if it demonstrates AV dissociation, AV block, or fusion or capture beats (Fig. 2–15). Unfortunately, in many cases, none of these findings is present, and it may be extremely difficult to distinguish VT from a supraventricular tachycardia with aberrant conduction. The surface electrocardiogram provides data that, although not diagnostic, are very suggestive of VT (Fig. 2–16). If the QRS duration is longer than 0.14 second, the arrhythmia is likely to be VT.[14] A QRS complex in V1 of the RSR′ pattern suggests the arrhythmia is supraventricular; all other QRS patterns in V1 argue for VT.[14] The absence of a RS pattern in any of the precordial leads is very suggestive of VT.[15] If the interval from the onset of the R wave to the nadir of the S wave is more than 0.1 second in any precordial lead, the arrhythmia is usually VT.[15]

The approach to therapy depends very much on the clinical setting in which the arrhythmia appears. In the patient with acute ischemia or with marked hemodynamic compromise, the treatment is usually a bolus of 50 to 100 mg of lidocaine, followed immediately by cardioversion. If cardioversion is unsuccessful or if the patient immediately reverts to tachycardia, another bolus of lidocaine is given and cardioversion is repeated. If the second attempt is unsuccessful, the patient is usually given intravenous procainamide, 5 to 15 mg/kg, at a rate of no more than 50 mg/min. If the patient fails to stabilize with procainamide, bretylium is usually employed. This agent is given in 5 mg/kg intravenous boluses to a maximum of 30 mg/kg; bretylium

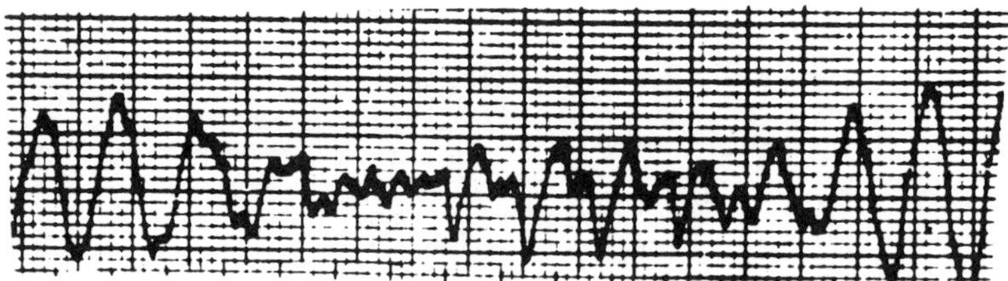

A

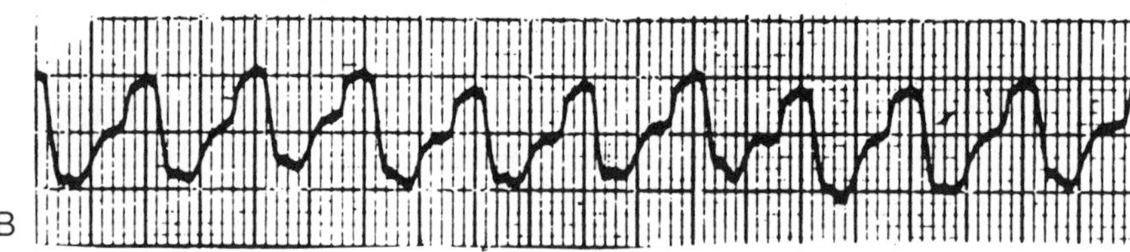

B

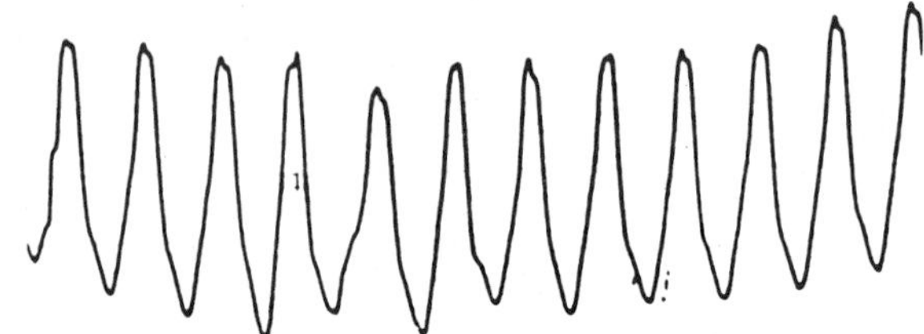

C

FIGURE 2–14. Torsades de pointes *(A)* demonstrates RR variation and varying R wave morphology and voltage. Ventricular tachycardia *(B)* is usually a regular rhythm. Atrial fibrillation with conduction via an accessory pathway *(C)* is distinguished from ventricular tachycardia by subtle variations in the QRS morphology as well as the RR interval irregularity and from torsades de pointes by the lack of the periodic variations in QRS morphology and voltage.

therapy may exacerbate digitalis toxicity and may produce profound hypotension. For patients who are better able to tolerate the rhythm disturbance, one might try several antiarrhythmic drugs before resorting to cardioversion.

Cardioversion of VT often can be accomplished with 10 watt-sec or less. Such low energies are hazardous if delivered during the vulnerable period, because they may induce ventricular fibrillation. If it is difficult to distinguish the QRS complex from the T wave, the energy should be delivered in the defibrillation mode, or energies of 100 to 150 watt-sec should be employed to minimize this hazard (Fig. 2–17). Cardioversion is extremely hazardous in the patient in whom VT is a manifestation of digitalis intoxication, because it may induce ventricular fibrillation.

The pharmacologic therapy of recurrent VT is often complex, and several drugs may be required, often in near-toxic doses. While procainamide, propranolol, quinidine, bretylium, tocainide, and disopyramide have all been beneficial in individual patients, no clear guideline exists to predict which patients will respond to each of these medications. Systematic testing of multiple drugs is often required, and one must be aware of the hazard of arrhythmia exacerbation by antiarrhythmic drugs in these patients.[11] Patients with life-threatening ventricular arrhythmias should be evaluated where electrophysiologic testing is available, because this technique has proved predictive of drug efficacy. Some patients may require an implantable defibrillator or surgery for rhythm control.[23]

PVT is a life-threatening arrhythmia that is often confused with VT.[24, 25] It is characterized by a periodic variation in QRS morphology and voltage that permits distinction of this arrhythmia from both VT and atrial fibrillation,

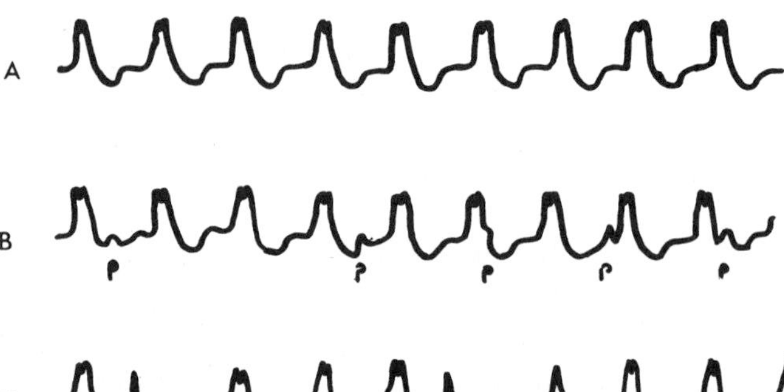

FIGURE 2–15. Ventricular tachycardia *(A)*. The rapid rate and wide QRS could also be seen in supraventricular tachycardia with intraventricular conduction delay. The diagnosis of ventricular tachycardia is established if one is able to demonstrate atrioventricular dissociation *(B)*, capture or fusion beats *(C)*, or ventriculoatrial block *(D)*.

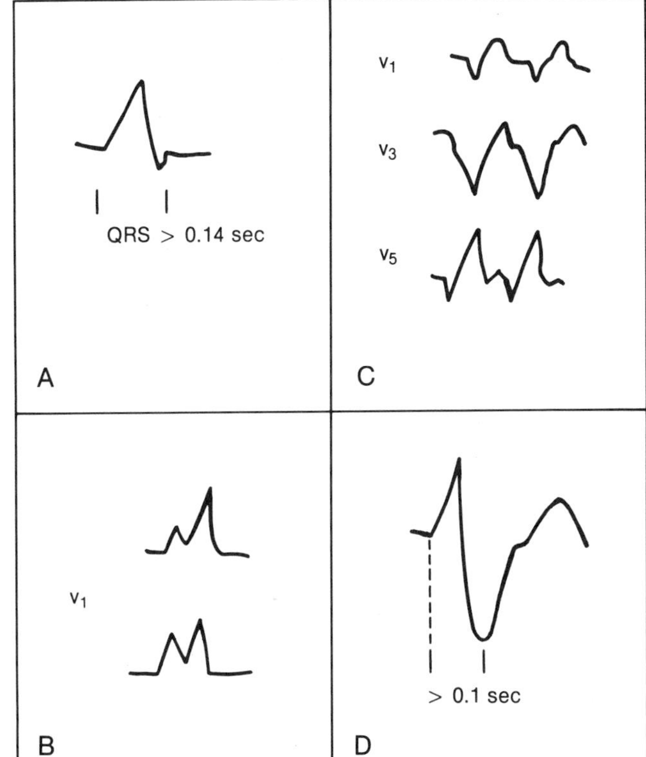

FIGURE 2–16. An electrocardiogram provides several patterns that suggest that a wide complex, regular tachycardia is ventricular tachycardia (VT) rather than a supraventricular tachycardia with a rate-related bundle branch block (SVT-RRBBB). A QRS with greater than 0.14 sec is more likely to be seen in ventricular tachycardia *(A)*. A QRS complex in V1, V2 of the RSR′ pattern is suggestive of SVT-RRBBB; other QRS patterns in V1 suggest VT *(B)*. The absence of an RS complex in the precordial leads suggests VT *(C)*. An RS interval (the onset of R wave to the nadir of the S wave) in a precordial lead that is greater than 0.1 second suggests that the arrhythmia is VT *(D)*.

with either pre-existing bundle branch block or AV conduction via an accessory pathway (see Fig. 2–14). PVT is often associated with QT prolongation; this variant, known as torsades de pointes, accounts for the vast majority of PVT seen in clinical practice. Quinidine, procainamide, disopyramide, phenothiazines, tricyclic antidepressants, lithium, terfenidine, pentamidine, erythromycin, hypokalemia, hypomagnesemia, and hypothyroidism—all of which increase the QT interval—have been implicated in causing torsades de pointes.

Recognition of this variant of VT is essential, because the treatment of torsades de pointes is different from that of VT; indeed, some of the classic medications used to treat VT are extremely hazardous in patients with torsades de pointes. Since quinidine-like drugs cause development of torsades de pointes, they are contraindicated in its treatment. Therapy for torsades de pointes is directed at shortening the prolonged QT interval by removing the precipitating drug, by correcting the electrolyte disorder, or by increasing the heart rate with a transvenous pacemaker. Intravenous magnesium (1 to 5 g of magnesium sulfate) often terminates torsades de pointes.[26] Patients with PVT and normal QT intervals often respond to type 1 antiarrhythmic drugs. Patients with congenital QT prolongation and a family history of sudden death may respond to sympatholytic therapy.

The patient with atrial fibrillation and an accessory pathway often presents with a rapid wide-complex tachycardia that is easily confused with VT. Subtle variations in the RR interval and in the QRS morphology are the clues that permit distinction of this arrhythmia from VT (see Fig. 2–14). Previous electrocardiograms that show a Wolff-Parkinson-White pattern are helpful in distinguishing this arrhythmia from VT; it must be remembered, however, that some patients have normal baseline tracings and are still able to conduct via an accessory pathway during atrial fibrillation.

Since the ventricular rate is often 180 to 250 during this arrhythmia, many patients tolerate it quite poorly. Therapy is directed toward reverting the arrhythmia with emergency cardioversion or to slowing the AV conduction with medications. Quinidine, procainamide, and the other type 1 antiarrhythmic agents, which slow conduction through the accessory pathway, may be used in the acute treatment of this arrhythmia. Digitalis drugs and verapamil, which accelerate conduction through the accessory pathway, are contraindicated in the treatment of this arrhythmia and may be life-threatening.

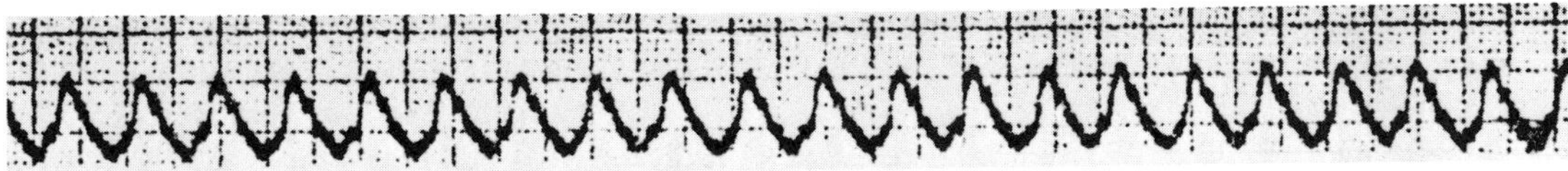

FIGURE 2–17. Ventricular tachycardia. It is impossible to distinguish with certainty the QRS complex and T waves. If electrical reversion is attempted with a synchronized discharge, there is a 50% chance of shocking the vulnerable period and, if the level of energy delivered is low, producing ventricular fibrillation. If low-energy electrical revision is attempted, it should be done with an unsynchronized (defibrillation mode) discharge. High-energy stimuli (>150 watt-sec) are unlikely to produce ventricular fibrillation even if delivered during the vulnerable period.

Although chronic therapy with a type 1 antiarrhythmic drug or amiodarone has been employed in the treatment of patients with atrial fibrillation and conduction via an accessory pathway, these drugs are hazardous when used over prolonged periods, and the arrhythmia is likely to recur if patients have compliance problems. The availability of radiofrequency ablation, with a high likelihood of therapeutic efficacy and a relatively low incidence of significant morbidity, has made definitive therapy with this modality the treatment of choice for patients with this problem.

The patient with multiple ventricular premature beats (VPBs) often seeks or is referred for treatment. VPBs had been considered a relatively benign finding until the coronary care unit experience demonstrated that they were often harbingers of more severe ventricular arrhythmia and that suppressing VPBs could prevent potentially lethal arrhythmias. Subsequent studies have shown that VPBs are a risk factor for sudden death and myocardial infarction in ambulatory patients.[27–29]

VPBs are almost ubiquitous, and 70 to 90% of adults have at least one during a 24-hour monitoring session. Many drugs, including digitalis, the antiarrhythmic drugs, phenothiazines, tricyclic antidepressants, sympathomimetics, theophylline, caffeine, and alcohol increase VPBs in some individuals. The risk associated with VPBs is very much a function of the presence or absence of underlying heart disease. In young patients without heart disease, the risk is minimal, if any.[30–32] In patients who have recently recovered from myocardial infarction, the risk is considerable, especially if, in addition to simple VPBs, there are more complex ventricular arrhythmias, such as bigeminy, couplets, brief salvos of VT, or early VPBs that interrupt the preceding T waves (the R-on-T phenomenon). VPBs occurring immediately postinfarction have little prognostic significance, but those occurring 2 weeks to 6 months postinfarction are useful in identifying patients at greater risk of sudden death.[28, 29, 33, 34] While it is clear that patients with severely damaged ventricles are at maximum risk, VPBs are a significant, independent indicator of the risk of cardiac death in all patients with ischemic heart disease.[35]

Unfortunately, no data exist to support the hypothesis that suppression of VPBs in the ambulatory patient will produce the marked decrease in arrhythmic deaths achieved in the coronary care unit. The Coronary Arrhythmia Suppression Trial (CAST) demonstrated significantly increased mortality in patients with VPB postmyocardial infarction who were treated with antiarrhythmic drugs, even though these drugs had been effective in suppressing VPBs in patients in the study.[36]

Patients who have recovered from ventricular fibrillation or life-threatening VT clearly need antiarrhythmic therapy and are probably best served by being referred to a center where electrophysiologic testing and implantable defibrillators are available. Patients with complex VPBs and organic heart disease are clearly at increased risk of sudden death; at present no therapy has been shown effective in reducing this risk. The hazards of antiarrhythmic therapy in patients with normal hearts and asymptomatic VPBs exceed the potential benefits, and such patients are best served by being treated with vigorous reassurance.

Atrial Fibrillation. Atrial fibrillation is a common arrhythmia that is usually seen in patients with organic heart disease. It is also seen in patients without known underlying heart disease after alcohol ingestion, in those with thyrotoxicosis, in association with sleep apnea syndrome, and in patients with pulmonary problems, including pneumonia, pulmonary embolic disease, and following pneumonectomy. Medications are not a common cause of atrial fibrillation, although the arrhythmia has been reported with nicotine chewing gum and with fluoxetine. Although the arrhythmia may be well tolerated, it is often complicated by congestive heart failure due to the poor rate control and the loss of atrial preload. Systemic arterial embolization is a common complication of atrial fibrillation of any cause.

Both atrial and ventricular activity are irregular in atrial fibrillation. The atrial activity is continuous (Fig. 2–18) and is often appreciated best in V1 or V2; the atrial voltage decreases as the atrial fibrillation becomes more chronic. Occasionally carotid sinus massage, which increases AV block, is useful in demonstrating the underlying atrial activity. The ventricular activity is usually completely irregular, although there is a tendency for a slight regularization at very fast heart rates. Regularization of ventricular activity at slow rates suggests either heart block from AV nodal disease or digitalis toxicity (Fig. 2–19); this may also be seen with verapamil therapy.[37]

In approaching the treatment of a patient with atrial fibrillation, it is essential that thyrotoxicosis and underlying valvular heart disease be ruled out. Patients with a slow ventricular response in the absence of any therapy do very poorly with either pharmocologic or electrical intervention; anticoagulation alone may be the optimal therapy for these patients. The treatment of atrial fibrillation may be directed at reversing the arrhythmia or at increasing the AV block, thus slowing the ventricular rate. Cardioversion is the treatment of choice for the patient with an acute myocardial infarction and hemodynamic deterioration or

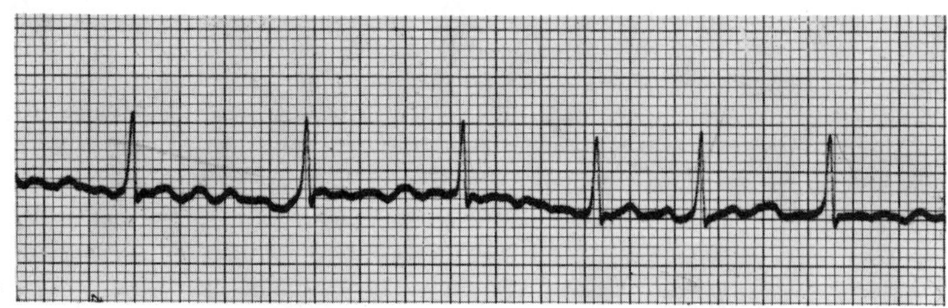

FIGURE 2–18. Atrial activity in atrial fibrillation *(A)* is chaotic and continuous; multifocal atrial tachycardia *(B)* is characterized by an isoelectric baseline with multiple P morphologies and varying PR and RR intervals.

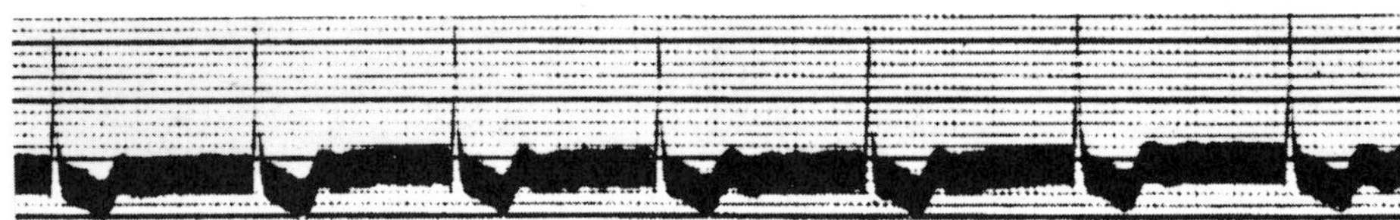

FIGURE 2–19. Atrial fibrillation. The marked ventricular regularization is the result of digitalis toxicity. Verapamil in therapeutic doses also may regularize the ventricular rhythm in atrial fibrillation.

continuing pain; antiarrhythmic drugs would be used to decrease the possibility of subsequent reversion to atrial fibrillation. Quinidine and digoxin are usually employed to prevent subsequent recurrences in stable patients; quinidine is hazardous when given intravenously, thus often intravenous procainamide is used before cardioversion in acutely ill patients. Cardioversion energies in excess of 50 watt-sec are usually required. If a question of digitalis intoxication exists, test doses of 1 to 2 watt-sec can be used; increased ventricular rate or ventricular irritability would be consistent with the diagnosis of digitalis toxicity.

In a less urgent situation, one would treat the patient pharmacologically in the hope that slowing the ventricular rate would permit clearing of underlying congestive heart failure and spontaneous reversion to sinus rhythm. A digitalis drug is given at regular intervals until the desired degree of slowing is achieved or toxic manifestations appear. The therapeutic endpoint is a controlled heart rate following mild exercise; often a patient whose resting rate has been slowed may still have an excessive rate upon mild exertion. In patients who develop signs of digitalis toxicity prior to achievement of adequate slowing (Fig. 2–20), verapamil, diltiazem, or a β-blocker may be employed to achieve greater AV block (Fig. 2–21). Verapamil seems to be especially effective in controlling the ventricular rate during exercise and may be employed alone if the patient does not require the positive inotropy provided by digitalis. Verapamil, 20 to 40 mg, three or four times daily, or propranolol, 5 to 20 mg, three or four times daily, is usually effective for chronic therapy; in the acutely ill patient, the ventricular rate can be slowed with intravenous verapamil, 5 to 20 mg in 1- to 2-mg increments, or with intravenous propranolol, 3 to 7 mg in 0.5- to 1-mg increments, given while carefully monitoring ventricular rate and blood pressure.

Patients who fail to revert to sinus rhythm with rate control and treatment of congestive heart failure may benefit from elective cardioversion. The improved rate control and a 10 to 20% increase in cardiac efficiency resulting from a return to normal sinus rhythm may be crucial to patients with limited cardiac reserve. If a clear cause for the fibrillation has been identified, such as pneumonia or thyrotoxicosis, cardioversion should be delayed until this has been treated, since cardioversion is often unsuccessful if performed prior to correction of the medical problem. In addition, after treatment of the precipitating medical problem, the arrhythmias often revert spontaneously. If fibrillation has lasted for more than a few days, anticoagulation should be instituted for at least 2 weeks prior to elective reversion to decrease the chance of an arterial embolism. Quinidine, 200 to 300 mg every 6 hours, is usually begun 18 to 24 hours before cardioversion; this achieves a return to sinus rhythm in 15% of patients and also increases the likelihood that the patient will remain in sinus rhythm after cardioversion. Quinidine interacts with both warfarin sodium (coumadin) and digoxin, increasing both the prothrombin time and the serum digoxin level. Adjustments of the dose of both digoxin and warfarin sodium are often required after a patient is started on quinidine. Procainamide or another type 1 agent may be used in patients who tolerate quinidine poorly. Studies have demonstrated the risks associated with the chronic use of type 1 antiarrhythmic medication. Low-dose amiodarone has been suggested as an equally potent but possibly less risky alternative in patients with chronic atrial fibrillation. This hypothesis is now being tested clinically. Patients who revert to atrial fibrillation soon after cardioversion should not undergo cardioversion again, unless the underlying medical condition has improved or the antiarrhythmic medications have been changed.

Systemic embolization is a frequent complication of atrial fibrillation. Of patients with chronic atrial fibrillation, 15% eventually have an embolic stroke. This risk increases with age. Several studies have demonstrated that anticoagulation with coumadin can safely reduce the risk of such strokes by 60 to 80%.[38, 39] Aspirin has a protective effect in younger patients but has not proved effective in older patients who are at the greatest risk of an embolic complication.

Multifocal Atrial Tachycardia. Multifocal atrial tachycardia (MAT) is a relatively uncommon arrhythmia

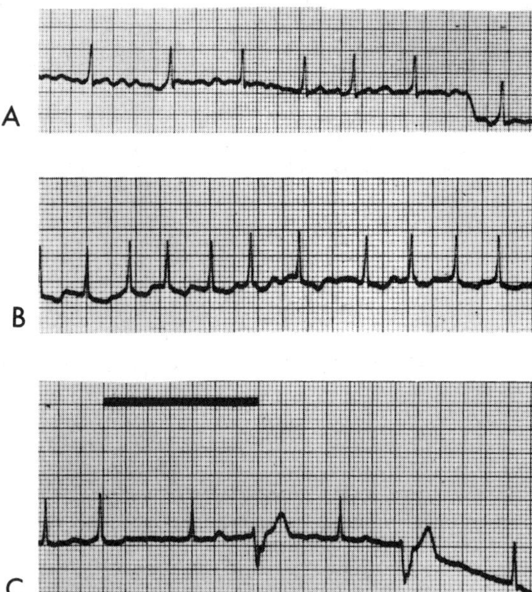

FIGURE 2–20. Resting ventricular rate was 80 *(A)* in this 54-year-old nurse with mitral stenosis and chronic atrial fibrillation. With a few sit-ups, the heart rate increased to 160 *(B)*, which is a response that is usually indicative of inadequate digitalization. However, carotid sinus pressure *(C)* consistently elicited slowing of the rate and brief runs of bigeminy, suggestive of early digitalis toxicity. Propranolol, 5 mg three times daily, controlled postexercise tachycardia and increased exercise tolerance.

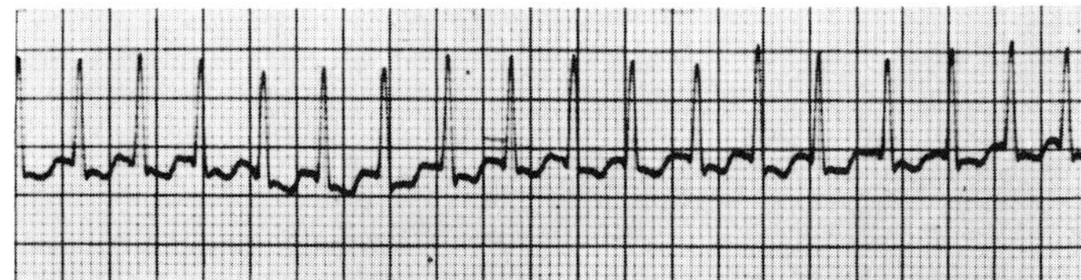

INDERAL 0.5 mg IV

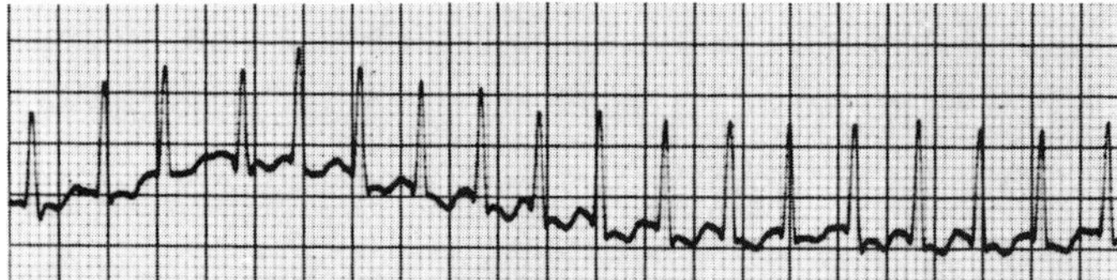

INDERAL 0.5 mg IV

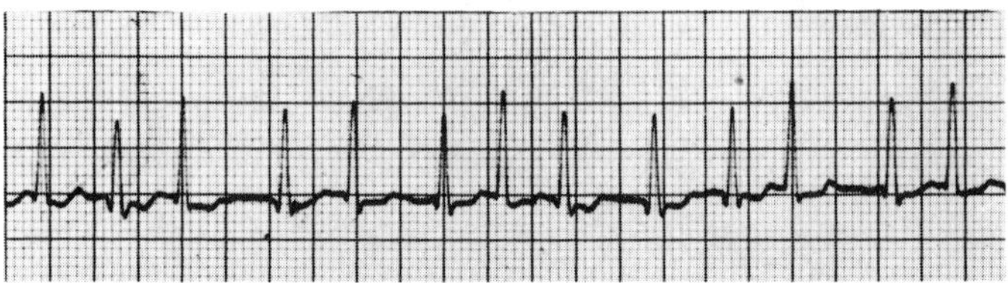

INDERAL 1.0 mg IV

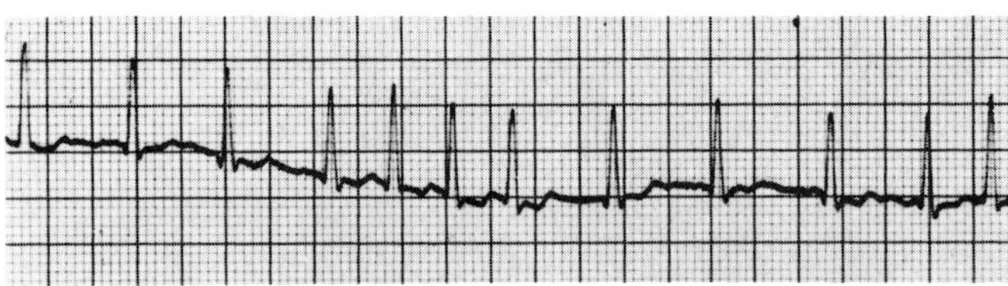

INDERAL 1.0 mg IV

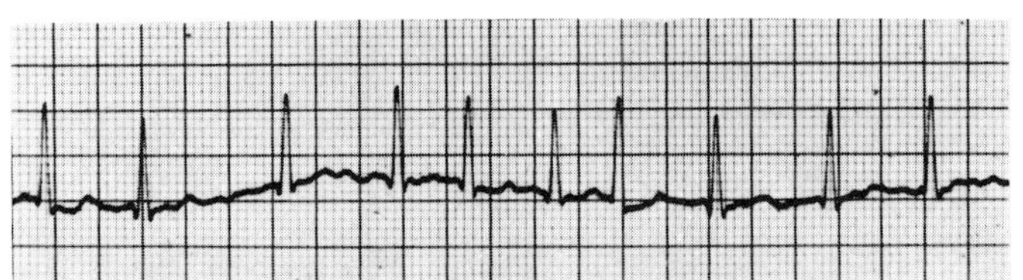

FIGURE 2–21. Atrial fibrillation with a rapid ventricular rate, hypotension, and cerebral and renal hypoperfusion developed after lobectomy in a 19-year-old student. Propranolol given intravenously in increments of 0.5 to 1.0 mg at 2- to 3-minute intervals produced prompt ventricular slowing and restored normal blood pressure.

that is usually seen in patients with advanced pulmonary insufficiency. It is often confused with atrial fibrillation.[40,41] The ventricular rate is usually between 100 and 200. To establish the diagnosis, one must demonstrate at least three different atrial pacemakers with variations in both P wave morphology and PR interval. P waves are separated by an isoelectric baseline and this, as well as the distinct atrial pacemakers (see Fig. 2–18), distinguishes it from atrial fibrillation. MAT has long been considered a manifestation of severe pulmonary disease rather than a primary rhythm disturbance. More recent studies suggest that in many patients it is due to theophylline sensitivity or to magnesium deficiency.[42] Initial therapy should always include repleting magnesium as well as tapering or discontinuing theophylline. The classic antiarrhythmic drugs are not efficacious in the treatment of MAT; verapamil is often effective in slowing the rate and in the minority of patients causing reversion to sinus rhythm.[43] Digitalis neither causes nor is effective in treating MAT and must be used with great caution since many of the patients with MAT are likely to develop toxicity with low serum digoxin levels.

Bradyarrhythmias

Heart rates of less than 55 beats/min may be a normal finding or may be a sign of underlying conduction system disease at either the sinoatrial or the AV node. As in the case of the tachyarrhythmias, their clinical significance very much depends on the patient's underlying cardiac status.

Sinus Bradycardia. Sinus bradycardia is a normal finding in a well-conditioned athlete or can result from sinus node dysfunction or increased vagal tone. It is common in patients who are taking β-blockers or calcium channel blockers. It is also seen in patients taking parasympathomimetic or sympatholytic medications and in those with hypothyroidism.[44] Vagally mediated bradycardia also occurs in patients with increased intracranial pressure and with carotid sinus sensitivity.

Most patients with sinus bradycardia are asymptomatic and do not require therapy. Occasionally, when this arrhythmia is associated with hypotension or cerebral hypoperfusion, restoration of normal heart rate is indicated. In patients with acute myocardial infarction, bradycardia may predispose to ventricular arrhythmias. Atropine, 0.2 to 0.3 mg given intravenously, is often successful in restoring a normal rate and is less likely to cause uncontrollable tachycardia than is the initial dosage of 0.5 to 1 mg that is usually recommended. If this initial dose is unsuccessful, additional increments may be given every few minutes up to a maximum of 1 mg intravenously. Isoproterenol, 1 to 2 μg/min by intravenous infusion, can be tried in the patient who does not respond to or who is unable to tolerate atropine. Occasionally, insertion of a transvenous pacemaker may be necessary.

Sinus Node Dysfunction. Sinus arrest may be manifested either as an occasional absent P wave or as prolonged pauses that are often terminated by junctional escape beats (Fig. 2–22). A somewhat similar cardiogram can be seen in the patient with blocked atrial premature contractions. Sinus node dysfunction may also be manifest as an exit block from the sinus node; repetitive groups of P waves with a gradually decreasing PP interval, followed by a pause in P wave activity, are seen in this disorder.

Both sinus arrest and sinus exit block are more likely to represent underlying heart disease than is sinus bradycardia. Occasionally, these disorders are a manifestation of drug toxicity, especially in patients taking digitalis or lithium.[45, 46] Treatment is not indicated unless these disturbances are associated with some degree of hemodynamic compromise or increased ventricular irritability. Atropine or isoproterenol, or both, can be tried; often transvenous pacemakers are required.

Atrioventricular Block. First-degree AV block is defined as a PR interval greater than 0.2 second in which every P wave is followed by a QRS complex (Fig. 2–23). It may be seen in patients without underlying heart disease and is common in the patient taking digitalis. It has no other clinical significance except as an indicator of the possibility of more advanced heart block.

In second-degree AV block, some of the P waves are not conducted to the ventricle. Although it is possible to subdivide patients with second-degree block according to the ratio between P waves and QRS complexes (i.e., 2:1, 3:1, or 3:2 AV block), this is much less useful clinically than a division into Wenckebach and Mobitz type II blocks (see Fig. 2–23).

Wenckebach AV block is characterized by a gradual prolongation of the PR interval, culminating in a P wave that is not followed by a QRS complex. It is usually a manifestation of AV nodal dysfunction and may be seen in the setting of digitalis toxicity or as a complication of myocardial infarction, especially inferior myocardial infarction. Progression to complete heart block is often gradual rather than sudden, and when complete heart block occurs, the

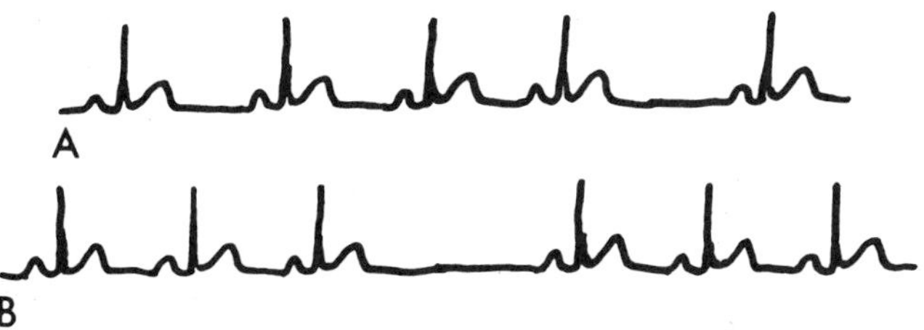

FIGURE 2–22. In sinus exit block *(A)* the PP interval gradually decreases until a P wave is blocked. This pattern is due to the underlying, gradually increasing sinus node–atrial block, similar to Wenckebach block at the AV node. In contrast, in the patient with sinus arrest *(B)*, the PP interval does not change prior to the dropped P wave, analogous to Mobitz type II AV block.

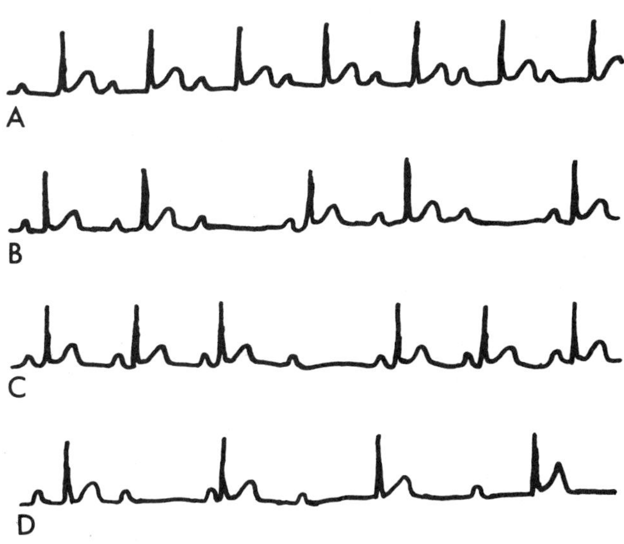

FIGURE 2–23. In first-degree atrioventricular (AV) block *(A)*, the PR interval is prolonged, but all the P waves are followed by a QRS complex. In Wenckebach AV block *(B)*, the PR interval gradually increases until a QRS complex is blocked. In Mobitz type II block *(C)*, the PR interval remains constant prior to the blocked QRS. In complete heart block *(D)*, there is no relationship between atrial and ventricular activity.

junctional pacemaker often maintains a heart rate that is sufficient to avoid severe hemodynamic compromise. Atropine may improve AV conduction and restore a more normal rate. Isoproterenol may also be effective.

In Mobitz type II AV block, the PR interval is constant and does not increase prior to the blocked QRS. It is usually a manifestation of disease in the conducting system below the AV node. When complete heart block develops, the ventricular pacemaker that assumes the pacing function often has a rate of 25 to 35, and severe hypotension or congestive heart failure may develop suddenly. The patient who develops complete heart block from an underlying Mobitz type II mechanism frequently does not respond well to either atropine or isoproterenol and often requires a transvenous pacemaker to maintain an adequate heart rate. This arrhythmia is also seen in patients with bifascicular block. A small percentage of ambulatory patients with right bundle branch block and either right or left axis deviation or left bundle branch block, especially in the presence of first-degree AV block, may progress to complete heart block annually.

In the setting of acute myocardial infarction, this is a more ominous pattern, and the development of Mobitz type II block or bifascicular block is an indication for a temporary transvenous pacemaker. If such patients progress even transiently to complete heart block during a myocardial infarction, they require a permanent pacemaker because of the high incidence of subsequent sudden death.[47]

In third-degree or complete heart block, there is no relationship between the P waves and the QRS complexes (see Fig. 2–23). The ventricular pacemaker may be either junctional, in which case the rate is likely to be in the range of 40 to 60 beats/min, or ventricular, in which case the QRS complex is likely to be wider than 0.11 second and the rate below 40. Some patients with junctional pacemakers and no significant underlying heart disease may tolerate complete heart block well, and neither pharmacologic nor pacemaker therapy is appropriate for these patients. Other patients with a similar pattern of heart block but with underlying cardiac disease may experience congestive heart failure, syncope, or extreme ventricular irritability, and pacemaker therapy may be lifesaving. Most patients with complete heart block and wide QRS complexes require permanent pacemakers.

REFERENCES

1. Walter PF, Reid SD, and Wenger NK: Transient cerebral ischemia due to arrhythmia. Ann Intern Med 72:471, 1970.
2. McAllen PM and Marshall J: Cardiac dysrhythmia and transient ischaemic attacks. Lancet 1:1212, 1973.
3. Jonas S, Klein I, and Dimant J: Importance of Holter monitoring in patients with periodic cerebral symptoms. Ann Neurol 1:470, 1977.
4. Stern S, Ben-Schacher G, Tzivoni D, et al: Detection of transient arrhythmias by continuous long-term recording of electrocardiograms of active subjects. Israel J Med Sci 6:103, 1970.
5. Wood P: Polyuria in paroxysmal tachycardia and paroxysmal atrial flutter and fibrillation. Br Heart J 25:273, 1963.
6. Luria MH, Adelson EI, and Lochaya S: Paroxysmal tachycardia with polyuria. Ann Intern Med 65:461, 1966.
7. Thomas FB, Mazzaferri EL, and Skillman TG: Apathetic thyrotoxicosis: A distinctive clinical and laboratory entity. Ann Intern Med 72:679, 1970.
8. Forfar JC, Miller HC, and Toft AD: Occult thyrotoxicosis: A correctable cause of "idiopathic" atrial fibrillation. Am J Cardiol 44:9, 1979.
9. Singer K and Lundberg WB: Ventricular arrhythmias associated with the ingestion of alcohol. Ann Intern Med 77:247, 1972.
10. Greenspan AJ, Stang JM, Lewis RP, et al: Provocation of ventricular tachycardia after consumption of alcohol. N Engl J Med 301:1049, 1979.
11. Velebit V, Podrid P, Lown B, et al: Aggravation and provocation of ventricular arrhythmias by antiarrhythmic drugs. Circulation 65:886, 1982.
12. Schweitzer P and Teichholz LE: Carotid sinus massage—its diagnostic and therapeutic value in arrhythmias. Am J Med 78:645, 1985.
13. Bass EB, Curtiss E, et al: The duration of Holter monitoring in patients with syncope: Is 24 hours enough? Arch Intern Med 150:1073, 1990.
14. Wellens HJJ, Bar FWHM, and Lie KI: The value of the electrocardiogram in the differential diagnosis of a tachycardia with a widened QRS complex. Am J Med 64:27, 1978.
15. Brugada P, Brugada J, Mont L, et al: A new approach to the differential diagnosis of a regular tachycardia with a wide QRS complex. Circulation 83:1649, 1991.
16. Stewart RB, Bardy GH, and Greene HL: Wide complex tachycardia: Misdiagnosis and outcome after emergent therapy. Ann Intern Med 104:766, 1986.
17. Mehta D, Ward DE, Wafa S, and Camm AJ: Relative efficacy of various physical maneuvers in the termination of junctional tachycardia. Lancet 5:28, 1988.
18. Adenosine or verapamil for the acute treatment of supraventricular tachycardia [Editorial]. Ann Intern Med 114:513, 1991.
19. Calkins H, Sousa J, El-Atassi R, et al: Diagnosis and cure of the Wolff-Parkinson-White syndrome or paroxysmal supraventricular tachycardias during a single electrophysiologic test. N Engl J Med 324:1612, 1991.
20. Johnson JC, Flowers NC, and Horan LG: Unexplained atrial flutter: A frequent herald of pulmonary embolism. Chest 60:29, 1971.
21. Vassaux C and Lown B: Cardioversion of supraventricular tachycardias. Circulation 39:791, 1969.
22. Lown B, Wyatt NF, and Levine HD: Paroxysmal atrial tachycardia with block. Circulation 21:129, 1960.
23. Manolis A, Rastegar H, and Estes NA: Automatic implantable cardioverter defibrillator. JAMA 262:1362, 1989.
24. Kay GN, Plumb VJ, Arciniegas JG, et al: Torsades de pointes: The long-short initiating sequence and other clinical features: Observations in 32 patients. J Am Coll Cardiol 2:806, 1983.
25. Smith WM and Gallagher JJ: "Les torsades de pointes": An unusual ventricular arrhythmia. Ann Intern Med 93:578, 1980.
26. Tzivoni D, Banai S, Schuger C, et al: Treatment of torsades de pointes with magnesium sulfate. Circulation 77:392, 1988.
27. Chiang BN, Perlman LV, Ostrander LD, et al: Relationship of premature systoles to coronary heart disease and sudden death in the Tecumseh Epidemiologic Study. Ann Intern Med 70:1159, 1969.
28. Coronary Drug Project Research Group: Prognostic importance of premature beats following myocardial infarction. JAMA 223:1116, 1973.
29. Ruberman W, Weinblatt E, Goldberg JD, et al: Ventricular premature beats and mortality after myocardial infarction. N Engl J Med 297:750, 1977.
30. Rodstein M, Wollock L, and Gubner NS: Mortality study of the significance of extrasystoles in an insured population. Circulation 44:617, 1971.
31. Fisher FD and Tyroler HA: Relationship between ventricular premature contractions on routine electrocardiography and subsequent sudden death from coronary heart disease. Circulation 47:712, 1973.
32. Kennedy HL, Whitlock JA, Sprague MK, et al: Long-term follow-up of asymptomatic healthy subjects with frequent and complex ventricular ectopy. N Engl J Med 312:193, 1985.
33. Vismara LA, Amsterdam EA, and Mason DT: Relation of ventricular arrhythmias in the late hospital phase of acute myocardial infarction to sudden death after hospital discharge. Am J Med 59:6, 1975.
34. Moss AJ, Davis HT, DeCamilla J, et al: Ventricular ectopic beats and their relation to sudden and nonsudden cardiac death after myocardial infarction. Circulation 60:998, 1979.
35. Schultze RA, Strauss HW, and Pitt B: Sudden death in the year following myocardial infarction. Am J Med 62:192, 1977.
36. Echt DS, Liebson PR, Mitchell LB, et al: Mortality and morbidity in patients receiving encainide, flecainide, or placebo. N Engl J Med 324:781, 1991.
37. Schwartz JB, Nielsen AP, and Griffin JC: Concentration-dependent enhancement of junctional pacemaker activity by verapamil in man. Circulation 71:450, 1985.
38. Peterson P, Boysen G, Godtfredsen J, et al: Placebo-controlled randomized trial of warfarin and aspirin for prevention of thromboembolic complications in chronic atrial fibrillation. Lancet 1:175, 1989.
39. Special Report: Stroke prevention in atrial fibrillation study group investigators: Preliminary report of the stroke prevention in atrial fibrillation study. N Engl J Med 322:863, 1990.
40. Shine KI, Kastor JA, and Yurchak PM: Multifocal atrial tachycardia: Clinical and electrocardiographic features in 32 patients. N Engl J Med 279:344, 1968.
41. Lipson MJ and Naimi S: Multifocal atrial tachycardia (chaotic atrial tachycardia). Circulation 62:397, 1970.
42. Levine JH, Michael JR, and Guarnieri T: Multifocal atrial tachycardia: A toxic effect of theophylline. Lancet 1:12, 1985.
43. Levine JH, Michael JR, and Guarnieri T: Treatment of multifocal atrial tachycardia with verapamil. N Engl J Med 312:21, 1985.
44. Scheinmann MM, Strauss HC, Evans GT, et al: Adverse effects of sympatholytic agents in patients with hypertension and sinus node dysfunction. Am J Med 64:1013, 1978.
45. Wellens HJ, Cats VM, and Duren VR: Symptomatic sinus node abnormalities following lithium carbonate therapy. Am J Med 59:285, 1975.
46. Wilson JR, Kraus ES, Bailas MM, et al: Reversible sinus node abnormalities due to lithium. Med Intell 294:1223, 1976.
47. Hindman MC, Wagner GS, JaRo M, et al: The clinical significance of bundle branch block complicating myocardial infarction. Circulation 58:689, 1978.

3

Angina Pectoris

THOMAS B. GRABOYS, MD
BERNARD LOWN, MD

Over 200 years ago Heberden expertly described the syndrome of angina pectoris and coined the term. "Angina" is derived from the Greek word *anchein*—to choke—and shares derivation with words such as "anxiety" and "anguish." Angina pectoris is a unique discomfort in the chest, usually indicating a diseased coronary arterial system. The most rewarding procedure in its diagnosis remains the unhurried interview with the patient, because today, as in Heberden's 18th century England, the diagnosis is made almost exclusively on the basis of history. Physical examination, electrocardiography, exercise testing, radionuclide imaging, and even coronary angiography may support or diminish the likelihood that angina is present, but the history is the decisive factor.

DIAGNOSIS

The History

Type of Discomfort. One can fail to detect angina during the first encounter with the patient by inappropriately phrasing the question regarding discomfort. If the patient is asked whether he or she experiences pain in the chest, the response may be negative because the symptom is not pain. A more accurate statement will usually be elicited if the patient is asked whether there is any sensation or discomfort in the chest and then is requested to describe it. The sensation is invariably a sense of fullness, constriction, tightness, pressure, or burning rather than pain. It is constant, never throbbing, and is deep rather than superficial. Frequently the patient is at a loss for words to provide adequate description, though manifesting intelligence and possessing great linguistic fluency. There may be a momentary introspection and a look of uncertainty as the patient responds that he or she is unable to describe this sensation. Such a response should increase suspicion that the condition troubling the patient is indeed angina pectoris. If the patient begins to tighten a fist over the midsternum—the so-called Levine sign—while struggling to describe the feeling in the chest, in most cases the problem is angina pectoris. This is also the case when the patient lays the flat of the hand over the breastbone and squeezes or curls the fingers or presses both sides of the chest wall with the palms toward the center of the sternum. If no such gestures are elicited, an attempt to misdirect should be made by asking the patient to *point* with a *finger* to where the *pain* is located. If the patient then points to one area or another, it is unlikely that angina is the problem. If the pain is described in great detail with location precisely defined, especially if the patient refers to it as being "over the heart" and points to the left subpectoral region, one is probably dealing with a noncardiac complaint.

Location, Radiation, and Duration. The location is retrosternal rather than precordial. At times there is also a tight sensation in the throat that may reach the lower jaw. The discomfort may radiate down one or another arm to the wrist or between the shoulder blades. When the patient has had a condition such as bursitis or cervical arthritis, angina may localize in the previously involved area; the sorting out of symptoms is then a challenge. Attention to the factors that produce or relieve the discomfort helps to reveal the true nature of the condition. A distinctive attribute of angina is that the discomfort rarely persists for more than 2 to 3 minutes. The intensity as well as the duration is significant. Following strenuous activity or intense emotional stress, angina is more likely to be severe and long-lasting. Generally, angina does not recur immediately once it has abated. If the patient indicates that the chest discomfort lasts for many hours and that the condition has been present for several years, angina pectoris is not likely to be the cause.

The response to the chest sensation is another important factor. If truly afflicted with angina, the patient stops what he or she is doing. With other types of discomforts, one may move, shift positions, or thrash about as with a colic; with angina the individual desists from activity and remains quiet.

Time of Onset. Time of onset of anginal discomfort is another significant clue to diagnosis. One might intuitively expect an attack of angina at the end of the day when fatigue has set in and the threshold for pain is low; actually, the reverse is true. Angina occurs most frequently when the individual is fully rested, after first arising in the morning, or while going to work in the morning rather than upon returning from work. Angina is also more likely to occur at the start of any activity rather than when it has been continued for a long time. For example, many patients begin to walk vigorously but are compelled to stop after less than a block; following several minutes of rest, when walking is resumed, they can maintain a faster pace over many city blocks or even miles. Many golfers with angina pectoris have also commented on this phenomenon. Angina may occur immediately after the individual tees off at the first hole; thereafter, the game can be pursued with greater vigor for the remaining 17 holes without further discomfort. Angina is particularly provoked when the arms are used, for example, while forcefully drying oneself with a towel after a shower or while carrying packages.

Type of Exertion That Precipitates Anginal Pain. This line of inquiry is sometimes rewarding. The patient who has been conditioned over a period of years to a specific type of activity may experience little or no discomfort from that task, although it may involve considerable exertion. By contrast, a new job to which the patient is unaccustomed or one in which he or she is not well trained may constitute a serious psychological stress and predispose to frequently recurring anginal attacks. Exertion to which one is accustomed over a lifetime is unlikely to provoke angina. When the work, however, is unpleasant, unwanted, frustrating, or exasperating, this does not hold true. The physician who is unaware of this fact, however, will urge a patient who has an arduous job to change to some sedentary work only to find that the anginal attacks then become more frequent and difficult to control.

Where the patient is when the chest discomfort occurs provides an important clue. Patients may be able to conduct virtually unlimited activity indoors but will have attacks when walking only a half block outdoors. This phenomenon is unrelated to the ambient temperature, as it is observed during all seasons of the year. One of the great clinical cardiologists of our era, S. A. Levine of the Peter Bent Brigham Hospital, was especially perceptive about the nuances of this syndrome. At times his history-taking with regard to this phenomenon was limited to but a single question: "Do you experience discomfort behind the breastbone while hurrying out of doors?"

Posture. Noting the effect of posture on the intensity of pain assists in the differential diagnosis. Although many discomforts are mitigated by recumbency, the converse is true with angina pectoris. The patient prefers to sit or stand and "lean into" the discomfort. The physician working in an exercise stress laboratory will frequently observe that after the test the patient dreads lying down. This may lead to confusion, for such a response is associated with the presence of hiatus hernia. An error in diagnosis is likely when, in addition, the sensation is described as indigestion or a burning in the epigastrium made worse by eating, assuaged by belching, and relieved by sitting up. This constellation of symptoms often leads the physician to suspect a gastrointestinal problem, especially hiatal hernia, and the patient is then subjected to an expensive and unwarranted work-up.

Angina sometimes occurs when the patient first gets into bed. This may result not only from the recumbent posture but also from the exercise of undressing and the encountering of cold bed sheets.

Relation to Digestion. More needs to be said about the digestive system and angina pectoris. It was not so long ago that sudden death was ascribed to acute indigestion. The patient with angina commonly describes symptoms as though they had their origin in the gut; he or she may complain of bloating, gas bubbles, burning relieved by belching, a sense of fullness in the stomach, and postprandial flatulence and may note that relief is afforded by antacids, especially when this promotes burping. Heberden already appreciated this association 2 centuries ago: "Those who are afflicted with it are seized while they are walking and *soon after eating* with a pain, an almost disagreeable sensation in the breast which seems as if it would extinguish life if it were to increase or to continue, but the moment they stand still this uneasiness vanishes." A meal will not necessarily bring on discomfort, but it will diminish the level of activity required to cause distress. The size of the meal is a decisive factor. In one particular patient, a modest meal of tea and toast precluded playing tennis, which he could do readily without discomfort after fasting for 24 hours.

Role of Emotion. When angina pectoris was first described as a syndrome, the role of psychological stress in bringing on angina was already appreciated. The redoubtable surgeon and Heberden's contemporary John Hunter, who was afflicted with angina, used to say "my life is in the hands of any scoundrel who chooses to put me in a passion." As a matter of fact, in line with his own prediction, he died in a fit of temper in 1793 while arguing with the Board of Trustees of St. George's Hospital in London. Even pleasurable emotion may cause angina; the unexpected quality and the intensity of the gratifying event are the key factors. A less-recognized fact is that the waxing and waning in frequency, intensity, or intractability of anginal discomfort may parallel the occurrence and severity of psychological depression. In the middle-aged man whose angina has become aggravated without an apparent cause, a coexistent depression can often be discovered. A loss of interest in work, indifference to socializing, decrease in frequency of sexual intercourse or actual impotence, decreased taste for palatable cuisine, change in sleep pattern, and a brooding and introspective manner should alert the physician to the fact that the angina is only a component of a profound psychological disturbance. The concurrence of angina pectoris and psychological depression is a grave augury of sudden cardiac death.

The psychological triggering of angina relates to behavioral conditioning. This is suggested by a number of observations. At times, seemingly innocuous stimuli, minor psychological stresses, or minute expenditures of effort may set off anginal episodes, whereas more arduous exertions may be well tolerated. Customary work, as stated previously, although strenuous, seldom triggers angina. One striking experience that bears on this issue has been reported.[1] A 40-year-old man with significant coronary artery disease consistently had anginal pain and exhibited 2 mm or more of ST segment depression after 44 crossings during a Master two-step test. When the number of times traversed over the two steps was miscounted so that the exercise was less, the pain occurred at the precise count of 44 and he showed the same profound degree of ST segment depression. However, when the count was accurate and he made only 32 crossings, he had neither pain nor ST segment deviation at the reduced exercise level.

The physician frequently needs to determine whether the complaint of chest pain is purely of functional origin. If the patient has been living with a close relative who has had angina, it is hard to detect whether the symptoms have been learned by exposure or have been actually experienced. The presence or absence of dyspnea is helpful in this respect. When the patient describes the sensation as choking or as breathlessness or admits to dyspnea in the presence of chest pain, the problem may well be psychological rather than cardiac in origin. This is especially true in the absence of any signs of heart disease. Dyspnea occurring simultaneously with bona fide angina pectoris is noted in less than 15% of patients.

Predisposing Factors. Of all the factors contributing to angina pectoris, none are more critical than time pressure and the intensity of the tempo of an activity. When performed against the clock, walking at a usually comfortable pace may precipitate angina. Being late for an appointment, having to do more than can be performed in the allotted time, or having overcommitted oneself to a tight schedule of appointments produces stress, which predisposes to angina. The patient is well tutored when he or she can moderate tempo and accomplish an objective in 12 seconds rather than in 10 seconds. The 2 seconds may be the determining factor of whether angina will develop. Sexual relations are among the many activities predisposing to angina, but they relate to a psychological state rather than to the actual physical expenditure of energy, which, in the middle-aged or elderly couple, is at most equivalent to climbing but a single flight of stairs. Other concurrent disease states that can increase the risk of angina must be considered—for example, anemia of whatever origin, thyrotoxicosis, cardiac arrhythmia, aortic valvular disease, hypertension, Paget's disease, and a host of other conditions that increase the workload of the heart.

Role of Carotid Sinus Pressure

When a patient who may be having an attack of angina pectoris is encountered, the carotid sinus pressure test provides decisive information. Pressure on the carotid sinus bulb will abolish anginal discomfort but is generally ineffective for pains in the chest that are unrelated to the coronary circulation. This response was already known to clinicians a half century ago, but it was S. A. Levine who gave this maneuver clinical applicability. The carotid sinus test is best performed when the patient first meets the physician, because this is the very time and perhaps the only time that angina will be experienced when the two people are together. It should be done expeditiously without having the patient go to an examining room or disrobe. In the case of a male patient, ask him to open his shirt, pull up his undershirt, and then rotate his neck a little to the left side. One should easily feel the right carotid bulb. The patient holds the physician's stethoscope against his own cardiac apex while the physician supports the chin with one hand and briskly massages with the other hand for 2 or 3 seconds.

Once a slowing in rate is detected, the physician then asks the patient whether the discomfort has become worse.* This question is vital. If one were to ask if the pain has become better, the patient is likely to agree with the physician, because the patient presupposes that the intent of the maneuver is to alleviate rather than aggravate the discomfort. If the patient is asked whether the pain has been made worse, the individual with angina responds in a typical manner. There will generally be a pause and a puzzled, introspective look; then after some hesitation, the patient will say that the pain or discomfort has gone away or is better. If the patient responds that the discomfort has become worse as a result of the maneuver, angina is not the problem. The high degree of suggestibility indicates a significant functional component.

In this test it is important to induce adequate slowing of the heart rate. If this cannot be achieved by carotid pressure on one side, it is worthwhile to repeat the test on the other side, since occasionally there is a difference in response between the two carotid sinuses. Because there are so few pains in the chest that are alleviated by the carotid sinus pressure maneuver, a positive response helps to confirm the diagnosis of angina pectoris.

*This diagnostic tool is a contribution of Dr. S. A. Levine.

Physical Examination

The physical examination generally is not decisive in helping with the diagnosis; it may, however, provide evidence of the severity of the underlying vascular disease and the presence of substantial impairment in myocardial function. For example, younger patients with familial forms of hyperlipidemia may exhibit arcus senilis, xanthelasmas, or tendon xanthomas. The patient with a previous myocardial infarction may demonstrate abnormal precordial movements, such as a discrete or diffuse area of paradoxic systolic motion. When hypertension has been present, a sustained ventricular impulse or a palpable apical presystolic tap (corresponding to the fourth heart sound) may be detected. At times, aortic stenosis—a condition commonly associated with exertional chest discomfort—predisposes to anginal pain. Occasionally, when the patient is examined during an anginal episode, certain findings are suggestive and even helpful. The heart rate accelerates, and blood pressure increases. The rhythm becomes irregular as a consequence of ventricular ectopic activity and rarely may be punctuated with bursts of ventricular tachycardia. A systolic paradoxic bulge may herald the presence of an ischemic dyssynergic area. The second sound splits paradoxically and becomes widened. A third or fourth sound not previously appreciated now is easily detected. At times a systolic murmur becomes intense and is evidence of papillary muscle dysfunction, an expression of malperfusion. As the anginal episode subsides, these findings rapidly disappear, thus indicating the cardiac source of the discomfort.

Observation of an anginal episode may be helpful in focusing on problems that were previously unsuspected. For example, the patient developing ventricular premature beats during angina requires antiarrhythmic therapy. The patient with clinically significant mitral regurgitation occurring only during episodes of angina may best be protected with long-acting nitrates; otherwise, these episodes, if they often recur, may cause cardiomegaly, which predisposes to pulmonary congestion.

Exercise Stress Testing

The diagnosis of angina pectoris is made almost exclusively on the basis of a detailed and careful history. This suffices for most patients. At times, however, the physician is faced with a history of atypical chest pain with variable provocative or precipitating factors, or the presence of other symptoms that make the diagnosis of angina pectoris uncertain. In these situations, exercise testing is of diagnostic help. Exercise testing also provides valuable information on the patient with an established diagnosis of coronary heart disease. It defines the extent of exercise that brings on anginal discomfort: It also demonstrates the accompanying changes in heart rate and blood pressure, the magnitude of electrocardiographic ischemia, and the occurrence of atrioventricular and intraventricular conduction defects. Rarely, exercise testing may precipitate a supraventricular tachycardia and thus divulge the cause of unidentified symptoms; but, most important, it may expose repetitive ventricular arrhythmia that may constitute an augury of sudden cardiac death.[2,3]

A number of reviews have analyzed the specificity and sensitivity of exercise testing for the diagnosis of coronary artery disease.[4–6] The proper technique for performing this test has also received exhaustive analysis.[7–9]

The association of ST segment depression with angina pectoris was first noted by Feil and Siegel in 1928.[10] The reversal of such findings with the administration of nitroglycerin suggests an ischemic basis for the ST segment changes. The commonly acceptable criterion for a "positive" response (and thus the diagnosis of coronary heart disease) is 1 mm or more of planar or downsloping ST segment depression recorded at 80 msec beyond the electrocardiographic "J" point. It is worth emphasizing that ST segment depression is a functional sign and does not provide proof of coronary artery disease. A myriad of factors may be responsible for false-positive ST segment depression, among which are electrolyte abnormalities (particularly hypokalemia); the taking of digitalis drugs, diuretics, psychotropic agents, chlorpromazine hydrochloride (Thorazine), and diazepam; and a variety of conditions such as anemia, myocardial hypertrophy, valvular heart disease, mitral valve prolapse, and so on. Both Kattus and Ellestad cite lack of conditioning and inadequate warm-up periods as additional causes for false-positive ST segment changes.[11,12] There is also a high incidence of positive results among women and asymptomatic persons undergoing exercise stress testing.[13,14]

A number of factors in exercise testing relate to prognosis. In a population with coronary artery disease, the critical variables include the duration of exercise; the peak heart rate achieved; the deviation in systolic and diastolic blood pressure; the development of angina pectoris; the extent of ST segment depression, the time of its first occurrence, and its duration; and changes in amplitude of the R wave. When considered in combination, these factors provide information on the state of left ventricular function. It is our view that the state of the myocardium rather than the cineangiographically demonstrated anatomy of the coronary vasculature is of greater value in determining length of survival.

Recent work from our laboratory is of interest in this regard.[15] Among 122 patients with coronary artery disease who had equal to or greater than 2 mm of ST segment depression and who were followed for a median time of 44 months on a medical regimen, annual mortality was less than 1%. The average heart rate and blood pressure for this group were 144 beats/min and 142/80 mm Hg, respectively, and duration of exercise was 7.2 minutes. The finding of severe ST segment depression, although perhaps indicative of multivessel coronary disease, did not indicate an adverse prognosis among these patients. The hemodynamic indices and duration of exercise achieved reflected adequate ventricular function, which, as already noted, is probably the single best predictor of survival.

Role of Noninvasive Techniques

Radionuclide thallium or dipyridamole (Persantine) scanning, echocardiography, and two-dimensional sector scanning are all noninvasive techniques that can be used in the patient with angina pectoris. They assist in defining the state of left ventricular function, focal wall motion abnormalities, and fixed versus reversible defects during radionuclide imaging. These techniques complement but do not substitute for a meticulously obtained history.

Coronary Spasm (Variant Angina)

As long as a century ago, coronary spasm had already been considered as the cause of angina pectoris,[16] but in 1959 Prinzmetal and colleagues determined that coronary spasm produced a syndrome distinct from angina pectoris.[17] This so-called variant form of angina has a number of unique features. Unlike classic angina, the pain occurs when the patient is at rest, frequently at the same time of the day; nocturnal pain is common, especially during the early morning, when it wakes the individual from a sound sleep. It tends to be cyclic in this respect, but it also may have a rhythmic quality, a waxing and waning. Its transient duration and prompt relief by nitroglycerin simulates the classic syndrome. However, what is remarkable is that these patients may exert themselves arduously without provoking discomfort.

The electrocardiogram, when recorded during a period of pain, is distinctive. At the onset of pain, T waves increase in amplitude and, if inverted, may become upright. Simultaneously, there is a remarkable degree of ST segment elevation, which rapidly increases in extent and may assume the configuration of a monophasic action current. The R wave grows in amplitude in the leads that have changes in repolarization. If the ST segment alterations are observed in leads II, III, and aVF, there will be reciprocal changes in lead I and at times in the left precordial leads. At the peak of the attack of pain, ventricular premature beats occur in as many as 50% of cases. Rarely, bouts of ventricular tachycardia have resulted in syncope or even death. Generally, with the onset of pain, the heart rate, instead of accelerating, as is true with angina pectoris, may slow. Heart rates as slow as 30 beats/min have been recorded. Advanced degrees of heart block and Adams-Stokes seizures have been noted in patients with currents of injury in the inferior leads, implicating spasm in the right coronary artery. Between attacks of pain, the electrocardiogram may be entirely normal. With cessation of pain, all these ominous changes disappear rapidly and completely.[18,19]

In the 3 decades since Prinzmetal's description, a spectrum of patients fulfilling some, all, or none of the original description have been described, yet in whom the underlying pathophysiology remains coronary vasospasm. We now realize that patients with or without associated coronary disease may demonstrate such spasm. This may reflect alterations in autonomic neural tone or the effects of local metabolites upon α or β receptors localized within the coronary vessels.[20,21] Agents that alter coronary vascular neural tone or inhibit smooth muscle contraction may offer specific or adjunctive therapy for the patient with angina.[22]

The role of coronary vasospasm as a cause of the diverse manifestations of ischemic heart disease requires resolution. Suffice it to say that vasospasm is probably a more common occurrence among coronary artery disease patients than previously believed.[23]

MANAGEMENT OF THE PATIENT WITH STABLE ANGINA PECTORIS

The physician generally derives great satisfaction from managing the patient with angina pectoris. Only rarely does the condition not respond to medical measures. Factors that are implicated in triggering an attack at times can be obviated entirely or need only be modified slightly to make the patient completely free of pain. The establishment of a trusting, caring relationship between the patient and the doctor is crucial and is usually achieved during the first interview. In this context, "management" rather than "therapy" is the appropriate term, because the control of angina does not depend on the dispensing of one or another medication but rather on the coordination of many measures taken over a prolonged period that lasts for years or even decades.

The goal of management is to keep the patient pain-free with a minimal modification in usual lifestyle. The initial principle in managing angina is to foster in the patient a sense of self-reliance, which is a key factor in sustaining confidence and optimism in the face of a long-lasting illness. Attention to details is decisive. For example, consider the patient who awakens late each morning, is in a mad rush to shower, shave, dress, and have breakfast before racing down to the automobile, and then experiences angina while reaching for the ignition key. Counseling such a patient to arise 5 to 10 minutes earlier may eliminate this pattern of angina. Simply slowing the tempo of activity still allows the patient to reach the planned destination but prevents chest discomfort.

If the patient exercises on an empty stomach, angina will be prevented, and there will be no need to give up a favored activity. If getting into bed on a wintry night brings on chest discomfort, the use of an electric blanket will frequently prove prophylactic. If showering immediately after awaking causes angina, postponing this activity until bedtime is likely to prevent chest discomfort. The imaginative, caring physician can find ingenious but nontaxing solutions to a myriad of other similar problems.

Use of Drugs

Nitroglycerin. Nitroglycerin is a most remarkable remedy for angina pectoris and is the pharmacologic mainstay of medical management. The patient is advised to keep it close at hand at all times. The mechanism of action involves diminution of coronary arterial spasm with redistribution of flow to nonperfused areas. Other salutary hemodynamic actions include reduced peripheral vascular resistance and venous pooling, which lower cardiac preloading and afterloading. The result is reduced ventricular volume and wall tension, which are the determinants of myocardial oxygen requirement (Table 3–1).

The patient should be urged to take the first dose of nitroglycerin in the physician's presence. At this point it is explained that a slight stinging under the tongue indicates onset of drug action, and a healthy pounding and throbbing in the head is a good sign that the drug is potent and is having the desired effect. We begin with a dose of 0.3 mg. The patient is encouraged to take nitroglycerin without hesitation at the first sign of discomfort. Although it may be possible that the discomfort is not anginal, no harm is done by taking extra nitroglycerin.

TABLE 3–1. MAJOR DETERMINANTS OF MYOCARDIAL OXYGEN CONSUMPTION (MVO_2) AND EFFECTS OF AGENTS THAT REDUCE MVO_2*

	Nitrates	β-Adrenergic Blockage
Intramyocardial systolic tension	↓	↓
Heart rate	↑	↓
Contractility	↑	↓

*Modified from Mason DT, Spann JF Jr, Zelis R, et al: Physiologic approach to the treatment of angina pectoris. N Engl J Med 281:1225, 1969. Reprinted with permission from the *New England Journal of Medicine.*

The patient generally resists taking nitroglycerin, even though the most careful instruction has been given by the physician. There are a number of reasons for recalcitrance. Perhaps a major factor relates to the denial of illness. Generally, in the patient's mind there is an association between the number of pills taken and the severity of the underlying problem; it is felt, wrongly, that the fewer pills consumed, the less one is afflicted with coronary artery disease. There is also anxiety about habituation and loss of drug effectiveness with repeated use. Some people are deterred by headaches. The patient also quickly learns that the discomfort is promptly alleviated by stopping activity, and this seems preferable to reliance on a drug.

It is best if the patient learns to reach for nitroglycerin reflexly. Thus, the mark of a properly instructed patient is that, when asked how many pills have been taken, the patient is uncertain because their number is ignored. The nitroglycerin is taken not only at the very onset of an episode but also in anticipation of discomfort. Taking nitroglycerin liberally permits the patient with angina to live a full life without undue restriction and without other medications for control of discomfort.

The first therapeutic measure is administration of nitroglycerin. It makes little sense to initiate therapy with some longer-acting coronary vasodilators to be taken a number of times a day when a single nitroglycerin tablet once or twice daily proves adequate. The patient learns to adapt the use of this remarkable agent to highly individual and varying needs and can take it only when needed. Why should one be taking an agent, the exclusive function of which is to allay discomfort, when there may be weeks when no discomfort whatsoever is experienced? Knowing that this remedy is instantly within reach may itself constitute an antidote to coronary pain by instilling confidence in the patient.

If angina continues undiminished after three nitroglycerin tablets have been taken 3 to 5 minutes apart, the patient is advised to report to the closest hospital emergency room for further attention. The patient is, of course, urged to seek advice promptly when there has been a change in frequency, severity, or duration of anginal attacks.

Longer-Acting Vasodilators. The decision to employ longer-acting coronary vasodilators is determined by the frequency or unpredictability of angina episodes. It is our practice first to instruct the patient in the proper use of nitroglycerin. If frequent episodes of angina occur despite adequate use of TNG, a longer-acting nitrate preparation is added. Isosorbide dinitrate taken orally in dosages ranging from 20 to 80 mg twice daily is a reasonable regimen. A sustained-release oral preparation may be helpful, particularly for the patient experiencing nocturnal angina. Studies have demonstrated increased efficacy of oral nitrates administered at 8- to 12-hour intervals.

There has been renewed interest in nitrate ointment. For the patient who experiences pain at night or when at rest, 1 to 2 inches applied to the chest, shoulder, or arm may produce a sustained effect for up to 6 hours. Cosmetic problems (staining of clothes) are a deterrent to its use in many patients, although this may be minimized with the use of a transparent plastic covering. Rarely, nitroglycerin paste may cause a contact dermatitis. Nitroglycerin sustained-release patches may be substituted for oral preparations but should be removed for at least 8 hours to avoid nitrate tolerance.

The combination of a long-acting nitrate, 6- to 8-inch blocks to raise the head of the bed, and the availability of nitroglycerin at the bedside does much to assuage the patient's fears of awakening with chest discomfort. Indeed, these simple practical measures will frequently suffice to control the condition in most patients with nocturnal angina.

The use of long-acting nitrate preparations may have a salutary effect on other aspects of the anginal patient's cardiac status. The vasodilatation that results from their administration reduces blood pressure and thus decreases impedance to left ventricular outflow (afterload). For patients with reduced left ventricular function or particularly for those with mitral regurgitation, improvement in cardiac output may be noted.

It is now apparent that most patients experiencing daily episodes of angina will also exhibit so-called silent ischemia. It has been our practice to incorporate long-acting anti-ischemic medications in the majority of these patients.

Why Do Patients Avoid Taking Nitroglycerin? Only a rare patient will be unable to tolerate nitroglycerin, and yet the physician frequently encounters patients who are reluctant to use it. This feeling may have been fostered by the well-meaning physician who warns that a headache may occur with the use of these agents. We choose to moderate the patient's response by indicating that the warm flush that is felt relates to the increased blood supply to the heart and brain. If the physician is present when the patient first takes nitroglycerin, a positive conditioned response can occur.

β-Adrenergic Blocking Agents. Propranolol was introduced in 1964 by Black and coworkers after a decade of searching for drugs to block the effect of sympathomimetic amines upon myocardial β-adrenergic receptors.[24] This class of agents reduces cardiac output by a direct negative chronotropic and inotropic effect. Arterial pressure is lowered secondary to a decrease in cardiac output. The reduction of heart rate and cardiac contractility results in lessened myocardial oxygen consumption (MVO_2), which permits the heart to perform its work within the capacity of the narrowed arterial system to deliver oxygen and nutrients. The result is beneficial for angina.

In patients with cardiomegaly, a previous history of congestive heart failure, or symptoms suggestive of limited ventricular functional reserve (exertional breathlessness and occasional paroxysmal nocturnal dyspnea or orthopnea), the use of propranolol may cause cardiac decompensation or frank heart failure. In such patients, daily measurements of body weight, the judicious intermittent use of diuretics, digitalization, or any combination of these will often allow the concomitant use of β-adrenergic blocking agents. In our experience, approximately 15% of patients are unable to tolerate β-adrenergic blocking agents.

The desired effect of any β-receptor antagonist is to decrease the resting heart rate. Most often patients receiving propranolol exhibit heart rates between 50 and 60 beats/min. A true β-antagonist effect of the drug will result in both a reduced heart rate and blood pressure response during exercise.

Physicians frequently become concerned when a patient receiving both calcium channel drugs and β-blocking agents exhibits heart rates less than 50 beats/min. This may be particularly noticeable during sleep, when physiologic vagotonia occurs and heart rates may be in the 40 to 45 beats/min range. These slow rates usually constitute no hazard for the anginal patient who has normal ventricular function.

Dosage of the β-blockers must be individualized, but they need not be administered more than twice or three times daily. We typically employ a daily dose of 180 to 240 mg of propranolol, 100 to 200 mg of metoprolol, or 100 mg of atenolol.

Adverse Reactions. The most common and troublesome reactions to β-adrenergic blocking agents include undue fatigue, lessening of drive and ambition, and sexual impotence in men. As indicated elsewhere, precipitation of congestive heart failure is a well-known adverse reaction. Other less common problems encountered in clinical practice are bronchospasm, nausea, and decreased sympathetic response to hypoglycemia in the diabetic patient. Rarely, these agents may worsen angina. This occurs in the patient experiencing coronary vasospasm in whom β-adrenergic blockade induces exaggerated coronary α-receptor tone. The availability of cardioselective β-adrenergic blocking agents will minimize a number of these side effects, but this will be a function of dose, for no completely cardioselective agent has been developed.

Calcium Channel Agents. The introduction of drugs that block the slow channel calcium current of the action potential has been a major advance in the treatment of patients with ischemic heart disease. Initially introduced for coronary vasospasm, this group of drugs is now used routinely in the pharmacotherapy of angina in concert with nitrates and β-adrenergic blocking agents. Drugs such as diltiazem, nifedipine, and verapamil are the prototype of the potent coronary vasodilators that have been found to be effective in patients with coronary spasm. These agents may have a more universal application to the anginal patient in whom there is an element of variable spasm superimposed upon fixed coronary lesions. Recently their clinical pharmacology was reviewed extensively.[36–38] Nifedipine was reported to completely or significantly abolish chest pain caused by variant angina in more than 80% of patients and also to improve symptoms of angina in most patients with classic angina pectoris. About 10% of patients are reported to worsen, however, possibly because these drugs reduce myocardial contractility and are peripheral as well as coronary arterial vasodilators. While calcium channel drugs are most effective for the treatment of angina, a multicenter study assessing the effect of diltiazem on mortality after a myocardial infarction did not demonstrate improved survival in this patient subset.[39]

Side Effects of Calcium Channel Agents. In general, these drugs are well tolerated. However, a number of side effects specific to a given agent occur. For example, nifedipine, because of its potent peripheral vasodilation, is more likely to produce leg edema than either verapamil or diltiazem. Verapamil is more likely to produce heart block. The physician employing these agents should be alert to the following notable side effects that may occur with these drugs: peripheral edema, constipation, dizziness, gastritic pain, increased insulin requirements, bradyarrhythmia or advanced atrioventricular block, and exfoliative dermatitis.

Antiplatelet Agents. Interest has developed in the use of drugs that inhibit platelet function. A randomized double-blind trial of aspirin (325 mg four times daily) in 555 patients hospitalized for unstable angina showed significant reductions in cardiac deaths (56%) and all deaths (43%) when analyzed by intention-to-treat after 18 months.[26] It is our practice to recommend that patients with active coronary disease take 325 mg/day of aspirin.

Summary of the Medical Management of Angina Pectoris

Nitroglycerin or some form of nitrate therapy remains the mainstay of initial management for patients experiencing angina pectoris. The availability of calcium channel and β-adrenergic blocking agents allows latitude in the decision regarding a secondary agent if symptoms warrant. In the setting of normal ventricular function, it is our practice to institute a β-adrenergic blocking agent in concert with a long-acting nitrate program. In the setting of clinical heart failure or reduced ventricular function, we initiate a calcium channel drug (nifedipine or diltiazem) as a second-line agent. For patients whose angina is not controlled by β-blockers, we have the option of adding a calcium channel drug to the nitrate–β-blocker program. Patients who are begun on nifedipine are also tutored in the use of this agent sublingually. Thus, chewing a nifedipine capsule or breaking it to allow the liquid to be absorbed sublingually is an extremely effective means of controlling chest discomfort that is not relieved by one or two sublingual nitroglycerin tablets.

The choice of which calcium channel agent to utilize in part becomes a function of each individual practitioner's experience with a given agent. We have found diltiazem and nifedipine to have approximately equal efficacy in individuals with exertional fixed obstructive angina. Among patients with coronary vasospasm, verapamil in our experience has proved equally efficacious.

Exercise Conditioning

A program of regular exercise may be therapeutic for the patient with angina pectoris. Prior to the initiation of such exercise programs, it has been our practice to have the patient with angina undergo a graded exercise tolerance test. This defines the patient's aerobic capacity as well as indicating whether the onset of angina pectoris or ischemic electrocardiographic changes are accompanied by either hypotension or serious arrhythmia. Exercise-induced ventricular arrhythmia in the patient experiencing angina pectoris may be an omen of sudden cardiac death and thus warrants aggressive therapy.

We encourage patients to pursue aerobic types of activities such as swimming, brisk walking, and stationary bicycle riding. Ordinarily, four 15- to 20-minute exercise periods weekly will achieve aerobic conditioning. In one commonly used program, the patient pedals for 5 minutes at 15 to 20 miles/hr, rests for 1 to 3 minutes, followed by an additional 5 minutes of pedaling, with "sprinting" the final 30 seconds of each 5-minute period. Alternatively, walking 1 mile in 15 minutes is a fitness program that could be carried out on a year-round basis. Isometric exercise should be discouraged because there is a rise in blood pressure secondary to increased peripheral resistance, without accompanying increases in heart rate.

Physical conditioning programs have been demonstrated to reduce the occurrence of angina pectoris. This has been noted for well over 2 decades.[27–29] It is presumed that such improvement occurs in part secondary to an improved circulatory system with an overall decrease in heart rate and blood pressure, which reduces myocardial oxygen requirement.[29] A number of studies, including work by Ferguson and colleagues,[30] have documented that although the pressure rate product at any level of exertion (heart rate × blood pressure) decreases following exercise programs, usually there are no changes in left ventricular hemodynamic indices. Rather, improved exercise tolerance is due to the reduced myocardial blood flow requirements at the given workload that previously had caused angina pectoris. Many of the hemodynamic changes effected by a regular exercise program are similar to those engendered when sympathetic nervous impulses are annulled by β-adrenergic blocking agents.

Regular daily exercise promotes self-reliance in the patient and permits him or her to play an active role in treatment; it also boosts morale for the patient frightened by the diagnosis of coronary artery disease. Other beneficial effects of an exercise program include a decrease in sympathetic tone, a means for the release of psychological stress and tension, and perhaps a reduction in the lability of blood pressure.

Hyperlipidemia and Weight Control

Patients with angina pectoris who demonstrate only modest elevations in serum cholesterol level generally are receptive to recommendations on modifying dietary cholesterol. Lipid-lowering agents are numerous and are generally quite effective.

For the anginal patient, redistribution of daily calories may reduce episodes of chest discomfort. For example, the typical daily diet for the middle-aged coronary patient is heavily weighted toward the evening meal. He or she rarely eats breakfast, may skip lunch, and then ingests a large dinner, which is followed by postprandial angina pectoris. Rather than this "fast or feast" dietary sequencing, we urge such patients to eat three moderate-sized meals with a nearly equal division of calories.

Control of Contributing Conditions

Hypertension. Modification of this risk factor for coronary heart disease is important for the patient with angina pectoris. Indeed, even borderline blood pressures of 150/90 mm Hg in these patients should be treated. The occurrence of angina pectoris is frequently, although not invariably, accompanied by a pressor response.[1, 31] Protracted hypertension results in elevation of afterload and may accelerate the intensity and frequency of the anginal episode. The hypertensive patient with cardiomegaly who has angina only nocturnally may in fact be experiencing left ventricular failure, and the "choking" represents congestion rather than angina. Digitalization, which does not assuage angina, may in this case prevent such nocturnal symptoms.

Arrhythmias. Ambulatory monitoring for 24 hours exposes at least some ventricular ectopic activity in close to 90% of patients with coronary artery disease.[32] The decision to utilize antiarrhythmic agents is based on the characteristics of the ventricular premature beats exposed, the extent of left ventricular dysfunction, the presence of symptoms, and the time relationship to acute myocardial infarction.[33] The presence of complex ventricular ectopic activity during angina pectoris may augur sudden death and may be an indication for antiarrhythmic therapy; increased anti-ischemic medication, or invasive intervention.

Anemia. Anemia from whatever etiology, particularly acute blood loss, in the coronary patient may cause a transient or sustained ischemic event, an increase in the frequency of anginal episodes, or myocardial infarction. It is our practice to transfuse with packed red blood cells when the hematocrit is 30 ml/dl or below. The improved hemodynamics not only decreases the frequency of angina but also improves left ventricular performance.

Thyrotoxicosis. Rarely, the patient with angina shows evidence of thyrotoxicosis. This is a welcome finding, for if the thyroid is indeed hyperactive, the angina can be completely alleviated or delayed in its recurrence for at least a decade. S. A. Levine believed that these patients had coronary artery disease but that the "thermostat" had been set back; once thyrotoxicosis is controlled, the myocardial demand is reduced commensurately with the diminished yet still adequate coronary blood flow. A warm palm on handshake, a flood of language in explaining symptoms, undue fatigue or angina without effort, and especially nocturnal angina may first alert the physician to the possibility of thyrotoxicosis. Finding on examination a forceful heartbeat, an accentuated first heart sound though the PR interval is full, a scratchy systolic murmur in the pulmonic area, a tachycardia when the patient is at rest, or a wide pulse pressure also suggests such a diagnosis. The physician must overestimate the possibility of thyrotoxicosis in order not to miss it, even though its occurrence with angina pectoris is rare.

Social, Psychological, and Economic Considerations

The patient should be urged to have the spouse accompany him or her to the initial visit with the physician. The seasoned practitioner may then gain some idea of marital tensions and perceive incompatibilities that may contribute to angina. A key area to be explored is work. The majority of middle-aged American men find their jobs difficult, unrewarding, or even distasteful. They feel entrapped in a situation over which they have little control. They often experience a sense of alienation and a growing feeling of inadequacy and lack of accomplishment. The physician is largely helpless in changing the social environment; however, interest and sympathy can help to alleviate the patient's anxieties and fears.

If it can be arranged, the patient should be encouraged to interrupt the working week with an afternoon away from stressful responsibilities. Taking off for a long weekend periodically is also beneficial and may contribute to a better, if not a longer, life. Engaging in a modest, satisfying exercise program is helpful in allaying psychological tension. It is wrong to encourage the patient to retire from a job unless there are interesting and viable alternatives. Having no job is worse than having a poor job. In addition, the physician must not be insensitive to the economic constraints of premature retirement, especially in an inflationary age. The physician, though not trained to function as a social engineer, must nonetheless become involved in numerous such problems for the sake of the patient's well-being.

Indications for Hospitalization

Most patients with angina pectoris can be managed with a judicious medical program. Occasionally, patients experience a change in their typical anginal symptoms. An increased frequency of attacks, lack of relief from nitroglycerin, decubitus angina or angina when the patient is at rest, and prolonged chest pain are all indications of a transitional phase in the patient's condition and require hospitalization. Close examination for factors that may be accountable for the change in symptoms is important. Approximately 10 to 15% of such patients develop an acute myocardial infarction in the ensuing 6 months.

Indications for Coronary Angiography and Myocardial Revascularization

There exists a fundamental controversy over coronary angiography and myocardial revascularization. The basis of the controversy is not the usefulness of this procedure, which has a definite role in the management of angina pectoris, but rather its indiscriminate application to patients who have coronary artery atherosclerosis.

We believe that coronary angiography should be performed primarily in patients in whom the physician contemplates coronary artery bypass graft surgery (CABG) or coronary angioplasty. Thus, subjecting a patient to cardiac catheterization merely to define that individual's coronary anatomy in order to determine a prognosis is unjustified. The intent is clearly to ascertain whether critical lesions exist, the repair of which could prolong life. This issue is dealt with by McIntosh and Garcia in an extensive review of the subject.[34] They contend that "despite a decade of experience in aortocoronary bypass grafting, embracing 300,000 or more operations, indications for its use remain controversial and no proof has been provided that life is prolonged." Persistent controversy reflects a lack of adequate controls with which to compare the clinical course of patients operated on; only 1248 have been reported who have been studied in a carefully controlled and random manner.[34] Surgical experience with low mortality in one institution cannot be extrapolated to all hospital facilities currently undertaking coronary revascularization.[35]

There is no doubt that revascularization consistently reduces or completely alleviates anginal discomfort, but there is still no conclusive evidence that myocardial revascularization prevents myocardial infarction or sudden cardiac death. The benefit of alleviating angina must be weighed against a 1 to 6% mortality and a 5 to 15% incidence of intraoperative myocardial infarction.

The completion of the coronary artery surgery study (CASS) randomized trial has shed light on this area. The 6-year follow-up of 780 patients randomized to either medical or surgical therapy demonstrated a cumulative survival of 90 and 92%, respectively.[40] The CASS data were somewhat at odds with the European Coronary Surgery Study (ECSS), which found a significant advantage to surgical therapy over a 5-year follow-up.[41] Nonetheless, neither study demonstrated any data to conclude that bypass surgery protects from risk of myocardial infarction. It does appear, however, that bypass surgery offers improved survival in two subsets of patients with *active* ischemic heart disease: those patients with left main coronary stenosis and those with left ventricular dysfunction and reduced ejection fractions (<40%). We note that the entry of patients into all three prospective randomized trials (CASS, ECSS, and VA Study) antedated the introduction of calcium channel agents and the widespread use of "triple therapy" for angina pectoris.

In our experience, the prime indication for this type of surgery is for the patient with chronic angina pectoris who continues to experience limiting chest pain despite an intensive medical program. We have recently reported on our experience with patients seeking a second opinion for either coronary bypass surgery or the need for coronary angiography.[42, 43] The majority of such patients were deemed stable and able to continue on medical therapy with an annualized mortality of 1.1% over a 47-month follow-up. A small group of patients whose symptoms have worsened require coronary bypass; indications for surgery include the presence of angina decubitus, angina unrelieved by nitroglycerin that is experienced when the patient is at rest, electrocardiographic evidence of profound subendocardial ischemia associated with pain at rest, exercise-induced exertional hypotension at low levels of exercise associated with profound ST segment depression, or evidence of medically refractory coronary vasospasm. The physician must carefully scrutinize patients with crescendo angina and exclude those with acute myocardial infarction. Intraoperative mortality is greatly increased in the patient with an acute infarct. Additionally, selected patients in whom a highly stressful lifestyle or drug intolerance does not permit adequate medical therapy may be considered for operation.

Coronary Angioplasty. With the widespread availability of coronary angioplasty, the number of individuals undergoing this procedure has increased tenfold over the past decade to approximately 300,000 patients. To date, there is no prospective trial comparing angioplasty to medical therapy, except for one study examining exercise tolerance and degree of angina for patients with single-vessel disease.[44] However, no data support a superior advantage of angioplasty compared with medical therapy. Our indications for this procedure are similar to those for CABG, that is, the patient with refractory or unstable angina deemed anatomically suitable for balloon dilatation.

REFERENCES

1. Lown B: Verbal conditioning of angina pectoris during exercise testing. Am J Cardiol 40:630, 1977.
2. Udall JA and Ellestad MH: Predictive implications of ventricular premature contractions associated with treadmill testing. Circulation 56:985, 1977.
3. Lown B and Graboys TB: Sudden death: An ancient problem newly perceived. Cardiovasc Med 2:219, 1977.
4. Fortuin NJ and Weiss JL: Exercise stress testing. Circulation 56:699, 1977.
5. Zohman LR and Kattus AA: Exercise testing in the diagnosis of coronary heart disease: A perspective. Am J Cardiol 40:243, 1977.
6. Bruce RA: Value and limitations of exercise electrocardiography. Circulation 50:1, 1974.
7. Sheffield LT and Roitman D: Stress testing methodology. Progr Cardiovasc Dis 19:33, 1976.
8. Faris JV, McHenry PL, and Morris S: Concepts and applications of treadmill exercise testing and the exercise electrocardiograph. Am Heart J 95:102, 1978.
9. Chaitman BR, Bourassa MG, Waigniart P, et al: Improved efficiency of treadmill exercise testing using a multiple lead ECG system and basic hemodynamic exercise response. Circulation 57:71, 1978.
10. Feil H and Siegel ML: Electrocardiographic changes during attacks of angina pectoris. Am J Med Sci 175:255, 1928.
11. Kattus AA: Exercise electrocardiography: Recognition of the ischemic response, false positive and negative patterns. Am J Cardiol 33:721, 1974.
12. Ellestad MH: Stress Testing—Principles and Practice. Philadelphia, FA Davis, 1975, pp 95–120.
13. Linhart JW, Laws JG and Satinsky JD: Maximum treadmill exercise electrocardiography in female patients. Circulation 50:1173, 1974.
14. Borer JS, Brensike JR, Redwood DR, et al: Limitations of the electrocardiographic response to exercise in predicting coronary artery disease. N Engl J Med 293:367, 1975.
15. Podrid PJ, Graboys TB and Lown B: Prognosis of medically treated patients with ≥2 mm of exercise-induced ST segment depression. Circulation 56(Suppl III):193, 1977.
16. Latham P: Collected Works, Vol 1, London, New Sydenham Society, 1876.
17. Prinzmetal M, Kennamer R, Merliss R, et al: Angina pectoris. I: A variant form of angina pectoris. Am J Med 27:375, 1959.
18. Siegel M and Feil H: Electrocardiographic studies during attacks of angina pectoris and of other paroxysmal pain. J Clin Invest 10:795, 1931.
19. Parkinson J and Bedford P: Electrocardiographic changes during brief attacks of angina pectoris. Lancet 1:15, 1931.
20. Gianelly R, Mugler F and Harrison DC: Prinzmetal's variant of angina pectoris with only slight coronary atherosclerosis. Calif Med 108:129, 1968.
21. Hillis LD and Braunwald E: Coronary artery spasm. N Engl J Med 299:695, 1978.
22. Goldberg S, Reichek N, Wilson J, et al: Nefedipine in the treatment of Prinzmetal's (variant) angina. Am J Cardiol 44:804, 1979.
23. Lown B: Introduction: Symposium on nifedipine and calcium flux inhibition in the treatment of coronary arterial spasm and myocardial ischemia. Am J Cardiol 44:780, 1979.
24. Black JW, Crowther AF, Shanks RG, et al: A new adrenergic beta-receptor antagonist. Lancet 1:1080, 1964.
25. The Anturane Reinfarction Trial Research Group: Sulfinpyrazone in the prevention of sudden death after myocardial infarction. N Engl J Med 302:250, 1980.
26. Cairns JA, Gent M, Singer J, et al: Aspirin, sulfinpyrazone, or both in unstable angina: Results of a Canadian multicenter trial. N Engl J Med 313:1369, 1985.
27. Battock DJ, Alvarez H and Chidsey CA: Effects of propranolol and isosorbide dinitrate on exercise performance and adrenergic activity in patients with angina pectoris. Circulation 39:157, 1969.
28. Frick MH and Katila M: Hemodynamic consequences of physical training after myocardial infarction. Circulation 37:192, 1968.
29. Epstein SE, Redwood DR, Goldstein RE, et al: Angina pectoris: Pathophysiology, evaluation and treatment. Ann Intern Med 75:263, 1971.
30. Ferguson RJ, Cote P, Gauthier P, et al: Changes in exercise coronary sinus blood flow with training in patients with angina pectoris. Circulation 58:41, 1978.
31. Ronghgarden JW: Circulatory changes associated with spontaneous angina pectoris. Am J Med 41:947, 1966.
32. Ryan M, Lown B and Horn H: Comparison of ventricular ectopic activity during 24 hour monitoring and exercise testing in patients with coronary heart disease. N Engl J Med 292:224, 1975.
33. Lown B and Graboys TB: Ventricular premature beats and sudden cardiac death. *In* McIntosh H (ed): Baylor Cardiology Series, Vol 3, No 1, 1980.
34. McIntosh HD and Garcia JA: The first decade of aortocoronary bypass grafting, 1967–1977: A review. Circulation 57:405, 1978.
35. Favaloro RG: Direct myocardial revascularization: A ten year journey. Am J Cardiol 43:109, 1979.
36. Antman EM, Stone PH, Muller JE, et al: Calcium channel blocking agents in the treatment of cardiovascular disorders. I: Basic and clinical electrophysiologic effects. Ann Intern Med 93:875, 1980.
37. Stone PH, Antman EM, Muller JE, et al: Calcium channel blocking agents in the treatment of cardiovascular disorders. II: Hemodynamic effects and clinical applications. Ann Intern Med 93:886, 1980.
38. Lazzara R and Scherlag B: Treatment of arrhythmias by blocking slow current (Editorial). Ann Intern Med 93:919, 1980.
39. Multicenter Diltiazem Post Infarction Trial Research Group: The effect of diltiazem on mortality and reinfarction after myocardial infarction. N Engl J Med 319:385, 1988.
40. CASS Principal Investigators and Associates: Coronary Artery Surgery Study (CASS): A randomized trial of coronary artery bypass surgery. Survival data. Circulation 68:939, 1983.
41. European Coronary Surgery Study Group: Long-term results of prospective randomized study of coronary artery bypass surgery in stable angina pectoris. Lancet 2:1173, 1982.
42. Graboys TB, Headley A, Lown B, et al: Results of a second opinion option program among candidates for coronary bypass graft surgery. JAMA 258:1611, 1987.
43. Graboys TB, Biegelsen B, Lampert S, et al: Results of a second opinion trial among patients recommended for coronary angiography. JAMA 268:2537, 1992.
44. Parisi AF, Folland ED, Hartigan P, et al: A comparison of angioplasty with medical therapy in the treatment of single vessel coronary artery disease. N Engl J Med 326:10, 1992.

4

Noninvasive Tests in Cardiology

THOMAS H. LEE, Jr, MD
LEE GOLDMAN, MD

Clinicians increasingly have relied on noninvasive tests to aid in the diagnosis, management, and estimation of prognosis in patients with cardiac signs or symptoms. This chapter emphasizes the use of these tests for *diagnostic* purposes, with the understanding that diagnosis frequently may have therapeutic and prognostic implications as well.

Three types of patients are considered: the patient suspected of having angina pectoris, the patient with a systolic murmur, and the patient suspected of having congestive heart failure. For these types of patients, noninvasive diagnostic tests—exercise electrocardiograms, stress thallium procedures, two-dimensional echocardiograms, and resting left ventricular function studies—are often used as substitutes for the accepted diagnostic gold standard, namely cardiac catheterization. Although the results of these noninvasive tests all correlate with cardiac catheterization, the correlations range from excellent, such as that of resting radionuclide ventriculography with left ventricular angiography, to reasonable but far from perfect, such as that of exercise electrocardiography with coronary angiography. In the latter situation, the clinician must interpret and use the results of the surrogate technology, that is, the noninvasive test that substitutes for the more expensive or morbid catheterization, with the understanding that the test result may affect the probability of a diagnosis but can neither absolutely establish it nor absolutely rule it out. This challenge of interpreting and using the results of surrogate technologies has stimulated development of the field of quantitative clinical decision-making, in which the concepts of epidemiology, probability, and cost-effectiveness may guide the clinical application of the new technologies.

When deciding whether or not to order a diagnostic test, the clinician should ask the following questions: what is the pre-test probability that the patient has the condition; how much higher or lower would that probability have to be for the diagnostic or therapeutic approach to be changed and what is the likelihood that the diagnostic test being considered will move the probability across this threshold; and, finally, how bad would it be to miss the diagnosis in question or mistakenly to treat the patient as if the condition were present even though it is not?

EVALUATION OF THE PATIENT SUSPECTED OF HAVING ANGINA PECTORIS

Angina pectoris is usually suspected or considered in a patient with chest pain or discomfort. The differential diagnosis of chest pain includes noncardiac conditions such as musculoskeletal chest pain, esophageal discomfort and other gastrointestinal abnormalities, and some neurologic disorders (see Chapter 3). No single clinical feature is perfectly predictive of the presence of coronary artery disease but, in sum, clinical assessment can give a good approximation of the likelihood of disease.

Depending on such issues as the character of the chest discomfort, its reproducibility or lack thereof by local palpation, its relationship to exercise, its location and sites of radiation, its response to rest and nitroglycerin, and its usual duration, a clinician can usually classify chest pain syndromes into one of three categories: (1) typical for angina pectoris, (2) atypical for angina pectoris but consistent with the diagnosis, or (3) clearly noncardiac chest pain. This clinical judgment is crucial, since the proper interpretation of the result of any diagnostic test in a patient with suspected angina pectoris depends on the pretest likelihood that the patient has coronary artery disease.

The patient with so-called "typical" chest pain has at least an 80% probability of coronary artery disease. Among patients with "atypical" angina who come to catheterization because of persistent complaints and often because of some abnormalities on diagnostic testing, the probability of coronary artery disease is usually in the 40 to 50% range. Among patients with noncardiac chest pain, the probability of coronary artery disease is only about 5%, which is little if any higher than the prevalence of asymptomatic coronary artery disease in age-matched control patients.

The diagnostic procedures that have been used traditionally for noninvasive assessment of patients with suspected angina pectoris have relied on physical exercise (usually walking on a treadmill) to increase the heart's workload in an attempt to unmask ischemia. The means of detecting

ECG Patterns indicative of Myocardial Ischemia

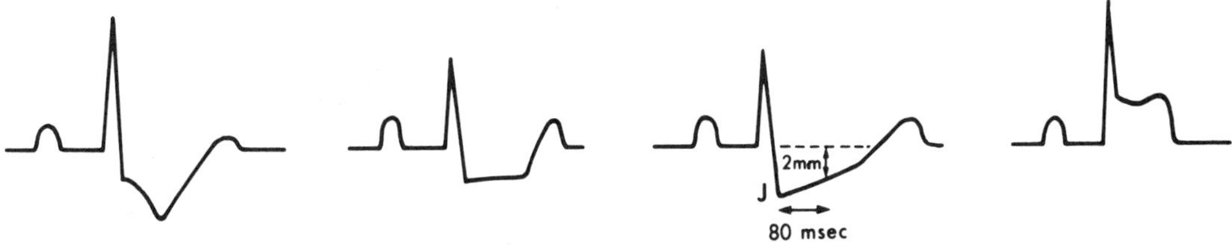

ECG Patterns not indicative of Myocardial Ischemia

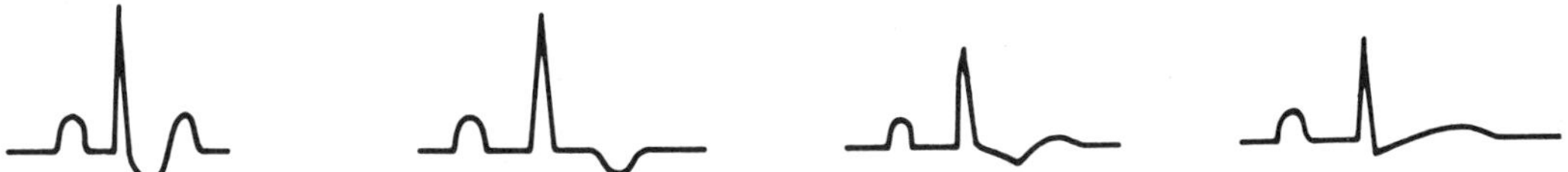

FIGURE 4–1. Electrocardiographic criteria suggestive of myocardial ischemia consist of at least 1 mm of J point depression with downsloping or horizontal ST segments; slowly upsloping ST segment depression, defined as 2 mm of ST depression measured 80 msec from the J point; and ST segment elevation. (Reproduced with permission, from Goldschlager N: Use of the treadmill test in the diagnosis of coronary artery disease in patients with chest pain. Ann Intern Med 97:383–388, 1982.)

ischemia during exercise include electrocardiography, scintigraphy with ^{201}Tl and other radionuclide agents, radionuclide ventriculography, and echocardiography. In recent years, new testing technologies have been developed that permit evaluation of patients who are unable to perform treadmill exercise. Some of these newer tests use pharmacologic agents such as dipyridamole, adenosine, and dobutamine to stress the heart in an attempt to induce ischemia. Another approach is ambulatory ischemia monitoring, in which a portable electrocardiographic monitor is used to record ST segments, usually for a period of 24 hours. Regardless of which technology is used, the clinician must have a basic understanding of each test's methodology and accuracy.

Exercise Electrocardiography

The most common protocol, the Bruce Protocol,[1] includes seven stages of 3 minutes each on a treadmill, and advances from 1.7 mph and a 10% elevation or grade (stage I) to 6 mph at a 22% elevation (stage VII). Although correlations between exercise tolerance on treadmill testing and classification of the severity of angina pectoris by the New York Heart Association criteria,[2] the Canadian Cardiovascular Society criteria,[3] or Specific Activity Scale criteria,[4] are imperfect, in general a patient is considered to be in class II if he or she can complete stage I of the Bruce Protocol and is considered class I if he or she can complete stage II of the Bruce Protocol. Since the Bruce Protocol is rather insensitive at lower levels of exercise capacity, a variety of modified protocols have been proposed. For example, the Naughton Protocol[5, 6] remains at 2 mph for the first four stages, with elevations of from 3.5% at stage I to 10.5% at stage IV.

Depending on the exercise laboratory, one might monitor 1, 2, or all 12 electrocardiographic leads during and after exercise testing. If only one lead is used, it usually corresponds approximately to lead V_5 on a standard electrocardiogram. However, data suggest that it is preferable to have at least two anterior precordial leads and one inferior electrocardiographic lead during exercise and then to have a full 12-lead electrocardiogram immediately after the completion of exercise.[7]

The interpretation of an exercise electrocardiogram depends principally on the amount of ST segment displacement during and after exercise (Fig. 4–1).[7] For ST depression to be considered important, it must persist for at least 0.08 second after the completion of the QRS complex. Depression at the J point, which is at the very conclusion of the QRS complex, is not usually considered to be of diagnostic importance, especially if the ST segment slopes upward to, or nearly to, baseline by 0.08 second later. ST segment elevation is also an abnormal response to exercise,[6–8] and it can be consistent with localized transmural ischemia, coronary artery spasm of the Prinzmetal type, or the provocation of regional dyskinesis in a patient with a true or functional aneurysm, usually as the residue of a previous myocardial infarction. In some patients, an increase in the amplitude of the R wave during exercise may be a reflection of left ventricular dysfunction and, by extrapolation, of ischemia caused by coronary artery disease.[9]

Several situations may greatly affect the electrocardiographic response to exercise testing.[6] For example, digitalis may cause resting abnormalities of the ST segment that may be exacerbated by exercise even in the absence of underlying coronary artery disease. Tricyclic antidepressants are also commonly associated with false-positive results on exercise testing. Patients whose ventricles are activated in an abnormal sequence, especially patients with left bundle branch block or with bypass tracts, such as in the Wolff-Parkinson-White syndrome, may have abnormal ST segments at rest and may have marked ST segment changes with exercise in the absence of coronary disease. Finally, β-adrenergic blocking agents may blunt the chronotropic response to exercise and thus make it more difficult to precipitate an ischemic electrocardiographic response.

The normal response to exercise is an increase in heart rate and in systolic blood pressure, often but not always with a decrease in diastolic blood pressure. The failure of the systolic pressure to rise with exercise suggests an inadequate increase in cardiac output, such as when cardiac

TABLE 4–1. TERMS MOST COMMONLY USED TO EVALUATE NONINVASIVE CARDIAC DIAGNOSTIC TESTS

	Patient Status	
Test Result	*Diseased (Abnormal)*	*Nondiseased (Normal)*
+ *(Abnormal)*	*a*	*c*
− *(Normal)*	*b*	*d*
Sensitivity	$\frac{a}{a + b}$	If the patient has the disease, how likely is a positive test result?
Specificity	$\frac{d}{c + d}$	If the patient does not have the disease, how likely is a negative test result?
Positive predictive value	$\frac{a}{a + c}$	If a test result is positive, how likely is it that the patient has the disease?

output cannot increase sufficiently to compensate for the vasodilatation that occurs in skeletal muscle.

Exercise testing is usually thought to be contraindicated in patients with unstable angina pectoris, probable acute myocardial infarction, severe aortic stenosis, severe hypertension, or uncontrolled cardiac arrhythmias. In patients without such contraindications, the mortality rate is about three to 10 per 100,000 exercise tests, with the morbidity rate of about 20 per 100,000, including such nonfatal complications as prolonged chest pain, cardiac arrhythmias, or myocardial infarction.[6, 10]

Interpretation of the Results of Exercise Testing. A standard nomenclature has been developed for expressing the usefulness of test results (Table 4–1). In general, one would like a sensitive test if one were trying to screen for the presence of disease. In such a circumstance, a negative result on a very sensitive test would essentially rule out the disease. One must be careful to distinguish sensitivity and specificity, which are characteristics of the test itself, from predictive value, which depends to a great extent on the prevalence of disease in the population being tested. For example, if the prevalence of disease is very high, more of the positive test results will be true positives, thus elevating the predictive value. Conversely, the sensitivity and specificity of a test do not depend on the prevalence of disease in the population being tested. Sensitivity and specificity, however, depend on the spectrum of diseased and nondiseased patients who are tested.[11] For example, if one tried to determine the sensitivity and specificity of an exercise test by evaluating 50 patients with severe three-vessel disease and 50 normal male medical students, one would obtain a rather high sensitivity and specificity. On the other hand, if the test was evaluated on 100 subjects of both sexes, 50 of whom had coronary disease but all of whom had chest pain syndromes and some type of cardiac condition, both the calculated sensitivity and specificity might be much lower because the spectrum of patients being tested would be different. Exactly such a phenomenon has been noted in exercise radionuclide ventriculography,[12] in which changes in the spectrum of patients undergoing the test have resulted in a marked decline in the calculated specificity of that test.

When determining the sensitivity and specificity of exercise electrocardiography, the situation is further complicated because there is no definitive distinction between a normal response versus an abnormal response. For example, if one were trying to use a very sensitive definition of abnormal to screen patients for the possible presence of coronary artery disease, one might call any ST segment depression an abnormal response. However, such a sensitive definition would result in many false-positive tests, thus either falsely labeling patients as having coronary disease or stimulating the ordering of a number of additional procedures. In deciding about a normal versus an abnormal response, one must therefore consider the intrinsic trade-off between increasing sensitivity and decreasing specificity (Fig. 4–2). In essence, if one wishes to increase sensitivity by calling a test abnormal even if there is minimal ST segment change, the specificity will decline, thus resulting in more false-positive results.[13] On the other hand, if one insists on a high specificity to eliminate false-positive results, sensitivity will decline and many truly diseased patients may be missed.

Using a definition of abnormal of 1 to 2 mm or more of ST depression, most recent studies have reported sensitivities in the 50 to 80% range if the patient achieves at least 85% of the predicted maximal heart rate.[6, 7] For detection of multivessel coronary artery disease, pooled data suggest that the sensitivity of the exercise test is about 81% and the specificity is about 66%, but the sensitivity for detecting single-vessel disease may be as low as 25 to 30%.

Integration of Test Result with the Prior Probability of Disease. As stated earlier, the predictive value, which is the likelihood that the patient has coronary artery disease after the test result is known, is a function not only of sensitivity and specificity but also of the prior, or pretest, probability that the patient has the disease. In clinical decision-making analyses, the post-test probability has usually been calculated using Bayes' theorem. In its most clinically applicable form, Bayes' theorem states that the post-test odds of having a disease can be calculated as the product of the pretest odds multiplied by the likelihood ratio of the test. In this calculation, the pretest odds are another way of expressing the prior probability, or prevalence. For example, if a patient has an 80% pretest probability of coronary disease, the pretest odds are 4:1. The likelihood ratio is the test's sensitivity divided by [1 − the test's specificity]. Thus, if a particular exercise test result has a sensitivity of 60% for diagnosing coronary artery disease and a specificity of 90%, such a test result would carry a likelihood ratio of [0.6] divided by [1−0.9]=6. Therefore,

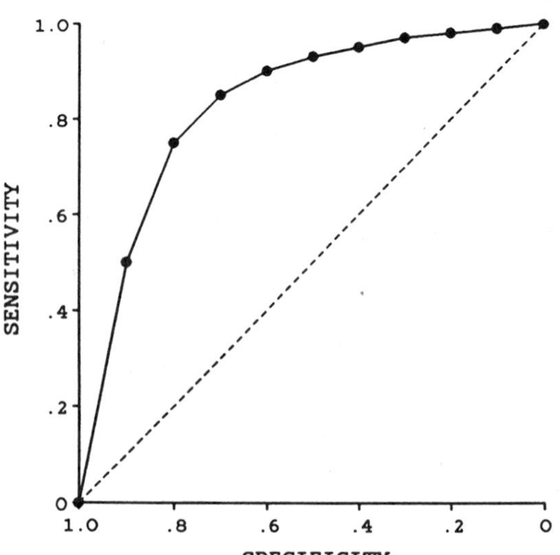

FIGURE 4–2. The points on the curve correspond to different choices of the boundary between normal and abnormal for a hypothetic test result. This type of curve has been termed a receiver-operating characteristic (ROC) curve.

this particular test result would increase the odds of having the disease sixfold, thus converting a pretest probability of 80% (odds of 4:1) into a post-test probability of 96% (a post-test odds of 24:1).

Using the available published data, Rifkin and Hood plotted a series of curves showing how the prior, or before-test, probability of coronary artery disease could be converted into a posterior, or after-test, probability of coronary artery disease by knowing the exercise test result (Fig. 4–3).[15]

The importance of the prior probability can best be understood by considering three types of patients with different pretest probabilities. First, a patient with a typical anginal syndrome may have about an 80% probability of coronary artery disease, based on history alone. The presence of 2 mm or more of ST segment depression by exercise electrocardiography would increase that probability to well above 95%. By comparison, if a patient had atypical symptoms that were perhaps consistent with angina pectoris but by no means classic for it, the pre-exercise test probability of coronary artery disease may be about 40%. In such a patient, 2 mm of ST depression would increase the probability of coronary disease to about 90%. Finally, in an asymptomatic patient, in whom the prevalence of asymptomatic coronary artery disease may be about 5%, the same 2 mm or more of ST segment depression would increase the probability only to about 50%. As can be inferred from Figure 4–3, exercise tests showing less than 1.5 mm of ST depression produce little or no change in the calculated probability of coronary artery disease; this implies that such mildly "abnormal" test results do little to establish a diagnosis in patients who lack the classic symptoms.

The calculation of a pre-exercise test probability of coronary artery disease may be formidable if one wishes to be more accurate than the rough approximations of 80% for typical angina, 40% for atypical angina, and 5% for asymptomatic persons. One can be more precise by knowing risk factor status, such as systolic blood pressure, cholesterol level, and smoking habits.[16, 17] A commercially available approach known as CADENZA has been used to calculate pre-exercise and postexercise test probabilities, and also for the integration of additional test results to the modification

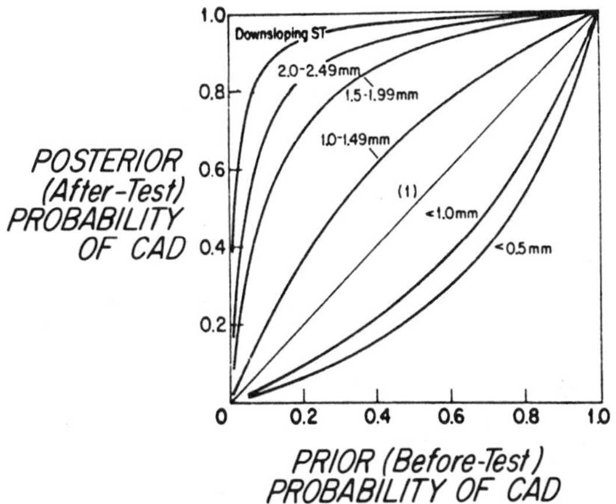

FIGURE 4–3. These curves show the posterior (after-test) probability as a function of the prior (before-test) probability for different results of the exercise electrocardiogram. Note that 1 mm or more of ST segment depression increases the probability of disease, whereas less than 1 mm of ST segment depression is associated with a modest reduction in the probability of disease. (From Rifkin RD and Hood WB: Bayesian analysis of electrocardiographic exercise stress testing. N Engl J Med 297:681–686, 1977. Reprinted by permission from the *New England Journal of Medicine.*)

of probability.[17] It is emphasized that the theoretical calculations by Bayes' theorem have been remarkably similar to the actual results found when large populations of patients are subjected to exercise testing,[18] thus indicating that these theoretical computations have true clinical relevance.

Threshold Approach to Test Utilization. As emphasized by Figure 4–2, Bayesian calculations result in larger changes in the probability of disease when the pretest probability is close to 50%. When the pretest probability is closer to the extremes, the changes in probabilities are often smaller, unless the test is very highly abnormal in someone with a very low prior probability of disease, which of course would be a rather unlikely test result.

One must distinguish, however, between large absolute changes in probability and the implications of such a change. For example, changing the probability of coronary artery disease from 30 to 70% may be a very impressive change in probability, but one may argue that a 70% probability of coronary artery disease does not establish the diagnosis any more than a 30% probability of coronary disease excludes the diagnosis. In the threshold approach to decision-making, a test result is important only if it is sufficiently positive or negative to move the patient's probability of disease across a diagnostic or therapeutic threshold.

If it is highly unlikely that a diagnostic test, such as exercise electrocardiography, could move a patient across a threshold regardless of its result, then the test usually should not be ordered, unless one would argue that it would be so bad to miss the diagnosis that one must order even low-yield tests. For example, one might argue that a lumbar puncture is a very low-yield test, but the implications of missing bacterial meningitis are so serious that such a test would be indicated. In most circumstances, however, very low yield noninvasive or surrogate tests are not useful unless they are extremely sensitive. In general, when it is absolutely necessary to exclude a diagnosis, the preferred approach is going directly to the gold standard test: for example, a lumbar puncture if one is ruling out meningitis or coronary arteriography if one must rule out coronary artery disease. As can be seen from Figure 4–3, in a patient with a 40% probability of coronary artery disease, a negative exercise test result does not rule out coronary disease. On the other hand, a strongly positive exercise electrocardiogram essentially establishes the presence of coronary artery disease in someone with typical symptoms and makes it very likely, although not certain, in someone with a 40 to 50% pretest probability.

Exercise Testing to Predict the Severity of Coronary Disease or to Estimate Prognosis. Independent of its role for diagnosing the presence or absence of coronary artery disease, exercise testing has been used for prognostic purposes and also for estimating the severity of coronary disease. In this latter mode, a variety of investigators have examined the value of the exercise test for diagnosing left main coronary artery disease, a condition for which surgical therapy clearly appears to improve survival.[19] Surgery also appears to prolong survival in patients who have mild symptoms or who are asymptomatic after a myocardial infarction and who have both three-vessel disease *and* mild-to-moderate left ventricular dysfunction.[20] Thus, an argument can be made for using the exercise electrocardiogram to detect left main coronary artery disease or three-vessel disease in patients who have mild symptoms.

Although left main coronary artery disease is more common in patients who are older and who have typical anginal symptoms, it is extremely difficult to predict its presence from clinical features alone.[21] In pooled data from the literature, about 87% of patients with left main coronary artery disease have at least 1 mm of ST segment depression, and 82% have 2 mm or more of ST depression. At 2 mm of ST depression, the exercise test has a specificity of 66% and a positive predictive value of 23% for left main coronary artery disease.[21] Left main coronary artery disease is also more common in patients whose exercise duration is less than 3 minutes or who develop exertional hypotension, but these two criteria are less sensitive than the amount of ST segment depression.[21] In an average patient with mildly symptomatic definite or probable angina, 2 mm or more of ST depression on exercise testing will increase the probability of left main coronary artery disease to about 17% and would yield a post-test probability of three-vessel disease or left main coronary artery disease of about 60% in men and about 35% in women. In patients with mild anginal symptoms, cost-effectiveness analyses suggest that a screening exercise tolerance test, with subsequent cardiac catheterization if it reveals 2 mm or more of ST depression, would be cost-effective in patients aged 40 to 70 years with typical anginal symptoms.[22]

The exercise test also may be used to estimate prognosis. Even in asymptomatic subjects, exercise test abnormalities correlate with the future development of coronary heart disease events.[23, 24] However, present data do not suggest that such screening is cost-effective, and, in general, exercise-test screening of asymptomatic subjects is not recommended,[25] except perhaps in the sedentary subject who now wishes to begin a vigorous exercise program. In patients with known heart disease, and especially in survivors of an acute myocardial infarction or unstable angina, exercise performance correlates with prognosis,[26, 27] and it appears to add prognostic information principally in patients who might otherwise seem to be at low risk.[28] Among patients with angina, good exercise tolerance predicts a benign short-term prognosis even in the presence of 2 mm or more of ST depression.[29]

^{201}Tl Scintigraphy

Myocardial perfusion scintigraphy is based on the principle that a radioactive tracer such as ^{201}Tl will be distributed in the myocardium in a manner that is proportional to the amount of blood flow.[30] Thus, with exercise, a well-perfused area of myocardium will have a greater uptake of ^{201}Tl than a poorly perfused area.

Thallium has a wash-out half-life of about 4 hours. By that time, there is also rapid wash-in into the ischemic zone. Therefore, repeat scintigraphy about 4 hours after a single intravenous injection results in a "redistribution" image, similar to an image that would have been obtained if the original intravenous injection had been made at rest. If a defect is shown only with the exercise scintiscan and is not present at rest, then this reversible defect is presumably due to transient ischemia in viable myocardium. If the scintiscan defect at exercise persists on the redistribution scintiscan 4 hours later, this fixed defect is consistent with nonviable myocardium, usually as the result of a prior myocardial infarction. However, studies indicate that not all such "fixed" defects represent permanent damage. A second injection of thallium during the rest period may be useful for detecting areas of myocardium that appear to be irreversibly damaged on the initial exercise and redistribution scans, but are in fact still viable.[31] Second thallium injections are not performed routinely in everyone with a fixed defect on both the exercise and redistribution scan, but such injections may be especially helpful if the patient has angina and no reversible defects or has no other prior evidence to suggest a myocardial infarction in that location.

False-positive exercise thallium scintigraphy can occur in patients with aortic stenosis and with other conditions that cause exercise-induced subendocardial ischemia in the absence of coronary artery disease. Fixed defects at both exercise and rest have also been described in patients with infiltrative myocardial diseases, congestive cardiomyopathy, and hypertrophic obstructive cardiomyopathy. False-positive test results also appear to be more common in women, perhaps because overlying breast tissue may attenuate thallium activity measurement.[30]

Thallium imaging can be used to help diagnose the presence or absence of coronary artery disease, to estimate the extent of disease, or to evaluate whether atypical chest pain in a patient with known coronary disease, such as the post-coronary artery bypass surgery patient, is associated with observable myocardial ischemia. The following discussion concentrates on thallium imaging principally to diagnose the presence or absence of coronary disease.

A variety of laboratories have investigated the sensitivity and specificity of ^{201}Tl scintigraphy, using a transient exercise-related defect as a definition of a positive test result in patients without prior myocardial infarction. Pooled data suggest that the sensitivity of thallium scintigraphy for detecting any coronary artery disease is about 84% and the specificity is 87%.[30] As is the case with exercise electrocardiography, the sensitivity of this test is influenced by the severity of coronary disease. Thus, the sensitivities for detecting one-, two-, and three-vessel disease are 78%, 89%, and 92%, respectively.[30] Such data allow generation of a graph depicting the way in which a pretest probability may be transformed into a post-test probability based on the exercise thallium result (Fig. 4–4), much as has been done for exercise electrocardiography (see Fig. 4–3).

Using Bayes' theorem as described previously, one can analyze the sequential value of exercise electrocardiography and exercise thallium scintigraphy by starting with a pretest probability, calculating a postexercise test probability from Figure 4–3, using the post-test probability from Figure 4–3 as the pre-thallium scintigraphy probability for Figure 4–4, and calculating a post-thallium probability

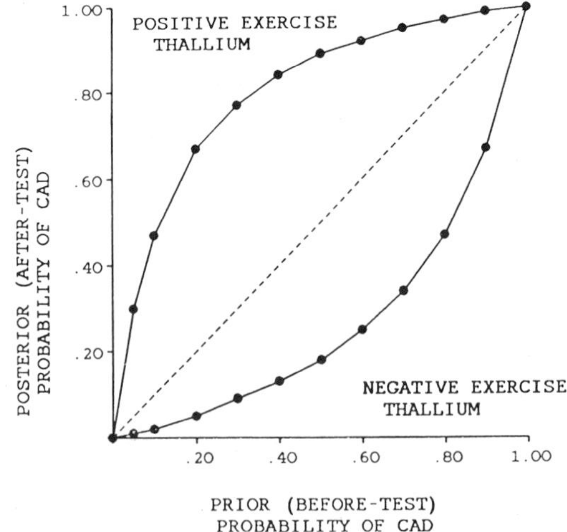

FIGURE 4–4. These curves show the posterior (after-test) probability as a function of the prior (before-test) probability for positive versus negative results on exercise thallium scintiscans, defined as a perfusion defect that is produced by exercise and resolves with rest. The before-test probability could be estimated from the clinical presentation or could be a postexercise electrocardiogram probability derived from Figure 4–3.

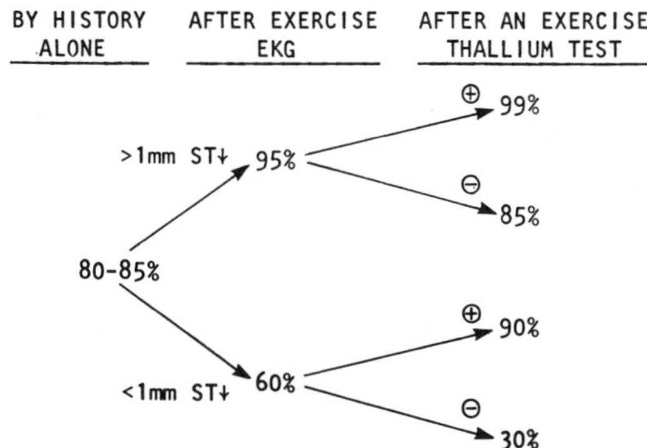

FIGURE 4–5. Approximate probability of coronary artery disease before and after noninvasive testing in a patient with typical angina pectoris. These percentages demonstrate how the sequential use of an exercise electrocardiogram and an exercise-thallium test may affect the probability of coronary artery disease in a patient with typical angina pectoris.

from Figure 4–4. Alternatively, one can estimate the value of exercise electrocardiography and exercise thallium testing in sequence for affecting the probability of coronary artery disease in patients with typical angina pectoris (Fig. 4–5), atypical angina (Fig. 4–6), or in asymptomatic patients in the coronary artery disease age range (Fig. 4–7). Although these theoretical calculations may be formidable for the unsophisticated clinician, the availability of computerized algorithms such as CADENZA[17] has allowed many referral laboratories to provide probability estimates as part of their routine interpretation of the results of these diagnostic tests. Furthermore, it is emphasized that these theoretical calculations correspond remarkably closely with the actual observed probabilities of disease in patients who have undergone both tests plus coronary angiography,[18] thus emphasizing the practical application of bayesian calculations.

Exercise thallium scintigraphy has a higher overall accuracy for diagnosing coronary disease than exercise electrocardiography, especially when the patient has an abnormal resting electrocardiogram.[30] Thallium scintigraphy is more expensive and time-consuming for the patient than exercise electrocardiography, and whether it should be used routinely as the initial noninvasive test for ischemic heart disease is controversial.

Hlatky and associates have shown that cardiologists' accuracy for predicting coronary disease in patients who had already undergone exercise testing was improved by the availability of thallium scintigraphy results.[32] Other studies have shown that exercise thallium data are superior to

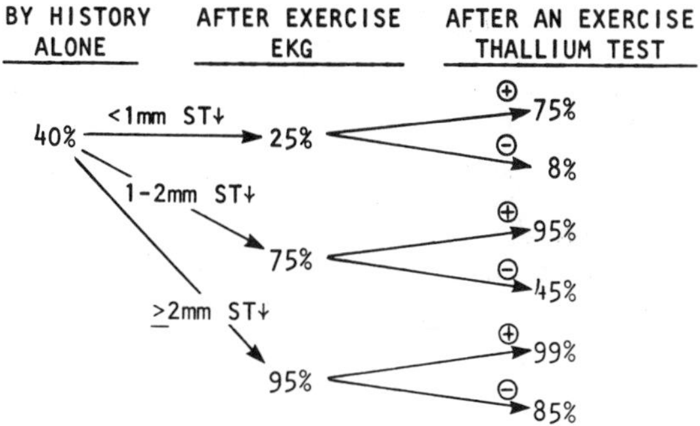

FIGURE 4–6. Approximate probability of coronary artery disease before and after noninvasive testing in a patient with atypical anginal symptoms.

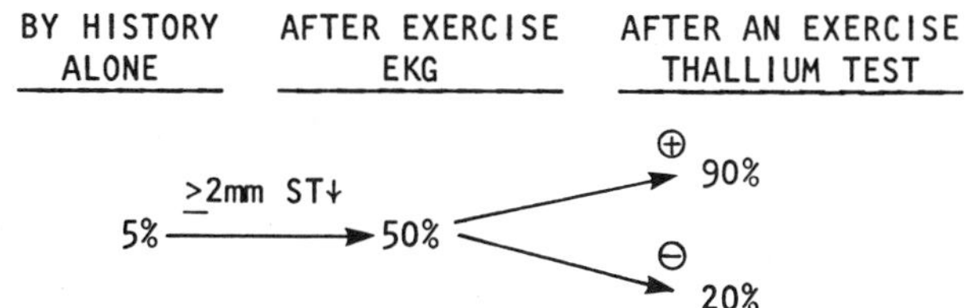

FIGURE 4–7. Approximate probability of coronary artery disease before and after noninvasive testing in an asymptomatic subject in the coronary artery disease age range.

data from both exercise testing alone and cardiac catheterization data alone for predicting future complications,[33] and that the combination of clinical plus thallium data is superior to the combination of clinical plus coronary angiographic data for predicting prognosis.[34]

However, exercise electrocardiography is usually much more readily available and less expensive. Furthermore, a negative result on an exercise electrocardiogram in a patient who has clearly noncardiac chest pain will result in a very low post-test probability of coronary disease. In patients with atypical angina, however, Figures 4–3 and 4–6 emphasize that a negative result on an exercise electrocardiogram is not adequate to exclude the possibility of coronary disease. If the patient with atypical angina has negative results on both an exercise electrocardiogram and an exercise thallium test with an adequate exercise tolerance, the probability of coronary artery disease is reduced to below 10%. Although this probability does not entirely rule out the possibility of coronary disease, it may be sufficiently reassuring in many patients. Of course, if one must rule out the disease with certainty, coronary angiography is required and the surrogate noninvasive diagnostic test should not be ordered.

Other Radionuclide Tests

At some medical centers, exercise radionuclide ventriculography is used not only for the assessment of left ventricular function but also to detect coronary artery disease. This test was initially proposed as a reasonably sensitive and specific test for detecting segmental wall motion abnormalities and a decrease in left ventricular ejection fraction with exercise in patients with coronary artery disease.[35]

However, whereas truly normal volunteers rarely have abnormal exercise responses, abnormal exercise responses are remarkably common in patients with chest pain and those with noncoronary cardiac conditions, so the specificity of exercise radionuclide ventriculography in the types of patients who are likely to undergo this diagnostic procedure appears to be as low as 36 to 49%.[12] The test, therefore, is not specific enough to substitute for cardiac catheterization in patients with chest pain or in those with other noncoronary cardiac diseases, such as restrictive cardiomyopathy, nonobstructive hypertrophic cardiomyopathy, constrictive pericarditis, or valvular heart disease.

Several studies indicate that a new radionuclide agent, known as ^{99m}Tc MIBI, may replace ^{201}Tl in the future at least in part. Tc-MIBI scanning provides images of superior quality compared with thallium scintigraphy, with fewer artifactual defects due to soft tissue attenuation.[36] Furthermore, this agent permits simultaneous assessment of left ventricular wall function, thus providing information that might otherwise require an additional test (e.g., echocardiogram or radionuclide ventriculogram) besides a myocardial perfusion scan. Further research is needed to define its clinical role.

Recommendations

Current data indicate that noninvasive diagnostic testing is not usually helpful for determining the presence or absence of coronary artery disease in patients with typical angina. Even if one or a combination of these test results are negative, the probability of disease remains too high for the patient or the physician to be reassured. However, exercise testing may prove to be helpful in such patients for the prediction of the probability of left main coronary artery disease or for the estimation of prognosis.

For patients with atypical anginal symptoms, negative results on an exercise test reduce the probability of coronary artery disease to about 25% and may indicate a relatively benign prognosis if exercise capacity is good. Negative results on both an electrocardiographic and a thallium exercise test will reduce the probability of coronary artery disease to below 10%, which often will be sufficiently reassuring in patients who have an excellent exercise tolerance. Of course, if one wants to rule out the disease with certainty, coronary arteriography is required.

In patients who have clearly nonanginal symptoms or who are asymptomatic, a negative result on an exercise electrocardiogram further lowers the probability of coronary disease to well below 5%. However, if the result of the exercise electrocardiogram is positive in such patients, a subsequent negative exercise thallium test does not certify that the exercise electrocardiogram was a false-positive result, although data suggest that such patients do have a favorable prognosis. If the goal is to exclude coronary disease, further testing will be required. In general, exercise electrocardiography is not recommended in asymptomatic subjects.

ASSESSMENT OF THE PATIENT WHO CANNOT PERFORM TREADMILL EXERCISE

Because of noncardiac conditions such as arthritis and peripheral vascular disease, many patients with suspected coronary artery disease are unable to perform treadmill exercise. This problem is especially common among patients undergoing noncardiac surgery, such as patients having peripheral vascular surgery or lower extremity joint replacements. In such cases, cardiovascular risk assessment can often be based on data from the history and physical alone, but coronary angiography is sometimes required for the evaluation of a chest pain complaint.

Several technologies can be used for the noninvasive assessment of patients who cannot perform exercise with their lower extremities. One test that does not actively attempt to precipitate ischemia is *ambulatory ischemia monitoring.* This technology uses a modification of the traditional ambulatory electrocardiographic monitor that is usually ordered to evaluate arrhythmias, but these monitors are able to detect shifts in the ST segment due to myocardial ischemia. An ambulatory ischemia monitor is usually worn for 24 hours, after which it is returned for computerized interpretation. This test is not useful for patients whose ST segments are abnormal on baseline electrocardiographic tracings.

The role of ambulatory ischemia monitoring in the diagnosis and management of coronary artery disease is currently unclear, since the relationship between the results from this test and exercise electrocardiography appears highly variable.[37] However, this technology is the best available method for detecting asymptomatic ischemia in patients with coronary artery disease, and research has shown that episodes of "silent" ischemia may be useful as a predictor of future complications, particularly in survivors of acute myocardial infarction.[38]

Ambulatory ischemia monitoring has also been shown to improve predictions of the risk of perioperative cardiac complications in patients undergoing vascular surgery. As is true of dipyridamole thallium scintigraphy, patients who have negative ambulatory ischemia monitor results have a very low risk for complications. The positive predictive value of an abnormal test result in one study was 38%[39]; that is, 38% of patients with ischemia detected by the monitor subsequently had major cardiac complications.

This high rate of complications suggests that patients who have ambulatory ischemia monitoring sessions positive for ischemia should be followed very closely during the perioperative period. If evidence of active ischemia is detected, these patients warrant aggressive medical therapy, such as administration of intravenous nitroglycerin. Patients who are undergoing major procedures such as operations involving the aorta may be considered for coronary angiography and possible revascularization via either angioplasty or coronary artery bypass graft surgery.

Other technologies attempt to provoke ischemia in patients with coronary artery disease by using physical exertion other than treadmill exercise or pharmacologic agents. Some cardiology laboratories offer arm ergometry, during which patients perform exercise with their upper extremities, usually upon a modified bicycle apparatus. When electrocardiography is used to detect ischemia, arm ergometry has a poor sensitivity (50%) for detecting coronary artery disease, but one study indicates that the use of thallium scintigraphy leads to a sensitivity of 80%.[40] A major limitation of arm ergometry is that the arms of many patients tire quickly. Women and elderly patients achieve significantly lower power outputs than men and younger patients, respectively.[41]

In recent years, there has been intense investigative interest in pharmacologic agents as a method of inducing ischemia in patients with coronary disease. The two most commonly used agents are dipyridamole and adenosine. Dipyridamole and adenosine are believed to precipitate ischemia by causing arteriolar vasodilatation. When these drugs are administered to a patient with critical coronary stenoses, flow is redistributed toward coronary arterial beds without stenoses, resulting in a "coronary steal."

After administration of one of these agents, thallium scintigraphy or, less often, echocardiography is used to detect evidence of ischemia. The alterations in coronary blood flow may result in an initial perfusion defect on thallium scintigraphy because of diminished uptake of the radionuclide. During follow-up scanning 2.5 to 4 hours later, the perfusion defect will resolve if the myocardium is ischemic but still viable. Sometimes handgrip exercise or low-level treadmill exercise is combined with these pharmacologic stresses to accentuate coronary blood flow redistribution.

The thallium defects precipitated by exercise have been shown to be similar in extent and location to those induced by dipyridamole.[42] Pooled data from published studies of patients undergoing dipyridamole thallium scintigraphy indicate that the sensitivity and specificity for detecting coronary artery disease are about 85% and 90%, respectively. Dipyridamole thallium scintigraphy also appears useful for predicting risk for future cardiac complications, particularly in patients undergoing peripheral vascular or aortic surgery. Multiple studies indicate that patients who have negative dipyridamole thallium scintiscans before vascular surgery have a very low risk for cardiac complications. However, because of the test's high sensitivity for detecting lesser degrees of coronary disease, only about 25% of patients who have positive test results have major complications during subsequent vascular surgery. Because of this low positive predictive value, dipyridamole thallium scintigraphy does not improve risk stratification for patients with no clinical risk factors for complications.[43] Noncardiac surgeries other than vascular procedures generally carry a lower risk for complications than vascular surgery; therefore, the role of dipyridamole thallium scintigraphy in these patient populations remains uncertain.

Although there have been fewer published studies using adenosine to induce ischemia, adenosine thallium scintigraphy appears to have a sensitivity and specificity for detecting coronary disease similar to those of exercise thallium scintigraphy.[44] The short half-life of adenosine may be an important advantage, because ischemia and other side effects (e.g., dyspnea, flushing, nausea, and headache) of adenosine usually resolve within less than 1 minute. Dipyridamole precipitates similar side effects that may persist for several minutes, and intravenous aminophylline is often required to hasten their resolution.

Either of these pharmacologic agents can also be used with echocardiography as a means of diagnosing coronary artery disease. In stress echocardiography, ischemia is detected by the development of a transient regional wall motion abnormality. Because a considerable amount of myocardium must be ischemic before such an abnormality becomes visible, stress echocardiography is probably less sensitive for detecting *any* coronary artery disease than the other technologies described earlier. However, some data suggest that stress echocardiography, with dipyridamole, adenosine, or dobutamine, may be a useful test for *severe* coronary artery disease and may therefore be an appropriate test for risk stratification of patients with probable coronary disease who are scheduled for elective noncardiac surgery.[45]

EVALUATION OF THE PATIENT WITH A SYSTOLIC MURMUR

The most common systolic murmur is a benign, functional flow murmur that is usually heard best at the left sternal border. Such murmurs occur in patients with fever, anemia, thyrotoxicosis, and other causes of increased cardiac output. They also are seen in pregnancy and in some young, healthy individuals. Such murmurs are usually soft in quality, are grade I or II/VI in intensity and thus are not accompanied by a thrill. They commonly are heard best in early systole but sometimes in midsystole. Benign flow murmurs should not be holosystolic nor radiate to the axilla nor loudly into the carotid arteries. The carotid upstroke should be normal, the second heart sound should be normally split, and there should be no accompanying diastolic murmurs. The electrocardiogram and chest radiograph will commonly be normal as well. Although such functional flow murmurs were thought to originate in the pulmonic outflow track, intracardiac recordings suggest that many are actually related to a flow across the aortic valve itself. In contrast, the murmur of valvular aortic stenosis, which is harsher in quality, late peaking, and often loudest in the right second intercostal space, is in large part caused by turbulence distal to the aortic valve.

The differential diagnosis of various causes of systolic murmurs in valvular heart disease is discussed in detail (see Chapter 5). However, without eliminating the possibility that a murmur may be caused by such unusual conditions as a subaortic membrane, a ventricular septal defect, a patent ductus arteriosus, an atrial septal defect, pulmonic stenosis, or tricuspid regurgitation, in adults the most common causes of systolic murmurs, other than functional flow murmurs, are murmurs across the aortic outflow track and murmurs of mitral regurgitation. Among the murmurs across the aortic outflow track, the most common are related to abnormalities of the aortic valve, ranging from mild sclerocalcific changes without important stenosis to critical aortic stenosis that requires urgent surgery. Hypertrophic obstructive cardiomyopathy, one form of which is called idiopathic hypertrophic subaortic stenosis, may sometimes mimic valvular aortic stenosis, although a careful physical examination usually distinguishes between the two. Mitral regurgitant murmurs can usually be distinguished from aortic outflow murmurs by their characteristic apical location, holosystolic timing, and radiation to the axilla, although in some elderly patients the murmur of aortic stenosis may actually be loudest at the apex.

In evaluating the patient with systolic murmur, noninvasive testing will help to localize the cause of the murmur, and if it localizes the murmur to the aortic valve region, it will help to estimate the likelihood of critical aortic valve stenosis requiring surgery. The principal noninvasive test for this evaluation is echocardiography, usually supplemented by Doppler analysis of blood flow turbulence.

Echocardiogram

The echocardiogram is the first-line diagnostic test in patients whose systolic murmurs may indicate important valvular heart disease. When used in this way, the echocardiogram is a highly accurate test and frequently has an impact on diagnostic decision-making.[46]

In evaluating the possibility that a systolic murmur may be caused by important valvular aortic stenosis, the echocardiogram is an exceptionally sensitive test; in other words, virtually always it will show some abnormality of the aortic valve in patients who have aortic valve stenosis. In most laboratories, an aortic valve opening of 2 cm or more is considered to be normal. This makes echocardiography useful in ruling out severe aortic stenosis, but, unfortunately, diminished aortic valve leaflet excursion can be misleading in estimating the severity of aortic stenosis when present. Many patients with mild or moderate aortic stenosis also may have markedly diminished aortic valve leaflet motion by echocardiography, often because multiple echoes reverberate in areas of calcification, thus making the aortic valve orifice appear to be smaller than it may actually be.

There are no specific echocardiographic findings for mitral regurgitation, although echocardiography is sometimes helpful in determining the cause of the regurgitation. Mitral regurgitation itself is usually suspected based on evidence of left ventricular volume overload and left atrial enlargement. Often, rheumatic mitral regurgitation is accompanied by echocardiographic abnormalities suggestive of rheumatic thickening of the mitral valve, perhaps associated with some degree of mitral stenosis. Mitral regurgitation from mitral valve prolapse is commonly associated with characteristic echocardiographic findings.

Echocardiography is the preferred method for diagnosing obstructive hypertrophic cardiomyopathy, and catheterization is usually not required to make this diagnosis. In addition, many patients have symmetric hypertrophy of the left ventricle, but the physiology is one of outflow obstruction, even though they do not have the classic asymmetric septal hypertrophy. If the resting echocardiogram shows hypertrophy without signs of obstruction, provocative maneuvers (see Chapter 5) can be used in an attempt to produce the echocardiographic signs of obstruction: systolic anterior motion of the mitral valve and the typical "spike and dome" carotid pulse morphology.

Doppler Echocardiography

A tool that has greatly enhanced the noninvasive evaluation of murmurs is Doppler echocardiography.[47] This is based on the principle of the Doppler shift, in which an ultrasonic wave is altered when reflected from a moving object so that the difference in frequency between the ultrasound that is transmitted and that which is returned depends on the speed of the reflecting interface and the angle at which the ultrasonic beam intersects with the object. Using Doppler echocardiography, one can distinguish laminar flow from turbulent flow. In laminar flow, the velocity of all blood particles in a given instance is similar, and a Doppler recording will show a relatively homogeneous tracing. In turbulent flow, in which blood cells may be moving in various directions, multiple velocities and directions will be recorded as scattered Doppler signals both above and below the baseline. The Doppler probe can be localized to a specific area by echocardiography, and thus flow in a localized area can be determined. In such a way, Doppler echocardiography can demonstrate mitral regurgitation or even the site of ventricular septal defect, as well as show the turbulence across an abnormal aortic valve.

Data from several centers indicate that continuous wave Doppler echocardiography can accurately measure the pressure gradient across an aortic valve, and this measurement may be used to estimate the aortic valve gradient and area noninvasively. Although these estimations of valve gradient and area have not been perfectly accurate to date, this technique is an excellent screening test to exclude significant aortic stenosis. Doppler echocardiography can substitute for left heart catheterization when it is difficult or dangerous to pass a catheter across the aortic valve and in some younger patients who do not require coronary angiography prior to valve replacement.

Recommendations

In virtually all patients with a heart murmur, an electrocardiogram and chest radiograph are indicated. The electrocardiogram is useful for determining the presence of left or right ventricular hypertrophy or of conduction system abnormalities that may accompany some causes of systolic murmurs. The chest film is useful for evaluating the possibility of ventricular or atrial dilatation, congestive heart failure, or changes in pulmonary blood flow to suggest a left-to-right shunt. After the physical examination, electrocardiogram, and chest radiograph have been performed, certain recommendations can be made to guide further noninvasive testing:

1. The patient who probably has a functional flow murmur. If an asymptomatic patient's physical examination is consistent with an innocent flow murmur and the electrocardiogram and chest radiograph do not suggest other causes of the murmur, then further cardiac evaluation with echocardiography is not commonly indicated. In these patients, however, it is important that a provocative maneuver such as the Valsalva maneuver or auscultation with standing be performed to demonstrate that the murmur is not suggestive of obstructive hypertrophic cardiomyopathy. Of course, when a flow murmur is diagnosed, the physician must consider the possibility that a noncardiac condition such as anemia, fever, or thyrotoxicosis has increased cardiac output and thus represents the underlying cause of the flow murmur.

2. The patient with probable mitral valve prolapse. If the patient has classic physical findings for mitral valve prolapse, including an isolated midsystolic click or a midsystolic click followed by a late systolic murmur, confirmation of the diagnosis by echocardiography is not required if the patient has a normal-sized heart by chest radiograph, no evidence of left ventricular hypertrophy by electrocardiogram, and no cardiac symptoms of congestive heart failure. It must be remembered that the echocardiogram is not absolutely definitive for mitral valve prolapse: some patients with classic physical findings may not have echocardiographic findings of prolapse, whereas some patients without murmurs or clicks may have an echocardiographic suggestion of prolapse.[47]

An echocardiogram is indicated if the physical examination is suggestive of mitral valve prolapse but is not classic. For example, if the patient has a mid- or late systolic murmur but no click, one may suspect that the murmur represents papillary muscle dysfunction if the patient also has some suggestion of coronary disease. Distinguishing between these two conditions may help the clinician to decide whether medications for ischemic heart disease are appropriate. In some young patients, it may be difficult to distinguish mitral valve prolapse from hypertrophic obstructive cardiomyopathy; hence, murmurs that increase with the Valsalva maneuver or standing but that are not accompanied by a definite click warrant echocardiography.

3. The patient with findings that might suggest valvular aortic stenosis. If the clinician suspects valvular aortic stenosis, principally because of the characteristics of the murmur or of the carotid upstroke, further noninvasive evaluation is strongly urged and is absolutely mandatory if the patient has any symptoms of angina, congestive heart failure, dizziness, or syncope. The echocardiogram, as noted earlier, is a remarkably sensitive test: It will show abnormalities in essentially every adult with valvular aortic stenosis. Thus, the finding of a normal echocardiogram or of a virtually normal aortic valve opening essentially rules out important aortic stenosis.

Definitive guidelines cannot be drawn for the use of the echocardiogram in a patient in whom the murmur is consistent with aortic valvular stenosis but in whom there are no symptoms. In the asymptomatic person, one would not normally consider aortic valve replacement. Nevertheless, it seems prudent to perform an echocardiogram when the carotid upstroke seems delayed, the murmur peaks after midsystole, or other findings suggest true valvular aortic stenosis. If aortic valve disease is established in an asymptomatic patient, one would prescribe prophylactic antibiotics for procedures and would sensitize the patient to the need for reporting immediately any symptoms that would then lead the physician to expedite further evaluation and therapeutic maneuvers.

4. Other findings that would suggest the need for a noninvasive work-up. In patients whose findings suggest that the murmur is not a functional flow murmur or do not allow it to be diagnosed definitively as mitral valve prolapse, further noninvasive evaluation may often be appropriate. Such an evaluation is indicated in patients with findings suggestive of hypertrophic obstructive cardiomyopathy or with the murmur of mitral regurgitation who lack classic features of mitral valve prolapse. Echocardiography is also indicated in any patient who has a holosystolic mitral regurgitation murmur, fixed splitting of the second heart sound, an increased pulmonic sound, a regurgitant murmur that increases with inspiration, a diastolic or continuous murmur, or a murmur that raises the question of a ventricular septal defect, atrial septal defect, pulmonic stenosis, tricuspid regurgitation, or patent ductus arteriosius. This evaluation commonly begins with the echocardiogram and Doppler echocardiography, with further evaluation guided by its results.

NONINVASIVE APPROACH TO THE PATIENT WITH CARDIOMEGALY OR CONGESTIVE HEART FAILURE

Apparent cardiomegaly as seen on physical examination or the chest radiograph may be caused by dilatation of cardiac structures or by pericardial fluid. Occasionally, other mediastinal shadows may simulate cardiomegaly.

In approaching the patient with a large heart, the clinician should have several objectives: to rule out valvular heart disease, to rule out congenital anomalies such as an atrial septal defect, to rule out a pericardial effusion, and, if the left ventricle is dilated, to distinguish between ischemic and nonischemic causes of a congestive cardiomyopathy. In some situations, congestive heart failure may be present with little or no cardiomegaly and no evidence of valvular heart disease; in such circumstances, a restrictive or hypertrophic cardiomyopathy may be present, and the clinician must evaluate the patient sufficiently to be sure that there is no potentially reversible cause.

For the evaluation of cardiomegaly, the noninvasive test of choice is echocardiography. Although exact normal ranges vary from one laboratory to another, in general the right ventricular end-diastolic diameter should not be more than about 2.3 cm and the left ventricular end-diastolic diameter should not be more than about 5.6 cm.[47] Individual laboratories usually have well-defined standards, which commonly are indexed by dividing the measurement by the patient's body surface area. Echocardiography is also an accurate way to measure wall thickness, but hypertrophy of the ventricular walls will rarely cause cardiomegaly except when associated with concomitant chamber dilatation.

If echocardiography demonstrates dilated cardiac chambers, it may also be helpful in estimating the reason for the dilatation. Severe heart failure is commonly associated with marked dilatation and focal or generalized hypokinesis of the left ventricle. Conversely, the volume overload that is associated with valvular regurgitant lesions or intracardiac shunts is often associated with good left ventricular systolic function until end-stage congestive heart failure ensues. Conditions such as an atrial septal defect or tricuspid regurgitation will cause dilatation of the right ventricle on echocardiography, commonly associated with paradoxic motion of the ventricular septum during systole.

Echocardiography also is the most sensitive and specific way to diagnose a pericardial effusion. Normal subjects harbor about 20 to 60 ml of pericardial fluid and echocardiography can identify pericardial fluid when as little as 50 ml is present. Thus, it is not surprising that small pericardial effusions have been noted in up to 10% of patients undergoing routine echocardiography. The size and clinical significance of the pericardial effusion can be estimated echocardiographically; large effusions are usually seen anteriorly as well as posteriorly.

If noncardiac structures, especially tumors, are simulating cardiomegaly, echocardiography is a reliable way to demonstrate normal-sized cardiac chambers, to identify any coexisting pericardial fluid, and sometimes to localize the metastases directly. In some cases, a large posterior pleural effusion may be confused with a pericardial effusion, but the absence of anterior pericardial fluid or fluid between the left atrium and the descending thoracic aorta is a helpful differential diagnostic sign.

It is important to emphasize that not all patients who have symptoms suggestive of congestive heart failure will have cardiomegaly upon chest radiography. In fact, abnormal diastolic compliance, even in the presence of normal or supernormal systolic function, may be the cause of symptoms of pulmonary congestion. In one series, 40% of patients with clinical congestive heart failure had normal systolic function, usually in the presence of pre-existing systemic hypertension, and appeared to be symptomatic because of poor left ventricular diastolic compliance.

In some patients with abnormal diastolic function, ventricular wall hypertrophy will be present, consistent with the syndrome of nonobstructive hypertrophic cardiomyopathy. In these patients, one may see evidence of abnormal diastolic function by echocardiography, radionuclide angiography, or Doppler echocardiography. Echocardiography may reveal that patients with abnormal diastolic function may have a prolonged left ventricular isovolumic relaxation time, a reduced peak rate of increase of left ventricular dimensions during diastole, or a reduced peak rate in posterior diastolic wall thinning. Radionuclide angiography may reveal a reduction in the peak diastolic filling rate. Doppler echocardiography may show a prolongation of the rapid diastolic filling phase, a shortened diastasis period between the rapid filling phase and atrial contraction, and enhanced filling during atrial systole. Many patients also will have left ventricular wall hypertrophy and normal or supernormal ejection fractions to document their excellent systolic function. In some cases, end-systolic volumes actually may be markedly reduced.

Unfortunately, assessment of abnormal diastolic function may be difficult because most of the measurements currently used have not undergone wide-scale prospective clinical trials. Nevertheless, in experienced noninvasive laboratories, one should often be able to document the noninvasive characteristics of restrictive or hypertrophic physiology in patients with symptoms of congestive heart failure and left ventricular wall hypertrophy. In patients with normal left ventricular wall size, one must rely more heavily on the noninvasive indices of diastolic function, or in some cases on cardiac catheterization, in which characteristics of the diastolic filling pattern can help to differentiate the physiology of a restrictive cardiomyopathy from that of constrictive pericarditis.

Recommendations

Echocardiography is the diagnostic test of choice if a patient has unexplained heart failure or cardiomegaly or has symptoms of heart failure in the absence of cardiomegaly. M-mode echocardiography is a reliable method for excluding valvular or congenital abnormalities or pericardial effusion as the principal cause of a dilated heart. If one wishes to distinguish an ischemic cardiomyopathy, which commonly causes regional left ventricular wall motion abnormalities, from a congestive cardiomyopathy, in which left ventricular contraction will be symmetrically impaired, a two-dimensional echocardiogram is required, and in some cases a radionuclide ventriculogram will be helpful.

Serial echocardiograms or radionuclide ventriculograms are not required in patients with established congestive heart failure. However, in patients with aortic or mitral insufficiency, echocardiography is a reliable method for determining progressive changes in left ventricular cavity size. Although precise recommendations cannot be made at this time, an end-systolic diameter above 55 mm, especially if it represents a change from prior echocardiograms, is indicative of worrisome left ventricular dilatation in patients with aortic insufficiency.[48] Such chamber dilatation is certainly an indication that the patient should be followed closely for the development of symptoms. In the presence of symptoms of heart failure, such chamber dilatation is commonly believed to represent an indication for aortic valve replacement (see Chapter 5). Although fewer data are available for patients with mitral insufficiency, a reasonable recommendation is that surgery usually should be performed in symptomatic patients with marked regurgitation, a diminished ejection fraction, and advanced or progressive left ventricular dilatation. In mitral insufficiency, a reduction in ejection fraction is worrisome, since the regurgitant lesion tends to increase the ejection fraction (see Chapter 5).[49] Patients with mitral regurgitation generally have problems before their left ventricular volumes become as large as those that are sometimes well tolerated in aortic insufficiency.[50] If left ventricular function becomes severely compromised because of far-advanced mitral regurgitation, valve replacement may be contraindicated because the ventricle may not be able to function without the low-pressure "run-off" that the regurgitation provides.

If a patient has a symmetric dilated cardiomyopathy of unclear etiology, experts differ about the recommended diagnostic approach. In patients with amyloidosis, which may cause either a dilated or a nondilated cardiomyopathy, the echocardiogram often shows a "granular sparkling" appearance of the myocardium[51]; when such a pattern is seen, biopsy of other appropriate organs often will document amyloidosis. In other cardiomyopathies, no diagnostic appearance will be noted. Further evaluation may require invasive procedures such as endomyocardial biopsy.

REFERENCES

1. Bruce RA: Exercise testing of patients with coronary heart disease. Ann Clin Res 3:323, 1971.
2. The Criteria Committee of the New York Heart Association, Inc: Diseases of the Heart and Blood Vessels; Nomenclature and Criteria for Diagnosis, 6th ed. Boston, Little, Brown, 1964.
3. Campeau L: Grading of angina pectoris. Circulation 54:522, 1975.
4. Goldman L, Hashimoto B, Cook EF, et al: Comparative reproducibility and validity of systems for assessing cardiovascular functional class: Advantages of a new specific activity scale. Circulation 64:1227, 1981.
5. Patterson JA, Naughton J, Pietras RJ, et al: Treadmill exercise in assessment of the functional capacity of patients with cardiac disease. Am J Cardiol 30:757, 1982.
6. Sheffield LT: Exercise stress testing. *In* Braunwald E (ed): Heart Disease: A Textbook of Cardiovascular Medicine. Philadelphia, WB Saunders, 1984, pp 258–278.
7. Goldschlager N: Use of the treadmill test in the diagnosis of coronary artery disease in patients with chest pain. Ann Intern Med 97:383, 1982.
8. Longhurst JC and Kraus WL: Exercise-induced ST elevation in patients without myocardial infarction. Circulation 60:616, 1979.
9. Bonoris PE, Greenberg PS, Castellanet MJ, et al: Significance of changes in R wave amplitude during treadmill stress testing: Angiographic correlation. Am J Cardiol 41:846, 1978.
10. Rochmis P and Blackburn H: Exercise tests: A survey of procedures, safety, and litigation experience in approximately 170,000 tests. JAMA 217:1061, 1971.
11. Hlatky MA, Pryor DB, Harrell FE Jr, et al: Factors affecting sensitivity and specificity of exercise electrocardiography. Am J Med 77:64, 1984.
12. Rozanski A, Diamond GA, Berman D, et al: The declining specificity of exercise radionuclide ventriculography. N Engl J Med 309:518, 1983.
13. McNeil BJ, Keeler E, and Adelstein SJ: Primer on certain elements of medical decision making. N Engl J Med 293:211, 1975.
14. Detrano R, Gianrossi R, Mulvihill D, et al: Exercise-induced ST segment depression in the diagnosis of multivessel coronary disease: A meta analysis. J Am Coll Cardiol 14:1501, 1989.
15. Rifkin RD and Hood WB: Bayesian analysis of electrocardiographic exercise stress testing. N Engl J Med 297:681, 1977.
16. Goldman L, Cook EF, Mitchell N, et al: Incremental value of the exercise test for diagnosing the presence or absence of coronary artery disease. Circulation 66:945, 1982.
17. Diamond GA, Staniloff HM, Forrester JS, et al: Computer-assisted diagnosis in the noninvasive evaluation of patients with suspected coronary artery disease. J Am Coll Cardiol 1:444, 1983.
18. Weintraub WS, Madeira SW, Bodenheimer MM, et al: Critical analysis of the application of Bayes' theorem to sequential testing in the noninvasive diagnosis of coronary artery disease. Am J Cardiol 54:43, 1984.
19. Chaitman BR, Fisher LD, Bourassa MG, et al: Effect of coronary bypass surgery on survival patterns in subsets of patients with left main coronary artery disease: Report of the Collaborative Study in Coronary Artery Surgery (CASS). Am J Cardiol 48:765, 1981.
20. Passamani E, Davis KB, Gillespie MJ, et al: A randomized trial of coronary artery bypass surgery: Survival of patients with low ejection fraction. N Engl J Med 312:1665, 1985.
21. Lee TH, Cook EF, and Goldman L: Prospective evaluation of a clinical and exercise-test model for the prediction of left main coronary artery disease. Med Decis Making 6:136, 1986.
22. Lee TH, Fukui T, Weinstein M, et al: Cost-effectiveness of screening strategies for left main disease in patients with stable angina. Med Decis Making 8:268, 1989.
23. Rautaharju PM, Prineas RJ, Eifler WJ, et al: Prognostic value of exercise electrocardiogram in men at high risk of future coronary heart disease: Multiple Risk Factor Intervention Trial experience. J Am Coll Cardiol 8:1, 1986.
24. Gordon DJ, Ekelund L, Karon JM, et al: Predictive value of the exercise tolerance test for mortality in North American men: The Lipid Research Clinics mortality follow-up study. Circulation 74:252, 1986.
25. Sox HC Jr, Littenberg B, and Garber AM: The role of exercise testing in screening for coronary artery disease. Ann Intern Med 110:456, 1989.
26. Wilcox I, Freedman SB, Allman KC, et al: Prognostic significance of a predischarge exercise test in risk stratification after unstable angina pectoris. J Am Coll Cardiol 18:677, 1991.
27. DeBusk RF, Blomqvist CG, Kouchoukos NT, et al: Identification and treatment of low-risk patients after acute myocardial infarction and coronary artery bypass graft surgery. N Engl J Med 314:161, 1986.
28. DeBusk RF, Kraemer HC, Nash E, et al: Stepwise risk stratification soon after acute myocardial infarction. Am J Cardiol 52:1161, 1983.
29. Podrid PJ, Graboys TB, and Lown B: Prognosis of medically treated patients with coronary artery disease with profound ST segment depression during exercise testing. N Engl J Med 305:1111, 1981.
30. Kotler TS and Diamond GA: Exercise thallium-201 scintigraphy in the diagnosis and prognosis of coronary artery disease. Ann Intern Med 113:684, 1990.

31. Dilsizian V, Rocco TP, Freedman NMT, et al: Enhanced detection of ischemic but viable myocardium by the reinjection of thallium after stress-redistribution imaging. N Engl J Med 323:141, 1990.
32. Hlatky M, Botvinick E, and Brundage B: The independent value of exercise thallium scintigraphy to physicians. Circulation 66:953, 1982.
33. Kaul S, Finkelstein DM, Homma S, et al: Superiority of quantitative exercise thallium-201 variables in determining long-term prognosis in ambulatory patients with chest pain: A comparison with cardiac catheterization. J Am Coll Cardiol 12:25, 1988.
34. Pollock SG, Abbott RD, Boucher CA, et al: Independent and incremental prognostic value of tests performed in hierarchical order to evaluate patients with suspected coronary artery disease: Validation of models based on these tests. Circulation 85:237, 1992.
35. Borer JS, Kent KM, Bacharach SL, et al: Sensitivity, specificity and predictive accuracy of radionuclide cineangiography during exercise in patients with coronary artery disease: Comparison with exercise electrocardiography. Circulation 60:572, 1979.
36. Kahn JK, McGhie I, Akers MS, et al: Quantitative rotational tomography with ^{201}Tl and ^{99m}TC 2-methoxy-isobutyl-isonitrile: A direct comparison in normal individuals and patients with coronary artery disease. Circulation 79:1282, 1989.
37. Panza JA, Quyyumi AA, Diodati JG, et al: Prediction of the frequency and duration of ambulatory myocardial ischemia in patients with stable coronary artery disease by determination of the ischemic threshold from exercise testing: Importance of the exercise protocol. J Am Coll Cardiol 17:657, 1991.
38. Nabel EG, Rocco MB, Barry J, et al: Asymptomatic ischemia in patients with coronary artery disease. JAMA 257:1923, 1987.
39. Raby KE, Goldman L, Creager MA, et al: Correlation between perioperative ischemia and major cardiac events after peripheral vascular surgery. N Engl J Med 321:1296, 1989.
40. Balady GJ, Weiner DA, Rothendler JA, and Ryan TJ: Arm exercise-thallium imaging testing for the detection of coronary artery disease. J Am Coll Cardiol 9:84, 1987.
41. Balady GJ, Weiner DA, Rose L, and Ryan TJ: Physiologic responses to arm ergometry exercise relative to age and gender. J Am Coll Cardiol 16:130, 1990.
42. Varma SK, Watson DD, and Beller GA: Quantitative comparison of thallium-201 scintigraphy after exercise and dipyridamole in coronary artery disease. Am J Cardiol 64:871, 1989.
43. Eagle KA, Singer DE, Brewster DC, et al: Dipyridamole-thallium scanning in patients undergoing vascular surgery: Optimizing preoperative evaluation of cardiac risk. JAMA 257:2185, 1987.
44. Gupta NC, Esterbrooks DJ, Hilleman DE, and Mohiuddin SM: Comparison of adenosine and exercise thallium-201 single-photon emission computed tomography (SPECT) myocardial perfusion imaging. J Am Coll Cardiol 19:248, 1992.
45. Tischler MD, Lee TH, Hirsch AT, et al: Prediction of major cardiac events after peripheral vascular surgery using dipyridamole echocardiography. Am J Cardiol 68:593, 1991.
46. Goldman L, Cohn PF, Mudge GH Jr, et al: Clinical utility and management impact of M-mode echocardiography. Am J Med 75:49, 1983.
47. Feigenbaum H: Echocardiography. *In* Braunwald E (ed): Heart Disease: A Textbook of Cardiovascular Disease, 4th ed. Philadelphia, WB Saunders, 1992, pp 64–115.
48. Henry WL, Bonow RO, Rosing DR, et al: Observation on the optimum time for operative intervention for aortic regurgitation. II: Serial echocardiographic evaluation of asymptomatic patients. Circulation 61:484, 1980.
49. Ross J: Left ventricular function and the timing of surgical treatment in valvular heart disease, Part I. Ann Intern Med 94:498, 1981.
50. Borow KM, Green LH, Mann T, et al: End-systolic volume as a predictor of postoperative left ventricular performance in volume overload from valvular regurgitation. Am J Med 68:655, 1980.
51. Nicolosi GL, Pavan D, Lestuzzi C, et al: Prospective identification of patients with amyloid heart disease by two-dimensional echocardiography. Circulation 70:432, 1984.

5

Valvular Heart Disease

JOSHUA WYNNE, MD
LEWIS DEXTER, MD

Major recent technologic advances have greatly aided the management of valvular heart disease. Transesophageal echocardiography and color-flow Doppler recordings[1,2] have expanded our ability to noninvasively diagnose a variety of forms of heart disease, and percutaneous balloon valvuloplasty has permitted the nonthoracotomy treatment of valvular stenosis, often obviating the need for anesthesia and surgery.[3]

Management of valvular heart disease hinges on an accurate anatomic diagnosis and correct assessment of the attendant pathophysiologic abnormalities. Perhaps more than in any other sphere of cardiology, valvular diseases require the proper integration of the history, physical examination, and laboratory findings to arrive at the correct management strategy.

History. The appearance and progression of symptoms is of critical value in determining the timing of interventions (especially surgical) in the management of valvular lesions, particularly stenotic ones. Symptoms may be of less value in the volume overload lesions (e.g., aortic and mitral regurgitation), in which surveillance for presymptomatic deterioration of ventricular function with noninvasive testing is of particular importance. Differentiation should be made between symptoms reflecting a reduced cardiac output (fatigue, lethargy), those due to pulmonary congestion (paroxysmal nocturnal dyspnea, orthopnea, cough), and those of right heart failure (peripheral edema, ascites). The course of the disease often can be ascertained by the patient's account of dyspnea produced by a given amount of exertion performed at a certain speed. This can serve as a yardstick of disability.

Physical Examination. The examination supplies data on the anatomic abnormality of one or more valves. It may indicate the severity of the process and can certainly reveal whether or not congestive heart failure is present.

Routine laboratory work-up for anyone with a murmur suspected of being organic may include the following items.

Anteroposterior and Lateral Radiographs of the Heart. Although a useful first step in assessing cardiac enlargement (Fig. 5–1), the chest film has been surpassed by echocardiography in evaluating specific cardiac chamber or great artery enlargement. The chest film remains of major importance in assessing the pulmonary vasculature for evidence of congestion.

Electrocardiography. The electrocardiogram (ECG) is useful in detecting evidence of left ventricular hypertrophy (LVH) and right ventricular hypertrophy (RVH), although it is unreliable for assessing chamber size. The ECG is of incalculable value for revealing cardiac rhythm.

Echocardiography. Two-dimensional echocardiography is of inestimable value in evaluating valves, chamber sizes, cardiac output, and myocardial function, such as ejection fraction (Fig. 5–2). A normal two-dimensional study is of particular value; it *excludes* hemodynamically significant valvular stenosis. Doppler ultrasound, often supplemented with a color display, has expanded the information available from echocardiographic studies. By detecting the frequency shift from moving red blood cells within the heart, Doppler ultrasound can measure intracardiac flow velocities and help to identify and quantify valvular stenosis and regurgitation.[2]

Cardiac Catheterization. Cardiac catheterization is generally performed in patients who are being considered for surgical correction. Often but *not* invariably necessary preoperatively, it is especially needed (1) to evaluate the severity of one or more valve lesions, particularly when there is any discrepancy between the findings from the history, physical examination, or noninvasive testing, (2) to measure pressures being generated by the left or right ventricle, and (3) to evaluate coronary vessels for atherosclerotic narrowings, especially in patients complaining of chest discomfort. The recent success of percutaneous balloon valvuloplasty for treating valvular stenosis (particularly of the pulmonary and mitral valves) has expanded cardiac catheterization from a merely diagnostic procedure to an often therapeutic procedure.[3,4]

All the information obtained from noninvasive evaluations should, and usually does, fit into a pattern if only one valve is involved. When two or more valves are diseased, it may be difficult to estimate the severity of each valvular lesion. When any of the information from noninvasive techniques is contradictory and not definitive, cardiac catheterization may be required to clarify it.

Therapy of patients with valvular heart disease is first medical and then interventional (percutaneous balloon val-

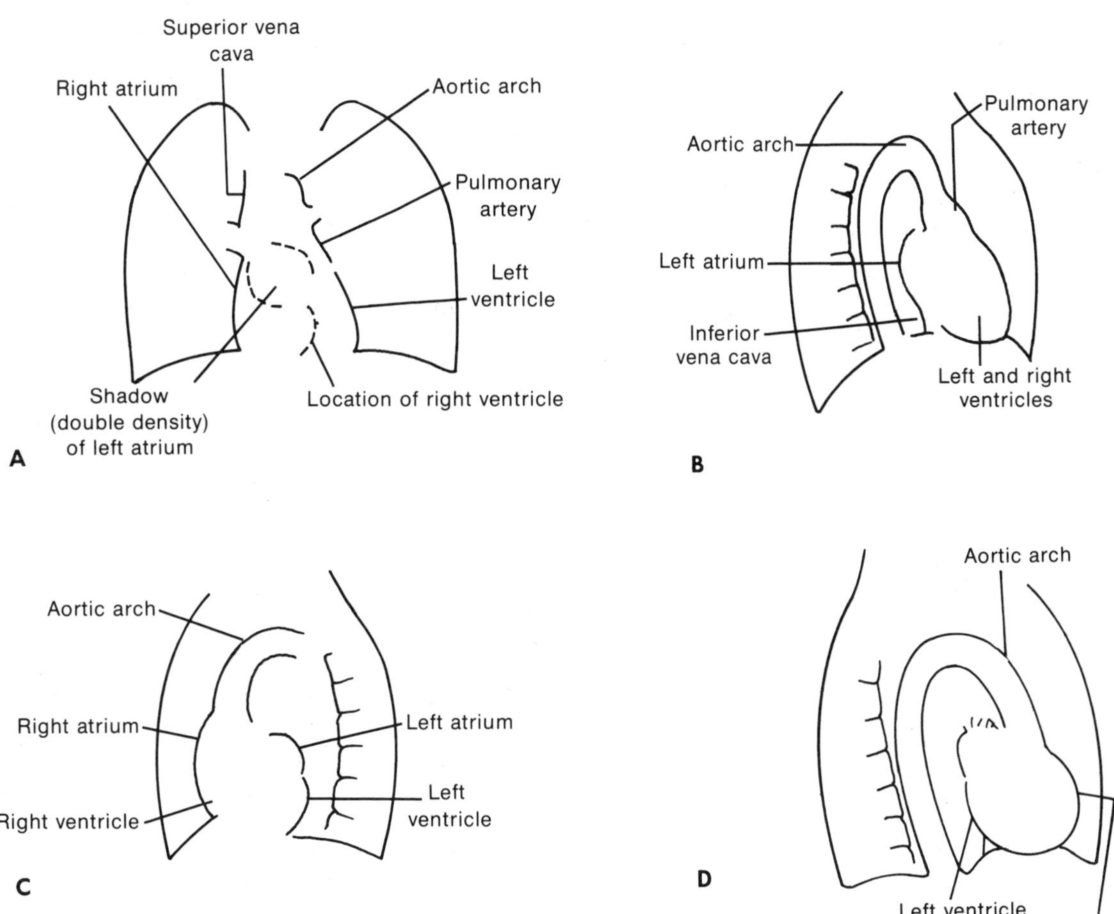

FIGURE 5–1. Cardiac contours in the standard radiographic projections. *A,* Posteroanterior projections: Left or right ventricular enlargement may enlarge the left heart border. Right atrial enlargement may cause bulging of the right heart border. Left atrial enlargement produces a double density and causes elevation of the left main bronchus. *B,* Right anterior oblique projection: Left atrial enlargement may be demonstrated posteriorly by indentation of a barium-filled esophagus. *C,* Left anterior oblique projection: Right ventricular enlargement causes the heart to bulge anteriorly. Right atrial enlargement also may cause anterior bulging. *D,* Right lateral projection: The left ventricle is seen posteriorly. (Adapted from Weens HS and Gray BB Jr: Radiologic examination of the heart. *In* Hurst JW and Logue RB [eds]: The Heart, New York, McGraw-Hill, 1966, pp 148–163.)

vuloplasty or surgery). The task of the primary care physician, usually in consultation with a cardiologist, includes deciding when intervention is desirable, that is, when the surgical outlook is more favorable than the medical outlook. Later on in this chapter, an attempt is made to define this issue.

RHEUMATIC HEART DISEASE

Acute rheumatic fever (ARF) is found mainly in school-aged children and occurs 1 to 2 weeks after a β-hemolytic streptococcal infection. There has been a progressive decline in its occurrence in manifest forms since the early

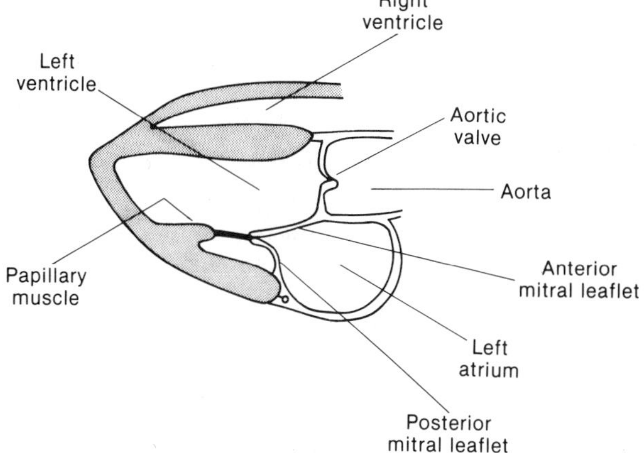

FIGURE 5–2. Normal two-dimensional echocardiographic findings. Two-dimensional echocardiographic study in long axis view. Abnormalities of the aortic and mitral valve can be identified. The size and function of the left ventricle can be evaluated, and left atrial and right ventricular enlargement can be noted.

years of this century, although the last decade has witnessed focal outbreaks of ARF in the military and civilian populations, associated with the reappearance of highly virulent streptococcal strains.[5] Although the progressive disappearance of symptomatic rheumatic fever was undoubtedly related to the use of antimicrobials, beginning with sulfa drugs in the late 1930s, the trend toward mildness of ARF had begun previously and is probably best explained by a change in streptococcal serotype and virulence, along with effects due to an overall improvement in housing, sanitation, and cleanliness.[5]

One to 3 weeks after a β-hemolytic streptococcal sore throat, ARF may occur. It is characterized by fever, polyarticular arthritis, and in one third to one half of ARF patients, carditis. All layers of the heart become involved—valves (endocarditis), muscle (myocarditis), and pericardium (pericarditis)—with, respectively, the appearance of regurgitant murmurs, heart failure, and pericardial friction rubs.

The clinical course of ARF lasts for months and sometimes years. It may run its course as a single cycle or it may be polycyclic. Eventually, ARF subsides. The myocarditis, pericarditis, and arthritis disappear without residua, but in many patients murmurs persist. Even though the patient is on penicillin prophylaxis and the antistreptolysin titer and throat cultures remain normal on repeated examination, valvular deformity progresses with time.

The most common valve involved in chronic rheumatic heart disease is the mitral, followed by the aortic, then the tricuspid, and very rarely the pulmonic. The valves may become stenotic or regurgitant. The following sections describe the different valvular lesions resulting from rheumatic fever, as well as those due to other causes.

MITRAL REGURGITATION

Mitral regurgitation (MR) may be caused by disorders of the mitral valve leaflet (commonly due to myxomatous degeneration, bacterial endocarditis, and, occasionally, rheumatic fever); disorders of the mitral annulus (secondary to calcification or dilatation of the ring); disorders of the chordae tendineae (with idiopathic rupture, or rupture due to myxomatous degeneration or bacterial endocarditis); and disorders of the papillary muscle (the result of myocardial ischemia or infarction, myocardial infiltration, or left ventricular dilatation).

The clinical manifestations of MR differ greatly, depending on whether the process is acute or chronic. In acute MR, a nondilated left atrium is flooded by the regurgitant flow, resulting in high pressures and symptoms of pulmonary congestion. In chronic MR, the left atrium and left ventricle dilate, often resulting in lowering of the filling pressures; the symptoms are often those of low forward cardiac output rather than those of pulmonary congestion (Table 5–1).

TABLE 5–1. CHRONIC MITRAL REGURGITATION

Etiology:	Mitral valve prolapse Calcified annulus Endocarditis Ruptured chordae tendineae Rheumatic heart disease
Clinical Course:	Prolonged asymptomatic period Onset of congestive heart failure in 4th to 6th decade Downhill course over ~10 years
Symptoms and Complications:	Slowly progressive congestive heart failure Systemic embolization Bacterial endocarditis
Indications for Surgery:	Clearly indicated when in NYHA Class III To be considered when cardiothoracic ratio >30% enlarged or LV ejection fraction <50%

Chronic Mitral Regurgitation

The most common causes of chronic MR are the mitral valve prolapse (MVP) syndrome, coronary artery disease with papillary muscle dysfunction, and infective endocarditis. Rheumatic heart disease used to be a common cause of chronic MR but is now less common.[6]

Mitral Valve Prolapse

MVP probably is the most commonly recognized valvular heart disorder. It has been reported under a number of names: click-murmur syndrome, floppy valve syndrome, prolapsing mitral valve leaflet syndrome, billowing mitral leaflet syndrome, and Barlow's syndrome. The prevalence of this disorder has been reported to be as high as 15%, but is probably found in about 5% of the adult population.

Etiology. Although associated with a wide variety of conditions, MVP is most commonly caused by redundancy of the mitral valve leaflets and by myxomatous degeneration of the mitral valve tissue. The posterior leaflet is usually more affected than the anterior leaflet. The mitral valve annulus is enlarged, and the chordae tendineae may be elongated. The valve tissue contains excessive amounts of mucopolysaccharides.

Mitral valve prolapse is said to be most common in women from 14 to 30 years of age. It has been reported in children as well as in the elderly. There may be an increased familial incidence, suggesting an autosomal dominant form of inheritance.

Clinical Aspects and Course. Most individuals with this syndrome are asymptomatic. The first indication of MVP may be when the click and late systolic murmur are heard on routine physical examination. A certain number of these patients have palpitation or chest pain. Many have arrhythmias revealed by 12- or 24-hour ECG monitoring. Arrhythmias include atrial and ventricular premature beats and supraventricular and ventricular arrhythmias. Arrhythmias not present on the resting ECG may be brought out by exercise. Chest pain typically is atypical—stabbing; not substernal; brief or prolonged; bearable or incapacitating; and related or not related to exertion, emotion, or meals. At times, it is suggestive of angina pectoris, and indeed there may or may not be coexisting coronary artery disease. Severe mitral regurgitation, often due to associated rupture of chordae tendineae, may produce congestive heart failure.

The long-term natural course of this disorder is usually benign, but important problems may develop, including sudden death, bacterial endocarditis, and heart failure from progressive worsening of mitral regurgitation.[7] There is also the suggestion that patients with MVP may be subject to systemic embolization, particularly in young patients. However, an understanding of the overall true natural course is hampered by inadequate data.

Physical Examination. Two findings on auscultation lead to the recognition of this syndrome (Fig. 5–3). The first is the systolic click, which typically is midsystolic and single but is occasionally multiple, best heard at the apex and at the lower left sternal border. It reflects the sudden tensing of the redundant leaflets and elongated chordae. It is a high-frequency snapping, clicking, or popping sound.

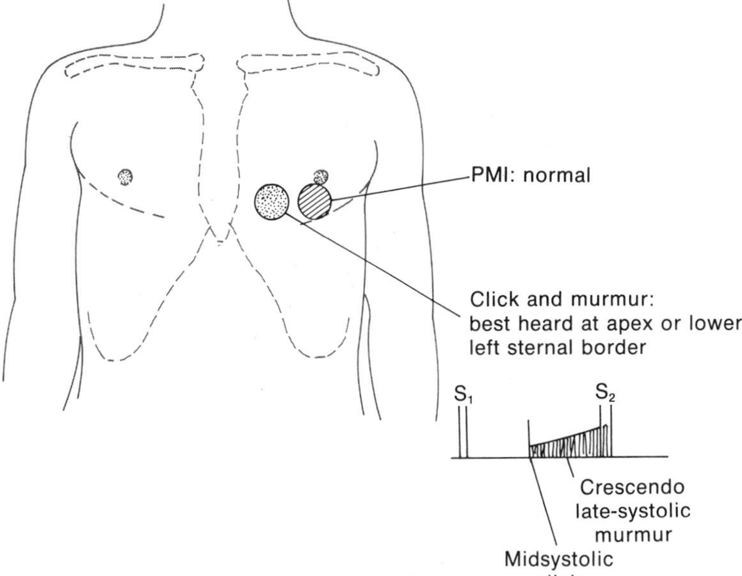

FIGURE 5–3. Typical findings on physical examination in mitral valve prolapse.

The second finding is the late systolic murmur, beginning after or at the time of the click. It is usually a crescendo murmur ending at the second sound. Occasionally, the murmur may be early in systole and ejection in quality, or it may be holosystolic. The click and murmur are quite sensitive to physiologic and pharmacologic interventions. They become accentuated and occur earlier in systole during amyl nitrite inhalation and on standing and become less loud and later on squatting.

Electrocardiography. Many patients, particularly those who are asymptomatic, have a normal resting ECG. Nonspecific ST and T wave abnormalities may occur in leads II, III, and aVf and the midprecordial leads, suggesting inferior wall ischemia, and occasionally anterior wall ST-T changes may occur. These changes correlate poorly with chest pain.

Supraventricular arrhythmias (particularly paroxysmal supraventricular tachycardia) are the most common sustained arrhythmias seen in MVP, although ventricular arrhythmias, sinus node dysfunction, and conduction defects are also found. The relationship between sudden death and MVP is still controversial; the QT interval is prolonged in some patients.

Echocardiography. The diagnosis of MVP is most definitively confirmed on two-dimensional echocardiography, which reveals the typical systolic bulging of one or both mitral valve leaflets into the left atrium (Fig. 5–4).[7] In addition to evaluating the degree of prolapse, echocardiography is useful in determining the degree of thickening and redundancy of the valve, the size and function of the left ventricle, and whether any associated prolapse of the tricuspid and aortic valves occurs, which may happen in one fifth of patients with MVP. Concomitant Doppler ultrasound recordings are useful to quantitate the severity of associated MR.

Treatment. Patients with murmurs or redundant mitral leaflets on echocardiography should receive antibiotic prophylaxis for dental and surgical procedures; whether those with clicks alone should also is unclear (Table 5–2 and see also Chapter 75).[7] Because sudden death is rare, patients with MVP who have no symptoms of arrhythmia and have no ectopic activity in the resting ECG do not usually require further evaluation. However, any symptoms suggestive of a serious arrhythmia, particularly syncope, or a family history of sudden death should prompt an exercise ECG and 24-hour Holter monitoring. If atrial or ventricular arrhythmias are detected and need to be treated, the drug of choice is a β-blocker. However, their long-term effectiveness in this syndrome is still uncertain. If mitral regurgitation leads to refractory symptoms of heart failure, mitral valve repair or replacement is indicated (Table 5–3). Suspicion of a transient cerebral ischemic attack in a young patient warrants a search for MVP and, if it is present, probably the institution of platelet-active drugs. Routine follow-up is indicated in most patients with MVP, and all those with murmurs.

Papillary Muscle Dysfunction

Papillary muscle dysfunction is defined as MR with structurally normal mitral valve leaflets, but with abnormal papillary muscles or chordae tendineae.

The papillary muscles, chordae tendineae, and mitral annulus comprise a dynamic group that ordinarily work together to prevent MR, but are very susceptible to disease.

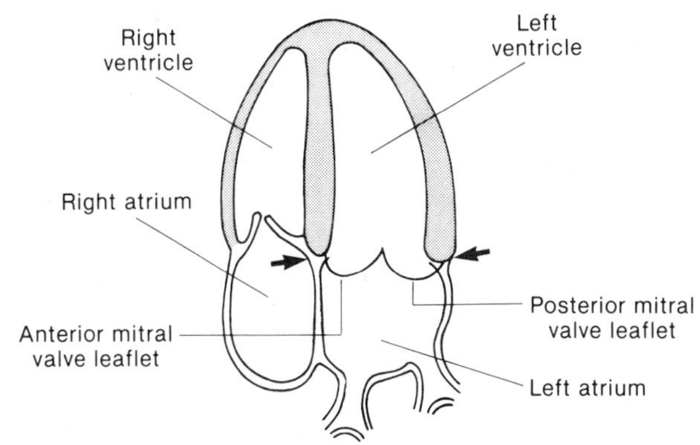

FIGURE 5–4. Echocardiographic mitral valve pattern in mitral valve prolapse. Two-dimensional echocardiographic study in the apical four-chamber view, demonstrating prolapse with bulging of both the anterior and posterior leaflets posterior to the annulus (*arrows*) into the left atrium.

The chordae may rupture because of degeneration or infection. The papillary muscles may contract poorly because of diseases affecting the myocardium, particularly coronary artery disease. The result is that the valve may herniate into the left atrium in systole if the papillary muscle does not contract enough or into the left ventricular cavity in systole if the length of papillary muscle–chordal apparatus has been shrunken by fibrosis. If the ventricular wall at the site of attachment of the papillary muscle contracts poorly because of disease, especially coronary artery disease, the papillary muscle contraction is ineffectual. Finally, if the left ventricle dilates and becomes considerably enlarged, the papillary muscles and their chordae simply are not long enough to keep the mitral valve tightly closed in systole, and the annulus may not contract adequately as it normally does during systole, resulting in MR.

MR may be quite severe and develop suddenly in patients with ruptured chordae tendineae but, when due to dysfunction of the papillary muscles, often is mild and of little hemodynamic significance (Table 5–4).

Symptoms. Symptoms, such as angina pectoris, are largely those of the underlying coronary artery disease. Symptoms directly related to papillary muscle dysfunction are mainly those of heart failure when MR is severe.

Physical Examination. The first sound is often normal but may be diminished. An apical systolic murmur is characteristic, but its timing is variable; holosystolic or late-systolic murmurs are common. Its intensity is variable and is maximal at the apex. It is sometimes heard all over the precordium and may even be transmitted into the carotid arteries, where it is then easily mistaken for the murmur of aortic stenosis. Usually, however, the murmur is not so widely transmitted. An atrial gallop (S_4) is always present, and a ventricular gallop (S_3) is variably present (Fig. 5–5).

Radiography. Radiographs of the heart initially may show little, if any, enlargement of the left ventricle and left atrium. With time or when regurgitation is severe, these chambers may enlarge, along with findings of pulmonary congestion.

Electrocardiography. Changes in the ECG are often but not invariably those of an old myocardial infarction.

Echocardiography. There are no specific structural abnormalities of the mitral valve echocardiogram, although malcoaptation of the leaflets often can be identified, along with MR on Doppler ultrasound recordings. Left atrial enlargement and abnormal left ventricular contraction patterns may be present.

Treatment. Medical therapy is directed at two types of symptoms: (1) angina pectoris and (2) exertional dyspnea and other manifestations of heart failure. If these symptoms are not satisfactorily controlled, regardless of the exact cause of mitral valve dysfunction, surgical intervention should be considered. This requires cardiac catheterization for evaluation of left ventricular function by recording of left ventricular pressure, left ventricular angiography to determine the contractility characteristics of the left ventricle and the degree of mitral regurgitation, and especially coronary angiography to determine the location and extent of the coronary artery narrowings. Surgery consists of mitral valve replacement and coronary artery bypass grafting.

Rheumatic Mitral Regurgitation

Severe MR may occur during but more commonly follows subsidence of ARF. The presence of the murmur of MR is compatible with a variably long life. In most cases, symptoms do not develop until the fourth to sixth decade of life,

TABLE 5–2. PROPHYLAXIS OF BACTERIAL ENDOCARDITIS IN THE ADULT

Dental/Respiratory Tract Procedures	
Preferred:	Amoxicillin 3 g orally 1 hour before procedure; then 1.5 g 6 hours after initial dose
Alternate:	Ampicillin 2 g IM or IV 30 minutes before procedure; then ampicillin 1 g IM or IV or amoxicillin 1.5 g orally 6 hours after initial dose
Penicillin allergy:	Erythromycin ethylsuccinate 800 mg or erythromycin stearate 1 g orally 2 hours before procedure; then half dose 6 hours after initial dose or Clindamycin 300 mg orally 1 hour before procedure; then 150 mg 6 hours after initial dose
High-risk patients†:	Ampicillin 2 g IM or IV plus gentamicin 1.5 mg/kg (not to exceed 80 mg) IM or IV 30 minutes before procedure; then amoxicillin 1.5 g orally 6 hours later. Alternatively, parenteral regimen may be repeated once 8 hours after initial dose
Penicillin allergy†:	Vancomycin 1 g IV over 1 hour, starting 1 hour before procedure; no repeat dose necessary
Genitourinary/Gastrointestinal Procedures	
Preferred:	Ampicillin 2 g IM or IV plus gentamicin 1.5 mg/kg (not to exceed 80 mg) 30 minutes before procedure; then amoxicillin 1.5 g orally 6 hours after initial dose. Alternatively, parenteral regimen may be repeated once 8 hours after initial dose
Alternative for low-risk patients:	Amoxicillin 3 g orally 1 hour before procedure; then 1.5 g 6 hours after initial dose
Penicillin allergy:	Vancomycin 1 g over 1 hour plus gentamicin 1.5 mg/kg (not to exceed 80 mg) IM or IV 1 hour before procedure; may be repeated once 8 hours after initial dose

*Adapted from Dajani AS, Bisno AL, Chung KJ, et al: Prevention of bacterial endocarditis: Recommendations by the American Heart Association. JAMA 264:2919–2922, 1990. Copyright 1990, American Medical Association.

†Those with prosthetic valves and surgical systemic-pulmonary shunts or conduits who require parenteral prophylaxis.

IM = intramuscular; IV = intravenous.

TABLE 5–3. MITRAL VALVE PROLAPSE

Etiology:	Congenital redundancy or myxomatous degeneration of valve leaflets
Clinical Course:	May remain asymptomatic
Symptoms or Complications:	Atrial or ventricular arrhythmias Sudden death from ventricular fibrillation Bacterial endocarditis Congestive heart failure
Indications for Surgery:	Severe mitral regurgitation

TABLE 5–4. PAPILLARY MUSCLE DYSFUNCTION

Etiology:	Ventricular dilatation of any etiology Ineffectual contraction in coronary artery disease
Clinical Course:	That of the underlying disease
Symptoms or Complications:	Progressive congestive heart failure or coronary artery disease
Indications for Surgery:	If severe mitral regurgitation is present in a symptomatic patient with preservation of global ventricular function.

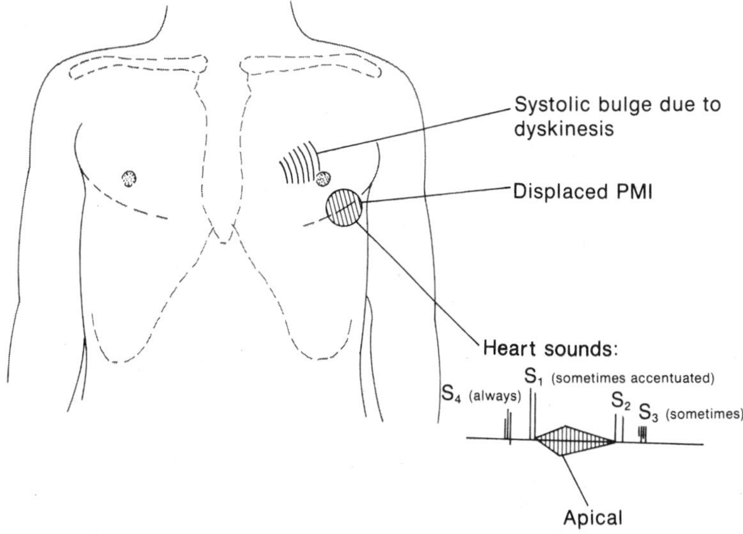

FIGURE 5–5. Typical findings on physical examination in papillary muscle dysfunction due to coronary artery disease.

but they may appear much earlier if the regurgitation is severe. After the appearance of symptoms, there is a slow and intermittent downhill course lasting on the average for about 10 years (see Table 5–1).

Physical Examination. The point of maximal impulse (PMI) is usually displaced laterally and is diffuse. The murmur with rheumatic MR is holosystolic and apical in location with transmission to the axilla and toward the sternum; it is usually grade 3 or more, and its intensity is uninfluenced by respiration (Fig. 5–6). In nonrheumatic MR, the murmur may be early, late, or holosystolic. An S_3 occurring up to 0.18 second after S_2 is commonly audible. Left ventricular dilatation may be followed by right ventricular dilatation, producing a sternal heave. With left ventricular failure, rales appear in the lungs and are often accompanied by signs of right ventricular failure (distended neck veins, enlarged liver, and edema). There is usually an accompanying murmur of mitral stenosis in rheumatic MR.

Radiography. The left ventricle and left atrium are enlarged, and valvular calcification is frequent. The lungs become congested as the left ventricle fails.

Electrocardiography. Atrial fibrillation is common. When sinus rhythm is present, P-mitrale is present. A left ventricular hypertrophy pattern may be seen on ECG.

Echocardiography. The value of echocardiography includes delineation of the cause of MR (whether leaflet, anular, chordae tendineae, or papillary muscle abnormality); assessment of left atrial size and left ventricular size and function; and documentation of the presence or absence of associated valvular abnormalities. The presence of regurgitation and a semiquantitative estimate of the degree of regurgitation can be determined by Doppler ultrasound studies.[2]

Natural Course of Chronic Mitral Regurgitation

The hemodynamic effect of chronic MR of any cause is enlargement of the left ventricle and left atrium. The left ventricle ejects part of its contents into the aorta and part back through the mitral valve into the left atrium. The amount going out the aorta is less than normal. This produces the symptoms of easy tiring and decrease of energy,

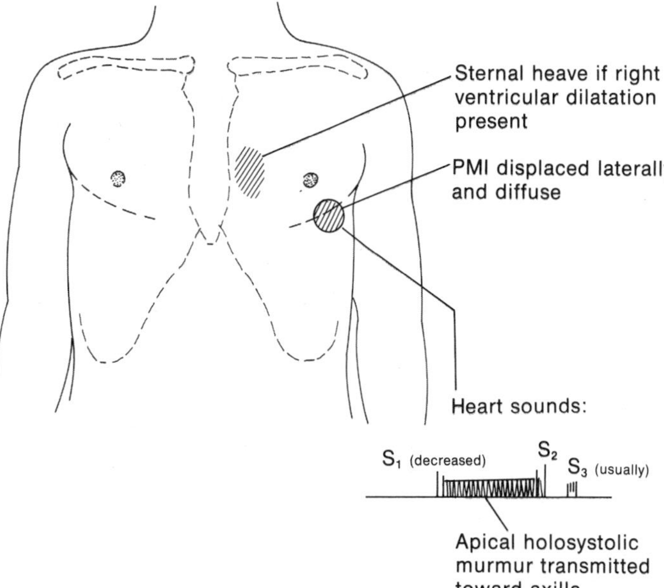

FIGURE 5–6. Typical findings on physical examination in chronic mitral regurgitation.

which may be the principal symptoms for years. The dilated left ventricle may function well for years, its diastolic pressure remaining quite normal. Eventually, as the regurgitation progresses, it dilates further and fails.[8] Its diastolic pressure rises. The left atrial and pulmonary capillary pressures rise to a similar degree. With exertion, the diastolic pressure may surpass the pulmonary edema threshold of about 25 mm Hg. This is associated with dyspnea, at first exertional and finally occurring when the individual is at rest, and orthopnea appears.

The left atrium is enlarged early in the course of mitral regurgitation and at times enlarges to a mammoth degree, with a capacity of 2 and even 3 liters.

Atrial fibrillation is common and correlates with the age of the patient, duration of the disease, and its severity.

Complications. These include *arterial embolism* and *bacterial endocarditis.* Arterial embolism occurs particularly in those who fibrillate. It is less common in these patients than in those with predominant mitral stenosis, but it is a dreaded complication. Anticoagulant prophylaxis is indicated when atrial fibrillation occurs, as discussed under Mitral Stenosis. Bacterial endocarditis produces further destruction of the valve and can rather abruptly increase the regurgitation and lead to acute congestive heart failure. Prophylaxis against endocarditis is mandatory.

Medical Management. Appropriate prophylaxis against rheumatic fever, at least until the age of 35 years, is mandatory in all patients with rheumatic valvular disease (Table 5–5).[9] Antibiotic prophylaxis against endocarditis is also required in all patients with MR of whatever cause (see Table 5–2).[10] It must be emphasized that the doses of antibiotics used for rheumatic fever prophylaxis are *inadequate* to provide adequate protection against endocarditis, and additional antibiotics are mandatory.

Symptoms of fatigue and dyspnea and the development of cardiac enlargement are indications for digitalization. Diuretic therapy and salt restriction are indicated when symptoms and signs of heart failure appear.

Restoration to normal sinus rhythm should be attempted when atrial fibrillation is of recent origin but is usually unsuccessful if it has been present for 6 months to 1 year or more. Immediate and long-term control of the ventricular rate in atrial fibrillation may be achieved with the use of digitalis glycosides, or if congestive heart failure is absent, with β-adrenergic blockers or verapamil. Vasodilator therapy may be useful in the management of severe or refractory heart failure as a temporary means of improving cardiac function prior to surgery, although its long-term role is not established.

Surgical Therapy. The problem of when to intervene surgically is not always easy to decide.[8] On the one hand, affected patients can be managed medically for a prolonged time, and if activities are sufficiently restricted they may remain relatively asymptomatic. On the other hand, if surgery is too long delayed, irreversible myocardial damage may result in minimal or no improvement following mitral valve replacement. The downhill clinical course in chronic MR is often slow and insidious, and indications of deteriorating left ventricular function may be subtle.

Mitral valve repair or replacement is clearly indicated when the patient becomes symptomatic with excessive fatigue, shortness of breath, or fluid retention, that is, when New York Heart Association (NYHA) functional class III or IV has developed, as long as left ventricular function is relatively preserved (i.e., ejection fraction > 40%). It is also clear that patients are all too often maintained on medical therapy too long. Irreparable left ventricular damage may occur despite the fact that the symptoms are only of class II severity. Postoperatively, improvement may be less than satisfactory owing to the myocardial damage that has occurred.

There currently is no sure way of assessing myocardial dysfunction preoperatively. Some recommend that surgery be performed irrespective of symptoms when cardiac size by cardiothoracic ratio exceeds 30% enlargement, when the ejection fraction falls below 50%, or when the ventricle is dilated in both end-diastole and end-systole (i.e., end-diastolic dimension greater than 75 mm and end-systolic dimension greater than 55 mm in transverse diameter by echocardiography).[11] However, these surgical indications are still being verified; nevertheless, it is tragic to subject a patient to surgery only to attain little benefit because the decision for surgery was too long delayed.[12]

The risk of surgery in skilled hands varies from 2 to 10%. The incidence of thromboembolic complications in recent years has been greatly reduced in those with prosthetic valves to an average of 5 emboli per 100 patient years. These patients must take anticoagulants for life. With biosynthetic valves (porcine xenografts), embolic complications are fewer, and patients do not have to take anticoagulant medication permanently unless they are chronic fibrillators. Causes of late death in follow-up have been embolism or thrombosis of the prosthetic valve, continued congestive heart failure, bacterial endocarditis, particularly with prosthetic valves, and incidental complications unrelated to valve replacement (e.g., pneumonia and carcinoma).

TABLE 5–5. PROPHYLAXIS (PREVENTION OF RECURRENT ATTACKS) OF RHEUMATIC FEVER IN THE ADULT*

Preferred:	Intramuscular benzathine penicillin, 1,200,000 units every 4 weeks
Alternate:	Oral penicillin V, 250 mg twice a day
Penicillin allergy:	Sulfadiazine, 1 g once a day
	Erythromycin, 250 mg twice a day (appropriate dose not definitively established)

*Adapted from Dajani AS, Bisno AL, Chung KJ, et al: Prevention of rheumatic fever: A statement for health professionals by the committee on rheumatic fever, endocarditis, and Kawasaki Disease of the Council on Cardiovascular Disease in the Young, the American Heart Association. Circulation 78:1082, 1988.

Acute Mitral Regurgitation

The most common causes of acute MR are the following:

1. Ruptured chordae tendineae
2. Ruptured papillary muscle
3. Valve destruction by bacterial endocarditis

With all these acute-onset MR, there is the sudden appearance of a mitral regurgitant murmur and clinical deterioration.

Ruptured Chordae Tendineae

Etiology. The majority of patients with ruptured chordae tendineae have no apparent underlying heart disease.[6] In many, however, there is a past history of systolic murmur that has usually been considered functional; it probably represents MVP in many. Bacterial endocarditis is the next most common cause. Chordal rupture also occurs in patients with rheumatic mitral valve disease and hypertrophic cardiomyopathy (HCM), or as a result of trauma (Table 5–6). Since the chordae are avascular structures, ischemic heart disease does not produce their rupture, al-

TABLE 5–6. RUPTURED CHORDAE TENDINEAE

Etiology:	Spontaneous (possibly related to mitral valve prolapse)
	Bacterial endocarditis, rheumatic mitral valve disease, trauma
Clinical Course:	Variable
	Acute onset of congestive heart failure in some
Symptoms and Complications:	Rapid progression into intractable congestive heart failure if mitral regurgitation severe
Indications for Surgery:	Severe mitral regurgitation or symptoms of congestive heart failure

though it may produce papillary muscle rupture as well as dysfunction.

Natural Course. If mitral regurgitation is slight, the patient may lead a normal life for decades. If it is moderate, there may be a clinical deterioration from fatigue and breathlessness, but the patient survives on more limited activity than previously. If the mitral regurgitation is severe, there is the sudden onset of dyspnea that is rapidly progressive. The patient rapidly progresses into intractable heart failure.

Physical Examination. When acute MR is severe, the apex impulse is overactive but not laterally displaced (Fig. 5–7). The systolic murmur may be pansystolic but is often early systolic, and it is frequently of the ejection type (crescendo-decrescendo). It thus can mimic the murmurs of valvular aortic stenosis or hypertrophic/obstructive cardiomyopathy. There is often an S_3 gallop. With less severe degrees of mitral regurgitation, the physical signs of left ventricular overload are less impressive. In all cases, however, there has been the sudden onset of an increase of the intensity of the murmur.

Radiography. With MR of recent onset, the left atrium is usually not enlarged, which is in striking contrast to its enlargement in chronic MR. The left ventricle and cardiac silhouette may be normal or enlarged. The lung fields are congested if the MR is severe.

Electrocardiography. This is usually normal, there not being time for the development of abnormal P waves or the pattern of left ventricular hypertrophy.

Echocardiography. In acute MR, echocardiography usually identifies the cause of the leak. One or both leaflets may be flail with ruptured chordae tendineae or papillary muscle. The left atrium and ventricle are not dilated to a significant degree in acute MR.

Therapy. If the MR is mild to moderate, the patients may respond well to digitalization, diuretics, and a low-salt diet. In most cases, however, the MR is severe, and mitral valve repair or replacement may be required on an emergency or semiemergency basis.

Ruptured Papillary Muscle

This occurs most frequently in the setting of an inferolateral myocardial infarction. Less severe mitral regurgitation is seen if only one or more papillary muscle heads are avulsed due to myocardial necrosis; massive MR results from rupture of the body of a papillary muscle. It must be differentiated from rupture of the interventricular septum, the other principal cause of a new murmur in the setting of acute myocardial infarction. Differentiation of the two is achieved noninvasively by echo/Doppler studies, or at right heart catheterization by demonstrating a left-to-right shunt in the case of an acquired ventricular septal defect.

Valve Destruction from Bacterial Endocarditis

This occurs particularly from acute bacterial endocarditis caused by a destructive organism such as the *Staphylococcus.* Valve leaflets are destroyed, and chordae may rupture.

The course is much the same as that described under Ruptured Chordae Tendineae, since the ensuing MR may be mild, moderate, or severe, and the clinical picture and course depend almost entirely on the severity of the MR. However, there is another factor—the bacterial endocarditis itself with its array of manifestations (fever; emboli to skin, spleen, kidneys, and brain). Early diagnosis and therapy with an appropriate antibiotic are mandatory. When the organism is virulent, microabscesses may be seeded all over the body. Some may be in areas where antibiotics cannot reach them, or abscesses become too large for antibiotics to be effective. Thus, there are two problems: the regurgitation and the infection. It may be necessary to perform mitral valve replacement in the presence of active

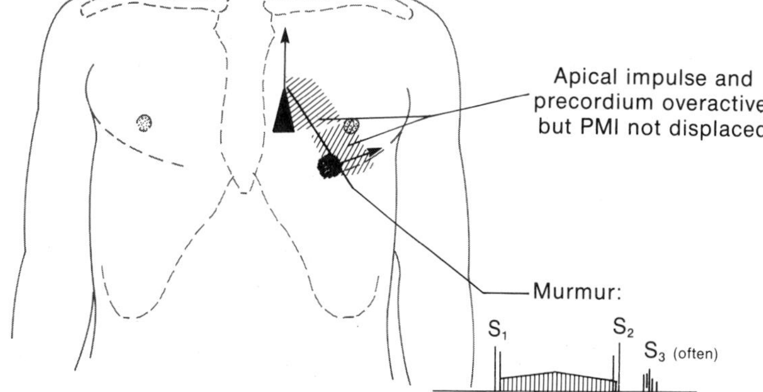

FIGURE 5–7. Typical findings on physical examination in ruptured chordae tendineae.

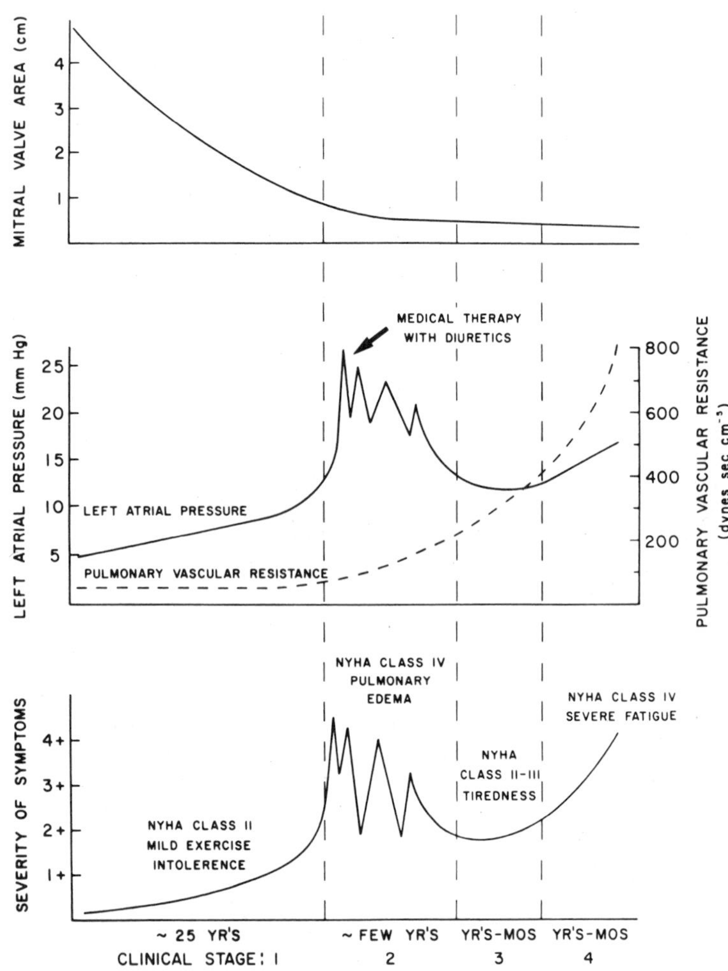

FIGURE 5–8. The clinical course of mitral stenosis. Stage 1: As mitral valve orifice narrows to about 1 cm^2, the patient develops mild exercise intolerance (NYHA classes I and II). Stage 2: When the critical valve area of about 1 cm^2 is reached, left atrial and pulmonary capillary pressures increase rapidly, especially if stress such as pregnancy, infection, or onset of atrial fibrillation is superimposed; the patient experiences rather abrupt onset of symptoms related to pulmonary congestion (NYHA classes III and IV). Stage 3: As pulmonary symptoms are controlled by diuretics, the pulmonary vascular resistance also is rising, which may tend to protect the patient from further increases in pulmonary capillary pressure but causes decreased cardiac output and right ventricular failure (NYHA class III). Stage 4: Further increases in pulmonary vascular resistance lead to a further decline in cardiac output. This terminal stage culminates in the picture of venous distention, edema, hepatomegaly, dyspnea, and cardiac cachexia (NYHA class IV).

endocarditis if the MR is life-threatening or if the appropriate antibiotic does not control the fever and infection promptly.

MITRAL STENOSIS

Diagnosis. The clinical diagnosis of mitral stenosis (MS) is based on the presence of an apical diastolic rumble and enlargement of the left atrium. Other disorders sometimes accompanied by an apical diastolic rumble are atrial septal defect, ventricular septal defect, patent ductus arteriosus, thyrotoxicosis, ball valve thrombus of the left atrium, and left atrial myxoma. Because of associated clinical features, these diseases can be easily differentiated from mitral stenosis.

Etiology. Congenital mitral stenosis is rare. Most cases result from rheumatic fever.

Natural Course of Rheumatic Mitral Stenosis. The classic studies of Oleson[13] and Roy and Gopinath[14] indicate that the average natural course of mitral stenosis begins with acute rheumatic fever at about 8 years of age. On recovery, patients feel well and may or may not have a murmur of mitral stenosis, but eventually some do. At the age of 31 years, they slow down compared with their peers. At 45 years they are very symptomatic. They die at about age 48 years. This description of the natural course is only general and gives little information about any one individual; the patient may die in the teens or die of something altogether different at the age of 90 years (Table 5–7).

Pathologic Physiology.[15] As the mitral valve narrows, pressure rises in the left atrium, with corresponding increases in the pulmonary veins, capillaries, and arteries (Fig. 5–8). When the orifice shrinks from the normal size of about 4.5 cm^2 to about 1 cm^2, pressures in the left atrium

TABLE 5–7. MITRAL STENOSIS

Etiology:	Rheumatic heart disease
Clinical Course:	*Stage 1:*
	Asymptomatic for ~20 years, gradual reduction in exercise tolerance for ~3–5 years
	Stage 2:
	Onset of pulmonary congestion related to infection, pregnancy, arrhythmia or other stress
	Stage 3:
	Development of pulmonary hypertension
	Stage 4:
	Progressively severe state of low cardiac output
Symptoms and Complications:	Hemoptysis of bright red blood
	Atrial fibrillation
	Systemic embolization
	Episodic pulmonary congestion early in the course (stage 2)
	Progressive fatigability later in the course (stages 3–4)
Balloon Valvuloplasty or Indications for Surgery:	Onset of pulmonary congestion (stage 2) (earliest manifestation is the development of dyspnea after climbing one flight of stairs)
	RVH (stage 3)

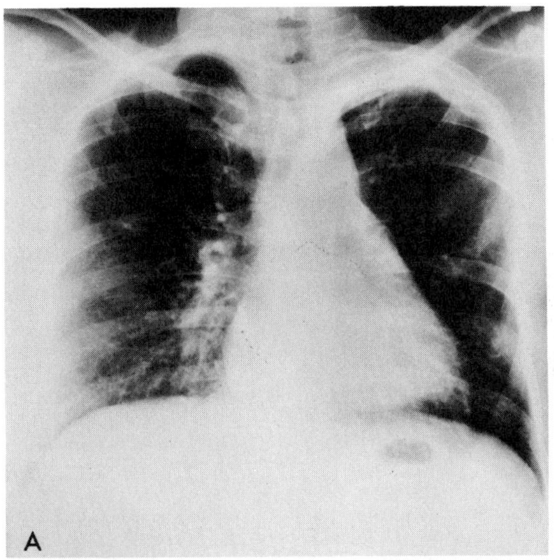

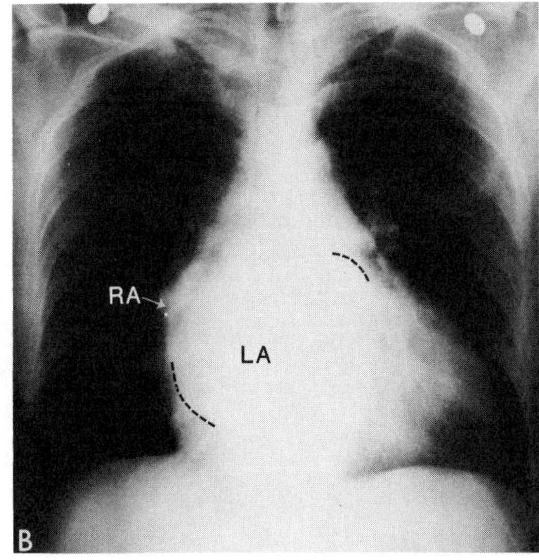

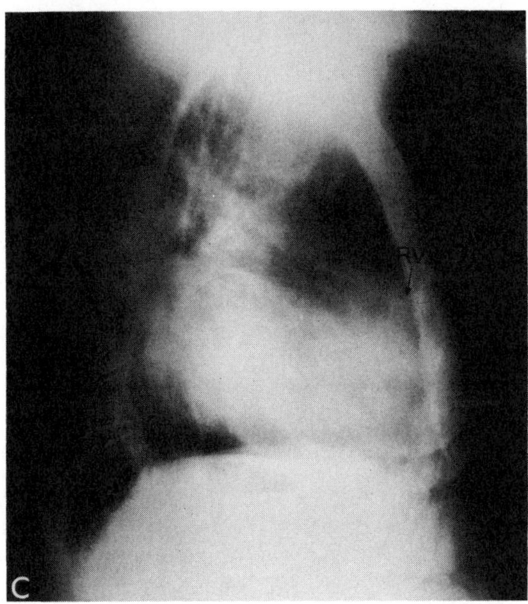

FIGURE 5–9. *A,* Chest radiograph of a patient with mitral stenosis who developed pulmonary edema when stressed by infection. The heart is normal in size, but the left atrium is dilated. The patient's symptoms were controlled by medication, and she has remained in stage 2 and in NYHA class II during 3 years of follow-up. *B* and *C,* Chest films of a patient with mitral stenosis whose only symptom was exercise intolerance. The patient was in stage 3 and in NYHA class II. The films show right ventricular and atrial enlargement in addition to left atrial enlargement. The patient's fatigability gradually increased during 2 years of follow-up until he was almost completely incapacitated (NYHA class IV). Mitral valve replacement was attempted at that point, but the patient failed to survive the operation.

Illustration continued on following page

and pulmonary capillaries when the patient is at rest rise from a normal value of 5 to 8 mm Hg to about 25 mm Hg. The natural history of a typical patient with MS may be divided into four stages. During stage 1, the patient has begun to slow down in physical activities and has thus remained relatively asymptomatic, even though the orifice of the mitral valve has become quite narrow. Cardiac index, which is cardiac output expressed as liters per minute per meters squared of body surface area, will have fallen from a normal resting value of 3.1 to about 2.7.

At the point of critical valve narrowing ($\sim$1 cm^2), patients enter stage 2 and become very symptomatic, particularly from exertional dyspnea, orthopnea, paroxysmal nocturnal dyspnea, and recurrent upper respiratory infections, which are, in fact, a mixture of infection and pulmonary edema. The onset of this very symptomatic stage is often seemingly abrupt, although careful history-taking will always document a long preceding period of reduced physical activity. The resistance of the pulmonary vessels (pulmonary vascular resistance) is normal or practically normal. Stage 2 of mitral stenosis may be ushered in by such events as an arrhythmia (e.g., atrial fibrillation), a salt "binge" (e.g., Thanksgiving dinner or Labor Day celebration), a period of bereavement, or the third trimester of pregnancy.

In any event, stage 2 is characterized by the patient's being very symptomatic and represents class IV of the NYHA classification. It has been described as tight mitral stenosis with a normal-sized heart (Fig. 5–9*A*).

At this time, changes begin to occur in the pulmonary vasculature that are in part histologic narrowing of the small muscular arteries (the resistance vessels) and mainly vasoconstriction. Thus, there is a stenosis not only of the mitral valve but also of the precapillary vessels of the lung. The latter now colors the whole clinical picture with the development of pulmonary artery hypertension, which ushers in the next stage of MS.

Stage 3 of mitral stenosis occurs when the mitral valve orifice is less than 1 cm^2 and the pulmonary vascular resistance rises to between 400 and 800 dyne-sec cm^{-5}, which is about 5 to 10 times greater than normal. The left atrial pressure will have remained in the region of 25 mm Hg; it cannot be much higher for any length of time without producing death from pulmonary edema. The cardiac index will have fallen further to the general level of 2.4 l/min/m^2.

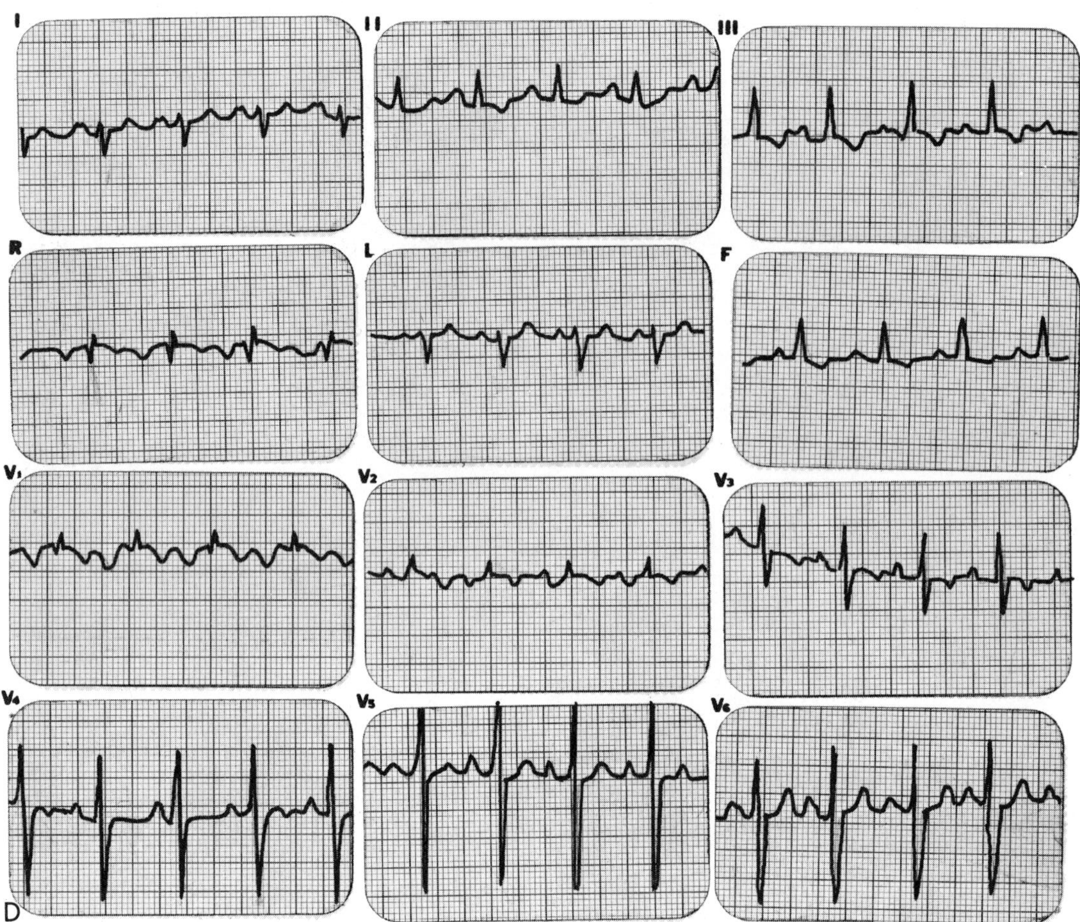

FIGURE 5–9 *Continued. D,* Electrocardiogram showing RVH and P-mitrale in the patient whose radiographs are shown in *B* and *C.* (Radiographs courtesy of Department of Radiology, Brigham and Women's Hospital, Harvard Medical School, Boston, MA.)

About half of these patients remain very short of breath, but in the other half exertional dyspnea becomes strikingly reduced. The chief complaint of this latter group of patients is easy fatigability. The fatigue syndrome is curious. Fatigue, a negative complaint, is a lack of energy that is poorly described by the patient. Close questioning may be necessary to elicit the fact that formerly the patient was meticulous in housework and now sweeps dust under the rugs; that formerly the children's clothes were always clean and in good repair but now are a bit unkempt with a button missing here and there; that formerly the patient kept a tidy desk, but now has a messy one, and so on. At this stage the radiograph and ECG have taken on striking changes (see Fig. 5–9*B–D*). The heart is always enlarged, there is prominence in the region of the pulmonary artery at the left hilum, and in the oblique view the right ventricle is enlarged. The ECG always shows the pattern of RVH. Stage 3 can be a clinically misleading one. The patient may be relatively asymptomatic (class II of the NYHA), but the x-ray film, ECG, and echocardiogram indicate clearly that the mitral stenosis is severe and pulmonary vascular complications are already advanced, and surgical intervention is indicated before the pulmonary vascular process advances further.

In stage 4 the patient becomes dyspneic again, but with associated findings of right ventricular failure as a consequence of sustained pulmonary artery hypertension. Dyspnea, orthopnea, paroxysmal nocturnal dyspnea, venous distention, hepatomegaly, edema, and finally cachexia are present. The patient is at the limit of circulatory reserve, with the reappearance of class IV symptoms of the NYHA.

Through an analysis of symptoms, signs, radiographs, ECG, and echocardiogram, the stage of the patient's disease can usually be quite accurately assessed. Since the narrowing of the mitral valve and the pulmonary vascular process are always progressive, it can never be anticipated that the disease will spontaneously improve. By examining the history, one can get a fairly good idea of how fast the disease is progressing and in this way have an idea of the individual patient's longevity. However, this is not the therapeutic issue. The problem is to decide when to intervene surgically or with balloon valvuloplasty.

Physical Examination. The typical findings of mitral stenosis are a loud S_1, an opening snap, an apical diastolic rumbling murmur with presystolic accentuation transmitted toward the axilla, and a quiet precordium on palpation (Fig. 5–10). The rhythm may be normal sinus or atrial fibrillation. If it is the latter, the presystolic accentuation of the murmur may be absent.

Associated findings may be those of pulmonary or systemic congestion (stages 2 and 4) and a sternal lift if right ventricular hypertrophy is present (stages 3 and 4).

Radiography. As soon as the murmur of mitral stenosis appears, the left atrium is enlarged, best seen on plain film in the right anterior oblique projection with a barium-filled esophagus.

Echocardiography. Two-dimensional echocardiography and Doppler ultrasound are extremely reliable in the

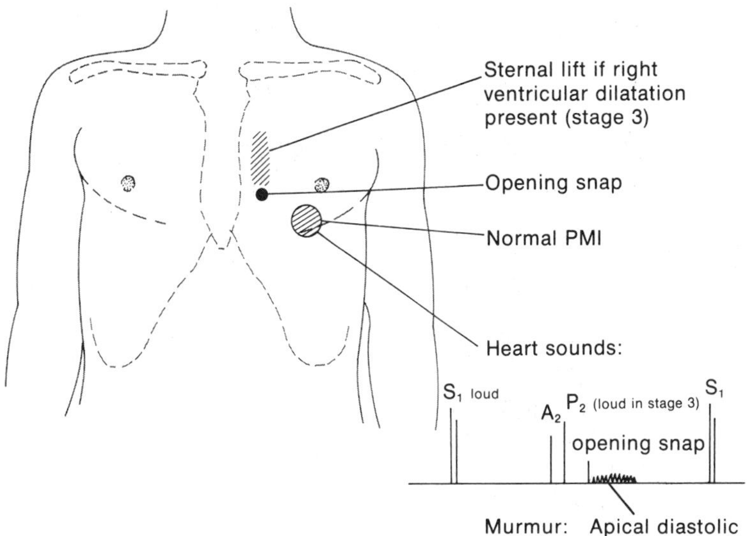

FIGURE 5–10. Typical findings on physical examination in mitral stenosis.

detection and estimation of severity of mitral stenosis. The reliability of the echocardiographic assessment of mitral stenosis is so great that in appropriately selected subjects (i.e., those without suspicion of associated coronary artery disease or other valvular abnormality), patients may be referred directly for mitral valve surgery without the need for routine preoperative cardiac catheterization.

Cardiac Catheterization. This is indicated when the patient is in stage 2, 3, or 4 and when other lesions—mitral regurgitation, aortic or tricuspid valve disease, coronary artery disease, or hypertension—cloud the issue. If none of these is suspected and the manifestations of mitral stenosis are typical for stage 2, 3, or 4, cardiac catheterization may not be necessary, although with the advent of percutaneous balloon valvuloplasty, most patients with MS undergo catheterization (with or without balloon valvuloplasty).

Complications. Several complications may incapacitate the patient.

Atrial Fibrillation. Patients with mitral stenosis occasionally develop atrial fibrillation before the valve becomes critically narrow. Others may have critically narrow mitral stenosis—stages 2, 3, and 4—and remain in normal sinus rhythm. It is easy to control the rate of atrial fibrillation with digitalis, verapamil, or β-adrenergic blockers, but if untreated, the rapid rate may precipitate acute pulmonary edema. Furthermore, atrial fibrillation increases the propensity to arterial embolization.

Arterial Embolization. This can be a tragic complication if it results in paralysis, aphasia, or loss of mentality. All patients with atrial fibrillation must take long-term anticoagulant medication, whether or not surgical replacement of the mitral valve is performed. We usually advocate anticoagulant therapy in *all* good risk patients with mitral stenosis who are over 35 years old, whether the rhythm is normal or abnormal, because, of those who embolize, two thirds are in atrial fibrillation and one third are in normal sinus rhythm. The mortality resulting from cerebral embolism approximates 50% and increases with subsequent emboli. If, following a stroke, surgery is to be performed, it is generally recommended that mitral valve replacement be delayed for 6 to 8 weeks to allow the central nervous system to stabilize.

Bacterial Endocarditis. Prophylactic antibiotics are mandatory in MS to reduce the risk of endocarditis. Bacterial endocarditis usually converts a stenotic valve into one with varying degrees of regurgitation due to destruction of valve substance. Occasionally, it is not possible to eradicate bacterial endocarditis with antibiotics. There should be no hesitation to intervene surgically if this occurs or if the patient's hemodynamic status deteriorates.

Complications in Pregnant Patients. Many patients with mitral stenosis become severely symptomatic during pregnancy. If they were asymptomatic before pregnancy, the chances are good that they can be managed medically through pregnancy. This requires close supervision, with emphasis on salt restriction, diuretics, restriction of physical activities, and control of tachycardia. Those who were symptomatic before pregnancy usually do badly during pregnancy and may require mitral valve surgery or balloon valvuloplasty during pregnancy; there is usually no need to terminate the pregnancy. There is no evidence that the risk to the mother from surgery is any higher than that for the nonpregnant woman, although the risk to the fetus has been reported to be about 33%.

Indications for Mechanical Intervention. Surgical intervention or percutaneous balloon mitral valvuloplasty (PBMV) is indicated in stage 2. Before this time (stage 1), it is difficult to predict when the patient will become symptomatic. However, a good rule of thumb is that when the patient develops dyspnea climbing one flight of stairs at a normal rate of ascent and feels that he or she must rest before ascending a second flight, mechanical intervention is indicated. At this stage, the patient's activities are restricted, cardiac reserve is small, and should the patient contract pneumonia, require surgery of any type, become pregnant, or have to exert himself or herself unduly because of circumstances beyond control, intractable and even lethal pulmonary edema might ensue.

Stage 3 can be difficult to detect because of the relative lack of complaints. The clue, however, is that radiography reveals the heart to be 20% or more enlarged, and the ECG shows right ventricular hypertrophy. These patients should undergo mechanical intervention because otherwise they will progress to stage 4, in which the risks are higher and the results are not as beneficial as when undertaken at an earlier stage (see Fig. 5–9B, C). Pulmonary artery hypertension is *not* a contraindication to intervention in severe mitral stenosis, since it will resolve to a large degree in the early postoperative period.

The results depend on the interventional procedure. Surgical mitral valvuloplasty or commissurotomy generally gives improvement of symptoms for an average of 7 years with less than 10% necessity of reoperation at 9 or 10 years.[16] A few patients have had a return to practically full activity sustained for 2 decades or more. This operation is now being performed less frequently, but when it is done, the commissurotomy is usually performed under direct vision rather than with the heart beating, as was done previously.[16, 17] If the valve cannot be repaired, the alternative is replacement with a prosthesis.

Excellent early and intermediate term results have been achieved with balloon valvuloplasty.[3, 4] In this technique one or two balloons are positioned across the mitral valve and then inflated after percutaneous insertion during cardiac catheterization. Results are comparable with those achieved with surgical commissurotomy, with a doubling of mitral valve area. Particularly suited for pliable nonregurgitant valves, PBMV is an excellent alternative to surgery.

VALVULAR AORTIC STENOSIS

Etiology. The three principal forms of valvular aortic stenosis (AS) are rheumatic, congenital, and acquired calcific. In patients with aortic stenosis between 15 and 65 years of age, most valves are congenitally deformed and usually bicuspid, with rheumatic heart disease as the second most common cause. When rheumatic AS is present, invariably there is concomitant mitral valve involvement; hence *isolated* rheumatic aortic valve disease is quite uncommon. The situation is totally different in patients over 65 years of age; more than 90% of these patients have acquired calcific aortic stenosis.

Natural Course. The course of aortic stenosis is a slow one until symptoms develop; then the course is rapidly downhill (Table 5–8). The average age at death in untreated patients is 58 years, with a wide variation from one patient to another.[18] As the orifice of the valve narrows, systolic pressure in the left ventricle rises and the left ventricle hypertrophies. These changes produce no symptoms. The size of the aortic orifice is normally about 4 cm^2, and not until it becomes 0.7 cm^2 or less do symptoms appear. Then there is a malignant downhill course.

The symptoms that usher in the malignant downhill course are angina pectoris, syncope, and congestive heart failure; the average survival is 5 years once angina pectoris appears, 3 years after syncope, and 2 years after the onset of congestive failure.

Angina Pectoris. About two thirds of patients with symptomatic AS develop angina pectoris, and in about half of these patients it is caused by the valve disease alone; in the other half, there is concomitant coronary artery disease.[19] It often is not possible to decide how much of each is present except by cardiac catheterization and coronary angiography.

Syncope. This occurs either in relation to exercise or as the result of arrhythmia. Most commonly it is due to hypoperfusion resulting from exercise-induced vasodilatation in the setting of a fixed cardiac output.

Arrhythmias of any sort produce an inefficient left ventricular contraction, and ectopic beats may not raise the left ventricular pressure sufficiently to open the stenotic aortic valve. Syncope results after only a few seconds of inadequate cerebral perfusion.

Congestive Heart Failure. Dyspnea is the most common complaint in patients with AS and usually results from impaired diastolic filling of the hypertrophied (and stiff) left ventricle. More overt findings of congestive heart failure are found in some patients, and systolic dysfunction may develop in addition to diastolic dysfunction. The significance of left ventricular failure is that the future downhill course is rapid and becomes more and more refractory to medical therapy. It has a more malignant downhill course than any of the other valvular diseases, the average duration of life being 2 years.[18] In marked contrast to other valvular conditions, there is usually a striking improvement in left ventricular function after aortic valve replacement, even if the left ventricle is severely impaired preoperatively (ejection fraction as low as 10 to 20%).

Physical Examination. Diagnosis depends on the presence of the murmur, which is an ejection type of murmur, starting just after the first sound, extending to but not past the second sound, and being loudest in midsystole (Fig. 5–11). It is usually loudest along the upper sternal borders and is likewise heard over the carotid arteries. Sometimes it is loudest at the apex. The intensity of the murmur gives no indication of the degree of the narrowing of the aortic valve, but the aortic component of the second heart sound is almost never distinctly audible in significant calcific aortic stenosis. An S_4 gallop is usually present. There are two associated signs. First is an apex impulse, which is frequently forceful in character. For years it remains in the fifth intercostal space in the midclavicular line. As the left ventricle fails and dilates, the apex impulse becomes more diffuse and lateral to the midclavicular line. Second, as the aortic valve narrows, the carotid pulse changes from a brisk upstroke and downstroke of good volume to the so-called plateau pulse: The upstroke and downstroke of the pulse are relatively slow and prolonged, the volume of pulsation is less than normal, and a shudder may be appreciated while palpating the carotid.

Radiography. It is not until fairly late in the course of AS that cardiomegaly, calcification of the valve, and poststenotic dilatation of the ascending aorta occur.

Electrocardiography. The pattern of left ventricular hypertrophy is often but not invariably present.

Echocardiography. This may yield information about thickening and calcification of the aortic valve and decreased mobility of the leaflets. These findings should be accompanied by the discovery of a thickened septum and free wall of the left ventricle. The size of the orifice of the aortic valve has been accurately demonstrated by two-dimensional echocardiography only in children. Doppler ultrasound has added a further dimension to the noninvasive evaluation of the severity of AS[2]; although it may underestimate the severity of aortic stenosis (especially in low flow states), it does not overestimate severity.

Cardiac Catheterization. This is currently the most precise method of determining not only the exact size of the aortic orifice but also associated left ventricular function and the state of the coronary arteries. The latter is particularly necessary in aortic stenotic patients with angina pectoris.

The main differential diagnosis of aortic stenosis in the

TABLE 5–8. VALVULAR AORTIC STENOSIS

Etiology:	Rheumatic heart disease Congenital (bicuspid valve) Acquired calcific
Clinical Course:	Prolonged asymptomatic period (till 5th to 6th decade) Rapid deterioration at onset of symptoms
Symptoms and Complications:	Syncope Angina pectoris Left ventricular failure
Indications for Surgery:	Earliest appearance of symptoms: decrease in exercise tolerance, dizziness, chest discomfort

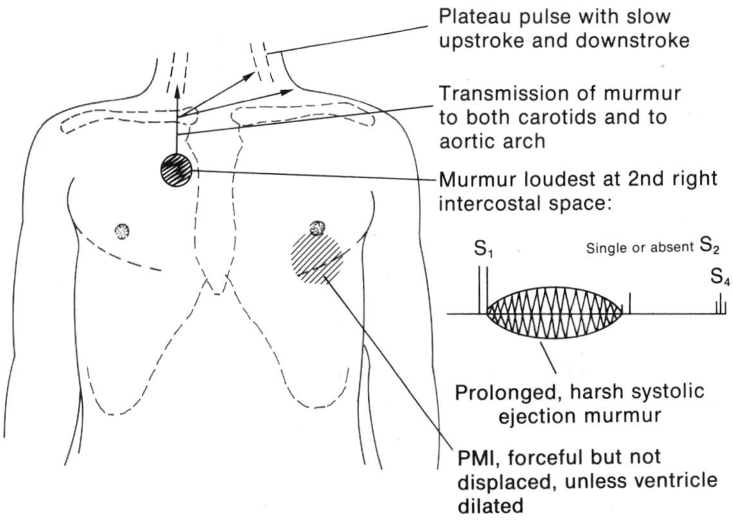

Plateau pulse with slow upstroke and downstroke
Transmission of murmur to both carotids and to aortic arch
Murmur loudest at 2nd right intercostal space:
S_1 Single or absent S_2 S_4
Prolonged, harsh systolic ejection murmur
PMI, forceful but not displaced, unless ventricle dilated

FIGURE 5–11. Typical findings on physical examination in valvular aortic stenosis.

older age group is atherosclerosis. Cerebrovascular disease can produce transient ischemic attacks (TIAs) and syncope. Coronary artery disease can produce angina pectoris and congestive heart failure. As patients grow older, it becomes increasingly difficult to decide how much of their disability results from AS and how much from associated atherosclerosis. For this reason cardiac catheterization should be performed in many of these patients prior to surgery.

Medical Management. Asymptomatic patients with aortic valve disease should be seen periodically and followed with noninvasive testing.[20, 21] The appearance of symptoms should prompt more detailed evaluation (i.e., consideration of cardiac catheterization).[22] Otherwise, prophylaxis for subacute bacterial endocarditis should be emphasized and diuretics and/or beta adrenergic blockers used with caution for fear of reducing cardiac output.

Surgical Indications. Until patients develop angina, syncope, or congestive heart failure, the medical outlook is excellent, and it is difficult to predict when these symptoms will develop. It is generally accepted that the occurrence of any one of this triad of symptoms is an indication to consider surgical intervention. Aortic valve replacement is sometimes considered in the asymptomatic patient with hemodynamically critically severe aortic stenosis.

The earliest appearance of shortness of breath on activities previously well tolerated, of dizziness, which usually precedes syncope, and of chest discomfort can be clues to the appearance in the near future of cardiac failure, syncope, and angina. If any of these early symptoms appear, the patient should then be considered a candidate for aortic valve replacement. The aortic valve area will be calculated to be less than or equal to 0.7 cm^2 in most of these patients.

In good risk patients the operative mortality is less than 5%, with an expected 5-year survival rate of about 85%. Once overt heart failure is present, the operative mortality rises to 10 to 15% or more, and the long-term functional status of survivors is impaired.[23] The occurrence of arterial embolism averages about 3 per 100 patient years in those with prosthetic valves who are taking anticoagulant medication, and about two per 100 patient years in those with porcine valves who were not taking anticoagulant medication.

Percutaneous balloon valvuloplasty is at best a palliative procedure in adult patients, as it typically enlarges the aortic valve orifice only modestly, and for a limited period of time.[24–26] One can expect the transaortic gradient to fall by half, but half the patients develop restenosis within 6 months.[27–29] It is most commonly employed as a "bridge" to eventual aortic valve replacement in critically ill patients with aortic stenosis.[29]

Congenital Aortic Stenosis in Childhood

Special consideration should be given to congenital aortic stenosis in the pediatric age group. These patients have the same symptoms, signs, ECG, and x-ray findings as do adults. However, there is one difference. Adults have enough "sense" to slow down, but children do not. It has been found that sudden death in children is almost always preceded by the presence of left ventricular hypertrophy and strain on the ECG and rarely occurs in the absence of LVH. Therefore, it is recommended that children be referred immediately for surgery as soon as the ECG shows the voltage criteria of LVH. In those individuals who have not attained their growth, valvulotomy is performed. Unfortunately, aortic insufficiency of some degree is not a rare complication of valvulotomy. The role of percutaneous balloon aortic valvuloplasty in congenital aortic stenosis continues to be studied and may evolve into an important therapeutic option in the future.

Hypertrophic Cardiomyopathy

The clinical diagnosis of hypertrophic cardiomyopathy (HCM) is often difficult. Echocardiography has made its recognition easy, provided that this diagnostic tool is considered. Its treatment is completely different from that of any other form of heart disease.

Hypertrophic cardiomyopathy[30] is a disorder characterized by marked hypertrophy of the left ventricle. Asymmetric septal hypertrophy with disproportionate involvement of the interventricular septum compared with the posterior wall is the characteristic feature, but other forms of hypertrophy (apical, concentric, free wall) are not rare.[31] During systole, the anterior leaflet of the mitral valve may abut the hypertrophied septum and narrow this region sufficiently to produce obstruction to left ventricular ejection. MR is often present owing to abnormal anterior displacement of the mitral valve. The primary pathophysiologic abnormality in HCM is increased stiffness of the left ventricle as a consequence of the hypertrophy; this results in impaired diastolic filling.

TABLE 5–9. HYPERTROPHIC CARDIOMYOPATHY

Etiology:	Congenital
Clinical Course:	Onset of symptoms in 3rd to 4th decade Episodic manifestations
Symptoms or Complications:	Exertional dyspnea Angina pectoris Postural dizzy spells
Indications for Surgery:	Severe angina or syncope unresponsive to β-adrenergic blocker

Etiology. It appears to be genetically transmitted as a nonsex-linked autosomal dominant in most cases. When this condition is discovered in a patient, other members of the family and offspring should be examined and have an echocardiogram performed for HCM even though they are currently asymptomatic.

Clinical Features. Most patients with HCM are asymptomatic; those who become symptomatic typically do so in the third and fourth decades, but this varies from infancy to the ninth decade. The presenting complaints are exertional dyspnea and angina pectoris; less often, postural dizzy spells and occasionally syncope and palpitation. These symptoms tend to be absent for years, then they may become unpredictably episodic, and finally in some patients fairly stable, rarely culminating in chronic congestive heart failure (Table 5–9). Regardless of prior symptoms, sudden death may occur. The occurrence of atrial fibrillation may result in the development or worsening of symptoms.

This rather variable and unpredictable course in the group as a whole, as well as in any individual patient, is generally unrelated to the outflow tract obstruction, which is quite dynamic and may be evanescent. In HCM, left ventricular contraction is characteristically vigorous. At end-systole, the chamber is almost completely emptied. During ejection, there may be a pressure gradient across the aortic outflow tract. Factors or agents that increase outflow obstruction are the following:

1. Inotropic agents, like digitalis and isoproterenol, and the Valsalva maneuver
2. Agents that decrease preload, such as diuretics
3. Factors that decrease afterload, such as taking isoproterenol, amyl nitrite, and nitroglycerin; exercise; a post-exercise state; and assumption of the upright position

Factors or agents that tend to abolish outflow obstruction are the following:

1. Pressor agents: methoxamine and phenylephrine
2. β-Blockers: propranolol
3. Increase of preload: recumbent position with the legs elevated and administration of intravenous fluids

One of the unique features of HCM is the variability in the severity of the obstruction occurring over brief intervals. For example, a sizable pressure gradient across the outflow tract at the beginning of cardiac catheterization may spontaneously disappear a half hour later. Debate continues whether the pressure gradient represents true obstruction or is merely an expression of the abnormal systolic flow dynamics in this condition. Regardless of the mechanism, it is now known that most subjects with HCM have the "nonobstructive" form and do not have an outflow pressure gradient. Symptoms in these patients thus are the result of abnormalities in diastolic and not systolic function.

Physical Examination. The heart may be enlarged with a left ventricular lift and a double apical impulse on the basis of an atrial as well as a ventricular component. In patients with obstruction, an ejection type of aortic systolic murmur is heard along the left sternal border and at the apex but is poorly transmitted to the carotids

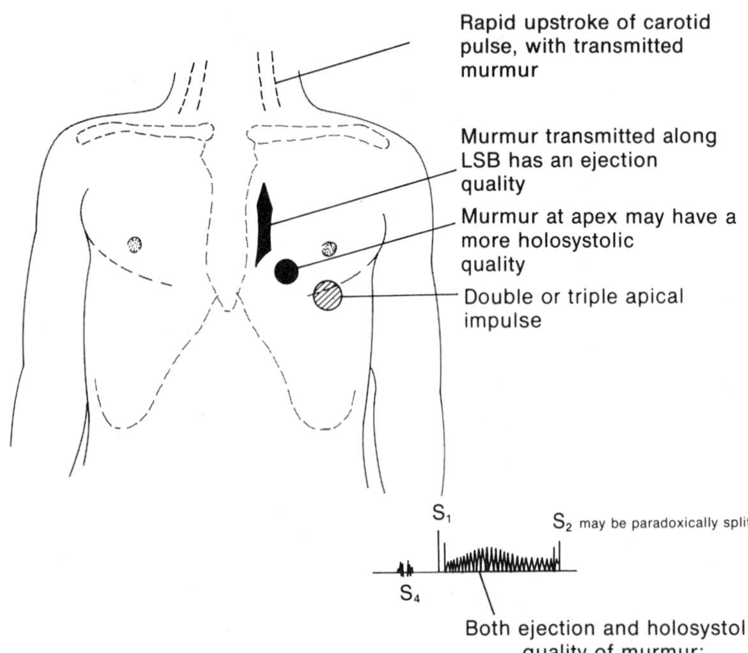

FIGURE 5–12. Typical findings on physical examination in the patient with hypertrophic cardiomyopathy.

(Fig. 5–12). An apical pansystolic murmur of MR is often present. The murmur may be observed to become louder during the Valsalva maneuver and to diminish transiently following Valsalva release (Table 5–10). The upstroke of the carotid pulse is rapid, not plateau, such as in valvular aortic stenosis. An S_4 is often present. Paradoxic splitting of the second heart sound is frequent in patients with outflow gradients.

Radiography. The cardiac silhouette is usually prominent with prominence in the region of the left ventricle. No poststenotic dilatation of the aorta and no intracardiac calcification are present.

Electrocardiography. In most instances, the pattern is of left ventricular hypertrophy. Commonly, deep, broad Q waves are found in leads II, III, and aVF and in the left precordial V leads, suggesting ischemic heart disease, but they are probably due to the hypertrophied septum.

Echocardiography. This is invaluable for diagnosis and for screening relatives. The characteristic abnormality is inappropriate left ventricular hypertrophy. Most patients demonstrate disproportionate hypertrophy of the septum, with septal thickness more than 30% greater than that of the posterior left ventricular wall. Hypertrophy of other portions of the ventricle may be noted, including the apex and left ventricular free wall, and a pattern of concentric hypertrophy. There is abnormal anterior motion of the anterior leaflet of the mitral valve during systole when obstruction is present, and an abnormally anterior position of the mitral valve in diastole.

Cardiac Catheterization. This technique[30] has allowed excellent studies of the nature and behavior of HCM but now is rarely necessary to perform because echocardiography, particularly when combined with Doppler recordings, gives most of the essential information noninvasively. Those agents and maneuvers, listed previously, that worsen and lessen the outflow obstruction can be studied echocardiographically, as can the therapeutic response to medical or surgical therapy.

Treatment. The therapeutic regimen of these individuals is almost exactly the opposite of that prescribed for all other types of heart disease. Digitalis aggravates the outflow obstruction and is contraindicated except for rate control when atrial fibrillation appears. Diuretics, leading to a reduction of blood volume, aggravate the condition and should be prescribed with caution. Use of nitroglycerin and nitrates for angina is contraindicated in HCM. Even in asymptomatic patients, strenuous physical activity is inadvisable because of a risk, though small, of sudden death.

Propranolol has been considered the drug of choice for medical treatment. As a β-adrenergic blocking agent, it produces bradycardia and blocks sympathetic activity. In doses of 20 to 80 mg four times a day, it may reduce the frequency and severity of angina pectoris and palpitation and possibly of episodes of syncope and arrhythmia, although the response to therapy is often disappointing. Calcium channel blocking agents, particularly verapamil, are useful agents for symptomatic HCM; they appear to exert their beneficial effect by improving the filling of the ventricle and thus reducing diastolic pressure.[31]

Management of the arrhythmias is a major challenge in HCM. Propranolol and even the routine antiarrhythmic agents apparently do not protect against sudden death. Whether any of the newer agents (such as amiodarone) will be effective remains to be established.

TABLE 5–10. EFFECTS OF MANEUVERS ON HEART MURMURS

		Auscultatory Findings			
Maneuver	**Physiologic Effect**	*HCM*	*Valvular Aortic Stenosis*	*Mitral Regurgitation*	*Mitral Valve Prolapse**
Valsalva straining	↓ Venous return ↓ Cardiac output ↓ Left ventricular volume	↑ Intensity of murmur	↓ Intensity of murmur	↓ Intensity of murmur	Click occurs earlier in systole; murmur is more prolonged
Valsalva release	↑ Venous return ↑ Cardiac output ↑ Left ventricular volume	↓ Intensity of murmur	↑ Intensity of murmur	↑ Intensity of murmur	Click occurs later in systole; murmur is less prolonged
Squatting†	↑ Venous return ↑ Cardiac output ↑ Left ventricular volume	↓ Intensity of murmur	↑ Intensity of murmur	↑ Intensity of murmur	Click occurs later in systole; murmur is less prolonged
Immediate standing	↓ Venous return ↓ Cardiac output ↓ Left ventricular volume	↑ Intensity of murmur	↓ Intensity or no change in murmur	↓ Intensity of murmur	Click occurs earlier in systole; murmur is more prolonged
Handgrip without Valsalva‡	Venous return unchanged ↑ Peripheral resistance ↓ Cardiac output ↑ Left ventricular volume	↓ Intensity of murmur	↓ Intensity or no change in murmur	↑ Intensity of murmur	Click occurs later in systole; murmur is less prolonged
Amyl nitrite§	↑ Venous return ↓ Peripheral resistance ↑ Cardiac output ↓ Left ventricular volume	↑ Intensity of murmur	↑ Intensity or no change in murmur	↓ Intensity of murmur	Click occurs earlier in systole; murmur is more prolonged

*Intensity of murmur depends upon left ventricular systolic pressure, but its duration is governed by left ventricular volume; reduced volume causes leaflet prolapse to occur earlier in systole.

†Also distinguishes HCM (diminished intensity) from ventricular septal defect (very much louder).

‡Distinguishes valvular aortic stenosis (diminished) from mitral regurgitation (louder).

§Distinguishes mitral regurgitation (diminished) from tricuspid regurgitation and pulmonic stenosis (louder).

Surgical therapy should be reserved for those with heart failure caused by obstruction or with disabling angina and syncope unresponsive to propranolol. The operation consists of partially excising the muscle obstructing the left ventricular outflow tract. In experienced hands, the risk of surgery is less than 5%. Operative survivors are often substantially improved, with reduced symptoms and improved exercise capacity.

AORTIC REGURGITATION

There are two types of aortic regurgitation (AR): acute and chronic. The two pose different problems of presentation and treatment and will therefore be considered separately.

Chronic Aortic Regurgitation

Etiology. Chronic AR results from diseases of the valve leaflets themselves, or of the aortic root. Common causes of valve dysfunction include rheumatic heart disease, infective endocarditis, congenital deformity, and degeneration.[32] Root abnormalities include severe systemic hypertension and annuloaortic ectasia. Less common forms are those associated with ankylosing spondylitis, Reiter's syndrome, psoriasis, congenital perforation of cusps, and that associated with ventricular septal defect and coarctation of the aorta. Irrespective of cause, the course is much the same, and therefore all these are considered under one heading.

Pathophysiology and Clinical Course. Since the valve leaflets do not approximate closely in diastole, there is a regurgitation of blood from the aorta into the left ventricle. Thus, the amount of blood ejected into the aorta in systole consists of that which continues to flow out the aorta plus that which regurgitates. The total stroke output of the left ventricle becomes larger for the simple reason that in addition to the regurgitated volume, the amount of blood going out the aorta to the body remains normal for years. The left ventricle dilates and hypertrophies to meet this challenge. The amount of blood that regurgitates depends mainly on the size of the regurgitant orifice but also on the level of the diastolic blood pressure in the aorta minus that in the left ventricle in diastole. In cases of free aortic regurgitation, the left ventricle may become enormous—the so-called cor bovinum, or beef heart. Because of the large left ventricular stroke output, the left ventricular systolic pressure, and therefore the arterial systolic pressure, rises. Because of the run-off back through the aortic valve from the aorta to the left ventricle in diastole, the aortic or arterial diastolic pressure falls. Thus, there is a wide pulse pressure. In cases of free aortic regurgitation, systolic blood pressures often are 180 to 200 mm Hg, and diastolic pressures of zero measured by blood pressure cuff can be recorded, although they are actually higher. Arterial pulses are very full and quick—the so-called Corrigan or water-hammer pulse. When pressure by blood pressure cuff is zero, pistol shot sounds can be heard over the large arteries without inflating the cuff.

It is surprising how well these patients do for many years, even in the presence of wide-open aortic regurgitation. Occasionally, one encounters severe aortic regurgitation in athletes, emphasizing that exercise intolerance is uncommon in compensated aortic regurgitation. There comes a time, however, when the patient develops a decrease in exercise tolerance. This period may continue for years, or it may rapidly progress. Eventually, the left ventricle "wears out."[33] This is partly because of excessive dilatation of the left ventricle, partly because of excessive overwork, and partly because the demands for coronary blood flow to provide the excessively overworked myocardium with nutrients exceed that which can be supplied. In any event, the left ventricle fails. Dyspnea, which previously occurred on excessive exertion, and then on less and less exertion, now is present when the individual is at rest. Orthopnea, paroxysmal nocturnal dyspnea, and pulmonary congestion, as indicated by rales, appear. At this point, one can anticipate a 50% mortality in 2 years. Another symptom of dire import is typical angina pectoris, which can occur in these patients in the presence as well as in the absence of coronary artery disease. It implies a 50% mortality in 6 years.

The natural course of this disease is, therefore, such that the patient at first is completely asymptomatic, then slows down but still lacks symptoms, and then slows down further because of exertional dyspnea, and finally experiences dyspnea at rest, that is, heart failure (Table 5–11). During this long course, the heart is susceptible to enlargement. One of the problems in medicine currently is how to assess and recognize irreversible cardiac damage before the advent of symptomatic breakdown. There is currently no clear-cut answer to this problem. What is apparent, however, is that if one waits for congestive heart failure or angina pectoris to occur before performing aortic valve replacement, there may already have been so much cardiac damage that postoperatively the patient is little improved owing to pre-existing cardiac damage. On the other hand, up to one half of individuals with huge hearts and moderately severe impairment of left ventricular function may respond to aortic valve replacement with substantial postoperative improvement; this is in contrast to the poorer outlook for mitral regurgitation.

Diagnosis. The diagnosis is made by the discovery of the typical murmur, which is a highpitched, decrescendo diastolic murmur best heard along the left sternal border (Fig. 5–13). Associated findings are water-hammer pulses in all parts of the body and a wide pulse pressure. Many names are attached to various physical signs in free aortic regurgitation: Quincke's pulses (pulsating capillaries in nail beds), DeMusset's sign (pulsatile bobbing of the head and pulsation of the uvula), Duroziez's sign (diastolic murmur over arteries that are slightly compressed with the stethoscope), and Corrigan's pulses (water-hammer pulse). The point of maximal apex impulse is displaced downward and

TABLE 5–11. CHRONIC AORTIC REGURGITATION

Etiology:	Rheumatic heart disease Syphilis Spondylitic syndromes Hypertension Congenital perforation of cusps Endocarditis
Clinical Course:	Prolonged asymptomatic period Period of decreased exercise tolerance Onset of overt congestive heart failure followed by progressively downhill course
Symptoms and Complications:	Pulmonary congestion Angina pectoris Dizziness
Indications for Surgery:	Definitely indicated when congestive heart failure or angina is present Must be considered if cardiothoracic ratio >30% enlarged, LV ejection fraction <50%, or end-systolic volume increasing progressively above normal

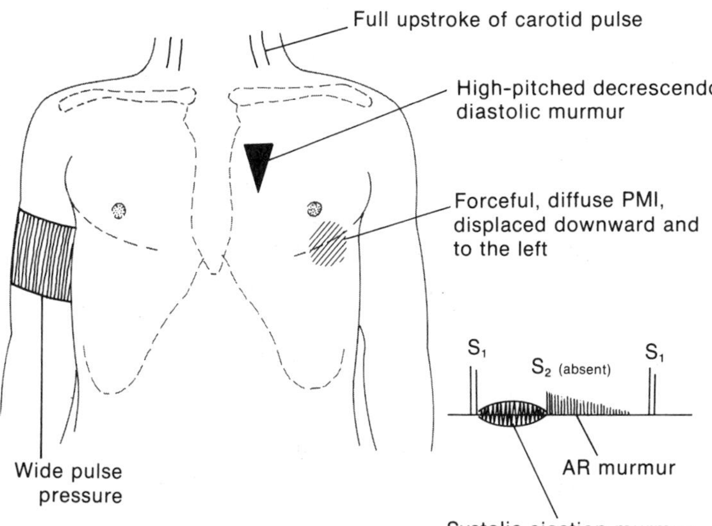

FIGURE 5–13. Typical findings on physical examination in patients with chronic aortic regurgitation.

to the left; it becomes forceful and diffuse as the left ventricle dilates. The blood pressure is characterized by elevation of the systolic and depression of the diastolic pressure, with a resultant wide pulse pressure.

Radiography. The heart becomes enlarged downward and outward owing mainly to enlargement of the left ventricle (Fig. 5–14 *B,C*).

Electrocardiography. Eventually, the pattern of LVH and strain develops (Fig. 5–14*A*).

Echocardiography. The echocardiographic appearance of the aortic leaflets may be normal or may show a specific abnormality (e.g., vegetation) that accounts for the regurgitation. Doppler studies document the presence of aortic regurgitation and offer a semiquantitative guide to the severity of the leak.[2]

Echocardiography is particularly useful for following asymptomatic patients with normal or mildly impaired left ventricular function. Patients whose serial echocardiographic studies demonstrate a deterioration of left ventricular function should be considered for valve replacement to prevent the development of irreversible left ventricular damage.

Nuclear Studies. The failure of the ejection fraction to rise appropriately during an exercise radionuclide ventriculographic study has been suggested as an indicator of incipient left ventricular dysfunction. Because of the multiple physiologic effects of exercise, however, we currently do not advocate the use of these data as independent determinants for the timing of valve surgery, particularly in minimally symptomatic patients.

Cardiac Catheterization. This is indicated when the patient clinically becomes a potential candidate for surgery. This technique allows semiquantification of the magnitude of aortic regurgitation, assessment of left ventricular function and, if indicated, of the coronary anatomy, and identification of associated valvular disorders.

Medical Therapy. Asymptomatic patients without cardiac enlargement should be seen periodically and followed with serial noninvasive testing, watching for any signs of reduced ventricular performance (at which point consideration should be given to surgical intervention). Symptomatic patients or those with severe aortic regurgitation may profit from digitalis and afterload reduction therapy. All patients require prophylaxis for subacute bacterial endocarditis.[10]

Surgical Indications. There is no question that the surgical outlook is much more favorable than the medical when either left ventricular failure or angina pectoris occurs in these patients. The surgical risk in the best of hands is similar to that for aortic stenosis (<5%). It is becoming increasingly apparent, however, that if one waits for these two symptoms to appear before recommending surgery, the results of surgery will not be optimal because of the cardiac damage that has already occurred, although usually ventricular function improves postoperatively even in the presence of moderate preoperative dysfunction. In general, surgical intervention must be considered even though the patient is not particularly symptomatic, when the heart is over 30% enlarged by the cardiothoracic ratio or when the left ventricular ejection fraction is moderately impaired (ejection fraction of 0.25 to 0.49), as measured by echocardiography, particularly if serial noninvasive testing has demonstrated progressive deterioration of left ventricular function.

Acute Aortic Regurgitation

Acute aortic regurgitation is very different from the chronic form. Time is too short for ventricular enlargement or hypertrophy to occur. Depending on the nature of the process, regurgitation may be overwhelming so that death occurs rapidly.

Because the ventricle has not had time to dilate, the pulse pressure is narrow and the physical examination is in marked contrast to that in chronic aortic regurgitation: the diastolic murmur is short and often quiet; there are no peripheral stigmata of a wide pulse pressure (i.e., normal blood pressure, no Quincke's sign); and the first heart sound is usually quiet or absent.

Bacterial endocarditis, particularly if it is due to a virulent organism such as the *Staphylococcus,* may erode or destroy a valve very rapidly and is a common cause of acute aortic regurgitation. The advent of left ventricular failure in these individuals results in almost a 100% mortality in 1 year. With the onset of symptoms or signs of left ventricular failure, aortic valve replacement should be performed on an emergency or nearly emergency basis, even in the presence of active infection.

Traumatic aortic regurgitation may result from a fall or a stab wound. It occurs occasionally in normal individuals but more often in those already having aortic valve disease.

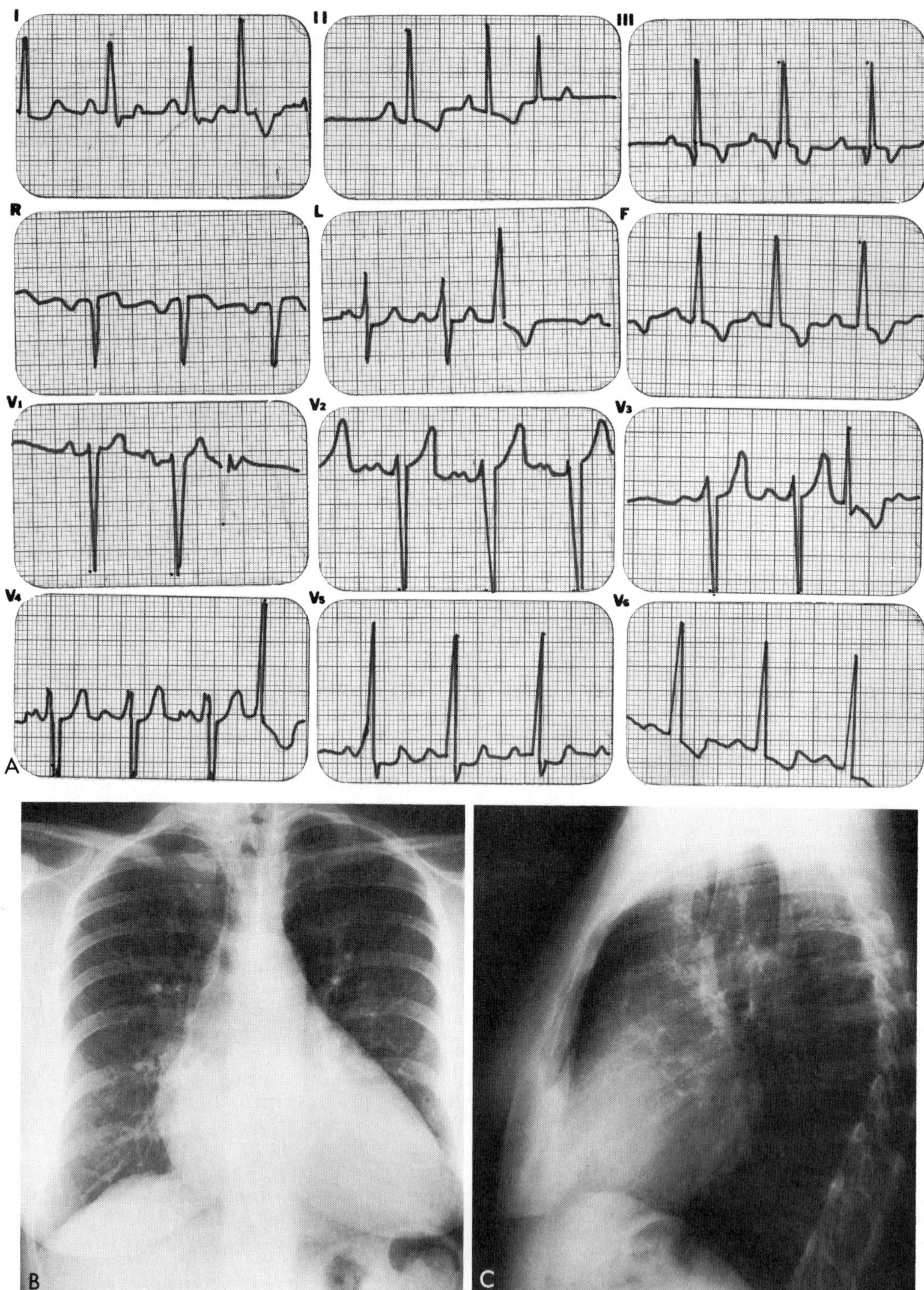

FIGURE 5–14. The patient with severe chronic aortic regurgitation is characterized by a widely increased pulse pressure, a pattern of left ventricular hypertrophy and strain on an electrocardiogram (ECG) and dilated LV on a chest radiograph. This patient was judged to have moderately severe, stable, asymptomatic AR. The blood pressure was 130/60. *A,* The ECG shows LVH and strain, as well as ventricular premature depolarizations. *B* and *C,* The chest film reveals a moderately severely dilated ventricle.

TABLE 5–12. VALVULAR PULMONIC STENOSIS

Etiology:	Congenital Rarely rheumatic or related to carcinoid
Clinical Course:	Asymptomatic if stenosis mild Symptoms of decreased cardiac output and right ventricular failure if severe
Symptoms and Complications:	Exertional fatigue Syncope Stasis cyanosis Distended neck veins and congestive hepatomegaly
Indications for Balloon Valvuloplasty:	Onset of symptoms Lack of normal growth in a child Cardiomegaly

It occurs almost exclusively in men. The condition is usually disastrous enough to require emergency valve replacement if time suffices.

Dissecting aneurysms of the ascending aorta may dissect along the media of the aorta and rupture into the pericardial cavity, resulting in rapid death. Such rupture is frequently preceded by a disturbance of aortic valve function. The appearance of the murmur of aortic regurgitation in a patient who has tearing chest pain accompanied by dilatation of the ascending aorta, as detected by radiography, should be considered as an emergency situation requiring surgical repair of the aorta to prevent the final perforation of the vessel. Aortic valve replacement is also necessary in many cases.

VALVULAR PULMONIC STENOSIS

With rare exceptions, isolated pulmonic stenosis (PS) is congenital. A rheumatic cause is very rare. Also rare is its occurrence in relation to the malignant carcinoid syndrome manifested by cutaneous flushing, telangiectasia, intestinal hypermotility, and bronchoconstriction.

Clinical Course and Manifestations.[34] The clinical course depends on the degree of narrowing of the orifice of the pulmonic valve (Table 5–12). The stenotic orifice does not enlarge with age. Therefore, an asymptomatic individual may become symptomatic, especially during the period of rapid growth.

Pulmonic stenosis produces an obstruction to blood flow from the right ventricle to the pulmonary artery. This results in a reduction of cardiac output and an increase of right ventricular systolic pressure. If the pulmonic stenosis is mild, these pressure and flow changes are unimportant, the patient is asymptomatic even on strenuous activity, and the ECG and heart size are essentially normal.

With increasingly severe pulmonic stenosis, symptoms develop that are referable to the decrease of cardiac output and right ventricular failure. Thus, the patient slows down, has exertional dyspnea (but not from pulmonary congestion), is underdeveloped, and may have syncopal attacks, stasis cyanosis, and manifestations of right ventricular failure such as distended neck veins, right upper quadrant discomfort from congestive hepatomegaly, and edema.

Physical Examination. The characteristic murmur is a harsh crescendo-decrescendo systolic murmur, loudest in the second and third left intercostal space and not transmitted or else poorly transmitted into the carotids. With mild-to-moderate pulmonic stenosis, the murmur reaches peak intensity in midsystole and ends at or before S_2. With increasing severity, the peak of the murmur is later, and S_2 becomes inaudible. A systolic click is heard just before the murmur in almost all except the severest cases. A fourth heart sound usually denotes severe obstruction. Right ventricular hypertrophy is denoted by a right ventricular heave. Prominent A waves are seen in the jugular veins (Fig. 5–15*A*).

Radiography. Radiographic findings are normal in mild PS. With increasing severity, the characteristic findings are an increase of size of the right ventricle, poststenotic dilatation of the proximal arteries, and oligemic-appearing lung fields (Fig. 5–16).

Electrocardiography. The mildest cases show no abnormalities. With increasing severity, the pattern of RVH appears—right axis deviation; tall, peaked P waves in leads II, III and V_1; tall R waves in lead V_1; and finally, inverted T waves and ST depression in lead V_1.

Echocardiography. Doppler ultrasound provides a reliable estimate of transpulmonic gradient and is usually performed at the same time as two-dimensional echocardiography.

Treatment. In the asymptomatic patient without cardiomegaly, the only real complication is bacterial endocarditis. Prophylactic antibiotics should be given for surgery and dental work.[10]

If there are any symptoms, lack of normal growth, or cardiomegaly, the patient should be considered for percutaneous balloon valvuloplasty, which has surpassed surgical resection as the treatment of choice for most patients with congenital valvular pulmonic stenosis.[35]

A postprocedure murmur of PR should give no cause for alarm. PR unlike aortic regurgitation, is well tolerated because of the low pressures in the pulmonary artery. With relief of PS, the patients are almost routinely restored to normal health. They must still use prophylaxis during surgery and dental work because bacterial endocarditis is a continued threat.[10]

PULMONIC REGURGITATION

Of all valve lesions, PR is the most unimportant from a hemodynamic standpoint. The reason is that the pulmonary artery diastolic pressure is so low that the amount of blood regurgitated is too small to have much hemodynamic significance (Table 5–13).

The murmur of PR is the same as that of aortic regurgitation—a soft, high-pitched decrescendo diastolic murmur along the left sternal border (see Fig. 5–15*B*). This murmur is likely to be encountered in two situations:

1. The murmur is associated with severe pulmonary hypertension from any cause; this is the most frequent cause of PR. The term Graham Steell's murmur has been used for that heard in connection with severe mitral stenosis. Usually, this murmur has in reality turned out to be due to AR.
2. After surgical or balloon pulmonary valvotomy for congenital pulmonic stenosis, there often is a murmur of

TABLE 5–13. PULMONIC REGURGITATION

Etiology:	Secondary to pulmonary hypertension Following valvotomy for congenital pulmonic stenosis
Clinical Course:	Generally benign
Symptoms and Complications:	Usually none Bacterial endocarditis if postvalvotomy
Indications for Surgery:	Generally unnecessary

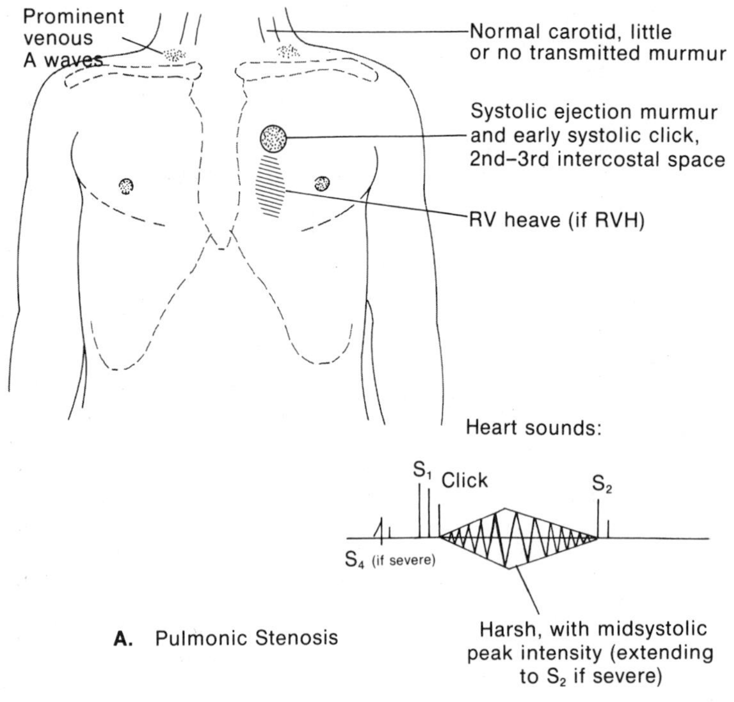

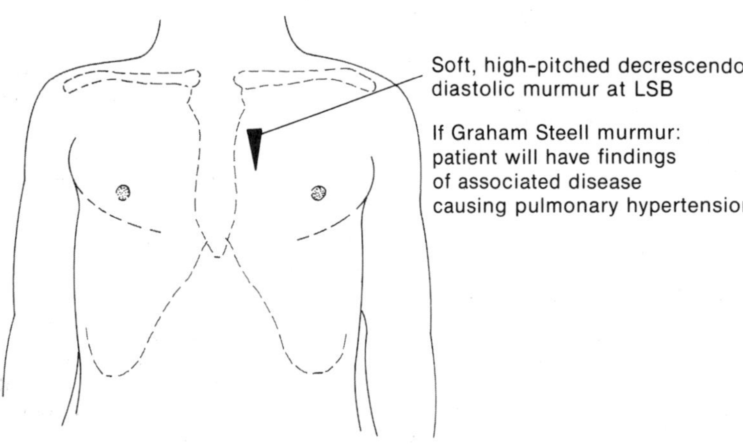

FIGURE 5–15. Typical findings on physical examination in (*A*) valvular pulmonic stenosis and (*B*) pulmonic regurgitation.

PR. As noted previously, it is clinically of no import except that prophylaxis against bacterial endocarditis must be taken for surgery and dental work.

TRICUSPID STENOSIS

Etiology. Tricuspid stenosis is usually caused by rheumatic fever but is rarely congenital or associated with the carcinoid syndrome. When the cause is rheumatic, there is always associated mitral stenosis and often aortic valve disease as well.

Course. Blockage at the tricuspid valve reduces cardiac output and in diastole produces a higher pressure in the right atrium than in the right ventricle. The elevated right atrial pressure necessitates a corresponding rise of venous pressure. If the stenosis, which is a fixed, obstructive lesion slowly progressing over months and years, is untreated surgically, chronic venous engorgement becomes the paramount manifestation (Table 5–14). It produces advanced cardiac cirrhosis of the liver, jaundice, cachexia in part from poor liver function and in part from malabsorption in the gut, ascites, and refractory edema. These occur when the venous pressure exceeds about 10 mm Hg. Venous and right atrial pressures rise further with the onset of atrial fibrillation. Peripheral manifestations of edema are out of proportion to those in the lung. Characteristically, symptoms of mitral stenosis are negligible, and pulmonary congestion is absent, as are paroxsymal nocturnal dyspnea, hemoptysis, or episodes of acute pulmonary edema.

Physical signs in addition to the findings just described are a diastolic rumble similar to that of mitral stenosis that increases in intensity on deep inspiration. It is best heard adjacent to the xiphoid process and is transmitted toward the apex (Fig. 5–17*A*).

Radiography. Characteristic changes are those of a large right atrium without significant engorgement of the lung fields.

Electrocardiography. Tall, peaked P waves in the absence of a pattern of RVH are characteristic. An almost

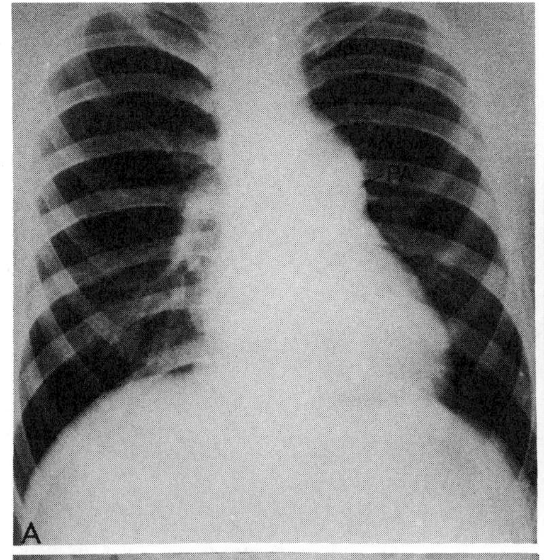

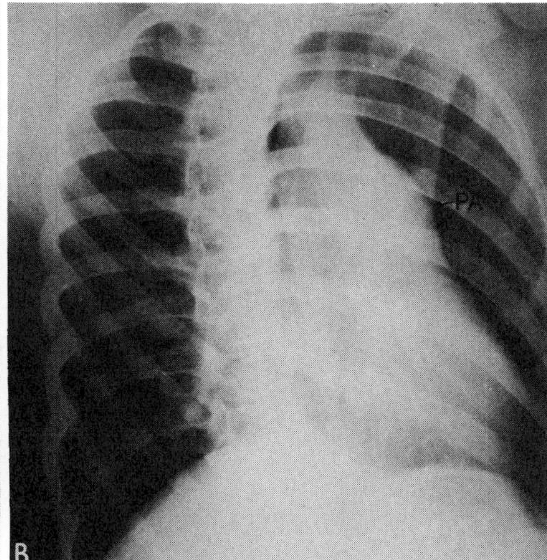

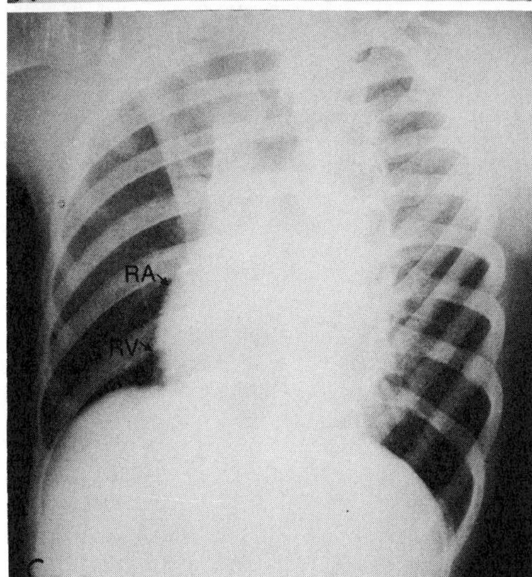

FIGURE 5–16. Chest films of patient with pulmonic stenosis. The posteroanterior view (*A*) reveals a dilated pulmonary artery segment, also revealed by the right anterior oblique view (*B*). The left anterior oblique view (*C*) shows the right border of the heart, although right ventricular dilatation is not clearly present. The lung fields are relatively oligemic. (Radiographs courtesy of Department of Radiology, Brigham and Women's Hospital, Harvard Medical School, Boston, MA.)

unique pattern for tricuspid stenosis is a small QRS complex of rsR′ configuration in leads V_1 and V_2 associated with a P wave of greater amplitude than the QRS complex.

Echocardiography. The pattern of motion of the stenotic tricuspid valve is similar to that of the mitral valve in mitral stenosis.

Cardiac Catheterization. The fundamental diagnostic finding is a higher right atrial than right ventricular diastolic pressure. The cardiac output is low. Critical valve narrowing, as for the mitral valve, is 1 cm^2 or less.

Treatment. Medical therapy has limited value. Diuretics and salt restriction are about the only effective treatment, unless the patient has atrial fibrillation, in which case digitalization is indicated to control the ventricular rate. Tricuspid valve replacement is highly effective and is clearly indicated when peripheral manifestations appear. Percutaneous balloon valvuloplasty may be an alternative in some patients.[36]

TABLE 5–14. TRICUSPID STENOSIS

Etiology:	Usually rheumatic Occasionally congenital or associated with carcinoid
Clinical Course:	Slowly progressive chronic venous engorgement Associated mitral stenosis
Symptoms and Complications:	Atrial fibrillation Severe edema Cardiac cirrhosis Only mild manifestations of the mitral valve disease
Indications for Surgery:	Appearance of peripheral manifestations

TRICUSPID REGURGITATION

Etiology. Pulmonary hypertension of any etiology results in right ventricular dilatation and failure, and dilatation of the right ventricular chamber results in functional tricuspid regurgitation (TR) in the same way that papillary muscle dysfunction of the left ventricle produces mitral regurgitation. The commonest underlying causes of functional tricuspid regurgitation produced by pulmonary hypertension are, in addition to primary pulmonary hypertension, mitral stenosis or regurgitation or both, aortic stenosis, and chronic obstructive pulmonary disease. Less commonly, tricuspid regurgitation results from rheumatic disease of the valve. When tricuspid regurgitation is caused by rheumatic disease, mitral stenosis always coexists, and there may also be aortic valve involvement.

Acute bacterial endocarditis involving the tricuspid valve

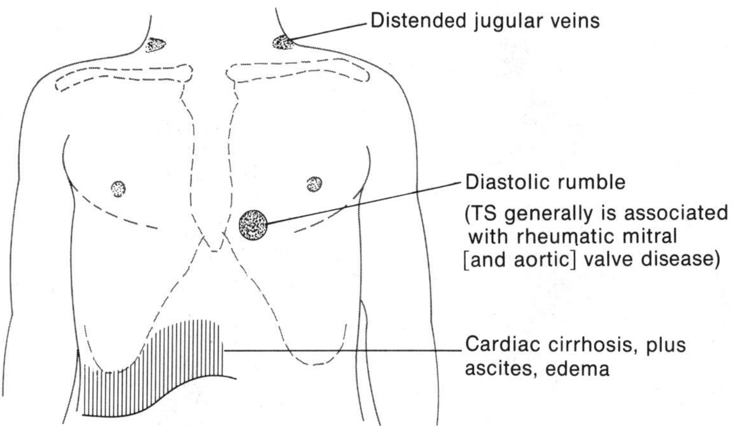

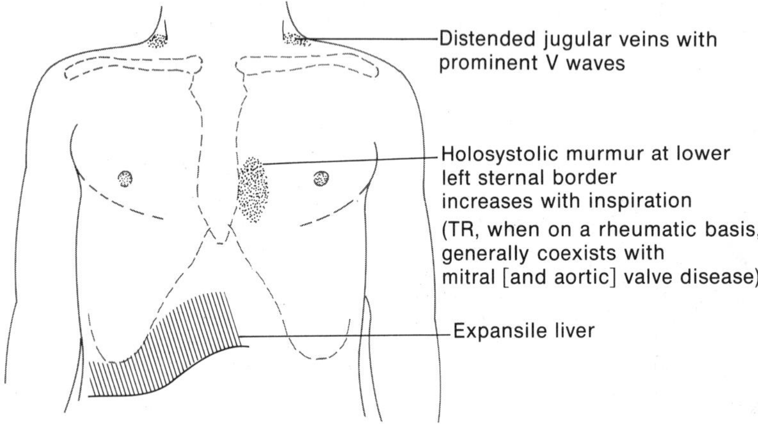

FIGURE 5–17. Typical findings on physical examination in (*A*) tricuspid stenosis and (*B*) tricuspid regurgitation.

is not infrequently seen in intravenous drug abusers. This is usually due to *Staphylococcus* or other virulent organisms that can produce rapidly incapacitating tricuspid regurgitation.

The malignant carcinoid syndrome may produce either tricuspid stenosis or TR, or both, and may be recognized by distinctive echocardiographic features. Ebstein's anomaly of the tricuspid valve is the commonest congenital cause of TR.

Clinical Picture. The patient is usually either a middle-aged woman with severe mitral stenosis or a narcotic addict presenting with fever. Symptoms are not distinctive but include fatigue and dyspnea related to a low cardiac output. As with tricuspid stenosis, pulmonary congestive symptoms are characteristically minimal, and systemic congestion (ascites and edema) is prominent (Table 5–15).

Physical Examination. Atrial fibrillation occurs in over 80% of patients with chronic TR. Prominent V waves in jugular veins are usually but not always present and by themselves are not diagnostic. The liver may be pulsatile. The most important physical sign is the murmur (see Fig. 5–17*B*). This is holosystolic and is best heard along the lower left sternal border. It is diagnostic of TR when it increases in intensity on deep inspiration. Unfortunately, this change on inspiration is not always present owing to a fixed stroke output. As the right ventricle dilates and fails, its diastolic pressure rises, as does that in the systemic veins. When venous pressure exceeds 10 mm Hg, edema and ascites appear.

Radiography. Both the right atrium and the right ventricle are enlarged. The overall size is often great, owing in part to coexisting valve lesions. Lung fields are characteristically not congested, even when there is coexisting severe mitral stenosis (Fig. 5–18).

TABLE 5–15. TRICUSPID REGURGITATION

Etiology:	Secondary to pulmonary hypertension Rheumatic deformity of the valve Acute bacterial endocarditis Malignant carcinoid syndrome Ebstein's anomaly of the tricuspid valve
Clinical Course:	Slowly progressive chronic venous engorgement and symptoms of low cardiac output Associated mitral stenosis
Symptoms and Complications:	Atrial fibrillation Severe edema Cardiac cirrhosis Fatigue and dyspnea related to low cardiac output Minimal pulmonary congestive symptoms
Indications for Surgery:	Symptomatic disability and pulmonary artery systolic pressure <60 mm Hg, indicating that free tricuspid regurgitation is due to valve deformity rather than secondary to pulmonary hypertension Continued fever or refractory right ventricular failure in a patient with endocarditis of the tricuspid valve

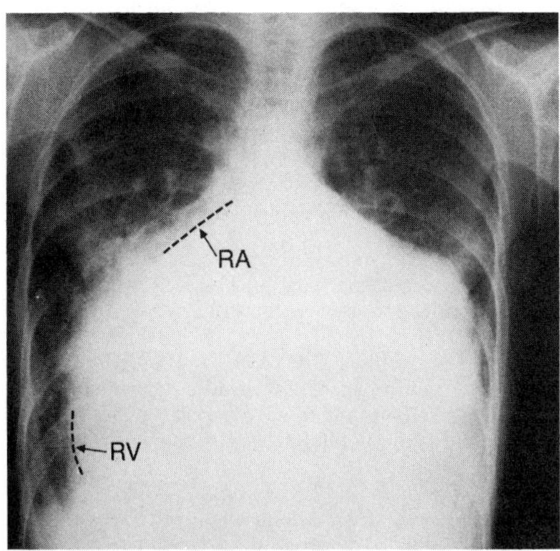

FIGURE 5–18. Posteroanterior view of the chest in a patient with severe tricuspid regurgitation. The right heart border is grossly enlarged owing to dilatation of the right atrium and right ventricle. The right mainstem bronchus is seen to be displaced upward by the dilated right atrium. The patient also has severe mitral regurgitation so that left ventricular and atrial enlargement are present as well. (Courtesy of Department of Radiology, Brigham and Women's Hospital, Harvard Medical School, Boston, MA.)

Electrocardiography. About half the patients with TR have right bundle branch block, an unusual pattern in mitral and aortic valve disease. Atrial fibrillation is customary.

Echocardiography. This is useful in distinguishing structural causes of TR (manifested by an abnormality of the valve) from functional abnormalities (normal-appearing tricuspid valve leaflets).

Doppler ultrasound is extremely reliable for detecting the presence of TR, although quantitation of the severity of TR is approximate at best.

Cardiac Catheterization. Injection of contrast medium into the right ventricle through a catheter often produces factitious TR because the catheter interferes with tricuspid valve closure. A large V wave may be detected in the right atrial pressure tracing. There is currently no satisfactory way of evaluating TR quantitatively, but by measuring the right ventricular and pulmonary artery pressures, it is possible to decide whether the TR is caused by an anatomically deformed valve or is secondary to pulmonary hypertension—in other words, whether the tricuspid valve, as well as the mitral valve, needs to be replaced.

Medical Therapy. This may produce dramatic improvement if the tricuspid regurgitation is functional (i.e., secondary to pulmonary hypertension). Bedrest, diuretics, salt restriction, and digitalization may result in loss of edema and ascites, production of quieter heart action, and diminution, if not disappearance, of the murmur of TR.

When TR has an organic etiology with valve deformity (rheumatic fever and bacterial endocarditis), the response is less dramatic but may still be effective.

Surgical Intervention. This is usually implemented because of disability resulting from the tricuspid regurgitation plus that produced by the presence of the associated valve lesions (mitral and aortic). If severe pulmonary hypertension is present (a right ventricular systolic pressure of over 60 mm Hg), it can be anticipated that the TR will become inconsequential following mitral valve replacement because of the immediate postoperative fall of pulmonary artery and right ventricular systolic pressures to almost normal levels. If the pulmonary artery systolic pressure is less than 60 mm Hg, one can assume that free TR is due in part or mainly to anatomic deformity of the valve. Tricuspid valve repair or replacement is then mandatory, along with mitral and maybe aortic valve replacement.

When TR results from bacterial endocarditis tricuspid valve replacement may become mandatory either for hemodynamic reasons or because of continued fever. Severe TR can be life-threatening because of refractory right ventricular failure. In some cases, it may be necessary to replace the tricuspid valve during the acute phase of the infection to make the process responsive to antibiotics. Delay in making the decision to operate may result in abscess formation throughout the body. These abscesses may not respond to antibiotic therapy and are one of the main causes of death in such patients.

REPAIR AND REPLACEMENT OF VALVES

Surgery. Surgical repair of damaged valves is becoming increasingly popular, although usually successful only with stenotic or regurgitant lesions of the mitral or tricuspid valve.[8, 16, 17, 37] When repair is not feasible, a prosthetic valve is inserted.[12] Several different design types are available. Of the currently available mechanical prostheses, the models include tilting disc, caged ball, and bileaflet valves. Alternatively, a bioprosthesis may be employed, most commonly consisting of a porcine aortic valve mounted on a supporting apparatus. Mechanical prostheses are more durable than porcine valves, but require lifelong anticoagulation (which can be avoided in most patients with porcine valves not in atrial fibrillation).

Balloon Valvuloplasty. An increasingly popular alternative to surgery for relief of valvular stenosis is percutaneous balloon valvuloplasty.[36] In this procedure, one or more balloons are placed across the stenotic valve during cardiac catheterization and then inflated, resulting in an improvement in orifice size. It has become widely accepted as an alternative to surgery for pulmonic and mitral stenosis, although its long-term efficacy in aortic stenosis is limited.[3, 29, 35]

REFERENCES

1. Omoto R, Kyo S, Matsumura M, et al: Evaluation of biplane color Doppler transesophageal echocardiography in 200 consecutive patients. Circulation 85:1237, 1992.
2. Slater J, Gindea A, Freedberg R, et al: Comparison of cardiac catheterization and Doppler echocardiography in the decision to operate in aortic and mitral valve disease. J Am Coll Cardiol 17:1026, 1991.
3. Turi ZG, Reyes VP, Raju BS, et al: Percutaneous balloon versus surgical closed commissurotomy for mitral stenosis. Circulation 83:1179, 1991.
4. Lefevre T, Bonan R, Serra A, et al: Percutaneous mitral valvuloplasty in surgical high risk patients. J Am Coll Cardiol 17:348, 1991.
5. Stollerman GH: Rheumatogenic group A streptococci and the return of rheumatic fever. Ann Intern Med 35:1, 1990.
6. Olson LJ, Subramanian R, Ackermann DM, et al: Surgical pathology of the mitral valve: A study of 712 cases spanning 21 years. Mayo Clin Proc 62:22, 1987.
7. Marks AR, Choong CY, Chir MBB, et al: Identification of high-risk and low-risk subgroups of patients with mitral-valve prolapse. N Engl J Med 320:1031, 1989.
8. Cohn LH: Surgery for mitral regurgitation. JAMA 260:2883, 1988.

9. Dajani AS, Bisno AL, Chung KJ, et al: Prevention of rheumatic fever: A statement for health professionals by the committee on rheumatic fever, endocarditis, and Kawasaki disease of the Council on Cardiovascular Disease in the Young, the American Heart Association. Circulation 78:1082, 1988.
10. Dajani AS, Bisno AL, Chung KJ, et al: Prevention of bacterial endocarditis: Recommendations by the American Heart Association. JAMA 264:2919, 1990.
11. Ross J Jr: Afterload mismatch in aortic and mitral valve disease: Implications for surgical therapy. J Am Coll Cardiol 5:811, 1985.
12. Crawford MH, Souchek J, Oprian CA, et al: Determinants of survival and left ventricular performance after mitral valve replacement. Circulation 81:1173, 1990.
13. Oleson K: The natural history of 271 patients with mitral stenosis under medical treatment. Br Heart J 24:349, 1962.
14. Roy SB and Gopinath N: Mitral stenosis. Circulation 38(Suppl 5):68, 1968.
15. Dexter L: Profiles in valvular heart disease. *In* Grossman W (ed): Cardiac Catheterization and Angiography. Philadelphia, Lea & Febiger, 1980, p 305.
16. Cohn LH, Allred EN, Cohn LA, et al: Long-term results of open mitral valve reconstruction for mitral stenosis. Am J Cardiol 55:731, 1985.
17. Farhat MB, Boussadia H, Gandjbakhch I, et al: Closed versus open mitral commissurotomy in pure noncalcific mitral stenosis: Hemodynamic studies before and after operation. Thorac Cardiovasc Surg 99:639, 1990.
18. Ross J Jr and Braunwald E: Aortic stenosis. Circulation 38(Suppl 5):61, 1968.
19. Vandeplas A, Willems JL, Piessens J, et al: Frequency of angina pectoris and coronary artery disease in severe isolated valvular aortic stenosis. Am J Cardiol 62:117, 1988.
20. Pellikka PA, Nishimura RA, Bailey KR, et al: The natural history of adults with asymptomatic, hemodynamically significant aortic stenosis. J Am Coll Cardiol 15:1012, 1990.
21. Kelly TA, Rothbart RM, Cooper CM, et al: Comparison of outcome of asymptomatic to symptomatic patients older than 20 years of age with valvular aortic stenosis. Am J Cardiol 61:123, 1988.
22. Kennedy KD, Nishimura RA, Holmes DR, et al: Natural history of moderate aortic stenosis. J Am Coll Cardiol 17:313, 1991.
23. Lund O: Preoperative risk evaluation and stratification of long-term survival after valve replacement for aortic stenosis: Reasons for earlier operative intervention. Circulation 82:124, 1990.
24. Isner J and the Mansfield Scientific Aortic Valvuloplasty Registry Investigators: Acute catastrophic complications of balloon aortic valvuloplasty. J Am Coll Cardiol 17:1436, 1991.
25. Holmes DR, Nishimura RA, and Reeder GS: In-hospital mortality after balloon aortic valvuloplasty: Frequency and associated factors. J Am Coll Cardiol 17:189, 1991.
26. McKay RG (for the Mansfield Scientific Aortic Valvuloplasty Registry Investigators): Overview of acute hemodynamic results and procedural complications. J Am Coll Cardiol 17:485, 1991.
27. Bashore TM, Davidson CJ, and the Mansfield Scientific Aortic Valvuloplasty Registry Investigators: Follow-up recatheterization after balloon aortic valvuloplasty. J Am Coll Cardiol 17:1188, 1991.
28. Nishimura RA, Holmes DR, Michela MA, et al: Follow-up of patients with low output, low gradient hemodynamics after percutaneous balloon aortic valvuloplasty: The Mansfield Scientific Aortic Valvuloplasty Registry. J Am Coll Cardiol 17:828, 1991.
29. Kuntz RE, Tosteson ANA, Berman AD, et al: Predictors of event-free survival after balloon aortic valvuloplasty. N Engl J Med 325:17, 1991.
30. Braunwald E, Lambrew CT, Rockoff SD, et al: Idiopathic hypertrophic subaortic stenosis: Description of the disease based upon an analysis of 64 patients. Circulation 29(Suppl 4):1, 1964.
31. Wynne J and Braunwald E: The cardiomyopathies and myocarditides: Toxic, chemical, and physical damage to the heart. *In* E Braunwald (ed): Heart Disease. Philadelphia, WB Saunders, 1992, pp 1394–1450.
32. Olson LJ, Subramanian R, and Edwards WD: Surgical pathology of pure aortic insufficiency: A study of 225 cases. Mayo Clin Proc 59:835, 1984.
33. Krayenbuehl HP, Hess OM, Monrad ES, et al: Left ventricular myocardial structure in aortic valve disease before, intermediate, and late after aortic valve replacement. Circulation 79:744, 1989.
34. Johnson LW, Grossman W, Dalen JE, et al: Pulmonic stenosis in the adult: Long-term follow-up results. N Engl J Med 287:1159, 1972.
35. Stanger P, Cassidy SC, Girod DA, et al: Balloon pulmonary valvuloplasty: Results of the Valvuloplasty and Angioplasty of Congenital Anomalies Registry. Am J Cardiol 65:775, 1990.
36. Turi ZG: Valvuloplasty. *In* Frankl WS and Brest AN (eds): Cardiovascular Clinics. Philadelphia, FA Davis, 1992, pp 293–326.
37. Stewart WJ, Currie PJ, Salcedo EE, et al: Intraoperative Doppler color flow mapping for decision-making in valve repair for mitral regurgitation: Technique and results in 100 patients. Circulation 81:556, 1990.

6

Congestive Heart Failure

EUGENE BRAUNWALD, MD

Heart failure, a clinical syndrome with characteristic symptoms and physical signs, is the condition in which an abnormality of *cardiac* function is responsible for the failure of the heart to pump blood in an amount commensurate with the requirements of the metabolizing tissues, or for its ability to do so only from an abnormally elevated filling pressure.[1] It may result from a primary abnormality of the heart muscle (e.g., in a cardiomyopathy); it may be secondary to ischemia (e.g., in coronary artery disease); or it may result from an extramyocardial abnormality that interferes with cardiac filling or emptying by placing an excessive burden on the heart (e.g., in hypertension or valvular heart disease). In some patients with heart failure, there is no detectable abnormality in the function of the heart muscle, per se. This occurs in two circumstances: (1) when the normal heart is suddenly presented with a load that exceeds its capacity, such as an acute hypertensive crisis, rupture of an aortic valve cusp, or massive pulmonary embolism and *myocardial* (but not heart) failure has not yet occurred; and (2) when there is impairment of ventricular filling. The latter can be caused by a variety of conditions, including tricuspid or mitral stenosis, constrictive pericarditis or cardiac tamponade, or endocardial fibrosis without myocardial involvement.

Pathophysiology

The clinical manifestations of heart failure result from an inadequate cardiac output (forward failure) or from the damming of blood behind one or both ventricles (backward failure) or from both.[1,2] Two fundamental pathophysiologic abnormalities have been described in heart failure: (1) *systolic failure,* in which an inadequate volume of blood is ejected from the ventricle, leading to a compensatory rise of ventricular end-systolic and end-diastolic volumes, and to a reduction of the fraction of ventricular end-diastolic volume that is ejected during each beat, that is, of the ejection fraction. Systolic failure is the typical form of heart failure in chronic valvular regurgitation, chronic ischemic heart disease after myocardial infarction, and dilated cardiomyopathy; and (2) *diastolic failure,* in which the ventricle relaxes slowly or inadequately during diastole, leading to an elevation of ventricular diastolic pressure without an increase in ventricular diastolic volume; this form of heart failure is quite common, is typical of acute ischemia and of severe ventricular hypertrophy, and occurs in a variety of conditions including systemic hypertension, valvular aortic stenosis, hypertrophic cardiomyopathy, and constrictive pericarditis.

In many patients, both systolic and diastolic failure occur simultaneously. Both systolic and diastolic heart failure cause (1) an elevation of volume and pressure in the atrium and venous and capillary beds upstream to it, that is, behind the failing ventricle; (2) an increase in transudation of fluid from the capillary bed into the interstitial space; and (3) an augmentation of extracellular fluid volume, resulting in edema (pulmonary edema in the case of left ventricular failure and peripheral edema in the case of right ventricular failure).

The symptoms characteristic of heart failure result from an increase in fluid in the interstitial spaces of the lungs, liver, subcutaneous tissues, and serous cavities and/or from a reduced cardiac output, which results in diminished perfusion of vital organs. Organs that may have diminished perfusion include the brain (leading to confusion), the skeletal muscles (leading to weakness), and the kidneys (producing sodium and water retention and contributing to the development of edema).

Fluid retention in heart failure is due, in part, to activation of the renin-angiotensin-aldosterone system.[3] Reduced cardiac output increases the elaboration of renin, which, acting through the activation of angiotensin, induces the release of aldosterone. Initially, abnormally retained fluid localizes behind the specific cardiac chamber that is affected. Thus, at first, symptoms secondary to pulmonary congestion predominate in patients with infarction of the left ventricle, hypertension, and aortic and mitral valve disease. However, with the passage of time pulmonary hypertension develops; the right ventricle fails; fluid accumulation becomes generalized; and ankle edema, congestive hepatomegaly, ascites, and pleural effusion occur.

The clinical manifestations of heart failure depend on a variety of factors, including the patient's age, the cause of the heart failure, the extent and rate of development of the impaired cardiac performance, and the precipitating causes of heart failure. The rapidity with which the syndrome develops is of particular importance. Thus, when a previously normal person suddenly develops a large myocardial infarction, rupture of a valve secondary to infective endocarditis, occlusion of a large segment of the pulmonary vascular bed by a pulmonary embolus, an arrhythmia with a very slow (<40/min) or rapid (>180/min) rate, serious heart failure characterized by a sudden reduction in cardiac output with symptoms due to inadequate organ perfusion or acute congestion of the venous bed behind the affected ventricle occurs. However, if the same abnormality develops gradually, the patient adjusts to and tolerates it more readily.

In most forms of heart disease—that is, congenital, valvular, rheumatic, hypertensive, ischemic, and cardiomyopathic—heart failure is characterized by a low cardiac output. However, a number of high-output states, including anemia, pregnancy, thyrotoxicosis, arteriovenous fistulas, beriberi, and Paget's disease of bone, may lead to heart failure as well. Low-output heart failure is characterized by peripheral vasoconstriction and cold, pale, and cyanotic extremities, and in late stages by a decline in stroke volume and narrowing of the pulse pressure. In high-output heart failure, on the other hand, the extremities are usually warm and flushed, and the pulse pressure is normal or widened.

CAUSES OF HEART FAILURE

The causes of heart failure can be usefully divided into three separate categories.

Fundamental Causes. These are the biochemical and physiologic mechanisms responsible for an impairment of cardiac contraction.

Underlying Causes. These are the congenital or acquired structural abnormalities that affect the peripheral and coronary vessels, myocardium, or cardiac valves and are responsible for the increased hemodynamic burden or the myocardial dysfunction that leads to heart failure. It is vital to recognize the underlying causes of heart failure, since appropriate management, for example, surgical correction of a congenital heart defect or of an acquired valvular abnormality or pharmacologic management of hypertension, may prevent the development or recurrence of heart failure.

Precipitating Causes. These are the specific causes or incidents responsible for approximately 50% of episodes of clinical heart failure. Since treatment of the precipitating cause usually rapidly terminates an episode of heart failure and may be lifesaving, it is as important to be cognizant of the precipitant as of the underlying causes.

Inappropriate Reduction of Therapy. Probably the most common (yet most readily avoidable) precipitating cause of heart failure is the inappropriate relaxation of the intensity of treatment. Many patients with serious underlying heart disease may be asymptomatic or only mildly symptomatic for as long as they adhere to their treatment regimen. Without proper, detailed, and explicit instructions, the patient who is doing well clinically may incorrectly assume that his or her underlying condition has been cured and may voluntarily diminish the intensity of therapy and thus precipitate a bout of congestive heart failure. Dietary excesses of sodium, often indulged in on vacations or holidays or when the person responsible for preparing the patient's meal is unavailable, are frequent causes of cardiac decompensation.

Arrhythmias. Cardiac arrhythmias occur commonly in patients with structural heart disease and commonly precipitate heart failure. *Tachyarrhythmias* impair cardiac function by reducing the time available for ventricular filling; this is of particular importance in patients with mitral stenosis, marked ventricular hypertrophy, and obstructive coronary artery disease. *Bradyarrhythmias* in patients with underlying myocardial disease often depress cardiac output since the stroke volume cannot increase, and these arrhythmias may intensify or precipitate heart failure. In addition to disturbances of heart rate, many arrhythmias result in a dissociation between atrial and ventricular contraction, which causes loss of the atrial booster pump mechanism and impairment of ventricular filling. This lowers cardiac output and raises atrial pressure. Atrioventricular dissociation is particularly troublesome in patients with a stiff ventricle and diastolic failure in whom the atrial booster pump mechanism is especially important. The abnormal intraventricular conduction that occurs in many arrhythmias, such as ventricular tachycardia, results in a loss of the normal synchronicity of ventricular contraction, which in turn may also precipitate or intensify heart failure.

Systemic Infection. Any serious infection may induce cardiac failure as a consequence of increased total metabolism, resulting from fever and discomfort, both of which increase the hemodynamic burden on the diseased heart. Patients with left ventricular failure and pulmonary congestion are particularly susceptible to pulmonary infections, which, in turn, may intensify heart failure.

Pulmonary Embolism. This is a frequent complication in patients with congestive heart failure, especially when they are confined to bed and in turn often intensifies the severity of heart failure. Pulmonary emboli may increase the hemodynamic burden on the right ventricle by elevating right ventricular systolic pressure and cause fever, tachypnea, and tachycardia.

Physical, Environmental, and Emotional Excesses. Severe fatigue, intense exertion, and severe climatic changes—particularly excessive heat and humidity—commonly increase the hemodynamic burden placed on the left ventricle and precipitate cardiac failure.

Systemic Hypertension. The rapid elevation of arterial pressure, which may occur in some instances of hypertension of renal origin or upon discontinuation of antihypertensive medication, may cause cardiac decompensation.

Myocardial Infarction. In patients with chronic but compensated ischemic heart disease, a new infarct, sometimes silent clinically, may further impair ventricular function and precipitate heart failure.

Cardiac Infection and Inflammation. The development of acute rheumatic fever and a variety of allergic or infectious processes affecting the myocardium may further impair myocardial function in patients with pre-existing heart disease. The anemia, fever, additional valvular damage, and myocarditis that may develop as a consequence of infective endocarditis are important precipitants of heart failure.

High-Output States. Although the normal heart is capable of augmenting its output, this is often not the case for the diseased heart; therefore, heart failure may be precipitated in patients with underlying heart disease who are compensated but who develop a hyperkinetic circulatory state, such as pregnancy, anemia, or hyperthyroidism.

Development of an Unrelated Illness. Heart failure may also be precipitated in patients with compensated heart disease who develop an unrelated illness, such as renal failure, prostatic obstruction, or parenchymal liver disease. The administration of blood transfusions, corticosteroids, nonsteroidal anti-inflammatory agents, or estrogens with sodium-retaining properties for treatment of a noncardiac illness may also cause heart failure in patients with compensated heart disease.

A cardinal principle in the management of patients with heart failure is to carry out a careful and systematic search for one or more of the aforementioned precipitating causes. Failure of recognition of the precipitating cause of heart failure may be responsible for otherwise refractory heart failure. However, if appropriate measures are taken to avoid the recurrence of these precipitating factors, heart failure may not recur for years.

SYMPTOMS OF HEART FAILURE

Respiratory Distress. Breathlessness is a cardinal manifestation of left ventricular failure.[4] In mild heart failure, exertional dyspnea may simply represent an aggravation of the breathlessness that normally occurs during activity. Typically, a specific task that a patient may have been able to carry out without difficulty evokes more breathlessness than previously. With progressive left ventricular failure, the intensity of exercise resulting in breathlessness declines.

Orthopnea is defined as dyspnea that develops upon assuming the recumbent position and that is relieved by sitting or standing. Its severity may be estimated from the number of pillows required to prevent nocturnal breathlessness. Patients often report that they awaken short of breath if their head has slipped off their pillows and that they may find relief from sitting in front of an open window. Orthopnea may be so severe that the patient cannot lie down at all and must spend the entire night in a sitting position, characteristically at the edge of the bed and slumped over a bedside stand. Patients with heart failure often have a nonproductive cough that is caused by pulmonary congestion and occurs during exertion or recumbency; such a cough has the same pathophysiologic and clinical significance as exertional dyspnea and orthopnea.[6]

Attacks of *paroxysmal cardiac dyspnea* usually occur at night.[5] Typically the patient awakens with a feeling of suffocation, sits bolt upright, and gasps for breath, but in contrast to orthopnea, paroxysmal nocturnal dyspnea often persists even when in the upright position. Bronchospasm is a common complicating factor; hence, *cardiac asthma* is an alternative name for this condition.

Full-blown *pulmonary edema* is characterized by extreme dyspnea and easily audible wet rales, rhonchi, and wheezes. Typically, the patient is anxious and perspires freely, and the sputum is frothy and blood-tinged. Gas exchange is severely compromised. Without effective treatment, progressive acidemia, hypoxemia, and respiratory arrest may ensue.

The various grades of dyspnea described above are clinical expressions of pulmonary venous hypertension and capillary congestion. Exertional dyspnea and orthopnea are caused by vascular and perivascular congestion, which is intensified by physical activity or recumbency. Paroxysmal nocturnal dyspnea is caused by interstitial edema. Pulmonary edema is caused by alveolar edema with transudation and expectoration of blood-tinged fluid.

Cheyne-Stokes respiration is characterized by alternating periods of hyperpnea and apnea and is secondary to the combination of depression of the sensitivity of the respiratory center to carbon dioxide and left ventricular failure.[7] Cheyne-Stokes respiration is caused by the combination of a cerebral lesion such as cerebral arteriosclerosis or stroke and left ventricular failure; the latter causes a prolongation of the circulation time from the lung to the brain and is responsible for the oscillations between hyperpnea and apnea.

Differential Diagnosis of Dyspneas.[4] The differentiation between cardiac and pulmonary dyspnea is an important clinical challenge. Most patients with dyspnea have obvious clinical evidence of disease of *either* the heart or the lungs, but sometimes differentiating between the two may be quite difficult. Patients with chronic obstructive lung disease may awaken at night with dyspnea, like patients with cardiac dyspnea, but this is usually associated with sputum production; the dyspnea is relieved after the patient rids himself or herself of secretions, rather than specifically by sitting up.

Acute *cardiac asthma* may be differentiated from acute *bronchial asthma* by the presence of diaphoresis, more bubbly airway sounds, and the more common occurrence of cyanosis in the former. However, the difficulty in distinguishing between cardiac and pulmonary dyspnea may be compounded by the coexistence of diseases involving both organ systems. The results of pulmonary function testing are often helpful in determining whether dyspnea is produced by heart or lung disease (Table 6–1). Reductions of vital capacity, maximum breathing capacity, forced expiratory flow rate, and pulmonary compliance occur characteristically in heart failure, whereas the resistance to air flow is usually only moderately increased. In addition, the patient with heart failure may have hyperventilation when at rest, with slight reductions both in the arterial P_{CO_2} and P_{O_2}.

It is often important to distinguish cardiac dyspnea on the one hand from dyspnea that has its basis in anxiety neurosis and in malingering on the other. With these latter two forms of shortness of breath, the complaint may be accompanied by the appearance of effortless or irregular respiration during an exercise test. Patients with anxiety neurosis often exhibit sighing respirations, dyspnea at rest, and difficulty in taking a deep breath, but their respiration is not rapid and shallow, as it is in cardiac dyspnea.

Other Symptoms. *Fatigue and weakness,* often accompanied by a feeling of heaviness in the limbs, are generally related to poor perfusion of the skeletal muscles in patients with a lowered cardiac output. *Nocturia* is characteristically a symptom that occurs early in the course of congestive heart failure. It is due to suppression of urine formation during the day when the patient is upright and active, with reversal of this pattern at night. In contrast, in renal failure there is no diurnal pattern of urine flow. *Impairment of memory,* headache, confusion, nightmares, and occasionally disorientation may occur, particularly in elderly patients with advanced heart failure, as a consequence of reduced cerebral perfusion.

In *right heart failure,* breathlessness, a cardinal manifestation of left ventricular failure, is uncommon because pulmonary congestion is usually absent. However, fatigue and a sense of heaviness of the limbs and anorexia are common symptoms in patients with predominant right heart failure. *Congestive hepatomegaly* may produce a dull ache or heaviness in the right upper quadrant or epigastrium that may be severe when the liver enlarges rapidly, such as in acute right heart failure. Anorexia, nausea, and a sense of fullness after meals occur as a consequence of congestion of the liver and the gastrointestinal tract.

Physical Examination

Extracardiac Findings. Patients with heart failure usually exhibit no distress when at rest but are often obviously dyspneic when observed during or immediately after activity. Patients with severe heart failure may ap-

TABLE 6–1. COMPARISON OF PULMONARY FUNCTION IN PATIENTS WITH CARDIAC AND PULMONARY DYSPNEA OF COMPARABLE SEVERITY*

Pulmonary Function Test	Chronic Obstructive Pulmonary Disease, Emphysema	Chronic Heart Disease	
		Left Ventricular Failure	*Mitral Stenosis*
Lung volumes			
VC	Considerably ↓	↓	↓
TLC	Considerably ↑	↓	↓
RV	Markedly ↑	Normal or slightly abnormal	Normal or slightly ↑
Ventilation			
Rest	↑	↑	↑
Exercise	Strikingly ↑	↑	↑
Dead space	Considerably ↑	↑	↑
Distribution of inspired gas	Abnormal	Normal or slightly abnormal	Normal or slightly abnormal
Distribution of ventilation-perfusion ratios	Uneven	Uneven to variable degree	Normal or somewhat uneven
Diffusing capacity			
Rest	↓	↓	Normal or ↓
Exercise	↓	↓	Normal or ↓
Carbon dioxide tension	↑	Normal or slightly ↓	Normal or slightly ↓
Oxygen tension, breathing air	Severely ↓	Normal or slightly ↓	Normal or slightly ↓
Breathing oxygen	Remains abnormal	Normal	Normal
Lung mechanics			
Compliance	↓	↓	Normal or ↓
Resistance (e.g., reflected by MBC, FEV)	Strikingly ↑	↑	Normal or ↑

*From Sieber EN and Katz LN: Heart Disease. New York, Macmillan, 1975, p 453.

VC = vital capacity; TLC = total lung capacity; RV = residual volume; MBC = maximum breathing capacity; FEV = forced expiratory volume; ↑ = increased; ↓ = decreased. Reduction roughly parallels the degree of heart failure.

pear anxious and exhibit signs of air hunger. Patients with the recent onset of heart failure are usually well nourished, whereas those with chronic, severe cardiac failure may appear malnourished and may even be cachectic.

The reduction of stroke volume when the patient in severe heart failure is at rest is reflected in a diminished pulse pressure and dusky discoloration of the skin. Increased activity of the adrenergic nervous system supports the circulation in heart failure and is responsible for peripheral vasoconstriction, presenting as pallor and coolness of the extremities and cyanosis of the digits. In addition, there may be diaphoresis, tachycardia, and distention of the peripheral veins secondary to venoconstriction. Arterial pressure is often slightly elevated.

Moist rales, commonly heard over the lung bases and often accompanied by dullness to percussion, are characteristic of congestive heart failure of at least moderate severity. Coarse, bubbling rales and wheezes heard over both lung fields and accompanied by the expectoration of frothy, blood-tinged sputum are present in acute pulmonary edema. Congestion of the bronchial mucosa or bronchospasm may produce rhonchi and wheezes.

Systemic venous hypertension can be detected by inspection of the jugular veins, which provides a useful index of right atrial pressure. Normally, the jugular venous pressure declines on exertion, but it usually rises in patients with right heart failure. In this condition, the liver usually enlarges *prior* to the development of edema, and often it remains enlarged when other symptoms of right heart failure have disappeared. The epigastrium may appear full, and there may be dullness on percussion of the right upper quadrant. The liver is usually tender if hepatomegaly has occurred rapidly and recently. In patients with mild right heart failure, the jugular venous pressure may be normal when the patient is at rest but rises to abnormal levels with compression of a congested liver, a sign known as the *hepatojugular reflux.* To elicit this sign, the liver should be compressed firmly, gradually, and continuously for 1 minute and the veins of the neck observed. Expansion of the jugular veins during and immediately after compression represents a positive test result and usually reflects the combination of a congested liver and inability of the right side of the heart to accept the transiently increased venous return.

Edema is a principal manifestation of congestive heart failure, but it does not correlate well with the height of the systemic venous pressure. Since a gain of extracellular fluid volume of about 5 liters is necessary before peripheral edema is evident, edema may take some time to develop after the onset of heart failure. Edema usually occurs first in the dependent portions of the body and is usually symmetric. In ambulatory patients cardiac edema is usually first noted in the feet or ankles at the end of the day and generally resolves after a night's rest. It is most commonly found over the sacrum in bedridden patients. Edema may become massive and generalized (anasarca) late in the course of heart failure, when it may involve the upper extremities, the thoracic and abdominal walls, and particularly the genital area. Long-standing edema results in pigmentation, reddening, and induration of the skin of the lower extremities, usually over the dorsum of the feet and the pretibial areas.

Hydrothorax usually occurs in patients with hypertension of both the systemic and the pulmonary venous beds, but it may also develop when there is very marked elevation of pressure in either venous bed. Hydrothorax is often bilateral; when it is confined to the right side of the chest, it is usually due to severe systemic venous hypertension. Less commonly, hydrothorax is limited to the left side, and in this case it is most commonly secondary to pulmonary venous hypertension. Hydrothorax usually intensifies dyspnea because it reduces vital capacity further.

Ascites occurs when the pressure in the hepatic veins and in the veins draining the peritoneum increases. It usually reflects long-standing systemic venous hypertension, and it may be more prominent than subcutaneous edema in patients with organic tricuspid valve disease and chronic constrictive pericarditis.

Intestinal absorption of fat may be impaired in heart failure[9] and rarely a protein-losing enteropathy may develop.[10] An increase in total metabolism may also occur in patients with heart failure. The combination of increased caloric expenditure and reduced caloric intake may lead to weight loss and in some cases to cardiac cachexia,[11] which may be severe enough to suggest the presence of a disseminated malignancy.

A low-grade temperature elevation (<37.7°C [100°F]) resulting from cutaneous vasoconstriction may occur in severe heart failure and usually subsides when compensation is restored.

Cardiac Findings. *Cardiomegaly* is a nonspecific finding and occurs in most patients with chronic heart failure. Protodiastolic sounds occurring 0.13 to 0.16 second after the second heart sound are common findings in healthy children and young adults. However, such sounds are rarely audible in healthy persons after 40 years of age but occur in patients of all ages with heart failure, in whom they are referred to as protodiastolic gallops or S_3 gallops. Thus, they generally signify the presence of heart failure in older adults. Gallop sounds emanating from the left ventricle are best heard at the apex with the patient in the left lateral recumbent position and are frequently palpable. They are usually louder *following* inspiration, in contrast to protodiastolic gallop sounds originating from the right ventricle, which are best heard *during* inspiration. Gallop sounds may sometimes be elicited by a brief bout of exercise.

Pulsus alternans is characterized by a regular rhythm with alternation of strong and weak contractions and must be distinguished from the alternation of strong and weak beats that occurs in pulsus bigeminus caused by coupled ventricular extrasystoles, in which the weak beat follows the strong beat by a shorter time interval than the strong beat follows the weak. Pulsus alternans may be detected either by palpation of the peripheral arteries, particularly the femoral artery, or by sphygmomanometry. Pulsus alternans (1) occurs most commonly in heart failure secondary to hypertension and aortic stenosis, coronary atherosclerosis, and cardiomyopathy; (2) is frequently associated with ventricular protodiastolic gallop sounds; (3) usually signifies the presence of advanced myocardial disease; (4) often disappears with treatment of heart failure; (5) is more commonly present during tachycardia; and (6) is often initiated by a premature beat.

With the development of left ventricular failure, pulmonary artery pressure rises and the sound of pulmonic valve closure (P_2) becomes accentuated. Systolic murmurs due to the mitral or tricuspid regurgitation, which may occur secondary to ventricular dilatation, are common in heart failure. Often these murmurs and the accentuation of P_2 diminish or disappear when cardiac compensation is restored.

Laboratory Findings

A high specific gravity of the *urine* and proteinuria are common in patients with overt heart failure. The blood urea nitrogen and creatinine levels are often moderately elevated, secondary to reductions in renal blood flow and glomerular filtration rate. The erythrocyte sedimentation rate may be unusually low. *Serum electrolyte* values are generally normal prior to treatment, even in cases of severe heart failure. However, prolonged rigid sodium restriction combined with intensive diuretic therapy, as well as the inability to excrete water, may lead to dilutional hyponatremia, which occurs despite an expansion of extracellular fluid volume and an increase in total body sodium. The serum potassium level is usually normal, although the prolonged administration of kaliuretic diuretics, such as the thiazides or loop diuretics, may result in hypokalemia. In terminal heart failure with secondary renal insufficiency, hyperkalemia may be present.

Congestive hepatomegaly and cardiac cirrhosis are often associated with impaired hepatic function, characterized by abnormal levels of serum glutamic oxaloacetic transaminase (SGOT) and other liver enzymes.[12] Increases in both the direct and indirect reacting bilirubins are common, and in severe cases of acute right ventricular failure, frank jaundice may occur.

Chest Roentgenogram

The size and shape of the cardiac silhouette provide important information concerning the precise nature of the underlying heart disease, and the plain chest film serves as a useful, though not very sensitive, screening test for heart failure. In the presence of normal pulmonary capillary pressure with the subject in the erect position, the lung bases are better perfused than the apices, and the vessels to the lower lobes are significantly larger than are those to the upper lobes. When the pulmonary capillary pressure is slightly elevated (i.e., ~13 to 17 mm Hg), the pulmonary vessels in the lower lobes become compressed, and there is an equalization in the size of the vessels to the apices and bases. There is further constriction of the vessels to the lower lobes and dilatation of the vessels to the upper lobes, that is, pulmonary vascular redistribution, with greater pressure elevation (~18 to 23 mm Hg). When pulmonary capillary pressures exceed approximately 20 mm Hg, interstitial pulmonary edema develops (Fig. 6–1); this may be manifest as Kerley's lines, that is, sharp linear densities of interlobular interstitial edema most prominent at the lung bases. In addition, there may be a loss of sharpness of central and peripheral vessels and spindle-shaped accumulations of fluid between the lung and adjacent pleural surface. Alveolar edema characterized by diffuse haziness of the lung fields and large pleural effusions usually occurs when the pulmonary capillary pressure exceeds 25 mm Hg.

Radionuclide Ventriculography and Echocardiography

Ventricular function can be conveniently assessed noninvasively by these methods. In radionuclide angiography, red blood cells labeled with ^{99m}Tc are rapidly injected intravenously, and their initial transit through the circulation is recorded (first-pass method) by means of a scintillation camera. Alternatively, in the equilibrium method, the changes in counts within the ventricle that occur during a series of cardiac cycles are determined. These two methods provide measurement of ejection fractions of both ventricles. Modifications of the method allow measurement of end-diastolic and end-systolic volumes. With systolic failure of the ventricle (discussed earlier), end-diastolic and end-systolic volumes rise while ejection fraction falls; pure diastolic failure has little effect on these measurements. Serial estimation of ejection fraction may be useful in following the course of patients with heart failure, as well as their response to therapy.

Two-dimensional echocardiography is equally useful (and less expensive) in assessing ventricular volume and ejection fraction. In addition, this technique provides measure-

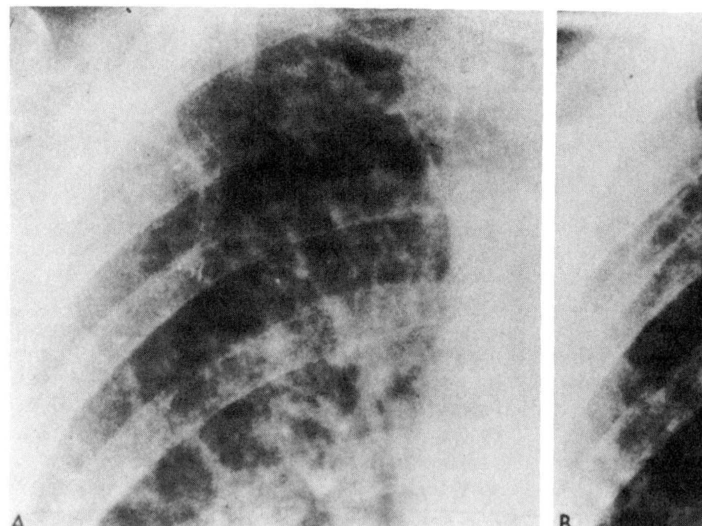

FIGURE 6–1. Interstitial pulmonary edema. *A,* Portable film made shortly after admission for an acute myocardial infarction. The vessels in the right upper lung are prominent and congested. However, their shadows can be delineated. At this time the patient was relatively asymptomatic. *B,* The following day the patient became tachypneic. The portable film shows an increase in the random shadows within the lung, obscuring the outlines of the pulmonary vessels. (From Rabin CB and Baron MG: Radiology of the Chest. Baltimore, Williams & Wilkins, 1979.)

ments of regional wall motion, ventricular wall thickness, and atrial size. When combined with Doppler ultrasonography, valve function can also be assessed.

TREATMENT

Three general approaches are employed in the treatment of heart failure. The first consists of removal of the underlying cause; whenever applicable, this is obviously the most desirable approach. It may involve surgical correction of structural abnormalities responsible for heart failure, such as congenital malformations and acquired valvular lesions, or correction of conditions such as infective endocarditis or hypertension by means of pharmacologic treatment. The second consists of the identification and removal of any precipitating cause.

The third general approach involves control of the congestive heart failure state. The three cornerstones of this approach are to (1) improve the pumping performance of the heart; (2) reduce the workload placed on the heart; and (3) control excessive salt and water retention. The vigor with which each of these measures is pursued in any individual patient should depend on the severity of the heart failure.

A condition as variable in etiology and clinical expression as congestive heart failure cannot be treated according to a simple formula.[7] The precise nature of the underlying condition and the rapidity of its progression, the presence of associated illnesses, and the patient's age, occupation, personality, family setting, and ability and motivation to cooperate with treatment must all be taken into account. Tables 6–2 and 6–3 are general guides to the therapy of adult patients with chronic congestive heart failure.

The general approach is to utilize, first, relatively simple means, such as mild restriction of physical activity, and reduction of dietary sodium intake. Treatment of heart failure should be begun when the first symptoms of diminished cardiac reserve occur, usually dyspnea during heavy exertion. Intense physical exertion, such as heavy labor and competitive or exhausting sports, are discontinued. Obese patients should be encouraged to lose weight, and systemic hypertension, if present, must be treated vigorously. If symptoms of heart failure persist despite these measures, an angiotensin-converting enzyme inhibitor and a digitalis glycoside are given. If symptoms secondary to extracellular fluid accumulation are present, a diuretic is added.

When a patient becomes symptomatic on ordinary exertion, such as shopping or cleaning the home, certain of the measures already taken are intensified. Full-time work or its equivalent is reduced, the patient is advised to take rest periods during the day, and a more powerful diuretic—furosemide, ethacrynic acid, or bumetanide—is substituted for the thiazide or thiazide equivalent.

In patients who are symptomatic at rest or with minimal activity, confinement to the home is necessary, and the dose of the cardiac glycoside is cautiously raised to achieve the maximum level consistent with an adequate margin of safety. All salt is eliminated at the table and in cooking, and a potassium-sparing diuretic that acts on the distal

TABLE 6–2. CONTROL OF CONGESTIVE HEART FAILURE*

1. Reduction of workload
   - (A) Physical and emotional rest
   - (B) Treatment of obesity
   - (C) Vasodilator therapy
   - (D) Assisted circulation
2. Improvement of pumping performance
   - (A) Digitalis glycoside
   - (B) Sympathomimetic agents
   - (C) Other positive inotropic agents
   - (D) Pacemaker
3. Control of excessive salt and water retention
   - (A) Low-sodium diet
   - (B) Diuretics
   - (C) Mechanical removal of fluid
     - (1) Thoracentesis
     - (2) Paracentesis
     - (3) Dialysis
     - (4) Ultrafiltration

*From Smith TW and Braunwald E: The management of heart failure. *In* Braunwald E (ed): Heart Disease: A Textbook of Cardiovascular Medicine. Philadelphia, WB Saunders, 1992, p 464.

TABLE 6–3. OUTLINE OF TREATMENT OF OVERT CHRONIC CONGESTIVE HEART FAILURE

1. Restriction of physical activity
   (A) Discontinue exhausting sports and heavy labor
   (B) Discontinue full-time work or equivalent activity, introduce rest periods during the day
   (C) Confine to house
   (D) Confine to bed, chair
2. Restriction of sodium intake
   (A) Eliminate saltshaker at table (Na = 1.6 to 2.8 g)
   (B) Eliminate salt in cooking and at table (Na = 1.2 to 1.8 g)
   (C) Institute A and B above plus low-sodium diet (Na = 0.2 to 1.0 g)
3. Diuretics
   (A) Moderately effective diuretics (thiazide†)
   (B) Loop diuretic (ethacrynic acid, furosemide, or bumetanide)
   (C) Loop diuretic plus distal tubular (potassium-sparing) diuretic
   (D) Loop diuretic plus thiazide and distal tubular diuretic
4. Vasodilators
   (A) ACE inhibitor, or combination of hydralazine plus isosorbide dinitrate
   (B) Intensification of oral vasodilator regimen
   (C) Intravenous nitroprusside
5. Digitalis glycosides
   (A) Usual maintenance dose
   (B) Maximum tolerable dose
6. Other inotropic agents (dopamine, dobutamine, amrinone)
7. Special measures
   (A) Cardiac transplantation
   (B) Dialysis
   (C) Assisted circulation (intraaortic balloon, left ventricular assist device, artificial heart)

*From Smith TW and Braunwald E: The management of heart failure. *In* Braunwald E (ed): Heart Disease: A Textbook of Cardiovascular Medicine. Philadelphia, WB Saunders, 1992, p 465.

†Thiazide or a diuretic of approximately equal potency, such as metalazone.

tubule, such as spironolactone or triamterene, is added to the "loop" diuretic. Any further deterioration usually requires hospitalization, during which physical activity is drastically curtailed, a low-sodium (200 mg) diet is instituted, the number and dose of diuretics are increased, an intravenous vasodilator is added to the angiotensin-converting enzyme inhibitor, and administration of sympathomimetic agents and the application of special measures such as the physical removal of fluid (thoracentesis, paracentesis, or dialysis) are considered.

Using the approach to the treatment of chronic heart failure outlined earlier, restriction of physical activity is carried out in a manner that disturbs the patient's lifestyle as little as possible; similarly, restriction of salt intake need be only mild initially, unless heart failure is severe. The judicious use of potent diuretics allows the patient to eat a nutritious and palatable diet for the major portion of the course of the disease.

General Measures

Restriction of Physical Activity. Restriction of physical activity is helpful in the treatment of heart failure by reducing the workload of the heart. Its intensity should depend, of course, on the severity of the heart failure. If, for instance, dyspnea occurs only while the patient is moving furniture or carrying large bundles of groceries, he or she should be advised to discontinue such activities. Competitive or exhausting sports should certainly be discouraged. However, physical activity to a level that does not regularly produce symptoms can and probably should be maintained. Often relatively minor adjustments in activity will allow a patient with mild heart failure to remain gainfully employed or be a homemaker. For instance, many women with mild-to-moderate congestive heart failure can cook, clean the home, and take care of their children, but they may experience difficulty in carrying bundles up several flights of stairs. Those tasks that are symptom-provoking should be avoided. Minor adjustments, such as the use of a golf cart, may allow the patient many hours of pleasurable activity. Patients with more severe heart failure are usually unable, and should not be permitted, to work full-time even at a relatively sedentary job. This should not mean, however, that total unemployment is necessary (or desirable). An adjustment of the work schedule, such as a reduction of the working day from 8 to 5 hours, with two mandatory 1-hour rest periods or a 4-day work week, with a day in the middle of the week during which the patient rests at home, is frequently helpful. Evening activities should be curtailed but need not be discontinued. Even some patients who are symptomatic on minimal activity and are therefore confined to the home are often able to lead more satisfying and productive lives by working for 2 or 3 hours a day at a desk.

Physical activity should be rigidly restricted in patients with acute or severe heart failure. Hospitalization of such patients is usually desirable, because this facilitates the search for a precipitating cause and allows adjustment of medication and institution of additional therapeutic measures while the patient is under observation. Physical rest, which is so important in the treatment of acute heart failure, does not mean complete bedrest in the recumbent position. Patients are often more comfortable and the preload is lower when they are in the sitting rather than the supine position. Patients should not be forced to use the bedpan, and trips to the bathroom can usually be allowed. The hazards of phlebothrombosis and pulmonary embolization should be recognized, and deep-breathing exercises, leg exercises, and use of elastic stockings are advisable. The use of anticoagulants should be considered in patients with severe heart failure, particularly those with a previous history of thromboembolic disease.

Emotional and mental rest are as important as physical rest for the patient with heart failure. Hospitalization is often beneficial, since it may remove the patient from a situation at home or at work that is anxiety-provoking. The physician should serve as a thoughtful, sympathetic listener and be available to discuss a variety of problems. It is often helpful to emphasize to the patient that if a precipitating cause of heart failure can be identified (and this is frequently the case), acute cardiac decompensation does not signify a hopeless outlook. It is important that the patient sleep well each night, and the use of flurazepam, 15 to 30 mg, as a hypnotic may be advisable. Diazepam, 2 to 5 mg twice a day, may be helpful as well in patients with marked anxiety.

Diet. It is possible to recommend only modest restriction of sodium intake in most patients with heart failure, with intensification of the diuretic regimen to prevent accumulation of extracellular fluid until the late stages of heart failure. The sodium content of the unrestricted American diet ranges from 3 to 6 g; simple elimination of the saltshaker at the table and of a few common foods such as pretzels, popcorn, salted nuts, and potato chips will reduce this to approximately half. Potassium chloride (substitute salt) may be used in place of ordinary table salt. There is no need to eliminate the salt in cooking and to make the diet unpalatable unless fluid retention occurs despite intensive use of diuretics. Indeed, the monotony and unpalatability of a low-sodium diet has caused unnecessary hardship to patients and their families and has often interfered with adequate nutrition.

Eliminating all salt from cooking will reduce sodium intake to approximately 1.5 g/day. Many common foods must be eliminated if it is necessary to reduce the sodium intake to 0.2 g/day in patients with severe congestive heart failure. Spices and herbs may be used to flavor the food in place of sodium chloride, and as wide a variety of foods as possible should be employed to diminish the monotony.

The patient may adjust water intake according to his or her own desire. However, in far-advanced congestive heart failure, the ability to excrete a free-water load may be impaired, with resultant dilutional hyponatremia. Only then is it desirable to restrict water intake so that the serum sodium concentration does not fall below approximately 130 mEq/l.

Oxygen. Oxygen inhalation, most conveniently performed by means of nasal prongs at 4 to 6 l/min, should be employed in patients with severe, acute congestive heart failure if the arterial oxygen saturation falls below 90%. This form of therapy is particularly useful in patients with heart failure precipitated by pulmonary infection or pulmonary infarction.

Digitalis

By stimulating the contractile function of the heart, digitalis improves ventricular emptying; that is, it augments the ejection fraction, increases cardiac output, promotes diuresis, and reduces the elevated diastolic pressure and volume of the failing ventricle with consequent reduction of symptoms resulting from pulmonary vascular congestion and increased central venous pressure.

Digitalis is usually effective in the common forms of chronic systolic, low-output heart failure associated with an excessive hemodynamic burden, such as hypertension and valvular heart disease, as well as in chronic ischemic heart disease. It is particularly valuable in the treatment of patients with atrial fibrillation or atrial flutter and rapid ventricular rates. The slowing of the ventricular rate, combined with the improved inotropic state of the myocardium, often causes striking and rapid clinical improvement. However, even in patients with sinus arrhythmia, digitalis may produce clinical improvement as a consequence of its positive inotropic action.[8, 9]

Cardiac glycosides are less effective or ineffective in cardiogenic shock, in the toxic and infectious myocarditides, in the various forms of cardiomyopathy, and in heart failure precipitated by infections, fever, anemia, thyrotoxicosis, beriberi, acute rheumatic fever, complete atrioventricular block, cor pulmonale, and in diastolic heart failure, especially constrictive pericarditis. Digitalis is contraindicated in patients with second-degree or unstable atrioventricular block, unless a pacemaker has been inserted, and in patients with hypertrophic obstructive cardiomyopathy.

Digitalis intoxication is a common, serious, and potentially fatal complication. The lethal dose of most glycosides is only about twice the dose that produces minor toxic manifestations, and the therapeutic-to-toxic ratios are identical for all cardiac glycosides. Advanced age, acute myocardial infarction or ischemia, hypoxemia, magnesium depletion, renal insufficiency, and hypothyroidism all reduce the tolerance of the patient to the digitalis glycoside or may provoke latent digitalis intoxication.

Anorexia, nausea, and vomiting, which are among the earliest signs of digitalis intoxication, are not of gastrointestinal origin but are caused by direct stimulation of centers in the medulla. Premature ventricular beats and bigeminal rhythm are the most frequent disturbances of cardiac rhythm caused by digitalis. Atrioventricular block of varying degrees of severity and nonparoxysmal atrial tachycardia with variable atrioventricular block are also characteristics of digitalis intoxication. The most serious arrhythmias are ventricular tachycardia and fibrillation. Withdrawal of the drug is of paramount importance. When tachyarrhythmias result from digitalis intoxication, treatment with a β-blocker, lidocaine, or phenytoin is indicated. Potassium should be administered if hypokalemia is present. In life-threatening tachyarrhythmias, the Fab fragments of high affinity cardiac glycoside specific antibodies are often quite effective.

Serum digoxin levels have a limited role in practice, because within the range of approximately 0.7 to 2.2 ng/ml, the level does not differentiate well between a therapeutic, a near-toxic, or a toxic state in an individual patient. It is necessary, therefore, to depend on clinical findings in deciding whether to increase, maintain, or decrease a patient's digoxin dose. In outpatient management, however, obtaining a routine serum digoxin level occasionally can be useful. An extremely low level (<0.5 ng/ml) may indicate noncompliance or the potential for achieving additional therapeutic benefit by increasing the dose. A high level (>2.2 ng/ml) in a clinically stable patient could indicate a state of near-toxicity, and, again depending on the clinical situation, may lead one to lower the dose.

Diuretics

In patients with mild heart failure, almost all diuretic agents are effective (Fig. 6–2). In the more severe forms of heart failure, the selection of diuretics is more difficult, and any existing abnormalities in the serum electrolyte levels must be taken into account. Overtreatment and resultant hypovolemia must be avoided, since excessive reduction of blood volume may reduce cardiac output, interfere with renal function, and produce profound weakness and lethargy.[10, 11]

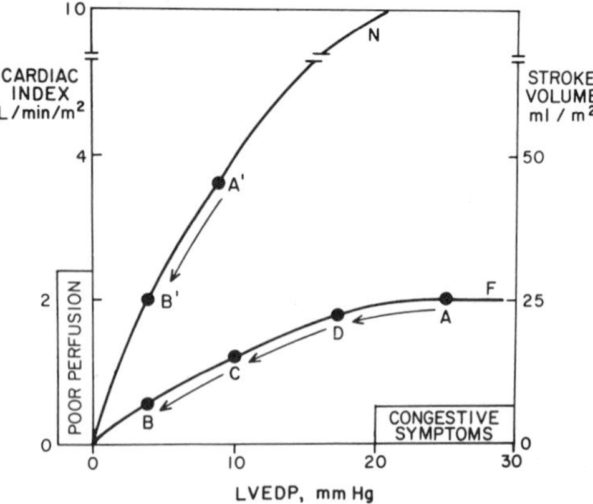

FIGURE 6–2. Effect of venodilator or diuretic therapy in a normal (N) subject (A′ → B′) and in patients with heart failure (F) and markedly elevated left ventricular filling pressure (A → D), and normal filling pressure (C → B). In all instances venodilators or diuretic therapy results in a decline in filling pressure; except in the patient with marked elevation of filling pressure, cardiac output declines. (From Smith TW and Braunwald E: The management of heart failure. *In* Braunwald E [ed]: Heart Disease. Philadelphia, WB Saunders, 1984, p 504.)

Thiazide Diuretics. These are widely used in clinical practice because of their effectiveness when administered orally and low cost. The administration of these drugs diminishes the need for very rigid dietary sodium restriction in patients with chronic heart failure. Many thiazide derivatives are available but differ principally in dosage and duration of action and therefore offer few significant advantages over the parent compound. They are well absorbed following oral administration and reduce the tubular reabsorption of sodium. Thiazide use results in the excretion of a hypertonic urine and may contribute to dilutional hyponatremia. Since they increase sodium-potassium exchange in the distal nephron, hypokalemia may result. Thus, potassium depletion is the chief adverse effect following prolonged administration and may enhance the likelihood of digitalis intoxication. Hypokalemia may be prevented by the oral supplementation of potassium chloride. Alternatively, intermittent dosage schedules, for example, omitting the diuretic every third day, and the addition of a potassium-retaining diuretic, such as spironolactone or triamterene, may be preferable.

Furosemide, Ethacrynic Acid, and Bumetanide. These so-called "loop diuretics" reversibly inhibit reabsorption throughout the nephron but especially inhibit active chloride reabsorption in the thick ascending limb of the loop of Henle. The major side effects of these potent agents result from their marked diuretic potency, which may produce circulatory collapse and reductions in the renal blood flow and glomerular filtration rate. A large increase in the urinary excretion of chloride, hydrogen, and potassium ions may cause alkalosis.

These drugs are readily absorbed orally and are excreted in the bile and urine. They are useful in all forms of heart failure, particularly in otherwise refractory heart failure including pulmonary edema. Their effectiveness may be potentiated by spironolactone, triamterene, or thiazide diuretics.

Potassium-Sparing Diuretics. The aldosterone antagonists, as well as triamterene and amiloride, act on the distal renal tubule by blocking the exchange between sodium and both potassium and hydrogen in the distal tubules and collecting ducts. These agents produce a sodium diuresis, but in contrast to the thiazides and loop diuretics, they tend to result in potassium retention.

The maximal effects of these agents are not observed for approximately 4 days. They are weak diuretics when used alone but may be quite effective when used in combination with a thiazide or loop diuretic in severe heart failure.

Vasodilator Therapy

Left ventricular afterload is increased in heart failure as a consequence of many influences that constrict the peripheral vascular bed in this condition. As ventricular end-diastolic volume rises, myocardial wall tension (afterload) rises further. In the presence of severely impaired cardiac function, the increase in afterload may also elevate myocardial oxygen consumption and left ventricular end-diastolic and pulmonary capillary pressures to levels that can produce pulmonary congestion and pulmonary edema. In many patients with heart failure, the ventricle is already operating on the flat portion of its Starling curve where any additional increase in afterload will reduce stroke volume. Conversely, a reduction of afterload will elevate the stroke volume of the failing ventricle.[12] Conventional vasodilators do not exert a direct effect on the heart, but their ability to relax vascular smooth muscle can result in profound improvement in both the clinical and hemodynamic state of the patient.

Venodilators cause a redistribution of the blood volume. Since the capacity of the venous bed is large, a relatively small reduction in venous tone can result in the pooling of substantial quantities of blood in this bed and its redistribution from the pulmonary to the systemic circuit. The hemodynamic effects of a pure venodilator resemble those of a diuretic (see Fig. 6–2). In the patient with heart failure and a markedly elevated filling pressure, venodilatation reduces filling pressure and thus relieves symptoms of pulmonary congestion without depressing cardiac output. Such agents should not be administered to patients in whom the preload or filling pressure has already been restored to normal by means of diuretic therapy or dietary sodium restriction or both.

Since the arterial vascular bed (just like the venous bed) is inappropriately constricted in patients with congestive heart failure, *arteriolar dilators* (afterload-reducing agents) are capable of augmenting stroke volume (and cardiac output) in patients with heart failure, and in this manner they reduce symptoms caused by poor perfusion (Fig. 6–3). The reduction in vascular resistance induced by afterload-reducing agents may be offset by an increase in cardiac output, and arterial pressure may decline only slightly or not at all. In normal subjects or patients with heart disease without heart failure, the reduction of systemic vascular resistance induced by afterload-reducing agents is associated with only small increases in cardiac output.

Arteriolar dilators may be particularly useful in patients with acute heart failure due to myocardial infarction and valvular regurgitation, as well as in patients with pulmonary edema secondary to hypertension. In patients with both acute and chronic intractable heart failure secondary to coronary artery disease or cardiomyopathy who are treated with arterial dilators, cardiac output increases substantially, the pulmonary wedge pressure falls, and the

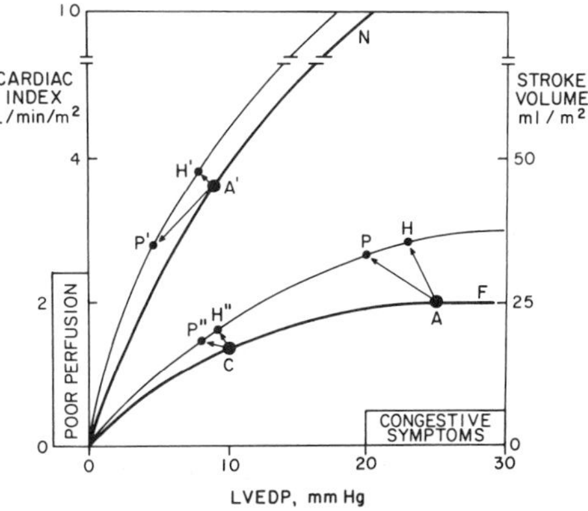

FIGURE 6–3. Effects of various vasodilators on the relationship between left ventricular end-diastolic pressure (LVEDP) and cardiac index or stroke volume in normal (N) and failing (F) hearts. H represents hydralazine or any other pure arterial dilator. It produces only a minimal increase in cardiac index in the normal subject (A′ → H′) or in the patient with heart failure with normal LVEDP (C → H″). In contrast, it elevates output in the patient with heart failure and elevated LVEDP (A → H). P represents a balanced vasodilator, such as sodium nitroprusside or prazosin. It reduces filling pressure in all patients, elevates cardiac output in patients with heart failure and elevated LVEDP (A → P), and has little effect on cardiac output in heart failure patients with normal filling pressures (C → P″). (From Smith TW and Braunwald E: The management of heart failure. *In* Braunwald E [ed]: Heart Disease. Philadelphia, WB Saunders, 1992, p 495.)

signs and symptoms of heart failure are relieved with only mild reduction of arterial pressure.

A number of vasodilators act on both the arterial and the venous beds (so-called "balanced" vasodilators), and their actions are intermediate between those of pure venous and pure arterial dilators (see Fig. 6–3). Most patients with heart failure display favorable reactions to these agents with augmentation of cardiac output and reduction of pulmonary capillary pressure but little decline in arterial pressure or elevation of heart rate.

Several vasodilators are available; they vary in their hemodynamic effects, locus and duration of action, and mode of administration. Hydralazine acts predominantly on the arterial bed, whereas nitroglycerin acts exclusively, or almost so, on venous circulation. Some agents, such as sodium nitroprusside, must be administered by continuous intravenous infusion. Nitroglycerin requires administration in ointment form when a prolonged effect is desired but is also useful when administered as a continuous infusion in patients with severe heart failure. Isosorbide dinitrate can be administered by the sublingual or oral routes.

For the treatment of *acute* heart failure, sodium nitroprusside is the ideal vasodilator. It has a rapid onset and brief duration of action, but continuous monitoring of arterial pressure is necessary.

Angiotensin-converting enzyme inhibitors have emerged as the best tolerated and most useful vasodilators.[13, 14] Their effectiveness has been established in rigorously defined randomized clinical trials in patients with heart failure across a wide spectrum, ranging from asymptomatic patients with left ventricular dysfunction to patients with end-stage heart failure. These drugs are "balanced" vasodilators.

The selection of the specific agent or combination of agents for any given patient should depend on the pathophysiologic state. For example, when the primary defect is a reduction of cardiac output or mitral regurgitation or both, an arterial vasodilator, such as hydralazine or the infusion of sodium nitroprusside (a balanced vasodilator) may be the drugs of choice; when pulmonary congestion is the principal defect, a venodilator, such as isosorbide dinitrate, is preferable. Nitroglycerin ointment applied prior to retiring is particularly useful in patients who have paroxysmal nocturnal dyspnea. In most patients, the clinician desires both to elevate cardiac output and to reduce pulmonary vascular pressures. An agent that acts on both the arterial and venous beds, such as a converting enzyme inhibitor, is indicated. These drugs have been shown to prolong life in patients with severe heart failure.

Sympathomimetic Amines

When heart failure persists and leads to hospitalization despite use of a combination of all the therapeutic measures described previously—restriction of physical activity and salt intake, cardiac glycosides, diuretics, and vasodilators—consideration should be given to the use of sympathomimetic amines.

Four sympathomimetic amines that act largely on β-adrenergic receptors—epinephrine, isoproterenol, dopamine, and dobutamine—are capable of improving myocardial contractility in various forms of heart failure. Dopamine and dobutamine appear to be most effective, since they increase cardiac output substantially. In low doses that are sufficient to augment contractility they exert relatively little effect on peripheral resistance. They must be administered by intravenous infusion and are useful in intractable heart failure, particularly in patients who have undergone cardiac surgery, and in some cases of myocardial infarction and shock or pulmonary edema. Although they improve the hemodynamics in these conditions, it is not clear whether they improve survival.

Dopamine, the naturally occurring immediate precursor of norepinephrine, has a combination of actions that makes it particularly useful in the treatment of a variety of hypotensive states and congestive heart failure. At very low doses—1 to 2 μg/kg/min—it dilates mesenteric and renal arterioles through stimulation of specific dopaminergic receptors, thus augmenting renal and mesenteric blood flow and sodium excretion. In the range of 2 to 10 μg/kg/min, dopamine stimulates myocardial β-adrenergic receptors but induces little tachycardia, whereas at higher doses it also stimulates α-adrenergic receptors, causes vasoconstriction, and elevates arterial pressure.

Dobutamine is a synthetic catecholamine that acts primarily on β-adrenergic receptors.[15] Consequently, it exerts a potent inotropic action. It has only a modest cardioaccelerating effect and lowers peripheral vascular resistance, but since it raises cardiac output, it has little effect on systemic arterial pressure. Given in continuous infusions, it is useful in the treatment of acute heart failure without hypotension. Like other sympathomimetic amines, it may be particularly valuable in the management of patients requiring relatively short-term inotropic support[16]—up to 1 week—in conditions that are reversible, such as the cardiac depression that sometimes follows open heart surgery, or in patients with acute heart failure who are being prepared for operation.

REFERENCES

1. Braunwald E: Pathophysiology of heart failure. *In* Braunwald E (ed): Heart Disease, 4th ed. Philadelphia, WB Saunders, 1992, pp 393–418.
2. Katz AM: Cardiomyopathy of overload: A major determinant of prognosis in congestive heart failure. N Engl J Med 322:100, 1990.
3. Packer M: Neurohormonal interactions and adaptations in congestive heart failure. Circulation 77:721, 1988.
4. Braunwald E and Grossman W: Clinical aspects of heart failure. *In* Braunwald E (ed): Heart Disease, 4th ed. Philadelphia, WB Saunders, 1992, pp 444–463.
5. Rees PJ and Clark TJH: Paroxysmal nocturnal dyspnea and periodic respiration. Lancet 2:1315, 1979.
6. Smith TW, Braunwald E, and Kelly RA: The management of heart failure. *In* Braunwald E (ed): Heart Disease, 4th ed. Philadelphia, WB Saunders, 1992, pp 464–519.
7. Poole-Wilson PA and Buller NP: Causes of symptoms in chronic congestive heart failure and implications for treatment. Am J Cardiol 62:31A, 1988.
8. Thomas R, Gray P, and Andrews J: Digitalis: Its mode of action, receptor and structure-activity relationships. *In* Testa B (ed): Advances in Drug Research, Vol 19. New York, Academic Press, 1989.
9. Antman EM and Smith TW: Pharmacokinetics of digitalis glycosides. *In* Smith TW (ed): Digitalis Glycosides. Orlando, FL, Grune & Stratton, 1985, p 45.
10. Hollenberg N: Diuretics in congestive heart failure. *In* Messerli FH (ed): Cardiovascular Drug Therapy. Philadelphia, WB Saunders, 1990.
11. Wilcox CS: Diuretics. *In* Brenner BM and Rector FC (eds): The Kidney, 4th ed. Philadelphia, WB Saunders 1991, pp 2123–2147.
12. Cohn JN (ed): Drug Treatment of Heart Failure, 2nd ed. Seacaucus, NJ, ATC International, 1988.
13. The SOLVD investigators: Effect of the angiotensin converting enzyme inhibitor enalapril on survival in patients with re-

duced left ventricular ejection fraction and congestive heart failure. N Engl J Med 325:293, 1991.
14. Stone CK, Uretsky BF, Linnemeier TJ, et al: Congestive heart failure: Hemodynamic effects of lisinopril after long-term administration in congestive heart failure. Am J Cardiol 63:567, 1989.
15. Majerus TC, Dasta JF, Bauman JL, et al: Dobutamine: Ten years later. Pharmacotherapy 9:245, 1989.
16. Stecy P and Gunnar RM: Is intermittent dobutamine infusion useful in the treatment of patients with refractory congestive heart failure? *In* Cheitlin M (ed): Dilemmas in Clinical Cardiology. Philadelphia, FA Davis, 1990, pp 277–289.

7

Hyperlipidemia

FRANK M. SACKS, MD

Despite intensive basic and clinical investigation of the role of plasma lipoproteins in atherosclerosis, many fundamental questions remain to be answered on selection of patients and appropriate therapy of abnormal plasma lipoprotein levels. In this chapter, a clear distinction is made between knowledge that is firmly established, that which comes from extrapolation, and that which is in the early stages of investigation. This chapter discusses common lipoprotein disorders that are linked to atherosclerosis and pancreatitis.

Plasma Lipoprotein System. For a review that is oriented to the nonexpert clinician, the reader is referred to Mahley and associates' article.[1] Lipoproteins provide the means by which fat-soluble molecules can be transported from one part of the body to another. Cholesterol (either unesterified or esterified), phospholipid, triglyceride, and the fat-soluble vitamins are located in blood within lipoprotein particles. Each type of lipoprotein particle requires the combination of a protein and phospholipid to form a hydrophilic outer coat that "surrounds" hydrophobic cholesterol esters and triglycerides (Fig. 7–1). The lipoproteins interact with each other, with plasma and cell surface-bound enzymes, and with cellular receptors in complex groupings of metabolic pathways. Lipoprotein metabolism in humans is still only rudimentarily understood, and much investigation is underway that is likely to provide new levels of sophistication in knowledge. It is worthwhile for a clinician to be aware of three metabolic pathways for lipoproteins: (1) chylomicron metabolism (postprandial lipoprotein metabolism), (2) the very low density lipoprotein (VLDL) to low-density lipoprotein (LDL) pathway, and (3) the high-density lipoprotein (HDL)/triglyceride pathway.

Chylomicrons are the largest lipoprotein particles. These globules of dietary fat are synthesized in intestinal cells, secreted into lymphatics, and transported into the systemic circulation. The principal protein on a chylomicron is apolipoprotein B48, which serves a structural role. Chylomicrons deliver their fat to muscle and adipose tissue by interacting with lipoprotein lipase, an enzyme that resides on the capillary endothelium. As the triglyceride is hydrolyzed, the chylomicron particle shrinks markedly and becomes what is termed a "remnant." A critical event in the conversion of chylomicrons to remnants is the acquisition of apolipoprotein E (apo E) by chylomicrons from HDL. Apo E provides the means by which the chylomicron remnant binds to receptors on hepatocytes and are removed from the circulation. Apo B48, unlike apo B100 on VLDL and LDL, is not capable of binding to cellular lipoprotein receptors. The most common reason for chylomicronemia is impaired activity of lipoprotein lipase. A structural mutation in apo E that impairs binding to receptors is a less common reason. Accumulation in blood of partially metabolized chylomicrons may contribute to atherosclerosis, since they are relatively rich in cholesterol ester and may be susceptible to oxidation.

VLDLs are synthesized in the fasting and postprandial state by hepatocytes. The major structural protein is apo B100 which also has a critical functional property of binding to cellular LDL receptors. Like chylomicrons, VLDL are triglyceride-rich and deliver the triglyceride to cells by

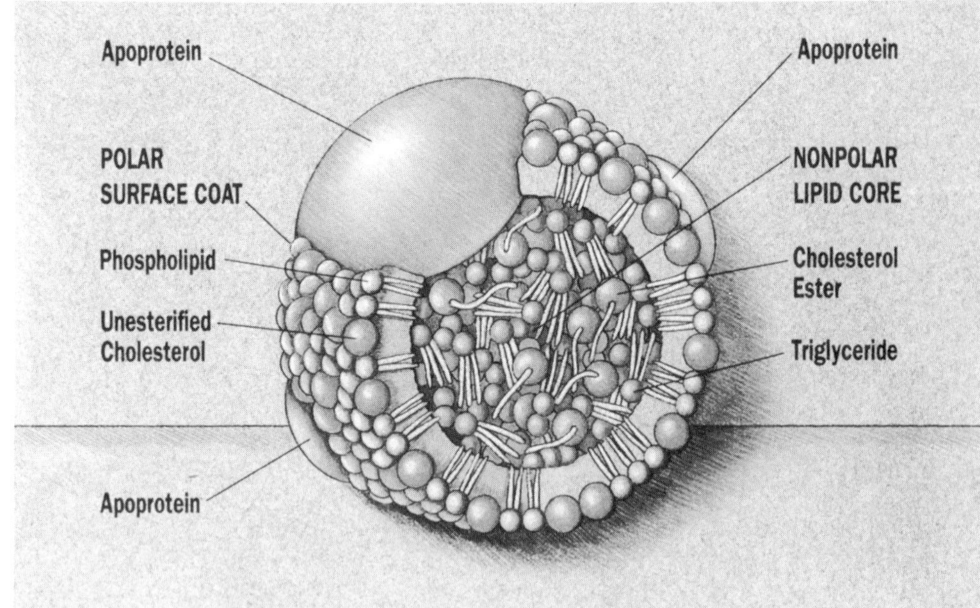

FIGURE 7–1. Basic structure of lipoproteins. (From Grundy SM: Slide Atlas of Lipid Disorders. New York, Gower Medical Publishing, 1990.)

means of lipoprotein lipase. During this process, VLDL shrink and become LDLs (Fig. 7–2). LDLs are then cleared from the circulation by the liver (~50%), steroidogenic tissues, and other tissues. An alternative route for the metabolism of VLDL particles is similar to that of chylomicrons. As VLDL is hydrolyzed, it can acquire apo E from HDL, bind to cells, and be removed from the circulation. Even without apo E, VLDL can employ apo B100 for cell binding and uptake, although less efficiently than LDL. VLDL particles that are destined to be removed directly without conversion to LDL are called "remnants." Impaired or inadequate lipolysis can cause accumulation of VLDL remnants as well as chylomicron remnants. Even if lipolysis is normal, overproduction of VLDL particles, as with alcohol or saturated fat intake, can cause accumulation of VLDL remnants if the rate of entry of VLDL into the circulation overwhelms the capacity of lipoprotein lipase.

HDLs are synthesized by the intestine and liver as discs of apolipoprotein A-I and phospholipid (Fig. 7–3). Nascent discoidal HDL rapidly become spherical, like other lipoproteins, as they "fill up" with cholesterol from other lipoproteins and cells. HDL induces cells to release cholesterol from intracellular vesicles and plasma membranes. This cholesterol can then be available for removal from the circulation by uptake by liver, kidney, adrenals, and gonads.

Critical to understanding the importance of HDL is the link with triglyceride metabolism. Impaired triglyceride (chylomicron and VLDL) metabolism is associated with low

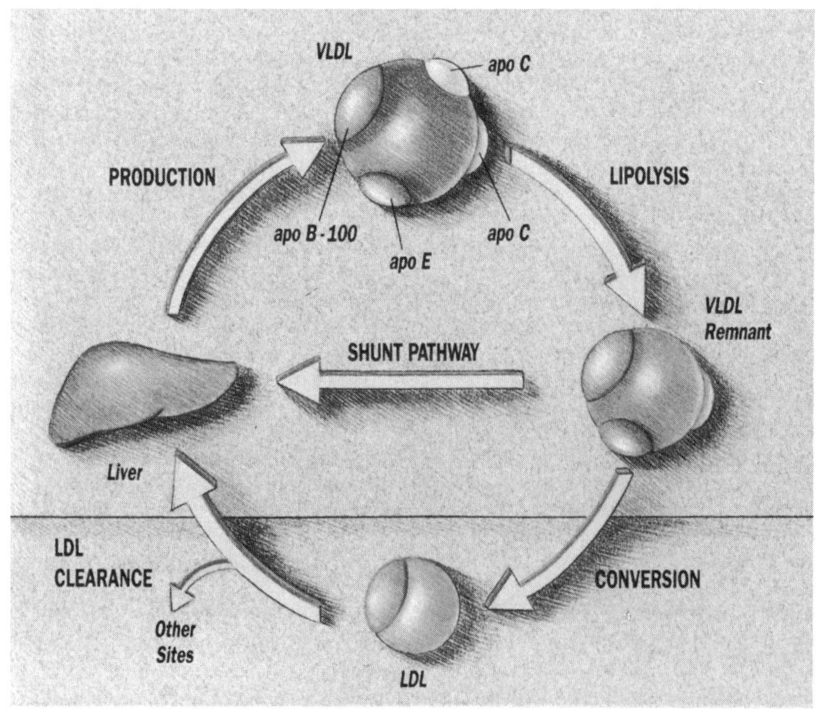

FIGURE 7–2. Basic pathways of the origins and fates of serum low-density lipoprotein. (From Grundy SM: Slide Atlas of Lipid Disorders. New York, Gower Medical Publishing, 1990.)

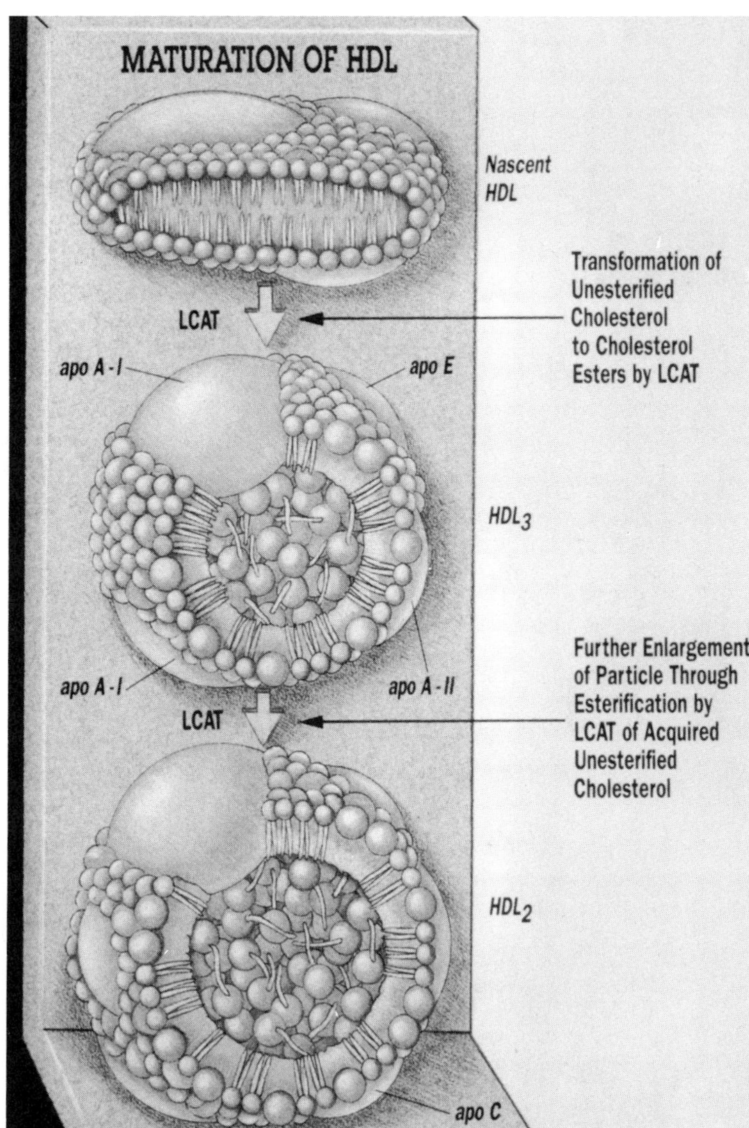

FIGURE 7–3. Basic steps in the maturation of high-density lipoprotein. (From Grundy SM: Slide Atlas of Lipid Disorders. New York, Gower Medical Publishing, 1990.)

HDL levels. HDL receives phospholipid and cholesterol from chylomicrons and VLDL that are undergoing lipolysis in the circulation. Nascent HDL can also be formed during this process. Thus when lipolysis is impaired, so is formation and expansion of HDL. In addition, for unknown reasons, impaired triglyceride metabolism is associated with accelerated removal of HDL from the circulation leading to low plasma HDL concentrations. Therefore, when hypertriglyceridemia results from impaired lipolysis, such as in obesity or diabetes, HDL levels are often low, and potentially atherogenic remnants are present. On the other hand, when hypertriglyceridemia results from overproduction of VLDL without impaired lipolysis (e.g., in oral estrogen therapy or alcohol intake), HDL levels are not decreased and can even be markedly increased, and atherogenic remnants may not be present.

LIPOPROTEIN RISK FACTORS

Total Cholesterol and Low-Density Lipoproteins. Worldwide, plasma cholesterol levels in a geographic area strongly correlate with the prevalence of coronary heart disease (CHD).[2] (The term "plasma" is used here to be synonymous with "serum" or "blood" lipoprotein levels.) This relationship represents the association of LDL levels with CHD, because LDL carries most of the plasma cholesterol in humans. CHD is unusual in populations in which the average plasma cholesterol level of adults is in the 160 mg/dl (4.1 mmol/l) range. Within single populations, this relationship begins at about 160 mg/dl (Fig. 7–4).[3–5] As plasma cholesterol increases, the relative risk of CHD increases consistently until hypercholesterolemia levels of 260 mg/dl (6.7 mmol/l) are reached. Then, CHD rates increase markedly. Thus to extrapolate this epidemiologic relationship to the effects of intervention, it would be expected that a greater proportionate benefit on CHD would result from lowering the cholesterol levels of patients with hypercholesterolemia than with average or mildly above average levels. This does seem to be true when effect of hypolipidemic therapy is examined in subgroups of patients in major clinical trials.[6]

High-Density Lipoproteins. Within populations, HDL levels are inversely associated with CHD (Fig. 7–5).[5, 7, 8]

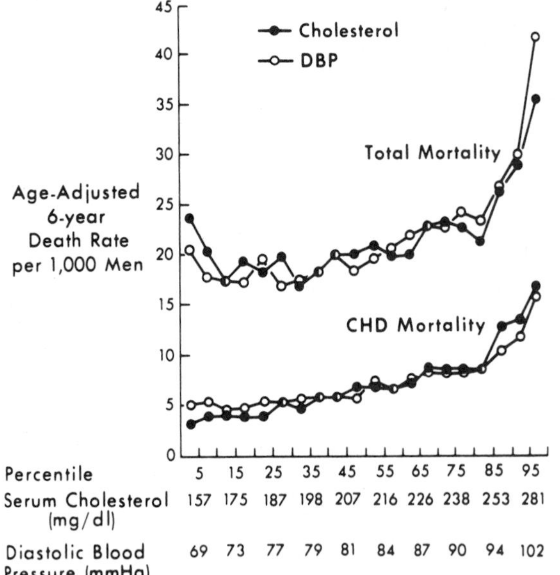

FIGURE 7–4. Age-adjusted coronary heart disease and total 6-year death rate per 1000 men screened for MRFIT according to serum cholesterol or diastolic blood pressure percentiles. (From Martin MJ, et al: Serum cholesterol, blood pressure, and mortality: Implications from a cohort of 361,662 men. Lancet 2:933, 1986.)

The adverse effect on CHD increases exponentially as HDL decreases to low levels (e.g., <30 mg/dl [0.8 mmol/l]). Worldwide, however, the apparent protective effect is not clear because a low-fat diet lowers HDL as well as LDL,[9] and populations with low-fat diets usually have low rates of CHD.[2]

Ratios. The total cholesterol to HDL cholesterol ratio (or LDL to HDL) is a convenient way to combine the opposing effects on CHD of these two lipoproteins (Fig. 7–6). The steep, high-risk range begins above about 6. The LDL to HDL ratio is no more predictive than total cholesterol to HDL.

Lipoprotein Subfractions and Apolipoproteins. The Physicians' Health Study, an ongoing United States trial of aspirin and β-carotene, studied prospectively the predictiveness for myocardial infarction (MI) of *HDL subfractions* and *apolipoproteins*.[8] In contrast to previous retrospective studies that are subject to bias and confounding because the lipids are measured after the MI has occurred, prospective studies measure the blood lipids before the patient is diagnosed with CHD. Total cholesterol and HDL cholesterol were the measurements that predicted risk of MI. Among the standard HDL subfractions, HDL_3 was more protective than HDL_2. Since alcohol intake raises HDL_3 rather than HDL_2 levels,[10] this apparent protective effect of HDL_3 supports the association of moderate intake of alcohol on decreased rates of CHD.[11]

Apo B100 was a significant predictor of CHD when considered in univariate analysis, but it was not an independent risk factor with total cholesterol and HDL in multiple regression analysis. Similar results were found for apo A-I, which is the principal protein of HDL.

Screening Persons for Risk of CHD. The total cholesterol and HDL cholesterol, but not HDL subfractions or apolipoproteins, should be measured. Nonfasting blood samples are acceptable for screening. However, if the cholesterol level is elevated, a fasting lipid profile that includes triglycerides and calculated LDL cholesterol is necessary.

Small, Dense LDL Subfractions. The prevalence of LDL particles that are small and dense (cholesterol depleted) is associated with risk of CHD.[12] Small, dense LDL is more prevalent in men than in women, and in patients who have low HDL and high triglyceride levels. Because of the coexistence of low HDL and high triglycerides, small dense LDL is not convincingly established as an independent risk factor, and its measurement is confined to research laboratories.[13]

Lipoprotein (a). Lp(a) is an LDL-like particle that contains a thrombogenic protein, apo (a), bound to apo B100.[14] Retrospective studies show an association of Lp(a) with MI. The main reasons that Lp(a) measurement is not ready for clinical use are the lack of *prospective* studies that investigated Lp(a), and the lack of an accepted standard assay procedure.

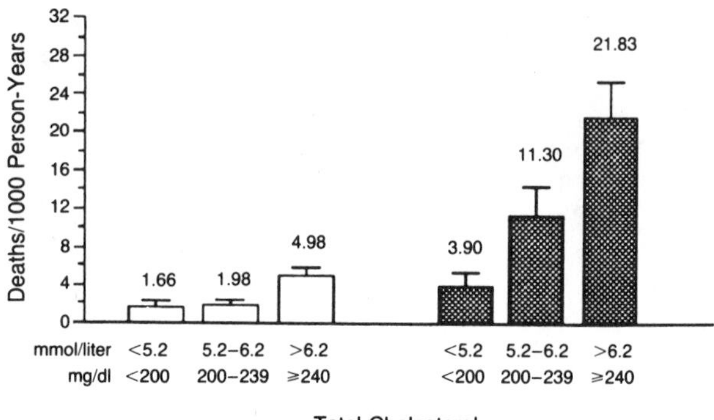

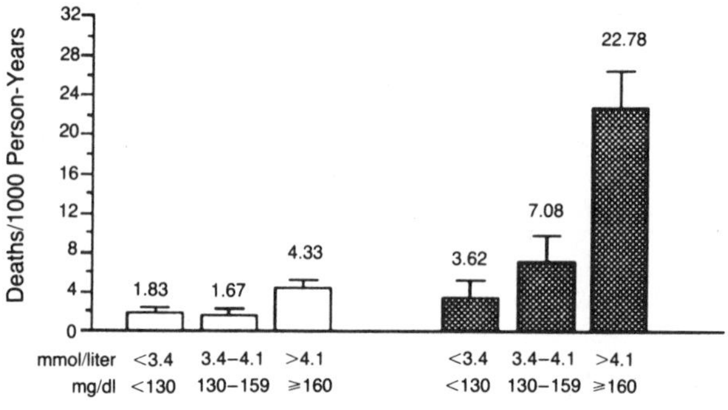

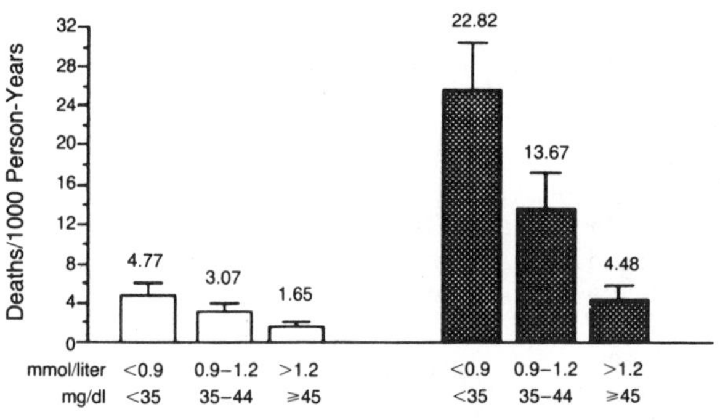

FIGURE 7–5. Age-adjusted rates of death from cardiovascular disease per 1000 person-years of follow-up, according to lipid level, for men with and without evidence of cardiovascular disease at base line. Men without cardiovascular disease at baseline are represented by open bars, and men with evidence of cardiovascular disease by shaded bars. The T bars indicate the standard errors. (From Pekkanen J, Linn S, Heiss G, et al: Ten-year mortality from cardiovascular disease in relation to cholesterol level among men with and without pre-existing cardiovascular disease. N Engl J Med 322:1700, 1990. Reprinted by permission from the *New England Journal of Medicine*.)

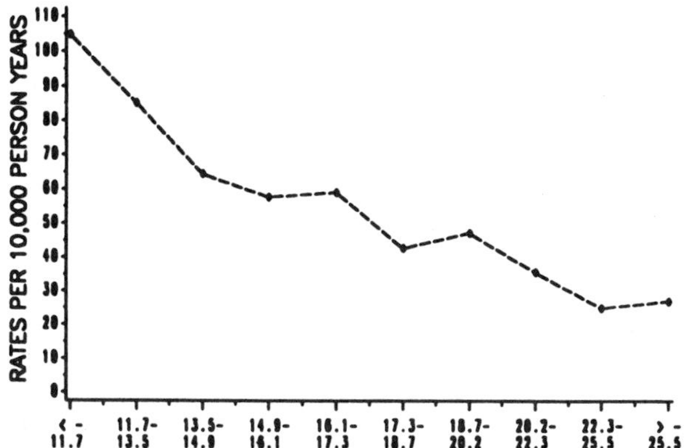

FIGURE 7–6. Twenty-three year coronary heart disease mortality in deciles by percentage of cholesterol (TC) in high-density lipoprotein cholesterol (HDLC) (age-adjusted rates per 10,000 person years). (From Goldbourt U and Yaari S: Cholesterol and coronary heart disease mortality: A 23-year follow-up study of 9902 men in Israel. Arteriosclerosis 10:512, 1990.)

TRIGLYCERIDES

Prospective epidemiologic studies found that triglycerides are significantly predictive of CHD independently of total cholesterol or LDL.[13, 15, 16] In contrast, when HDL-cholesterol is added in multiple regression analysis, the predictiveness of triglycerides weakens or disappears completely. The reason is that a high triglyceride level often coexists with a low HDL level, as discussed previously. However, as discussed, a high triglyceride level could indicate the presence of abnormal "remnant" forms of VLDL that can stimulate atherogenic and thrombotic processes. Generally, HDL is concomitantly low. In my opinion, a moderately high triglyceride level with normal or high HDL levels, as occurs with oral estrogen therapy, alcohol intake, and therapy with bile acid binding resins, is unlikely to be atherogenic.

GENDER CONSIDERATIONS

An important reason for the higher incidence of CHD in men than in women is that men have higher average levels of plasma total cholesterol and LDL and lower levels of HDL.[17] When men and women with similar cholesterol-to-HDL ratios are compared, the gender difference in the incidence of CHD is substantially narrowed, indicating that women are protected by their favorable average lipid levels. Thus women with adverse LDL or HDL levels should be considered at nearly as high risk as men.

PATIENTS WITH PRE-EXISTING CORONARY HEART DISEASE

A once popular notion was that cholesterol levels are not important in patients who already have CHD. It was reasoned that the outcome in such patients is determined more by the left ventricular ejection fraction and the propensity for arrhythmias than by their cholesterol level. But we now know that cholesterol and HDL levels are important predictors of recurrent coronary events.[3, 5] In fact, the current guidelines have lower thresholds and more aggressive treatment goals for patients with CHD compared with persons who do not have manifestations of CHD.[18]

BENEFIT OF INTERVENTION

Lowering LDL Cholesterol Levels. Primary prevention trials (studies in patients who initially do not have CHD) tested the effects of diet, cholestyramine resin, and the fibric acid derivatives, clofibrate and gemfibrozil, on CHD. These interventions produced a modest (~10%) reduction in the total cholesterol level and in the aggregate reduced CHD by 24%.[19] Thus, coronary disease incidence was lowered by about 2% for every 1% decrease in cholesterol level. This relationship has been confirmed in trials in patients with pre-existing CHD.[5, 19]

Raising HDL. Clinical trials suggest that raising a low HDL level contributes to the atherosclerosis regression process and to a lower CHD event rate. In coronary arteriographic trials, increases in HDL were associated with improvement in atherosclerosis independently of decreases in LDL cholesterol.[20, 21] Patients whose disease worsened while on therapy had low HDL levels that averaged 35 mg/dl, whereas those who had stable atherosclerosis had mean HDL levels of 40 to 45 mg/dl.[22, 23] In the Coronary Primary Prevention Trial (CPPT)[19] and the Helsinki Heart Study[24] that used cholestyramine or gemfibrozil respectively, the magnitude of increases in HDL in response to therapy was associated with decreases in the CHD event rates independently of the equally important effect of decreases in LDL. Among the patients who received gemfibrozil, reduction in CHD occurred primarily in those with pretreatment HDL below 42 mg/dl.[25] Therefore, it may be hypothesized that patients with low HDL are the primary beneficiaries of drug therapy that increases HDL.

Lowering Triglycerides. There is no direct evidence that lowering plasma triglyceride levels decreases the incidence of CHD. In the CPPT,[19] CHD rates were decreased despite increases in triglyceride levels caused by cholestyramine, and in the Helsinki Heart Study,[24] decreases in triglyceride levels with gemfibrozil had no association with reduced coronary events.

NATIONAL GUIDELINES

New guidelines for cholesterol screening and treatment from the National Cholesterol Education Program are shown in Figures 7–7 to 7–9 and Table 7–1.[18]

Screening. The major change from the previous guidelines in regard to screening is the inclusion of an HDL cholesterol measurement for all adults (Fig. 7–7). When the serum cholesterol is at least 240 mg/dl in any patient (Fig. 7–8), or over 200 mg/dl in patients with CHD or two or more additional risk factors (Figs. 7–8 and 7–9), a fasting blood sample is obtained for lipoprotein analysis for measurement of LDL. Any patient, regardless of the total cholesterol level, who has an HDL cholesterol level <35 mg/dl should also undergo lipoprotein analysis. All patients who have coronary heart disease should have lipoprotein analysis on two separate occasions to establish a baseline for therapy. Finally, a high HDL level, defined as ≥60 mg/dl, is considered to be protective and cancels out the presence of an adverse risk factor.

Therapy. The recommendations for therapy continue to be based on LDL cholesterol levels (Table 7–1). Dietary treatment is recommended when LDL is ≥160 mg/dl in patients who do not have CHD and who have no more than one additional risk factor; ≥130 mg/dl in patients without CHD who have two or more other risk factors; and >100 mg/dl in patients with CHD. The treatment goals for diet therapy are to decrease the LDL cholesterol level to below

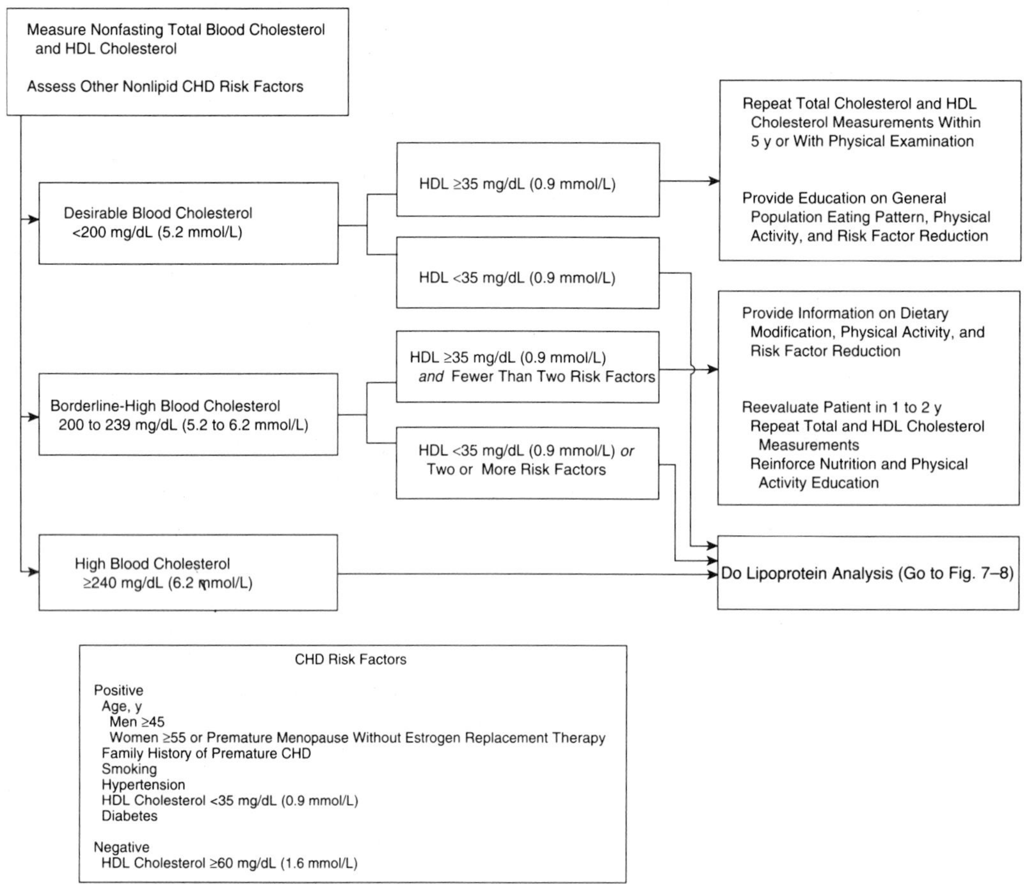

FIGURE 7–7. Primary prevention in adults without evidence of CHD. Initial classification is based on total cholesterol and HDL cholesterol levels. (From Expert Panel on Detection, Evaluation, and Treatment of High Blood Cholesterol in Adults: Summary of the Second Report of the National Cholesterol Education Program [NCEP]. JAMA 269:3015–3023, 1993. Copyright 1993, American Medical Association.)

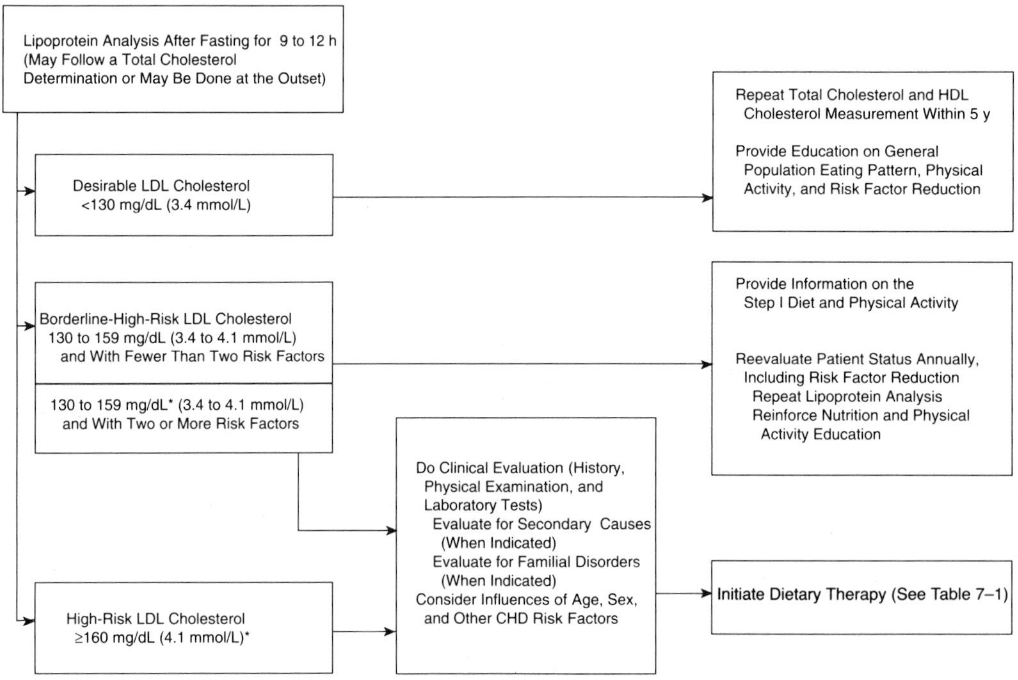

FIGURE 7–8. Primary prevention in adults without evidence of CHD. Subsequent classification is based on LDL cholesterol level. (From Expert Panel on Detection, Evaluation, and Treatment of High Blood Cholesterol in Adults: Summary of the Second Report of the National Cholesterol Education Program [NCEP]. JAMA 269:3015–3023, 1993. Copyright 1993, American Medical Association.)

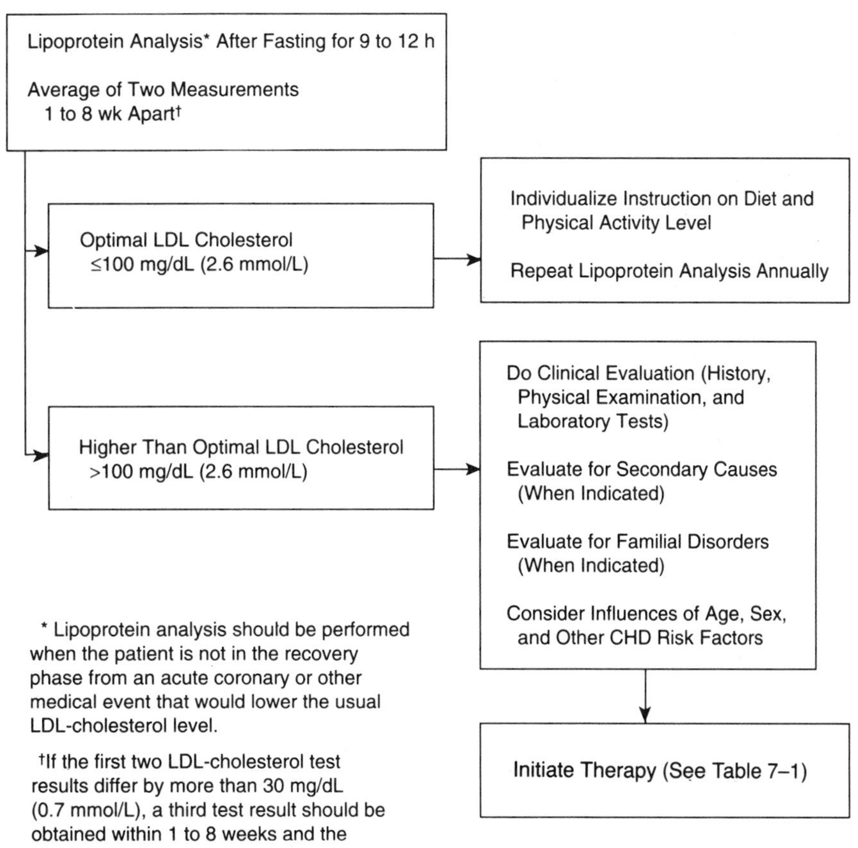

FIGURE 7–9. Secondary prevention in adults with evidence of CHD. Classification is based on low-density LDL cholesterol level. (From Expert Panel on Detection, Evaluation, and Treatment of High Blood Cholesterol in Adults: Summary of the Second Report of the National Cholesterol Education Program [NCEP]. JAMA 269:3015–3023, 1993. Copyright 1993, American Medical Association.)

the respective thresholds for initiating diet therapy. The thresholds for drug treatment in each patient category are 30 mg/dl higher than for diet treatment. The treatment goals are the same as for diet therapy.

These guidelines should be adapted to the individual patient's clinical picture. For example, the physician might refrain from drug therapy in a healthy patient who has an LDL level that is moderately above the treatment threshold but who has better than average risk factors (e.g., he or she is lean, is physically active, or has a high HDL level). On the other hand, therapy that is more aggressive than the guidelines recommend may be appropriate for a patient with multiple abnormal risk factors in addition to hypercholesterolemia.

The guidelines have been criticized on several grounds. First, no clinical trial in primary or secondary prevention has been performed that demonstrated reduction in CHD in patients with LDL levels in the lower part of the drug treatment range (e.g., 130–160 mg/dl). Second, HDL levels are not used integrally in the treatment algorithms. Third, achieving the treatment goal of 100 mg/dl for LDL cholesterol in patients with CHD often requires administration of two or more hypolipidemic drugs, which can involve substantial additional cost and presents the risk of side effects.

TREATMENT FOR NORMOLIPIDEMIC PERSONS, WOMEN, AND THE ELDERLY

Pharmacologic therapy has not been proved to benefit patients with normal or only moderately elevated serum

TABLE 7–1. TREATMENT DECISIONS BASED ON LDL CHOLESTEROL LEVEL*

Patient Category	Initiation Level	LDL Goal
	Dietary Therapy	
Without CHD and with fewer than two risk factors	≥160 mg/dL (4.1 mmol/L)	<160 mg/dL (4.1 mmol/L)
Without CHD and with two or more risk factors	≥130 mg/dL (3.4 mmol/L)	<130 mg/dL (3.4 mmol/L)
With CHD	>100 mg/dL (2.6 mmol/L)	≤100 mg/dL (2.6 mmol/L)
	Drug Treatment	
Without CHD and with fewer than two risk factors	≥190 mg/dL (4.9 mmol/L)	<160 mg/dL (4.1 mmol/L)
Without CHD and with two or more risk factors	≥160 mg/dL (4.1 mmol/L)	<130 mg/dL (3.4 mmol/L)
With CHD	≥130 mg/dL (3.4 mmol/L)	≤100 mg/dL (2.6 mmol/L)

*LDL indicates low-density lipoprotein; and CHD, coronary heart disease.

(From Expert Panel on Detection, Evaluation, and Treatment of High Blood Cholesterol in Adults: Summary of the Second Report of the National Cholesterol Education Program [NCEP]. JAMA 269:3015–3023, 1993. Copyright 1993, American Medical Association.)

cholesterol levels. Thus, the justification for treating the coronary disease patient who has total cholesterol in the low to mid 200s or LDL in the mid- to high-100s (mg/dl) is extrapolation from trials in hypercholesterolemic patients. Although the Helsinki Heart Study suggests that raising low HDL levels decreases CHD,[24] there has been no clinical trial that specifically tests the HDL-raising theory, particularly in patients who do not have coexistent hypercholesterolemia or hypertriglyceridemia. Also, because so few women have been included in the clinical trials performed to date, it is not clear whether this group as a whole would derive any benefit from such treatment. Whether lipid-lowering drugs are effective in patients over 60 years of age also remains to be determined.

CLASSIFICATION OF LIPID DISORDERS
(Table 7–2)

The system of phenotypes of hyperlipidemia of Fredrickson, Levy and Lees (types I to V) is giving way to a simplified classification for elevated VLDL and LDL and to specific enzymic or cofactor deficiencies.[26] For a review of pathophysiology of these disorders, refer to reference 1, and to the slide atlas referred to in Figures 7–1 to 7–3.

Hypercholesterolemia (Type IIa Hyperlipidemia). Elevated total and LDL cholesterol levels are due to decreased or defective LDL receptors.[27] A defective apo B that cannot bind to LDL receptors has been identified.[1] In addition, overproduction of LDL is usually present.[28] Triglyceride and VLDL cholesterol levels are normal. HDL may be at any level.

Hypertriglyceridemia (Type IV Hyperlipidemia). Increased triglyceride and VLDL levels occur without increased LDL cholesterol. HDL is usually low. The cause may be either primary (genetic) or secondary to obesity or medications. Delayed catabolism of VLDL by lipoprotein lipase is often the cause, and production of VLDL may be somewhat elevated.[29, 30] Catabolism of LDL is enhanced, producing low plasma LDL levels. The total cholesterol level may be elevated from elevated VLDL cholesterol, not from LDL cholesterol.

Combined Hyperlipidemia (Type IIb Hyperlipidemia). This involves elevated total and LDL cholesterol, elevated triglyceride, and VLDL cholesterol levels. HDL cholesterol is usually low. Obesity, hypertension, and diabetes mellitus are often present. The metabolic abnormality results from primary (genetic) or secondary factors that cause the liver to overproduce VLDL and LDL particles.[31] Decreased activity of lipoprotein lipase may contribute to severely elevated triglyceride levels. LDL catabolism may be delayed probably from decreased cellular LDL receptors.

TABLE 7–2. CLASSIFICATION OF HYPERLIPIDEMIA

	Total Cholesterol	Triglycerides	VLDL	LDL	HDL
Hypercholesterolemia (Type 2a)	↑↑	↔	↔	↑↑	↑, ↓ ↔
Hypertriglyceridemia (Type 4)	↔ or ↑	↑	↑	↓	↓
Combined Hyperlipidemia (Type 2b)	↑	↑	↑	↑	↓
Chylomicronemia (Types 1, 3, 5)	↔ or ↑	↑↑↑	↑↑↑	↓	↓

↑ = elevated; ↓ = decreased; ↔ = normal; HDL = high-density lipoprotein; LDL = low-density lipoprotein; VLDL = very low density lipoprotein.

Chylomicronemia (Types I, III, or V Hyperlipidemia).[32] There should be no chylomicrons in fasting plasma. Chylomicronemia is most often caused by superimposing a secondary stimulus to triglyceride production such as alcohol or obesity on a genetic defect in triglyceride catabolism. Deficient (but not absent) lipoprotein lipase is usually present. Thus the usual forms of chylomicronemia (types III and V) could be considered variants of hypertriglyceridemia. HDL is usually very low. Type III hyperlipidemia denotes a defective apolipoprotein E (E2) that cannot bind to LDL receptors.[1] This slows the catabolism of chylomicrons and VLDL. The cholesterol content of VLDL is high in this disorder. Type I hyperlipidemia denotes a rare genetic disease resulting from absent lipoprotein lipase or its cofactor apo C-II. In this disorder, fasting triglyceride levels are in the thousands, and the risk of pancreatitis is high.

Low High-Density Lipoproteins (Hypoalphalipoproteinemia). A low HDL level (e.g., <35 mg/dl) may be either an isolated abnormality or coexistent with hypertriglyceridemia, combined hyperlipidemia, or obesity.

SECONDARY CAUSES OF HYPERLIPIDEMIA

Elevated LDL and triglycerides are caused by hypothyroidism. Hyperlipidemic patients should be screened for hypothyroidism with a thyrotropin (TSH) measurement. An elevated TSH should be evaluated further with a thyroxine level. If the thyroid hormone level is in the lower portion of the normal range, and TSH is mildly elevated, then plasma lipid levels could be affected. Thyroid hormone replacement should be prescribed with caution in the patient with CHD because of adverse effects in a clinical trial.

Nephrotic syndrome and chronic renal failure produce multiple abnormalities in the plasma lipoprotein profile, including elevated triglyceride, low HDL, and high LDL levels.[34] Usually the high triglyceride/low HDL pattern is more prominent than hypercholesterolemia. Patients who have received a renal transplant often have lipoprotein abnormalities that reflect transplant rejection, mild chronic renal failure, and corticosteroid and cyclosporine use. Plasma LDL levels are elevated by the immunosuppressive drug therapy.[35]

Autoimmune disease can cause chylomicronemia when antibodies against lipoprotein lipase are present.[36]

TREATMENT

Diet Therapy (Tables 7–3 and 7–4)

Initial therapy for any hyperlipidemia involves diet therapy. Diet therapy, to be successful, needs the active support of an enthusiastic physician, a dietitian who establishes a bond with the patient, and willingness of the patient. The physician and the dietitian must openly acknowledge the difficulty of diet therapy. An encouraging, nonjudgmental attitude is much preferable to scare tactics.

I advocate teaching the patient to make major rather than moderate dietary changes since the lipid response is directly proportional to the extent of dietary change. Patients need to know what is the ideal and that anything less than ideal is a compromise. However, both physician and dietitian must acknowledge to the patient that adherence will sometimes fall short and that this is to be ex-

TABLE 7–3. THERAPY OF LIPID DISORDERS

Hypercholesterolemia
Low saturated fat and cholesterol diet
Cholestyramine or colestipol
Nicotinic acid
HMG CoA reductase inhibitors (lovastatin, pravastatin, simvastatin)
Oral estrogen (postmenopausal women):
Conjugated equine estrogens, micronized estradiol
Hypertriglyceridemia, Chylomicronemia
High complex carbohydrate diet
Exercise, weight loss, diabetic control
Gemfibrozil
Nicotinic acid
Fish oil
Low High-Density Lipoprotein
Weight loss, exercise, diabetic control
Gemfibrozil
Nicotinic acid
Oral estrogen (postmenopausal women)

pected and accepted. In fact, I advocate a "binge" of a totally unrestricted single meal every other week.

There are two opinions among experts on the ideal total fat intake. Some experts advocate that fat intake should be as low as possible (<10% of the total energy intake).[37] Low-fat, high-carbohydrate diets are traditionally eaten in East Asia, where CHD rates are very low. An alternative to a low-fat diet that lowers LDL just as well is a high liquid vegetable oil diet.[38] Since decreased saturated fat and cholesterol produces the LDL changes, substitution of unhydrogenated vegetable oil for saturated fat is as effective as substituting carbohydrate. People in traditional cultures in Greece and other Mediterranean countries eat much olive oil but little animal fat and have as low CHD and cancer rates as the Asian populations who eat a very low fat diet.[2] Moreover, the use of oil allows a much wider range of cuisine than does a very low fat diet and enhances long-term compliance.

Nonpharmacologic Therapy for Elevated LDL Cholesterol (Types IIa or IIb)

(The effect of nutrients on plasma lipoproteins is reviewed in references 39 and 40.)

Decrease Intake of Saturated Fatty Acids. Saturated fat is the most potent LDL-raising nutrient and acts by increasing the production of LDL, and by diminishing the activity of LDL receptors. Saturated fatty acids are found in meat, eggs, poultry, and coconut and palm kernel oil. Lauric, myristic, and palmitic acids (with 12, 14 and 16 carbons, respectively) raise LDL cholesterol levels. Stearic acid (18 carbon atoms) does not raise LDL. However, stearic acid is a minor component of the fat in beef and chocolate.

TABLE 7–4. THERAPY FOR COMBINED HYPERLIPIDEMIA

1. **Initial therapy**
   - Diet, exercise, weight loss
   - Correct glucose intolerance, if present
2. **If the triglyceride abnormality is severe (e.g., >1000 mg/dl)**
   - Start with gemfibrozil (preferably) or nicotinic acid
   - Fish oil is an alternative

   If LDL remains elevated
   - Add cholestyramine or colestipol, or an HMG-CoA reductase inhibitor
3. **If the LDL elevation is severe and the triglycerides are mildly elevated**
   - Start with nicotinic acid or an HMG-CoA reductase inhibitor to lower LDL
   - Add gemfibrozil if needed

The Keys Equation predicts the change in serum cholesterol from changes in dietary fats.[41] The predicted change in serum cholesterol = 2.7 × change in saturated fat (% kcal). For example, if saturated fat decreases from 20 to 10% (a change from a high to a moderate dietary level), then the average person's serum cholesterol decreases by 27 mg/dl.

The saturated fat should be replaced with monounsaturated or polyunsaturated fat and carbohydrate. Monounsaturated fat (oleic acid) is the predominant fatty acid in olive oil and canola (rapeseed) oil. Polyunsaturated fat (linoleic acid) predominates in safflower, sunflower, and corn oils. Monounsaturated fat and polyunsaturated fat lower LDL when substituted for saturated fat.

Decrease Dietary Cholesterol

1 egg = 240 to 300 mg; meats = 100 mg/4 oz

Cholesterol is not needed in the diet since endogenous synthesis meets the body's needs. Serum cholesterol is much more responsive to dietary cholesterol in the low range of intakes (0 to 300 mg/day) than in a higher range, which is suggested by the following equation:[41]

$$\text{Change in serum cholesterol} = 1.5\,(\text{change in dietary cholesterol})^{\frac{1}{2}}$$

When dietary cholesterol is increased, hepatic synthesis of cholesterol decreases. But in most people, this compensation is insufficient to balance the dietary increase and the net production of cholesterol and LDL increases.

Shrimp and other carnivorous shellfish such as crab and squid have cholesterol, but they appear to raise LDL less than the same of amount of egg cholesterol (probably because of ω-3 polyunsaturated fatty acids in shrimp).[42, 43] Mollusks (e.g., oysters, clams, scallops) have virtually no cholesterol.

***Trans*-Unsaturated Fatty Acids.** Mammals synthesize and metabolize unsaturated fatty acids with double carbon bonds in the *cis* conformation. The human diet contains a small amount of *trans* isomers of oleic and linoleic acids produced by bacterial metabolism in ruminants, but most *trans* fatty acids come from partially hydrogenated vegetable oils in baked goods, fried foods in restaurants, potato chips, and so forth. *Trans* isomers of unsaturated fatty acids are metabolized differently than are *cis* isomers and share some characteristics of saturated fatty acids. *Trans*-unsaturated fatty acids raise serum cholesterol in the same way as saturated fatty acids; however, unlike saturated fatty acids, the *trans* isomers lower HDL.[44, 45] Margarine lowers LDL compared with butter, but not as much as unhydrogenated natural vegetable oil. Current dietary guidelines need to be modified. At present, I recommend avoiding the hydrogenated oils as much as possible.

Fiber. Water-soluble, gummy fiber such as pectin and guar at very high amounts as pure dietary supplements lower serum LDL cholesterol.[46] Psyllium seed (Metamucil), 1 to 2 teaspoons daily, is effective.[47] However, the independent LDL-lowering effect of dietary fiber as supplied by foods such as oats and fruit has been overrated and can be discounted at practical amounts of intake. For example, three packets of instant oats have a direct cholesterol-lowering effect of approximately 2%.[48] Much of the effect of fiber-rich foods is caused by their substituting for fatty foods.[49]

Caffeine and Coffee. *Caffeine* does not affect plasma lipoprotein levels. *Coffee* contains a lipid substance that raises LDL. This lipid is extracted into the drink by boiling the beans or by some other processing step.[50] Coffee brewed by pouring hot water over ground beans in a filter does not increase LDL.[51]

Exercise. Exercise may lower LDL either independently (small effect) or by causing a change in the diet.

Cigarette smoking may increase LDL by an unknown mechanism.

Nonpharmacologic Therapy for Low HDL Levels

Some experts do not advocate specific treatment for raising HDL. To the contrary, I will treat low HDL particularly in selected persons at particularly high risk of cardiovascular disease or with pre-existing disease. I think that any agent that raises HDL (except for dietary saturated fat) is likely to be antiatherogenic. This conclusion is based on epidemiologic studies of different HDL-raising interventions including physical activity, alcohol and estrogen, and on clinical trials of prevention of cardiovascular disease using nicotinic acid and gemfibrozil, which raise HDL.[52] A consensus panel of the National Heart, Lung and Blood Institute that met in February, 1992, advocated nonpharmacologic therapy to raise HDL that is less than 35 mg/dl. The panel suggested that drug therapy be considered for low HDL in selected patients with multiple risk factors including pre-existing CHD.

Except for alcohol, the effect of any agent on HDL levels is small compared with the major effects of diet and drugs on VLDL and LDL. However, even a small change in HDL of 10% can be considered clinically important because it could lower risk of cardiovascular disease by 20 to 30%.[19, 24]

Dietary Fat Versus Carbohydrate. HDL decreases on a high-carbohydrate, low-fat diet, but on a percentage basis HDL will decrease less than the amount that LDL will decrease.[9] Saturated and monounsaturated fats raise HDL slightly more than polyunsaturated fats.[40] Simple sugars may lower HDL more than complex carbohydrates. Since a diet rich in unsaturated fats will lower LDL as much as a low-fat diet but not lower HDL, some experts advocate a moderate intake of vegetable oils, primarily monounsaturated oils such as olive oil.[38]

Alcohol. Alcohol exerts a potent graded effect to raise HDL levels beginning at one-half drink per day.[10] Increased HDL levels are probably one mechanism for the decreased CHD incidence with moderate alcohol intake.[11]

Weight Loss, Smoking, and Exercise. HDL increases modestly after weight loss is stabilized.[53] However, during the period of weight loss, HDL often declines. Cigarette smoking lowers HDL. Aerobic exercise raises HDL substantially only at extreme activity, such as marathon running or mountaineering.[54] Moderate exercise raises HDL by up to 15%.[53] Weight-lifting also increases HDL perhaps by increasing muscle mass rather than from raising maximum oxygen uptake (aerobic conditioning).

Nonpharmacologic Therapy for Hypertriglyceridemia

Saturated fatty acids raise the plasma triglyceride concentration by increasing the production of VLDL particles. Sugar also raises triglyceride levels. Compared with saturated fat, polyunsaturated fatty acids lower triglyceride levels with fish oil being the most potent, followed by linoleic acid–rich oils such as corn, sunflower, soy, and safflower oils. Monounsaturated fatty acids as in olive or canola oils have little triglyceride-lowering effect. For severe chylomicronemia, a very low fat–high starch diet is necessary to eliminate chylomicron production. However, if the overall diet is changed to decrease saturated and increase polyunsaturated fat, then the chylomicronemia that results when fat intake is superimposed on endogenous hypertriglyceridemia may become mild.

Weight loss and exercise are important in lowering triglyceride levels.

Alcohol is a potent inducer of triglyceride production and VLDL secretion by the liver. Restriction of alcohol intake is most important, since it could exert a synergistic effect with hypertriglyceridemia to induce pancreatitis.

DRUG THERAPY BY LIPID DISORDER

(see Tables 7–3 and 7–4)

If nonpharmacologic measures are not successful, lipid-lowering drug therapy will be needed.

Hypercholesterolemia: Elevated LDL (see Table 7–3). Drugs that have major LDL-lowering effects are bile acid–sequestering resins, nicotinic acid, oral estrogens, HMG-CoA reductase inhibitors, and probucol. Gemfibrozil is mildly effective.

Hypertriglyceridemia: Elevated VLDL (see Table 7–3). Drug therapy is not indicated unless there is a serious risk of pancreatitis (e.g., triglycerides >1000 mg/dl or perhaps with lower triglyceride levels and substantial alcohol use). Some experts advocate treating the triglyceride level in high-risk patients even when triglycerides are only mildly elevated (e.g., >250 mg/dl), particularly when HDL is concomitantly low. However, almost all serum triglyceride-lowering drugs also raise HDL levels. When total cholesterol is also elevated, it is necessary to determine whether the increase is from VLDL-cholesterol or from LDL-cholesterol. High VLDL-cholesterol levels can indicate the presence of potentially atherogenic remnants. Treatment with HMG-CoA reductase inhibitors or resins are ineffective or even detrimental. Gemfibrozil is the most effective and convenient agent to lower triglyceride and VLDL levels. Nicotinic acid and fish oil are alternatives. Both gemfibrozil and nicotinic acid also raise HDL. Gemfibrozil and fish oil mildly raise LDL levels in severe hypertriglyceridemia.

Combined Hyperlipidemia: Elevated VLDL and LDL (see Table 7–4). This disorder poses a diagnostic problem and is often treated inappropriately. When total cholesterol and triglyceride levels are together elevated, it must be established whether the cholesterol is elevated due to high VLDL or to high LDL. Combined hyperlipidemia is induced by exogenous influences such as abdominal obesity, adult-onset diabetes, and a poor diet superimposed on a genetic susceptibility. Nonpharmacologic therapy is often very effective. The initial choice of drug depends on whether the hypertriglyceridemia or hypercholesterolemia (elevated LDL levels) is the more serious abnormality. If triglycerides are severely elevated, then gemfibrozil is the best initial therapy. If LDL remains elevated, then a second agent that lowers LDL such as nicotinic acid or an HMG-CoA reductase inhibitor may be needed. If the triglyceride level is very well controlled (e.g., <250 mg/dl), then the bile acid–sequestering resins may be used. However, since resins raise triglyceride levels, their use may complicate the control of hypertriglyceridemia. The combination of gemfibrozil and an HMG-CoA reductase inhibitor accentuates the very low risk of each agent alone for myopathy.[55] This combination should be restricted to high-risk patients who can reliably report early symptoms of muscle weakness or myalgia. Since the myopathic effect of the reductase inhibitor is dose-dependent,[56] it is advisable to keep the dose of lovastatin or pravastatin at 10 to 20 mg rather than at 40 to 80 mg, or simvastatin at 5 to 10 mg. Theoretically, pravastatin could offer an advantage since uptake is very low in extrahepatic tissues.[57]

Decreased High-Density Lipoproteins (see Table 7–3). Low HDL levels often accompany hypertriglyceridemia but can be present as the sole lipoprotein abnormality. The NCEP classifies a low HDL as less than 35 mg/dl. Drug therapy with nicotinic acid, gemfibrozil, or oral estrogen (for postmenopausal women) may be considered for patients who are at particularly high risk of CHD events.

DRUG THERAPY—INDIVIDUAL AGENTS

Nicotinic Acid (Niacin). This drug is effective for elevated cholesterol or LDL; elevated triglycerides or VLDL; and low HDL.

Mechanism of Action. Nicotinic acid decreases the production of VLDL and most likely also decreases LDL production.[58] LDL receptors do not seem to be affected. The mechanism of raising HDL is decreased catabolism.[59]

Nicotinic acid, although a vitamin, affects plasma lipids only at pharmacologic doses of 1.5 g/day.[60, 61] Regular release nicotinic acid may be prescribed up to 6 g/day. At these doses it must be considered a drug. However, the FDA classifies nicotinic acid as a vitamin (food supplement), thus it can be obtained without prescription. The regulation of quality and efficacy of nicotinic acid preparations is minimal. Nicotinic acid has been used for at least 25 years to treat hyperlipidemia and *may be considered safe with medical supervision. It is the only lipid-lowering drug that has increased longevity in patients with CHD.*[62] *Relative contraindications to niacin are diabetes, hyperuricemia, gout, and hepatic disease.*

Cutaneous flushing is the adverse reaction that limits adherence. Even a low initial dose of 100 mg can produce flushing. Episodes last 30 to 60 minutes. Pretreatment with aspirin prevents or lessens this reaction. Tolerance develops over weeks of gradual increments, and eventually the flushing usually abates and the patient becomes used to the mild effect.

New types of slow-release nicotinic acid have greatly increased acceptability and drug effectiveness (Enduracin, Endurance Products Co., Portland, OR; Slo Niacin, Upsher-Smith, MN).[61] These tablets are formulated differently from the time-release capsules (Nicobid and generics) and produce little flushing and gastric irritation at 1.5 g/day in divided doses. The maximum dose should be lower than regular-release nicotinic acid and should not exceed 3 g/day. Severe hepatotoxicity has occurred with much higher doses. Adverse symptoms do occur with the time-release tablets: mild cutaneous flushing, rash, gastric upset, fatigue (check liver function tests), and body odor. In addition, elevated serum hepatic enzymes, hyperuricemia, and hyperglycemia due to insulin resistance occur.

Niacin "Hepatitis." In the usual presentation, the patient shows an asymptomatic increase of the serum glutamic-oxaloacetic transaminase (SGOT) or serum glutamic-pyruvic transaminase (SGPT). This usually occurs during upward titration of the dose. When these tests exceed three times the upper limit of normal, then the dose should be decreased. Hepatomegaly, fatigue, and malaise, alone or with a dramatic drop in serum cholesterol levels, may occur occasionally and unpredictably. Hyperbilirubinemia occurs rarely. The syndrome reverses within days after discontinuing the drug.

HMG-CoA Reductase Inhibitors. Lovastatin (Mevacor), pravastatin (Pravachol), and simvastatin (Zocor) are approved drugs in the class of inhibitors of hydroxy methyl glutaryl coenzyme A reductase (HMG-CoA reductase), a rate-limiting enzyme in cholesterol synthesis. The primary action of this class of drugs is to decrease plasma LDL levels. The mechanism is decreased production of VLDL and LDL and increased removal of LDL from plasma due to upregulation of hepatic LDL receptors.[63–65] Since serum triglycerides are only slightly reduced (<10%), these agents should not be used for hypertriglyceridemia. HDL levels increase slightly by an unknown mechanism.

The initial dose of lovastatin and pravastatin is 10 mg, and the initial dose for simvastatin is 5 mg. Lovastatin and pravastatin are equipotent. Simvastatin is about 1.5 times as potent as lovastatin or pravastatin, but its maximal efficacy is the same.[66] Lovastatin or pravastatin, 10 mg/day, lowers LDL by an average of 20%, which increases to 25% when the dose is doubled to 20 mg.[56, 67] Lovastatin or pravastatin, 40 mg/day, produces an average 30% decrease in LDL levels. The maximum decrease of LDL is approximately 35% with pravastatin or lovastatin (80 mg).

Adverse symptoms from these drugs are unusual. Myositis is a rare, but potentially serious, complication of lovastatin and occurs more when lovastatin is used with gemfibrozil, niacin, or cyclosporine.[55] Myalgia and weakness are early symptoms. Liver enzymes may increase mildly, and, as in the case of nicotinic acid, the dose should be decreased if the SGOT or SGPT exceeds three times the upper limit of normal.

Pravastatin is a hydrophilic drug in contrast to lovastatin and simvastatin, which are hydrophobic drugs. In experimental models, pravastatin has little effect on extrahepatic cells[57] and therefore has less potential to cause adverse reactions. Pravastatin does not cross the blood-brain barrier as does lovastatin.[68] However, these drugs have not been directly compared for the incidence of myositis.

Gemfibrozil. Gemfibrozil (Lopid) is a fibric acid derivative that lowers plasma triglycerides substantially and raises HDL and lowers LDL each by about 10%.[24, 25, 69] HDL may increase by 25 to 35% in patients with combined hyperlipidemia or with low HDL levels. Gemfibrozil decreases the hepatic production of triglycerides and VLDL particles and increases the clearance of triglycerides by lipoprotein lipase. The dose is 300 to 600 mg twice daily. In moderately to severely hypertriglyceridemic patients who usually have low LDL levels, LDL levels increase.[69] Gemfibrozil was most effective in lowering CHD in patients with hypertriglyceridemia and low HDL or with combined hyperlipidemia.[24] Thus the mild increase in LDL that occurs in these patients is probably not important. Gemfibrozil was ineffective in lowering CHD in patients with hypercholesterolemia without hypertriglyceridemia (type IIa).[24] Side effects are infrequent and include myositis.

Resins. Cholestyramine (Questran) and colestipol (Colestid) are approved bile acid–sequestering resins that increase the excretion of bile acids. Since the enterohepatic circulation of bile acids is diminished, hepatocyte cholesterol concentrations are depleted to replenish the bile acid pool. This causes the hepatocyte to upregulate its LDL receptors to take in additional cholesterol. Therefore, blood cholesterol and LDL concentrations decrease. HDL slightly increases by an unknown mechanism. Triglycerides increase mildly in patients with normal triglyceride levels but often substantially in patients with hypertriglyceridemia.

The effective dose of these resins is two to six packets or scoops per day (8 to 24 g/day). The dose response effect on LDL levels is linear.[19]

Taste and gastrointestinal side effects limit patient acceptability, although side effects tend to diminish after several months of use.

Cholestyramine decreased the rate of CHD in patients with hypercholesterolemia.[19]

Fish Oil. Fish oil is effective for the treatment of severe hypertriglyceridemia. Fish oil produces a dose-dependent decrease in triglycerides and VLDL concentrations beginning at 3 g/day of the n-3 fatty acids, eicosapentaenoic (EPA) and docosahexaenoic (DHA).[70] Commercial varieties include Promega (50% n-3), and Max-Epa (25% n-3). The main side effect is fishy-tasting belches. At very high doses, clinical thrombocytopenia can occur.

Probucol (Lorelco). Probucol is not much utilized in the United States because it decreases HDL more than it decreases LDL concentrations. Probucol is also an antioxidant that reduces atherosclerosis in animal models.[71] However, there is no clinical trial of probucol in humans to determine whether the drug improves coronary atherosclerosis or CHD incidence.

Antihypertensive Medications and Plasma Lipid Levels.[72] Thiazides increase triglycerides and LDL, but the adverse effects of low doses may be minimal.[73] β-Adrenergic blockers increase LDL and triglycerides and decrease HDL.[74] There is no difference in the lipid effects of selective and nonselective antagonists; on the other hand, β-blockers with intrinsic sympathomimetic activity do not affect plasma lipid levels. Combined α-/β-blockers also have no net effect on plasma lipids. Prazosin, an α-adrenergic antagonist, decreases triglyceride and LDL levels and increases HDL levels. Surprisingly, other α-adrenergic antagonists such as doxazosin have not produced consistent improvement in lipid levels in various trials. Calcium channel blockers and angiotensin-converting enzyme inhibitors probably do not adversely affect plasma lipids.

Exogenous Sex Hormones

Oral Contraceptives.[75, 76] Contemporary low-dose products that do not have norgestrel probably do not alter plasma lipid levels (e.g., Demulen, Ortho Novum 1/35 or 7/7/7 or Ovcon-35). These preparations do raise plasma triglycerides, which could be a problem in women who have hypertriglyceridemia. Norgestrel-containing products (e.g., Ovral) lower HDL and triglyceride levels and raise LDL levels. I would avoid products with norgestrel in women who have risk factors for CHD.

Postmenopausal Estrogens. Oral estrogens such as conjugated equine estrogens (Premarin) or micronized 17-β-estradiol (Estrace) decrease LDL and increase HDL, each by about 15%, whereas transdermal estrogen (Estraderm) has little effect on LDL and HDL.[17, 77] Oral but not transdermal estrogens increase VLDL and triglycerides by approximately 25%. Conjugated estrogens, 0.625 mg and 1.25 mg, have the same effect on LDL and HDL levels.[77] However, the higher dose proportionately raises triglycerides. The incidence of cardiovascular disease is less in postmenopausal women who are taking oral estrogens than in nonusers.[78, 79]

Because estrogen in the absence of a progestin (unopposed estrogen) induces endometrial hyperplasia, which can lead to endometrial carcinoma, concomitant administration of a progestin is recommended. Women without a uterus do not need a progestin. Medroxyprogesterone acetate (Provera and generics) (5 mg/day for 10 days per month) or continuous administration of 5 mg are alternative regimens. It is not established that continuous administration of 2.5 mg will prevent endometrial hyperplasia. Continuous administration produces atrophic endometrium after 6 to 9 months which usually does not bleed, whereas cyclic administration causes monthly withdrawal bleeding. Unfortunately, medroxyprogesterone acetate lessens the beneficial effects of estrogens on HDL.[17] Some experts recommend omitting the progestin since the incidence of endometrial cancer is much less than that of cardiovascular disease. Also, endometrial cancer that arises in women receiving estrogen is curable by hysterectomy, and survival is similar to women who do not have cancer. Progestins also cause premenstrual syndrome and diminish compliance to the entire hormonal replacement regimen. However, if a progestin is not used, most gynecologists recommend an endometrial biopsy or transvaginal uterine ultrasound before treatment and at the annual gynecologic examination. A compromise is to administer medroxyprogesterone acetate 10 mg/day for 14 days every 3 or 4 months, thus lessening adverse effects.

TABLE 7–5. DRUG TREATMENT OF HYPERLIPIDEMIA: COST AND EFFECTIVENESS*

	ΔLDL	ΔHDL	ΔTG	Cost/Yr†
Niacin (1.5–3 g/day)	↓10–20%	↑10–20%	↓25%	$50–200
Pravastatin, Lovastatin (10–20 mg/day)	↓25–30%	↑5%	↓10%	$550–750
Cholestyramine, Colestipol (10–20 g/day)	↓10–20%	↑3–5%	↑10%	$500–1100
Gemfibrozil (1200 mg/day)	↓10%	↑10–20%	↓35%	$700
Estrogen (oral) (Conjugated equine estrogens, 0.625 mg/day, or micronized 17 β-estradiol, 1–2 mg/day)	↓15%	↑15%	↑25%	$125

*From F. Sacks, Brigham and Women's Hospital.
†Average wholesale price.

Economic Concerns (Table 7–5). Unfortunately, there is no ideal lipid-lowering agent—highly effective, well-tolerated, and inexpensive. Nicotinic acid would be ideal were it not for its adverse effects, since it favorably affects all lipoprotein levels. If drug-induced increases in HDL are considered together with decreases in LDL, oral estrogen therapy is quite cost-effective. The HMG-CoA reductase inhibitors are not priced linearly with dose. For example, 10 mg of pravastatin costs nearly as much as 20 mg. Although simvastatin is more potent than the other two agents, its cost is approximately double. For an LDL-lowering action, the reductase inhibitors are more cost-effective than the bile acid–binding resins.[80] Overall, low doses of the reductase inhibitors were particularly cost-effective in high-risk patients with hypercholesterolemia and CHD.[81] It is difficult to compare the cost-effectiveness of gemfibrozil with the reductase inhibitors since their indications do not overlap.

REFERENCES

1. Mahley RW, Weisgraber KH, Innerarity TL, and Rall SC: Genetic defects in lipoprotein metabolism: Elevation of athero-

genic lipoproteins caused by impaired catabolism. JAMA 265:78–83, 1991.
2. Keys A: Seven Countries. Cambridge, MA, Harvard University Press, 1980.
3. Rose G, Reid DD, Hamilton PJ, et al: Myocardial ischemia, risk factors and death from coronary heart disease. Lancet 1:105–109, 1977.
4. Martin MJ, Hulley SB, Browner WS, et al: Serum cholesterol, blood pressure, and mortality: Implications from a cohort of 361,662 men. Lancet 2:933–936, 1986.
5. Pekkanen J, Linn S, Heiss G, et al: Ten-year mortality from cardiovascular disease in relation to cholesterol level among men with and without preexiting cardiovascular disease. N Engl J Med 322:1700–1707, 1990.
6. Sacks FM, Pfeffer MA, Moye L, et al: Rationale and design of a secondary prevention trial of lowering normal plasma cholesterol levels after acute myocardial infarction: The Cholesterol and Recurrent Events Trial (CARE). Am J Cardiol 68:1436–1446, 1991.
7. Goldbourt U and Yaari S: Cholesterol and coronary heart disease mortality: A 23-year follow-up study of 9902 men in Israel. Arteriosclerosis 10:512–519, 1990.
8. Stampfer MJ, Sacks FM, Salvini S, et al: A prospective study of lipids, apolipoproteins and risks of myocardial infarction. N Engl J Med 325:373–381, 1991.
9. Sacks FM, Handysides GH, Marais GE, et al: The effect of a low fat diet on plasma lipoproteins in normal adults. Arch Intern Med 146:1573–1577, 1986.
10. Taskinen M-R, Nikkila EA, Valimaki M, et al: Alcohol-induced changes in serum lipoproteins and in their metabolism. Am Heart J 113:458–464, 1987.
11. Rimm EB, Giovannucci EL, Willett WC, et al: Prospective study of alcohol consumption and risk of coronary disease in men. Lancet 338:464–468, 1991.
12. Austin MA, Breslow JL, Hennekens CH, et al: Low density lipoprotein subclass patterns and risk of myocardial infarction. JAMA 260:1917–1921, 1988.
13. Krauss RM: The tangled web of coronary risk factors. Am J Med 90(Suppl 2A):36S–41S, 1991.
14. Rader DJ and Brewer HB: Lipoprotein(a): Clinical approach to a unique atherogenic lipoprotein. JAMA 267:1109–1112, 1992.
15. Avins AL, Haber RJ, and Hulley SB: The status of hypertriglyceridemia as a risk factor for coronary heart disease. Clin Lab Med 9:153–168, 1989.
16. Austin MA: Plasma triglycerides as a risk factor for coronary heart disease: The epidemiologic evidence and beyond. Am J Epidemiol 129:249–259, 1989.
17. Sacks FM and Walsh BW: The effects of reproductive hormones on blood lipoproteins and blood pressure: Unresolved issues in biology and clinical practice. Ann N Y Acad Sci 592:272–285, 1990.
18. Expert Panel on Detection, Evaluation, and Treatment of High Blood Cholesterol in Adults: Summary of the Second Report of the National Cholesterol Education Program [NCEP]. JAMA 269:3015–3023, 1993.
19. Lipid Research Clinics Program: The Lipid Research Clinics Coronary Primary Prevention Trial Results. II: The relationship of reduction of incidence of coronary heart disease to cholesterol lowering. JAMA 251:365–374, 1984.
20. Brown G, Albers JJ, Fisher LD, et al: Regression of coronary artery disease as a result of intensive lipid-lowering therapy in men with high levels of apolipoprotein B. N Engl J Med 323:1289–1298, 1990.
21. Levy RI, Brensike JF, Epstein SE, et al: The influence of changes in lipid values induced by cholestyramine and diet on progression of coronary artery disease: Results of NHLBI Type II Coronary Intervention Study. Circulation 69:325–327, 1984.
22. Nikkila EA, Viikinkoski P, Malle M, and Frick MH: Prevention of progression of coronary atherosclerosis by treatment of hyperlipidemia: A seven year prospective angiographic study. BMJ 289:220–223, 1984.
23. Arntzenius AC, Kromhout D, Barth JC, et al: Diet, lipoproteins, and the progression of coronary atherosclerosis: The Leiden Intervention Trial. N Engl J Med 312:805–811, 1985.
24. Manninen V, Elo O, Frick H, et al: Lipid alterations and decline in the incidence of coronary heart disease in the Helsinki Heart Study. JAMA 260:641–651, 1988.
25. Manninen V, Huttunen JK, Heinonen OP, et al: Relation between baseline lipid and lipoprotein values and the incidence of coronary heart disease in the Helsinki Heart Study. Am J Cardiol 63:42H–47H, 1989.
26. Fredrickson DS, Levy RI, and Lees RS: Fat transport in lipoproteins—an integrated approach to mechanisms and disorders. N Engl J Med 276:234–281, 1967.
27. Brown MS and Goldstein JL: Familial hypercholesterolemia. *In* Scriver CR, Beaudet AL, Sly WS, and Valle D (eds): The Metabolic Basis of Inherited Disease, 6th ed. New York, McGraw-Hill, 1989, pp 1215–1250.
28. James RW, Martin B, Pometta D, et al: Apolipoprotein B metabolism in homozygous familial hypercholesterolemia. J Lipid Res 30:159–169, 1989.
29. Packard CJ, Munro A, Lorimer R, et al: Metabolism of apolipoprotein B in large triglyceride-rich very low density lipoproteins of normal and hypertriglyceridemic subjects. J Clin Invest 74:2171–2192, 1984.
30. Kesaniemi YA and Grundy SM: Dual defect in metabolism of very low density lipoprotein triglycerides. JAMA 251:2542–2547, 1984.
31. Teng B, Sniderman AD, Soutar AK, and Thompson GR: Metabolic basis of hyperapobetalipoproteinemia. J Clin Invest 77:663–672, 1986.
32. Brunzell JD and Bierman EL: Chylomicronemia syndrome. Med Clin North Am 66:455–468, 1982.
33. The Coronary Drug Project Research Group: The Coronary Drug Project: Findings leading to further modifications of its protocol with respect to dextrothyroxin. JAMA 220:996–1008, 1972.
34. Grundy SM: Management of hyperlipidemia of kidney disease. Kidney Int 37:847–853, 1990.
35. Henkin Y, Como JA, and Oberman A: Secondary dyslipidemia: Inadvertent effects of drugs in clinical practice. JAMA 267:961–968, 1992.
36. Kihara S, Matsuzawa Y, Kubo M, et al: Autoimmune hyperchylomicronemia. N Engl J Med 1255–1259, 1989.
37. Ornish D, Brown SE, Scherwitz LW, et al: Can lifestyle changes reverse coronary heart disease? The Lifestyle Heart Trial. Lancet 336:129–133, 1990.
38. Sacks FM and Willett WC: More on chewing the fat; the good fat and the good cholesterol. N Engl J Med 325:1740–1742, 1991.
39. Denke MA and Grundy SM: Dietary influences on serum lipids and lipoproteins. J Lipid Res 31:1149–1172, 1990.
40. Mensink RP and Katan MB: Effect of dietary fatty acids on serum lipids and lipoproteins: A meta-analysis of 27 trials. Arterioscler Thromb 12:911–919, 1992.
41. Keys A, Anderson JT, and Grande F: Serum cholesterol response to changes in the diet. Metabolism 14:747–786, 1965.
42. Childs MT, Corsett CS, King IB, et al: Effects of shellfish consumption on lipoproteins in normolipidemic men. Am J Clin Nutr 51:1020–1027, 1990.
43. Nestel PJ: Fish oil attenuates the cholesterol induced rise in lipoprotein cholesterol. Am J Clin Nutr 43:752–757, 1986.
44. Mensink RP and Katan MB: Effect of dietary trans fatty acids on high density and low density lipoprotein cholesterol levels in healthy subjects. N Engl J Med 323:439–445, 1990.
45. Nestel P, Noades M, Belling B, et al: Plasma lipoprotein lipid and Lp(a) changes with substitution of elaidic acid for oleic acid in the diet. J Lipid Res 33:1029–1036, 1992.
46. Jenkins DA, Leeds AR, Newton C, and Cummings JH: Effect of pectin, guar gum, and wheat fibre on serum-cholesterol. Lancet 1:1116–1117, 1975.
47. Bell LP, Hectorne K, Reynolds H, et al: Cholesterol-lowering effects of psyllium hydrophilic mucilloid. JAMA 261:3419–3423, 1989.
48. Ripsin CM, Keenan JM, Jacobs DR, et al: Oat products and lipid lowering: A meta-analysis. JAMA 267:3317–3325, 1992.
49. Swain JF, Rouse IL, Curley CB, and Sacks FM: Comparison of the effects of oat bran and low fiber wheat on serum lipoprotein levels and blood pressure. N Engl J Med 322:147–152, 1990.
50. Zock PL, Katan MB, Merkus MP, et al: Effect of a lipid-rich fraction from boiled coffee on serum cholesterol. Lancet 335:1235–1237, 1990.

51. Bak AA and Grobbee DE: The effect on serum cholesterol levels of coffee brewed by filtering or boiling. N Engl J Med 321:1432–1437, 1989.
52. Sacks FM: Desirable serum total cholesterol with low HDL cholesterol levels: An undesirable situation in coronary heart disease. Circulation 86:1341–1344, 1992.
53. Wood PD, Stefanick ML, Williams PT, and Haskell WL: The effects on plasma lipoproteins of a prudent weight-reducing diet, with or without exercise, in overweight men and women. N Engl J Med 325:461–466, 1991.
54. Nestel PJ, Pidkolinski M, and Fidge NH: Marked increase in HDL in mountaineers. Atherosclerosis 34:193–196, 1979.
55. Pierce LR, Wysowski DK, and Gross TP: Myopathy and rhabdomyolysis associated with lovastatin-gemfibrozil combination therapy. JAMA 264:71–75, 1990.
56. Bradford RH, Shear CL, Chremos AN, et al: Expanded clinical evaluation of lovastatin (EXCEL) study results. Arch Intern Med 151:43–49, 1991.
57. Koga T, Shimada Y, Kuroda M, et al: Tissue-selective inhibition of cholesterol synthesis in vivo by pravastatin sodium, a 3-hydroxy-3-methylglutaryl coenzyme A reductase inhibitor. Biochim Biophys Acta 1045:115–120, 1990.
58. Grundy SM, Mok HY, Zech L, and Berman M: Influence of nicotinic acid on metabolism of cholesterol and triglycerides in man. J Lipid Res 22:24–36, 1981.
59. Shepherd J, Packard CJ, Patsch JR, et al: Effects of nicotinic acid therapy on plasma high density subfractions and composition and on apolipoprotein A metabolism. J Clin Invest 63:858–867, 1979.
60. Figge HL, Figge J, Souney PF, et al: Nicotinic acid: A review of clinical use in the treatment of lipid disorders. Pharmacotherapy 8:287–294, 1988.
61. Alderman JD, Pasternak RC, Sacks FM, et al: Effect of a modified, well-tolerated niacin regimen on serum total cholesterol, high density lipoprotein cholesterol and the cholesterol to high density lipoprotein ratio. Am J Cardiol 64:725–729, 1989.
62. Canner PL, Berge KG, Wenger NK, et al: Fifteen year mortality in Coronary Drug Project patients: Long-term benefit with nicain. J Am Coll Cardiol 8:1245–1255, 1986.
63. Arad Y, Ramakrishnan R, and Ginsberg HN: Lovastatin therapy reduces LDL apo B levels in subjects with combined hyperlipidemia by reducing the production of apo B-containing lipoproteins: Implications for the pathophysiology of apo B production. J Lipid Res 31:567–582, 1990.
64. Vega GL, Krauss RM, and Grundy SM: Pravastatin therapy in primary moderate hypercholesterolaemia: Changes in metabolism of apolipoprotein B-containing lipoproteins. J Intern Med 227:81–94, 1990.
65. Reihner E, Rudling M, Stahlberg D, et al: Influence of pravastatin, a specific inhibitor of HMG-CoA reductase, on hepatic metabolism of cholesterol. N Engl J Med 323:224–228, 1990.
66. Stein E, Kreisberg R, Miller V, et al: Effects of simvastatin and cholestyramine in familial and nonfamilial hypercholesterolemia. Arch Intern Med 150:341–345, 1990.
67. Hunninghake DB, Mellies MJ, Goldberg AC, et al: Efficacy and safety of pravastatin in patients with primary hypercholesterolemia. Atherosclerosis 85:219–227, 1990.
68. Triscari J, Pan H, DeVault A, et al: Pravastatin and lovastatin concentrations in cerebrospinal fluid of healthy subjects following oral administration (Abstract). Clin Pharmacol Ther 49:147, 1991.
69. Leaf DA, Connor WE, Illingworth DR, et al: The hypolipidemic effects of gemfibrozil in type V hyperlipidemia. JAMA 262:3154–3160, 1989.
70. Harris WS: Fish oils and plasma lipid and lipoprotein metabolism in humans: A critical review. J Lipid Res 30:785–807, 1989.
71. Witztum JL and Steinberg D: Role of oxidized LDL in atherogenesis. J Clin Invest 88:1785–1792, 1991.
72. Lardinois C and Neuman SL: The effects of antihypertensive agents on serum lipids and lipoproteins. Arch Intern Med 148:1280–1288, 1988.
73. Pollare T, Lithell H, and Berne C: A comparison of the effects of hydrochlorothiazide and captopril on glucose and lipid metabolism in patients with hypertension. N Engl J Med 321:868–873, 1989.
74. Sacks FM and Dzau VJ: Adrenergic effects on plasma lipoprotein metabolism: Speculation on mechanisms of action. Am J Med 80 (2A):71–81, 1986.
75. Wahl P, Walder C, Knopp R, et al: Effect of estrogen/progestin potency on lipid/lipoprotein cholesterol. N Engl J Med 308:862–867, 1983.
76. Godsland IF, Crook D, Simpson R, et al: The effects of different formulations of oral contraceptive agents on lipid and carbohydrate metabolism. N Engl J Med 323:1375–1381, 1990.
77. Walsh BW, Schiff I, Rosner B, et al: Effects of postmenopausal estrogen replacement on the concentrations and metabolism of plasma lipoproteins. N Engl J Med 325:1196–1204, 1991.
78. Bush TL, Barrett-Connor E, Cowan LD, et al: Cardiovascular mortality and noncontraceptive use of estrogen in women: Results from the Lipid Research Clinics Program Follow-up Study. Circulation 75:1102–1109, 1987.
79. Stampfer MJ, Colditz GA, Willett WC, et al: Postmenopausal estrogen therapy and cardiovascular disease: Ten-year followup from the Nurses Health Study. N Engl J Med 325:756–762, 1991.
80. Schulman KA, Kinosian B, Jacobson TA, et al: Reducing high blood cholesterol level with drugs: Cost-effectiveness of pharmacologic management. JAMA 264:3025–3033, 1990.
81. Goldman L, Weinstein MC, Goldman PA, and Williams LW: Cost-effectiveness of HMG-CoA reductase inhibition for primary and secondary prevention of coronary heart disease. JAMA 265:1145–1151, 1991.

8

Exercise for Primary Prevention or Rehabilitation in Heart Disease

L. HOWARD HARTLEY, MD

Exercise conditioning is associated with good cardiovascular health and leads to physiologic benefits. Because of exercise, physical working capacity increases, and heart rate, blood pressure, and circulating catecholamines are reduced, which in turn decreases the myocardial oxygen uptake. In the conditioned person, the circulatory system is more efficient. In view of these impressive effects, it is not surprising that exercise conditioning equates with good health.

The results of most studies that examined the relationship between physical activity and cardiovascular health have shown beneficial effects of exercise. No controlled studies have suggested that exercise is harmful. In studies of adverse event rates for exercising populations, benefits have exceeded the risks, with the possible exception of high-intensity (and unsupervised) exercise for individuals who have heart disease.[1] All available studies of physical activity and cardiovascular health were reviewed by the Centers for Disease Control (CDC) and the results published in 1987.[2] After carefully reviewing papers for adequacy of study design, an analysis of scientifically sound data showed that inactivity is a major risk factor for coronary disease. The risk ratio was 1.7, which is similar to the risk ratio for cholesterol, blood pressure, and cigarette smoking. Somewhat of a dose-response curve was noted for physical activity and health, with more protection as levels of activity increased and with a minimal beneficial amount of 20 minutes of exercise three times per week. Since the number of sedentary individuals in the United States of America is actually greater than the number with other risk factors, the potential for positively affecting health is actually greater with physical activity than with any of the other risk factors.

After the onset of cardiac disease, physicians take measures intended to restore the patient to activity and productivity as soon as possible. This process is called cardiac rehabilitation. When viewed in the broad sense, cardiac rehabilitation employs drugs, surgery, exercise, diet, and counseling. Although all these treatments are important, this chapter is devoted to physical activity.

Strict bedrest was the rule for management of patients with heart disease until the 1950s. At that time, early ambulation of patients after myocardial infarctions was suggested as not only harmless but also beneficial.[3]

There have been 22 randomized controlled trials of cardiac rehabilitation programs that use exercise as a principal component. Only one of these studies has shown a statistically significant reduction in mortality.[4] Of these studies, 10 were examined in a meta-analysis in 1988 by Oldridge,[5] which included the results of 4357 patients with a mean follow-up period of 3.5 years. The pooled odds ratio in the cardiac rehabilitation was 0.76 for all causes of mortality and 0.75 for cardiovascular mortality (both statistically significant). Later 22 studies were examined by O'Connor and associates, and 4554 patients were included with a mean follow-up of 3 years.[6] The odds ratios were 0.80 for total mortality and 0.78 for cardiovascular mortality in the exercising groups. In neither of these two meta-analyses were frequency of recurrent myocardial infarctions significantly changed.

A major consideration for prescribing physical activity to individuals with heart disease is to be certain that exercise does no harm. No studies have suggested that mortality or morbidity is increased by regular physical activity. Recent uncontrolled studies did suggest that ventricular function deteriorated in individuals with anterior myocardial infarctions. However, more recent controlled trials have found no decrease in ejection fraction associated with regular physical activity.[7]

Other benefits can accrue from participating in regular physical activity. Physical working capacity increases, and an increment occurs regardless of age, the initial physical working capacity, or the use of β-blockers. Although some studies suggest that physical activity programs can lead to the occurrence of angina at a higher heart rate–pressure product,[8] this finding is unusual. Most individuals with angina pectoris have increased physical working capacity because the heart rate–pressure product is reduced during exercise as a result of conditioning.

One of the fields of expanding use for exercise rehabilitation is the rehabilitation of patients with congestive heart failure. Although congestive heart failure was once considered a contraindication for exercise, several studies have shown that not only is physical activity safe, but it is also beneficial. Most of the early reports were uncontrolled, but recent, well-controlled studies have shown improved working capacity with exercise conditioning and no adverse effects on ventricular function.[9]

Risk factors for the progression of coronary disease are better controlled in individuals who participate in exercise programs. Our studies have shown that individuals who employ both diet and exercise are more likely to control body weight and blood lipids than with exercise alone.[10] The caloric costs of exercise are fairly modest, although they may become substantial over time. At the rate of 100 kcal/mile, one needs to walk or jog 35 miles to lose 1 lb of weight. Also, the effect of regular exercise on the blood lipids is modest. In studies of middle-aged normal men who participated in a vigorous activity program, significant reductions of 10% in cholesterol[11] and about 15% in triglycerides have been noted.[12] An important aspect of reducing blood lipids is to lower body weight.[13] Exercise and diet together are the best approaches to weight loss, in our experience.

Reductions in blood pressure also occur as a result of endurance training, especially if the value is high initially. Although weight loss is effective for reducing the levels of arterial pressure, physical activity also has been effective, in our experience.[14] Most workers now agree that physical activity is a reasonable initial approach to the management of mild hypertension.[15]

Finally, the psychological effects of regular physical activity are marked.[16] Depression is common with cardiac disease, particularly after a myocardial infarction[17] and is a major cause of noncompliance and poor prognosis.[18] One of the most powerful regimens for combatting depression is regular physical activity. Several studies have shown reductions in depression scores on standard psychological tests in those who exercise. The mechanism of the reduced depression is not clear. In our studies, lessening of depression does not seem to correlate with the amount of increased physical working capacity.[19] However, most workers in the field are impressed with the improved confidence and mood that physical activity engenders in cardiac patients.

Although the benefits of exercise outweigh the risks, there are certain precautions that can reduce the risks even further. The risks of vigorous exercise are higher in individuals with heart disease than in normal people. This higher risk can be avoided by moderating physical activity. Guidelines published by the American Heart Association have placed emphasis on determining if the individual has cardiovascular disease, and if disease is found or suspected, restricting activity to moderate levels.[1]

PHYSICAL ACTIVITY FOR APPARENTLY NORMAL PATIENTS

The major concern in screening apparently normal individuals who wish to exercise is to determine if they are in fact normal. Obviously, a careful history and physical examination should precede any decision for medical clearance. A history of known heart disease indicates that the person has increased risk for a complication during vigorous exercise. If the examination discloses a heart murmur, possibly indicative of valvular heart disease, or if the resting electrocardiogram is abnormal, a full medical work-up including an exercise tolerance test, should be performed. Only if there is no significant disease found and if the exercise tolerance test has a normal result, can vigorous exercise be encouraged.

The decision to perform an exercise test depends in part on the likelihood of finding an abnormality. Individuals younger than 30 years of age, with no signs or symptoms of heart disease, have almost no probability of having an abnormal test[20]; therefore it makes little sense to perform tests in that age group. The American Heart Association recommends that individuals 40 years of age or older with risk factors for coronary disease should have an exercise test if contemplating vigorous exercise.[21] Of course if the individuals are willing to restrict their activity to walking, then an exercise test is probably not necessary. Encouraging patients to call at any point that symptoms develop should also be stressed.

The type of exercise that normal individuals will perform after medical clearance depends on their wishes. A simple program for normal persons includes walking to "warm up" for 10 minutes, then jogging at a comfortable pace—defined as one at which it is possible also to converse easily with another person—for 20 minutes, and then gradually ceasing to exercise by walking for 5 to 10 minutes. This should be done at least three times weekly to maintain good cardiovascular fitness. Many lay books and manuals are available, and we recommend that patients be referred to those sources for more details of exercise techniques.

PHYSICAL ACTIVITY FOR CORONARY DISEASE PATIENTS

Conditions that would make physical activity inadvisable include congestive heart failure, unstable chest pain, a changing pattern on the electrocardiogram, or any other condition that might be worsened by exercise. An important guideline is to be certain that the patient's condition is stable. Hence, physical activity may begin soon after a heart attack, but if the patient's chest discomfort persists, then the activity should be delayed until the situation is resolved and the condition stabilizes. If the result of the electrocardiogram is abnormal, the individual should be followed until the pattern is stable. Although controlled trials have not been performed in such individuals, there are anecdotal reports of severe adverse reactions, including heart failure and cardiogenic shock, in exercise tests performed in individuals with unstable ischemic disease.

The exercise test provides a cornerstone for exercise prescription to patients with coronary disease. Especially useful information includes detection of hazardous conditions that cannot be discovered in any other way, determination of the endpoints for physical activity, assessment of physical working capacity, determination of the conditioning workloads, and provision of a basis for comparison as improvement occurs. During the exercise test either high-grade ventricular ectopic rhythm disturbances or severe ischemic episodes can be precipitated without symptoms. Ventricular tachycardia is particularly worrisome. The main concern is that ischemia and ventricular arrhythmias set the stage for ventricular fibrillation.[22] Thus, prescribing physical activity at an intensity that avoids occurrence of these arrhythmias seems to be a logical goal. In our experience the rhythm disturbances have been quite reproducible at a given heart rate, thus maintenance of a physical activity intensity below that required to induce the rhythm abnormality works out quite well.

Severe ischemia includes marked ST displacement—usually more than 2 mm—multilead electrocardiographic changes, fall in blood pressure, and occurrence of either pain or ST displacement at low work intensities. These changes are known to have a high association with either multivessel or proximal left main disease.[23] Ischemia therefore tends to be global and leads to hemodynamic instability and pump failure. The high mortality and morbidity in severe coronary disease justifies surgical intervention in many cases. However, some patients either are not candidates for surgery or are failures of operative treatment. In these patients, rehabilitation programs are an important part of the management. Physical activity can be carried out by such individuals provided great care is exerted in exercise prescription. The level of activity should be regulated carefully so that severe ischemia is not induced and enough follow-up is provided to ensure that the level is well tolerated. In such cases we have found an improvement in physical working capacity and an increase in confidence of the patients that is very gratifying. However, this type of rehabilitation program is time consuming and cannot easily be managed in an office practice; referral of such patients to a rehabilitation center is probably desirable.

Studies have shown that if exercise is judiciously prescribed and conscientiously performed, physical working capacity will improve with no risk to the patients with poor ventricular function. Ventricular function neither deteriorates nor improves. A major benefit is to increase the patient's understanding of how to perform various activities with only limited working capacities.

Complications of Physical Activity. The most common complications are orthopedic.[24] The incidence of musculoskeletal injuries increases with age and intensity of exercise. However, careful planning and moderate exercise will prevent most of those injuries.

Experience with programs for patients who have coronary disease suggests that participation in strenuous physical activity (e.g., jogging) leads to ventricular fibrillation in 1 in 6000 man-hours of exercise.[1] If medical personnel are present when the complication occurs, the arrhythmia can usually be successfully treated. However, if exercise is performed in an unsupervised setting, the rhythm disturbance will probably be fatal. This underscores the importance of encouraging patients with cardiovascular disease to perform vigorous activity in the presence of trained medical personnel.

We recommend the following guidelines for exercise for patients with heart disease: (1) careful medical evaluation; (2) vigorous physical activity only with medical supervision; (3) moderate physical activity without medical supervision, provided it is prescribed under controlled conditions.

HOW IS PHYSICAL ACTIVITY PRESCRIBED FOR CORONARY PATIENTS?

The principles of selecting a tolerable work intensity, observing the patients during the activity, and increasing the activity as tolerated are essentially the same for all activities. For the *inpatient,* activity usually begins when the patient's condition is stable—that is, electrocardiographic changes, symptoms, and physical signs do not suggest worsening of the disease process. Supervisory personnel should carefully inquire about symptoms and measure heart rate and blood pressure before and after the activity. Of special interest is the occurrence of chest discomfort, dyspnea, or faintness. An inordinate increase in heart rate (over 120 beats/min) or fall in blood pressure with activity suggests marginal cardiovascular status. However, after prolonged bedrest these signs or symptoms could also be due to blood volume reduction. In the case of hypovolemia, the patients may have to gradually adapt to the upright position and may need restriction of diuretics and increased fluid consumption.

The series of activities that are used for the gradual increase in the patients' activity varies depending on available facilities. A usual regimen is to start with sitting in a bedside chair, followed by daily increments of walking in the room, walking in the hallway, and finally walking as desired. Each change in activity level should be accompanied by questioning the patient about symptoms and measuring the heart rate and blood pressure.

Predischarge submaximal exercise tests have been useful both for identifying patients who are at particularly high risk of early mortality and for identifying those with clinically significant angina pectoris.[1] Also, the amount of activity to be prescribed can be gauged by the level of activity achieved on the exercise test.

Outpatient exercise for the first few weeks should be geared to the intensity of activity being performed during the hospitalization. Walking is recommended as the mainstay of physical activity during this period of convalescence. The patient should walk for 10 minutes twice a day, then he or she should gradually increase the exercise to 30 minutes twice a day. Usually we do not prescribe arm exercise during this period of time. More intense activity and arm exercise are usually prescribed after a full, symptom-limited exercise test has been performed about 2 to 4 weeks after discharge.

USE OF THE EXERCISE TEST FOR ACTIVITY PRESCRIPTION

A symptom-limited exercise test consists of monitoring by inquiring about symptoms, measuring the blood pressure, and observing the electrocardiogram during increasing intensities of activity until the exercise is stopped because of fatigue or because a clinical reason for stopping supervenes. The test supplies the following information that can be used for the exercise prescription: peak work intensity, peak heart rate, and signs or symptoms that limit exercise. The usual procedure is to prescribe activity based on heart rate.

We recommend that individuals regulate conditioning exercise by counting the pulse or using a heart rate monitor. The heart rate provides a linear response to exercise intensity, expressed as a percentage of maximal oxygen uptake. This is the rationale for using the formula: (220 − the patient's age) × 0.7 as the target heart rate for normal individuals, since that provides an estimate of oxygen uptake approximately 80% of predicted maximum, which is an effective load for conditioning purposes. However, using 70% of predicted maximal heart rate is not suitable for cardiac patients. The heart rate tolerated during exercise is too variable in cardiac patients to use a calculation, and the prescription for activity must be based on an exercise test.

The method of calculating the heart rate goal for conditioning in cardiac patients depends on the reason that the exercise test was stopped. If the individual stopped because of fatigue, the heart rate used as a target for conditioning is as follows: [(peak heart rate − resting heart rate) × 0.5] + resting heart rate. This is within the tolerance of most patients. We recommend an activity session lasting for 30 minutes. The patient warms up for 5 minutes with little or no resistance and cools down at the end for 5 minutes with little or no resistance. The 20-minute conditioning session is carried out at the target heart rate. After the patient has demonstrated that he or she tolerates the work well, a higher heart rate may be tried until either fatigue or a clinical reason for stopping the activity intervenes. As conditioning occurs, the individual will be able to exercise at a higher work intensity, but the heart rate for that activity will remain the same (unless the medications are changed). This approach is appropriate even if the individual is on β-blockers.

If the exercise was stopped because of a clinical event, such as chest discomfort or arrhythmia, we usually prescribe activity at an intensity that is 10 beats less than that at the occurrence of the clinical event (e.g., angina). The individual is then carefully monitored during the activity for signs of intolerance.

The two most common activities in our programs are riding a stationary bicycle ergometer or walking. If the bicycle ergometer is used, the individual should either be able to set the work intensity (from the exercise test) or count the pulse during exercise. We recommend 5 minutes of activity at no resistance to warm up, 20 minutes at an intensity that will increase the heart rate to the target range, and 5 minutes of cool-down at the end. Ideally, walking speed can be prescribed by determining the step rate at which the target heart rate is reached on a treadmill. Individuals can usually safely exercise at 100 steps/min.

If the individual wants to do more intense exercise (e.g., jogging or tennis), then the activity should be started in the presence of medical supervision since programs that allow such activity have found ventricular fibrillation to occur once for each 6000 man-hours of activity, which is clearly more frequent than in normal persons. That rhythm disturbance, which almost surely would be fatal without treatment, is almost always successfully treated in the presence of medical supervision. If an individual successfully participates in such a program for 3 to 6 months, it is probably safe to continue outside the program. However, the participant should know that a small possibility of either heart attack or sudden death is still present, even though the likelihood is so low that the risk is probably acceptable. If the individual has evidence of medical problems (arrhythmias, chest discomfort) during the program, then activity should be supervised indefinitely.

Follow-Up

Regular follow-up sessions should include inquiry regarding symptoms, physical examination, measurement of body weight, review of medications, and observations during exercise. Initially, once per week is probably enough. Later, as the individual demonstrates tolerance of the exercise program and understanding of all aspects of the rehabilitation program, the amount of follow-up can decrease. The follow-up sessions should be directed toward (1) determining whether the patient's disease has progressed, (2) determining the effectiveness of the program, (3) reviewing diet and medications, and (4) revision of activity or dietary prescription. An exercise test should be performed after 3 months in the program and at 6- to 12-month intervals thereafter. If medications are changed so that heart rate may be affected, the exercise test should be repeated.

Guidelines for the Patient

The following guidelines are recommended for individuals with coronary heart disease who are beginning an exercise program:

1. Exercise regularly at the prescribed level at least 3 nonconsecutive days/wk.
2. Follow directions carefully, and if you do not understand or have questions, restrict your exercise to walking until you check with your physician.
3. Begin each exercise session with a warm-up for 5 minutes and conclude with 5 minutes or more of cool-down. This allows the circulatory system to adjust to the changes in activity.
4. Decrease the intensity of your activity, and do not resume that intensity until you have discussed it with your physician if you have shortness of breath, chest or other upper body discomfort that occurs with activity, or nausea, faintness, or excessive fatigue during the remainder of the day. It is expected that you will feel slightly tired as a result of the activity. You may also note that your heart beats more quickly—that also is normal. If you have palpitations—an awareness of your heartbeat being unusual in rate or rhythm—please report it to your physician. This is usually no cause for alarm but may mean that your medication or diet needs to be changed.
5. We recommend walking, bicycling, or similar exercise. We do not recommend swimming for conditioning because of difficulties in regulating intensity. Arm exercises are helpful for improving the upper extremity strength and tone; however, that activity should be prescribed by professionals who can monitor your response. As a rule, we recommend that loads should be restricted to under 20 to 25 lb, unless special monitoring has demonstrated that heavier loads are safe for you.

CORONARY BYPASS GRAFT SURGERY

Patients who have undergone coronary bypass graft surgery should also follow the guidelines just listed. Protection of the chest incision should be emphasized. In particular, exercise that stresses the sternum should be avoided. Usually in the first 2 to 3 weeks after surgery, activities are restricted to leg exercise and light, no-resistance arm exercise. Caution about tension in the chest incision during the activity is usually sufficient to ensure safety.

REFERENCES

1. Fletcher GF, Froelicher VF, Hartley LH, et al: Exercise standards: A statement for health professionals from the American Heart Association. Circulation 82:2286, 1990.
2. Progress in chronic disease prevention: Protective effect of physical activity on coronary heart disease. MMWR 36:426, 1987.
3. Paffenbarger RS, Wing AL, and Hyde RT: Physical activity as an index of heart attack risk in college alumni. Am J Epidemiol 108:161, 1978.
4. Kallio V, Hamalainen H, Hakkila J, et al: Reduction in sudden deaths by a multifactorial intervention programme after acute myocardial infarction. Lancet 2:1091, 1979.
5. Oldridge NB, Guyatt GH, Fischer ME, and Rimm AA: Cardiac rehabilitation after myocardial infarction: Combined experience of randomized clinical trials. JAMA 260:945, 1988.
6. O'Connor GT, Buring JE, Yusuf S, et al: An overview of randomized trials of rehabilitation with exercise after myocardial infarction. Circulation 80:234, 1989.
7. Jette M, Heller R, Landry F, and Blumchen G: Clinical investigation: Randomized 4-week exercise program in patients with impaired left ventricular function. Circulation 84:1561, 1991.
8. Sim DN and Neill WA: Investigation of the physiological basis

for increased exercise threshold for angina pectoris after physical conditioning. J Clin Invest 54:763, 1974.
9. Coats AJS, Adamopoulos S, Meyer TE, et al: Medical science: Effects of physical training in chronic heart failure. Lancet 335:63, 1990.
10. Ribeiro JP, Hartley LH, Sherwood J, et al: The effectiveness of a low lipid diet and exercise program in the management of coronary artery disease. Am Heart J 108:1183, 1984.
11. Kihlbom A, Hartley LH, Saltin B, et al: Medical evaluation of the effects of physical conditioning on middle-aged men. Scand J Clin Lab Invest 24:315, 1969.
12. Holloszy JO, Skinner J, Toro G, et al: Effects of a 6 months program of endurance exercise on the serum lipids of middle-aged men. Am J Cardiol 14:753, 1964.
13. Olefsky J, Reaven GM, and Farquhar JW: Effects of weight reduction on obesity: Studies of lipid and carbohydrate metabolism in normal and hyperlipoproteinemic subjects. J Clin Invest 53:64, 1974.
14. Choquette G and Ferguson RJ: Blood pressure reduction in borderline hypertensives following physical training. Can Med Assoc J 108:699, 1973.
15. Joint National Committee on Detection, Evaluation, and Treatment of High Blood Pressure: The 1984 Report. Arch Intern Med 144:1045, 1984.
16. Hellerstein HK: Exercise therapy in coronary disease. Bull N Y Acad Med 44:1028, 1984.
17. Garrity TF and Klein RF: Emotional response and clinical severity as early determinants of 6-month mortality after myocardial infarction. Heart Lung 4:730, 1984.
18. Hackett TP, Cassem NH, and Wishnie HA: The coronary care unit: An appraisal of its psychologic hazards. N Engl J Med 279:1365, 1968.
19. Sherwood J and Hartley LH: Optimal frequency of follow-up for rehabilitation after myocardial infarction. Circulation 68:111, 1983.
20. Hartley LH, Herd JA, Day WC, et al: An exercise testing program for large populations. JAMA 241:269, 1979.
21. Committee on Exercise: Exercise Testing and Training of Apparently Healthy Individuals: A Handbook for Physicians. Dallas, TX, American Heart Association, 1972.
22. Adgey AA, Devlin JE, Webb SW, et al: Initiation of ventricular fibrillation outside hospital in patients with acute ischaemic heart disease. Br Heart J 47:55, 1982.
23. Dash H, Massie BM, Botvinick EH, et al: The noninvasive identification of left main and 3 vessel coronary artery disease by myocardial stress perfusion scintigraphy and treadmill exercise electrocardiography. Circulation 60:276, 1979.
24. Pollock ML and Wilmore JH (eds): Exercise in Health and Disease: Evaluation and Prescription for Prevention and Rehabilitation, 2nd ed. Philadelphia, WB Saunders, 1990.

9

Tobacco Use

HARRY L. GREENE, MD

Epidemiologic studies conducted since the 1940s have clearly established the association of tobacco use and numerous diseases and conditions (Table 9–1).[1] In fact, each year more people in the United States die of smoking and smoking-related diseases than from acquired immunodeficiency syndrome (AIDS), alcohol, car accidents, cocaine, fires, heroin, homicide, and suicide combined.[2] The magnitude of smoking-related illness establishes it as the single most alterable risk factor for premature morbidity and mortality in the United States. There has been considerable progress made, going from 42% of the American adult population smoking in 1964 to 29.1% in 1990, which is an annual decline of 0.5%/yr.[3] The epidemiology of smoking is changing in other ways, with a higher percentage of women than men expected to smoke in the year 2000 because of slower rates of cessation in women. Similarly, there are currently more black men than white men smoking, but the annual rate of decrease among black men is greater. In the United States almost 40% of Hispanic men continue to smoke, with rates in the 30% range for Puerto Rican women being highest for Hispanic women.[4]

Overall, nearly 50 million American citizens smoke, and 3.5 million of these people are teenagers.[5] Although progress is being made, the current statistics show that 31.7% of men and 26.8% of women are smokers.[6] If the current trend persists, by the year 2000, 23% of women and 20% of

TABLE 9–1. SOME DISEASES AND CONDITIONS ASSOCIATED WITH SMOKING

Cancer
Bladder
Esophagus
Kidney
Larynx
Lung
Oral cavity
Pancreas
Cardiovascular diseases
Aggravation of exercise-induced angina
Arteriosclerotic aneurysm of the aorta
Arteriosclerotic peripheral vascular disease
Myocardial infarction
Stroke
Sudden death
Thromboangiitis obliterans
Perinatal effects of maternal smoking
Increased mortality
Reduced birth weight
Sudden infant death syndrome
Miscellaneous
Alteration of drug metabolism
Cataracts
Erythrocytosis
Peptic ulcer disease
Peripheral blood leukocytosis
Pustulosis
Smoker's skin
Postmenopausal tooth loss
Osteoporosis
Male sexual dysfunction

men will continue to smoke.[3] Within these groups will be increasing percentages of less educated and theoretically less employable persons, thus producing disease in persons less likely to be covered by current health plans.

The burden of suffering associated with tobacco use is immense, with an estimated 434,000 people dying each year because of smoking-related diseases.[7] This loss of life is compounded by the $22 billion that is expended to treat smoking-related disease and another $43 billion lost due to decreased productivity of those stricken with these illnesses.[8]

Fortunately, much of the risk of smoking is reversible in persons who stop in time. Prospective studies have shown that the excess cardiac mortality due to smoking approaches that of nonsmokers after 10 years of abstinence.[9] Indeed the greatest drop (~ 50%) occurs after only 1 year of abstinence.[10] The risk of lung cancer for a 1 pack/day smoker drops from 137/100,000 to 72/100,000 at 5 years, and by 10 years approaches (but never reaches) that of the nonsmoker. The risk of dying due to stroke (twice that of nonsmokers) returns to near normal by about 5 years. There are also salutary effects of cessation on the rate of decline of lung function, incidence of respiratory infection, progression of peripheral vascular disease, risk of sudden death, and recurrent myocardial infarction. Most smokers are unaware of the studies that show increased life expectancy with smoking cessation, even when cessation takes place later in life (e.g., 3.3 extra years of life for a smoker who quits at age 65).[11]

The physician's role in smoking cessation is pivotal for many patients. Seventy-five per cent of adults in the United States visit the physician at least once per year, and those who smoke may do so from three to five times/yr. This provides an opportunity to convince the patient of the dangers of smoking and to personalize their risk by linking smoking to the patient's complaints or physical findings.[12]

A number of randomized studies have shown clearly that physicians' advice to quit smoking has a positive effect. In a meta-analysis utilizing 39 of these studies, it was shown that an overall cessation rate of 8.4% at 6 months was obtained with less than 5 minutes of advice to quit.[13] Other studies done more recently have shown quit rates up to 10%.[14] This simple advice is extremely cost-effective at $750/yr of life saved versus $65,000/yr of life saved in management of hypercholesterolemia.[15] Cessation rates increase if the physician provides brochures on smoking cessation,[16] personalizes the risk through carbon monoxide monitoring or pulmonary function testing,[17, 17a] arranges for follow-up visits to focus on smoking cessation, or counsels after a critical event, that is, myocardial infarction (50 to 63%) in the coronary care unit or newly diagnosed cancer.[18] The challenge of inducing change requires more time if the event is viewed as less threatening or is applied to persons with less perceived risk.[19] The physician's job is to facilitate change for the smoker no matter at what point he or she is in the behavior change continuum.

At any point in time the smoker may be at any one of three points in a Behavior Change Paradigm. These stages of change have been defined by Diclemente and associates and are precontemplation, contemplation, and action.[20]

The patient who is in the precontemplation phase is not thinking about quitting. The physician's role here should be to make the patient aware of the health consequences and indicate that smoking is injurious to health. The physician should give firm advice to quit and provide supporting written material. A follow-up visit may be scheduled to discuss the issue further. The goal is to make a person who is not thinking about quitting, begin considering it.

Planting the idea that smoking is dangerous and that it may already have started to damage the patient's body would be the goal of a first visit with a patient who had not considered quitting. This, combined with advice to quit and the offer of support, is an excellent start for those who are reticent to quit. For the person contemplating quitting, the following approach is appropriate, because it is for the person who is ready to quit!

Most smokers (90%) express an interest in quitting, 60% have already made one or more serious attempts at quitting, and 66% express health concerns about smoking-related illness.[21] One way to remember the physician's role in smoking cessation comes from Cummings[14]:

ASK
MOTIVATE
SET A QUIT DATE

and we would add follow-up. A kit (Helping Smokers Quit) is available to all physicians from the Department of Health and Human Services.[21] Table 9–2 provides a synopsis of the Department of Health and Human Services' approach to office-based cessation, and we have supplemented these with suggestions from other programs.[23] This approach is straightforward. Identify the smoker and tell him or her about how smoking is affecting his or her health. Ask if the person would be willing to try to quit if you try to help. Help to motivate him or her to expect success. Let the person discuss what "went wrong" in previous cessation attempts. Use these barriers to brainstorm a new plan (e.g., against craving-nicotine replacement and against a relapse while using alcohol). The person should avoid drinking during the early stages of cessation and also should avoid cig-

TABLE 9–2. SYNOPSIS FOR PHYSICIANS: HOW TO HELP YOUR PATIENTS STOP SMOKING

1. **Ask** about smoking at every opportunity.
   a. "Do you smoke?"
   b. "How much?"
   c. "How soon after awakening do you have your first cigarette?"
   d. "Are you interested in stopping smoking?"
2. **Advise** all smokers to stop.
   a. State your advice clearly, for example: "As your physician, I must advise you to stop smoking now."
   b. Personalize the message to quit. Refer to the patient's clinical condition, smoking history, family history, personal interests, or social roles.
3. **Assist** the patient in stopping.
   a. Set a quit date. Help the patient pick a date within the next 4 weeks, acknowledging that no time is ideal.
   b. Provide self-help materials. The smoking cessation coordinator or support staff member can review the materials with the patient if desired (for example, call 1-800-4-CANCER for NCI's *Quit for Good* materials).
   c. Consider prescribing nicotine gum, especially for highly addicted patients (those who smoke one pack a day or more or who smoke their first cigarette within 30 minutes of waking).
   d. Consider signing a stop-smoking contract with the patient.
   e. If the patient is not willing to quit now:
      • Provide motivating literature (for example, call 1-800-4-CANCER for NCI's *Why Do You Smoke?* pamphlet).
      • Ask again at the next visit.
4. **Arrange** follow-up visits.
   a. Set a follow-up visit within 1–2 weeks after the quit date.
   b. Have a member of the office staff call or write the patient within 7 days after initial visit, reinforcing the decision to stop and reminding the patient of the quit date.
   c. At the first follow-up visit, ask about the patient's smoking status to provide support and help prevent relapse. Relapse is common; if it happens, encourage the patient to try again immediately.
   d. Set a second follow-up visit in 1–2 months. For patients who have relapsed, discuss the circumstances of the relapse and other special concerns.

arettes provided by others at work or home. The person should let others know that he or she is quitting and should ask for help. For the smoker who wants to quit, ask him or her to pick a quit day and sign a quitting contract with you, the physician, signing as a witness. For the majority of addicted smokers the nicotine withdrawal symptoms will have played a major role in relapse in the past.[24] These symptoms include craving, irritability, frequent awakening, anxiety, decreased concentration, restlessness, drowsiness, impatience, confusion, increased appetite, and slow reaction time.

Some of these symptoms have been managed successfully by using pharmacologic therapy. The agents that are approved for these indications are nicotine replacement via, for example, nicotine Polacrilex gum and nicotine-containing transdermal patches.

Nicotine Polacrilex is available in 2-mg and 4-mg strengths and is the first agent proven efficacious in a number of controlled studies.[25] The majority of the nicotine is absorbed from the buccal mucosa (approximately half) and depends on the oral pH. Using acid beverages, colas, tea, or coffee lowers the pH and decreases absorption.[26] This fact, combined with the observation that blood levels of nicotine with the 2-mg dose do not approach that of smoking, may lead to decreased efficacy in relieving cravings.[27] Experience has shown that in order for patients to obtain the high cessation rates quoted in the literature (28% at 2 years versus 9.4% for placebo), they need to be carefully instructed in the use of the gum. They should use enough gum, 15 pieces/day, and take it in conjunction with a behavioral program.[28] A further important factor is the continuation of gum use for 3 to 6 months before starting to taper the amount taken.[29] It is also clear that simply prescribing the gum without the aforementioned components results in no improvement in cessation rates (8% nicotine gum versus 13% placebo gum).[30]

Nicotine via transdermal patches has been approved and is now being widely marketed in the United States. The level of nicotine delivered by these devices is lower but comparable with that obtained by smoking[31] and is higher than levels seen with the 2-mg nicotine gum. The symptoms of withdrawal are better controlled with the patches, although some patch wearers will still have some degree of symptoms. The cessation rates for studies that have had follow-up for at least 3 months vary from 17% using the patch versus 4% in the placebo group to 48% using the patch versus 13% in the placebo group.[32–36]

In clinical trials the adverse effects of transdermal nicotine rarely caused discontinuation of the drug (6 to 7%).[37] The most frequently observed adverse reaction was skin irritation, which included localized erythema, edema, or pruritus and did not lead to discontinuation of patch use. One study showed an allergic reaction to nicotine beginning between the 6th and 28th day of patch application in 3.2% of subjects tested.[38] The other described effects are similar to those seen in patients undergoing nicotine withdrawal. Patients commonly commented on a change in dreaming while on the higher-dose patches. The patches are designed to be used by those who are quitting smoking. It is not recommended for pregnant patients, although it is probably better for the mother and the fetus than if the mother continues to smoke. The patches should be kept away from children and pets, since the higher-dose patches could cause nicotine toxicity. Other side effects are shown in Table 9–3. ***One must not continue to smoke and use the patches!***

Different formulations include Nicoderm (Marion Merrill Dow), Habitrol (Basel Ciba Geigy), PROSTEP (Ledere), and Nicotrol (Parke-Davis). PROSTEP is the largest of the patches and delivers 22 mg/day. Habitrol is intermediate in size (30 cm^2) and contains 52.5 mg of nicotine, with Nicoderm being the smallest size (22 cm^2) containing 114 mg of nicotine. Nicotrol patches deliver 15 mg, 10 mg, or 5 mg/16 hours, depending on the patch size. The Nicoderm

TABLE 9–3. SIDE EFFECT PROFILE FOR THE NICOTINE PATCH*

Effect	Reported Frequency
Short-lived erythema, pruritus or burning	35–54
Local erythema	7–22
Local edema	3–8
Cutaneous hypersensitivity	2–3
Mild to moderate insomnia	1–23
Diarrhea	1–9
Dyspepsia	1–9
Myalgia	3–9
Nervousness	3–9
Somnolence	1–9
Abnormal dreams	1–9
Arthralgia	1–9
Abdominal pain	1–3
Dry mouth	1–3
Sweating	1–3

*From Fiore MC, Jorenby DE, Baker TB, et al: Tobacco dependence and the nicotine patch. JAMA 268:2690, 1992.

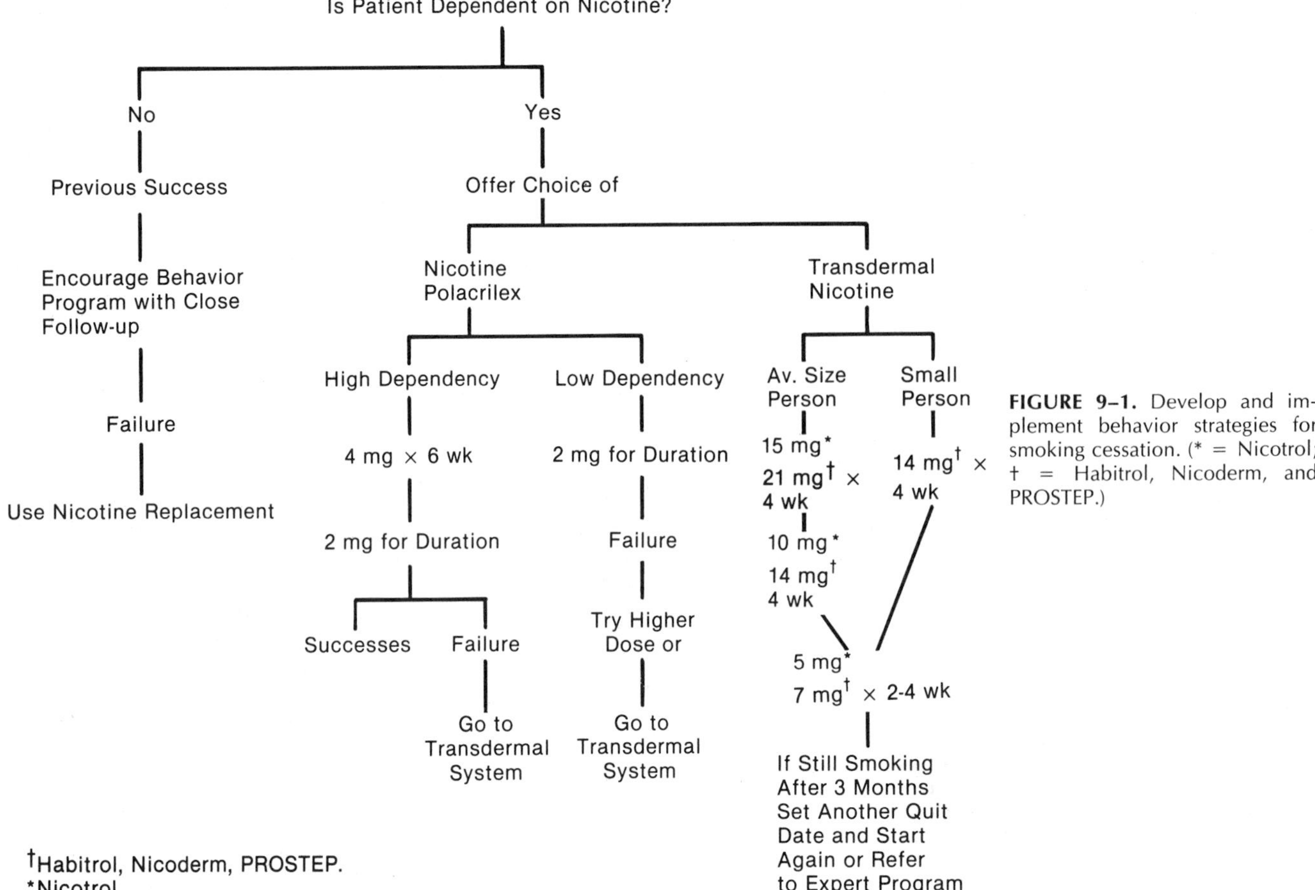

FIGURE 9–1. Develop and implement behavior strategies for smoking cessation. (* = Nicotrol; † = Habitrol, Nicoderm, and PROSTEP.)

and Habitrol patches are designed to deliver 21 mg/24 hr. All four products come with "behavioral kits" that supply patient information, a quitting contract, advice to spouses or support personnel, and two products supply a relaxation and motivation audio tape from the American Lung Association (Habitrol, Nicotrol).

These products vary in their advice regarding the dose and how to taper off the dose. Nicoderm is recommended for 6 weeks at the 21-mg dose, with a taper at 2 weeks to 14 mg followed by 2 weeks at 7 mg. Habitrol is used in a 4-week 21-mg program, 4-week 14-mg program, then 2- to 4-week 7-mg program. PROSTEP is recommended for a shorter interval. Nicotrol recommendations are for 15 mg for 2–4 weeks, 10 mg for 2 weeks, and 5 mg for 2 weeks. Decreased doses may be needed for smaller individuals or for those smoking less than 15 cigarettes/day.

There are no data to show an advantage of one product over another, and all have similar early cessation rates. The cost for 1 month of therapy approximates $100 to $120, and 10 weeks of therapy costs from $250 to $300. There have been no published trials comparing the various suggested weaning strategies.[39]

If patients cannot quit smoking after 4 weeks of therapy, the patch should be discontinued because in the controlled trials those who continued to smoke for this length of time were unlikely to quit. The patches can be reinstituted after a greater commitment is demonstrated and a new quit date is selected.

Nicotine replacement therapy is contraindicated, or at best would be used cautiously, in those in whom its presence might worsen their condition (e.g., recent myocardial infarction, accelerated hypertension, life-threatening arrhythmias, peptic ulcers, hyperthyroidism, esophagitis, vasospastic disease, pheochromocytoma, and diabetes). In the face of pregnancy, behavioral methods should probably be used, although some suggest that nicotine replacement may have a role. If one chooses to do this, we would advise getting informed consent from the patient.

Patients who fail on an office-based attempt may require a more expert or more individualized program. These expert programs usually include a physician, psychologist, psychiatrist, or experienced counselor and should have a low ratio of patients to therapist. Many of these programs are in academic centers where smoking cessation research is continuing. Most experts in the United States do not believe that acupuncture offers any additional benefit over counseling. The use of hypnosis has mixed reviews, and when it is shown to have an effect, it is usually in the context of a counseling program.

Although smoking cessation rates have been low in the past, recent office-based programs that include identifying the smoker, advising him or her to quit, working with him or her to identify and overcome any barriers, using nicotine replacement to combat withdrawal, and scheduling regular follow-up visits have put the promise of success within reach for the 50 million people who continue to smoke but would like to join the 30 million others who have already quit.[40]

An algorithm for office-based smoking cessation is shown in Figure 9–1.[41]

REFERENCES

1. Greene HL, Goldberg RJ, and Ockene JK: Cigarette smoking: The physician's role in cessation and maintenance. J Gen Med 3:75–87, 1988.
2. Centers for Disease Control: Cigarette Smoking among Adults—United States 1990. MMWR 1992 41:354–355, 1992.
3. Pierce JP, Fiore MC, Novotny TE, et al: Trends in cigarette smoking in the United States: Projections to the year 2000. JAMA 261:61–65, 1989.
4. Escobedo LG, and Remington PL: Birth cohort analysis of prevalence of cigarette smoking among Hispanics in the U.S. JAMA 261:66–69, 1989.
5. Greydanus DE: Routing a modern pied-piper of Hamelin. JAMA 261:99–100, 1989.
6. Fiore MC: Methods used to quit smoking in the United States. JAMA 263:2760–2765, 1990.
7. Smoking—Attributable Mortality and Years of Potential Life Lost—United States, 1988. HHS Publication No. (CDC) 91-8017. Atlanta, GA, Centers for Disease Control, 1991.
8. US Department of Health and Human Services: Smoking Tobacco and Health: A Fact Book. DHHS Publication No. (CDC) 87-8397 (revised 10/89).
9. Friedman GD, Petitti DB, Bawol RD, et al: Mortality in cigarette smokers and quitters. N Engl J Med 304:1407, 1981.
10. Health Benefits of Smoking Cessation: A Report of the Surgeon General—1990. U.S. Department of Health and Human Services, Public Health Service, Centers for Disease Control, Center for Chronic Disease Prevention and Health Promotion, Office of Smoking and Health. DHHS Publication number (CDC) 90-8416, 1990.
11. Sachs DP: Advances in smoking cessation treatment. *In* Simmons DH. (ed): Current Pulmonology. Chicago, Year Book Medical Publishers, 1991, pp 139–198.
12. Stone S and Perlmutter KJ: Methods for stopping cigarette smoking. Ann Intern Med 105:281–291, 1986.
13. Kottke TE, Battista RN, Defriese GH, et al: Attributes of successful smoking cessation intervention in medical practice: A meta-analysis of 39 controlled trials. JAMA 259:2882–2889, 1988.
14. Cummings SR, Coates TJ, Richard RJ, et al: Training physicians in counseling about smoking cessation: A randomized trial of the "Quit for Life" Program. Ann Intern Med 110:640–647, 1989.
15. Cummings SR, Rubin SM, and Oster G: The cost-effectiveness of counseling smokers to quit. JAMA 261:75–79, 1989.
16. Russell MAH, Wilson C, Taylor C, et al: The effect of general practitioner's advice against smoking. BMJ 2:231–235, 1979.
17. Jamrozik K, Vessey M, Fowler G, et al: Controlled trial of three different anti-smoking interventions in general practice. BMJ 288:1499–1502, 1984.

17a. Risser NL and Belcher DW: Adding spirometry, carbon monoxide and pulmonary symptom results to smoking cessation counseling: A randomized trial. J Gen Med 5:15–22, 1990.

18. Croog SH and Richards NP: Health beliefs and smoking pattern in heart patients and their wives: A longitudinal study. Am J Public Health 67:921–930, 1977.
19. Rose G and Hamilton PJS: A randomized controlled trial of the effect on middle-aged men of advice to stop smoking. J Epidemiol Community Health 36:102–108, 1982.
20. Diclemente C, Prochaska JO, Farithurst SK, et al: The precess of smoking cessation: An analysis of precontemplation, contemplation and preparation stages of change. J Consult Clin. Psychiatry 59:295–304, 1991.
21. Orleans CT: Understanding and promoting smoking cessation: Overview and guidelines for physician intervention. Ann Rev Med 36:51–61, 1965.
22. National Cancer Institute: Helping Smokers Quit. Bethesda, MD, Office of Cancer Communication, 1987.
23. Cocores JA: The Clinical Management of Nicotine Dependence. New York, Springer-Verlag, 1991.
24. Henningfield JE and Nemeth-Coslett R: Nicotine dependence: Interface between tobacco and tobacco-related disease. Chest 93(Suppl):37S–55S, 1988.
25. Ferno O, Lichtneckert S, and Lundgren C: A substitute for tobacco smoking. Psychopharmacology 31:201–204, 1973.
26. Benowitz NL, Jacob P, and Savanapridi C: Determinants of nicotine intake while chewing nicotine polacrilex gum. Clin Pharmacol Ther 41:467–473, 1987.
27. Smoking and Health: A National Status Report; HHS/PHS/CAC 87-8396. Rockville, MD, US Department of Health and Human Services, Public Health Service, 1986.
28. Tonnesen P, Fryd V, Hansen M, et al: Effect of nicotine gum in combination with group counseling and the cessation of smoking. N Engl J Med 318:15–18, 1988.
29. Lam W, Szn C, Sacks HS, et al: Meta-analysis of randomized controlled trials of nicotine chewing-gum. Lancet 2:27–30, 1987.
30. Schneider NG, Jarvik ME, Forsythe AB, et al: Nicotine gum in smoking cessation: A placebo controlled, double-blind trial. Addict Behav 8:256–261, 1983.
31. Mulligan SC, Masterson JG, Devone JG, et al: Clinical and pharmacokinetic properties of a transdermal nicotine patch. Clin Pharmacol Ther 47:331–337, 1990.
32. Abelin T, Buehler A, Mueller P, et al: Controlled trial of transdermal nicotine patch in tobacco withdrawal. Lancet i:7–10, 1989.
33. Buchkremer G and Minniker E: Efficiency of multimodal smoking cessation therapy combining transdermal nicotine substitution with behavioral therapy. Methods Find Exp Clin Pharmacol 11:215–218, 1989.
34. Daughton DM, Heatley SA, Prendergast JJ, et al: Effect of transdermal nicotine delivery as an adjunct to low-intervention smoking cessation therapy: A randomized, placebo-controlled, double-blind study. Arch Intern Med 151:749–752, 1991.
35. Hurt RD, Lauger GG, Offord KP, et al: Nicotine replacement therapy with use of a transdermal nicotine patch: A randomized double-blind placebo controlled trial. Mayo Clin Proc 65:1529–1537, 1990.
36. Tonnessen P, Norregaard J, Simonsen K, et al: A double blind trial of 16 hour transdermal nicotine patch in smoking cessation. N Engl J Med 325:311–315, 1991.
37. Rose JE: Transdermal nicotine and nasal nicotine administration as smoking-cessation treatments. *In* Cocores JA (ed): The Clinical Management of Nicotine Dependence. New York, Springer Verlag, 1991.
38. Eichelberg E, Stolze P, Block M, et al: Contact allergies induced by TTS treatment. Methods Find Exp Clin Pharmacol 11:223–225, 1989.
39. Rose JE: Transdermal nicotine and nasal nicotine administration as smoking-cessation treatments. *In* Cocores JA (ed): The Clinical Management of Nicotine Dependence. New York, Springer Verlag, 1991, p. 202.
40. Jaffe JH: Tobacco smoking and nicotine dependence. *In* Wonnacott S, Russell MAH, and Stolerman IP (eds): Nicotine Psychopharmacology. Oxford, Oxford University Press, 1990.
41. Greene HL and Garcia LA: Smoking cessation. *In* Greene HL, Johnson WP, and Maricic MJ (eds): Decision Making in Medicine. St. Louis, Mosby–Year Book, 1992.

10

Hypertension

ROBERT C. GOLDSZER, MD
HAROLD S. SOLOMON, MD

Hypertension is the most common diagnosis for physician visits and for prescription medications.[1] The prevalence in the United States is currently estimated at 30 million.[2] The benefits of treatment to public and individual health have been demonstrated beginning with the VA Cooperative Study Groups on antihypertensive agents in 1967.[3] Hypertension is an independent risk factor for all cardiovascular diseases,[4] and treatment is beneficial in decreasing vascular complications. Patients with mild to moderate hypertension (90 to 114 mm Hg diastolic pressure) or severe hypertension (>115 mm Hg diastolic pressure), and the elderly with systolic hypertension, all show decreased vascular events with lowering blood pressure.[5] In 1990, Collins and associates published a meta-analysis of 14 trials involving 37,000 subjects. Blood pressure was decreased an average of 5 to 6 mm Hg. Mortality from all vascular causes was reduced by 21%, the incidence of stroke was decreased by 42%, and the incidence of myocardial infarction was reduced by 15%.[6]

Public awareness of the adverse consequences of hypertension has grown dramatically and has undoubtedly helped to increase the number of patients being treated. Newer medications allow lower dosages and once-a-day treatment in many patients. However, side effects and costs remain significant barriers to effective treatment, and the same questions remain unanswered.

The role of nonpharmacologic treatments of hypertension remains controversial. Data demonstrating their efficacy in decreasing vascular complications are nonexistent, but studies demonstrate that blood pressure is decreased with weight loss, exercise, and reduction in alcohol intake.[7, 8] Nonpharmacologic instructions in conjunction with medications are now recommended as part of the initial therapy.

The question of which antihypertensive agent to use first has become more complex for the physician but beneficial for the patient. The physician can now select the single agent that may best treat the patient's pathophysiology. We have called this select-care and monotherapy, rather than step-care. No single class of agents is the initial choice for all patients. Each of the classes of agents is beneficial in certain patients, and we frequently employ diuretics, β-blockers, or angiotensin-converting enzyme inhibitors as initial therapy.

The level of blood pressure at which the risk of treatment exceeds the risk of cardiovascular consequences is not known. Adverse effects of the medications used must be considered. The Multiple Risk Factor Intervention Trial raised questions about the safety of diuretic therapy for patients with mild hypertension who also have an abnormal electrocardiogram. Although the findings were not striking and thus are unlikely to cause major upheavals in our views of treatment, they nevertheless underscore our need for more information about who needs treatment and what such treatment ought to be.[9]

A newly recognized problem that demands attention is the presence of elevated blood pressure levels among children. It is becoming apparent that essential hypertension is more common in children than was once thought and that children whose parents have hypertension tend to have higher blood pressures than do their peers. Unfortunately, the question of whether to treat the majority of these children who have marginally elevated blood pressure remains unanswered.

At What Level of Blood Pressure Should Treatment Be Initiated?

According to the recommendations of the Joint National Committee on Detection, Evaluation, and Treatment of High Blood Pressure, all patients with sustained diastolic pressures greater than 105 should definitely receive treatment.[10] At the other end of the spectrum, "normal" blood pressure is defined as less than 140/85. For a pressure between 90 and 104 mm Hg—that group called "mildly high"—individualization of therapy is recommended. It has been our policy to treat with pharmacotherapy the usual middle-aged hypertensive patient whose diastolic blood pressure reproducibly exceeds 90 mm Hg. This may be an aggressive approach, although our experience is that practically all physicians prescribe medications for diastolic pressure in excess of 95 and most do so as well for those between 90 and 95.

The Hypertension Detection and Follow-Up Program (HDFP),[11] the Australian Therapeutic Trial,[12] and the VA Study[3] all showed decreased stroke, left ventricular hypertrophy, and congestive heart failure in treated hypertensives. The HDFP showed decreased coronary events, as did the MRC study in male patients.[13] Conversely, the Multiple Risk Factor Intervention Trial[14] has raised a question of benefits of treatment in a group of patients whose diastolic pressures were persistently 90 to 95 and in whom diuretics were used as the first-step drug. Upon further scrutiny, these patients were found to have an abnormal electrocardiogram in addition to mild hypertension. Diuretics may have been a suboptimal or wrong choice of therapy in this population.

The decision to treat must be individualized. If the diastolic pressure is labile—that is, sometimes 90 to 95 and sometimes below—treatment may be postponed or nonpharmacologic approaches employed (see subsequent discussion). Patients for whom hypertension is the least serious of other concomitant illnesses may be observed rather than treated. We tend to treat those younger patients (<35 years of age) in whom systolic pressure repeatedly exceeds 160 mm Hg without diastolic elevations and generally favor treating borderline patients if other coronary risk factors, such as family history of premature vascular disease, lipid abnormalities, smoking, or diabetes, are present. The importance of not smoking needs to be emphasized; the relatively modest benefit of treating mild hypertension (2.1 [in men] and 1.0 [in women] fewer cardiovascular events, chiefly strokes, per 1000 patient-years in the MRC study[13]) is far outweighed by the risk of continued smoking.

Once the decision to treat has been made, drug therapy is instituted. Once the patient has achieved successful blood pressure control with adequate doses of tolerated medications, and once the patient is comfortable in our practice, we then also initiate lifestyle alterations such as weight loss, physical activity, and smoking cessation. The message is that there is an added benefit to lifestyle changes and that medications might be decreased or discontinued if they are successful.

The goal of therapy, which should be clearly explained to the patient, should be to maintain blood pressures as low as possible without side effects from medication, certainly below 90 mm Hg diastolic or 140 mm Hg systolic. In general, if a specified dose of medication causes diastolic pressure to fall to as low as 70 mm Hg, for example, with no perceptible adverse effects, the dosage should remain at that level rather than be reduced.

YOUNG, ASYMPTOMATIC, HYPERTENSIVE INDIVIDUAL

If one arbitrarily selects a sustained diastolic blood pressure above 90 mm Hg as the level at which treatment should begin, most patients with essential hypertension will have achieved that level by 35 years of age. At this age, people are often busy pursuing economic and social goals or raising young children and, in general, pay little attention to matters of health. This lack of concern combined with the fact that hypertension in its earliest stages is usually without significant symptoms places a great burden on the physician, who must convince asymptomatic, vigorously active persons that they should take steps to improve their health. The lack of immediate adverse consequences if these steps are not taken, the absence of symptoms, and the complex regimens offered by some physicians encourage noncompliance.

How can the physician maximize the patient's motivation to reduce this health risk and to maintain a therapeutic program? The most important determinant of success in treatment of the patient with hypertension is how seriously he or she perceives the condition to be. The initial visits to the physician are critical in this regard. The first obligation to the physician is to turn the "person" into a "patient," that is, someone who thinks of health every day and performs certain related activities (e.g., taking medication). Since the patient must depend upon health personnel (physicians, nurses, nutritionists) for advice and guidance about the activities of daily living, the patient may sense a loss of control over his or her own life. Thus, if the physician immediately imposes numerous restrictions and changes in the patient's normal behavior with respect to diet, smoking, exercise, medication, and office visits, the likelihood of compliance will be jeopardized. Another major consideration is cost versus benefit; if an individual perceives the value of therapy to be great and the cost not excessive, he or she will "buy" the treatment.

Therefore, many factors affect a patient's decision to continue care, and different combinations of motivators of and deterrents to compliance will apply in each individual case (Fig. 10–1). In our model (derived from the literature and personal experience), positive numbers represent "contributors" to compliance and negative numbers represent "detractors"; zero makes no contribution. For a given patient, the magnitude of the positive or negative number determines the level of importance of a given category in enhancing patient compliance. The higher the total positive number, the more likely the patient would be to comply.

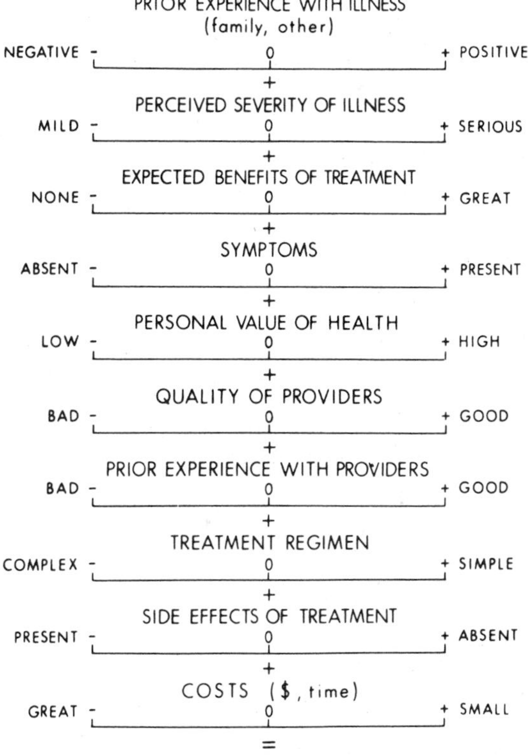

FIGURE 10–1. Factors involved in a patient's decision to comply with treatment based on cost versus benefit. (From Solomon HS: How to improve patient compliance. *In* Lasagna L [ed]: Controversies in Therapeutics. Philadelphia, WB Saunders, 1980, p 569.)

The essential ingredients to ensure compliance are minimizing the changes in lifestyle and providing a treatment plan that builds on successful completion of each step. Of all the desired health behavioral changes mentioned, the simplest is the taking of medication. So, once the physician decides that *blood pressure is sustained at a high enough level to require treatment,* pharmacotherapy is the first step. The patient will then perceive that the initial "cost" is minimal, requiring only that he or she take the medication and return for follow-up visits. Once blood pressure has been controlled by means of standard antihypertensive regimens, usually within the first 2 months of care, one may seek to reduce medications and improve the patient's total cardiovascular risk profile.

It is likely that most cigarette smokers in the United States are already aware of the potential hazards of this habit. Thus, the approach should not be simply to reinforce a patient's guilt and anxiety about smoking but must include teaching the skills that will help the patient achieve this health behavioral goal. The same approach can be taken to implement changes in nutrition. Encouraged by the control of blood pressure achieved with antihypertensive medication, the patient will be more likely to accept dietary changes to promote weight loss and to lower serum cholesterol levels.

Patients are more likely to adhere to a treatment regimen when they sense that the physician is concerned about whether or not they comply. The amount of time and effort spent in instructing the patient is certainly important. Other simple measures include phoning patients to remind them of appointments, minimizing office waiting time, and providing a courteous and helpful staff. One should reasonably expect that 80% of the hypertensive population will successfully pursue their treatment goals. Among the other 20% of patients, alcoholism, severe depression, and other psychiatric disorders, as well as denial, may present obstacles that are difficult to overcome.[15]

STANDARD TREATMENTS FOR HYPERTENSION

Pharmacologic Treatment

Blood pressure can be determined by multiplying cardiac output by the peripheral vascular resistance. Cardiac output depends on plasma volume, heart rate, and myocardial contractility. Of these factors, plasma volume is determined by the state of hydration, plasma protein concentrations, sodium intake, the state of the venous system, and the renin-angiotensin-aldosterone system; heart rate and myocardial contractility are regulated predominantly by the β-adrenergic nervous system. Peripheral vascular resistance is influenced by the α-adrenergic system, angiotensin, bradykinins, and prostaglandins. The function of the various cardiovascular reflex mechanisms is to maintain adequate blood pressure at all costs.

Generally, sustained hypertension is associated with normal cardiac output and increased peripheral resistance. The cardiovascular system responds as though elevated blood pressure were a normal state in this setting, so that if peripheral vascular resistance is reduced (with vasodilators), cardiac output increases. Conversely, if one decreases cardiac output either by acutely depleting blood volume or by giving a β-adrenergic blocking agent, the response will be a reflex increase in peripheral vascular resistance. Most drugs that lower blood pressure, except angiotensin-converting enzyme inhibitors (ACEI), activate aldosterone secretion, which prompts sodium retention and thus reduces the effect of the antihypertensive agent. These compensatory reflexes, however, usually are not as efficient as is the primary effect of the medications, so that a net decrease in blood pressure will occur.

Choice of Medications

Antihypertensive medications can be most conveniently divided into three categories based on their pharmacologic effect: (1) diuretics; (2) sympathoactive drugs, and (3) peripheral vasodilators. Uncomplicated hypertension has traditionally been treated initially with a diuretic. Our policy is to use β-blockers or ACEIs more often as initial therapy in the usual uncomplicated patient, because of questions of the long-term safety of diuretics, specifically hypokalemia, hyperlipidemia, hyperglycemia, and insulin resistance. Factors associated with a more beneficial response to β-blockers are young age, male sex, white race, abnormal baseline electrocardiogram (ECG), and nonsmoking, but in the absence of contraindications β-blockers or ACEIs can be tried in most patients. If a second agent is required, we then select a thiazide or other diuretic. If the combination of thiazide diuretic and β-blocker or ACEI does not satisfactorily control blood pressure, a third agent (ACEI or β-blocker depending on which was chosen first) is added.

If the pressure normalizes with addition of the third agent, the diuretic will be stopped. The patient is seen at frequent intervals to assess blood pressure and side effects and to communicate with the patient. As blood pressure stays normal, the agents will slowly be decreased in dosage in an attempt to achieve monotherapy with as low a dose as possible.

Classes of Drugs, Effects, and Dosage

Diuretics. Three types of diuretics are currently in use: the benzothiadiazides (thiazides) and thiazide-like drugs; the more potent "loop" diuretics, furosemide, ethacrynic acid, and bumetanide; and the potassium-sparing agents, spironolactone, triamterene, and amiloride (Table 10–1).

Thiazide Diuretics. These agents have been available for over 30 years and are still a cornerstone of therapy. Clinical observation indicates that none of the thiazides or thiazide-like drugs is superior to the least expensive generic hydrochlorothiazide preparations, in terms of either

TABLE 10–1. DIURETICS, SYMPATHOLYTICS, AND VASODILATORS

Diuretics	Usual Dosage Range*
Hydrochlorothiazide	25–50 mg
Chlorthalidone	25–100 mg
Furosemide	20–100 mg
Bumetanide	0.5–1 mg
Spironolactone	25–100 mg
Amiloride	50–100 mg
Triamterene	100–200 mg
Sympathoactive Agents	
Methyldopa	0.5–3 g
Clonidine	0.2–2 mg
Rauwolfia alkaloid	0.25–0.50 mg
Guanethidine	10–100 mg
Guanadrel	10–80 mg
Guanabenz	8–32 mg
Peripheral Vasodilators	
Hydralazine	50–200 mg
Minoxidil	5–30 mg
Prazosin	2–20 mg

*Dosage per 24 hours.

potassium-sparing or antihypertensive potency of the maximally tolerable dose.

Initially the thiazides inhibit sodium reabsorption in the cortical segment of the ascending limb of the loop of Henle. As a result, plasma volume falls, reducing cardiac output. After 1 to 2 weeks of therapy, plasma volume returns to nearly normal levels, and peripheral resistance decreases. It is likely that this effect on peripheral vascular resistance—through an as yet unknown mechanism—contributes to the sustained reduction of blood pressure.[16] The extent of this reduction depends on the diastolic pressure level at which therapy is begun, but in general ranges from 5 to 15 mm Hg. Unless salt intake increases, thiazides continue to be effective for an indefinite period of time.

Usually one starts with a single 25-mg dose of hydrochlorothiazide. Titration to 50 mg may be necessary, or reduction to lower dosages, 12.5 mg, may be successful. Although the natriuretic effect of hydrochlorothiazide persists for less than 12 hours, blood pressure reduction requires only a single daily dose. Side effects are usually mild; patients may complain of nonspecific fatigue, muscle cramps, gastrointestinal disturbances, and, rarely, impotence or decreased libido. Although fatigue and muscle cramps are sometimes attributed to hypokalemia, often these symptoms do not disappear with correction of potassium deficiency. Other effects of thiazide therapy include hypokalemia, hyperuricemia, hyperglycemia, and hyperlipidemia. Less frequent complications are hypercalcemia, severe hyponatremia, thrombocytopenia, granulocytopenia, vasculitis, liver disease, pancreatitis, and photosensitive skin eruptions.[17]

Hypokalemia. In most cases, thiazide therapy reduces serum potassium, with levels falling below 3.5 mEq/l in about 10% of patients. A reasonable approach is to monitor serum potassium levels at 3- to 6-month intervals during therapy. Traditional means of supplementing the diet with bananas or dried fruits are ineffective. If the patient is taking digitalis or is predisposed to cardiac arrhythmia, potassium supplementation is usually employed initially. For those with potassium values of 3.5 mEq/l or less, a combination of thiazide and potassium-sparing diuretic may be substituted, or potassium chloride (Slow-K tablets, Kay Ciel Elixir, K-Lyte, K-Lor) may be given in doses of 40 to 70 mEq/day. Although serious complications of hypokalemia may occur, including cardiac arrhythmias, renal structural changes with inability to concentrate the urine, electrocardiographic changes, and altered carbohydrate tolerance, such complications are probably rare and do not justify use of expensive or unpleasant supplements for every patient.[18] Among 332 of our own patients, 48% are taking potassium-wasting diuretics, whereas only 8% are using potassium supplements, and 18% are on combinations of thiazides with potassium-sparing diuretics.

Hyperuricemia. Hyperuricemia occurs in perhaps two thirds of patients taking thiazides. Overt gout develops less frequently. Thiazides interfere with the excretion of urate but have no effect on its rate of production, so that serum but not urinary uric acid levels increase. Uric acid stone formation is therefore not a concern. It is usually not necessary to treat mild hyperuricemia (<10 mg/dl); however, when levels exceed 10 mg/dl or if patients experience overt gouty attacks, uricosuric drugs or allopurinol may be employed in conjunction with thiazide therapy.

Hyperglycemia. Carbohydrate intolerance can occur with thiazide therapy, and pre-existing maturity-onset diabetes may become more difficult to control. Insulin-dependent diabetics, on the other hand, are usually not adversely affected by thiazides. Several mechanisms probably account for the development or exacerbation of hyperglycemia: hypokalemia inhibits insulin release, thiazides may have a direct effect on insulin release, and the uptake of glucose by peripheral cells may be reduced. The appearance of increased blood sugar levels is not in itself an absolute indication for discontinuing thiazide therapy. If a patient is already receiving insulin or an oral hypoglycemic agent, simple dosage adjustments will often correct the hyperglycemia. An exception to this rule would be the maturity-onset diabetic whose condition is well controlled with dietary restrictions alone but who must begin taking medication as a consequence of thiazide therapy; in this case an alternative to thiazides should be sought. Furosemide is less diabetogenic than are the thiazides.

Hyperlipidemia. Thiazide diuretics have been demonstrated to have an adverse effect on lipid metabolism by increasing plasma triglycerides, total cholesterol, and low-density lipoprotein cholesterol.[19] The mechanism of these elevations has not been determined. These elevated lipid levels could tend to increase the risk of coronary heart disease,[20] blunting somewhat the benefits of blood pressure reduction. Patients on therapy should have baseline lipids measured and regular monitoring thereafter.

Less Common Adverse Reactions. The relatively mild side effects of thiazide use just discussed are usually not serious enough to warrant discontinuation of therapy. However, the development of more serious side effects such as cholestatic jaundice, pancreatitis, deteriorating renal or liver function, thrombocytopenia, or photosensitive cutaneous eruptions represents an absolute indication for cessation of this therapy.

"Loop" Diuretics. The potent diuretic agents furosemide, ethacrynic acid, and bumetanide have sometimes been used in the treatment of hypertension. There is evidence that although these agents are more potent diuretics, their antihypertensive effect is not any greater than that of the thiazides. As mentioned earlier, this may suggest that whereas the thiazides work as peripheral vasodilators as well as diuretic agents, loop diuretics act by means of volume reduction alone. Occasional patients tolerate these agents when thiazides have caused serious adverse reactions. Otherwise, they are rarely chosen for treating hypertension, except in patients with renal insufficiency, in whom thiazides inadequately control hypervolemia and may worsen azotemia.

Potassium-Sparing Diuretic Agents. In addition to their mild diuretic effects, spironolactone (Aldactone), triamterene (Dyrenium), and amiloride act to prevent potassium wasting. Spironolactone is a competitive inhibitor of aldosterone, thus blocking the exchange of sodium and potassium in the distal tubule of the kidney. Its antihypertensive effects are similar to those of the thiazides, and it may be useful in combination with these drugs to prevent potassium wasting. Side effects include gynecomastia, impotence, and gastrointestinal disturbances. Triamterene and amiloride inhibit potassium wasting by direct inhibition in the distal nephron. They have a slight blood pressure lowering effect alone, diminish magnesium wasting, do not adversely influence sexual functioning, but rarely are associated with renal calculi and possibly nitrogen retention or interstitial nephritis.

Sympathoactive Drugs. Sympathoactive agents are the initial choice for control of hypertension in young white men and in patients who also have coronary artery disease or an abnormal baseline ECG. They operate within the sympathetic nervous system, acting either peripherally to block receptor neuronal-releasing sites or centrally to inhibit the α or β outflow tracts. Since clinical selection is not based on the cellular mechanism of action, however, a detailed description of such action for each of these drugs does not seem warranted here. Side effects include depression, lethargy, and sleep disturbances as well as changes in sexual potency.

β-Adrenergic Blocking Agents. Each year the roster of available β-blockers increases. They have similar mechanisms of action, but each has specific theoretical advantages and disadvantages. In general, their differences can be stated according to (1) duration of action, (2) selectivity for β_1-(cardiac) receptors; and (3) other sympathetic effects (α-blockade or intrinsic sympathomimetic activity) (Table 10–2).

The initial effect of β-blockers is to reduce blood pressure by reducing cardiac output, myocardial contractility, and heart rate. This reduced cardiac output results initially in a reflex increase in peripheral vascular resistance but later this progressively falls to lower than pretreatment level. Thus, the long-term effect of β-blockers is a balanced reduction in both cardiac output and peripheral vascular resistance. β-Blockers also suppress β-receptor activity in the kidney, inhibiting renin release, although this is probably not a long-term effect and does not correlate well with reductions in blood pressure. The antihypertensive effect of β-blockers is not usually associated with postural hypotension. In contrast to older antihypertensive agents, β-blockers tend to work better as time passes, often allowing the clinician to reduce dosages after 6 months to 1 year. The β-blockers have great value in patients with concomitant coronary artery disease, angina pectoris, and a history of cardiac arrhythmias, especially atrial tachycardias. Caution needs to be exercised in treating patients who have slow resting heart rates or are on concomitant medications that may cause bradycardia (verapamil) or have bronchospastic pulmonary diseases. A small group of patients may have a paradoxic hypertensive effect when begun on β-blockers. This is most frequently seen in those with excess sodium retention and thus low renin activity.

Patients need to be cautioned about the abrupt cessation of therapy, which may result in palpitations, tachycardia, angina, and even myocardial infarction. If a patient is to discontinue moderate doses of β-blockers, we reduce the dosage every 3 days until a minimum dose is achieved and then discontinued. Most surgeons and anesthesiologists suggest that patients stay on their β-blockers for surgery.

Our choice of specific drug is individualized for each patient. Characteristics such as side effects from prior medications and renal, pulmonary, or peripheral vascular disease are important. Cost and dosage frequency also are important for compliance.

In patients with pulmonary disease (asthma or chronic obstructive pulmonary disease), we try to avoid use of β-blockers; however, if the patient has been resistant to other antihypertensive agents we may try low doses of the cardioselective agents metoprolol or atenolol. Propranolol has been shown to decrease the glomerular filtration rate, thus we try to avoid this drug in patients with renal insufficiency. Nadolol has been demonstrated as not detrimental to renal function. In patients with significant peripheral vascular disease, we may choose pindolol, because of its intrinsic sympathomimetic activity, or labetolol, which has α-blocking activity, although adverse effects on claudication are probably minimal using any of the β-blockers.[21] Our agent of first choice for the routine patient with essential hypertension and no other complications is nadolol or atenolol, which can be given once daily.

β-Blockers are valuable in combination with vasodilators. Although propranolol and hydralazine was classically the combination used, similar antihypertensive effects are seen when β-blockers are used with ACEIs and calcium channel blockers.

Adverse consequences of β-blocker therapy are relatively uncommon. In our experience, therapy is discontinued in about 3% of patients; others have reported up to 10%. Side effects that usually require discontinuation include bronchospasm, severe claudication or Raynaud's phenomenon, and congestive heart failure. Additional side effects include sleep disturbances, fatigue, cold extremities, diminished exercise tolerance, gastrointestinal disturbances, depression, and impotence.[22–25]

β-Blockers may be used in insulin-dependent diabetics, but with caution. These agents inhibit insulin release from the pancreas, making maturity-onset diabetes worse, and block autonomic manifestations of hypoglycemia. The patient may be at risk of not being aware that blood sugar has dropped. Diabetics should watch for excessive hunger as a sign of hypoglycemia, since there may be no tachycardia or diaphoresis.

Methyldopa. This drug has been a useful antihypertensive for over 40 years. Investigations indicate that methyldopa has a central antihypertensive effect. Blood pressure is lowered through a reduction in peripheral resistance, with minor decreases in heart rate and cardiac output. Because sodium retention frequently occurs with methyldopa therapy, this drug is often combined with diuretic therapy. Dosage is between 0.5 and 3 g/day, divided into two to four doses. It has been shown to be especially useful in patients with renal insufficiency, congestive heart failure, and pulmonary disease. The drug is excreted by the kidney.

Side effects include depression, fatigue, and sleepiness, all of which should occur at the beginning of therapy and often dissipate within the first week. More troublesome side effects include the frequent occurrence of impotence as well as dry mouth, a positive direct Coombs' test (in 20% of

TABLE 10–2. CURRENTLY AVAILABLE β-ADRENERGIC BLOCKERS FOR TREATMENT OF HYPERTENSION

Medication	Half-Life (hours)	Cardioselective	Adrenergic Effects	Dosage (mg)	~Monthly Cost (dollars)
Propranolol	2–3	–		20–200 b.i.d.	10.24
Inderal-LA	10	–		120 q.d.	15.17
Nadolol	20–24	–		20–400 q.d.	12.54
Metoprolol	3–4	+		50–200 b.i.d.	11.40
Atenolol	6–9	+		25–200 q.d.	12.56
Timolol	3–4	–		10 b.i.d.–20 q.i.d.	15.68
Pindolol	3–4	–	ISA	5 b.i.d.–20 q.i.d.	13.43
Acebutolol	3–4	+	ISA	400 q.d.	11.87
Labetalol	3–5	–	α-blocker	100–600 b.i.d.	15.44

ISA = intrinsic sympathomimetic activity.

patients, with clinical hemolysis present in less than 1%), and serious liver dysfunction; the drug must be discontinued in the event of these last two adverse reactions. Methyldopa also interferes with the measurement of urinary catecholamines, vanillylmandelic acid (VMA), and metanephrines. If methyldopa therapy is abruptly withdrawn, an occasional patient will experience tachycardia, agitation, and insomnia—reactions that may be hazardous to patients with angina.

Rauwolfia Alkaloids. The most widely used of the rauwolfia agents, reserpine, has been available for many years. Reserpine works both centrally and peripherally to decrease sympathetic tone, resulting in a slow heart rate, reduced myocardial contractility, and lower peripheral resistance. Reserpine is an equally potent antihypertensive agent compared to methyldopa or propranolol. Its main advantage is once-a-day dosing. The usual effective dosage is 0.25 to 0.5 mg/day, although the higher of these dosages is frequently associated with side effects. Tablets that combine reserpine with thiazide diuretics can be obtained and can be especially convenient for patients whose required doses of each drug match the combinations offered.

Serious side effects include sedation, agitated depression, accentuation of gastric acid secretion with ulcer disease, diarrhea, weight gain due to increased appetite, and nasal congestion.

Clonidine. Clonidine (Catapres), like methyldopa and reserpine, works in the central nervous system to lower blood pressure. It is a centrally active α-receptor blocker. It is similar to methyldopa in its side effects and effectiveness. About one third of patients given clonidine complain of dry mouth and fatigue or drowsiness, but these effects are usually transient. Sudden cessation of clonidine therapy has caused an "overshoot" of blood pressure to higher than pretreatment levels. This response is unusual, however, and probably occurs rarely after methyldopa or propranolol therapy as well. The initial dosage of clonidine is 0.1 mg twice daily but may be increased gradually up to 1 mg twice daily, and much higher amounts have been used. Clonidine may be particularly useful in the elderly hypertensive patient. A once-daily dose, given at bedtime, in combination with a thiazide diuretic given in the morning, has been well tolerated and effective in our practice. A form of clonidine for transdermal delivery is available which has a prolonged half-life and need be given only once per week. We find that this medication is useful for patients who cannot take pills, have significant gastrointestinal malabsorption, or are taking nothing by mouth postoperatively. It may also be useful for control of symptoms related to alcohol, cigarette, or drug withdrawal.

Guanabenz. Guanabenz (Wytensin) is another centrally active sympatholytic agent that appears to be as effective as methyldopa or clonidine and to have similar side effects. The usual dosage is 4 mg twice daily (up to 16 mg twice daily).

Guanethidine. Because of the frequent occurrence of intolerable side effects at therapeutic levels, guanethidine (Ismelin) is usually reserved for cases that are most severe and difficult to control. Guanethidine's action is almost exclusively peripheral. It may be useful in patients with moderate hypertension who have experienced severe central nervous system depression or sleepiness when using other sympathoactive drugs. The tricyclic antidepressants, however, block the peripheral uptake of guanethidine and impair its antihypertensive function. Guanethidine acts to reduce heart rate and decreases stroke volume, predominantly by impeding venous return. It also produces a modest decrease in peripheral vascular resistance, but this, together with the diminution in venous compliance, results in a prominent and limiting postural hypotension. Guanethidine has a wide dose-response range, so that doses from 10 to 200 mg have been used.

Since the effects of guanethidine are slow and cumulative, the dose should only be increased every 3 to 5 days. Initial dosage should be 10 mg/day, with subsequent 5-mg increases once or twice weekly until the drug has taken effect. Its effectiveness is enhanced in combination with diuretics and vasodilators.

Guanadrel sulfate (Hylorel) is an agent similar in efficacy to guanethidine with similar but less frequent side effects. We have found this agent useful as a second choice in patients intolerant to β-blockers.

Blood pressure should be measured when the patient is both supine and upright, the upright pressure being the limiting factor. Patients with very high blood pressures when supine and normal blood pressures when upright should probably be counseled to sleep with the head of the bed elevated and to rise slowly from sitting and lying positions. One way to minimize the postural effect is to prescribe pressure-gradient–type elastic stockings.

Adverse consequences of guanethidine or guanadrel therapy are impotence, postural hypotension, and fluid retention. Patients should be cautioned against sitting in an automobile or a bus for too long a period without moving their extremities, and they should not remain standing without walking about.

α-Blocking Agents. Prazosin (Minipress), terazasin (Hytrin) and doxazosin are currently available for treatment of hypertension. They are mild antihypertensive agents, probably equivalent to reserpine or methyldopa in effectiveness. Although they predominantly effect peripheral vasodilation, they differ from the predominantly arterial vasodilators, hydralazine and minoxidil, in that they significantly reduce venous tone; the net effect of these other arterial vasodilators is to *increase* cardiac output, whereas α-blockers cause no net change in cardiac output.

α-Blockers should be administered cautiously to the hypertensive patient, since idiosyncratic reactions may occur. Initial doses as low as 1 mg have caused serious hypotension, even syncope, in about 10% of patients. It is best to give the first dose when the patient is about to retire for the evening, with the advice that he or she should arise slowly the following morning. Tachyphylaxis may develop. Side effects, in addition to first-dose collapse, include nausea, headache, nervousness, and dizziness, but the drugs are usually well tolerated. α-Blockers can be used in conjunction with β-blockers and other antihypertensive agents, but hydralazine and guanethidine should be avoided because of their additional postural hypotensive effect. Terazasin is also used for men with prostatic hypertrophy and symptoms of bladder spasticity.[26]

Peripheral Vasodilators. The agents for oral use that act predominantly as vasodilators include hydralazine, prazosin (discussed earlier), minoxidil, angiotensin-converting enzyme inhibitors, and calcium channel blockers.

Hydralazine. Although available for many years, hydralazine was seldom used until the β-blocker propranolol was introduced. This is because the reduced peripheral resistance due to vasodilatation often causes reflex tachycardia and increased cardiac output, with consequent headaches, palpitations, tachycardia, and symptoms of coronary insufficiency in patients with borderline coronary artery disease. Concomitant use of a β-blocker to counteract the increase in cardiac output prevents these worrisome adverse effects and may preclude angina or myocardial infarction. The dosage of hydralazine is 25 to 100 mg twice daily.

TABLE 10–3. CURRENTLY AVAILABLE ANGIOTENSIN-CONVERTING ENZYME INHIBITORS

	Usual Dosage Range (mg)*
Benezepril	10–80
Captopril	25–300
Enalapril	5–40
Fosinopril	10–80
Lisinopril	5–40
Quainapril	10–80
Ramipril	2.5–20

*Dosage per 24 hours.

Prolonged use of large doses of hydralazine (>200 mg/day) is frequently associated with the appearance of a positive test for lupus erythematosus, a side effect that is almost always reversible upon discontinuation of the drug.

Minoxidil. This is a potent, long-acting vasodilator with serious long-term consequences, including hirsutism and perimyocarditis.[27] Its use has been restricted to patients whose blood pressure cannot be controlled by conventional therapy, especially those with severe renal failure, for whom it seems to be particularly suitable. Patients with otherwise uncontrollable hypertension may respond to minoxidil, but risks of long-term consequences limit its use.

Angiotensin-Converting Enzyme Inhibitors. There are currently six angiotensin-converting enzyme inhibitors available for treatment of hypertension (Table 10–3). They differ chiefly according to half-life. The angiotensin-converting enzyme inhibitors block the conversion of angiotensin I to angiotensin II, thus decreasing the activity of this potent vasoconstrictor, which is also a stimulator of aldosterone secretion.[28] They also increase the level of the vasodilator bradykinin by decreasing its degradation. This, along with elevation of vasodilator prostaglandins, contributes to the hypotensive action of ACEI. The drugs are excreted by the kidneys.

ACEI should be initiated cautiously in patients who may be hypovolemic. Captopril is begun in doses of 6.2 mg to 12.5 mg tid. The usual maintenance dose is 12.5 to 50 mg tid, with the maximum being 400 mg/day. Enalapril is begun in a dosage of 5 mg once daily and may be increased to 40 mg/day. The ACEI may be particularly suited for the patient with hypertension plus heart failure or those intolerant of sympathoactive agents. They are also used for initial therapy in some patients. Those with diabetes mellitus, hyperlipidemia, and central nervous system medication intolerance are particularly good candidates. These agents are also gaining acceptance for use in treatment of early renal failure and proteinuria because of beneficial intrarenal hemodynamic changes.[29, 30]

Side effects include altered taste, skin rash, proteinuria, hyperkalemia (especially if given with potassium-sparing diuretics), acute renal failure, hepatitis, neutropenia, and aplastic anemia. These problems are uncommon using low doses in patients with normal renal function.

Calcium Channel Blockers (Table 10–4). These agents (nifedipine, verapamil, diltiazem, isradapine, and felodipine) are vasodilators. They were designed for patients with angina pectoris; however, because of their direct vasodilator capacity they are effective in decreasing peripheral resistance. They are effective in patients with hypertension and coronary artery disease, in resistant hypertension, and in the elderly hypertensive. Side effects and cost have limited their usage. We do not recommend them as initial therapy agents. Common side effects include headache, palpitations, edema and flushing with the nifedipine-type agents, and bradycardia, constipation, and decreased left ventricular function with verapamil.

Nutritional Treatments

Weight Control. Most investigators believe that excessive body weight and hypertension are causally related.[31] In our series of 57 individuals who lost a mean of 67 lb and were successful at keeping it off for an average of 7 months, 17 of 29 previously hypertensive patients became normotensive. None required more antihypertensive agents.[32]

Ideally, obesity among hypertensive patients should be eradicated; however, the physician should consider two important observations: First, few patients will lose weight in response to instructions from someone else; weight reduction will be attained only when the individual is self-motivated. Second, weight loss supervision in the medical setting has produced dismal results, whereas nonmedical weight reduction centers, such as Weight Watchers and Diet Workshop, claim great success, probably owing to the patient's voluntary participation. Hypertension, especially if fairly mild, is usually not perceived by the patient as a serious illness, whereas weight reduction is often viewed as an unappealing and difficult change in health behavior. Thus the physician should probably encourage patients to consider weight loss only after it has become evident that they will stay in care. Weight loss and other nonpharmacologic therapies can be the initial approach when the blood pressure is borderline or minimally elevated. We encourage obese patients whose blood pressure is high enough to justify pharmacologic treatment to take medication until such time as they have lost a significant amount of weight.

Sodium Restriction. Diuretics have replaced dietary salt restriction as a means of controlling blood pressure. It is now clear that the American diet contains high levels of sodium chloride, and it is possible that this is related in some way to the prevalence of high blood pressure levels in the population.[33] The benefits of sodium restriction as a treatment for hypertension, however, are not so clear. Moderate salt restriction seems to lower diastolic blood pressures in some patients to about the same degree as thiazide diuretics do, while in other patients there is no effect.[34]

Other Nonpharmacologic Treatments

Various biofeedback techniques and relaxation therapies such as yoga, transcendental meditation, autogenic training, and evocation of the "relaxation response" have all been shown by their proponents to have significant, albeit modest, effects on blood pressure. In one review of behavioral treatments for hypertension,[35] the investigators concluded that relaxation techniques were more effective than was biofeedback conditioning, although none of the treat-

TABLE 10–4. CURRENTLY AVAILABLE CALCIUM CHANNEL BLOCKERS

	Usual Dosage Range (mg)*
Diltiazem	120–360
Felodipine	5–20
Isradipine	5–20
Nicardipine	60–120
Nifedipine	30–120
Verapamil	120–480

*Dosage per 24 hours.

ments was believed to have wide applicability or a confirmed long-term benefit. A major drawback of these techniques is that they all require a considerable investment of time compared with medical treatments. When asked by a patient whether or not such therapy is indicated, one probably should not dismiss the suggestion entirely but should instead offer the patient reliable sources of information. Most patients we have followed report increased feelings of well-being but show minimal or no significant changes in blood pressure. Although the few studies that have been undertaken to assess the relation between exercise and reductions in elevated blood pressure have been poorly controlled and unconvincing,[36] the physician's response to patients' questions about exercise should also be positive. Exercise generally increases feelings of well-being, and weight loss may be enhanced by this additional energy expenditure. The risk of coronary disease may be reduced by mild-to-moderate exercise.[5]

Reduction of intake of alcohol has been shown to decrease blood pressure in some patients. The precise mechanism is unclear, but there may be less catecholamine stimulation, less tachycardia, and weight loss.[37] We recommend minimal alcohol use with a maximum of 1 to 2 oz/day.

EVALUATION

Less than 5% of the hypertensive population has a secondary, and therefore potentially curable, form of hypertension (Table 10–5). Secondary forms may be obvious (e.g., hypertension related to the third trimester of pregnancy) or may be quite subtle and devoid of clinical features, such as some forms of renovascular hypertension.

TABLE 10–5. KNOWN CAUSES OF SECONDARY HYPERTENSION

Renal vascular diseases
- Atherosclerosis (60%, older male patients)
- Fibrous dysplasias: intimal (5%, younger patients), medial (30%, younger female patients), subadventitial (5%, younger female patients)

Renal parenchymal diseases
- Chronic glomerulonephritis
- Polycystic kidney disease

Renin-secreting tumors
- Juxtaglomerular cell tumors
- Nephroblastoma (Wilms' tumors)

Primary aldosteronism
- Adenoma
- Hyperplasia

Pheochromocytoma (20% are associated with other lesions—neurocutaneous syndromes, MEA II)

Pregnancy; estrogen-containing contraceptive pills

Cushing's syndrome

Congenital adrenal hyperplasia
- 11-Hydroxylase deficiency—virilizing; ↑ 17 KS, 17 OHCS, and DOC; responds to cortisol therapy
- 17-Hydroxylase deficiency—nonvirilizing; ↑ DOC; responds to cortisol therapy

Coarctation of the aorta (occurring in young patients, delayed or diminished femoral pulse, bruits)

Hypothyroidism (narrow pulse pressure, which improves with thyroid hormone replacement)

Miscellaneous
- Burns
- Myocardial revascularization surgery
- Aortic stenosis surgery
- Increased intracranial pressure
- Cerebellar tumors

KS = ketosteroids; OHCS = hydroxycorticosterone; DOC = desoxycorticosterone.

The initial evaluation of the hypertensive patient should be directed toward simple screening for secondary forms, including urinalysis and serum creatinine and potassium determinations, and toward detecting other conditions that might influence the choice of drug therapy (e.g., asthma, congestive heart failure, diabetes, hyperlipidemia, and asymptomatic hyperuricemia). Thus, for most hypertensive individuals with diastolic blood pressures lower than 110 mm Hg, the first visit should consist of a careful history and physical examination, urinalysis, appropriate blood tests, and an ECG. By means of blood chemistry profiles, one should evaluate the patient's renal, hepatic, and hematologic status and should measure the serum cholesterol level. Routine use of lipoprotein phenotyping and cholesterol fractionation does not seem warranted. Although some investigators persist in advocating "renin profiling" as a screening test,[38] we—as do most others—find this procedure unnecessary for empiric treatment of hypertensive patients. Most patients can be instructed to measure their own blood pressures.

Indications For More Extensive Diagnostic Evaluation

Findings That Suggest Secondary Hypertension. Before proceeding with additional diagnostic tests, the physician should determine whether invasive forms of treatment would be feasible. If these are not deemed possible, further testing is not indicated. If a patient presents with vasomotor symptoms suggestive of pheochromocytoma, this diagnosis should obviously be investigated. Diminished femoral pulses may suggest coarctation of the aorta. Absence of a family history of hypertension or premature cardiovascular disease suggests the possibility of a secondary form. In patients not receiving diuretic therapy, unprovoked hypokalemia (serum potassium < 3.4 mEq/l without diuretics) warrants evaluation for primary aldosteronism. Chronic renal failure is the most common secondary form of hypertension.

Treatment Failure. If the clinician is satisfied that the patient is in fact taking the appropriate medications, and the medications have failed to reduce significantly elevated blood pressures, evaluation for secondary forms is indicated. History and laboratory studies should be reviewed for clues. Renovascular hypertension is by far the most common curable form of hypertension.

Extremes of Age. Usually, men with essential hypertension will begin to show persistently elevated blood pressure by 35 years of age and women by 40 to 45 years of age. Although essential hypertension is becoming a more recognized cause of blood pressure elevations in patients younger than 25 years of age, secondary forms are still more common causes of hypertension in this population. Thus, in a 19-year-old patient with sustained hypertension, a careful investigation for secondary forms should be undertaken. Likewise, if a person with lifelong documented normal blood pressures suddenly experiences serious blood pressure elevations after 55 years of age, a secondary form should be considered. The most common curable secondary form of hypertension in the elderly is atherosclerotic renovascular disease.

Side Effects from Antihypertensive Medications. An occasional patient presents with multiple allergies or intolerable and variable side effects due to the medications chosen. In some patients, side effects are a consequence of severe anxiety, whereas in others, documented cutaneous eruptions, serologic changes, and other disturbances may occur. The end result, however, is the same—a patient whose blood pressure cannot be controlled by usual therapy. For this patient, too, a more comprehensive evaluation should be done, not because there is greater likelihood of a secondary form but because failure to find a curable form is associated with such a poor prognosis.

Malignant or Accelerated Hypertension. Patients with malignant or accelerated hypertension (i.e., diastolic blood pressure of 125 mm Hg), should be evaluated. Those with the highest blood pressures will benefit most from surgical therapy.

COMMON SECONDARY FORMS OF HYPERTENSION

Renovascular Hypertension

As mentioned previously, indications for work-up of renovascular hypertension are (1) onset of stubborn hypertension in the elderly (older than 60 years of age) population, (2) onset of hypertension in people younger than 25 years of age, especially without family histories, (3) hypertension that is unusually severe or resistant to tolerated therapies, and (4) hypertension associated with unexplained progressive renal failure. The only physical finding helpful to the diagnosis is the presence of abdominal bruits. These tend to be both systolic and diastolic and are heard best in the upper outer abdominal quadrants or the flank. Because of the rarity of renovascular hypertension (~ 5% of hypertensive patients), most patients with abdominal bruits have essential hypertension.

Before we initiate a diagnostic work-up for renovascular hypertension, even in the patient with one of the aforementioned indications, we must be convinced that we will act on a positive finding. If the patient is a suspect for renal artery stenosis but not otherwise a candidate for treatment, we do not even initiate the diagnostic procedures. We recommend a renal arteriogram and a renal vein renin assay as initial tests in most patients. These are performed during a 1-day or overnight stay. If the patient is elderly, blood pressure is very elevated, or there are bleeding or allergic complications, the patient stays overnight. These two tests provide anatomic and physiologic screening for renovascular hypertension.[39] If there is a renal artery stenosis and elevated renin secretion from the affected kidney, the chance of improvement in hypertension is 80 to 90%.[40] Even if the renal vein renins do not lateralize to the stenotic side, the chance is still about 40 to 50% that the patient will improve after correction. Vascular stenoses may be corrected in the absence of renin lateralization, depending on the nature of the case.[41]

The decision for angioplasty (percutaneous transluminal angioplasty [PTA]) is made during the procedure. Patients with fibromuscular hyperplasia are often very responsive to PTA, in the range of 90%. Those with atherosclerotic lesions are somewhat less likely to respond, and lesions at the ostium of the renal artery are least likely to respond.[42] A vascular surgeon is on standby prior to PTA in case of complications like arterial rupture, embolization, or dissection. Serious complications are quite rare. Although some dissection of the renal artery occurs often, this usually is not a serious complication.

Surgical management of patients with renovascular hypertension is highly effective in those in whom PTA has been unsuccessful or with ostial lesions. Mortality for patients who have atherosclerotic disease has decreased from 9 to less than 5% but is still considerable because of the often concomitant occurrence of coronary and carotid disease.[43]

In some hospitals, angiography is not well developed or radiologists lack extensive experience. Alternative procedures, including isotope renograms and magnetic resonance imaging (MRI) of the renal arteries, are reasonable as screening tests. Good predictors of subsequent surgically curable renovascular disease are (1) a greater than 1.5-cm difference in kidney length, (2) late appearance, and (3) late hyperconcentration of contrast medium in the involved kidney. The combination of MRI and isotope renogram have not been studied extensively as predictors of cure; however, if both studies are normal, it would be uncommon that a patient could have a significant stenosis. For diabetic and renal failure patients in whom large volumes of contrast agent are contraindicated, one may employ the isotopic renogram and MRI as initial screens and, if positive, then proceed directly to arteriography and PTA.

Pheochromocytoma

Pheochromocytomas are rare tumors of the chromaffin cells, which embryologically arise from the sympathetic nerve cell precursors of the neural crest and neural tube. The tumors can occur wherever there are sympathetic nerve plexuses. The adrenal medulla is the most common site, but tumors have been found in the carotid body; the renal bladder; the posterior cranial fossa; the organ of Zuckerkandl; and the sympathetic chains in the cervical, thoracic, and lumbosacral areas. More than 95% occur within the abdomen and pelvis. Of affected patients, 80% have a single benign tumor, but as many as 20%, especially those with associated endocrinopathies, have multiple primary sites. Less than 10% of pheochromocytomas are malignant. All pheochromocytomas contain norepinephrine, but only about 50% synthesize epinephrine as well. If there is evidence of epinephrine secretion, an adrenal origin is suggested. These tumors tend to occur within families and are also seen in association with the phakomatoses or neurocutaneous syndromes such as von Recklinghausen's neurofibromatosis, von Hippel-Lindau's cerebroretinal angiomatosis, and multiple endocrine adenomatosis (MEA) type II.

Evaluation. The vigor with which one tests for pheochromocytoma is determined by the level of clinical suspicion. Biochemical tests for urinary catecholamines or their metabolites are the key to diagnosis.

Twenty-four-hour excretion of metanephrines is the most reliable clue to the presence of pheochromocytoma. Determination of the level of total plasma catecholamines is also suggestive: according to Bravo and Gifford, a value over 2000 pg/ml confirms the presence of pheochromocytoma.[44] In the patient with suggestive symptoms, we analyze one or more 24-hour urine collections for metanephrines, VMA, and total catecholamines. If any of these levels are persistently elevated, we proceed to localization of the tumor by computed tomography (CT) scan. If the urine collection is equivocal and suspicion is still high, we measure total plasma catecholamines in the fasting supine state, then proceed to CT scan.

Normal levels of VMA, metanephrine, or urinary free catecholamines will exclude the diagnosis to a confidence level of about 95%, with metanephrine and catecholamine levels being somewhat more sensitive than VMA levels.[44]

An exception is illustrated by one of our patients with paroxysmal episodes of severe hypertension, unprovoked sweating, and severe orthostatic hypotension, in whom 31 total measurements of VMA, metanephrine, and catecholamines performed on 11 urine samples resulted in only three abnormal determinations. Because clinical suspicion was great, however, arteriography was performed and revealed a left adrenal pheochromocytoma.

The triad of unprovoked sweating, pounding headaches, and episodic palpitations was noted in approximately 90% of patients with pheochromocytoma in one series, and in only approximately 6% of hypertensives without pheochromocytoma.[44] Occasionally, patients have facial pallor, anxiety, tremor, weight loss, nausea, and cardiomyopathy. Pheochromocytomas can mimic hyperthyroidism, menopausal symptoms, and a host of other diseases with vasomotor symptomatology. Many patients with labile hypertension and the hyperdynamic β-adrenergic state behave as though they have pheochromocytomas, but diagnostic tests prove negative.

When clinical suspicion is high and urinary metabolite determinations are abnormal, the physician must try to locate the tumor; in most cases tumors arise in the abdomen. Abdominal CT has become the diagnostic test most relied on for determining the location and extent of the tumor. Arteriography occasionally may be necessary to define the vascular anatomy, but this causes considerable risk of severe hypertension. In the patient with a clinical suspicion, biochemical evidence of norepinephrine excess, and a mass on CT scan, we recommend that the next step be exploration by an experienced surgeon after appropriate preparation, as described later.

We no longer perform pharmacologic manipulations, such as the phentolamine (Regitine), histamine, tyramine, or glucagon tests, all of which have received some attention in the past. If a pheochromocytoma is indeed present, these pharmacologic manipulations confer unnecessary risk in addition to producing high false-positive and false-negative rates. In rare cases when the tumor cannot be localized, plasma catecholamines can be measured in blood samples drawn from different sites along the inferior and superior vena cava. Increased levels of plasma catecholamines may indicate the location of the tumor and will help direct the surgeon.

Therapy. Prior to undertaking studies that require large amounts of contrast agents or performing surgery, one must protect the patient from the possibility of excessive norepinephrine release by treatment with phenoxybenzamine (Dibenzyline). Preoperatively, blood pressure should be controlled by gradually increasing the dose of phenoxybenzamine to 40 to 80 mg/day as tolerated, and contracted plasma volume should be replenished with a high-salt diet, together with volume expanders such as albumin if needed. Heart rate usually does not require control, except for the occasional patient who releases large amounts of epinephrine, in whom tachycardias must be regulated with propranolol. Patients should always be given phenoxybenzamine first and propranolol subsequently.

If a pheochromocytoma is located, it should be excised; the surgeon should be aware of the sometimes complex vascularization of these tumors. Induction of anesthesia is particularly difficult in patients with pheochromocytomas, often resulting in prominent reductions in blood pressure; entering the peritoneum and handling the tumor, on the other hand, may cause dramatic increases in blood pressure, even in the carefully prepared patient. Most cases should be referred to a center with anesthesiologists experienced in treating this disorder. Postoperatively, the patient should be counseled that there is a 15 to 40% chance of tumor recurrence, so that follow-up care is essential.

Mineralocorticoid Excess and Hypokalemia

Any patient with pronounced hypokalemia who is not receiving diuretics and who is not experiencing gastrointestinal losses of potassium should be considered to have mineralocorticoid excess. Aldosterone, the principal mineralocorticoid secreted by the adrenal cortex, acts in the nephron to promote potassium loss at the distal tubule sodium-potassium exchange site while reabsorbing sodium. Experimentally, mineralocorticoid administration leads to the retention of 250 to 400 mEq of sodium followed by the reestablishment of a new steady state based on an increased total body sodium content. This "desoxycorticosterone acetate (DOCA) escape" phenomenon explains why autonomous hyperactivity of the mineralocorticoid system does not usually result in fluid retention to edematous levels.

The most difficult problem confronting the physician with a hypertensive patient who has a low serum potassium level will be distinguishing between primary and secondary aldosteronism. Primary aldosteronism results from the secretion of excessive amounts of aldosterone due to autonomous hyperfunction of the adrenal cortex either by an adrenal cortical adenoma (common) or by bilateral adrenal hyperplasia (rare). Secondary aldosteronism is defined as aldosterone production responsive to stimuli such as diminished blood volume (hemorrhage), diminished "effective" blood volume (congestive heart failure or hypoalbuminemia due to nephrosis or cirrhosis), or an activated renin-angiotensin system (renovascular hypertension, accelerated hypertension, or chronic renal parenchymal disease). Of course, hypokalemia commonly results from treatment with thiazide diuretics, thus one must be very careful to determine recent thiazide or loop diuretic use before any further evaluation is undertaken.

Evaluation. When the patient is not acutely ill, the initial screening can be done in the office. History should include questions about licorice ingestion (since glycyrrhizic acid, contained in licorice, has an aldosterone-like effect) and steroid or diuretic therapy. Nocturia and polyuria result from the effect of hypokalemia on the renal-concentrating mechanism. The physical examination is usually not productive, and laboratory studies, if primary aldosteronism is present, will reveal hypokalemia with a metabolic alkalosis. Serum sodium concentration is usually normal or slightly elevated. Hypertension is usually mild.

In *secondary* forms of aldosteronism, renin activity is usually very high, whereas in *primary* aldosteronism renin is suppressed and generally cannot be stimulated by normal mechanisms. This distinction forms the basis of the ambulatory screen. Potassium chloride, 80 to 120 mEq/day for 3 days, should be given followed by furosemide, 40 mg administered the day before and the morning of the renin assay. The volume depletion brought about by furosemide is mild, and having the patients upright, either standing or walking, for 90 minutes prior to obtaining blood for the renin assay further stimulates maximum renin secretion. Patients with primary hyperaldosteronism usually have low renin values despite these maneuvers, but many patients with essential hypertension may also have low renin values. Patients with secondary hyperaldosteronism will have high renin values.

Renin specimens generally require special handling techniques, for example, in some laboratories, blood must be drawn into chilled tubes containing edetate (EDTA), and plasma must be separated in a cold centrifuge prior to assay. Falsely low renin activity may be determined unless these instructions are followed carefully. Note that renin measurement advocated in this section is carried out only after the occurrence of unprovoked hypokalemia, not as a routine screening procedure.

Some confusion exists over the term "low-renin essential hypertension," a form of *essential* hypertension with suppressed renin activity. In this condition, aldosterone and serum potassium levels are normal. In mineralocorticoid excess, both hypokalemia and suppressed renin activity are present. Conversely, hypokalemia alone with high or normal renin activity suggests parenchymal renal disease, renovascular hypertension, or "high-renin" essential hypertension, in each of which the hypokalemia is induced by hyperaldosteronism that is secondary to the increased renin.

Once the presumptive diagnosis of mineralocorticoid excess has been confirmed by means of the ambulatory screen, the patient should be hospitalized and brought into "balance" on a diet of 10 mEq of sodium and 100 mEq of potassium for 4 or 5 days, which will maximally stimulate renin secretion. Aldosterone secretion rates and renin assays are determined under these circumstances, after which one gives the patient a saline load (2 liters over 8 hours) and again measures renin and aldosterone levels.[45]

In patients with primary aldosteronism who are on a low-salt diet and who receive saline infusions, renin activity will be suppressed, whereas aldosterone secretory rates will be elevated or unchanged by these maneuvers. In patients with secondary aldosteronism, renin activity and aldosterone levels are increased in the low-salt state and are suppressed after saline infusion. If these results confirm those obtained during the outpatient screen, the next step is to differentiate between a primary adrenal adenoma and bilateral adrenal hyperplasia by means of CT.

Therapy. Therapy is primarily surgical, either bilateral or unilateral adrenalectomy. Recurrence of hypertension is fairly common (20 to 40% in our experience) in patients with primary aldosteronism even after the tumor has been resected, and one should counsel the patient that blood pressure elevations may recur.

SPECIAL PROBLEMS IN MANAGEMENT

Elderly Hypertensive Patient

The patient over 65 years of age who develops hypertension needs special consideration. If predominantly systolic, blood pressure elevations may represent arteriosclerotic stiffness of the arterial tree. However, systolic as well as diastolic elevations are associated with subsequent cardiovascular mortality in elderly patients as well as in younger patients,[46, 47] and neither systolic nor diastolic levels should be ignored. The stress of an office examination may be sufficient to cause an inordinate increase in systolic pressure (170 to 180 mm Hg) in elderly patients who under normal circumstances have only moderately elevated systolic pressure. Blood pressure levels measured at home by visiting nurses or the patient's family may, instead, be as low as 130 to 140 mm Hg systolic, and these patients should not be treated.

Although treatment is recommended for the elderly patient with both systolic and diastolic pressure elevations, caution is necessary. In older patients, the aorta is less elastic and baroreceptor sensitivity may be diminished, rendering them more sensitive to antihypertensive medication and more likely to develop postural hypotension; thus, one should proceed slowly when prescribing antihypertensive drugs. In addition, the elderly hypertensive patient may be institutionalized or may have meals served by family members, with no attention given to the adequacy of water and salt intake. In these patients, diuretics should be used with caution, since hyponatremia, renal insufficiency from dehydration, and hypokalemia may be particularly hazardous consequences.

The goals of therapy for the elderly hypertensive patient should probably be liberalized. Initially, it might be reasonable to attempt nondrug therapy, such as salt restriction and weight reduction, since these patients are at high risk for developing side effects from medication. In addition, agents that may cause psychological depression in younger patients can create symptoms indistinguishable from dementia in the elderly population.

In a patient whose initial blood pressure is 180/105 mm Hg, reduction of this level to 150/95 mm Hg with diuretic therapy may be considered adequate. When a second drug is needed to supplement diuretic therapy, methyldopa or a β-blocker is usually chosen. Although risks include postural hypotension and central nervous system depression, these drugs are usually better tolerated, are effective, and are less expensive than the newer agents.

The published results of the systolic hypertension in the elderly (SHEP) trial support treatment of the elderly hypertensive. Treatment with a diuretic and low-dose β-blocker, if necessary, resulted in a significant decrease in stroke, myocardial infarction, and mortality, without prohibitive side effects.[47]

Unresponsive Hypertensive Patient

With each succeeding generation of antihypertensive medications, fewer patients are actually "unresponsive." But at all stages of hypertension, from mild to malignant, for some patients medical therapy does not completely control blood pressure, and for a few individuals medical therapy is of no benefit whatever. However, in *all* cases in which medications do not seem to lower blood pressure, patients should be suspected of noncompliance. Generally, this will not be easy for a patient to admit. Rather than confronting a patient directly, one might encourage a discussion of this issue by asking the patient whether he or she has any difficulty remembering to take the medication as prescribed. If the patient does not admit to noncompliance, one must still be alert for the absence of expected pharmacologic responses. For example, a patient taking a thiazide diuretic whose serum potassium level is 4.7 mEq/l and uric acid level is 4.5 mg/dl is possibly noncompliant. If the patient is taking propranolol at dosages of 160 to 320 mg/day and the heart rate has not begun to decrease below baseline levels, the patient is most likely not taking this medication. However, some noncompliance is to be expected, and it is a mistake to overprescribe medications. Most patients with adequate blood pressure control take only 80% of prescribed medications.[48]

If noncompliance is not the problem, failure to achieve blood pressure control in patients with mild or moderate hypertension is an indication for a complete diagnostic evaluation. Such patients should be considered for admission to hospital, where blood pressure levels may be observed, diagnostic studies can be obtained, and pharmacologic intervention can be begun under supervised conditions. A few patients have severe hypertension that cannot be controlled. Since these patients may have diastolic pressures greater than 125 mm Hg, grade III retinopathy and

TABLE 10–6. EMERGENCIES INVOLVING HYPERTENSION

Malignant hypertension—fundi reveal papilledema
Hypertension with acute pulmonary edema
Hypertensive encephalopathy
Cerebrovascular accident, including hemorrhage and infarction, associated with severe hypertension
Aortic dissection
Pheochromocytoma with severe hypertension
Hypertension following tyramine ingestion in patients taking monoamine oxidase inhibitors
Severe toxemia or eclampsia

TABLE 10–7. URGENT CONDITIONS ASSOCIATED WITH HYPERTENSION

Accelerated hypertension—fundi reveal hemorrhage and exudates
Severe hypertension in a patient with myocardial infarction or severe angina
Occlusive stroke or transient ischemic attack in a hypertensive patient
Renal failure or significant renal impairment in a hypertensive patient
Marked hypertension associated with burns, acute glomerulonephritis, or preeclampsia
Severe hypertension in patients with postoperative bleeding
New cardiovascular or neurologic symptoms in the patient with hypertension
New patient with diastolic blood pressure >130 mm Hg

gradually deteriorating renal function, serious consideration must be given to transferring them to a center where drugs not yet approved are under investigation. There are also rare patients with malignant hypertension and renal insufficiency for whom the only treatment is bilateral nephrectomy and hemodialysis. In our institution, this has been done extremely rarely, and unsuccessful medical management is unusual.

Emergencies Involving Hypertension

Clinical situations associated with hypertension for which hospitalization is essential and parenteral antihypertensive therapy may be necessary may be classified as either urgent or emergent. Emergent situations are those requiring parenteral antihypertensives to reduce an immediate threat of morbidity and mortality due to the elevated blood pressure itself (Table 10–6). In urgent situations, hypertension may be contributing to a clinical condition for which hospitalization, observation, and antihypertensive therapy are indicated but for which immediate intravenous antihypertensive treatment is not required. (Table 10–7). These situations are treated with high-dose oral medications given at frequent intervals. Clonidine, hydralazine, captopril, and nifedipine are effective, potent, rapid agents.

For emergent situations the rational choice of a parenteral agent depends on (1) the desired hemodynamic effect, (2) the rate of blood pressure reduction required, and (3) familiarity with the agent and the ability of the hospital staff to monitor its effectiveness. Parenteral antihypertensives can be divided into two categories: (1) the vasodilators—nitroprusside, diazoxide, and hydralazine; and (2) drugs acting predominantly on the sympathetic nervous system—trimethaphan, labetalol, methyldopa, phentolamine, and propranolol. Table 10–8 shows the proper selection of parenteral antihypertensive agents for specific clinical settings. In general, nitroprusside and trimethaphan have the most rapid onset and dissipation of effects, and either one should be used when the potential benefit of drug therapy is uncertain. Thus, if an adverse reaction ensues, the medications can be discontinued and the undesirable reaction readily stopped. Table 10–9 shows the route, the adult dose, and the onset and duration of certain antihypertensive agents. A detailed discussion of this topic is beyond the scope of this chapter but can be found elsewhere.[49]

Hypertension Associated with Renal Disease

Renal parenchymal disease may be a cause of hypertension or may result from untreated or accelerating hypertension. In one series, about 5% of hypertensive patients had renal parenchymal disease.[50] Judging from this study, it is by far the most common secondary cause of hypertension, and uncontrolled hypertension may be especially detrimental in patients with renal disease.

In most cases fluid retention is an element of renal insufficiency, thus diuretic therapy and salt restriction should be the initial therapeutic measures. Potent diuretics such as furosemide or ethacrynic acid generally are necessary when blood urea nitrogen (BUN) exceeds 30 mg/dl or the serum creatinine level is higher than 2 mg/dl (see also Chapter 36). A small number of patients with hypertension and renal failure do not benefit from volume restriction. Renin activity is much higher in this group. Methyldopa, used in low doses because it is excreted by the kidney, has been useful in many such patients. β-Adrenergic blockers

TABLE 10–8. SELECTION OF PARENTERAL ANTIHYPERTENSIVE AGENTS FOR SPECIFIC CLINICAL SETTINGS

Agent	Pulmonary Edema	Encephalopathy	Chest Pain, Aneurysms	CVA	Malignant Hypertension (Including Renal)	Pheochromocytoma	MAO Inhibitors	Toxemia/ Eclampsia
Vasodilators								
Nitroprusside	1	1	3	1	1	2	2	4
Diazoxide	3	2	X	2	2	2	2	2
Hydralazine	3	3	X	2	3	3	3	2
Sympathoactive Drugs								
Trimethaphan	2	2	1	1	1	2	2	X
Labetalol	0	2	2	2	3	3	3	1
Methyldopa	3	X	2	3	3	3	3	3
Phentolamine	0	0	0	0	0	1	1	0
Propranolol	X	0	2	0	2	2	2	3

X = usually contraindicated; 0 = of no value; 1 = usual first choice for acute cases; 2 = of frequent value in acute cases; 3 = of occasional value in acute cases or for longer-term therapy; 4 = not known, no opinion.

TABLE 10–9. ROUTE, ADULT DOSE, AND TIMING OF PARENTERAL ANTIHYPERTENSIVES

Agent	Route	Dose	Onset	Duration
Vasodilators				
Nitroprusside	IV continuous	25–300 μg/min	<1 min	Minutes
Diazoxide	IV rapid bolus	3 mg/kg	1 to 3 min	4 to 18 hr
Hydralazine	IV; IM	5–20 mg	15 min	2 to 6 hr
Enalapril	IV	1.25–5 mg	15 min	6 hr
Nicardipine	IV	5–10 mg	10 min	1 hr
Sympathoactive Agents				
Trimethaphan	IV continuous	1–15 mg/min	<1 min	minutes
Labetalol	IV	20–80 mg	5–10 min	4 to 8 hr
Methyldopa	IV	250–1000 mg	1 to 3 hr	4 to 8 hr
Phentolamine	IV	5–15 mg	<1 min	1/4 to 2 hr
Propranolol	IV slowly	1–5 mg	<1 min	1 to 2 hr

(often combined with hydralazine) have been effective for controlling blood pressures in patients with renal failure, but they are not the drug of first choice because they may lead to increased azotemia. Other useful agents include labetalol and angiotensin-converting enzyme inhibitors. These patients need to have frequent surveillance of their serum potassium levels and renal function for possible deleterious effects. The decision for dialysis in hypertensive patients is made for the same clinical reasons as in nonhypertensive patients, but in a very small number of cases bilateral nephrectomy is performed as therapy for uncontrolled hypertension in patients already requiring dialysis.[51]

Diabetic Hypertensive Patient

Because of their added risk of vascular and renal disease, diabetic patients with even borderline hypertension generally should be treated (see Chapter 46). Currently the use of angiotensin-converting enzyme inhibitors is in favor because of good control of blood pressure and beneficial effects on renal hemodynamics. These agents may also improve insulin resistance and, thus, may diminish carbohydrate intolerance.[29, 52] β-Blockers and thiazide diuretics may be used, but with monitoring of glucose control and hypoglycemic episodes.

Oral Contraceptive Pills and Pregnancy

Estrogens increase the availability of angiotensinogen produced in the liver, thus allowing more angiotensin to circulate. Most patients who use oral contraceptives containing estrogen will have slightly higher than average blood pressure.[53] In 4 to 5%, diastolic blood pressures are elevated to hypertensive levels (>90 mm Hg),[54] rarely, accelerated or malignant hypertension occurs. Any hypertensive woman receiving oral contraceptives probably should stop taking them for at least 6 months to determine whether pressures will normalize. Even if the effect of the estrogens is only unmasking essential hypertension, discontinuation of the contraceptive may postpone treatment for many years.

Hypertension associated with pregnancy requires careful consideration, since our understanding of this relationship has changed during the past few years. If a patient is known to have hypertension before pregnancy, she should be treated similarly to any other hypertensive individual, with some precautions. In patients with mild hypertension who are attempting to become pregnant, antihypertensive medications should be discontinued up to and during the first trimester of pregnancy. Since careful monitoring is required for such circumstances, measuring blood pressure at home is particularly useful. After the first trimester, thiazide diuretics, methyldopa, and hydralazine have been shown to be quite safe. These same agents may not be unsafe during the first trimester, but it is an accepted general principle to withhold as many medications as possible during this time. Propranolol, lopressor, and labetalol have been shown to be safe and well tolerated during pregnancy.[55] However, at the time of delivery, neonates with bradycardia and hypoglycemia have been reported. We taper and stop β-blockers before delivery and replace them with methyldopa.

Therapy recommendations have changed for a patient who develops hypertension and proteinuria during the last trimester of pregnancy (i.e., preeclampsia). These patients are no longer treated with sodium restriction or with diuretics.[56] The most effective therapy seems to be hospitalization on an intermediate care floor, where patients continue to pursue normal activities of daily living. Their salt intake is mildly restricted. Patients are monitored carefully for progressive organ or fetal deterioration. Delivery is the treatment of choice if there is any fetal jeopardy or major organ involvement. If the hypertension requires therapy, the drugs of first choice are hydralazine and methyldopa.

REFERENCES

1. Kaplan NM: Clinical Hypertension. Baltimore, Williams & Wilkins, 1990, pp 1–25.
2. Rowland M and Roberts J: National Center for Health Statistics advance data: Vital health statistics of the National Center for Health Statistics, No. 84. Washington, DC, US Department of Health and Human Services, 1982.
3. Veterans Administration Cooperative Study on Antihypertensive Agents: Effects of treatment on morbidity in hypertension: Results in patients with diastolic blood pressure averaging 115 through 129 mm Hg. JAMA 202:116, 1967.
4. McMahon S, Peto R, Cutler J, et al: Blood pressure, stroke and coronary heart disease. 1: Prolonged differences in blood pressure: Prospective observational studies corrected for the regression dilution bias. Lancet 335:765–774, 1990.
5. Mason J, Tosteson H, Ridker P, et al: The primary prevention of myocardial infarction. N Engl J Med 326:1406–1416, 1992.
6. Collins R, Peto R, Macmahon S, et al: Blood pressure, stroke, and coronary heart disease. 2: Short term reduction in blood pressure: Overview of randomized drug trials in their epidemiologic context. Lancet 335:827–838, 1990.
7. Goldszer R and Solomon H: Non-pharmacologic treatment of hypertension: Medical Update, Brigham and Women's Hospital, Vol 4, No 2, 1991, pp 1–5.

8. Stamler R, Grim R, Dyer A, et al: Cardiac status after four years in a trial on nutritional therapy for high blood pressure. Arch Intern Med 149:661–665, 1989.
9. Alderman MH: Which antihypertensive drug first and why. JAMA 267:2786–2787, 1992.
10. 1988 Report of the Joint National Committee on detection, evaluation, and treatment, of high blood pressure. Arch Intern Med 148:1023–1038, 1988.
11. Hypertension Detection and Follow-up Program Cooperative Group: The effect of treatment on mortality in mild hypertension. N Engl J Med 307:976, 1983.
12. Australian therapeutic trial in mild hypertension: Report of the management committee. Lancet 1:1261, 1980.
13. Medical Research Council Working Party: MRC trial of treatment of mild hypertension: Principal results. BMJ 291:97, 1985.
14. Multiple Risk Factor Intervention Trial Research Group: Multiple Risk Factor Intervention trial. JAMA 248:1465, 1982.
15. Finnerty FA, Shaw L, and Himmelsbach CK: Hypertension in the inner city. II: Detection and follow-up. Circulation 47:76, 1973.
16. Lund JP: Hemodynamic changes in long-term diuretic therapy of essential hypertension: A comparison study of chlorthalidone, polythiazide, and hydrochlorthiazide. Acta Med Scand 187:509, 1970.
17. Gifford RW: The role of diuretics in the treatment of hypertension, Am J Med 77:102, 1984.
18. Kassirer JP and Harrington JT: Fending off the potassium pushers. N Engl J Med 312:785, 1985.
19. Grimm RH, Leon AS, Hunninghake DB, et al: Effects of thiazide diuretics on plasma lipids and lipoproteins in mildly hypertensive patients: A double blind controlled trial. Ann Intern Med 94:7, 1981.
20. Cutler R: Effect of antihypertensive agents on lipid metabolism. Am J Cardiol 51:628, 1983.
21. Hiatt WR, Stoll S, and Neis A: Effect of beta-adrenergic blockers on the peripheral circulation in patients with peripheral vascular disease. Circulation 72:1226, 1985.
22. Greenblatt DJ, Koch-Weser J: Adverse reactions to beta-adrenergic receptor blocking drugs: A report from the Boston Collaborative Drug Surveillance Program. 7:118–129, 1974.
23. Frishman WH: Beta adrenoreceptor antagonists: New drugs and new indications. N Engl J Med 3052:500, 1981.
24. Medical Research Council Working Party: Adverse reactions to bendrofluazide and propanolol for the treatment of mild hypertension. Lancet 2:539, 1981.
25. Schoenberger JA, Croog SH, Sudilovsky A, et al: Self-reported side effects from antihypertensive drugs: A clinical trial. Am J Hypertension 3:123–132, 1990.
26. Khoury AF and Kaplan NM: Alpha blocker therapy for hypertension. JAMA 266:394, 1991.
27. Linas SL and Nies AS: Minoxidil. Ann Intern Med 94:61, 1981.
28. Hollenberg NK: Pharmacologic interruption of the renin angiotensin system. Ann Revu Pharmacol 19:559, 1979.
29. Laragh J: A decade of angiotensin converting enzyme (ACE) inhibitors. Am J Med 92(4B)3s–7s, 1992.
30. Hermans MP, Brichard SM, Colin I, et al: Long-term reduction of microalbuminuria after 3 years of angiotensin converting enzyme inhibitor by perindopril in hypertensive insulin treated diabetic patients. Am J Med 92(4B):102s–107s, 1992.
31. Reisin E, Abel R, and Modan M: Effect of weight loss without salt restriction on the reduction of blood pressure. N Engl J Med 298:1, 1978.
32. Solomon HS, Lindewall D, and Goldszer RC: Effects of sustained weight loss and exercise on cardiac risk factors in an obese population. Washington DC, National Conference on High Blood Pressure Control, 1983, p 73.
33. Freis ED: Salt, volume, and the prevention of hypertension. Circulation 53:589, 1976.
34. Moore TJ, Malarick C, Olmedo A, and Klein R: Salt restriction lowers resting blood pressure but not 24 hour ambulatory blood pressure. Am J Hypertension 4:410, 1991.
35. Shapiro AP, Schwartz GE, Ferguson DC, et al: Behavior methods in the treatment of hypertension: A review of their clinical status. Ann Intern Med 86:626, 1977.
36. Martin JE, Dubbert PM, and Cushman WC: Controlled trial of aerobic exercise in hypertension. Circulation 81:1560, 1990.
37. MacMahon S: Alcohol consumption and hypertension. Hypertension 9:111, 1987.
38. Laragh J, Letcher RL, and Pickering TG: Renin profiling for diagnosis and treatment of hypertension. JAMA 241:151, 1979.
39. Vaughn ED: Renal artery stenosis. *In* Brenner BM and Stein JH (eds): Contemporary Issues in Nephrology. 8; Hypertension. New York, Churchill-Livingstone, 1981, pp 247–269.
40. Ying CY, Tift CP, Gavras H, et al: Renal revascularization in the azotemic hypertensive patient resistant to therapy. N Engl J Med 341:1070, 1984.
41. Marks LS, Maxwell MH, Varady PD, et al: Renovascular hypertension: Does the renal vein renin ratio predict operative results? J Urol 115:365, 1976.
42. Sos T, Pickering TG, Sniderman K, et al: Percutaneous transluminal renal angioplasty in renovascular hypertension due to atheroma or fibromuscular dysplasia. N Engl J Med 309:274, 1983.
43. Dean R, Krueger T, Whiteneck JM, et al: Operative management of renovascular hypertension: Results after a follow up of fifteen to twenty-three years. J Vasc Surg 1:234, 1984.
44. Bravo EL: Pheochromocytoma: New concepts and future trends. Kidney Int 40:544–556, 1991.
45. Cain JP, Tuck ML, Williams GH, et al: The regulation of aldosterone secretion in primary aldosterone, Am J Med 53:627–637, 1972.
46. Rutan GH, Kuller LH, Neaton JB, et al: Mortality associated with diastolic hypertension and isolated systolic hypertension among men screened for the Multiple Risk Factor Intervention Trial. Circulation 77:504–514, 1988.
47. SHEP Cooperative Research Group: Prevention of stroke by antihypertensive drug treatment in older persons with isolated systolic hypertension. JAMA 265:3255–3264, 1991.
48. Sackett DL, Haynes RB, Gilson ES, et al: Randomized clinical trials of strategies for improving medication compliance in primary hypertension. Lancet 1:1205, 1975.
49. Ramos O: Malignant hypertension. Kidney Int 25:209, 1984.
50. Gifford RW Jr: Evaluation of the hypertensive patient with emphasis on detecting curable causes. Milbank Memorial Fund Q 47:170, 1969.
51. Acosta JH: Hypertension in chronic renal disease. Kidney Int 22:702, 1982.
52. Taguma Y, Kitaamoto Y, and Futaki G: Effect of captopril on heavy proteinuria in azotemic diabetics. N Engl J Med 313:1617, 1985.
53. Weir RJ, Briggs E, Mack A, et al: Blood pressure in women taking oral contraceptives. BMJ 1:533, 1974.
54. Fisch IR and Frank J: Oral contraceptives and blood pressure. JAMA 237:2499, 1977.
55. Rubin PC: Beta-blockers in pregnancy. N Engl J Med 305:1323–1326, 1981.
56. Lindheimer MD and Katz AI: Hypertension in pregnancy. N Engl J Med 313:675–680, 1985.

11

Intermittent Claudication

ANTHONY D. WHITTEMORE, MD
MAGRUDER C. DONALDSON, MD
JOHN A. MANNICK, MD

Charcot used the term *intermittent claudication* in 1858 to describe a syndrome in horses that were subsequently proved to have an obstruction of the iliac artery.[1] His terminology derives from the Latin *claudicare,* which strictly defined, means "to limp; be halt or lame." This relatively specific symptom has been appropriately described as pain, discomfort or fatigue that occurs in a muscle or muscle group after repetitive use.[2] Equally characteristic, and most important diagnostically, is the intermittent nature of true claudication in that it must subside promptly with rest. In the overwhelming majority, claudication is the net result of critical atherosclerotic stenosis of a major artery, which reduces distal blood flow and therefore oxygen delivery to such an extent that spontaneous collateral vasculature can no longer provide sufficient compensation. The onset of claudication represents a late manifestation of atherosclerosis, as evidenced by the observation that two thirds of the working population with documented peripheral arterial occlusions are asymptomatic and remain so for some 10 years.[3] Of the 4030 subjects completing the 14-year Framingham Study, 79 men and 46 women developed intermittent claudication, yielding an annual incidence of 2.6 men and 1.2 women per 1000 population at risk. This overall 2:1 sex ratio diminishes with age, however, such that within the 65- to 74-year age group, in which claudication reaches its peak incidence, the rate becomes 6.1 men and 5.4 women per 1000.[4] The patient prompted by claudication to seek medical advice presents the physician with a broad challenge, as born out in the Framingham group, in which patients with claudication emerged with twice the mortality of the claudication-free population. Although 75% of these deaths result from cardiovascular disorders, not one could be attributed directly to claudication. Thus, claudication represents merely the peripheral manifestation of a systemic disease. Although individual series differ, particularly when comparing operative to nonoperative series, the incidence of coronary heart disease is two to five times that observed in a claudication-free population and is clinically evident in as many as 50% of patients in surgical series. The coincidence of claudication and cerebrovascular disease may be clinically apparent in as many as 45% of patients managed surgically.[5, 6] At least one third of patients with intermittent claudication are hypertensive, and the prevalence of diabetes mellitus, previously overestimated in this group, ranges from 10 to 15%.[7]

Thus, the evaluation and subsequent management of the patient with intermittent claudication must be tempered by the fact that claudication is not the life-threatening problem. It is the management and ultimate evolution of the associated coronary or cerebrovascular disease that not only determines longevity but also may contribute substantially to the degree of palliation achieved with treatment of claudication.

CLINICAL ANATOMY

Since a basic understanding of the distal arterial anatomy is required for an appreciation of intermittent claudication, a brief review is presented. As shown in Figure 11–1, the arterial system distal to the origin of the renal arteries may be divided into three major sections: aortoiliac, femoropopliteal, and tibioperoneal.

The aortoiliac division originates just below the level of the renal arteries and terminates with the origin of the common femoral artery in the groin. Initial atheromatous plaque formation with subsequent stenoses occurs most frequently at the aortic and common iliac bifurcations. A third common site is located within the distal external iliac artery as it traverses the inguinal ligament. The occlusive process with associated thrombus formation may then extend proximally from each site in a progressive manner, such that the entire aortoiliac system below the renal arteries may become occluded.

The femoropopliteal system originates at the inguinal ligament with the common femoral artery and terminates distally as the popliteal artery bifurcates into the anterior tibial artery and the common tibioperoneal trunk. Although atherosclerotic occlusive disease may occur along the entire length of the superficial femoral or popliteal vessels, the most common site is the segment within Hunter's canal, with maximal disease occurring at the adductor hiatus.

The final major division originates at the bifurcation of the popliteal and extends to the plantar arches. Although

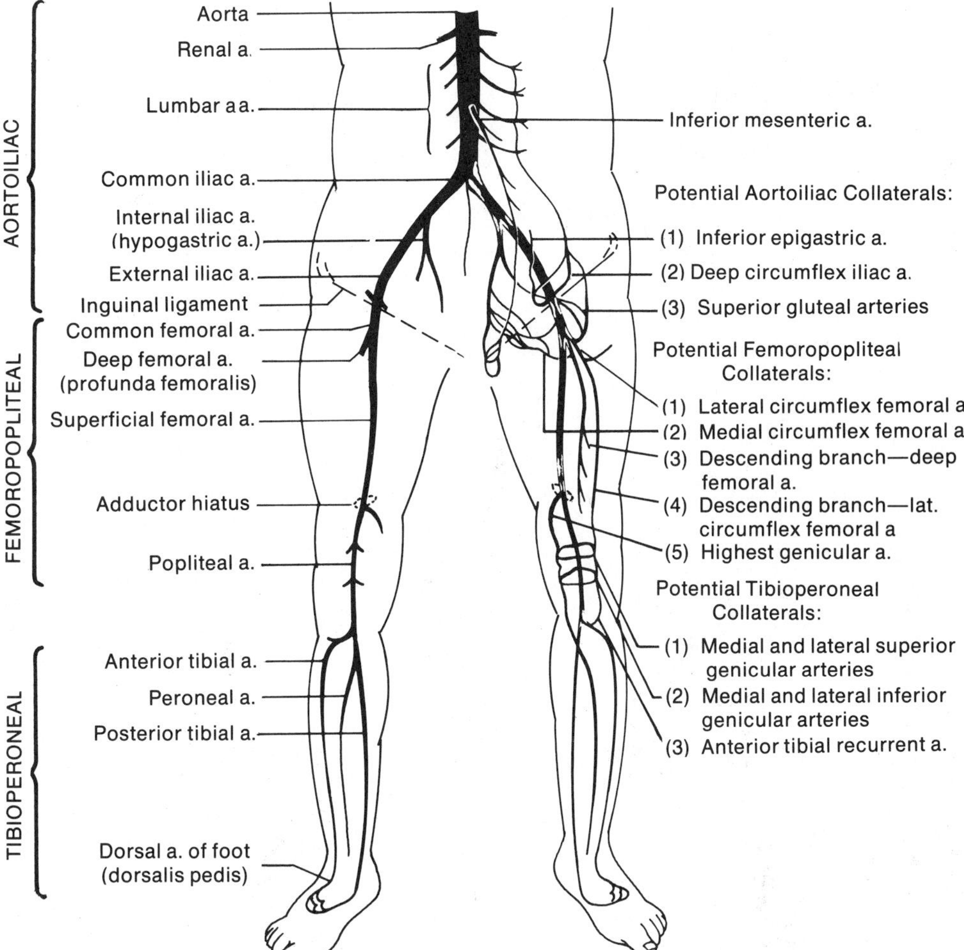

FIGURE 11–1. The aortoiliac, femoropopliteal, and tibioperoneal systems are shown on the left. Potential collateral vessels are shown on the right. Areas often involved by stenoses are indicated by showing narrowing in the figure.

the entire length of these vessels may be severely diseased, especially in diabetics, the predilection is again at the bifurcations.

The major collateral pathways available to the diseased aortoiliac system originate primarily from the inferior mesenteric artery and from the lumbar vessels. Both sources of collateral are capable of dilating dramatically to accommodate increased blood flow. Similar spontaneous collateral may effectively bypass an occluded superficial femoral artery through pathways that take origin from the profunda femoris. Occlusion of the proximal popliteal may be bypassed with flow through the highest genicular artery via anastomoses with medial genicular vessels. An anterior tibial artery occluded at its origin may be reconstituted by retrograde flow derived from the genicular anastomoses. Although potential collateral pathways are by no means limited to those just described, it is apparent that the more distal the occlusive process, the more limited will be the available collateral. Thus, the more proximal the disease, the better will be the prognosis.

CLINICAL PRESENTATION

Intermittent claudication may be the presenting symptom of several entities that fall into three general categories: (1) atherosclerotic occlusive disease, (2) nonatherosclerotic occlusive disease, and (3) mechanical compression syndromes. Of the three, atherosclerotic occlusion is by far the most frequently encountered.

Atherosclerotic Occlusive Disease

Femoropopliteal Disease. Intermittent claudication most commonly results from atherosclerotic occlusive disease involving the superficial femoral and popliteal arteries (Fig. 11–2). While most patients are in their seventh decade, the occlusive process may remain asymptomatic for many years, and most patients do not seek medical intervention until their physical activities become severely curtailed several years after the onset of symptoms. Both lower extremities are usually diseased, but claudication in the presenting limb often precedes contralateral symptoms by 2 or 3 years. The limitations imposed upon exercise intolerance by the affected limb often preclude claudication in the less diseased opposite limb.

The character of femoropopliteal claudication is often described as cramping pain, soreness, or a tightening sensation in the posterior calf musculature. When the occlusive process is confined to the superficial femoral artery or prox-

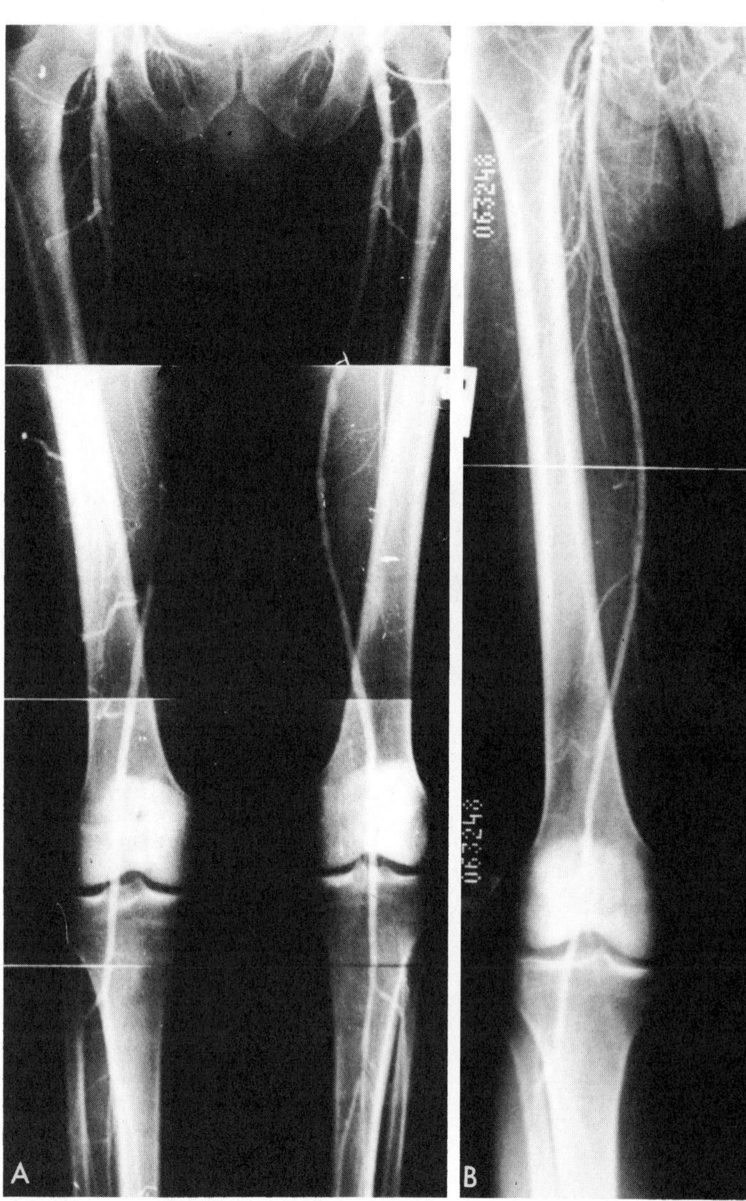

FIGURE 11–2. Femoropopliteal occlusive disease. *A,* Occlusion of all but the most proximal segment of the superficial femoral artery within the adductor canal. The popliteal artery is reconstituted, with retrograde flow through the highest genicular artery, which appears stenotic at its origin. *B,* Occlusion of the proximal popliteal artery, with reconstitution of the distal popliteal via the patent highest genicular artery.

imal popliteal artery, calf claudication is usually the only symptom. Associated stenosis of the profunda femoris or tibioperoneal system may, however, compromise collateral circulation to such an extent that symptoms of more advanced ischemia appear. The affected person then complains of numbness or tingling, coldness, discoloration, or nonhealing ulcerations of the toes or foot. These symptoms of more advanced disease are especially prominent in the patient whose activities have been so restricted by concurrent systemic illness that claudication may only rarely have been apparent.

The limb of a patient presenting with claudication usually appears adequately nourished, without the trophic changes classically associated with more severe peripheral ischemia. The femoral pulse is normal, but the popliteal pulse is diminished or absent, depending on collateral flow. The posterior tibial and dorsalis pedis pulses in the foot are also either entirely absent or markedly diminished and, if perceptible at rest, frequently disappear with repetitive exercise. Doppler ankle pressures obtained with the cuff at calf level while listening over the posterior tibial or dorsalis pedis arteries demonstrate systolic pressures in the range of 60 to 80 mm Hg and ankle brachial indices (ABI) between 0.5 and 0.9.

More extensive occlusive disease in the individual with claudication associated with ischemic symptoms is reflected by finding trophic changes of varying degrees of hair loss, attenuation of skin and subcutaneous tissue, and muscular atrophy. The foot is usually cool and may exhibit blanching on elevation and hyperemia (rubor) when dependent. Doppler ankle pressures are usually between 40 and 60 mm Hg, with ABI ranging between 0.2 and 0.5.

Aortoiliac Disease. Intermittent claudication as the result of more proximal aortoiliac occlusive disease accounts for only 10 to 15% of the affected population (Fig. 11–3). The clinical presentation differs considerably from that associated with more distal disease, its onset characteristically occurring a decade earlier. The syndrome associated with thrombotic occlusion of the aortic bifurcation was classically described by Leriche and Morel in 1948:

> In the male: inability to keep a stable erection, the blood flow being insufficient to fill the spongious processes.

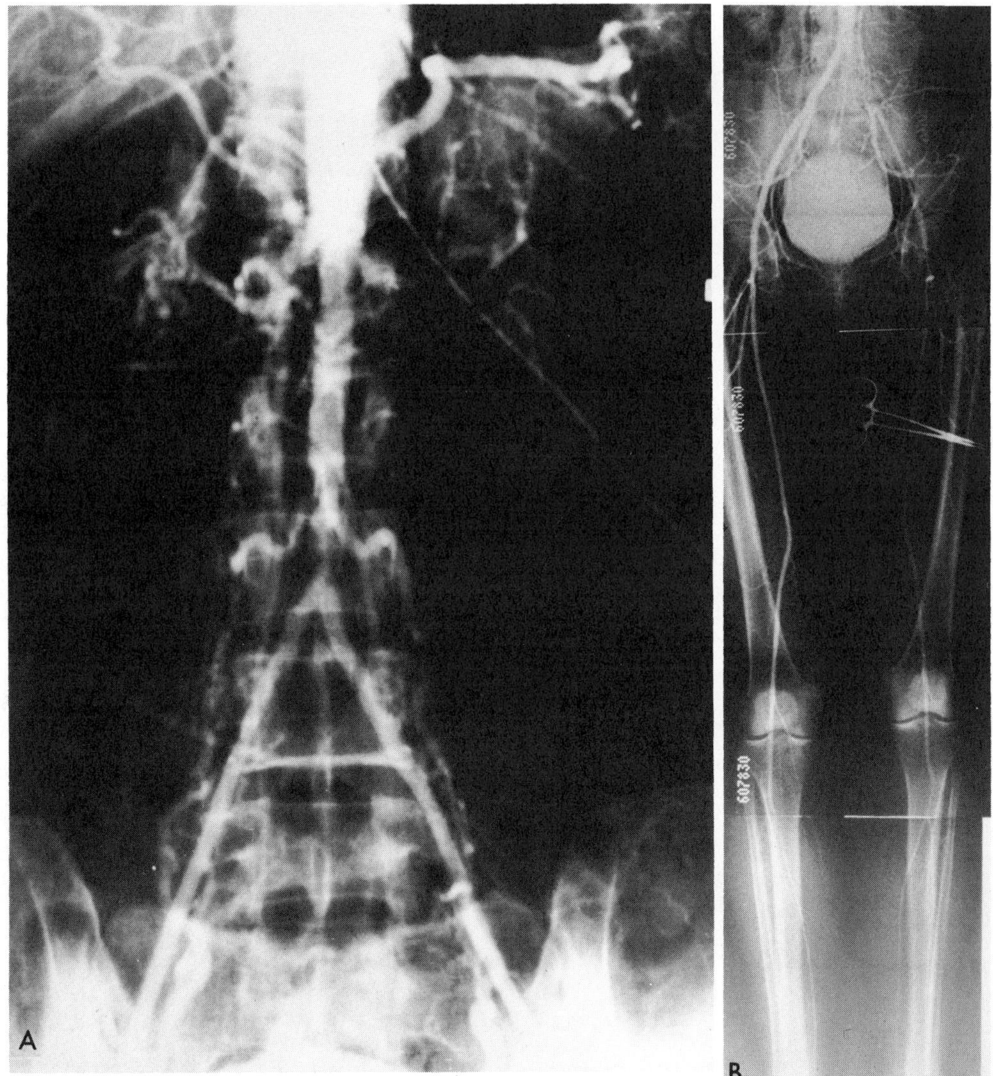

FIGURE 11–3. Aortoiliac occlusive disease. *A,* Extensive disease involving the terminal aorta and both iliac arteries. The well-developed retroperitoneal collateral allowed reconstitution of the distal iliofemoral system. *B,* Unilateral occlusion of the left common iliac artery with reconstitution of both internal and external iliacs via extensive collateralization. Of particular note is the prominent deep iliac circumflex branch of the distal external iliac.

> Extreme liability to fatigue of both lower limbs. It is not well-known "intermittent claudication," but an extreme weariness, which comes quickly on walking, sometimes even in ordinary standing position.
>
> Usually a global atrophy of both lower limbs, which is difficult to appreciate, as a normal limb lacks as a term of comparison.
>
> No trophic changes, either of the skin, or the nails. Toes look normal. It is difficult to believe that circulation is severely impaired.
>
> Pallor of legs and feet, even when standing. At rest the limb looks as if a Martin rubber bandage had just been released.[8]

This blatant description, of course, represents the extreme of aortoiliac occlusive disease but serves to point out several salient features. Although typical calf claudication is indeed present in the majority, about half the patients complain predominantly of hip and thigh claudication, described not as pain but as a tightening sensation or heaviness of the entire lower extremity accompanied by extreme fatigue or weariness. Proximal fatigue becomes especially apparent as the hip, buttock, and thigh muscles are used in climbing stairs. The severity of the proximal claudication depends on the relative status of the collateral bed, which is potentially more extensive than that available with more distal occlusion. In some cases, collaterals are sufficiently developed to preclude claudication entirely, as typified by the occasional asymptomatic individual with absent femoral pulses.

Physical examination may reveal disproportionately small limbs, but diffuse pallor is rarely evident, and trophic changes typically absent. Femoral and distal pulses are commonly diminished, rather than absent, owing to extensive collateralization. A bruit over the common femoral artery confirms the diagnosis. Doppler ankle pressures are frequently in the range of 80 to 110 mm Hg at rest with ABIs, of 0.7 to 1.0. It is important to emphasize that the paucity of findings at rest do not correlate reliably with either the extent of disease or its clinical disability. Moderate exercise with repetitive dorsiflexion of the elevated foot, however, frequently elicits symptoms associated with diminished pulses, Doppler pressures, and ABI.

Tibioperoneal Disease. Most patients with intermittent claudication from occlusive disease isolated at or distal

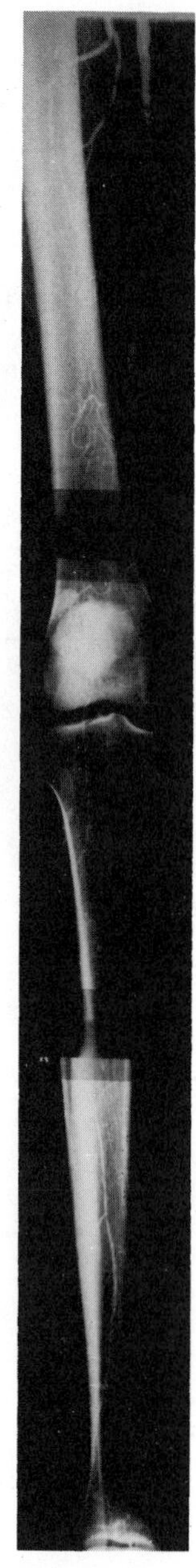

FIGURE 11–4. Tibioperoneal disease: occlusion of the entire popliteal artery plus the anterior and posterior tibial arteries. Collaterals fill the peroneal artery at midcalf, the only major artery patent below the knee.

to the popliteal bifurcation are overt or latent diabetics (Fig. 11–4). Painful claudication of the metatarsal arch is the most frequent presentation, but with insufficient genicular collateralization, calf symptoms may also develop. Numbness, tingling, burning paresthesias, and mild pain at rest, indicative of advanced disease, are more frequently present in this group but may be either masked or exacerbated by diabetic neuropathy. On physical examination, trophic changes or cutaneous ulceration may be apparent, particularly in the presence of peripheral neuropathy. In isolated tibioperoneal disease, the popliteal pulse remains palpable, but all distal pulses are usually absent. Pedal edema results from prolonged dependency, reflecting the patient's attempt to seek relief from more advanced ischemic rest pain. Doppler ankle pressures are markedly diminished, although such pressures may be spuriously elevated owing to circumferentially calcified and therefore rigid arterial walls.

Combined Arterial Disease. The presence of significant stenoses at more than one level, so-called "tandem lesions," often produces variations in the clinical presentation. A strong femoral pulse associated with foot claudication or severe trophic changes and absent pedal pulses suggests femoropopliteal disease with collateral vasculature comprised by concurrent tibioperoneal or profunda femoris occlusion (Fig. 11–5*A*). A diminished or absent femoral pulse with marked trophic changes is indicative of aortoiliac stenosis combined with significant distal disease (see Fig. 11–5*B*). Bilateral symptomatology does not necessarily correlate with symmetric lesions. Proximal iliac obstruction

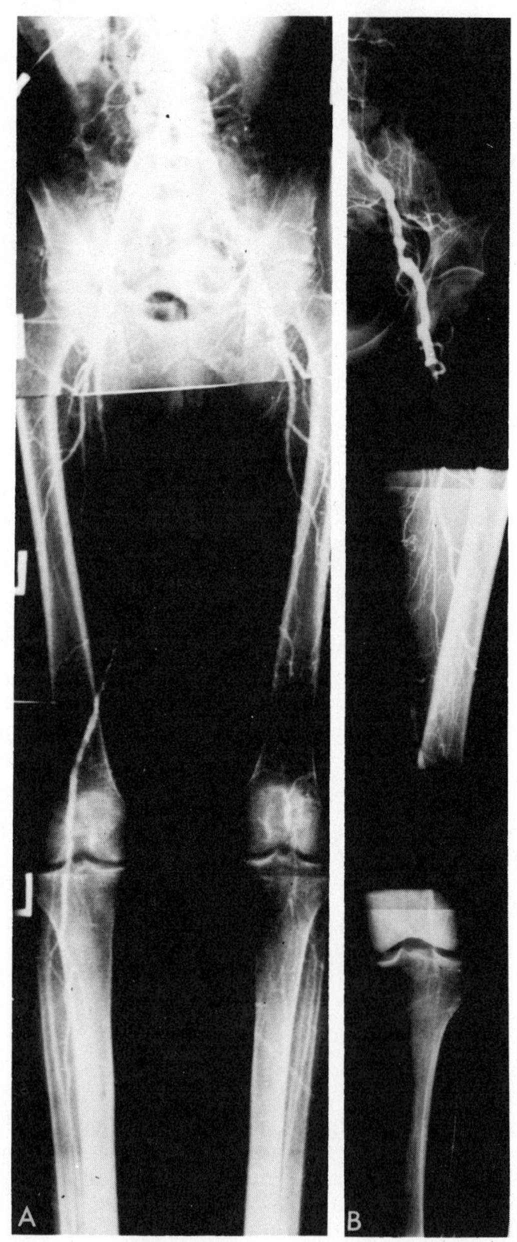

FIGURE 11–5. Combined arterial disease. *A,* Extensive disease has occluded both superficial femoral and distal popliteal arteries on the left. The resultant isolated popliteal segment is demonstrated at the level of the femoral condyles. *B,* Tandem lesions of both iliac and superficial femoral arteries.

may be the responsible lesion in one limb and the more distal disease in the other.

Nonatherosclerotic Occlusive Disease

Thromboangiitis Obliterans. Buerger's disease most commonly causes intermittent claudication of the metatarsal arch and, less frequently, of the calf musculature. Buerger's disease remains quite rare but is generally accepted as a discrete entity distinct from distal atherosclerosis.[9] Thromboangiitis should be considered in a young, heavy smoker with instep claudication and varying degrees of trophic changes, especially when associated with upper extremity involvement (absent ulnar pulse), migratory superficial phlebitis, vasospastic phenomena, and a normal glucose tolerance curve. The angiogram frequently confirms the suspicion by revealing characteristic segmental disease, exceptional tortuosity of smaller arteries, and absence of atheromata in larger vessels.

Adventitial Cysts. Adventitial cysts are an exceedingly rare cause of intermittent claudication.[10] The lesion is usually located in the popliteal artery and, as with Buerger's disease, typically affects men in the fourth decade. The cyst is located between the media and adventitia, thus compromising the lumen of the vessel. Arteriography reveals a characteristic curvilinear stenosis isolated in the midpopliteal artery.

Mechanical Compression Syndromes

Popliteal Entrapment. Occasionally, the origin of the medial head of the gastrocnemius or the plantaris muscle is aberrant such that muscular bundles with associated fibrous bands compress the popliteal artery during contraction. This compression produces temporary arterial occlusion, and repeated trauma may lead to aneurysm or plaque formation. This syndrome occurs in young men in their twenties, and although acute thrombotic occlusion may occasionally necessitate urgent surgical intervention, patients more commonly complain of typical intermittent claudication. A physical examination demonstrates obliteration of distal pulses with any maneuver causing contraction of the calf muscles and dorsiflexion of the foot. Arteriography carried out in conjunction with these maneuvers reveals an isolated occlusion of the popliteal artery, but the diagnosis can be established noninvasively with a duplex scan and more precisely with magnetic resonance imaging (MRI).[11]

Retroperitoneal Fibrosis. Although ureteral obstruction or peripheral edema associated with caval compression is a more frequent mode of presentation, isolated aortic or iliac arterial compression can occur in retroperitoneal fibrosis and presents with claudication resembling aortoiliac atherosclerosis.[12] Bipolar arteriography is needed to detect the compression that exerts its force in the anteroposterior direction.

DIFFERENTIAL DIAGNOSIS

Musculoskeletal or neuropathic symptoms are not usually confused with claudication, except when the peripheral pulses are diminished by concurrent peripheral vascular disease. It is important to re-emphasize that claudication becomes apparent only with exercise, occurs intermittently at regular fixed intervals, and subsides promptly with rest.

Arthritis. Patients with degenerative arthritis of the hip may have thigh and buttock pain, and those with arthritis of the knee not infrequently develop calf pain. Although such pain may be exacerbated by walking, it is usually more pronounced at rest or with prolonged standing. Appropriate radiologic studies help to confirm the diagnosis, as does the patient's response to medical therapy.

Degenerative Disc Disease. Herniated nucleus pulposus of the L4–L5 intervertebral disc characteristically produces episodic pain along the dermatome of the fifth lumbar nerve root. This pain is thus located along the anterolateral aspect of the leg and is frequently present at rest, though it is aggravated by exercise. Associated peripheral vasospasm may occasionally result in diminished distal pulses. The appropriate diagnosis is suggested by the loss of lumbar lordosis, marked paravertebral muscular spasm, diminished dorsiflexion and ankle reflexes, reduced sensation, and pain on straight leg raising (see Chapter 51).

Neurogenic Claudication. Neurogenic claudication (pseudoclaudication) is the result of intermittent ischemia of the lower spinal cord or cauda equina, usually secondary to bony spinal stenosis but occasionally due to a prolapsed intervertebral disc.[13] Lower extremity pain in this syndrome occurs more often with changes in position rather than during exercise. When symptoms are associated with exercise, however, they occur at progressively shorter intervals, and a prolonged period of rest is required for relief. Although absent at rest, neurologic signs may be elicited immediately after positional changes or exercise.

Restless Legs Syndrome. The cause of this syndrome is unknown, but it is not related to obstructive or vasospastic disease. The symptoms are not painful, are most pronounced at rest, and are characterized by a poorly defined, restless, twisting, achiness or crawling sensation of the lower limbs. The net result is an irresistible urge to exercise the extremity, an urge that may become so overwhelming that sleep is seriously impaired.[14]

Muscle Cramps. Painful muscular spasm usually affecting the gastrocnemius is common following extreme exercise even in young individuals without vascular disease. Nocturnal cramps frequently awaken such patients with an exquisitely painful muscular contraction that subsides slowly with massage or exercise. The muscle usually remains sore for several days following the acute episode. The cause remains obscure in most patients, but a commonly encountered cause is the subtle hypokalemia of the patient taking diuretics. Such cramps may also occur in thyroid disorders, uremia, pregnancy, hypomagnesemia, and occasionally during clofibrate therapy.[15] When muscular cramps become frequent and impair sleep, quinine sulfate or diazepam has offered relief.

Venous Claudication. An occasional patient with deep venous insufficiency or thrombosis will complain of pain suggestive of arterial claudication, but some degree of discomfort is present at rest. The edema of venous stasis is usually obvious in severe cases, and the symptoms respond to therapy directed toward reducing that edema.

McArdle's Syndrome. Patient's with congenital deficiency of muscle phosphorylase have muscle pain on exertion, and this pain may appear at any age.[16] Although the pain associated with this syndrome may mimic claudication, it is typically provoked with minimal muscular effort and affects both upper and lower extremities. The diagnosis can be confirmed by finding increased amounts of muscle enzymes without elevated venous lactic acid levels following exercise of the upper extremity.

Anterior Compartment Syndrome. This rare entity is

produced by marked edema within the anterior tibial compartment, resulting in compression of muscular and neurovascular structures between bone and the equally unyielding compartmental fascia. The presentation is more frequently acute than chronic, and it usually follows a period of excessive exercise.

The acute presentation is characterized by a dull, aching pain in the anterior compartment adjacent to the tibia; it is refractory to rest and analgesics. The overlying skin becomes attenuated, and the entire compartment is tensely distended and tender. Peroneal nerve palsy may develop with progressive loss of toe, then foot, dorsiflexion. Finally, loss of the dorsalis pedis pulse reflects ongoing compression. Progressive nerve or arterial compression mandates surgical intervention with fasciotomy in order to prevent muscle necrosis and foot drop.

The chronic syndrome is rare and consists of repetitive episodes of anterior tibial muscle pain that occurs on exertion and resolves with rest.[17] The discomfort along the anterolateral aspect of the lower leg therefore mimics that produced by isolated anterior tibial arterial occlusion, but the pain requires a longer period of rest for relief, and the dorsalis pedis pulse is usually present on examination. Signs and symptoms may be provoked by repetitive dorsiflexion of the foot against resistance, resulting in the characteristic pain and a firm bulging of the anterior compartment. Bilateral elective fasciotomy has provided relief for these patients.

Shin Splints. This relatively common problem may be related in part to the anterior compartment syndrome, but neuromuscular function is not seriously jeopardized. It is the nemesis of athletes beginning a vigorous training schedule as well as tourists unaccustomed to walking or climbing long distances. The dull ache is located more directly over the tibia, compartmental swelling is not obvious, and pedal pulses are present. The pain begins during exercise but persists even with rest. An initial period of rest followed by a graduated exercise program is usually sufficient therapy.[18]

SPECIAL DIAGNOSTIC TECHNIQUES

Angiography

Angiography is chiefly of value for defining the surgical anatomy and should be reserved for those claudicators with indications for surgical reconstruction. Intra-arterial digital subtraction angiography is frequently used because it minimizes the volume of contrast required.[19]

Visualization of the arterial system allows the vascular surgeon and interventional radiologist to plan the most appropriate procedure. The suspected lesion is confirmed, other significant lesions are demonstrated, collateral vessels are visualized, and associated abnormalities such as renal or mesenteric artery stenosis or aberrant visceral arterial anatomy are defined.

Serious major complications are fortunately rare, with an incidence well under 1%.[20] These complications include allergic reactions and hypotension, pseudoaneurysm formation within a residual hematoma, and laceration of the arterial wall. Catheter dissection of the intima or dislodgement of plaque may result in subsequent thrombosis or embolization. Frank perforation of an arterial wall can produce life-threatening hemorrhage.

Vascular Laboratory

Doppler ultrasound and plethysmographic techniques are now available for initial diagnosis and following patients on a chronic basis to assess medical or surgical therapy.

Transcutaneous Doppler (Pressure Measurements). This method utilizes a small hand-held Doppler instrument applied to the skin overlying a blood vessel. The emitted ultrasonic beam is partially deflected by moving particles in the blood stream, and is recorded by a receiving crystal. The simplest application of this instrument is the direct measurement of systolic pressures as carried out in the office setting. Systolic pressures are obtained from the sphygmomanometer by listening over the dorsalis pedis or posterior tibial arteries as the cuff is deflated. Normal individuals at rest have a systolic ankle pressure equal to or higher than the brachial artery pressure. The ankle-to-brachial artery index is, therefore, normally in excess of 1.0. Claudicators usually demonstrate lower pressures in the range of 60 to 100 mm Hg, with ABI ranging from 0.5 to 1.0 at rest. One can obtain an objective assessment of the location of significant occlusive lesions by recording the pressure at different levels.

Since resting pressures may be normal in some claudicators, the sensitivity of the Doppler technique can be increased by measurements made immediately after exercise or on a treadmill. Ankle pressure may actually increase in the normal individual but diminishes significantly in the patient with peripheral occlusive disease.

A significant limitation of this technique pertains to diabetic patients whose arterial walls may be so rigidly calcified that they are relatively incompressible with the cuff. This factor, when present, yields spuriously high pressures, and in 10% of the diabetic population ankle pressures cannot be determined at all by the Doppler technique.[21]

Waveform Analysis (Flow Measurements). Pulsatile flow may also be determined by pulse volume recordings (PVR) obtained with an air plethysmograph. The volume changes at several levels in the extremity concurrent with arterial inflow are transduced and usually correlate well with pressure measurements obtained with the Doppler technique. PVR is most useful in interpreting the pressures from diabetic limbs. Although incompressible arteries may result in spuriously high pressures, the dampened amplitude of PVRs will identify patients with significant arterial insufficiency.

Neither Doppler pressures nor waveform analysis are sufficiently standardized to isolate candidates for surgery; an individual with claudication and systolic ankle pressures of less than 40 to 45 mm Hg is most appropriately treated surgically. But pressure and waveform recordings allow long-term repetitive evaluation of both medical and surgical management.[22] Successful medical management is indicated by either stability or a gradual improvement in these parameters, whereas sudden deterioration should prompt consideration of surgical reconstruction even in the absence of increasing symptoms. Similarly, a diminished ankle pressure occurring postoperatively in a patient who has had a bypass indicates a progression of disease distal to the bypass or mechanical stenosis of the graft itself, either of which indicates that further surgery may be required.

SPECIAL CLINICAL PROBLEMS

Prior to a general consideration of the management of intermittent claudication, two special clinical problems warrant discussion. The onset of ischemia at rest and development of sudden arterial occlusion are recognizable as specific entities, each with major therapeutic implications.

Ischemic Pain at Rest

Patients with intermittent claudication who have or subsequently develop ischemic symptoms at rest manifest far-advanced occlusive disease with a poor prognosis if untreated. The atherosclerotic process has become so extensive that collateral blood flow cannot maintain minimal nutritional requirements of the tissues, even in the basal resting state. Although pain in the toes, arch, or heel at rest is the most common symptom, it is important to recognize that numbness or paresthesias, if caused by vascular insufficiency, have the same significance.

Most commonly, patients with ischemic pain at rest have multisegment arterial disease, with occlusion of the superficial femoral artery as the common denominator. The onset of symptoms usually occurs when either the run-off (tibioperoneal system) or the source of collateral (profunda femoris) becomes critically inadequate. Ischemic pain is distinctly unusual in isolated aortoiliac disease. Symptoms at rest may develop, however, with isolated distal tibioperoneal occlusions especially in diabetic patients.

A physical examination of the involved limb reveals marked trophic changes and deep rubor when the limb is dependent. In an effort to improve blood flow and relieve pain, patients often maintain the leg in a dependent position, which results in considerable edema. Pulses are absent, and Doppler examination may reveal continuous nonpulsatile flow with ankle pressures not infrequently less than 40 mm Hg. Patchy cellulitis, nonhealing ulcers, and incipient or frank gangrene of the toe tips are not uncommon.

In the differential diagnosis of pain at rest, absent pulses, dependent rubor, and a cool foot are important indicators of an ischemic etiology. Peripheral neuropathy usually follows the distribution of a specific nerve, but ischemic neuritis can be a component of pain at rest as well. Causalgia (see Chapter 52) refers to pain following trauma of any nature that presents or persists long after the specific lesion has healed.[23] It is thought to result from a reflex arc mediated by afferent pain fibers and efferent sympathetics—hence the alternate term "post-traumatic reflex sympathetic dystrophy," which may become so chronically debilitating as to result in osteoporosis (Sudeck's atrophy). Erythromelalgia is an obscure condition, occasionally familial, characterized by episodic attacks of burning pain and redness of one or both feet.[24] These attacks are associated with exposure to warm temperatures, exertion, or occasionally dependency. Although it is not usually difficult to distinguish these conditions from ischemic pain at rest, ankle pressure measurements usually differentiate confusing cases.

Once ischemic symptoms are present at rest, amputation is virtually ensured unless revascularization can be carried out. Advocates of early amputation argue that although the mortality associated with revascularization is not much higher than that with primary amputation, the debility imposed by subsequent morbidity and prolonged hospitalization and the necessity for repeated operations argue against salvage operations except under the most favorable conditions. In view of our initial experience with 240 patients operated on for limb salvage, this argument seems unjustified.[25] Although primary amputation was carried out in 6% of such patients because of extensive gangrene, distal arterial anatomy unsuitable for reconstruction, or concurrent systemic illness precluding anesthesia, the majority (94%) were revascularized. More recently, this aggressive approach toward reconstruction for limb salvage yielded an 81% 5-year cumulative salvage rate with an acceptable 2% operative mortality in nearly 300 patients operated on in our service.[26]

Sudden Arterial Occlusion

The individual with intermittent claudication may occasionally present with sudden occlusion of a diseased vessel when acute arterial thrombosis occurs in the absence of well-developed collateral. The majority of sudden arterial occlusions, however, result from peripheral embolization, usually in patients without antecedent claudication. Such emboli originate from the heart or from ulcerated plaques of the aorta and proximal arteries. A representative review of 124 patients with arterial embolization revealed that 87% of the emboli originated in the heart.[27] The underlying process in half of these patients was atherosclerotic heart disease, and half of these had recent myocardial infarction with subsequent mural thrombus formation. Rheumatic heart disease was present in 27% of this group; all except one had concurrent atrial fibrillation.

The site of acute arterial occlusion is usually the bifurcation of larger vessels, and the severity of ischemic symptoms and signs depends on the availability of collateral. Thus, embolic phenomena involving the upper extremity are frequently unrecognized because of the extensive collateral available. Conversely, emboli to the lower extremity are usually obvious.

Most patients present with the abrupt onset of excruciating pain accompanied by paresthesias. However, symptoms may occasionally develop more slowly, over a period of 24 to 36 hours.[28] A line of color and temperature demarcation is evident distal to the occlusion, distal pulses are absent, and peripheral veins are collapsed. Although acute thrombosis of an atherosclerotic artery may produce a similar picture, an embolic etiology is suggested by the presence of a source, by normal contralateral pulses, and by the lack of antecedent claudication.

The site of lodgement in approximately one half of patients with embolic occlusion is the bifurcation of the common femoral artery. The line of demarcation is usually located at the midcalf level, and popliteal and tibial pulses are absent. In the remaining patients, the site is equally distributed among the bifurcations of the aorta, iliac, popliteal, and brachial arteries. With occlusion of the aortic bifurcation (saddle embolus), symptoms and signs are bilateral; demarcation may occur as high as the umbilicus; and nausea, vomiting, and hypotension frequently present.

Microemboli consisting of atheromatous debris or cholesterol crystals that originate from an ulcerated plaque or aneurysm may occlude smaller arteries or arterioles. Particles may lodge within the distribution of either an isolated digital artery or multiple vessels of similar caliber, producing a "shower" effect. An acutely painful, dusky toe from microemboli may be a presenting symptom of a popliteal aneurysm. A cool, painful extremity with tender muscles and a petechial or maculopapular eruption is suggestive of a shower of such emboli. Peripheral pulses are frequently preserved.[29]

Following acute occlusion, the clinical course is dictated by the subsequent behavior of available collateral, which, if adequate, allows warmth and normal color to return over a 2- to 4-hour period. Conversely, the intensification of pallor, pain, and coldness is an ominous sign of impending gangrene, and with the onset of anesthesia or paralysis, frank muscle necrosis becomes inevitable within 4 to 6 hours. In either situation, systemic heparinization should be initiated. Angiography is generally unnecessary in case of arterial embolus but may be of value when the site of lodgement is uncertain. Prompt embolectomy less than 4 to 6 hours after the onset clearly takes precedence over arteriography. Similarly, surgery should not be delayed for exhaustive medical evaluation and preparation, as embolectomy is expeditiously carried out with balloon catheters through a small groin incision with the patient under local anesthesia.

When acute thrombosis occurs in the claudicant with antecedent atherosclerosis, arteriography should be performed, if possible, to determine the extent of pre-existing disease. The information thus acquired allows appropriate reconstruction to be performed at the time of thrombectomy. Nevertheless, this study should be omitted if surgery would be delayed 4 to 6 hours from the onset of anesthesia or paralysis. On-the-table arteriography following initial thrombectomy is a satisfactory alternative. Thrombolytic agents (see later on) may be used in high-risk patients or in those with distal small vessel occlusion. Finally, when the acute occlusion is secondary to microemboli, surgery is generally less urgent and arrangements for arteriography can be made.

The overall prognosis for the group of patients with arterial emboli is grim.[27] The hospital mortality of patients undergoing embolectomy approaches 30%, primarily because of concomitant myocardial infarction. Although prompt embolectomy within 24 hours of the onset of symptoms yielded an immediate limb salvage rate of 81%, only half of these patients survived for 2 years.

MANAGEMENT

Natural History

The intelligent management of patients with intermittent claudication must be based on an understanding of the natural course of atherosclerotic peripheral vascular disease. The Framingham Study showed that although the mortality of those with claudication is twice that of an unaffected population, the underlying systemic atherosclerosis, not its peripheral manifestations, is the lethal factor.[4] In 1962 Boyd reported his observations in a group of 1476 patients with intermittent claudication (Table 11–1). Although the majority (73%) of such individuals in the 55- to 64-year age group survived for 5 years, only 38% survived the ensuing decade.[30] In these patients, who have very high mortality rates from stroke and myocardial infarction, the role of surgery for intermittent claudication is palliative.

The threat of limb loss imposed by the presence of claudication is not great. Table 11–1 shows that major amputation was required in 7.2% of patients at 5 years and 12% at 10 years in one series[30] and in 5.8% in another, the majority of which occurred in individuals with less than one block tolerance and distal tibioperoneal disease.[31] McAllister found a similar amputation rate and observed that as diabetics were excluded, the rate diminished to 1%.[5] No limb was lost in the Framingham group during the 14-year study period.[4]

TABLE 11–1. NATURAL HISTORY OF INTERMITTENT CLAUDICATION WITHOUT SURGERY

Series	No. of Patients	Mean Follow-up Interval (yr)	Survivors (%)	Amputation (%)	Stable/ Improved (%)
Boyd (1962)	1476	5	73	7.2	80
		10	38	12.0	60
Imparato (1975)	104	2.5	—	5.8	79
McAllister (1976)	100	6	89	7.0	78

Another important factor in the natural history is that the symptom itself is not necessarily progressive. On the contrary, both McAllister and Imparato found progressive disability in only 20% of their patients. Eighty per cent either improved or remained stable during the follow-up periods. Once pain at rest or nonhealing ulcerations become established, however, amputation becomes inevitable unless arterial reconstruction is carried out.

Medical Management

It is clear from the natural course of intermittent claudication that most patients managed medically will either improve or achieve stability, and in the event that surgical reconstruction proves necessary, continuous medical supervision remains essential for optimal results. Ideally, such care should be directed primarily at arrest or reversal of the underlying disease process and secondarily at preventing complications and alleviating symptoms. The association of coronary artery disease with risk factors such as obesity, hypertension, hyperlipoproteinemia, tobacco consumption, and a sedentary lifestyle is well known,[32–39] and a similar association with peripheral vascular disease is evident.[40–43] Most important is the fact that coronary artery disease often coexists with and usually limits the life expectancy of the individual with claudication.

General Measures. Intermittent claudication associated with poorly compensated congestive heart failure or chronic obstructive pulmonary disease is sometimes improved by rigorous treatment of the systemic illness. Management of polycythemia should maintain the hematocrit below 55%, not only to avoid thromboses but also to reduce blood viscosity. Although the sequelae of systemic hypertension mandate strict control, the diastolic pressure should probably be maintained at about 90 mm Hg to maximize collateral flow. Since obesity increases the work and oxygen consumption of exercising muscle, thus aggravating claudication, weight reduction with exercise and dietary therapy is helpful. Although there is objective evidence that treatment of the rare type III hyperlipoproteinemia results in attenuation of symptomatic peripheral vascular disease,[44] only preliminary data are available with respect to claudication in patients with the more common types of hyperlipoproteinemia.[45] Nevertheless, it seems logical for claudicants with hyperlipoproteinemia to undergo drug and diet therapy similar to that recommended for patients with coronary artery disease (see Chapter 7).

Local Measures. Because ischemic tissue is unduly susceptible to injury, delayed healing, and infection, local measures are directed at preventing trauma. Ischemic skin should be lubricated daily to prevent drying and cracking with subsequent infection. Nails must be trimmed horizontally to avoid ingrowth, a complication that must be conservatively treated with a cotton twist under the corner of the nail. Shoes should be meticulously fitted to ensure adequate protection of toes to minimize chafing. Trauma of any nature must be carefully avoided, since minimal injury may result in subsequent ulceration and gangrene. This is particularly true of the diabetic whose peripheral neuropathy may preclude recognition of mechanical or thermal injury. The care of the ischemic limb of a patient confined to bed for other reasons is often overlooked with disastrous consequences. It is a simple matter to avoid elastic (Ace) wraps or stockings and to place sheepskin under heels, lamb's wool between toes, and a cradle to support linen.

Exercise. Exercise programs of varying intensity have been used for the treatment of intermittent claudication and are based on both experimental data and empiric observations. It has been taught that exercise induces maximal development of collateral, yet proof that this is the mechanism responsible for increased exercise tolerance is wanting. In fact, xenon isotope and venous occlusion plethysmographic studies fail to substantiate any increased blood flow in the exercised ischemic limb.[46, 47] Nevertheless, there are studies supporting the empiric observation that claudicant individuals do increase walking distance with regular exercise and may do so to the extent that their disability is no longer incapacitating.[48] Thus, an exercise program consisting of frequent daily walks to the point of tolerance is generally recommended. Continued walking beyond the onset of ischemic pain, however, serves no useful purpose and frequently results in a discouraged patient with persistently sore muscles. Such an exercise program is suggested for a trial period of 3 to 6 months, especially for relatively sedentary claudicant patients. Substantial improvement cannot be expected, however, in the individual who already exercises to tolerance in performing the routine tasks of his or her vocation. In addition to decreasing disability, regular exercise is a useful adjunct to other measures designed to reduce weight, curtail tobacco consumption, and alter dietary habits.

Use of Tobacco. Recent evidence suggests that cigarette smoking promotes atherogenesis through a variety of interrelated mechanisms.[49] Tobacco consumption exerts its deleterious effects by producing vasoconstriction of cutaneous blood vessels, direct injury to endothelium, elevation of fatty acids, enhanced platelet aggregation, diminished production of prostacyclin associated with increased thromboxane levels, and elevation of red and white blood cell counts. The person with intermittent claudication from reduced muscle blood flow cannot necessarily expect symptomatic relief with abstinence from tobacco alone, yet the subsequent risk of amputation is tenfold higher among patients who fail to abstain.[50]

Pharmacologic Measures. These measures include the use of vasodilators, anticoagulation, fibrinolysis, and antiplatelet therapy.

Vasodilators. α-Lytic agents, such as tolazoline (Priscoline), or drugs that stimulate β-receptors, such as nylidrin (Arlidin), produce vasodilatation by interfering with autonomic regulation. Other agents (e.g., cyclandelate [Cyclospasmol]) act directly to relax arterial smooth muscle. Isoxsuprine (Vasodilan) is primarily β-adrenergic but may also exert part of its effect through direct muscle relaxation. Studies supporting the use of these agents are voluminous, but most lack objectivity and adequate controls. None of the agents studied to date is consistently effective in significantly prolonging walking time prior to the onset of symptoms, and thus they remain of questionable value.[51, 52]

Pentoxifylline (Trental). Intermittent claudication has been treated with pentoxifylline, based on small clinical trials documenting its efficacy in increasing walking distance. The drug is thought to improve capillary blood flow by increasing red blood cell deformity and decreasing red blood cell and platelet aggregation. Although it is well tolerated, its benefits remain equivocal and may result from concomitant exercise training.[53]

Anticoagulation. Although the final thrombotic occlusion of a stenotic arterial segment may be forestalled with anticoagulation, the progression of existing lesions is probably not altered.[54] Since the complications of this therapy are not insignificant, the use of anticoagulants, like vasodilators, is not routinely recommended at present.

Fibrinolysis. Clinical studies employing thrombolytic plasminogen activators such as streptokinase, urokinase, and recombinant tissue plasminogen activator have achieved success in restoring flow through recently occluded vessels, yet remain much less successful in treating chronic occlusions.[55–57] The most favorable results have been obtained with intra-arterial infusion of plasminogen activators directly into the thrombus, in contrast to the less successful outcome obtained with inducing a systemic lytic state intravenously.[57] Surgery remains preferable to thrombolytic therapy in most cases at present, yet the combination of thrombolysis followed by percutaneous transluminal angioplasty remains an attractive approach for managing critical ischemia in high-risk patients and when surgical results are poor. The hemorrhagic complications associated with thrombolytic therapy and the time required for its administration must be weighed carefully against potential benefits when compared with immediate surgical intervention.

Antiplatelet Therapy. Among several potential mechanisms underlying atherogenesis, it has been postulated that atheromatous plaques result from abnormal healing of injured endothelium.[58] Following endothelial injury and subsequent exposure of subendothelial connective tissue, platelets adhere to the denuded surface and release a variety of factors that stimulate smooth muscle cell proliferation. Smooth muscle cells then migrate centrally to produce a luminal surface that is many times thicker than the original endothelium.

The administration of an antiplatelet drug such as aspirin or dipyridamole has a firm theoretical basis, and both are reasonably well tolerated. Although further clinical studies are needed to justify its continued use, it has become common to use antiplatelet therapy in the chronic management of the atherosclerotic patient.

Surgical Management and Percutaneous Transluminal Angioplasty

Indications. Revascularization of the lower limb in patients with intermittent claudication is indicated when the symptom becomes incapacitating, rapidly progressive, or associated with ischemia of the foot at rest. Because of the natural history of claudication and the fact that reconstruction does not alter progression of the process, such intervention remains both elective and palliative. Successful palliation with restoration of a functional limb can be anticipated, along with dramatic improvement in the quality of life remaining for these individuals. Whether or not claudication qualifies as an incapacitating disorder in a given patient is a matter of clinical judgement. There is little hesitation to recommend intervention for the mail carrier or construction worker whose vocation demands functional limbs. Conversely, reconstruction is hardly warranted in the sedentary individual content with a daily excursion to the mailbox or limited by concurrent systemic disease. Most individuals with claudication, however, lie somewhere between these extremes, and it is the practice of most vascular surgeons to recommend surgery or percutaneous transluminal angioplasty (PTA) following a trial of conservative management when claudication jeopardizes vocation or proves truly incapacitating.

Although the severity of symptoms does not necessarily correlate with the extent of disease and is not a reliable prognosticator, rapid progression of symptoms is another relative indication for reconstruction, particularly applicable to the diabetic population.[59] Insulin-requiring diabetics are more likely to have distal tibioperoneal occlusive disease, and the amputation rate is at least four times higher than in nondiabetics. Thus, rapid acceleration of symptoms and the least suggestion of ischemia at rest should prompt serious consideration of reconstruction in diabetics. Considerable clinical judgement is required for nondiabetics with worsening symptoms because the state of collateralization is less predictable and may allow significant improvement during a period of a few weeks with conservative management.

Ischemic signs and symptoms at rest, including numbness and parethesias as well as frank pain, are ominous and presage the eventual onset of gangrene. As mentioned in the preceding section, intervention at this point becomes mandatory if amputation is to be avoided.

Endovascular Intervention

Percutaneous Transluminal Angioplasty. PTA has clearly achieved a place in the palliation of atherosclerotic disease for lesions limited to short segments (<5cm) of proximal vessels. The most favorable results have been obtained in patients with aortoiliac occlusive disease. Localized stenoses of the common or external iliac arteries have been successfully treated, as demonstrated by Gruntzig's original series that documented an initial success rate of 91% and a subsequent cumulative patency rate of 87% after 2 years.[60] Our own experience with more than 200 such patients confirmed these initially favorable results and documented a 5-year patency rate of 75%. Although not quite as durable as surgical reconstruction, PTA provides an expeditious initial first approach for many patients with aortoiliac disease. If unsuccessful, PTA may be followed by conventional aortoiliac reconstruction.

Results obtained with PTA in patients with femoropopliteal disease have been less encouraging. Of 184 such procedures initially carried out by Gruntzig, the cumulative patency rate after 2 years was 72%. Our more recent experience with approximately 100 claudicant patients documented a 5-year patency rate of only 60%. These results are less favorable than conventional bypass in keeping with a much larger Canadian experience and suggests that femoropopliteal PTA be reserved for highly selected individuals with short segment focal lesions.[61]

PTA offers several advantages, especially for high-risk patients with appropriate lesions who can be effectively palliated without the rigors of anesthesia and major surgery. That a successful procedure is cost effective is unquestioned, since a patient may be discharged from the hospital the day following dilatation after a short course of intravenous anticoagulation. This advantage is quickly negated, however, in patients who sustain early occlusion and ultimately require surgery. In an effort to improve durability of angioplasty, a variety of intraluminal stents are currently being used as an adjunct to PTA and results await further investigation.

Endovascular Techniques. In addition to intraluminal stents, a variety of laser techniques and rotary atherectomy devices are currently available for peripheral arterial application. Results with both generic modalities have to date been disappointing with respect to providing durable revascularization. Their role seems limited to highly selected individuals with limb-threatening ischemia or severely disabling claudication in patients without a vein available for a conventional bypass who seek a short-term solution.[62, 63]

Surgical Reconstruction of Femoropopliteal Disease. When intermittent claudication secondary to femoropopliteal occlusive disease becomes severely disabling or threatens limb viability, the procedure of choice is still the femoropopliteal bypass graft utilizing the autogenous saphenous vein, either reversed as originally described by Kunlin in 1949 or in situ (Fig. 11–6).[26, 64] Because femoropopliteal bypass is limited to an extremity and can be carried out under regional anesthesia, operative mortality (2 to 3%) and serious morbidity are acceptable. Whereas early patency rates approximate 95% at discharge from the hospital, the long-term prognosis must remain guarded. Fifteen years ago, patient survival was limited to 50% after 5 years and 25% after 10 years. Corresponding graft patency rates were only 60% and 40%, respectively. Because of improvements in the management of concurrent cerebrovascular and cardiac disease, our more recent experience demonstrates that 70% of patients survive 5 years with overall graft patency rates of 80%. In general, the more proximal the location of the distal anastomosis, the more favorable will be the results. In addition, an autogenous vein provides better long term patency than any prosthetic material. Thus, an above-knee vein graft results in a 90% 5-year

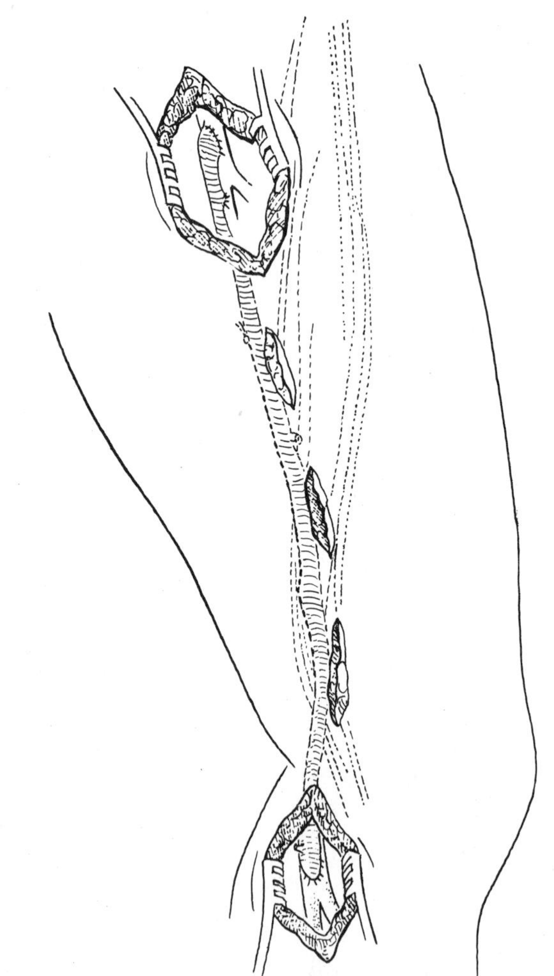

FIGURE 11–6. Femoropopliteal bypass graft illustrating the reversed autogenous saphenous vein technique as described by Kunlin. Bypass has been completed with proximal anastomosis to the common femoral artery and distal anastomosis to the distal popliteal artery.

patency rate in contrast to a lower 60% rate achieved with a prosthetic material. Below the knee, vein maintains a 75% patency rate, whereas prosthetic material diminishes to 35% after 5 years.[65] Most important, amputation following femoropopliteal reconstruction for claudication occurs infrequently (< 2%), identical to the rate anticipated from the natural history of the disease.

Aortoiliac Reconstruction. Surgical reconstruction in the patient with intermittent claudication due to isolated aortoiliac occlusive disease is effectively achieved with aortoiliac endarterectomy or bypass graft.[66–69] With the addition of certain technical modifications, effective palliation is also provided for the claudicant patient with tandem lesions, the most proximal of which is hemodynamically significant aortoiliac stenosis.[66] Both limited endarterectomy and bypass graft yield similar long-term results.[67] Endarterectomy avoids extensive retroperitoneal dissection and the use of prosthetic material but is limited to occlusive lesions confined to a short segment. Such lesions in the iliac arteries are more expeditiously treated with PTA. Endarterectomy may still be useful for short-segment aortic lesions most commonly found in the young female smoker. Aortoiliac disease, however, usually involves several segments of the vessels in a more diffuse pattern, and a bypass graft with prosthetic material is required (Fig. 11–7). The risk of infection and pseudoaneurysm formation has declined with use of newer prosthetic grafts and perioperative antibiotics. The 30-day operative mortality ranges from 2 to 7%, and most deaths are attributed to systemic cardiopulmonary complications. Major operative morbidity occurs in approximately 10% of cases and consists primarily of myocardial infarction, respiratory insufficiency, and occasionally renal failure. The immediate graft limb patency rate is approximately 99%, and 90% of patients are initially rendered asymptomatic or clearly improved.[68]

These impressive early results, however, are tempered by long-term complications and by progression of disease distally. While 80 to 90% are asymptomatic or improved after 5 years, only 50% remain in this category after 10 years.[68] This deterioration results primarily from graft thrombosis associated with progressive distal disease. Less commonly, infection or pseudoaneurysm (2%) result in failure. Most discouraging, of course, is the overall high mortality from systemic vascular disease. Although 80% survive for 5 years, only 50% survive 10 years after surgery.[69]

Major advances in perioperative management have reduced the mortality and morbidity of aortoiliac bypass graft to acceptable levels. Nevertheless, an occasional patient with combined tandem disease and a threatened limb will require aortoiliac reconstruction but will not survive a major transabdominal procedure under prolonged deep general anesthesia. The presence of intra-abdominal sepsis or multiple adhesion may also preclude conventional aortoiliac surgery. Fortunately, alternative methods allow revascularization of the femoral vessels with subcutaneous bypass procedures (Fig. 11–8). The axillobifemoral bypass graft takes origin from the proximal axillary artery and is tunneled subcutaneously to the ipsilateral femoral artery. An additional limb, originating from the axillofemoral graft, is tunneled suprapubically to the contralateral femoral vessel. The procedure requires about the same operating time as conventional aortofemoral bypass but can be carried out with minimal anesthesia. In similar fashion, unilateral iliac occlusion can be palliated with a femorofemoral bypass graft. Although mortality tends to be higher (3 to 4%) with extra-anatomic reconstruction because these patients are more often critically ill, the long-term results for survivors approach those achieved with conventional bypass. After 5 years, 70% of axillofemoral grafts and 90% of femorofemoral grafts remain patent, yielding a 90% limb salvage.[70, 71]

Reconstruction for Combined Disease. PTA or proximal aortoiliac reconstruction with repressurization of the deep femoral artery usually achieves effective palliation in patients with distal superficial femoral or tibioperoneal lesions. The majority of such patients are adequately managed in this fashion, but some 20% require distal femoropopliteal bypass within 5 years.

An occasional individual with claudication, but more frequently a patient with resting ischemia, presents with femoropopliteal disease combined with more distal occlusions of one or more of the tibial arteries. Such patients, often diabetics, have not been the best candidates for reconstructive surgery because high peripheral resistance resulted in

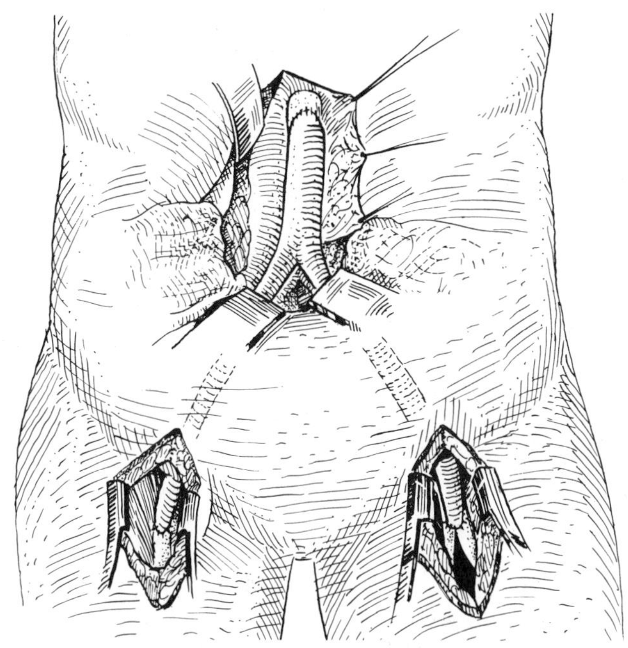

FIGURE 11–7. Aortofemoral bypass completed with an end-to-side anastomosis to the common femoral artery on the right and a similar end-to-side anastomosis on the left but extended distally into the profunda femoris to effect an angioplasty.

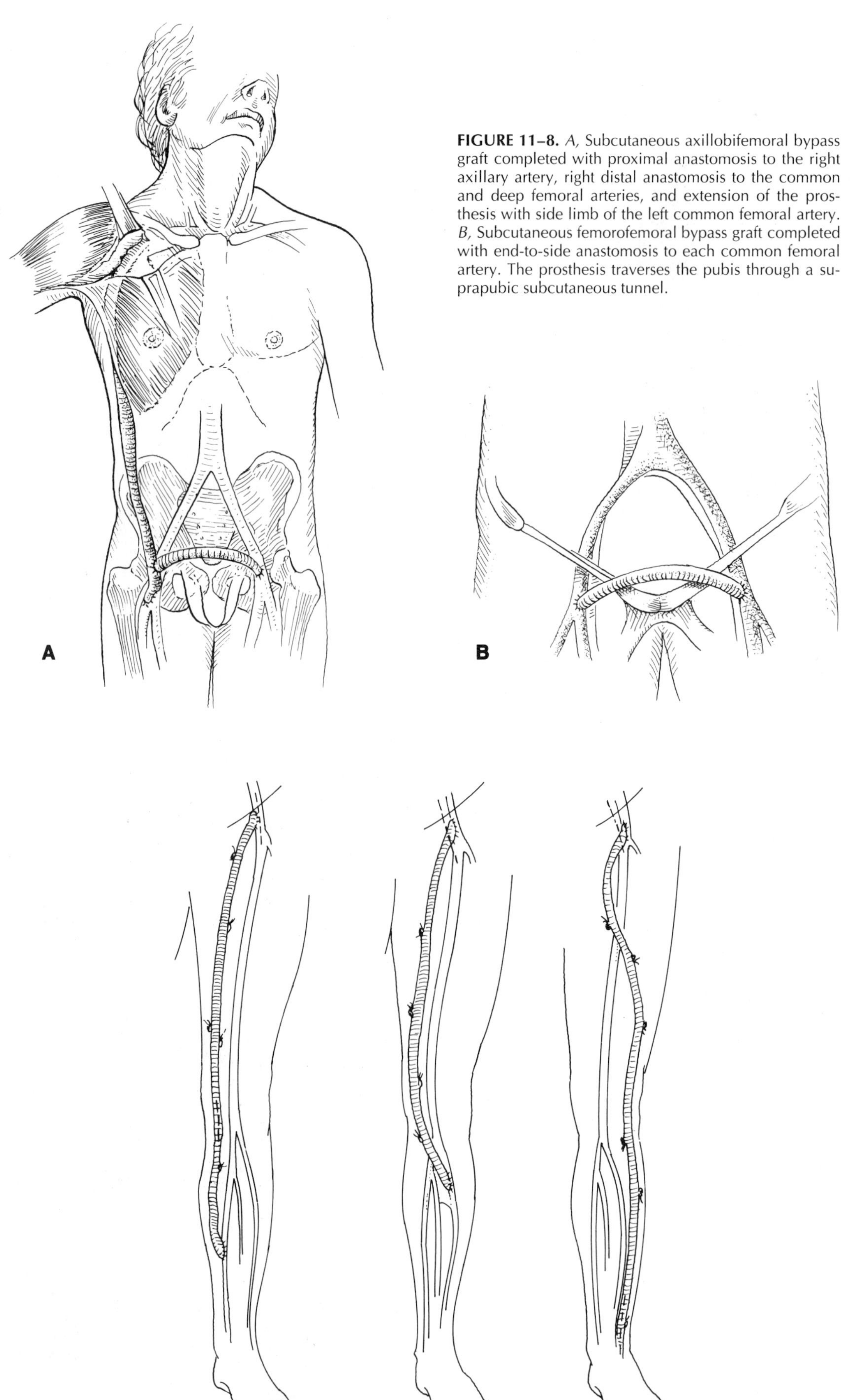

FIGURE 11–8. *A,* Subcutaneous axillobifemoral bypass graft completed with proximal anastomosis to the right axillary artery, right distal anastomosis to the common and deep femoral arteries, and extension of the prosthesis with side limb of the left common femoral artery. *B,* Subcutaneous femorofemoral bypass graft completed with end-to-side anastomosis to each common femoral artery. The prosthesis traverses the pubis through a suprapubic subcutaneous tunnel.

FIGURE 11–9. Three examples of the long femorotibial bypass vein graft. *A,* Femoral-to-posterior tibial artery. *B,* Femoral-to-anterior tibial artery. *C,* Femoral-to-distal anterior tibial artery.

thrombosis of the proximal femoropopliteal graft. Fortunately, this is not necessarily the case at present.[26, 72] Bypass vein grafts can be readily extended into the common tibioperoneal trunk or to any one of the three vessels in the calf (Fig. 11–9). Such long femorotibial or femoroperoneal vein grafts are nearly exclusively carried out in patients who have pain at rest or impending gangrene. With such extensive disease, the results are acceptable from the perspective of limb salvage. It has been shown that a cumulative graft patency rate of 60 to 70% may be anticipated at 5 years, with a limb salvage rate of 70% among survivors.[26]

REFERENCES

1. Charcot JM: Sur la claudication intermittente observée dans un cas d'obliteration complète de l'une des artères iliaques primitives. Mem Soc Biol 1:225, 1858.
2. Cranley JJ: Vascular Surgery, Vol 1. Hagerstown, MD, Harper & Row, 1972, p 4.
3. Widmer LK, Greensher A, and Kannel WB: Occlusion of peripheral arteries. Circulation 30:836, 1964.
4. Kennel WB, Skinner JJ Jr, Schwartz MJ, et al: Intermittent claudication: Incidence in the Framingham Study. Circulation 41:857, 1970.
5. McAllister FF: The fate of patients with intermittent claudication managed nonoperatively. Am J Surg 132:593, 1976.
6. Malone JM, Moore WS, and Goldstone J: Life expectancy following aortofemoral arterial grafting. Surgery 81:551, 1977.
7. Barker WF: Peripheral Arterial Disease, 2nd ed. Philadelphia, WB Saunders, 1975, p 77.
8. Leriche R and Morel A: The syndrome of thrombotic obliteration of the aortic bifurcation. Ann Surg 127:193, 1948.
9. McKusick VA, Harris WS, Ottesen OE, et al: Buerger's disease: A distinct clinical and pathological entity. JAMA 181:5, 1962.
10. Flanigan DP, Burnham SJ, Goodreau JJ, and Bergan JJ: Summary of cases of adventitial cystic disease of the popliteal artery. Ann Surg 189:2, 1979.
11. diMarza L, Cavallaro A, Sciacca V, et al: Diagnosis of popliteal artery entrapment syndrome: The role of duplex scanning. J Vasc Surg 13:434, 1991.
12. Snow N, Kursh E, DePalma RG, et al: Peripheral ischemia due to retroperitoneal fibrosis. Am J Surg 133:640, 1977.
13. Karayannacos PE, Yashon D, and Vasko JS: Narrow lumbar spinal canal with "vascular" syndromes. Arch Surg 111:803, 1976.
14. Parrow A and Werner I: The treatment of restless legs. Acta Med Scand 180:401, 1966.
15. Layzer RB and Rowland LP: Cramps. N Engl J Med 285:31, 1971.
16. McArdle B: Myopathy due to a defect in muscular glycogen breakdown. Clin Sci 10:13, 1951.
17. Mavor GE: The anterior tibial syndrome. J Bone Joint Surg 388:513, 1956.
18. O'Donoghue DH: Treatment of Injuries to Athletes, 3rd ed. Philadelphia, WB Saunders, 1976, pp 686–687.
19. Kubal WS, Crummy AB, and Turnipseed WD: The utility of digital subtraction arteriography in peripheral vascular disease. Cardiovasc Intervent Radiol 6:241, 1983.
20. Sigstedt B and Lunderquist A: Complications of angiographic examinations. Am J Roentgenol 130:455, 1978.
21. Raines JK, Darling RC, Both J, et al: Vascular laboratory criteria for the management of peripheral vascular disease of the lower extremities. Surgery 79:21, 1976.
22. Darling RC, Raines JK, Brener BJ, et al: Quantitative segmental pulse volume recorder: A clinical tool. Surgery 72:873, 1972.
23. Baker AG and Wineganner FG: Causalgia: A review of 28 treated cases. Am J Surg 117:690, 1969.
24. Babb RR, Alarcon-Segovia D, and Fairbairn JR II: Erythermalgia: Review of 51 cases. Circulation 29:136, 1964.
25. Maini BS and Mannick JA: The effect of arterial reconstruction on limb salvage—A ten year appraisal. Presented at the 26th Scientific Meeting of the International Cardiovascular Society, Los Angeles, June, 1978.
26. Donaldson MC, Mannick JA, and Whittemore, AD: Femoral-distal bypass with in situ greater saphenous vein. Ann Surg 213:457, 1991.
27. Hight DW, Tilney NL, and Couch NP: Changing clinical trends in patients with peripheral arterial emboli. Surgery 79:172, 1976.
28. Haimovici H: A study of 330 unselected cases of embolism of the extremities. Angiology 1:20, 1950.
29. Moldveen-Geronimus M and Merriam LC Jr: Cholesterol embolization: From pathological curiosity to clinical entity. Circulation 35:946, 1967.
30. Boyd AM: The natural course of arteriosclerosis of the lower extremities. Proc R Soc Med 55:591, 1962.
31. Imparato AM, Kim G, Davidson T, et al: Intermittent claudication: Its natural course. Surgery 78:795, 1975.
32. Kannel WB, Dawber TR, Friedman GD, et al: Risk factors in coronary artery disease. Ann Intern Med 61:888, 1964.
33. Paterson D and Slack J: Lipid abnormalities in male and female survivors of myocardial infarction and their first degree relatives. Lancet 1:393, 1972.
34. Kannel WB, Castelli WP, Gordon T, et al: Serum cholesterol lipoproteins and the risk of coronary heart disease. Ann Intern Med 74:1, 1971.
35. Cox FC, Rifkind B, Robinson J, et al: Primary hyperlipoproteinemia in myocardial infarction. *In* Peeters H (ed): Protide of the Biological Fluids, Vol 19. New York, American Elsevier, 1972, p 279.
36. Doyle JT, Dawber TR, Kannel WB, et al: The relationship of cigarette smoking to coronary heart disease: The second report of the combined experience of the Albany, NY, and Framingham, MA, studies. JAMA 190:886, 1964.
37. Oberman A, Harlan WR, Smith M, et al: The cardiovascular risk associated with different levels and types of elevated blood pressure. Minn Med 52:1283, 1969.
38. Strong JP and Eggen DA: Risk factors and atherosclerotic lesions. *In* Jones RJ (ed): Atherosclerosis: Proceedings of the Second International Symposium. New York, Springer-Verlag, 1970, pp 355–364.
39. Paul O: Physical inactivity: The associated cardiovascular risk. Minn Med 52:1327, 1969.
40. Sirtori CR, Baisi G, Vercello G, et al: Diets, lipids and lipoproteins in patients with peripheral vascular disease. Am J Med Sci 268:325, 1974.
41. Vogelberg KH, Berchtold P, Berger H, et al: Primary hyperlipoproteinemias as risk factors in peripheral artery disease documented by arteriography. Atherosclerosis 22:271, 1975.
42. Greenhalgh RM, Rosengarten DS, Mervant I, et al: Serum lipids and lipoproteins in peripheral vascular disease. Lancet 2:947, 1971.
43. Criqui MH, Langer RD, Fronek A, et al: Mortality over a period of 10 years in patients with peripheral arterial disease. N Engl J Med 326:381, 1992.
44. Zelis R, Mason DT, Braunwald E, et al: Effects of hyperlipoproteinemias and their treatment on the peripheral circulation. J Clin Invest 49:1007, 1970.
45. O'Connor J, Ballantyne D, Pollack JG, et al: Limb blood flow in treated hyperlipoproteinemic patients with peripheral vascular disease. Atherosclerosis 27:325, 1977.
46. Larsen OA and Lassen NA: Effect of daily muscular exercise in patients with intermittent claudication. Lancet 2:1093, 1966.
47. Blumchen G, Landry F, Kiefe H, et al: Hemodynamic responses of claudicating extremities. Cardiology 55:114, 1970.
48. Skinner, JS and Strandness DE Jr: Exercise and intermittent claudication. II: Effect of physical training. Circulation 36:23, 1967.
49. Krupski WC: The peripheral vascular consequences of smoking. Ann Vasc Surg 5:291, 1991.
50. Juergens JL, Barker NW, and Hines EA Jr: Arteriosclerosis obliterans. Circulation 21:188, 1960.
51. Coffman JD and Mannick JA: Failure of vasodilator drugs in arteriosclerosis obliterans. Ann Intern Med 76:35, 1972.
52. Coffman JD: Vasodilator drugs in peripheral vascular disease. N Engl J Med 300:713, 1979.

53. Pentoxifylline. Med Lett 26:103, 1984.
54. Tillgren C: Obliterative arterial disease of the lower limbs. IV: Evaluation of long term anticoagulant therapy. Acta Med Scand 178:203, 1965.
55. Sharma GVRK, Cella G, Parisi AF, et al: Thrombolytic therapy. N Engl J Med 306:1268, 1982.
56. Marder VJ and Sherry S: Thrombolytic therapy: Current status (First of Two Parts). N Engl J Med 318:1512, 1988.
57. McNamara TO and Fisher JR: Thrombolysis of peripheral arterial and graft occlusions: Improved result using high dose urokinase. AJR 144:769, 1985.
58. Ross R and Gloset JA: The pathogenesis of atherosclerosis. N Engl J Med 295:369, 1976.
59. Strandness DE Jr and Stahler C: Atherosclerosis obliterans: Manner and rate of progression. JAMA 196:1217, 1966.
60. Gruntzig A: Die perkutane transluminale rekanalization chronisher Arterienverschlusse mit einer neuen Dilatationstechnik. Baden-Baden, G. Witzstrock Verlag, 1977.
61. Johnson KW, Rae M, Hogg-Johnston SA, et al: Five year results of a prospective study of percutaneous transluminal angioplasty. Ann Surg 206:403, 1987.
62. White RA, White GH, Mehringer MC, et al: A clinical trial of laser thermal angioplasty in patients with advanced peripheral vascular disease. Ann Surg 212:257, 1990.
63. Ahn SS, Yeatman LR, Eton D, et al: Intraopertive peripheral rotary atherectomy: Early and late clinical results. J Vasc Surg 1993 (In press).
64. Kunlin J: Le Traitement de l'arterite obliterante par la greffe veineuse. Arch Mal Coeur 42:371, 1949.
65. Whittemore AD, Kent KC, Donaldson MC, et al: What is the proper role of polytetrafluoroethylene grafts in infrainguinal reconstruction? J Vasc Surg 10:299, 1989.
66. Royster TS, Lynn R, and Mulcare RJ: Combined aortoiliac and femoropopliteal occlusive disease. Surg Gynecol Obstet 143:949, 1976.
67. Darling RC and Linton RR: Aortoiliofemoral endarterectomy for atherosclerotic occlusive disease. Surgery 55:184, 1964.
68. Malone JM, Moore WS, and Goldstone J: The natural history of bilateral aortofemoral bypass grafts for ischemia of the lower extremities. Arch Surg 110:1300, 1975.
69. Malone JM, Moore WS, and Goldstone J: Life expectancy for aortofemoral arterial grafting. Surgery 31:551, 1977.
70. Eugene J, Goldstone J, and Moore WS: Fifteen-year experience with subcutaneous bypass grafts for lower extremity ischemia. Ann Surg 186:177, 1977.
71. LoGerfo FW, Johnson WC, Corson JD, et al: A comparison of the late patency rates of axillobilateral femoral and axillounilateral femoral grafts. Surgery 81:33, 1977.
72. Kaufman JL, Whittemore AD, Couch NP, et al: The fate of bypass grafts to an isolated popliteal artery segment. Surgery 92:1027, 1982.

12

Venous Disease of the Lower Extremities

MARK A. CREAGER, MD

VENOUS ANATOMY

Veins are thin-walled capacitance blood vessels that contain more than 70% of the total blood volume. The histology of veins is easily distinguished from that of arteries. The tunica intima is lined with endothelial cells. The subendothelial layer is thin or absent. The tunica media comprises small bundles of smooth muscle cells as well as reticular and elastic fibers. Numerous thin, filamentous bicuspid valves, formed of endothelial folds, are located within the veins to ensure unidirectional flow.

Leg veins can be categorized as either superficial or deep (Fig. 12–1). The superficial veins are located subcutaneously, superficial to the deep fascia. They include the greater and lesser saphenous veins and their tributaries. The greater saphenous vein originates on the dorsal surface of the foot and ascends anterior to the medial malleolus, traversing the medial aspect of the calf, passing posterior to the medial femoral condyle at the knee, and ascending

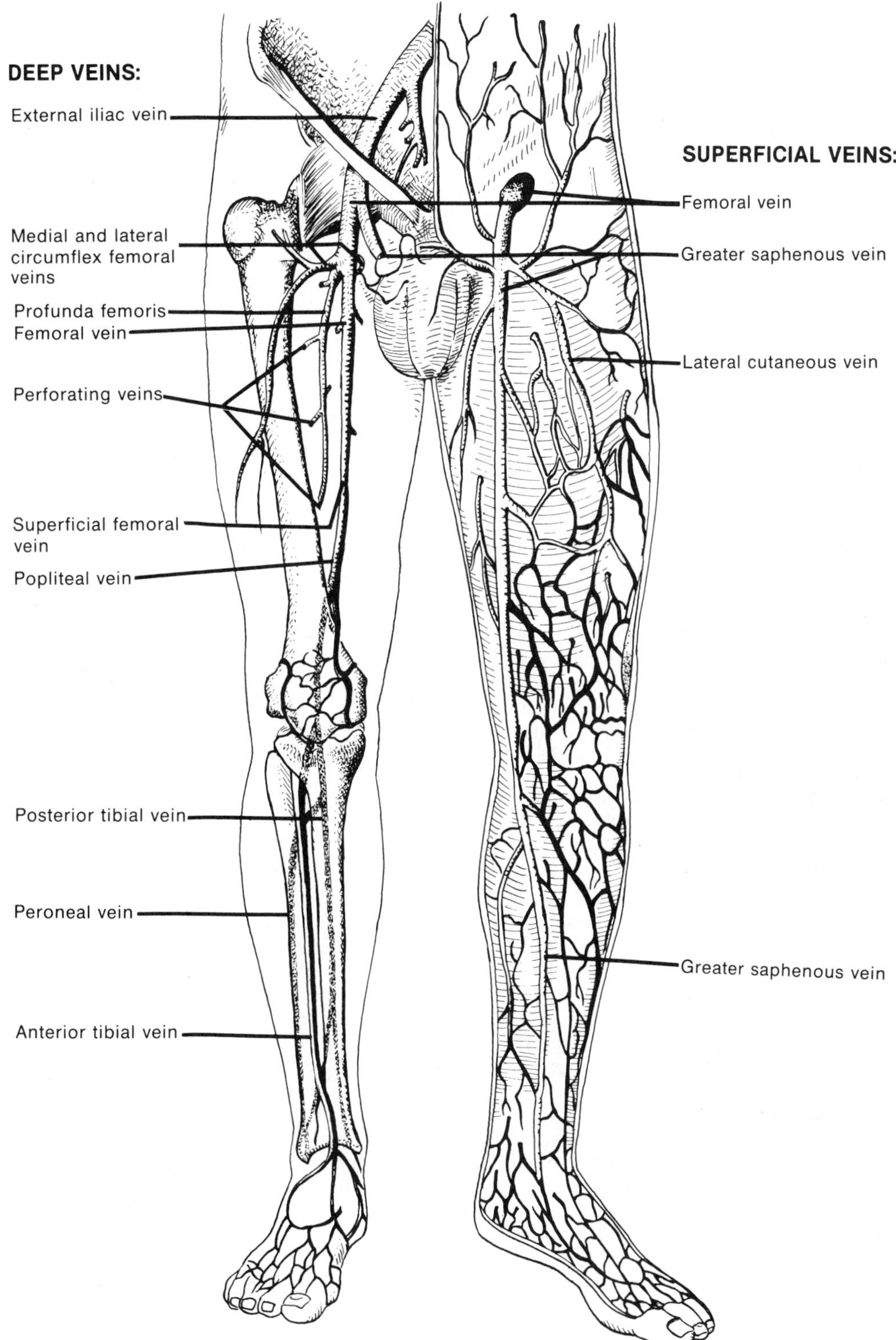

FIGURE 12–1. The leg veins with the deep system depicted in the right leg and the superficial system in the left. The former system lies deep to the muscle fascia, whereas the latter is superficial thereto.

the medial aspect of the thigh to the groin where it merges with the common femoral vein. The lesser saphenous vein begins posterior to the lateral malleolus, ascends the posterolateral aspect of the calf, and merges with the popliteal vein. The deep veins are located beneath the muscular fascia. Their location and nomenclature relates closely to the major arteries of the leg. In the calf there are three pairs of veins, each running parallel to a single artery. These include the anterior tibial, posterior tibial, and peroneal veins. These veins coalesce to form the popliteal vein. Several groups of small muscular veins, including the gastrocnemius and soleus venous plexi, join the tibioperoneal and popliteal veins. As the popliteal vein enters the adductor canal it becomes the superficial femoral vein (also designated the "femoral vein"). The superficial femoral vein ascends the thigh and is joined near the groin by the deep femoral vein to form the common femoral vein. As the common femoral vein passes superiorly to the inguinal ligament, it becomes the external iliac vein, which merges with the internal iliac vein to form the common iliac vein. Left and right common iliac veins merge to become the inferior vena cava. Communicating veins, also called perforating veins, connect the superficial and deep venous systems. Valves within the communicating veins direct the flow from the superficial to the deep veins.

Venous blood from the lower extremities is directed centrifugally toward the heart by force created from the pressure gradient between the left ventricle and the right atrium and also by the pumping action of contracting leg muscles. Venous flow is also influenced by changes in intrathoracic and intra-abdominal pressures that occur during respiration. With inspiration venous flow diminishes, and with expiration it increases.

VENOUS THROMBOSIS

The presence of a thrombus within a superficial or a deep vein and the accompanying inflammatory response in the vein wall is called thrombophlebitis or phlebothrombosis. These terms are synonymous and are often used interchangeably. At first, the thrombus is comprised primarily of fibrin and platelets. Thereafter, red blood cells become interspersed with the fibrin. The pathologic changes in the vein wall can be minimal or extensive and include loss of endothelium, granulocyte infiltration, and edema. Thrombi usually propagate in the direction of blood flow. They may decrease or obstruct flow or become dislodged and fragment to create emboli. In the legs, venous thrombi are classified by location as either superficial venous thrombi or deep venous thrombi.

The factors that predispose to venous thrombosis were described initially by Virchow and include the triad: stasis, vascular damage, and hypercoagulability.[1] Stasis contributes to venous thrombosis by disrupting laminar flow and enabling platelets to come into contact with the endothelium. Trauma may precipitate venous thrombosis by injuring blood vessels, disrupting the endothelium, and impairing local release of factors that inhibit platelet aggregation and facilitate thrombolysis. A hypercoagulable state is broadly defined but includes situations in which there may be decreased production of coagulation inhibitors, excessive production of coagulation factors, reduced thrombolytic activity, or platelet abnormalities promoting adhesion and aggregation. The clinical conditions associated with venous thrombosis are listed in Table 12–1. Each of these conditions usually includes one or more factors of Virchow's triad.

Surgery is among the most common clinical situations associated with venous thrombosis. If prophylactic measures are not undertaken, venous thrombosis occurs in approximately 50% of patients undergoing orthopedic procedures, in 10 to 30% of patients following most genitourinary procedures (>30% in patients with gynecologic malignancy), and in 30% of patients undergoing general abdominal surgical procedures.[2, 3] Venous thrombosis occurs in relatively immobile individuals, particularly in those placed at bed rest as the result of myocardial infarction, congestive heart failure, or stroke. Neoplasms, particularly pancreatic, lung, stomach, breast, and genitourinary tract cancers are associated with venous thrombosis.[4, 5] Trousseau's syndrome, a disorder characterized by recurrent venous thrombi, affecting multiple veins, has been described in patients with cancer.[4, 6]

Venous thrombosis is also associated with pregnancy, although the overall incidence is low, approximating 1 per 2000 pregnancies.[2, 7] It occurs most frequently in the third trimester and in the first 3 to 4 weeks post partum. Contributing factors include stasis caused by gravid uterus compressing the left iliac vein and possibly initiation of hypercoagulable state at the time of delivery. The risk of venous thrombosis is increased also in individuals who use oral contraceptives.[8] Conditions in which the endothelium is damaged may promote thrombosis. These include insertion of intravenous catheters, previous venous thrombosis, and inflammatory disorders such as the venulitis that occurs in thromboangiitis obliterans and Behçet's syndrome.[9, 10] A variety of disorders of coagulation are associated with venous thrombosis. These include deficiencies of antithrombin III, protein S, and protein C.[11–13] Furthermore, the presence of antiphospholipid antibodies such as the "lupus anticoagulant" are associated with venous thrombosis.[14]

Superficial Vein Thrombosis

Superficial vein thrombi are designated as such because they occur in the greater and lesser saphenous veins and their tributaries. These thrombi occur frequently at sites of superficial venous varicosities. Superficial vein thrombi produce symptoms locally and rarely cause pulmonary emboli.

The clinical features of superficial vein thrombosis include pain at the site of the thrombus, a tender cord, and localized erythema, warmth, and edema (Table 12–2). The diagnosis is made by physical examination. The examiner should be able to palpate a tender, superficial cord. Therapy is primarily supportive and depends, in part, on the location and severity of the superficial vein thrombus. Often, patients benefit from a short course of bedrest with leg elevation and application of warm compresses. Nonsteroidal anti-inflammatory drugs will reduce inflammation but may obscure evidence of clot propagation. Accordingly, they should be avoided if a superficial vein thrombus occurs in the thigh, since it may not be possible to detect progression towards the groin and into the deep system. If a greater saphenous vein thrombus propagates into the common femoral vein, a deep vein, there is significant potential for pulmonary embolism. Anticoagulant therapy should be considered if the thrombus threatens to extend into the common femoral vein.

Deep Vein Thrombosis

Deep vein thrombosis of the lower extremities afflicts approximately 10 per 10,000 individuals each year.[15–17] This accounts for an annual incidence in the United States of approximately 300,000 cases. The incidence increases exponentially with age. The importance of diagnosing and treating acute vein thrombosis is underscored by the potentially lethal consequence of this disorder, pulmonary embolism. Furthermore, deep venous thrombosis damages the delicate venous valves and leads to the long-term morbidity associated with post-phlebitic syndrome (i.e., chronic venous insufficiency).

Deep venous thrombi are usually, but not always, occlusive. They occur in the following order of frequency: calf > popliteal > femoral > iliac veins. It is useful to classify

TABLE 12–1. CLINICAL CONDITIONS ASSOCIATED WITH VENOUS THROMBOSIS

Surgery
Orthopedic, thoracic, abdominal, and genitourinary procedures
Trauma
Fractures of the spine, pelvis, femur, and tibia
Immobilization
Acute myocardial infarction, congestive heart failure, stroke, and postoperative convalescence
Neoplasms
Pancreas, lung, genitalia, urinary tract, breast, and stomach
Pregnancy
Estrogen use
Venulitis
Thromboangiitis obliterans, Behçet's disease, and homocysteinemia
Previous deep vein thrombosis
Hypercoagulable states
Deficiencies of antithrombin III, protein C, or protein S; lupus anticoagulant; myeloproliferative disease, dysfibrinogenemia; disseminated intravascular coagulation

deep venous thrombosis of the legs into two categories: (1) proximal, involving the iliac, femoral, or popliteal veins and (2) calf, involving the anterior tibial, posterior tibial, peroneal, gastrocnemius, and soleal veins. Patients with deep vein thrombosis present with leg discomfort. They often describe a pain or ache, particularly in the calf, which is aggravated by standing or walking and is relieved by rest. Many, particularly, those with proximal deep vein thrombosis, have unilateral leg swelling, with or without associated discomfort. An examination of patients with proximal deep vein thrombosis frequently leads to the diagnosis (Fig. 12–2, see also Table 12–2). The physical findings include unilateral leg swelling, warmth, and erythema. The examiner can often elicit tenderness over the involved vein. A cord may be palpable, particularly along the course of the superficial femoral vein as it ascends from the adductor canal along the anteromedial thigh, or along the course of the common femoral vein as it crosses the groin. Additional signs include distention of superficial veins and the presence of prominent venous collaterals. In patients with iliac vein thrombosis, for example, venous collaterals may be evident along the sides of the pelvis and the lower abdomen. Cyanotic discoloration of the leg may result from deoxygenated hemoglobin in stagnant veins, a condition designated phlegmasia cerulea dolens. Phlegmasia alba dolens refers to a tense, massively edematous leg that impairs capillary flow, causing pallor and ultimately skin necrosis.

TABLE 12–2. CLINICAL FEATURES OF VENOUS THROMBOSIS

Superficial vein thrombosis
Localized pain
Perivenous erythema and warmth
Tender cord
Deep vein thrombosis, proximal
Calf or thigh discomfort
Circumferential edema
Warmth (± erythema)
Tenderness along course of deep vein
Cord
Distention of superficial veins
Prominent venous collaterals
Deep vein thrombosis, calf
Calf pain
Posterior calf tenderness
Increased tissue turgor (± edema)
Cord, rarely

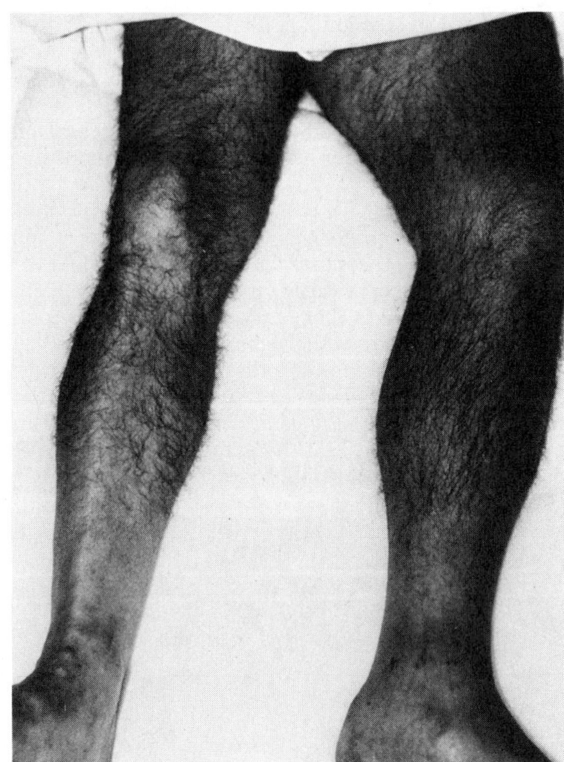

FIGURE 12–2. A patient with proximal deep vein thrombosis of the left leg. In comparison with the right leg, the left thigh, calf, and ankle are swollen.

In contrast to proximal deep vein thrombosis, the diagnosis of calf deep vein thrombosis is difficult to make at the bedside. This is because only one of multiple veins may be involved, allowing adequate venous return via the remaining patent vessels. An examination may elicit posterior calf tenderness, increased tissue turgor, modest swelling, warmth, and rarely a cord. Homans' sign, described originally as calf pain and resistance to active dorsiflexion of the foot, is sensitive but nonspecific.

Noninvasive Diagnostic Tests

A variety of noninvasive tests have been used to evaluate patients suspected of having deep vein thrombosis. These tests include duplex venous ultrasonography, Doppler ultrasonography, plethysmography, and ^{125}I fibrinogen scanning (Table 12–3).

Venous duplex ultrasonography is currently the most frequently used noninvasive test to diagnose deep vein thrombosis. It utilizes both B-mode (i.e., gray scale) imaging and pulse wave Doppler measurements to examine the veins of

TABLE 12–3. DIAGNOSTIC TESTS FOR DEEP VEIN THROMBOSIS

Duplex ultrasonography
Includes gray-scale imaging and pulse-wave Doppler examination ±Color Doppler
Plethysmographic techniques
Impedance plethysmography
Phleborheography
^{125}I fibrinogen scanning
Venography

the leg, hence the term duplex ultrasonography. With high-resolution ultrasound units, it is possible to image the proximal and distal deep veins of most individuals. The pulse Doppler component is used to evaluate blood flow within the veins. Many ultrasound units incorporate color Doppler capability, which provides a visual image of venous flow.

Several criteria are used to diagnose deep vein thrombosis by ultrasound.[18, 19] These include: (1) apposition of the vein walls (i.e., collapse of the vein) during compression; (2) visualization of the thrombus; and (3) loss of normal venous flow patterns with provocative maneuvers (see Fig. 12–1). Normally, the sonographer can cause a vein to collapse, enabling the opposing walls to come in contact with each other, simply by applying pressure on a probe (Fig. 12–3). This is because a low venous pressure is easily overcome by light manual pressure. It is usually not possible to visualize a thrombus because it has the same echogenic properties as flowing blood. If a thrombus is present within the vein, it will not collapse during a direct compressive maneuver. Occasionally, however, it is possible to visualize a thrombus within a vein, because changes in its composition impart echoic properties that can be detected by ultrasound imaging. In addition, a nonobstructive thrombus may be detected by use of color Doppler, since flow is seen coursing around it. A Doppler shift signal can be graphically displayed or qualitatively assessed by color imaging. Pulse Doppler interrogation assesses changes in venous flow during respiration or maneuvers that accelerate or impede venous flow. In the absence of thrombus, venous flow from the legs increases during expiration and decreases during inspiration. If a proximal vein thrombus is present, respiratory variation in venous flow is no longer apparent. Manual compression of the calf accelerates venous flow through the proximal veins. Flow augmentation will not take place if an intervening thrombus is present between the site of compression and the position of the scanner.

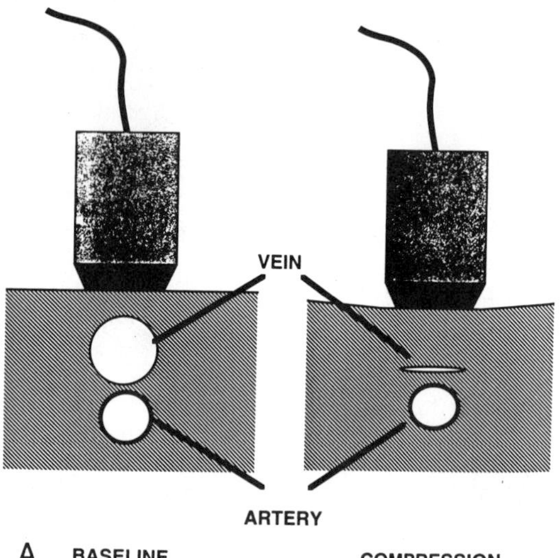

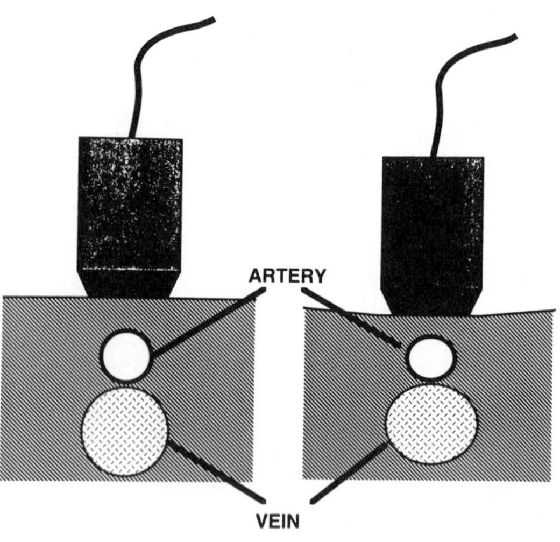

FIGURE 12–3. *A* and *B*, Schematic of a venous ultrasound examination. The probe is positioned to obtain cross-sectional views of the artery and vein. *A*, With compression, the vein easily collapses, resulting in apposition of the anterior and posterior walls. *B*, In the presence of venous thrombosis, manual compression is no longer able to collapse the vein.

The predictive value of venous duplex ultrasonography has been assessed by using contrast venography as the "gold standard." Both the sensitivity and specificity of venous ultrasound testing for diagnosing symptomatic proximal deep vein thrombosis approximates 95%.[20–22] It is more difficult to visualize calf veins than proximal veins, and less information is available about the predictive value of venous ultrasonography for diagnosing calf deep vein thrombosis. Whereas the specificity is relatively high, approximating 95%, the sensitivity is lower, ranging from 50 to 80%.[23, 24] Also, ultrasonography may exhibit less sensitivity when used in screening for asymptomatic DVT.

Some laboratories utilize plethysmographic techniques as noninvasive diagnostic tests for deep vein thrombosis. These include impedance plethysmography and phleborheography.[25, 26] These techniques detect changes in limb volume during respiration or other maneuvers that affect venous flow. Changes in limb volume are related inversely to changes in venous flow. With inspiration and the subsequent increase in intra-abdominal pressure, venous return from the legs diminishes and leg volume increases. With expiration, abdominal pressure decreases, venous flow accelerates, and leg volume decreases. Impedance plethysmography (IPG) employs two electrodes that are placed on the calf. The change in voltage across these two electrodes is measured while a small amount of electrical current is transmitted, and impedance is determined. Impedance is inversely proportional to leg volume. Inflation of a sphygmomanometric cuff placed on the thigh is used to impair venous return and increase calf volume. Normally, with cuff deflation, blood exits through a patent venous system and calf volume decreases. In the presence of a proximal deep vein thrombosis, thigh cuff inflation and subsequent deflation result in only a modest increase and decrease in calf volume, respectively. Phleborheography uses air displacement transducers to assess changes in leg volume during maneuvers similar to that described for pulsed Doppler ultrasonography. Air displacement cuffs are placed along the limbs to detect changes in leg volume during respiration. Normal respiratory changes in volume will not occur if a thrombus is present in a proximal deep vein. Compression of the foot or calf normally propels blood through the deep system without affecting volume. If a thrombus is present in a proximal vein, compressive maneuvers in the foot or calf will increase leg volume. The sensitivity and specificity for plethysmographic techniques for the diagnosis of proximal deep vein thrombosis approximate 85%.[25, 26] These tests are not reliable for diagnosing calf deep vein thrombosis.

^{125}I fibrinogen scanning is based on the principle that fibrinogen is incorporated into a propagating thrombus. Thus, a growing thrombus can be detected by nuclear scanning. Scanning must be performed daily, since it takes at least 24 to 72 hours for radiolabeled fibrinogen to be incorporated into a growing thrombus. The sensitivity and specificity of ^{125}I fibrinogen scanning to diagnose calf deep vein thrombosis approximate 80% and 75%, respectively.[27, 28] It is less specific for the diagnosis of proximal deep vein thrombosis. It has been used to complement plethysmographic techniques, enabling the examination of the entire leg for proximal and calf deep vein thrombosis. This technique is not available in most noninvasive laboratories.

Venography is indicated in patients in whom noninvasive studies fail to confirm or definitely exclude the presence of proximal deep vein thrombosis, especially if strongly suspected clinically. The technique entails injection of a radioopaque contrast agent into a dorsal pedal vein.[29] Using fluoroscopic guidance, posteroanterior and lateral x-ray images of the veins are obtained at the levels of the calf, knee, thigh, and pelvis. A venogram is considered positive for venous thrombosis if a discrete filling defect or an abrupt vessel cutoff is seen in multiple views (Fig. 12–4).

Treatment

Deep vein thrombosis is treated to prevent pulmonary embolism. Treatment with anticoagulants or inferior vena caval filters is indicated in all patients with proximal deep vein thrombosis, since pulmonary embolism may occur in approximately 50% of untreated individuals.[30–32] Treatment of acute calf deep vein thrombosis is controversial. Propagation of thrombus into the proximal veins occurs in approximately 10 to 20% of patients with deep calf vein thrombosis.[33, 34] The reported incidence of pulmonary embolism in patients originally presenting with deep calf vein thrombosis ranges from 5 to 20%.[30, 31] Some have advocated treating calf deep vein thrombosis with anticoagulants.[35] Others favor a more conservative approach and withhold anticoagulants unless serial noninvasive examinations, conducted over a 2-week period, demonstrate propagation of the thrombus into proximal veins.[30, 36, 37]

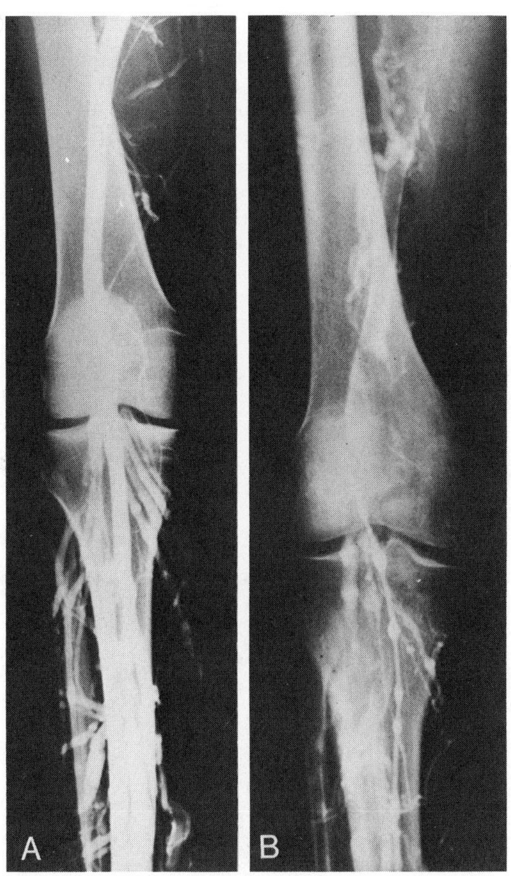

FIGURE 12–4. *A* and *B*, Contrast venography to diagnose deep vein thrombosis. *A*, Normal venogram. *B*, Deep vein thrombosis. There is an absence of filling of multiple calf veins. In the thigh, an extensive thrombus is outlined by contrast material in the superficial femoral vein.

Anticoagulant treatment is initiated with intravenous heparin, preferably given via a constant infusion. Patients initially receive an intravenous bolus of 5000 to 10,000 USP units of heparin followed by a continuous infusion of heparin. The constant infusion is administered initially at a rate of 1000 to 1500 units/hr. The activated partial thromboplastin time (APTT) should be measured approximately 4 hours after beginning the heparin infusion and thereafter at 4- to 6-hour intervals. The infusion dose should be adjusted to achieve a therapeutic APTT in a range of 1.5 to 2.5 times the normal control value.[38] Adjusted subcutaneous heparin may be as effective as continuous intravenous heparin in the initial treatment of proximal deep vein thrombosis.[39, 40] Recent data suggest that fixed-dose subcutaneous low molecular weight heparin also may be effective.[41] Anticoagulant treatment should be continued for at least 3 to 6 months after the initial episode of proximal deep vein thrombosis. Individuals with recurrent deep vein thrombosis, and those in whom a predisposing clinical condition persists, should be treated indefinitely.

Treatment with warfarin is initiated during the first week of treatment with heparin and may be started as early as the first day of heparin treatment.[42] The dose of warfarin is adjusted to achieve a prothrombin time equivalent to an international normalized ratio (INR) of 2.0 to 3.0. The INR permits uniform reporting of prothrombin times and eliminates the considerable variability that exists among laboratories that use different thromboplastins to assess the prothrombin time.[43] Once a therapeutic prothrombin time is achieved, it is important to continue the coadministration of heparin with warfarin for at least 3 days. This will ensure adequate oral anticoagulation by inhibition of all vitamin K–dependent coagulation factors (II, VII, IX, and X) and avoid the initial thrombogenic potential of warfarin that occurs as a result of its ability to decrease protein C and protein S levels. Long-term anticoagulation may also be achieved with subcutaneous heparin, given twice daily, and adjusted to achieve a therapeutic APTT.[44] This approach may be useful in patients who cannot take warfarin, such as pregnant women needing to avoid the teratogenic effects of the oral anticoagulant.

The efficacy of thrombolytic drugs in the treatment of isolated deep vein thrombosis has not been established. The potential advantages of thrombolytic therapy include rapid dissolution of thrombus, decreased likelihood of pulmonary embolism, and preservation of venous valves thus preventing the subsequent development of postphlebitic syndrome. To date, limited studies have been conducted with several thrombolytic agents, including streptokinase, urokinase, and recombinant human tissue-type plasminogen activator (rt-PA).[45, 46] Thrombolytic drugs have been shown to cause more rapid lysis of deep vein thromboses than heparin; however, there is a greater risk of hemorrhage. Sample sizes in individual studies have been inadequate to determine whether or not the risk of pulmonary

TABLE 12–4. PROPHYLACTIC MEASURES FOR DEEP VENOUS THROMBOSIS

Low-dose heparin
Thoracic, abdominal, and genitourinary procedures
Immobilization, acute myocardial infarction, congestive heart failure, and stroke
Adjusted-dose warfarin
Orthopedic procedures and fractures
Intermittent pneumatic compression stockings
Neurosurgery and genitourinary procedures
Contraindication to anticoagulants

embolism is less with thrombolytic drugs than with heparin. Similarly, it is not yet known whether or not early treatment with thrombolytic agents prevent postphlebitic syndrome.

Patients with proximal deep vein thrombosis who cannot be treated with anticoagulants require placement of a filter in the inferior vena cava to prevent pulmonary embolism.[47] Inferior vena cava filters are inserted percutaneously via the internal jugular or common femoral vein and are advanced to the inferior vena cava just below the renal veins. Important factors in choosing a specific inferior vena cava filter among the several that are marketed include its ability to effectively prevent a pulmonary embolism, its lack of thrombogenicity, thus preserving inferior vena cava patency, and low complication rate following placement.

Prevention of Venous Thrombosis

A variety of nonpharmacologic and pharmacologic interventions are available to prevent deep vein thrombosis in patients at risk for its development (Table 12–4). Nonpharmacologic methods include graduated compression stockings and intermittent pneumatic compression boots. Pharmacologic means of prophylaxis include low-dose subcutaneous heparin, low molecular weight heparin, and adjusted dose warfarin. In most studies, aspirin has not been shown to be an effective prophylactic agent. Decisions regarding which specific intervention should be used to prevent deep vein thrombosis depend on established efficacy and potential risk of bleeding with each clinical situation. In many situations, both nonpharmacologic and pharmacologic preventive measures can be employed.

Table 12–1 provides a list of clinical conditions that are associated with deep vein thrombosis. Prophylactic treatment should be considered in each of these situations. Low-dose heparin is effective in preventing deep vein thrombosis because it inhibits the coagulation cascade prior to the amplification process that occurs once thrombus has formed. Low-dose heparin substantially reduces the incidence of pulmonary embolism in patients undergoing general abdominal and thoracic surgery.[3, 48] These patients should receive 5000 units of heparin subcutaneously 2 hours before surgery and every 8 hours thereafter for approximately 1 week. Low-dose heparin should also be administered to patients placed at prolonged bedrest, including patients with acute myocardial infarction, congestive heart failure, and stroke.

Low molecular weight heparin has been shown to be an effective agent to prevent deep vein thrombosis in patients who undergo abdominal and hip surgery.[49, 50] The molecular weight of low molecular weight heparin is approximately 4000 to 5000 daltons. The molecular weight of conventional heparin is 12,000 to 16,000 daltons. Low molecular weight heparin is reported to have greater bioavailability, greater efficacy, and a lower frequency of bleeding than conventional heparin. It is administered only once daily.

Adjusted-dose warfarin is an effective method of preventing deep vein thrombosis in patients who have sustained bone fractures or have undergone an orthopedic surgical procedure.[48] Warfarin is administered on the night before surgery and is continued throughout the hospitalization. The initial dose is 5 to 10 mg. Thereafter, the dose is adjusted to achieve an INR of approximately 2.0. Warfarin should be continued for approximately 1 month after discharge from the hospital.

Low-dose heparin is effective as a prophylactic agent for patients undergoing genitourinary surgical procedures but may cause excessive bleeding in these individuals.[3] Also, anticoagulants are relatively contraindicated in patients undergoing neurosurgical procedures. Therefore, nonpharmacologic preventive measures, such as intermittent pneumatic compression, may be used in these patients.[51] Intermittent pneumatic compression boots reduce venous stasis and may activate the endogenous fibrinolytic system. These boots intermittently apply graduated compression to the ankle, calf, and thigh, thus increasing venous blood flow velocity. In selected situations, combination of intermittent pneumatic compression boots and pharmacologic agents (e.g., low-dose heparin) may have a more beneficial effect in preventing deep vein thrombosis than either modality when used alone.

VARICOSE VEINS

Varicose veins are dilated tortuous components of the superficial venous system (Fig. 12–5). Approximately 10 to 20% of the population develop varicose veins. Varicose veins are caused by intrinsic weakness of the venous wall, defective structure and function of venous valves, or increased intraluminal pressure. Varicosities can occur in both the greater and lesser saphenous veins and their tributaries. Histologically, varicose veins have subintimal fibrosis, vascular smooth muscle hypertrophy, and elastin

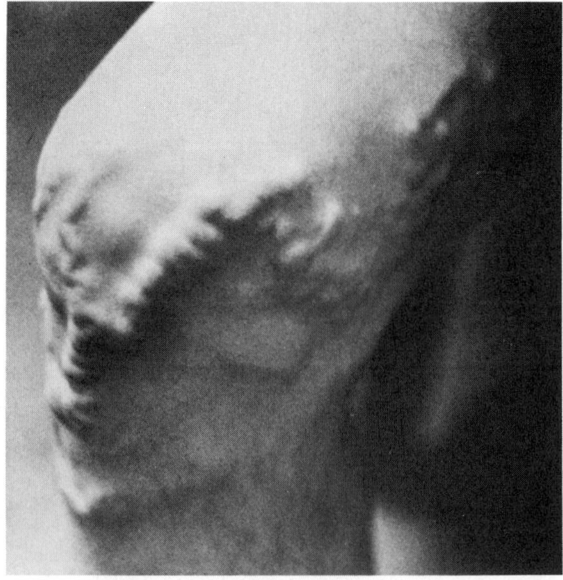

FIGURE 12–5. Extensive superficial venous varicosities are affecting the right leg.

degeneration. Valvular deformities are common, and intraluminal thrombi occur.

Varicose veins can be classified as either primary or secondary. Primary varicose veins originate in the superficial venous system. They occur three times more frequently in women than in men. Approximately 50% of individuals with primary venous varicosities have a family history of varicose veins.[52] This implicates an inherited defect in vein structure or function. Additional factors that contribute to the development of primary varicose veins include pregnancy, prolonged standing, and obesity. In individuals with inherent weakness of the vein wall, high venous pressure caused by these conditions may contribute to the development of varicose veins. The development of varicose veins is a progressive process. Initially, a dilated segment of vein causes valvular incompetence and reflux of blood. The increased hydrostatic pressure promotes vein dilatation and elongation. This process alters the normal alignment of the bicuspid valve leaflets, causing progressive valvular incompetence. The process continues distally in each vein, ultimately involving peripheral branches and perforating veins.

Secondary varicose veins occur as a consequence of deep venous insufficiency or occlusion and incompetent perforating veins.[53] Blood is preferentially channeled to superficial veins, which act as collateral channels. Consequently, the increased blood volume and pressure causes enlargement of superficial veins. Varicose veins should be distinguished from spider veins (i.e., venous telangiectases or spider hemangiomas). Spider veins are small cutaneous veins that are characterized by serpiginous branches in a caput medusa pattern. They may be isolated, or they may occur in small clusters.

Symptoms of varicose veins include a dull ache or pressure sensation in the legs that occurs after prolonged standing and is relieved with leg elevation. Ankle edema develops occasionally. Skin ulceration near the ankle can occur in patients with extensive varicosities because the high venous pressure contributes to interstitial edema. This reduces nutritional blood supply, making the tissue vulnerable to injury. Superficial vein thrombosis occurs in venous varicosities, probably as a consequence of blood stasis. Occasionally, trauma may cause a thin wall of venous varicosity to rupture and bleed. Most patients with varicose veins are asymptomatic. Some of these seek medical attention because of cosmetic concerns.

Varicose veins can be diagnosed by inspection and palpation. Patients should be examined with the legs in the dependent position, so that the veins distend and are both visible and easily palpated. It is possible to distinguish primary from secondary causes of venous varicosities using the Brodie-Trendelenburg and Perthes' tests.[54] After the leg is elevated, a tourniquet is placed just above the knee, thus preventing reflux of blood through proximal superficial veins. The leg is then placed in a dependent position. If the varicose veins have occurred secondary to deep venous insufficiency and incompetent perforating veins, the varicosities will distend promptly. If this does not occur, but the veins fill promptly after removal of the tourniquet, the varicose veins are categorized as primary since the problem originates in the superficial venous system.

Treatment

Most varicose veins can be treated conservatively. Patients who are asymptomatic or those with minor symptoms of leg discomfort should be reassured. Graduated compression stockings should be fitted to prevent distention of superficial venous varicosities with standing and walking. Walking or running exacerbates venous reflux through incompetent venous valves. Patients should be instructed to wear compressive hose during these activities.

Ablative procedures, such as sclerotherapy or surgery, should be considered in patients who are severely symptomatic, have recurrent superficial vein thrombosis, or manifestations of venous insufficiency such as edema, or skin ulceration. On occasion, ablative procedures may be used in individuals who are asymptomatic but distraught because of the cosmetic implications of varicose veins. Sclerotherapy is used to treat local venous varicosities.[55] This entails injection of a sclerosing solution into the varicose vein, resulting in inflammation and ultimately fibrosis. Surgical treatment involves ligation and stripping of the varicose veins.[56] Extensive varicosities may be treated by ligation and stripping of both greater and lesser saphenous veins. Removal of superficial veins is contraindicated in patients with obstruction of the deep venous system, since the superficial veins serve as important collaterals for venous return from the legs.

Chronic Venous Insufficiency

Chronic venous insufficiency is a disorder characterized by venous valvular insufficiency or persistent venous thrombosis resulting in chronic leg edema. Chronic venous insufficiency occurs as a primary disorder in some individuals, in whom elongated, redundant venous valves fail to coapt normally. The most common secondary cause is deep vein thrombosis, and the term postphlebitic syndrome is used interchangeably with chronic venous insufficiency in these patients. There are several sequelae to deep venous thrombosis that adversely affect venous competence.[53, 57] Thrombus may persist and become adherent to the vein wall causing chronic obstruction. Alternatively, the thrombus may lyse, causing partial or complete recanalization, leaving venous function impaired. The vein walls and the venous valves scar, retract, and reflux. As a result, veins are less capable of antegrade flow toward the heart. Venous reflux through incompetent valves increases distal hydrostatic pressure. This causes distal, previously undamaged, components of the vein to dilate, preventing apposition of normal venous valves, and promoting further reflux. This process repeats itself, affecting most of the deep venous system and the perforating veins.

Symptoms include a dull ache or discomfort in the calf that is worsened by standing and walking and is relieved with leg elevation. Muscular contraction during ambulation increases the severity of reflux, increasing venous hydrostatic pressure and subsequently extravasation of fluid into the interstitial space and muscular compartments. Venous claudication should be distinguished from claudication that occurs secondary to peripheral arterial occlusive disease.[58] The most common physical finding is leg swelling. The severity of edema progresses with prolonged dependency and ambulation. Conversely, edema is less in the morning after the patient has slept, particularly if the leg is kept elevated. Venous varicosities develop because retrograde flow through incompetent perforating veins increases venous return via superficial veins, often causing these veins to dilate and elongate (see earlier). Chronic edema and increased interstitial pressure impair capillary perfusion and reduce nutrient supply to the skin and subcutaneous tissue. This often results in skin breakdown and ulceration, particularly near the medial and lateral malleoli (Fig. 12–6). The

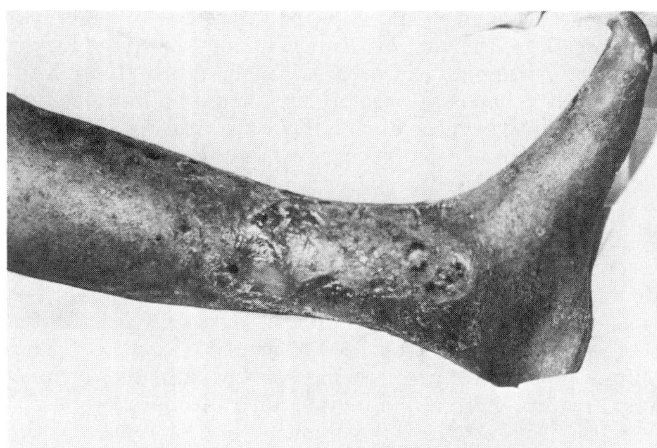

FIGURE 12-6. Chronic venous insufficiency is characterized by leg swelling, venous stasis pigmentation, and a superficial ulceration near the left medial malleolus.

edges of the ulcer are usually irregular, and its base is composed of granulation tissue. The ulcer may be covered by cellular debris and eschar. The skin may appear erythematous and shiny and sometimes may mimic cellulitis. Chronic inflammation causes subcutaneous fibrosis, which is clinically detected as induration. Local deposition of hemosiderin, caused by the lysis of red blood cells, imparts a brownish pigmentation to the skin. This is particularly evident over the pretibial region and near the ankles.

Chronic venous insufficiency must be distinguished from other clinical entities that cause leg swelling such as lymphedema, cellulitis, and arteriovenous fistulas. The differential diagnosis in patients with bilateral leg edema includes congestive heart failure, hypoalbuminemia caused by cirrhosis, nephrotic syndrome, or malabsorption syndrome, inferior vena cava obstruction, and bilateral lymphedema. In patients with a previous history of deep vein thrombosis who present with recurrent leg swelling, it may not be possible to distinguish postphlebitic syndrome from acute deep vein thrombosis that has developed at a site of previous venous thrombosis.

Several noninvasive laboratory studies are useful in evaluating patients suspected of having postphlebitic syndrome. Color-assisted duplex ultrasonography demonstrates features that are characteristic of previous deep vein thrombosis.[19] This includes thickened vein walls, persistent echogenic thrombi, partially recanalized thrombi, and deep venous collateral channels. Pulse and color Doppler techniques detect retrograde venous flow when patients perform a Valsalva maneuver or when the examiner compresses the leg muscles. Plethysmographic techniques can be used to demonstrate venous reflux in incompetent perforating veins.[59, 60] Venography is rarely indicated to diagnose chronic venous insufficiency but could be performed if acute deep vein thrombosis is suspected. Venographic evidence of chronic venous insufficiency includes partially recanalized veins, venous collaterals, and valvular reflux. Often, however, it is not possible to determine if a venous obstruction is caused by acute or previous deep vein thrombosis, particularly if features of chronic venous insufficiency are evident on the venographic examination.

Chronic venous insufficiency is treated to improve patient comfort and preserve skin integrity. Patients should be instructed to elevate their legs frequently, particularly at night. The leg should be positioned higher than the chest to facilitate venous return. Graduated compression stockings, applying an extrinsic pressure of at least 30 to 40 mm Hg at the ankle, should be worn when patients are seated or ambulating to prevent extravasation of fluid into the interstitial tissue. Custom-made stockings are available for those with severe venous insufficiency. A moisturizing cream should be applied to the legs to prevent dryness and cracking. Venous ulcers should be identified and treated promptly. When ulcers develop, patients should be placed at bedrest with the leg elevated. Wet to dry to dressings should be applied three to four times each day. Saline-soaked gauze is applied for approximately 20 minutes. This is replaced with dry gauze. The dry gauze débrides the ulcer by removing cellular debris at the time of the next dressing change. If the ulcer is complicated by cellulitis, the patient should be treated with systemic antibiotics. In selected individuals, venous ulcers can be treated while the patient remains ambulatory. Commercially available dressings employing antiseptic solutions and compressive bandages can be applied and left in place. These dressings are changed weekly until healing has occurred. Persistent large venous ulcers may require skin grafting. Recurrent venous ulceration can often be prevented by identifying and surgically interrupting local incompetent perforating veins.[61] In selected situations, venous reconstruction procedures may be used to treat chronic venous insufficiency, but long-term efficacy has not been established in rigorous trials.[62, 63] These procedures include autologous and prosthetic venous bypass grafts for chronic venous obstruction and venous valve repair and autologous valve transplantation in patients with valvular incompetence.

REFERENCES

1. Virchow R: Gesammelte abhandlungen zur wissenschafflichen medizin. Frankfort-am-Main, Von Meidinger Sohn, 1856.
2. Paltier G: Epidemiology of venous thromboembolism. *In* Leclerc JR (ed): Venous Thromboembolic Disorders. Philadelphia, Lea & Febiger, 1991, pp 141–165.
3. Collins R, Scrimgeour A, Yusuf S, and Peto R: Reduction in fatal pulmonary embolism and venous thrombosis by perioperative administration of subcutaneous heparin. N Engl J Med 318:1162–1173, 1988.
4. Trousseau A: Phlegmasia alba dolens: Clinique médicale de l'Hotel-Dieu de Paris. London, The New Sydenham Society, 1865.
5. Gore JM, Appelbaum JS, Greene HL, et al: Occult cancer in patients with acute pulmonary embolism. Ann Intern Med 96:556–560, 1982.
6. Sack GH, Levin J, and Bell WR: Trousseau's syndrome and other manifestations of chronic disseminated coagulopathy in patients with neoplasms: Clinical pathophysiologic, and therapeutic features. Medicine 56:1–37, 1977.
7. Jeffries WS and Bochner F: Thromboembolism and its management in pregnancy. Med J Aust 155:253–258, 1991.
8. Realini JP and Goldzieher JW: Oral contraceptives and cardiovascular disease: A critique of the epidemiologic studies. Am J Obstet Gynecol 152:729–798, 1985.
9. Olin JW, Young JR, Graor RA, et al: The changing clinical spectrum of thromboangiitis obliterans. Circulation 82:IV-3–IV-8, 1990.
10. Lie JT: Vascular involvement in Behçet's disease: Arterial and venous vessels of all sizes. J Rheumatol 19:341–343, 1992.
11. Vikydal R, Korninger C, Kyrle PA, et al: The prevalence of heredity antithrombin-III deficiency in patients with a history of venous thromboembolism. Thromb Haemost 54:744–745, 1985.
12. Clouse LH and Comp PC: The regulation of hemostasis: The protein C system. N Engl J Med 314:1298–1304, 1986.
13. Engesser L, Broekmans AW, Briet E, et al: Hereditary protein S deficiency: Clinical manifestations. Ann Intern Med 106:677–682, 1987.
14. Elias M and Eldor A: Thromboembolism in patients with the

"lupus"-type circulating anticoagulant. Arch Intern Med 144:510–515, 1984.
15. Coon WW, Willis PW, and Keller JB: Venous thromboembolism and other venous disease in the Tecumseh community health study. Circulation 43:839–846, 1973.
16. Gillum RF: Pulmonary embolism and thrombophlebitis in the United States, 1970–1985. Am Heart J 114:1262–1264, 1987.
17. Anderson FA Jr, Wheeler HB, Goldberg RJ, et al: A population-based perspective of the incidence and case fatality rates of venous thrombosis and pulmonary embolism: The Worcester DVT study. Arch Intern Med 151:933–938, 1991.
18. Creager MA, O'Leary DH, and Doubilet PM: Noninvasive vascular testing. *In* Loscalzo J, Creager MA, and Dzau VJ (eds): Vascular Medicine. Boston, Little Brown, 1992, pp 419–451.
19. Polak JF: Peripheral Vascular Sonography. Baltimore, Williams & Wilkins. 1992.
20. Lensing AW, Prandoni P, Brandjes D, et al: Detection of deep-vein thrombosis by real-time B-mode ultrasonography. N Engl J Med 320:342–345, 1989.
21. White RH, McGahan JP, Daschbach MM, and Hartling RP: Diagnosis of deep-vein thrombosis using duplex ultrasound. Ann Intern Med 111:297–304, 1989.
22. Becker DM, Philbrick JT, and Abbitt PL: Real-time ultrasonography for the diagnosis of lower extremity deep venous thrombosis: The wave of the future? Arch Intern Med 149:1731–1734, 1989.
23. Polak JS, Cutler SS, and O'Leary DH: Deep veins of the calf: Assessment with color Doppler flow imaging. Radiology 171:481–485, 1989.
24. Yucel EK, Fisher JS, Egglin TK, et al: Isolated calf venous thrombosis: Diagnosis with compression US. Radiology 179:443–446, 1991.
25. Hull R, Taylor DW, and Hirsch J: Impedance plethysmography: The relationship between venous filling and sensitivity and specificity for proximal vein thrombosis. Circulation 58:898–902, 1979.
26. Cranley JJ, Canos AJ, Sull WT, et al: Phleborheographic technique for diagnosing deep venous thrombosis of the lower extremities. Surg Gynecol Obstet 141:331–339, 1975.
27. Flanc C, Kakkar VV, and Clarke MB: The detection of venous thrombosis in the legs using ^{125}I-labelled fibrinogen. Br J Surg 55:742–747, 1968.
28. Harris WH, Salzman EW, Athanasoulis C, et al: Comparison of ^{125}I-fibrinogen count scanning with phlebography for detection of venous thrombi after elective hip surgery. N Engl J Med 292:665–667, 1975.
29. Rabinov K and Paulin S: Roentgen diagnosis of venous thrombosis in the leg. Arch Surg 104:134–144, 1972.
30. Moser KM and Lemoine JR: Is embolic risk conditioned by location of deep venous thrombosis? Ann Intern Med 94:439–444, 1981.
31. Huisman MV, Buller HR, ten Cate JW, et al: Unexpected high prevalence of silent pulmonary embolism in patients with deep venous thrombosis. Chest 95:498–502, 1989.
32. Kistner RL, Ball JJ, Nordyke RA, and Freeman GC: Incidence of pulmonary embolism in the course of thrombophlebitis of the lower extremities. Am J Surg 124:169–176, 1972.
33. Kakkar VV, Howe CT, Flanc C, and Clarke MB: Natural history of postoperative deep vein thrombosis. Lancet 2:230–232, 1969.
34. Hirsch J, Genton E, and Hull R: Venous Thromboembolism. New York, Grune & Stratton, 1981, pp 234–318.
35. Lagerstedt CI, Olsson C-G, Fagher BO, et al: Need for long-term anticoagulant treatment in symptomatic calf-vein thrombosis. Lancet 2:515–518, 1985.
36. Huisman MV, Buller HR, ten Cate JW, and Vreeken J: Serial impedance plethysmography for suspected deep vein thrombosis in outpatients: The Amsterdam General Practicioner Study. N Engl J Med 314:823–828, 1986.
37. Hillner BE, Philbrick JT, and Becker DM: Optimal management of suspected lower-extremity deep vein thrombosis. Arch Intern Med 152:165–175, 1991.
38. Cruickshank MK, Levine MN, Hirsh J, et al: A standard heparin nomogram for the management of heparin therapy. Arch Intern Med 151:333–337, 1991.
39. Doyle DJ, Turpie AGG, Hirsch J, et al: Adjusted subcutaneous heparin or continuous intravenous heparin in patients with acute deep vein thrombosis. Ann Intern Med 107:441–445, 1987.
40. Hommes DW, Bura A, Mazzolai L, et al: Subcutaneous heparin compared with continuous intravenous heparin administration in the initial treatment of deep vein thrombosis. Ann Intern Med 116:279–284, 1992.
41. Prandoni P, Lensing AWA, Buller HR, et al: Comparison of subcutaneous low-molecular-weight heparin with intravenous standard heparin in proximal deep-vein thrombosis. Lancet 339:441–445, 1992.
42. Hull RD, Raskob GE, Rosenbloom D, et al: Heparin for 5 days as compared with 10 days in the initial treatment of proximal venous thrombosis. N Engl J Med 322:1260–1264, 1990.
43. Bussey HI, Force RW, Bianco TM, and Leonard AD: Reliance of prothrombin time ratios causes significant errors in anticoagulation therapy. Arch Intern Med 152:278–282, 1992.
44. Hull R, Delmore T, Carter C, et al: Adjusted subcutaneous heparin versus warfarin sodium in the long-term treatment of venous thrombosis. N Engl J Med 306:189–194, 1982.
45. Goldhaber SZ: Thrombolysis in venous thromboembolism: An international perspective. Chest 94:176S–181S, 1990.
46. Turpie AGG, Levine MN, Hirsch J, et al: Tissue plasminogen activator (rt-PA) vs. heparin in deep vein thrombosis: Results of a randomized trial. Chest 97:172S–175S, 1990.
47. Grassi CJ: Inferior vena caval filters: Analysis of five currently available devices. Am J Roentgenol 156:813–821, 1992.
48. Turpie AGG and Leclerc JR: Prophylaxis of venous thromboembolism. *In* Lecler JR (ed): Venous Thromboembolic Disorders. Philadelphia, Lea & Febiger, 1991, pp 303–345.
49. Kakkar VV and Murray WJG: Efficacy and safety of low-molecular-weight heparin (CY216) in preventing postoperative venous thrombo-embolism: A cooperative study. Br J Surg 72:786–791, 1985.
50. Turpie AGG, Levine MN, Hirsh J, et al: A randomized controlled trial of a low-molecular weight heparin (Enoxaparin) to prevent deep-vein thrombosis in patients undergoing elective hip surgery. N Engl J Med 315:925–929, 1986.
51. Nicholaides AN, Miles C, Hoare M, et al: Intermittent sequential pneumatic compression of the legs and thromboembolism deterrent stocking in the prevention of postoperative deep venous thrombosis. Surgery 94:21–24, 1983.
52. Lofgren EP: Present-day indications for surgical treatment of varicose veins. Mayo Clin Proc 41:515–523, 1966.
53. O'Donnell TF Jr: Chronic venous insufficiency and varicose veins. *In* Young JR, Graor RA, Olin JW, and Bartholomew JR (eds): Peripheral Vascular Diseases. St. Louis, Mosby Year Book, 1991, pp 443–480.
54. Dodd H and Crockett FB: The Pathology and Surgery of the Veins of the Lower Limb. Edinburgh, Livingstone, 1976.
55. Bergan JJ: Varicose veins: Chronic venous insufficiency. *In* Moore WS (ed): Vascular Surgery: A Comprehensive Review. Philadelphia, WB Saunders, 1991.
56. Villaviciencio JL: Excision of varicose veins. *In* Ernst CB and Stanley JC (eds): Current Therapy in Vascular Surgery. Philadelphia, BC Decker, 1991.
57. Donaldson MC: Chronic venous disorders. *In* Loscalzo J, Creager MA, and Dzau VJ, (eds): Vascular Medicine. Boston, Little Brown, 1992.
58. Killewich LA, Martin R, Cramer M, et al: Pathophysiology of venous claudication. J Vasc Surg 1:507–511, 1984.
59. Barnes RW: Noninvasive tests for chronic venous insufficiency. *In* Bergan JJ and Yao JST (eds): Surgery of the Veins. Philadelphia, Grune & Stratton, 1985.
60. Cikrit DF, Nichols WK, and Silver D: Surgical management of refractory venous stasis ulceration. J Vasc Surg 7:473–478, 1988.
61. Nicolaides AN, Christopoulous D, and Vasdekis S: Progress in the investigation of chronic venous insufficiency. Ann Vasc Surg 3:278–292, 1989.
62. Bergan JJ, Yao JST, Flinn WR, and McCarthy WJ: Surgical treatment of venous obstruction and insufficiency. J Vasc Surg 3:174–181, 1986.
63. Gloviczki P and Merrell SW: Surgical treatment of venous disease. *In* Spittell JA Jr (ed): Contemporary issues in peripheral vascular disease. *In* Brest AN (ed): Cardiovascular Clinics. Philadelphia, FA Davis, 1992, pp 81–100.

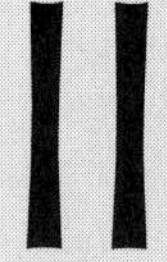

Diseases of the Respiratory Tract

13

Pharyngitis, Coryza, and Related Infections in Adults

ANTHONY L. KOMAROFF, MD

Infections of the upper respiratory tract constitute the commonest problem for which patients seek medical attention. Most disease is acute in onset, of relatively short duration, and self-limited. However, so many millions of people experience these usually brief illnesses that they constitute a major social cost, in dollars spent on medical care and time lost from work. The primary function of the physician in most cases is to establish the cause of the infection and to decide what drug to select if antimicrobial therapy is needed. In a relatively small number of instances, he or she must manage problems arising from complications, some of which may be severe, possibly life-threatening: acute rheumatic fever, acute glomerulonephritis, chronic pyogenic paranasal sinusitis, bacterial meningitis, and acute otitis media with or without suppurative mastoiditis.

Clinical Anatomy

The anatomy of the head and neck and the common sites of disease involving these areas are illustrated in Figure 13–1. Symptoms associated with disorders in these sites may indicate the presence of either infectious or noninfectious processes.

A detailed anatomy of the nose, mouth, and pharynx is presented in Figure 13–2. The septum separates the two sides of the nasal cavity. The inferior, middle, and superior

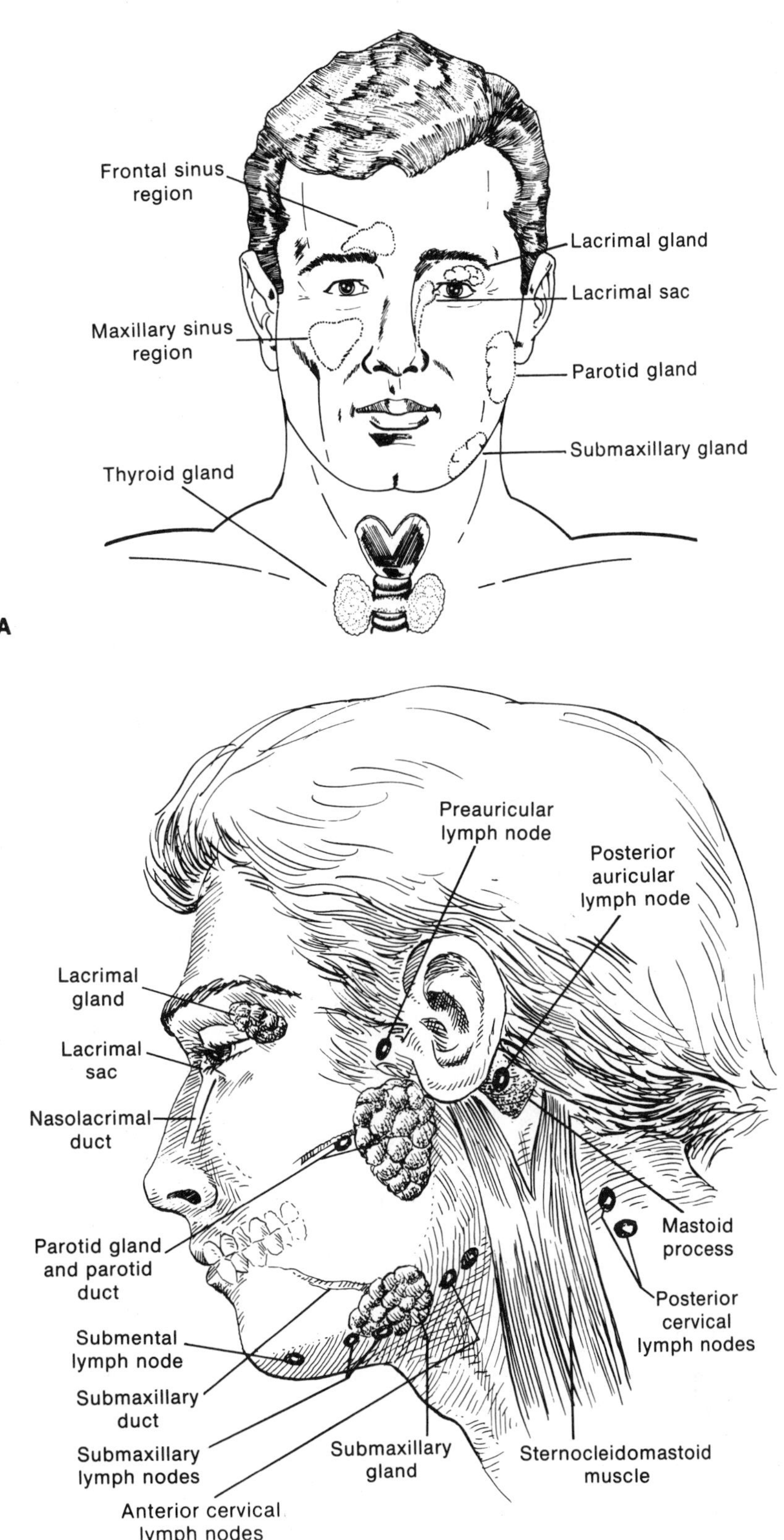

FIGURE 13–1. General anatomy of the head and neck. *A,* Anteroposterior view. *B,* Lateral view.

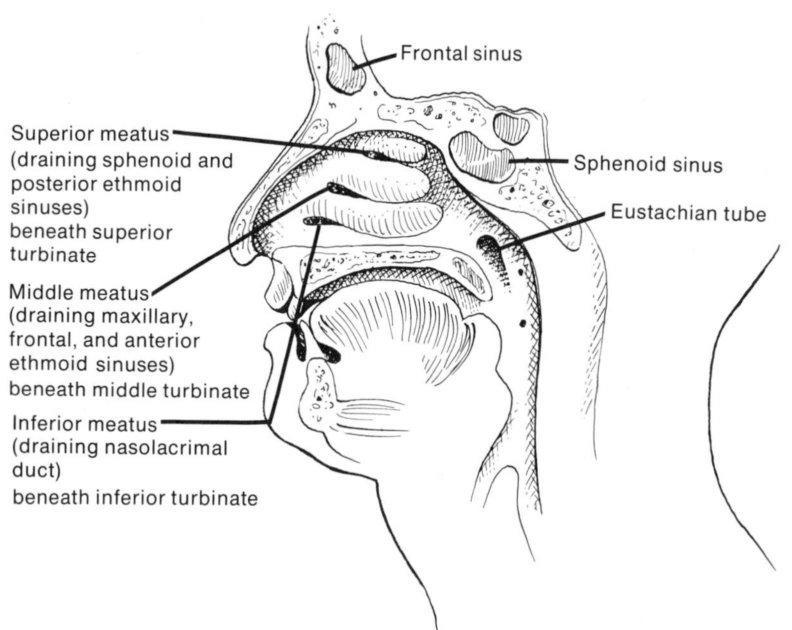

FIGURE 13–2. Lateral wall of the nose showing the nasal turbinates and sites of sinus drainage.

turbinates are situated laterally. Between them are the three meatal passages. The inferior meatus drains the nasolacrimal duct; the middle meatus empties the frontal, maxillary, and anterior ethmoid sinuses; and the superior meatus drains the posterior ethmoid and sphenoid sinuses. The nose warms and moistens inhaled air and acts as an air conditioner. It also traps small particles and provides a mucous and ciliary blanket for removal of dust and bacteria. The turbinates are normally hyperemic, and they enlarge and shrink in a physiologic sequence that, in general, serves to regulate the flow of air through first one and then the other side of the nose. Exposure to cold usually leads to contraction of these structures; re-entry into a warm environment produces hyperemia and swelling, which is often accompanied by the appearance of a thin, watery nasal discharge.

The anatomy of the pharynx, including the tonsils, is shown in Figure 13–3. A view of the hypopharynx, including the epiglottis and vocal cords, as seen with a laryngeal mirror, is provided in Figure 13–4. Details of the anatomy of the paranasal sinuses and ear are presented in a later chapter.

PHARYNGITIS SYNDROME

The pharyngitis syndrome consists of a predominant sore throat, fever, malaise, generalized myalgia, sometimes cough (depending on the etiologic agent), and minimal or absent coryza.

The management of patients with pharyngitis is often thought to be straightforward: the cause is thought to be either a viral or streptococcal infection, a culture is assumed to distinguish reliably between the two, and penicillin is assumed to be effective treatment when the culture is "positive" for the streptococcus. It is not that simple, however. For one thing, various rare forms of bacterial infection besides streptococcal pharyngitis have long been recognized in the differential diagnosis of pharyngitis; many of these

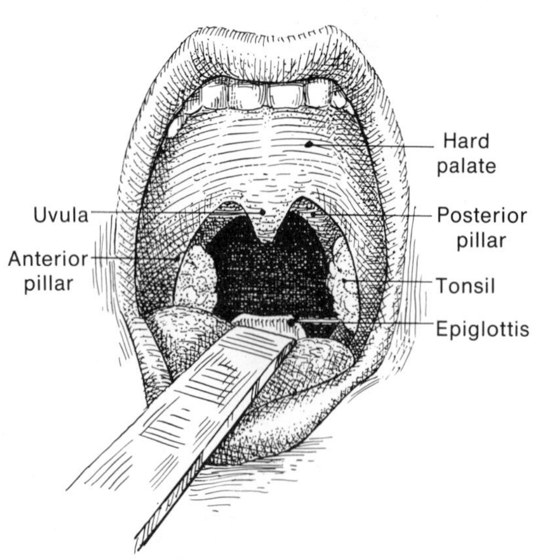

FIGURE 13–3. The pharynx and tonsils.

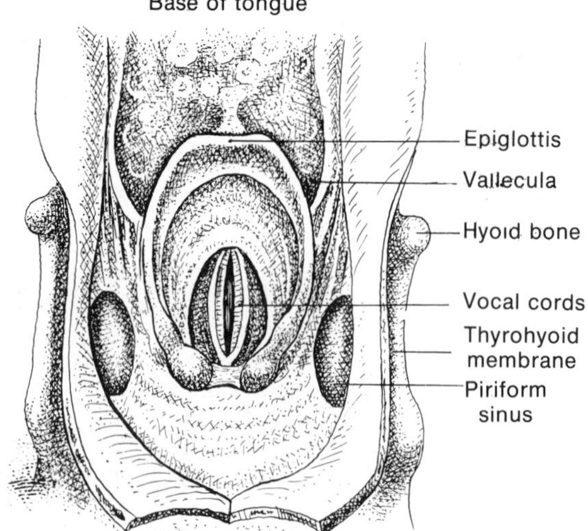

FIGURE 13–4. The supraglottic larynx, including the epiglottis and vocal cords.

are discussed in this chapter. Moreover, studies suggest that other forms of nonviral pharyngitis may be more common than previously suspected and that the management of possible streptococcal infection is not as clear-cut as once it was thought to be.

Viral Pharyngitis

Clinicians often assume that most patients with pharyngitis have a viral infection. However, several studies employing culture or serologic diagnostic tests fail to support this assumption, revealing evidence of viral infection in only 17 to 25% of children (>2 years of age) and adults.[1,2]

The most common viral causes of pharyngitis are rhinovirus, influenza virus, parainfluenza virus, adenovirus, respiratory syncytial virus, the enteroviruses, cytomegalovirus, Epstein-Barr virus, and herpes simplex virus. Infection with the latter two agents are discussed separately later.

The respiratory tract viral pathogens usually cause self-limited illness in otherwise healthy patients, but several of them may produce serious and life-threatening lower respiratory tract infection on occasion.

Currently no treatment is of proven clinical usefulness for any of these forms of viral pharyngitis, although new agents (e.g., intranasal α_2-interferon prophylaxis for rhinovirus) are being investigated. Antiviral drugs (amantadine, acyclovir) are of demonstrated efficacy against more serious infections with influenza virus and the herpes viruses.

Group A Streptococcal Pharyngitis

The group A streptococcus is the best known and best studied cause of bacterial pharyngitis. Group A streptococcal pharyngitis has long been of particular concern to clinicians because of its recognized association with nonsuppurative sequelae, primarily acute rheumatic fever, and acute glomerulonephritis.

The group A streptococcus produces both sporadic and epidemic pharyngitis. The incubation period in streptococcal infection of the upper respiratory tract may be as short as 18 hours or as long as 7 days, but the average is 48 to 72 hours.

Clinical Findings. The clinical findings of group A streptococcal pharyngitis range from mild to severe and overlap with the findings produced by other infectious forms of pharyngitis. It is not possible to predict perfectly whether a patient has streptococcal pharyngitis from the clinical findings (or from the laboratory findings, for that matter). However, clinical findings can be quite useful in separating patients with a very low probability of streptococcal pharyngitis from those with a moderate or relatively high probability. As is discussed later, estimates of the probability of streptococcal pharyngitis in an individual patient allow the clinician to alter or individualize the approach to diagnosis and treatment.

The earliest symptoms are soreness of the throat, generalized malaise, and fever ranging from 37.2 to 40° C (99 to 104° F). In severe cases, nausea, vomiting, and diarrhea may be present; in a few cases, mono- or polyarthralgia may be a striking component. Pharyngeal pain may be so intense that swallowing sputum is difficult. Discrete collections of yellow exudate are present in the crypts of the reddened, swollen tonsils and on the surface of the submucosal collections of lymphoid tissue in the pharynx; these wipe off readily and leave no areas of bleeding or ulceration (Fig. 13–5*A*).

A number of very useful studies of the probability of group A streptococcal pharyngitis in patients with different symptoms and signs have been published.[3–7] A simple formula based on three clinical findings is summarized in

A. Exudative pharyngitis
Tonsils enlarged and inflamed with yellow patchy exudate
B. Diphtherial pharyngitis
Firmly attached, bluish-white membrane with sharply defined borders surrounded by inflammation of the mucosa; the membrane is not confined to the tonsils

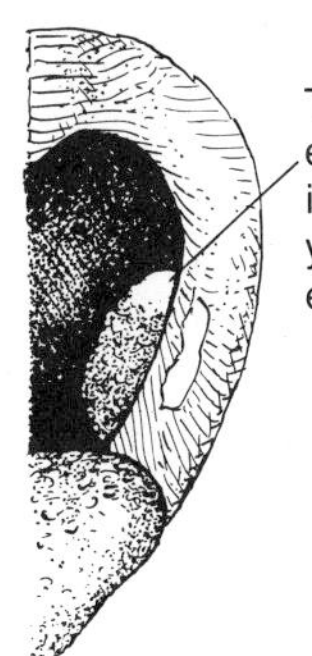

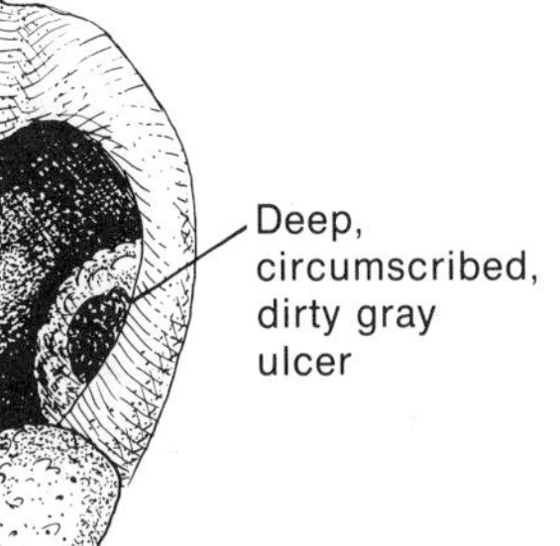

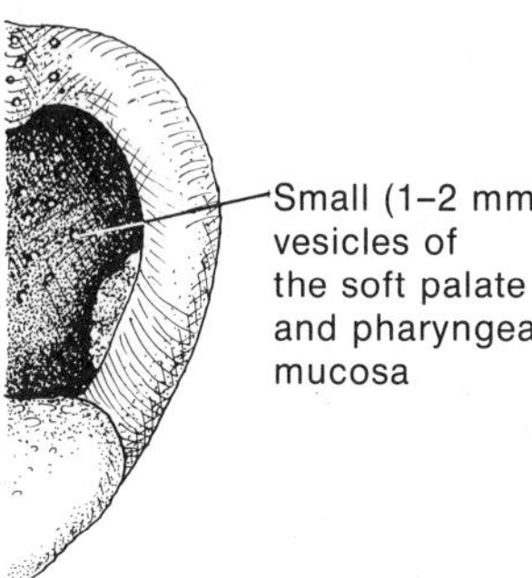

FIGURE 13–5. *A,* Typical features of exudative pharyngitis due to streptococcal or viral disease. *B,* Diphtheria involving the tonsils and soft palate. *C,* Plaut-Vincent ulcer of the tonsil. *D,* Herpangina of the pharynx and soft palate.

TABLE 13–1. USING CLINICAL FINDINGS TO ESTIMATE THE PROBABILITY OF GROUP A STREPTOCOCCAL ISOLATION IN ADULT PATIENTS

Clinical Findings	Probability of + Culture* (%)	Probability of + Culture and Antibody Rise* (%)	Recommended Action
Temperature <37.8°C (100°F) *and* No tonsillar exudate *and* No anterior cervical adenitis	3.4	0.4	No culture, no treatment: A false-positive culture could lead to unnecessary and potentially risky treatment
Temperature >37.8°C (100°F) *or* Tonsillar exudate *or* Anterior cervical adenitis	13.5	5.6	Culture, and treat patients with positive cultures
Temperature >37.8°C (100°F) *and* Tonsillar exudate *and* Anterior cervical adenitis	42.1	16.5	Treat immediately: A false-negative culture could prevent necessary treatment
	Special "Risk Factors"		
Past history of acute rheumatic fever		*or*	Treat immediately:
Documented strep exposure in past week		*or*	Patient is at special risk from strep throat
Known strep epidemic in community		*or*	
Patient is diabetic or otherwise immunocompromised		*or*	
Patient has scarlatiniform rash			

*From Komaroff AL, Pass TM, Aronson MD, et al: The prediction of streptococcal pharyngitis in adults. J Gen Intern Med 1:1, 1986.

Table 13–1. A slightly more accurate formula employing a "streptococcal score" (Table 13–2) derived from a statistical analysis of findings in nearly 700 adult patients can be used by referring to a nomogram (Fig. 13–6).

Throat Culture. Culture of the pharynx and tonsils is the basis for diagnosing streptococcal pharyngitis. For proper isolation of group A streptococci, two cotton or Dacron swabs should be rubbed firmly, under direct vision, over the tonsils and posterior pharyngeal wall. Use of a liquid transport medium preserves the specimen for at least 48 hours before culturing. The conventional culture medium is sheep-blood agar, although studies indicate that blood agar plates with trimethoprimsulfamethoxazole may be superior. With both types of agar, non-group A streptococci and other pharyngeal saprophytes may produce β-hemolysis (a clear hemolytic zone). Plates should be kept under relatively anaerobic conditions to enhance β-hemolysis.

The throat culture is not perfectly accurate. It may be "falsely negative" due to sampling error: a second swab will yield group A streptococci when the first swab has not in about 10 to 20% of patients. Occasionally, the culture will truly be falsely negative: some group A streptococci will not produce β-hemolysis.

The throat culture can also be falsely positive, in several senses. First, a substantial fraction of β-hemolytic colonies will not be group A. This well-recognized cause of a false-positive result is largely avoided by use of a bacitracin disc, which inhibits the growth of those β-hemolytic colonies that are group A (with rare exceptions). Also, a fluorescent antibody technique is widely used; it is rapid, simple, and accurate (with rare exceptions).

Next, and more important, the throat culture may be falsely positive in another sense. Thirty to fifty per cent of adult patients with pharyngitis and a positive culture may be only streptococcal carriers: some other agent may be responsible for the pharyngitis.[1, 3, 8] These patients are thought not infected because they do not demonstrate an antibody response to streptococcal antigens; therefore, they are commonly considered to be examples of the *carrier state* (a positive culture without an antibody response). The most commonly measured evidence of an antibody response has been a fourfold or greater increase in the tube dilution level of antistreptolysin O (ASLO) on convalescent serum obtained 1 to 6 months later. The ASLO titer in the acute serum specimen is of no value in diagnosing the presence of current infection.[9]

Rapid Antigen Detection Tests. The problem with the throat culture, of course, is that it cannot give an immediate answer, thus being of little use in decision-making at the time of the patient's visit. For that reason, the development of "rapid" tests (minutes to hours) for identifying group A streptococcal antigen promised to be a major diagnostic advance.

These tests have not proved to be as useful as had been expected, however. For one thing, they have not proved to be highly accurate. The initial studies that compared the results of different rapid test kits with throat culture found sensitivities ranging from 77 to 95% (i.e., false-negative rates ranging from 5 to 23%) and specificities ranging from 86 to 100% (i.e., false-positive rates from 0 to 14%).[10] However, more recent and methodologically stronger studies find much lower sensitivity, ranging from 31 to 50%, with no improvement in specificity.[11]

A second problem with the rapid tests is that a negative result may lead the clinician to conclude that antibacterial therapy must be unnecessary. However, this is not the case. The test often has false-negative results. Also, group A streptococcal infection is not the only cause of pharyngitis

TABLE 13–2. CALCULATING THE "STREP SCORE" BY DISCRIMINANT ANALYSIS*†

Clinical Predictor	Score
Marked tonsillar exudate‡	+2
Pinpoint tonsillar exudate‡	+1
Enlarged tonsils	+1
Tender anterior cervical adenopathy	+1
Myalgias	+1
Positive throat culture in past year	+1
Itchy eyes	−1

*From Komaroff AL, Pass TM, Aronson MD, et al: The prediction of streptococcal pharyngitis in adults. J Gen Intern Med 1:1, 1986.

†See Figure 13–6 for nomogram.

‡No patient can have a tonsillar exudate described as *both* "pinpoint" and "marked."

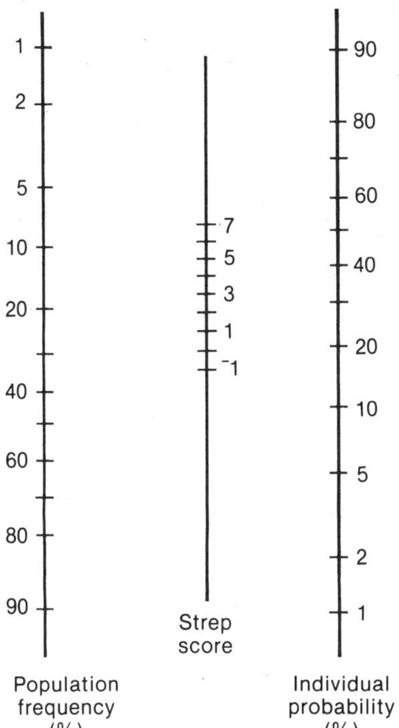

FIGURE 13–6. Nomogram for predicting probability of group A streptococcal pharyngitis. To use the nomogram, determine the overall prevalence of positive cultures among adult patients presenting with sore throat at the site. Second, add the points based on the clinical findings to arrive at a strep score for an individual. Third, place a ruler on the figure so that it crosses the left line at the site prevalence and the center line at the strep score value. The point where the ruler crosses the right line is then the probability of a positive culture for that patient.

As an example, if 20% of adult patients with sore throat at a site typically have positive cultures and a patient in this group has a strep score of 5, then a straight line connecting 20% on the left line with 5 points on the center line crosses the right line at a value of 55%, indicating that this is the likelihood of a positive culture for this patient.[10]

that is theoretically treatable by antibacterials, as noted later.

Thus, in our view, the role of currently available rapid antigen detection tests remains uncertain.

Treatment. Because a throat culture or rapid diagnostic test for group A streptococcus can be falsely positive (i.e., can indicate a carrier state), and because penicillin treatment prescribed on the basis of a false-positive culture can produce more suffering than it can be expected to eliminate, a good case can be made that patients who have a low probability of streptococcal pharyngitis, based on clinical findings, do not require a throat culture or diagnostic testing.

Risk-benefit and cost-benefit analyses performed by our group suggest that, when the probability is below 3%, a throat culture can be avoided. As can be seen in Table 13–1, clinical findings can be used to estimate such a low probability. (This recommendation does not apply to patients who have special "risk factors" for streptococcal disease, as summarized in Table 13–1.)

Conversely, since a throat culture or rapid diagnostic test for group A streptococcus can also have a false-negative result, treatment without resorting to culture is usually indicated in patients with a relatively high probability of streptococcal pharyngitis: greater than 40%. As can be seen in Table 13–1, clinical findings can be used to identify patients with such a high probability.

Table 13–3 displays appropriate treatment regimens for adults. Although some studies suggest that cephalosporins might be slightly superior to penicillin in eradicating the streptococcus, this does not justify routine use of cephalosporins: The added expense and generation of cephalosporin-resistant organisms are too great a price to pay to achieve a possible slight benefit in eradication rate.

Management of Contacts. The following contacts of patients with documented or highly probable streptococcal pharyngitis should be cultured: (1) Those who become symptomatic, and (2) Asymptomatic contacts who are at high risk from streptococcal pharyngitis—for example, because of a past history of acute rheumatic fever.

Follow-Up. It is not necessary (or typically possible) to obtain post-treatment follow-up cultures in every patient who has been treated for presumed streptococcal pharyngitis. However, patients who are at high risk for streptococcal sequelae, or who live in close contact with those who are at high risk, probably should have follow-up cultures.

A prolonged carrier state (2 to 3 weeks) may be a problem in untreated patients after they have apparently fully recovered from pharyngitis. Streptococci may spread to family members and close contacts. The organism is more likely to be disseminated if it is carried in the nose. Whether or not asymptomatic carriers should be treated is presently controversial. However, if an asymptomatic carrier is known to have been the source of pharyngitis in others, or is likely to come in contact with a person who has had rheumatic fever, therapy should be initiated.

Local Suppurative Complications. The local suppurative complications of infection of the upper respiratory tract include obstruction of drainage from the paranasal sinuses or middle ear, or both, local extension of a bacterial infection (peritonsillar cellulitis or abscess), and spread of disease into the lower respiratory tract (bronchitis, pneumonia). Each of these, except peritonsillar infection, is described in other chapters.

Peritonsillar abscess is the most common suppurative complication of bacterial pharyngitis. The organism involved is often a group A (β-hemolytic) streptococcus. However, staphylococcus, pneumococcus, or members of the normal microflora of the pharynx may be responsible for this complication. The disease usually starts with a sore throat, followed by increasing unilateral pain referred to the ear and difficulty in swallowing for several days. The patient may hold the mouth open and drool. The voice is muffled because of the inability to clear secretions. Unilateral swelling involves the tonsil, anterior pillar, and its adjacent soft palate (Fig. 13–7). Persons with peritonsillar abscess should be hospitalized and given antimicrobial therapy intravenously. Because of the frequency with which gram-positive cocci are involved, oxacillin (8 to 12 g/day) is probably the drug of first choice. A fluctuant mass may need to be surgically drained. In some instances, if aspiration by needle has failed to reveal localized pus, medical therapy alone resolves the problem.

Parapharyngeal space abscess is characterized by an increase in the fever associated with the pharyngitis, protrusion of the tonsil on the involved side toward the midline,

TABLE 13–3. RECOMMENDED TREATMENT REGIMENS FOR STREPTOCOCCAL PHARYNGITIS IN ADULTS

1. Penicillin G, benzathine (Bicillin), 1.2 million units IM
2. Penicillin V, 250 mg q.i.d. for 10 days*
3. Erythromycin, 250 mg q.i.d. for 10 days*

*Treatment for less than 10 days results in unacceptably high recurrence rates.

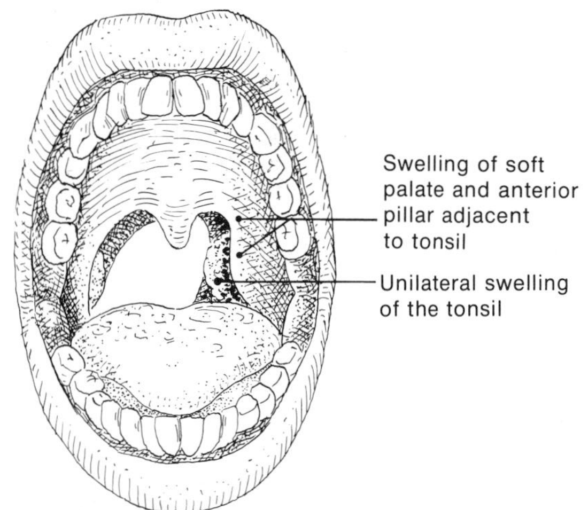

FIGURE 13–7. Peritonsillar abscess. The tonsil is pushed forward, downward, and toward the midline. Tense swelling is apparent in the anterior tonsillar pillar and adjacent soft palate. Pus is localized between the tonsil and fascia behind the tonsil covering the superior constrictor muscle.

and tenderness at the angle of the jaw on the same side. Thrombosis of the tonsillar vein in these patients may extend to the jugular vein. Once this has occurred, the disease becomes life-threatening because of bacteremia, multiple pulmonary infarcts with the formation of abscesses, and metastatic infections at other sites.

Nonsuppurative Sequelae of Streptococcal Infections. The clinical features of the nonsuppurative sequelae of streptococcal infections—acute rheumatic fever and post-streptococcal glomerulonephritis—are discussed in Chapters 5 and 30. It has been demonstrated unequivocally that treatment of streptococcal pharyngitis with penicillin reduces the incidence of acute rheumatic fever.[12] Furthermore, it has been reported that the availability of comprehensive health care in a community may decrease the attack rate by almost two thirds.[13] The evidence that therapy of streptococcal infection reduces the frequency with which glomerulonephritis occurs is equivocal, but because it would no longer be ethical to withhold treatment deliberately, we are likely never to know the answer to this question.

The risk of developing a primary attack of acute rheumatic fever in untreated cases of streptococcal pharyngitis has diminished markedly in the developed nations. An attack rate of 3% was recorded in an epidemic of severe exudative pharyngitis studied 40 years ago.[12] Today, using data provided by the National Center for Health Statistics, I estimate that the risk is approximately 1 in 10,000 among untreated adults and approximately 1 in 100,000 among treated adults. However, in the mid-1980s, rheumatic fever attack rates began rising in the United States, due to virulent new strains of streptococci.[14]

The risk of a *recurrence* of rheumatic fever is substantial with subsequent streptococcal infections. This justifies continuous prophylaxis with penicillin (200,000 units twice a day) or sulfadiazine (1 g every 12 hours) administered orally. For individuals in whom compliance may be poor, it has been recommended that 1.2 million units of benzathine penicillin be administered intramuscularly once a month.[15] There is no age at which prophylaxis can be discontinued with complete safety. However, because the risk seems to diminish with age, continued prophylaxis beyond the age of 50 years is not mandatory. In general, those at increased risk of developing rheumatic fever (e.g., schoolteachers, medical personnel, mothers of young children, and individuals who have had previous episodes of rheumatic carditis or who are in the lower socioeconomic groups) should be treated more aggressively with prophylactic regimens.

Non-Group A Streptococcal Pharyngitis

Many of the important early investigations of streptococcal pharyngitis demonstrated that non-group A streptococci could often be isolated from the pharynx in patients with pharyngitis. Because the non-group A streptococci were only rarely associated with nonsuppurative complications and infrequently produced increases in antistreptococcal antibodies, they were for many years thought not to be important pharyngeal pathogens.

Evidence suggests, however, that this may not be true. Non-group A streptococci are isolated more frequently than are the group A streptococci from the throats of adults seeking medical care for the complaint of sore throat.[16, 17] The isolation rate of non-group A streptococci among patients with symptomatic pharyngitis is much higher than among patients of comparable age and sex seeking medical care at the same medical facilities at the same time for conditions other than pharyngitis. Furthermore, strong anecdotal experience, not yet confirmed by a controlled clinical trial, suggests that patients with pharyngitis from whom non-group A streptococci are isolated respond to antibacterial therapy.

Therefore, while it has not yet been firmly established, it is quite possible that non-group A streptococci can produce pharyngitis that clinically is similar to the pharyngitis produced by group A streptococci and that is responsive to appropriate therapy.

Mycoplasmal Pharyngitis

It has been well established that patients who have bronchopulmonary infection with *Mycoplasma pneumoniae* often have an antecedent pharyngitis.[2, 18–21] (Other members of the *Mycoplasma* family besides *M. pneumoniae* are not established pharyngeal pathogens.)

Recent serologic evidence suggests that *M. pneumoniae* may indeed be a common cause of pharyngitis: serologic evidence of infection was found in 11% of adult patients (ranging in age from 16 to 70 years) seeking primary care for a sore throat.[1] Many of these patients had bronchopulmonary symptoms, in contrast to patients with streptococcal pharyngitis. Unlike the case in epidemic mycoplasmal infections,[21] bullous myringitis seems to be a rare finding in patients with sporadic mycoplasmal pharyngitis.

Diagnostic testing for *M. pneumoniae* is difficult. Special culture techniques are required, and the organism is fastidious. Cold agglutinin tests lack sensitivity and specificity. Specific *Mycoplasma* serologic techniques are useful only when paired sera are obtained. A rapid test for mycoplasmal nucleic acid has been introduced, but is not yet widely used.

The efficacy of antibacterial treatment, with either tetracycline or erythromycin, in mycoplasmal pneumonia has been demonstrated in controlled trials.[22, 23] There are as yet no published controlled trials of antibacterial therapy in mycoplasmal pharyngitis. Nevertheless, in the patient who is significantly symptomatic with what may be mycoplasmal infection, treatment is probably indicated. Appropriate regimens include erythromycin or tetracycline hydrochloride, 250 to 500 mg four times a day for 10 days.

Chlamydial Pharyngitis

Research suggests that chlamydial organisms may be a pharyngeal pathogen in adults.[1, 24–26] A recently discovered species, *Chlamydia pneumoniae, strain TWAR,*[27–29] appears to be the most important chlamydial pathogen in patients with pharyngitis.[26] *C. pneumoniae* is an important cause of community-acquired pneumonia. As might be expected, *C. pneumoniae* appears to be a much more likely cause of pharyngitis when the patient also has symptoms of *lower* respiratory tract infection.[27–29] Therefore, it appears that *C. pneumoniae* is a pharyngeal pathogen; one study indicates that it may explain 9% of cases of pharyngitis.[26]

A second chlamydial organism, *C. trachomatis,* may also occasionally produce pharyngitis.[1, 24, 25] The role of this organism is controversial. A role for *C. trachomatis* in pharyngitis is plausible: It is an established and important respiratory tract pathogen in newborn babies[30] and may be a cause of community-acquired pneumonia in adults.[31] In one study, *C. trachomatis* was isolated from the throat of 5% of patients seeking primary care for the complaint of pharyngitis.[24]

At this time, diagnostic testing for both *C. pneumoniae* and *C. trachomatis* is impractical for the physician in office practice. As with *M. pneumoniae,* serologic testing is useful when a fourfold increase in antibody levels is demonstrated in paired sera. The clinical utility of IgM antibody against either chlamydial organism in the acute phase serum is currently unknown. Isolation of both organisms requires cell culture; at the time of this writing, very few laboratories are experienced in culturing *C. pneumoniae.* The role of rapid diagnostic tests for *C. trachomatis* in pharyngitis is unstudied.[32] There currently are no available rapid tests for diagnosing *C. pneumoniae.*

Treatment for presumed or documented chlamydial pharyngitis has unproven value. Nevertheless, in a patient with persistent pharyngitis and symptoms of lower respiratory tract infection, who does not have a positive streptococcal throat culture or who does not respond to penicillin therapy, treatment with erythromycin probably is justified. This is especially true if the patient has associated symptoms of bronchopulmonary infection or of genitourinary infection.

Haemophilus influenzae Pharyngitis

Haemophilus influenzae may cause pharyngitis in 1 to 2% of adults.[32, 33] Both encapsulated and nonencapsulated *H. influenzae* have been found with greater frequency in patients with pharyngitis than in control patients. *Haemophilus* pharyngitis should be suspected in an adult with concomitant symptoms or signs of otitis media. Cough may also occur. Heavy growth of *H. influenzae* on throat culture is strong evidence that this organism is responsible for the pharyngitis.

A successful treatment regimen is ampicillin or amoxicillin, 250 to 500 mg, four times a day for 10 days.

Epstein-Barr Virus Infection

Nearly 90% of people have been infected with Epstein-Barr virus (EBV) by 40 years of age. New primary infection with EBV is often entirely asymptomatic. Sometimes it produces a mild respiratory tract infection syndrome. New EBV infection may be the cause of pharyngitis in 1 to 6% of young adults, although it only rarely is the cause of pharyngitis in adults older than 40 years of age.[34] Only a quarter of patients with new EBV infection seeking medical care for pharyngitis manifest the complete infectious mononucleosis syndrome: Most are clinically indistinguishable from patients with other forms of viral pharyngitis and have a similarly brief and benign clinical course.

Clinical Findings. Several clinical findings are seen significantly more often in patients with new EBV infections, as suggested by a positive heterophil antibody titer. These are listed in Table 13–4. With the full-blown infectious mononucleosis syndrome, a severe exudative tonsillopharyngitis often is present, as is splenomegaly. Even with milder cases, sore throat rather than fatigue and malaise is often the presenting complaint.

Laboratory Findings. The diagnosis of infectious mononucleosis is suggested if: (1) the absolute lymphocyte count is greater than 4000 per mm^3 (or the relative count is greater than 50%); (2) over 10% of the cells are "atypical lymphocytes." Most patients with pharyngitis due to new EBV infection do not have atypical lymphocytosis, however.[34] A small number of atypical lymphocytes are present in the blood of individuals with other viral infections.

The horse-cell agglutination test (Monospot) for heterophil antibody is helpful in establishing the presence of the disease: It is as sensitive and specific as the standard Paul-Bunnell sheep-cell test.[35] However, results of this test usually do not become positive until 7 to 14 days after the onset of symptoms. Furthermore, the horse-cell test results may stay positive for much longer than in the sheep-cell test; thus, it can produce false-positive results in future episodes of pharyngitis caused by other organisms.

Treatment. No definitive antiviral therapy is yet available for EBV infections; acyclovir may have some utility during periods of active viral replication, although several clinical trials of acyclovir in mononucleosis do not demonstrate benefit convincingly. Symptomatic therapy for the pain of pharyngitis may be required. In unusual cases, when tonsillar swelling is so great as to threaten the airway, steroid therapy is sometimes used. Steroids should be reserved only for such unusual cases, in light of theoretic concerns about using steroids at a time of new infection with a virus that seems to play a role in human oncogenesis.

Gonococcal Pharyngitis

The gonococcus may be the cause of pharyngitis in 1% of adult patients seeking primary care for a sore throat.[36] In

TABLE 13–4. CLINICAL FINDINGS SUGGESTING NEW EPSTEIN-BARR VIRUS INFECTION*

	Predictive Value Positive†	Likelihood Ratio‡
Palatine petechiae	.11	5.8
Posterior auricular adenopathy	.19	12.0
Marked axillary adenopathy	.33	21.0
Inguinal adenopathy	.06	2.9
Palatine petechiae, posterior auricular adenopathy, or marked axillary adenopathy	.11	6.3

*Reproduced with permission, from Aronson MD, Komaroff AL, Pass TM, et al: Heterophil antibody in adults with sore throat: Frequency and clinical presentation. Ann Intern Med 96:505, 1982.

†Predictive value positive is the fraction of all patients with a particular physical examination finding who have heterophil antibody.

‡Likelihood ratio: true positive rate/false positive rate.

some patient populations, especially in homosexual men and female contacts of men with genital gonorrhea, pharyngeal gonorrhea may be much more common, although it often is asymptomatic.[37–40]

Clinical Findings. Gonorrhea can be passed to the pharynx by fellatio and possibly by cunnilingus.[38, 39] Pharyngeal gonorrhea, when symptomatic, may be mild to severe, with a protracted pharyngitis characterized by pain, fever, and the presence of abundant yellow exudate on the posterior pharynx and in the tonsillar crypts. No known symptoms or signs help to distinguish gonococcal pharyngitis from any other kind of pharyngitis, except for a history of fellatio.[36, 38]

Laboratory Findings. Culture for suspected gonococcal pharyngitis requires a specimen obtained from the throat, planted on warmed Thayer-Martin or New York City medium[41] agar plates, inserted directly into a candle jar, and incubated at 37°C for as long as 48 hours; *Neisseria gonorrhoeae* is identified by Gram stain, positive oxidase test, and sugar fermentation patterns.

Given the low frequency of gonococcal pharyngitis in most patients seeking primary care for a sore throat, routine throat cultures for gonorrhea cannot be justified. However, cultures seem justified in several circumstances. First, culture should be obtained in the male patient with pharyngitis who is known or presumed to be gay.[37] Even in this group the yield will not be large: only one of eight homosexuals attending a venereal disease clinic and complaining of sore throat had a pharyngeal culture positive for *N. gonorrhoeae.*[40] Second, a culture should be obtained in patients with sore throats who have intercurrent symptoms of dysuria, urethral discharge, vaginal discharge, pelvic pain, or proctitis. Third, patients with sore throats who have had recent sexual exposure to contacts with gonococcal infection should be cultured. Finally, the patient with persistent sore throat who has been treated for presumptive streptococcal pharyngitis should be cultured, since the antibacterial drugs prescribed have probably been inadequate in type or dosage to eliminate pharyngeal gonorrhea. For the same reason, culture may be justified in a patient with persistent sore throat that is "culture-negative" for the streptococcus.

Possibly, heterosexual men seeking care for a sore throat should be routinely asked about the practice of cunnilingus and should have specimens cultured for *N. gonorrhoeae* if they respond affirmatively.

Treatment. Several treatment regimens are effective for gonococcal pharyngitis:

1. Ceftriaxone, 250 mg, as a single intramuscular injection (also effective against penicillin-resistant strains).
2. Ciprofloxacin, 500 mg, as a single oral dose.
3. Cefixime, 800 mg, as a single oral dose.

UNUSUAL BUT IMPORTANT CAUSES OF PHARYNGITIS

Unusual Forms of Bacterial and Fungal Pharyngitis

Diphtheria. Although rare, diphtheria still occurs in the United States, and in recent years an epidemic form has been reported in the Pacific Northwest and the Southwest.[42] Patients with this disease usually have only mildly sore throats, unless simultaneous infection with *C. diphtheriae* and β-hemolytic streptococcus is present. Diphtheria commonly causes only minor to moderate degrees of fever, but the patients appear weak and pale and have a rapid, thready pulse.

The classic diphtheritic "pseudomembrane" is bluish-white and homogeneous; its borders are sharply defined from the uninvolved areas of the tonsils and pharynx. A narrow zone of reddened pharyngeal mucosa surrounds the membrane, which may be limited to the posterior wall of the pharynx or extend to cover the tonsils, uvula, and the entire surface of the naso-, oro-, and hypopharynx. It is firmly attached to the underlying tissue and, when removed, leaves small areas of bleeding (see Fig. 13–5*B*). It is emphasized that a pseudomembrane resembling that of diphtheria may be present occasionally in other types of pharyngitis, especially in infectious mononucleosis.

Diphtheria is diagnosed by removing a piece of the pseudomembrane and staining it with Mallory's methylene blue. *C. diphtheriae* appears as a pleomorphic rod that contains dark-staining metachromatic granules. Cultures made on Loeffler's medium often yield the organism within 12 to 18 hours. However, if a patient has received even a small dose of antibiotic to which the organism is sensitive, growth may be delayed for as long as 5 days or be absent.

Antimicrobial therapy of diphtheria is without benefit in either altering the course of the local disease or preventing the cardiac and neurologic complications. However, it is very effective in eradicating the carriage of the organism, a common problem that may persist for weeks to months after recovery or become permanent. The antibiotic of choice is erythromycin: 2 g/day (0.5 g every 6 hours) orally for 10 to 14 days. Some strains of *C. diphtheriae* are resistant to penicillin. The only potential therapeutic modality for the management of diphtheria is antitoxin, which must be given immediately (after testing for sensitivity): delay of treatment for more than 48 hours is associated with an increased incidence of complications and death. When the pharyngeal membrane extends downward to involve the larynx and trachea, threatening obstruction of the airway, tracheostomy is often necessary.

Unimmunized contacts of patients with diphtheria should be given antitoxin. It has been argued that all patients should be reimmunized against diphtheria approximately once every 10 years, because of evidence that only about 80% of adults in the United States have protective titers of antibody, with lower levels seen in certain high-risk groups, including the chronically ill elderly.[43]

Plaut-Vincent Angina. This infection has been referred to, in the past, as fusospirochetal angina. The primary agent responsible for it is *Fusobacterium plauti-vincenti,* an anaerobic, nonsporulating, gram-negative bacillus. Invasion of the tonsils and pharynx by fusobacteria is occasionally primary, especially in immunosuppressed individuals; however, it also develops secondary to acute gingivitis ("trench mouth") caused by the same organism.

The characteristic lesion in the throat or on the tonsils is a gray membrane, which, when removed, reveals an ulcer (see Fig. 13–5*C*). The membrane may be extensive, covering the tonsils and entire pharyngeal mucosa, or may be present on only one tonsil. There is an odor typical of the growth of anaerobes. The temperature may be only mildly elevated but may reach as high as 39.4 to 40° C (103 to 104° F) when extensive and severe infection is present. Such cases of severe infection may be potentially life-threatening: Extensive necrosis of pharyngeal tissue may occur and be followed by perforation of the carotid artery and death from exsanguination. Other complications result from the spread of the organisms into the lung, with development of anaerobic pulmonary abscess, or to the genitalia, producing gangrenous balanitis or vulvovaginitis.

The diagnosis of Plaut-Vincent angina is established by the demonstration of large numbers of thin, cigar-shaped, gram-negative rods in Gram-stained smears or by the growth of large numbers of *F. plauti-vincenti* on anaerobic cultures.

F. plauti-vincenti is sensitive to penicillin G and the tetracycline compounds. Mild cases can be successfully treated by the oral administration of either of these antibiotics. Patients in whom the infection involves the pharyngeal tissues extensively, and who appear severely ill, should be hospitalized. Treatment is with 10 to 20 million units of penicillin G given intravenously or, if the patient is allergic to penicillin, with 2 g/day of a tetracycline compound (intravenous administration may be necessary when the disease is very severe). The eating utensils used by patients must be boiled to avoid spread to other members of a group or family.

Ludwig's Angina. This infection, caused by streptococci and oral anaerobes, is characterized by fever; tense, brawny swelling of the neck or submandibular tissues, which may develop a "woody" consistency; elevation and tenderness of the floor of the mouth; and, in severe cases, progressive obstruction of the airway as the tongue is pushed toward the roof of the mouth by the swelling of the sublingual tissues. Maintenance of the airway is the most important aspect of management and often requires tracheostomy. Although antibiotics must be given, incision and drainage of the submandibular areas is usually needed.

Others. *N. meningitidis* may produce infection restricted to the pharynx; about 50% of patients with meningococcal bacteremia or meningitis have a sore throat for between 2 and 10 days before the meningeal symptoms and signs become apparent. Note, however, that isolation of *N. meningitidis* from the pharynx is not diagnostic of infection: a carrier state is not uncommon.

Syphilis may produce pharyngitis. The primary luetic lesion, the painless chancre, may be present on the posterior wall of the pharynx in patients who kiss people with syphilitic oral lesions or who engage in fellatio with individuals with genital lesions. During the secondary stage of infection, characteristic "mucous patches"—silver-gray erosions surrounded by a red border—may be present on the buccal mucosa, pharyngeal mucosa, tongue, and palate.

Tuberculosis may produce multiple pale or white shallow ulcers of the pharynx or larynx, usually as a complication of pulmonary disease.

Staphylococcus aureus is not responsible for acute pharyngitis in normal individuals. Rarely, it may produce disease in immunosuppressed patients, especially those with severe granulocytopenia.

Diplococcus pneumoniae is a rare cause of pharyngitis. Recovery of this organism in a culture of the pharynx does not establish its involvement in infection, because the carrier rate may be quite high, especially during the colder months of the year.

Gram-negative enteric bacteria such as *Escherichia coli, Klebsiella pneumoniae,* and *Pseudomonas aeruginosa* may be isolated from the throats of patients treated with various antibiotics. The presence of such bacteria usually indicates a change in the pharyngeal microflora induced by an antimicrobial agent, *not* a true suprainfection. It is very difficult, in fact, to prove that these organisms ever are responsible for acute pharyngitis.

Yersinia enterocolitica has been associated with pharyngitis in a large multistate epidemic of milk-borne yersiniosis.[44] The patients were all adults and did not have prominent enteritis. Most patients were febrile and had a leukocytosis, an erythematous or exudative pharyngitis, and anterior cervical adenitis. Some strains of *Yersinia* grow on MacConkey's agar. Others may be more fastidious.

Candidiasis may produce acute stomatopharyngitis in immunocompetent persons treated with antimicrobial agents, especially broad-spectrum ones. Candidiasis of the oral cavity may be an early sign of the acquired immunodeficiency syndrome (AIDS).[45] The characteristic lesions are very shallow ulcers covered with a white exudate; they may be quite painful.

Corynebacterium hemolyticum was the etiologic agent in 0.4% of cases of pharyngitis in one large series from Seattle.[46] In most cases, a scarlatiniform rash involving the trunk and extremities was seen. Thus, in the rare patient presenting with pharyngitis and a scarlatiniform rash, *C. hemolyticum* as well as the streptococcus must be considered as possible agents. *C. hemolyticum* is sensitive to penicillin and erythromycin.

Unusual Forms of Viral Pharyngitis

Acute pharyngitis may be produced by a variety of viruses in addition to those commonly causing upper respiratory tract infections. Coxsackievirus type A causes *herpangina,* which is most often found in children. The disease is characterized by a cluster of small vesicles (1 to 2 mm) often limited to one area of the soft palate or pharynx (see Fig. 13–5*D*). When the lesions rupture, small, shallow ulcers with gray centers and red margins remain.

Vesicular lesions are also present in *hand-foot-and-mouth disease,* also caused by a coxsackievirus type A. The lesions of this infection are larger than those of herpangina. They usually do not appear on the pharyngeal mucosa but are widely distributed on the tongue, mouth, gingiva, and soft and hard palates. As indicated by the name of the disease, similar vesicles develop on the skin over the dorsal and periungual areas of the fingers and toes. Both herpangina and hand-foot-and-mouth disease are self-limited and are characterized by fever, malaise, sore throat, coryza, and nausea; an exanthem is present in some instances.

Herpesvirus infection may produce diffuse gingivostomatopharyngitis. In the affected patient, many vesicles are present on the pharyngeal mucosa, buccal mucosa, gingiva, and tongue. Pain is often very severe. Fever is consistently present and may be as high as 40.5° C (105° F). Severe dysphagia occurs in some cases and is related to involvement of the esophagus, in which vesicular lesions are also present. Encephalitis is an occasional complication. If *uncomplicated,* herpetic gingivostomatopharyngitis usually lasts for about 1 week. The value of acyclovir is not well established but seems appropriate in severe cases (see Chapter 69).

The cause of *aphthous ulcers* has not been established. These lesions are initially vesicular and rapidly rupture, producing shallow, red, and very painful ulcers. Recurrences are common. Fever is usually low grade or, most often, absent.

Oral Lesions That Should Be Distinguished from Pharyngitis

Lingual tonsillitis, a clinical variant of streptococcal infection, is characterized by severe discomfort on swallowing, especially on moving the tongue; however, no sore throat or physical evidence of pharyngitis is present. This disease is due to infection of the lymphoid tissue situated on the most posterolateral aspects of the tongue. Pulling the tongue forward will disclose swollen, reddened lingual tonsils, in the crypts of which yellow, soft exudate is present. Uncommonly, viral infection may produce the same syndrome.

Diseases of the gingiva—including periodontal disease and gingival hyperplasia—that result from any longstanding irritation (e.g., from the use of phenytoin or ill-fitting dentures) should not be overlooked (see Chapter 14). Periodontal disease begins with a nonspecific gingivitis manifested by bleeding or swollen gums and may progress to pyorrhea with regression of the gums, exposing the roots of teeth. Dental intervention for periodontal disease is effective when appropriate management is instituted early.

It is important not to overlook tumors and leukoplakia when examining patients complaining of oral lesions (see Chapter 14). White lesions of the buccal mucosa, gingiva, lips, or tongue that are thick and plaque-like and that can be palpated represent *leukoplakia.* These need to be distinguished from the painless, lace-like, white lesions of the buccal mucosa that occur in *lichen planus.* As for *tumors,* oropharyngeal carcinomas most often involve the lower lip, the side or undersurface of the tongue, the palate, the tonsils, and the tonsillar pillars. Slow-growing and often multicentric, nodular, or ulcerative, the lesions usually are visible on inspection but sometimes are palpable only as an indurated area.

Postnasal drip from rhinitis or infected sinuses may cause chronic irritation of the pharynx. One should not mistake gray streaks in the mucus in the posterior pharynx for an exudate. In fact, postnasal drip is more common than asthma, chronic bronchitis, or gastroesophageal reflux as a cause of persistent unexplained cough.[47]

Pharyngitis of Unknown Cause

A number of studies have failed to demonstrate a bacterial or viral cause of pharyngitis in 15 to 40% of patients with symptoms severe enough to seek medical care.[1, 2, 26]

Viral infections, in particular, are likely to have been more common than was suggested by these studies. Although the serologic tests employed are more sensitive than cultures for many viral causes of respiratory infection, false-negative results may occur. Furthermore, serologic methods are inadequate for diagnosing infection with the rhinoviruses, enteroviruses, and coronaviruses. Nevertheless, many of these studies also employed viral cultures and still failed to isolate a viral agent.

My suspicion is that currently unrecognized or undiscovered infectious respiratory pathogens may cause pharyngitis. Also, noninfectious causes of pharyngeal inflammation may produce the symptom of a sore throat. Such causes could include physical agents—through a direct irritative effect. This could occur from mouth breathing, hyperventilation, smoking, or excessive coffee intake. Other noninfectious causes may include a local allergic response to inhaled allergens and systemic vasculitis. Indeed, one report highlights the fact that a sore throat (along with cough and hoarseness) may be an associated symptom in 9% and the presenting symptom in 4%, of patients with giant cell arteritis.[48] It is thought that this symptom is a manifestation of inflammation in the arteries supplying the pharyngeal tissues, just as the symptoms of headache, jaw claudication, and scalp tenderness in giant cell arteritis are attributed to a similar pathogenetic process.

CORYZA SYNDROME

Many episodes of upper respiratory tract infection consist of coryza: rhinorrhea, sneezing, low-grade fever, moderate malaise, and occasionally diffuse myalgias. A cough usually represents clearing of upper respiratory tract secretions, which are colorless, thin, and translucent, rather than lower respiratory tract infection. The patient may have a sore throat but often does not.

The agents responsible for coryza are almost always viral: the rhinoviruses (the commonest cause of the "common cold"), coronaviruses, respiratory syncytial virus, and adenovirus. The clinical features of viral infections may include exudative pharyngitis, enlarged and tender cervical lymph nodes, fever (as high as 39.4° C [103° F] in some cases), generalized myalgia, and fatigue. However, in most instances, and especially in adults, the clinical picture consists only of moderate-to-severe nasal congestion with watery discharge (coryza), "scratchy" sore throat, low-grade or no fever, and mild headache and myalgia. The incubation period is 24 to 72 hours. High-grade fever and severe exudative pharyngitis are prominent features of respiratory infection produced by adenovirus. Bronchitis occurs in 1 to 2% of adults with antecedent upper respiratory tract infections. Invasion by parainfluenza virus tends to cause hoarseness and cough (laryngotracheobronchitis) that persist for a longer period than the 3 to 4 days characteristic of respiratory infection produced by other viruses. Bronchiolitis and bronchopneumonia are much more common in children than in older individuals.

LARYNGOTRACHEITIS

Most cases of laryngotracheitis are viral in origin (see Chapter 17). The primary symptoms of laryngotracheitis are hoarseness, a "croupy" cough, and, if the disease is severe, inspiratory stridor. Such stridor generally is absent in adults, whose main problem may be an episode of choking on waking from sleep; this is usually caused by a plug of thick, viscous sputum in the trachea or larynx. Fever of appreciable degree is not typical of viral infection of the larynx and trachea. Treatment of children with humidified air and oxygen usually suffices. Almost all adults with laryngotracheitis recover spontaneously; however, hoarseness and irritative coughing may persist for several weeks. Tracheostomy is rarely required in adults and is only occasionally necessary in children.

ACUTE EPIGLOTTITIS (Supraglottitis)

The bacterium that most often causes acute epiglottitis (supraglottitis) (see Chapter 17), especially in children, is type B *H. influenzae;* however, *Diplococcus pneumoniae, Streptococcus pyogenes,* and *Staphylococcus aureus* occasionally may also produce epiglottitis.

In acute epiglottitis, hoarseness develops quickly and is followed by rapidly progressing symptoms of airway obstruction. The patient's temperature usually is elevated and may reach as high as 40° C (104° F). The patient will not respond to a humidified environment. Because obstruction of the airway may become life-threatening with dramatic suddenness, the patient with epiglottitis must be watched constantly. The most diagnostic finding is direct visualization of the epiglottis on depressing the tongue; the epiglottis will be seen to be inflamed and enlarged and to protrude up into the hypopharynx (sometimes called the "rising sun sign").

A significant number of patients will require an airway because of the tremendous swelling of the tissues. Endotracheal intubation may be difficult, though it can usually be accomplished (see Chapter 17); manipulation of the epiglottis by a laryngoscope, a tube, or even a culture swab may provoke laryngeal spasm, asphyxia, and cardiac arrest. Radiographic study of the neck may help diagnostically by revealing the enlarged epiglottis (Fig. 13–8). Parenteral treatment with antibiotics is mandatory. Chloramphenicol, ampicillin, or cephalothin are all acceptable antimicrobial agents, with chloramphenicol clearly superior in some communities.

It may be difficult to distinguish early acute epiglottitis from early acute laryngotracheitis, particularly when only hoarseness or stridor, with little elevation of temperature, is present. If the diagnosis is suspected but not definitely confirmed by physical examination or by radiography, direct laryngoscopy may be performed in an operating room after all preparations have been made for intubation or, if necessary, tracheostomy.

ALGORITHMS FOR INITIAL MANAGEMENT OF A PATIENT WITH A SORE THROAT

In the preceding discussion, we have considered separately each of the disease entities that may produce a sore throat. However, the clinician seeing a patient with sore throat of uncertain cause must employ a management strategy that considers all possible causes of pharyngitis, orders diagnostic tests efficiently, and makes initial treatment decisions (before diagnostic test results have returned) wisely.

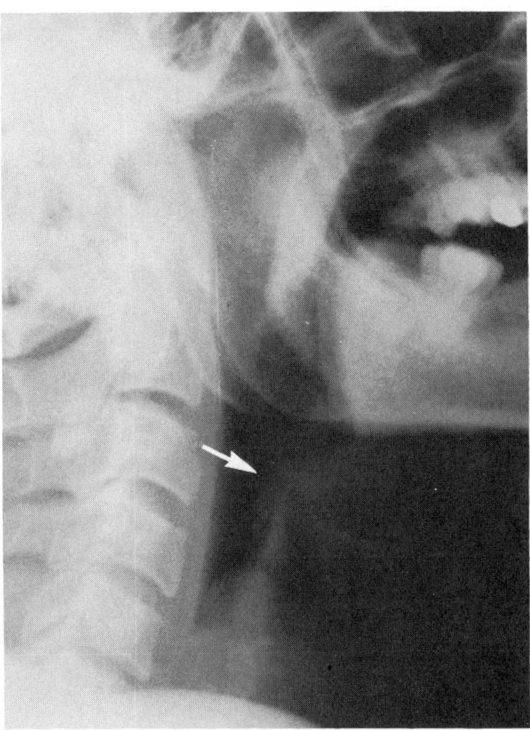

FIGURE 13–8. Acute epiglottitis. A lateral radiograph of the neck reveals massive swelling of the epiglottis in a patient with acute epiglottitis caused by *Haemophilus influenzae*.

Figures 13–9, 13–10 and 13–11 present three algorithms that serve as a generally applicable guide to the care of most patients. Of course, no such algorithms should be binding in the care of an individual patient. These algorithms attempt a synthesis of many of the key points made earlier. First (see Fig. 13–9), the clinician is advised to consider unusual, high-risk causes and complications of pharyngitis. Then (see Fig. 13–10), the clinician is advised to consider several more common causes of pharyngitis, which frequently may be overlooked. Finally (see Fig. 13–11), the clinician is provided with a simple strategy for the diagnosis and treatment of group A streptococcal pharyngitis.

Symptomatic Treatment. When no treatable form of infection is suspected, and the patient is not sufficiently ill to warrant further diagnostic tests or observation, symptomatic therapy may be indicated.

Painful sore throat or fever generally can be treated with acetylsalicylic acid (aspirin) or acetaminophen (Tylenol). Patients may be advised to gargle with warm salt water (1 level teaspoon of salt in 1 pint of warm water) for symptomatic relief and to rest at home until they feel improved. Except for those with laryngotracheo-bronchitis, which may persist for several weeks, most patients with infections of the upper respiratory tract experience their illness for only a few days.

Decongestants should be prescribed when there is a history of intermittent pain in the paranasal sinuses or "stuffiness" of the ears. Systemic decongestants have the advantage of longer duration of action and less rebound. Longer-acting, systemic decongestants such as phenylephrine and phenylpropanolamine (Dimetapp), given twice daily for 1 or 2 weeks, may be required when severe congestion, otitis media, or purulent sinusitis is present. Antihistamines (chlorpheniramine, 4 mg orally four times a day, or brompheniramine [in Dimetapp], 4 mg twice daily) are also commonly administered to reduce congestion, sneezing, and nasal discharge. Results of a randomized study in which one group of patients was given chlorpheniramine and another group a placebo revealed that the use of chlorpheniramine produced a statistically significant improvement in sneezing, nasal discharge, and blowing of the nose. However, the clinical benefits of such use for individual patients with infections of the upper respiratory tract were limited because the symptoms had decreased sharply in both groups of patients after 36 hours.[49]

Topical decongestants are rapidly effective and generally do not aggravate hypertension or arrhythmias; however, if used for longer than a week, they may produce *rhinitis medicamentosa* owing to rebound congestion. For patients with mild nasal congestion, it is reasonable to prescribe a 2- to 3-day course of oxymetazoline hydrochloride nasal spray (Afrin) three times daily. Patients should be instructed to inhale the drug, wait for 1 minute, and then reinhale a second dose of the drug; the first dose shrinks the partially congested turbinates sufficiently to permit the second dose to reach the nasopharynx.

ACKNOWLEDGMENTS

I am deeply grateful to my colleagues Louis Weinstein, MD, and William T. Branch Jr, MD. They wrote this chapter in the first edition, and I have borrowed liberally from

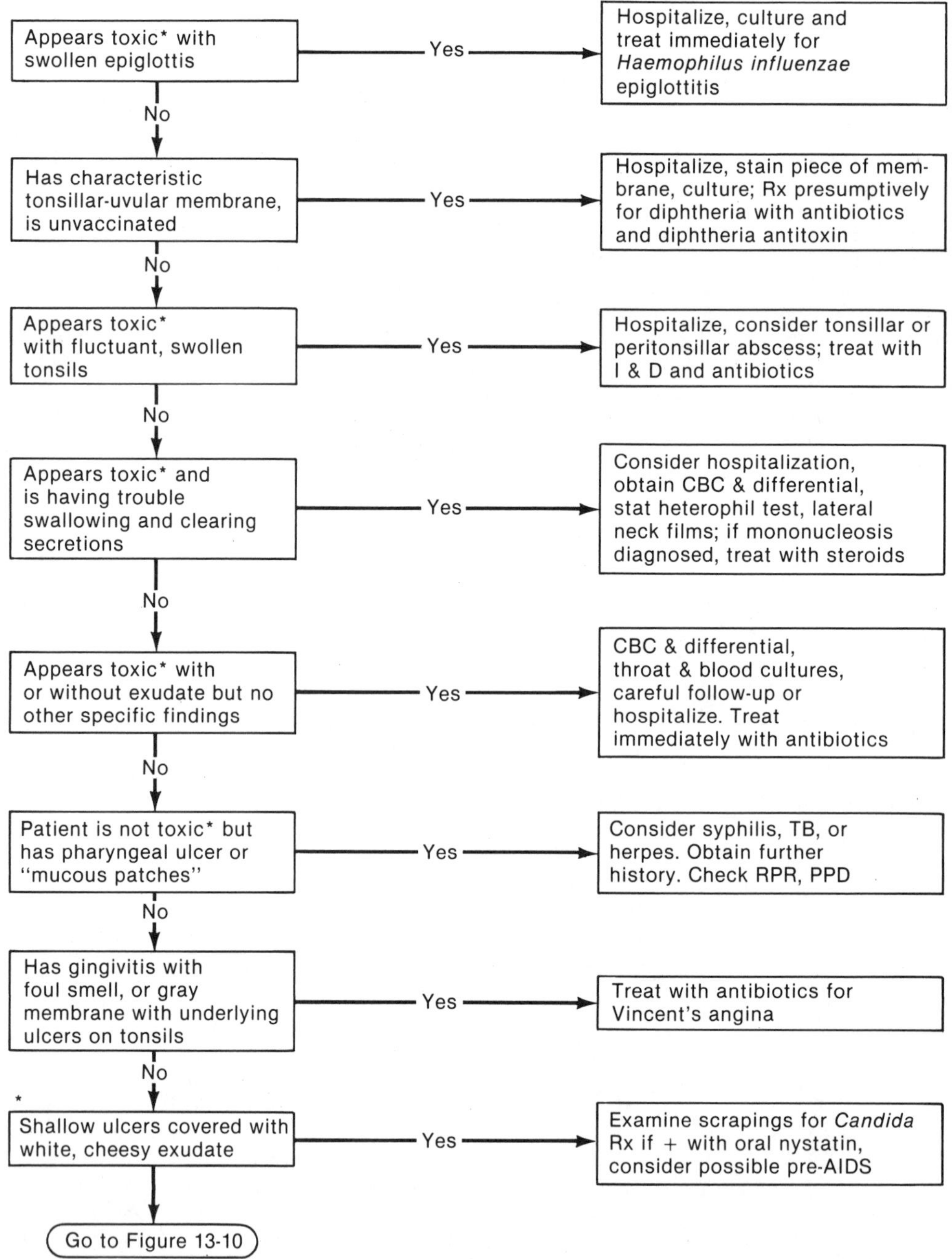

FIGURE 13–9. Algorithm describing an evaluation for unusual, high-risk conditions.* *Toxic* refers to the finding of high fever, prostration, tachycardia, thready pulse, and so on. (Immediate treatment is preferred for those individuals whose throat culture results will not be complete for 9 days into the illness, since treatment after that time has not been shown to be protective against rheumatic fever.)

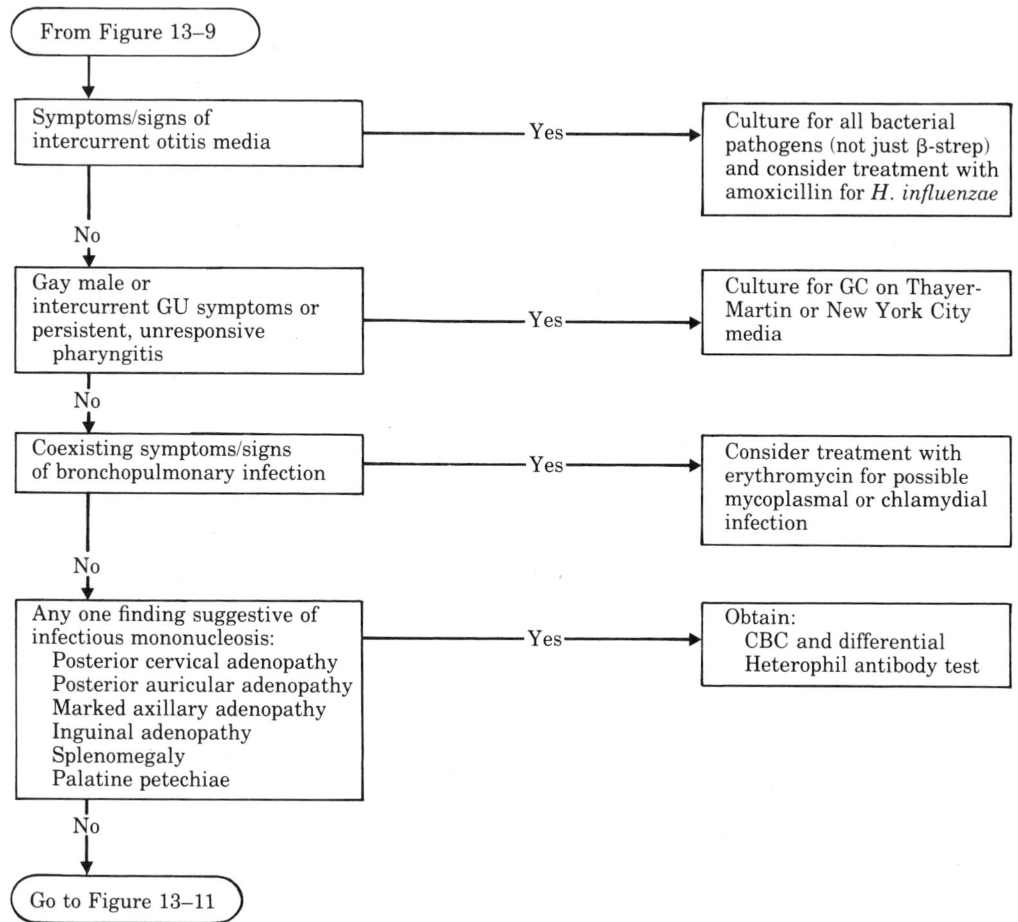

FIGURE 13–10. Algorithm describing an evaluation of more common nonstreptococcal causes of pharyngitis.

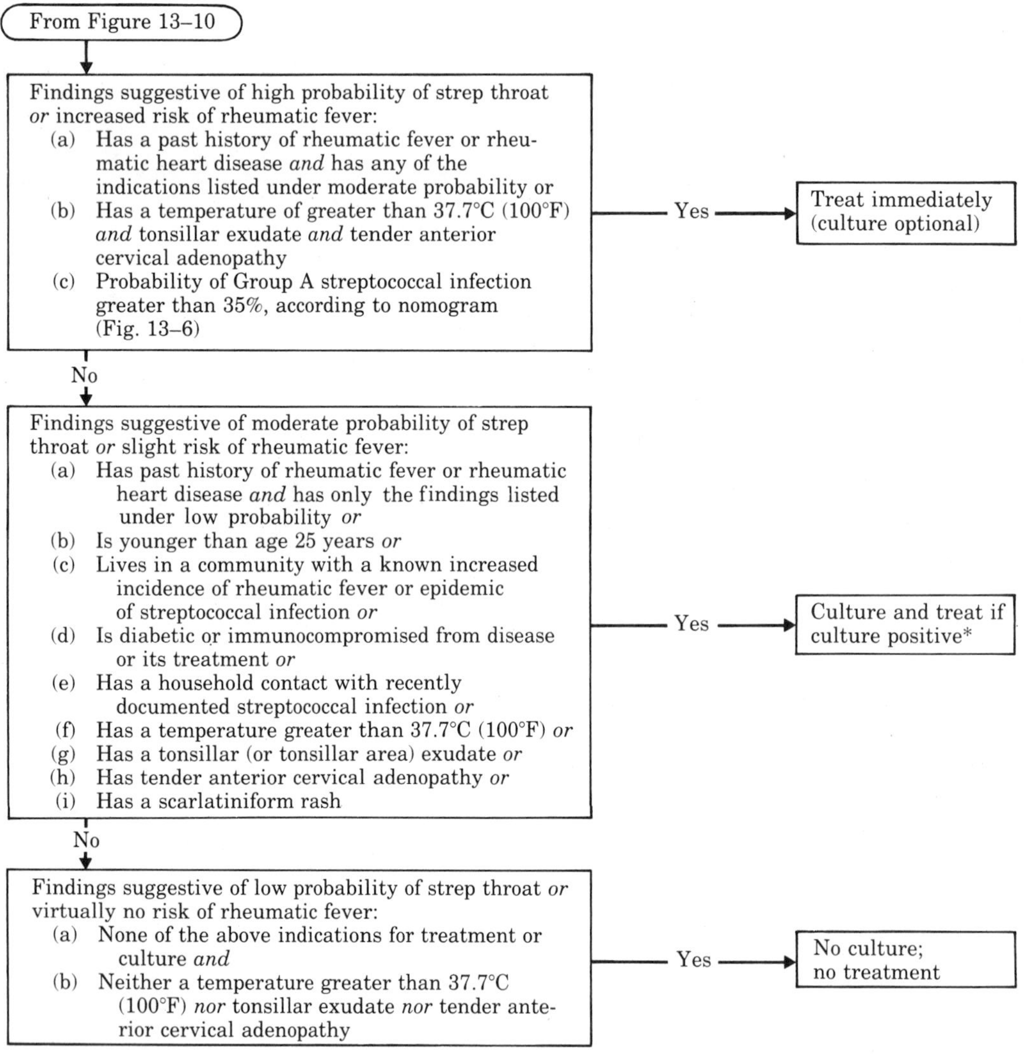

FIGURE 13–11. Algorithm describing an evaluation of the probability of group A streptococcal pharyngitis and the risk of developing acute rheumatic fever.

their vivid descriptions of the uncommon causes and complications of this common syndrome.

REFERENCES

1. Komaroff AL, Aronson MD, Pass TM, et al: Serologic evidence of chlamydial and mycoplasmal pharyngitis in adults. Science 222:927, 1983.
2. Glezen WP, Clyde WA, and Senior RJ: Group A streptococci, mycoplasmas, and viruses associated with acute pharyngitis. JAMA 202:455, 1967.
3. Kaplan EL, Top FH, and Dudding BA: Diagnosis of streptococcal pharyngitis: Differentiation of active infection from the carrier state in the symptomatic child. J Infect Dis 123:490, 1971.
4. Crawford G, Brancato F, and Holmes KK: Streptococcal pharyngitis: Diagnosis by Gram stain. Ann Intern Med 90:293, 1979.
5. Centor RM, Witherspoon JM, Dalton HP, et al: The diagnosis of strep throat in adults in the emergency room. Med Dec Making 1:239, 1981.
6. Walsh BT, Bookheim WW, Johnson RC, et al: Recognition of streptococcal pharyngitis in adults. Arch Intern Med 135:1493, 1975.
7. Komaroff AL, Pass TM, Aronson MD, et al: The prediction of streptococcal pharyngitis in adults. J Gen Intern Med 1:1, 1986.
8. Komaroff AL: A management strategy for sore throat. JAMA 239:1429, 1978.
9. Bisno AL and Stollerman GH: Laboratory Diagnostic Procedures in the Rheumatic Diseases. Boston, Little Brown, 1975.
10. Rapid office diagnostic tests for streptococcal pharyngitis. Med Lett 27:49, 1985.
11. Wegner DL, Witte DL, and Schrantz RD: Insensitivity of rapid antigen detection methods and single blood agar plate culture for diagnosing streptococcal pharyngitis. JAMA 267:695, 1992.
12. Denny FW, Wannamaker LW, Brink WR, et al: Prevention of rheumatic fever. JAMA 143:151, 1950.
13. Gordis L: Effectiveness of comprehensive care programs in preventing rheumatic fever. N Engl J Med 289:331, 1973.
14. Bisno AL: Group A streptococcal infections and acute rheumatic fever. N Engl J Med 325:783, 1991.
15. Kaplan EL, Bisno A, and Derrick W: Prevention of rheumatic fever. Circulation 55:51, 1977.
16. Meier FA, Centor RM, Graham L, and Dalton HP: Clinical and microbiological evidence for endemic pharyngitis among adults due to Group C streptococci. Arch Intern Med 150:825, 1990.
17. Turner JC, Hayden GF, Kiselica D, et al: Association of Group C β-hemolytic streptococci with endemic pharyngitis among college students. JAMA 264:2644, 1990.
18. Govil MK, Agrawal BD, Lal MM, et al: A study of acute respiratory diseases with special reference to *Mycoplasma pneumoniae* infections. J Assoc Phys India 23:297, 1975.
19. Mogabgab WJ: *Mycoplasma pneumoniae* and adenovirus respiratory illnesses in military and university personnel, 1959–1966. Am Rev Respir Dis 97:345, 1968.
20. Evans AS, Allen V, and Sueltmann S: *Mycoplasma pneumoniae* infections in University of Wisconsin students. Am Rev Respir Dis 96:237, 1967.
21. Evatt BL, Dowdle WR, Johnson M, et al: Epidemic mycoplasmal pneumonia. N Engl J Med 385:372, 1971.
22. Shames JM, George RB, Holliday WB, et al: Comparison of antibiotics in the treatment of mycoplasmal pneumonia. Arch Intern Med 125:680, 1970.
23. Wenzel RP, Hendley JO, Dodd WK, et al: Comparison of josamycin and erythromycin in the therapy of *Mycoplasma pneumoniae.* Antimicrob Agents Chemother 10:899, 1976.
24. McDonald CJ, Tierney WM, Hui SL, et al: A controlled trial of erythromycin in adults with nonstreptococcal pharyngitis. J Infect Dis 152:1093, 1985.
25. Jones RB, Rabinovitch RA, Katz BP, et al: *Chlamydia trachomatis* in the pharynx and rectum of heterosexual patients at risk for genital infection. Ann Intern Med 102:757, 1985.
26. Huovinen P, Lahtonen R, Ziegler T, et al: Pharyngitis in adults: The presence and coexistence of viruses and bacterial organisms. Ann Intern Med 110:612, 1989.
27. Grayston JT, Kuo C, Wang S-P, et al: A new *Chlamydia psittaci* strain, TWAR, isolated in acute respiratory infections. N Engl J Med 315:161, 1986.
28. Marrie TJ, Grayston JT, Wang S-P, et al: Pneumonia associated with the TWAR strain of chlamydia. Ann Intern Med 106:507, 1987.
29. Grayston JT, Campbell LA, Kuo C-C, et al: A new respiratory tract pathogen: *Chlamydiae pneumoniae strain TWAR.* J Infect Dis 161:618, 1990.
30. Beem MO and Saxon EM: Respiratory-tract colonization and a distinctive pneumonia syndrome in infants infected with *Chlamydia trachomatis.* N Engl J Med 296:306, 1977.
31. Komaroff AL, Aronson MD, and Schachter J: *Chlamydia trachomatis* infection in adults with community-acquired pneumonia. JAMA 245:1319, 1981.
32. Tam MR, Stamm WE, Handsfield HH, et al: Culture-independent diagnosis of *Chlamydia trachomatis* using monoclonal antibodies. N Engl J Med 310:1146, 1984.
33. Bridger RC: *Haemophilus influenzae:* The relationship to upper respiratory tract infection. N Z Med J 80:19, 1974.
34. Aronson MD, Komaroff AL, Pass TM, et al: Heterophil antibody in adults with sore throat: Frequency and clinical presentation. Ann Intern Med 96:505, 1982.
35. Evans AS, Niederman JC, Cenabre LC, et al: A prospective evaluation of heterophil- and Epstein-Barr virus–specific IgM antibody tests in clinical and subclinical infectious mononucleosis: Specificity and sensitivity of the tests and persistence of antibody. J Infect Dis 132:546, 1975.
36. Komaroff AL, Aronson MD, Pass TM, et al: Prevalence of pharyngeal gonorrhea in general medical patients with sore throat. Sex Transm Dis 7:116, 1980.
37. Wiesner PJ, Tronca E, Bonin P, et al: Clinical spectrum of pharyngeal gonococcal infection. N Engl J Med 288:181, 1973.
38. Bro-Jorgensen A and Jensen T: Gonococcal pharyngeal infections. Report of 110 cases. Br J Vener Dis 49:491, 1973.
39. Wiesner PJ: Gonococcal pharyngeal infection. Clin Obstet Gynecol 18:121, 1975.
40. Shahidullah M: Pharyngeal gonorrhea in homosexuals. Br J Vener Dis 52:168, 1976.
41. Granato PA, Schneible-Smith C, and Weiner LB: Use of New York City medium for improved recovery of *Neisseria gonorrhoeae* from clinical specimens. J Clin Microbiol 13:963, 1981.
42. McCloskey RV, Eller JJ, Green M, et al: The 1970 epidemic of diphtheria in San Antonio. Ann Intern Med 75:495, 1971.
43. Sargent RK, Rossing TH, Dowton SB, et al: Diphtheria immunity in Massachusetts—A study of three urban patient populations. Am J Med Sci 287:37, 1984.
44. Tacket CO, Davis BR, Carter GP, et al: *Yersinia enterocolitica* pharyngitis. Ann Intern Med 99:40, 1983.
45. Klein RS, Harris CA, Small CB, et al: Oral candidiasis in high-risk patients as the initial manifestation of the acquired immunodeficiency syndrome. N Engl J Med 311:354, 1984.
46. Miller RA, Brancato F, and Holmes KK: *Corynebacterium hemolyticum* as a cause of pharyngitis and scarlatiniform rash in young adults. Ann Intern Med 105:867, 1986.
47. Irwin RS, Corrao WM, and Pratter MR: Chronic persistent cough in the adult: The spectrum and frequency of causes and successful outcome of specific therapy. Am Rev Respir Dis 123:413, 1981.
48. Larson TS, Hall S, Hepper NGG, et al: Respiratory tract symptoms as a clue to giant cell arteritis. Ann Intern Med 101:594, 1984.
49. Howard JC, Kantner TR, Lilienfeld LS, et al: Effectiveness of antihistamines in the symptomatic management of the common cold. JAMA 227:1278, 1979.

14

Lesions of the Mouth

STEPHEN T. SONIS, DMD, DMSc

EXAMINATION OF THE MOUTH

Examination of the mouth should be performed in a comfortable environment with adequate lighting. An orderly, step-by-step routine minimizes the chances of forgetting some aspect of the examination. After the lips, buccal and labial mucosa, and hard and soft palate, the oral pharynx is examined. This is most easily accomplished by having the patient relax the tongue and then pushing it down and forward with a tongue blade. Such a technique offers an excellent view of the oral pharynx and minimizes the likelihood of the patient's gagging.

The tongue and floor of the mouth are best examined by grasping the tongue with a 2 × 2-inch gauze sponge and pulling it gently forward, upward and laterally. Both areas should also be palpated bimanually by placing one hand within the mouth while the other hand provides opposing pressure. The salivary glands should be palpated, and the ducts should be observed for clear, copious, painless salivary flow. Breath odor should be noted.

The extraoral examination should include observation of facial symmetry. The submental, submandibular, and cervical areas should be palpated for lymphadenopathy. This can be done easily from either the front or the rear of the patient's head.

Following examination of the soft tissues, the gingiva and teeth should be evaluated to identify periodontal disease, caries, or developmental problems. Normal gingiva is firm, pink, and stippled and does not bleed spontaneously or on provocation. Gingival swelling, edema, rolling, or drainage is a sign of periodontal disease. Tooth mobility may be checked by gently trying to rock each tooth against a tongue blade placed firmly against the teeth. Mobility or flaring of the teeth suggests periodontal disease. A lack of attached gingiva predisposes to gingival recession and alveolar bone loss. The presence of high frenula, especially in children, should be noted as these may cause orthodontic problems later; early intervention may prevent this.

An assessment of oral hygiene should be established. Poor oral hygiene is the most frequent cause of periodontal disease and is associated with increased frequency of a variety of other oral diseases, including carcinoma. Gingival inflammatory changes or periodontal disease in the absence of local factors such as bacterial plaque or calculus strongly suggests a systemic component to the oral condition. Any sign of periodontal disease warrants referral to a general dentist or periodontist.

Teeth should be observed for overall alignment. Caries appears as brownish areas and can destroy large areas of the teeth. Normal teeth are not sensitive to percussion. Thus, if a periapical abscess is suspected, tapping on the tooth with a tongue blade usually elicits pain. The orifices of draining fistulas are often present high in the mucobuccal fold near the apex of the roots of infected teeth. Caries, percussion sensitivity, or fistulas require definitive dental therapy.

ADJUNCTIVE TECHNIQUES FOR DIAGNOSIS

Biopsy

Most oral lesions can be definitively diagnosed by histologic examination. This is a requirement when dealing with suspected malignancy. The pathologist's expertise is also valuable in diagnosing vesiculobullous diseases, specific infections, and white and pigmented lesions. With few exceptions, a biopsy of an oral lesion is a safe, easy, and reliable way to assist in making a definitive diagnosis. The risks of biopsy are minimal and are far outweighed by the consequences of an incorrect or inadequate diagnosis. Almost all diagnostic biopsies are technically within the realm of the general dental practitioner, although it may be prudent to refer the patient to a specialist for biopsies of lesions involving the floor of the mouth or a salivary duct.

Exfoliative Cytology

Cytologic smears have limited value in the diagnosis of oral lesions. If a lesion is suspicious enough for a smear, it should be biopsied; one study demonstrated a 15% false-negative rate of smears of patients with malignancies proved by biopsy. Cytologic smears can be used as a screening device when many patients are examined over a short period. Smears may also be helpful in the diagnosis of viral or fungal infections and certain vesiculobullous diseases, such as pemphigus vulgaris.

Immunofluorescence

Immunofluorescent testing, using sera or biopsies, may play a significant role in the diagnosis and assessment of autoimmune diseases, including pemphigus vulgaris, pemphigoid, systemic lupus erythematosus, and lichen planus.

DEVELOPMENTAL LESIONS AND NORMAL VARIANTS

A number of developmental anomalies affect the oral cavity. Most are of little or no pathologic or clinical significance and require no treatment. Frequently a patient will notice the presence of one of these conditions and become alarmed. The practitioner's role is to identify the lesions and inform and reassure the patient. The exceptions are anomalies that affect function or appearance, such as clefts. In this discussion, only the most common anomalies are mentioned.

Lip Pits. These are unilateral or bilateral areas of indentation at the commissures of the mouth and are considered hereditary in origin. They have no clinical significance unless they represent the extension of a fistula, in which case drainage may be present. Treatment is not generally required unless infection occurs; surgery is curative.

Ankyloglossia. An absent or short lingual frenum results in partial or complete ankyloglossia (Fig. 14–1). The former is most common. Lingual motion may be limited; the degree depends on the extent of the frenum. Speech may be compromised, especially the ability to pronounce consonants. Surgical separation of the frenum is simple and curative.

Bifid Uvula. This results from incomplete fusion of the posterior portion of the soft palate, which could indicate incomplete closure of the posterior border of the hard palate, resulting in a submucosal cleft palate. This defect can be diagnosed by having the patient say "ahh" to constrict the muscles over the posterior hard palate, thus allowing visualization of the underlying bone architecture. The major clinical significance of submucosal cleft palate lies in the potential difficulty of the patient to clear the eustachian tubes, which may result in frequent middle ear infections.

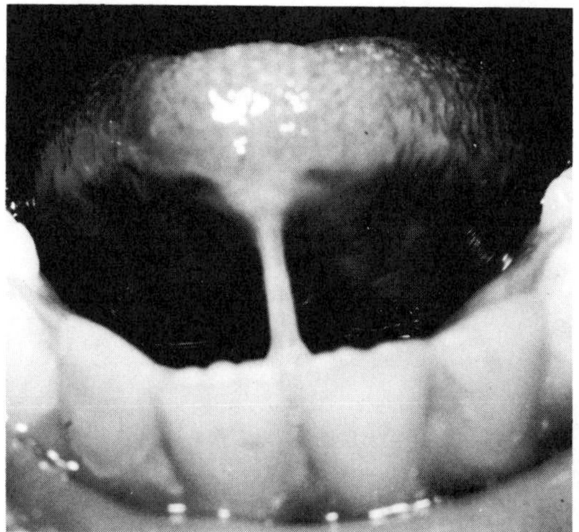

FIGURE 14–1. Ankyloglossia due to a lingual frenum, which severely inhibits motions of the tongue.

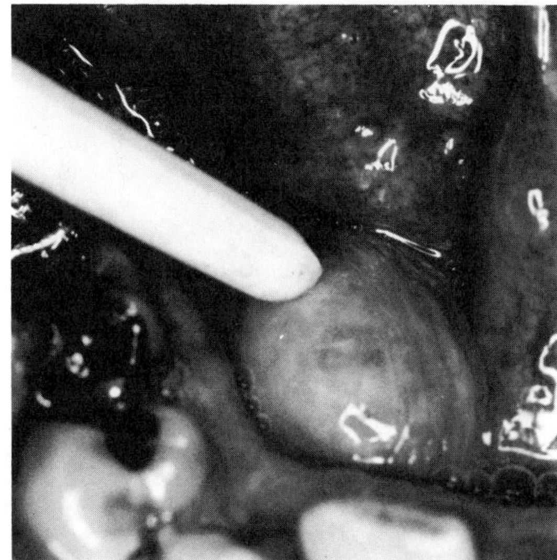

FIGURE 14–2. Torus mandibularis is demonstrated at the tip of the pointer.

Torus Palatinus and Torus Mandibularis. Tori are relatively frequent bone protuberances that occur most often on the lingual surfaces of the mandible and on the midline of the palate. They represent bone exostoses that are non-neoplastic developmental malformations. The overlying mucosal is normal but may sometimes be traumatized. Torus palatinus occurs in approximately 20% of the population. Clinical presentations vary widely, ranging from subtle bone enlargements of the midline of the hard palate to large knob-like protuberances in the same area.

Torus mandibularis (Fig. 14–2) is less common and occurs in only 6% of the population. Mandibular tori usually present as bilateral symmetrical enlargements on the lingual surfaces of the mandibular canines or premolars and range in appearance from subtle small nodules to large knob-like hard lobules.

Neither anomalies are of clinical significance unless the patient requires a prosthesis, in which case the tori may require surgical removal.

Glossitis Areata and Glossitis Migrans (Geographic Tongue). This is an inflammatory form of glossitis of unknown etiology. Localized areas of filiform papillae are rapidly lost and replaced by uneven areas of smooth lingual mucosa, which is often erythematous owing to hyperemia. The most common area of involvement is the dorsal surface of the tongue, although the lateral borders may be affected (Fig. 14–3). The fungiform papillae are exaggerated. The borders of the lesions are uneven, giving a geographic appearance, and may appear raised and whitish. No specific therapy exists, although palliation in the form of sprays, ointments, or rinses may be helpful in symptomatic cases.

Fissured Tongue. Fissuring of the tongue is a relatively common occurrence, in which congenital deep furrowing or fissures run trench-like on the dorsal surface of the tongue (Fig. 14–4). Frequently, fissured tongue is associated with geographic tongue. Fissures vary significantly in depth. The major clinical significance of fissuring is that debris can collect in the depths and create a chronic, slightly inflammatory condition that may manifest clinically as sensitivity to certain spicy foods. There is no specific therapy.

Fordyce Granules. These are common congenital "le-

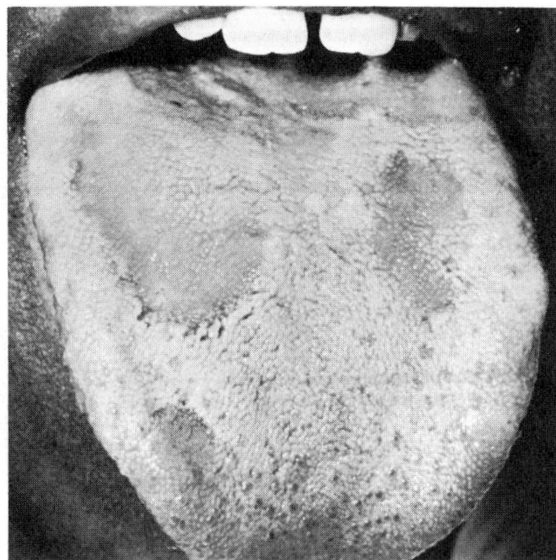

FIGURE 14–3. Geographic tongue. An irregular area of lost filiform papillae is noted on the dorsal surface of the tongue.

sions" caused by ectopic sebaceous glands on the buccal mucosa. Most commonly, the lesions are bilateral. They are generally asymptomatic and appear as raised, papillate, yellowish clumps on the mucosa (Fig. 14–5). They have no clinical significance.

Median Rhomboid Glossitis. This is a benign congenital defect thought to represent remnants of the tuberculum impar on the posterior midline of the tongue. Two clinical variations of median rhomboid glossitis have been described: One appears as a slightly depressed, oval or rhomboid reddish area on the posterior midline of the tongue; the other appears as a raised, tumor-like mass that is often pebbly and pinkish. The lesion is totally asymptomatic and is frequently incidentally recognized by the patient. No treatment is required once diagnosis has been made.

PERIODONTAL DISEASE

Anatomically, the periodontium consists of four structures that function to support teeth: the cementum, the periodontal ligament, the alveolar bone, and the gingiva (Fig. 14–6). Cementum is a bone-like mesenchymal substance that covers the surfaces of the roots of teeth. Collagenous fibers of the periodontal ligament attach to the cementum and thus bind the tooth to its socket in alveolar bone. Covering the alveolar bone is the gingiva, which also surrounds the necks of the teeth in a collar-like arrangement. The gingiva, which consists of squamous keratinized or parakeratinized epithelium and underlying fibrous connective tissue, attaches directly to the tooth at a level just below the junction of the crown and the root. The integrity of this attachment plays a major role in limiting the progression of gingival and periodontal disease.

Periodontal disease is one of the most common diseases in the United States, affecting approximately three of four adults. There are two major forms of the disease: gingivitis and periodontitis. Gingivitis represents the inflammatory response of the marginal and papillary gingiva to the local accumulation of tooth-borne bacteria (plaque). Gingivitis may be present alone or seen in conjunction with periodontitis in which there is destruction of bone and periodontal ligament. While bacteria play the major etiologic role in periodontitis, the disease process is multifactorial; it has been hypothesized that tooth-borne bacteria act as nonspecific polyclonal activators and cause lymphocyte proliferation and the release of a variety of biologically active cytokines, which result in the destruction of the periodontal ligament and the alveolar bone. The gingival attachment breaks down; its attachment follows the height of the alveolar bone. A pocket is thus formed, which prevents adequate removal of the bacterial plaque. The flora of the periodontal pocket undergo changes so that in the longstanding periodontal lesion, a variety of virulent endotoxin-producing organisms, is present.

The clinical manifestations of gingivitis are predominantly associated with the vascular changes accompanying inflammation. The most consistent symptom of gingivitis is bleeding on provocation, usually following eating or brushing. Additionally, edematous enlargement of the marginal and papillary tissue and sensitivity and loss of normal gingival architecture may be noted. The chronic presence of gingival inflammation may lead to fibrosis of the gingiva.

The soft tissue appearance of early periodontitis may be identical to that of gingivitis. Generally, early periodontitis is painless, although as the disease progresses sensitivity to sweets and thermal changes may develop as recession of gingiva exposes the sensitive root surface. Patients also may have a dull, throbbing discomfort after eating or upon

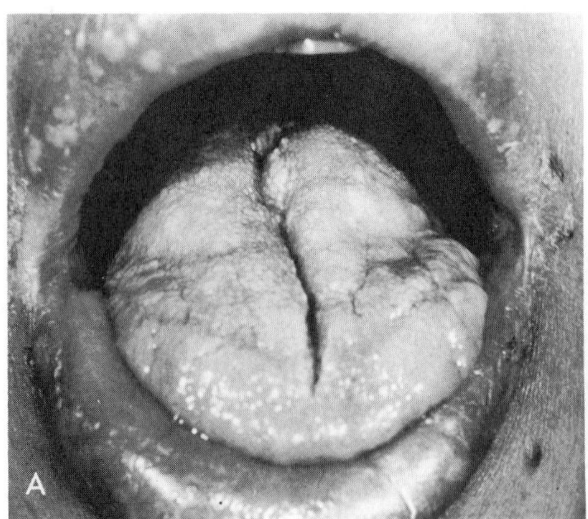

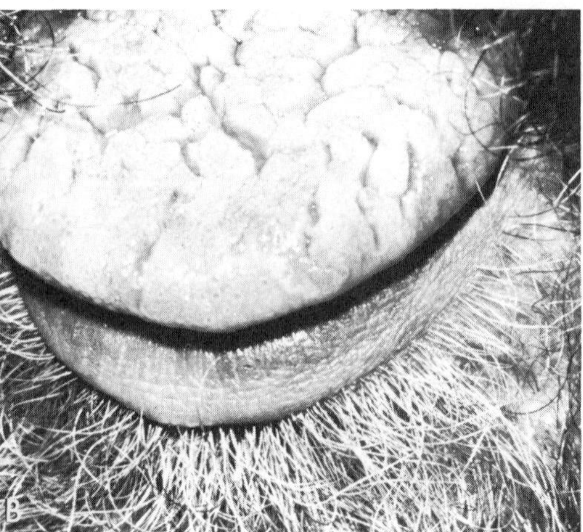

FIGURE 14–4. Fissured tongue.

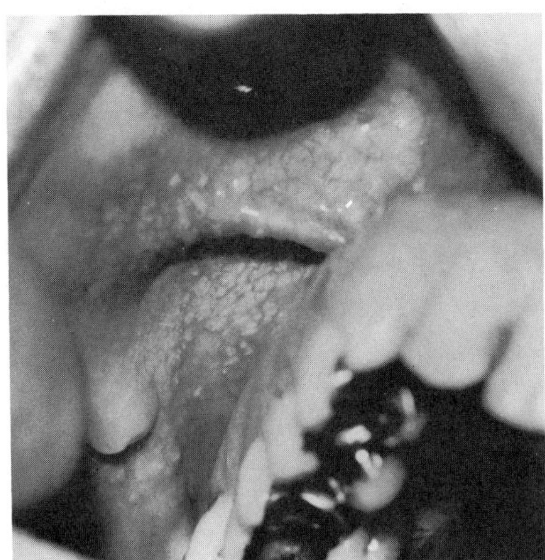

FIGURE 14–5. Fordyce granules: ectopic sebaceous glands.

arising. With loss of alveolar bone, tooth mobility may be noted. As pocket formation progresses, suppuration often develops, as well as halitosis or bad taste. Abscess formation may also be present. Ultimately, spontaneous tooth loss may occur.

The two most consistent factors related to the prevalence and severity of periodontal disease are the level of oral hygiene and age. A number of social factors such as race, sex, education, and income have been implicated in the epidemiology of periodontal disease, but their relevance is probably to patients' oral hygiene, diet, and access to dental care. The most important factor in the establishment and progression of periodontal disease is poor oral hygiene. Recent evidence suggests that cigarette use accelerates the progression of periodontal disease.

A strong correlation exists between the prevalence and severity of periodontal disease and age. Gingival inflammatory changes may be noted as early as 5 years of age and demonstrate a sudden increase in both severity and frequency with the eruption of the permanent dentition. Although wide variations exist in the reported frequency of gingivitis in children (from 11 to 90%), there is general agreement that most adolescents are affected by the disease.

Few adults are totally unaffected by periodontal disease. Evidence suggests that the destructive phase of periodontal disease (periodontitis) begins at approximately 35 years of age and takes about 20 years to reach the advanced phase without intervention. The severity increases with advancing age. The frequency of periodontitis with loss of periodontal attachment has been reported to be 20% in patients at age 15 years and 99% by age 50 years. Of the American adult population, it has been estimated that 75% have some form of periodontal disease and 25% demonstrate the destructive phase of the disease.

Recognition of periodontitis can be made most easily by observing the color and texture of the gingiva, by determining the mobility of the teeth simply by trying to rock them gently between two tongue blades, and by noting the level of oral hygiene and the presence of any oral suppuration. It is clear that effective removal of bacterial plaque at the early stages of the disease prevents its progression. Once the lesion of periodontal disease has been established, progressive loss of alveolar bone occurs. Tooth loss follows.

Treatment

Treatment of periodontitis is usually divided into three major phases: etiotropic, surgical, and maintenance.

The etiotropic phase is aimed at assessment and control of systemic factors that may affect the progression of disease, oral hygiene instruction that will allow the patient to control the accumulation of dental plaque, the removal of hard accretions from the root surfaces, elimination of gross occlusal disharmonies, and, at times, provisional stabilization of loose teeth. Such approaches are the mainstay for treatment of all forms of periodontal disease.

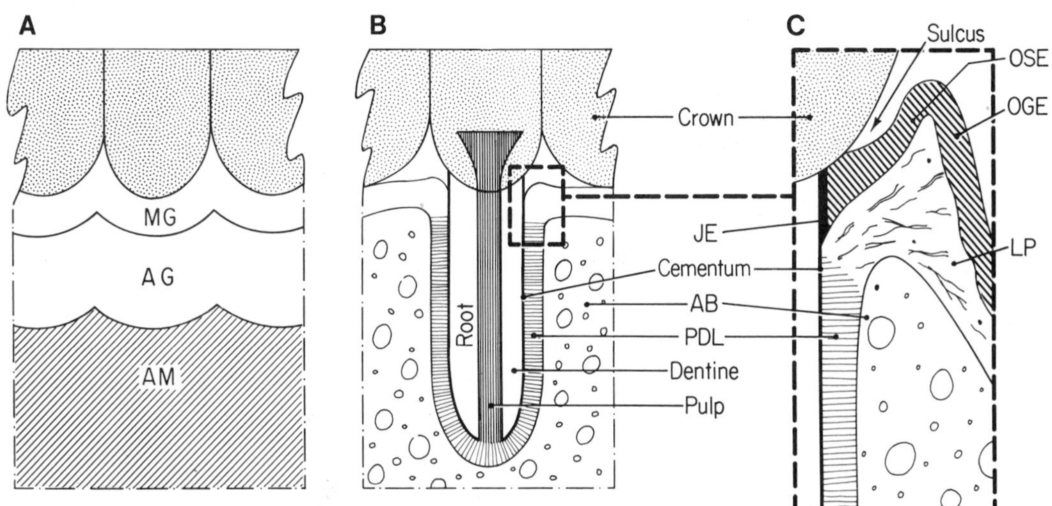

FIGURE 14–6. The normal periodontium. *A,* Frontal view demonstrating the relationship between the marginal or free gingiva *(MG),* the attached gingiva *(AG),* the alveolar mucosa *(AM),* and the crown. *B,* Frontal section of a mandibular incisor showing the position of the tooth in bone and its relationship to the periodontium. The tooth is attached to the alveolar bone *(AB)* by fibers of the periodontal ligament *(PDL). C,* Sagittal enlargement of the boxed area in *B.* The gingival attachment to the tooth, by junctional epithelium *(JE),* occurs at the base of the sulcus and demarcates the marginal gingiva from the attached gingiva. The sulcus is lined by oral sulcular epithelium *(OSE).* The exposed surface of the gingiva is covered by oral gingival epithelium *(OGE).* Fibrous connective tissue constitutes the underlying lamina propria *(LP).*

Surgical treatment aims to eliminate diseased periodontal pockets and establish a physiologically sound supporting apparatus that can be maintained by the patient. Curettage, gingivectomy, and the gingival flap are used. In the curettage technique, the lining wall of the pocket is removed without direct visualization of the involved tissue. Although absolute pocket reduction is not immediately achieved, shrinkage of edematous tissue often occurs with a decrease in pocket depth. The curettage technique is most often used for moderate disease or as an initial approach to severe periodontitis.

The gingivectomy technique is the most direct resective technique used for pocket elimination. A continuous incision is made at the depths of the periodontal pocket, and the tissue is excised. The applicability of the gingivectomy is determined by the adequacy of the attached gingiva and by the pattern of alveolar bone loss. At present, gingivectomy is generally confined to excision of hyperplastic, fibrotic tissue, such as that caused by phenytoin (Dilantin), cyclosporine, or nifedipine.

The gingival flap procedure offers a number of advantages over other resective techniques for advanced periodontitis. In this technique, the involved portion of the gingiva (pocket lining) is resected. Gingival flaps are then elevated from the underlying alveolar bone, which permits direct visualization of the affected areas after the removal of granulomatous tissue. All accretions are removed from the root surface. Osteotomy or ostectomy may be performed, although the trend seems to be away from routine surgical modification of alveolar bone. The flap margins are then placed at the crest of bone, which permits the establishment of adequate levels of attached gingiva and closure of the wound.

Regeneration of alveolar bone may occur with the use of osteoinductive or osteconductive materials to fill defects. Additionally, the temporary placement of an obstructive membrane between the soft tissue flap and underlying bone has been beneficial in permitting bony fill of certain periodontal defects.

Free gingival grafting may be performed to eliminate isolated mucogingival defects with inadequately attached gingiva. The cause of these defects is unresolved, but congenital anomalies, orthodontics, overzealous brushing, and tooth-grinding habits have all been implicated. Inflammatory changes of the marginal gingiva with communication between the sulcus and the underlying mucosa are generally regarded as an indication for free gingival grafting. The objective is to replace mucosal tissue with keratinized tissue, and this is usually accomplished by grafting of autologous intraoral tissue from the palate.

The long-term success of periodontal treatment can be assessed by the survival of the dentition. Pocket depth, bleeding, length of connective tissue attachment, and bone height are also criteria for success. The effectiveness of surgical therapy depends on adequate débridement of the affected area and aggressive postoperative maintenance.

ACUTE NECROTIZING ULCERATIVE GINGIVITIS

Acute necrotizing ulcerative gingivitis (ANUG) is a unique bacterial infection that characteristically affects the marginal and papillary gingiva. The disease has been documented since the time of the early Romans. Outbreaks of ANUG among the armies of the world have been reported regularly, and its presence during World War I led to the name "trench mouth" for the condition. ANUG has also been referred to as Vincent's disease in recognition of the individual who originally documented it. Unlike conventional periodontal disease, ANUG is most often observed in young adults in their early twenties. It is the only periodontal disease in which bacterial invasion of the gingival tissue has been observed.

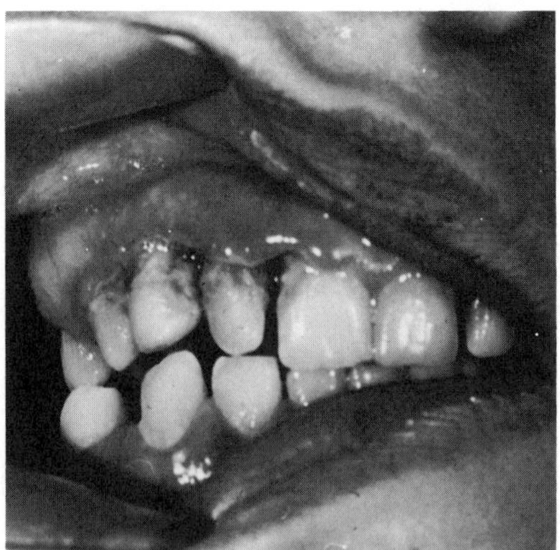

FIGURE 14–7. Acute necrotizing ulcerative gingivitis.

Clinically, ANUG is characterized by the sudden onset of local or diffuse gingival pain, with the former being more common. Patients also note gingival bleeding, bad taste, and fetor oris. Fifty per cent of patients experience systemic manifestations of infection, which may include malaise, fever, and lymphadenopathy.

The clinical appearance of ANUG is unique (Fig. 14–7). Gingival examination reveals local or general areas of papillary and marginal necrosis. The disease usually begins between the teeth and then spreads laterally (Fig. 14–8). The necrotic areas form a pseudomembrane overlying an inflammatory base. There is complete loss of the interdental papillae, which appear to be punched-out and craterlike. The tissue is friable and may bleed spontaneously or on the slightest provocation. The patient usually feels miserable.

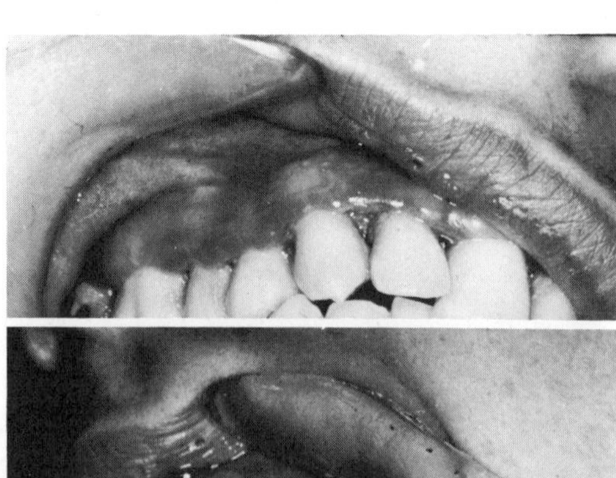

FIGURE 14–8. Two views of acute necrotizing ulcerative gingivitis.

The bacterial flora associated with ANUG has been described as a fusospirochetal complex that includes *Fusobacterium fusiforme,* vibrios, streptococci, diplococci, and filamentous forms. *Treponema vincentii* is the most common spirochete associated with the lesion. Since many of the organisms are normal inhabitants of the oral cavity, smears are of little value in establishing a diagnosis of ANUG.

Although once thought to be communicable, the disease cannot be transmitted by the transfer of organisms from one individual to another. It is believed that a localized reduction in tissue resistance, often precipitated by stress, produces an environment in which the organisms proliferate.

The diagnosis is made on the basis of the patient's age, history, and clinical appearance. ANUG is most commonly confused with herpetic gingivostomatitis (see Chapter 13), which occurs in a younger age group, is preceded by a viral prodrome, and is characterized by the presence of mucosal vesicular lesions, in addition to gingivitis.

The aims of treatment are to reduce the presence of local bacterial accumulations and to eliminate the systemic effects of infection. Most causative organisms are penicillin sensitive. Following a 1-g loading dose of penicillin V (Pen-Vee K), 500 mg four times daily for 1 week is recommended. In addition, the lesions should be gently débrided with cotton pellets soaked with 3% USP hydrogen peroxide. The patient should be referred to a dentist for definitive débridement.

Dental Caries

Dental caries or tooth decay is a common infection that is a major cause of tooth loss. Caries results from bacterial acid production following the fermentation of carbohydrates, most often sucrose. Consequently, demineralization and destruction of tooth structure occur. Two major forms of caries exist: classification is based on the site of infection. Coronal caries affect the crown of the tooth and occur most often in the grooves and fissures on the occlusal posterior of the tooth or on the smooth interproximal surfaces. Primary lesions are most common in children, adolescents, and young adults and are primarily caused by *Streptococcus mutans*.

Alternatively, *Actinomyces* may cause caries of exposed root surfaces. Hence, these are most notable in adults, especially those with gingival recession.

Not all patients are at equal risk for caries. High levels of caries-causing bacteria, poor or unbalanced nutrition, and xerostomia are factors that predispose to caries.

Overwhelming data exist to support the contention that caries is largely a preventable disease. Water fluoridation has been repeatedly demonstrated to be the most cost-effective preventive measure available. When water fluoridation is not available, nutritional supplements of fluoride should be used. Patients at high risk of caries, particularly those receiving radiation therapy in which the salivary glands are included in the field, should receive daily self-administered fluoride applications.

INFECTION

Dental infection arises from two major sources: pulpal necrosis with subsequent infection as a result of carious exposure or periodontal infection as a consequence of bacterial proliferation within a deepened gingival sulcus (Fig. 14–9). For the physician, treatment of dental infection is likely to occur in an emergent setting. Therefore, a generic diagnosis of odontogenic infection is all that is required for appropriate treatment. Since neglected dental infection can have serious and occasionally fatal consequences, the ability to assess the severity of dental infection and its potential for spread is critical.

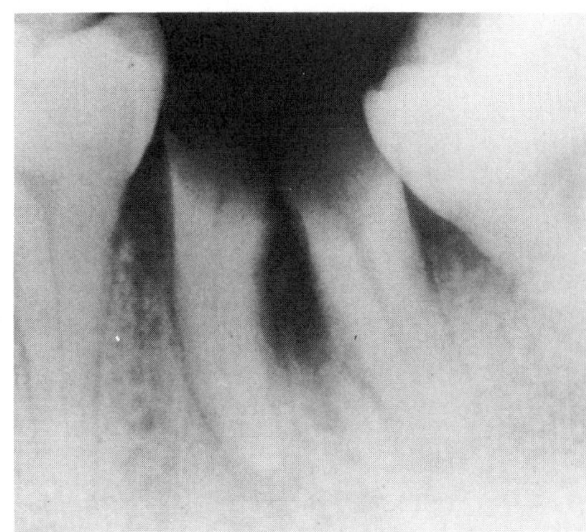

FIGURE 14–9. Odontogenic infection from decay of the crown of a tooth, which has spread into the space between the roots (furcation).

Most often, dental infection presents as either diffuse or local swelling. The degree of pain varies from dull aches to tear-rendering throbbing. Lymphadenopathy may be present. Leukocytosis and fever are often present with diffuse infection but are frequently absent even in the presence of large intraoral abscesses. The affected tooth or teeth are generally exquisitely tender to percussion and may demonstrate mobility. Suppuration may sometimes be noted at the gingival margin.

Spreading infection is also frequently encountered in dentistry. These infections, if uncontrolled, can pose a major physiologic threat to the patient, in the form of either septicemia or extension into an anatomic area so as to compromise function. The patient with a spreading infection (cellulitis) is generally sick and feels poorly. Patients often have a variety of symptoms: fever, chills, malaise, diffuse swelling, anorexia, and lymphadenopathy. Tachycardia may be noted, often proportional to the level of fever. Since spread of infection may occur via tissue planes or septic embolization or along lymphatic channels, the anatomic site of infection is important.

In assessing the patient with an oral cellulitis, four points should be considered:

1. Is the airway obstructed or does the patient have difficulty swallowing?
2. Is there evidence of deleterious change in mental status?
3. Is there closure of the eye?
4. Is the nasolabial fold intact?

A positive answer to the first question may suggest retropharyngeal spread of infection or Ludwig's angina (see Chapter 13).

Spread of infection through the facial veins may involve the cavernous sinus, resulting in neurologic signs and symptoms. Similarly, direct spread of infection may result in a brain abscess. This is most frequently reported after extraction of infected teeth but may also occur as a consequence of chronic suppurative periodontitis.

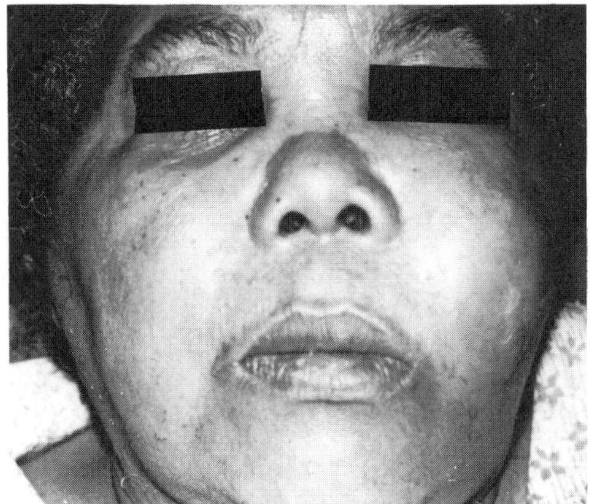

FIGURE 14–10. Spreading cellulitis involving the left side of the patient's face. Note the lack of the nasolabial fold, swelling of the cheeks, and suborbital edema.

Periorbital edema or loss of the nasolabial fold indicates localized cellulitis (Fig. 14–10). Since this occurs in the anterior facial area, the potential for spread to the central nervous system via the valveless facial veins must be considered.

Microbiology of Oral Infections

Most oral infections are caused by a mixture of organisms, of which the streptocci are the most frequent isolates. Of these, *Streptococcus viridans* is the most common. Almost all streptococcal isolates are sensitive to penicillin, ampicillin, or cephalothin. *Staphyloccus aureus* is often found in oral infections as either a pure isolate or as a component of mixed infection. Of staphylocci isolated from oral infection, 20% appear to be resistant to penicillin and 50% to erythromycin. Gram-negative anaerobes may contribute to infection of periodontal origin.

Management of Patients with Dental Infection

A patient with dental infection must be assessed for a patent airway, systemic spread of infection, or cerebral complications (Fig. 14–11). Hospital admission and supportive care are indicated for any patient with the potential for life-threatening complications as a result of treatment. Patients who have an actual or potential inability to deal physiologically with infection (underlying systemic disease) must clearly be dealt with more aggressively.

Patients with localized oral infection require dental care. If an area of localized fluctuance is observed, a stab incision following a few drops of infiltrated local anesthesia may be performed by the physician in the emergency room as an interim treatment. The patient should be treated concurrently with an antibiotic (penicillin, 500 mg every 6 hours), advised to use warm salt rinses, and told to seek dental care within 12 hours.

Patients with non–life-threatening spreading infections require localization of the infection. In addition to antibiotic therapy, warm salt rinses are advised. The application of heat to the skin is to be *avoided* as it could lead to the development of a skin fistula (Fig. 14–12). Pain medication may be required. The patient should be advised to seek dental care within 24 hours. If constitutional symptoms are marked, blood cultures for aerobic and anaerobic organisms are advisable.

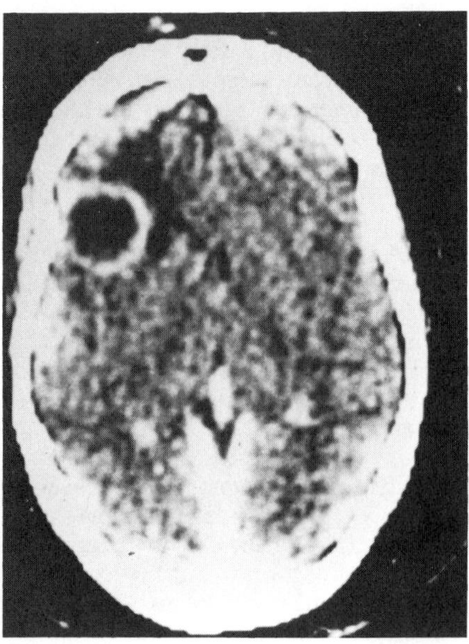

FIGURE 14–11. Brain abscess demonstrated by a computed tomography scan. This infection resulted from direct spread of periodontally involved maxillary teeth.

As noted, life-threatening infections require hospitalization and intravenous antibiotic therapy and fluid support.

Choice of Antibiotic. Penicillin is the antibiotic of choice for the treatment of oral infection. When a choice exists between penicillin and other antimicrobials, the former should be used. For oral infection, potassium phenoxymethyl penicillin is recommended in a therapeutic range of 250 to 500 mg given four times daily for 10 to 14 days.

Erythromycin is usually the first alternative to penicillin V for oral infection. Unfortunately, more than 50% of oral staphylococci are resistant to erythromycin. It can be used as a second-order antibiotic in penicillin-allergic patients.

In patients who have a gastrointestinal intolerance to erythromycin or in whom periodontal infection is suspected, clindomycin (150 to 300 mg) every 8 hours may be substituted.

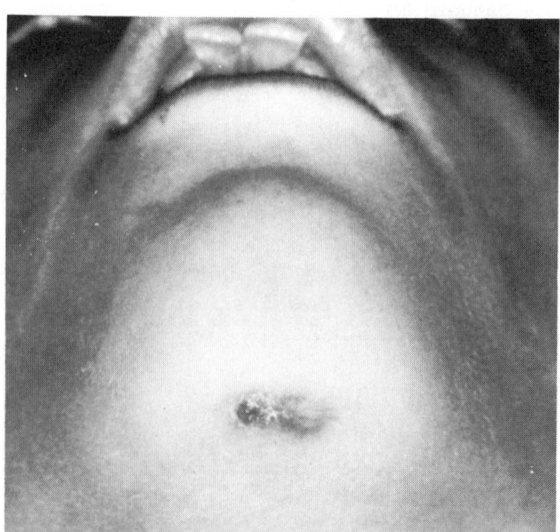

FIGURE 14–12. Fissured opening to the skin from an infected mandibular incisor.

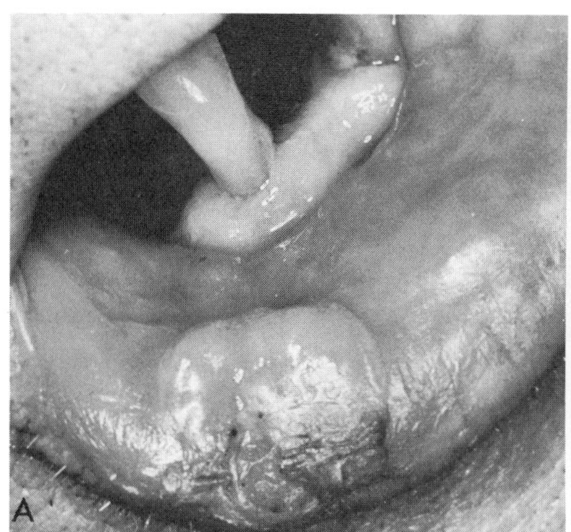

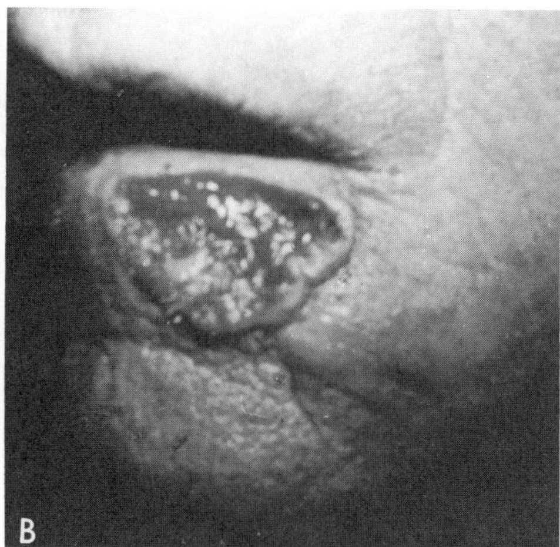

FIGURE 14–13. Two views of squamous cell carcinoma of the lower lip.

MALIGNANCIES OF THE ORAL CAVITY

Cancer of the mouth accounts for 4% of all cancers in men and 2% in women. There were 30,500 new cases of oral cancer in 1990. Statistics cannot describe the tremendous impact on lifestyle caused by oral cancer. The patient's ability to communicate, eat, and be socially acceptable to family, friends, and colleagues is often altered by the disease. More than 90% of oral cancers are epidermoid or squamous cell carcinomas.

The most consistent factor in the development of oral carcinoma is tobacco usage in the forms of cigarette smoking and snuff dipping. Alcohol consumption appears to be an important cofactor to cigarette smoking. Individuals who are both heavy drinkers and smokers develop oral and pharyngeal cancer at six times the rate of individuals who do neither. The role of viruses, particularly papillomaviruses, in the induction of oral cancer remains unresolved.

Oral carcinoma is predominantly a disease of white men. Fifty-seven per cent of cancers occur during the fifth and sixth decades of life. However, a trend toward higher incidence at younger ages is evident. About 11% of all oral cancers are seen in patients younger than 39 years of age.

Squamous cell carcinoma of the mouth most commonly presents as an asymptomatic nonhealing ulcer (Fig. 14–13) or an area of leukoplakia or erythroplasia (areas of speckled erythema and keratosis). However, exophytic and scirrhous forms also occur. Palpation to detect induration is an essential part of the examination of all suspicious areas. The lower lip is the most common site for oral carcinoma; the posterior lateral border of the tongue is the second most common site, with nonhealing ulcers being the most frequent form. Other sites of the mouth may also be involved (Fig. 14–14; Table 14–1).

Given the clinical presentation of carcinoma in the mouth, **biopsy is mandatory** for keratotic white lesions and nonhealing ulcers (ulcer present more than 14 days) (Fig. 14–15). For most sites, a biopsy is easily accomplished by the general dentist. For sites involving the floor of the mouth or salivary ducts, the patient should be referred to an oral surgeon. Cytologic smears of oral carcinoma yield a 15% false-negative rate and therefore should be reserved for mass screenings.

Squamous cell carcinomas of the mouth spread by local invasion and metastasize to regional lymph nodes via lymphatic channels. Distant metastases are rare.

Survival and morbidity, including disfigurement, are favorably related to early diagnosis and treatment.

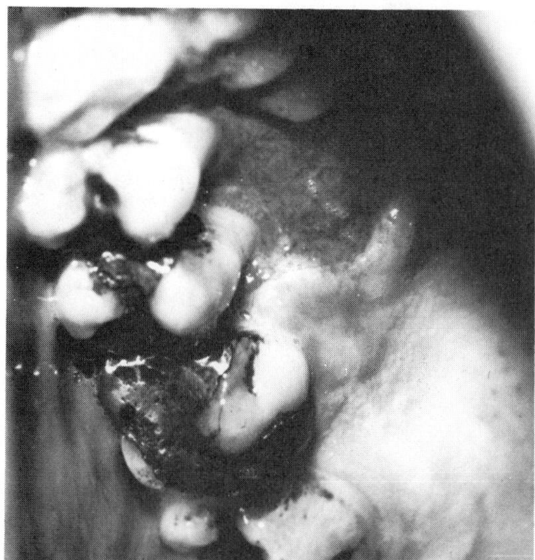

FIGURE 14–14. Squamous cell carcinoma presenting as an ulcerative area of the palatal mucosa.

TABLE 14–1. DISTRIBUTION OF ORAL CARCINOMA*

Anatomic Site	No. of Patients	%
Lower lip	5399	38
Tongue	3117	22
Floor of mouth	2479	17
Gingiva	923	6
Palate	786	5.5
Tonsil	673	5
Upper lip	553	4
Buccal mucosa	245	2
Uvula	78	0.5

*From Krolls SO and Hoffman S: Squamous cell carcinoma of the oral soft tissues: A statistical analysis of 14,253 cases by age, sex, and race of patients. J Am Dent Assoc 92:571, copyright © 1976. Reprinted by permission of ADA Publishing Co., Inc.

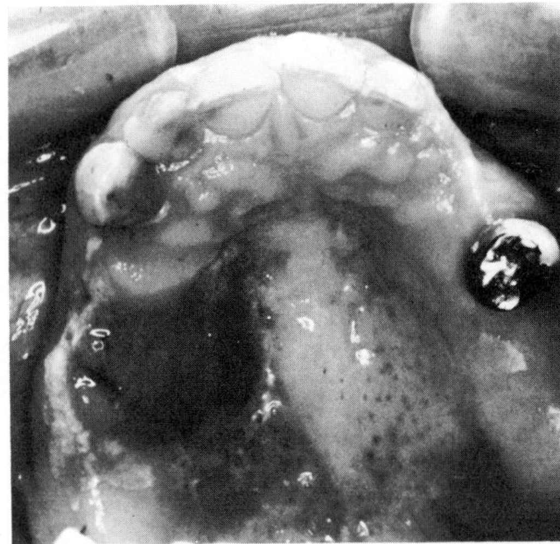

FIGURE 14–15. Squamous cell carcinoma of the mucosa affecting the maxillary ridge, presenting as a combined area of ulceration and leukoplakia.

Nonsquamous Cell Malignant Neoplasms

These may be either primary lesions or lesions metastatic to the oral cavity. Primary nonsquamous cell malignancies are most often of mesenchymal origin and include fibrosarcoma, lymphoma, chondrosarcoma, rhabdomyosarcoma, and melanoma. Fibrosarcoma and chondrosarcoma are most often seen in or about the jaws rather than in soft tissue. Patients complain of a unilateral, progressive, painless enlargement of the jaw, which is frequently accompanied by paresthesia. The overlying mucosa may be normal in appearance. **Any patient presenting with the combination of progressive swelling of the jaw with paresthesia should be presumed to have a malignancy** (Fig. 14–16) and should be referred for radiographic and histologic studies. Malignant neoplasms of soft tissue may also present as nonhealing ulceration. It is clinically impossible to differentiate these lesions from squamous cell carcinoma. A biopsy is required in order to make a diagnosis.

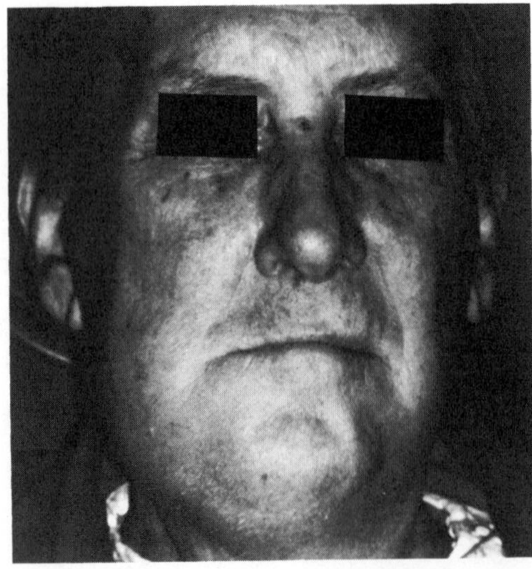

FIGURE 14–16. Clinical presentation of osteogenic sarcoma of the right side of the mandibula. The patient complained of a painful enlargement of his jaw and paresthesia.

Metastases to the oral cavity are unusual. Most of these lesions metastasize to the mandible, but soft tissue lesions may also arise. Tumors of breast, lung, and kidney are most likely to metastasize to the mouth and present as nonhealing ulceration or radiolucencies of the jaws. Neither form is usually symptomatic, but paresthesia may be noted in mandibular lesions.

Benign Neoplasms

A wide variety of benign neoplasms may be seen in the mouth; most may represent developmental anomalies rather than true neoplasms. These lesions commonly have a raised appearance and well-circumscribed borders; they are usually freely movable and asymptomatic (Fig. 14–17). Surgical excision is the treatment of choice.

ULCERS

Ulcers of the oral mucosa are common. Although the overwhelming majority are due either to trauma or aphthous stomatitis, serious diseases may also present as ulceration. Benign ulcerations of the oral mucosa due to trauma (Fig. 14–18) or aphthous stomatitis, are impossible to differentiate based on appearance (Fig. 14–19). They have yellowish, depressed centers with an erythematous border and are universally painful. Lymphadenopathy may be present. In traumatic ulceration, a specific event may be obtained from the history or an irritating filling or prosthesis may be noted. Aphthous stomatitis, commonly called canker sores, usually follows a recurrent pattern and may present as either solitary or multiple lesions. Both these forms of ulcers heal spontaneously and without scarring in 10 to 14 days. Palliation may be achieved with an ointment like Orabase with benzocaine or lidocaine (Xylocaine), 2.5%. Topical steroid ointments (e.g., triamcinalone oretonide in Orabase) may reduce inflammation and help palliation.

Oral ulceration may also represent a stage of vesiculobullous disease in which the intact vesicle has ruptured. This is true of viral infections as well as lichen planus, pemphigus vulgaris, pemphigoid, and erythema multiforme. Unlike aphthous, traumatic lesions, or virally induced ulcers,

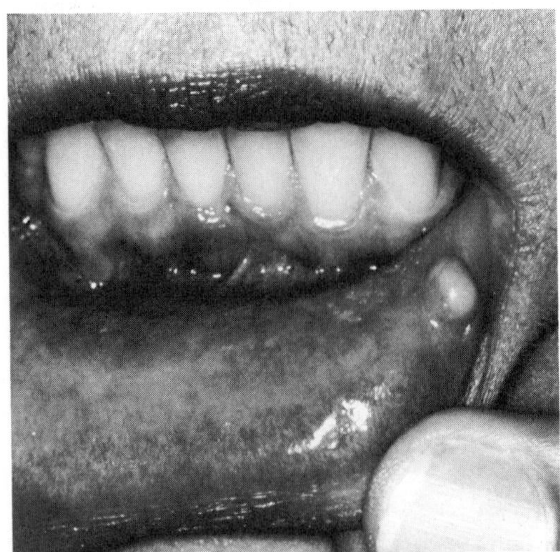

FIGURE 14–17. Fibroma, the most common benign lesion of the oral soft tissue.

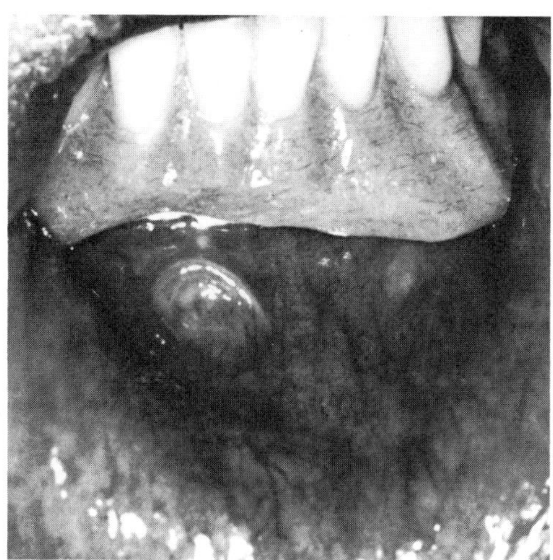

FIGURE 14–18. Traumatic ulcer secondary to an irritating denture flange.

lesions caused by the diseases mentioned earlier fail to heal in 10 to 14 days. Additionally, since oral ulceration may represent manifestations of primary syphilis, tuberculosis, or carcinoma, biopsy of nonhealing oral ulcers is mandatory.

VESICULOBULLOUS DISEASES

Five major vesiculobullous diseases or conditions affect the mouth: pemphigus vulgaris, mucous membrane pemphigoid, bullous lichen planus, erythema multiforme, and certain drug eruptions.

Diagnosis of vesiculobullous disease is usually based on history, clinical examination, and biopsy. Incisional biopsies that include a portion of noninvolved tissue are most effective. Cytologic smears may be useful in the diagnosis of pemphigus vulgaris.

Pemphigus Vulgaris. Pemphigus is noted most often among women of Mediterranean or Middle Eastern background older than 60 years of age. An autoimmune mechanism is suggested by the finding of antibodies in lesions of skin and mucosa localized in the intercellular spaces between epithelial cells.

Oral lesions are present in virtually all cases of pemphigus vulgaris and often precede skin involvement. Any area of the mouth may be involved, including mucosal surfaces and gingiva (Fig. 14–20). Pemphigus vulgaris may manifest as a desquamative gingivitis. In severe cases, virtually the entire oral mucosa may be affected, with vesiculobullous lesions in various stages of development, regression, and healing. The oral lesions are the last to heal, and minor oral involvement may persist with periodic exacerbation and regression of lesions even after relatively successful therapy of severe widespread pemphigus. Development of oral lesions can be stimulated by traumatic influences, such as mucosal abrasion by hard food fragments. Bullae can be produced simply by rubbing the mucosa with the thumb (a positive Nikolsky sign).

Mucous Membrane Pemphigoid. This is thought to be of autoimmune etiology, in which antibodies directed against the basement membrane cause separation of the epithelium from the underlying connective tissue and the formation of subepithelial bullae. The oral cavity is almost always involved in mucous membrane or cicatricial pemphigoid, with reported frequencies ranging between 90 and 100%. This lesion appears to have a predilection for women. It is seen over a broad age range, with peak frequency between 50 and 60 years of age.

Lesions are initially vesiculobullous but usually become erosive. Keratinized gingiva are almost exclusively affected, appearing red and eroded with areas of necrotic white slough causing a desquamative gingivitis. Interspersed bullae formation may be noted. Although edentulous areas are not often affected, lesions may be seen and are aggravated and made painful by removable prostheses. It is rare to observe intact bullae, because these usually rupture prior to presentation. Secondary surface infection of areas of necrosis is not uncommon and appears clinically as ulcers with yellowish centers surrounded by regions of erythema. These lesions generally heal in about 2 weeks. It is not uncommon to have lesions at different stages in the same mouth.

The major goal in diagnosis of mucous membrane pemphigoid is to differentiate it from pemphigus vulgaris, since the former has a more benign course. A biopsy is critical to make a diagnosis.

No specific therapy is available. Treatment should aim for palliation, preventing serious complications, and reducing local irritation since this aggravates the condition. Periodontal disease should be eliminated. Palliative mouth-

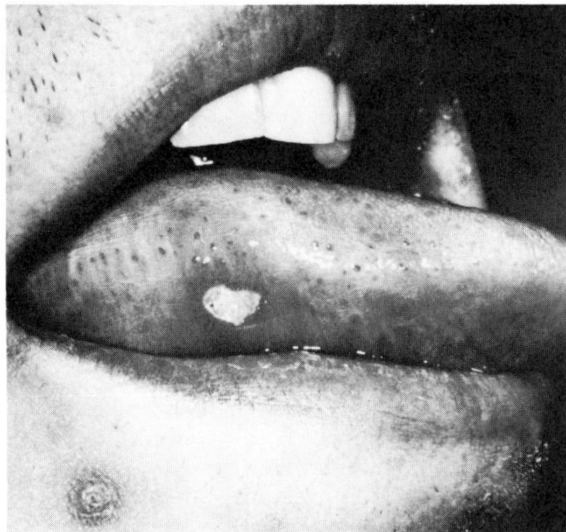

FIGURE 14–19. Aphthous stomatitis.

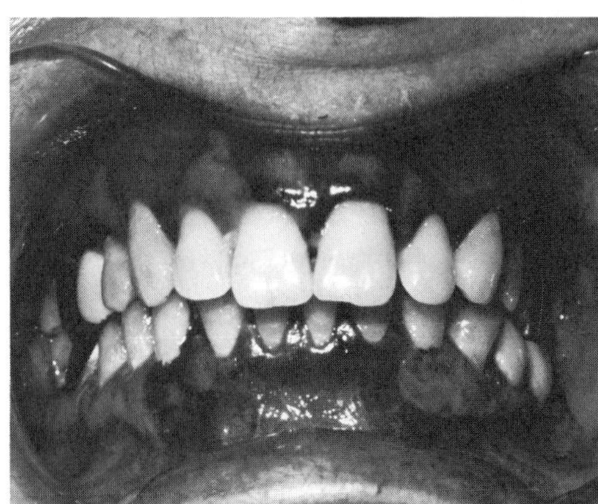

FIGURE 14–20. Pemphigus vulgaris.

washes can be recommended, but commercial rinses containing alcohol or other irritating compounds should be eliminated. Topical steroids in ointment or paste form can be applied for local control of inflammation and reduction of discomfort. Their usefulness in controlling the disease is variable. Orabase with benzocaine, lidocaine (Xylocaine Viscous), diphenhydramine hydrochloride (Benadryl) and Kaopectate in a 50–50 suspension, or dyclonine hydrochloride (Dyclone) may be used to soothe sore tissues. In extremely symptomatic patients, systemic corticosteroids may be utilized to control the disease.

Mucous membrane pemphigoid often runs a chronic, protracted course. Patients should be reassured but also realistically appraised of the drawn-out nature of this disease.

Bullous Pemphigoid. Unlike mucous membrane pemphigoid, bullous pemphigoid is predominantly a disease of skin; oral involvement is noted in only one fifth of patients with the disease. Bullous pemphigoid tends to affect elderly individuals, most commonly after 60 years of age. Oral involvement generally is noted after cutaneous lesions are present.

The most consistent oral finding in bullous pemphigoid is a diffuse, painful, desquamative gingivitis. The lesions appear on attached gingiva and demonstrate areas of redness and bleeding. Lesions at different stages of development are often seen simultaneously. The margins of the lesions may actually be noted to peel away. Other areas of the oral mucosa may also be involved. A definitive diagnosis is made by histologic examination. As with the other vesiculobullous diseases, immunofluorescent tests are also helpful.

Lichen Planus. One of the clinical manifestations of lichen planus is an erosive or bullous form (Fig. 14–21). Usually, this lesion appears along with the hyperkeratotic form of the disease in which linear striations of oral mucosal surfaces are noted.

Clinically, patients are usually uncomfortable and complain of burning, pain, and sensitivity to spices. An examination may demonstrate the presence of bullae of varying sizes. Rarely are bullae intact, however. Rather, one observes large, open, raw, eroded areas that are frequently bordered by lichenoid areas of leukoplakia. The borders of these lesions are usually uneven, and the bases may be erythematous. Areas of hyperkeratotic striae are often evident in other parts of the mouth. Frequently, bullous or erosive lichen planus involves the buccal mucosa, ventral surface of the tongue, or attached gingiva. In most instances, lesions are distributed bilaterally and often symmetrically. The flexor surfaces of the arms may concurrently demonstrate the skin lesions of lichen planus.

A diagnosis usually can be based on the appearance of the lesions. However, because lichen planus may resemble other conditions, a biopsy is strongly recommended.

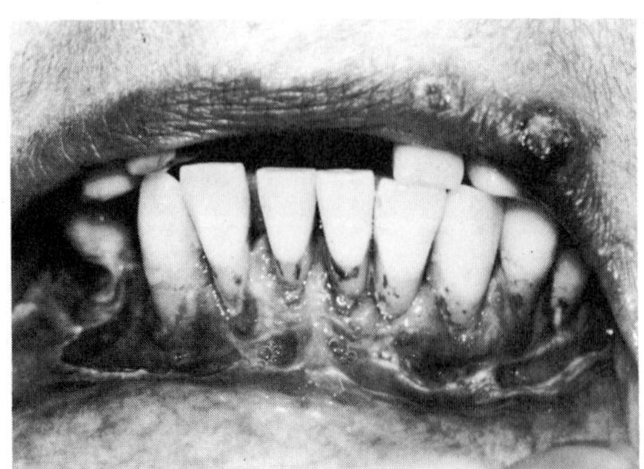

FIGURE 14–21. Erosive lichen planus.

There is no cure. Patients who are uncomfortable may receive symptomatic relief through the use of palliative mouth rinses or ointments. Topical steroid ointments or creams have been reported effective in some patients. For patients who are constantly uncomfortable, a short course of systemic steroids may be prescribed. Patients should be advised to avoid spicy foods. Any source of oral irritation should be eliminated.

Over the past few years, the issue of whether patients with lichen planus are predisposed to oral squamous cell carcinoma has been raised. The conclusions of a number of studies are conflicting.

Erythema Multiforme. This is an acute mucocutaneous disease with extreme clinical variability. Although usually grouped with the vesicubullous diseases, it may also present as ulcerative, erythematous, or erosive lesions. The etiology is not well understood, and a variety of causes have been suggested. Erythema multiforme has been reported following bacterial, viral, and fungal infections; as many as 70% of cases have been associated with herpes simplex infection. A variety of drugs have also been implicated as having a role in this condition, including quinidine, gold salts, digitalis, phenylbutazone, heavy metals, antibiotics, and oral contraceptives.

It seems likely, based on the explosive onset of the disease and the suggestion of a multiagent cause, that some form of humoral autoimmune reaction is responsible for the development of the disease.

Unlike other forms of oral vesiculobullous diseases, erythema multiforme is noted most frequently in young adults, with a male sex predilection. Children may also be affected.

Clinically, erythema multiforme has an acute onset. A detailed history often reveals one of the aforementioned agents. The disease may affect skin or mucosa; both types of tissue may be simultaneously involved. Skin lesions of erythema multiforme present a unique picture, consisting of a central region of vesiculation surrounded by a circumferential band of erythema. Because of the concentric ring appearance, the lesions are commonly referred to as "target lesions."

The oral lesions are more variable in appearance than the skin lesions. Almost all are painful. Any area of the mouth may be involved. The severity of the lesions also varies; some areas may demonstrate only subtle mucosal erythema. In contrast, large hemorrhagic vesiculobullous lesions may extend from the mouth beyond the mucocutaneous junction to involve the lips (Fig. 14–22). Lesions tend to be symmetric. The onset of erythema multiforme tends to be sudden. Although healing may occur spontaneously, particularly in young patients, lesions may become chronic, with periods of remission and exacerbation.

Effective treatment of erythema multiforme has been reported most often with steroid therapy, although some cases heal without treatment. Additionally, immunomodulatory treatment with levamisole has demonstrated efficacy. It is interesting that while prednisone apparently decreases the severity of oral lesions, it may not affect the frequency of attacks. In addition, palliation of oral lesions with topical agents is often effective in controlling symptoms. When oral lesions can be correlated with drug intake, the offending agent should be discontinued. Supportive care may be required, especially in youngsters with severe oral lesions in whom fluid and food intake are compromised. Such patients may require hospitalization so that intravenous fluids and nutrition may be supplied. Systemic analgesics may also be used if needed.

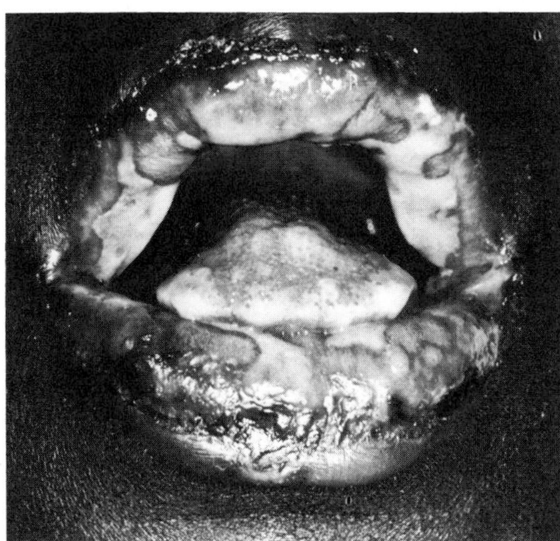

FIGURE 14–22. Erythema multiforme.

Stevens-Johnson Syndrome. In 1922, Stevens and Johnson described an entity in children that they called an "eruptive fever associated with stomatitis and ophthalmia." The condition they described had a number of unique features that differentiated it from more common forms of erythema multiforme. Since that time, severe cases of hemorrhagic erythema multiforme in which patients have a specific set of concurrent findings, including either fibromembranous or papulovesicular conjunctival involvement, skin and mouth lesions, fever, and leukopenia, are referred to as Stevens-Johnson syndrome. Other mucous membranes may also be affected, especially the external genitalia. Ocular lesions may be especially severe and, if untreated, can lead to blindness.

Oral Manifestations of Human Immunodeficiency Virus Infection

The mouth is a common site of a number of conditions that are associated with human immunodeficiency virus (HIV) infection. These changes often herald the conversion from the asymptomatic to the symptomatic phases of the disease. For the most part, the oral changes associated with HIV infection represent opportunistic infections or malignant disease.

Candidiasis is a frequent and early finding in patients with symptomatic HIV infection. While many patients present with raised, white or yellowish, curdy lesions of pseudomembranous thrush on their palates, three other forms of candidiasis may also be observed. The erythematous or atrophic variety is most often noted on the dorsal surface of the tongue or hard palate. It presents as a reddish patch that may be sensitive. A hyperplastic form has been described as appearing as a nonscrapable white lesion on the buccal mucosa. Its appearance resembles other forms of leukoplakia. Angular cheilitis may be caused by the fungus. A diagnosis is based on clinical findings with confirmation by culture. Treatment with nystatin, fluconazole, or chlortrimazole is generally effective. For patients with angular cheilitis or in patients with palatal lesions and who wear dentures, Mycolog ointment may be used.

Herpes simplex type 1 infections may produce dramatic vesiculobullous and ulcerative intraoral eruptions in the patient with HIV infection. These lesions are painful and usually occur on the movable mucosa. Most often multiple lesions are present and have a bilateral distribution on the movable mucosa. Clinically, lesions may resemble aphthous lesions; a diagnosis is made by taking a culture. Systemic acyclovir is the treatment of choice.

Intraoral lesions of herpes zoster may be seen in the patient with HIV infection. Intraoral herpes zoster infections usually present as croppy vesicular or ulcerative lesions with a unilateral distribution usually following the distribution of a branch of the fifth cranial nerve. Systemic acyclovir is the treatment of choice.

Hairy leukoplakia is the term given to a common lesion among patients with HIV infection. It is often a precursor of the conversion from asymptomatic HIV infection to acquired immunodeficiency syndrome (AIDS). Lesions present as asymptomatic white, nonscrapable plaques, most often, of the lateral borders of the tongue. Although they usually have a bilateral distribution, they may be unilateral and may occur on the buccal mucosa. The cause of hairy leukoplakia is thought to be viral, and both papillomavirus and Epstein-Barr virus have been implicated. There is no need for treatment.

Among the intraoral HIV-related neoplasms, Kaposi's sarcoma is the most common. Lesions of intraoral Kaposi's sarcoma may present as a purplish plaque of the mucosa, of the palate, or as a raised pigmented mass. The latter are commonly noted on the gingiva. Alternatively, submucosal Kaposi's sarcoma arising from the bone may present as a mass with a normal-appearing overlying mucosa. A biopsy is required to make a diagnosis. Asymptomatic macular lesions generally do not require therapy. Enlarging lesions of the gingiva that impede function or that have esthetic ramifications may be excised. Intralesional infiltration with vinblastine or low-dose radiation therapy have also been successful in the control of intraoral Kaposi's sarcoma.

Lymphomas are also noted intraorally in patients with HIV infection. Generally, these are of the B cell variety and present as enlarging mucosal masses. The lesions are fairly firm, but they are not rock-hard as one might expect of a carcinoma. A biopsy is indicated to make a diagnosis.

Periodontal changes have been reported to varying degrees in patients with HIV infection. Of these, a form of necrotizing gingivitis is most common. Like lesions of ANUG, patients present with painful gingiva, loss of the normal gingival architecture, and necrosis of the epithelium. Fever and lymphadenopathy may be present. Like ANUG, the cause of these lesions is bacterial, and patients respond well to penicillin (500 mg, every 6 hours). Antimicrobial mouth-rinses of povidine iodine or chlorhexidine gluconate may also be beneficial.

HIV-associated periodontitis is an entity that has been described, but one in which its existence has been questioned. Rapidly progressing alveolar bone loss and the presence of necrotizing gingival changes have been described as the two predominant components. There have not been any findings to suggest that the bacterial flora of HIV-associated periodontal lesions is unique.

Aphthous-like ulcerations are a relatively common finding among patients with symptomatic HIV infection. Although these lesions present with a similar appearance and symptoms as those of typical aphthae, their clinical course is protracted. Whereas healing would normally occur in 7 to 14 days, HIV-related aphthae are often present for much longer periods. Topical or intralesional injections of steroids may help. Thalidomide has been suggested as being efficacious but is unavailable in the United States. It is most important to make a correct diagnosis. A culture for herpes simplex virus and a biopsy of lesions that have been present for more than 2 weeks is mandatory.

15

Allergic Rhinitis and Other Diseases of the Nose

LAWRENCE M. Du BUSKE, MD
ALBERT L. SHEFFER, MD

The nose participates in a variety of functions that maintain an equilibrium between the upper respiratory tract and the ambient atmosphere. The nose modifies ambient humidity and temperature, chiefly by engorgement of venous sinuses within the inferior turbinates, which causes the swelling necessary to diminish patency for heat conservation (Fig. 15–1). Normally, there is a cycle of alternating congestion and decongestion in each nares. Although the dimensions of the nasal chambers may change, the total resistance afforded by both nasal passages remains constant. The turbinates also provide a significant surface area for trapping particles and bacteria, which are deposited on the viscous glycoprotein-rich mucus on columnar ciliated epithelium found on the posterior nasal pharynx.[1]

Following the application of a suitable decongestant, a detailed examination of the nose can be accomplished (Fig. 15–2). The anterior nasal septum can be examined for deviation, perforation, and ulceration. Other common pathologic conditions such as nasal polyps are easily identified. Polyps, representing hypertrophic or localized swelling of the mucosa, arise most often from the ethmoid sinuses. Hypertrophic turbinates may have a similar appearance but resist motion and are more sensitive on palpation. Malignancies seldom mimic benign nasal polyps and are usually friable and bleed easily.

The character of the nasal discharge may aid in defining the underlying pathology. Purulent discharge usually indicates infection. Allergic rhinitis is associated with a clear, occasionally thick mucoid rhinorrhea. Unilateral recurrent epistaxis signifies a localized process, possibly neoplasia, especially if there is no associated trauma. Clear unilateral rhinorrhea may indicate a leakage of cerebrospinal fluid (CSF).

The most common nasal symptoms are obstruction and irritation. Obstruction or nasal "stuffiness" accompanies a myriad of disorders affecting the nose. The most common causes of "stuffiness" are viral respiratory infections, bacterial infections including purulent rhinitis or acute suppurative sinusitis, allergic rhinitis, perennial nonallergic rhinitis, nasal polyposis, vasomotor rhinitis, and rhinitis produced by medications, both systemic and topical. Mucous membrane atrophy occurs in the elderly or following extensive sinus surgery and may cause an incapacitating sensation of nasal "stuffiness."

DIFFERENTIAL DIAGNOSIS OF RHINITIS

Nasal Vestibulitis and Cellulitis

A nasal furuncle most often presents as an erythematous, indurated, firm lesion of the nasal tip. It can be surrounded by a region of cellulitis and is most often caused by a staphylococcal infection originating in the nasal vibrissae. The infection should be treated with an antibiotic that provides staphylococcal coverage (e.g., dicloxacillin, 500 mg four times a day). Warm soaks should be applied locally. Incision and drainage most often are not required and should not be performed unless appropriate antibiotic coverage has been instituted to avoid bacterial seeding.

Nasal Polyposis and Nonallergic Rhinitis with Eosinophilia

Nonallergic rhinitis with eosinophilia (NARES) begins with nasal congestion and discharge occurring at first intermittently but gradually becoming more persistent during the second or third decade of life. Ultimately, patients develop hyperplasia of the nasal mucosa, often culminating in nasal polyposis and hyperplastic sinusitis due to intolerance (Fig. 15–3).[2] A few patients with nasal polyposis have associated allergic rhinitis. About 70% of patients with nasal polyposis have bronchial asthma as well, which also is nonallergic in type.[3]

The syndrome of nasal polyposis, aspirin intolerance, and asthma has been called the "aspirin triad." Among all asthmatics, the incidence of aspirin sensitivity is between 10

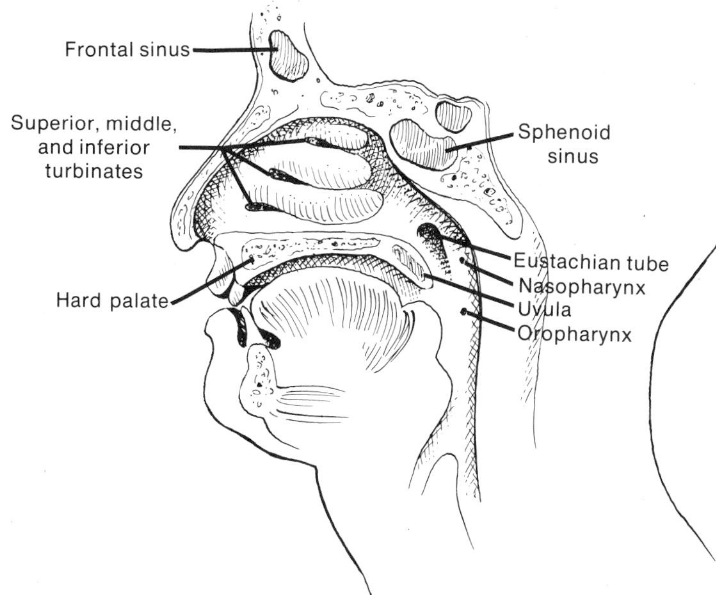

FIGURE 15–1. The lateral wall of the nose showing the turbinates and nasopharynx.

and 20%, and the incidence of nasal polyps is less than 10%, whereas among those asthmatics who have aspirin-induced bronchospasm, the incidence of nasal polyps is 70%.[4] Up to 33% of patients with nasal polyposis are intolerant of aspirin and nonsteroidal anti-inflammatory drugs (NSAIDs).[3] Patients often tolerate medications that lack significant cyclooxygenase inhibitory ability, such as choline magnesium trisalicylate or acetaminophen, but high doses of medication may give some symptoms of rhinosinusitis.[5, 6]

Treatment consists of avoidance of aspirin and NSAIDs, plus a brief course of corticosteroids administered orally, followed by chronic therapy using topical corticosteroid sprays. Avoidance of yellow dyes such as tartrazine has not been found to be useful, because these compounds possess no activity as cyclooxygenase inhibitors.[7] Immunotherapy is ineffective as a primary treatment for nasal polyposis.

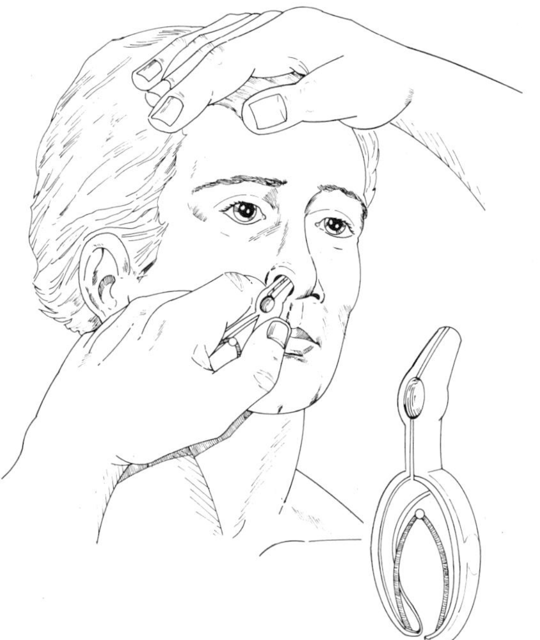

FIGURE 15–2. Use of the nasal speculum. The speculum is held in the left hand and stabilized by placing a finger upon the patient's nose. It is inserted about 1 cm and opened to avoid traumatizing the septum. A penlight or head mirror should be used for illumination.

Patients who do not respond to medical therapy frequently can benefit from nasal polypectomy. This may be done initially as an outpatient procedure. Success rates of up to 80% have been reported when a thorough intranasal ethmoidectomy is done in conjunction with a sphenoidotomy.[8] However, nasal mucosa must be conserved to reduce the occurrence of atrophic rhinitis.

Inhaled nasal corticosteroids are particularly effective in diminishing the recurrence of polyps after polypectomy. Patients treated with beclomethasone after polypectomy showed a significant decline in the mean score of polyp symptom severity and frequency of polyp recurrence compared with patients who did not receive beclomethasone treatment after polypectomy.[9, 10] Triamcinolone and flunisolide appear to be equally effective.

Vasomotor Rhinitis

Vasomotor rhinitis represents an abnormality in the parasympathetic nerve stimulus to the nasal mucosa. It results in an exaggerated response to nasal nonspecific alteration. Manifested by nasal mucosal swelling, profuse rhinorrhea, and congestion with ambient temperature fluctuation, vasomotor rhinitis occasionally leads to marked obstruction in response to environmental pollutants. Additional precipitating factors may include ingestion of highly seasoned food or alcohol, inhalation of odors or perfumes, and exposure to air conditioning.

Most patients have mild symptoms. Antihistamines or intranasal steroids sprays may be beneficial. Nasal irrigation is not at all helpful, and decongestant sprays should be avoided. Most patients seen in primary care practice respond to conservative measures plus an explanation of the symptoms.

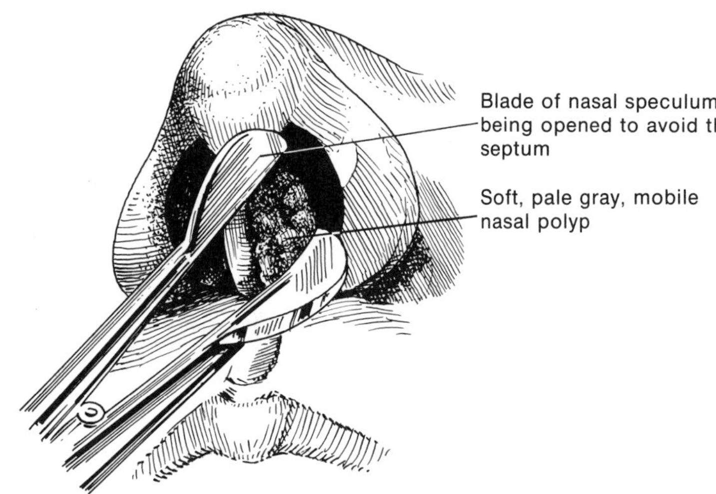

FIGURE 15–3. Use of a nasal speculum to demonstrate a nasal polyp. The speculum may be used with a head mirror or penlight. Its blades are inserted about 1 cm into the nasal vestibule and opened widely in the anteroposterior direction to avoid the septum. Polyps are soft, pale gray, smooth, pedunculated tumors, which, unlike the nasal turbinates, are moveable and nontender.

Purulent Rhinitis

Purulent rhinorrhea induced by a bacterial infection of the nasal mucosa may be confined to the anterior nasal septum and vestibule. Common respiratory pathogens are *Staphylococcus,* and rarely *Haemophilus influenzae.* The disorder is often superimposed on other sources of rhinitis. In patients afflicted with cystic fibrosis or Kartagener's syndrome in which the natural ciliary motility is restricted, repeated episodes of purulent rhinitis may occur concurrently with nasal polyposis and sinusitis.

Antihistamines are of no benefit in nasal infections. Cultures of nasal mucosa correlate poorly with the etiology but may lead to narrowing the field of antibiotic therapy when all else fails. Attention focused only on the rhinitis and not an associated sinusitis may lead to failure. An evaluation of the sinuses by a computed tomography (CT) scan may be required. Endoscopic inspection of sinus ostia and an evaluation for osteomeatal outflow tract obstruction is often helpful in both the diagnosis and treatment of chronic rhinosinusitis.

Rhinitis Medicamentosa

This disorder occurs after prolonged use of topical vasoconstrictors. Pathologically, stasis of mucus secretions is produced and the natural function of the respiratory epithelium is altered. Ciliary motility is halted. The groundwork is set for recurrent superimposed infection. After only a few days of topical vasoconstrictor therapy, a rebound phenomenon occurs in which resulting mucosal congestion may supersede the original pathology. Topical nasal steroids such as beclomethasone are frequently beneficial and help the patient to eliminate usage of vasoconstrictor sprays, which should be discontinued and avoided in the future.

Atrophic Rhinitis (Ozena)

The cause of atrophic rhinitis is obscure. It is associated with an offensive nasal odor, epistaxis, anosmia, nasal obstruction, and purulent nasal crusting. The frequent complaint of a sensation of nasal congestion is due to decreased nasal resistance to airflow in a hyperpatent nasal chamber and not to true congestion. An examination discloses nasal crusting, atrophy of the turbinates, and enlargement of the nasal cavity. Overaggressive nasal surgery and resection may lead to a similar problem. Medical therapy consists of nasal irrigations with isotonic saline. Topical ointments have no prolonged benefit.

Other Causes of Rhinitis

Endocrinologic disturbances as well physiologic responses alter the nasal mucosa. These include such common situations as pregnancy and hypothyroidism. The nasal mucosa is sensitive to alterations in blood supply as well as to changing hormone levels in the body. Similar obstructive rhinitis can be induced by the use of oral contraceptives having high estrogen content, antihypertensive agents including reserpine, β-adrenergic blocking agents, and α-methyldopa; cholinergic agents; phenothiazines; alcohol; and cocaine.

A unilateral obstruction in any patient older than 40 years of age is suggestive of a malignancy. More commonly, however, septal deviations or nasal polyps can cause unilateral nasal airway obstruction. In the child or mentally incompetent patient, unilateral purulent rhinorrhea suggests the presence of a foreign body. The first step in any diagnostic sequence is a careful intranasal examination. Often, nasal endoscopic examination and CT scans of the sinuses and nasal pharynx may be required to establish a definitive diagnosis of the anatomic cause of nasal obstruction.

Allergic Rhinitis

Almost 22% of Americans have symptoms of possible upper respiratory allergy. The average patient with allergic rhinitis has symptoms for nearly 20 weeks/yr and requires medication for 40% of the time that symptoms occur.[11] In studies ranging from 5 to 25 years of follow-up, rates of remission for allergic rhinitis are remarkably low and are generally between 5 and 10% of patients studied.[12] Almost 40% of patients with allergic rhinitis have had some episode of asthmatic bronchospasm.[11–13]

Allergic rhinitis may be seasonal, such as tree, grass, or ragweed pollen-induced rhinitis; perennial, such as rhinitis associated with mold, animal dander, dust mite, or cockroach exposure; or episodic, such as rhinitis associated with intermittent animal dander exposure.

Pathophysiology of Allergic Rhinitis

A current hypothesis of the natural history of allergic sensitization is that this condition results from the interaction of a specific allergen with an antigen-presenting cell such as a macrophage that processes the allergen for presentation to a helper T cell,[14] which then induces B cell differentiation into plasma cells capable of producing immunoglobulin E (IgE). Antigen-specific IgE enters the circulation and is avidly bound to receptors on mast cells and basophils, which are both found in association with the nasal mucosa.[15] Activation of these cells causes the immediate release of preformed mediators stored in secretory granules (including histamine), which cause microvascular leak, mucous secretion, and vasodilatation.[16] Concomitant with mast cell degranulation is the generation of newly formed mediators of inflammation derived from arachidonic acid metabolism, most notably leukotriene LTB_4, a potent chemotactic factor; LTC_4, a bronchoconstrictor; and PGD_2, a potent vasoactive agent.

The early phase of allergic inflammation induced by mast cell and basophil activation is associated with symptoms including rhinorrhea, sneezing, lacrimation, pruritus, and bronchospasm. These symptoms are evident within 1 to 5 minutes of encounter with an allergen and generally will last for no more than 30 minutes to 1 hour in experimental allergen challenges.[17] A late phase of allergic inflammation may also occur, beginning 2 to 6 hours after the initial allergic response.[17] This late phase is associated with the infiltration of a variety of inflammatory cells into the site of the allergic response, including eosinophils, neutrophils, basophils, macrophages and lymphocytes.[18, 19]

During late-phase allergic inflammation general hyperresponsiveness to a variety of nonspecific stimuli may occur wherein symptoms of allergic rhinitis are elicited by irritants at a threshold lower than would be the case if allergic inflammation were not present. Additionally, late-phase inflammation causes priming of allergy reactive cells, such that lower allergen doses are required to induce allergic inflammation.[17] It has been observed that higher antigen challenge dosages induce greater release of inflammatory mediators and greater tendency to produce late-phase inflammation.[20] Repetitive antigen challenge induces greater mediator release and enhanced symptoms, with progressively lower antigen challenge being required to induce an equivalent allergic response. The net effect of chronic and repetitive antigen challenge, which clinically occurs with chronic high allergen exposure, is the production of perennial and debilitating symptoms of rhinitis that are often associated with complications, including sinusitis and asthma.

Therapy for allergic rhinitis aims at either eliminating mast cell activation through allergen avoidance or modifying the subsequent consequences of mast cell activation by utilization of treatment modalities that either inhibit allergic inflammation or inhibit the effects of inflammatory mediators.

Diagnosis of Allergic Rhinitis

The diagnosis of allergic disease is made through a correlation of the allergy history and an examination of the patient with results of testing of the patient for presence of allergy done either by in vivo skin testing using allergen extracts applied to the skin as a means of demonstrating mast cell reactivity to selected allergens or done by in vitro testing for detection of allergen-specific IgE in the patient's serum.

Allergy History

The patient history is essential for the establishment of the diagnosis of allergic rhinitis. Important factors in the allergy history include: (1) the previous occurrence of allergic disease such as hay fever, asthma, eczema, or hives in the patient; (2) the presence of a family history of allergic disease; and (3) the patient's exposure to cigarette smoke. A thorough allergy history should include an assessment of the patient's indoor environment both at home and at work for potential allergens and irritants. It is especially important to document the type of heating system with reference to the use of a forced hot air furnace or a wood burning stove in the home environment. The presence of animals, cockroach infestation, and carpeting, particularly in damp and moldy areas in the home, should also be noted. Documentation of exposure to allergens in the bedroom is critical, including the presence or absence of animals in the bedroom, the type and age of the mattress and box spring, the type and age of pillows that are present, and the presence or absence of bed coverings. In addition, careful attention should be given to the timing as well as to the location of symptoms of allergic rhinitis.

Seasonal Versus Perennial Allergic Rhinitis

Seasonal allergic rhinitis produces symptoms of nasal itching, watery rhinorrhea, nasal congestion, and sneezing that is often associated with conjunctival injection and ocular itching due to seasonal pollen exposure in the Eastern United States. Tree pollen typically induces symptoms from March to early June, whereas grass pollens induce symptoms from late May to early July, and ragweed and other weed pollens induce symptoms from mid-August through early October. Mold spores may induce allergy symptoms throughout the spring, summer, and early fall.

Patients with perennial allergic rhinitis have nearly continuous symptoms of nasal itching, obstruction, rhinorrhea, and sneezing. "Vacuum" sinus headaches, caused by mucosal edema obstructing sinus drainage ostia, are common in these patients. Chronic serous otitis media due to obstruction of the eustachian tube may also occur. Typical allergens inducing perennial allergic rhinitis are house dust mites, mold spores, or animal danders. In many patients who have perennial allergic rhinitis, some degree of seasonal exacerbation may occur with exposure to pollen.

Examination of the Allergic Patient

Among the physical examination findings often noted in individuals with allergic rhinitis are: (1) an "allergic crease" running horizontally across the bridge of the nose secondary to constant rubbing of the nose in an upward fashion; (2) the presence of "allergic shiners," dark shadows about the eyes; (3) the presence of sinus tenderness on palpation; and (4) the presence of oral breathing.

An intranasal examination of the anterior nasal pharynx using an otoscope with speculum will reveal mucosal edema, a bluish-white pallor, and some degree of nasal obstruction in most patients with allergic rhinitis. A thin, watery serous discharge is typically present, although in perennial rhinitis or in cases in which secondary infection has occurred, more tenacious, thickened, or even frankly purulent secretions may be noted. Among those individuals with perennial symptoms, nasal polyps may occasionally be seen.

An examination of the eyes of the allergic patient may reveal increased conjunctival vascularity and conjunctival edema consistent with allergic conjunctivitis. An ear examination may reveal some degree of chronic inflammation of the tympanic membrane with slight bulging of the tympanic membranes associated with acute allergic serous otitis media, or retraction of the tympanic membranes due to chronic serous otitis media. A lung examination may reveal, in some individuals, increased expiratory phase on forced expiration or even mild wheezing consistent with allergy-associated asthmatic bronchospasm.[21] Factors that help to discriminate the patients with allergic rhinitis from the patients with infectious rhinitis include the presence of conjunctival pruritus and the absence of fever in the typical patient with allergic rhinitis. The diagnosis of allergic rhinitis depends on the proper correlation of symptoms with exposure to a given allergen.

Allergy Skin Testing

The most frequently used in vivo tests for IgE-mediated disease is the allergy skin test. In general, allergy skin testing is done by utilizing the prick/puncture methodology as the primary diagnostic testing modality, with intradermal tests done towards selected allergens to which the patient has signs of clinical allergic disease but towards which the patient fails to show reactivity in prick/puncture tests.

The prick/puncture method of skin testing involves application of a 1:10 or 1:20 weight/volume allergen extract solution to the skin as a small drop, which is then pricked through utilizing a solid-bore needle. Both a positive control using a dilute solution of histamine and a negative control using a diluent identical to that of the allergen extract should always be applied. This testing method is safe, rapid, and causes little discomfort. Results correlate well with the occurrence of allergic disease. Although false-negative reactions are possible, false-positive reactions are rare.

Intradermal skin testing is performed by injection of approximately 0.05 ml of a 1:500 to 1:1000 weight/volume allergen extract into the skin, using a fine-gauge needle to place a small "bleb" of extract intradermally. Intradermal tests are more reproducible and are approximately 1000-fold more sensitive than are prick/puncture skin tests, but false-positive reactions are possible.[22]

A variety of factors may influence the results of allergy skin testing, such as the patient's age; time of day; and presence of antihistamines, including medications such as tricyclic antidepressants and phenothiazines that have antihistaminic properties. As B_2-antagonists may inhibit the treatment of anaphylaxis that could occur as an adverse consequence of allergy skin testing, for individuals for whom discontinuation of such medication is impossible, utilization of in vitro assessment of serum antigen-specific IgE may be required as the safest and most reliable method of allergy diagnostic testing.

Laboratory Testing for Allergenic Disease

The laboratory assessment of allergic rhinitis may at times include determinations of the total IgE level, the percentage of eosinophils in the white blood cell differential, and the presence of antigen-specific IgE levels. The presence of elevated levels of total serum IgE or increased total peripheral eosinophil count does not, in itself, constitute the diagnosis of allergy.[23, 24] Additionally, test results indicating merely the presence of antigen-specific IgE in the serum do not necessarily indicate that the patient has clinical disease related to exposure to this antigen. All test results must be interpreted in the context of the patient's allergy history, and laboratory tests should not be used as the sole criteria for establishment of the diagnosis of allergy.

In vitro assessment for the presence of allergen-specific IgE antibody can be done utilizing the radioallergosorbent test (RAST) or enzyme allergosorbent test (EAST). In these tests, the antigen to be evaluated has been coupled to a solid phase to which is added the patient's serum, which contains the antigen-specific IgE antibody. This IgE antibody from the patient's serum binds to the antigen and is detected by adding a second antibody, an anti-IgE antibody to which is bound a tracer, either a radioactive label in the RAST test or an enzyme label in the EAST test. Results are reported as semiquantitative classes. Sensitivity and specificity of these tests vary depending on the particular antigen to be evaluated, ranging from 50 to 80% of the sensitivity and from 85 to 95% of the specificity of allergy skin prick/puncture testing.[25] Newer methods such as the CAP system, utilizing a matrix solid phase, have enhanced sensitivity.[26]

Allergen-specific IgE tests have some advantages over allergy skin testing, including a lack of significant risk to the patient of an allergic reaction and a lack of interference of test results by concomitant medications[24] and are the methods of choice in select groups such as infants, elderly patients with cardiovascular disease, patients unable to discontinue antidepressant medications, patients with severe skin diseases, and patients with dermatographism, which is a condition that afflicts 5 to 10% of adults who form hives upon stroking the skin.[24]

Basophil Histamine Release

In an attempt to achieve an in vitro allergy testing method that more closely resembles in vivo allergic events, basophil histamine release tests have been developed.[27] A recently developed glass fiber whole blood leukocyte histamine-release test possesses sensitivity and specificity approaching that of skin prick testing for some selected inhalant allergens.[27, 28] As the sensitivity of this assay may be affected by the intrinsic ability of individual patient basophils to release histamine and by sample transportation time and conditions, leukocyte histamine release technology is still considered investigational as a method for the diagnosis of allergic disease.

Treatment of Allergic Rhinitis

There are three general methods of treatment of allergic rhinitis. The primary treatment is allergen avoidance. The second form of treatment is the use of pharmacologic therapy including antihistamines, decongestants, topical corticosteroids, and topical cromolyn. In cases in which antigen avoidance and pharmacologic therapy fail, immunotherapy utilizing parenteral administration of allergenic extracts may be required.

Allergen Avoidance

An essential treatment for dust allergy and animal dander allergy is allergen avoidance. Significant improvement in symptoms from mold allergy and pollen allergy may also be achieved through simple avoidance modalities. Most American homes are infested with dust mites. These microscopic organisms serve as scavengers of flecks of human skin, ingesting the skin shed into clothing, furniture, and bedding. Dust allergen exposure increases with the presence of high humidity and seasonally exacerbates from June to October due to increased seasonal propagation of dust mites in humid conditions. Activities, such as vacuuming, bed making, lying on a carpet, or sleeping in a bed that has only been intermittently used may enhance dust mite exposure.

To decrease dust mite allergen exposure, it is essential to keep the relative humidity to less than 45% inside the home. In this regard, dehumidifiers are helpful, whereas humidifiers are detrimental. The use of air conditioners during the summer will both dry and cool the air, thus decreasing dust mite propagation. Environmental controls, such as eliminating carpeting and clutter from the home, eliminating stuffed furniture, and most important, utilizing plastic-lined mattress and pillow covers to encase bedding completely, may significantly decrease exposure to dust mite allergens.

A variety of agents are currently available to control dust mite infestation, including an application of tannic acid that is sprayed on carpeting or the application of benzyl benzoate used as a moist powder applied to carpeting and furniture. These treatments may effectively diminish either dust mite antigenicity or dust mite growth but must be applied frequently, generally every 3 months.

Animal allergen exposure can cause significant allergic rhinitis. Animal dander, saliva, and urine may all contribute unique allergens that can induce rhinitis in persons sensitive to animals. The most efficacious method of treating animal dander allergy is to eliminate the animal from the home environment and to eliminate circumstances that lead to exposure to animals.

Mold allergen exposure increases seasonally in the early spring, midsummer, and early autumn, especially on days with relatively hot weather and breezy winds that allow dissemination of mold spores. Outdoor activities such as hiking, lawn mowing, or leaf raking and indoor exposure to cool mist ultrasonic humidifiers, vaporizer reservoirs, house plants, fish tanks, old paper products, and poorly ventilated areas may exacerbate mold-induced symptoms. The mold-sensitive individual can diminish mold growth by decreasing the humidity through the use of a dehumidifier or air conditioner.

Pollen allergen exposure increases from 4 AM to 9 PM on warm, dry days with brisk winds that allow dissemination of pollen into the air. Exposure to pollen allergen may be diminished by simply closing windows, thus prohibiting pollen from entering the home area as the pollen settles to the ground overnight. Air conditioning the home environment may also significantly diminish pollen exposure.

Pharmacologic Therapy for Allergic Rhinitis

When environmental modification and avoidance modalities fail to control symptoms of allergic rhinitis, pharmacologic therapy must be utilized. Antihistamines, which compete with the H_1 receptor site for histamine, are indicated for the treatment of rhinorrhea and sneezing. Oral sympathomimetic agents such as pseudoephedrine, phenylpropanolamine, or phenylephrine that act as α-adrenergic agonists are indicated for the treatment of nasal obstruction. Symptoms, such as "vacuum sinus" headaches, often respond to the use of an oral sympathomimetic agent and not to an antihistamine, because sinus ostium obstruction may induce these headaches.

Persistent or refractory symptoms of nasal congestion may require the use of topical anti-inflammatory medications such as intranasal steroids or intranasal cromolyn. Intranasal steroids may safely be used for the long-term treatment of perennial allergic rhinitis and, in general, are more effective than intranasal cromolyn in such cases. Both intranasal steroids and intranasal cromolyn effectively ameliorate the symptoms of seasonal allergic rhinitis; cromolyn being particularly effective if only intermittent therapy is required, such as immediately prior to exposure in cases of episodic animal dander-induced allergic rhinitis.

Antihistamine Therapy

Antihistamines, which block the H_1 histamine receptors, have traditionally been categorized according to their chemical structure into several classes. "Ethanolamine-class" antihistamines include agents such as diphenylhydramine HCl, carbinoxamine maleate, phenyltoloxamine citrate, and clemastine fumarate. These agents are potent H_1 antagonists but have a significant sedative effect. The "alkylamine class" antihistamines are among the most commonly used antihistamines in nonprescription medications, including chlorpheniramine maleate, and brompheniramine maleate. Although very effective for allergic rhinitis, sedation and dry mouth are common undesirable effects of these agents.

Chronic therapy with antihistamines may be associated with an apparent loss of clinical efficacy that is often due to a significant decline in compliance consequent to side effects. Classic H_1 antihistamines may induce a variety of adverse reactions, such as central nervous system sedation or paradoxic stimulation, especially in children. A variety of anticholinergic side effects may also be seen, including the occasional occurrence of urinary retention, especially in elderly men with prostate disease; constipation; mucosal dryness; and rarely, development of tachycardia.

The most important development in antihistamine therapy has been the advent of nonsedating antihistamines in the 1980s.[29] Terfenadine was the first nonsedating antihistamine made available in the American market. A study comparing terfenadine with chlorpheniramine for the treatment of fall and spring allergic rhinitis demonstrated that both drugs were equally efficacious, with peak efficacy achieved by 2 to 3 days of therapy.[30] Approximately 50% suppression of symptom scores are noted.[29, 30] The degree of sedation seen in the terfenadine group was not statistically different from that found in the placebo group. Terfenadine is efficacious within 4 hours after dosing, making it an appropriate agent for occasional or chronic use as therapy for allergic rhinitis. Studies have demonstrated terfenadine not only to be nonsedating but also to have no significant effect on cognitive performance in complicated tasks as measured by reaction time and visual-tracking skills.[31] Other studies that evaluate long-term use of terfenadine have demonstrated no tachyphylaxis with chronic use.[32]

Although terfenadine is considered an extraordinarily safe medication in most clinical circumstances, rare instances of cardiac arrhythmias, including ventricular tachycardia and torsades de pointes, have been reported in patients who have a QT interval prolongation that may be exacerbated by high levels of terfenadine,[33] such as in terfenadine overdoses, in patients with hepatic disease and in cases in which the use of systemic antifungal agents such as ketoconazole or macrolide antibiotics such as erythromycin inhibit hepatic metabolism of terfenadine. Terfenadine, therefore, should not be used in doses greater than the recommended dose of 60 mg bid.

Astemizole was the next nonsedating antihistamine made available in the United States. Astemizole is capable of suppression of cutaneous reactivity to histamine for up to 1000 hours.[30] Astemizole is rapidly absorbed, with plasma levels peaking in 1 hour and declining to zero by 4 days after dosing. Its desmethyl derivative allows for a significant antihistamine effect to be present for up to 6 weeks after the cessation of astemizole.[34,35] Whereas agents such as terfenadine may more rapidly occupy H_1 receptors, but decline to 50% of maximum occupation by 12 hours, astemizole will ultimately achieve 80% occupancy of H_1 receptors that persists for more than 1 week.

Clinically, the administration of astemizole at a dose of 10 mg/day is associated with the achievement of peak efficacy after approximately 4 days of treatment, whereas a 60-mg dosage of terfenadine will achieve peak efficacy in 24 hours, with significant efficacy seen in 2 to 12 hours. Although a loading dose of astemizole, 20 to 30 mg/day at the initiation of therapy will significantly enhance the rapidity of the initial relief of allergic symptoms, this form of astemizole loading is no longer recommended due to the occurrence of ventricular tachyarrhythmias that have been reported to occur at daily doses as low as 20 mg/day. The kinetics of astemizole efficacy do not make this agent appropriate for occasional use but rather suggest that it be reserved for situations in which daily antihistamine therapy is required to control allergic rhinitis. In long-term therapy for allergic rhinitis, astemizole and terfenadine are roughly equivalent in their relief of the symptoms of sneezing and nasal stuffiness, astemizole being somewhat superior for the relief of rhinitis and nasal pruritus.

The main common adverse reaction noted with astemizole has been a mild weight gain. The incidence of sedation produced by astemizole is no different than that produced by placebo. Astemizole taken in excessive doses or in the setting of hepatic disease may induce cardiac arrhythmias, including serious ventricular tachyarrhythmias such as torsades de pointes.[36] Unlike terfenadine, no drug interactions have been reported with astemizole as a cause of cardiac arrhythmias. Daily astemizole dosing should not exceed 10 mg.

Evidence indicates that some antihistamines including cetirizine and loratadine, two investigational antihistamines possessing minimal sedative effects, may also have anti-inflammatory properties beyond their effect as H_1-blocking agents. Cetirizine inhibits eosinophil infiltration into the site at late-phase allergic events, and both loratadine and terfenadine have been found to suppress basophil histamine release.

Topical Inhaled Cromolyn Therapy

Topical application of cromolyn sodium, as a liquid nasal spray, has been found to be an effective treatment for seasonal and perennial allergic rhinitis. Cromolyn inhibits IgE-dependent mast cell but not basophil activation in humans. Cromolyn is also capable of inhibiting eosinophil and neutrophil cytotoxicity. Cromolyn is available as a 4% solution liquid spray containing 5.2 mg of cromolyn sodium per spray, generally administered as 2 sprays in each nostril before allergen exposure and up to every 3 to 4 hours throughout the day during allergen exposure.[37]

Administration of topical nasal cromolyn before antigen challenge has been demonstrated to significantly ablate the immediate rise in nasal airway resistance that normally occurs 2 to 20 minutes after allergen exposure.[38] Cromolyn also ablates the dual response to nasal allergen, which occurs in some individuals who show both an immediate-phase and a late-phase reaction occurring 6 to 12 hours after allergen challenge. The effect of cromolyn is critically dependent on the time it is administered prior to the allergen challenge.

The successful usage of cromolyn sodium is vitally dependent on having proper administration of the medication.[37] It is essential that the nasal airways be cleared in order to ensure a good response to nasal inhaled cromolyn. Typical acute doses of cromolyn are 1 to 2 sprays in each nostril immediately before allergen exposure. Chronic dosage is typically 1 to 2 sprays in each nostril every 3 to 4 hours, dependent on the degree of allergen exposure that the patient experiences. Positive responses to cromolyn therapy typically occur in patients with (1) episodic usage of cromolyn just prior to occasional allergen exposure; (2) seasonal allergic rhinitis; or (3) perennial allergic rhinitis who have many positive results on skin tests and high levels of antigen-specific IgE. Negative responses to cromolyn therapy often occur in patients with: (1) vasomotor rhinitis; (2) nasal polyposis; (3) NARES; and (4) marked congestion and intractable nasal edema.

Topical nasal cromolyn is an extraordinarily safe method of treatment for allergic rhinitis. Side effects of cromolyn sodium are minimal. Nasal irritation is the most significant side effect, and sneezing or throat irritation occurs rarely. Nasal bleeding is seen less commonly with cromolyn therapy than with aqueous beclomethasone usage.[39]

Topical Inhaled Corticosteroid Therapy

Topical corticosteroids are capable of suppressing many aspects of allergic inflammation, including anti-inflammatory mediator release. There are four corticosteroid preparations available for nasal administration, including dexamethasone sodium phosphate, flunisolide, beclomethasone dipropionate, and triamcinolone acetonide. The dexamethasone nasal spray contains 100 μg per spray of which approximately one third is absorbed systemically, significantly limiting its clinical utility since suppression of adrenal function occurs. The flunisolide nasal spray, which is available as a metered liquid spray containing 25 μg of flunisolide per spray, typically is given as 2 sprays in each nostril once per day. Beclomethasone is available as both a fluorocarbon-propelled spray and as an aqueous metered liquid spray, each of which contains 42 μg of beclomethasone diproprionate per spray. Typical daily dosing is 1 to 2 sprays in each nostril, two to four times per day. The aqueous preparation was developed to diminish the local irritation that may occur with the use of the fluorocarbon-propelled preparation.[37]

In studies of patients with seasonal allergic rhinitis, beclomethasone nasal spray achieves peak efficacy between 7 and 14 days of therapy, with significant efficacy noted by 4 days. In patients with seasonal rhinitis, treatment with beclomethasone nasal spray significantly diminishes nasal obstruction, rhinorrhea, sneezing, and nasal itch.[40] It is recommended that therapy be instituted at least 1 week before the beginning of a susceptible patient's allergy season.[9] The long-term efficacy of beclomethasone has been demonstrated to be 80% in a study of its use over a 5-year period.[41]

The triamcinolone spray, which uses a fluorocarbon propellant to deliver 55 μg of triamcinolone acetonide per spray, is recommended at starting dosages of 2 sprays in each nostril once a day. Symptoms improve in 4 to 7 days in two thirds of patients treated at this dosage, but if symptoms persist, the dosage can be advanced to 2 sprays twice a day.

Multiple studies have demonstrated that topical nasal corticosteroid therapy has greater clinical efficacy for the treatment of allergic rhinitis than has therapy with antihistamines, including comparisons of beclomethasone to terfenadine or flunisolide to astemizole.

Topical corticosteroid intranasal therapy is indicated for: (1) seasonal allergic rhinitis; (2) perennial allergic rhinitis; (3) nasal polyposis; and (4) NARES. In rhinitis medicamentosa and vasomotor rhinitis, modest efficacy of inhaled topical nasal corticosteroids has been noted.

The safety of inhaled nasal corticosteroids has been proved in several long-term studies. In a 6-year study of patients who received beclomethasone for perennial rhinitis, no significant changes were noted in mucosal biopsies or plasma cortisol levels during the treatment period.[42, 43]

Possible side effects of intranasal steroids include: (1) transient symptoms of nasal irritation, sneezing, sore throat, or rarely, loss of taste or smell; (2) nasal bleeding; (3) candidiasis of the nose; and (4) rare occurrence of atrophic changes including septal perforation, especially among patients who also covertly use topical sympathomimetic sprays. Adverse effects may occur when intranasal steroids are administered at higher concentrations or after prolonged use. Adrenal suppression has not been reported when inhaled topical nasal steroid medications are used at the recommended dosages.

Allergen Immunotherapy

Allergen immunotherapy is an appropriate treatment for patients with allergic rhinitis who have disease of significant severity and duration that induces debilitating symptoms not adequately controlled by allergen avoidance and pharmacologic therapy. Before the initiation of allergen immunotherapy, it is essential to document relevant allergen sensitivity by the performance of appropriate allergen skin tests or analysis of serum for allergen-specific IgE, the results of which are then correlated with the patient history and physical examination. A typical criterion for the initiation of allergen immunotherapy is treatment of rhinitis that has caused symptoms over two consecutive allergy seasons and that has not been sufficiently controlled with allergen avoidance and therapy using antihistamines, topical corticosteroid nasal sprays, or topical cromolyn nasal sprays.

Allergen extracts currently available are generally aqueous extracts that utilize glycerinated saline or human serum albumin as a diluent. The diluents generally contain phenol as an antibacterial agent, making local infections consequent to proper administration of allergen immunotherapy extremely rare. Advances in allergen immunotherapy have included the development of a variety of standardized extracts with reliable potency, which is expressed in standardized units.

Allergen immunotherapy programs may fail due to improper administration of the allergens, including inadequate amounts of the relevant antigen, using injection schedules that have too infrequent injections or using inappropriate antigens. It is essential never to design an immunotherapy regimen solely on the result of an allergen skin test or an allergen specific IgE blood test without considering the individual patient's clinical sensitivity.

Many placebo-controlled studies have demonstrated the efficacy of allergy immunotherapy for allergic rhinitis. Ragweed pollen, mountain cedar pollen, birch pollen, grass pollen, and dust mite–induced rhinitis have demonstrated significant improvement in patients receiving allergen immunotherapy. The failure of some earlier studies to demonstrate a significant effect of allergen immunotherapy may relate to a lack of standardization of the extracts and a lack of standardization of the allergen dosages administered in these studies. Studies that have employed lower doses of allergen immunotherapy have demonstrated less benefit among the allergen immunotherapy treatment groups compared with placebo treatment groups.

A variety of immunologic changes occur during the course of allergen immunotherapy, including an increase in antigen-specific serum and nasal secretion IgG and a gradual decline in antigen-specific IgE in nasal secretions. After only 12 weeks of allergen immunotherapy there is a significant decline in nasal secretion content of histamine, indicating that allergen immunotherapy rapidly decreases the production and appearance of mediators of allergic inflammation in nasal secretions. In addition to its effect on immediate mediator release, allergen immunotherapy is also particularly effective in suppressing late-phase allergic reaction.

The dose of allergen immunotherapy is critical, because the effect of allergen immunotherapy as an immunomodulating treatment is clearly dose-dependent. As the cumulative dose of allergen administered in immunotherapy rises, the daily patient symptom scores and nasal production of allergy mediators tend to significantly decrease.[44] Typically, patients treated for 2 years will have lower daily symptom scores than patients treated for only 1 year. Thus, high-dose immunotherapy administered by a schedule that allows for sufficiently frequent injections, generally given weekly for a significant period, is necessary to see an optimal immunologic response.

Complications may occur consequent to allergen immunotherapy, including anaphylaxis, exacerbation of allergy symptoms, and local reactions at the site of immunotherapy. Allergen immunotherapy should be given as subcutaneous injections, not intramuscular, to achieve maximum benefit and safety. Caution must be employed that errors in the dose administered do not occur. Changes in dose should follow an established protocol, and consideration should be given to the patient's degree of symptoms at the time of immunotherapy administration.

In a retrospective study of patients receiving allergen immunotherapy, systemic reactions occurred in less than 3%.[45] Allergy immunotherapy should not be administered to patients who are having a significant increase in symptoms at the time of immunotherapy. New evidence clearly indicates that patients with asthma are at particular risk for serious and life-threatening reactions to immunotherapy.[46] A survey of 27,806 allergy injection visits revealed 143 systemic reactions, including rhinoconjunctivitis, urticaria, angioedema, cough, wheeze, abdominal pain, and hypotension. Seventy-two per cent of the systemic reactions appeared within 30 minutes, 8% appeared in 30 to 60 minutes, and 8% appeared after 2 hours.[46] Fifty per cent of the patients who had systemic reactions had asthma; 45% had a prior history of systemic reactions; 14% had reactions due to injections given later than had been scheduled; and 7% had reactions associated with new extract preparations being administered.

A review of fatalities consequent to allergen immunotherapy revealed only 24 deaths over approximately a 40-year period of reported adverse events related to allergen injections.[47] However, one study has indicated that ten deaths occurred from allergy immunotherapy administered in the USA from 1989 to 1991 and that 70% of the deaths were among asthmatic patients.[48] Careful evaluation of asthmatics, including questioning regarding symptoms and examining results of either peak flow measurement readings or pulmonary function testing results, should be part of the routine management of asthmatics who receive allergen immunotherapy.[49]

Patients who receive allergen immunotherapy should stay in a physician's office for a minimum of 30 minutes after immunotherapy is administered. Patients should also be warned of the possibility of exacerbation of asthma or the development of urticaria consequent to allergen immunotherapy. The patient should be advised that late systemic reactions can occur, and they should be properly warned to seek the immediate advice of a physician if such an event arose.

Due to the complications that can ensue consequent to the allergen immunotherapy, it is essential that this treatment only be administered in the presence of physicians and staff who are able to recognize reactions to immunotherapy, including anaphylaxis, and who are cognizant of the proper therapy for such catastrophes. Physicians should have available injectable sympathomimetic agents, preferably adrenaline, and should have ready access in the office to other forms of therapy for anaphylaxis.[50]

Several clinical circumstances modify the risk of administration of allergen immunotherapy. The increased risk involved in treating anaphylaxis in the pregnant patient mitigates against instituting immunotherapy or accelerating an ongoing allergen immunotherapy in such patients. Allergen immunotherapy is not associated with increased risk of fetal morbidity or sensitization, and maintenance of ongoing immunotherapy regimens at somewhat attenuated dosages is permissible during pregnancy. Significant underlying cardiovascular disease precludes the initiation or continuation of allergen immunotherapy due to the risks entailed in treatment of anaphylaxis in such patients.

Although the use of β-adrenergic blocking drugs does not enhance the risk of development of anaphylaxis, the concomitant usage of β-adrenergic blocking medications may make difficult the treatment of anaphylaxis consequent to allergen immunotherapy. For patients who require allergen immunotherapy, substitutes for β-adrenergic blocking medications should be sought, such as utilization of calcium channel blocking agents that do not have the same adverse impaction on therapy for anaphylaxis.

In summary, allergen immunotherapy should only be administered in clinical settings in which physicians are present who can rapidly recognize and treat potential anaphylaxis and other adverse consequences of immunotherapy.

REFERENCES

1. Kaliner M, Marom Z, Patow C, and Shelhamer J: Human respiratory mucus. J Allergy Clin Immunol 73:318, 1984.
2. Moneret-Vautrin DA, Hsieh V, Wayoff M, et al: Nonallergic rhinitis with eosinophilia syndrome—a precursor of the triad: Nasal polyposis, intrinsic asthma, and intolerance to aspirin. Ann Allergy 64:513, 1990.
3. Settipane GA and Chafee FH: Nasal polyps in asthma and rhinitis: A review of 6037 patients. J Allergy Clin Immunol 59:17, 1977.
4. Gryglewska-Rzymowska J, Roznieck J, Szmidt M, and Kowalski ML: Asthma with aspirin intolerance: Clinical entity or coincidence of nonspecific bronchial hyperreactivity and aspirin intolerance. Allergol Immunopathol 9:533, 1981.
5. Ogino S, Harada T, Okawachi I, et al: Aspirin-induced asthma and nasal polyps. Acta Otolarnygol (Stockh) 430 (Suppl): 21, 1986.
6. Stevenson DD and Lewis R: Proposed mechanisms of aspirin sensitivity reactions (Editorial). J Allergy Clin Immunol 70:788, 1987.
7. Stevenson DD, Simon RA, Lumry WR, and Mathison DA: Adverse reactions to tartrazine. J Allergy Clin Immunol 78:182, 1986.
8. Friedman WH, Katsantonis GP, Slavin RG, et al: Sphenoidethmoidectomy: Its role in the asthmatic patient. Otolaryngol Head Neck Surg 90:171, 1982.
9. Karlsson G and Rundcrantz H: A randomized trial of intranasal beclomethasone dipropionate after polypectomy. Rhinology 20(3):144, 1982.
10. Virolainen E and Puhakka H: The effect of intranasal beclomethasone diproprionate on the recurrence of nasal polyps after ethmoidectomy. Rhinology 18:9, 1980.
11. Meltzer EO: Evaluating rhinitis: Clinical, rhinomanometric, and cytologic assessments. J Allergy Clin Immunol 82:900, 1988.
12. Smith JM: Epidemiology and natural history of asthma, allergic rhinitis, and atopic dermatitis (eczema). *In* Middleton E, et al (eds): Allergy—Principles and Practice, 3rd ed. St. Louis, CV Mosby, 1988, p 891.
13. Turkeltaub PC and Gergen PJ: Prevalence of upper and lower respiratory conditions in the US population by social and environmental factors: Data from the second National Health and Nutrition Examination Survey, 1976 to 1980 (NHANES II). Ann Allergy 67:147, 1991.
14. Naclerio RM: Drug therapy: Allergic rhinitis. N Engl J Med 325(12):860, 1991.
15. Hastie R, Heroy JH III, and Levy DA: Basophil leukocytes and mast cells in human nasal secretions and scrapings studied by light microscopy. Lab Invest 40:554, 1979.
16. Schwartz LB, Atkins PC, Fleekoppe P, et al: Release of tryptase and histamine during cutaneous challenge with allergen. J Allergy Clin Immunol 77:246, 1986.
17. Kaliner M: Hypotheses on the contribution of late-phase allergic responses to the understanding and treatment of allergic disease. J Allergy Clin Immunol 73:311, 1984.
18. Naclerio RM, Proud D, Togias AG, et al: Inflammatory mediators in late antigen-induced rhinitis. N Engl J Med 313:65, 1985.
19. Svensson C, Andersson M, Persson CGA, et al: Albumin, bradykinins, and eosinophil cationic protein on the nasal mucosa surface in patients with hay fever during natural allergen exposure. J Allergy Clin Immunol 85:828, 1990.
20. Iliopoulos O, Proud D, Adkinson NF Jr, et al: Relationship between the early, late and rechallenge reaction to nasal challenge with antigen: Observations on the role of inflammatory mediators and cells. J Allergy Clin Immunol 86:851, 1990.
21. Altounyan REC: Changes in histamine and atropine responsiveness as a guide to diagnosis and evaluation of therapy in obstructive airways disease. *In* Pepys S and Frankland AW (eds): Disodium Chromoglycate in Allergic Airways Disease. London, Butterworths, 1970, pp 47–53.
22. Bousquet J: In vivo methods for study of allergy: Skin tests, techniques, and interpretation. *In* Middleton E, et al (eds): Allergic Principles and Practice, 3rd ed. St Louis, CV Mosby, 1988, pp 419–636.
23. Weltman JK: Laboratory tests for total and allergen-specific immunoglobulin E. N Engl Reg Allergy Proc 9(2):129, 1988.
24. Yunginger JW: Clinical significance of IgE. *In* Middleton E, et al (eds): Allergy Principles and Practice, 3rd ed. St Louis, CV Mosby, 1988, pp 849–860.
25. Eriksson NE and Ahlstedt S: Diagnosis of reaginic allergy with house dust, animal dander and pollen allergens in adult patients. V: A comparison between the enzyme-linked immuno-

sorbent assay(ELISA), provocation tests, skin tests and RAST. Int Arch Allergy Appl Immunol 54:88, 1977.
26. Kelso JM, Sodhi N, Gosselin VA, and Yunginger JW: Diagnostic performance characteristics of the standard Phadebas RAST, modified RAST, and Pharmacia CAP system versus skin testing. Ann Allergy 67:511, 1991.
27. Nolte H, Schiotz PO, and Stahl Skov P: A new glass microfibre-based histamine analysis for allergy testing in children. Allergy 42:366, 1987.
28. Nolte H, Storn K, and Schiotz PO: Diagnostic value of a glass fibre-based histamine analysis for allergy testing in children. Allergy 45:213, 1990.
29. Buckley CE III, Klemawesch SJ, and Lucas SK: Treatment of allergic rhinitis with a new selective H_1 antihistamine, terfenadine. N Engl Reg Allergy Proc 6:63, 1985.
30. Kaliner MA: Non-sedating antihistamines. Allergy Proc 9:649, 1988.
31. Gaillard AW, Gruisen A, and de Jong R: The influence of antihistamines on human performance. Eur J Clin Pharmacol 35(3):249, 1988.
32. Simons FE, Watson WT, and Simons KJ: Lack of subsensitivity to terfenadine during long-term terfenadine treatment. J Allergy Clin Immunol 82(6):1068, 1988.
33. Monahan BP, Ferguson CL, Killeavy ES, et al: Torsades de pointes occurring in association with terfenadine use. JAMA 264:2788, 1990.
34. Heykants J: The pharmacokinetics and metabolism of astemizole in man. *In* Heykants J (ed). Astemizole: A New Non-sedative, Long-acting H_1 Antagonist. Oxford, The Medicine Publishing Foundation, 1984, pp 25–34.
35. Lantin JP, Huguenot C, and Pecoud AR: Effect of astemizole on skin tests with histamine, codeine and allergens (Abstract). J Allergy Clin Immunol 81:213, 1988.
36. Simons FER, Kesselman MS, Giddins NG, et al: Astemizole-induced torsade de pointes. Lancet 1:624, 1988.
37. Mabry RL: Uses and misuses of intranasal corticosteroids and cromolyn. Am J Rhinol 5:121, 1991.
38. Pelikan Z and Pelikan-Filipek M: The effects of disodium cromoglycate and beclomethasone diproprionate on the immediate response of the nasal mucosa to allergen challenge. Ann Allergy 49:283, 1982.
39. Morrow-Brown H, Jackson FA, and Pover GM: A comparison of beclomethasone dipropionate aqueous nasal spray and sodium cromoglycate nasal spray in the management of seasonal allergic rhinitis. Allergol Immunopathol (Madr) 12:355, 1984.
40. Kobayashi RH, Tinkelman DG, Reese ME, et al: Beclomethasone diproprionate aqueous nasal spray for seasonal allergic rhinitis in children. Ann Allergy 62:205, 1989.
41. Brown HM, Storey G, and Jackson FA: Beclomethasone dipropionate aerosol in treatment of perennial and seasonal rhinitis: A review of five years' experience. Br J Clin Pharmacol 4 (Suppl 3):283S, 1977.
42. Holopainen E, Malmberg H, and Tarkiainen E: Experience of treating allergic rhinitis with intra-nasal beclomethasone diproprionate: Short-term trials and long-term follow-up. Acta Allergol 32:263, 1977.
43. Malm L and Wihl JA: Intra-nasal beclomethasone dipropionate in vasomotor rhinitis. Acta Allergol 31:245, 1976.
44. Creticos PS: Immunologic changes associated with immunotherapy. Immunol Allergy Clin North Am 12:13, 1992.
45. Hepner MJ, Ownby DR, Anderson JA, et al: Risk of systemic reactions in patients taking beta-blocker drugs receiving allergen immunotherapy injections. J Allergy Clin Immunol 86:407, 1990.
46. Matloff SM, Bailit IW, Parks P, et al: Systemic reactions to immunotherapy (Abstract). J Allergy Clin Immunol 89:273, 1992.
47. Lockey RF, Benedict LM, Turkeltaub PC, et al: Fatalities from immunotherapy (IT) and skin testing (ST). J Allergy Clin Immunol 79:660, 1987.
48. Stewart GE II, and Lockey RF. Editorial: Systemic reactions from allergen immunotherapy. J Allergy Clin Immunol 90:567–578, 1992.
49. DuBuske LM, Ling CJ, and Sheffer AL: Special problems regarding allergen immunotherapy. Immunol Allergy Clin North Am 12:145, 1992.
50. Norman PS and Van Metre TE Jr: The safety of allergenic immunotherapy. J Allergy Clin Immunol 85:522, 1990.

16

Pain or Congestion of the Paranasal Sinuses

MARSHALL STROME, MD, MS

Acute sinusitis is the most common cause of symptoms referable to the paranasal sinuses. In many cases, congestion resulting from an upper respiratory infection or allergic rhinitis predisposes to bacterial infection by obstructing sinus drainage. The most common symptoms once infection supervenes are dull pain over the area of the sinus, stuffy nose, and purulent nasal discharge. Low-grade fever may be present but most adults with sinusitis are afebrile.[1]

The most important task for the clinician is to recognize and treat adequately all cases of acute sinusitis, thus preventing complications or persistence as chronic sinusitis. Complications are rare but must be recognized, because they can be life threatening. An acute sinusitis must be distinguished from other sinus pathology, including chronic sinusitis, other inflammatory conditions, carcinoma, and mucocele. Most of the latter disorders have clinical presentations that differ from those of acute sinusitis (Table 16–1). The major symptoms of chronic sinusitis are persistent, often painless, purulent discharge and cough. Unilateral nasal obstruction, bloody or serosanguineous discharge, anesthesia in the area of the infraorbital nerve, or persistent pain suggests carcinoma of the nose or the sinus. Mucoceles are slowly enlarging cystic structures within a completely obstructed sinus and can cause an insidious swelling most often identified clinically in the frontal sinus beneath the supraorbital ridge.

Clinical Anatomy. The maxillary sinuses are located in the maxilla and over the hard palate. The ethmoid sinuses are multiple thin-walled cavities located medial to the wall of the orbit; these are divided into anterior and posterior groups. The frontal sinuses are located medially above the orbits in the frontal bone and generally are asymmetric; some adults have only one and a few have no frontal sinuses. The sphenoid sinuses lie behind the upper portion of the nasal cavities. These relationships are illustrated in Figures 16–1 and 16–2. Each of the sinuses drains into the nasal cavity, either at the middle meatus, located between the middle and inferior turbinates, or at the superior meatus, located between the superior and middle turbinates (see Fig. 16–2). The maxillary, anterior ethmoid, and frontal sinuses drain into the middle meatus, whereas only the sphenoid and posterior ethmoid sinuses drain into the superior meatus.

The maxillary sinuses are adjacent to the teeth, so that symptoms may result from periapical dental abscesses as well as from blockage of sinus drainage. The ethmoid and frontal sinuses are more closely associated to the orbit, the optic nerve, and the dura covering the frontal lobes, whereas the sphenoid sinuses are contiguous to the cavernous sinuses and cranial nerves III to VI. Venous pathways from these sinuses extend to the meninges via dural veins.

TABLE 16–1. COMMON PRESENTING SYMPTOMS OF PARANASAL SINUS DISEASES

Disease	Symptoms
Acute suppurative sinusitis	Dull, persistent pain over the sinus Low-grade fever Stuffy nose Purulent nasal discharge
Chronic suppurative sinusitis	Persistent, purulent drainage, cough, halitosis
Carcinoma	Recurrent unexplained rhinosinusitis Unilateral nasal obstruction Bloody or serosanguineous discharge Infraorbital anesthesia Persistent, unexplained pain
Mucocele	Rubbery mass, usually beneath the supraorbital ridge
Complications of sinusitis	High fever, shaking chills Periorbital edema Visual blurring, diplopia, loss of bulbar mobility Severe, persistent retrobulbar pain Generalized headache Vomiting, convulsions, or change in mental status

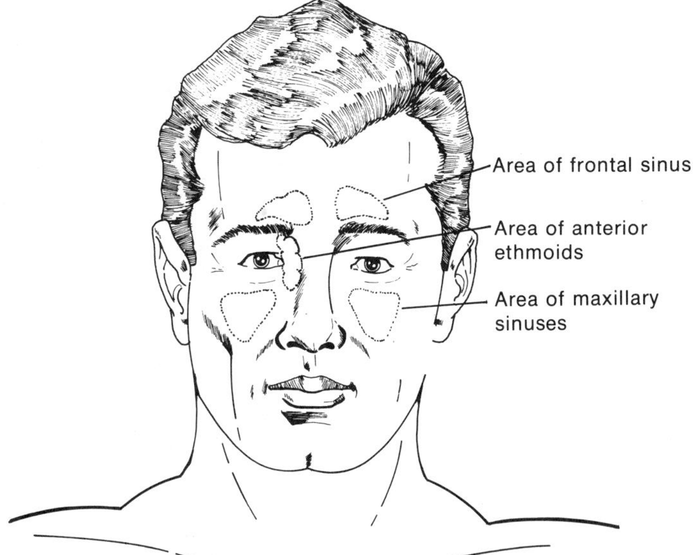

FIGURE 16–1. Areas of the face beneath which paranasal sinuses are located.

Acute Suppurative Sinusitis

Suppurative infection of the sinuses can be distinguished from intermittent congestion, which occurs in the course of upper respiratory infections and rhinitis, on the basis of the patient's pain and the nature of the nasal discharge. There is a persistent, dull ache instead of just intermittent fullness, and the nasal discharge becomes purulent instead of clear or mucoid. The infection is confined to the closed space; thus, fever is absent or low grade; shaking chills or fevers above the range of 38.3 to 38.8° C (101 to 102° F) are not expected in uncomplicated cases.

Pain related to sinusitis usually can be distinguished from that caused by headache, because the former is perceived locally rather than generalized, is worse on bending over, and is generally steady and dull rather than throbbing, sharp, or "band-like." Maxillary, frontal, and ethmoid sinusitis usually cause local pain perceived at the cheek, at the frontal region, and beneath the nasal bones medial to the orbit, respectively. Occasionally, ethmoid sinusitis causes pain radiating to the temporal region, but temporal pain is usually due to another cause, such as temporomandibular joint dysfunction or cranial arteritis.

Sphenoid sinusitis may be difficult to distinguish from headache or temporal pain. Whereas headache radiating to the vertex may suggest this diagnosis, most patients have unilateral temporal, vertex, occipital or retro-orbital pain.[2] Sphenoid sinusitis should be considered when such a pain or headache persists for weeks to months unrelieved by minor analgesics and typically interferes with sleep.[2] Paresthesias of the periorbital region, nose, teeth or cheeks (nerve V regions) suggest this diagnosis. Similar symptoms in association with photophobia and tearing occur in migraine, but if associated with sphenoid sinusitis, this complex suggests early spread to the cavernous sinus.[2]

Most commonly, sinusitis involves the maxillary sinus. To examine, one presses or percusses beneath the maxilla, or above the orbit for frontal sinusitis, to detect tenderness. The fact that sinuses filled with fluid will not transilluminate also may be helpful diagnostically. Transillumination requires a bright light source within a completely dark room. If transillumination of the maxillary sinus is sought, the light is aimed at the inferior rim of the orbit and the hard palate is observed with the patient's mouth open (Fig. 16–3); or the light source may be placed at the superior rim of the orbit to outline the frontal sinuses. Complete failure of the maxilla to transilluminate does suggest fluid in patients with acute symptoms, although the maxillary sinus is not always completely filled with fluid in sinusitis, so that "dull" transillumination cannot be interpreted[3]; failure to outline a frontal sinus is not conclusive because the sinus is commonly absent or varies in size.

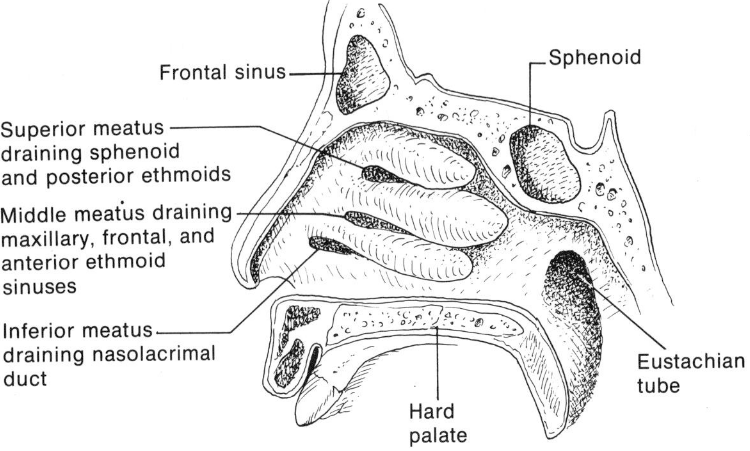

FIGURE 16–2. Relationships of paranasal sinuses to the lateral wall of the nose.

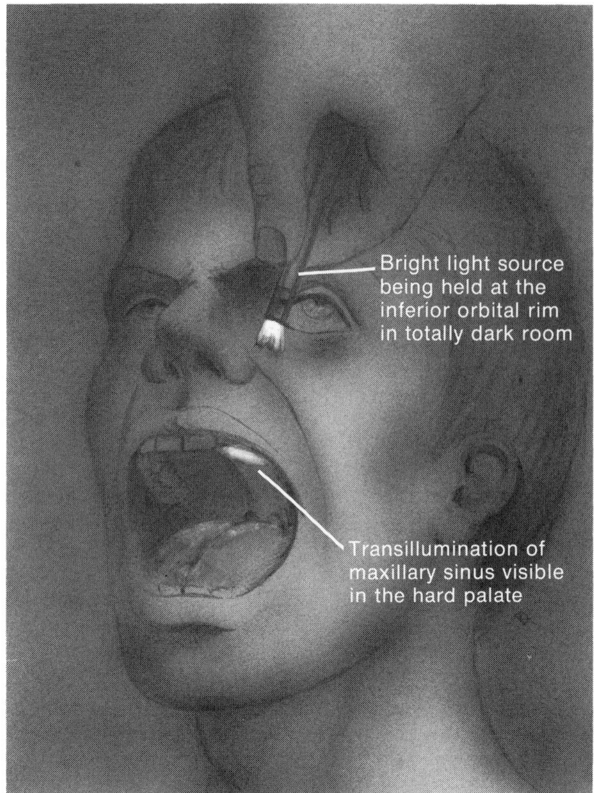

FIGURE 16–3. Transillumination of the maxillary sinus.

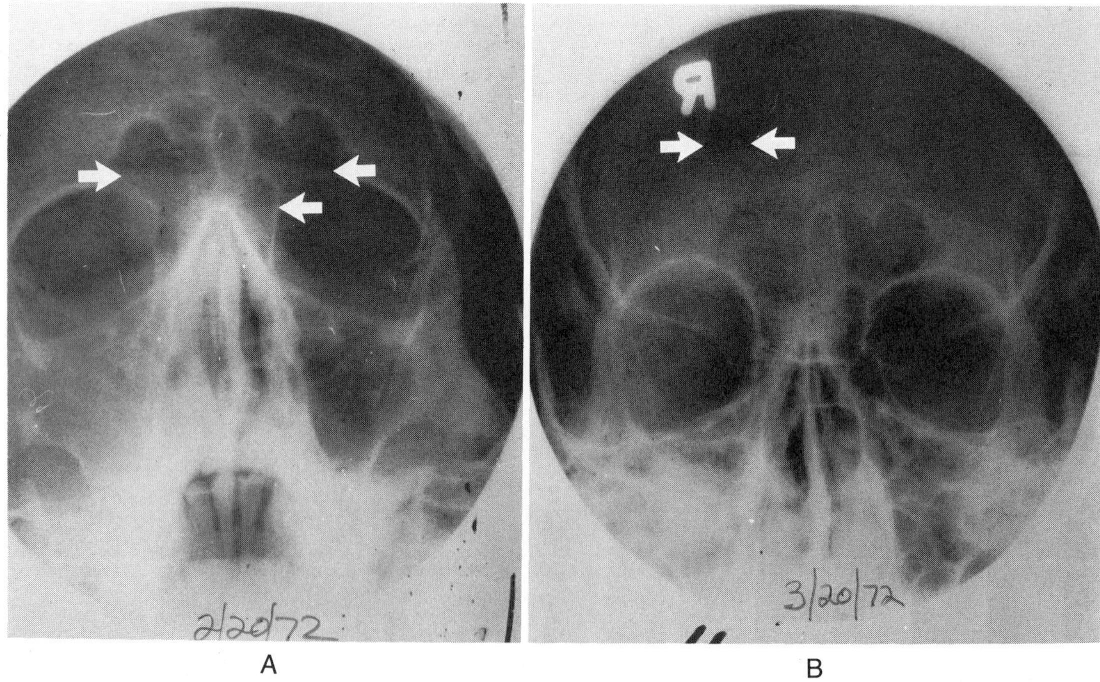

FIGURE 16–4. Radiographic findings in acute suppurative sinusitis. *A,* The Waters view, taken with the head at an angle, reveals an opaque right maxillary antrum and air-fluid levels *(arrows)* in an anterior ethmoidal sinus on the left and in both frontal sinuses. *B,* The Caldwell view, taken head-on, 1 month later reveals continued opacification of the right maxillary sinus and of the right frontal sinus. The patient had received an inadequate course of therapy with antibiotics. Arrows in the Caldwell view point to an area of frontal osteomyelitis developing as a complication.

The usual x-ray series includes three views of the sinuses (Fig. 16–4). The Caldwell view, taken head-on, shows the frontal and ethmoid sinuses, but the maxillary sinuses are partially obscured by the temporal bones in this view. The Waters view, taken with the head at an angle, shows the maxillary sinuses clearly, as well as the orbits, frontal sinuses, and nasal septum, and is as accurate as the entire series for diagnosing maxillary sinusitis.[2a] Lateral films are best for viewing the sphenoid sinuses and posterior walls of the frontal sinuses. A basal view also may be obtained and provides additional information on the status of the posterior ethmoid, sphenoid, and maxillary sinuses. Acute or chronic inflammation within a sinus produces a haziness or radiopaque appearance because of fluid or mucosal thickening. If high-quality radiographs are obtained, a completely normal appearance is thought to be good evidence against the presence of sinus disease. However, unless air-fluid levels are noted in addition to mucosal thickening, the diagnostic usefulness of radiographs is limited by false-positive findings in many asymptomatic individuals, who possibly had previous allergies or episodes of sinusitis. Computed tomography (CT) scans are essential to assess recurrent or persistent symptomatology.

The history and clinical findings are usually sufficient to diagnose acute sinusitis. Maxillary toothache (specific but not highly sensitive), abnormal transillumination, poor response to decongestants, and purulent or colored nasal discharge correlate with sinusitis, although the physician's overall clinical impression is diagnostically more accurate than any one finding.[2b] Radiographic studies, which are expensive and often result in nonspecific findings, are not necessary, except in unusually severe, persistent, or complicated cases. Sphenoid sinusitis is often more difficult to diagnose than infection involving the other sinuses; a CT scan of the head is the preferred method to confirm this diagnosis, when necessary.[2]

Otolaryngologists can gain valuable information by anesthetizing and vasoconstricting the nasal cavity and then performing an endoscopic-endonasal evaluation in an office setting.

Cultures of the nose or nasopharynx are often misleading unless obtained from the draining sinus ostium (Fig. 16–5). Throat cultures have no value in diagnosing sinusitis. In one study in which the nose was prepared with povidone-iodine (Betadine) and the maxillary antrum was punctured using a sterile technique, purulent aspirates containing bacteria and more than 1000 white blood cells per cubic millimeter were found in 17 of 24 adult patients with symptoms suggestive of sinusitis.[3] *Streptococcus pneumoniae* and *Haemophilus influenzae* were the organisms most commonly isolated, together accounting for more than half the cases, but a variety of other organisms were also recovered. The frequency with which various bacteria are likely to be encountered has been estimated in Table 16–2 on the basis of published series.[3–5] Staphylococci are isolated frequently from acutely infected sphenoid sinuses.[2] In general, purulent secretions grow bacteria if properly cultured, whereas nonpurulent secretions are usually sterile. Anaerobic bacteria rarely, if ever, are isolated in the presence of the aerobic pathogens, such as the pneumococcus or *H. influenzae,* and are thought to be secondary invaders that predominate and replace other organisms once oxygen tension has fallen within an infected antral space.[4, 5]

TABLE 16–2. BACTERIOLOGY OF ACUTE SUPPURATIVE SINUSITIS[3–5]

Bacteria	Frequency of Occurrence (%)
Streptococcus pneumoniae	50
Anaerobic organisms derived from the upper respiratory tract: *Streptococcus intermedius, Peptostreptococcus micros, Peptococcus magnus, Streptococcus constellatus*	20–30
Haemophilus influenzae, usually nontypable	10–15
Group A β-hemolytic streptococcus	5–7
Staphylococcus aureus, Staphylococcus epidermidis, and *Moraxella catarrhalis*	3–5
Aerobic, gram-negative bacilli	1
No growth	5

Treatment of acute suppurative sinusitis consists of administering antibiotics and decongestants. Because of the difficulty in obtaining reliable cultures, the antibiotic should be chosen on clinical grounds in most cases (see discussion in Chapter 19). Augmentin, which achieves high tissue concentrations and is effective against most nontypable strains of *H. influenzae,* may be the drug of choice. Newer erythromycins, such as clarythromycin, trimethaprim/sulfamethoxazole (co-trimoxazole), and cephalosporins, are alternative considerations. In diabetics or those with isolated frontal or sphenoid sinusitis, an antistaphylococcal agent, such as one of the semisynthetic penicillins, should be considered.

Topical nasal decongestants are most effective initially in establishing drainage and should be prescribed for the first few days but not for longer than 1 week. An oral decongestant also can be started and continued for several weeks. The oral drug pseudoephedrine (Sudafed) diminishes mucosal congestion within 30 minutes and continues to have effect for 4 hours.[6] Guaifenesin should be considered for thinning secretions. Antihistamines dry nasal se-

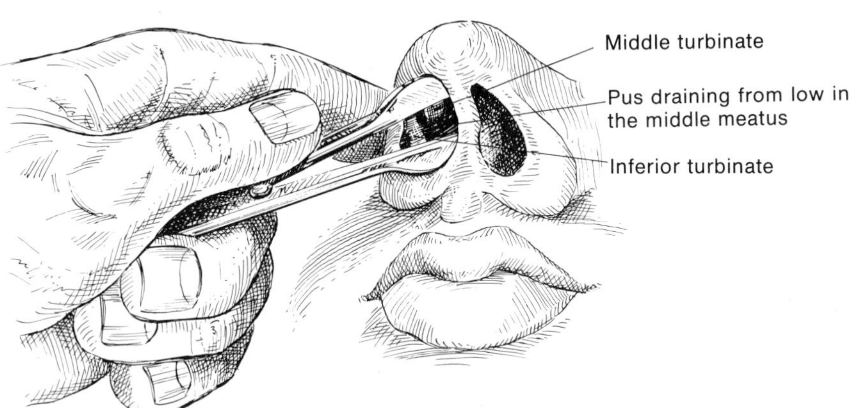

FIGURE 16–5. Demonstration of pus draining from low in the middle meatus between the middle and inferior turbinates in maxillary sinusitis.

cretions and generally are to be avoided in acute suppurative sinusitis.

Rest with the head elevated to decrease congestion, adequate hydration and humidity, and analgesic medications all help diminish symptoms in patients with acute sinusitis. Patients with sinusitis should also avoid alcohol, smoking, and exposure to cold, which may cause mucosal swelling.

It is generally believed that persistence of infection leads to mucosal thickening or ostial scarring, culminating in a poorly draining sinus and chronic sinusitis. In some cases, a purulent exudate remains within the sinus following treatment, although the patient is asymptomatic. For these reasons, antibiotics and oral decongestants probably should be continued for a minimum of 2 weeks, followed by an additional 10 days if purulent drainage persists.

In acute cases, it is important not to manipulate the natural ostium, because there is a risk of causing permanent scarring that may interfere with drainage. Effort should not be made, in most cases, to puncture the wall of the antrum. In ordinary acute sinusitis, in which drainage can be achieved by using decongestants, antral puncture increases the incidence of osteomyelitis without hastening symptomatic resolution. The only acute cases in which antral punctures are indicated are those involving acute empyema—that is, cases in which a sinus is filled with pus that fails to drain, causing severe, persistent pain and rendering treatment for infection inadequate.

If it becomes necessary to drain a maxillary sinus, a No. 18 gauge needle can be passed beneath the inferior turbinate (not at the middle meatus) after preparation with 5% cocaine; the cavity is entered, and when pus has been obtained, one may irrigate gently with normal saline to help re-establish mucosal ciliary action (Fig. 16–6).

Subacute or Chronic Suppurative Sinusitis. Purulent discharge, stuffy nose, and intermittent discomfort persist for more than 3 weeks in 10% or less of patients with acute suppurative sinusitis. Some of these have so-called hyperplastic sinusitis associated with allergic or nonallergic perennial rhinitis. In hyperplastic sinusitis, the mucous membrane lining the nose and paranasal sinuses becomes markedly hypertrophic and is subject to polyposis, chronic vasomotor instability, and inadequate drainage.[7] Presumably, in patients who have chronic suppurative sinusitis, the ciliated columnar epithelium lining the sinuses is damaged by continuous infection and is replaced by goblet cells or squamous cells (metaplasia). The primary symptoms are persistent purulent drainage, cough, and halitosis, although bouts of congestion and superimposed infections may occur. Irreversible chronic suppuration can persist despite adequate medical therapy but is uncommon. Patients with nasal stuffiness or postnasal drip are more likely to have vasomotor, perennial, or allergic rhinitis than chronic sinusitis, and the correct diagnosis is suggested by the history and examination. When chronic sinusitis is suspected, axial and coronal CT scans of the sinuses are indicated. The status of the mucosa, sinus ostea, and any aberrant bone architecture are defined by this imaging modality. Routine sinus films are no longer recommended in this setting.

Therapy of subacute and chronic sinusitis consists of antibiotics and decongestants administered in 2-week courses to eradicate infection, establish drainage, and allow the mucosa to return to normal with ciliary action restored. Perennial hyperplastic rhinosinusitis should be treated additionally with measures designed for allergic or nonallergic rhinitis (see Chapter 15). In one series in which cultures were obtained by strictly aseptic techniques at the time of sinus surgery, 23 of 28 specimens from cases of chronic sinusitis yielded a pure, heavy growth of anaerobes and only three showed pure, heavy growth of aerobes.[8] These anaerobic organisms derived from mouth flora generally are sensitive to penicillin. Clindamycin and tetracycline derivatives are alternatives.

For patients with persistent, subacute disease, as opposed to those with acute infections, antral puncture can be useful to obtain cultures and irrigate the sinus.

Surgery is indicated for patients who fail to respond to conservative management, presumably because persistent mucosal swelling or infection are compromising normal drainage and aeration. Limited endonasal fiberoptic sinus surgery has replaced more traditional approaches (e.g., external ethmoidectomy and Caldwell-Luc approaches). Enhanced visualization enables the sinus ostea to be enlarged and surrounding diseased mucosa to be removed. Even cases formerly considered advanced can respond to this conservative surgery. A success rate of 80% is to be anticipated in nonasthmatic patients. In some cases, even the frontal sinus ostia can be approached endoscopically.

Complications of Sinusitis

Suppurative complications of sinusitis resulting from local or hematogenous spread, usually in inadequately or

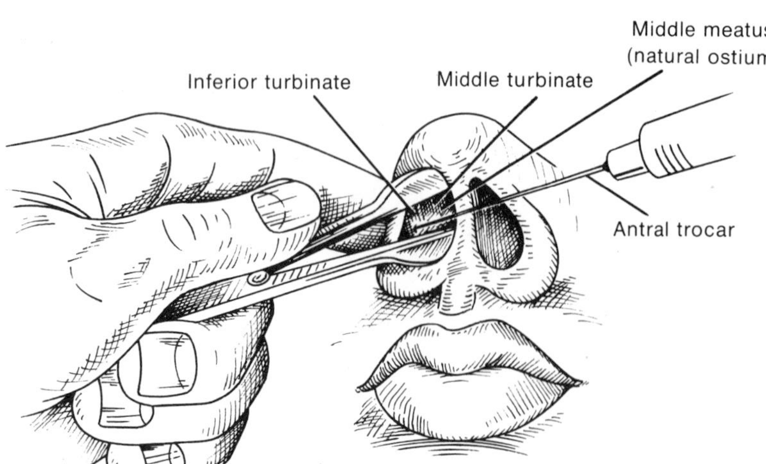

FIGURE 16–6. Irrigation of the maxillary sinus. The trocar is inserted under the inferior turbinate and enters the maxillary antrum through the lateral wall of the nose. The sinus can be irrigated with normal saline, and the irrigations are washed back into the nose through the natural ostium in the middle meatus.

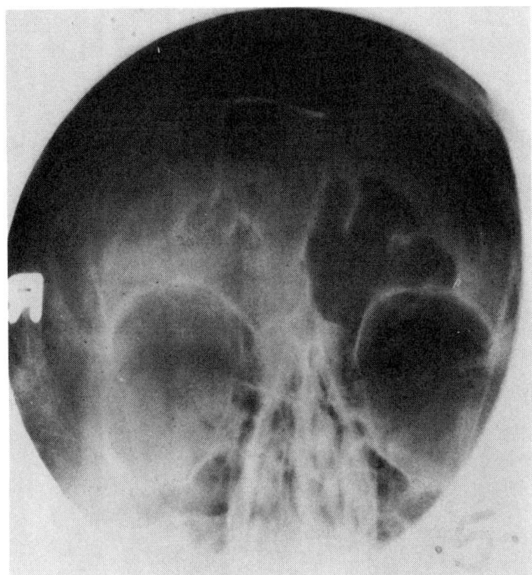

FIGURE 16–7. Frontal osteomyelitis. A Caldwell view of the frontal bone and sinuses reveals patchy lucency of the bone above an opacified right frontal sinus. The patient had complained of increasingly severe right frontal headaches, tenderness, and soft tissue swelling over a period of 6 weeks.

partially treated cases, are uncommon but potentially lethal. In frontal osteomyelitis, low-grade persistent fever and dull headache are accompanied, over a period of weeks, by doughy, cool swelling of the frontal periostium and edema of the eyelids (Pott's puffy tumor). In some cases, frontal osteomyelitis may develop abruptly and follow a more fulminant course (Fig. 16–7). CT scans may reveal opacification within the sinus, together with an indistinct superior margin or radiolucency within the frontal bone. Periostitis of the orbit or subperiosteal abscess arises by extension of ethmoid sinusitis through the lateral ethmoidal plate (Fig. 16–8). Manifestations include fever, pain on motion of the eyes, edema at the inner canthus, and mild chemosis. As this progresses into orbital cellulitis, chills and fever, periorbital edema, diminished bulbar mobility, proptosis, and advanced chemosis accompany the symptoms of sinusitis.[9] Cavernous sinus thrombosis results from septic thrombophlebitis via the ethmoidal vein or from extension of infection from sphenoid sinusitis. Its manifestations begin with chills, fever, and progressive severe retrobulbar pain and progress to retinal engorgement and loss of vision, frequently accompanied by a selective orbital palsy (third, fourth, or sixth nerve) that precedes severe edema and fixation of the eye, delirium, and coma. Meningitis develops from septic thrombophlebitis of the dural veins. In this illness, the patient, who often has purulent sinusitis of abrupt onset, may have a chill followed by persistent headache and vomiting. Fever, stiff neck, and altered sensorium develop as later manifestations. Finally, brain abscess or epidural or subdural abscess may develop in the presence of acute or chronic purulent sinusitis. In one series, a third of patients with brain abscess had accompanying sinusitis.[10] Abscesses usually involve the "silent" frontal lobe and present chiefly with recurrent, progressively worsening headaches that eventually are accompanied by mood or personality changes.[10] Papilledema is a late manifestation. Subdural or epidural empyema should be suspected when there is an abrupt onset of headache, vomiting, and high fever, later followed by alterations of consciousness and signs of meningeal irritation. Focal neurologic signs or convulsions occur only very late in the course of the illness.

The diagnosis of intracranial suppurative complications is best established by computed tomography or magnetic resonance imaging (MRI). Lumbar puncture must be considered when meningitis is suspected. Burr holes may be necessary as a life-saving measure in critically ill patients with subdural empyema.[11]

Complications are reported to be frequent in sphenoid sinusitis. However, the diagnosis of sphenoid sinusitis undoubtedly is not made in many mild cases that spontaneously resolve or respond to antibiotic therapy; thus, the true incidence of complications remains unknown. In one series of 30 cases, complications included five patients with cavernous sinus thrombosis and six with acute meningitis.[2] The location of the sphenoid sinus and the delay in diagnosing infections within it no doubt account for some complications. Twenty of these 30 patients required surgical drainage of the sinus in addition to antibiotic therapy.[2]

An important point to emphasize about the suppurative complications of sinusitis is that their initial manifestations may be nonspecific—that is, chills, fever, vomiting, generalized headache, personality alterations, or periorbital edema—but none of these is expected in uncomplicated cases of sinusitis. Ordinarily, acute sinusitis is a local infection without systemic symptoms other than low-grade fever and malaise. Patients who appear to be in a toxic state or who have any of the manifestations detailed earlier should be hospitalized and treated parenterally with antibiotics under close medical observation even when specific signs of meningitis, brain abscess, empyema, or osteomyelitis are absent.

Meningitis in adults generally is caused by the pneumococcus, whereas brain abscesses and other intracranial suppurative complications usually result from a mixture of organisms, including anaerobic streptococci.[12] Neverthe-

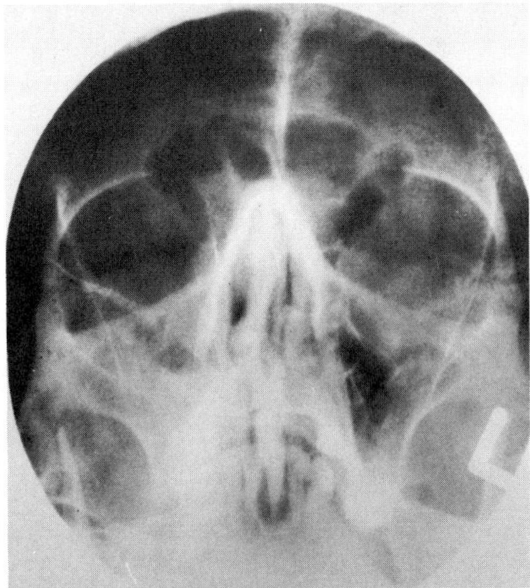

FIGURE 16–8. Periostitis of the orbit. A 50-year-old diabetic woman complained of pain over the left eye. Her symptoms had begun 5 days previously with an upper respiratory infection and nasal congestion. Three days later, she had fevers to 38.8° C (102° F) and a sense of fullness over the left eye. She then developed persistent pain over the eye with swelling at the inner canthus and orbit. The radiograph (Waters view) reveals opacification of the right maxillary and bilateral ethmoidal sinuses. She was hospitalized and received intravenous antibiotics. There was no loss of bulbar mobility, and the patient recovered fully without requiring surgery.

less, until the results of cultures are known, broad-spectrum coverage should be planned for most patients suspected of having complications of sinusitis. Intravenously administered clindamycin remains an excellent initial drug, having good sinus penetrability, and can be combined with others as the need arises. Further treatment may include complete exenteration of the frontal sinus and removal of areas of diseased frontal bone in frontal osteomyelitis, if the process fails to resolve on antibiotics alone; drainage of localized pus in periorbital abscess; surgical drainage if there is loss of bulbar mobility, deterioration of vision, or failure to respond to antibiotic therapy within 24 to 48 hours in periorbital cellulitis or periostitis of the orbit; heparinization, even though not proved to be beneficial, in cavernous sinus thrombosis; and neurosurgical drainage of brain abscesses or subdural or epidural empyemas, with use of antibiotics.

Tumors, Growths, and Other Disorders of the Sinuses

More than one half of malignant tumors of the sinuses are squamous cell carcinomas and involve the maxillary sinus.[13, 14] The annual incidence of all sinus malignancies is only 1.5 to 3.5 per 100,000, mostly occurring in individuals above 35 to 40 years of age[14]; about one half of the cases are related to occupational exposures to dusty environments from work with hardwoods, rubber, or shoe leather.[15]

There are no symptoms until the tumor causes obstruction, bleeding, or pain from bony invasion. Then, the most common manifestation is recurrent, chronic rhinosinusitis that fails to resolve as expected, indicating obstruction of the middle meatus.[13] On occasion, proptosis, diplopia, infraorbital anesthesia, or looseness of the maxillary teeth from erosion by a tumor may be the initial symptom (see Table 16–1). A mass may be apparent radiographically within the sinus cavity and constitutes the most important diagnostic finding (Fig. 16–9). Bone destruction is a more specific finding, suggesting tumor. Bony sclerosis is a nonspecific finding. An abnormality on plain films or clinical features suggesting malignancy are indications for CT scanning with enhancement. When a tumor is suspected a biopsy, using a Caldwell-Luc or other incision, is mandatory, is easily accomplished, and provides definitive information. CT scanning and MRI jointly are helpful for planning surgery and/or radiation therapy. The MRI can differentiate a tumor from obstructed ostia with retained secretions. Chemotherapy may be considered as an up-front adjunct for advanced lesions.

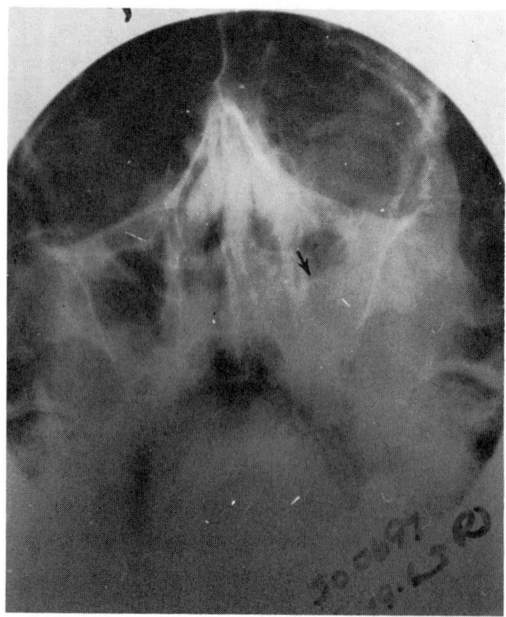

FIGURE 16–9. Squamous cell carcinoma of the maxillary antrum. The patient had a fever and pain in the left maxilla for 3 weeks. A plain radiograph (Waters view) reveals a mass within the sinus. A biopsy of the mass through a Caldwell-Luc incision was necessary to establish the diagnosis.

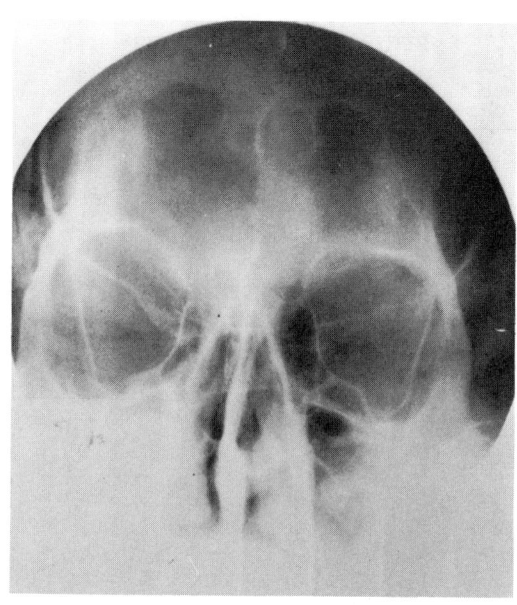

FIGURE 16–10. Mucocele of the right frontal sinus. The patient complained of frontal headaches, and swelling of the right eyelid was noted. On plain film (Caldwell view), a soft tissue mass is visible within the right frontal sinus. The mass has eroded into the superior rim of the orbit and into the left frontal sinus.

Mucoceles are late complications of sinusitis. They may gradually enlarge and eventually produce erosion caused by accumulation of mucus in a completely blocked sinus. The frontal sinus is most commonly affected. Often, there is a history of prior intranasal surgery with older techniques. Facial trauma is another predisposing factor. Patients present with headache, swelling of the eyelid, and a rubbery mass beneath the supraorbital ridge. Radiographs show that the bone margins of the sinus are indistinct (Fig. 16–10), which can be confirmed by tomography; a soft tissue mass may be demonstrable. The management is with surgery. The external approach is still preferred in this setting.

Benign tumors of the sinuses include osteomas and chondromas, which may be removed if they cause obstruction. Antral cysts noted radiographically are of no clinical import unless they cause osteal obstruction or pressure symptoms based on size. Choanal polyps, arising from the maxillary sinus, pass through the meatus and may obstruct the nasopharynx (choana). They are amenable to endoscopic surgical techniques.

Lethal midline granuloma, Wegener's granulomatosis, reticulum cell sarcoma, and fungal infections represent chronic inflammatory or destructive conditions of the nose and sinuses. All may be associated with a mass effect or bone erosions mimicking carcinoma. Aspergillosis is usually confined to a single maxillary sinus and presents with unilateral nasal obstruction and greenish, firm, gelatinous material that is found in the nasal cavity or on antral irrigation.[17] Patients generally are afebrile, and the disease follows a chronic course marked by little or no obtainable pus and failure to improve after antral lavages.[18] Rhinocerebral mucormycosis has a more fulminant, progressive course marked by headache, fever, lethargy, facial swelling, and a black, necrotic appearance to the tissue. The diagnosis is established most reliably by transnasal biopsy.[19] Whereas aspergillosis may occur when no underlying chronic illness is present,[18] mucormycosis is associated with immunosuppression from varied etiologies and diabetic ketoacidosis. *Candida albicans* also produces an opportunistic maxillary sinusitis in diabetic patients or in those who have had maxillary trauma.[20] In rare cases with chronic or necrotizing involvement of the nose or sinuses, the question of vasculitis, granulomatous disease, or lymphoma arises. A biopsy will establish the diagnosis of Wegener's granulomatosis by demonstrating a necrotizing vasculitis. The pathologic distinction between granuloma (lethal midline granuloma) and lymphoma may be difficult.[21]

REFERENCES

1. Mulbury PE: Medical management of sinusitis. Ear Nose Throat J 63:151, 1984.
2. Lew D, Southwick FS, Montgomery WW, et al: Sphenoid sinusitis: A review of 30 cases. N Engl J Med 309:1149, 1983.

2a. Williams JW, Roberts L Jr, Distell B, et al. Diagnosing sinusitis by x-ray: Is a single Waters view adequate? J Gen Intern Med 7:481. 1992.

2b. Williams JW, Simel DL, Roberts L Jr, et al. Clinical evaluation for sinusitis. Making the diagnosis by history and physical examination. Ann Intern Med 117:705, 1992.

3. Evans FO Jr, Sydnor JB, Moore WEC, et al: Sinusitis of the maxillary antrum. N Engl J Med 293:735, 1975.
4. Carenfelt C, Landberg C, Nord CE, et al: Bacteriology of maxillary sinusitis in relation to quality of the retained secretion. Acta Otolaryngol (Stockh) 86:298, 1978.
5. Landberg C, Carenfelt C, Engquist S, et al: Anaerobic bacteria in the maxillary sinus. Scand J Infect Dis 19(Suppl):74, 1979.
6. Roth RP, Cantekin EI, Bluestone CD, et al: Nasal decongestant activity of pseudoephedrine. Ann Otol Rhinol Laryngol 86(Part 1):235, 1977.
7. Wilson M: Chronic hypertrophic polypoid rhinosinusitis. Neuroradiology 120:609, 1976.
8. Frederick J and Braude AI: Anaerobic infection of the paranasal sinuses. N Engl J Med 290:135, 1975.
9. Mann W, Beck CH, and Rover J: Surgical or conservative treatment for orbital complications of sinus inflammations. HNO 26:296, 1978.
10. Carey ME, Chou SN, and French LA: Experience with brain abscesses. J Neurosurg 36:1, 1972.
11. Kaufman DM, Miller MH, and Steigbigel NH: Subdural empyema: Analysis of 17 recent cases and review of the literature. Medicine 54:485, 1975.
12. Yue A and Sasaki CT: Intracranial complications of sinusitis. Conn Med 41:70, 1977.
13. Weber AL, Tadmor R, Davis R, et al: Malignant tumors of the sinuses: Radiological evaluation including CT scanning with clinical and pathologic correlation. Neuroradiology 16:443, 1978.
14. Bridges MWM, Beale FA, and Bryce DP: Carcinoma of the paranasal sinuses—a review of 158 cases. J Otolaryngol 7:379, 1978.
15. Acheson ED: Nasal cancer in the furniture and boot and shoe manufacturing industries. Prev Med 5:295, 1976.
16. Parsons C and Hudson N: Computed tomography of paranasal sinus tumors. Radiology 32:641, 1979.
17. Warder FR, Chikes PG, and Hudson WR: Aspergillosis of the paranasal sinuses. Arch Otolaryngol 101:683, 1975.
18. Jahrsdoerfer RA, Ejercito VS, Johns MME, et al: Aspergillosis of the nose and paranasal sinuses. Am J Otolaryngol 1:6, 1979.
19. Pillsbury HC and Fischer ND: Rhinocerebral mucormycosis. Arch Otolaryngol 103:600, 1977.
20. Chapnik JS and Bach MC: Bacterial and fungal infections of the maxillary sinus. Otolaryngol Clin North Am 9:43, 1976.
21. Michaels L and Gregory MM: Pathology of nonhealing (midline) granuloma. J Clin Pathol 30:317, 1977.

17

Hoarseness and Diseases of the Larynx

MARSHALL STROME, MD, MS
MARVIN FRIED, MD

The larynx begins as an outgrowth of the pharyngeal floor at approximately the third week of gestation. After initial laryngeal development, secondary proliferation of the lining obliterates the central tract. Canalization normally occurs via reabsorption; however, when it does not, developmental anomalies frequently become clinically significant.[1, 2]

Phylogenetically, the most important function of the larynx is to protect the airway. A common misconception is that the epiglottis is most important in this regard. However, the strong sphincteric action of the true vocal cords, aided by the false cords and aryepiglottic folds, functionally has more significance. In addition to phonation, the larynx participates in the process of deglutition, respiration, and the act of coughing.[3]

CLINICAL ANATOMY

The superior margin of the larynx is the tip of the epiglottis, and the inferior border is considered to be the undersurface of the cricoid cartilage. The two vocal folds (true vocal cords) form the glottis. The area above the glottis to the tip of the epiglottis is defined as the supraglottic larynx (Fig. 17–1), whereas the area below the vocal folds to the inferior border of the cricoid cartilage and trachea is considered subglottic.

The blood supply to the larynx is derived from both the superior and inferior thyroid arteries via the laryngeal vessels. The nerve supply is bilateral and is from both the superior and inferior laryngeal nerves.[3]

DIAGNOSIS AND HISTORY

The two most common laryngeal symptoms are hoarseness and dyspnea or stridor. The onset of each should be noted for duration and change in severity. Often they are insidious in nature with no definable starting point. The cause of hoarseness is most commonly infection but can be trauma, malignancy, or vocal cord paralysis from a disorder of the recurrent laryngeal nerve. Of diagnostic import are the patient's age, the duration of the hoarseness, and the association of obstructive respiratory symptoms or other symptoms, such as hemoptysis, dysphagia, and local or referred pain. The physician should determine the location of pain and assess whether it is associated with speaking or swallowing.

Trauma may be associated with laryngeal derangement. This may be external, as by motor vehicle accident, or internal due to intubation at the time of surgery. Foreign bodies must be considered, especially in children. Systemic pathology, such as rheumatoid cricoarytenoid arthritis, may present initially as localized laryngeal disease.

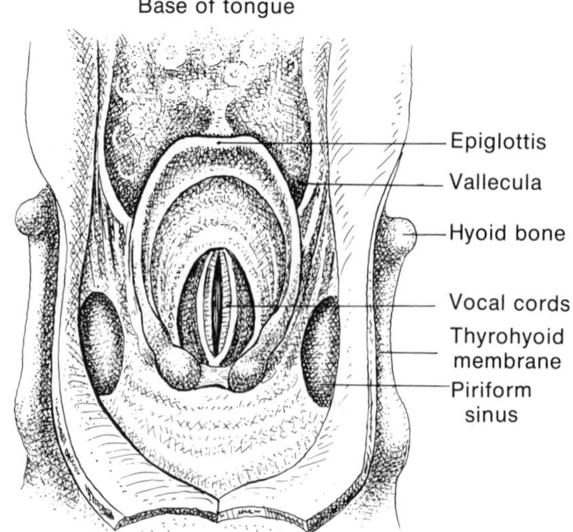

FIGURE 17–1. The supraglottic larynx, including the epiglottis and vocal cords, seen from above.

Hoarseness lasting longer than 2 weeks absolutely requires visualization of the larynx by direct or indirect techniques.

PHYSICAL EXAMINATION—LARYNGEAL EXAMINATION

Observing the respiratory pattern, phonatory effort, and vocalization will help with the differential diagnosis. Standard initial examination involves the use of the laryngeal mirror. A bright light source is directed by the physician's head mirror toward the anatomic region to be examined. Positioning of the mirror during phonation affords good visualization in most instances of not only the larynx but also the hypopharynx and tongue base. Mirrors with increased magnification are available, affording better visualization of pathology. Children younger than 4 years of age will not tolerate this technique because of the associated tongue manipulation necessary for detailed visualization. For this age group the 3-mm or less flexible laryngoscope can now be used safely in most cases without anesthesia in an outpatient setting (Fig. 17–2).

Rigid right-angle telescopes are becoming more common in the office. Since they are distal illuminating, they may be easier to master by the novice than indirect laryngoscopy; they are passed orally into the pharynx and allow exceptional visualization in the cooperative patient.

Anterior-posterior radiographs of the neck as well as lateral views provide information about altered soft tissue anatomy. In selected cases, computed tomography can provide additional detailed and specific anatomic information.

In the child with completely normal respiration and persistent minor phonatory abnormalities, the larynx may not be readily visualized indirectly. A period of observation may be rewarded by the ability to perform a satisfactory outpatient examination at a later date. This conservative approach in most instances eliminates the need for general anesthesia. When the history or physical examination suggests respiratory obstruction or increasing dyspnea, however, direct visualization is mandatory. With the improvements in endoscopic instrumentation and anesthesia techniques, most direct laryngoscopies in all age groups are performed with general anesthesia. The relaxation afforded allows introduction of a large enough laryngoscope for routine use of the operating microscope. Telescopes enable excellent functional assessment of the subglottic space and trachea and preclude the need for formal bronchoscopy in many instances.[4]

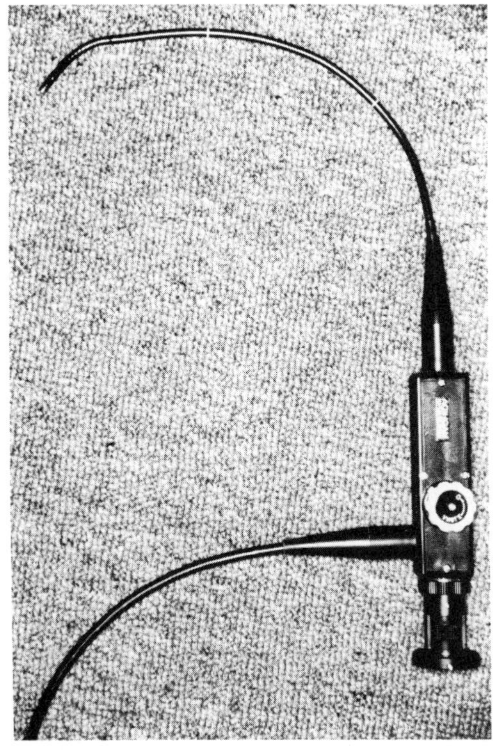

FIGURE 17–2. Fiberoptic flexible nasopharyngolaryngoscope, which allows full visualization of the upper airway when passed nasally.

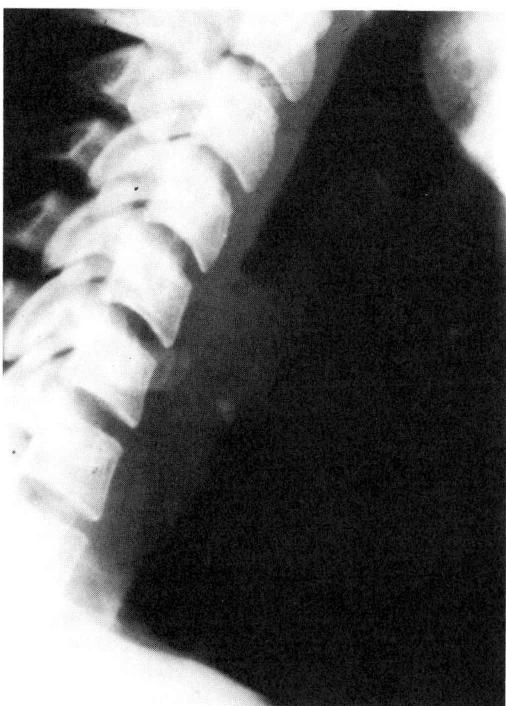

FIGURE 17–3. Plain soft tissue lateral radiograph of the larynx, depicting a blunted and edematous epiglottis (supraglottitis) in an adult.

Radiology

Plain Films

Although these may be limited by the superimposition of the cervical spine on laryngeal architecture, the anterior-posterior view is useful when evaluating air-fluid levels (as found in laryngoceles) or assessing subcutaneous emphysema as well as distortion of the upper airway. The lateral view of the neck is particularly useful in evaluating the epiglottis, the retropharynx, or the parapharyngeal space (Fig. 17–3). The nasopharynx also can be included in this projection. Radiopaque foreign bodies can be easily demonstrated in both the anterior-posterior and lateral plain films (Fig. 17–4).[5]

Fluoroscopy

Fluoroscopy allows the dynamic visualization of the airway, evaluating the functions of both respiration and phonation.

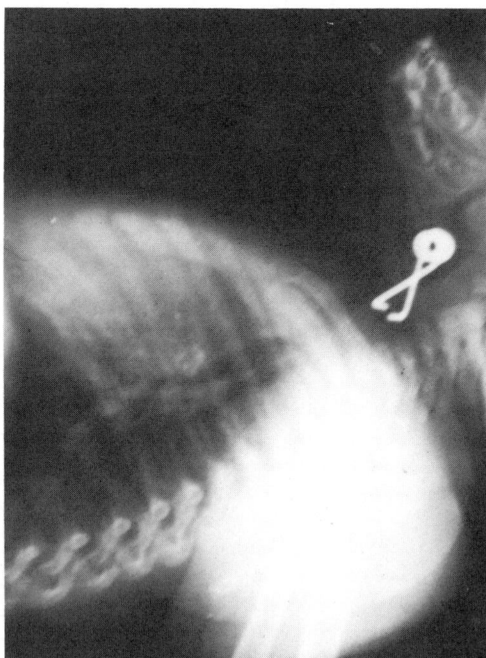

FIGURE 17–4. Lateral neck projection showing a foreign body (clothespin clip) lodged at the level of the larynx.

Barium Swallow

This study is of particular value when radiolucent foreign bodies are suspected in the upper airway or esophagus. It also may assist in delineating neoplastic processes within the hypopharynx and surrounding area. Often there is some degree of aspiration of the barium in patients with upper airway dysfunction, which coats the intralaryngeal structures (Fig. 17–5).[5] This technique also helps in assessing upper airway anomalies in the infant and should be considered prior to direct examination of the larynx.

Computed Tomography

This technique is the definitive radiographic analysis of the larynx. It allows visualization of the architecture and soft tissue densities when other radiographic techniques fail. It can delineate destruction of both bone and cartilage as well as distortion of the airway and is now the most precise noninvasive method of viewing the upper airway (Fig. 17–6).[6]

Magnetic Resonance Imaging

Magnetic resonance imaging (MRI) is an excellent modality to evaluate the soft tissues and vascular cervical structures but offers no benefit in imaging the larynx. Future use of three-dimensional reconstruction may prove beneficial but is currently not routinely available.

DIFFERENTIAL DIAGNOSIS

Hoarseness has multiple causes. Although the underlying pathology may be suspected on the basis of duration of symptoms and vocal quality, no specific characteristics of hoarseness are definitely diagnostic. Infectious diseases cause the majority of cases seen in primary care practice.

Infectious and Inflammatory Etiologies

Acute Laryngitis. Acute laryngitis is the most frequent cause of hoarseness in the adult; supraglottitis (epiglottitis), croup (subglottitis), and laryngotracheobronchitis are more often seen in children. Acute laryngitis is usually viral in etiology. The patient has hoarseness and inflammation of the larynx. Influenza and adenoviruses are the most frequently recognized pathogens. Rare causes, seen in patients with unusually severe or protracted courses, include diphtheria and herpes simplex. Symptoms associated with acute laryngitis include malaise, rhinitis, and pharyngalgia (pharyngeal pain). Frank hoarseness and in many instances transient aphonia can be correlated clinically with significant erythema and edema of the vocal cords.

Bacteria, most often *Streptococcus pneumoniae, Haemophilus influenzae*, β-hemolytic streptococcus, and staphylococcus, rarely produce a fulminant form of laryngitis in the adult. In this entity, epithelial sloughing associated with fibrinopurulent exudate can organize and lead to an obstructing pseudomembrane.

For management of the commonly encountered viral laryngitis, voice rest, humidification, reduced physical activity, and analgesics are warranted. Secondary bacterial infections are best managed with antibiotic therapy chosen to cover the most common pathogens. Fulminant pseudomembranous laryngitis presents with stridor and necessitates hospitalization with hydration, humidification, and high doses of intravenously administered antibiotics. Often, if the airway is significantly obstructed, the tenacious crusts must be endoscopically removed.[7]

Laryngeal abscesses are rare complications of acute bacterial laryngitis and are encountered more frequently following endotracheal intubation, as a consequence of an infected field or laryngeal trauma. Differentiating features of this entity include severe pharyngalgia, associated odynophagia (painful swallowing), significant fever, and signs of

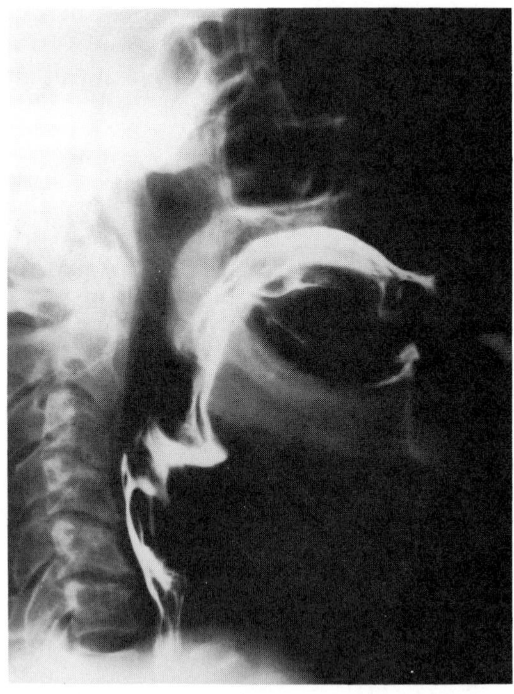

FIGURE 17–5. Barium swallow, outlining a deformity at the level of the larynx, suggestive of a neoplastic process.

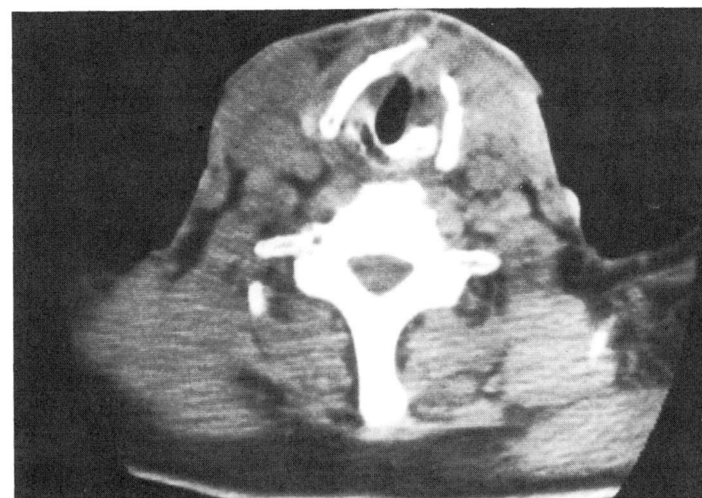

FIGURE 17–6. Computed tomogram of a carcinoma of the larynx, showing fullness of the vocal cord and thyroid cartilage destruction. (Same patient as shown in Figure 17–5.)

systemic toxicity. Pain is often reproduced by lateral motion of the larynx. Respiratory distress is expected. If a response to high-dose intravenous antibiotics providing coverage for *Staphylococcus, Pseudomonas*, and *Proteus* does not result in improved symptoms within 48 hours, a tracheotomy followed by drainage of the abscess is essential.

Croup Syndromes (Subglottic Inflammations). We prefer to use the term *laryngotracheobronchitis* for viral or bacterial infection with cough that involves the larynx, trachea, and bronchi. *Croup* refers to a syndrome of subglottic space inflammation, usually with hacking cough and stridor, most often encountered in neonates and infants, usually viral but possibly bacterial, and spasmodic or traumatic in etiology.[7,8] The subglottic space in infants is small enough so that 1 mm of edema reduces air passage by as much as 40%. Boys under 3 years of age are most often affected. An acute upper respiratory infection usually antedates the subsequent hoarseness, barking cough, and, ultimately, respiratory obstruction. Progression of symptoms varies according to the anatomy and virulence of the invading organism but may be rapid.

Adults can get infections of the subglottic space with similar symptoms. The syndrome in adults also occurs following prolonged endotracheal intubation.

Racemic epinephrine administered with intermittent positive pressure often gives dramatic relief of respiratory distress. Several cycles of therapy may be necessary. When this treatment is used the patient must be hospitalized; deaths have occurred after a single treatment was administered and the patient was sent home.[8] Cardiac monitoring is advised for adults. Humidification assists in thinning tracheal secretions and is the hallmark of any treatment program. Use of antibiotics and steroids is controversial, but most laryngologists believe that they have merit. If despite medical management, respiratory obstruction increases, or if a patient presents in extremis, judicious intubation is warranted for a short interval only. If intubation for this condition is needed for longer than 72 hours, consideration must be given to performing a tracheotomy. Repeated episodes of "croup" in the child raise the question of an underlying congenital anomaly, and bronchoscopy should be performed.

Supraglottitis (Epiglottitis). Acute supraglottitis (epiglottitis) involves not only the epiglottitis but usually all the laryngeal structures above the vocal folds. Although more common in children, this condition also affects adults. In the classic form, it is a life-threatening illness.[9] Though less common than laryngitis or laryngotracheobronchitis, milder variants of supraglottitis probably occur more frequently than is recognized and pass for a severe sore throat.

In adults, supraglottitis is most often viral in etiology. In children, usually 2 to 5 years of age, bacterial infection, particularly *Haemophilus influenzae* type B, is most frequent. Patients are usually quite symptomatic. The child may sit with the head erect and forward; drooling is associated; and if the spoken word is audible, the voice will be muffled as opposed to hoarse. The adult usually complains of severe pharyngalgia and has a normal-appearing oropharynx, associated drooling, and a muffled voice. A lateral soft tissue film of the neck can be confirmatory (see Fig. 17–3). Indirect laryngoscopy reveals inflammation of the supraglottic larynx, but this procedure is hazardous as it may precipitate respiratory obstruction. However, the fiberoptic laryngoscope, when placed transnasally, can visualize the supraglottis without approaching the tip of the epiglottis. Hypoxic patients, whenever possible, should not be manipulated until they are in the operating room or if in extremis when the equipment and surrounding facilities permit an emergency tracheotomy.

If the adult has been symptomatic for more than 8 hours, has a white blood cell count within the range of normal, and is afebrile, intervention of any type is unlikely to be necessary. Such a patient may be hospitalized for observation for a 24-hour period, although most patients, with careful explanation, can be managed as outpatients.[10] The febrile adult with an elevated white blood cell count must be hospitalized. The child with supraglottitis absolutely must be hospitalized. If there are any signs of respiratory obstruction, and these do not respond within 2 hours to intravenously administered antibiotics and steroids, intubation is essential. During the period of medical trial in pediatric patients, an expert bronchoscopist must remain with the patient.[11]

Today, intubation is the management of choice for both adults and children when respiratory obstruction supervenes. A tracheotomy is rarely necessary. Prior to the antibiotic era, supraglottitis was observed to resolve spontaneously in 5 to 7 days.[12] If steroids are used in conjunction with antibiotics, at most a 3-day period of intubation is warranted.

Internal Trauma

Emergent or inexpert intubations can cause contusions of the vocal cords, lacerations anywhere within the larynx, arytenoid cartilage dislocations, and transient associated vocal cord paralysis. Prolonged intubation, in both adults and children, has been associated with ulceration and subsequent dissolution of the vocal processes of the arytenoids, since all such tubes rest primarily in the posterior glottic area. These patients will persist in having a breathy vocal quality upon extubation. If too large a tube is used, secondary infection occurs, and stenosis of the subglottic space can be a sequela.

External Trauma

Most often the neck hyperextends in automobile accidents, and the larynx or upper trachea impacts upon the steering wheel. In neck trauma, hoarseness, respiratory distress, flattening of the thyroid ala, and crepitation suggesting subcutaneous emphysema indicate that a laryngeal fracture should be considered. Immediate indirect laryngoscopy and palpation should establish the diagnosis. Once made, an emergency tracheotomy must be considered. Subsequent repair should be performed as soon as the patient's general physical condition permits general anesthesia.[13] Chronic laryngeal stenosis can usually be avoided in adults if the operation is performed within the first 10 days after injury.[14, 15]

Hemmorhage

Hemorrhage within the substance of the vocal cords is uncommon but can occur secondary to anticoagulant therapy, bleeding diathesis, or trauma. The diagnosis rests upon visualization of the larynx. Although hemorrhage may be localized, the bleeding and subsequent swelling may be progressive, as evidenced by diffuse ecchymosis of the glottic and the supraglottic structures. Any underlying bleeding diathesis should be corrected. The condition is usually of limited duration; however, in the presence of airway compromise, hospitalization is mandatory. Intubation must precede any consideration of a tracheotomy.

Allergies

Allergic involvement of the larynx is uncommon in the conventional sense. Many substances as well as inhalants have been implicated. In childhood, foods are the most common cause and are not uncommon in the adult. Dust affects not only the nasal mucosa but also the tracheobronchial tree. The associated swelling of nasal structures may lead to a confusing picture of hyponasality in combination with hoarseness. Indirect laryngoscopy will reveal erythema, usually mild, and swelling of the free margin of the vocal folds. Appropriate allergic management, including avoidance of the offending agents and desensitization, is frequently rewarded with cessation of the symptoms. Newer steroid sprays (beclomethasone, flunisolide) are frequently beneficial and can be used in the older child and adult for short intervals. Dysphonia associated with giant urticaria can lead to respiratory obstruction.

Cigarette smoke has a definite effect on a child's larynx. In the past 8 years, we have seen a significant number of children with erythema of the vocal folds for whom the only significant history was that of parental smoking.

Nonhereditary angioneurotic edema can occur in any region of the larynx as a response to a wide range of provokers, the most common of which are foods, inhalants, and medication. There is typically a family history of allergic disorders, including asthma, hay fever, and eczema. The use of aspirin is commonly noted; however, other sensitivities have been identified, including bee stings, house dust, cosmetics, and beef. Aniline dye ingestion, tetanus antitoxin, and other vaccines may produce a similar response. Laryngeal edema can occur after the administration of penicillin, either oral or parenteral, as much as 1 to 4 hours after the initial exposure. The acute response is an anaphylactic reaction that can involve the epiglottis, arytenoids, ventricular bands, true vocal cords, or subglottis. The diagnosis is established by obtaining the appropriate history of an antecedent exposure. An examination of the larynx discloses a pale, boggy edema of the regions involved. In the early stages, therapy is based on the use of subcutaneous epinephrine usually with a rapid resolution. The supplemental use of an antihistamine (diphenhydramine, 25 to 50 mg IV) or a corticosteroid (dexamethasone, 5 to 10 mg IV) merits consideration. If a rapid response does not occur, then the airway must be secured by endotracheal intubation.

Hereditary angioneurotic edema is a genetic disease of autosomal dominant inheritance, in which there is a deficiency of the inhibitor of the first component of complement. Usually the attacks begin in childhood, occur frequently, and diminish with age. Mortality has been reported to vary from approximately 5 to 50%. Hereditary angioneurotic edema differs from other forms because of the presence of associated gastrointestinal symptoms (intermittent abdominal pain, nausea, vomiting, diarrhea); peripheral edema; poor response to standard epinephrine, steroid, and antibiotic therapy; and more pronounced laryngeal involvement. Attacks are often brought on by trauma, stress, or anxiety, or aggravated by pregnancy and menstruation.

The laboratory measurement of C1 esterase is abnormally low and confirms the diagnosis of this disorder. Also, C4 and C2 levels (other components of the complement system) may be depressed. Allergens per se are not involved. An examination of the larynx discloses the same features of swelling that are noted in other forms of allergic edema. The edema may be slow to progress and may continue to do so for 24 to 48 hours, in contrast with the more rapidly progressing allergic variant.

Securing the airway is essential, whether by intubation or tracheotomy. The trauma of intubation may aggravate the local allergic swelling. Topical steroids, antihistamines, and epinephrine do *not* provide benefit. Acute episodes respond to a purified C1 esterase, which may not be universally available but appears to be the most effective treatment. Long-term therapy is directed toward reversing the suppressed production of C1 esterase. Epsilon-aminocaproic acid (EACA) has this benefit as does its analog, tranexamic acid. Both these agents have been used as short- or long-term therapy. Androgens, such as danazol, have also been used as long-term treatment.[16]

Sicca Syndrome

The sicca syndrome may be acute or chronic. The acute phase is evidenced after surgery, with inadequate hydration. In the chronic phase, diminished mucous production occurs with a similarly diminished salivary flow. An associated dryness of the eyes and mucous membranes, with salivary gland enlargement, suggests Sjögren's syndrome.

Persistent dryness of the laryngeal mucosa leads to chronic laryngitis, which is often later associated with atrophy. Other causes of laryngeal dryness include radiation therapy and medications such as antihistamines, antispasmodics, thiazides, and tricyclic antidepressants. Therefore, a detailed documentation of pertinent medications is important. Arthritis, urethritis, or swelling of the salivary glands similarly must be investigated.

On examination the oral mucosa is frequently dry, and extremely thick saliva may be expressed from the salivary ducts. The vocal cords are often structurally unaltered, yet a tenacious mucus in strands is almost always observed throughout the larynx.

Therapy is directed toward elimination of offending medications; if this is not efficacious, only symptomatic treatment is available. Humidification and hydration are essential. Steroid therapy offers little in this disorder.

Endocrinopathy

Hypothyroidism causes hoarseness as a result of hypertrophy of the vocalis muscle.[12] Mucopolysaccharides may be deposited subepithelially, limiting vocal cord mobility. Thus there is associated thickening of the vocal cords and, on occasion, demonstrable polyposis. Hyperthyroidism has been associated with increased respiratory rate, increased vocal pitch, and fatigue.

Hypogonadal syndromes have been associated with the persistence of a juvenile, high-pitched vocal quality in males. Virilizing tumors may cause a premature masculinization.

Increased adrenal function leads to virilization from hypersecretion of androgenic hormones—again, associated with a lowered vocal register. Conversely, more rarely, estrogenic hypersecretion is associated with feminization and elevation of pitch. Addison's disease is associated with vocal weakness secondary to muscular asthenia, with speech being somewhat listless and indistinct.

Acromegaly causes an accelerated growth of the laryngeal framework with hyperplasia of the mucosa. This is associated with a deep phonatory quality. The hoarseness is accentuated when the cricoarytenoid joint is involved. With pituitary hypofunction, an immature, high-pitched voice is characteristic.

Neoplasia

Benign. Squamous papillomas are the most common benign laryngeal childhood neoplasms; however, they can occur at any age. They are suspected to be of viral etiology and are often multiple, occurring anywhere in the upper respiratory tract. An association has been noted with maternal vaginal condyloma acuminata. Hoarseness is the most frequent symptom. Progressive respiratory obstruction may occur. The diagnosis is confirmed by laryngoscopy and biopsy. The current management is microsurgical removal, which can be aided by the laser or other modalities such as cryosurgery. The goal of treatment is to remove the papillomas without altering laryngeal function. Spontaneous regression may occur as the child grows older.

Small mucus-retention cysts may occur anywhere within the larynx and are caused by obstruction of minor glands within the respiratory epithelium. They are rarely found on the free edge of the vocal cords, occur most often in the laryngeal ventricle, and can involve other supraglottic structures. An uncommon laryngeal cyst that can attain massive proportions is the laryngocele. It arises secondary to an obstruction of the vestigial ventricular saccus and can cause obstruction if it presents endolaryngeally. On occasion, a laryngocele may present externally as a neck mass after penetrating the thyrohyoid membrane. As with other neoplasias of the larynx, the most common symptom is hoarseness. The diagnosis and management of this disorder are surgical. Other benign lesions of the larynx may occur, including chondroma, hemangioma, and neurofibroma.[2]

Malignant. Statistically, carcinoma of the larynx remains among the most curable of malignancies. With early detection, cure rates upward of 90% can be attained. The prognosis with advanced disease is significantly diminished. Alteration of the vocal quality is most frequently the first symptom associated with carcinoma. Others include pharyngalgia, with referred otalgia secondary to an ulcerative lesion; a cough that does not respond to conservative management may signify decreased cordal mobility secondary to invasion by tumor with concomitant aspiration; dyspnea suggests a more extensive lesion, as does dysphagia. Adenopathy associated with hoarseness must be considered to represent spread from the primary malignancy.

Histologically, squamous cell carcinoma is the predominant cell type, others being distinctly uncommon. The most identifiable, consistent, predisposing epidemiologic factor associated with this tumor is cigarette smoking. Heavy smokers have more than three times the risk of nonsmokers. Alcohol acts synergistically with tobacco in elevating cancer risk. The most common occupational exposure is asbestos.[17]

Indirect laryngoscopy is usually diagnostic. There is no single characteristic appearance of squamous cell carcinoma of the larynx, but the lesion may present as a white plaque, granulomatous thickening, or ulceroinfiltrative area. Hospitalization is arranged after identification of suspected malignancy by indirect laryngoscopy. The biopsy by direct laryngoscopy should be the last in a series of studies designed to adequately assess the dimensions of the lesion, thus affording appropriate staging (Table 17–1).[18]

The computed tomographic scan has proved to be a most valuable adjunct in assessing the magnitude and extension of the lesion as well as cartilaginous invasion.[19] It must be performed prior to biopsy, because postoperative swelling would negate most of its efficacy. A barium swallow aids in assessing extension and helps to rule out second primaries involving the esophagus. The necessity for a chest film is obvious.

Routine blood study should include blood counts and chemistry profile. Thyroid function baselines are particularly important because, following combined cancer therapy, thyroid dysfunction is frequent. When alcoholism is a consideration, a coagulation profile is warranted. A nutritional status evaluation must be considered in selective cases. Pulmonary function studies are essential if conservation surgery (partial laryngectomy) is a consideration.

The liver scan has not proved beneficial unless the alkaline phosphatase level is elevated. Lung and bone scans are indicated only when clinical or routine radiologic evaluations are suggestive of metastatic disease.

Laryngoscopy and esophagoscopy remain essential for mapping and to rule out small secondary esophageal primaries. The reported low yield associated with routine bronchoscopy and washings has led some to conclude that

TABLE 17–1. STAGING OF LARYNGEAL CANCER: DEFINITIONS*

Primary Tumor (T)
[ ] TX Primary tumor cannot be assessed
[ ] T0 No evidence of primary tumor
[ ] Tis Carcinoma in situ

Supraglottis
[ ] T1 Tumor limited to one subsite of supraglottis with normal vocal cord mobility
[ ] T2 Tumor invades more than one subsite of supraglottis or glottis, with normal vocal cord mobility
[ ] T3 Tumor limited to larynx with vocal cord fixation and/or invades postcricoid area, medial wall of piriform sinus, or pre-epiglottic tissues
[ ] T4 Tumor invades through thyroid cartilage, and/or extends to other tissues beyond the larynx, e.g., to oropharynx, soft tissues of neck.

Glottis
[ ] T1 Tumor limited to vocal cord(s) (may involve anterior or posterior commissures) with normal mobility
  [ ] T1a Tumor limited to one vocal cord
  [ ] T1b Tumor involves both vocal cords
[ ] T2 Tumor extends to supraglottis and/or subglottis, and/or with impaired vocal cord mobility
[ ] T3 Tumor limited to the larynx with vocal cord fixation
[ ] T4 Tumor invades through thyroid cartilage and/or extends to other tissues beyond the larynx, e.g., oropharynx, soft tissues of neck

Subglottis
[ ] T1 Tumor limited to the subglottis
[ ] T2 Tumor extends to vocal cord(s) with normal or impaired mobility
[ ] T3 Tumor limited to larynx with vocal cord fixation
[ ] T4 Tumor invades through cricoid or thyroid cartilage and/or extends to other tissues beyond the larynx, e.g., oropharynx, soft tissues of neck

Lymph Node (N)
[ ] NX Regional lymph nodes cannot be assessed
[ ] N0 No regional lymph node metastasis
[ ] N1 Metastasis in a single ipsilateral lymph node, 3 cm or less in greatest dimension
[ ] N2 Metastasis in a single ipsilateral lymph node, more than 3 cm but not more than 6 cm in greatest dimension, or multiple ipsilateral lymph nodes, none more than 6 cm in greatest dimension or bilateral or contralateral lymph nodes, none more than 6 cm in greatest dimension
  [ ] N2a Metastasis in a single ipsilateral lymph node more than 3 cm but not more than 6 cm in greatest dimension
  [ ] N2b Metastasis in multiple ipsilateral lymph nodes, none more than 6 cm in greatest dimension
  [ ] N2c Metastasis in bilateral or contralateral lymph nodes, none more than 6 cm in greatest dimension
[ ] N3 Metastasis in a lymph node more than 6 cm in greatest dimension

Distant Metastasis (M)
[ ] MX Presence of distant metastasis cannot be assessed
[ ] M0 No distant metastasis
[ ] M1 Distant metastasis

*From American Joint Committee on Cancer, 4th ed. Philadelphia, JB Lippincott Co., 1992, pp. 39–44.

it is not essential. For the expert endoscopist, however, the minimal additional investment in time and the minimal morbidity warrant performing bronchoscopy in most cases. Immediately following endoscopy, the lesion is diagrammed and clinically staged (Fig. 17–7; see also Table 17–1).

The therapeutic regimen is predicated on a positive biopsy result and on accurate staging. Modern management necessitates a team approach, a competent head and neck surgeon, a radiotherapist well versed in head and neck anatomy and malignancies, and a medical oncologist with a regional interest. Preoperative consultations with each are essential, and the final therapeutic decision remains a cooperative effort between the medical team, the patient, and the family. The status of the dentition, particularly when radiation therapy is being contemplated, must be assessed by a dental colleague. A speech pathologist should consult the patient preoperatively, discussing the rehabilitative choices available. A good esophageal speaker can prove to be an invaluable reassurance for the surgical candidate. The complications of all the therapeutic modalities to be employed must be stressed to the patient.

The biologic behavior of squamous cell carcinoma depends on the site, tumor extent, and the influences of nodal metastases. Radiotherapy has its greatest curative effect as a single therapeutic modality for the smaller lesion. Whereas surgery generally fails in the neck, radiotherapy fails at the primary site, and thus the combined approach is used for larger lesions.

Early lesions are usually treated either by radiation therapy or conservation surgery. Advanced lesions require total laryngectomy plus possible radiation therapy; occasionally, extended partial laryngectomy with radiation therapy postoperatively may salvage a serviceable larynx. Very advanced lesions require preoperative chemotherapy, followed by surgery and irradiation therapy. The role of chemotherapy followed by radiation with attempts at laryngeal preservation is currently being evaluated, but definitive outcome is as yet not established.

Followup stresses abstinence from alcohol and smoking, as well as monthly evaluations for the first 2 years. Frequent examinations are especially important during this time interval when most recurrences are detected. Subsequently, the patient is followed annually for life because of the increased incidence of second primaries in this population.

Functional Hoarseness

Occasionally some vocal disturbances have no detectable physical aberration. Some of these may be psychogenic in origin; for others no specific basis can be discerned. Often associated emotional problems, if they are allowed to proceed without intervention, may lead to organic lesions such as vocal nodules and polyps.

Dysphonia plicae ventricularis is a disorder of phonation caused by vocalization with the false vocal cords. The voice tends to have a low pitch and is obviously hoarse with lack of projection. This disorder often occurs after laryngitis, as a compensatory mechanism. On examination, the ventric-

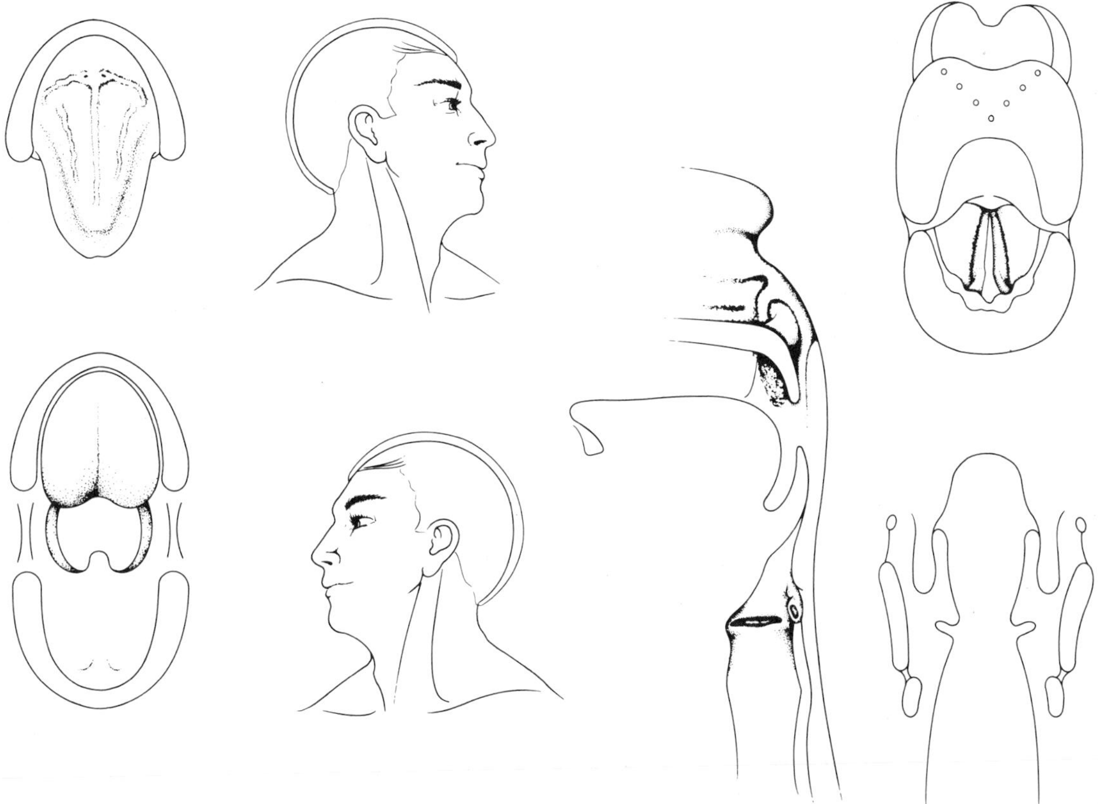

FIGURE 17–7. Diagrams used to stage primary head and neck malignancies, including the location and size of involved nodes.

ular folds can be seen to oppose and override the true vocal cords. Speech therapy may help reverse this process.[20]

Psychogenic aphonia represents a total loss of voice and is often associated with a traumatic emotional episode. Other associated symptoms of emotional distress are frequent. On examining the larynx, discrete pathology is not in evidence. The vocal folds are seen to move but do not approximate the midline. In this circumstance, psychiatric consultation is warranted.[20]

Myasthenia laryngis is a disorder of weakness of the voice, which may be due to fatigue, emotional tension, anxiety, distress, or even aging. Many patients lose their capability to phonate in response to stressful situations. Occasionally, the fear of cancer may give rise to this disorder. Prior to the diagnosis, however, other neuromuscular abnormalities must be excluded, including myasthenia gravis, amyotrophic lateral sclerosis, or a primary myopathy. In myasthenia laryngis, the vocal quality is breathy and weak. On examination the larynx appears normal. However, in the elderly the vocal cords may appear atrophic. The patients must be reassured that no organic pathology exists, and speech therapy is often mandatory.

Laryngeal spasm is due to hyperkinetic muscle tone and may be either emotional or neuromuscular in origin. Spasmodic dysphonia, although presently idiopathic appears to be related to the group of dystonias. The voice is cracking and harsh, with the patient often straining to produce any sound whatsoever. When extreme, stridor may occur. With true spasmodic dysphonia, sound production is staccato in nature. Associated facial grimacing may occur. It is surprising that on laryngeal examination no discrete pathology is noted. Although psychiatric and speech therapies have often been used, resolution of this process is not frequent. Current therapy is the endolaryngeal injection of botulism toxin. This treatment must be repeated at intervals but has proved to be very effective in most patients.[21]

Vocal Cord Paralysis

With damage to the recurrent laryngeal nerve, there is a resultant paralysis of the ipsilateral vocal cord, which then attains a median or paramedian position. Initially the voice is breathy and remains so until the paralyzed cord migrates to the midline or the unaffected cord compensates by approaching the paralyzed cord during phonation. With injury to both recurrent nerves, the cords may be sufficiently close to the midline to cause significant respiratory distress. If one or both cords is in a lateral position, the protective function of the laryngeal sphincter is in jeopardy.

In most instances, vocal cord paralysis results from a peripheral nerve injury, with only 10% being due to central nervous system pathology. The diagnosis is made by observing cord mobility. This can be accomplished radiographically or by indirect endoscopic techniques. In patients older than 40 years of age, if the cause is not readily apparent, laryngoscopy, bronchoscopy, and esophagoscopy are essential to rule out malfunction of the cricoarytenoid joint and malignancy. Iatrogenic vocal cord paralysis can occur following surgical procedures in the neck and chest or following endoscopy. Thyroidectomy still ranks as the most frequent iatrogenic cause in adults. It can also occur following cardiac or intrathoracic surgery. Anterior approaches to cervical spine pathology may result in nerve injury. Prolonged and traumatic intubation are known precursors.

Within the mediastinum, the recurrent laryngeal nerve may be involved by aneurysmal dilatation of the aortic arch. Most frequently, however, carcinoma of the lung or breast with metastatic nodes causes a disruption of function. Similarly, this can occur from lymphomas or other neoplasms including thyroid malignancies.

Peripheral neuropathies causing laryngeal paralysis may be associated with diabetes mellitus, chronic alcoholism, toxicity from metals like lead or mercury, or inflammatory processes such as syphilis or tuberculosis. Viral infections, such as herpes simplex or zoster, influenza, or coxsackievirus are other precursors. Guillain-Barré syndrome is sometimes associated with laryngeal paralysis. Very advanced carcinoma of the larynx may limit vocal cord motion by infiltration of the recurrent laryngeal nerve. Lesions of the skull base and nasopharynx, metastases, trauma, and congenital deformities may involve the tenth nerve, as may parapharyngeal space neoplasms, deep lobe parotid tumors, carotid body tumors, or involvement from carcinogenic spread.[22]

Central nervous system disorders affecting cordal function can arise from pathology in the cerebral cortex or brain stem. Space-occupying lesions, trauma, cerebrovascular accidents and thrombosis, as well as a myriad of diffuse neurologic disturbances, such as syringomyelia, multiple sclerosis, Friedreich's ataxia, and poliomyelitis, are but a few of the possible considerations.

When the aforementioned possibilities have been considered and ruled out, there remain approximately 30% of patients for whom the diagnosis cannot be established.

Although not entirely specific,[23] the central versus the peripheral origin of vocal cord paralysis can be suspected in part from the nature of the position and configuration of the vocal cord as viewed by laryngoscopy. Then the appropriate additional diagnostic procedures can be ordered.

Treatment of vocal cord paralysis must be individualized. Often unilateral cord involvement requires no treatment. Most patients seem to compensate within 6 months to 1 year after onset. With the aid of a speech pathologist, the vocal quality achieved thereafter is quite acceptable. If, however, the paralysis is bilateral or the larynx has not regained adequate function and the symptoms of hoarseness, breathiness, ineffective cough, and aspiration occur, further therapy should be considered. One therapeutic modality is injection of Teflon into the substance of the vocal cord to gain bulk. This allows the contralateral, normally mobile vocal cord to abut against a firm structure, improving vocal quality.[23] Surgical medialization (thyroplasty) of the vocal cord can be performed if breathiness is a significant complaint. Reinnervation of the paralyzed larynx using nerve-muscle pedicles has been attempted but has not gained universal acceptance or success.

REFERENCES

1. Crelin ES: Development of the upper respiratory system. Clin Symp 28: 1, 1976.
2. Fried MP (ed): The Larynx: A Multidisciplinary Approach. Boston, Little, Brown, 1988.
3. Meller SM: Functional anatomy of the larynx. Otolaryngol Clin North Am 17:30, 1984.
4. Strome M: Common laryngeal disorders in children. *In* Filter MD (ed): Phonatory Voice Disorders in Children. Springfield, IL, Charles C Thomas, 1982, pp 3–20.
5. Weber AL: Radiology of the larynx. *In* Fried MP (ed): The Larynx: A Multidisciplinary Approach. Boston, Little, Brown, 1988, pp 93–111.
6. Mancuso AA and Hanafee WN: Larynx, hypopharynx and cervical nodes—malignant tumors. *In* Computed Tomography of the Head and Neck. Baltimore, Williams & Wilkins, 1982, pp 26–65.
7. Vrabec DP and Davison FW: Inflammatory disease of the larynx. *In* English GM (ed): Otolaryngology, Vol 3. Hagerstown, MD, Harper & Row, 1990.
8. Fried MP: Controversies in the management of supraglottitis and croup. Pediatr Clin North Am 26:931, 1979.
9. Crockett DM, McGill TJ, Healy GB, and Friedman EN: Airway management of acute supraglottitis at the Children's Hospital, Boston, 1980–1985. Ann Otol Rhinol Laryngol 97:114, 1988.
10. Mustoe T and Strome M: Adult epiglottitis. Am J Otolaryngol 4:393, 1983.
11. Pillsbury HC III and Sasaki CT: Granulomatous diseases of the larynx. Otolaryngol Clin North Am 15:539, 1982.
12. Fried MP and Shapiro J: Acute and chronic laryngeal infections. *In* Paparella MN, Shumrick DA, Gluckman JL, and Myerhoff WL (eds): Otolaryngology. 3rd ed. III: Head and Neck. Philadelphia, WB Saunders, 1991, pp 2245–2256.
13. Snow JB Jr: Surgical therapy for vocal dysfunction. Otolaryngol Clin North Am 17:91, 1984.
14. Cohn AM and Larson DL: Laryngeal injury. Arch Otolaryngol 102:166, 1976.
15. Potter CR, Sessions DG, and Ogura JH: Blunt laryngeal trauma. Otolaryngol Head Neck Surg 86:909, 1978.
16. Fineman SN: Urticaria and angioedema. *In* Lawlor GJ Jr and Fischer TJ (eds): Manual of Allergy and Immunology, 2nd ed. Boston, Little, Brown, 1988, pp 214–224.
17. Rothman KJ, Cann CI, Flanders D, et al: Epidemiology of laryngeal cancer. Epidemiol Rev 2:195, 1980.
18. American Joint Committee for Cancer Staging and End Results Reporting: Manual for Staging of Cancer, 3rd ed. Philadelphia, JB Lippincott, 1988, pp 39–44.
19. Sagel SS, Auflerheide JF, Aronberg DJ, et al: High resolution computer tomography in the staging of carcinoma of the larynx. Laryngoscope 91:292, 1981.
20. Hart CW: Functional and neurological problems of the larynx. Otolaryngol Clin North Am 3:609, 1970.
21. Blitzer AB, Brin MF, Fahn S, and Lovelace RE: Localized injections of botulinum toxin for the treatment of focal laryngeal dystonia (spastic dysphonia). Laryngoscope 98:193, 1988.
22. Tyler HR: Neurology of the larynx. Otolaryngol Clin North Am 17:75, 1984.
23. Tucker HM: Management of the patient with an incompetent larynx. Am J Otolaryngol 1:47, 1979.

18

The Painful or Discharging Ear

DAVID M. VERNICK, MD
WILLIAM T. BRANCH, Jr., MD

Ear pain (otalgia) and ear drainage (otorrhea) are common complaints. Acute otitis externa, acute otitis media, serous otitis media, and chronic otitis media can present in any age group. Their incidence varies from children to adults. Children tend to have acute otitis media much more often than do adults. Adults have more chronic otitis media. Otitis externa occurs about equally in all age groups. The differential diagnosis and subsequent treatment, however, vary little between children and adults.

Figure 18–1 provides a general overview of the approach to patients with symptoms related to ear disease. One begins by noting that the diagnosis usually conforms to the presenting complaint. Patients with acutely painful ears usually have acute purulent otitis media or external otitis, whereas those who complain of subacute hearing loss more often have serous or mucoid otitis media. Chronic suppurative otitis media usually manifests as chronic hearing loss or as painless drainage from the ear. In most cases, it is then possible to confirm the diagnosis by carefully examining the external canal and tympanic membrane. If the results of the ear examination are normal, one must consider that the pain may be referred to the ear. Diseases of the nose, nasopharynx, paranasal sinuses, mouth, hypopharynx, larynx, and neck can all refer pain to the ear. Dental caries, pharyngitis, temporomandibular joint dysfunction, cervical adenopathy, acute sinusitis, and tonsillitis as well as tumors of the head and neck can all cause otalgia. A thorough head and neck examination must be performed to identify the source of pain any time that the ear is normal.

Figure 18–2 outlines the clinical anatomy of the ear and its contiguous structures. The eustachian tube connects the middle ear cavity with the nasopharynx. Blockage of the eustachian tube creates a vacuum within the middle ear that may result in the transudation of fluid. Conversely, infected secretions from the nasopharynx may reflux through the eustachian tube and thus contaminate the middle ear. Sound striking the tympanic membrane is concentrated through a chain of ossicles (malleus, incus, and stapes) to the oval window; hence, blockage or disruption of the tympanic membrane or ossicles leads to conductive hearing loss. Figure 18–3 provides a diagram of the middle ear cavity as viewed from within. The ossicles are shown to be located within the middle ear cavity; this is connected to the mastoid antrum. Thus, infection of the middle ear cavity may involve the mastoid antrum and may spread to the main mastoid cell tract. The proximity of the middle ear cavity and the mastoid air cells explains why acute mastoiditis can follow from otitis media.

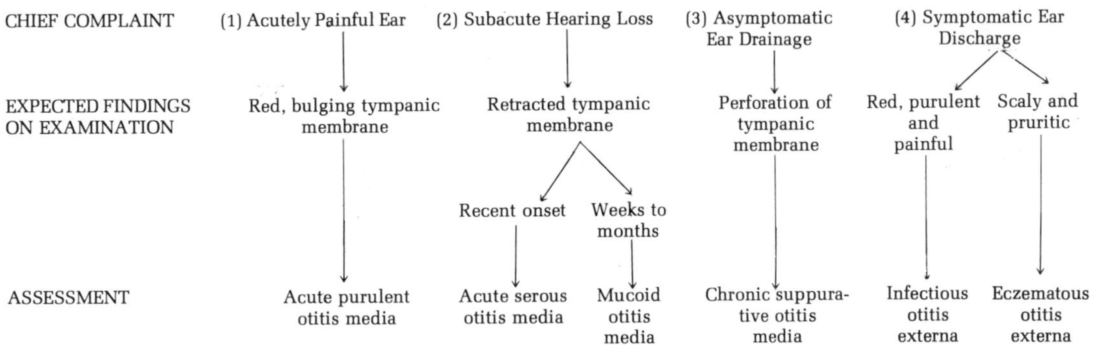

FIGURE 18–1. Schematic representation of the approach to patients with otitis.

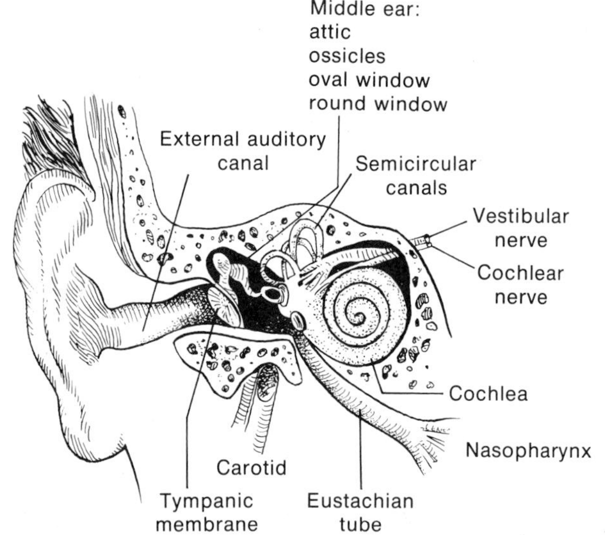

FIGURE 18–2. Clinical anatomy of the middle ear and related structures.

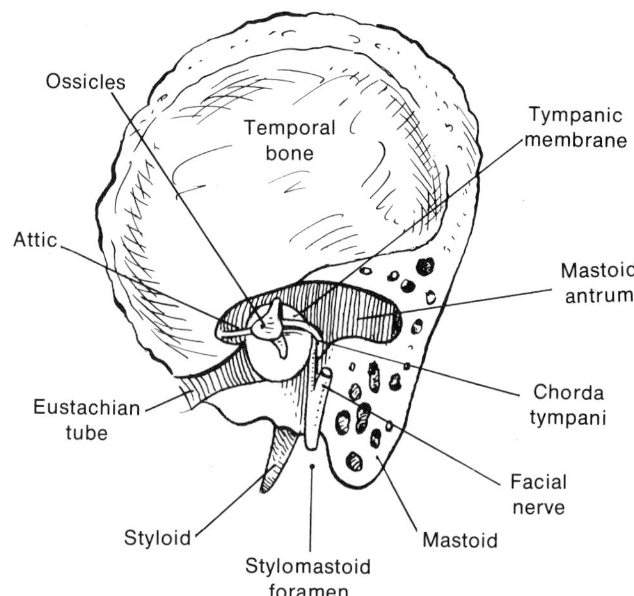

FIGURE 18–3. The middle ear cavity and temporal bone as seen from within.

ACUTE PURULENT OTITIS MEDIA

Pain in the ear is the key presenting symptom of acute purulent otitis media. Patients generally do not appear to be in a septic state, but they may have fever and a leukocytosis. The diagnosis can be confirmed by finding a red, bulging tympanic membrane. Figure 18–4 illustrates the landmarks of the tympanic membrane. Often in acute suppurative otitis media these are obscured by bulging. (Fig. 18–5). Hearing is usually decreased. If the tympanic membrane perforates, there may be otorrhea. The ear canal, however, is usually not swollen and tender as it is in otitis externa.

The natural history of this disease is well documented in the pediatric population.[2, 3] Two thirds of all children have at least one episode of acute otitis media, most frequently before the age of 2 years.[4] Of these children, one third have a second episode and one third of these, a third episode; a small number have numerous recurrences.[5]

Allergic rhinitis is implicated in some cases. Studies have failed to document immunodeficiency in most patients, even in those with repeated episodes. Although the majority of patients with acute otitis media have been shown to carry pathogenic bacteria within the nasopharynx, it remains unclear whether this factor alone can account for the episodes.[6] Most controversy centers on the relative importance of eustachian tube obstruction from hypertrophied adenoids in children versus poor eustachian tube function secondary to developmental delay. Adenoidectomy might be beneficial in the former case but might not be beneficial in the latter case. A variety of conservative measures to establish drainage of the middle ear are discussed in more detail in the section on management of mucoid otitis media. In adults (older than 40 years of age) with unilateral recurrent otitis media, carcinoma of the nasopharynx must also be considered.

Management. Management of the acute episode is relatively straightforward.[7] Table 18–1 summarizes bacteriologic findings from cases of acute purulent otitis media in teenagers and adults.[8–10] Only 1 to 2% of cases are due to *Staphylococcus aureus* or gram-negative bacilli and 1 to 5% to group A β-hemolytic streptococci. Most known cases in adults are caused by *Pneumococcus,* which is readily susceptible to penicillin. *Haemophilus influenzae* is reported in up to 12% of patients older than 7 years old.[10] Penicillin concentrations within the middle ear are not sufficient to

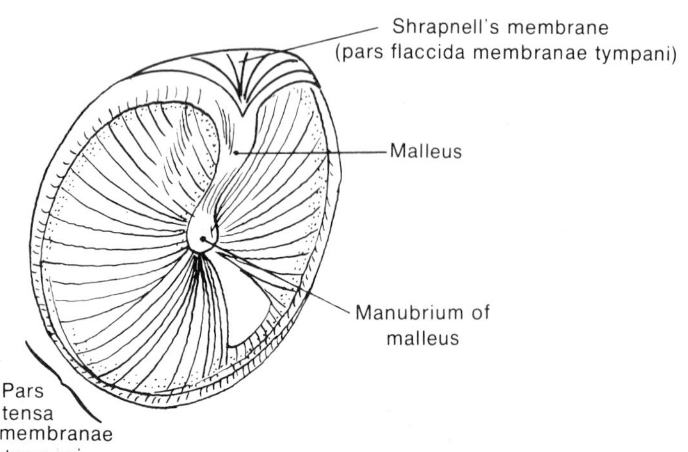

FIGURE 18–4. The tympanic membrane.

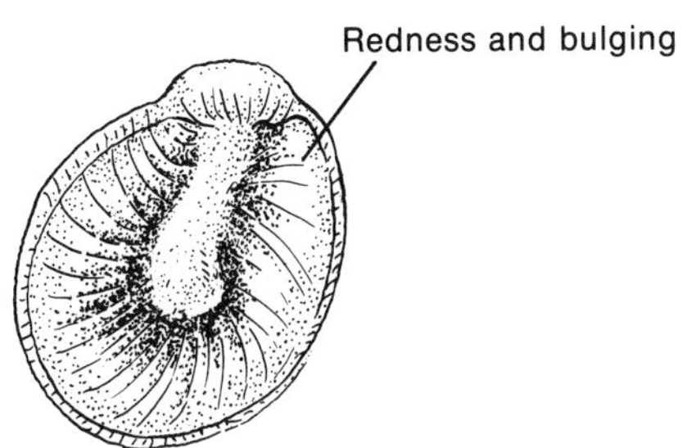

A. Acute purulent otitis media—
redness of entire drum or hyperemia of vessels across the drum
bulging with obscuring of landmarks

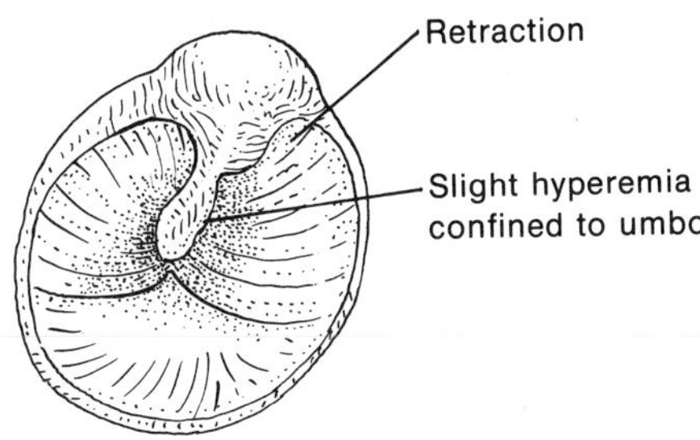

B. Serous otitis media—
retraction of drum
vessels along the handle of the malleus may be dilated but hyperemia does not involve vessels extending across the entire drum
air fluid level (amber) or air bubbles may be visible

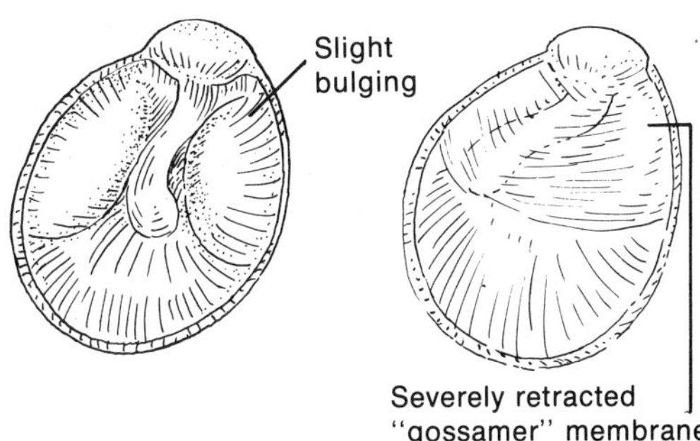

C. Mucoid otitis media—
mild bulging (or retraction) may be present
membrane is gray or minimally red
ear is not acutely painful
bubbles or air fluid level may be seen

FIGURE 18–5. Characteristics of the tympanic membrane in acute purulent otitis media (*A*), serous otitis media (*B*), and mucoid otitis media (*C*).

inhibit the growth of the organism. Furthermore, up to 35% of *H. influenzae*, including both type B and nontypable strains, are now resistant to ampicillin in some communities.[11] It is known, however, that 70 to 85% of adult cases of acute purulent otitis media resolve spontaneously *without* antibiotics when treated by myringotomy alone.[1, 12, 13] It has been demonstrated in several controlled trials that the outcome is even more satisfactory when penicillin is employed as therapy.[9, 10, 14, 15] Resistant *H. influenzae* accounted for about half of the small percentage of treatment failures in most trials, with failure to obtain adequate drainage or the presence of another resistant organism such as *M. catarrhalis* or *S. aureus* accounting for the rest.[16]

A reasonable strategy is to treat mild cases of acute otitis media in adults initially with phenoxymethyl penicillin (500 mg, taken 4 times daily by mouth for 7 to 10 days). More severe cases and those that fail to respond within 2 days can be treated with amoxicillin. In communities with resistant *H. influenzae*, nasopharyngeal cultures can be obtained before beginning therapy. These have good predictive value for detection of ampicillin-resistant *H. influenzae* and other resistant organisms if predominant growth by a single pathogen is noted after plating the culture immediately onto solid agar to avoid overgrowth.[17] Resistant *M. catarrhalis* or *H. influenzae* can be treated with amoxicillin and clavulanic acid (Augmentin), co-trimoxazole, or cefaclor (Ceclor).

Data from controlled trials have shown no or only slight benefit (in terms of somewhat fewer treatment failures) when antihistamines are prescribed in addition to antibiotics.[10, 18] Although no controlled trial has demonstrated efficacy,[18] nasal decongestants should be considered if nasal congestion is present.

Using standard therapy, about 5% of all patients will have intractable pain that is not relieved within 24 hours by the antibiotics. Another 3 to 10% of cases fail to resolve after 7 to 10 days of antimicrobial therapy, as manifested by either persistent fever and ear ache or tympanic membrane abnormalities and hearing loss.[8, 18] Further management is needed for these patients.

If a culture is necessary, aspiration of middle ear fluid using a small needle inserted in the central inferior portion of the tympanic membrane can be performed. This allows drainage of pus, as well as providing material for cultures (Fig. 18–6). This procedure is beneficial with intractable pain or when antibiotics fail to resolve the infection. The actual fluid may take several weeks to resolve after the infection has cleared. Persistence of the fluid beyond this point should lead to (1) therapy to remove the fluid either by aspiration or ventilation tube insertion, and (2) evaluation of the nasopharynx to rule out eustachian tube obstruction. In practice, about half of these patients have a positive middle ear culture with resistant organisms, whereas the other half do not, and presumably their persistent manifestations are related to inadequate drainage.[16]

Two controlled trials have demonstrated efficacy for pro-

TABLE 18–1. BACTERIOLOGY IN ADULTS WITH ACUTE SUPPURATIVE OTITIS MEDIA

Bacteria	Frequency of Occurrence (%)
Streptococcus pneumoniae	25–50
Sterile or nonpathogenic	20–30
Moraxella catarrhalis	10
Haemophilus influenzae	1–12
β-Hemolytic streptococcus	1–5
Staphylococcus aureus	1–2
Gram-negative bacilli	1
Mycoplasma pneumoniae or viral otitis	Rare

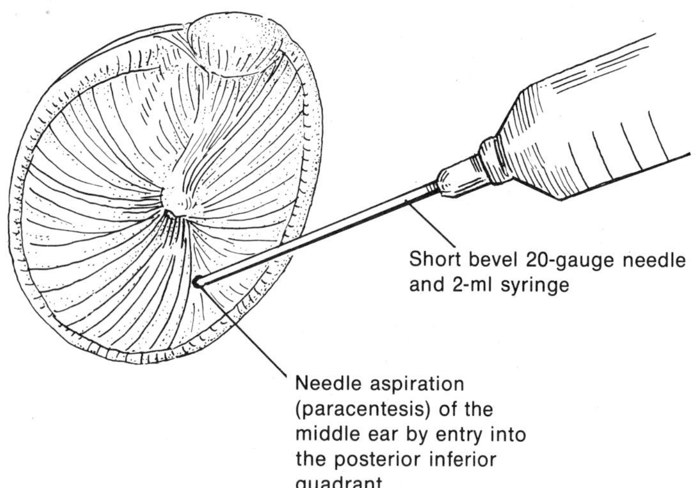

FIGURE 18–6. Paracentesis of the middle ear, using a 20-gauge needle.

phylactic antimicrobial therapy in preventing recurrences in children; one used ampicillin (one tablet daily for 6 months)[19] and the other, sulfisoxazole (twice daily for 1 year).[20] Experience with prophylaxis is not yet extensive in adults. It is unclear whether prophylaxis will be effective in preventing recurrences beyond a 6- to 12-month period. Thus, use of prophylactic antimicrobials should be reserved for patients with many recurrences who do not respond to other measures designed to promote drainage via the eustachian tube.

Recurrences are less common in adult patients than in children. Most cases in adults are sporadic, apparently related to upper respiratory infections with temporary obstruction of the eustachian tube or reflux of infected secretions into the middle ear cavity. Data indicate that in children viral infections precede bacterial ear infections in a large percentage of cases.[21] Permanent conductive hearing loss (15 db) probably occurs infrequently in adults, although it was reported in as many as 12% of children with a history of recurrent otitis media.[22] There is concern about its effect on acquisition of language skills and social development.[23] Although the extent of permanent hearing loss after otitis media in adults is probably low, we recommend follow-up after treatment to detect any residual hearing impairment, which might result from persistence of fluid within the middle ear.

Complications. The incidence of suppurative complications from acute otitis media has diminished since the advent of antimicrobial therapy[24] and is now estimated at from 0.2 to 0.4% of patients.[25] Acute mastoiditis is manifested by pain, fever, and tenderness elicited by pressure over the mastoid process, which may develop abruptly or 1 to 2 weeks after an inadequately treated initial episode of acute otitis media. Mastoiditis can also present as persistent drainage, which may be bloody or putrid, from a perforated tympanic membrane. The diagnosis is a clinical one. Radiographic signs of mastoiditis may be subtle or may not develop for 7 to 10 days after the onset of symptoms. When radiographs of the diseased and the normal side are compared, the diagnosis sometimes can be confirmed by showing cloudiness and loss of clear cell outlines within the mastoid air cells. Treatment requires cultures from the middle ear and parenteral antibiotic therapy sufficient to eradicate the infection. Mastoidectomy may be necessary in severe cases or when antibiotic therapy fails. Occasionally acute mastoiditis presents with a subperiosteal abscess that is palpable as a fluctuant, tender mass behind the auricle. Other infrequent complications with mastoiditis include thrombophlebitis of the sigmoid sinus, epidural abscess, serous labyrinthitis, and paralysis of the seventh cranial nerve.

Acute meningitis associated with otitis media may develop early in the disease within a day or two via thrombotic spread of the infection through venous anastomoses with the dura.[26] Late occurrence of meningitis, so-called otogenic meningitis, may occur after a week or two via spread from osteitis in the mastoid process. *Pneumococcus* is the most common pathogen, although recent reports in children list an increasing proportion of acute cases due to *H. influenzae*, type B.[24] The cardinal manifestations of meningitis are continuous headache and vomiting. (The pain is localized to the ear in otitis media.) The importance of recognizing the distinction between acute meningitis and otogenic meningitis lies in the fact that patients with otogenic meningitis often require mastoidectomy in addition to therapy with antimicrobial agents.[26]

SEROUS AND MUCOID (SECRETORY) OTITIS MEDIA

Serous otitis media usually presents with subacute hearing loss. Patients may have a "popping" or "fullness" within the ear. Many have an erroneous impression that the external canal is occluded by cerumen. Pressure in the ear is common. Pain, if present, is often mild or intermittent, and the patient is afebrile.

The pathogenesis of this syndrome involves dysfunction of the eustachian tube. Blockage may be due to viral upper respiratory infection, travel in partially unpressurized airliner cabins, hypertrophy of the adenoids, carcinoma of the nasopharynx, or, perhaps, excessive "floppiness" with collapse of the tube on negative pressure.[27] Allergic rhinitis is found in only 3 to 4% of chronically affected children.[28] Residual effusions within the middle ear have been noted, during the recovery phase of patients following acute otitis media.[29]

With obstruction of the eustachian tube, oxygen is absorbed from the middle ear cavity, leaving a partial vacuum within which a serous transudate forms. This early process is called *acute serous otitis media*. The tympanic membrane is retracted, making the handle of the malleus easily visible. At times, a fluid level is present. Congestion of vessels around the umbo may give the tympanic membrane a pink appearance, although bulging does not occur.

As the process continues, metaplasia of the mucosa within the cavity of the middle ear creates goblet cells secreting a thick, tenacious mucus difficult to drain. At this chronic stage, the process is termed *mucoid* or *secretory otitis media*. The tympanic membrane then may appear amber or yellow, thick, and possibly even bulging. At times, more severe retraction gives the appearance of a gossamer membrane collapsed around the ossicles or adhesive within the middle ear. If drainage can be established, this metaplasia subsides over time and the membranes usually return to normal.[30] Otherwise, thick mucus, adhesive to the ossicles, may result in permanent conductive hearing loss. Collapse and pouch formation of a flaccid membrane may also occur and lead to the migration of squamous epithelium into the middle ear cavity and mastoid with cholesteatoma formation. This process is the most common cause of severe (35 db) hearing loss in children.[31]

It is usually possible to differentiate serous otitis media from acute purulent otitis media because of the lack of pain and the retracted appearance of the tympanic membrane in the former (see Fig. 18–5). In cases in which there is a question of erythema or thickening and bulging of the membrane, one may resort to an empirical trial of antibiotic therapy. A few colonies of bacteria, often mixed aerobic and anerobic organisms, including *Pseudomonas* in many cases, have been found on aspiration in about one half of the patients with mucoid otitis media; hence, there may be justification for antibiotic therapy.[32–34] If it is essential to establish a precise diagnosis, the middle ear cavity may be aspirated with a spinal needle and the fluid cultured.

Another, perhaps more frequently encountered problem for the clinician is distinguishing a normal tympanic membrane from a slightly retracted one caused by serous otitis in the patient with questionable symptoms. An attempt to estimate the mobility of the tympanic membrane may be made by applying pressure with the pneumatic otoscope. If unpracticed with this technique, one may utilize the Weber test, which, though diagnostically insensitive, can detect conductive hearing loss in full-blown cases. Otherwise, tympanometry, which measures the compliance of the tympanic membrane by an impedance device, is capable of distinguishing a normal from an abnormally stiff tympanic membrane, such as that caused by fluid within the middle ear cavity, in 70% of cases.[35]

Management. Acute serous otitis media is initially managed in a child with low-dose antibiotics. Antihistamines and decongestants have not shown any benefit in controlled trials. In adults, decongestants and antihistamines may be used if the patient has symptoms of nasal congestion. Nasal sprays such as Neosynephrine may be used in adults for a few days, but prolonged use can result in rhinitis medicamentosa and counteract any good that they might have done. Eustachian tube "exercises" such as chewing gum, swallowing, or performing a Valsalva maneuver may hasten the recovery by aerating the middle ear. Progress in clearing the effusion can be documented using audiometry or tympanometry.[36]

Additional management involves the use of tympanostomy tubes (grommets). These are small drainage tubes inserted through the central inferior portion of the tympanic membrane. They create constant equalization of pressures and have been left in place for as long as 3 years.[37] Immediate hearing improvement can be achieved with the use of grommets, and this may prompt their early use in those who have hearing disabilities or are in the initial ages of speech and language development (ages 2 to 5). Some believe that long-term irreversible changes in the ear can be avoided by appropriate ventilation.[38] An adenoidectomy has been shown to be of benefit in those requiring a second set of grommets.[47]

In adults, standard practice is first to allow drainage of effusions by short courses of decongestants and antihistamines and by eustachian tube "exercises" before resorting to external drainage.

CHRONIC SUPPURATIVE OTITIS MEDIA

Chronic suppurative otitis media usually prevents with asymptomatic, painless discharge that may be persistent or episodic. In virtually every case, the patient has a permanent perforation of the tympanic membrane, although there are sporadic reports (≤2%) of cholesteatoma behind an intact tympanic membrane.[39] Cholesteatoma is the chief complication of chronic suppurative otitis. It refers to the migration of squamous epithelium into the middle ear and mastoid cavity with subsequent proliferation into a slowly expanding mass of cells, keratin, and debris. Over a period of years, this acts as a locally invasive process that may destroy bone, expose the labyrinth, or impinge on the seventh cranial nerve.

Most cases seem to have begun either with an acute episode of ear pain with subsequent discharge (in 50%) or with the insidious onset of ear drainage or hearing loss (about 40%).[40] Trauma is involved in 4% of the cases, and the rest have no known cause. Half the cases begin before age 10, but many are of 10 to 15 years' duration when brought to medical attention. The contralateral ear also is involved in 15 to 20% of cases. It seems likely that cases with an acute onset result from inadequately treated acute purulent otitis media, whereas those with an insidious onset probably are sequelae of mucoid otitis media.

Management. Chronic otitis media is separated into two major divisions—those with central perforations and those with marginal or attic perforations (Fig. 18–7). Although the bacteria isolated from such ears are quite varied (Table 18–2),[33, 41] patients with central perforations can usually

TABLE 18–2. BACTERIAL ISOLATES IN ADULTS WITH CHRONIC OTITIS MEDIA

Bacteria	Frequency of Occurrence (%)
Gram-positive cocci	10
Staphylococcus aureus (5%)	
Streptococcus pneumoniae	
α-Hemolytic streptococci	
Gram-negative aerobic bacilli	50–60
Pseudomonas aeruginosa (35%)	
Proteus sp. (7%)	
Escherichia coli	
Klebsiella pneumoniae	
Serratia marcescens	
Citrobacter diversus	
Providentia sp.	
Anaerobic organisms	30–40
Peptococcus (20%)	
Peptostreptococcus	
Bacteroides fragilis (5%)	
Bacteroides corrodens	
Bacteroides melaninogenicus	
Clostridium sp.	
Mixed infections	~50
Aerobic organisms only	~40
Anaerobic organisms only	~10

Type I

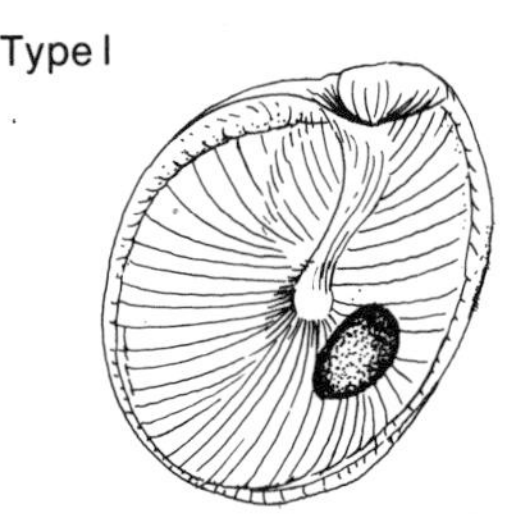

Anterior perforation characterized by thin, mucoid discharge from the eustachian tube.

Type II

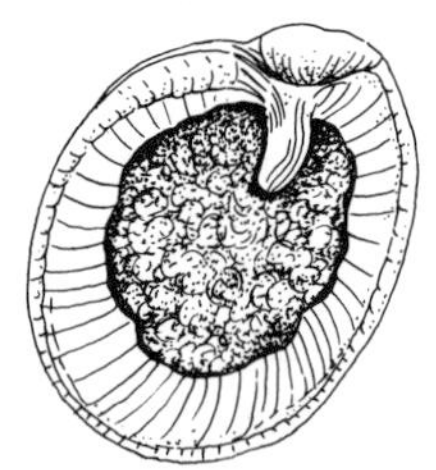

Large central perforation characterized by filling of the middle ear with mucopurulent fluid, granulation tissue, and polyps.

Type III

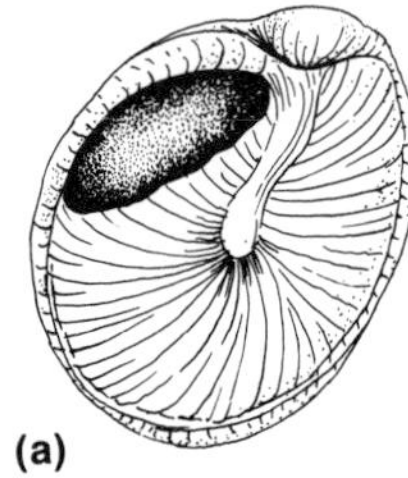

(a)

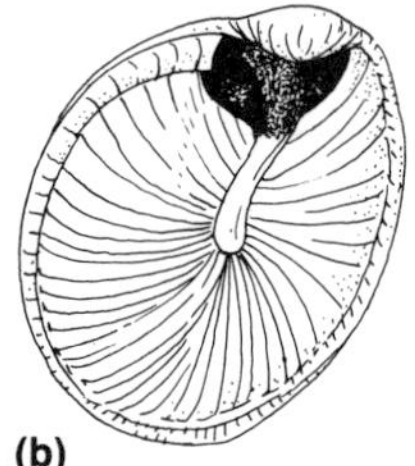

(b)

(a) Posterior marginal perforation or
(b) attic (pars flaccida) perforation, usually associated with cholesteatoma.

Type IV

Any of the above (usually III) with additional signs of extension into the labyrinth, meninges, brain, or seventh cranial nerve. Cholesteatoma is always suspected.

FIGURE 18–7. Types of chronic suppurative otitis media.

achieve a "dry" ear through the use of eardrops and occasional oral antibiotics. Since the perforation does not involve the margin of the tympanic membrane, ingrowth of skin with cholesteatoma formation is infrequent. Erosions of the ossicles resulting in a conductive hearing loss and recurrent infections, however, are common and may lead one to consider repair of the perforation. If granulation tissue is present and does not clear with medical therapy, an underlying cholesteatoma should be suspected and surgery entertained. Any patient with a perforated eardrum should avoid getting water in the ear as this will result in infection.

When the perforation involves the margins of the eardrum or the attic area, growth of skin into the middle ear and mastoid with cholesteatoma formation is much more likely. Treatment of the infection is the same as for central perforations. However, if the infection does not clear, a microscopic examination of the ear should be undertaken in the office to check for cholesteatoma (Fig. 18–8). If cholesteatoma is present, surgery usually is necessary to clear up the infection. Even if the infection clears, however, patients with marginal perforations either should be followed closely if they are poor surgical candidates or should undergo repair of the drum, as the likelihood of eventually developing trouble is high.

Complications. The cholesteatoma may invade the bony labyrinth, producing a labyrinthine fistula.[25] Vertigo is the key symptom. It may be reproduced by pressure with the pneumatic otoscope, the so-called "fistula test." Such vertigo in the presence of chronic suppurative otitis media requires immediate consideration of surgery, since it implies invasion of the labyrinth by a cholesteatoma. A second complication of chronic suppurative otitis media is purulent labyrinthitis with labyrinthogenic meningitis.[25] In these patients, the labyrinth has become infected by a suppurative process that proceeds in virtually all cases to invade the meninges. Fever and headache accompany the vertigo.

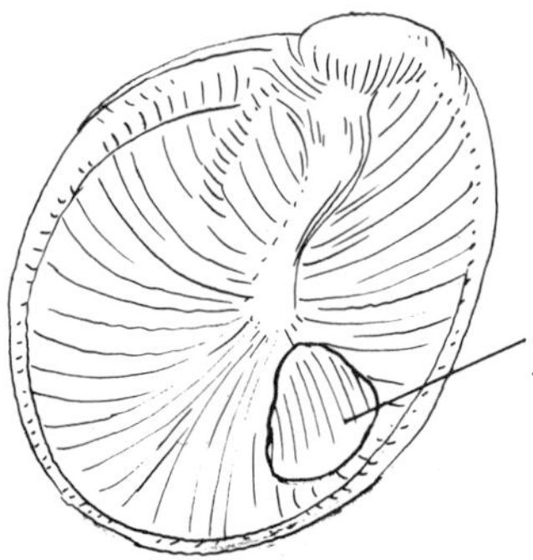

A. Healed perforation

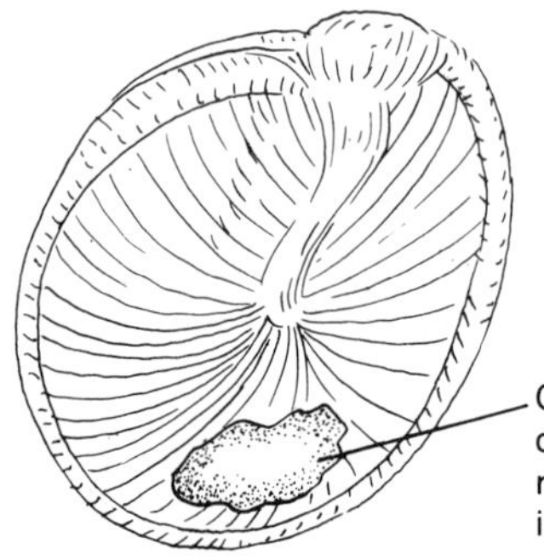

B. Tympanosclerosis

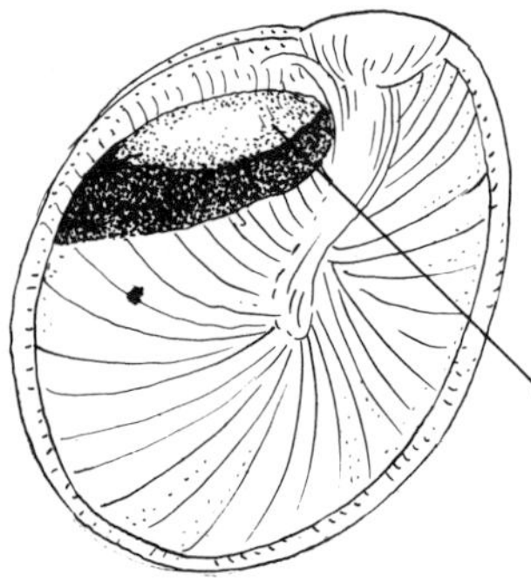

C. Cholesteatoma

FIGURE 18–8. Distinguishing among healed perforation, tympanosclerosis, and cholesteatoma on examination of the tympanic membrane. The former two are benign, incidental findings; the latter is slowly invasive and generally leads to complications.

None of these symptoms is present in uncomplicated chronic otitis media. Thus, any patient with unexplained vertigo, fever, pain, or generalized headache who has a permanent perforation of the tympanic membrane should be approached as an otologic emergency.

Paralysis of the seventh cranial nerve can also occur with some cases of chronic otitis media. Other less frequent complications include brain abscess of the temporal lobe, which is usually manifested by progressively worsening headaches in the mornings followed by drowsiness and changes in mental status; progressive, rarefying mastoiditis manifested by cloudiness, loss of trabeculation, and sclerosis of the mastoid air cells; lateral sinus thrombosis, manifested by septic fevers, chills, and headache, but sometimes inducing a pseudotumor cerebri; and petrositis, manifested chiefly by persistent deep pain behind the orbit.[42]

In these cases, surgical intervention is mandatory to relieve the cause and prevent progression of the symptoms.

OTITIS EXTERNA

Types of otitis externa are listed in Table 18–3. *Acute infectious otitis externa* generally occurs when there is maceration of tissues within the external ear canal. Factors leading to maceration include trapping of water within the canal and excessive heat and humidity. "Swimmer's ear" results when trapped water is contaminated with *Pseudomonas aeruginosa.* Other patients become infected via trauma, often induced by efforts to clean the canal using Q tips or match sticks; or infection may be superimposed upon a chronic eczematous process at the stage of crusting and cleft formation. The bacteriology (Table 18–4) is similar to that seen in chronic suppurative otitis media. Key clinical symptoms are acute otalgia with purulent drainage; a red, swollen canal; and pain that can be reproduced by movement of the auricle.

The first step in assessment is to clean the external canal thoroughly by gentle suctioning under direct vision. A view of the eardrum is always necessary, either on initial examination or on a follow-up visit, since middle ear disease can sometimes present as secondary otitis externa. Treatment should include antimicrobial otic drops such as a polymyxin B-hydrocortisone combination or sulfacetamide. When soft tissue swelling prevents adequate therapy, a wick of cotton or merocel should be placed within the canal and moistened continuously with antibiotic drops for several days.[43, 44] Adequate pain medication should be given to those requiring it.

Very exquisite tenderness on motion of the tragus may imply a *staphylococcal carbuncle,* which may be visible as an erythematous swelling. If severe, the carbuncle should be treated using an orally administered antibiotic; if the condition does not resolve spontaneously, consideration of incision and drainage or ovaspiration is in order. If inflammation spreads beyond the superficial tissue of the external canal and involves a portion of the pinna, therapy should always include antibiotics taken by mouth or given parenterally.

TABLE 18–3. DIFFERENTIAL DIAGNOSIS OF OTITIS EXTERNA

Infectious otitis externa; bacterial, fungal, herpetic
Staphylococcal carbuncle
Malignant otitis externa
Eczematous otitis externa; contact dermatitis, eczematous dermatitis, seborrheic dermatitis, psoriasis
Trauma, iatrogenic or foreign body

TABLE 18–4. BACTERIAL ISOLATES IN ADULTS WITH INFECTIOUS OTITIS EXTERNA

Bacteria	Frequency of Occurrence (%)
Staphylococcus	20
Pseudomonas, Klebsiella, Proteus, and other aerobic, gram-negative bacilli	61
Anaerobic organisms or no growth	15
Candida or *Aspergillus*	4

Eczematous otitis externa presents as a more indolent process without purulent drainage but with pruritus rather than pain as the key manifestation. Patients with this condition may have contact dermatitis, idiopathic eczema, psoriasis, or seborrheic dermatitis. The canal may appear weepy, swollen, or scaly. Treatment usually involves corticosteroid drops or ointment, plus antibiotics when secondary infection is suspected. Once the acute stage is over, intermittent use of a desquamative agent such as VōSol or VōSol HC may help to prevent recurrences.

Malignant otitis externa is a syndrome generally noted in elderly (90% over the age of 55 years) or diabetic (80%) patients who have pain and purulent discharge from the external canal. Cases are reported in immunocompromised and AIDS patients. The majority of these have a *Pseudomonas* infection, which is bilateral in 27% of cases.[45] Clinical investigation reveals bacterial invasion through clefts in the cartilage of the external canal to involve the deep soft tissues around the stylomastoid foramen and in the retroparotid space. Thus, cranial nerve VII is paralyzed early in the course of the infection. Multiple other cranial nerve palsies (of X, XI, XII, and, eventually, V and VI) may develop. The bacteria invade the base of the skull and produce meningitis as a late manifestation. One cannot rely on the presence of fever or leukocytosis for detection of this process. It should be suspected in any elderly or diabetic patient when otitis externa is associated with pain that is unusually severe and constant. Radiographs may reveal nothing abnormal except soft tissue swelling.

Treatment for early disease involves débridement of the ear canal and oral antipseudomonal drug therapy like ciprofloxin. In advanced cases intravenous drug therapy, usually with two drugs such as tobramycin and ticarcillin, is necessary. Extensive surgical exenteration of the soft tissue may be necessary except in patients who clearly improve within a few days after receiving antibiotics.[46] In spite of therapy, mortality rates up to 20% are reported in most series.[46] Because of this poor prognosis, the physician should seek consultation with an otolaryngologist whenever deep soft tissue invasion is suspected in elderly or diabetic patients with otitis externa.

REFERENCES

1. Halstead C, Lepow ML, Balassanian N, et al: Otitis media: Clinical observations, microbiology, and evaluation of therapy. Am J Dis Child 115:512, 1968.
2. Bluestone CD: Otitis media in children: To treat or not to treat? N Engl J Med 306:1399, 1982.
3. Farquer BD and Linthium FH Jr: Middle ear effusion in children: Report of treatment in 500 cases. West J Med 137:370, 1982.
4. Howie VM: Natural history of otitis media. Ann Otol Rhinol Laryngol 84(Suppl 19):67, 1975.
5. Taylor C and Onion D: The first six months after otitis media. J Maine Med Assoc 60:280, 1975.

6. Branefors-Helander P, Dahlberg T, and Nylen O: Acute otitis media. Acta Otolaryngol (Stockh) 80:399, 1975.
7. Sooh AJ, Blackwelder WC, and Kaslow RA: Treatment of acute otitis media. JAMA 248:1071, 1982.
8. Rose DS: Acute suppurative otitis media. Pediatrics 56:285, 1975.
9. Laxdal OE, Merida J, and Jones RH: Treatment of acute otitis media: A controlled study of 142 children. Can Med Assoc J 102:263, 1970.
10. Stickler GB, Rubenstein MM, McBean JB, et al: Treatment of acute otitis media in children. IV: A fourth clinical trial. Am J Dis Child 114:123, 1967.
11. Schwartz R, Rodriguez W, Khan W, et al: Increasing incidence of ampicillin-resistant *Haemophilus influenzae*: Cause of otitis media. JAMA 239:320, 1978.
12. Lowe JF, Bamforth JS, and Pracy R: Acute otitis media: One year in a general practice. Lancet 2:1129, 1963.
13. Townsend EH Jr: Otitis media in pediatric practice. NY J Med 64:1591, 1964.
14. Lorcacy P and Hougten P: Treatment of acute suppurative otitis media. J Laryngol Otol 91:331, 1977.
15. Meistrop-Larsen KI, Sorensen H, and Johnsen NJ: Two vs. seven days' penicillin treatment for acute otitis media. Acta Otolaryngol 96:99, 1983.
16. Bass JW, Cashman TM, Frostad AL, et al: Antimicrobials in the treatment of acute otitis media. Am J Dis Child 125:397, 1973.
17. Schwartz R, Rodriguez WJ, Mann R, et al: The nasopharyngeal culture in acute otitis media: A reappraisal of its usefulness. JAMA 241:2170, 1979.
18. Chilton LA and Skipper BE: Antihistamines and alpha-adrenergic agents in treatment of otitis media. South Med J 72:953, 1979.
19. Maynard JE, Fleshman JK, and Tschopp CF: Otitis media in Alaskan Eskimo children: Prospective evaluation of chemoprophylaxis. JAMA 219:597, 1972.
20. Perrin JM, Charney E, MacWhinney JB Jr, et al: Sulfisoxazole as chemoprophylaxis for recurrent otitis media: A double-blind crossover study in pediatric practice. N Engl J Med 291:664, 1974.
21. Henderson FW, Collier AM, Sanyal M, et al: A longitudinal study of respiratory viruses and bacteria in the etiology of acute otitis media with effusion. N Engl J Med 306:1377, 1982.
22. Olmstead RW, Alvarez MC, Moroney JD, et al: The pattern of hearing following acute otitis media. J Pediatr 65:252, 1964.
23. Kaplan GJ, Fleshman JK, Bender TR, et al: Long-term effects of otitis media: A 10-year cohort study of Alaskan Eskimo children. Pediatrics 52:577, 1973.
24. Gower D and McGuirt F: Intracranial complications of acute and chronic infectious ear disease: Problem still with us. Laryngoscope 93:1028, 1983.
25. Juselius H and Kaltiokallio K: Complications of acute and chronic otitis media in the antibiotic era. Acta Otolaryngol 74:445, 1972.
26. Brydoy B and Ellekjaer EF: Otogenic meningitis: A five-year study. J Laryngol Otol 86:871, 1972.
27. Bluestone CD, Berry QC, and Andrus WS: Mechanics of the eustachian tube as it influences susceptibility to and persistence of middle ear effusions in children. Ann Otol Rhinol Laryngol 83(Suppl 11):27, 1974.
28. Rahko T, Koivikko A, and Silvonniemi P: The occurrence of secretory otitis media in allergic children. Clin Otolaryngol 4:267, 1979.
29. Shurin PA, Pelton SI, Donner A, et al: Persistence of middle-ear effusion after acute otitis media in children. N Engl J Med 300:1121, 1979.
30. Tos M: Secretory otitis media: Pathology and pathogenesis related to clinical picture. Acta Otolaryngol 82:286, 1976.
31. Eliachar I: Audiologic manifestations of otitis media. Otolaryngol Clin 11:769, 1978.
32. Boodey RJ and Bowers M: Antibiotic treatment of secretory otitis media assessed by impedance audiometry. N Z Med J 82:187, 1975.
33. Brook I: Bacteriology and treatment of chronic otitis media. Laryngoscope 89:1129, 1979.
34. Brook I and Finegold SM: Bacteriology of chronic otitis media. JAMA 241:487, 1979.
35. Paradise JL: Testing for otitis media: Diagnosis ex machina (Editorial), N Engl J Med 296:445, 1977.
36. Paradise JL: Tympanometry (Editorial). N Engl J Med 307:1074, 1982.
37. Gundersen T and Tonning FM: Ventilation tubes in the middle ear. Arch Otolaryngol 102:198, 1976.
38. Aviel A and Ostfeld E: Acquired irreversible sensorineural hearing loss associated with otitis media with effusion. Am J Otolaryngol 3:217, 1982.
39. Pratt LL: Management of mastoid air cell system in chronic otitis media. Myringoscope 86:674, 1976.
40. Sade J and Halevy A: The natural history of chronic otitis media. J Laryngol Otol 90:743, 1976.
41. Jokipii AMM, Karma P, Kauko O, et al: Anaerobic bacteria in chronic otitis media. Arch Otolaryngol 103:278, 1977.
42. Lund WS: A review of fifty cases of intracranial complications from otogenic infection between 1961 and 1977. Clin Otolaryngol 3:495, 1978.
43. Taylor JS: Otitis externa: Treatment using a new expandable wick. South Med J 68:698, 1975.
44. Walike JW: Management of acute ear infections. Otolaryngol Clin 11:439, 1979.
45. Zaky DA, Bentley DW, Lowy K, et al: Malignant external otitis: A severe form of otitis in diabetic patients. Am J Med 61:298, 1976.
46. Chandler JR: Malignant external otitis: Further consideration. Ann Otol Rhinol Laryngol 86:417, 1977.
47. Gates GA, Avery CA, Prihoda TJ, and Cooper JC Jr: Effectiveness of adenoidectomy and tympanostomy tubes in the treatment of chronic otitis media with effusion. N Engl J Med 317:1444, 1987.

19

Community-Acquired Pneumonia

JAMES L. BREELING, MD

Pneumonia is the sixth leading cause of death in the United States, with a rate of 24.1 deaths per 100,000 population.[1] Mortality rates are low for children and young adults and increase with age, ranging from 5 to 40%. However, even in children and young adults, the morbidity of a febrile respiratory illness can be measured in 150 million days lost from work, 75 million physician visits, and $10 billion in costs for medical care.[1] Although treatment based on a specific microbiologic diagnosis is preferable, the dilemma for the practitioner is that such a diagnosis cannot be obtained in many cases. Classic descriptions of pneumonia syndromes are not helpful in assisting the practitioner in the three major clinical challenges: (1) making a triage decision when confronted with a febrile patient with a cough; (2) obtaining a microbiologic diagnosis; and (3) offering specific therapy in an ambulatory or hospital setting.

TRIAGE DILEMMA

In most cases (the very young and very old are occasional exceptions), the primary presenting symptom of pneumonia is cough, whether productive or nonproductive. The presence of fever with a cough helps to differentiate other causes of cough such as asthma, chronic obstructive lung disease, congestive heart disease, pulmonary embolus, or spontaneous pneumothorax, although any of these conditions may be associated with fever as well. Most patients with chronic bronchitis cough productively (by definition) for several months of the year, and fever and a *change* in the amount and quality of sputum produced is often used to clinically suspect superimposed pneumonia. A variety of upper respiratory tract conditions (e.g., sinusitis, postnasal drip, common colds) can also be associated with a cough, but other symptoms and physical findings help to direct the practitioner away from pneumonia as a diagnosis.

The common cold is usually manifested by sneezing, a watery discharge from the nose (which may become thick and semipurulent), scratchiness of the throat, and a feeling of malaise. Influenza-like illnesses are similar with more extensive malaise, myalgias, fever, and cough. Bronchitis usually involves a productive cough without fever and a history of lung disease. Pneumonia can usually be thought of as a triad of fever, cough, and lung consolidation. The morbidity of pneumonia is distinctly different from the other respiratory conditions (Table 19–1).

The differential diagnosis of a cough is simplified if the clinician finds evidence of lung consolidation on examination with the stethoscope. The findings of dullness to percussion, bronchial breath sounds, crepitant rales, decreased chest expansion, or increased tactile fremitus are the classic findings of pneumonia and should be searched for diligently, although the sensitivity and specificity of each finding is unknown. One study suggested that rapid respiratory rate and chest retractions were sensitive and specific for children younger than 36 months of age,[2] but no such studies exist to guide the diagnosis in adults.

Routine chest radiology has been criticized for elective hospital admission, for routine admission of patients with exacerbations of chronic obstructive lung disease,[3] and has been questioned as a diagnostic tool to confirm or exclude pneumonia in adults with acute respiratory complaints[4] (only 16 to 28% of x-rays show pneumonia in patients presenting to an emergency ward). Heckerling and associates proposed a clinical prediction rule based on an evaluation set of 1134 patients and a validation set of 302 patients at three clinical settings.[5] The findings of temperature higher than 37.8° C, a pulse greater than 100 beats/min, *rales* or *locally decreased breath sounds*, and the absence of asthma each significantly and independently increased the probability of the patient having pneumonia seen on a chest x-ray. Because the study made no attempt to standardize pulmonary examination techniques, interobserver variation in detecting pulmonary signs may have even underestimated the predictive power of the lung findings, suggest-

TABLE 19–1. FREQUENCY AND SEVERITY OF UPPER AND LOWER RESPIRATORY TRACT INFECTION IN ADULTS*

Condition	Episodes per 100 Persons per Year	Average Duration of Restricted Activity (days)
Common cold	41.4	2.8
Influenzas	49.7	3.8
Bronchitis	2.8	6.0
Pneumonia	1.5	16.2

*From 1981 National Health Interview Survey.

TABLE 19–2. TREATMENT OF PNEUMONIA IN ADULTS AT HOME

Patient Criteria	Instructions
Young patients (<45 yr)	Fluids
Capable of taking pills by mouth	Antipyretics
Breathing comfortably	Cough suppressant
No serious underlying illness	Call provider in
No dehydration	24–48 hours

TABLE 19–3. TREATMENT OF PENUMONIA IN THE HOSPITAL

Patient Criteria	Admission Testing
Older than 45 years	CBC/differential
Nausea, vomiting	Chest x-ray
Severe pleurisy or hemoptysis	Blood gas
Dehydration	Sputum Gram Stain
	Sputum culture
	Blood culture

ing that each practitioner should work to gain confidence in his or her own clinical skills as the best way to achieve cost-effective medicine.

However, Singal and associates used a set of "low-yield" criteria derived from the clinical history and physical examination and concluded that they were not able to improve the physician's ability to predict pneumonia.[6]

Most patients with community-acquired pneumonia seen in a primary care setting do not require hospitalization.[7] Clinicians evolve a sense of severity of illness based on experience that suggests that some patients with fever, cough, focal findings in the chest, or a pulmonary infiltrate seen on x-ray can be treated with oral antibiotics. Little clinical research has been done to confirm this experience, but criteria can be suggested for an ambulatory candidate (Table 19–2). Routine laboratory testing should include at a minimum a complete blood count (CBC) to exclude patients with very low or very high white blood cell counts, a chest x-ray to exclude patients with multilobe pneumonia, empyemas, or cavities, and if possible, a sputum Gram stain and culture. Oral therapy is usually successful in young adults; however, since mortality is high among the elderly, especially with pneumococcal disease, it is imperative that the provider contact the patient after 24 to 48 hours of therapy to be certain of the response. The development of confusion, dehydration, dyspnea, hemoptysis, rigors, or new fever would all constitute a reason for the patient's admission to the hospital.

Fine and associates performed a prospective observational study of 280 ambulatory patients with pneumonia to assess all potential morbid complications and 6-week mortality.[8] Appropriateness of admission was judged using the Appropriateness Evaluation Protocol (AEP) of six indicators for admission (a severe vital sign abnormality, altered mental status, suppurative complication, hypoxemia, acute coexistent medical problem, severe laboratory abnormality).[9] Most common indications for admission included arterial hypoxemia or a severe vital sign abnormality, occurring in 110 patients (39%). The remaining 170 patients (61%) did not have an indication for admission at presentation, but 38% developed complications during inpatient treatment. Five independent predictors of complicated hospital courses were identified: (1) age greater than 65 years, (2) comorbid illness such as diabetes, renal insufficiency, or congestive heart failure, (3) temperature higher than 38.3° C, (4) immunosuppression, or (5) high-risk etiology such as staphylococcal, gram-negative rod, aspiration, or postobstructive pneumonia. If validated, this model may be useful in identifying a low-risk group of patients who could safely be managed in the ambulatory setting.

Criteria requiring admission for treatment include nausea, vomiting, inability to take pills, severe pleurisy or hemoptysis, or dehydration as judged by orthostatic blood pressure or serum sodium or blood urea nitrogen. Hospitalization may be necessary if the patient is elderly or unreliable or has no home support system. The requirement for oral antibiotics may be influenced in the future by the development of broad-spectrum antibiotics that can be given once or twice daily via intramuscular or intravenous (IV) route and also by home infusion technology and support services required to delivery parenteral therapy at home.

Several attempts have been made to derive clinical prediction rules for hospitalization of ambulatory patients with pneumonia. Black and associates retrospectively reviewed 141 patients with pneumonia and unclear clinical indication for admission (Table 19–3).[10] Patients with a serious comorbid illness, pre-existing lung disease, multilobar lung involvement, and observed or likely aspiration were found to predict a higher risk group and had more frequent complications.

The British Thoracic Society (BTS) conducted a prospective multicenter study in 1982 to 1983 that involved 25 centers and 453 patients with community-acquired pneumonia. A microbiologic cause was identified in 67% of patients, with pneumococcal pneumonia being most frequent. The analysis found several risk factors that identified a group of patients with a 10- to 21-fold increased mortality (Table 19–4). This prediction rule has the advantage of relying on easily assessable clinical values and not on the microbiologic diagnosis. A retrospective study by Farr and associates of 245 patients and a prospective study by Karalus and coworkers of 92 patients confirmed the predictive power of this rule, suggesting its value in identifying a high-risk group of patients.[11, 12] Fine and associates used different methods to identify five similar variables predictive of greater mortality (pleuritic chest pain, mental status changes, a severe vital sign abnormality, neoplastic disease, and a "high-risk" pneumonia etiology—either staphylococci or gram-negative bacteria), but their prediction rule relies somewhat on microbiologic data that may not be available at presentation.[13]

The practitioner, therefore, can resolve the first dilemma in the treatment of pneumonia by conducting a careful history and examination with special attention to focal findings in the chest and by basing the decision for a chest radiograph on these findings. The decision to admit a patient to the hospital or pursue ambulatory therapy can be made independently of the microbiologic diagnosis, relying on purely clinical parameters such as vital signs, age, underlying illness, mental status, hypoxemia, dehydration, leukopenia, or leukocytosis.

TABLE 19–4. PREDICTION RULE FROM THE BRITISH THORACIC SOCIETY

Diastolic blood pressure < 60 mm Hg
Respiratory rate > 30 breaths/min
Confusion
Previous history of congestive heart failure
Age > 60 years
P_{O_2} < 60 mm Hg on admission
White blood cell count < 4.0 or > 30.0 on admission
Blood urea nitrogen > 70 mg/dl

TABLE 19–5. TYPES OF PNEUMONIA BASED ON CLINICAL SETTING

Category	Common Organisms
Community-acquired pneumonia	Pneumococci, *Mycoplasma*, viruses, *Legionella*
Community-acquired aspiration	Anaerobic bacteria (mouth flora)
Postinfluenzal pneumonia	Staphylococci, pneumococci
Underlying chronic bronchitis	*Haemophilus influenzae*, *Moraxella catarrhalis*
Alcoholism	*Klebsiella*, other gram-negative bacteria
Nursing home patient	Gram-negative bacteria, staphylococci, influenzas, tuberculosis

TABLE 19–7. ETIOLOGIES OF COMMUNITY-ACQUIRED PNEUMONIAS ENCOUNTERED IN OUTPATIENTS

Pathogen	%
Bacterial	70–80
Streptococcus pneumoniae	60–75
Haemophilus influenzae	4–5
Legionella sp.	2–5
Staphylococcus aureus	1–5
Gram-negative bacilli	Rare
Anaerobes	Rare
Atypicals	10–20
Mycoplasma	5–18
Chlamydia	5–10
Viruses	10–20
Influenzas	8–18
Other viruses	2–8

DIAGNOSTIC DILEMMA

The second major dilemma for the practitioner is to obtain a microbiologic diagnosis for the patient with pneumonia. With easy availability of broad-spectrum effective oral and parenteral drugs, and the low mortality of many pneumonias, especially "atypical" pneumonia in the young adult, the effort to obtain sputum and multiple other microbiologic tests seems fruitless. The BTS study used several diagnostic tools including blood and sputum cultures, sputum Gram stain, and serologic examination for *Legionella* and *Mycoplasma* and respiratory viruses. Follow-up analysis by Farr and associates found that sputum was not available in one third of patients on admission to the hospital, and in one third of patients the cause was never determined.[14] Fang and coworkers found that prior antibiotic administration was significantly associated with an undetermined etiology.[15] Woodhead and associates observed clinical practice in two British hospitals and found that blood cultures were obtained in 81% of patients,[16] whereas sputum was examined in 45% and complete serologic tests were done in only 28% of cases. A microbial diagnosis could be reached in only 26% of cases, suggesting that outside of prospective studies the microbial evaluation of pneumonia is not pursued, even though methodology could have defined the cause in two thirds of cases.

Most practitioners recognize the clinical setting of the patient as being related to the type of pneumonia (Table 19–5). Alternatively, two principal clinical patterns are sometimes relied on to determine the microbial source (Table 19–6). Although this type of information may assist the practitioner in making a "best guess," it does not reliably predict the microbiology in all cases. For example, many elderly dehydrated patients with pneumococcal pneumonia may have a nonproductive cough and ill-defined infiltrate that could be mistaken for an "atypical" agent. Conversely, *Legionella* pneumonia frequently presents as multilobar consolidation like the more "typical" bacterial agents.

TABLE 19–6. TWO PRINCIPAL CLINICAL PATTERNS FOR COMMUNITY-ACQUIRED PNEUMONIA

Feature	Classical Pneumonia	Atypical Pneumonia
Onset	Abrupt	Gradual
Fever >103° F	Common	Less common
Chills	Common	Uncommon
Pleuritic pain	Common	Uncommon
Tachycardia >130/min	Frequent	Rare
Consolidation	More common	Less common
Pleural effusion	More common	Less common
Sputum volume	Abundant	Minimal
Sputum character	Thick, purulent, "rusty"	Thin, mucoid
Sputum Gram stain	"Single predominant organism" Many polys	No polys, some monos Scattered normal flora

Epidemiologic studies of ambulatory and hospitalized patients with pneumonia have also been used to estimate the frequency of various agents as causes of disease. One estimate is shown in Table 19–7.[17] Several methodologic problems prevent comparisons of these studies, including (1) incomplete microbiologic investigation for newer "atypical" agents (especially *Legionella* and *Chlamydia*) in older surveys[18–20]; (2) reporting on pneumonia in hospitalized patients versus ambulatory patients[21, 22]; and (3) lack of follow-up prevalence surveys in the same community during different years, making more likely the appearance of "mini epidemics" of influenza, *Mycoplasma*, or other agents that circulate with high attack rates in communities, only to disappear during other seasons.[23, 24]

In a relevant 5-year prospective Canadian study that ended in 1987, 719 adults (mainly elderly) were admitted to an acute care hospital and had the "classic" diagnostic approach of sputum, blood, and pleural fluid cultures and serology for *Legionella, Mycoplasma, Chlamydia, Coxiella,* and viruses.[25] The cause could be demonstrated in 53% of patients, with *Pneumococcus* (10.3%) most common, followed by staphylococci (4%), *Haemophilus* (3.7%), gram-negative bacteria (3%), and *Legionella* (1.9%). The overall mortality was 21%. None of the bacteremic patients had received antibiotics prior to admission, compared with 34% of nonbacteremic patients.

The importance of the microbiologic diagnosis is emphasized by the BTS multicenter study that found that none of the patients who died of pneumococcal, staphylococcal, or *Mycoplasma* (Table 19–8) pneumonia had received appropriate antibiotics before admission to the hospital. Torres and associates found an odds ratio predictive of mortality of 20.7% in patients with severe community-acquired pneumonia who received the incorrect antibiotic.[26] Although the ideal situation of knowing the cause of pneumonia rarely applies when a patient first presents with acute pneumonia, a "best guess" based on an understanding of the likely pathogens in particular settings, followed by empiric therapy and appropriate microbiologic investigation is the standard of practice.

The resolution of this diagnostic dilemma still rests with obtaining a sample of deep respiratory secretions.[27] A properly coached and encouraged patient will produce a deep sample within a short time. The role of the provider as

TABLE 19–8. VALUE OF *MYCOPLASMA* DIAGNOSTIC TESTS

Test	Sensitivity (%)	Specificity (%)	Positive Predictive Value (%)
Cold agglutinins	56	96	65
Complement fixation > 4-fold rise	68	100	—
Mycoplasma-specific IgG > 4-fold rise	40	100	—
Mycoplasma-specific IgM > 4-fold rise	74	99	97
Antigen ELISA*	80	98	—
DNA probe	76	95	82

*ELISA = *e*nzyme-*l*inked *i*mmuno*s*orbent *a*ssay.

coach is emphasized by the study of Fine and associates in which house staff were significantly more likely to obtain a purulent sample compared with the nursing staff.[28] A dry cough in a well-hydrated patient should be used as diagnostic information in considering "atypical" agents. Sputum "scoring" systems have been advocated to improve sensitivity and specificity of sputum Gram stain and culture results.[29, 30] Specimens containing more than 25 leukocytes per ×100 field and less than 10 epithelial cells per ×100 field should be examined for a single predominant organism and sent for culture. Culture of specimens that are contaminated with oral bacteria (>25 epithelial cells and <25 leukocytes) should be discouraged since the results will be misleading.

Several strategies exist for obtaining deep respiratory secretions via more invasive techniques. These strategies include transtracheal aspiration,[31–33] percutaneous needle aspiration,[34] and fiberoptic bronchoscopy with lavage and quantitative bacteriology.[35, 36] Only one study of community-acquired pneumonia that compares invasive techniques has been done.[37] Because of the increased morbidity and sometimes mortality associated with these techniques, they are often reserved for the more seriously ill patient in whom the diagnosis is critical or in patients who fail to respond to empiric therapy.

Community-Acquired Bacterial Pneumonias

Streptococcus pneumoniae remains the most common cause of community-acquired bacterial pneumonia, with one general hospital reporting 62% of the persons being treated as inpatients for pneumonia that was found to be pneumococcal pneumonia.[38] Clinical features of pneumococcal pneumonia are typical of bacterial pneumonias and include an abrupt onset of fevers and chills, acute pleuritic chest pain, and cough productive of "rusty" sputum that turns purulent with time. Preceding upper respiratory tract symptoms are usually absent. The radiologic infiltrate is homogeneous and involves all or part of a lobe, usually with an air bronchogram. The margins of the spreading infiltrate typically appear smooth and well defined. The sensitivity and specificity of the sputum Gram stain and culture have been variably reported in different settings. The BTS study reports a sensitivity of 15% for the Gram stain but used nonrigorous criteria for gauging the quality of the specimen. Others,[39] using more rigorous criteria to reject inadequate samples, find a sensitivity of 62% and a specificity of 85%, with a positive predictive value of 90% when more than 10 gram-positive lancet-shaped diplococci per oil immersion field (×1000) are found. The study by Fine and associates found that house staff read Gram stains with a 90% sensitivity for *Pneumococcus*. The BTS study reported a sensitivity of 24% for sputum culture in pneumococcal pneumonia, but others found that culture was more sensitive,[40] especially if recovery was enhanced by anaerobic incubation as well as by a plate bile test and optochin disk on a primary blood agar plate. Results of blood cultures may be positive in 26% of patients and predict serious sequelae such as meningitis, empyema, endocarditis, arthritis, and peritonitis.[41] An approach that encourages sputum Gram stain, sputum culture, and blood cultures on hospitalized patients with pneumonia could be expected to correctly diagnose two thirds of those patients with pneumococcal pneumonia. Most cases with a classic lobar presentation and negative results of cultures prove to be pneumococcal, especially if the patient received oral antibiotics prior to hospitalization. A diagnostic test using the gene *lyt*A as a DNA probe for pneumococci has been suggested as a promising rapid diagnostic method,[42] which may allow diagnosis in such situations.

The role of Gram stain, sputum culture, and blood culture is less well understood for the other "classic" bacterial pneumonias. For example, Gram stains with *Haemophilus influenzae* are notoriously difficult to read (the study by Fine and associates gives a sensitivity of 58% for house-staff-read Gram stains in *Haemophilus* pneumonia), and results of sputum cultures have been positive in as few as 50% of patients with bacteremic *Haemophilus* pneumonia.[28, 43] A few colonies of nontypable *H. influenzae* recovered from the sputum may indicate an asymptomatic carrier state and not an established diagnosis of pneumonia, not a justification for changing antibiotics if the patient's clinical condition is improving. *H. influenzae* pneumonia is more common in children, the elderly, alcoholics, immunocompromised adults, and individuals with chronic lung disease. Typical lobar or bronchopneumonia patterns are similar to pneumococcal disease. Commercial antigen detection kits for *Haemophilus influenzae* in cerebrospinal fluid have been used to detect urinary antigen in children suspected of having *Haemophilus* pneumonia. At present, the kits lack the necessary sensitivity and specificity, but a modified counterimmunoelectrophoresis technique to detect urinary antigen may be useful.[44]

Community-acquired staphylococcal pneumonia is of most concern during major influenzal epidemics. Woodhead and coworkers found a preponderance of gram-positive cocci visible on stain for a sensitivity of 69%, and results of blood cultures were positive in 20% of cases.[45] Generally, the clinical picture is of a fulminant, toxic illness with high fever, bloody sputum, cyanosis, and prostration with a 30 to 40% mortality.[46]

In approximately 6% of patients who require hospitalization for pneumonia, a gram-negative organism is found to be the pathogen. Almost all cases of community-acquired, gram-negative bacillary pneumonia involve elderly or debilitated patients (e.g., nursing home residents or alcoholic patients) who are subject to aspiration. Gram-negative organisms can be cultured from the oropharynx in these patients, while few healthy adults harbor gram-negative bacilli, except transiently. One study of 73 elderly but ambulatory patients did not find an increased incidence of gram-negative pathogens, except for *Haemophilus*, which suggests that debility rather than age should be used in calculating an index of suspicion for gram-negative pneumonia.[47] Classic clinical features, such as the "bulging" lobar fissure or "currant jelly"–like sputum of *Klebsiella* pneumonia, are rare presentations. One modern review of bacteremic *Klebsiella* pneumonia failed to report bulging interlobar fissures or cavitation in any patient, with most cases occurring in immunocompromised hosts.[48] Sensitivity or specificity of clinical, radiographic, and microbiologic data are low,[49] especially since many of the elderly patients affected have an inadequate cough. Suspected staphylococcal or gram-negative pneumonia in the elderly or debilitated may be one indication for a more invasive approach to obtaining deep respiratory secretions.

Legionella pneumophila is a gram-negative non–acid-fast bacillus that is one of at least 20 different species in the genus *Legionella*. Almost all are free-living in the environment (soil or water), and most are capable of causing a febrile human illness, usually involving the respiratory tract. Transmission via the airborne route (e.g., air conditioning, water supplies, cooling towers) appears to be the source of contagion for humans. The severity of the illness may reflect the size of the inhaled inoculum.

The clinical picture in normal hosts is a spectrum from mild flu-like illness to severe, often progressive, pneumonia. When pneumonia occurs, it tends to be lobar or to rapidly develop into multilobar disease. Retrospective studies of the early epidemic cases in the Philadelphia legionnaires' convention emphasized the multisystemic problems of confusion, hyponatremia, diarrhea, liver function abnormalities, and proteinuria.[50] However, prospective studies found no consistent clinical or laboratory differences between legionnaires' pneumonia and other types of serious pneumonia (e.g. pneumococcal pneumonia).[51, 52] In the normal host, the presentation is most frequently a multilobar pneumonia, but in the immunocompromised host, especially if the disease is nosocomially transmitted, the initial infiltrate may be more "atypical."

Diagnostic testing for *Legionella* is underutilized by practitioners (Table 19–9). One report indicates that the organism may be visible using a Giemsa-stained smear on a bronchial aspirate examined by direct microscopy.[53] The diagnosis was suggested by the presence of violaceous intracellular and extracellular bacilli on Giemsa staining, despite the absence of immunofluorescence to *L. pneumophila* serogroup 1. The organism was isolated and shown to be *L. pneumophila* serogroup 6. A direct fluorescent antibody test performed on deep respiratory secretions is available for rapid results but requires a panel of fluorescently tagged antibody and a clinical laboratory with persons experienced in fluorescent microscopy. There is some concern that cross-reaction with other oral bacteria may limit the usefulness of this test on expectorated sputum. The serum indirect fluorescent antibody test also has acceptable sensitivity and specificity; however, a four-fold rise in titer must be observed and can take 6 to 8 weeks, making this test less useful in the acute setting but very useful for retrospective epidemiologic studies.

Most modern clinical microbiology laboratories now have experience in culturing *Legionella* on charcoal-yeast extract agar.[54] The organism grows readily in 5 to 7 days, thus making this test the "gold standard," especially if performed on deep respiratory secretions. Newer techniques such as antigen detection in the urine[55] (Access Medical Systems, uses monoclonal antibody to detect *L. pneumophila* serogroup 1 antigen) or sputum antigen by Enzyme-Linked Immunosorbent Assay (ELISA), and DNA probes[56] (Gen Probe, San Diego) will have widespread clinical usefulness in a few years. The DNA probe is especially interesting because it only requires 20 minutes and can detect *Legionella* DNA up to 8 days into antibiotic therapy, whereas direct fluorescent antibody and culture may rapidly become negative with empiric use of erythromycin.

In recent years the pathogenic potential of *Moraxella catarrhalis* (formerly *Branhamella catarrhalis*) has become clear.[57] This organism is now thought to be a reasonably frequent cause of otitis media, acute sinusitis, bronchitis and pneumonia in smokers and patients with chronic lung disease and is also found in immunocompromised patients. Its clinical presentation is similar to *Haemophilus influenzae* infection with bronchopneumonia or patchy transient infiltrates.[58] A sputum Gram stain may reveal abundant intra-cellular and extracellular gram-negative diplococci. Since this organism frequently expresses a β-lactamase gene product, therapy with the usual β-lactams is problematic.

Pulmonary abscess, empyema, and necrotizing pneumonia constitute a group of suppurative pulmonary diseases that can be "community-acquired" but are different in terms of clinical presentation. Most frequently sequelae of aspiration or loss of consciousness, the causative organisms may include *Bacteroides* sp., *Fusobacterium* sp., and other anaerobic organisms that are usually part of the oral flora.[59] Most patients have underlying conditions such as alcoholism, seizure disorders, cerebrovascular accidents, general anesthesia, drug overdose or addiction, dysphagia, mental retardation, and dementia. The hallmark is copious production of a putrid sputum with gradual onset over 1 week to several weeks. The patient frequently has weight loss, anemia, fever, and leukocytosis. Cavitation in the posterior segments of the upper lobes or the superior segments of the lower lobes occurs with aspiration in the recumbent position. Tuberculosis and cancer must be considered as part of the differential diagnosis but usually can be excluded by examination of a sputum Gram stain, acid-fast smear, and cytologic preparations. In some cases, fine needle aspiration of the cavity may be necessary to confirm its microbiology.

TABLE 19–9. VALUE OF *LEGIONELLA* DIAGNOSTIC TESTS

Test	Sensitivity (%)	Specificity (%)	Positive Predictive Value (%)
Serum antibody	75	90–95	—
Direct fluorescent antibody			
Sputum	50	90	—
Lung tissue	80–90	99	—
Culture			
Sputum	70	100	100
Lung tissue	90	100	100
Blood	10	100	100
Urine antigen	80–90	87	—
DNA probe	94	97	99

Community-Acquired "Atypical" Pneumonia

Mycoplasmal pneumonia has a fairly low but constant incidence during the 12 months of the year. Cases tend to be clustered in the summer and fall, when the frequency of pneumonias due to adenovirus and influenzae declines. Community-wide epidemics can occur with a periodicity of every 4 to 7 years, affecting mostly young children between the ages of 8 and 10 years and young adults aged 20 to 40 years.[60, 61] Family clustering is common. Disease in the elderly is uncommon, with the most common cause of "atypical" pneumonia in the elderly being influenza. Holmberg and associates constructed a prediction equation that suggests that younger patients with normal white blood cell counts and higher serum lactate dehydrogenase values are more likely to have mycoplasmal pneumonia than pneumococcal disease.[62]

The clinical manifestations of mycoplasmal pneumonia are a relatively low-grade fever (38.3 to 38.8° C), malaise, headache, pharyngitis with little rhinitis, congestion or fullness in the ear, and a dry, persistent cough. Extrapulmonary manifestations have been noted but are rare and should not be relied on when making a diagnosis.[63] The radiograph usually shows a patchy pneumonitis, with lobar consolidation in less than 10% of cases.[64] The patient usually looks less ill, and the chest examination is usually less impressive than the radiographic infiltrate.

The clinical microbiology laboratory can offer several methods of diagnosis (see Table 19–8). A fourfold rise in complement-fixation antibody or *Mycoplasma*-specific IgG occurs after 2 weeks of illness and therefore is not useful in making the diagnosis at the time of presentation. Cold agglutinins should not be used since they are nonspecific and usually peak during the third week after the infection. Newer techniques, such as ELISA for specific anti-*Mycoplasma* IgM,[65] detection of *Mycoplasma* antigen directly in the sputum by ELISA,[66] or use of DNA probes (Gen Probe, San Diego), offer the best strategy for making the diagnosis of *Mycoplasma* in the acute setting while the patient is sick.[67, 68] These techniques will become widely commercially available in the near future.

Chlamydia pneumoniae (formerly *Chlamydia* TWAR) has recently been recognized as a third species of *Chlamydia*.[69] The other two *Chlamydia* sp. are *C. trachomatis* (the organism involved in sexually transmitted urethritis and cervicitis), and *C. psittaci* (the agent of psittacosis, which is a respiratory infection transmitted to humans from infected birds). The clinical spectrum and epidemiology of *C. pneumoniae* infection is just beginning to be understood. Apparently, like many other respiratory pathogens, most patients are relatively asymptomatic or have symptoms that are too mild to lead them to seek medical attention. Fever and sore throat, especially with hoarseness, may be the most early common symptom, with sinusitis-type complaints occurring in 5% of cases. The illness may then progress over 5 to 7 days to bronchitis, with nonproductive cough or asthmatic wheezing lasting for several weeks. In some, abnormal breath sounds herald pneumonia. The chest radiograph usually demonstrates a single, subsegmental infiltrate in milder cases and more extensive or bilateral pneumonitis in hospitalized cases.[70] The leukocyte count may be normal, although the sedimentation rate is generally elevated. A complete recovery is slow, even with appropriate antibiotics and cough, and malaise may persist for many weeks.

The frequency and severity of *C. pneumoniae* infection varies with age, with most disease seen in children between 5 and 14 years of age and in young adults, much like *Mycoplasma* infection. Disease is rare in older adults but can occur and may be more severe. Country-wide epidemics have occurred in Finland, Denmark, Sweden, and Norway. Retrospective studies of banked serum indicate a mycoplasma-like periodicity of 4- to 6-year cycles. Reinfection can apparently occur in older adults since the immunity seems to wane with time.

Culture and isolation of *C. pneumoniae* still involves a special technique that requires tissue-culture facilities and is not generally useful in the clinical setting. Serologic methods are now commercially available for the detection by microimmunofluorescence of specific IgG and IgM directed against the elementary body antigen. IgM appears 2 to 4 weeks after the onset of symptoms, and IgG appears at 6 to 8 weeks, making diagnosis in the acute setting difficult at the present time. A more widely available *Chlamydia* complement fixation antibody test can detect an antibody directed against *C. pneumoniae* and also *C. trachomatis* and *C. psittaci*. Pneumonia due to *C. pneumoniae* may respond to either erythromycin or tetracycline.[71]

Most other "atypical" pneumonia acquired in the community is viral in origin. Viruses associated with pneumonia include influenza, parainfluenza, respiratory syncytial virus, and adenovirus,[72] with measles, varicella, and the herpes viruses as rare causes. During epidemics of influenza, 3 to 5% of patients have developed pneumonia manifested by a pulmonary infiltrate.[73] In population-based studies, influenza and parainfluenza are more frequent causes of pneumonia in the elderly than either *Mycoplasma* or *Chlamydia*.

The pulmonary complications of influenza include bronchitis, primary viral pneumonias, and secondary bacterial pneumonias.[74] Mortality in primary viral pneumonia due to influenza is associated with more diffuse involvement and underlying disease, such as mitral stenosis or chronic obstructive lung disease. Secondary bacterial pneumonias are most frequently pneumococcal, but the incidence of community-acquired staphylococcal pneumonia is increased during years with particularly virulent influenza strains.

Parainfluenza virus is an important cause of croup and bronchitis in children and occasionally pneumonia in children and adults. Respiratory syncytial virus causes bronchiolitis in infants and tracheobronchitis in young children. When families are infected with these viruses, most members develop signs of upper respiratory tract infection, with nasal congestion and cough as the most common signs. Adults with underlying lung disease can develop airway hyperreactivity, exacerbations of bronchitis, or influenza-like illness and pneumonia. In the elderly and institutionalized, outbreaks of respiratory syncytial virus infection have been associated with a particularly high proportion (between 50 and 60%) developing bronchopneumonia.[75, 76]

Viral diagnostic testing has improved beyond culture techniques. Most modern hospital virology laboratories now have the capability to directly examine nasopharyngeal secretions by immunofluorescence, DNA probe, or ELISA.[77–79] Sensitivity and specificity compare well with older and slower culture methods. These tests have also utility in adults and should be utilized in settings where viral pneumonia can be considered (e.g., a family cluster of pneumonia/respiratory disease or in institutional outbreaks of respiratory illness and pneumonia in the elderly).

Other organisms may be encountered by the practitioner as rare causes of community-acquired pneumonia. Such diseases as psittacosis, Q fever (*Coxiella*), tularemia, plague, actinomycosis, primary histoplasmosis, primary coccidioidomycosis, and primary tuberculosis should be suspected when the patient has not responded to the usual therapeutic strategy and attempts at microbiologic diagnosis of the aforementioned organisms have not yielded a result.

ANTIBIOTIC TREATMENT DILEMMA

The initial, often empiric antibiotic choices for community-acquired pneumonia depends on the microbiologic cause indicated by the clinical setting and by any rapid diagnostic information available to the practitioner (including but not limited to sputum Gram stain). Other factors such as drug allergies, local situations (e.g., mycoplasma or influenza epidemics, high incidence of ampicillin-resistant *H. influenzae*), drug costs, and personal clinical experience must also be considered in the increasingly large choice of oral antibiotics.

Unfortunately, almost all clinical information on the efficacy of drugs used to treat pneumonia is *deficient* in one of several ways. Randomized and blinded comparisons of oral agents that enroll sufficient numbers of seriously ill patients, with confirmed microbiologic causes for their pneumonia, are rare. In vitro studies and single drug/open label trials are common. One's conclusion is that many regimens are therapeutically equivalent and that one drug or a group of drugs may be preferred for reasons of patient tolerance and antibiotic costs.

Oral Therapy

Oral antibiotics continue to be the mainstay of the practitioner's pharmacopeia because they are generally safe, economical, and convenient. The fact that most patients have few side effects from this practice has led many physicians to overprescribe. The occasional treatment failure has encouraged the practice of prescribing additional courses of more "advanced" and costly oral drugs (Table 19–10). In general, oral drugs should be readily absorbed from the gastrointestinal tract, have a long enough half-life to allow convenient dosing intervals, have a pharmacology that allows good tissue levels in the lungs/sputum, and be easily tolerated by the patient.

Oral Penicillins

Penicillin VK, ampicillin, and amoxicillin are the older penicillins that, for many reasons, are still among the most widely used oral antibiotics. In the treatment of lower respiratory tract infection, ampicillin and amoxicillin may be preferred because of the superior absorption from the gastrointestinal tract. Both are active against most bacteria sensitive to penicillin G (especially *Pneumococcus*) plus some gram-negative bacteria (*E. coli, Proteus mirabilis*, and approximately 80% of *H. influenzae* depending on local prevalence of *H. influenzae* β-lactamase production). Both drugs are acid-stable, and a common adult dosage is 500 mg every 6 hours (8-hourly for amoxicillin). The peak drug level occurs 2 hours after an oral dose, and the drug is still detectable in the serum at 6 hours (8 hours for amoxicillin). Amoxicillin has greater bioavailability than does ampicillin—the same 500-mg dose of amoxicillin gives twice the peak serum level of ampicillin (10 to 12 μg/ml versus 5 to 6 μg/ml), and this is not impaired by food in the stomach. The most common toxicities of both drugs are hypersensitivity reactions since they are "cross-allergenic" with penicillin and rashes (5 to 7%, but perhaps 65% in patients with mononucleosis). Nausea and diarrhea are usually not serious but occur in 5 to 20% of adults who take either drug. Because amoxicillin is better absorbed from the gastrointestinal tract, diarrhea occurs in 2% of patients. Both drugs are effective in chronic bronchitis despite relatively low bronchial levels, probably because most of the usual pathogens are very sensitive. Amoxicillin produces higher levels in purulent and mucoid sputum than does ampicillin. Pneumococcal lobar pneumonia is well treated by either drug, but both are ineffective for *M. pneumoniae* and *Legionella*. Causative agents in sinusitis and otitis are *S. pneumoniae*, *H. influenzae*, and other *Neisseria* and *Streptococcus* spp. Both conditions respond well to the usual oral doses. Since

TABLE 19–10. COST OF ORAL ANTIBIOTICS

Drug	Daily Dosage	Cost of 7 Days of Treatment ($)*
Amoxicillin		
Generic	500 mg tid	6.02
Amoxil (Beecham)	500 mg tid	8.82
Amoxicillin-clavulanic acid	500 mg tid	38.34
Augmentin (Beecham)		
Ampicillin		
Generic	500 mg qid	3.79
Amcill (Parke-Davis)	500 mg qid	5.04
Polycillin (Bristol)	500 mg qid	9.24
Cefaclor		
Ceclor (Lilly)	500 mg tid	50.18
Cefuroxime axetil		
Ceftin (Glaxo)	500 mg bid	50.18
Cephalexin		
Keflex (Dista)	500 mg qid	40.02
Cephradine		
Anspor (SKF)	500 mg qid	32.80
Velosef (Squibb)	500 mg qid	37.88
Norfloxacin		
Noroxin (Merck)	400 mg bid	28.42
Sulfisoxazole		
Generic	1 g qid	2.24
Gantrisin (Roche)	1 g qid	6.55
Tetracycline		
Generic	1 g/day	.91
Achromycin (Lederle)	1 g/day	1.82
Trimethoprim		
Generic	100 mg bid	2.58
Trimpex (Roche)	100 mg bid	5.38
Trimethoprim-Sulfamethoxazole		
Generic–double strength	1 tablet bid	2.82
Bactrim DS (Roche)	1 tablet bid	9.02
Septra DS (Burroughs-Wellcome)	1 tablet bid	9.02
Ciprofloxacin		
Cipro (Miles)	750 mg bid	48.72
Cefixime		
Suprax (Lederle)	400 mg/day	Not available
Cefadroxil		
Duricef (Princeton)	500 mg bid	25.55

*Average wholesale price in *Red Book 1988.*

M. catarrhalis produces a β-lactamase, these drugs may be ineffective when pneumonia is caused by this agent.

Dicloxacillin is perhaps the most widely used oral semisynthetic penicillin. All drugs of this class are active against most *Staphylococcus* and *Streptococcus* spp., except for *S. fecalis* (now called *Enterococcus fecalis*). However, there is no activity against gram-negative pathogens including *Haemophilus*. The drug is acid stable but should be administered 1 hour before meals for optimal absorption. The usual dose is 500 mg every 6 hours, but the dose can be doubled in severe infection if tolerated by the patient's gastrointestinal tract. Peak levels of 8 to 10 μg/ml are reached after 1 hour, and the drug is excreted renally. Penicillinase-producing *S. aureus* has a median minimal inhibitory concentration (MIC) of 0.12 μg/ml. The drug is highly protein-bound, and the MICs may be 20-fold higher if the test is performed in the presence of serum, but even then they are still within the peak serum level. Like ampicillin or amoxicillin, it is "cross-allergenic" to penicillin and causes gastrointestinal upset that only occasionally necessitates cessation of treatment. Dicloxacillin would be a reasonable choice for the treatment of staphylococcal pneumonia or as treatment of a patient with lobar pneumonia who presents during a viral influenza season.

Amoxicillin/clavulanic acid is a combination drug linking amoxicillin to a naturally occurring β-lactamase inhibitor. Clavulanic acid has only weak antibacterial activity by itself but readily inhibits β-lactamase produced by staphylococci, *H. influenzae*, and *M. catarrhalis*. It is also active against the β-lactamase produced by the *Enterobacteriaceae* and *Bacteriodaceae*, whether carried by plasmids or chromosomally. However, it is not active against the *Serratia/Pseudomonas* group of chromosomally mediated β-lactamases that are inducible and important causes of resistance to third-generation cephalosporins. Methicillin-resistant *S. aureus* and *S. epidermidis* are also resistant to the combination.

The dosage forms are fixed as 250 mg amoxicillin plus 125 mg of clavulanic acid or 500 mg amoxicillin/125 mg of clavulanic acid, which are both given every 8 hours. Serum levels of clavulanic acid are unaffected by meals or the fasting state; however, if this drug is taken just before meals, the side effects of nausea or vomiting are less notable. Both drugs are well distributed in the body, except for the cerebrospinal fluid, and excreted by the urine. Nausea and vomiting occur in 3 to 5% of patients, and rashes occur in 1 to 4% of patients. Mucosal candidiasis occurs in 1% of patients—more commonly than with ampicillin or co-trimoxazole.

The combination is useful in upper and lower respiratory tract infection, especially against β-lactamase–producing *H. influenzae* (which occurs in 10 to 40% of isolates depending on the area surveyed) or *M. catarrhalis*. It offers no advantage over penicillin or ampicillin in pneumococcal-, streptococcal-, or penicillin-sensitive anaerobic infection. It has no activity against *Mycoplasma, Legionella*, or the respiratory *Chlamydia*. If the pathogen has been identified, older, cheaper, and more narrow-spectrum antibiotics are usually indicated.

Oral Cephalosporins

Cephalexin can be regarded as an oral form of the parenteral cephalothin. It is active against all *Streptococcus* sp. and against *Staphylococcus* sp. sensitive to penicillin or dicloxacillin. β-Lactamase–producing strains of *Staphylococcus* vary in their degree of susceptibility (some MICs range from 1.6 to 100 μg/ml, with a median of 12.5 μg/ml), but methicillin-resistant staphylococci are resistant to cephalexin. Like ampicillin, cephalexin has some activity against *E. coli, P. mirabilis*, and *Klebsiella* but has less activity against *H. influenzae*. The usual dose is 250 to 500 mg four times a day for mild to moderate infections. Cephalexin is almost completely absorbed after oral administration, with the peak level (18 to 20 μg/ml) occurring at 1 hour and high urinary excretion levels for most of the dosing interval. Diarrhea, emesis, and pseudomembranous colitis all have been reported but are not common. Only 6 to 9% of penicillin-allergic patients will have a cross-allergy to cephalexin.

Cephalexin is an alternate to penicillin or ampicillin for streptococcal and pneumococcal disease, especially for mildly allergic patients. However, it is less active than either of the penicillins and, because of its cost, is not a first-line agent. It has been used for bronchitis, otitis, sinusitis, and pneumonia but poor results may occur, especially if *H. influenzae* is involved. Cephradine is another oral cephalosporin similar to cephalexin in all respects.

Cefaclor and cefadroxil are similar in many ways to cephalexin and cephradine, except that cefaclor may be more active in vitro against some strains of *H. influenzae*. (The letter "f" replaced "ph" in the spelling of cephalosporins named after 1975; therefore, these are "newer" but not of a different "generation"). Cefadroxil has a long serum half-life and can be given every 8 to 12 hours instead of dosing with cefaclor every 6 hours. The peak serum levels of both drugs are slightly lower than for cephalexin, and both are renally excreted. Toxicity is also similar to that of cephalexin, except that eosinophilia, a positive result on a Coombs test, and serum sickness–like reactions have been described for cefaclor.

The indications for use of cefaclor and cefadroxil are similar to those for using cephalexin, except that these drugs may be more useful in sinusitis, otitis, and bronchitis when *H. influenzae* is a pathogen. Because of their cost, they are not considered first-line agents in the treatment of most community-acquired pneumonia. Generic trimethoprim/sulfamethoxazole would be a vastly less expensive treatment for *Haemophilus* infection.

A new oral cephalosporin known as cefprozil has an in vitro spectrum of activity that is similar to cefaclor but has a longer half-life and thus can be given twice daily.[80] It offers no significant advantage in terms of rate of clinical response or cost.

Cefuroxime axetil is a second-generation agent because it has increased resistance to β-lactamase produced by gram-negative bacteria that inactivate older cephalosporins. It is an ester of the parenteral drug cefuroxime. The ester linkage is cleaved in the intestine yielding the parent drug. The parent drug has activity against the same spectrum of gram-positive microorganisms as cephalexin and is active against many *E. coli, Klebsiella, H. influenzae, M. catarrhalis*, and most *Proteus*. It is not active against *Pseudomonas, Serratia*, and *Acinetobacter*. Its bioavailability is variable (25 to 45%), making it a less useful drug to treat serious gram-negative infections outside of the urinary tract and limiting its use in serious gram-negative respiratory infections, which would be better treated by the parenteral drug cefuroxime. Because of its extended gram-negative spectrum, diarrhea with *C. difficile* may be more of a problem as a side effect. In one trial, cefuroxime axetil was equivalent to amoxicillin in treating lower respiratory tract infections. Its cost limits its use to pneumonia involving *H. influenzae* or *M. catarrhalis* when other cheaper drugs cannot be used. One use may be in follow-up treatment of pneumonia once a clinical response to parenteral cefuroxime was established and an oral agent would be needed to complete a 10- to 14-day course. However, amoxicillin or trimethoprim/sulfamethoxazole may also serve this purpose unless the microbiologic cause of pneumonia was resistant.

Cefixime is advertised as a third-generation oral antibiotic because it is more active than other oral cephalosporins against the *Enterobacteriaceae*, excluding *Pseudomonas* and *Acinetobacter*. Almost 90% of the susceptible isolates are inhibited at concentrations less than 1 μg/ml. However, bioavailability is relatively poor (40 to 52%), and peak serum levels are correspondingly low (3 to 5 μg/ml after a dose of 400 mg). At these levels almost all staphylococci are considered to be resistant to cefixime, which severely limits its use. One advantage is that cefixime can be dosed every 12 to 24 hours to allow once or twice-a-day dosing. Despite this in vitro broad-spectrum activity, it has been very difficult to show clinical superiority versus co-trimoxazole or amoxicillin/clavulanic acid in various clinical settings such as acute bronchitis, sinusitis, otitis media, or pneumonia.

A troubling side effect in one study comparing amoxicillin with cefixime in acute otitis was a 16% incidence of diarrhea resulting in a significant number of patients stopping therapy.

Trimethoprim/Sulfamethoxazole

Trimethoprim/sulfamethoxazole (generic brand is co-trimoxazole) is a combination drug (a 1:5 ratio) with a wide range of antibacterial activity, including *S. pneumoniae*, most *Enterobacteriaceae*, and *H. influenzae*, including ampicillin-resistant strains. The MICs against *S. aureus* can be as low as 0.2 μg/ml. Resistance in community-acquired infection is uncommon, although in-hospital acquisition of plasmid-mediated resistance factors may occur. Both components of this drug are well absorbed after oral administration (the usual dose is two single-strength tablets every 12 hours or 160 mg of trimethoprim/800 mg of sulfamethoxazole). If the individual dose of co-trimoxazole is increased, even up to 12 tablets/day, peak serum levels of these drugs are increased linearly and their half-lives for elimination through the urine are prolonged. The availability of a pediatric suspension and the capability of giving higher doses (5 to 15 mg/kg/day) especially to tube-fed elderly patients makes this drug an excellent and cheap broad-spectrum agent in the treatment of pneumonia. The 1:5 ratio of administered drug gives a peak serum level in 2 hours with a drug ratio of 1:25—a ratio at which maximum synergy occurs against many organisms. Both drugs are rapidly and widely distributed in body tissues, especially sputum.

Rashes occur in 2 to 8% of patients, with an increased incidence in patients with acquired immunodeficiency syndrome (AIDS). Gastrointestinal side effects are less common; nausea occurs in 3% and diarrhea occurs in 0.5%. Because of its mode of action, co-trimoxazole may interfere with human folate metabolism, especially if large doses are given over a long period. Reported abnormalities include aplastic anemia, neutropenia, and thrombocytopenia. Patients with pre-existing bone marrow disorders are more susceptible to this effect, and several large studies of otitis media and urinary tract infection have shown rare marrow depression in normal individuals.

Co-trimoxazole is effective against most bacteria that cause superinfection in patients with chronic bronchitis, including pneumococci, *Klebsiella, H. influenzae*, and *M. catarrhalis*. It has been used extensively and is as effective as amoxicillin for acute bronchitis, bacterial pneumonia, and otitis media/sinusitis. It is also effective against *S. aureus* in many settings, but dicloxacillin may be preferred for known *Staphylococcus* infections. The low cost of the generic drug makes it a desirable choice for broad-spectrum empiric therapy of lower respiratory tract infections.

Oral Macrolides

Erythromycin is probably the safest of all currently available antibiotics (Table 19–11). Erythromycin is highly active against streptococci and staphylococci, including β-lactamase–producing strains (median MIC for sensitive staphylococci is 0.5 μg/ml). This drug has limited activity against gram-negative organisms but has activity against some *H. influenzae* and is the most useful agent for *Legionella* sp. In addition *M. pneumoniae* is very susceptible. The usual adult dose is 500 mg every 6 hours. Bioavailability and resultant serum concentrations vary to a greater degree than do any other agent discussed earlier. Erythromycin base is destroyed by acid in the stomach, thus most formulations are enteric coated to dissolve in the duodenum. Despite this, many individuals may have an undetectable peak serum level, and average peaks (0.3 μg/ml) may be below the MIC for staphylococci or *Legionella*.[81] Erythromycin stearate is less readily destroyed in the stomach, but peak serum levels appear to be the same as with the base, and the marked individual variation in levels remains the same. Two forms of erythromycin that are acid stable and yield consistently high peak serum levels (1.5 μg/ml to 2.5 μg/ml) are erythromycin estolate and erythromycin ethyl succinate. There are data to show that the estolate is more effective in streptococcal pharyngitis than the ethyl succinate form in children because of higher peak levels, more sustained serum levels, and better penetration into tonsilar tissues. More children had post-treatment throat cultures that showed positive results for streptococci with the ethyl succinate form. There are no comparable data in adults indicating clinical failure in any disease state for either drug. Excretion occurs through the kidneys, bile, and by an unknown process of tissue inactivation.

TABLE 19–11. COST OF ORAL ERYTHROMYCINS

Drug	Dosage	Cost of 7 Days of Treatment ($)
Erythromycin base		
Generic–enteric coated	500 mg qid	9.60
E-mycin (Upjohn)	500 mg qid	16.24
Erythromycin stearate		
Generic–film coated	500 mg qid	6.86
Erythrocin (Abbott)	500 mg qid	9.42
Erythromycin estolate		
Generic	500 mg qid	15.76
Ilosone (Dista)	500 mg qid	23.48
Erythromycin ethylsuccinate		
Generic	400 mg qid	14.16
E.E.S. (Abbott)	400 mg qid	19.32

Gastrointestinal intolerance is the chief side effect of oral erythromycin. Abdominal cramps, nausea, vomiting, or diarrhea occur in 15 to 45% of patients. The epigastric distress can be diminished by taking the drug with meals, but this lowers peak serum levels for all forms except the estolate. In some studies, up to 20% of patients stop taking their prescribed course because of gastrointestinal intolerance. The practitioner would have no way of knowing about patient compliance unless the original symptoms of infection persisted, and most patients with sore throat, bronchitis, and so forth improve without further antibiotics.

A mild, reversible, chemical hepatitis can occur with all forms of erythromycin. The estolate form has been associated with an occasionally protracted cholestatic jaundice in adults treated for more than 14 days, but symptoms and jaundice usually subside rapidly once the drug is withdrawn and no progression to chronic liver disease or fatalities have ever been reported. Because of its hepatic excretion, erythromycin can lead to a 20 to 25% increase in theophylline half-life, leading to potentially toxic accumulation. This drug interaction should be monitored in all patients with chronic lung disorders who are taking erythromycin for "bronchitis" or the clinical suspicion of *Mycoplasma* infection. Other drugs with reported interaction include oral anticoagulants, digoxin, methylprednisolone, carbamazepine, terfenadine, and cyclosporin.

Erythromycin is an effective alternate to penicillin for the treatment of pneumococcal pneumonia. It is effective in acute bronchitis, sinusitis, and otitis when the usual pathogens are streptococci and pneumococci. However, since erythromycin does not reach adequate levels in the sinuses and middle ear to exceed the MIC against *H. influenzae*, amoxicillin or co-trimoxazole are preferred. In cases of pneumonia due to *Mycoplasma*, erythromycin effectively reduces the length of illness, but mycoplasmas may often persist in respiratory tract secretions both during and after therapy, leading to a 10 to 15% relapse rate. Erythromycin is the drug of choice for Legionnaires' disease. A total daily dose of 2 g/day may be adequate for mild disease, but the erratic bioavailability of some forms makes oral therapy risky in moderately or severely ill patients. These patients should be given IV erythromycin 4 to 6 g/day, and the most severely ill patients may only respond to the addition of rifampin.

Two second-generation macrolides have been approved for use in lower respiratory tract infection. Clarithromycin is an acid-stable analog of erythromycin with improved bioavailability, improved gastrointestinal tolerance, and activity against *Streptococcus, Haemophilus, Moraxella, Bordetella, Mycoplasma, Legionella*, and *Chlamydia*. It may be four times more active against *Legionella* than erythromycin.[82, 83] Clinical trials in pneumonia show similar usefulness in treating most causes of lower respiratory tract infection at a dosage of 250 mg orally twice daily, except for *H. influenzae* in which dosages of 500 mg twice daily were needed to achieve similar cure rates with agents such as cefixime, cefuroxime axetil, and cefaclor.[84] In one comparison between clarithyromycin 250 mg twice daily and erythromycin 250 mg or 500 mg given four times daily, cure rates for pneumonia were similar, but clarithromycin was better tolerated.[85] Another study comparing clarithromycin with erythromycin found similar clinical outcomes in cases of proven mycoplasmal pneumonia.[86] Apparently the 14-hydroxy metabolite is twice as potent against *Haemophilus* as the parent drug.[87] The role of clarithromycin in the treatment of community-acquired pneumonia remains to be determined by larger clinical experience.

Azithromycin is another second-generation macrolide with the unique property of increased uptake in polymorphonuclear leukocytes and macrophages when compared with erythromycin,[88] making it especially appealing in the treatment of cell-associated and intracellular pathogens such as *Chlamydia, Mycoplasma*, and *Legionella*. Its exceptionally long half-life[89] makes it a candidate for once-a-day dosing; it has been approved by the Federal Drug Administration (FDA) for single-dose treatment of genital *Chlamydia* infection. Azithromycin has been given as a 500-mg dose once, then 250 mg/day for the next 4 days (a total of 5 days of therapy) and has similar response rates to ampicillin/clavulanate for 10 days[90] or erythromycin 500 mg four times daily for 10 days[91] or cefaclor 500 mg three times daily[92] in chronic bronchitis. No clinical trials in pneumonia have yet been reported, but azithromycin may make "short-course" pneumonia therapy a possibility.[93] One open-label, randomized trial comparing 3-day versus 5-day therapy with azithromycin in atypical pneumonia (*Mycoplasma, Chlamydia*, and *Coxiella*) found most patients afebrile by 48 hours of therapy and all patients "cured" by the fifth day of therapy.[94] Clinical experience to date indicates that it is generally better tolerated than erythromycin,[95] but its exact role in the treatment of community-acquired pneumonia remains to be determined by larger clinical trials. Both clarithromycin and azithromycin are more expensive than are the older erythromycins and would need to be proved better tolerated or more effective in order to replace the older first-line drugs.

Oral Quinolones

The quinolones are the cause of much excitement in the field of oral antibiotic therapy, particularly when gram-negative pathogens are suspected or confirmed. They are bacteriocidal drugs that act on DNA gyrase, an enzyme needed in bacterial replication. They are active against a broad spectrum of gram-positive and gram-negative bacteria.

Ciprofloxacin is readily absorbed from the gastrointestinal tract and reaches higher peak serum levels than does norfloxacin (2 to 5 μg/ml), making it useful outside of the urinary tract or gastrointestinal tract. Its activity includes many of the *Enterobacteriaceae, H. influenzae*, and *M. catarrhalis*. It is active but less so against *Pseudomonas aeruginosa* and staphylococci, and resistance to ciprofloxacin has emerged during therapy when these pathogens are involved. Many streptococci are more susceptible to penicillin. Neither norfloxacin nor ciprofloxacin covers anaerobic bacteria. Side effects include nausea, headache, and dizziness. Quinolones are not recommended for pregnant or nursing mothers, because cartilage deterioration and arthropathy have been observed in young animals. Occasionally tremors, confusion, *Candida* superinfection, and elevations of serum aminotransferase activity and creatinine have been reported. Important drug interactions with theophylline and caffeine have been reported, causing toxic elevations when these drugs are given in combination.

Oral ciprofloxacin offers an acceptable alternative to parenteral therapy for many serious infections, including complicated respiratory tract infections, except when streptococci, staphylococci, and oral anaerobes are a factor, and for some deep-seated gram-negative infections. Several well-documented failures in cases of pneumococcal pneumonia highlight ciprofloxacin's weakness against streptococcal infection.[96] For this reason, it should not be used when pneumococcal pneumonia is suspected. However, especially in the elderly, it may be useful when *Haemophilus* or other gram-negative pneumonia is suspected but is not clearly superior to co-trimoxazole.

Several new quinolones are now available for the treatment of pneumonia. Ofloxacin has a higher bioavailability than ciprofloxacin and higher peak serum levels for longer periods. It may have greater activity against streptococci and staphylococci than ciprofloxacin[97] and is active against *Legionella, Chlamydia*, and *Mycoplasma* in vitro. Because it is not hepatically metabolized, there is no interaction with theophylline. The efficacy of ofloxacin (400 mg twice daily for 7 to 10 days) has been studied in six clinical trials[98] with similar results to ampicillin, trimethoprim/sulfamethoxazole, and erythromycin, although ofloxacin is more expensive than the older agents. Ofloxacin seems to have activity in pneumococcal pneumonia,[99] but with small numbers of patients reported, a penicillin is still the drug of choice.

Lomafloxacin is a newly approved quinolone antibiotic that inhibits most *Enterobacteriaceae, Haemophilus*, and *Moraxella* at 1 μg/ml, and *S. pneumoniae* and staphylococci at 2 μg/ml. Achievable serum levels at peak are near 3.5 μg/ml. Clinical studies to date, mainly of chronic bronchitis, have suggested that lomafloxacin is similar to ciprofloxacin. Larger numbers of patients will need to be studied before the drug becomes a first-line agent when pneumococci are considered likely.[100] The role of the newer quinolones may be in the elderly or debilitated, in whom gram-negative pathogens may play a larger role.

Parenteral Therapy

The wide variety of oral antibiotics has revolutionized the ambulatory therapy of community-acquired pneumonia. The advances in IV therapy for home delivery of parenteral antibiotics have also been effective. Outpatient IV antibiotic therapy for children and adults at home or in an infusion center makes it feasible and practical for some patients to complete their entire course of therapy in an outpatient setting.[101, 102] For the elderly or institutionalized patient, an episode of pneumonia may not require that the person be transferred to an acute care facility but may instead involve parenteral therapy without the patient having to leave his or her institution.[103]

Two innovations have allowed such changes: (1) the development of IV access technology that allows long-term venous delivery with low risk of infection, and (2) the development of broad-spectrum antibiotics with prolonged elimination half-lives that allow once daily dosing. Ceftriaxone,[104, 105] cefonicid, and ceftazidime are examples, but newer programmable pump technology[106] makes possible administration of older drugs like penicillin. IV formulations of newer drugs like cefuroxime, ofloxacin, and lomafloxacin make it easier to switch from IV to oral drug administration.

Criteria and patient-training guidelines have been proposed.[107] The patient with community-acquired pneumonia should be stable or improving, without congestive heart failure or other conditions that would require careful fluid management, and without features that would predict fatal outcome as outlined earlier. A brief hospitalization may precede the home parenteral therapy or the first dose may be given in an infusion center.

REFERENCES

1. Garibaldi RA: Epidemiology of community-acquired respiratory tract infection in adults. Am J Med 78(Suppl 6B):32–37, 1985.
2. Cherian T, John TJ, Simoes E, et al: Evaluation of simple clinical signs for the diagnosis of acute lower respiratory tract infection. Lancet 2:125–128, 1988.
3. Sherman S, Skoney JA, and Ravikrishnan KP: Routine chest radiographs in exacerbations of chronic obstructive pulmonary disease. Arch Int Med 149:2493–2496, 1989.
4. Heckerling PS: The need for chest roentgenograms in adults with acute respiratory illness: Clinical predictors. Arch Intern Med 146:1321–1324, 1986.
5. Heckerling PS, Tape TG, Wigton RS, et al: Clinical prediction rule for pulmonary infiltrates. Ann Intern Med 113:664–670, 1990.
6. Singal BM, Hedges JR, and Radack KL: Decision rules and clinical prediction of pneumonia: Evaluation of low yield criteria. Ann Emerg Med 18:37–44, 1989.
7. Woodhead MA, MacFarlane JT, McCracken JS, et al: Prospective study of the aetiology and outcome of pneumonia in the community. Lancet 1:671–674, 1987.
8. Fine MJ, Smith DN, and Singer DE: Hospitalization decision in patients with community-acquired pneumonia: A prospective cohort study. Am J Med 89:713–721, 1990.
9. Gertman P and Restuccia J: The appropriateness evaluation protocol: A technique for assessing unnecessary days of hospital care. Med Care 19:855–871, 1981.
10. Black ER, Mushlin AI, Griner PF, et al: Predicting the need for hospitalization of ambulatory patients with pneumonia. J Gen Intern Med 6:394–400, 1991.
11. Farr BM, Sloman AJ, and Fisch MJ: Predicting death in patients hospitalized for community-acquired pneumonia. Ann Intern Med 115:428–436, 1991.
12. Karalus NC, Cursons RT, Leng RA, et al: Community-acquired pneumonia: Aetiology and prognostic index evaluation. Thorax 46:413–418, 1991.
13. Fine MJ, Orloff JJ, Arisumi D, et al: Prognosis of patients hospitalized with community-acquired pneumonia. Am J Med 88 (Suppl 5N):1N–8N, 1990.
14. Farr BM, Kaiser DL, Harrison BDW, and Connolly CK: Prediction of microbial aetiology at admission to hospital for pneumonia from the presenting clinical features. Thorax 44:1031–1035, 1989.
15. Fang GD, Fine M, Orloff J, et al: New and emerging etiologies for community-acquired pneumonia with implications for therapy: A prospective multicenter study of 359 cases. Medicine 69:307–316, 1990.
16. Woodhead MA, Arrowsmith J, Chamberlain-Webber R, et al: The value of routine microbial investigation in community-acquired pneumonia. Respir Med 85:313–317, 1991.
17. MacFarlane JT: Treatment of lower respiratory infection. Lancet 2:1446–1449, 1987.
18. Mufson MA, Chang V, Gill V, et al: The role of viruses, mycoplasmas and bacteria in acute pneumonia in civilian adults. Am J Epidemiol 86:526–544, 1967.
19. Fiala M: A study of the combined role of viruses, mycoplasmas and bacteria in adult pneumonia. Am J Med 257:44–51, 1969.
20. Lepow ML, Balassanian N, Emmerich J, et al: Interrelationships of viral, mycoplasmal and bacterial agents in uncomplicated pneumonia. Am Rev Respir Dis 97:533–545, 1968.
21. Sullivan RJ, Dowdle WR, Marine WM, and Hierholzer JC: Adult pneumonia in a general hospital. Arch Intern Med 129:935–942, 1972.
22. Dorff GJ, Rytel MW, Farmer SG, and Scanlon G: Etiologies and characteristic features of pneumonias in a municipal hospital. Am J Med Sci 266:349–358, 1973.
23. Denny FW, Clyde WA, and Glezen WP: *Mycoplasma pneumoniae* disease: Clinical spectrum, pathophysiology, epidemiology, and control. J Infect Dis 123:74–92, 1971.
24. Foy HM, Cooney MK, McMahn R, and Grayston JT: Viral and mycoplasmal pneumonia in a prepaid medical care group during an eight-year period. Am J Epidemiol 97:93–102, 1973.
25. Marrie JT, Durant H, and Yates L: Community-acquired pneumonia requiring hospitalization: 5-year prospective study. Rev Infect Dis 11:586–599, 1989.
26. Torres A, Serra-Batilles J, Ferrer A, et al: Severe community-acquired pneumonia: Epidemiology and prognostic factors. Am Rev Respir Dis 144:312–318, 1991.
27. Gleckman R, DeVita J, Hibert D, et al: Sputum Gram stain assessment in community-acquired bacteremic pneumonia. J Clin Microbiol 26:846–849, 1988.
28. Fine MJ, Orloff JL, Rihs JD, et al: Evaluation of housestaff physician's preparation and interpretation of sputum Gram stains for community-acquired pneumonia. J Gen Intern Med 6:189–198, 1991.
29. Bartlett RG: Medical Microbiology: Quality, Costs and Clinical Relevance. New York, John Wiley & Sons, 1974, pp 24–31.
30. Murray PR and Washington JA: Microscopy and bacteriologic analysis of expectorated sputum. Mayo Clin Proc 50:339–344, 1975.
31. Bartlett JG, Rosenblatt JE, and Finegold SM: Percutaneous transtracheal aspiration in the diagnosis of anaerobic pulmonary infection. Ann Intern Med 79:535–540, 1973.
32. Pecora DV: A method of securing uncontaminated tracheal secretions for bacterial examination. J Thorac Surg 37:653–654, 1959.
33. Hahn HH and Beaty HN: Transtracheal aspiration in the evaluation of patients with pneumonia. Ann Intern Med 72:183–187, 1970.
34. Zavala DC and Schoell JE: Ultrathin needle aspiration of the lung in infectious and malignant disease. Am Rev Respir Dis 123:125–131, 1981.
35. Thorpe JE, Baughman RP, Frame PT, et al: Bronchoalveolar lavage for diagnosing acute bacterial pneumonia. J Infect Dis 155:855–861, 1987.
36. Torres A, Puig de la Bellacasa J, Xaubet A, et al: Diagnostic value of quantitative cultures of bronchoalveolar lavage and telescoping plugged catheters in mechanically ventilated patients with pneumonia. Am Rev Respir Dis 85:499–506, 1989.
37. Davidson M, Tempest B, and Palmer DL: Bacteriologic diagnosis of acute pneumonia: Comparison of sputum, transtracheal aspirates, and lung aspirates. JAMA 235:158–163, 1976.

38. Sullivan RJ, Dowdle WR, and Marine WM: Adult pneumonia in a general hospital. Arch Intern Med 129:935–938, 1972.
39. Rein MF, Gwaltney JM, O'Brien WM, et al: Accuracy of Gram's stain in identifying pneumococci in sputum. JAMA 239:2671–2673, 1978.
40. Drew WL: Value of sputum culture in diagnosis of pneumococcal pneumonia. J Clin Microbiol 6:62–65, 1977.
41. Austrian R and Gold J: Pneumococcal bacteremia with special reference to bacteremic pneumococcal pneumonia. Ann Intern Med 60:759–771, 1964.
42. Pozzi G, Oggioni MR, and Tomasz A: DNA probe for identification of *Streptococcus pneumoniae*. J Clin Microbiol 27:370–372, 1989.
43. Wallace RJ, Musher DM, and Martin RR: *Haemophilus influenzae* pneumonia in adults. Am J Med 64:87–90, 1978.
44. Rusconi F, Rancilio L, Assael BM, et al: Counterimmunoelectrophoresis and latex particle agglutination in the etiologic diagnosis of presumed bacterial pneumonia in pediatric patients. Pediatr Infect Dis 7:781–784, 1988.
45. Woodhead MA, Radvan J, and MacFarlane JT: Adult community-acquired staphylococcal pneumonia in the antibiotic era: A review of 61 cases. Q J Med 64:783–790, 1987.
46. Kaye MG, Fox MJ, Bartlett JG, et al: The clinical spectrum of *Staphylococcus aureus* pulmonary infection. Chest 97:788–792, 1990.
47. Venkatesan P, Gladman J, MacFarlane JT, et al: A hospital study of community acquired pneumonia in the elderly. Thorax 45:254–258, 1990.
48. Korvick JA, Hackett AK, Yu VL, and Muder RR: *Klebsiella* pneumonia in the modern era: Clinicoradiographic correlations. South Med J 84:200–204, 1991.
49. Carpenter JL: *Klebsiella* pulmonary infections: Occurrence at one medical center and review. Rev Infect Dis 12:672–682, 1990.
50. Fraser DW, Tsai TF, Orenstein W, et al: Legionnaires' disease: Description of an epidemic of pneumonia. N Engl J Med 297:1189–1192, 1977.
51. Grandos A, Podzamczer D, Gudiol F, and Manresa F. Pneumonia due to *Legionella pneumophila* and pneumococcal pneumonia: Similarities and differences on presentation. Eur Respir J 2:130–134, 1989.
52. Helmes CM, Viner JP, Sturm RH, et al: Comparative features of pneumococcal, mycoplasmal and legionnaires' disease pneumonias. Ann Intern Med 90:543–546, 1979.
53. Reitano M, Engler HD, and Bottone EJ: *Legionella pneumophila*: Initial detection through evaluation of Giemsa-stained smears of a bronchial aspirate. Diagn Microbiol Infect Dis 10:125–130, 1988.
54. Zuravleff JJ, Yu VL, Shonnard JW, et al: Diagnosis of legionnaires' disease: An update of laboratory methods with new emphasis on isolation by culture. JAMA 250:1981–1983, 1983.
55. Saphapatayavongs B, Kohler RB, Whear LJ, et al: Rapid diagnosis of legionnaires' disease by urinary antigen detection: Comparison of ELISA and radioimmunoassay. Am J Med 72:576–579, 1982.
56. Pasculle AW, Veto GE, Krystofiak S, et al: Laboratory and clinical evaluation of a commercial DNA probe for the detection of *Legionella* species. J Clin Mirobiol 27:2350–2358, 1989.
57. Yuen KY, Seto WH, and Ong SG: The significance of *Branhamella catarrhalis* in bronchopulmonary infection: A case-control study. J Infect Dis 19:251–256, 1989.
58. Nicotra B, Rivera M, Luman JI, and Wallace RJ: *Branhamella catarrhalis* as a lower respiratory tract pathogen in patients with chronic lung disease. Arch Intern Med 146:890–893, 1986.
59. Lorber B and Swenson RM: Bacteriology of aspiration pneumonia: A prospective study of community- and hospital acquired cases. Ann Intern Med 81:329–331, 1974.
60. Foy HM, Kenny GE, and Cooney MK: Long-term epidemiology of infections with *Mycoplasma pneumonia*. J Infect Dis 139:681–685, 1979.
61. Ponka A and Ukkonen P: Age-related prevalence of complement-fixing antibody to *Mycoplasma pneumoniae* during an 8-year period. J Clin Microbiol 17:571–575, 1983.
62. Holmberg H, Bodin L, J'onsson I, and Krook A: Rapid aetiological diagnosis of pneumonia based on routine laboratory features. Scand J Infect Dis 22:537–545, 1990.
63. Murray HW, Masur H, and Senterfit LB: The protean manifestations of *Mycoplasma pneumoniae* infection in adults. Am J Med 58:229–232, 1975.
64. Putman CE, Curtis AM, and Simeone JF: *Mycoplasma pneumoniae*: Clinical and roentgenographic patterns. Am J Roentgenol 124:417–421, 1975.
65. Vikerfors T, Brodin G, Grandien M, et al: Detection of specific IgM antibodies for the diagnosis of *Mycoplasma pneumoniae*: A clinical evaluation. Scand J Infect Dis 20:601–612, 1988.
66. Kok TW, Varkanis G, Marmion BP, et al: Laboratory diagnosis of *Mycoplasma pneumoniae* infection. I: Direct detection of antigen in respiratory exudates by enzyme immunoassay. Epidemiol Infect 101:669–684, 1988.
67. Tilton RC, Dias F, Kidd H, and Ryan RW: DNA probe versus culture for detection of *Mycoplasma pneumoniae* in clinical specimens. Diagn Microbiol Infect Dis 10:109–112, 1988.
68. Hata D, Kuze F, Mochizuki Y, et al: Evaluation of DNA probe test for rapid diagnosis of *Mycoplasma pneumoniae* infections. J Pediatr 116:273–276, 1990.
69. Grayston JT, Wang SP, Kuo CC, and Campbell LA: Current knowledge on *Chlamydia pneumoniae* strain TWAR, an important cause of pneumonia and other acute respiratory diseases. Eur J Clin Microbiol Infect Dis 8:191–202, 1989.
70. Grayston JT, Diwan VK, Cooney M, and Wang SP: Community- and hospital-acquired pneumonia associated with *Chlamydia* TWAR infection demonstrated serologically. Arch Intern Med 149:169–173, 1989.
71. Atmar RL and Greenberg SB: Pneumonia caused by *Mycoplasma pneumoniae* and the TWAR agent. Semin Respir Infect 4:19–31, 1989.
72. Luby JP: Pneumonias in adults due to *Mycoplasma, Chlamydia*, and viruses. Am J Med Sci 294:45–64, 1987.
73. Oswald NC, Shooter RA, and Curwen MP: Pneumonia complicating Asian influenzae. BMJ 2:1305–1307, 1958.
74. Hers JFPH, Masurel N, and Mulder J: Bacteriology and histopathology of the respiratory tract and lungs in fatal Asian influenzae. Lancet 2:1141–1143, 1958.
75. Mathur U, Bentley DW, and Hall CB: Concurrent outbreaks of respiratory syncytial virus and influenza A/Texas/77 infection in the institutionalized elderly and chronically ill. Ann Intern Med 90:49–53, 1980.
76. Garvie DG and Gray J: Outbreak of respiratory syncytial virus infection in the elderly. BMJ 281:1253–1255, 1980.
77. Salomon HE, Grandien M, Avila MM, and Pettersson CA: Comparison of three techniques for detection of respiratory viruses in nasopharyngeal aspirates from children with lower acute respiratory infections. J Med Virol 28:159–162, 1989.
78. Bruckova M, Grandien M, Pettersson CA, and Kunzova L: Use of nasal and pharyngeal swabs for rapid detection of respiratory syncytial virus and adenovirus and antigens by enzyme-linked immunosorbent assay. J Clin Microbiol 27:1867–1869, 1989.
79. Vandyke RB and Murphy-Corb M: Detection of respiratory syncytial virus in nasopharyngeal secretions by DNA-RNA hybridization. J Clin Microbiol 27:1739–1743, 1989.
80. Eliopoulos GM, Reiszner E, Wennersten C, et al: In vitro activity of BMY-28100, a new oral cephalosporin. Antimicrob Agents Chemother 31:653–656, 1987.
81. Yakatan GJ, Rasmussen CE, Reis PJ, et al: Bioinequivalence of erythromycin ethylsuccinate and enteric-coated erythromycin pellets following multiple oral doses. J Clin Pharmacol 25:36–42, 1985.
82. Jones RN and Barry AL: The antimicrobial activity of A-56268 (TE-031) and roxithromycin (RU965) against *Legionella* using broth microdilution method. J Antimicrob Chemother 19:841–842, 1987.
83. Hamedani P, Ali J, Hafeez S, et al: The safety and efficacy of clarithromycin in patients with *Legionella pneumoniae*. Chest 100:1503–1506, 1991.
84. Hardy DJ, Guay DRP, and Jones RN: Clarithromycin, a unique macrolide: A pharmacokinetic, microbiological, and clinical overview. Diagn Microbiol Infect Dis 15:39–53, 1992.
85. Anderson G, Esmonde TS, Coles S, et al: A comparative

safety and efficacy study of clarithromycin and erythromycin stearate in community-acquired pneumonia. J Antimicrob Chemother 27 (Suppl A): 117–124, 1991.

86. Cassell GH, Drnec J, Waites KB, et al: Efficacy of clarithromycin against *Mycoplasma pneumoniae.* J Antimicrob Chemother 27 (Suppl A):47–59, 1991.
87. Jorgensen JH, Maher LA, and Howell AW: Activity of clarithromycin and its principal human metabolite against *Haemophilus influenzae.* Antimicrob Agents Chemother 35:1524–1526, 1991.
88. Ishiguro M, Koga H, Kohno S, et al: Penetration of macrolides into human polymorphonuclear leukocytes. J Antimicrob Chemother 24:719–729, 1989.
89. Foulds G, Shepard RM, and Johnson RB: The pharmacokinetics of azithromycin in human serum and tissues. J Antimicrob Chemother 25(Suppl A):73–82, 1990.
90. Balmes P, Clerc G, Dupont B, et al: Comparative study of azithromycin and amoxicillin/clavulanic acid in the treatment of lower respiratory tract infections. Eur J Clin Microbiol Infect Dis 10:437–439, 1991.
91. Daniel R: Simplified treatment of acute lower respiratory tract infection with azithromycin: A comparison with erythromycin and amoxicillin. J Intern Med 19:373–383, 1991.
92. Dark D: Multicenter evaluation of azithromycin and cefaclor in acute lower respiratory tract infections. Am J Med 91(3A):31S–35S, 1991.
93. Morris DL, DeSouza A, Jones JA, and Morgan WE: High and prolonged pulmonary tissue concentrations of azithromycin following a single oral dose. Eur J Clin Microbiol Infect Dis 10:859–861, 1991.
94. Schonwald S, Skerk V, Petricevic I, et al: Azithromycin pharmacodynamics. Eur J Clin Microbiol Infect Dis 10:877–880, 1991.
95. Hopkins S: Clinical toleration and safety of azithromycin. Am J Med 91(3A):40S–45S, 1991.
96. Cooper B and Lawlor M: Pneumococcal bacteremia during ciprofloxacin therapy for pneumococcal pneumonia. Am J Med 87:475–480, 1989.
97. Bellido F and Pechere JC: Laboratory survey of fluoroquinalone activity. Rev Infect Dis 11 (Suppl 5):S917–924, 1989.
98. Ashby BL: Treatment of pneumonia: New strategies for changing pathogens. Clin Ther 13:637–649, 1991.
99. Sanders WE, Morris JF, Alessi P, et al: Oral ofloxacin for the treatment of acute bacterial pneumonia: Use of a nontraditional protocol to compare experimental therapy with "usual care" in a multicenter clinical trial. Am J Med 91:261–266, 1991.
100. Thys JP, Jacobs F, and Byl B: Role of quinolones in the treatment of bronchopulmonary infections, particularly pneumococcal and community-acquired pneumonia. Eur J Clin Microbiol Infect Dis 10:304–315, 1991.
101. Dagan R, Phillip M, Watemberg NM, and Kassis I: Outpatient treatment of serious community-acquired pediatric infections using once daily intramuscular ceftriaxone. Pediatr Infect Dis 6:1080–1084, 1987.
102. Rehm SJ and Weinstein AJ: Home intravenous antibiotic therapy: A team approach. Ann Intern Med 99:388–92, 1983.
103. Mulligan T: Parenteral antibiotic therapy for patients in nursing homes. Rev Infect Dis 13 (Suppl 2):S180–S183, 1991.
104. Brown R: Once-daily ceftriaxone in the treatment of lower respiratory tract infections. Chemotherapy 37 (Suppl 3):11–14, 1991.
105. Leibovitz E, Tabachnik E, Fliedel O, et al: Once-daily intramuscular ceftriaxone in the outpatient treatment of severe community-acquired pneumonia in children. Clin Pediatr 29:634–639, 1990.
106. Williams DN, Gibson JA, and Bosch D: Home intravenous antibiotic therapy using a programmable infusion pump. Arch Intern Med 149:1157–1160, 1989.
107. Brown RB: Selection and training of patients for outpatient intravenous antibiotic therapy. Rev Infect Dis 13(Suppl 2):S147–S151, 1991.

20

Obstructive Lung Disease

E. R. McFADDEN, Jr., MD

This chapter deals with the ambulatory therapy of patients with obstructive lung disease, including asthma, chronic bronchitis, and emphysema. Although the in-hospital management of conditions such as severe, life-threatening asthma and acute-on-chronic respiratory failure will not be emphasized, the factors commonly precipitating these conditions, as well as the features of the illnesses that lead the physician to these diagnoses, are dealt with in some detail. Emphasis has been placed on the known pathophysiologic bases of clinical features and response to treatment, since such a basic understanding is fundamental to the management of patients with airway obstruction.

DRUG THERAPY

The drugs commonly used to treat airway obstruction can be grouped into five major categories: *methylxanthines, β-agonists, anticholinergics, mast cell stabilizing agents,* and *glucocorticosteroids.*

Methylxanthines

The methylxanthines (caffeine, theophylline, and theobromine) are naturally occurring alkaloids. Theophylline, the only methylxanthine routinely used, is a bronchodilator of medium potency, and improvement in lung function is directly related to plasma concentrations.[1] Although efficacious, the methylxanthines are not as potent as the adrenergic stimulants, and they have a narrower therapeutic-toxic window.

The mechanism responsible for the bronchodilator effect of the methylxanthines is unknown. It was formerly thought that theophylline produced its effect by increasing the intracellular levels of cyclic adenosine monophosphate through the inhibition of phosphodiesterase, but is now known that this is not the case. Three potential areas of action of theophylline have been suggested: (1) smooth muscle relaxation; (2) inhibition of mediator release from tissue mast cells; and (3) inhibition of leukocyte proteolytic enzyme release. The relative importance of each of these factors in improving airway obstruction remains to be determined. It has also been suggested that theophylline can reduce experimentally induced diaphragmatic fatigue, and lower pulmonary arterial pressures in patients with chronic obstructive lung disease. The clinical importance of these effects remains to be defined, and is probably minor.

Theophylline is rapidly and completely absorbed in the digestive tract from both liquid and plain uncoated tablet preparations. The rate of absorption can be slowed somewhat by the presence of food and magnesium-containing antacids,[1] but the delay is not clinically significant. Absorption may be slower at night.[2]

Approximately 85% of a dose of theophylline is degraded in the liver, and 15% or less is excreted free in the urine. Because of the latter, little adjustment of dosage is required in renal failure. Theophylline clearance and thus dosage requirements are decreased importantly in neonates, the elderly, and those with acute and chronic hepatic dysfunction, cardiac decompensation, and cor pulmonale.[1] Clearance is also decreased during febrile illnesses and with the use of erythromycin and H_2 blockers like Tagamet. Clearance is increased in children, cigarette smokers, and in those ingesting a high-carbohydrate, low-protein diet.

Bolus injections of aminophylline should not be given, since there is considerable risk of cardiac arrhythmias and seizures if high peak plasma levels are attained. Thus, the loading dose should be given by infusion over 15 to 30 minutes rather than by syringe.[3]

The pharmacokinetic properties of aminophylline are such that typically four half-lives must occur before a steady state is achieved in the plasma drug concentration. In a young patient, this time approaches 24 hours, but if the half-life of the drug is prolonged, which occurs in patients with hepatic dysfunction, a steady state may not be achieved for several days. Since clearance of theophylline from the plasma may decrease at drug concentrations in the upper end of the therapeutic range, upward adjustments in the dosage of intravenous aminophylline therapy need to be made with caution if serious side effects are to be avoided, particularly in children, the elderly, and patients with decreased liver function.

For long-term management, both rapid- and sustained-release formulations are available, and the choice of product depends upon the therapeutic goal desired (Table 20–1). For the treatment of acute but nonemergent symptoms a rapidly absorbed compound such as uncoated tablets or liquids frequently will suffice. These formulations can rap-

TABLE 20–1. ABSORPTION PROFILES FOR REPRESENTATIVE FORMULATIONS OF THEOPHYLLINE

Theophylline Preparations	Product Example	Release Pattern	Time to Peak Serum Concentrations in Adults (hr)
Solutions	Theophylline elixir	Rapid	1.5
Uncoated tablets	Theophyl	Rapid	2
Sustained-release bead-filled capsules	Slo-phyllin Theophyl-SR	Gradual and consistent	5
Sustained release tablets			
Twice daily dosage	Theo-Dur	Gradual and consistent	6
Single daily dosage	Uniphyl Theo-24	Gradual and consistent	10

idly produce therapeutic blood levels. Since there are no important differences in their absorption characteristics, they can be used interchangeably. For chronic prophylaxis, however, serum concentrations may fluctuate widely with these formulations, thus necessitating unacceptably short dosing intervals. For example, in individuals with rapid elimination kinetics, it is frequently quite difficult to maintain therapeutic blood levels even with dosing schedules as short as 6 hours. To overcome this problem, a number of sustained-release formulations have been developed. These compounds allow for improved time-concentration profiles with very little variation between peak and trough serum levels and thus allow longer intervals between doses. Developments in the area of release kinetics have been reasonably rapid and in the last several years dosage schedules have been reduced, from 6 to 8 hours to twice a day, and now, to once every 24 hours. The obvious advantage of the sustained-release compounds is improved patient compliance and therefore better symptom control.

The available data suggest that most patients can be managed on daily or twice-daily regimens. However, in those with very rapid elimination a larger variation between peak and trough concentration may occur, and more frequent administration may be required. To determine the needs of any particular patient, measurement of steady-state theophylline serum concentrations is required.

The most common side effects of theophylline are nervousness, nausea, vomiting, anorexia, and headache. These symptoms appear to correlate with plasma concentrations, and levels greater than 20 μg/ml are frequently associated with these complaints. The risk of seizures and cardiac arrhythmias increases markedly at plasma levels greater than 30 μg/ml; however, it is important to note that gastrointestinal symptoms need not precede these more serious side effects.[4]

Adrenergic Stimulants

This class of bronchodilators can be subdivided into three types, based on their chemical structures, catechols, resorcinols, and saligenins.[5] They have their effect through stimulation of α- and β-adrenergic receptors. Activation of β-receptors causes smooth muscle relaxation in the respiratory tract and other organs and produces stimulation of the myocardium and of skeletal muscle, causing tremor. α-Adrenergic receptors increase peripheral vascular resistance but are not involved in bronchodilatation. There are two classes of β-receptors: β_1-agonists cause cardiac stimulation, and β_2-agonists cause bronchodilatation. Thus, the more "β_2-specific" a given adrenergic agent is, the fewer cardiac side effects it will produce.

The physiologic actions of the β-adrenergic drugs are probably mediated through the effects of increased intracellular cyclic adenosine monophosphate (AMP) on calcium flux produced by activating the enzyme adenylcyclase.

The adrenergic agonists are much more potent than the methylxanthines. The native catecholamines consist of dopamine, norepinephrine, and epinephrine, but only the latter is unequivocally efficacious in the treatment of airway obstruction. The analogs of epinephrine that have been synthesized are isoproterenol, isoetharine, rimeterol, and hexoprenaline. The last two drugs are not used in the United States. The catecholamines are rapid acting, potent bronchodilators. Their chief disadvantages are their short duration of action and their absolute or relative lack of β_2-selectivity.

Epinephrine is approximately equal in its α and β effects. Because of its significant cardiac effects, its use is limited to emergency situations. Isoproterenol is devoid of α effects and is produced by a simple substitution in the epinephrine structure. It is the most potent compound of this group but also has significant cardiac effects. Other agents that are more β_2-selective have been developed. Substitution in the isoproterenol moiety produces isoetharine, a drug less potent than isoproterenol but more β_2-selective. None of the catecholamines are effective orally and must be given either by inhalation or parenterally.

In a search for longer-acting agents with less cardiogenic activity, the catecholamine nucleus has been replaced with resorcinol and saligenin rings. These structural modifications circumvent the metabolic pathways used to degrade the catecholamines and give rise to moderately long-acting drugs with a high degree of airway selectivity that are effective by all routes of administration. The resorcinols used in clinical practice are metaproterenol, terbutaline, and fenoterol; the only saligenin available in the United States is albuterol (Table 20–2).

The catecholamines achieve peak bronchodilatation within 5 minutes of inhalation, but their effects are dissipated within 1 to 2 hours, depending on the dose that is used. The noncatecholamines are somewhat slower in onset but achieve near-maximal bronchodilatation within 10 to 15 minutes. Their half-lives vary from 3 to 6 hours depending on the dose. Like the methylxanthines, extremely long-acting compounds have been developed. One such agent, salmeterol, is due for release soon. It is reported to have a duration of action of 10 to 12 hours.

From a practical clinical standpoint, albuterol, terbutaline, and fenoterol probably are as potent as isoproterenol in relieving airway obstruction, with metaproterenol and the catecholamines being somewhat less effective. In terms of their cardiac effects, isoproterenol is the most active; isoetharine tends not to cause obvious cardiovascular problems in therapeutic doses. Of the saligenins and resorcinols, terbutaline and albuterol appear similar and somewhat more cardioselective than the others.

TABLE 20–2. ADRENERGIC STIMULANTS USED IN TREATMENT OF OBSTRUCTIVE AIRWAY DISEASE

Agent	Product Examples	Route of Administration			Relative Potency on Scale 1–4	Duration of Effect (hr)	Mechanism of Action		
		Injection	Inhalation	Oral			β_2	β_1	α
Ephedrine	Ephedrine	—	—	√	2	2–3	√	√	√
Epinephrine	Adrenaline	√	—	—	3	0.5–2	√	√	√
Isoproterenol	Isuprel	(IV)	√	—	4	2–3	√	√	—
Isoetharine	Bronkosol	√	√	—	2	2–3	√√	√	—
Metaproterenol	Alupent	—	√	√	3	3–5	√√	√	—
Terbutaline	Brethine; Bricanyl	√	√	√	4	4–6	√√	—	—
Fenoterol	Berotac	√	√	√	4	4–6	√√	—	—
Albuterol (salbutamol)	Ventolin, Proventil	√	√	√	4	4–6	√√	—	—

Based on all the available evidence, most authorities agree that the β_2-adrenergic agonists should be first-line therapy for acute episodes of asthma, and other forms of airway obstruction. These drugs produce three to four times more bronchodilatation acutely than does the intravenous administration of aminophylline.[6–8] To minimize side effects and promote the most rapid onset of action, these agents should be given by inhalation. A typical regimen for the treatment of acute asthma is to administer aerosolized albuterol by hand-held nebulizer every 20 minutes for 3 doses and then repeat at 2-hour intervals for 6 to 12 hours until the attack ends. There are some data to suggest that a metered-dose inhaler in combination with a spacer can be employed in place of the nebulizer without a loss of effectiveness.[9] It is important to appreciate that previous unsuccessful use of a β_2-agonist by the patient does not imply resistance nor prejudice against its use in emergency situations.[10]

One major problem encountered with use of the inhaled route of therapy is the inability of some patients to master the proper technique required with metered-dose inhalers, as well as the lack of physician knowledge in instructing them. It has been estimated that perhaps as many as 40 to 50% of patients using commercial nebulizers are unable to coordinate activation of the device and inhalation despite careful tuition and that as many as 60% of general internists may not know how to demonstrate the proper procedures or detect and correct improper ones.[11–14] Some pharmaceutical houses now market powder aerosol devices, such as Spinhalers and Rotahalers. Since these insufflators are patient triggered, they can readily be employed by anyone who cannot coordinate the activities required with a propellant-driven nebulizer.

Another approach has been to incorporate a spacer between the delivery system and the patient's mouth (e.g., InspirEase, Aerochamber, Breathancer), in an effort to maximize aerosol deposition in the airways. With a spacer the aerosol remains suspended for sufficient time to allow the patient to inhale at will. In patients who use metered-dose inhalers correctly, the addition of a spacer tends not to result in further increments in lung function. However, in those with impaired ability, spacers can increase the quantity of drug retained and thus the therapeutic response. The magnitude of improvement in pulmonary mechanics varies from one study to another, but on average one can expect peak flow or forced expiratory volumes to increase 8 to 10% over those seen with a standard nebulizer.

Anticholinergic Agents

The anticholinergic drugs currently available to treat airway disease are atropine sulfate, atropine methonitrate, and ipratropium bromide. Unlike atropine sulfate, the latter two drugs are quaternary ammonium compounds and therefore are long lasting, are poorly absorbed from mucosal surfaces when given locally, and do not readily penetrate the blood-brain barrier. Consequently, they have few of the undesirable side effects of atropine sulfate such as mydriasis, bladder obstruction, drying of secretions, precipitation of acute glaucoma in patients with narrow angles, palpitations, and central nervous system dysfunction. These drugs compete with acetylcholine on smooth muscle receptors and only inhibit acetylcholine on nicotine receptors at very high concentrations. Single-dose studies with atropine methonitrate and ipratropium bromide demonstrate that both are effective bronchodilators without major untoward effects when given in the usual therapeutic doses.[15] In most investigations, the anticholinergics have been found to be less potent than the sympathomimetics. However, the chief disadvantage of the parasympatholytics is their slow onset of action. Sixty to 90 minutes is frequently required before maximum bronchodilatation is achieved. Hence their use in acute situations has been superseded by more potent, faster-acting compounds like the sympathomimetics. Antimuscarinic agents are occasionally helpful in the treatment of asthma that has resisted other forms of therapy and frequently useful in cough variants. In addition, it has been suggested that patients with chronic bronchitis show greater bronchodilatation after inhaled antimuscarinics than after a sympathomimetic. In modern practice, it is rare to use atropine or its analogs as single therapy for acute disease. The literature suggests that the anticholinergics interact positively with both the β-agonists and methylxanthines. However, the effect tends to be one of increased duration rather than increased magnitude of bronchodilatation. It is important to remember that the parasympatholytics should be given only by inhalation, and even then it is prudent to check for the presence of narrow-angle glaucoma or bladder neck obstruction before administering them.

Some studies have implied that ipratropium bromide significantly adds to the effects of sympathomimetics in the acute treatment of asthma, but analysis of the data suggests that the response to the β-agonists was abnormally low.[16] This is a theme that frequently recurs in the literature on this subject.

Mast Cell Stabilizing Agents

Disodium Cromoglycate (Cromolyn Sodium)

Cromolyn sodium is an agent that is employed in the treatment of asthma to attenuate the bronchial narrowing that follows exposure to a variety of acute provocations and to reduce airway reactivity on a chronic basis. Cromolyn is extremely safe, and its low incidence of side effects and broad range of activities suggest that it can be employed effectively in individuals with recurrent symptoms, particularly if there is an allergic diathesis.[17] This drug has no bronchodilatory activity, and its chief mechanism of action is believed to be related to its ability to stabilize mast cells and thus ameliorate airway inflammation on an acute and chronic basis. Since other drugs with more potent mast cell–stabilizing properties have not worked in asthma,[19] only part of cromolyn's activity can be attributed to this factor. Cromolyn has no role in the management of patients with chronic bronchitis or emphysema.

The major role of cromolyn is prophylaxis. A single dose given 15 to 20 minutes before exercise, exposure to cold air, or antigen or industrial chemicals like diisocyanate will prevent acute airway obstruction from developing. When administered prior to an antigen, cromolyn will block both the early and late reactions and abolish any increase in airway reactivity. From a clinical standpoint, this means that a patient who has intermittent exposure to either antigenic or nonantigenic stimuli that provoke acute episodes of asthma need not use this drug on a continuous basis. Rather, such individuals can readily be protected by only taking cromolyn 15 to 20 minutes before contact with the precipitant. With stimuli such as exercise, cromolyn will interact positively with β-adrenergic agonists to produce a greater protective effect than either drug alone.

The effect of cromolyn on bronchial reactivity is variable and not all patients respond. This matter has been reviewed recently and approximately 80% of studies show a diminution in reactivity while the remainder do not show any benefit.[18] The reasons for this dichotomy are unknown. In the positive studies, patients have more symptom-free days and require less concomitant medication. It is of interest that this result occurs even though the changes in bronchial responsiveness that develop are quite small, again, suggesting an as yet undefined mechanism of action.

Cromolyn is most efficacious in atopic patients who have seasonal disease or who are experiencing perennial stimulation of their airways. It also works in some nonatopics, but since there is no prospective way of determining who will benefit, a therapeutic trial should be undertaken. If the goal is to reduce airway inflammation and thus promote long-range healing, the drug needs to be administered on a regular basis four times daily for at least one month.

Nedocromil Sodium

Nedocromil is an anti-inflammatory agent with a clinical activity similar to cromolyn. It is due to be released soon for use in the United States. This drug prevents immediate and late asthmatic responses to antigen, reduces nonspecific bronchial responsiveness, as well as asthma symptoms and the need for concomitant bronchodilator medications. It also protects against bronchial narrowing following acute exposures to a variety of asthma provocations.

Glucocorticosteroids

Glucocorticoids are commonly employed in the treatment of bronchial asthma and their efficacy has led to their widespread use in other types of obstructive lung disease even though scientific documentation of the efficacy in many circumstances has been lacking. Steroids significantly speed the rate of resolution of acute severe episodes of asthma in hospital and reduce the frequency of relapses of patients discharged from an emergency room.[18, 19] It is important to emphasize that the benefits from adding steroids are delayed and should not be anticipated for 6 to 12 hours following their administration.[18] Consequently, when treating acute disease, it is mandatory to continue vigorous bronchodilator therapy.

In chronic obstructive lung diseases such as chronic bronchitis the situation is less clearcut. Although glucocorticoids cannot be expected to relieve the obstruction that results from fixed pathologic lesions, data are available suggesting that other causes of impairment, such as inflammation with cellular infiltrate, can be affected. Methylprednisolone may be beneficial in some patients with chronic bronchitis and acute respiratory insufficiency. In one study pulmonary mechanics showed a greater improvement in those given glucocorticoids over a placebo-treated group.[20] Although few would disagree with such an approach, it is important to emphasize that the absolute changes in pulmonary mechanics observed in this study were quite small and that no differences were found in arterial blood gases.

Glucocorticoids are usually initiated in doses equivalent to 40 to 60 mg/day of prednisone and then tapered as quickly as possible—for example, by 5 to 10 mg every third to fourth day—until a dose equivalent to 15 mg/day of prednisone is achieved. Tapering is then continued more slowly until steroids are ultimately discontinued. In practice a 10- to 20-day treatment period has no effect subsequently upon the hypothalamic-pituitary adrenal axis. Continued long-term therapy with corticosteroids should not be undertaken in patients with acute or chronic airway obstruction unless objective evidence of their efficacy can be demonstrated with pulmonary function testing. If long-term therapy is deemed necessary, an alternate-day schedule with a medium-duration preparation (e.g., prednisone) will minimize the side effects of chronic steroid usage. Long-acting steroids should never be used in this form of therapy because they defeat the purpose of the alternate-day regimen.

An alternative approach is to employ one of the high-potency inhaled steroids with minimal systemic absorption such as beclomethasone (Vanceril, Beclovent), triamcinolone (Azmacort), or flunisolide (AeroBid) as systemic steroids are withdrawn.[21–24] Typically, these agents are begun when the oral dose reaches 15 to 20 mg/day of prednisone or its equivalent. These drugs can also be used rather than oral agents to initiate steroid therapy.

Steroid aerosols reduce the symptomatic manifestations of asthma and the severity of bronchial hyperresponsiveness over a period of weeks.[25] Airway reactivity falls as a function of duration of therapy and rises again when the drugs are stopped. The mechanism by which reactivity is lowered is unknown. Although this reduction in airway reactivity has received a great deal of attention, typically the changes reported are very minor, being on the order of one-half log or less.[25] Therefore, although these effects are statistically significant, their physiologic relevance is uncertain, and it is difficult to know what clinical value to place on them. Their size precludes them from being the sole cause of the improvements seen in the clinical state.

In Canada and many European countries, high-dose aerosolized steroids (i.e., two times or more than the conventionally recommended quantities) are commonly used for the control of unstable asthma.[26] Although this approach is effective in reducing the need for oral corticosteroids, it carries with it the risk for increasing side effects. The most common unwanted actions of aerosolized steroids are thrush, which occurs in 5 to 15% of adults and 1% of children, and dysphonia, which is rarer still. With increasing doses, there is greater systemic absorption of these agents, and suppression of adrenal function in both adults and children has been reported as well as cataract formation, interference with bone metabolism, decreased linear growth in children, purpura, and thinning of the skin.

ASTHMA

Asthma is a disease of the airways that is characterized by increased responsiveness of the tracheobronchial tree to a wide range of stimuli. The disease is typified by acute episodes of cough, wheezing, and dyspnea interspersed with symptom-free periods. The disease affects approximately 5% of the population in the United States and is equally prevalent in other countries. Although deaths from asthma are not common (~5000 deaths/yr), the mortality rate has been rising and its morbidity is considerable.

Although it has proved useful to classify asthma by the principal stimuli associated with acute episodes, it should be emphasized that the underlying asthmatic diathesis is a nonspecific increased irritability of the tracheobronchial tree. Hence, the classification of various forms of asthma may often be artificial, since the response in any given patient may be initiated by more than one type of stimulus. With this reservation in mind, asthma can be classified into two broad groups: allergic and idiosyncratic. *Allergic asthma* is associated with a personal or family history of allergic disorders (eczema, rhinitis, urticaria), positive skin reactions to extracts of airborne allergens, increased levels of IgE, bronchoconstriction in response to inhalation of specific antigens, or any combination of these factors. Allergic asthma is frequently seasonal but may be perennial if associated with antigens continually present in the environment. Patients with a negative family or personal history of allergy, negative skin tests, and normal serum IgE levels are said to have *idiosyncratic asthma.* Exacerbations of both types of asthma may be associated with *environmental factors* (e.g., cold air and airborne pollutants such as sulfur dioxide and oxides of nitrogen); *industrial factors* (e.g., reflex bronchospasm in patients with byssinosis and immunologically induced bronchospasm associated with the manufacturing of detergents and handling of flour); *physical exertion; emotional factors;* and *viral upper respiratory infections.*[27] In addition, it has been estimated that between 10 and 15% of patients with adult-onset asthma of the idiosyncratic type are sensitive to *aspirin.*[28] In its severest form, ingestion of as little as a single aspirin tablet may be associated with acute rhinitis, wheezing, flushing, urticaria, and hypotension. It is important to recognize this syndrome and the fact that patients who demonstrate aspirin intolerance may also exhibit intolerance to all the other nonsteroidal anti-inflammatory agents available as well as to tartrazine (a yellow dye widely distributed in food and pharmaceutical products).

The natural history of asthma has not been previously defined. Although some data suggest that a small number of patients may develop apparently irreversible changes in lung function with time, this is not the case in the vast majority. Asthma, unlike other airway diseases such as chronic bronchitis, cystic fibrosis, and bronchiectasis, is not progressive. Patients, even if untreated, do not inexorably move from mild to severe disease with time, rather their clinical course is characterized by exacerbations and remissions.

Relationship Between Pathophysiology and Clinical Features

The pathophysiologic hallmark of asthma is airway obstruction, secondary to bronchial smooth muscle contraction, vascular engagement with mucosal edema, and thick, tenacious secretions. The amount of obstruction can be quantitated by obtaining simple spirometric indices (forced expiratory volume in 1 second [FEV_1], maximum midexpiratory flow [MMF] rate) or airway resistance. When lung volumes are measured in patients with acute asthma, hyperinflation is invariably found to be present with elevation of residual volume, functional residual capacity, and occasionally total lung capacity. Even in the asymptomatic state, the patient frequently has compromized lung function with elevations of residual volume and decreases of flow rates in the midvital capacity range.[29]

The most common finding of the arterial blood gases during an acute exacerbation of asthma is a combination of arterial hypoxemia (usually moderate; Pa_{O_2}, 50 to 70 mm Hg), hypocapnia (Pa_{CO_2} < 40 mm Hg), and respiratory alkalosis.[30, 31] Since the airway obstruction is not uniformly distributed throughout the lungs in patients with asthma, topographic inequalities of ventilation and pulmonary blood flow are the major cause for the hypoxemia. Since arterial P_{CO_2} is inversely related to alveolar ventilation, patients with acute attacks of asthma hyperventilate in relation to metabolic demands possibly because of reflexes originating in the airways, lung parenchyma, or chest wall. A minority of patients develop hypercapnia during an attack of asthma. Since the arterial P_{CO_2} tends to normalize only when the FEV_1 (as a representative index of the severity of the degree of airway obstruction) falls to about 25% of predicted, the finding of a normal P_{CO_2} in an acutely ill asthmatic should be viewed as impending respiratory failure and treated as such. Occasionally, a patient is seen who develops acute hypercapnia despite only moderate airway obstruction. Studies of ventilatory control in asthma, though limited in number,[32] suggest that these patients may have a defect in ventilatory control and may have little ventilatory response to hypercapnia or hypoxemia induced in the laboratory. At present, there is no information concerning the frequency with which individuals with reduced responsiveness to chemical stimuli are seen in the asthmatic population, but such a possibility should be kept in mind for patients who repeatedly develop respiratory failure during attacks of asthma.

Detection of arterial hypoxemia and hypercapnia at the bedside is extraordinarily difficult. Cyanosis is a late sign, and there is wide inter- and intraobserver variability in its detection. The signs of hypercapnia, such as tachycardia, wide pulse pressure, and restlessness, occur too frequently with mild asthma and are too nonspecific to be relied on. The only acceptable way of assessing the adequacy of gas exchange during an attack of asthma is to measure oxygen and carbon dioxide tensions in the arterial blood.

Cough, dyspnea, and wheezing constitute the classic triad of symptoms in patients with acute asthma. A dry cough tends to occur early in the attack and then abates as airway obstruction worsens, with the production of wheezing and shortness of breath. Occasionally, cough is an asthmatic patient's only complaint. As the attack of asthma clears, cough frequently recurs and becomes productive of mucoid sputum. Discolored sputum does not necessarily indicate secondary bacterial infection, for the sputum of asthmatics may contain eosinophils, which can cause a change in sputum consistency and discoloration.

Conventionally, the severity of the wheezing heard in asthma is thought to reflect the degree of airway obstruction, with wheezing increasing in intensity as the attack worsens and decreasing as the attack abates. It is emphasized, however, that this pattern does not always occur, and, in particular, relatively quiet breathing in a dyspneic, tachypneic patient is a sign that the attack of asthma is very severe. Conversely, increased wheezing may accompany improvement in airway obstruction and thus should not necessarily be taken as a sign that the patient's condition is deteriorating.

Assessment of the Acutely Ill Asthmatic Patient

Examination of the relationship between clinical variables and physiologic abnormalities in a group of asthmatics undergoing treatment demonstrated that when patients considered their attacks had ended, marked hyperinflation and airway obstruction were still present.[29, 33, 34] When the physicians in attendance considered the patients to be well, residual volume was still about twice normal and moderate airway obstruction was still demonstrable. These findings indicate that the use of clinical variables alone to judge the severity of an attack of asthma or the success of therapy will frequently lead to serious underestimations of the abnormalities present in the lung. More and more it is becoming clear that an objective measure of lung function such as a peak flow is required to adequately assess the efficacy of acute and chronic therapy.

In acute situations, clues that an attack of asthma is likely to be severe may be obtained from the patient's history. The prior need for hospitalization or large amounts of corticosteroid therapy should alert the physician that the present attack is also likely to be severe. Two reliable signs of severe obstruction are use of the accessory muscles of respiration and pulsus paradoxus.[33, 34] Both of those findings indicate the presence of severe airway obstruction ($FEV_1 < 1$ liter) and marked hyperinflation of the chest.

Cyanosis, disturbance of consciousness, and a quiet chest in a tachypneic, dyspneic patient are grave findings that indicate acute respiratory failure. A chest x-ray film is absolutely essential in patients who have chest, shoulder, or neck pain or dysphagia to rule out the serious but fortunately uncommon complications of pneumothorax and pneumomediastinum. If these complications are present, use of positive pressure devices to deliver aerosolized bronchodilators is absolutely contraindicated. Acute changes in the electrocardiogram, such as p-pulmonale and right ventricular strain, also indicate severe asthma.[33]

Thus, the most severely ill patients can be quickly identified by history, physical examination, and some simple routine investigations. Since treatment of an attack of asthma of moderate severity usually results in the disappearance of accessory muscle use, pulsus paradoxus, and dyspnea within 30 minutes or so, failure to eliminate these problems indicates the need for objective monitoring. Measurements of arterial blood gases and of the degree of airway obstruction present (e.g., the FEV_1 or peak flow) should be obtained. If, after the administration of bronchodilators, spirometry does not improve by more than a few hundred milliliters, the patient will need frequent reassessment and vigorous therapy. Failure of spirometric values to improve over several hours despite repeated medications indicates the need to obtain serial measurements of arterial blood gases, for even if the initial blood gas assessments revealed the presence of hypocapnia, the danger that incipient hypercapnic respiratory failure will develop is now increasing. If the initial blood gas levels reveal eucapnia or mild hypercapnia, intensive therapy, including corticosteroids, should be started. Failure of the arterial P_{CO_2} to fall into the hypocapnic range indicates the need for hospitalization; a rising P_{CO_2} indicates that the patient should be transferred to a place that is able to supply ventilatory support.

Management Guidelines

The major goal of treatment is to bring the patient with asthma to a stable asymptomatic state with the best pulmonary function possible. Once this aim has been accomplished, the drugs should be withdrawn systematically, beginning with the most toxic, to find the lowest quantity of medication necessary to maintain the patient's well-being. Such an approach requires a close patient-physician relationship, patient education, and the objective monitoring of lung function.

To promote rapid improvement, first-line therapy should include an aerosol β_2-agonist. These drugs provide prompt bronchodilatation with a minimum of side effects. In patients who have difficulty in coordinating inhalation with activation of a metered-dose inhaler, a spacing device should be incorporated. If nocturnal complaints are a prominent feature, either a long-acting theophylline compound or a β_2-agonist may be included to provide sufficient medication to last the night through.

In patients whose disease is more active and who have unstable lung function as indicated by increasing or persistent symptoms despite adequate bronchodilator therapy, an attempt should be made to reduce the airway irritability by adding cromolyn or inhaled steroids. Since these drugs frequently take many weeks to produce this effect, one may also wish to employ a long-acting theophylline compound or a short but intense course of oral steroids to accelerate the remission. In such individuals it is essential to monitor peak flow and to base medication adjustments both on the patient's symptoms and on lung function measurements.

When symptoms stabilize, reduction of medication should be systematic and should be guided by close physician-patient communication and objective measures of disease activity. Oral drugs should be withdrawn first, followed thereafter by a diminution in the frequency of aerosols. If high-dose inhaled glucocorticoids have been used, they should be the first topical agent to be lowered. If the patient is going to get into difficulties, lung function will diminish prior to the onset of symptoms and there will be marked circadian changes in flow rates.[29] If these events occur, and the patient is asymptomatic, no further adjustments in therapy should be made until function normalizes. This may take several weeks. If the patient becomes symptomatic, reinstitution of the lowest effective quantities of medication should be undertaken.

In emergency situations, inhaled β_2-adrenergic agents are the first line of therapy.[35] If the response is slow, aminophylline is then given intravenously in a dosage tailored to the patient's history of recent drug ingestion, age, and presence of other disease. Failure to respond to these simple measures demands objective measurements of lung function and arterial blood gases. If symptoms or signs of severe asthma continue, intravenous corticosteroids are administered. Many dose schedules have been proposed, but we have found that intravenous hydrocortisone at 14 mg/kg over 24 hours[18] is adequate. After 24 to 48 hours, the intravenous steroids can be withdrawn and oral prednisone, 40 to 60 mg/day, may be started. There is no evidence that larger doses of steroids are more effective.

All sedatives must be avoided in the treatment of acute asthma. No matter how great a role anxiety appears to play in the patient's symptoms, there is no such thing as a safe tranquilizer or sedative. In the *uncommon* situation of worsening hypercapnia associated with obtundity of the patient, intubation and mechanical ventilation are indicated.

CHRONIC BRONCHITIS AND EMPHYSEMA

Chronic bronchitis and emphysema occur with or without airway obstruction. These two illnesses rank second only to coronary artery disease as causes of permanent disability in the adult population of many Western countries. *Chronic bronchitis* is defined clinically, based on a history of cough and sputum production during at least 3 consecutive months for more than 2 successive years, other causes of cough and sputum production having been excluded. *Emphysema* is defined in morphologic terms and thus can be diagnosed with certainty only by histologic examination of sections of whole lung fixed at full inflation. The disease is characterized by distention of air spaces distal to the terminal bronchioles accompanied by destruction of alveolar septa. The two disorders , despite being distinct entities, most frequently coexist, and this, together with the considerable difficulty that is encountered in establishing the diagnosis of emphysema with certainty during life, has led to the lumping of the two together under the heading *chronic obstructive pulmonary disease* (COPD).

The most commonly identified factor associated with chronic bronchitis and emphysema is cigarette smoking. Chronic bronchitis is four times more common among cigarette smokers than among nonsmokers, and smoking correlates well with the extent of emphysema found at autopsy. Cigarette smoking impairs pulmonary clearance mechanisms, provokes mucus secretion and possibly mucous gland hypertrophy, and leads to acute increases in airway resistance that are reflexly mediated, presumably by stimulation of submucosal irritant receptors located in the tracheobronchial tree. Other factors statistically related to the prevalence and morbidity of chronic bronchitis and emphysema include atmospheric pollution, socioeconomic class and occupation, and acute respiratory infections. Deficient or absent serum levels of the protease inhibitor, α_1-antitrypsin, are found in some patients with early onset of emphysema.[36] The emphysema is panacinar and occurs predominantly at the lung bases. It remains controversial whether individuals who are heterozygous for the genes associated with α_1-antitrypsin deficiency and who have intermediate levels of α_1-antitrypsin in their serum have abnormalities of lung function.[36, 37]

Since the discovery of homozygous α_1-antitrypsin deficiency, it has been postulated that emphysema results from an imbalance between proteases and antiproteases in the lung. The effects of elastases derived from neutrophils and macrophages are normally offset in the lung parenchyma by α_1-protease inhibitor and α_2-macroglobulin. The airways are protected by a compound called bronchial mucous inhibitor on secretory leucoprotease inhibitor (SLPI). Oxidants from cigarette smoke or activated macrophages and neutrophils may inactivate the antiproteases and thus interfere with controlled lung repair.[38]

This hypothesis has given rise to attempts to treat α_1-antitrypsin deficiency by infusing this compound into affected patients to protect against their own proteases. While this approach restores serum and bronchoalveolar lavage levels to normal, there is no evidence that it prevents the progression of emphysema.[39]

There is evidence to suggest that COPD may start in the periphery of the lung and interfere with the function of the peripheral airway lung before there are diagnostically interpretable symptoms or interference with routine lung function.[40] Once COPD is established, epidemiologic data demonstrate a slow and relentless diminution in ventilatory function. Although slow, the decrement in function with time far exceeds the rate of change seen with normal aging and it increases as a function of the number of years of smoking. Generally, in patients with mixed disease, dyspnea on exertion begins to develop when the FEV_1 falls below 50% of its predicted value, and dyspnea at rest is seen when the FEV_1 falls to 25% of normal. At this point cor pulmonale and carbon dioxide retention are common.

Relationship Between Pathophysiology and Clinical Features

The airway obstruction of chronic bronchitis and emphysema may be secondary to structural changes in the airways (mucosal edema, inflammation, fibrosis, and mucus secretion), bronchoconstriction, loss of lung elasticity, or dynamic collapse of airways during forced expiration. The symptoms of *chronic bronchitis* (cough, breathlessness on exertion) and signs (sputum, rhonchi) provide a poor guide to the severity of the problem unless considered in conjunction with functional impairment. If routine spirometry is recorded at the time of initial consultation, approximately 20% of patients with predominant bronchitis will have a normal vital capacity and FEV_1. In most of these patients, peripheral airway function is abnormal. These abnormalities may be detected by measurement of expiratory flow rates in the mid-to-low vital capacity range, closing volume or frequency dependence of dynamic compliance.[41] Characteristically, the patient is a smoker in early middle age, sputum production will occur early in the morning, and dyspnea, if present, will occur only with moderate to severe exercise. Initial consultation is usually sought because of an exacerbation of sputum production, secondary to an acute tracheobronchitis. If such a patient is persuaded to stop smoking, sputum production will decline, and functional deficits in pulmonary function may improve.

The remaining 80% of patients will have abnormal FEV_1 and flow rates on presentation, and this group of patients may be usefully subdivided into those with normal arterial blood gas values and those without. The former constitutes the largest group, and in these patients, FEV_1 is likely to range from 40 to 80% of the predicted value. Measurement of lung volumes frequently reveals hyperinflation with an elevation of residual volume, but total lung capacity is usually normal. Measurements of diffusing capacity of the lung for carbon monoxide are normal. Cessation of smoking at this stage may result in less sputum production, and there may be mild improvement of lung function and dyspnea.

The final group of patients with chronic bronchitis are those with abnormal spirometry and derangement of arterial blood gases. The majority of these patients will have severe airway obstruction with an FEV_1 around 25% of predicted; most will also have associated emphysema.[42] However, there is a small group of patients who develop chronic hypercapnic respiratory failure despite only moderate airway obstruction. As discussed in the section on asthma, it is likely that these patients have either an acquired or a congenital defect of ventilatory control. Since the ventilatory responses to carbon dioxide and hypoxia are determined in part by genetic factors, it has been postulated that patients who are born with decreased responsiveness to chemical stimuli may be the ones who go on to develop early-onset respiratory failure when lung disease supervenes. This hypothesis needs further testing, but it is interesting to note that family members of patients with chronic hypercapnic respiratory failure have been shown to have low responses to carbon dioxide and hypoxia.[43]

Once arterial blood gases become abnormal, cor pulmonale frequently develops.[44] Factors leading to the development of pulmonary hypertension, secondary right ventricular hypertrophy, and eventual right ventricular failure include pulmonary vascular constriction in response to alveolar hypoxia that is exacerbated by coexistent acidosis; obliteration of the pulmonary vascular bed secondary to coexistent emphysema; and, possibly, an increased rheologic load on the right ventricle secondary to erythrocytosis. The onset of peripheral edema in a patient with chronic bronchitis or emphysema is a poor prognostic sign. In general terms, patients with predominant chronic bronchitis may experience many episodes of acute-on-chronic respiratory failure and exacerbations of cor pulmonale from which recovery is frequent with proper management (see further on). By contrast, the development of acute-on-chronic respiratory failure and cor pulmonale in patients with predominant emphysema is frequently a terminal event.

Patients with chronic bronchitis may have wheezing and spasmodic attacks of shortness of breath in addition to their longstanding symptoms of cough and sputum production. In some of these patients, significant improvement in airway obstruction may occur after administration of bronchodilators. These patients have been said to have *chronic asthmatic bronchitis,* but a better term would be chronic bronchitis with a bronchospastic element.

Patients with predominant *emphysema* usually present in late middle age with a history of exertional dyspnea and minimal cough unless the emphysema is secondary to α_1-antitrypsin deficiency. Then the presentation will be at an earlier age. Characteristically, the physical signs are those of hyperinflation of the chest with a fixed or poorly expanding rib cage, tachypnea with prolonged expiration through pursed lips, and diminished breath sounds with high-pitched rhonchi late in expiration. The FEV_1 is commonly less than 40% of the predicted value when the patient presents, and measurements of lung volume reveal marked hyperinflation with elevations of total lung capacity and residual volume. The elastic recoil of the lung is severely reduced, as is the capacity of the lung to transfer carbon dioxide.[45] These abnormalities are not found in patients with predominant bronchitis and reflect underlying damage to the lung parenchyma. Arterial blood gas measurements frequently reveal an arterial P_{O_2} in the midseventies and an arterial P_{CO_2} that is normal to low. Thus, in contrast to many patients with predominant chronic bronchitis, patients with predominant emphysema choose to maintain an increased minute ventilation despite airway obstruction and high wasted ventilation ratios and thus maintain relatively normal blood gas levels at the expense of severe dyspnea. Patients with emphysema frequently have a deterioration of arterial oxygenation on exercise. Eventually, chronic hypercapnic respiratory failure and cor pulmonale supervene.

Management Guidelines

Smoking Cessation. Since cigarette smoking is one of the major factors contributing to the cause of COPD, the importance of cessation should be emphasized. This is true particularly in patients with mild to moderate airway obstruction. The less the severity of the obstruction, the more likely it is to improve or reverse completely when cigarettes are discontinued.

Physical Measures. Postural drainage and assisted coughing probably aid clearance of sputum from central airways, but there is no evidence that this improves the long-term outlook of patients with chronic bronchitis and emphysema. Similarly, evidence is scant that breathing exercises or muscle retraining improves ventilatory capacity in patients with chronic lung disease. Pursed-lip breathing is known to decrease the respiratory rate, increase tidal volume, lessen dyspnea, and improve gas exchange; thus, this maneuver can be usefully taught to patients who do not adopt it spontaneously. Other maneuvers such as "diaphragmatic breathing" may also result in changes in respiratory pattern and in lessening of dyspnea, but available evidence suggests that objective long-term benefits do not accrue. With regard to the respiratory muscles, studies suggest an objective improvement in diaphragmatic function when a patient with chronic airway obstruction adopts a posture of leaning forward with arms braced on knees; this maneuver, like pursed-lip breathing, is frequently intuitively adopted by patients. There is no evidence that positive-pressure devices either improve the delivery of bronchodilators or change the rate of decline of lung function in patients with chronic bronchitis and emphysema.

Exercise tolerance can be improved in patients with chronic bronchitis and emphysema who undertake a graded physical conditioning program. Pulmonary function does not improve, but maximal oxygen consumption increases, and minute ventilation and heart rate at any given workload decrease as training continues.[46] These changes are not specific for patients with lung disease and are seen in all subjects who improve physical fitness through a training program, and thus there is no improvement in prognosis. Since the effects of training are in part task-specific, and since stationary bicycles and treadmills are expensive, it seems advisable simply to encourage patients to increase their daily activity and undertake walks of increasing distances in an attempt to improve physical fitness.

Airway Obstruction. The pharmacologic agents used to treat airway obstruction in patients with chronic bronchitis and emphysema are the same as those used in the treatment of asthma discussed previously, and they are introduced in similar fashion. An inhaled sympathomimetic agent is administered at first, to which is added an oral methylxanthine or oral β-adrenergic agent or both if dyspnea is not improved. Clearly, patients in whom an acute improvement in airway obstruction can be demonstrated in the laboratory with administration of a bronchodilator are those who most predictably will derive benefit from these agents. However, bronchodilators should not be withheld if immediate responsiveness cannot be demonstrated, since even in these patients dyspnea frequently improves, and long-term therapy may actually improve lung function.[47] Under these circumstances, improved mucociliary transport may play a role. For example, β-adrenergic agents are known to change secretion volume and increase rates of mucociliary clearance.[48] Since patients are often elderly or have incipient or overt right ventricular failure, theophylline dosage should be adjusted cautiously, and measurements of plasma levels will greatly aid the planning of therapeutic regimes. The controversial role of corticosteroids in the treatment of patients with chronic bronchitis and emphysema has been noted previously. There is very little convincing evidence of their efficacy; however, there is some suggestion that patients with chronic bronchitis with reactive airways may derive benefit from a trial of steroids.[49, 50] If objective improvement of pulmonary function (>10% increase in FEV_1) is not demonstrable within 4 weeks of commencing corticosteroids, these agents should be discontinued.

Expectorants (e.g., saturated solution of potassium iodide, glycerol guaiacolate) are frequently employed in the management of patients with chronic bronchitis, but there is no convincing evidence of their efficacy. If the patient or physician finds these agents helpful, they can be continued. *N*-acetylcysteine (Mucomyst) may be administered by a hand-held nebulizer in an effort to thin secretions, but it can be quite irritating. If use of this agent is accompanied by bronchospasm, a β-adrenergic agent should be added to the aerosol mixture. Occasionally, the use of these agents together can provide dramatic improvements in lung function by facilitating the clearance of retained secretions. Although most agree that adequate hydration should be maintained in an effort to decrease sputum viscosity, there is no evidence that aerosol droplets delivered by ultrasonic nebulizers reach beyond the nasopharynx and upper airway. Although this may make the patient feel more comfortable, it is doubtful whether secretions are liquefied, as has been claimed.

Control of Infection. Acute respiratory tract infections may produce worsening airway obstruction with increased cough, sputum production, and shortness of breath and are a common precipitant of acute respiratory failure. Thus, antibiotics play an important role in the management of patients with chronic bronchitis and emphysema. Although more than 50% of episodes of acute tracheobronchitis are caused by nonbacterial agents, secondary infection is common. Gram stain and culture of the sputum are not necessary when initiating antibiotic therapy in patients with chronic airway obstruction, since mixed organisms without a specific pathogen will most commonly be found. Early use of antibiotics appears to reduce the frequency and severity of exacerbations of bronchitis; therefore, it seems wise to commence patients on a 10-day course of tetracycline or ampicillin at the first sign of respiratory infection. A trimethoprim-sulfamethoxazole combination (Bactrim) may be a useful alternative. Continuous prophylactic antibiotic use has not proved to be of benefit. Pneumovaccine and influenza vaccine should be routinely employed.

Oxygen Therapy. The primary indication for low-flow oxygen therapy in ambulatory patients is the presence of severe hypoxemia (Pa_{O_2} < 50 mm Hg). Additional indications are diminished mental function, provided that it can be clearly established that oxygen improves this situation, and decreased exercise tolerance such that the patient cannot undertake normal daily activities, provided that objective measurements reveal worsening hypoxemia on exercise and improvement of exercise performance with oxygen therapy. Dyspnea per se is not an acceptable indication for chronic oxygen administration because patients with emphysema, in whom this symptom is most marked, are not usually hypoxemic. A large multicenter trial has demonstrated that maximum effectiveness in decreasing pulmonary artery pressures and patient morbidity is achieved by continuous therapy for 24 hours/day.[51] Occasionally, a patient is seen who has poor-quality sleep. Since arterial desaturation is known to occur during sleep in patients with chronic respiratory failure, such a patient may benefit from nocturnal oxygen therapy. Significant worsening of hypercapnia is not usually a problem with chronic low-flow oxygen therapy, even in patients who develop worsening hypercapnia when oxygen is administered during episodes of acute respiratory failure. Low-flow oxygen for ambulatory patients is usually delivered via nasal prongs at flow rates of 1 to 2 l/min, utilizing either conventional tanks or liquid oxygen systems. A transtracheal catheter has been developed to replace the prongs. While this method clearly deceases the supplemental oxygen that needs to be delivered to the patient, it does occasionally produce complications that require its removal.[52]

Digitalis and Diuretics. Oxygen and measures directed at improvement of pulmonary function are the mainstays of therapy for cor pulmonale. With such therapy, afterload to the right ventricle is reduced, and patients frequently undergo a spontaneous diuresis. Diuretics, although effective in reducing peripheral edema, may induce hypochloremic alkalosis, leading to refractory hypercapnia. It is generally agreed that the combination of hypoxemia and electrolyte disturbance increases the hazards of digitalis therapy. Hence, caution should be exercised in using digitalis or diuretics in patients with COPD.

Conservative Management of Acute-on-Chronic Respiratory Failure. Acute-on-chronic respiratory failure is frequently precipitated by an acute exacerbation of bronchitis or pneumonia, sedative administration, excessive oxygen administration, and major surgery. In many cases no specific cause can be identified. Another possible cause of worsening, pneumothorax, is fortunately a rare complication; although if present, it may be exceedingly difficult to diagnose on clinical examination. Since many of these predisposing factors are potentially reversible, the aim of treatment of acute-on-chronic respiratory failure is to maintain adequate oxygenation while attempting to relieve the precipitating cause. Uncontrolled oxygen therapy is frequently hazardous, since progressive hypercapnia and obtundity of the patient may be anticipated to occur in approximately 30% of patients treated in this manner. Many patients with hypercapnic respiratory failure depend on the hypoxic drive to breathe in order to maintain ventilation, and removal of this drive by excessive oxygen administration may, therefore, lead to progressive hypercapnia. In addition, high inspired oxygen concentrations may worsen ventilation-perfusion ratios by causing complete atelectasis of poorly ventilating units. Owing to the shape of the oxyhemoglobin dissociation curve, a modest increase in arterial P_{O_2} to approximately 50 mm Hg will result in a considerable increase in oxygen content of the arterial blood (Fig. 20–1). Hence, controlled oxygen therapy via a Venturi mask (0.24 or 0.28 inspired oxygen concentration) or nasal prongs (1 to 2 l/min) will produce adequate oxygenation while causing a small tolerable increase in arterial P_{CO_2} in most patients. If the arterial P_{CO_2} rises progressively despite the use of controlled oxygen therapy, this treatment should never be abruptly discontinued. Returning the patient to breathing room air under these circumstances may result in a dangerous fall in alveolar and arterial P_{O_2} to levels lower than were present before oxygen therapy was instituted. A progressively rising P_{CO_2} that cannot be controlled with conservative measures and that is associated with obtundity of the patient, such that he or she is now no longer able to cooperate and cough effectively, indicates the need for endotracheal intubation and mechanical ventilation.

Principles of care of the acutely ill patient are otherwise the same as in the ambulatory patient; however, therapy is intensified. Physical therapy of the chest with postural drainage, intravenous hydration, aerosolized bronchodilators, and intravenous aminophylline are vigorously administered. Dosages and precautions are similar to those employed in the management of patients with acute asthma. Broad-spectrum antibiotic coverage is usually employed on an empiric basis, but few objective data exist to attest to

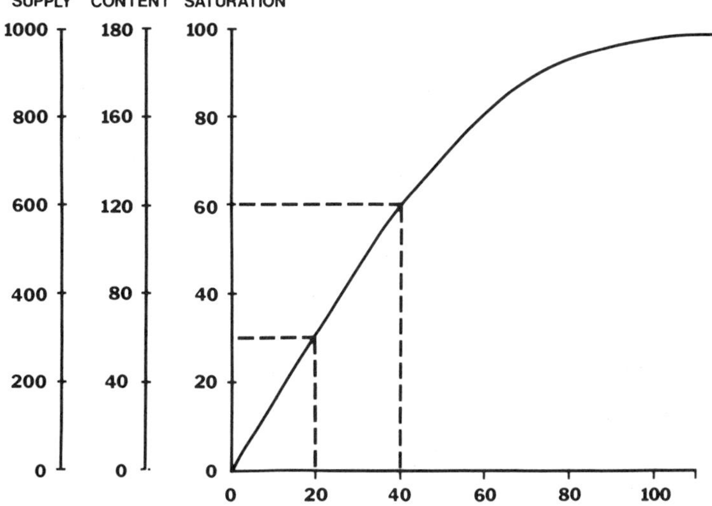

FIGURE 20–1. The oxygen-hemoglobin association-dissociation curve. PaO_2 signifies arterial oxygen pressure. The first vertical scale is arterial oxygen saturation (content ÷ capacity). The next scale gives the O_2 content per liter of blood, assuming a normal hemoglobin concentration and O_2 combining power. The supply scale gives the systemic O_2 flow per minute (cardiac output × content), assuming a cardiac output of 5 l/min. Note that increasing the partial pressure of O_2 only 20 mm Hg (from 20 to 40 mm Hg) results in a doubling of O_2 supply.

the efficacy of this approach in situations in which there is no bacterial pneumonia or tracheobronchitis.

REFERENCES

1. Hendeles L and Weinberger M: Theophylline. A "state of the art" review. Pharmacotherapy 3:2, 1983.
2. Isles AF, MacLeod SM, and Levison H: Theophylline: New thought about an old drug. Chest 82:495, 1982.
3. I.V. Dosage Guidelines for Theophylline Products. F.D.A. Drug Bulletin, Feb. 4, 1980.
4. Zwillich CW, Sutton FD, Neff TA, et al: Theophylline-induced seizures in adults: Correlation with serum concentrations. Ann Intern Med 82:784, 1975.
5. McFadden ER Jr: Beta$_2$-receptor agonist: Metabolism and pharmacology. J Allergy Clin Immunol 68:91, 1981.
6. Rossing TH, Fanta CH, Goldstein DH, et al: Emergency therapy of asthma: Comparison of the acute effects of parenteral and inhaled sympathomimetics and infused aminophylline. Am Rev Respir Dis 122:365, 1980.
7. Rossing TH, Fanta CH, and McFadden ER Jr: A controlled trial of the use of single versus combined-drug therapy in the treatment of acute episodes of asthma. Am Rev Respir Dis 123:190, 1981.
8. Fanta CH, Rossing TH, and McFadden ER Jr: Emergency room treatment of asthma: Relationships among therapeutic combinations, severity of obstruction and time course of response. Am J Med 72:416, 1982.
9. Fuglsang G and Pedersen S: Comparison of nebuhaler and nebulizer therapy of acute severe asthma in children. Eur J Respir Dis 69:109, 1986.
10. Rossing TH, Fanta CH, and McFadden ER Jr: Effect of outpatient treatment of asthma with beta agonists on the response to sympathomimetics in an emergency room. Am J Med 75:781, 1983.
11. Coady TJ, Stewart CJ, and Davies HJ: Synchronization of bronchodilator release. Practitioner 217:273, 1976.
12. Shim C and Williams MH: The adequacy of inhalation of aerosol from canister nebulizers. Am J Med 69:891, 1980.
13. Crompton G: Problems patients have using pressurized aerosol inhalers. Eur J Respir Dis 63(Suppl 119):101, 1982.
14. Kelling JS, Strohl KP, Smith RL, et al: Physician knowledge in the use of canister nebulizers. Chest 83:612, 1983.
15. Gross NJ and Skorodin MS: Anticholinergic antimuscarinic bronchodilators. Am Rev Respir Dis 129:645, 1984.
16. Murphy S and Kelly HW: Cromolyn sodium: A review of mechanisms and clinical use in asthma. Drug Intell Clin Pharm 21:22, 1987.
17. Hoag JE and McFadden ER Jr: Long-term effect of cromolyn sodium on nonspecific bronchial hyperresponsiveness: A review. Ann Allergy 66:53, 1991.
18. Fanta CH, Rossing TH, and McFadden ER Jr: Glucocorticoids in acute asthma: A critical controlled trial. Am J Med 74:845, 1983.
19. Fiel SB, Swartz MA, Glanz K, et al: Efficacy of short-term corticosteroid therapy in out-patient treatment of acute bronchial asthma. Am J Med 75:259, 1983.
20. Albert RK, Martin TR, and Lewis SW: Controlled clinical trial of methylprednisolone in patients with chronic bronchitis and acute respiratory insufficiency. Ann Intern Med 92:753, 1980.
21. Brogden RN, Heel RC, Speight TM, and Avery GS: Beclomethasone dipropionate: A reappraisal of its pharmacodynamic properties and therapeutic efficacy after a decade of use in asthma and rhinitis. Drugs 28:99, 1984.
22. Bernstein IL, Chervinsky P, and Falliers CJ: Efficacy and safety of triamcinolone acetonide aerosol in chronic asthma. Chest 81:20, 1982.
23. Rafferty P, Tucker LG, Frame MH, et al: Comparison of budesonide and beclomethasone dipropionate in patients with severe chronic asthma: Assessment of relative prednisolone-sparing effects. Br J Dis Chest 79:244, 1985.
24. Slavin RG, Izu AE, Bernstein IL, et al: Multi-center study of flunisolide aerosol in adult patients with steroid-dependent asthma. J Allergy Clin Immunol 66:379, 1980.
25. Haahtela T, Jarvinen M, Kava T, et al: Comparison of a β_2-agonist, terbutaline, with an inhaled corticosteroid, budesonide, in newly detected asthma. N Engl J Med 325:388, 1991.
26. Salmeron S, Guerin JC, Godard P, et al: High doses of inhaled corticosteroids in unstable chronic asthma: A multicenter, double-blind, placebo-controlled study. Am Rev Respir Dis 140:167, 1989.
27. McFadden ER Jr: Pathogenesis of asthma. J Allergy Clin Immunol 73:413, 1984.
28. Szczeklik A and Gryglewski J: Asthma and anti-inflammatory drugs. Mechanisms and clinical patterns. Drugs 25:533, 1983.
29. McFadden ER Jr: Pulmonary Structure, Physiology, and Clinical Correlates in Asthma. *In* Middleton E Jr, Busse W, Ellis E, Younger J, et al (eds): Allergy; Principles and Practice, 3rd ed. St. Louis, CV Mosby, 1993.

30. McFadden ER Jr and Lyons HA: Arterial blood gas tensions in asthma. N Engl J Med 278:1027, 1968.
31. Tai E and Read J: Blood gas tensions in bronchial asthma. Lancet 1:644, 1967.
32. Hudgel DW and Weil JV: Asthma associated with decreased hypoxic drive. Ann Intern Med 80:622, 1974.
33. Rebuck AS and Read J: Assessment and management of severe asthma. Am J Med 51:788, 1971.
34. McFadden ER Jr, Kiser R, and deGroot WJ: Acute bronchial asthma: Relations between clinical and physiologic manifestations. N Engl J Med 288:221, 1973.
35. Fanta CH, Rossing TH, and McFadden ER Jr: Treatment of acute asthma: Is combination therapy with sympathomimetics and methylxanthines indicated? Am J Med 80:5, 1986.
36. Kueppers F and Black LF: α_1-Antitrypsin and its deficiency. Am Rev Respir Dis 110:176, 1974.
37. Bruce RM, Cohen BH, Diamond EL, et al: Collaborative study to assess risk of lung disease in PiMZ phenotype subjects. Am Rev Respir Dis 130:386, 1984.
38. Snider GL, Lucey EC, and Stone PJ: State of the art: Animal models of emphysema. Am Rev Respir Dis 133:149, 1986.
39. Wewers MD, Casolaro A, Sellers SE, et al: Replacement therapy for α_1-antitrypsin deficiency associated with emphysema. N Engl J Med 316:1055, 1987.
40. McFadden ER Jr and Linden DA: A reduction in maximum midexpiratory flow rate: A spirographic manifestation of small airway disease. Am J Med 57:725, 1972.
41. McFadden ER Jr and Ingram RH Jr: Peripheral airway obstruction. JAMA 235:259, 1976.
42. Thurlbeck WM, Henderson JAM, Frazer RG, et al: Chronic obstructive lung disease: A comparison between clinical, roentgenologic, functional, and morphologic criteria in chronic bronchitis, emphysema, asthma, and bronchiectasis. Medicine 49:81, 1970.
43. Mountain R, Zwillich C, and Weil J: Hypoventilation in obstructive lung disease: The role of familial factors. N Engl J Med 298:521, 1978.
44. McFadden ER Jr and Braunwald E: Cor pulmonale. *In* Braunwald E (ed): Heart Disease, 4th ed. Philadelphia, WB Saunders, 1992, p 1581.
45. Macklem PT and Becklake MR: The relationship between the mechanical and diffusing properties of the lung in health and disease. Am Rev Respir Dis 87:47, 1963.
46. Pierce AK, Taylor HF, Archer RK, et al: Responses to exercise training in patients with emphysema. Arch Intern Med 113:28, 1964.
47. Ayres SM, Griesback SJ, Reimold F, et al: Bronchial component in chronic obstructive lung disease. Am J Med 57:183, 1974.
48. Wood RE, Wanner A, Hirsch J, et al: Tracheal mucociliary transport in patients with cystic fibrosis and its stimulation by terbutaline. Am Rev Respir Dis 111:733, 1975.
49. Shim C, Stover DE, and Williams MH Jr: Response to corticosteroids in chronic bronchitis. J Allergy Clin Immunol 62:363, 1978.
50. Mendella LA, Manfreda J, Warren CP, and Anthonisen NR: Steroid response in stable COPD. Ann Intern Med 96:17, 1982.
51. Nocturnal Oxygen Therapy Trial Group: Continuous or nocturnal oxygen therapy in hypoxemic obstructive lung disease: A clinical trial. Ann Intern Med 93:391, 1980.
52. Heimlich HJ and Carr GC: Transtracheal technique for pulmonary rehabilitation. Ann Otol Rhinol Laryngol 94:502, 1985.

21

Hemoptysis

CHRISTOPHER H. FANTA, MD

Hemoptysis always reflects pathology within the respiratory tract, although its etiology may vary from the benign and self-limited (e.g., bronchitis) to the more serious and potentially life-threatening (e.g., lung cancer or pulmonary vasculitis). Because diseases at either end of this spectrum of severity may manifest with only minor blood-streaking of the sputum, it is mandatory that every episode of hemoptysis be evaluated seriously, at least on its initial presentation. The chest radiograph is the pivotal diagnostic test. When an abnormality is detected on the chest film, the evaluation generally aims to explain the radiographic lesion. On the other hand, if the chest film is clear and no clinical feature in addition to the hemoptysis points to a specific diagnosis, a different series of diagnostic steps is indicated. The main question is often whether fiberoptic bronchoscopy is warranted in the attempt to identify the source of bleeding and to rule out occult lung cancer.

DIFFERENTIAL DIAGNOSIS

Forty to 50 years ago, hemoptysis was considered virtually synonymous with pulmonary tuberculosis. In recent years, with the reduced incidence of tuberculosis and the rapidly rising prevalence of cigarette smoking–related lung diseases—specifically, chronic bronchitis and lung cancer—the relative frequencies of these common causes of hemoptysis are changing. No etiologic information is available from a general medical practice in which extensive evaluations were performed and long-term follow-up undertaken. What is known comes from referral populations, which tend to favor cases of more extensive or prolonged hemoptysis. Table 21–1 displays the results of the evaluation of hemoptysis in four series reported both before and after the application of fiberoptic bronchoscopy.[1–4] In all, bronchitis or bronchiectasis and cancer of the lung accounted for most of the cases (48 to 77%). A minority of cases were due to tuberculosis (3 to 10%) or cardiovascular diseases like mitral stenosis, congestive heart failure, or pulmonary embolism (0 to 6%). A long list of miscellaneous diagnoses, including bacterial, fungal, and parasitic infections; benign tumors; vasculitides; bleeding dyscrasias; and vascular abnormalities, make up another 6 to 16% of cases. Finally, after complete evaluation, including bronchoscopic examination, some 10 to 20% of cases of hemoptysis are unexplained.

Another way to think of the differential diagnosis of hemoptysis is to consider the pathophysiologic mechanisms of bleeding. When one recalls that virtually the entire cardiac output passes through the pulmonary capillary bed separated from the alveolar air spaces by a membrane only 1-μm thick and approximately 70 m^2 in surface area, it is remarkable that hemorrhage into the tracheobronchial tree is not more common. In health, the low pressures of the pulmonary circulation are protective. However, if the pulmonary veins become engorged from left ventricular decompensation, such as in mitral stenosis or other causes of congestive heart failure, hemoptysis may result. The alveolar-capillary membrane itself may become disrupted, leading to diffuse alveolar hemorrhage, such as in Goodpasture's syndrome or idiopathic pulmonary hemosiderosis. Frank infarction and necrosis of lung tissue, which may occur in pulmonary embolism, necrotizing pneumonia, or vasculitis (e.g., Wegener's granulomatosis, polyarteritis nodosa, bronchocentric granulomatosis) lead to breakdown of vessel walls and bleeding into lung tissue.

The lung of course has a dual blood supply, with the bronchial circulation providing blood to the airway mucosa and tracheobronchial walls. Probably the majority of hemoptysis originates from the bronchial blood supply. The superficial vessels of the mucosal surface may become dilated and friable as part of the inflammatory process of chronic bronchitis, or they may be eroded by direct tumor invasion or by rupture of a broncholith (fragment of calcified lymph node eroding through to the bronchial lumen). Commonly, at the site of a chronic suppurative process, bronchial vessels proliferate and become dilated and tortuous; anastomoses may form to the pulmonary vessels. These hypervascularized areas are the source of bleeding in cavitary tuberculosis, lung abscess, and all forms of bronchiectasis, including cystic fibrosis, and are a common source of massive hemoptysis.

One unusual mechanism of hemoptysis is the ectopic growth of endometrial tissue in the tracheobronchial tree.[5] This pathology results in recurrent hemoptysis at the time of the menstrual period, called "catamenial hemoptysis."

CLINICAL ASSESSMENT

The first step in the evaluation of hemoptysis is to establish that the reported bleeding originates in the tracheobronchial tree. If the patient describes coughing the sample from deep in the chest or reports sputum mixed or streaked with blood, one can reliably assume a pulmonary source. When the specimen is simply cleared from the back of the throat or wells up into the mouth unexpectedly, the origin of the bleeding may be in doubt. A history of nosebleeds or gingival bleeding after tooth brushing may suggest an upper airway etiology, whereas associated vomiting or retching suggests hematemesis. Features said to favor true hemoptysis in confusing cases are "frothiness" or air bubbles mixed with at least a portion of the blood and the identification of alveolar macrophages on staining of the specimen.[6] Note that the demonstration of a small amount of blood in the stomach on gastric aspiration does not exclude the possibility of hemoptysis, since coughed blood is often swallowed rather than expectorated.

TABLE 21–1. ETIOLOGIES OF HEMOPTYSIS

	1966[1]	1979[2]	1981[3]	1991[4]
Number of patients	1024	70	129	264
Bronchitis/bronchiectasis	355 (35%)	26 (37%)	52 (40%)	64 (24%)
Neoplasia	136 (13%)	28 (40%)	31 (24%) Primary, 23 Metastatic, 8	78 (29%)
Tuberculosis	85 (8%)	6 (8%)*	4 (3%)	15 (6%)
Cardiovascular diseases	64 (6%)	2 (3%)	7 (5%) Congestive heart failure, 5 Pulmonary infarction, 2	1 (0.4%)
Unknown etiology	345 (34%)	1 (14%)	14 (11%)	57 (22%)
Miscellaneous etiologies†	59 (6%)	7 (10%)	21 (16%)	49 (19%)

*Includes tuberculosis plus fungal and bacterial pneumonias.
†Bleeding diathesis, necrotizing pneumonia, endometriosis, sarcoidosis, nonspecific bronchial granulomata, vasculitis (including Wegener's granulomatosis), lipoid pneumonia, occupational diseases (including silicosis, bagassosis, asbestosis, byssinosis), mycetoma (including aspergilloma), fungal pneumonia (including histoplasmosis, blastomycosis, coccidioidomycosis), parasitic infestation (including paragonimiasis, hookworm, strongyloidiasis, trichinosis, amebic abscess, ascariasis, hydatid cyst), hereditary telangiectasias, hamartoma, Loeffler's syndrome, and bronchopleural fistula.

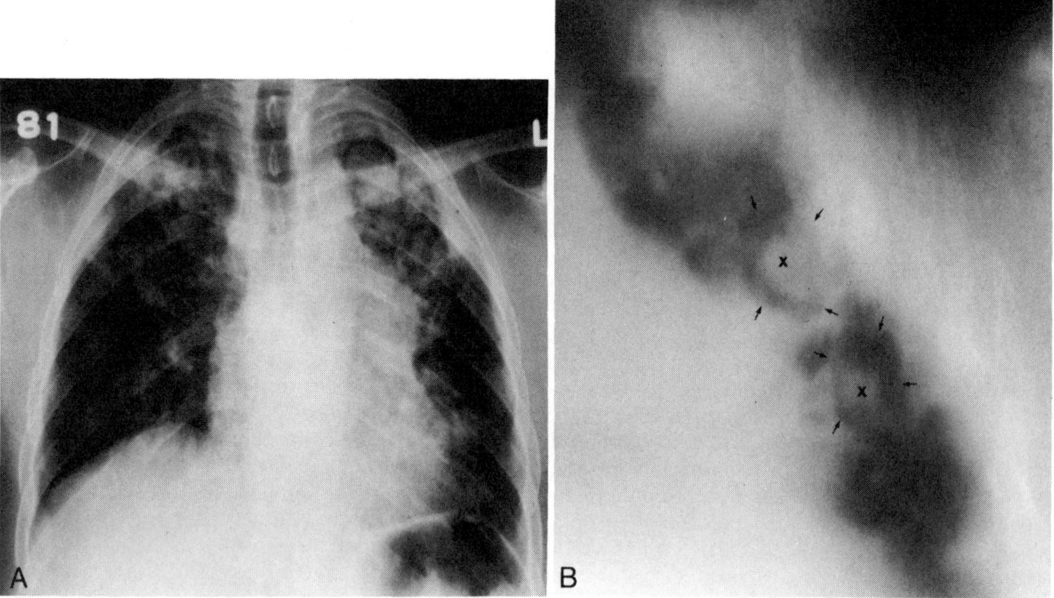

FIGURE 21–1. *A,* Posteroanterior chest radiograph of a patient with pulmonary sarcoidosis who developed hemoptysis. Close inspection reveals multiple upper lobe cavities. A tomographic cut of the left upper lobe *(B)* clearly delineates two rounded densities (marked with "X") (mycetomas or "fungus balls") within cavities (delineated with arrows).

In many cases the finding of hemoptysis is only one of a complex of symptoms and signs that readily point to the diagnosis. For instance, the previously healthy young patient with the sudden onset of fever, shaking chills, and purulent sputum production who reports small amounts of blood mixed with "rusty" sputum is likely to have an acute bacterial pneumonia. The older patient with a more subacute illness characterized by chronic cough with purulent sputum production, night sweats, weight loss, anemia, and repetitive bouts of hemoptysis may be suspected of having tuberculosis or perhaps a lung abscess; chest radiograph and sputum smears for bacteria and acid-fast bacilli are likely to establish the diagnosis and adequately explain the hemoptysis.

At times, however, cough and hemoptysis may be the only presenting symptoms volunteered by the patient. If the bleeding is massive (more than approximately 100 ml of blood at one time or 200 to 600 ml over 24 to 48 hours), then the patient should be hospitalized and emergent work-up and treatment should be undertaken in parallel. The problem of massive hemoptysis is further discussed later. In assessing the patient with lesser hemoptysis, certain historical points should be elicited.

History. The age of the patient is important, since chronic bronchitis and lung cancer are uncommon before 40 years of age and peak in incidence after 50 years of age. A history of no cigarette smoking virtually excludes chronic bronchitis as the etiology of hemoptysis and makes primary lung cancer much less likely. Bronchiectasis can be sought by inquiring about childhood pneumonia, recurrent or persistent childhood chest infections, daily cough with production of purulent sputum, and accompanying sinusitis. A history of rheumatic fever or a heart murmur raises consideration of mitral stenosis; recent prolonged bedrest, leg immobilization, childbirth, or prior documented deep venous thrombosis in the lower extremities puts the patient at risk for pulmonary embolism. A past history of pulmonary tuberculosis is also important since even adequately treated inactive tuberculosis can be a source of bleeding: hemoptysis may result from the "dry bronchiectasis" in areas of lung left scarred by the disease, from tuberculous cavities colonized by fungus (mycetoma), or from bronchial erosion by calcified lymph nodes (broncholiths). Finally, one should ask about bleeding from other sites, particularly from the nose or in the urine or stool, since hemoptysis may be only one manifestation of more generalized bleeding in vasculitides, bleeding dyscrasias, or hereditary telangiectasia.

Physical Examination. Among the common causes of hemoptysis, the physical examination is probably most useful to suggest lung cancer (hoarseness, clubbing, hard supraclavicular lymphadenopathy, or localized wheezing from obstruction or compression of a bronchus), bronchiectasis (focal inspiratory rales), and cardiac disease (signs of congestive heart failure or the opening snap and diastolic rumble of mitral stenosis). Occasionally, the astute clinician will be directed to the cause of hemoptysis by a subtle physical finding: nasal ulceration suggesting Wegener's granulomatosis; an accentuated pulmonic component of the second heart sound and a palpable impulse over the pulmonic area indicating pulmonary hypertension (primary pulmonary hypertension or recurrent pulmonary emboli may cause hemoptysis); or oral telangiectases pointing to the syndrome of hereditary telangiectasia.

Chest Radiograph. In most cases of hemoptysis, the chest radiograph is the critical diagnostic test and usually directs further work-up. Even when the cause of hemoptysis is readily explained by the clinical circumstances, such as in the setting of an acute tracheobronchitis complicating chronic bronchitis, a chest film should be obtained to exclude an alternative, comorbid disease, such as a new lung mass.

In some cases the chest film alone is virtually diagnostic. Figure 21–1 shows the posteroanterior chest radiograph of a woman with extensive pulmonary sarcoidosis. Her sarcoidosis caused extensive scarring and cavitation in her lungs, and the radiograph and tomograms document fungus balls within several of these cavities. Sputum cultures positive for *Aspergillus* confirmed the radiographic diagnosis of aspergillomas. Similarly, a middle-aged, cigarette-smoking patient with hemoptysis and a large, irregular central lung mass is likely to have a pulmonary neoplasm. Hemoptysis in this setting indicates an endobronchial tumor with tissue necrosis or erosion into the airway mucosa, and fiberoptic bronchoscopy is likely to give a tissue diagnosis. (The yield of fiberoptic bronchoscopy in diagnosing lung cancer when an endobronchial lesion is visualized is greater than 95%.[7]) If the chest film of a patient with hemoptysis shows atelectasis with segmental or lobar volume loss (Fig. 21–2), bronchoscopy, again, is the procedure of choice. An endobronchial obstructing lesion is likely, and the differential diagnosis includes bronchogenic carcinoma, bronchial adenoma, and aspirated foreign body.

Other examples of diseases in which the chest radiograph may strongly point to a specific diagnosis include tuberculosis, with upper lobe apical or posterior patchy infiltrates, with or without cavitation and retraction; bronchiectasis, in which the thickened bronchial walls cut longitudinally may appear as parallel linear densities called tram-lines, or where one may find a persistent segmental infiltrate with atelectasis; and mitral stenosis, suggested by calcification of the mitral valve, the left atrial "double density," and displacement upward of the left mainstem bronchus. The finding of multiple nodular densities or localized infiltration at least would raise the question of Wegener's granulomatosis and necessitate a search for sinus, nasal, and renal manifestations of the disease.

Heavy bleeding in the lung may itself cause an infiltrate (a "blood pneumonitis"), which does not shed light on the cause of the bleeding but rather is simply a manifestation of it. Similarly, a unilateral source of bleeding—for instance, a lung cancer in the left mainstem bronchus—easily may cause bleeding that appears as infiltrates in both lungs, since cough may move the blood centrally and then the next inhalation may redistribute it throughout the tracheobronchial tree—that is, the blood is "aspirated" into other pulmonary segments. In the absence of further bleeding, such a "blood pneumonitis" usually shows spontaneous radiographic resolution over 5 to 7 days.

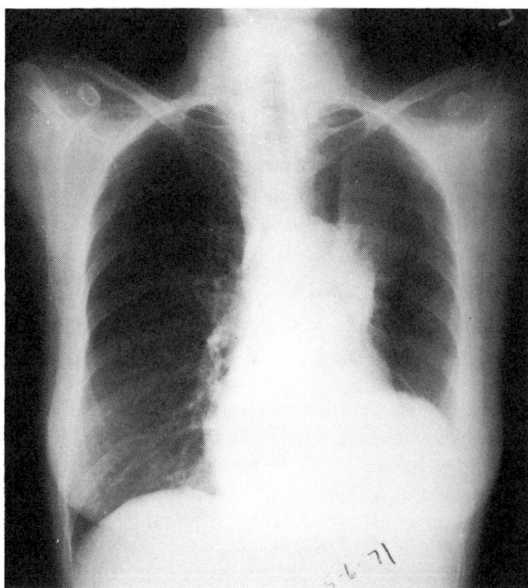

FIGURE 21–2. Posteroanterior chest radiograph of a 57-year-old cigarette smoker with hemoptysis. This film demonstrates left upper lobe collapse with the suspicion of a mass lesion in the region of the left mainstem bronchus. Fiberoptic bronchoscopy revealed that the source of bleeding was an endobronchial carcinoma completely occluding the left mainstem bronchus.

Finally, one cannot always assume that a radiographic abnormality in a patient with hemoptysis is in fact the source of the bleeding. A small peripheral lung nodule or apical pleural thickening, for instance, is almost certainly an incidental x-ray finding, and the cause of the hemoptysis must be sought elsewhere. In such a circumstance, the approach to the hemoptysis is the same as for the patient with a normal chest radiograph, as discussed next.

Hemoptysis with a Normal Chest Radiograph. In these patients, the most common diagnosis is tracheobronchitis (usually chronic bronchitis), although equally often no explanation can be found.[3, 8] A small percentage of patients with bronchiectasis will have a normal chest film, and bleeding may originate from this radiographically occult bronchial site. Bronchoscopy alone generally does not identify areas of bronchiectasis; computed tomography (CT) of the chest is necessary for this purpose. In most cases of hemoptysis with a normal chest film, bronchoscopy reveals either nonspecific findings of bronchial wall inflammation (in bronchitis or bronchiectasis) or no abnormality at all (when the lesion is beyond the range of vision of the bronchoscope or in cases of idiopathic hemoptysis).

The disturbing problem, however, is that lung cancer may also be the cause of hemoptysis with a negative result on a chest radiograph. Although in most cases of lung cancer hemoptysis is a late manifestation of an easily visible radiographic lesion, in a small percentage of patients early endobronchial cancer may cause bleeding when still too small to be detected by x-ray. Such a lesion could be easily detected with bronchoscopy and might represent a curable lung cancer. Other less common causes of hemoptysis with a clear chest film include laryngeal or nasopharyngeal carcinoma, mitral stenosis, pulmonary embolism, severe thrombocytopenia, and postoperative granulation tissue.

In addition to a careful history and physical examination, as outlined, the work-up of the patient with a normal chest radiograph who coughs up blood in most cases should include the following: blood for coagulation studies (prothrombin time, partial thromboplastin time, platelet count, and in some cases a bleeding time), ear, nose, and throat evaluation with indirect or direct fiberoptic laryngoscopy, and sputum samples for cytologic study. If the results of all these studies are normal or nondiagnostic, the next big question is whether fiberoptic bronchoscopy should be pursued.

FIBEROPTIC BRONCHOSCOPY

The introduction of the fiberoptic bronchoscope into the United States in 1971 revolutionized the practice of pulmonary medicine. The greater ease of the procedure compared with rigid bronchoscopy—for patients and operator alike—meant that many more procedures could be done, predominantly on an outpatient basis, and pulmonary physicians could perform them as well as thoracic surgeons. Furthermore, the extent of the tracheobronchial tree that could be visualized was extended far distally, to subsubsegmental bronchi and beyond.

Techniques used in performing fiberoptic bronchoscopy on ambulatory patients vary among bronchoscopists, both in terms of preparing the patient and passing the instrument. One commonly used approach is as follows: The fasting patient arrives in the endoscopy suite in the morning and receives premedication with parenteral meperidine or morphine and atropine. Then, with the patient reclining on a hospital bed, a 4% lidocaine solution is nebulized onto the nares and pharynx. Supplemental oxygen is given by way of a face mask. Through a hole cut in the face mask, the bronchoscope (with a diameter of 5 mm) is passed transnasally into the posterior pharynx and through the vocal cords into the tracheobronchial tree. Additional topical anesthesia (1% lidocaine) is delivered to the airways through the bronchoscope, and additional sedation with midazolam is given intravenously as needed. Detailed examination of all accessible bronchial branches in both lungs, with sampling of suspicious areas, takes an average time of approximately 20 to 40 minutes.

Specimens can be collected in the following manner: Saline can be lavaged through a central channel in the bronchoscope and then aspirated back by applying suction (bronchial washings and bronchoalveolar lavage). Also, a fine brush at the end of a long sheathed wire can be rubbed along the bronchial mucosa or surface of an endobronchial lesion; the material collected on the brush is then prepared for cytologic examination (bronchial brushings). Biopsies can be obtained by using a forceps device passed through the bronchoscope lumen (bronchial and transbronchial lung biopsies). Under special circumstances, reliable specimens for bacterial culture can be retrieved from the lung without contamination from nasopharyngeal flora using a double-sheathed sampling brush, and paratracheal or peribronchial lymph nodes or masses can be aspirated by a specially designed needle passed through the tracheal or bronchial wall.

Contraindications to bronchoscopy are an uncooperative patient, a refractory bleeding disorder, and uncorrectable hypoxemia. Relative contraindications include severe asthma, hypercapnia, and superior vena cava syndrome.

Several reports of the yield of fiberoptic bronchoscopy in evaluating the patient with hemoptysis describe a 70 to 90% success rate in establishing a specific diagnosis.[3, 8, 9] However, if the finding of "bronchitis" on inspection of the bronchial mucosa is not accepted as definitive diagnosis of the cause of hemoptysis, then the yield falls to below 50%.[2] In the subgroup of patients with hemoptysis and a normal chest radiograph, a specific diagnosis (other than "chronic bronchitis") is made in only 10 to 20% of the cases.[2] One is more likely to identify an active bleeding site or lung segment as a source of the bleeding when bronchoscopy is performed during or within 48 hours of active hemoptysis.[2] Even under these optimal circumstances, however, one fails to visualize the source of bleeding in most patients in whom hemoptysis is accompanied by no radiographic abnormality.

In most cases, then, the purpose of performing fiberoptic bronchoscopy routinely in patients with hemoptysis plus a clear chest film is primarily to find (or exclude) those with early and potentially curable endobronchial carcinomas. The frequency with which radiographically occult lung cancers are found in patients with hemoptysis has been reported in some series to be as high as 16 to 22%,[10, 11] but these figures are undoubtedly inflated by the selection bias of referral populations. One series reported no cancers found among 72 such patients examined.[12] The precise frequency of early malignancies among a general ambulatory population with hemoptysis and a normal or nonlocalizing chest x-ray is unknown, but it is likely to be significantly less than the 7% shown in Table 21–2, based on cumulative data from eleven reported series.[2, 3, 9–17]

The cost of fiberoptic bronchoscopy (based on the average reimbursement by third-party payers in Massachusetts in 1992) is approximately $700. The risk of the procedure is small. Large retrospective surveys of over 70,000 fiberoptic bronchoscopies revealed a mortality rate of approximately 0.01% with major complications occurring in 0.1 to 0.3% of cases.[18, 19] A smaller series in which data were collected prospectively gave higher mortality (0.1%) and morbidity (1.7% for major complications) rates.[20] Major complications included pneumonia, pneumothorax (>20%), severe airway obstruction, and respiratory arrest. High-risk patients (e.g., with asthma, a partially obstructed bronchus, or cardiac disease) accounted for a significant proportion of these complications. Pneumothorax is a potential complication of transbronchial lung biopsy or needle aspiration, procedures infrequently indicated in the evaluation of hemoptysis.

TABLE 21–2. YIELD OF FIBEROPTIC BRONCHOSCOPY IN HEMOPTYSIS AND A NEGATIVE RESULT ON A CHEST RADIOGRAPH

	No. of Patients with Hemoptysis and Normal Chest Radiograph	No. Found to Have Lung Cancer	(%)
Rath et al[9]	17	1	(6)
Zavala[10]	55	9	(16)
Weaver et al[2]	15	0	(0)
Kalenbach et al[11]	32	7	(22)
Gong et al[3]	42	3	(7)
Dreisin et al[13]	19	2	(11)
Donlan et al[12]	72	0	(0)
Peters et al[14]	26	0	(0)
Poe et al[15]	196	12	(6)
Lederle et al[16]	106	6	(6)
O'Neil et al[17]	119	6	(5)
TOTAL	699	46	7

With this information it is not possible to perform a precise cost-benefit analysis of fiberoptic bronchoscopy in the evaluation of hemoptysis in patients with normal chest radiographs. The cost of finding one occult lung cancer is probably at least $10,000 and may well be ten times as great. To find a curable lung cancer would be even more costly. On the other hand, the psychologic benefit to the patient who can be reassured about the absence of a malignant lesion must be factored into the equation as well. We conclude, as have others,[3] that selection of patients at increased risk for lung cancer by virtue of age (> 40 years), cigarette-smoking history, or persistence of bleeding beyond a day or two is likely to maximize the yield from fiberoptic bronchoscopy in this setting and justify its use as a case-finding tool.

MANAGEMENT

Only with large amounts of hemoptysis (e.g., a cupful of blood or more within 24 hours) or serious underlying cardiopulmonary disease is it necessary to hospitalize the patient for observation or emergent intervention. Most hemoptysis remains minor in amount, permitting time for the initial evaluation to begin in the physician's office. Besides a careful history and general physical examination, in most instances this work-up includes blood studies to assess for a bleeding disorder, a chest radiograph, and, as appropriate, sputum for cultures or cytologic study. Further evaluation is then made of abnormalities detected on these initial screening procedures, particularly an abnormal finding on chest radiograph. If the chest radiograph and the other studies are normal, fiberoptic bronchoscopy is probably indicated in patients over the age of 40 years, who have more than just a day or two of hemoptysis, have a history of cigarette smoking, or are unreliable with respect to medical follow-up. For patients failing to meet these criteria or who have a contraindication to the procedure, a chest CT scan can be useful in localizing the bleeding source.[21, 22] Alternatively, a follow-up chest film may be obtained after 6 weeks, 3 months, and 6 months to exclude the delayed radiographic appearance of a specific source of the bleeding, particularly a lung cancer. Circumstances meriting special and often individualized attention are discussed next.

Young Adult with Hemoptysis. In patients younger than 35 to 40 years of age, the cigarette-induced lung diseases of chronic bronchitis and cancer are uncommon, and thus the spectrum of diseases causing hemoptysis changes. Among the primary pulmonary diseases to consider, bronchiectasis and bronchial adenoma are probably the most common. Bronchiectasis usually develops in early childhood and manifests as chronic or recurrent cough with purulent sputum production. This is also true for cystic fibrosis, a condition characterized by generalized bronchiectasis. However, in some cases of bronchiectasis, symptoms may first develop or become troubling in early adulthood, and hemoptysis may be the presenting complaint. Bronchial adenoma typically grows as a polypoid lesion within central airways, causing a postobstructive pneumonia or lobar or segmental atelectasis due to proximal obstruction.

In this younger population, cardiac (e.g., mitral stenosis) and pulmonary vascular diseases (e.g., pulmonary emboli or primary pulmonary hypertension) are important considerations, as are the pulmonary-renal hemorrhage syndromes (e.g., systemic lupus erythematosus, Wegener's granulomatosis, and Goodpasture's syndrome). Toxic inhalations (e.g., "crack lung" due to inhaled freebase cocaine) may cause hemoptysis. Catamenial hemoptysis due to endometriosis, presenting as perimenstrual hemoptysis, is exceedingly rare.

Recurrent Hemoptysis. The patient with unexplained hemoptysis that recurs or persists over a period of weeks or months poses an especially puzzling clinical problem. In those with a chest film abnormality, special studies may help to elucidate the radiographic finding. In selected patients, lung scanning, chest CT scanning, or bronchial arteriography may be indicated. The role of repeated fiberoptic bronchoscopies was evaluated in one series of 14 patients.[23] In 4 of 14 patients (29%), a diagnosis of malignancy was established at repeat bronchoscopy performed 1 to 15 months after the original procedure. Strict guidelines on when and how often to repeat bronchoscopy in the patient with recurrent hemoptysis despite a normal chest radiograph and at high risk for lung cancer (i.e., the older cigarette smoker) cannot be given. Close follow-up with serial chest films is certainly warranted, along with collection of sputum specimens for cytologic study. A second fiberoptic bronchoscopy performed after 2 to 3 months, repeated one or more times, may be warranted in some patients.

Massive Hemoptysis. Management of the patient with massive hemoptysis (defined variously as more than 100 to 600 ml of blood expectorated within 24 hours) is entirely different from the approach to lesser amounts of hemoptysis. Massive hemoptysis poses a risk of sudden death from asphyxiation when aspiration of large amounts of blood occurs, often superimposed on severely compromised baseline lung function. The most common causes of massive hemoptysis in several modern-day reported series are tuberculosis, active or inactive, followed by bronchiectasis and necrotizing pneumonia or lung abscess.[24–26] Lung cancer and mycetomas may also cause life-threatening hemoptysis on occasion.

Patients with massive hemoptysis should be hospitalized, and a thoracic surgeon should be involved in their care quickly. It is desirable to localize the source of bleeding early. Fiberoptic bronchoscopy should be performed via an endotracheal tube to ensure adequacy of ventilation. In some cases, rigid bronchoscopy is needed for this purpose. Radionuclide lung scanning using ^{99m}Tc sulfur colloid or tagged erythrocytes has been shown to be effective in localizing the site of massive pulmonary hemorrhage.[27] This noninvasive technique may prove as useful as bronchoscopy if one's goal is simply to identify which lung is the source of bleeding.

Conservative treatment measures include bedrest with the patient positioned so as to have the bleeding lung dependent (to prevent aspiration of blood into the uninvolved lung) and with close monitoring of arterial blood gases and serial radiographs. Codeine may be used cautiously to suppress cough if bleeding seems triggered or exacerbated by paroxysms of coughing, but oversedation must be scrupulously avoided to prevent respiratory depression with "drowning" in intra-airway blood.

Immediate surgery in the operable patient with massive hemoptysis is debated. In one series of patients treated medically, the majority stopped bleeding within 4 days, and only one operable patient (2%) died of pulmonary hemorrhage.[26] However, others have reported a 50% or greater mortality with use of this conservative approach and strongly recommend surgical treatment.[24] Since explosive pulmonary hemorrhage may cause death within minutes and one cannot predict in whom this catastrophic event will occur, we too favor a surgical approach when localized resectable disease can be identified as the bleeding source.[28] In patients in whom diffuse disease, an unidentified bleeding source, or limited cardiopulmonary reserve precludes surgery, other measures have been used to control persistent hemorrhage. Most effective among these techniques is bronchial artery embolization, particularly in patients with bronchiectasis, but experienced angiographers are needed to perform the procedure, and a potential complication is spinal cord injury due to accidental spinal cord artery embolization.[30] Temporizing methods include endobronchial control with balloon tamponade (using a Fogarty catheter), topical thrombin,[29] iced saline lavage, or gauze packing. Measures thought not to be effective include systemic administration of pitressin, ϵ-aminocaproic acid, or estrogens.

REFERENCES

1. American Thoracic Society: The management of hemoptysis—a statement by the Committee on Therapy. Am Rev Respir Dis 93:471, 1966.
2. Weaver LJ, Solliday N, and Cagell DW: Selection of patients with hemoptysis for fiberoptic bronchoscopy. Chest 76:7, 1979.
3. Gong H Jr and Salvatierra C: Clinical efficacy of early and delayed bronchoscopy in patients with hemoptysis. Am Rev Respir Dis 124:221, 1981.
4. Santiago S, Tobias J, and Williams AJ: A reappraisal of the causes of hemoptysis. Arch Intern Med 151:2449, 1991.
5. Rodman MH and Jones CW: Catamenial hemoptysis due to bronchial endometriosis. N Engl J Med 266:805, 1962.
6. Lyons HA: Differential diagnosis of hemoptysis and its treatment. Basics Resp Dis 5:1, 1976.
7. Martini N and McCormick PM: Assessment of endoscopically visible bronchogenic carcinomas. Chest 73(Suppl):718, 1978.

8. Smiddy JF and Elliott RC: The evaluation of hemoptysis with fiberoptic bronchoscopy. Chest 64:158, 1973.
9. Rath GS, Schaff JT, and Snider GL: Flexible fiberoptic bronchoscopy: Techniques and review of 100 bronchoscopies. Chest 63:689, 1973.
10. Zavala DC: Diagnostic fiberoptic bronchoscopy: Technique and results of biopsy in 600 patients. Chest 68:12, 1975.
11. Kallenbach J, Song E, and Zori S: Hemoptysis with no radiological evidence of tumor—the value of early bronchoscopy. S Afr Med J 59:556, 1981.
12. Donlan CJ Jr, Foreman DR, and Klayton RJ: Fiberoptic bronchoscopy in nonhospitalized patients. Arch Intern Med 138:698, 1978.
13. Dreisin RB, Albert RK, Talley PA, et al: Flexible fiberoptic bronchoscopy in the teaching hospital: Yield and complications. Chest 74:144, 1978.
14. Peters J, McClung HC, and Teague RB: Evaluation of hemoptysis in patients with a normal chest roentgenogram. West J Med 141:624, 1984.
15. Poe RH, Israel RH, Marin MG, et al: Utility of fiberoptic bronchoscopy in patients with hemoptysis and a nonlocalizing chest roentgenogram. Chest 92:70, 1988.
16. Lederle FA, Nichol KL, and Parenti CM: Bronchoscopy to evaluate hemoptysis in older men with nonsuspicious chest roentgenograms. Chest 95:1043, 1989.
17. O'Neill KM and Lazarus AA: Hemoptysis: Indications for bronchoscopy. Arch Intern Med 151:171, 1991.
18. Credle WF Jr, Smiddy JF, and Elliott RC: Complications of fiberoptic bronchoscopy. Am Rev Respir Dis 109:67, 1974.
19. Suratt PM, Smiddy JF, and Bruber B: Deaths and complications associated with fiberoptic bronchoscopy. Chest 69:747, 1976.
20. Pereira W Jr, Kovnat DM, and Snider GL: A prospective cooperative study of complications following flexible fiberoptic bronchoscopy. Chest 73:813, 1978.
21. Haponik EF, Britt EJ, Smith PL, et al: Computed chest tomography in the evaluation of hemoptysis: Impact on diagnosis and treatment. Chest 91:80, 1987.
22. Naidich DP, Funt S, Ettenger NA, et al: Hemoptysis: CT-bronchoscopic correlations in 58 cases. Radiology 177:357, 1990.
23. Gong H Jr: Repeat fiberoptic bronchoscopy in patients with recurrent, unexplained hemoptysis. Respiration 44:225, 1983.
24. Crocco JA, Rooney JJ, Fankushen DS, et al: Massive hemoptysis. Arch Intern Med 121:495, 1968.
25. Conlan AA, Hurwitz SS, Krige L, et al: Massive hemoptysis: Review of 123 cases. J Thorac Cardiovasc Surg 85:120, 1983.
26. Bobrowitz ID, Ramakrishna S, and Shim Y-S: Comparison of medical versus surgical treatment of major hemoptysis. Arch Intern Med 143:1343, 1983.
27. Haponik EF, Rothfeld B, Britt EJ, et al: Radionuclide localization of massive pulmonary hemorrhage. Chest 86:208, 1984.
28. Thompson HB, Teschler H, and Rennard SI: Pathogenesis, evaluation, and therapy for massive hemoptysis. Clin Chest Med 13:69, 1992.
29. Tsukamoto T, Sasaki H, and Nakamura H: Treatment of hemoptysis patients by thrombin and fibrinogen-thrombin infusion therapy using a fiberoptic bronchoscope. Chest 96:473, 1989.
30. Rémy J, Arnaud A, Fardou H, et al: Treatment of hemoptysis by embolization of bronchial arteries. Radiology 122:33, 1977.

22

Solitary Pulmonary Nodule

CHRISTOPHER H. FANTA, MD

Decisions regarding the evaluation of solitary pulmonary nodules frequently fall within the domain of the primary health care provider. These "coin lesions" are generally asymptomatic; they are most often detected on chest radiographs obtained for reasons unrelated to the nodule, such as routine screening, trauma, or respiratory tract infection.[1] The first decision is probably the most crucial: whether to pursue further evaluation of the radiographic abnormality. The current epidemic of cancer of the lung has made this decision crucial. More than 170,000 new cases of lung cancer will be identified in the United States this year.[2] The 5-year survival for patients undergoing resection of a lung cancer presenting as a solitary nodule less than 2 cm in diameter exceeds 50%,[3, 4] the 5-year survival for unresectable lung cancer is less than 5%.[5] Phrased in another way, some solitary pulmonary nodules are lung cancers in a curable stage; if left untreated, they progress to become inoperable and fatal. Thus, virtually every pulmonary nodule, regardless of how small, must be evaluated for the possibility that it may represent bronchogenic carcinoma.

The extent of this work-up varies, from review of previous chest radiographs in some patients to diagnostic chest surgery in others, but it begins most importantly with the determination not to ignore a pulmonary nodule simply because it is asymptomatic. The work-up then focuses on two key questions: (1) Is the nodule a lung cancer?; and (2) if it is or may be a lung cancer, is it surgically resectable?

DIFFERENTIAL DIAGNOSIS

A solitary pulmonary nodule can be defined as a single, relatively well-circumscribed, rounded or oval density surrounded by aerated lung. Masses larger than 4 cm in diameter or invading chest wall, hilum, or mediastinum are generally excluded from this designation. A central nodule with smaller surrounding nodules, referred to as "satellite lesions," can be thought of under the same rubric, but multiple nodules scattered throughout the lung fields present a separate problem of differential diagnosis and management.

More than 80 different etiologies have been identified as causes of solitary lung nodules, but the major differentiation is between benign and malignant disease. Malignant solitary nodules are most often primary bronchogenic carcinomas; metastatic cancers make up only 5 to 10% of cases in most series.[1, 6] The relative frequencies of the major histologic types of lung cancer vary among different reports. In general, however, adenocarcinoma is the most frequently encountered cell type; small cell undifferentiated carcinoma (of which the oat cell type constitutes the majority) is the least common, being present only in approximately 5% of cases.[3] In the United States, benign solitary nodules are generally either granulomatous disease (e.g., tuberculoma) or benign neoplasms (e.g., hamartoma, bronchial adenoma). In areas of the country endemic for fungal infections, solitary nodules have an increased prevalence, with a preponderance of histoplasmomas or coccidioidomas. Elsewhere in the world (e.g., the Orient), echinococcal cysts are the first consideration in the differential diagnosis. A great many miscellaneous causes of benign solitary nodules exist, including lung abscess, arteriovenous malformation, intrapulmonary lymph node, mucoid impaction, round atelectasis, bronchogenic cyst, and dirofilariasis ("dog heartworm").

The differential diagnosis of solitary pulmonary nodules can be viewed in another, entirely pragmatic way, as a dichotomy between primary bronchogenic carcinoma and all other causes. The optimal treatment of the former in most cases is immediate surgical resection; management of all other conditions may be simple observation, medical therapy, or surgery. Even if the latter is indicated (as for bronchial adenoma, for example, because of its potential for local invasion and occasionally malignant degeneration), there is minimal risk in delay during a period of observation. Thus, the primary question in the differential diagnosis reduces to the following: Is the nodule—or could the nodule be—a primary lung cancer? The frequency of bronchogenic carcinoma among reported series of resected pulmonary nodules varies from less than 10% to over 50%.[1, 6–8] Three factors that influence the likelihood of lung cancer are (1) cigarette smoking or having quit smoking less than 15 years ago; if cigarette smoking is combined with significant asbestos exposure, the risk of developing a lung cancer rises astronomically; (2) increasing age; in patients younger than 35 years of age, less than 5% of solitary nodules are malignant, whereas in patients older than 60 years of age, more than 50% are malignant in at least some series[8, 9]; and (3) geographic location; as mentioned, the percentage of malignant nodules diminishes in areas endemic for certain fungal organisms.

DIAGNOSTIC EVALUATION—IS THIS SOLITARY NODULE A LUNG CANCER?

History and Physical Examination

The patient's clinical presentation only occasionally helps to suggest the benign or malignant cause of a newly discovered lung nodule. For instance, an alcoholic with poor oral hygiene and recent loss of consciousness who has fever, purulent sputum production, and a rounded opacity in the lower lobe that has ill-defined margins probably has an anaerobic lung abscess. On the other hand, if a left upper lobe nodule is associated with mediastinal widening in a middle-aged cigarette smoker who has cough, weight loss, and hoarseness, the most likely diagnosis is lung cancer with recurrent laryngeal nerve involvement. However, in most cases the patient is free of symptoms or has only nonspecific symptoms such as cough. In this circumstance, the history serves mainly to assign a "prior probability" that the patient does or does not have lung cancer, based on age, cigarette smoking history, asbestos exposure, and geographic location. This estimate of the likelihood of lung cancer will guide one's clinical approach to the solitary nodule, as outlined later.[10]

Finding clubbing of the fingers and toes on physical examination leads one to suspect a primary lung cancer, but this finding is by no means diagnostic since a variety of chronic inflammatory pulmonary conditions, such as bronchiectasis and idiopathic pulmonary fibrosis, may also cause clubbing. The role of the physical examination in the diagnostic evaluation of solitary nodules is primarily to search for evidence of an extrathoracic primary malignancy from which the lung nodule might be a solitary metastasis. For example, the finding of a large, hard breast mass increases the likelihood that a lung nodule on chest radiograph is metastatic adenocarcinoma and might lead to a different diagnostic strategy. Examination of skin, thyroid, breasts, testes, prostate, uterus, and ovaries is particularly important in this regard. A normal examination, combined with negative findings on laboratory studies for occult blood in urine and stool, makes metastasis an unlikely cause of a single lung nodule. It is our practice *not* to perform any additional diagnostic tests (e.g., intravenous pyelogram or barium studies of the gastrointestinal tract) to exclude an extrathoracic primary malignancy under these circumstances.

The Chest Radiograph

Two radiographic features of a solitary nodule can reliably exclude a diagnosis of lung cancer: calcification of the nodule in a characteristic pattern, and its failure to increase significantly in size over an extended time (usually defined as 2 years or more).

1. Calcification. Calcium is virtually never deposited into lung cancers in amounts visible by conventional radiography (and only rarely is apparent in certain metastatic neoplasms, such as osteogenic sarcoma and papillary adenocarcinoma of the thyroid). Thus, homogeneously calcified nodules (an example of which is the calcified lower lobe granuloma or Ghon lesion of previous primary tuberculosis) or nodules that display calcium deposited in a central nidus ("target" or "bull's eye" lesion), in a ring or laminated pattern, or in a collection of dense clumps ("popcorn ball" calcification) are usually granulomas or hamartomas and are reliably identified as benign. Rarely, a peripheral lung cancer may engulf a pre-existing calcified granuloma; the resultant malignant lung nodule will have a small, eccentric focus of calcium within it.[11] Therefore, small, peripherally located foci of calcium, though often a manifestation of benign disease, are not of sufficient specificity to exclude lung cancer as the cause of the nodule. The presence or absence of calcium within a pulmonary nodule is a subjective determination, and in ambiguous cases there may be considerable interobserver disagreement. Calcifications can be highlighted by low-kilovoltage chest radiographs, fluoroscopic spot films, or computed tomography (CT).

2. Radiographic Stability. The rate of growth of nodular lung cancers can readily be determined from serial chest radiographs, if available. It appears that in general lung cancers have a relatively constant exponential rate of growth; that is, their *volume* doubles at a relatively fixed interval. Calculations made from a number of lung cancers followed over time indicate that the doubling time for individual cancers varies from 10 to 460 days.[19] Despite reported exceptions, it is generally true that nodules that do not double their volume (i.e., increase diameter by 26%) in less than 460 days are benign. A conservative and useful application of this concept is that a nodule that has remained unchanged in size for at least 2 years is benign. At the other extreme, a nodule that doubles its volume in less than 10 days is likewise usually benign, such as a round pneumonia.

3. Other Radiographic Features. Certain aspects of the radiographic appearance of a nodule, particularly its size, margins, contour, and the presence or absence of satellite lesions, may favor a benign or malignant etiology. Table 22–1 lists these features and their relative significance in categorizing pulmonary nodules. These radiographic signs are not of sufficient predictive value, either singly or in combination, to establish a definitive diagnosis of benign or malignant disease, but they may influence the prior probability of lung cancer and thus may affect management decision. Thus, a large nodule with irregular margins and a notched or indented contour and no satellite lesions is most likely malignant, whereas a small (<2 cm) nodule with sharp margins and a smooth, rounded contour, especially in association with satellite nodules, is probably granulomatous. Predictions based on these radiographic features are at best only 75% accurate, however[20]; unlike patterns of calcification or rate of nodule growth they cannot be relied upon to establish definitively the benign etiology of any given lung nodule.

TABLE 22–1. SIGNIFICANCE OF RADIOGRAPHIC APPEARANCE OF SOLITARY PULMONARY NODULE

Radiographic Pattern		Favors Benign Disease	Favors Malignant Disease
Size:	≤2 cm	+	
	≥4 cm		+ +
Margins:	Sharp	+	
	Hazy or indistinct		+ +
Contour:	Smooth	+	
	Lobulated or irregular		+
Presence of satellite lesions		+ + +	
Presence of cavitation		—	—

4. Chest CT Scan. Using CT scanning one can distinguish among the densities or attenuations of pulmonary nodules to a greater degree than with chest radiography or conventional tomography. Some investigators have reported that among nodules noncalcified by conventional radiographic techniques, those with the greatest density (having a high calculated "attenuation coefficient") are reliably benign nodules, whereas those that are less dense may be benign or malignant nodules.[12] The technique of CT densitometry gave promise of being able to identify the benignity of a significant number of noncalcified lung nodules without invasive diagnostic procedures. However, other investigators found that the CT attenuation coefficients of benign and malignant nodules overlap completely and are not a useful discriminant.[13] Technical variation among different CT scanners appears to account to a large extent for these differences, so that criteria for benign nodules established on one machine are not applicable to the next.

In an attempt to overcome this technical variability, chest CT "phantoms" have been designed; these are epoxy resin models of transverse sections of the chest with a calcium carbonate (phantom) nodule of known CT density placed within them. If the patient's nodule is found to be denser than the reference nodule, the patient's nodule is said to be benign.[14] Impressive accuracy was demonstrated for this technique in a large, multicenter trial.[15] Nonetheless, a small but significant false-negative rate still exists; that is, CT densitometry using phantom nodules may give erroneous reassurance that a malignant pulmonary nodule is benign.[16] Because this technique can be used only to weigh the likelihood of a lesion being benign or malignant and cannot provide a definitive assessment, it has not found widespread use in routine clinical practice. Research continues into radiographic characteristics that might serve to differentiate benign from malignant lung nodules, including position emission tomography[17] and CT scanning using an iodinated contrast agent.[18]

Skin Testing

Intradermal skin testing to evaluate the delayed hypersensitivity response to tuberculin or fungal proteins has no diagnostic value in assessing lung nodules. Both positive and negative results are commonly found in patients with a lung cancer, thus the test cannot distinguish malignancy from granulomas.

Sputum Cytology

The yield of malignant cells found on cytologic examination of expectorated sputum varies from less than 1 to 34% among reported series of lung cancers presenting as solitary pulmonary nodules.[6, 21] The latter series (a 34% detection rate) included cytologic examination of bronchial secretions obtained at bronchoscopy and involved a group of particularly large nodules (the mean diameter of nodules with positive findings on cytologic examination was 4.8 cm).[21] Factors influencing the percentage of positive results include the number of sputum samples examined (three specimens optimize the yield), the care in preserving and preparing the specimens, the size of the nodule, and its proximity to the mainstem bronchi. Sputum cytology is rarely diagnostic in peripheral lesions less than 2 cm in diameter. In fact, if malignant cells are found in the sputum of a patient with a 1- to 2-cm peripheral lung nodule, serious consideration should be given to an alternative source for the neoplastic cells, such as an oropharyngeal or laryngeal cancer or a centrally located, radiographically occult lung cancer.

Percutaneous Needle Aspiration

In the hands of skilled operators, needle aspiration (with or without biopsy) will correctly identify 90 to 95% of peripheral lung cancers, with 5% or fewer false-positives.[22, 23] The greatest utility of a diagnostic test in the preoperative assessment of a lung nodule, however, is in establishing a definitive diagnosis of benignity, so that chest surgery can be avoided. Among a number of published reports, as shown in Table 22–2, the frequency with which needle aspiration establishes a specific etiology for benign nodules averages only about 20% (range: 0 to 45%). In one large series of 650 patients, benign lesions were accurately identified with a definitive diagnosis in 93 of 137 cases (68%). This experience remains the exception rather than the rule, however, being a tribute to the skill and expertise of the particular operator and associated pathologist and cytologist.[30]

In the remainder of benign lesions, a result of "nonspecific inflammatory cells" is usually obtained. Does "nonspecific inflammation" on needle aspiration reliably exclude a lung cancer? The answer may be *yes* if a highly experienced operator is confident that the aspirating needle entered the lung nodule, if the cytopathologist confirms that a sample of abnormal tissue was obtained, and if the procedure is repeated two or three times when a nonspecific result is first obtained.[22, 23] On the other hand, the answer is probably more often *no* given an operator of only average expertise, especially for small nodules more easily missed by the aspirating needle. In 25% or more instances, the nonspecific inflammatory cells will have been obtained from tissue surrounding a lung cancer and will represent a false-negative result.[24, 25, 28, 29] Thus, a finding of nonspecific inflammation on needle aspiration in most cases is best considered nondiagnostic.

Percutaneous needle aspiration is usually performed as an outpatient procedure. No premedication, other than perhaps some mild sedation, is needed. After sterile preparation of the skin and topical anesthesia, the sampling needle is advanced under fluoroscopic or CT scan guidance into the center of the nodule, and suction is applied to an attached syringe. The aspirate is both spread onto glass slides and spun down into a cellular pellet for cytologic examination. A variety of needles have been used in this procedure, with a recent tendency toward thinner needles (22- to 25-gauge) without a cutting edge; these have a lower risk of serious complications but less often provide a core of tissue for histologic examination (i.e., a biopsy). The most common complication is pneumothorax, which occurs in 10 to 30% of cases and is of sufficient magnitude to require drainage in approximately half of these. Serious hemoptysis is unusual.

Fiberoptic Bronchoscopy

The accuracy of fiberoptic bronchoscopy in diagnosing peripheral nodules is inferior to that of percutaneous needle aspiration.[27, 28] Using standard techniques, including bronchial washings, bronchial brushing, and fluoroscopically guided transbronchial lung biopsy, only approximately 60% of endoscopically nonvisible lung cancers will be correctly diagnosed by bronchoscopic sampling; the reported yield for peripheral lesions less than 2 cm in diameter ranges from 0 to 28%.[27, 31, 32] Equally important, the frequency of establishing a specific diagnosis of a benign disease is low, and a result demonstrating nonspecific benign inflammatory cells by no means excludes malignancy.

In patients with lung cancer, fiberoptic bronchoscopy can provide useful information independent of sampling from the nodule itself. First, by examining the bronchial anatomy, it can define the proximal extent of tumor spread and help to guide surgical resection margins, an indication relevant only to relatively large, centrally located cancers. Second, preoperative bronchoscopy can serve to rule out a second, radiographically invisible, synchronous primary lung cancer, admittedly an infrequently encountered problem but one that might alter the therapeutic approach. A separate diagnostic bronchoscopy is not warranted for these two indications alone; it can be performed in the anesthetized patient in the operating room by the thoracic surgeon immediately prior to pulmonary resection.

DIAGNOSTIC EVALUATION—IS THIS (POTENTIAL) LUNG CANCER RESECTABLE?

If a solitary pulmonary nodule has been proved to be a lung cancer, or if a definite benign diagnosis has not been established and thoracic surgery is contemplated for diagnosis, some assessment of the resectability of the lesion should be made prior to surgical referral. Because we are addressing here only nodules surrounded by aerated lung, contiguous spread by direct invasion into the diaphragm, chest wall, or mediastinum is not a consideration. However, nodular lung cancers can metastasize to hilar or mediastinal lymph nodes or to extrathoracic sites, particularly

TABLE 22–2. PERCUTANEOUS NEEDLE ASPIRATION: RESULTS IN BENIGN NODULES*

Reference	No. of Lesions	Specific Diagnosis (%)	Nonspecific Inflammation (%)	False-Positive for Malignancy (%)
Poe et al[24]	17	3 (18)	13 (76)	1 (6)
Zelch et al[25]	69	9 (13)	60 (87)	0 (0)
Johnson et al[26]	62	28 (45)	33 (53)	1 (2)
Wallace et al[27]	24	0 (0)	23 (96)	1 (4)
Mark et al[28]	20	2 (10)	18 (90)	0 (0)
Calhoun et al[29]	98	15 (15)	83 (85)	0 (0)
TOTAL	290	57 (20)	230 (79)	3 (2)

*Includes benign tumors.

liver, bone, brain, and adrenal glands. To what extent should nodal and extrathoracic metastases be sought before surgical resection of a pulmonary nodule?

In recent years the criteria for what constitutes surgically resectable lung cancer have been revised, largely as the result of observations that some patients with lung cancer and lymph node involvement can achieve long-term survival (cure) following resectional surgery. Reflecting this more aggressive surgical approach to lung cancer utilizing novel surgical procedures, a new staging system for lung cancer has been devised (Table 22–3),[33] and patients with ipsilateral mediastinal adenopathy (stage IIIa disease) are now considered to be potential operative candidates.

On the other hand, patients with spread of cancer to the contralateral hilar or mediastinal lymph nodes or to nodes or other sites outside the thorax remain inoperable (stage IIIb or stage IV disease). Experimental multimodality protocols are available for patients with stage IIIb disease in attempts to eliminate cancer outside the hemithorax with chemotherapy sometimes combined with radiation therapy, converting inoperable disease to potentially resectable disease.

History, Physical Examination, and Laboratory Studies

Significant weight loss should alert one to the possibility of disseminated disease even though a specific metastatic site may not be implicated. Hoarseness may indicate mediastinal spread of cancer with recurrent laryngeal nerve involvement. A new or unusual pattern of headaches or focal neurologic symptoms may suggest cerebral metastasis, while persistent skeletal pain may be a symptom of bone metastasis. The following signs should be sought on physical examination: hoarseness, hepatomegaly, focal neurologic abnormalities, and tenderness on percussion over the vertebrae and long bones. Chemical analyses that may give a clue to metastatic lung cancer are the serum calcium, alkaline phosphatase, and hepatic transaminase determinations. Symptoms, physical findings, or laboratory abnormalities that suggest possible metastatic disease need to be further evaluated with the appropriate radionuclide or radiographic imaging techniques before proceeding to thoracotomy.

TABLE 22–3. STAGING OF LUNG CANCER TNM DEFINITIONS (SIMPLIFIED VERSION)

T1	Tumor ≤3 cm in diameter, surrounded by lung or visceral pleura
T2	Tumor >3 cm in diameter; or Any tumor invading visceral pleura; or Any tumor with atelectasis or obstructive pneumonitis involving less than an entire lung.
T3	Any tumor with direct extension into the chest wall, diaphragm, mediastinal pleura, or pericardium.
T4	Any tumor with invasion into mediastinum, heart, great vessels, trachea, esophagus, vertebral body, or main carina; or Any tumor associated with a malignant pleural effusion.
N0	No metastasis to regional lymph nodes
N1	Metastasis to peribronchial or ipsilateral hilar lymph nodes
N2	Metastasis to ipsilateral mediastinal or subcarinal lymph nodes
N3	Metastasis to contralateral hilar or mediastinal lymph nodes; or Metastasis to scalene or supraclavicular lymph nodes
M0	No distant metastasis
M1	Distant metastasis present

	Stages of Lung Cancer		
Stage I	T1	N0	M0
	T2	N0	M0
Stage II	T1	N1	M0
	T2	N1	M0
Stage IIIa	T3	N0	M0
	T3	N1	M0
	T1-3	N2	M0
Stage IIIB	Any T	N3	M0
	T4	Any N	M0
Stage IV	Any T	Any N	M1

Mediastinal Evaluation

The frequency of malignant mediastinal lymph node involvement in bronchogenic carcinoma varies with cell type (most common in small cell undifferentiated cancer; adenocarcinoma and large cell undifferentiated cancer more common than squamous cell cancer), location (central greater than peripheral), and size of the primary lesion. Among non–small cell lung cancers in the lung periphery, less than 4 cm in diameter without evidence of mediastinal widening on plain chest film, malignant mediastinal lymph node involvement is uncommon (< 4%).[34] Chest CT scanning is the best noninvasive technique for assessing the spread of lung cancer to the mediastinum, with a sensitivity of approximately 90% and a low false-positive rate.[35] Thus, a chest CT scan is probably indicated in every patient with a solitary pulmonary nodule; it helps to evaluate calcification of the nodule, assess mediastinal lymph node enlargement, detect the presence of other nodules not detected on conventional radiography, and image the adrenal glands and most of the liver for possible distant metastases.

Whether or not to perform prethoracotomy mediastinoscopy is a surgical decision, and practices vary widely among thoracic surgeons. Without exploring the controversy in any depth, two points are worth making: First, in most cases in which a pulmonary nodule is associated with significant mediastinal adenopathy by CT scan, mediastinoscopy is indicated to exclude nonmalignant lymph node enlargement. A peripheral lung cancer may be associated with benign reactive mediastinal adenopathy, and a potentially curative lung resection should not be denied on the basis of the CT image alone. Second, if a mediastinoscopy is planned before thoracotomy, a CT scan is often useful to guide the surgeon in the selection of lymph nodes to be sampled.

Testing for Extrathoracic Metastases

Among patients undergoing what is thought to be "curative" resection for lung cancer and later succumbing to their cancer, distant metastases are the most common site of recurrence.[36] Although it is desirable to detect extrathoracic metastases preoperatively so as to avoid useless surgery, the value of routine scanning of liver, bones, brain, and adrenal glands in every patient with a peripheral pulmonary nodule has not been established, and practices vary widely. Some thoracic surgeons insist that the preoperative evaluation of every patient include a head CT scan, radionuclide bone scan, and abdominal CT scan (for complete visualization of the liver). Other practitioners do not perform routine multiorgan scanning, not simply for the purpose of cost savings but also because of the potential for false-positive results—such as bone infarcts and rib fractures on radionuclide bone scan or hyperplastic nodules and benign cysts on CT scan of the liver—that confound management. Thus, among patients being considered for resection of a solitary peripheral lung nodule, it may be reasonable to perform an abnormal CT scan only in those who have hepatomegaly or abnormal liver function tests on chemistry profile; to perform a head CT scan only if focal neurologic symptoms or signs are present; and to perform a radionuclide bone scan only in patients with bone pain or tenderness, hypercalcemia, or an elevated serum alkaline phosphatase level. If a diagnosis of lung cancer is known or strongly suspected, a decision to pursue all three types of scans may be made even in the absence of localizing signs of metastatic disease if (1) the large size (≥3 cm) of the nodule makes metastases more likely; (2) mediastinal adenopathy is present; or (3) systemic signs and symptoms (e.g., weight loss and anorexia) give suspicion of widespread disease.

PREOPERATIVE EVALUATION—ASSESSING CARDIOPULMONARY RESERVE

Before referring a patient for resection of a pulmonary nodule, it is the role of the medical physician to assess the patient's operative risk. In a young, otherwise healthy person who can run up several flights of stairs without stopping, no additional testing is necessary. On the other hand, an elderly cigarette smoker with coronary artery disease and chronic obstructive pulmonary disease may have a high risk of surgical morbidity and mortality. At a minimum, an electrocardiogram and pulmonary function testing should be performed, and often referral to a specialist is indicated to define precisely, and perhaps to minimize, the operative risk. As a general rule, patients with significant arterial carbon dioxide retention ($PCO_2 > 45$ mm Hg) or an anticipated postoperative 1-second forced expiratory volume (FEV_1) of less than 0.8 liter are considered inoperable.[38]

In recent years chest surgery has been revolutionized by application of endoscopic techniques for the purpose of lung biopsy and resection.[39] Thoracoscopy involves only three small chest incisions, one for the introduction of the thoracoscope with video camera to visualize the lung, the others for the passage of specially designed surgical instruments. The morbidity of the operation is much less than for traditional thoracotomy; hospitalization is reduced to as little as 2 days. Thoracoscopic surgery is particularly suited for wedge resection of peripheral lung nodules, making biopsy and removal of indeterminate lesions much safer. In addition, wedge resection of peripheral lung cancers, considered by some to provide long-term survival rates comparable with those achieved with lobectomy,[40] can be performed in patients with very limited pulmonary reserve.

CLINICAL APPROACH

The approach to the patient with a solitary pulmonary nodule varies, based on the prior probability that the nodule is a lung cancer and on the patient's surgical risk for chest surgery. Detailed management strategies have been specified in recent reviews.[41–43]

The following case example outlines a step-by-step management strategy for a typical patient at high-to-moderate risk for lung cancer but with good cardiopulmonary function: a 55-year-old asymptomatic cigarette-smoking construction worker whose chest radiograph is shown in Figure 22–1.

Step 1. Prior chest films should be assiduously sought and reviewed. Every attempt should be made to obtain the actual radiograph and not simply a descriptive report. If the nodule can be shown to have been present and of the same size 2 or more years earlier, it can be presumed to be benign. In this event the specific etiology of the nodule is unimportant, and no further evaluation is necessary. If chest films from 2 or more years earlier are not available or if the nodule can be shown to be new or enlarging, it should be presumed to be a lung cancer. This working diagnosis should not be altered on the basis of any radiographic features of the nodule, such as smooth margins or a rounded contour, despite the more common association of these findings with benign disease. In certain cases analysis of the rate of growth of the nodule will result in "gray" areas of decision making—for example, a prior chest film showing the nodule unchanged in size over 18 months but no earlier films available; or slight growth of the nodule over 2 years but less than a doubling in its volume—then choices will have to be tailored to individual cases. In general, if the likelihood of cancer is high, such as in this case example, the presumption that the nodule is a lung cancer should be maintained in borderline cases. In this patient, no previous chest films were available.

Step 2. If the plain film is at all suggestive of possible calcifications in the nodule, fluoroscopic spot films or tomography should be obtained. A small, peripherally located fleck of calcium does not alter the suspicion of lung cancer; any other pattern of calcification generally excludes malignancy and terminates the diagnostic work-up. In this case, no calcification was present in the lung nodule.

Step 3. The possibility of an extrathoracic malignancy with a solitary pulmonary metastasis should be sought by careful history-taking, physical examination, urinalysis, and stool analysis for occult blood. If such a cancer exists or was previously present, the likelihood of pulmonary metastasis needs to be assessed, based on a knowledge of the pattern and time course of metastatic spread of specific cancers. CT is the most sensitive technique to search for additional lung nodules that are not visible on the plain chest film. Remember that lung cancer may also occur in patients with other malignancies; in one series, solitary

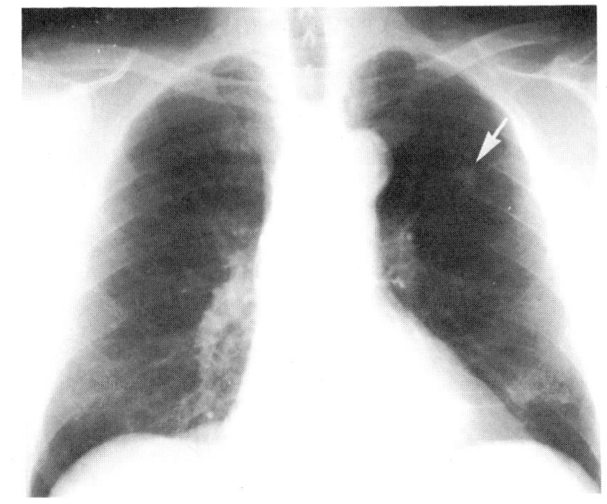

FIGURE 22–1. Posteroanterior chest radiograph of a 55-year-old asymptomatic, cigarette-smoking construction worker. A solitary pulmonary nodule is visible in the left upper lobe (*arrow*).

nodules in patients with prior malignancies were primary lung cancers more than twice as often as they were solitary metastases.[44] History and examination gave no evidence of extrathoracic malignancy in the patient presented here.

Step 4. A chest CT scan is obtained to assess for the presence of significant (>1 cm) mediastinal adenopathy. Enlarged lymph nodes accessible to the mediastinoscope will be sampled by mediastinoscopy or occasionally by transbronchial needle aspiration via the fiberoptic bronchoscope. In some centers, mediastinoscopy is routinely performed in all patients prior to thoracotomy or thoracoscopy for a pulmonary nodule.

Step 5. In the absence of hepatomegaly, abnormal liver function tests, skeletal pain, hypercalcemia, or elevated alkaline phosphatase, no abdominal CT scan or bone scan was obtained in this case example. No head CT scan was done because of the absence of neurologic symptoms or signs. In other patients, clinical or chemical abnormalities should be further evaluated with the appropriate radiographic or scanning procedures, and findings suggestive of metastases should be biopsied, when possible.

Step 6. A patient's cardiopulmonary reserve can be assessed most simply by taking a history, performing an electrocardiogram, and accompanying the patient up two flights of stairs. If no abnormal exercise limitation is apparent and the result of the electrocardiogram is normal (as in this case), no further testing is required. If the patient's activity is limited by dyspnea or chest pain, further evaluation is indicated, including pulmonary function studies and possibly an exercise stress test.

Step 7. This patient was next referred to a thoracic surgeon for a diagnostic and potentially curative surgical resection of his lung nodule. Percutaneous needle aspiration was not attempted because (1) the finding of malignant cells (other than small cell undifferentiated cancer) on the aspirate does not change the management; (2) small cell undifferentiated cancer is uncommonly a cause of peripheral nodules, is not reliably diagnosed cytologically, and in the opinion of some oncologists should be surgically resected if found as a small peripheral lung nodule; (3) a specific benign diagnosis is infrequently made by needle aspiration; and (4) a result of nonspecific inflammatory cells does not rule out lung cancer with sufficient accuracy in this high-risk patient to avoid diagnostic thoracic surgery. In the patient presented here, a large cell undifferentiated cancer was found at operation, and a lobectomy was performed.

Under other clinical circumstances, one may choose to perform needle aspiration prior to considering surgical resection. For instance, if radiographic stability of the nodule for more than 24 months or the presence of calcification cannot be demonstrated, percutaneous needle aspiration may help to avoid surgery in a young patient strongly suspected of having a benign diagnosis because of age, epidemiologic factors, or radiographic features of the nodule (e.g., no change in the nodule size over 12 months). In such a patient, the yield of specific benign diagnoses will be greater than in an unselected group, and nonspecific inflammation found on two or more aspirates may lead to a course of "watchful waiting" with serial follow-up chest films. Likewise, in a patient considered a marginal surgical candidate because of limited cardiopulmonary reserve, a definite preoperative diagnosis of lung cancer by needle aspiration often makes pulmonary resection for an asymptomatic lung nodule more acceptable to the patient and surgeon alike.

Thus, no single paradigm for the evaluation of solitary pulmonary nodules is applicable to all patients. The approach is modified according to the estimated likelihood that the nodule is a primary lung cancer.[10] The approach is further modified if the patient's general medical condition greatly exaggerates the morbidity and mortality of thoracic surgery. In the patient likely to have a primary lung cancer, one should expedite referral for resection if a contraindication (e.g., distant metastases, impaired cardiopulmonary function) cannot be found. In the patient unlikely to have a lung cancer (e.g., younger than 35 years old) or at high risk for surgical complications, every effort should be made to establish a diagnosis without resorting to immediate thoracic surgery, and in some of these cases watchful waiting with serial follow-up chest films may be appropriate.[45]

With this latter approach, radiographic stability of the lesion gives reassurance of its benign etiology, whereas enlargement on a follow-up chest x-ray necessitates the presumption that it is potentially malignant.

REFERENCES

1. Toomes H, Delphendahl A, Manke H-G, et al: The coin lesion of the lung: A review of 955 resected coin lesions. Cancer 51:534, 1983.
2. Boring CC, Squires TS, and Tong T: Cancer statistics, 1993. CA Cancer J Clin 43:7, 1993.
3. Jackman RJ, Good CA, Clagett OT, et al: Survival rates in peripheral bronchogenic carcinomas up to four centimeters in diameter presenting as solitary pulmonary nodules. J Thorac Cardiovasc Surg 57:1, 1969.
4. Steele JD and Buell P: Survival in bronchogenic carcinoma resected as solitary pulmonary nodules. Proc Natl Cancer Conf 6:835, 1970.
5. Mountain CF, Carr DT, and Anderson WAD: A system for clinical staging of lung cancer. Am J Roentgenol 120:130, 1974.
6. Steele JD: The solitary pulmonary nodule: Report of a cooperative study of resected asymptomatic solitary pulmonary nodules in males. J Thorac Cardiovasc Surg 46:21, 1963.
7. Ray JF III, Lawton BR, Magrim GE, et al: The coin lesion story: Update 1976. Chest 70:332, 1976.
8. Bateson EM: An analysis of 155 solitary lung lesions illustrating the differential diagnosis of mixed tumors of the lung. Clin Radiol 16:51, 1965.
9. Trunk G, Gracey DR, and Byrd RB: The management and evaluation of the solitary pulmonary nodule. Chest 66:236, 1974.
10. Cummings SR, Lillington GA, and Richard RJ: Estimating the probability of malignancy in solitary pulmonary nodules: A Bayesian approach. Am Rev Respir Dis 134:449, 1986.
11. O'Keefe ME Jr, Good CA, and McDonald JR: Calcification in solitary nodules of the lung. Am J Roentgenol 77:1023, 1957.
12. Siegelman SS, Zerhouni EA, Leo FP, et al: CT of the solitary pulmonary nodule. Am J Roentgenol 134:1, 1980.
13. Holle RH, Cairns J, Mack L, et al: CT scanning of the solitary pulmonary nodule in Seattle (Abstract). Am Rev Respir Dis 125(Part 2):78, 1982.
14. Zerhouni EA, Boukadoum M, Siddiky MA, et al: A standard phantom for quantitative CT analysis of pulmonary nodules. Radiology 149:767, 1983.
15. Zerhouni EA, Stitik FP, and Siegelman SS: CT of the pulmonary nodule: A cooperative study. Radiology 160:319, 1986.
16. Swensen SJ, Harms GF, Morin RL, et al: CT evaluation of solitary pulmonary nodules: Value of 185-H reference phantom. Am J Roentgenol 156:925, 1991.
17. Gupta NC, Frank AR, Dewan XIA, et al: Solitary pulmonary nodules: Detection of malignancy with PET with 2-[F-18]-fluoro-2-deoxy-D-glucose. Radiology 184:441, 1992.
18. Swensen SJ, Morin RL, Schueler BA, et al: Solitary pulmonary nodule: CT evaluation of enhancement with iodinated contrast material—a preliminary report. Radiology 182:343, 1992.
19. Nathan MH, Collins VP, Adams RA: Differentiation of benign and malignant pulmonary nodules by growth rate. Radiology 79:221, 1962.

20. Templeton AW, Jansen C, Lehr JL, et al: Solitary pulmonary lesions: Computer-aided differential diagnosis and evaluation of mathematical methods. Radiology 89:605, 1967.
21. Attar S, Naib ZM, Cowley RA: Exfoliative cytology in solitary peripheral lesions of the lungs. J Thorac Cardiovasc Surg 42:168, 1961.
22. Sinner WN: Transthoracic needle biopsy of small peripheral malignant lung lesions. Invest Radiol 8:305, 1973.
23. Westcott JL: Direct percutaneous needle aspiration of localized pulmonary lesions: Results in 422 patients. Radiology 137:31, 1980.
24. Poe RH, Tobin RE: Sensitivity and specificity of needle biopsy in lung malignancy. Am Rev Respir Dis 122:725, 1980.
25. Zelch JV, Lalli AF, McCormack LJ, et al: Aspiration biopsy in diagnosis of pulmonary nodule. Chest 63:149, 1973.
26. Johnson RD, Gobien RP, Valicenti JF Jr: Current status of radiologically directed pulmonary thin needle aspiration biopsy. Ann Clin Lab Sci 13:225, 1983.
27. Wallace JM, Deutsch AL: Flexible fiberoptic bronchoscopy and percutaneous needle lung aspiration for evaluating the solitary pulmonary nodule. Chest 81:665, 1982.
28. Mark JBD, Marglin SI, Castellino RA: The role of bronchoscopy and needle aspiration in the diagnosis of peripheral lung masses. J Thorac Cardiovasc Dis 76:266, 1978.
29. Calhoun P, Feldman PS, Armstrong P, et al: The clinical outcome of needle aspirations of the lung when cancer is not diagnosed. Ann Thorac Surg 41:592, 1986.
30. Khouri NF, Stitik FP, Erozan YS, et al: Transthoracic needle aspiration biopsy of benign and malignant lung lesions. Am J Roentgenol 144:281, 1985.
31. Radke JR, Conway WA, Eyler WR, et al: Diagnostic accuracy in peripheral lung lesions: Factors predicting success with flexible fiberoptic bronchoscopy. Chest 76:176, 1979.
32. McDougall JC, Cortese DA: Transbronchoscopic lung biopsy for localized pulmonary disease. Sem Resp Med 3:30, 1981.
33. Mountain CF: A new international staging system for lung cancer. Chest 89(Suppl. 4):225S, 1986.
34. Whitcomb ME, Barham E, Goldman AL, et al: Indications for mediastinoscopy in bronchogenic carcinoma. Am Rev Respir Dis 113:189, 1976.
35. Faling LJ, Pugatch RD, Jung-Legg Y, et al: Computed tomographic scanning of the mediastinum in the staging of bronchogenic carcinoma. Am Rev Respir Dis 124:690, 1981.
36. Matthews MJ, Kanhouwa S, Pickren J, et al: Frequency of residual and metastatic tumor in patients undergoing curative surgical resection for lung cancer. Cancer Chemother Rep 4(part3):63, 1973.
37. Chapman GS, Kumar D, Redmond J III, et al: Upper abdominal computerized tomography scanning in staging nonsmall cell lung carcinoma. Cancer 54:1541, 1984.
38. Tisi GM: Preoperative evaluation of pulmonary function: Validity, indications, and benefits. Am Rev Respir Dis 119:293, 1979.
39. McKeown PP, Conant P, and Hubbell DS: Thoracoscopic lung biopsy. Ann Thorac Surg 54:490, 1992.
40. Errett LE, Wilson J, Chin RC, et al: Wedge resection as an alternative procedure for peripheral bronchogenic carcinoma in poor-risk patients. J Thorac Cardiovasc Surg 90:656, 1985.
41. Swensen SJ, Jett JR, Payne WS, et al: An integrated approach to evaluation of the solitary pulmonary nodule. Mayo Clin Proc 65:173, 1990.
42. Lillington GA: Management of solitary pulmonary nodules. Dis Mon 37:271, 1991.
43. Midthun DE, Swensen SJ, and Jett JR: Clinical strategies for solitary pulmonary nodule. Annu Rev Med 43:195, 1992.
44. Cahan WG, Shah JP, and Castro EB: Benign solitary lung lesions in patients with cancer. Ann Surg 187:241, 1977.
45. Cummings SR, Lillington GA, and Richard RJ: Managing solitary pulmonary nodules: The choice of strategy is a "close call." Am Rev Respir Dis 134:453, 1986.

23

Screening, Prophylaxis, and Treatment of Tuberculosis

PHYLLIS JEN, MD

In this century until 1984, the number of newly diagnosed cases of active tuberculosis was declining by an average of 5%/yr. This was attributed to a higher standard of living, better nutrition, effective antituberculosis chemotherapy, and earlier recognition and isolation of new cases. However, with the emergence of acquired immunodeficiency syndrome (AIDS), there has been a reversal of this downward trend, and since 1985 there has been an annual 5 to 10% increase in the number of new cases.[1] The incidence in the United States of extrapulmonary tuberculosis has particularly increased in recent years from 7% of cases in 1963 to 18% in 1987.[2]

Epidemiology and Pathogenesis

Substantial differences exist in the rates of tuberculosis in different areas and population groups within the United States. Tuberculosis tends to be a disease of the elderly, minorities, the urban poor, and patients with immunosuppressive diseases. Tuberculosis has always demonstrated a bimodal age distribution, particularly affecting children and the elderly. Presently, tuberculosis among minorities occurs primarily in young adults, whereas in whites tuberculosis occurs more among the elderly. Since 1984, the greatest increase in cases has been in young men, who constitute the group that is at greatest risk for AIDS. Persons with AIDS may have a 170-fold greater risk of tuberculosis, with the highest risk among Haitians, blacks, Hispanics, and intravenous drug users. Patients who are both human immunodeficiency virus (HIV) and tuberculin skin test (PPD)–positive have a 50% chance of developing active tuberculosis (compared with a 3 to 5% chance in HIV-negative–PPD-positive individuals).[2,3]

An understanding of the epidemiology of tuberculosis depends on the recognition of tuberculosis as a two-stage process: (1) the acquisition of infection and (2) the development of disease. Each stage has distinctly different risk factors.

The first stage begins when airborne tubercle bacilli are inhaled by a tuberculin-negative individual. For the first 3 to 6 weeks after exposure, the bacteria multiply with little immunologic resistance and spread with little or no symptoms to lymph nodes. Hematogenous dissemination occurs, and further bacterial multiplication is favored in areas of high oxygen tension such as lung apices, renal parenchyma, and growing ends of long bones. This entire process constitutes the primary infection.

Within 6 weeks, cellular immunity and hypersensitivity in the T cell and macrophage system are activated in most infected individuals and limit further bacterial replication. At this point, tuberculin sensitivity can often be demonstrated by skin test (PPD) reactivity, but the infected host continues to have few or no symptoms, has no radiographic findings of tuberculosis, and has negative results on bacteriologic studies. Infection may then remain dormant for an indefinite period.

The second stage in the pathogenesis of tuberculosis, the progression to active disease, can occur in two ways:

(1) *Progression of primary infection to active tuberculosis disease.*

About 5% of newly infected persons are not able to control bacterial multiplication, and active disease becomes apparent within 1 or 2 years. The factors that increase risk of progression to active disease include HIV infection, early childhood, old age, size of inoculum, poor nutrition, and possibly race.

(2) *Reactivation of a remote tuberculosis infection.*

Dormant bacilli in old infected foci such as the lung apices can reactivate after a long and indefinite incubation period. The likelihood that active disease will develop decreases with time from infection. An untreated infected individual may develop active tuberculosis at any time, especially in the presence of HIV disease, steroid or immunosuppressive therapy, diabetes, silicosis, gastric resection, malnutrition, and possibly pregnancy.

In the United States, the majority (92%) of new cases of active tuberculosis result from reactivation of a remote tuberculosis infection. Approximately 60% of cases of reactivation tuberculosis occur in persons with previously normal chest radiographs with neither a history of active tuberculosis nor a history of skin test conversion within the past year. About 33% of cases occur in persons with abnormal chest radiographs with a history of untreated or inadequately treated tuberculosis.[4]

Only 8% of new cases of active tuberculosis represent primary infection, as evidenced by recent conversion of the tuberculin skin test to positive. Primary tuberculosis infection is most likely to be diagnosed in household contacts or in close associates of persons with newly diagnosed active tuberculosis. Because most individuals with primary tuberculosis have a self-limited course with little or no symptoms and do not develop progressive disease, new cases are frequently undetected. However, the risk of progression to active disease in a household contact is approximately 2.5 to 5% in the first year. For this reason, all contacts of patients with active tuberculosis should be examined.

In patients with HIV disease, tuberculosis is frequently the first serious infection, 85% of cases presenting before the time of diagnosis of HIV infection (Table 23–1).[5] The incidence of tuberculosis in patients with AIDS is increased nearly 500 times over the general population and is most frequently seen in patients with HIV who are intravenous drug users or who are from areas of high tuberculosis prevalence. The risk of an HIV-infected person with a positive tuberculin skin test result progressing to active tuberculosis is estimated to be 8%/yr (a 100- to 200-fold increase over patients without HIV disease).[6] Evidence of extrapulmonary involvement is significantly more common in patients with AIDS who have tuberculosis than in HIV-negative persons, occurring in 62% of cases in persons with AIDS compared with 17% in HIV-negative patients.[7] The 1993 CDC case definition for AIDS now includes HIV-infected persons with either pulmonary or extrapulmonary tuberculosis.

It is estimated that between 1930 and 1980 the prevalence of exposure to tubercle bacilli infection in the general population of the United States, as measured by positive results on tuberculin skin tests, decreased from 75% to 7%. Seventy per cent of tuberculin test reactors are now older than 35 years of age. The prevalence is 0.2% among 6 year olds and 0.7% among adolescents.[8]

For the general internist, control of tuberculosis in the community warrants the identification of two groups of individuals:

1. Individuals with active tuberculosis must be identified and rendered noninfectious to reduce the spread of infection, and
2. Asymptomatic infected individuals should be evaluated for possible therapy to prevent the development of active tuberculosis. Subpopulations within this group with increased risk of developing active disease include (a) household or close contacts of active cases, (b) HIV-positive individuals, (c) individuals from high prevalence areas such as Southeast Asia, (d) health care personnel exposed to active cases, and (e) persons with a positive result on a tuberculin test.

TABLE 23–1. CLINICAL PRESENTATION OF TUBERCULOSIS (TB) IN HIV-INFECTED PATIENTS*

Presentation of TB	AIDS/TB Patients	HIV⁺/TB Patients	HIV⁻/TB Patients
Time of TB Diagnosis			
Before AIDS†	(58%)	(88%)	
At AIDS†	(19%)	(12%)	
After AIDS†	(23%)		
Site of TB			
Any pulmonary	(74%)	(76%)	(92%)
Any extrapulmonary	(62%)	(34%)	(8%)
Chest X-Ray Pattern			
Diffuse infiltrate	(30%)	(22%)	
Focal infiltrate	(27%)	(62%)	
Cavitation	(12%)	(28%)	(77%)
Intrathoracic lymphadenopathy	(33%)	(15%)	(2%)
Tuberculin Skin Reaction			
Significant‡	(32%)	(56%)	(91%)
Not Significant	(68%)	(44%)	(9%)

*Adapted from Pitchenik AE and Fertel D: Tuberculosis and nontuberculous mycobacteria disease. Med Clin North Am 76(1):121, 1992.
†AIDS-defining disease other than tuberculosis (TB).
‡≥10 mm induration.

DIAGNOSIS OF ACTIVE TUBERCULOSIS

Tuberculosis is a multisystem disease with protean manifestations. The history, physical examination, radiologic tests, and skin tests are important; however, definitive diagnosis of tuberculosis requires microbiologic confirmation in secretions or tissue specimens. Occasionally, when the clinical picture is sufficiently suggestive of disease and culture results are pending, presumptive diagnosis of tuberculosis is justified and empiric treatment should be initiated.

History and Physical Examination

The clinical manifestations are varied, ranging from an indolent localized process to life-threatening multiorgan failure. Nonspecific symptoms such as fever, night sweats, malaise, anorexia, or weight loss can be present for weeks to months. A persistent productive cough, hemoptysis, or pleuritic chest pain is a more specific symptom suggestive of pulmonary involvement. Localized symptoms in sites such as bone, kidney, or lymphatics suggest extrapulmonary tuberculosis. Massive dissemination or miliary tuberculosis may also occur. Lymphatic and miliary tuberculosis are the most common extrapulmonary forms of tuberculosis in patients with HIV infection.

Physical examination may show signs of pulmonary consolidation, cavitation, pleural effusion, or lymphadenopathy. However, the results of the examination may be entirely negative, even with advanced disease noted on chest radiograph.

Laboratory

Tuberculin Skin Test. The Mantoux (PPD) test is the prototype of a cell-mediated delayed hypersensitivity reaction. The test consists of an intradermal injection of 0.1 ml of liquid PPD containing 5 tuberculin units (TU). The diameter (mm) of induration (not erythema alone) is measured at 48 to 72 hours. The skin test, however, is not entirely specific for tuberculosis infection and can result from cross-reactivity from atypical mycobacteria. Although reactions from atypical mycobacteria tend to be smaller, no absolute diameter separates the two infections (Fig. 23–1).

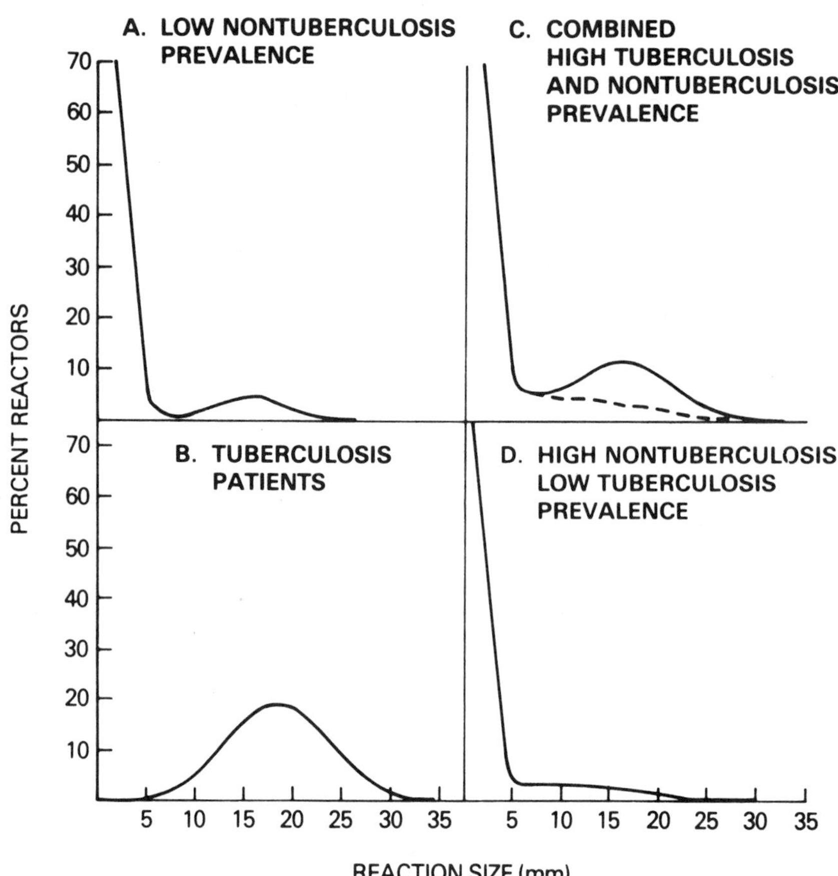

FIGURE 23–1. PPD reaction size for different population groups. Nontuberculosis is primarily atypical mycobacteria. (Adapted from Chaparas, SD: Immunity in tuberculosis. Bull WHO 60(4):447–462, 1982.)

The criteria for a "positive" PPD reaction as an indicator of tuberculosis infection are influenced by the risk of tuberculosis in the given population and the prevalence of atypical mycobacteria. Previously a reaction size of 10 mm or more was considered a positive finding. In 1990, the Centers for Disease Control and the American Thoracic Society issued new guidelines for the interpretation of the tuberculin reactor. The new classification has three size cut-offs of 5-, 10-, and 15-mm induration, for populations with high, medium and low risk of tuberculosis infection.[9]

⩾ 5-mm induration is a positive finding in:

1. Recent close contacts of active tuberculosis
2. HIV-infected and other immunosuppressed persons
3. Persons with previous untreated tuberculosis

⩾ 10-mm induration is a positive finding in:

1. Foreign-born persons from high-prevalence countries (e.g., Asia, Africa, Latin America)
2. Intravenous drug users
3. Low income populations, especially the homeless
4. Residents of correctional facilities and nursing homes
5. Persons older than 70 years of age and children younger than 15 years of age
6. Health care providers
7. Persons with medical conditions known to increase risk (e.g., diabetes, silicosis, malabsorption, postgastrectomy)

⩾15–mm duration is a positive finding in all other persons.

False-negative tests can occur, related to improper storage of the PPD or poor technique of administration and reading of the test. In addition, poor tuberculin reactivity may occur in patients with HIV or lymphoid diseases, immunosuppressive therapy (> prednisone 20 mg/day for > 2 weeks), recent live virus vaccinations, or viral or bacterial infections. Simultaneous skin testing for anergy using mumps or *Candida* antigen should be administered at the time of PPD testing in all HIV-infected persons. The presence of anergy varies inversely with the CD4 count, with 10% with anergy when CD4 count is >500, and 80% with anergy when the CD4 count is <50.[10] Patients with tuberculosis and early HIV disease will have a positive result on a tuberculin test in 56% of cases. As HIV disease advances, the ability to demonstrate hypersensitivity wanes, and in patients with AIDS the test result is positive in 33% (see Table 23–1).[11] Of note is that even in the pre-AIDS era overwhelming tuberculosis infection and occasionally uncomplicated tuberculosis infection resulted in a negative tuberculin test in as many as 17% of cases.[12] Some of these patients were elderly and debilitated and anergic to multiple antigens; however, in others, no etiology for the false-negative reaction can be found. Therefore, it is important to recognize that a negative result on a skin test does not totally exclude active tuberculosis. Use of either the 1 TU or 250 TU PPD adds no diagnostic information.

Vaccination with BCG (bacille Calmette-Guérin) results in development of variable tuberculin sensitivity, depending on the strain of BCG used. In a significant number of BCG vaccinees, a positive tuberculin reaction either never occurs or wanes with time after vaccination. Tuberculin reactivity rarely measures greater than 15 mm of induration without concomitant natural tuberculosis infection. It is therefore advisable to consider large reactions in BCG-vaccinated individuals as indicative of tuberculosis infection, especially if a chest x-ray shows evidence of previous infection.

Multiple puncture tests (e.g., the Tine test) have moderately high false-positive and false-negative rates and should be used only when ease of administration is essential, such as in large-scale screening in short periods. All positive reactions to multiple puncture methods should be verified with the Mantoux test.

In surveillance programs (e.g., for hospital employees), in which skin testing is repeated periodically, the *booster phenomenon* can interfere with the interpretation of the test. An individual, most commonly older than 50 years, with a remote tuberculous or atypical mycobacterial infection may demonstrate a false-negative reaction on the first testing and appear to convert to a positive reaction on subsequent testing. This, however, does not indicate a recent infection. The booster effect can best be evaluated by administering a second tuberculin test 1 week after the first test in persons older than 50 years of age or in those persons who may have had exposure to atypical mycobacteria. The result of the second test indicates the true tuberculin reactivity.[13]

Radiographic Features

Posteroanterior (PA) and lateral chest x-ray views should be obtained in all persons with a positive tuberculin skin test or a history suggestive of tuberculosis. Two thirds of chest x-rays will demonstrate a "typical" pattern of upper lobe disease with or without cavitation, while one third will show "atypical" patterns such as pleural effusion, hilar adenopathy, or lower lung interstitial disease. These atypical patterns are seen more commonly in HIV-infected patients as immunologic dysfunction progresses (see Table 23–1). If the results of the PA and lateral films are negative and clinical suspicion is high, apical lordotic views should be obtained. A negative result on a chest radiograph generally rules out active pulmonary tuberculosis.[14]

Smears and Cultures

If pulmonary tuberculosis is suspected, sputum specimens should be obtained, using aerosol induction (ultrasonic nebulization with normal saline) if necessary. Smears showing acid-fast bacilli on staining are highly suggestive of tuberculosis but could occasionally represent *Mycobacterium avium* or other mycobacterial infection. Positive cultures are usually definitive but require 4 to 8 weeks. Until results of culture and drug susceptibility testing are available, a positive smear can establish the presumptive diagnosis of tuberculosis. Morning gastric aspirates containing swallowed sputum may yield positive cultures in individuals unable to expectorate adequate amounts of sputum.

In patients who have negative sputum smears for acid-fast bacilli but who are still suspected of having tuberculosis, fiberoptic bronchoscopy, transbronchial biopsy, and postbronchoscopy sputum smears can improve the ability to document active disease. The sputum smear and culture have positive results in 30 to 90% of patients with tuberculosis, depending on the extent of the pulmonary disease. Patients with cavitary disease almost always have positive smears. The diagnostic yield of a sputum smear is lower in patients with severe HIV disease.

Other Tests

The complete blood count may demonstrate anemia of chronic disease; the white blood cell count may show monocytosis. Sterile pyuria suggests renal tuberculosis, and elevated liver function tests suggest disseminated disease. HIV testing should be done in all cases of active tuberculosis, since treatment of both tuberculosis and HIV may need to be adjusted.

Treatment

Treatment of active tuberculosis has undergone major changes in the decades since the introduction of streptomycin in 1941 and of isoniazid in 1952. Current chemotherapeutic regimens are designed to be shorter and simpler and take into account the recent emergence of drug-resistant tuberculosis. Multidrug resistance has occurred in several institutional outbreaks and has been found in 19% of new tuberculosis cases in New York City in 1991 and in 3% of cases nationwide. Drug-resistant tuberculosis has a mortality rate of greater than 75% and occurs more frequently in HIV-infected persons and in partially treated or recurrent cases. The risk of transmission to contacts, however, appears to be similar for drug-resistant and drug-susceptible organisms.

A four-drug regimen is now preferable for initial therapeutic treatment of tuberculosis until drug susceptibilities are available. The regimens listed below are recommended for initial treatment of tuberculosis (Table 23–2).[15, 15a]

1. Isoniazid (INH), rifampin (RIF), and pyrazinamide (PZA), daily for 8 weeks, then INH and RIF for 16 weeks, either daily or 2 to 3 times per week. Ethambutol (ETM) or streptomycin (SM) should be added to the initial regimen until susceptibility to INH and RIF is demonstrated unless the likelihood of drug resistance is very low.
2. INH, RIF, PZA, and ETM or SM daily for 2 weeks, then 2 times per week for 6 weeks. Then, INH and RIF 2 times per week, directly observed.
3. INH, RIF, PZA, and ETM, or SM 3 times per week for 6 months, directly observed.

Relapse rate with the above regimens is less than 3%. Patients who comply with therapy or are directly observed generally have an excellent prognosis with the following exceptions:

HIV-Infected Individuals. Response to standard antituberculosis drugs and relapse rates are comparable in both HIV-infected and normal individuals. Duration of treatment, however, should be prolonged to a minimum of 9 months or 6 months after cultures are negative.[16–18] Ethambutol should be added if disseminated or central nervous system disease is present.

Multidrug Resistance. In situations in which previous outbreaks of drug-resistant tuberculosis have occurred, regimens may need to include administration of 5 or 6 drugs as initial therapy.

Drug Toxicity. Several of the most effective antituberculosis drugs (INH, rifampin, and pyrazinamide) are potentially hepatotoxic, with additive effects when the drugs are given in combination. INH hepatotoxicity is discussed in more detail in the section on chemoprophylaxis of tuberculosis. Treatment of patients with concomitant liver disease or alcohol use requires a program with the least hepatotoxic drugs, reduced dosages, and careful monitoring.

The majority of treatment failures occur because of pa-

TABLE 23–2. TREATMENT OF MYCOBACTERIAL DISEASE IN ADULTS AND CHILDREN*

Commonly Used Agents	Dosage: *Daily Dose*	Dosage: *Twice Weekly Dose*	Most Common Side Effects	Tests for Side Effects	Drug Interactions	Remarks
Isoniazid	5 to 10 mg/kg up to 300 mg PO or IM	15 mg/kg PO or IM	Peripheral neuritis, hepatitis, hypersensitivity	SGOT/SGPT (not as a routine)	Phenytoin—synergistic Antabuse	Bactericidal to both extracellular and intracellular organisms. Pyridoxine, 10 mg, as prophylaxis for neuritis; 50 to 100 mg as treatment
Rifampin	10 mg/kg up to 600 mg PO	10 mg/kg up to 600 mg PO	Hepatitis, febrile reaction, purpura (rare)	SGOT/SGPT (not as a routine)	Rifampin inhibits the effect of oral contraceptives, quinidine, corticosteroids, coumadin, methadone, digoxin, and oral hypoglycemics; PAS may interfere with absorption of rifampin	Bactericidal to all populations of organisms; orange urine and other body secretions; discoloring of contact lens
Streptomycin	15 to 20 mg/kg up to 1 g IM	25 to 30 mg/kg	8th nerve damage, nephrotoxicity	Vestibular function, audiograms; BUN and creatinine	Neuromuscular blocking agents—may be potentiated to cause prolonged paralysis	Bactericidal to extracellular organisms. Use with caution in older patients or those with renal disease
Pyrazinamide	15 to 30 mg/kg up to 2 g PO	50 to 70 mg/kg	Hyperuricemia, hepatotoxicity	Uric acid, SGOT/SGPT		Bactericidal to intracellular organisms. Combination with an aminoglycoside is bactericidal
Ethambutol	15 to 25 mg/kg	50 mg/kg PO	Optic neuritis (reversible with discontinuation of drug; very rare at 15 mg/kg), skin rash	Red-green color discrimination and visual acuity. Difficult to test in a child under 3 years		Bacteriostatic to both intracellular and extracellular organisms, primarily used to inhibit development of resistant mutants. Use with caution with renal disease or when eye testing is not feasible

*From American Thoracic Society: Treatment of tuberculosis and other mycobacterial diseases. Am Rev Respir Dis 127:791, 1983.

tient noncompliance. Patients should be followed for 12 months after completion of chemotherapy since most relapses are likely to occur within this period.

CHEMOPROPHYLAXIS OF TUBERCULOSIS

Any person with tuberculosis exposure, as indicated by a positive PPD skin test, is at risk for developing tuberculosis at some time during his or her life. Evidence suggests that at any age the risk of developing active tuberculosis is greatest shortly after the initial exposure. In addition, the risk of developing active disease is especially high in individuals who are young, have had strong or recent exposure, or have immunologic dysfunction. This risk is reduced 60 to 90% by INH 300mg/day chemoprophylaxis for 6 months.[19, 20] INH therapy, however, is associated with some risk of toxicity, most significantly drug-induced hepatitis. In 10 to 20% of INH-treated persons, transient asymptomatic hepatic dysfunction as evidenced by serum glutamic-oxaloacetic transaminase (SGOT) elevations may occur. Although enzyme levels frequently return to normal despite continuation of INH, clinical hepatitis and progressive liver damage occasionally occur. Extensive studies on the incidence of INH hepatitis show that the frequency of progressive liver damage increases with age (Table 23–3). Daily use of alcohol may increase the risk of INH hypersensitivity, but the presence of alcoholic cirrhosis does not.[21]

TABLE 23–3. INCIDENCE OF ISONIAZID HEPATITIS VERSUS AGE*

Age	Incidence (%)
20–34	<0.3
35–49	<1.2
50–64	<2.3

*From Kopanoff DE, Snider DE, and Caras DJ: Isoniazid related hepatitis: A U.S.P.H.S. cooperative surveillance study. Am Rev Respir Dis 117:995, 1978.

Although every person infected with *M. tuberculosis* is at risk of developing active disease, it is not practical in low prevalence areas to identify and treat all persons with a positive result on a PPD skin test. Instead, the probability of developing tuberculosis must be weighed against the probability of INH hypersensitivity for each individual.[22] The American Thoracic Society and the Centers for Disease Control recommend that the benefits of INH chemoprophylaxis outweigh the risk of hepatitis in the following situations, in order of priority.[23]

1. Persons who have or who are suspected of having HIV infection (⩾5mm PPD)
2. Household and other close contacts of persons with newly diagnosed tuberculosis (⩾5mm). If the likelihood of infection is high, some contacts (especially children) should receive INH prophylaxis for 3 months even if the tuberculin test result is initially negative. If a repeat skin test 3 months after exposure is still negative, therapy may be discontinued.
3. Newly infected persons (recent converter) as demonstrated by skin test conversion within the past 2 years. Skin test is defined as an increase in induration of at least 10 mm for persons under age 35 and 15 mm for persons older than 35 years of age.
4. Persons with abnormal CXR that show fibrotic lesions likely to be old healed tuberculosis (⩾5mm).
5. Intravenous drug users who are HIV negative (⩾10mm).
6. Persons at increased risk because of corticosteroid therapy, immunosuppressive therapy, leukemia, Hodgkin's disease, diabetes mellitus, and silicosis, and those post-gastrectomy (⩾10mm).

In addition, tuberculin-positive persons under the age of 35 years who are not known to belong to any of the above groups should be considered for INH chemoprophylaxis, but this is controversial and has been challenged.[24] It is appropriate to recommend isoniazid in foreign-born persons from high-prevalence countries or in certain groups, such as low income populations, blacks, Native Americans, Hispanics, and residents of long-term care facilities (Table 23–4).[23] Recently some experts have recommended that HIV-infected individuals who are anergic and are from areas of high prevalence should also receive INH prophylaxis.

Risks of developing tuberculosis for each of these risk groups are summarized in Table 23–5. INH single-drug therapy should never be given until active tuberculosis has been excluded. All positive reactors should have a chest radiograph, and if abnormalities consistent with pulmonary tuberculosis are found further evaluation is necessary.

Patients with a previous reaction to isoniazid or who have acute liver disease of any etiology should not be given INH. Before taking INH, patients should be asked about a history of chronic liver disease and use of other drugs, including alcohol. Chemoprophylaxis of pregnant patients should be delayed until after delivery, although INH is not known to have any teratogenic effect.

Patients should be made aware of symptoms suggestive of hepatotoxicity, such as unexplained anorexia or nausea of greater than 3 days' duration, persistent dark urine, pruritus, icterus, or abdominal tenderness. Patients must be advised to report promptly for further evaluation if these symptoms develop.

The currently recommended chemoprophylaxis regimen for immunocompetent adults is INH, 300 mg/day for 6 months. For immunocompromised patients, 12 months of INH therapy is recommended. At present, no other drug has received large-scale testing as a chemoprophylactic agent, but if a patient is a known contact of an active case with INH-resistant tuberculosis, alternative therapies, possibly using rifampin, may be indicated.

The American Thoracic Society recommends that individuals receiving prophylaxis be seen at monthly intervals to evaluate signs or symptoms of adverse reactions. Routine monitoring of liver function tests is not recommended in the absence of clinical suspicion. Some authorities, however, recommend routine surveillance of SGOT levels in daily alcohol users, individuals with a history of liver disease, and those older than 35 years of age. If liver enzyme levels are greater than three to five times normal, the decision to continue therapy should be reconsidered. Often, these elevations are transient, but close monitoring is essential. At the conclusion of the prescribed period of therapy, patients should be instructed to report any symptoms suggestive of tuberculosis, but further routine follow-up is thought to be unnecessary.

TABLE 23–4. CRITERIA FOR DETERMINING NEED FOR PREVENTIVE THERAPY FOR PERSONS WITH POSITIVE TUBERCULIN REACTIONS, BY CATEGORY AND AGE GROUP*

Category	Age Group (Yr)	
	<35	*>35*
With risk factor†	Treat at all ages if reaction to 5TU purified protein derivative (PPD) ≥10 mm (or ≥5 mm and patient is recent contact, HIV-infected, *or* has radiographic evidence of old TB)	
No risk factor High-incidence group‡	Treat if PPD >10 mm	Do not treat
No risk factor Low-incidence group	Treat if PPD >15 mm§	Do not treat

*From The use of preventive therapy for tuberculosis infection in the United States: Recommendations of the Advisory Committee for Elimination of Tuberculosis. MMWR 39(RR-8):1, 1990.

†Risk factors include HIV infection, recent contact with infectious person, recent skin-test conversion, abnormal chest radiograph, intravenous drug abuse, and certain medical risk factors (see text).

‡High-incidence groups include foreign-born persons, medically underserved low income populations, and residents of long-term-care facilities.

§Lower or higher cut points may be used for identifying positive reactions, depending on the relative prevalence of *Mycobacterium tuberculosis* infection and nonspecific cross-reactivity in the population.

TABLE 23–5. RISK OF DEVELOPING ACTIVE TUBERCULOSIS

Group	Risk (%)	Reference
Household contact of new case		
Recent PPD conversion	2.5-4 in 1st year	(15)
PPD (−)	0.5 per 10 years	(19)
PPD (+), unknown duration	2.7 per 10 years	(19)
History of TB, inadequately treated	1.3 per year	(19)
Recent PPD conversion	3.3 in 1st year	(15)
PPD (+), abnormal chest radiography	0.8 per year	(15)
PPD (+), normal chest radiograph, age <35 years	0.03–0.08 per year	(28, 29)
PPD (+), HIV (+)	8 per year	(6)

The use of BCG vaccines as prophylactic therapy has declined in the United States. However, a significant number of people, especially immigrants from developing countries (e.g., Southeast Asia, the Caribbean), have received the vaccine. The various BCG vaccines have different immunogenic properties (varying from 0 to 80% efficacy) with different skin test reactivity making interpretation of the skin test difficult.[25] In the United States, where the incidence of tuberculosis is low, the ability to use the PPD as an indicator of disease outweighs the benefits of vaccination. The U.S. Public Health Service and the American Thoracic Society, however, continue to recommend the vaccine in certain situations: (1) in PPD-negative persons who have repeated exposure to sputum-positive pulmonary tuberculosis, or (2) in well-defined communities with an excessive rate of new infection.[26] BCG should not be given to HIV-infected individuals.

SCREENING

Screening to identify individuals with positive tuberculin skin tests and potential active disease should be directed to certain target groups. Screening is clearly warranted in groups in whom prevalence rates or exposure risk is high, such as (1) contacts of active cases; (2) patients with HIV disease; (3) persons living in areas or institutions where tuberculosis prevalence is high, such as nursing homes and long-term prisons; (4) persons from areas like Southeast Asia; and (5) specific occupational groups such as health care workers who are in contact with high-prevalence groups.[23] Routine tuberculin skin test screening in the American general population is currently not thought to be cost-effective. Periodic x-ray examinations of persons with positive tuberculin reactions are also nonproductive.[27]

REFERENCES

1. Centers for Disease Control: Tuberculosis mortality in the U.S.: Final data. MMWR 40:23, 1990.

2. Bloch AB, Reider HL, Kelly GD, et al: The epidemiology of tuberculosis in the U.S. Clin Chest Med 10:297, 1989.
3. Pitchenik AE, Fertel D, and Bloch AB: Mycobacterial disease: Epidemiology, diagnosis, treatment and prevention. Clin Chest Med 9:425, 1988.
4. Horwitz O, Edwards PQ, and Lowell AM: National tuberculosis control program in Denmark and the United States. Health Service Reports 88:493, 1973.
5. Centers for Disease Control: TB and acquired immunodeficiency syndrome—Florida. MMWR 35:587, 1986.
6. Selwyn PA Hartel D, Lewis VA, et al: A prospective study of the risk of TB among intravenous drug users with HIV infection. N Engl J Med 320:545, 1989.
7. Theur CP, Hopewell PC, Elias D, et al: HIV infection in TB patients. J Infect Dis 162:8, 1990.
8. Edwards PQ: Tuberculosis testing of children. Pediatrics 54:628, 1973.
9. American Thoracic Society: Diagnostic standards and classification of tuberculosis: Joint statement of American Thoracic Society and Centers for Disease Control. Am Rev Respir Dis 142:725, 1990.
10. PPD Anergy and HIV infection: Guidelines for anergy testing and management of anergic persons at risk of tuberculosis. MMWR 40 (No. RR-5):27, 1991.
11. Rieder HL, Cauthen GM, Bloch AB, et al: Tuberculosis and acquired immunodeficiency syndrome. Arch Intern Med 149:1268, 1989.
12. Holden M, Dubin MR, and Diamond PH: Frequency of negative intermediate-strength tuberculosis sensitivity in patients with active tuberculosis. N Engl J Med 285:1506, 1971.
13. Thompson NJ, Glassroth JL, Snider DE, et al: The booster phenomenon in serial tuberculosis testing. Am Rev Respir Dis 119:587, 1979.
14. Khan MA, Kornat DM, Bachus B, et al: Clinical and roentgenographic spectrum of pulmonary tuberculosis in the adult. Am J Med 62:31, 1977.
15. American Thoracic Society: Treatment of tuberculosis infection in adults and children. Am Rev Respir Dis 134:355, 1986.
15a. Initial Therapy for Tuberculosis in the Era of Multidrug Resistance: Recommendations of the ACET. MMWR 42 (No. RR-7):1–7, 1993.
16. Tuberculosis and HIV infection: Recommendations of the Advisory Committee for the Elimination of Tuberculosis (ACRT). MMWR 38:236, 1989.
17. Barnes PF, Bloch AB, Davidson PT, et al: Tuberculosis in patients with HIV infection. N Engl J Med 324(23):1644, 1991.
18. Small PM, Schecter GF, Goodman PC, et al: Treatment of tuberculosis in patients with advanced HIV infection. N Engl J Med 324:289, 1991.
19. Ferebee SH: Controlled chemoprophylaxis trials in tuberculosis: A general review. Adv Tuberc Res 17:29, 1969.
20. Comstock CW and Woolpert SF: Preventive therapy. *In* Kubica GP (ed): The Mycobacteria: A Sourcebook. New York, Marcel Dekker, 1984, p 1071.
21. Kopanoff DE, Snider DE, and Caras GJ: Isoniazid related hepatitis: A U.S.P.H.S. cooperative surveillance study. Am Rev Respir Dis 117:991, 1978.
22. Comstock GW and Edwards PQ: The competing risks of tuberculosis and hepatitis for adult tuberculin reactors. Am Rev Respir Dis 111:573, 1975.
23. Screening for tuberculosis in high-risk populations and the use of preventive therapy for tuberculous infection in the United States: Recommendations of the Advisory Committee for Elimination of TB. MMWR 39 (RR-8):1 1990.
24. Taylor WC, Aronson MD, and Delbanco TL: Should young adults with a positive tuberculosis test take isoniazid? Ann Intern Med 94:808, 1981.
25. Clemens JD, Chuong JJ, and Feinstein AR: The BCG controversy. JAMA 249:2362, 1983.
26. American Thoracic Society: BCG vaccines for tuberculosis. Am Rev Respir Dis 112:478, 1975.
27. Stead WW: Goals and productivity of tuberculosis screening. Chest 68:446, 1975.
28. Comstock GW, Woolpert SF, and Livesay VT: Tuberculosis studies in Muscogee County, Georgia: Twenty year evaluation of a community trial of BCG vaccination. Public Health Rep 91:276, 1976.
29. Horwitz O, Wilbek E, and Erickson PA: Epidemiological basis of tuberculosis eradication: Longitudinal studies on the risk of tuberculosis in the general population of a low prevalence area. Bull WHO 41:95, 1969.

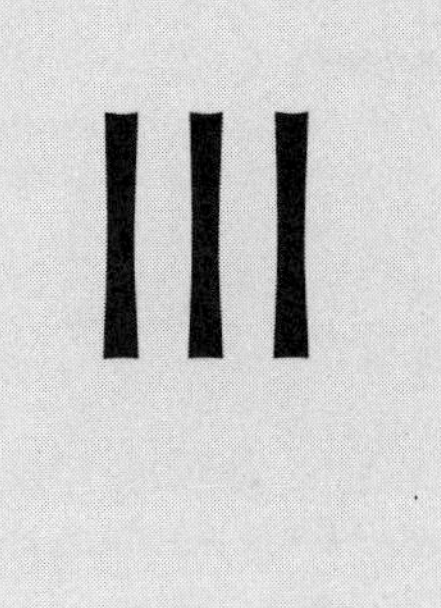

Diseases of the Digestive Tract

24

Dyspepsia and Upper Abdominal Pain

T. EDWARD BYNUM, MD
WILLIAM T. BRANCH, Jr., MD

INITIAL ASSESSMENT

The term *dyspepsia* applies to a variety of complaints encountered in conditions of the upper abdomen. Included are epigastric pain or burning, nausea, repeated belching and bloating, fatty food intolerance, or inability to complete a normal meal. It has been estimated that 2 to 3% of patients who consult a physician do so for upper abdominal pain or dyspepsia.[1]

Although there are many potential causes of dyspepsia, in practice a few major ones account for the majority of patients with recurring or chronic symptoms. More than 90% of these patients have one of the following four disorders: duodenal ulcer, gastric ulcer, gastric malignancy, or "functional" (nonulcer) dyspepsia.[2] Esophagitis (not included in the study just cited) is also clearly an important cause of dyspepsia, as are gallstone disease, pancreatitis, carcinoma of the pancreas, and a few other uncommon but relatively serious problems.

Differential Diagnosis

Duodenal Ulcer. From the clinical presentation in patients with duodenal ulcer disease, one often can suspect the diagnosis. Important features to consider are the course of the illness; the type, localization, and timing of pain; and the relation of pain to meals and antacids. The course is intermittent, but often lifelong, illness. Symptoms may begin at any age, but most frequently the onset is between ages 30 and 40 in men and slightly later in women. The natural history is characterized by periodic remissions and exacerbations of symptoms, the latter lasting weeks to months. In contrast, a history of sporadic, brief symptoms or onset of symptoms late in life is less suggestive of duodenal ulcer disease than of some of the other causes of dyspepsia.[2]

The primary site of pain in duodenal ulcer disease is almost always epigastric, although substernal heartburn is common as a secondary symptom (Fig. 24–1).[3] Classically, the pain is described as "burning" or "gnawing" and is well localized to the epigastrium. Its tendency to occur at night

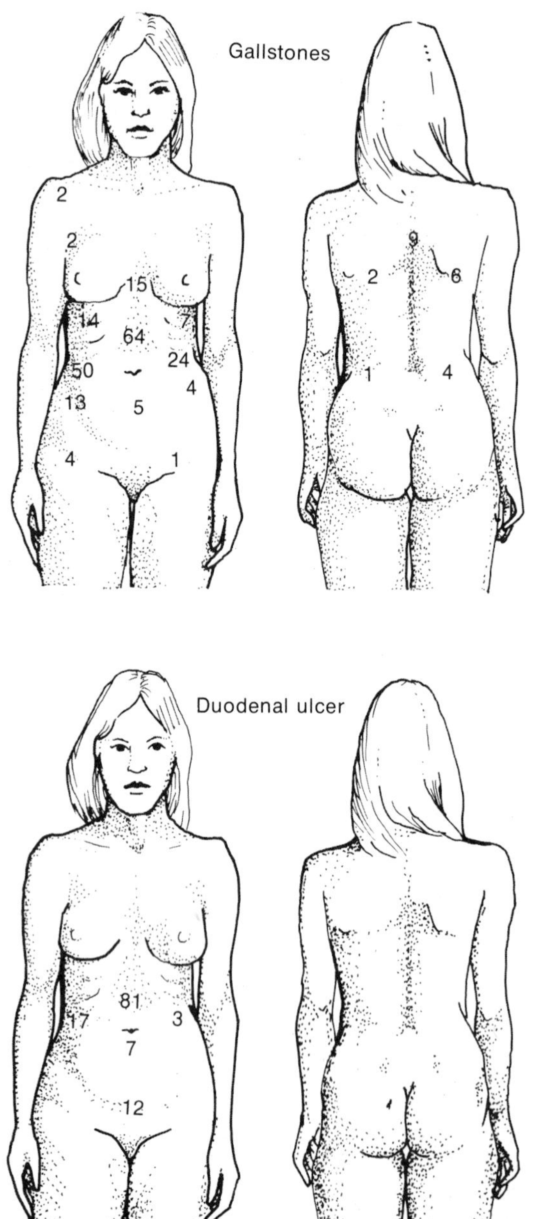

FIGURE 24–1. Sites of *primary* or *most severe pain* in patients with gallstones compared with those having duodenal ulcer disease. Shown is the percentage of patients experiencing pain at each site at some time. (Adapted from Gunn A and Keddie N: Some clinical observations on patients with gallstones. Lancet 2:239, 1972; and Earlam R: A computerized questionnaire analysis of duodenal ulcer symptoms. Gastroenterology 71:319, 1976.)

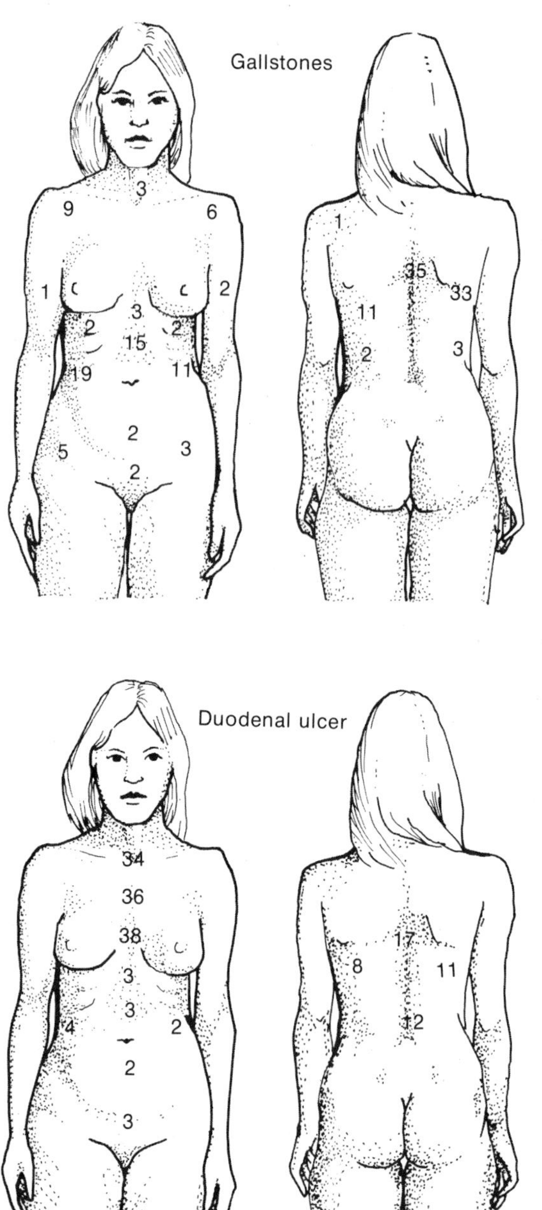

FIGURE 24–2. Sites of *secondary pain* or *radiation* of pain in patients with gallstones compared with those having duodenal ulcer disease. Shown is the percentage of patients experiencing radiation to each site at some time. (Adapted from Gunn A and Keddie N: Some clinical observations on patients with gallstones. Lancet 2:239, 1972; and Earlam R: A computerized questionnaire analysis of duodenal ulcer symptoms. Gastroenterology 71:314, 1976.)

is noted in 70% of patients.[2] Nausea may accompany the pain, although this occurs more commonly in gastric ulcer or malignancy; radiation to the back or shoulder occurs at some time in 26% of all patients with duodenal ulcer (Fig. 24–2).[2] Epigastric tenderness is often present.

Pain is usually most prominent 2 to 4 hours after a meal; less common is actual relief of pain by meals.[3] The adage that patients with duodenal ulcers increase their food consumption is not necessarily true; most patients report that symptoms cause them to eat less, and weight loss occurs in some.[2, 3] Relief by antacids is not so predictable as once thought. A minority of only 39% actually claim this[2]; however, the symptoms are relieved in almost all duodenal ulcer patients after intensive antacid therapy over a period of 4 weeks.[4]

Esophagitis. Heartburn is most characteristic of reflux esophogitis, but several other symptoms may help to confirm the diagnosis. Heartburn, or pyrosis, is characterized, first, by its substernal location and, second, by its quality of burning (e.g., "fire" coming up the chest) as opposed to pain. Other features of heartburn include association with recumbency, large meals, or intake of citrus juice and often relief 2 to 5 minutes after ingesting antacids. It is said to occur about 1 hour after meals and to be of variable duration. By itself, heartburn does not warrant a diagnosis of esophagitis, since this symptom also occurs in some patients with peptic ulcer disease, biliary disease, and other forms of dyspepsia.[3, 5, 6] It is possible that these patients also have esophagitis as a manifestation of associated reflux gastric acidity, but heartburn is not the most prominent symptom in these cases. The majority of normal people also experience heartburn at one time or another, but probably only 5% experience significant, recurrent symptoms.[5]

Regurgitation of sour acid material, typically occurring at night or when the patient is bending over, confirms the presence of reflux and may suggest that the patient's symptoms are related to esophagitis. Severe esophagitis, especially when associated with an esophageal ulcer, may cause a more persistent discomfort than heartburn. The patient frequently describes substernal aching that radiates to the midback, whereas relief by antacids is incomplete or inconsistent, or occurs only after several days of intensive therapy. Pain during swallowing (odynophagia) is more likely in patients with frank ulceration or severe esophagitis. In addition, dysphagia, perceived as the temporary arrest of a food bolus, may result from a transient motor dysfunction, causing spasm, or from actual scarring and stricture formation caused by inflammation. Less frequently, patients with reflux esophagitis describe sudden filling of the mouth by large quantities of a clear, slightly salty fluid. This is referred to as "water brash"; it also occurs in peptic ulcer disease and is due to an outpouring of salivary secretions.

Generally a constellation of the aforementioned symptoms, particularly sour acidic regurgitations associated with heartburn, allows one to make the clinical diagnosis of esophagitis. Whenever dysphagia is present, it is essential to exclude more serious esophageal disease, such as achalasia, benign stricture, or esophageal carcinoma, before assuming that dysphagia is transient and related to spasm caused by esophagitis.

Gastric Ulcer and Gastric Carcinoma. Gastric ulcer and gastric carcinoma share some common clinical features. Frequently, the presence of one or the other is suspected from the patient's history and the setting in which symptoms develop. Both occur most often in relatively elderly patients, usually in the age range of 40 to 70 years for gastric ulcer and 60 to 80 years for gastric malignancy.[2] The patient usually has a "nagging," "dull," or "aching" pain in the region of the epigastrium. Nausea is frequent; bleeding occurs relatively frequently; and the radiation of pain to the back or shoulder is common.[2] The pattern of pain is quite variable in relation to meals or antacids. It may be unrelated, worsened, or apparently relieved by food in either condition; relief by single doses of antacids was noted in only 36% of patients with gastric ulcers.[2] Weight loss is characteristic of both conditions, particularly gastric carcinoma, in which 85% of patients lost 7 lb (3.2 kg) or more.[2] Most ascribed their weight loss to anorexia rather than early filling.

In patients with gastric carcinoma, pain and other symptoms tend to be progressive and continuous rather than intermittent or periodic; taken as a whole, patients with either gastric ulcer or gastric carcinoma characteristically show progressively more severe pain, nausea, and weight loss over a period of months and tend to be older or even elderly patients. A long history of exacerbations and remissions is unusual.

In this setting, the diagnosis should be suspected, and the indications clearly are present to obtain an upper gastrointestinal series (UGIS) or upper endoscopy. Unfortunately, only a few patients with gastric carcinoma who have progressed to the point of developing the symptoms just described can be cured by surgical resection, and there is no currently available, practical method for detecting the disease at an earlier stage.

Gallstones. The symptoms of gallbladder disease most likely to be encountered in ambulatory practice are repeated attacks of pain. In the series of Horrocks and DeDombal, the incidence was most common between ages 40 and 80 years, and symptoms had generally been present for 1 to 3 years.[2] For the most part, symptoms are unrelated to meals, not relieved by antacids, often accompanied by nausea, and accompanied by weight loss in few cases. It is characteristic for the pain to occur in circumscribed attacks that last from hours to days, as opposed to a pattern of exacerbations weeks to months in duration or to a pattern of continuous, unremitting pain. Quite frequently, the pain radiates to the back or shoulder (77%) (see Fig. 24–2).[2] About one third of the patients are awakened at night by attacks.

The symptoms of biliary pain or colic are caused by an impacted calculus within the cystic duct or common duct. The duct becomes dilated, sometimes to three or four times the normal size, and pain develops that ultimately is relieved either when the stone passes into the common duct or duodenum or when it shifts proximally back into the dilated duct or into the gallbladder. By definition, patients with biliary pain have gallstones or at least biliary gravel. It has been claimed that there may be "functional" obstruction of the cystic duct, producing similar pain caused by impaired emptying of the gallbladder after a meal or cholecystokinin stimulation, but this is controversial. Almost as controversial, but now a well-established if very rare motility disorder, is *biliary dyskinesia.* Symptoms can mimic either functional dyspepsia or biliary pain and are due to high pressure muscle contraction at the ampullary sphincter.

Biliary colic is a steady visceral pain that generally increases in intensity over a period of 15 to 45 minutes, although it may be sudden in onset in one third of cases. Severe pain usually persists for several hours and then gradually resolves over a longer period. The term "colic" applied to this pain refers to its diffuse, dull, difficult to localize, visceral character, and not to its duration, because the pain is constant rather than crampy or intermittent.

It is important for the clinician to recognize how variable the location of biliary pain may be.[6] Although some patients do experience right upper quadrant pain, the primary site most often is epigastric. Left upper quadrant pain is not rare (see Fig. 24–1). Although radiation to the back or shoulder is characteristic, radiation can also occur to the upper or lower abdomen or neck (see Fig. 24–2). Patients with biliary colic generally do not have right upper quadrant tenderness on examination, although if the cystic duct remains obstructed, inflammation of the gallbladder (cholecystitis) will eventually develop. Rarely, a distended but noninflamed gallbladder will be palpable as a tender mass.

Patients with uncomplicated biliary colic are afebrile. Elevation of the serum amylase level sometimes accompanies the passage of gallstones, even in the absence of demonstrable inflammation within the pancreas; conversely, frank pancreatitis may develop in some cases.

Some patients with gallstones also complain of food intolerance, excessive belching, postprandial bloating, or heartburn. In rare patients, such vague symptoms of dyspepsia have been relieved after cholecystectomy was performed for biliary "colic" or cholecystitis. However, vague dyspepsia, in the absence of biliary pain or cholecystitis, should not serve as an indication for surgery. Epidemiologic studies have demonstrated that dyspepsia and fatty food intolerance have no specific association with gallbladder disease.[10]

"Functional" (Nonulcer) Dyspepsia and Other Causes of Abdominal Pain. Gastroenterologists use the term functional or nonulcer dyspepsia to refer to patients with chronic symptoms but negative diagnostic studies. In several reported series, a peptic ulcer eventually developed in from 3.5 to 12% of such patients,[11] whereas in a study of 35 patients with negative UGIS who had abdominal pain that was *not* thought to be typical of peptic ulcer disease, 7% could be found to have a gastric or duodenal ulcer at endoscopy.[12] Thus, some patients thought to have functional or nonulcer dyspepsia may have or will develop ulcers or other disease; however, the majority within this category have no recognizable lesion.

The question of whether or not this is a distinct clinical entity is unresolved.[13–15] Horrocks and DeDombal described 50 patients who, in addition to negative x-ray studies of the stomach, duodenum, and gallbladder, had been followed for 2 years without another diagnosis being established.[2] In most of their patients, the symptoms were unrelated to meals, were not relieved by antacids, and occurred in a pattern of sporadic or intermittent, brief episodes over a period of several years. They tended not to have exacerbations lasting for weeks that are typical in patients with peptic ulcer disease; nor did they have well-defined circumscribed attacks as did patients with biliary pain. However, some complained of being awakened at night by symptoms (32%), and many complained of nausea (60%) and of radiation of pain to the back or shoulder (36%).[2] Weight loss sometimes was present in these patients (32%) but was not progressive or substantial. Without endoscopy, including multiple biopsies of the esophageal mucosa, there is no absolute way to exclude the diagnosis of peptic disease of the esophagus, stomach, or duodenum in at least some of these patients. It seems likely, however, that the majority did have functional dyspepsia; although the symptomatology is complex, a few unifying factors appear to exist.

Two practical approaches to this problem can be entertained. First, there is a group of patients whose symptoms relate primarily to the upper abdomen but who have a specific psychogenic cause for the complaint: patients with anorexia caused by depression, with aerophagia and excessive belching caused by anxiety, or with abdominal pain due to hysteria and hypochondriasis. For these, the psychiatric diagnosis should be established positively, from observation of the patient's personality and behavior during the interview and from the history, in addition to the finding of negative gastrointestinal contrast studies. Second, there may be other patients with functional dyspepsia, defined by repeatedly negative studies, whose symptoms will tend to be atypical for peptic ulcer disease—that is, unrelated to meals and sporadic in occurrence. These patients may have upper abdominal symptoms analogous to the lower abdominal symptoms of the irritable bowel syndrome, which may not be entirely psychogenic but are produced in part by some functional abnormality, such as altered motility, in an otherwise healthy gastrointestinal tract. In our experience, the symptoms are mild, and most respond to reassurance plus empirically based therapy. However, these individuals should be reassessed if symptoms worsen, since some ultimately will develop peptic ulcer disease.

Among the many individuals with chronic abdominal pain or dyspepsia will be a few who have none of the common etiologies but are harboring a serious underlying disease. Acute abdominal conditions have not been considered in this discussion of dyspepsia but should be excluded in every patient with abdominal pain; likewise, diarrhea and lower abdominal pain are discussed in Chapters 26 and 27. Substernal fullness and "indigestion" can also be the presenting symptoms of coronary heart disease (see Chapter 3). Persistent pain, especially at night, and weight loss are the two manifestations that may alert the examiner to the presence of a serious disease process in patients with *chronic upper abdominal symptoms.* In *chronic pancreatitis*, there is often steady, boring, or aching pain, generally epigastric, with radiation to either upper quadrant or directly through to the back. This pain generally is persistent, noncrampy, and unrelated to gas, bowel movements, or intestinal activity, although perhaps aggravated by food or ethanol ingestion. Identical pain may occur in *carcinoma of the pancreas*, first as a dull or vague epigastric ache, then as episodic pain often following meals, but finally as persistent, severe pain radiating to the back. Leaking or expanding *abdominal aneurysms* may cause a steady mid-epigastric or back pain persisting for weeks prior to rupture; a tender, expansile mass is felt at the epigastrium or umbilicus. *Abdominal angina* is a rare condition seen in patients with more than 90% narrowing of at least two of the three major splanchnic arteries (celiac, superior mesenteric, or inferior mesenteric). Patients are elderly and often manifest marked weight loss in addition to the bruits and diminished pulses caused by extensive atherosclerotic vascular disease. Their pain occurs after eating; thus, it is fear of pain, rather than anorexia, that often leads to weight loss. In all these conditions, pain is usually more severe, steady, and persistent than that experienced by patients with the usual causes of dyspepsia.

Summary

Each of the commonly encountered causes of dyspepsia has characteristic manifestations; these are summarized in Tables 24–1 and 24–2. In practice, both biliary pain and reflux esophagitis usually have easily recognizable, usually distinguishing clinical features. In the other conditions that cause chronic dyspepsia, the patient's description of the symptoms is often suggestive but may not be specific enough to allow one to make the diagnosis accurately from the history alone. The problem for the physician in such cases is to decide whether radiographic studies or endoscopy is indicated. In this light, it seems reasonable to treat empirically, using antacids or sucralfate in young patients ($<$ 40 years old) with symptoms that are minor, short in duration, or infrequent. In older patients with new onset of symptoms or in those whose symptoms are persistent, lasting for more than a few weeks, or recurrent more than several times within a year, an effort should be made to document the diagnosis. This approach is outlined in Figure 24–3.

TABLE 24–1. DYSPEPSIA: USUAL PATTERNS OF SYMPTOMS*

	"Functional"	Symptomatic Cholelithiasis	Duodenal Ulcer	Gastric Ulcer	Gastric Cancer
Age	Any age	40–80 yr	30–60 yr	40–70 yr	60–80 yr
Duration of Symptoms	1–3 yr	1–3 yr	5–15 yr	2–4 mo	1–3 wk
Pattern of Symptoms	Intermittent or brief recurrences of symptoms	Attacks lasting hours to days	Episodes or exacerbations lasting weeks	Persistent or recurring symptoms	Persistent or continuously worsening symptoms
Back or Shoulder Pain (%)	36	77	29	42	14

*Adapted from Horrocks JC and DeDombal FT: Clinical presentation of patients with "dyspepsia." Detailed symptomatic study of 360 patients. Gut 19:19, 1978.

TABLE 24–2. DYSPEPSIA: CHARACTERISTICS OF SYMPTOMS*

	"Functional"	Symptomatic Cholelithiasis	Duodenal Ulcer	Gastric Ulcer	Gastric Cancer
Relation to Meals	Unrelated	Unrelated	Delayed after food	Any pattern	Any pattern
Immediate Relief by Antacids (%)	26	6	39	36	9
Accompanied by Nausea (%)	60	76	59	70	77
Awakened at Night by Pain (%)	32	34	70	32	16
>7-lb Weight Loss (%)	32	23	44	61	85

*Adapted from Horrocks JC and DeDombal FT: Clinical presentation of patients with "dyspepsia." Detailed symptomatic study of 360 patients. Gut 19:19, 1978.

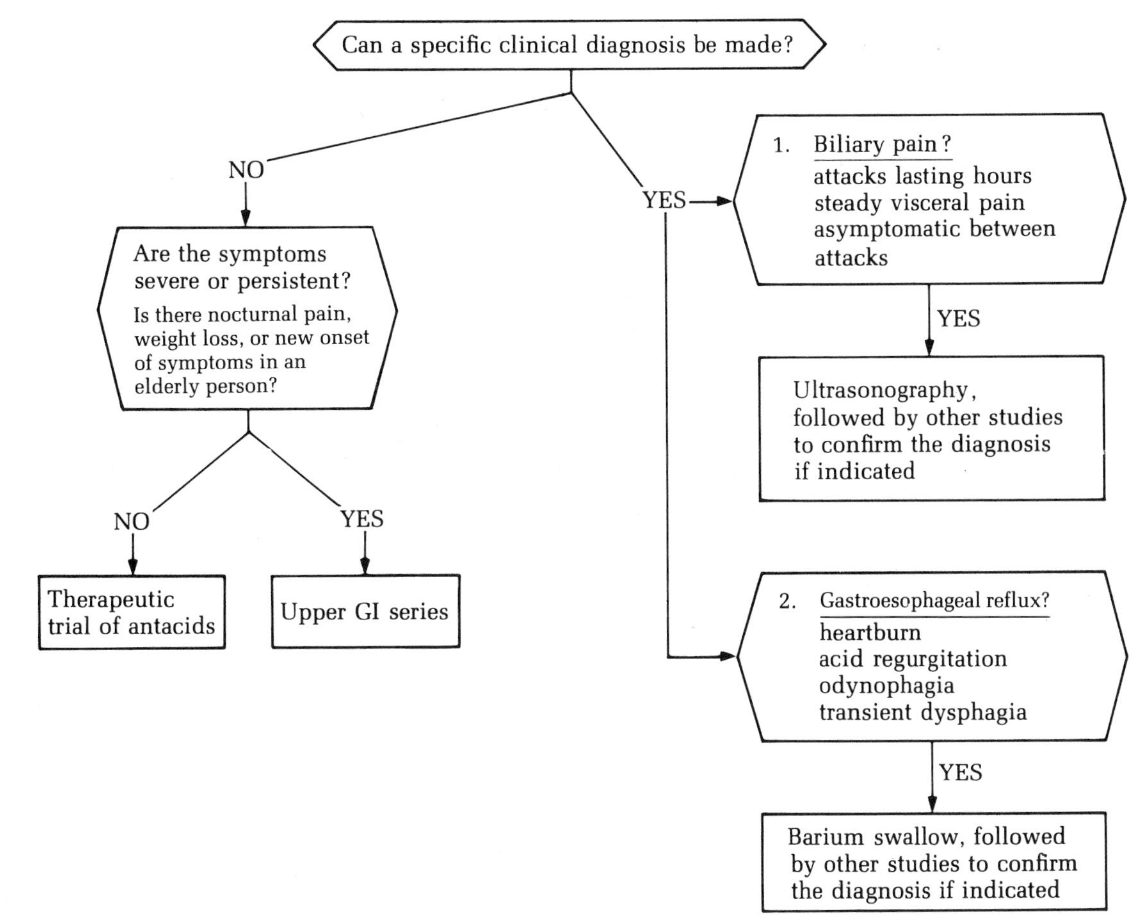

FIGURE 24–3. An initial approach for most patients with chronic dyspepsia and upper abdominal pain.

ESTABLISHING THE DIAGNOSIS AND TREATING THE CAUSES

Duodenal Ulcers

Diagnostic Studies and Approach to the Patient. UGIS, even when done by expert radiologists, are normal in 10 to 20% of patients with duodenal ulcer, demonstrable by endoscopy. For example, in the Mayo Clinic series, 15% of patients with ulcer-like symptoms but a normal UGIS were shown to have an ulcer on endoscopy.[12] This was a particular problem in patients with duodenal scarring and deformity, of whom 33% with no radiologically identifiable crater had an ulcer demonstrated by endoscopy.

The radiographic diagnosis of duodenal ulcer disease depends on demonstrating an ulcer niche that reproducibly fills with barium and remains filled during manual pressure to empty the duodenum. Folds may radiate from the ulcer niche in a spoke-like fashion, and a mound of edema may surround the ulcer in acute cases (Fig. 24–4).

Spiro has pointed out that even in patients with documented duodenal ulcer disease the symptoms do not always correlate with the presence or absence of an ulcer crater.[16] Endoscopists are now recognizing hemorrhagic mucosal lesions of the duodenum, often accompanied by superficial erosions. These are referred to as duodenitis; they do not always correspond to the hyperplastic duodenal folds sometimes referred to by radiologists as "duodenitis." In a small series of 13 patients with endoscopic findings of duodenitis, followed for 1 to 3.5 years, 6 eventually developed a documented ulcer, 2 remained symptomatic but without developing documented ulcers, and 5 became asymptomatic.[17] Furthermore, a carefully controlled study of antacid therapy showed that the symptoms of duodenal ulcer usually resolve after a period of weeks, even if the ulcer itself has not healed, whereas symptoms are persistent in other patients whose ulcers have healed according to endoscopic examination.[4] These data confirm Spiro's observation that the presence or absence of an actual ulcer crater does not always correlate with the symptoms of "duodenal ulcer disease."

If duodenal ulcer disease has been documented previously in a patient or a symptomatic patient's UGIS shows deformity of the duodenal bulb, even without an ulcer crater, it is easy to decide that a course of therapy is needed for exacerbations of typical symptoms. When the UGIS is normal, or a patient fails to respond to therapy, complications are suspected, or surgery is recommended but there is some diagnostic uncertainty, endoscopy needs to be considered.

Endoscopy at the time of an exacerbation will confirm the diagnosis of duodenal ulcer disease and is a much more sensitive test than UGIS. A reasonable approach in uncomplicated patients is to recommend endoscopy at that point when the patient's expense, in terms of time lost from work and suffering from the symptoms, begins to exceed the inconvenience, discomfort, and cost (currently ~ $350) of endoscopy. Using this approach, for example, one would not feel that it was always essential to have an endoscopically (or radiographically) proved diagnosis of duodenal ulcer disease before prescribing a trial of antacids or sucralfate. On the other hand, poor response to such a trial or early or multiple recurrences justifies the effort to base further treatment upon a firm diagnosis.

Management. When the patient's symptoms suggest ulcer recurrence, it is necessary to prescribe a 6- to 8-week course of therapy adequate to promote healing. On a longer-term basis, sufficient therapy should be prescribed to suppress symptoms while altering environmental factors when possible to minimize the likelihood of ulcer recurrences or complications. If symptoms tend to recur soon after completing each course of therapy, prescribing maintenance treatment that is adequate to prevent recurrences or advising surgery may be considered.

A realistic appraisal of the importance of *environmental factors* in the pathogenesis of duodenal ulcer disease is necessary. With regard to emotional stress, there is no proof that one can diminish the likelihood of ulcer recurrence through changes in work patterns or environment[18]; however, it is thought that complete removal from the work and home setting in the hospital can promote healing of active ulcers. A general principle is that sedatives or tranquilizers should be prescribed only for a patient's recognizable anxiety or other symptoms, not for the treatment of ulcer disease per se.

Evidence clearly associates cigarette smoking with increased incidence of ulcer development or recurrence.[19, 20] Thus it is mandatory to convince patients known to have duodenal ulcer disease to desist from smoking. The data conflict whether coffee, cola beverages, alcohol, and aspirin are associated with an increased risk of duodenal ulcer.[19–22] However, alcohol and aspirin may be associated with gastric ulcer or bleeding gastric erosions, particularly in individuals with underlying gastric hyperacidity,[23] and should be avoided by ulcer patients. The relationship of adrenal glucocorticosteroids (steroids) to peptic ulcer is highly controversial. One paper summarized a large amount of data and concluded that there was no increased risk of ulcer in patients receiving steroids for less than 30 days or a total dose of less than 100 mg of prednisone[7]; another paper concluded that there was a small increase in gastric ulcers among patients receiving moderate-to-large doses of steroids.[8]

There is no evidence that ulcers heal more rapidly on bland diets.[23] Milk, which is given routinely in most ulcer diets, has only a limited neutralizing effect on gastric acidity and is followed by increased acid secretion. Frequent small meals also have the adverse consequence of stimulating rebound gastric hyperacidity.

Antacids remain a mainstay of ulcer therapy. Since they are inorganic, unlike milk or other foods, they do *not* cause as much gastrin release and rebound hyperacidity, provided they do not contain calcium salts. Given in adequate dosage, they can increase gastric pH to a value above 3.3, at which the total amount of acid exposure of the duodenum is reduced by 99%.[24, 25] Furthermore, the activity of pepsin is diminished at a pH greater than 2.0, and pepsin is inactive at a pH greater than 3.5. A well-designed, randomized trial has demonstrated duodenal ulcer healing, proved by endoscopy, in 78% of patients after 4 weeks on high-dose liquid antacids (30 ml taken 1 and 3 hours after meals and once at bedtime), compared with healing in the same time period in 45% of patients receiving placebos.[4]

Preparations containing calcium carbonate (Tums, Titralac) stimulate gastrin release. When taken in large doses, they also may induce hypercalcemia with subsequent renal failure. Aluminum hydroxide–magnesium trisilicate preparations are constipating and may cause phosphate depletion, leading to osteoporosis over a prolonged period. Magnesium-aluminum hydroxide preparations are generally the most potent; their only adverse effects in normal people are diarrhea and interference with absorption of tetracycline and certain other medications. In patients with renal failure, however, Mg^{2+} may accumulate to toxic levels. Aluminum carbonate (Basaljel) and aluminum hydroxide

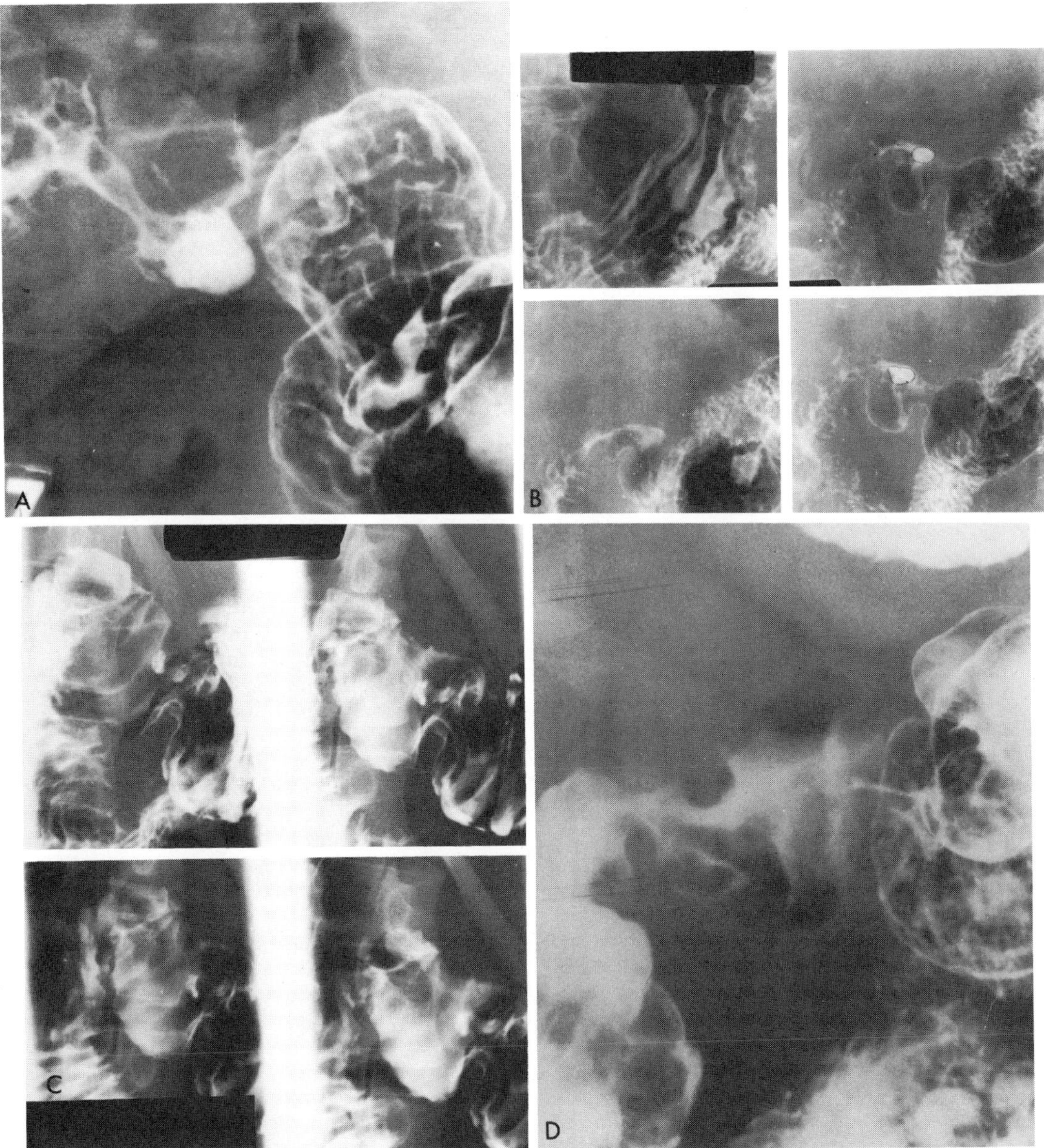

FIGURE 24–4. Radiographic features of duodenal ulcers. *A*, Barium is lodged in a niche in a posterior bulbar duodenal ulcer; folds can be seen radiating to the niche. The ulcer niche remains filled with barium during various maneuvers designed to remove barium from the remainder of the duodenal bulb. In *B*, a 1.5-cm ulcer niche is located at the posterosuperior aspect of the duodenal bulb. The bulb is deformed, with folds radiating to the ulcer crater. In *C*, the ulcer niche is surrounded by edema. *D*, The duodenal bulb is deformed, but no active ulcer crater can be identified. Deformity of the duodenal bulb suggests duodenal ulcer disease, although in many cases with deformity no ulcer crater is demonstrable radiographically. (Courtesy of Department of Radiology, Brigham and Women's Hospital, Harvard Medical School, Boston, Massachusetts.)

(AlternaGEL) are effective phosphate-depleting agents for patients with renal failure and do not contain magnesium. Maalox and Mylanta now have very low sodium content, as low or lower than Riopan, and have greater buffering capacity than does Riopan. Table 24–3 shows the acid-neutralizing capacities of various preparations.[24, 25]

Antacid tablets are less effectively distributed to the mucosa than are liquid suspensions. The most efficacious timing for doses is 1 hour after meals, when the antacid remains within the stomach longer. Thirty ml of magnesium-aluminum hydroxide (Maalox) given at this time will maintain intragastric pH above 3.5 for as long as 60 minutes.[24, 25] However, the best approach for controlling more refractory symptoms is to increase the frequency of antacid administration. In practice, a 2- to 4-week course of 30 ml of Maalox, Mylanta, or Mylanta-II taken 1 hour after each meal and at night before bed may be sufficient therapy for those with mild symptoms. For patients with more severe symptoms or documented presence of an ulcer crater, we recommend that 30 ml be prescribed 1 hour after meals, 3 hours after meals, and at night before bed (total of seven doses). This treatment should be continued until the patient has been free of pain for 2 weeks, at which point the dosage can be lowered to 30 ml four times daily (1 hour after meals and at bedtime) for an additional 4 weeks. If the patient remains pain-free, antacids can be discontinued but should be reinstituted promptly if symptoms recur.

An *H_2-receptor antagonist* appears to be a reasonable alterative to high-dose antacids for short-term therapy (no longer than 8 weeks). It has advantages over antacids,

TABLE 24–3. NEUTRALIZING CAPACITY OF COMMONLY USED ANTACIDS*

	Volume for Neutralizing 80 mEq Acid (ml)
Delcid (Magnesium-aluminum hydroxide)	11.3
Mylanta-II (Magnesium-aluminum hydroxide)	19.3
Maalox (Magnesium-aluminum hydroxide)	31.0
Mylanta (Magnesium-aluminum hydroxide)	33.6
Gelusil M (Aluminum hydroxide and magnesium trisilicate)	35.9
Riopan (Magaldrate)	36.2
Amphojel (Aluminum hydroxide)	41.4
Gelusil (Aluminum hydroxide and magnesium trisilicate)	60.1

*Adapted from Morrissey JF and Barreras RF: Drug therapy. Antacid therapy. N Engl J Med 290:550, 1974; and Littman A and Pine BH: Diagnosis and treatment: Drug spotlight program. Antacids and anticholinergic drugs. Ann Intern Med 82:544, 1975.

chiefly a longer duration of action and greater compliance. However, since antacids are equally effective in short-term therapy and have been found virtually free of serious toxicity after many years of experience, they should still be used in patients in whom the diagnosis is uncertain or who have minor symptoms or brief recurrences. Short-term treatment with an H_2 blocker might be reserved for patients who fail to respond adequately to antacids and for those in whom antacid therapy is not optimal owing to difficulty with compliance, frequent exacerbations, or side effects.

Cimetidine, the original H_2-receptor blocker, is effective in management of duodenal ulcer disease.[26] An oral dose of 400 mg of cimetidine after a meal produces a reduction in postprandial duodenal acid load equal to that produced by 30 ml of Maalox taken 1 and 3 hours after meals, although antacids cannot match the prolonged nocturnal inhibition of gastric acid secretion achieved with cimetidine taken at bedtime. Endoscopically controlled trials clearly demonstrate the superiority of short-term treatment with cimetidine over placebo or minimal therapy with antacids. Healing occurred in 70 to 80% of patients after 4 to 6 weeks on cimetidine compared with 30 to 40% of the controls.[27–30] These results are virtually identical to the results using high doses of liquid antacids.[4]

Occasional patients complain of nausea, which can be relieved by taking the drug with a small snack. Rather common are confusion, apathy, and sleep disturbances in elderly patients (and patients with renal or hepatic failure) and endocrine disturbances (manifested by erective difficulty, impotence, and gynecomastia) in men of all ages. Cimetidine interferes with hepatic oxidative metabolism of many drugs, including warfarin, propranolol, diazepam, phenytoin, lidocaine, theophylline, and verapamil; dosages of these agents need to be lower in patients concomitantly treated with cimetidine. Other toxic and side effects include skin rashes, decreased renal perfusion, interstitial nephritis, agranulocytosis, aplastic anemia, toxic hepatitis, drug cholestasis, and brachycardia; all are rare.[23, 28, 31, 32]

Rebound acid hypersecretion caused by increased gastrin release after discontinuance of cimetidine was not substantiated in a report of patients treated for 12 months. An increased gastrin response to meals while the patients were on cimetidine did not persist after the drug had been discontinued.

Ranitidine is an H_2-receptor antagonist that is more potent and has a longer duration of action than does cimetidine.[35, 36, 38] It will block acid secretion in some patients who are resistant to cimetidine. Ranitidine in usual dosages of 150 mg given twice daily has fewer side effects and less toxicity: very little crosses the blood-brain barrier, so there is less central nervous system problem in the elderly; pituitary-endocrine effects are negligible; there is less interference with hepatic metabolism.

The newest H_2-blockers are famotidine (Pepcid) and nizatidine. Famotidine[39] may be marginally better than its predecessors, while nizatidine can be considered almost identical to ranitidine with regard to efficacy and side effects.

Omeprazole stops acid secretion even more effectively than H_2-blockers, by inhibiting the parietal cells' proton pump. Although approved for use in duodenal ulcer,[40, 41] it should be restricted to only ulcers that defy endoscopic healing by any other agent, because of drawbacks that accompany such complete inhibition of acid secretion (discussed in greater detail later, under peptic esophagitis). Omeprazole is the pharmacologic therapy of choice for an ulcer due to Zollinger-Ellison syndrome and systemic mast cell disease.

Sucralfate (Carafate) is a sulfated aluminum hydroxide salt of sucrose with radial and linear polymerization, which has no effect on acid. It binds to ulcer craters, erosions, and intact mucosa, stimulating healing.[42–47] In all trials, sucralfate (1 g orally, four times or 2 gm bid) has been equal to cimetidine or any other H_2-blocker in healing 73 to 97% of duodenal and 71 to 75% of gastric ulcers after 4 to 6 weeks of therapy.[48] Sucralfate is more effective than H_2-blockers in patients who continue to smoke cigarettes. Cost exceeds cimetidine by 20% but is 20% less than ranitidine.[48] In contrast to H_2-receptor antagonists, sucralfate acts locally and very little is systemically absorbed, giving much lower side effects or toxicity. To date, the only adverse reaction reported has been mild-to-moderate constipation.

Doses of cimetidine used in practice (200 to 300 mg, four times daily) appear to be adequate for healing most duodenal ulcers but increase the mean gastric pH only from approximately 1.3 to 1.8.[49] In fact, many duodenal ulcers will heal completely even on placebo therapy.[50] Occasionally, however, patients are encountered whose *symptoms do not resolve* or recur despite the usual therapy. These individuals may have an inordinate lack of mucosal defenses against acid in the duodenum.[49] In addition, *Helicobacter pylori* may be involved (see further on), and a few of these patients may have massively elevated basal acid secretory rates.[51] Measurement of serum gastrin levels is required to exclude the Zollinger-Ellison syndrome in all refractory cases, but most patients with basal acid outputs greater than 15 mEq/hr have no obvious cause or have pyloric stenosis.[31]

The *natural history* of duodenal ulcer disease is probably quite variable. In studies of unselected patients who were followed for 10 to 13 years after an initial diagnosis, one half to two thirds had had no complications and either mild or no symptoms.[52, 53] However, there is clearly a subgroup with severe symptoms. In Fry's series, 43% of patients lost time from work because of recurrences or exacerbations during the first 5 years after the diagnosis was established, and 20% ultimately experienced complications.[53] It is interesting that only 2% of the patients continued to have severe symptoms 10 years following the diagnosis. The most difficult problem for clinicians are the patients who have frequent recurrences of ulcer disease; these are the individuals who most often are referred to gastroenterologists and have appeared in the published series of patients treated with cimetidine.[54–58] Repeated short courses of H_2-receptor antagonists resulted in an ultimate rate of ulcer recurrence, once the drug was discontinued, that was exactly the same as in patients on no therapy.[55]

Long-term therapy with H_2-blockers for selected cases reduces the incidence of endoscopically ascertained recurrence, during the time patients are maintained on the drug, from a 55 to 80% range down to 13 to 20%.[6, 56–58] A single bedtime dose of cimetidine (600 to 800 mg) or ranitidine (300 mg) or sucralfate (2 g) appears to be effective.[57]

At present, most patients with recurrent ulceration should be managed by repeated 6- to 8-week courses of antacids, sucralfate, or H_2-blockers. Longer-term omeprazole therapy can be recommended for those with the Zollinger-Ellison syndrome. Long-term maintenance therapy should be considered for patients with complicated cases, such as a history of previous ulcer bleeding or recurrences following surgery for peptic ulcer disease. It seems reasonable also to recommend that cigarette smokers, elderly individuals, and those at high risk for elective surgery be treated with long-term maintenance using sucralfate.[45] In the younger patient with uncomplicated peptic ulcer, the potential for very long-term toxicity from H_2-blockers (or omeprazole) outweighs the advantages of lifelong therapy with either form of acid suppression therapy.

Helicobacter pylori has the apparently unique ability to survive in the acid environment of the normally secreting stomach.[59–61] Its presence close to the surface of antral mucosa is strongly associated with duodenal ulcer (80 to 90%), gastric ulcer (~ 70%), and antral gastritis (>90%). *Helicobacter* is also common in the stomach of the general population (without ulcer, without dyspepsia) and increases with age to a peak of approximately 80% in the seventh decade. In some undeveloped countries where the incidence of peptic ulcer is very low, virtually 100% of adults harbor gastric *Helicobacter*. Experiments have shown that initial infection with *Helicobacter* can cause symptomatic acute antral gastritis (during which acid secretion falls to zero), sometimes leading to symptomatic chronic antral gastritis. Patients with functional or nonulcer dyspepsia have the same incidence of *Helicobacter* as an age-matched population without symptoms, and eradication of *Helicobacter* relieves dyspeptic symptoms no better than does placebo in these patients.

Our current perspective agrees with many experts, who believe that *Helicobacter* is a definite cause of chronic antral gastritis (usually without symptoms) and is not the sole cause of gastroduodenal ulcer but appears to interact with other factors, probably by adversely affecting mucosal defenses, to promote peptic ulcer. Bismuth compounds (e.g., Pepto-Bismol) alone or single antibiotics can suppress *Helicobacter*, but suppression affords no apparent long-term benefit. Simpler methods are being sought, but standard therapy for complete eradication of *Helicobacter* currently requires two broad-spectrum antibiotics (amoxicillin 500 mg qid [or tetracycline 500 mg qid in pen-allergic patients] for 2 weeks and metronidazole 250 mg qid for 10 days) plus a bismuth preparation (Pepto-Bismol, two tablets three times daily for 2 weeks). Eradication of *Helicobacter* combined with usual ulcer therapy offers no supplemental benefit for ulcer healing. However, if *Helicobacter* is eradicated, the time for a recurrence of a duodenal ulcer is significantly longer.[62] Thus, *Helicobacter* eradication is recommended when recurrence of duodenal ulcer is deemed likely.

The diagnosis of *Helicobacter* requires culture of endoscopically obtained biopsy specimens, properly handled, and/or histologic examination with Giemsa staining of multiple biopsy specimens when available. The urea breath test, in which labeled urea ingested orally can be detected as CO_2 in the breath, offers a noninvasive test on which treatment or follow-up may be based.

For non-ulcer dyspepsia, H_2-blockers (or antacids) are no more effective than placebo. (In non-ulcer dyspepsia, there is a greater than average favorable response to placebo therapy, similar to that in irritable bowel syndrome. This has prompted some to refer to non-ulcer dyspepsia as the irritable bowel syndrome of the upper gastrointestinal tract.) One study reported that sucralfate was superior to placebo in relieving symptoms in non-ulcer dyspepsia.[63]

The indications for *surgery* in duodenal ulcer are (1) a second episode of bleeding or massive, painless bleeding from a duodenal ulcer, (2) unrelenting obstruction, and (3) perforation. In all cases, definitive ulcer surgery is performed with the object of preventing a recurrence. The two standard antiulcer procedures are antrectomy and vagotomy, and vagotomy and drainage (pyloroplasty). After antrectomy and vagotomy, the recurrence rate of duodenal or marginal ulcers is as low as 0.6%, and the operative mortality of antrectomy and vagotomy is about 1.6%.[64] The operative mortality for vagotomy and drainage is about 0.9%, but recurrent ulceration within 5 years probably ranges from 6 to 12%.[65] The incidence of postgastrectomy symptoms such as diarrhea and malabsorption is substantially less after vagotomy and drainage than after antral resection.

"Intractable" symptoms have clinically constituted an indication for peptic ulcer surgery. Although elective operative mortality rates are low, up to 4% of patients may experience serious complications of vagotomy, including splenic rupture, esophageal perforation, and postoperative hemorrhage; leakage from the gastrojejunostomy or pyloroplasty suture line occurs in 2%.[65] In addition, many patients develop diarrhea, mild dumping, and nausea after surgery, particularly if gastric resection is performed. Up to half the patients have some steatorrhea, one third report a weight loss of more than 6 kg, and almost half are anemic.[65] When the operative mortality, serious operative complications, postoperative side effects, and incidence of recurrent ulcer in patients undergoing gastric resection or vagotomy and drainage are totaled, it appears that about 10% will experience poor results. This, together with the effectiveness of *Helicobacter* eradication or long-term treatments, and the continuous decline in the incidence of duodenal ulcers in recent years, explains why surgery is now performed less commonly than in the past and is not often needed for symptoms in the absence of complications.

There has been an effort to develop a better surgical procedure. Truncal vagotomy alone lowers basal acid secretion by 70 to 80%. (The pyloroplasty is performed to facilitate gastric emptying that otherwise would be inhibited by the vagotomy.) The addition of an antrectomy or hemigastrectomy to vagotomy further reduces both basal and histamine-stimulated acid secretion by 10 to 20% and will lead to fewer recurrent ulcers, as noted previously. Dumping and diarrhea probably are due to denervation of the stomach and of the small bowel, respectively, in addition to the absence of a physiologically functioning pyloric mechanism after surgically reconstructed drainage. Gastric mucosal atrophy with perhaps symptomatic gastritis occurs as a result of loss of antral gastrin.

In proximal gastric vagotomy, also called superselective vagotomy (Fig. 24–5), only those fibers of the vagus that actually supply the body and fundus (i.e., the parietal cell mass) of the stomach are resected. Since the nerve supply to the pylorus is not disrupted, there is no need for a drainage procedure. Likewise, the small bowel remains normally enervated. Acid secretion is reduced to a similar degree as after truncal vagotomy. In the hands of expert surgeons, the operative mortality has been low, and few complications have been reported. Ulcer recurrence rates are somewhat higher (10 to 15%) than has been experienced after truncal vagotomy and drainage (5 to 10%).[65, 67] Surgeons who perform the operation have reported less postoperative diarrhea, substantially less dumping, and nearly normal gastric emptying and small bowel transit.[67–70] Thus, proximal gastric vagotomy is now a standard elective operation for duodenal ulcer patients in selected medical centers.[67] It is also amenable to supplementation with another operation for patients who have recurrences. However, the operation is technically difficult, cannot be done in patients with pyloric obstruction, and requires that the patient be capable of withstanding prolonged anesthesia. At this time, most surgeons continue to perform traditional truncal vagotomy and drainage procedures.

GASTROESOPHAGEAL REFLUX AND OTHER BENIGN ESOPHAGEAL DISEASES

The symptoms of esophageal disease fall into two categories: pain and dysphagia. Dysphagia refers to the sensation of inability to pass food through the esophagus. This must be distinguished from globus hystericus (sensation of a lump in the throat), which is always a benign symptom, and from difficulty in initiating the act of swallowing, usually a neurologic symptom. Dysphagia always requires thorough investigation and should never be attributed to hysteria or emotional overlay. A spectrum of pain manifestations referable to the esophagus exists. Various pain syndromes have been described.

1. Heartburn (pyrosis): a "burning" substernal or high epigastric sensation often accompanied by sour regurgitation, with a tendency to occur nocturnally or 1 hour after meals.
2. Pain of chronic or severe reflux: persistent, substernal or midback, aching discomfort, less immediately or completely relieved by antacids, often worse with hot or spicy foods, and sometimes accompanied by dysphagia.
3. Odynophagia: pain that occurs during and immediately after swallowing, resulting from severe esophagitis, esophageal ulcer, candidal or herpetic esophagitis, or esophageal perforation.
4. Constrictive esophageal pain: an episodic substernal visceral sensation of tightness or constriction, often radiating to the back, neck, arm, or jaw, which can be accompanied by diaphoresis, may occur nocturnally, and sometimes is slowly relieved by nitroglycerin.

The two major categories of benign esophageal diseases are gastroesophageal reflux disease (GERD) and motility disorders. Esophagitis of variable severity and its complications—esophageal ulcers and benign strictures—are associated with reflux. Motility disorders include diffuse esophageal spasm, achalasia, and scleroderma. They typically present with constrictive esophageal pain, intermittent dysphagia for liquids and solids, and/or spontaneous regurgitation of food. Intermittent dysphagia also may be caused by an esophageal ring. Esophageal carcinoma must be carefully considered and excluded in every patient complaining of dysphagia. Miscellaneous conditions such as neuromuscular dysfunction, diverticula, and webs are uncommon and generally present as intermittent dysphagia or bouts of aspiration pneumonitis.

Gastroesophageal Reflux. Peptic esophagitis results from reflux of gastric (and perhaps duodenal) secretions into the esophagus. This occurs at least transiently in many normal individuals. Patients with esophagitis have more prolonged and more severe reflux. This is related to dysfunction of the lower esophageal sphincter (LES) and to inability to clear acid from the esophagus.[71] The LES, a physiologic mechanism for the prevention of reflux, normally is located 1 to 3 cm above the anatomic esophagogastric juncture (Fig. 24–6). Sphincter pressure is detected by

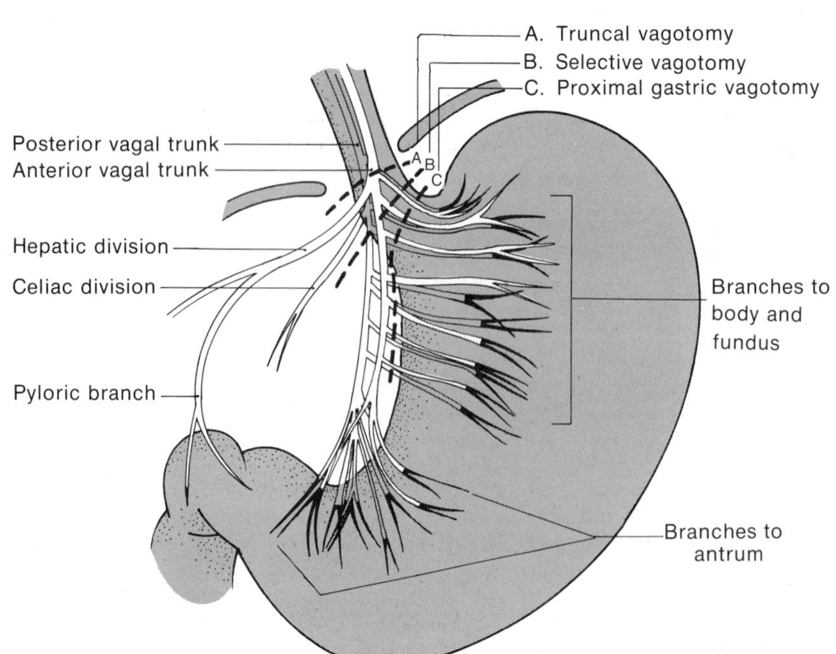

FIGURE 24–5. The vagus nerve and the levels of transection in various forms of vagotomy. (Adapted from Schrock TR: Progress in gastroenterology: Vagotomy in the elective treatment of duodenal ulcer. Gastroenterology 68:1615, 1975.)

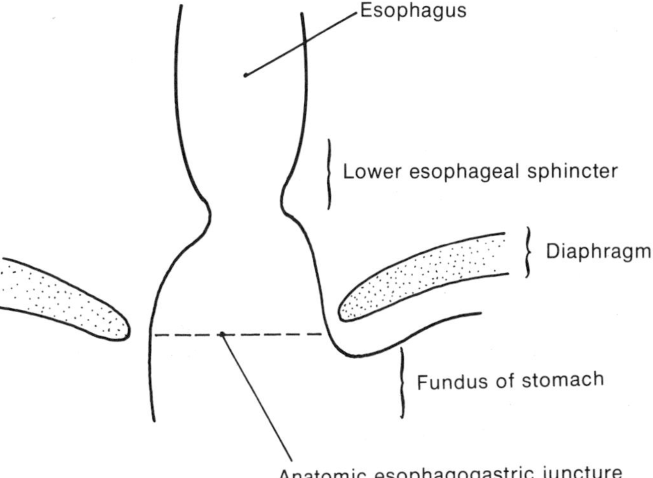

FIGURE 24–6. The lower esophageal sphincter (LES) and its relationship to the anatomic esophagogastric juncture.

manometry, although only very subtle anatomic differences in the smooth muscle have been identified at this location. Uncertainty remains concerning the relationship of esophagitis to the presence of a sliding hiatal hernia. The incidence of hiatal hernia varies from 30 to 75%, depending on the age of the population studied; however, severe reflux symptoms occur in a minority of these (~ 5%) and occur also in patients without hiatus hernias.[72,73] It is conceivable that hiatal hernias may contribute to reflux by interfering with LES function in some patients. Other factors known to promote reflux or to relax the LES include cigarette smoking, fatty foods, chocolate, anticholinergic, nitrate and calcium channel blocking drugs, obesity, pregnancy, oral contraceptive pills, and severe esophagitis per se.[74] Patients with peptic ulcer are also reported to experience heartburn.

Benign Strictures. Benign strictures result from scar formation induced by chronic reflux esophagitis; hence, most patients have had persistent heartburn and other manifestations of esophagitis of several years' duration. Some are silent, however, and dysphagia is reported without a previous history of heartburn. The exact incidence cannot be given, but in the practice of one gastroenterologist, 11% of 413 patients referred for esophagitis developed a stricture.[73] Benign fibrous strictures that cause dysphagia may also follow ingestion of corrosive substances, such as lye. The cardinal manifestation of the stricture itself is slowly progressive dysphagia for solid food. The dysphagia begins intermittently but progresses for many months or years; this is in contrast to most malignant strictures, in which dysphagia progresses more rapidly. Strictures of the midesophagus often have an associated columnar-lined Barrett's epithelium, acquired as a result of gastroesophageal reflux. Adenocarcinoma has been reported as a late sequela in as many as 8% of these individuals.[75] Hence, the major diagnostic problems in patients with strictures are to distinguish between benign and malignant ones at the outset and to detect those at risk for future malignancy.

Diffuse Esophageal Spasm. The symptoms of diffuse esophageal spasm are pain and intermittent dysphagia, not necessarily simultaneously. Pain is usually described as visceral tightness, constriction, or waves of pain experienced substernally and often radiating to the back. It can be severe and can be accompanied by diaphoresis. Its occurrence is often spontaneous, sometimes nocturnal, or possibly triggered by ingestion of very hot or cold liquids. Dysphagia is transient and not progressive and is also at times related to very hot or cold food.

Patients with diffuse spasm have normal peristalsis in the upper third of the esophagus (striated muscle), but in the lower two thirds (smooth muscle) the act of swallowing initiates uncoordinated movements. These occur simultaneously rather than following a peristaltic sequence. In about one third of such individuals, LES pressure is elevated, but the number of ganglion cells is not reduced as it is in achalasia.[76, 77] The muscle in the lower two thirds of the esophagus is diffusely thickened. However, of 600 patients referred for evaluation, only a small number had all three classic features of diffuse esophageal spasm, including a history of pain and dysphagia, typical manometric findings, and typical x-ray findings.[77] Much more frequently encountered were patients with intermittent pain or dysphagia that appeared related to less specific manometric abnormalities.

Achalasia. Dysphagia is the most common of a variety of symptoms in achalasia. Initially intermittent, this progresses to being constant and characteristically occurs with eating either solid or liquid food but is often provoked by rapid eating or emotional stress. Spontaneous regurgitation of retained esophageal contents is another prominent symptom; it may occur during positional changes or exertion. The regurgitated material consists of undigested food and lacks the sour, acid quality of reflux. A hazardous complication is aspiration pneumonitis. Odynophagia, colic, or spontaneous esophageal pain occurs also in some cases; a substantial number of patients may show features of achalasia and diffuse esophageal spasm concurrently.[78, 79]

The most characteristic pathophysiologic feature of achalasia is failure of the LES to relax its resting pressure with swallowing. Resting pressure may be increased or normal. Above the sphincter, the lower two thirds of the esophagus is characterized by aperistalsis, which becomes virtually total in advanced cases. In earlier cases, peristalsis ends at the aortic arch, below which there are aimless contractions.

Scleroderma. In advanced visceral scleroderma the LES is incompetent, occasionally with no measurable tone, and there is aperistalsis of the lower esophagus. Essentially, this results in free reflux and subsequent impaired clearance of refluxed gastric contents from the distal esophagus. The most common clinical manifestation is relentless heartburn, but dysphagia also occurs intermittently in 25% of patients.[77] Similar but less pronounced findings occur in some patients with Raynaud's phenomena, whether or not it is associated with a specific connective tissue disease.

Diagnostic Studies

Barium Swallow. This defines the anatomy of the esophagus. Peristalsis is observed by fluoroscopy. Reflux of barium is sought during maneuvers to increase intra-abdominal pressure. When reflux is obvious, the test is diagnostically helpful.[80] Unfortunately, fewer than half of patients with reflux demonstrated by other methods also have it on barum swallow. In addition, the barium swallow is not a sensitive means to detect the superficial mucosal ulcers often found in patients with peptic esophagitis—only deep, chronic ulcers are seen. With adequate barium to distend the esophagus, strictures should be noted. Benign peptic strictures have a smooth, tapered appearance, are of variable length, and usually occur in the distal one third of the esophagus. However, in general, one should not depend on radiographic features alone, without negative esophageal biopsies and cytology, to exclude malignancy in patients with strictures.

Normal findings on barium swallow were reported in 9% of 362 patients with esophageal carcinoma.[81] A later review describes no falsely negative barium swallows in patients with carcinoma, but the lesion was mistaken for an extrinsic mass, benign stricture, or ulcer in 12 to 30% of cases.[82]

The radiographic findings in diffuse esophageal spasm are of uncoordinated contractions of the lower two thirds, which may assume a "corkscrew" or "curling" pattern. Not every patient with esophageal pain and abnormal manometrics has the classic findings on barium swallow; likewise, patients with radiographically noted esophageal spasm can be asymptomatic.

In achalasia and scleroderma, it is important to examine the patient while he or she is recumbent, so as not to mistake a gravitational flow of barium for that due to peristalsis. Late findings of gross dilatation, absent peristalsis, and "beaking" of the distal esophagus are clearly diagnostic of achalasia, but in early cases, special attention should be paid to the lower two thirds of the esophagus, where normal peristalsis is replaced by weak or inconstant contractions. In advanced esophageal scleroderma, the barium swallow reveals aperistalsis, stasis of barium within the esophagus of the supine patient, and dilatation with free reflux. Cineradiography and special swallowing studies are helpful when there is suspicion of a lesion in the swallowing mechanism or upper esophagus.

Esophagoscopy. This is performed frequently in patients suspected of having esophagitis. However, in many cases, the mucosa is not frankly hemorrhagic, so that the esophagus may appear normal to the endoscopist in some patients with symptoms caused by reflux esophagitis. Hyperemia (redness) without ulceration is a nonspecific finding. Hence, suction biopsies usually are necessary to confirm the diagnosis. These reveal epithelial ulceration and inflammatory infiltrate in some patients. Patients without these findings generally meet other histologic criteria for the diagnosis. There is thickening of the basal epithelial layer (above 15% of total epithelial thickness) and extension of submucosal pegs toward the luminal surface. With a sufficient number of biopsies, virtually all patients with esophagitis should have these findings. Unfortunately, similar findings, particularly within 5 cm of the LES, are seen in many asymptomatic individuals and probably are caused by minor degrees of reflux. Thus, biopsies are very sensitive but not entirely specific.

Esophagoscopy may not detect mild narrowing due to stricture, but scarring is usually evident. Since negative results on biopsies (diagnostic accuracy, 94%) do not entirely rule out malignancy, brush or exfoliative specimens for cytologic study (diagnostic accuracy, 92%) should also be collected.[82] The procedures should be repeated, if necessary, to obtain sampling from the distal esophagus following therapeutic dilatations. Esophagoscopy is not useful in the diagnosis of esophageal motility disorders.

pH Monitoring in the Esophagus. In 80% of patients with severe symptoms of reflux, intraesophageal pH will decrease to less than 4.0 during the Valsalva maneuver, coughing, and other maneuvers designed to increase intra-abdominal pressure. This test is performed by withdrawing a pH probe 5 cm above the LES after filling the stomach with 300 ml of 0.1 normal hydrochloric acid. As many as 20% of asymptomatic individuals also have a positive test result.[83, 84]

Because of the nonspecificity of the standard acid reflux test, interest has centered on 24-hour pH monitoring in the esophagus. The patient keeps a diary recording symptoms of reflux and relating them to changes in posture or activity throughout the 24-hour period. A composite score is then derived from the intraesophageal pH and the patient's symptoms. More than 80% of patients with reflux are thought to have scores at least two standard deviations above the normal mean.[85, 86] This test, if available, is probably the most reliable way to determine the relationship of reflux to symptoms.

Acid Perfusion (Bernstein) Test. An effort is made to reproduce pain systematically by alternating infusions of 0.1 normal hydrochloric acid and saline. It is important to ascertain that the test reproduces the patient's symptoms exactly. The test result is positive in most patients with esophagitis but also in some control subjects and patients with peptic ulcers.[87]

Manometry. This is chiefly useful for investigating motility disorders. Patients with diffuse esophageal spasm have repetitive or simultaneous contractions of increased amplitude occurring with more than 30% of swallows. Those with achalasia tend to have aperistalsis and failure of relaxation of the LES after swallowing. LES pressure determined manometrically is elevated in many patients with achalasia ($\geqslant$ 40 mm Hg) but also in a subset of those appearing to have diffuse esophageal spasm.[76] In patients with features of both diffuse spasm and achalasia, the manometric features of spasm (high-amplitude, nonperistaltic contractions in the lower two thirds) coexist with dysphagia and esophageal retention resembling achalasia.[77, 78]

It is generally accepted that the LES pressure measured manometrically is diminished in most patients with reflux esophagitis when compared with a normal population. However, some patients have normal sphincter pressures ($\geqslant$10 mm Hg), so that the test is neither completely specific nor sensitive enough for routine diagnostic use.[80] Most of these patients have greatly increased frequency of spontaneous relaxations of the LES.[71]

Summary of the Approach to the Patient

When the symptoms are those of gastroesophageal reflux—chiefly heartburn and sour regurgitation without dysphagia—most clinicians will obtain a barium swallow and UGIS as a baseline study if symptoms are persistent and then treat the patient empirically. One cannot be so certain of the underlying problem in patients with spontaneous or persistent pain. In this case, the evaluation begins with a barium swallow with cineradiography if a motility disorder is suspected. In those with esophagitis, the study may be normal or may show reflux. In patients with motility disorders, some abnormality of the barium swallow or cinestudy should suggest spasm, achalasia, or scleroderma. A third category of patients have dysphagia. All require a barium swallow to exclude the presence of a stricture. In some, intermittent symptoms are explained adequately by finding an esophageal ring. All patients with a documented stricture, as well as those with persistent, unexplained dysphagia even if the result of the radiographic study is negative, require esophagoscopy with biopsies and brush cytology to exclude malignancy and to identify individuals with Barrett's epithelium, who are at increased risk of developing malignancy.

In patients with esophagitis, the role of diagnostic studies beyond the barium swallow depends on the clinical situation (Table 24–4). No additional studies are needed in patients without dysphagia who respond to treatment. If the symptoms are relatively severe but the diagnosis is questionable, esophagoscopy will determine whether the esophagus shows friability and ulceration, and multiple biopsies of the esophageal mucosa usually reveal histologic changes in patients with less severe esophagitis. If the patient has persistent or poorly controlled symptoms and antireflux surgery is being considered, it is essential to establish unequivocally that reflux exists and is causing the patient's problem. When this is uncertain despite esophagoscopy and biopsy, 24-hour pH monitoring should be performed if available. Manometry can also be useful preoperatively when it is uncertain whether the symptoms are caused by reflux or diffuse spasm. Findings of uncoordinated contractions with increased amplitude suggest a motility disorder as the diagnosis; an unexpectedly high LES pressure ($\geq$15 mm Hg) makes reflux unlikely in patients whose symptoms are so severe that surgery is being considered.

Another clinical problem occurs when the patient has undiagnosed chest pain. The acid perfusion (Bernstein) test is a practical way to prove that the pain could result from GERD, if the test reproduces the patient's symptoms exactly. However, neither the Bernstein test nor esophageal manometry is an appropriate screening test for patients with chest pain. In patients with chest pain selected because some features of their history suggested an esophageal disorder, the tests were unequivocally positive in only 10 to 15%, but many of these appeared *also* to have coronary artery disease.[88, 89] It seems best to make the diagnosis of esophageal or coronary artery disease from their respective specific features and to reserve acid perfusion and manometry tests for patients with atypical chest pain in whom an esophageal disorder is suspected; positive test results do not exclude concurrent coronary artery disease.

TABLE 24–4. MAJOR INDICATIONS FOR DIAGNOSTIC STUDIES IN ESOPHAGEAL DISEASE

Reflux Disorders
- Gastroesophageal reflux (with or without esophageal ulcer)
  - Barium swallow—baseline study
  - Esophagoscopy and biopsy—when necessary to establish diagnosis
  - pH monitoring—to confirm diagnosis preoperatively
  - Acid perfusion (Bernstein)—to investigate chest pain of unclear origin
- Benign stricture
  - Barium swallow—diagnosis of stricture
  - Esophagoscopy with biopsies and brush cytology—necessary to exclude malignancy

Motility Disorders
- Diffuse esophageal spasm
  - Barium swallow with cineradiography—for diagnosis
  - Manometry—confirmation of diagnosis when necessary or to determine the usefulness of dilatation in management
- Achalasia
  - Barium swallow with cineradiography—for diagnosis
  - Manometry—confirmation of diagnosis when necessary
  - Esophagoscopy with biopsy—exclusion of malignancy
- Scleroderma or Raynaud's phenomenon
  - Barium swallow with cineradiography—for diagnosis
  - Manometry—confirmation of diagnosis when necessary

For motility disorders, the barium swallow is usually sufficient to suggest a diagnosis. Those with achalasia who have advanced LES spasm creating an obstructive "beaked" appearance of the lower esophagus also require biopsies to exclude malignancy, because clinical features suggestive of achalasia may be associated with adenocarcinoma of the gastroesophageal juncture, whereas squamous cell carcinoma of the esophagus ultimately develops in 5 to 10% of patients with achalasia.[90]

Manometry is a somewhat more sensitive procedure than barium swallow to detect abnormal motility, especially early in the course of the disease. In clinical practice, manometry may be used to confirm the diagnosis when the result of the radiograph is questionable or negative in a patient with recurrent symptoms. In addition, dysphagia responds to dilatations in patients with achalasia and in the subgroup of those with diffuse spasm who also have increased LES pressures. In patients with relatively severe, persistent complaints that warrant resorting to dilatation, manometry may be of value in determining the course of management.

Management

Reflux Esophagitis. Patients with esophagitis should be advised to achieve an ideal body weight and to avoid tight-fitting garments that may increase intra-abdominal pressure. They should not eat within several hours of retiring in order to diminish gastric content and acid secretion during the night. Elevation of the head of the bed with 6- or 8-in. blocks or a large foam wedge (between mattress and innersprings) is very beneficial. Alcohol, chocolate, and fatty food intake is limited, if associated with symptoms, and smoking should be avoided.

Antacids given in the same dosages used for peptic ulcer disease are the mainstays of medical therapy. They should be continued for 6 to 12 weeks after each exacerbation, depending on the severity of the symptoms. Anticholinergics, which relax the LES, are contraindicated.

Patient compliance with the conservative program will vary, depending on the severity of symptoms. Palmer reported that the endoscopic signs of esophagitis cleared and recurred intermittently and unpredictably in his series of 413 patients. In about half, the esophagitis subsided. The other half remained the same or worsened.[73] In a more recent series, antacids were reported to control the symptoms in 75% of patients who had an exacerbation of esophagitis.[91]

H_2-blockers in patients with esophagitis have shown statistically significant decreases in the amounts of antacids used and in symptoms.[92, 93] Unfortunately, successful short-term therapy had no effect on the frequent exacerbations of esophagitis when treatment was stopped or on the LES pressure. Metaclopramide, given in doses of 10 mg twice daily, increased gradually to four times daily, increases LES sphincter pressure and reduces reflux, although its efficacy is limited by the frequent occurrence of central nervous system side effects.[90]

It is suggested that the initial therapy of patients with esophagitis should consist of antacids, dietary modification, weight loss, elevation of the head of the bed, and avoidance of cigarettes.[91] H_2-blockers or metaclopramide can be added in the 25% of patients that fail to respond to initial therapy.[94] For the subset of patients with severe esophagitis accompanied by endoscopically documented erosions or ulcers, omeprazole has achieved high rates of symptom relief and healing when all else has failed.[95–97] Unfortunately, the effectiveness of acid inhibition from omeprazole therapy leads to high levels of gastrin, which in turn has a trophic and proliferatory effect on gastrointestinal mucosa. This has led to carcinoid tumors of gastric mucosa in experimental animals, endocrine cell proliferation in human gastric mucosa, and a concern about stimulating neoplasia in the colon or in Barrett's epithelium. Omeprazole therapy should be limited to 12 weeks and should only be continued thereafter if serum gastrin remains normal. It takes about 6 months for the trophic effects to reverse after omeprazole is stopped.

Surgery is effective for patients with intractable symptoms. Antireflux operations provide an extrinsic pressure mechanism by surrounding the esophagus with a portion of the stomach. Vagotomy is avoided, since it interferes with gastric emptying. The classic anterior fundoplication procedure has been shown to increase resting LES pressures, although a physiologically functioning sphincter mechanism is not restored. Antireflux surgery appears to be effective for about 5 years, after which the symptoms may recur.[94] Controlled studies document symptomatic and objective improvement in about 80% of the patients following this procedure,[98, 99] compared with 25% of patients treated with antacids. A recent randomized trial showed that surgery was superior to continuous treatment with H_2-blockers, which were partially effective in controlling refractory symptoms as well as endoscopic signs related to GERD for up to 2 years.[102] Omeprazole, which is almost certainly as effective as surgery for short-term control of refractory symptoms, is not approved for long-term use.

Benign Stricture. If malignancy has been excluded by biopsies and the diagnosis confirmed by a repeat barium study after treatment for esophagitis, the general approach is to dilate by esophageal bougienage. Although the interval between dilatations can be gradually increased, generally the need persists indefinitely for at least occasional dilatations. Perforations have been reported to occur in about 3% of patients, and the risk is increased when bougienage is withheld until the stricture is very narrow.[100] Thus, it is important not to neglect early or mild strictures, since these frequently progress to become more difficult to manage.[101]

Most patients with dysphagia due to benign esophageal rings can be managed by providing a thorough explanation of the symptoms with instructions to eat and chew more slowly; a few severe cases require bougienage for relief of symptoms.

Motility Disorders. Dilatation is the mainstay of therapy for patients with achalasia. Relief by bougienage is usually transient but may be long-lasting in mild or early cases. Otherwise, pneumatic dilatation is preferred. If symptomatic relief is not obtained after two attempts at pneumatic dilatation, partial esophageal myotomy can be considered.[77] Good clinical and radiologic remission is achieved by this procedure in 80% of patients, but others develop reflux esophagitis postoperatively.

No specific pharmacologic therapy for diffuse esophageal spasm exists. Some patients respond to nitrates or nifedipine. Patients with persistent dysphagia accompanied by increased LES pressure may improve with dilatation. A long surgical myotomy has been reported to improve about two thirds of a small group who had severe dysphagia and weight loss.[103]

In patients with sclerodermal esophageal disease, treatment is directed at the reflux esophagitis. A vigorous treatment program should be adhered to indefinitely by the patient.

BENIGN AND MALIGNANT GASTRIC ULCERS

Both gastric ulcers and gastric carcinoma usually occur in patients with chronic atrophic gastritis, a condition characterized by thinning of the mucosa, atrophy of gastric glands, and lymphocytic infiltration of the lamina propria of the mucosa of the fundus and the body of the stomach.[104, 105] In the absence of an ulcer, chronic atrophic gastritis is asymptomatic or associated only with vague symptoms of dyspepsia.[106] A minority of patients also have parietal cell antibodies and may develop pernicious anemia.[107] Other types of gastritis are not usually associated with chronic ulcer or carcinoma. Acute hemorrhagic or erosive "gastritis," which can be related to stress, aspirin, or alcohol, may remain asymptomatic or be accompanied by hematemesis but is rarely found associated with gastric ulcer.[106] Radiologically noted enlargement of the gastric mucosal folds has been described in the Zollinger-Ellison syndrome in addition to granulomatous, lymphomatous, or carcinomatous infiltration of the stomach and a rare form of hypertrophic gastritis (Ménétrier's disease), characterized by achlorhydria, benign hyperplasia of surface epithelial cells, occasionally excessive leakage of plasma protein, and in some cases adenomatous polyps and adenocarcinoma of the stomach.[104, 106]

Gastric polyps also occur in the setting of chronic atrophic gastritis. They may be hyperplastic or, less commonly, adenomatous. Most invasive carcinomas associated with hyperplastic polyps occur at a different site within the stomach.[108]

The absolute risk of developing gastric carcinoma probably is low in an individual patient with chronic gastritis. A 10- to 15-year follow-up of 116 patients with chronic atrophic gastritis recorded nine cases of gastric carcinoma, an incidence of 0.5 to 0.8 new cases per 100 patients per year of follow-up.[109]

Diagnostic Studies and Approach to the Patient

The problem of detecting gastric carcinoma is difficult. Nevertheless, older individuals with chronic dyspeptic symptoms or new onset of dyspepsia should be considered for upper endoscopy. If upper gastrointestinal x-rays are chosen instead, a double-contrast study is preferable, because of its somewhat greater sensitivity in identifying either gastric ulcer or carcinoma (~ 90%, versus 80% by conventional single-contrast procedure).[110] Of all patients with carcinoma, however, less than 10% will survive for 5 years.[104] Occasionally, patients with a history suggestive of peptic ulcer disease will be found to have superficial carcinoma; the initial manifestation may mimic benign gastric ulcer owing to peptic digestion of the superficial cancer. Following surgical resection, the 5-year survival rate is 93% in these patients[104]; hence, it is worthwhile to identify and evaluate carefully all gastric ulcers, even though invasive—as opposed to superficial—ulcerating carcinomas have a poor prognosis.

On the upper gastrointestinal x-ray series, malignant ulcers may appear as depressions within a tumor mass extending into the lumen of the stomach. This mass surrounding the ulcer may be eccentric with uneven borders. The ulcer itself may not penetrate past the border of the lumen as defined by contrast agent. Normal gastric folds may not approach the ulcer margins in a concentric or a spoke-like fashion. When gastric ulcers have these radiographic features (Fig. 24–7), there can be little doubt that an aggressive approach is warranted.

Benign gastric ulcers are characterized radiographically by their central location within a smoothly contoured mound; although often a margin of edematous tissue surrounds the ulcer crater, the ulcer usually penetrates with a collar-button or mushroom-like shape past the border of the gastric lumen as defined by contrast. Gastric folds generally do radiate to the lips of the ulcer crater in a spoke-like fashion. An ulcer with these radiographic features is thought to be benign (Fig. 24–8). When some of the features are atypical or more suggestive of malignancy but most of the appearance is that of a benign ulcer, the ulcer is called indeterminate (see Fig. 24–8).

The VA Cooperative Study of Gastric Ulcers[111] reported 774 patients with benign or indeterminate gastric ulcers. Overall, only 3.3% of these were found to be malignant. Benign and malignant ulcers occurred on both curvatures of the stomach, slightly more often on the lesser curvature; thus ulcer location did not help to establish the diagnosis. The incidence of malignancy was lower when the gastric ulcer occurred concurrently with a duodenal ulcer or deformity (1.2%) and when a small gastric ulcer was less than 1.7 cm in diameter (2.2%); larger ulcers had a higher incidence of malignancy (10.7%), and ulcers with indeterminate rather than benign radiographic features were more likely to be malignant (9.4%). Pyloric channel ulcers were less likely to be malignant than were those of the body and fundus of the stomach. Clearly, no feature changes the probability sufficiently to exclude malignancy; nevertheless, large ulcers (>1.7 cm in diameter) and those with indeterminate radiographic features should be approached more aggressively.

Healing with treatment occurred in 50% of the benign ulcers within 3 weeks, in 75% within 6 weeks, and in 80% within 12 weeks, but 32% recurred within a year.[111] Three of the 25 malignant ulcers in the VA series initially seemed to have healed but reappeared on subsequent radiographic studies.

Endoscopy is sufficiently reliable so that if five or more adequate biopsy and brush cytology specimens can be obtained from the inner edges of an ulcer margin, it is most unusual to fail to establish the diagnosis in patients with malignancy. In one series, using such techniques, 166 (98%) of 168 total patients with malignancy were diagnosed accurately.[114] Thus, all patients with large or radiographically indeterminate ulcers should have endoscopy with biopsy. For others, especially those at greatest risk of gastric malignancy because they are over the age of 50 years, endoscopy provides diagnostic certainty without having to wait until the ulcer has healed. This may also reduce the number of diagnostic studies, such as repeat upper gastrointestinal series, that would otherwise be needed. Therefore, endoscopy is generally recommended in patients with gastric ulcer who are older than 50 years of age. Only a few of the small gastric ulcers are malignant, however, so that aged persons, those with chronic medical illnesses that may

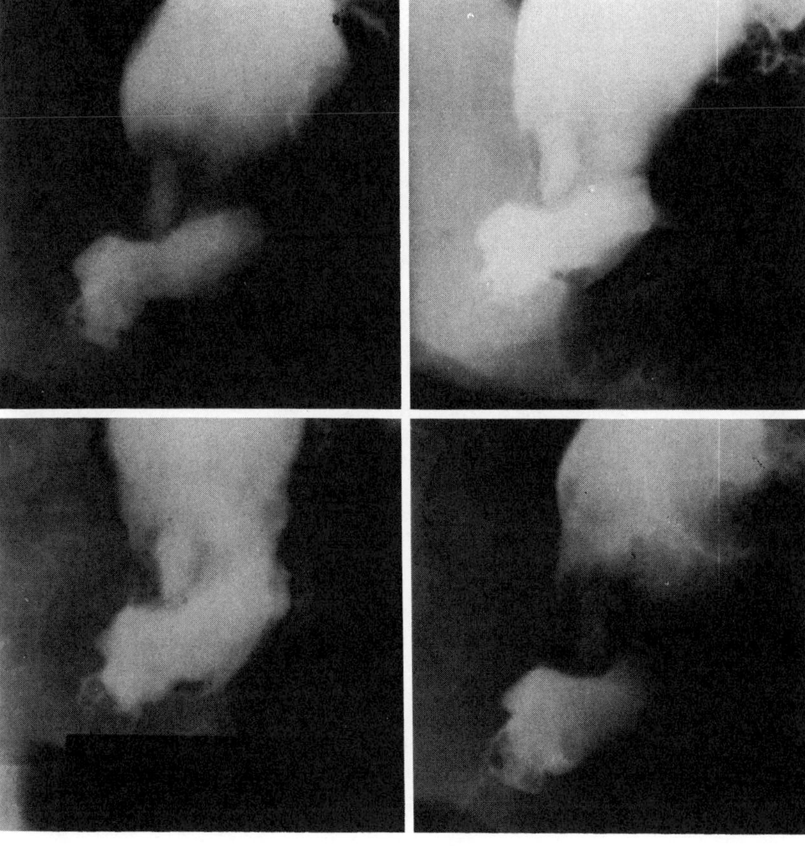

FIGURE 24–7. Malignant gastric ulcer. UGIS in an 85-year-old woman who had a positive result on a stool test for occult blood and iron deficiency anemia reveals an intraluminal mass involving the lesser curvature of the stomach. The mass has ragged borders and a central ulceration. This ulcer-like lesion has radiographic features of malignancy. The results of gastroscopy with biopsy were negative. Because of the highly suspicious radiographic features, the patient underwent surgery, and the lesion was found to be malignant. (Courtesy of Department of Radiology, Brigham and Women's Hospital, Harvard Medical School, Boston, Massachusetts.)

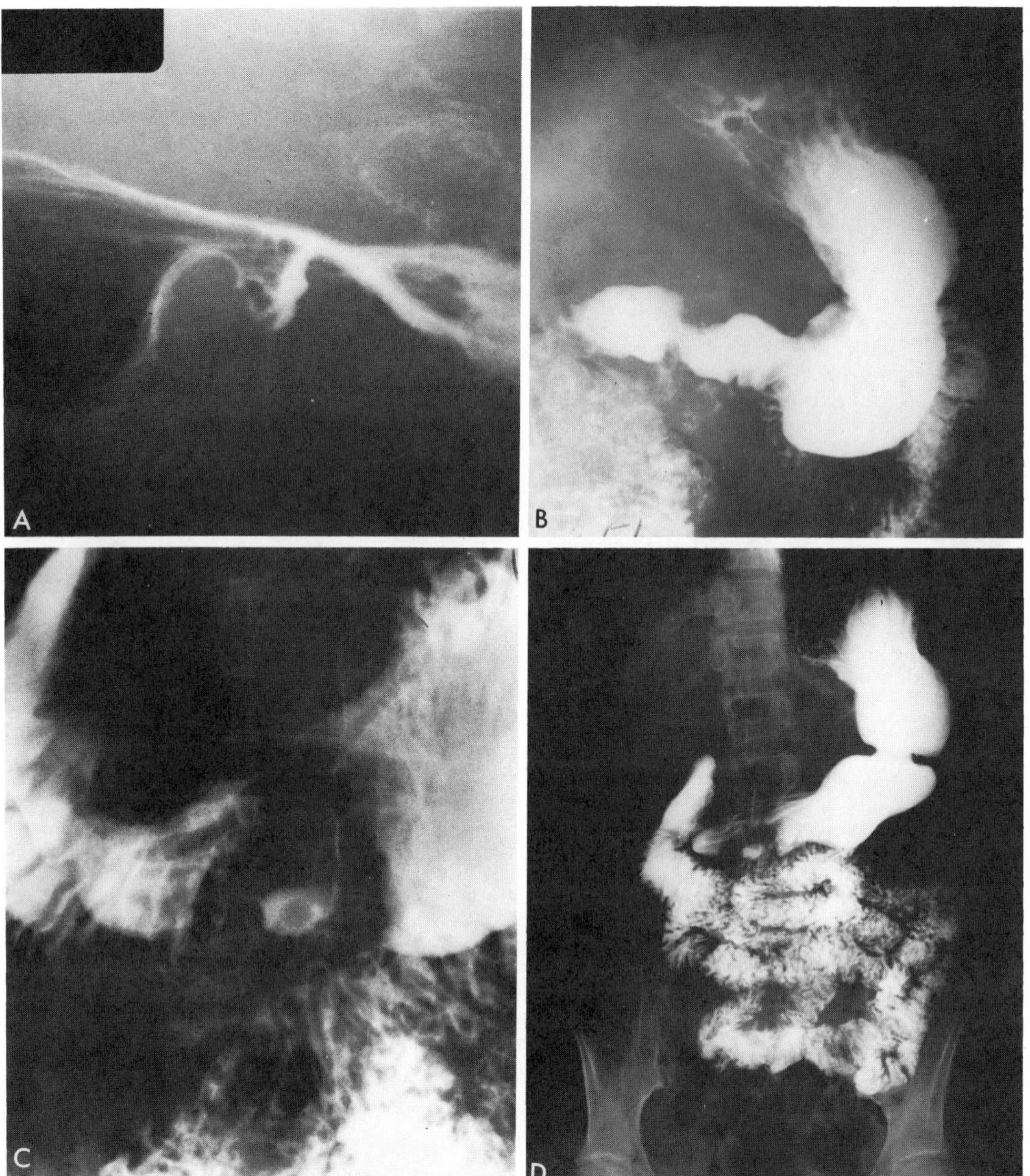

FIGURE 24–8. Radiographically benign and indeterminate gastric ulcers. *A,* This ulcer has radiographic features of a benign ulcer. It projects beyond the gastric lumen, it has a collar-button shape, and gastric folds radiate to the margins of the ulcer. *B,* This ulcer of the lesser curvature also has radiographic characteristics of a benign ulcer. It projects beyond the gastric lumen and does not appear to be located within a mass; nevertheless, the ulcer failed to heal on medical management, and results of gastroscopic biopsies revealed that it was malignant. *C,* An ulcer of the greater curvature that initially appeared as a 1-cm benign lesion within a smooth symmetric area of edema. This follow-up film shows that the ulcer has grown to 1.5 cm in diameter, and the edematous mass around the ulcer now appears to show an abrupt transition without smoothly radiating gastric folds; thus, radiographically, the ulcer has indeterminate features. Biopsies were performed and revealed that the ulcer was benign. *D,* This follow-up film was obtained 4 months after the initiation of treatment for a benign gastric ulcer. The film reveals that the ulcer has grown from 1 cm to 1.5 cm in size and is located within a symmetric edematous mound of the greater curvature. The mound, however, shows an abrupt transition from the gastric mucosa without radiating gastric folds; thus, the ulcer has indeterminate radiographic features. Biopsy specimens revealed that the ulcer was benign. (Courtesy of Department of Radiology, Brigham and Women's Hospital, Harvard Medical School, Boston, Massachusetts.)

cause endoscopy to be difficult, or those whose ulcers can be explained by a history of recent salicylate or other nonsteroidal anti-inflammatory drug ingestion can be treated medically if adequate follow-up is ensured. After 6 weeks, endoscopy or upper gastrointestinal series should be repeated. If the ulcer is more than 90% healed, medical management can be continued, but follow-up endoscopy or UGIS is necessary to document no sign of recurrence after 6 months.

Biopsies should be performed of any ulcer that recurs during follow-up or has greater than 10% of its original diameter after 6 weeks of intensive medical therapy. Larger ulcers require more time (average of 15 weeks) for complete healing.

Endoscopy with negative biopsy results and brush cytology is sufficiently reliable, when performed according to the recommendations just given, so that after it has been performed, one then may persist with medical management of slowly healing or recurrent ulcers and plan to recheck the endoscopy after an additional 6 to 12 weeks. Repeated biopsies or surgical exploration become necessary if the ulcer fails to heal completely.

Management

Antacids, H_2-blockers, and sucralfate are the mainstays of medical therapy. Although evidence is not conclusive that antacids promote healing of gastric ulcers, most authorities recommend treatment with doses adequate to partially neutralize gastric acidity. H_2-blockers and sucralfate have been shown to have a beneficial effect on the healing of gastric ulcers. Alcohol, cigarettes, high-dose (>80 mg/day of prednisone) corticosteroids, salicylates, and nonsteroidals should be avoided in patients with gastric ulcer. Hospitalization facilitates healing and formerly was a standard component of therapy. With the use of adequate doses of antacids and the addition of H_2-blockers or sucralfate, the additional expense of hospitalization usually can be avoided.

Benign ulcers recur in up to half of patients followed for 5 years. In itself, this is not an indication for surgery. The VA Study showed that 87% of recurrent gastric ulcers were healed by 12 weeks of medical management, and there was no increased incidence of bleeding or perforation in recurrent ulcers.[113] When surgery is required for benign gastric ulcers, the choice of procedure depends on whether it is a lesser curvature ulcer in an older patient or a prepyloric ulcer in a younger individual, since the latter may resemble duodenal ulcers in its pathophysiology. The standard procedure for lesser curvature ulcers is partial gastric resection, using either a gastroduodenostomy (Billroth I) or gastrojejunostomy (Billroth II) for the anastomosis, but without vagotomy. Recurrence rates are extremely low after these procedures for gastric ulcer. The pyloroplasty and vagotomy procedure has a higher recurrence rate but can be done in very elderly or poor-risk candidates.

TABLE 24–5. CAUSES OF PANCREATITIS

Alcohol abuse Gallstone-associated	Account for majority with known cause; relative frequency varies with population studied
Traumatic, postoperative, or post-ERCP pancreatitis	
Drug-induced:	
Thiazides and related diuretics	Azathioprine
Oral contraceptive pills	Sulfonamides
Corticosteroidal drugs	Tetracycline
Metabolic:	
Hyperlipoproteinemia	
Hypercalcemia	
Pregnancy	
Infections:	
Mumps	*Ascaris*
Hepatitis	*Mycoplasma*
Other viruses	
Vasculitis, including systemic lupus erythematosus and thrombotic thrombocytopenia purpura	
Obstruction of ampulla of Vater by tumor, diverticulum, or inflammation	
Renal failure and postrenal transplantation-induced pancreatitis	
Hereditary pancreatitis	
Cause not identified in 15–20% of reported cases, some of which may be related to factors listed above that were not documented	

SYMPTOMS CAUSED BY PANCREATIC DISEASE

Acute pancreatitis is characterized by epigastric or midabdominal pain, often radiating through to the back, accompanied by nausea, vomiting, and dehydration. Acute pancreatitis has 13 or 14 causes but more than 90% of cases are due to alcohol abuse or gallstone-associated biliary tract disease (Table 24–5). There are only two causes of chronic pancreatitis: repeated bouts of acute pancreatitis and familial pancreatitis.[114] More than 95% of all chronic pancreatitis is due to alcohol abuse.

Chronic pancreatitis has two major clinical manifestations: chronic abdominal pain and functional pancreatic insufficiency. Pancreatic insufficiency is *exocrine* (inadequate pancreatic enzymes, leading to an intraluminal defect type of malabsorption, resulting in weight loss and steatorrhea) or *endocrine* (lack of insulin and glucagon, leading to hyperglycemia). The pain of chronic pancreatitis is usually persistent (which may vary a little with meals and body position), dull, and boring, often radiating into the midback. It is one of the most difficult problems in clinical medicine. Diagnosis is relatively easy only when the pain is typical, alcohol abuse is known, and a plain film of the abdomen demonstrates scattered calcifications in the pancreas. When the situation is less certain, or when one wishes to confirm the diagnosis in typical cases, the endoscopic retrograde pancreatogram (ERCP) is helpful.[115, 116] The characteristic appearance is a dilated and irregular main pancreatic duct with dilated and knobbed side branches. Treatment for pancreatic insufficiency is replacement of pancreatic enzymes (4 to 6 capsules taken during and immediately after each meal) and administration of NPH insulin as needed. The relief of pancreatic pain is much more difficult; many of these patients become addicted to physician-prescribed narcotics (replacing their abuse of alcohol), while extensive surgery (including a 90% pancreatectomy, or even total pancreatectomy) fails to provide relief in a surprisingly high number of patients. Celiac plexus block is less hazardous than major pancreatic surgery and may be almost as successful.[117]

The incidence of pancreatic cancer is increasing. Malignant neoplasm of the pancreas must be considered in the diagnosis of mature adults with dyspepsia or chronic abdominal pain, particularly if they are more than 60 years old and have otherwise unexplained weight loss. Pancreatic cancer may present a clinical picture that mimics chronic pancreatitis.[118] CT scan may reveal a mass in the pancreas or an enlarged pancreatic head but fails to distinguish these changes in carcinoma from similar possibilities in chronic pancreatitis. Endoscopic pancreatography is also not entirely specific, although a rat-tail obstruction of an otherwise normal pancreatic duct is highly suggestive of cancer. Skinny needle aspiration of a pancreatic mass under ultrasound or CT guidance is very helpful if the result is positive for cancer, but a negative test result does not exclude malignancy. At present, the best diagnostic strategy is not clear or uniform for all suspected cases,[119] but a reasonable approach is outlined below (see Fig. 24–10). If pancreatic carcinoma is present, the 5-year survival rate is 1%.

The diagnosis of biliary dyskinesia, another condition with manifestations similar to pancreatitis, can ultimately be established only by performing biliary motility studies (done endoscopically, using techniques similar to ERCP) and finding elevated resting pressure at the sphincter of Oddi. However, elevated sphincter pressure (and subse-

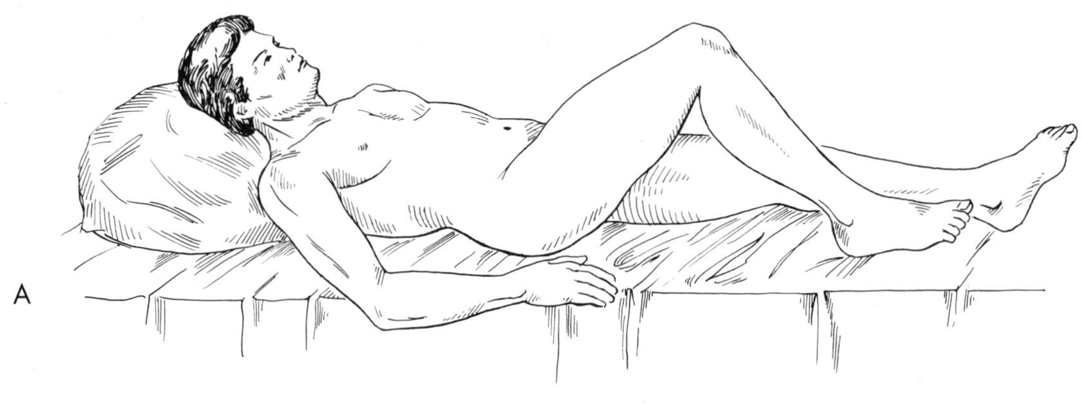

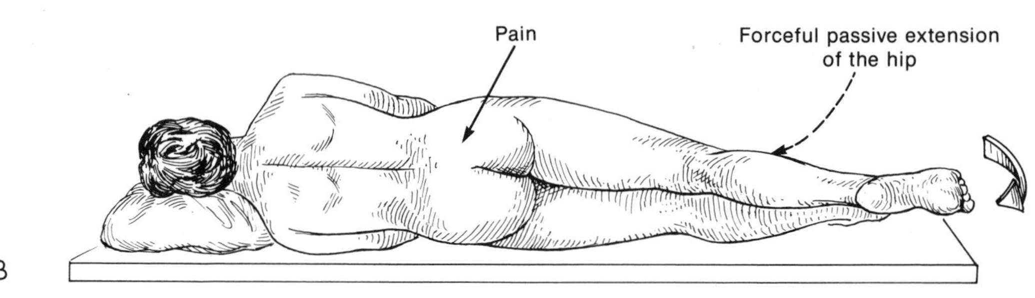

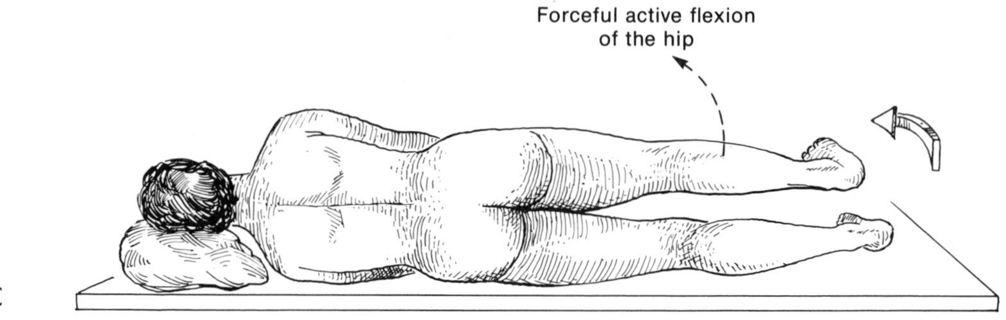

FIGURE 24–9. *A,* A patient with irritation and reflex rigidity of the iliopsoas muscle (possibly from perforation of an appendix lying in the iliac fossa) prefers to hold the right thigh flexed in order to relax the muscle. *B,* The patient experiences flank pain when the iliopsoas muscle is stretched by fully extending the right thigh (the psoas maneuver). *C,* Such a patient may also experience pain in the flank or groin if attempting to actively flex the thigh.

quent symptom relief by performing endoscopic sphincterotomy) is consistently predicted by the presence of elevated liver enzymes (the alkaline phosphatase most often) *and* bile duct dilatation on ultrasound, in addition to symptoms of abdominal pain or discomfort.

APPROACH TO THE PATIENT WITH UPPER ABDOMINAL PAIN OF UNKNOWN ORIGIN

Less than 5% of patients with chronic upper abdominal pain or dyspepsia do not have one of the previously discussed, commonly encountered conditions. Rather than attempting to characterize the numerous potential causes of such abdominal pain or referred pain to the abdomen, we will try to summarize a general approach to the patient that may be taken.

The onset and course of the illness should be described in detail. From the history, the clinician should be able to distinguish pain of intestinal origin from that caused by conditions affecting other organs within the abdomen. Colicky or crampy pain, especially if related to borborygmi, fluctuating abdominal distention, passage of flatus, or bowel movements, usually arises from diseases of the bowel (see Chapters 26 and 27). Conditions that chronically affect other organs within the abdomen generally cause more constant, noncolicky pain. Pain radiating to the back is characteristic of pancreatic disease as well as of biliary pain; radiation to the flank, sacrum, or genitalia may signify expansion of an abdominal aortic aneurysm as well as pain

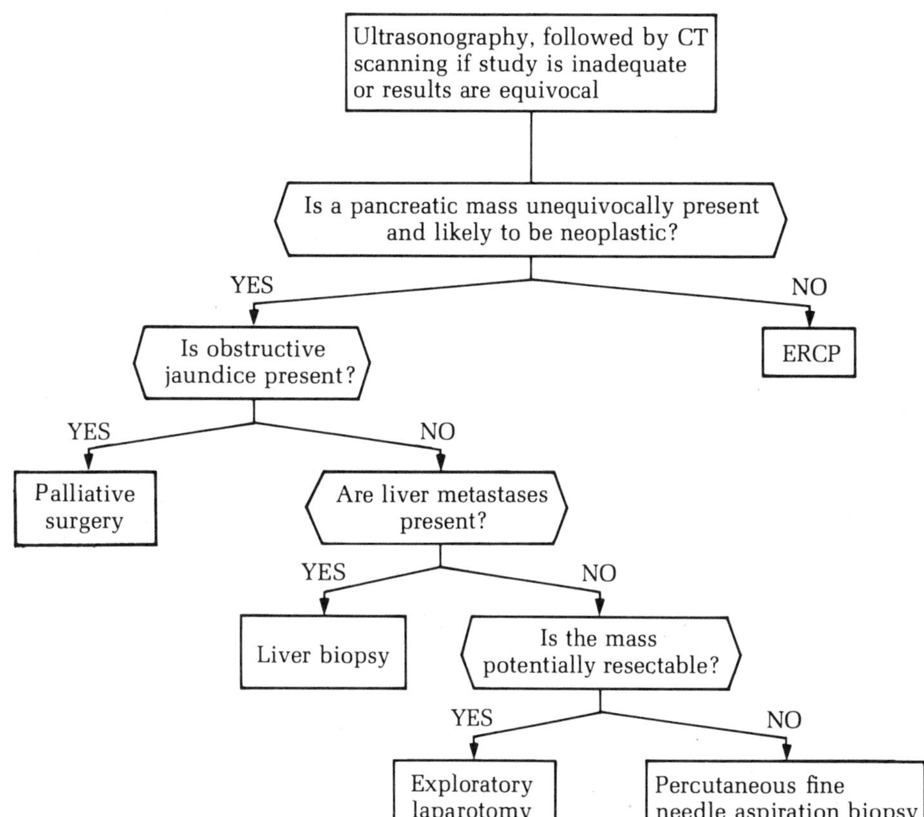

FIGURE 24–10. The approach to patients suspected of having a pancreatic mass that causes pain.

of renal or ureteral origin. Needless to say, a thorough examination of the abdomen, rectum, and genitalia, including a search for hernias, is essential. Palpation should be performed very gently to avoid alarming or discomforting the patient and thus adding to the difficulty of the examination. The examiner should seek to identify fluid or masses within the abdomen as well as direct and rebound tenderness. If one happens to observe the patient during an episode of pain, note that peritoneal inflammation usually causes people to avoid motion and lie quietly, whereas pain of other types, including that produced by gallstones and intestinal obstruction, is often accompanied by writhing and grimacing. In patients with flank or back pain, it is important also to perform the psoas maneuver, seeking to elicit discomfort by either maximal extension of the hip or flexion of the hip against resistance (Fig. 24–9). This may identify the source of subacute pain as a psoas abscess or hematoma.

It should be possible from the history and physical examination to distinguish pain caused by intra-abdominal diseases from referred pain to the abdomen. The former sometimes will be accompanied by positive findings on examination, for example, local areas of tenderness or tender loops of bowel; these are invariably *absent* in the latter. Pain elicited by cough, movement, or ambulation may signify peritoneal irritation, but if straining, coughing, and motion of the spine elicit a lancinating pain that comes and goes suddenly, one should suspect a spinal neurogenic source. True visceral pain is generally dull and diffuse, experienced as arising from deep within the abdomen, and difficult to localize. Causalgic pain due to nerve injury is characterized by its "burning" quality, limited distribution, and precipitation by such surface stimuli as touch or gentle palpation.[119] In pain referred to the abdomen, the musculature, if resistant, will relax when the patient exhales.

In most cases, the presence of the metabolic condition associated with an abdominal crisis, such as sickle cell anemia, other hemoglobinopathies, and diabetic ketoacidosis, will be readily apparent to the examiner. Occasionally, patients are encountered with the problem of unexplained, recurrent attacks of severe pain. If the history and examination suggest that these are manifestations of intestinal colic or of shifting peritonitis, lead toxicity, acute porphyria, and familial Mediterranean fever should be considered.

In patients with persistent, obscure pain of the upper abdomen, disease involving any organ system will be sought, but particular attention should be paid to the pancreas. For the diagnosis of pancreatic carcinoma, both ultrasonography and computed tomography (CT) scanning have approximately a 70 to 90% sensitivity.[120–129] The specificity of ultrasonography (64 to 97%) is reported to be as good as that of CT scanning (64 to 85%).[120–129] In practice, ultrasonography is frequently difficult to interpret in obese individuals, or when loops of bowel sonographically mimic a mass. False-positive results may occur with either technique.[121] Chronic pancreatitis may be identified by noting enlargement of the gland, calcifications, or a very small "echo-dense" atrophic gland.[121] The sensitivity of ultrasound or CT scanning for detecting this disorder is considerably less (~ 40%) than for detecting pancreatic carcinoma.[125] If the entire gland is enlarged, it may not be possible to distinguish noninvasively between pancreatic carcinoma and pancreatitis.[121]

Both ultrasound and CT scanning are highly reliable for detecting pancreatic pseudocysts and retroperitoneal processes.[121] For masses located outside the pelvis but within the peritoneal cavity, the sensitivity of either technique is only about 50%.[124] One report described the ability to diagnose accurately intra-abdominal abscesses by CT scanning in more than 90% of instances.[128] Neither ultrasonography nor CT can consistently identify lesions less than 2 cm in size.[127]

Other noninvasive approaches for making the diagnosis of chronic pancreatic disease have proved less fruitful. The specificity and sensitivity of the serum amylase to creatinine clearance ratio have not been established for patients with chronically, mildly elevated amylase values or for those with pancreatitis accompanied by a normal serum amylase value.[132] Calcifications in the pancreas can be identified on plain films in only 30% of patients with chronic pancreatitis,[123] and selenomethionine scanning has proved unreliable.[129] Although pancreatic function testing is quite sensitive for detecting pancreatic disease, it cannot distinguish between neoplastic and inflammatory processes, requires considerable expertise, and may fail to detect lesions in the body and tail of the pancreas.[129]

When ultrasonography or CT scanning suggests the possibility that the pancreas is the source of pain, one must consider ERCP, percutaneous fine needle aspiration biopsy, and exploratory laparotomy. The ERCP has approximately 90% sensitivity and specificity for detecting carcinoma of the pancreas. It can be accomplished successfully in 92% of patients and without complications in 97%, and it may identify a localized stricture of the pancreatic or common bile duct, possibly curable by operation, in a small number of patients with chronic pancreatitis.[120, 129, 133, 134] The percutaneous fine needle aspiration biopsy, done with a 15-cm 22-gauge needle under ultrasonic or CT guidance, has been reported to establish the diagnosis in about 80% of patients with pancreatic carcinoma and to entail essentially no false-positive results or major complications.[135, 136]

Small, resectable carcinomas of the pancreas are exceptional cases, and as a rule, although the physician should make every effort to identify accurately the source of chronic abdominal pain, a diagnosis of carcinoma of the pancreas implies only a 1% 5-year survival rate.[129] Most patients have unresectable disease by the time they present with symptoms; those who have resectable lesions have only 4 to 6% 5-year survival rates.[137]

The approach to the patient can be summarized as follows (Fig. 24–10): Patients in whom the diagnosis of pancreatic disease is equivocal should be approached by ERCP. Those thought to have hepatic metastases on ultrasound or CT studies should have a liver biopsy as the next diagnostic procedure. If the lesion is in the head of the pancreas, and the patient requires palliative surgery for obstructive jaundice, the diagnosis should be established intraoperatively without resorting to additional diagnostic studies. Otherwise, if the lesion is unresectable, the diagnosis can be established by percutaneous fine needle aspiration biopsy.

REFERENCES

1. Marsland DW, Wood M, and Mayo F: Content of family practice. I: Rank order of diagnoses by frequency. J Fam Pract 3:37, 1976.
2. Horrocks JC and DeDombal FT: Clinical presentation of patients with "dyspepsia." Detailed symptomatic study of 360 patients. Gut 19:19, 1978.
3. Earlam R: A computerized questionnaire analysis of duodenal ulcer symptoms. Gastroenterology 71:314, 1976.
4. Peterson WL, Sturdevant RAL, Frankl HD, et al: Healing of duodenal ulcer with an antacid regimen. N Engl J Med 297:341, 1977.
5. Hendrix TR: Does sliding hiatus hernia constitute a distinct clinical entity? Gastroenterology 57:442, 1969.
6. Gunn A and Keddie N: Some clinical observations on patients with gallstones. Lancet 2:239, 1972.
7. Hogan WJ and Geenan JE: Biliary dyskinesia. Endoscopy 20 (Suppl 1):179, 1988.
8. Conn HO and Blitzer BL: Nonassociation of adrenocorticosteroid therapy and peptic ulcer. N Engl J Med 294:473, 1976.
9. Messer J, Reitman D, Sacks HS, et al: Association of adrenocorticosteroid therapy and peptic ulcer disease. N Engl J Med 309:21, 1983.
10. Price WH: Gallbladder dyspepsia. BMJ 3:138, 1963.
11. Gregory DW, Davies GT, Evans KT, et al: Natural history of patients with x-ray-negative dyspepsia in general practice. BMJ 4:519, 1972.
12. Cameron AJ and Ott BJ: The value of gastroscopy in clinical diagnosis: A computer-assisted study. Mayo Clin Proc 52:806, 1977.
13. Brown C and Rees WD: Dyspepsia in general practice. BMJ 300:829, 1990.
14. Barbara L, Camilleri M, Corinaldesi R, et al: Definition and investigation of dyspepsia. Dig Dis Sci 34:1272, 1989.
15. Talley NJ: Drug treatment of functional dyspepsia. Scand J Gastroenterol 182 (Suppl):47, 1991.
16. Spiro HM: Visceral viewpoints. Moynihan's disease? The diagnosis of duodenal ulcer. N Engl J Med 291:567, 1974.
17. Thomson WO, Robertson AG, Imrie CW, et al: Is duodenitis a dyspeptic myth? Lancet 1:1197, 1977.
18. Sturdevant RA and Walsh JH: Duodenal ulcer. *In* Sleisenger MH and Fordtran JS: Gastrointestinal Disease: Pathophysiology, Diagnosis, Management, 2nd ed. Philadelphia, WB Saunders, 1978, pp 840–860.
19. Grossman MI (moderator), Guth PH, Isenberg JI, et al: UCLA Conference: A new look at peptic ulcer. Ann Intern Med 84:57, 1976.
20. Isenberg JI: Long-term management of duodenal ulcer. Hosp Pract 15:63, 1980.
21. Levy M: Aspirin use in patients with major upper gastrointestinal bleeding and peptic ulcer disease: A report of the Boston Collaborative Drug Surveillance Program. N Engl J Med 290:1158, 1974.
22. Chapman BG and Duggan JM: Aspirin and uncomplicated peptic ulcer. Gut 10:443, 1969.
23. Welsh JD: Diet therapy of peptic ulcer disease. Gastroenterology 72:740, 1977.
24. Morrissey JE and Barreras RF: Drug therapy: Antacid therapy. N Engl J Med 290:550, 1974.
25. Littman A and Pine BH: Diagnosis and treatment. Drug spotlight program: Antacids and anticholinergic drugs. Ann Intern Med 82:544, 1975.
26. Freston JW: Cimetidine. I: Developments, pharmacology, and efficacy. Ann Intern Med 97:573, 1982.
27. Binder HJ, Cocco A, Corssley RJ, et al: Cimetidine in the treatment of duodenal ulcer: A multicenter double blind study. Gastroenterology 74:380, 1978.
28. Bodemar G and Walan A: Cimetidine in the treatment of active duodenal and prepyloric ulcers. Lancet 2:161, 1976.
29. Malagelada J-R and Cortot A: Subject review: H-2 receptor antagonists in perspective. Mayo Clin Proc 53:184, 1978.
30. Winship DH: Cimetidine in the treatment of duodenal ulcer: Review and commentary. Gastroenterology 74:402, 1978.
31. Freston JW: Cimetidine II: Adverse reactions and patterns of use. Ann Intern Med 97:728, 1982.
32. Knapp AB, Grimshaw RS Jr, Goldfarb JP, et al: Cimetidine-induced anaphylaxis. Ann Intern Med 97:374, 1982.
33. Rudnick MR, Bastl CP, Elfenbein IB, et al: Cimetidine-induced acute renal failure. Ann Intern Med 96:180, 1982.
34. Forrest JAH, Fells MR, and McLoughlin GP: Effect of long-term cimetidine on gastric acid secretion, serum gastrin, and gastric emptying. Gut 20:404, 1979.
35. Domschke W, Lux G, Domschke S: Furan H_2 antagonist ranitidine inhibits pentagastrin-stimulated gastric secretion stronger than cimetidine. Gastroenterology 79:1267, 1980.
36. Korman MG, Hansky J, Merrett AC, et al: Ranitidine in duodenal ulcer. Dig Dis Sci 27:712, 1982.
37. Danilewitz M, Tim LO, Hirschowitz B: Ranitidine suppression of gastric hypersecretion resistant to cimetidine. N Engl J Med 306:20, 1982.
38. Collen MJ, Howard JM, McArthur KE, et al: Comparison of ranitidine and cimetidine in the treatment of gastric hypersecretion. Ann Intern Med 100:52, 1984.

39. Berardi RR, Tankanow RM, Nostrant TT: Comparison of famotidine with cimetidine and ranitidine. Clin Pharm 7:271, 1988.
40. Graham DY, McCullough A, Sklar M, et al: Omeprazole versus placebo in duodenal ulcer healing: The United States experience. Dig Dis Sci 35:66, 1990.
41. Lauritsen K, Rune SJ, Bytzer P, et al: Effect of omeprazole and cimetidine on duodenal ulcer: A double-blind comparative trial. N Engl J Med 312:958, 1985.
42. Martin F, Farley A, Gagnon M, et al: Comparison of the healing capacities of sucralfate and cimetidine in the short-term treatment of duodenal ulcer: A double-blinded randomized trial. Gastroenterology 82:401, 1982.
43. Richardson CT: Sucralfate. Ann Intern Med 97:269, 1982.
44. Rubin W: Medical treatment of peptic ulcer disease. Med Clin North Am 75:981, 1991.
45. Bynum TE and Koch GG: Maintenance therapy with sucralfate in duodenal ulcer. Am J Med 91 (2A):84, 1991.
46. Reese WD: Mechanisms of gastroduodenal protection by sucralfate. AMJ Med 91(A): 58, 1991.
47. Szabo S: The mode of action of sucralfate. Scand J Gastroenterol 185(Suppl):7, 1991.
48. Sucralfate for peptic ulcer—a reappraisal. Med Lett 26:43, 1984.
49. Fordtran JS: Placebos, antacids and cimetidine for duodenal ulcer (Editorial) N Engl J Med 298:1081, 1978.
50. Scheurer U, Witzel L, Halter F, et al: Gastric and duodenal ulcer healing under placebo treatment. Gastroenterology 72:838, 1977.
51. Kirkpatrick TM and Hirschowitz BI: Cause and effect of massive basal gastric acid hypersecretion not due to Zollinger-Ellison syndrome (Abstract). Gastroenterology 74:1049, 1978.
52. Greibe J, Bugge P, Gjorup T, et al: Long-term prognosis of duodenal ulcer: Follow-up study and survey of doctor's estimates. BMJ 2:1572, 1977.
53. Fry J: Peptic ulcer: A profile. BMJ 2:809, 1964.
54. Bardhan KD, Blum A, Gillespie G, et al: Long-term treatment with cimetidine in duodenal ulceration. Lancet 1:900, 1977.
55. Saunders JHB and Wormsley KG: Long-term effects and after-effects of treatment of duodenal ulcer with metiamide. Lancet 1:765, 1977.
56. Gray GR, Smith ILS, Mackenzie I, et al: Long-term cimetidine in the management of severe duodenal ulcer dyspepsia. Gastroenterology 74:397, 1978.
57. Blackwood WS, Mangdal DP, and Northfield TC: Prevention of relapse of duodenal ulcer by bed-time cimetidine, a double-blind clinical trial. Gut 18:A420, 1977.
58. Bronfield MW, Batchelor AJ, and Larkworthy W: Controlled trial of maintenance cimetidine in treatment of healed duodenal ulcer: Short- and long-term effects. Gut 20:526, 1979.
59. Clearfield HR: *Helicobacter pylori.* Med Clin North Am 75:815, 1991.
60. Peterson WL: *Helicobacter pylori* and peptic ulcer. N Engl J Med 324:1043, 1991.
61. Rabeneck L and Ransohoff DF: Is *Helicobacter pylori* a cause of duodenal ulcer? Am J Med 91:566, 1991.
62. Graham DY, Lew GM, and Klein PD: Effect of treatment of *Helicobacter pylori* infection on the long-term recurrence of gastric or duodenal ulcer: A randomized, controlled study. Ann Intern Med 116:705, 1992.
63. Kairaluoma MI, Hentilae R, Alavaikko M, et al: Sucralfate vs. placebo in treatment of non-ulcer dyspepsia. Am J Med 83:51, 1987.
64. Greco RS and Cahow C: Alternatives in the management of perforated duodenal ulcer. Am J Surg 127:109, 1974.
65. Schrock TR: Progress in gastroenterology: Vagotomy in the elective treatment of duodenal ulcer. Gastroenterology 63:1615, 1975.
66. Johnston D, Goligher JC, Pulvertaft CN, et al: The two to four year clinical results of highly selective vagotomy (parietal cell vagotomy) without a drainage procedure for duodenal ulcer. Gut 13:842, 1972.
67. Kelly KA: Which operation for duodenal ulcer? Mayo Clin Proc 55:5, 1980.
68. Johnston D, Humphrey CS, Walker BE, et al: Vagotomy without diarrhea. BMJ 3:788, 1972.
69. Wilkinson AR and Johnston D: Effect of truncal selective and highly selective vagotomy on gastric emptying and intestinal transit of a food-barium meal in man. Ann Surg 178:190, 1973.
70. Dorricott NJ, McNeish AR, Alexander-Williams J, et al: Prospective randomized multicenter trial of proximal gastric vagotomy or truncal vagotomy and antrectomy for chronic duodenal ulcer: Interim results. Br J Surg 65:152, 1978.
71. Dodds WJ, Dent J, Hogan WJ, et al: Mechanisms of gastroesophageal reflux in patients with reflux esophagitis. N Engl J Med 307:1547, 1982.
72. Wolf BS, Brahms S, and Khilonani MT: The incidence of hiatus hernia in barium meal examination. J Mount Sinai Hosp 26:598, 1959.
73. Palmer ED: The hiatus hernia-esophagitis-esophageal stricture complex: 20-year prospective study. Am J Med 44:566, 1967.
74. Dodds WJ, Hogan WJ, and Miller WN: Reflux esophagitis. Dig Dis Sci 21:49, 1976.
75. Naef A, Savary M, Ozzello L, et al: Columnar-lined lower esophagus: An acquired lesion with malignant predisposition: Report on 140 cases of Barrett's esophagus with 12 adenocarcinomas. J Thorac Cardiovasc Surg 70:826, 1975.
76. DeMarino AJ Jr and Cohen S: Characteristics of lower esophageal sphincter function in symptomatic diffuse esophageal spasm. Gastroenterology 66:1, 1974.
77. Pope CE: Motor disorders. *In* Sleisenger MH and Fordtran JS: Gastrointestinal Disease: Pathophysiology, Diagnosis, Management, 3rd ed. Philadelphia, WB Saunders, 1983, pp 424–448.
78. Castell DO: The spectrum of esophageal motility disorders. Gastroenterology 76:639, 1979.
79. Vantrappen G, Janssens J, Hellemans J, et al: Achalasia, diffuse esophageal spasms, and related motility disorders. Gastroenterology 76:450, 1979.
80. Pope CE: Gastroesophageal reflux disease (reflux esophagitis). *In* Sleisenger MH and Fordtran JS: Gastrointestinal Disease: Pathophysiology, Diagnosis, Management, 3rd ed. Philadelphia, WB Saunders, 1983, pp 449–475.
81. Applequist P: Carcinoma of the esophagus and gastric cardia. Acta Chir Scand 360 (Suppl):1, 1972.
82. Bruni HC and Nelson RS: Carcinoma of the esophagus and cardia: Diagnostic evaluation in 113 cases. J Thorac Cardiovasc Surg 70:367, 1971.
83. Thurer RL: The distal esophageal sphincter and its relationship to gastroesophageal reflux. J Surg Res 16:418, 1974.
84. Skinner DB and Booth DJ: Assessment of distal esophageal function in patients with hiatal hernia and/or gastroesophageal reflux. Ann Surg 172:627, 1970.
85. Johnson LF and DeMeester TR: Twenty-four hour pH monitoring of the distal esophagus. Am J Gastroenterol 62:325, 1974.
86. DeMeester TR, Johnson LF, Joseph GJ, et al: Patterns of gastroesophageal reflux in health and disease. Ann Surg 184:459, 1976.
87. Benz LJ: A comparison of clinical measurements of gastroesophageal reflux. Gastroenterology 62:1, 1972.
88. Areskog M, Tibbing L, and Wranne B: Oesophageal acid perfusion test as a complement to work test in patients with chest pain. Acta Med Scand 201:559, 1977.
89. Brand DL, Martin D, and Pope CE: Esophageal manometrics in patients with angina-like chest pain. Dig Dis Sci 22:300, 1977.
90. Cohen S: Motor disorders of the esophagus. N Engl J Med 301:184, 1979.
91. Castell DO: Medical therapy of reflux esophagitis. Ann Intern Med 93:926, 1980.
92. Behar J, Brand DL, Brown FC, et al: Cimetidine in treatment of symptomatic gastroesophageal reflux: A double-blind controlled trial. Gastroenterology 74:441, 1978.
93. Wesdorf E, Bargelsman J, Pope K, et al: Oral cimetidine in reflux esophagitis: A double blind controlled trial. Gastroenterology 74:821, 1978.
94. Brand DL, Eastwood IR, Martin D, et al: Esophageal symptoms, manometry and histology before and after antireflux surgery: Long-term follow-up study. Gastroenterology 76:1393, 1979.

95. Maton PN: Omeprazole. N Engl J Med 324:965, 1991.
96. Bardhan KD, Morris P, Thompson M, et al: Omeprazole in the treatment of erosive esophagitis refractory to high dose cimetidine and ranitidine. Gut 31:745, 1990.
97. Hetzel DJ, Dent J, Reed WD, et al: Healing and relapse of severe peptic esophagitis after treatment with omeprazole. Gastroenterology 95:903, 1988.
98. Behar J, Bianciani P, Spiro H, et al: Effect of an anterior fundoplication on lower esophageal sphincter competence. Gastroenterology 67:209, 1974.
99. Behar J, Sheahan DG, Bianciani P, et al: Medical and surgical management of reflux esophagitis: A 38-month report on a prospective clinical trial. N Engl J Med 293:263, 1975.
100. Sanderson DR, Ellis FH, and Olson AM: Achalasia of the esophagus: Therapy by dilatation. 1950–67. Chest 58:116, 1970.
101. Palmer ED: Practical gastroenterology: Neglected esophageal narrowing. JAMA 234:857, 1975.
102. Spechler JJ, et al: Comparison of medical and surgical therapy for complicated gastroesophageal reflux disease in veterans. N Engl J Med 326:786, 1992.
103. Ellis FH, Olson AM, Schlegel JF, et al: Surgical treatment of esophageal hypermotility disturbances. JAMA 188:862, 1964.
104. Brandborg LL: Polyps, tumors and cancer of the stomach. *In* Sleisenger MH and Fordtran JS: Gastrointestinal Disease: Pathophysiology, Diagnosis, Management, 2nd ed. Philadelphia, WB Saunders, 1978, pp 752–776.
105. Isenberg J, Richardson CT, and Fordtran JS: Pathogenesis of peptic ulcer. *In* Sleisenger MH and Fordtran JS: Gastrointestinal Disease: Pathophysiology, Diagnosis, Management, 2nd ed. Philadelphia, WB Saunders, 1978, pp 792–806.
106. Jeffries GH: Gastritis. *In* Sleisenger MH and Fordtran JS: Gastrointestinal Disease: Pathophysiology, Diagnosis, Management, 2nd ed. Philadelphia, WB Saunders, 1978, pp 733–743.
107. Strickland RG and Mackay IR: An appraisal of the natural history and significance of chronic atrophic gastritis. Am J Dig Dis 18:426, 1973.
108. Spiro HM: Tumors. *In* Spiro HM (ed): Clinical Gastroenterology. Toronto, Macmillan, 1977, pp 130–146.
109. Srurala M, Varis K, and Wiljasalo MP: Studies of patients with atropic gastritis: A 10–15 year follow-up. Scand J Gastroenterol 1:40, 1966.
110. Laufer IL: Clinical trends and topics: Assessment of the accuracy of double contrast gastroduodenal radiology. Gastroenterology 71:874, 1976.
111. Wenger J, Brandborg LL, and Spellman FA: The Veterans Administration Cooperative Study on Gastric Ulcer: Clinical aspects. Gastroenterology 61:598, 1971.
112. Dekker W and Tytgat GN: Diagnostic accuracy of fiberendoscopy in detection of upper intestinal malignancy. Gastroenterology 73:710, 1977.
113. Littman A and Hanscom DH: The Veterans Administration Cooperative Study of Gastric Ulcer: The course of recurrent ulcer. Gastroenterology 61:592, 1971.
114. Perrault J, Gross JB, King JE: Endoscopic retrograde cholangiopancreatography in familial pancreatitis. Gastroenterology 71:138, 1976.
115. Nagata A, Homma T, Tamai K, et al: A study of chronic pancreatitis by serial endoscopic pancreatography. Gastroenterology 81:884, 1981.
116. Braganza JM, Hunt LP, Warwick F: Relationship between pancreatic exocrine function and ductal morphology in chronic pancreatitis. Gastroenterology 82:1341, 1982.
117. Kune GA, Cole R, Bell S: Observations on the relief of pancreatic pain. Med J Aust 2:789, 1975.
118. Becker V: Carcinoma of the pancreas and chronic pancreatitis. Acta Hepato-gastroenterol 25:257, 1978.
119. Silen W: Abdominal pain. *In* Thorn GW, Adams RD, Braunwald E, et al (eds): Principles of Internal Medicine. New York, McGraw-Hill, 1977, pp 33–36.
120. Reber HA: Chronic pancreatitis. *In* Sleisenger MH and Fordtran JS: Gastrointestinal Disease: Pathophysiology, Diagnosis, Management. Philadelphia, WB Saunders, 1978, pp 1439–1456.
121. Johnson MD and Mack LA: Ultrasonic evaluation of the pancreas. Gastrointest Radiol 3:257, 1978.
122. Lawson T: Sensitivity of pancreatic ultrasonography in detection of pancreatic disease. Radiology 128:733, 1978.
123. Fraumeni JF Jr: Cancers of the pancreas and biliary tract: Epidemiological consideration. Cancer Res 35:3437, 1975.
124. Baker C and Way LW: Clinical utility of CAT body scans. Am J Surg 136:37, 1978.
125. Lawson T, Irani SK, and Stock M: Detection of pancreatic pathology by ultrasonography and endoscopic retrograde choledochopancreatography. Gastrointest Radiol 3:335, 1978.
126. DiMagno EP, Malagelada J-R, Taylor WF, et al: A prospective comparison of current diagnostic tests for pancreatic cancer. N Engl J Med 297:738, 1977.
127. Arikama J, Shirakabe H, and Ikenobe H: The diagnosis of resectable pancreatic carcinoma. Clin Radiol 28:437, 1977.
128. Koehler PR and Moss AA: Diagnosis of intra-abdominal and pelvic abscesses by computerized tomography. JAMA 244:49, 1980.
129. DiMagno E: Pancreatic cancer, a continuing diagnostic dilemma. Ann Intern Med 90:847, 1979.
130. Szego PK and Stein LA: Endoscopic retrograde choledochopancreatography: A review of the rewards and indications. Gastrointest Radiol 3:319, 1978.
131. Levitt MD and Johnson S: Is the C_{am}/C_{er} ratio of value for diagnosis of pancreatitis? Gastroenterology 75:118, 1978.
132. Farrar WH and Calkins G: Sensitivity of the amylase-creatinine clearance ratio in acute pancreatitis. Arch Intern Med 138:958, 1978.
133. Siegel JH: Endoscopic retrograde choledochopancreatography update: Diagnostic and therapeutic applications. Gastrointest Radiol 3:311, 1978.
134. Mullens JE: Endoscopic retrograde cholangiopancreatography (ERCP) in the diagnosis of chronic pancreatitis. Surgery 84:308, 1978.
135. Cloose ME, Gregg JA, McDonald DG, et al: Percutaneous fine needle aspiration biopsy of pancreatic carcinoma. Gastrointest Radiol 2:67, 1977.
136. Goldstein HM, Zornoza J, Wallace S, et al: Percutaneous fine needle aspiration biopsy of pancreatic and other abdominal masses. Diagn Radiol 123:319, 1977.
137. Freeney PC and Ball TJ: Rapid diagnosis of pancreatic carcinoma. An algorithmic approach. Radiology 127:627, 1978.

25

Gallstones

MICHAEL D. APSTEIN, MD
MARTIN C. CAREY, MD, DSc

Gallstones are a common problem in clinical medicine,[1, 2] probably affecting 15% of the United States (US) population, or 36 million individuals. They are newly diagnosed in approximately 1 million US patients each year, one half of whom undergo biliary tract surgery[1] at a cost of at least $5 billion.[3]

The results of epidemiologic and basic research have had an enormous impact on the management of gallstone patients. For example, 2 decades ago the proper management of patients with asymptomatic (silent) gallstones was highly controversial.[4] Now, because of reliable natural history data there is agreement that silent stones should be left alone in most patients.[5, 6] The appropriate treatment of patients following a single attack of biliary pain is a new focus of controversy, since its predictive value in terms of natural history, or even its specificity, is uncertain.[7]

The treatment of choice for the majority of gallstone patients with true symptoms or complications is still surgery,[5, 8] specifically, laparoscopic cholecystectomy. Curiously, even before the introduction of this new technique, rates of gallstone surgery were threefold higher in the US than in Western Europe, despite a somewhat lower gallstone prevalence in the US.[9] Another revolutionary improvement is the management of retained common bile duct gallstones following cholecystectomy with endoscopic retrograde cholangiopancreatography (ERCP) and sphincterotomy.[10]

This chapter focuses principally on the management of patients with gallstone disease seen in office practice. We will discuss the most expedient diagnostic "work-up" of each presenting syndrome, with special attention to the role of "state-of-the-art" diagnostic tests. We will base our recommendations on a critical review of the epidemiology, risk factors, and natural history of gallstones. We will discuss the dominant role of laparoscopic cholecystectomy and summarize the limited indications for medical therapy with oral bile acids with or without extracorporeal shock wave lithotripsy. We will mention some problems that are unique to patients who remain symptomatic after biliary tract surgery. Finally, we will examine the proven measures to prevent gallstones in those who are at very high risk: patients receiving very low-calorie diets for rapid weight loss,[11, 12] total parenteral nutrition (TPN),[13–15] or estrogen therapy for prostatic cancer.[16]

PREVALENCE

Prevalence of gallstones varies tremendously throughout the world.[9, 17] They are "epidemic" among certain South Western US Indians and are very rare in many "Third World" countries. Ultrasonography has facilitated the determination of true and clinical prevalence of gallstones in free-living populations.[7, 18–22]

In the largest study,[21] from Sirmione, Italy, the prevalence of symptomatic and asymptomatic cholesterol gallstones was determined in 2000 men and women aged 18 to 65, 70% of the town's population being enrolled. In women, gallstone prevalence increased linearly from 2.9% in the 18- to 29-year-old group to 27% in those aged 50 to 65. In men the corresponding rates were 1.1% and 11%. Of subjects with gallstones, 80% were unaware of their presence and had no history of biliary pain. Other ultrasonographic studies of British,[23] Danish,[18] Roman,[7, 22] and Norwegian[20] ambulatory populations have reported similar results.

Patients with all forms of chronic hemolysis are at unusually high risk for development of pigment gallstones. In sickle cell disease, one third of 226 juveniles and adolescents had sonographic evidence of gallstones or gallbladder sludge.[24] The prevalence of gallstones increased from 12% in 2 to 4 year olds to 43% in the 15 to 18 year olds. As in cholesterol stone patients, biliary tract pain or complications were infrequent, but women with stones were not at higher risk for symptoms.[24]

Based on age-adjusted autopsy data,[9, 17, 25] Chile has the highest age-adjusted prevalence of gallstones in the world (27%), followed by Northern Europe (15%), and the United States (15%). Nonindustrialized countries have a low prevalence of gallstone disease. For example, the nomadic Masai of East Africa are unique in having a zero prevalence.[9] There may be marked regional variations within large countries: the age-adjusted autopsy prevalence rate of gallstones in Northern India is 6%, compared with 1% in Southern India.[26] In countries with high prevalence rates, the overall female to male ratio is approximately 2:1, reflecting a predominance of cholesterol stones, but in countries with low prevalence, the sex ratio is 1:1, reflecting a predominance of pigment stones. Gallstone prevalence among Japanese and Chinese has changed markedly during this century.[25] Up until the end of World War II, both nations had a low prevalence of gallstones that were predominantly pigment stones.[5, 9, 27] During the last 40 years, the prevalence of cholesterol gallstones has increased markedly, especially in urban areas, and the prevalence of pigment gallstones has fallen, particularly in rural communities.[27]

PATHOGENESIS OF GALLSTONE DISEASE

Gallstones are classified by chemical composition, either composed of cholesterol monohydrate or pigment calcium bilirubinate salts: Patients have either one type or the other. In the US 80% of gallstone patients have cholesterol stones.[28] Since only cholesterol stones potentially can be treated with dissolution therapy or lithotripsy, identifying stone type is of practical significance.

The physical chemical sequences in the pathogenesis of both cholesterol and pigment gallstones have features in common.[5] They are, in chronologic order, supersaturation of bile, nucleation of insoluble molecules, and agglomeration of biliary precipitates forming macroscopic stones. Pathophysiologic events common to both stone types are: (1) relative hypersecretion (in some cases secondary to overproduction) of the otherwise insoluble molecules compared with that of the solubilizing agents, (2) mucin hypersecretion by the gallbladder mucosa, and (3) gallbladder stasis. Nonetheless, several important distinctions exist, depending on whether the major component of stones is cholesterol monohydrate or calcium bilirubinate.

Cholesterol Gallstone Formation

Patients who develop cholesterol gallstones typically have a "triple defect": (1) supersaturation of bile with cholesterol, (2) accelerated cholesterol nucleation, and (3) gallbladder hypomotility (i.e., increased fasting and residual volumes).[29]

Supersaturation of Bile with Cholesterol

The primary excretory route for cholesterol from the body is bile, an aqueous solution in which cholesterol is secreted as unesterified molecules and as its catabolic products, the bile salts. Cholesterol is insoluble in water but in health is effectively solubilized in bile by micelles and vesicles composed of bile salts and the phospholipid, lecithin.[29]

The physical-chemical setting for cholesterol gallstone formation requires an excess of cholesterol molecules compared with molecules of the solubilizing lipids. If this imbalance is not countered by other factors that stabilize supersaturation,[30] cholesterol molecules will not remain in solution, but nucleate, crystallize, and precipitate. In humans, this imbalance between cholesterol and bile salts plus lecithin is caused principally by an increase in biliary cholesterol secretion. A decrease in biliary bile salt secretion is rare. A deficiency of biliary lecithin has not been identified.[29]

There are many causes of hypersecretion of cholesterol into bile: increased hepatic uptake from plasma lipoproteins, increased synthesis, decreased conversion to form new bile salts, or decreased cholesterol ester synthesis. It is now believed that small bile salt pools in gallstone patients are secondary to the effect of lithogenic bile or gallstones themselves on gallbladder function. Furthermore, small bile salt pools are associated with increased recycling via the enterohepatic circulation so that bile salt *secretion* rates are still within the normal range.[31, 32]

Accelerated Cholesterol Nucleation

Bile supersaturated with cholesterol is not in itself a sufficient physical-chemical cause of cholesterol gallstone formation. Most humans have supersaturated bile for several hours each day, particularly during fasting when biliary bile salt secretion rates are physiologically low.[33] Therefore, factors that promote or inhibit nucleation and crystallization must be of critical importance because many biles that are highly enriched with cholesterol do not form stones.[30, 34] In lithogenic (stone-forming) bile, cholesterol crystallizes from solution about five times faster than in control bile for the same degree of supersaturation.[30] There are antinucleating[35] and pronucleating[36] proteins in bile. In addition, gelled gallbladder mucin plays a role in gallstone nucleation.[37] Animal studies suggest that lithogenic bile stimulates gallbladder mucin synthesis and secretion,[38] and drugs that inhibit mucin production can prevent gallstone formation despite the persistence of supersaturated bile.[39]

Gallbladder Hypomotility

Gallbladder "stasis" is an important contributory factor to cholesterol gallstone formation. Animals fed a lithogenic diet show decreased gallbladder smooth muscle contractility[40] and decreased gallbladder emptying[41] prior to gallstone formation. Furthermore, gallbladder muscle contractility is reduced in patients with cholesterol gallstones compared with those with pigment stones.[42] In cholesterol stone disease, incomplete gallbladder emptying allows cholesterol crystals to remain in the gallbladder, aggregate, and form stones.[29] Both accelerated nucleation and decreased gallbladder contractility may be secondary to, and mediated by, abnormal biliary lipid secretion acting on gallbladder mucosa and muscle.[29] The stimulus may be hypersecretion of cholesterol itself, changes in the molecular composition (species) of lecithin, or increased hydrophobicity of the bile salt pool.[31, 32]

The time interval between the development of lithogenic bile and nucleation in whites is not known. In Pima Indians, the average time between the appearance of "lithogenic" bile and macroscopic gallstones is 8 years.[43] In patients whose stones have been dissolved with medical therapy, 10% will form new stones within 1 year, and 50% within 5 years after discontinuing therapy.[44, 45] In contrast, the speed of stone formation can be reduced to weeks or months in patients with an acute spinal cord injury,[46] in obese patients ingesting very low calorie diets, or in patients who have undergone gastric stapling procedures.[11, 12, 47]

Pigment Gallstone Formation

There are two varieties of pigment gallstones, trivially named black or brown stones.[48] Black pigment stones are the more common pigment stones in Western populations and form principally in the gallbladder. In Western subjects, brown pigment stones usually form de novo in the bile ducts following cholecystectomy, but in the Orient these stones are often found in the gallbladder as well. Black pigment stones consist of bilirubin polymers and inorganic salts of calcium (carbonate, phosphate), whereas brown pigment stones consist principally of calcium bilirubinate and organic fatty acid (palmitate and stearate) salts of calcium.[48] On this account, most pigment stones formed in the gallbladder are radio-opaque, whereas those found in the bile ducts are radiolucent.[49–51]

Black pigment gallstones form as a result of overproduction of unconjugated bilirubin in the biliary tree from endogenous β-glucuronidase activity, increased biliary ionized calcium activity, and/or decreased bile salt secretion.[48] Excess biliary ionized calcium complexes with unconjugated bilirubin to form insoluble precipitate, which grows to form stones. Normally, bile salts both solubilize unconjugated bilirubin and bind to ionized calcium. Consequently, bile salt deficiency may promote pigment stone formation by making more unconjugated bilirubin and ionized calcium available for coprecipitation.[52]

Biliary tract infection is a prerequisite for brown pigment stone formation as evidenced by the presence of the monosaccharide rhamnose, which is unique to bacteria and bacterial cytoskeletons, in these gallstones.[53, 54] Patients with brown stones have high levels of unconjugated bilirubin in bile secondary to bacterial β-glucuronidase deconjugation of conjugated bilirubin and high levels of saturated fatty acids secondary to bacterial phospholipase α_2 hydrolysis of biliary lecithin. Although glucaro-1,4-lactone, an inhibitor of bacterial glucuronidase, is normally present in bile, its activity is quickly overcome by a β-glucuronidase–producing anaerobic bacterial infection.[55]

PUTATIVE RISK FACTORS FOR GALLSTONE FORMATION

Cholesterol Gallstones

Female Gender. Between puberty and menopause, women have twice the risk compared with men of developing cholesterol gallstones.[56] Bile is normally not saturated with cholesterol before puberty, but during puberty, it becomes 15% more saturated with cholesterol in females compared with males because of increased biliary cholesterol secretion.[43] Beyond menopause, women lose their increased risk of gallstone formation.[57]

Parity. Pregnancy is an independent risk factor for cholesterol gallstones[7, 21, 58] in proportion to parity, particularly among younger women.[7] Elevated estrogen and progesterone levels during pregnancy increase biliary cholesterol secretion and inhibit gallbladder motor function.

Obesity. Obesity increases the risk of cholesterol gallstone formation in proportion to total body fat.[7, 21, 57, 59] The development of symptoms from gallstones also increases with obesity.[60] More cholesterol is synthesized and secreted into bile in obese people compared with normal people and often results in bile that is greatly supersaturated with cholesterol.[61] If obese subjects achieve ideal body weight, biliary cholesterol saturation reverts to normal.[61]

Rapid Weight Loss. Obese patients undergoing rapid weight loss (~1 to 2% of body weight or 2 to 5 lb/wk), either by very low calorie diet[11, 12] or by gastric stapling,[47] have a 25 to 70% chance of developing gallstones within 4 months. When obese individuals begin to lose weight, biliary cholesterol saturation increases acutely as cholesterol is mobilized from adipose tissue. In addition, the low triglyceride content of these diets causes gallbladder hypomotility secondary to reduced cholecystokinin (CCK) release from the duodenum. Even less dramatic periods of weight loss, particularly in males, have been associated with gallstone formation.[62]

Native Americans. Gallstones are very common in Pima, Navejo, Hopi, Micmac, and Chippewa Indians, especially in young females. In the Pima study, gallstone prevalence in women was 73% in the 25- to 34-year-old group and 90% in those older than 65 years of age. In male Pimas, the corresponding rates were 4% and 70%. Approximately 40 to 50% of Pima women older than 35 years of age experienced symptoms or complications of gallstones, whereas Pima men, like whites, were usually asymptomatic.[63]

Gallbladder Stasis. Incomplete gallbladder emptying (i.e., increased residual volume) is associated with cholesterol gallstone formation in women during pregnancy,[64] and in patients with somatastatinoma[65] or receiving octreotide therapy,[66] and, to a lesser degree, all white patients with cholesterol gallstones.[67, 68]

Medications. Drugs (i.e., the fibric acids) that lower serum cholesterol by increasing biliary cholesterol secretion increase the risk of cholesterol gallstones.[69] Cholestyramine and other drugs that lower serum cholesterol by binding bile acids in the intestine and causing bile acid malabsorption do not increase the risk of gallstones, because the liver can compensate by increasing synthesis of bile salts to maintain normal bile salt secretion.[33] Drugs that competitively inhibit HMG CoA reductase, the rate-limiting enzyme of cholesterol synthesis (i.e., lovastatin, simvastatin, pravastatin), *decrease* biliary cholesterol saturation.[70]

Estrogen therapy in either men or women is associated with an increased risk of developing cholesterol gallstones.[71–73] Men receiving estrogen therapy for prostatic cancer have a 25% annual incidence of gallstone formation[16] because of up-regulation of the hepatic low-density lipoprotein (LDL) receptor and increased excretion of cholesterol into bile.[74]

Serum Lipids. The relation of serum and bile lipids is complex. Nonetheless, high-density lipoprotein (HDL) cholesterol levels are correlated inversely with both biliary cholesterol saturation index[75] and gallstone disease.[7, 76] Furthermore, there is a positive correlation between the biliary cholesterol saturation index, gallstone prevalence, and plasma triglyceride concentrations especially when combined with low HDL cholesterol levels.[7, 21, 75, 77] In addition, there is an increased prevalence of gallstones in patients with types IIb and IV hyperlipoproteinemia (elevated very low density lipoprotein [VLDL] triglyceride)[7, 21, 78] because of increased biliary cholesterol secretion.[79]

Diet. There are little reliable data concerning diet and cholesterol gallstone disease. Increased intake of calories,[80] refined carbohydrate (e.g., sucrose[81]), cholesterol,[82] and saturated fats[83] have all been implicated in gallstone formation. However, these effects may not be independent of obesity. Decreased meal frequency may also be a risk factor.[81] On the other hand, a diet high in bran[84] or containing moderate amounts of alcohol[85] has been reported to protect against gallstone formation. However, with the exception of obesity and weight loss, there is no conclusive evidence that dietary habits influence cholesterol gallstone formation.

Primary Biliary Cirrhosis. Patients with primary biliary cirrhosis also probably have an increased risk of cholesterol gallstone disease.[86–88] Although stone composition has not been studied in these patients, biliary cholesterol saturation is increased, suggesting that these are cholesterol stones and not pigment stones.[88]

Diabetes Mellitus. Patients with diabetes have increased total body cholesterol synthesis and increased biliary cholesterol secretion independent of obesity.[89] In addition, some diabetics have incomplete gallbladder emptying.[90] Nevertheless, diabetes mellitus, per se, does not appear to be an independent risk factor for cholesterol gallstone disease.[5, 21, 57] Most older epidemiologic studies of diabetics that described such a correlation fail to separate the effects of obesity and hypertriglyceridemia.[91] Only autopsy studies, which are inherently biased, have suggested diabetes is a risk factor for gallstone disease.[92]

Pigment Gallstones

The major identifiable physiologic derangements of importance in pigment gallstone formation are (1) delivery of increased bilirubin loads to the liver and bile, (2) gallbladder stasis and incomplete emptying, and (3) anaerobic bacterial invasion of the biliary tree.

Chronic Hemolysis. Inherited hemolytic anemias, sickle cell disease,[24] spherocytosis,[93] thalassemia,[94] chronic hemolysis associated with artificial heart valves,[95] and malaria[96] dramatically increase the risk of pigment gallstone formation. The mechanism probably relates to an increased biliary excretion of bilirubin conjugates. Although the fraction (~1%) of unconjugated bilirubin in bile of patients with chronic hemolysis is not greater than in normal people, the absolute concentration of unconjugated bilirubin may be increased 10-fold.[97]

Alcoholic Cirrhosis. Patients with alcoholic cirrhosis[98–100] or alcoholism[100] have an increased prevalence of pigment gallstones that increases steadily with advancing age[99, 100] and severity of liver disease.[101, 102] Autopsy and prospective studies indicate that 30 to 60% of alcoholic cirrhotics have gallstones; almost half of these are pigment stones.[98, 99] Possible mechanisms for this increased risk include (1) subclinical hemolysis,[99, 102] (2) defective bilirubin conjugation,[103] (3) alcohol-induced secretion of unconjugated bilirubin into bile,[104] and defective bile salt synthesis associated with liver disease.[105]

Age. Increasing age is a risk factor for pigment gallstone formation.[93, 99, 100] Interestingly, patients with pigment gallstones undergo cholecystectomy at a later age than do patients with cholesterol gallstones.[106] This suggests that pigment stones either form later in life than cholesterol stones or that they remain asymptomatic for longer periods.

Ileal Disease, Resection, or Bypass. Patients with ileal disease, resection, or bypass have a strikingly increased risk for developing gallstones[107–110] that is directly proportional to the length of ileum involved or resected.[110, 111] Thirty per cent of patients with ileal Crohn's disease have gallstones.[107–110] Heretofore, it was believed that ileal disease led to only cholesterol stone formation. However, better studies now confirm that these patients are at risk for pigment stones.[112] Following an ileal bypass operation performed for treatment of obesity, gallstones can develop within 6 months and by 2 to 4 years, the incidence reaches 20 to 60%.[113] The true distribution of cholesterol or pigment stones in these patients is unknown.

Biliary Infection. Pigment stones are frequently found in the intrahepatic bile ducts in the Orient and are nearly always associated with bacterial infection (usually *Escherichia coli*) or parasitic infestation (e.g., *Chlonoreis sinensis, Ascaris lumbricoides*).[114] In Western patients, intraductal stones developing after cholecystectomy are associated with stasis and/or biliary tree infection[5, 115] and, thus, are almost invariably brown pigment stones, even in patients whose original gallstones were cholesterol stones.[115, 116]

There is a strong association between diverticula near the ampulla of Vater and the presence of pigment gallstones in the gallbladder.[117–119] These patients frequently have β-glucuronidase–producing bacteria in their biliary tract.[120] An attractive working hypothesis is that decreased muscular tone and contractility of the sphincter of Oddi and the common bile duct secondary to the physical presence of the diverticulum allows the biliary tract to become infected with anaerobic bacteria from the diverticulum.

Gallbladder Stasis Syndromes

Total Parenteral Nutrition. TPN dramatically increases the likelihood of pigment gallstone formation.[13–15] Although TPN of itself promotes gallstone formation, the true frequency depends on the underlying illness for which TPN was instituted. Routine ultrasonographic screening of adults on TPN for a mean of 23 months has shown a 35% incidence of gallstone formation.[13] Of these, stones developed in 39% of patients with, and 25% of patients without, ileal disease.[13] In a prospective study using ultrasonography, 43% of children on TPN for a mean of 21 months developed gallstones.[14] All patients had ileal disease or resection, and over half required cholecystectomy. There is evidence suggesting that 100% of patients on TPN for more than 6 weeks develop biliary sludge, a prestone condition,[37] in their gallbladders.[121] The pathogenesis of gallstone formation during TPN is mainly a result of decreased gallbladder motility and poor gallbladder emptying in the setting of cholesterol or calcium bilirubinate supersaturated bile. The daily intravenous administration of CCK-octapeptide in animals[122] or in humans[123] corrects the motility defect and prevents stone formation.

Vagotomy. There is probably a four- to sixfold increase in gallstone formation after truncal vagotomy.[124, 125] Although stone composition in these patients has not been studied, gallbladder stasis[126] and pathophysiologic evidence[127, 128] suggest that these stones should be pigment, rather than cholesterol gallstones. Also, in an animal model, truncal vagotomy caused biliary "sludge" and pigment stones to develop.[129]

DIAGNOSIS OF CHOLELITHIASIS

Epidemiologic data have suggested that biliary pain, which is defined as at least one episode of continuous pain in the right hypochondrium or epigastrium lasting for at least 30 minutes, has a relatively low specificity (80%), sensitivity (35%), and predictive value (10%) for the diagnosis of gallstones.[7] Therefore, since the physical examination is generally normal, the physician must rely on one or more diagnostic tests for a definitive diagnosis of gallstones.

Oral cholecystography and real-time ultrasonography are both excellent methods for detecting cholelithiasis. Both have a specificity of approximately 98% with a sensitivity of approximately 95%.[130, 131] Both tests have unique advantages. However, ultrasonography has now become the initial diagnostic procedure of choice since it does not involve patient preparation, potential side effects of radiocontraast administration, or x-ray irradiation and is simple to perform and interpret. However, oral cholecystography demonstrates gallbladder concentrating and contractile function and allows a more accurate assessment of the number, size, and density of stones, which is crucial information if dissolution therapy with oral bile acids is contemplated.

Both oral cholecystography and ultrasonography are associated with a small percentage of false-negative examinations. Therefore, if one of these diagnostic tests has a negative result for stones and the clinical suspicion of gallstone disease is high, the alternate diagnostic test should be employed.

The clinician is frequently faced with an abdominal ultrasonographic report that describes gallbladder "sludge."[37] This is the description of multiple weak echoes without acoustic shadowing in the dependent part of the gallbladder or, rarely, observed diffusely throughout the gallbladder.[132] Biliary sludge can form during prolonged fasting in debilitated, hospitalized patients or during hyperalimentation,[121] and in patients with extrahepatic biliary obstruction, or in 40% of women just after pregnancy.[133] Gallbladder sludge consists of a mixture of mucin glycoproteins and microprecipitates of calcium bilirubinate, liquid crystals of bile lipids, and solid cholesterol monohydrate crystals.[134] Mucin glycoproteins accumulate in the gallbladder during gallbladder stasis and in response to the presence of lithogenic bile[37] and can entrap microprecipitates of calcium bilirubinate and, less frequently, liquid crystals and solid cholesterol crystals.[134]

The natural history of biliary sludge is unpredictable. In many patients, gallbladder sludge may be innocuous and disappears soon after delivery[133, 135] or oral refeeding.[121] In others, however, biliary sludge may cause biliary pain, acute cholecystitis, or pancreatitis.[136–139] The clear evolution of biliary sludge to gallstones has been documented.[133, 134] Today it is believed that biliary sludge represents an early, but still reversible, stage of gallstone formation.

CLINICAL SYNDROMES

At least two thirds of individuals with gallstones remain asymptomatic all of their lives ("silent stones").[7, 21] If the gallstones or biliary sludge transiently block the cystic duct, biliary pain (misnamed "colic") may occur. Prolonged obstruction of the cystic duct results in infection behind the obstruction, giving rise to acute cholecystitis. Stones or biliary sludge migrate from the gallbladder through the cystic duct into the common bile duct frequently and may cause biliary pain, jaundice, cholangitis, or pancreatitis. Rarely, a gallstone erodes through the gallbladder directly into the stomach or small intestine to cause small bowel obstruction, "gallstone ileus." Adenocarcinoma of the gallbladder, though rare, is epidemiologically associated with long-standing gallstone disease.[140]

Asymptomatic Gallstones

By definition, patients with asymptomatic (silent) stones have never had biliary pain. Their gallstones are usually discovered incidentally during abdominal surgery or radiographic or ultrasonographic studies performed for nonbiliary tract indications.

A retrospective Mayo Clinic study from 1948 analyzed 112 patients who had asymptomatic gallstones that were discovered incidentally during surgery 10 to 20 years previously.[141] Of these patients, 55% had no abdominal symptoms and 26% had developed nonspecific abdominal symptoms: "gaseous indigestion, intolerance to certain specific foods, and heartburn" now known to be unrelated to gallstones. Only 19% developed true biliary symptoms, that is, biliary pain or jaundice. Three other retrospective studies of patients with silent stones gave similar results.[6, 142, 143] A long-term prospective study followed 123 individuals (mostly male college professors) with asymptomatic gallstones discovered by oral cholecystographic screening for 11 to 24 years.[144] Only 13% developed biliary tract pain, and typically this occurred within the first 5 years. A 5-year prospective evaluation of the original Sirmione cohort showed similar results.[145]

The epidemiologic literature indicates that (1) most gallstones, whether cholesterol or pigment in type, are asymptomatic; (2) patients who develop symptoms usually do so within the first 5 years of diagnosis; and (3) in more than 90% of patients who develop symptoms, the initial symptom is biliary pain rather than a complication (acute cholecystitis, cholangitis, or pancreatitis).[144]

Treatment of Patients with Asymptomatic Gallstones

Because of the benign course of patients with asymptomatic gallstones (only a 1% chance per year of developing symptoms), the physician needs only to reassure and follow the patient. If patients develop biliary pain, they should be re-evaluated for surgery or medical dissolution therapy at that time. A recent decision analysis supports this approach and has demonstrated that prophylactic cholecystectomy for men with asymptomatic gallstones resulted in a *loss* of 4 to 18 days of life, depending on age.[146]

Whether diabetics with asymptomatic gallstones should undergo prophylactic cholecystectomy is still controversial. It is clear from both older[147–149] and recent[151, 152] studies that diabetics with acute cholecystitis have a worse prognosis than do age-matched gallstone patients: operative mortality rates vary from 11 to 20% compared with less than 5% in nondiabetics. However, two recent retrospective studies have shown that diabetes is not an *independent* risk factor for operative mortality or serious postoperative complications in patients with acute cholecystitis.[153, 154] An important unanswered question is, how often do diabetics with gallstones have complications? Anecdotal evidence suggests that diabetic patients are more likely to develop acute cholecystitis and other complications of gallstones without prior episodes of biliary pain. Unfortunately, the natural history of gallstones in diabetic patients is not known. Despite a decision analysis that concluded prophylactic cholecystectomy resulted in 2 to 8 months of *shorter* life span regardless of patient age,[155] the issue remains unsettled because of the assumptions used in the model.[156]

Role of Prophylactic Cholecystectomy. There are several groups of asymptomatic gallstone patients for whom prophylactic cholecystectomy is recommended.

Otherwise healthy patients who, because of their occupation, do not have easy access to high-quality medical care (e.g., crew members of nuclear submarines, missionaries, or public health field workers in developing countries) should undergo elective cholecystectomy at a convenient time to avoid the very small, but real, risk of developing symptoms or complications under inauspicious conditions. Medical dissolution therapy in these patients would not be advisable because of the length of therapy and the risk of recurrence (see later).

There are subgroups of gallstone patients who have an increased risk of developing gallbladder cancer (four- to sevenfold higher than gallstone controls): Native-American women[157–159] and patients with solitary stones that exceed 3 cm in diameter.[140, 160] Medical therapy to dissolve gallstones would not be appropriate in these settings since the gallstones per se may not necessarily be the causative or even the promoting factor for cancer. The risk of surgery in the average Western gallstone patient, albeit small, outweighs the chance of developing gallbladder cancer.[5, 9, 140]

Patients with any one of the following four conditions, all of which are associated with gallbladder cancer, should undergo a prophylactic cholecystectomy: "porcelain" gallbladders[161]; large (>10 mm) gallbladder polyps[162]; anomalous pancreaticobiliary ductal junction[163]; and *Salmonella typhosa* infection.[164]

Porcelain gallbladder is a result of precipitation of salts of calcium phosphate in the gallbladder mucosa and, although rare, is associated with an extremely high (20 to 60%) prevalence of gallbladder cancer. The diagnosis is made on an abdominal flatplate x-ray by observing patchy calcification of the gallbladder wall.[165] Patients with porcelain gallbladders must be distinguished from patients with "milk of calcium" bile (limy bile), in which calcium carbonate and calcium oxalate precipitates within the gallbladder lumen.[51, 166] The diagnosis of "milk of calcium" bile is made by observing an "opacified" gallbladder on abdominal flatplate x-ray examination without ingestion of radiocontrast material. These patients have a clinical course that is no different from gallstone patients in general. In fact, "milk of calcium" bile often disappears spontaneously but may be recurrent.[167]

Prevention of Gallstones

Prevention of gallstones is possible in two groups of patients at high risk for stone formation. Patients receiving TPN for longer than 3 months invariably develop biliary sludge in their gallbladders.[121] These patients have more complications—usually acute cholecystitis—than would be expected in conventional populations with cholelithiasis.[137] The opinion of many experts is that, if a patient is undergoing laparotomy for a condition that is likely to require long-term TPN (i.e., massive small bowel resection or severe Crohn's disease), a prophylactic cholecystectomy should be performed even though there are no stones in the gallbladder.[137] Alternatively, the daily administration of intravenous cholecystokinin-octapeptide (CCK-OP) to patients receiving TPN prevents gallbladder stasis, biliary sludge, and gallstone formation.[123]

Ursodiol (8 to 10 mg/kg/day), taken during the weight loss period by obese patients undergoing rapid weight loss, completely prevents gallstone formation.[11] A lower ursodiol dose, or the inclusion in the diet of at least 10 g/day of long-chained trigylceride (e.g., corn or canola oil), may be effective as well.[168] Whether there is sufficient risk of gallstone formation in patients undergoing more moderate weight loss to justify ursodiol prophylaxis is unknown.

Symptomatic Gallstones

Biliary Pain

Biliary tract pain (misnamed "colic") most often results when a gallstone transiently obstructs the cystic duct or the common bile duct. It is not a "colicky" (intermittent) pain but a steady pain. It has an interesting circadian periodicity that is most frequent, *not* after meals, but rather 1 to 2 hours after the patient goes to bed.[169] Typically, the pain starts gradually, builds to a plateau of intensity over 15 to 30 minutes, remains constant for several hours, and gradually disappears.[5, 9] Occasionally, both the onset and termination of biliary pain are abrupt. Biliary pain is most frequently localized to the epigastrium or the right upper quadrant, although pain can occur in the left upper quadrant, subxiphoid region, or in the back.[5, 9] In approximately 50% of patients, biliary pain radiates to other parts of the abdomen or back, classically to the right shoulder or right subscapular region. Nausea and vomiting may occur during an attack of biliary pain but are often absent.

The time intervals between attacks of biliary pain are highly variable, ranging from months to years, or very rarely, daily. Despite anecdotal reports by patients, there is no evidence that ingestion of fatty or rich food, overeating, exercise, straining, or stress precipitates biliary pain.[170, 171] Nevertheless, patients with frequent attacks of biliary pain should expect continued and frequent attacks in the future.[143, 172]

Traditionally, a group of vague, ill-defined "dyspeptic" symptoms have been frequently associated with gallstones: particular food (usually fatty) intolerance, postprandial bloating, indigestion, flatulence, or abdominal discomfort.[173, 174] These symptoms occur periodically in the general population in the absence of organic disease. Since the prevalence of gallstones in Western populations is high, it is not surprising to find these symptoms in many patients with gallstones. Large-scale prospective studies of ambulatory women and of hospitalized patients showed that these ill-defined "dyspeptic" symptoms occurred frequently (34 to 50%), but no more frequently in gallstone patients than in controls.[7, 21, 170, 171]

Physical examination of a patient during an acute attack of biliary pain is usually normal. Nevertheless, the patient is frequently restless in a vain attempt to find a position that relieves discomfort. Occasionally, tenderness is present in the right upper quadrant. More important, neither fever nor leukocytosis is present during an attack of biliary pain, unless a complication is developing. If the patient becomes febrile, with or without laboratory evidence of infection, then progression to acute cholecystitis should be suspected and appropriate studies should be performed (see later).[5, 9]

The natural history of patients with biliary pain is less benign than that of patients with asymptomatic gallstones. The annual cholecystectomy rate in (placebo-treated) patients who were monitored with biliary pain was 2% during the 2 years of the National Cooperative Gallstone Study.[172] Recurrent pain will develop in 30 to 60% of patients during a 5 to 20-year period.[6, 142, 143, 175–177] The incidence of biliary complications increases linearly with time at a rate of approximately 1%/yr.[6, 177] The risk of recurrent pain or complications is higher in women[175, 177] and in those with a nonfunctioning gallbladder revealed by oral cholecystography.[177]

Treatment of Patients with Symptomatic Gallstones

There are now several options, both surgical and medical, for treatment of symptomatic gallstone patients. Cholecystectomy is still the so-called "gold" standard, but now it is usually carried out laparoscopically rather than via laparotomy.

It is controversial whether cholecystectomy should be performed after only the first attack of biliary pain or delayed until repeated attacks have occurred. It is also not clear what role medical dissolution therapy should play in patients who have mild symptoms versus those with severe symptoms.

Medical Dissolution Therapy. The earliest medical dissolution studies were based on the hypothesis that the chronic ingestion of any bile salt would expand the bile salt pool, increase bile salt secretion rates, desaturate bile with cholesterol, and dissolve cholesterol gallstones. However, bile salt feeding does not appreciably expand the total bile salt pool[178] nor increase bile salt secretion rates.[179] Furthermore, a contracted bile salt pool is known now to be secondary to the presence of gallstones in the gallbladder and incomplete gallbladder emptying. The primary reason that administration of ursodeoxycholic acid (ursodiol [Actigall]), a naturally occurring bile acid, is effective in desaturating bile and dissolving cholesterol gallstones[179] is that it decreases cholesterol secretion into bile,[180] in part, by decreasing cholesterol absorption.[181] Unsaturated bile plucks cholesterol molecules, literally one by one, from the surfaces of gallstones and redissolves them in micellar or vesicular solution, and gallbladder contraction discharges the dispersed cholesterol into the duodenum.

Medical dissolution treatment with ursodiol is effective in treating mildly symptomatic patients with small (<1 cm in diameter) cholesterol (but not pigment or calcified) gallbladder stones.[8] In addition, patients who refuse or who would tolerate surgery poorly may be candidates for medical therapy. The applicability of this treatment is limited critically by the character and sizes of stones and by the severity of symptoms. The major disadvantages are that gallstones dissolve slowly (1 mm shrinkage in radius per month)[182] and will reform in 50% of patients within 5 years of discontinuing therapy.[44]

Ursodiol completely dissolves small (<5 mm) gallstones in up to 80% of highly selected patients.[183] Prior to the initiation of treatment with ursodiol, stone size, number, and calcium content need to be evaluated with ultrasonography and abdominal flat plate. If small, noncalcified stones are demonstrated, ursodiol therapy at 8 mg/kg/day in two divided doses in the morning and at bedtime can be started. Computed tomography (CT) scanning is a sensitive way to measure calcium content but may not be cost effective.[184]

Reassessment of stone size, either by oral cholecystography (OCG) or by ultrasonography, after 6 months of therapy is the only follow-up required. Ursodiol should be continued for 3 months after complete stone dissolution has been confirmed by ultrasonography, not by OCG.[185] Although some patients with nonopacified gallbladders on initial OCG have responded to ursodiol, in general, such patients are not considered candidates for this therapy. The development of a nonvisualized OCG during therapy predicts dissolution failure. Therefore, either the development of a nonvisualized OCG or the lack of dissolution at follow-up should prompt the physician to discontinue therapy. In addition, if, during therapy, frequent attacks of biliary pain occur (an uncommon event), a delay in definitive treatment is unacceptable and such patients require surgery.

After successful dissolution, patients should be re-evaluated for recurrent gallstones only if symptoms of biliary tract disease recur. Secretion of lithogenic bile resumes in all patients within 1 week of discontinuing oral bile salt therapy.[186] Surveillance ultrasonography for gallstone recurrence is not recommended. Maintenance therapy with either low-dose ursodiol at bedtime or dietary manipulations (low cholesterol, high-fiber diet) might prevent gallstone recurrence[187] but cannot be recommended at this time. Ursodiol, unlike its predecessor, chenodiol, is remarkably free of side effects. It does not cause hepatic injury, diarrhea, or elevation of serum cholesterol.[188] However, patients should be advised that the drug is expensive and that a second course of therapy for symptomatic recurrence may be required.

Lithotripsy. Extracorporeal shock wave lithotripsy (ESWL) is still investigational and should be considered as an adjuvant to ursodiol treatment to accelerate dissolution of cholesterol stones only.[189, 190] Focusing shock waves on gallstones causes fragmentation, transforming a large stone into myriads of small stones that can either migrate into the duodenum without obstruction or dissolve in unsaturated bile more rapidly. Symptomatic patients with a single radiolucent stone, 1 to 2 cm in size, are the best candidates for combination ESWL and ursodiol therapy.[8]

ESWL has limited overall applicability because only 10 to 15% of gallstone patients have a solitary, 1- to 2-cm noncalcified stone in a functioning gallbladder. Other exclusion criteria include all complications of gallstones, inability to target the gallstones while avoiding bone, lung, cysts or aneurysms, and pregnancy. Nevertheless, appropriately selected patients have an 80 to 90% chance of complete stone and fragment dissolution after ESWL and 1 year of ursodiol therapy.[191, 192]

The newer lithotriptors that employ piezoceramic technology are painless and well tolerated by patients. The procedure can be done in an outpatient setting without intravenous lines or analgesics.[192] Severe side effects are related to transient obstruction of the cystic or common bile ducts, resulting in acute cholecystitis or pancreatitis in 4% and 2%, respectively, usually within 48 hours of ESWL.[191] Biliary pain occurs in 30 to 70% of patients during the first 3 months after lithotripsy, and diarrhea may be more frequent than with ursodiol treatment alone.[189, 191]

Cholecystectomy. Cholecystectomy is the treatment of choice for most patients with symptomatic gallstones or gallstone complications.[8] It relieves symptoms in more than 88% of patients.[193] Treatment failure almost always results from an operation being performed for inappropriate reasons, usually abdominal symptoms not caused by gallstones.[174] Elective, traditional cholecystectomy is very safe.[194] Mortality is related to age, sex, pre-existing medical conditions, and presence of biliary complications of gallstones. The National Halothane Study of 27,600 cholecystectomies performed in the early 1960s revealed that operative mortality for women in good health ranged from 0.05% of women younger than 50 years of age to 0.3% for women who were 70 years of age.[194] Severe pre-existing systemic illness increased operative mortality to 1.3% and 1.7%, respectively. The operative mortality in men was twice that of women, probably because of concomitant atherosclerotic disease. Furthermore, operative mortality doubled with emergency operations and quadrupled when the common bile duct was explored. The most serious morbidity was bile duct injury, which occurred in 0.2% of patients. Large surveys in the 1980s suggest that US mortality and morbidity rates from open cholecystectomy are less than 1% and 5%, respectively.[195]

Laparoscopic cholecystectomy has almost replaced traditional cholecystectomy worldwide, with more than 85% of elective operations being performed via this approach.[8, 196] Regrettably, no studies have compared the safety of the two approaches. Clear advantages of laparoscopic cholecystectomy include: (1) much smaller scars, (2) reduced hospital stay (1 to 2 versus 5 to 6 days), and (3) earlier return to normal activities (7 versus 40 to 60 days).[196] Early results suggest a higher rate of bile duct injury (0.8%) than during traditional cholecystectomy but less overall morbidity.[196]

Although biliary physiology is profoundly altered following cholecystectomy,[33] there is no malabsorption of fat and no special diet is ever indicated. The bile salt pool is not sequestered during an overnight fast, thus there is continuous recirculation eliminating low fasting bile salt secretion rates and consequently high cholesterol saturation. The lack of sequestration explains the absence of recurrent cholesterol stone formation in the biliary ducts following cholecystectomy.[5, 9] Continuous recirculation of the bile salt pool causes a mild increase in bile salt malsorption and results in mild diarrhea in 5% of patients after cholecystectomy.[197]

Overall Treatment Strategy

Patients with more than one attack of biliary pain should be treated definitively to prevent (1) repeated attacks of biliary pain and (2) the complications of gallstones, acute cholecystitis, cholangitis, and pancreatitis. Patients with "dyspepsia" should not expect resolution of those symptoms after treatment for gallstones.

Male or female gallstone patients under 50 years of age who are otherwise in good health and who have *recurrent* attacks of biliary pain should have an elective cholecystectomy while the operative risk is small (<0.1%).[146] Although 50% of these patients may have only infrequent attacks of pain during the next 20 years, at least 20% will develop complications of their gallstones and have significantly higher operative risks at that time. We believe that medical dissolution therapy has a very small role in young, symptomatic patients.

Diabetic patients should have an elective cholecystectomy, even if they experience only one episode of biliary pain.

The management of nondiabetic patients after only one episode of biliary pain is controversial. In young, otherwise healthy patients, cholecystectomy is reasonable. Similarly, an expectant "watch and wait" approach to observe the frequency of attacks and confirm that they are definitely due to gallstones is also rational. Patients with small, noncalcified stones, especially if they developed during weight loss, recent pregnancy, or use of medications, would be ideal candidates for ursodiol therapy during the period of observation. Clearly a proportion of these patients will fail medical therapy or will develop accelerated symptoms and require surgery.

Older symptomatic patients present the most difficult therapeutic dilemma, since they are likely to have a concomitant medical problem that influences operative mortality and life expectancy. The physician needs to balance the risks of waiting and possibly being forced to perform surgery under adverse conditions versus the chance that the patient will die of other causes before gallstones cause complications. For example, a man with his first attack of biliary pain at 65 years of age might be treated surgically if he were otherwise healthy and expected to live an additional 20 years. On the other hand, if the patient were a poor surgical risk, either symptomatic (expectant) treatment or a trial of medical therapy might be appropriate.

Expectant management or medical therapy are the only therapeutic possibilities in symptomatic patients who refuse surgery.

BILIARY COMPLICATIONS OF GALLSTONES

Acute Cholecystitis

Acute cholecystitis is an acute inflammation of bile as well as the gallbladder wall.[5, 9] More than 90% of cases are secondary to an obstruction of the cystic duct by gallstones. Acalculous cholecystitis occurs occasionally, usually in otherwise severely ill hospitalized patients,[198] and may be due to biliary sludge occluding the cystic duct. The precise sequence of events from cystic duct obstruction to acute inflammation of the gallbladder is not understood. It is believed that the earliest events (first 24 to 48 hours) are probably secondary to chemical inflammation of the gallbladder and are not bacterial in origin. In animal experiments, stones in the gallbladder (with or without cystic duct obstruction) can cause the gallbladder wall to secrete fluid probably via a prostaglandin-mediated pathway.[199, 200] The net result is a dramatic increase in intraluminal pressure.[199] Bacteria can be cultured from gallbladder bile in only 35% of cases during the first day of an attack.[201] However, after 4 days of acute cholecystitis, cultures are positive in 80% of patients.[201]

Clinical Manifestations. The usual attack of acute cholecystitis begins in an identical fashion to an attack of biliary pain.[5, 9] The pain localizes rapidly to the right hypochondrium and is associated with anorexia, nausea, and vomiting. The range of physical findings depends on the extent of the inflammatory process. Some patients have only mild direct, but not rebound tenderness and low-grade fever. Others will have marked tenderness with rebound and guarding and a fever up to 102° F. In the first attack of acute cholecystitis, the gallbladder may become palpable, but this finding has no prognostic significance. Laboratory values are abnormal in all cases of acute cholecystitis. In the early stages, the white blood cell count is elevated to 10,000 to 15,000 cells/mm^3.[5] Higher values suggest empyema or perforation of the gallbladder. Transaminases are usually less than 250 IU. Mild to moderate jaundice (serum bilirubin <7 mg/dl) occurs in approximately 20% of patients, even in the absence of common duct stones.[202] The mechanism is unknown but may be a result of absorption of bilirubin across an inflamed gallbladder wall or secondary to transient obstruction of the common bile duct by edema and inflammation from the contiguously inflamed gallbladder.[202, 203] Serum levels of alkaline phosphatase or amylase can be elevated occasionally during an episode of acute cholecystitis alone. To every physician, hyperbilirubinemia, elevation of alkaline phosphatase or amylase in the clinical setting of acute cholecystitis should raise the possibility of a common bile duct gallstone or pancreatitis.[5, 202–204] A normal urinary amylase/creatinine clearance ratio may be helpful in excluding pancreatitis.[205, 206]

Diagnosis. The diagnosis of acute cholecystitis should always be considered in patients with abdominal pain, fever, and upper abdominal, especially right upper quadrant, tenderness. Radiographic studies are usually necessary to confirm the diagnosis. An abdominal flatplate and upright x-ray should be examined for calcified gallstones, air in the biliary system, or free air in the peritoneal cavity.

An oral cholecystogram is *never* an appropriate diagnostic test in this setting because of overnight patient preparation; radiocontrast material may not be absorbed secondary to vomiting and gastric retention; and hepatic dysfunction may prevent adequate excretion of the contrast agent into the biliary tract.[5, 9] Abdominal ultrasonography can be highly suggestive of acute cholecystitis if, in the presence of gallstones, either a thickened gallbladder wall, or localized pericholecystic fluid collection, is demonstrated.[207–211] Because of the frequency of gallstones in the general population, the presence of stones alone in the gallbladder does not make the diagnosis of acute cholecystitis.

Biliary scintigraphy with a ^{99}Tc-labeled iminodiacetic acid derivative (HIDA, PIPIDA, DISIDA) is the test of choice to confirm the diagnosis of suspected acute cholecystitis.[212–218] These compounds, when injected intravenously, are excreted rapidly in high concentrations into bile even in patients whose serum bilirubin levels are 10 to 20 mg/dl. After injection, the radionuclide normally appears in the biliary tree within 15 to 30 minutes and in the duodenum within 45 minutes. Cholescintigraphy obtained at this time will outline the hepatic bile ducts, gallbladder, common bile duct, and duodenum. In patients with acute cholecystitis, surface counting of radioactivity will outline the bile ducts and duodenum, but since the cystic duct is occluded, the gallbladder will not be visualized. Such a "positive scan" is consistent with, but does not absolutely prove, that acute cholecystitis is present. However, a great deal of worldwide experience suggests that acute cholecystitis is extremely unlikely if the gallbladder is seen during such a scan.[212–218] Moreover, in patients with acalculous cholecystitis, cholescintigraphy is almost always positive because the cystic duct, although not obstructed by a stone, becomes occluded by edema, viscous mucin, and inflammatory exudate.[219] In some very jaundiced patients (serum bilirubin >20 mg/dl), sufficient radioactivity may not be excreted into the biliary tract to allow an adequate determination of gallbladder filling. Such a scan should be labelled "nondiagnostic." False-positive scans may occur in some alcoholics and in some patients receiving TPN.[220]

Treatment of Acute Cholecystitis. The treatment for acute cholecystitis is early cholecystectomy. Surgery should be performed within the first 72 hours of the onset of the attack (called "early cholecystectomy") rather than 6 to 8 weeks after the patient has fully recovered from the acute episode ("late cholecystectomy").[221] Bile acid therapy has no role in the management of acute cholecystitis.

During the diagnostic "work-up," the patient should have a nasogastric tube attached to suction and should be stabilized with intravenous fluids and electrolytes. While surgery is being scheduled, it is common practice to administer intravenously antibiotics that have high biliary excretion rates (i.e., ampicillin or cephalosporin). However, their usefulness is probably restricted to diabetic patients and to very old or debilitated patients.[5]

Several controlled and prospective studies have demonstrated the advantage of early, rather than late, cholecystectomy.[221–226] Mortality, overall morbidity, complications of cholecystitis, rupture, abscess (empyema), recurrent pain, and cholangitis are all reduced. Early operation also reduces the total length of hospitalization and the total economic cost to the patient and society.[226]

The acute treatment of some patients with severe concomitant medical illness (e.g., respiratory failure, myocardial ischemia, renal failure) will take priority over that of biliary surgery. Cholecystectomy should be delayed in these high-risk patients until they have been stabilized. If surgery cannot be delayed because of clinical deterioration in the patient's biliary condition, then a temporizing cholecystostomy may be necessary.[5] This operation can be performed under local anesthesia. The gallbladder is decompressed, and the stones are removed. Depending on the patient's subsequent recovery and management of other underlying diseases, a definitive biliary operation should be performed when possible.

The natural history of patients with a prior episode of acute cholecystitis who have not undergone a cholecystectomy is poor. Recurrences of biliary colic and complications are common, occurring in 50% of patients within 5 years.[143, 176] A nonfunctioning gallbladder by oral cholecystography doubles the risk of future complications in these patients.[176]

An occasional patient in the high surgical risk category may still have a functioning gallbladder after recovery from acute cholecystitis. Chronic therapy with ursodeoxycholic acid might be tried in this situation, although successful stone dissolution before another attack of cholecystitis is unlikely.

Choledocholithiasis (Common Duct Stones)

Stones in the common bile duct originate in one of two ways. They either migrate from the gallbladder (95%) or form de novo in the common duct (5%).[227, 228] The migratory stones, having originated in the gallbladder, are cholesterol stones in 80% of patients and black pigment stones in the remainder. The prevalence of common bile duct stones that have migrated from the gallbladder increases with the age of the patient. Between 20 and 60 years of age, 8 to 15% of patients with gallbladder stones have common bile duct stones. This figure increases exponentially to more than 50% in patients who are 60 years of age and older.[229, 230] Therefore, the longer time that stones are present in the gallbladder, the greater is the chance that they will not only migrate into the common bile duct (a common event) but will also remain there.

The mechanisms by which stones form de novo in the common duct after cholecystectomy are poorly defined. Since the stones consist mainly of calcium bilirubinate plus calcium salts of long-chain fatty acids, it is likely that stasis and infection play a major role.[5, 53, 231] Stasis from biliary strictures or other anatomic changes are usually not found in such patients. Motor abnormalities of the sphincter of Oddi or in the common bile duct itself may be responsible initially for brown stone formation.[232]

CLINICAL SYNDROMES OF CHOLEDOCHOLITHIASIS

The clinical syndromes and natural history associated with common bile duct stones are highly variable[233] and unpredictable.[228] At least 10% of patients with multiple stones in the gallbladder frequently pass their stones "silently" into the common duct and out into the intestines and feces.[234, 235] In long-term (20-year) follow-up studies utilizing oral cholecystography, 7% of patients with multiple stones can even empty their gallbladders completely, only to reform stones at a later date.[236] Stones that remain lodged in the bile ducts may remain asymptomatic for months to several years.[237] Others present with: (1) cholangitis; (2) intermittent or persistent obstructive jaundice, with or without pain; (3) acute pancreatitis; and (4) biliary pain without other complications.

Cholangitis

Cholangitis is a bacterial infection of the bile ducts and bile. Bile duct obstruction does not invariably produce cholangitis, but cholangitis *cannot* occur without obstruction from a stone, stricture, or neoplasm. Interestingly, the risk of cholangitis is not related to the degree of bile duct obstruction: With a malignant obstruction bile cultures are positive in 36% of cases, but they are positive in 72% of patients with obstructing calculi.[238] As such, progressive high-grade obstruction from neoplasms is associated with only approximately a 10% risk of cholangitis[239] compared with a 33% risk in patients with common duct stones.[233]

The clinical manifestations of cholangitis are protean.[240, 241] Some patients have a mild, self-limited illness characterized by fever, chills, abdominal pain, and dark urine. Others, especially the elderly, debilitated, or immunosuppressed patients, present with sepsis and shock without specific signs that are referable to the biliary tract. The usual patient presents with jaundice, chills, and fever (Charcot's triad) and abdominal pain.[240] Jaundice may be clinically absent in 20% of patients.[242, 243] Unlike biliary pain, the abdominal pain associated with cholangitis is generally mild; severe pain should raise the possibility of acute cholecystitis or pancreatitis.

The physical findings in patients with cholangitis are also variable. Abdominal tenderness is frequent but is not invariable. Rebound tenderness or guarding are uncommon because peritoneal irritation is not a prominent feature. Hypotension and mental confusion occur in approximately 15% of cases and forebode an ominous outcome.[241]

Laboratory tests in the diagnosis of cholangitis are not pathognomonic. Leukocytosis, occasionally as high as 40,000/mm^3, may occur. Elevations of serum bilirubin, alkaline phosphatase, transaminases, and amylase are common but do not distinguish cholangitis from acute cholecystitis or pancreatitis.[244] In the presence of normal liver function tests, cholangitis is extremely unlikely. Bacteremia, which arises most commonly with *E. coli* and *Klebsiella*,[238] occurs in 40% of patients.[244] In addition, in approximately 15% of patients, anaerobes are found in the biliary tract.[238, 245]

Radiographic studies are generally nondiagnostic. Abdominal plain films can show air in the biliary tree if gas-producing organisms are present, but more often the results are normal or show a nonspecific small bowel ileus. Abdominal ultrasonography may show a dilated common bile duct, with or without a stone. However, its specificity is low (approximately 25%) because cholangitis can occur without ductal dilatation.[246–248] Furthermore, stones in the common duct are difficult to visualize by way of ultrasonography and have false-negative rates of 40%.[246, 248]

Treatment of cholangitis is a medical and surgical emergency. The patient should be stabilized quickly, with intravenous hydration and antibiotics followed, not by surgery, but by prompt *endoscopic* decompression of the common bile duct. We recommend intravenous triple therapy with ampicillin or a third-generation cephalosporin, clindamycin or metronidazole, and an aminoglycoside, or any combination that is effective against anaerobes as well as *E. coli* and *Klebsiella*. With proper medical therapy, patients should show signs of clinical improvement within 12 hours and become afebrile within 2 to 3 days.

If the patient with cholangitis deteriorates or even fails to improve and stabilize within 24 hours on appropriate medical therapy, the biliary tree should be decompressed *immediately* via ERCP.[241, 249–251] If ERCP fails or is unavailable, other options for emergency decompression, albeit with higher morbidity and mortality, include laparotomy and T tube drainage of the common bile duct,[241, 249, 250] or percutaneous placement of a transhepatic catheter.[252] Decompression should not be delayed because "the patient is too sick" since drainage of the biliary tree will produce beneficial results immediately.

After the patient has recovered from the acute attack of cholangitis, a definitive procedure to correct the bile duct obstruction should be performed. The approach depends on (1) the cause of the ductal obstruction, and (2) whether the gallbladder is present. Prior to definitive surgical or endoscopic therapy, the anatomy of the biliary tree and the nature of the ductal obstruction should be delineated by direct cholangiography, preferably by ERCP. Patients with common bile duct stones and an intact gallbladder should have their bile ducts cleared of stones via ERCP, followed within 24 to 48 hours by laparoscopic cholecystectomy if they are suitable candidates. An open cholecystectomy with exploration and removal of stones from the common bile duct and T tube drainage is a reasonable alternative. For patients without *gallbladder* stones or symptoms referable to the gallbladder, or for patients who are poor operative risks, an endoscopic sphincterotomy with removal of the common duct stone is an acceptable alternative.[253–255] The risk of cholecystitis or recurrent choledocolthiasis in patients thus treated is only 10%.[256, 257] Medical dissolution therapy of stones is contraindicated in patients with cholangitis.

The treatment of choice for benign biliary strictures is surgical resection (see later). Obstructing neoplasms of the pancreatic or bile duct can be resected in a minority but usually must be bypassed via endoscopic or percutaneous transhepatic placement of an internal stent through the area of obstruction.[258, 259] Failing this, a percutaneous transhepatic catheter can be attached permanently to external drainage.[260, 261] Unfortunately, the risk of recurrent cholangitis or catheter occlusion following all of these manipulations is high.[262, 263] Surgical bypass with a cholecystoduodenostomy or choledochojejunostomy is an alternative, especially if there is a need for a tissue diagnosis.

"Painless" Intermittent or Persistent Jaundice

Common duct stones are the cause of obstruction in approximately 10% of patients who present with "painless jaundice."[264] Although a gallstone etiology of intermittent or persistent jaundice can often be inferred by history, physical examination, and routine laboratory tests, the extrahepatic biliary tree should be visualized by ERCP to confirm the diagnosis and to provide precise delineation of the anatomy for definitive management. The degree of elevation of serum bilirubin is often proportional to the degree of biliary tract obstruction. Since common duct stones usually cause low-grade, intermittent obstruction, serum bilirubin levels rarely exceed 10 to 15 mg/dl.[243] Elevation of alkaline phosphatase is less useful, although almost always abnormal, varying from less than five times normal (80% of patients) to more than 1000 IU.[243]

The simplest and fastest, but unfortunately the least reliable, method to initially evaluate the patient with suspected choledocholithiasis is abdominal ultrasonography. The ultrasonogram is extremely useful if the result is positive; however, nonvisualization of stones or a normal-sized common bile duct does not exclude the presence of stones. Ductal dilatation may be prevented if hepatic cirrhosis or sclerosing cholangitis is present.[265] More important, ductal dilatation may not occur because of the low-grade, intermittent character of the obstruction.[265]

ERCP is the procedure of choice for visualizing the biliary tree. In addition, ERCP allows the physician to visualize the periampullary region of the duodenum and the pancreatic ducts and to perform sphincterotomy with stone extraction or stent placement. Reported success rates in visualizing the desired duct are higher than 85%.[266–268] ERCP can be performed even in patients who have Billroth II anastomoses,[269] mild bleeding disorders, or allergy to iodinated contrast agents. ERCP is contraindicated in uncooperative patients. In skilled hands, complication rates of ERCP are approximately 1% with sepsis and pancreatitis being the most frequent causes of morbidity.[267, 268] If ERCP fails or is unavailable, transhepatic cholangiography (THC) can be attempted. Success rates with THC range from 75 to 98% in patients with nondilated and dilated ducts, respectively,[270, 271] but major complications (e.g., sepsis, bleeding) occur in approximately 4% of patients.[270–272] Contraindications to THC include coagulaopathy, ascites, and an uncooperative patient.

Gallstone Pancreatitis

Alcohol abuse and gallstones are the leading causes of acute pancreatitis in industrialized societies.[273] Gallstones migrating from the gallbladder through the biliary tree and into the duodenum are the primary event in causing gallstone pancreatitis.[234, 235, 274–277] After an attack of acute gallstone pancreatitis, recurrent pancreatitis occurs in 36 to 92% of patients in whom the biliary tree is not cleared of stones; in patients who have undergone cholecystectomy and adequate common duct exploration, the risk is 2 to 7% (which is the risk of retained common duct stones).[204, 274–276] Following gallstone pancreatitis, gallstones can be recovered from 10-day collections of stool in 92% of patients, compared with 12% in patients with cholelithiasis alone.[234, 277] Approximately 33% of patients with gallstone pancreatitis are found to have stones in the common bile duct at surgery or autopsy.[234, 278] In contrast, only 11% of patients with uncomplicated gallbladder stones also have choledocholithiasis.[229]

Up to 60% of patients with so-called "idiopathic pancreatitis" have pancreatitis induced by biliary sludge. Biliary sludge causes pancreatitis as particulate matter or cholesterol crystals pass through the common bile duct.[138, 139] If the ultrasonogram of the gallbladder is unrevealing, the diagnosis can be made by examining a sample of duodenal bile by microscopy for cholesterol crystals or calcium bilirubinate granules.

An acute attack of gallstone pancreatitis is indistinguishable from an episode of acute pancreatitis from any other cause, except that its mortality (8%) and morbidity rate (25%) are higher.[279] Gallstone pancreatitis very rarely results in chronic pancreatitis or pancreatic insufficiency,[275] even after recurrent attacks. In contrast, alcoholic pancreatitis is a chronic, progressive, or relapsing disease that often results in chronic pancreatitis and pancreatic insufficiency.[280]

The immediate medical treatment of acute gallstone pancreatitis is the same as that for acute pancreatitis of any other cause. If the patient with suspected gallstone pancreatitis fails to improve within 24 to 48 hours, emergency ERCP and sphincterotomy to remove the impacted stone is mandatory.[281]

An abdominal ultrasonogram or CT scan only detects the common duct gallstone directly in 15 to 50% of patients, respectively.[246] Lack of stones in the gallbladder is not helpful in excluding the diagnosis. A dilated common bile duct is also not helpful in establishing that a stone is impacted, because dilatation of the bile ducts secondary to external compression can be seen in acute or chronic pancreatitis of any etiology.[282]

After recovery from an acute attack of gallstone pancreatitis, the patient should have the common bile duct cleared of gallstones via ERCP, followed promptly by an elective cholecystectomy if gallbladder stones are present. If cholecystectomy is delayed, 25% of patients will have another attack of potentially fatal acute pancreatitis within 30 days and 50% within 11 months.[278, 283, 284] Endoscopic sphincterotomy and removal of common duct stones leaving a diseased gallbladder in place is a reasonable alternative in patients with high operative risks. If biliary sludge is the cause, medical dissolution treatment with ursodiol is an acceptable alternative.[139]

Biliary Tract Pain Without Other Complications

The pain from uncomplicated choledocholithiasis is indistinguishable from biliary pain due to gallbladder stones. However, biliary pain secondary to gallbladder stones without cholecystitis never causes abnormal liver function tests. Therefore, biliary pain alone without signs of inflammation in the setting of elevated bilirubin, alkaline phosphatase, or amylase should raise the suspicion of choledocholithiasis. ERCP is the diagnostic test of choice because of the low sensitivities of ultrasonography or CT scanning. Cholescintigraphy does not have sufficient resolution to delineate the bile ducts.

GALLSTONE ILEUS

Small bowel obstruction secondary to an impacted gallstone is called gallstone ileus. It usually results from a large gallstone eroding through the gallbladder wall and into the small bowel. In the nondiseased small bowel, the gallstone becomes impacted at the ileocecal valve. However, in patients with small bowel disease or previous surgery, the gallstone can become impacted at any site. Clinically, gallstone ileus should be suspected in any elderly patient presenting with small bowel obstruction. The treatment of gallstone ileus is surgical removal of the impacted gallstone. Generally, the cholecystoduodenal fistula does not need repair because it will rarely cause symptoms.[285]

Although gallstone ileus often occurs in the setting of longstanding clinical gallbladder disease, 30% of patients give no antecedent clinical history of cholelithiasis. Most (85%) patients experience vomiting, whereas only half have right upper quadrant tenderness. The abdominal plain film is crucial in making the diagnosis. Air in the biliary tree is present in at least 60% of patients, and in nearly half of these patients a radiopaque gallstone is seen outside the gallbladder.[285]

PROBLEMS FOLLOWING CHOLECYSTECTOMY

Three problems, often intractable, that can arise after cholecystectomy are: (1) retained common duct stone, (2) biliary stricture, and (3) the so-called "postcholecystectomy syndrome."

Retained Common Duct Stone

Despite careful intraoperative cholangiography and surgical exploration of the bile ducts, gallstones are retained in the common bile duct after 1 to 8% of surgical explorations.[229, 231, 286, 287]

With the widespread use of endoscopic sphincterotomy, the management of retained common duct stones is now less hazardous because reoperation can be avoided in almost all patients. Even in patients with a postoperative T tube, we suggest an endoscopic sphincterotomy rather than an attempt at Dormia basket retrieval via the T tube, which would necessitate an 8- to 12-week wait for a fibrous tract to develop.[5] During this waiting period, cholangitis or other complications could occur.

Endoscopic sphincterotomy is safe and effective. In this setting it has a mortality rate of approximately 1%, and stones can be removed in more than 85% of cases.[288, 289] Relative contraindications include stones larger than 2 cm, bile duct stricture proximal to the ampulla, an ampulla situated in a duodenal diverticulum, and significant coagulopathy. Mechanical or extracorporeal shock-wave lithotripsy (with the "renal" lithotriptor) to crush a large stone will allow almost all retained stones to be removed endoscopically. If ERCP fails, medical dissolution therapy with ursodeoxycholic acid could be tried in the occasional patient if the following conditions are rigorously adhered to[290]: (1) there is incomplete, not total, obstruction of the common duct; (2) there is no evidence of biliary tract infection; and (3) the patient's stones, removed at cholecystectomy, contain predominantly cholesterol. Surgical removal and exploration of the common bile duct should be considered as the last resort. However, if endoscopic papillotomy fails, surgery should be done promptly in the setting of a patient with an infected or obstructed biliary tree.

We do not recommend attempted dissolution of retained common duct stones with T tube infusion of cholesterol solvents, such as methyl *tert*-butyl ether (MTBE), monooctanoin (Capmul), or sodium cholate. To date, no controlled trials have shown that these agents are safe or effective in treatment of common duct stones.[5] MTBE, an investigational agent, can be safely instilled into the gallbladder by experienced investigators,[291] but its use in the common duct is probably hazardous. Sodium cholate is toxic to the biliary tree and should not be used.[292] Use of monooctanoin is associated with a high incidence of side effects including abdominal pain, nausea, vomiting, and diarrhea.[293] Furthermore, it causes tissue damage in the biliary tree, stomach, and duodenum.[293, 294]

Biliary Stricture

In most patients, benign biliary stricture is caused by inadvertent trauma during cholecystectomy.[295] Most occur during a "routine" cholecystectomy rather than during a difficult operation or exploration of the common bile duct. It occurs more commonly during cholecystectomy performed via the laparoscopic route than via laparotomy. Injuries causing strictures include complete or partial transection of the common bile duct, a tear in the wall, or complete or partial occlusion secondary to a suture. In addition, subhepatic infections can cause fibrosis and stricturing of the extrahepatic bile ducts. One third of the injuries become manifest within 30 days of the operation. The remainder usually present within 2 years, but a symptom-free period of 25 years has been reported.[295] The most common presenting signs are intermittent jaundice or cholangitis.[295, 296] The major entity that needs to be excluded is a retained stone. Cholangitis appearing more than 5 years after cholecystectomy is most likely to be secondary to retained or newly formed stones rather than a biliary stricture.[297] The diagnosis of biliary stricture is made by ERCP or THC. There is no role for oral or intravenous cholangiography or biliary scintigraphy in this setting. An abdominal CT scan or ultrasonogram may show dilated ducts but will rarely be able to distinguish a stricture from a retained stone.

Surgical repair should be attempted as soon as the stricture is identified and the patient has recovered from acute cholangitis. The long-term complications of a biliary stricture are secondary biliary cirrhosis, portal hypertension, and liver failure.[295] Therefore, an attempt should be made to correct surgically all biliary strictures. Even if the patient has had previously unsuccessful attempts to repair the stricture, there is a 75% chance that a surgeon who specializes in reconstructive biliary tract surgery can make a successful repair.[298] If the patient is not a surgical candidate, it may be possible to perform percutaneous transhepatic balloon dilatation of certain strictures.[299] However, the long-term outlook for these patients is unknown.

Postcholecystectomy Syndrome

Cholecystectomy relieves biliary tract pain in at least 88% of patients.[193] Since dyspepsia is not a specific symptom of biliary tract disease, it is not surprising that 30% of patients continue to have dyspepsia after cholecystectomy.[300] Nonetheless, patients with any abdominal pain or discomfort following cholecystectomy are often given the diagnosis of postcholecystectomy syndrome.

A systematic approach is needed to diagnose the *specific* cause responsible for the discomfort in these patients; labeling them with postcholecystectomy syndrome does not aid in management. Four possible explanations for the patient's symptoms exist: (1) an operative error has produced biliary tract pathology (i.e., biliary stricture); (2) new biliary tract disease has developed (i.e., choledocholithiasis); (3) a true motor dysfunction of the sphincter of Oddi exists; or most commonly (4) the symptoms that prompted the cholecystectomy were *not* related to gallstones.

Patients with severe symptoms (e.g., episodic severe pain, jaundice, or cholangitis) usually have some readily identifiable abnormality of the biliary system. On the other hand, patients with mild upper right quadrant discomfort, continuous pain, or dyspeptic symptoms are less likely to have a distinct abnormality of the biliary tree to explain their symptoms.[301]

Bile duct dyskinesia or abnormalities of the sphincter of Oddi (ampullary stenosis) have been implicated as a cause of symptoms after cholecystectomy.[302] In fact, some suggest that cholecystectomy itself, by removing a pressure-buffering reservoir, can increase bile duct pressures and cause pain.[303] With the advent of endoscopic manometry of the biliary tree,[304, 305] patients have now been described with spasm of the sphincter of Oddi,[306, 307] altered responsiveness of sphincter pressure to CCK,[308] and abnormal contractions of the common bile duct.[232, 309] One study has suggested that 17% of patients with postcholecystectomy syndrome had abnormalities of the sphincter of Oddi.[309]

Before the clinical significance of sphincter of Oddi dysfunction as an explanation for abdominal pain after cholecystectomy is known, natural history studies and the results of long-term surveillance of patients treated for the disorder need to be evaluated. The patient with abdominal distress persisting after cholecystectomy should have a thorough evaluation, and special attention should be paid to the biliary tree. Abdominal ultrasonography and determination of serum chemistries (bilirubin, alkaline phosphatase, transaminases, and amylase) are important screening tests. However, these patients usually need to undergo ERCP to exclude structural disease of the biliary tract. Biliary tract manometry may also be necessary. The morphine-neostigmine provocative test for ampullary stenosis is not specific and should be avoided.[310] Patients with abnormal sphincter of Oddi manometry should undergo endoscopic sphincterotomy only if they have recurrent pain and abnormalities in liver chemistries.

REFERENCES

1. Cohen S and Soloway RD (eds): Gallstones. New York, Churchill Livingstone, 1985.
2. Capocaccia L, Ricci G, Angelico F, et al (eds): Epidemiology and Prevention of Gallstone Disease. Lancaster, MTP Press, 1984.
3. Mack E: Role of surgery in the management of gallstones. Semin Liver Dis 10:222–231, 1990.
4. Glenn F and Small DM: Management of gallstones, particularly the silent variety. *In* Ingelfinger RV, Finland M, and Relman AS (eds): Controversy in Internal Medicine II. Philadelphia, WB Saunders, 1974, pp 531–559.
5. Apstein MD and Carey MC: Biliary tract stones and associated disease. *In* Stein JH (ed): Internal Medicine, 4th ed. Boston, Little Brown. (In press.)
6. McSherry CK, Ferstenberg H, Calhoun WF, et al: The natural history of diagnosed gallstone disease in symptomatic and asymptomatic patients. Ann Surg 202:59–63, 1985.
7. Rome group for the epidemiology and prevention of cholelithiasis (GREPCO): Prevalence of gallstone disease in an Italian adult female population. Am J Epidemiol 119:796–805, 1984.
8. Sauerbruch T and Paumgartner G: Gallbladder stones: Management. Lancet 338:1121–1124, 1991.
9. Carey MC and O'Donovan MA: Gallstone disease: Current concepts on the epidemiology, pathogenesis and management. *In* Petersdorf RG, Adams RD, and Braunwald E (eds): Harrison's Principles of Internal Medicine: Update V. New York, McGraw-Hill, 1984, pp 139–168.
10. Sherman S, Hawes RH, and Lehman GA: Management of bile duct stones. Semin Liver Dis 10:205–221, 1990.
11. Broomfield PH, Chopra R, Sheinbaum RC, et al: Effects of ursodeoxycholic acid and aspirin on the formation of lithogenic bile and gallstones during loss of weight. N Engl J Med 319:1567–1572, 1988.
12. Liddle RA, Goldstein RB, and Saxton J: Gallstone formation during weight-reduction dieting. Arch Intern Med 149:1750–1753, 1989.
13. Pitt HA, King W III, Mann LL, et al: Increased risk of cholelithiasis with prolonged total parenteral nutrition. Am J Surg 145:106–112, 1983.
14. Roslyn JJ, Berquist WE, Pitt HA, et al: Increased risk of gallstones in children on total parenteral nutrition. Pediatrics 71:784–789, 1983.
15. Roslyn JJ, Pitt HA, Mann LL, et al: Gallbladder disease in patients on long-term parenteral nutrition. Gastroenterology 84:148–154, 1983.
16. Henriksson P, Einarsson K, Eriksson A, et al: Estrogen-induced gallstone formation in males: Relation to changes in serum and biliary lipids during hormonal treatment of prostatic carcinoma. J Clin Invest 84:811–816, 1989.
17. Lowenfels AB: Gallstones and the risk of cancer. Gut 21:1090–1092, 1980.
18. Jorgensen T: Prevalence of gallstones in a Danish population. Am J Epidemiol 126:912–921, 1987.
19. Jensen KH and Jorgensen T: Incidence of gallstones in a Danish population. Gastroenterology 100:790–794, 1991.
20. Glambek I, Kvaale G, Arnesjo B, and Soreide O: Prevalence of gallstones in a Norwegian population. Scand J Gastroenterology 22:1089–1094, 1987.
21. Barbara L, Sama C, Labate AMM, et al: A population study on the prevalence of gallstone disease: The Sirmione study. Hepatology 7:913–917, 1987.
22. The Rome Group For Epidemiology And Prevention Of Cholelithiasis (GREPCO): The epidemiology of gallstone disease in Rome, Italy. Part I: Prevalence data in men. Hepatology 8:904–906, 1988.
23. Heaton KW, Braddon FEM, Mountford RA, et al: Symptomatic and silent gallstones in the community. Gut 32:316–320, 1991.
24. Sarnaik S, Slovis TL, Corbett DP, et al: Incidence of cholelithiasis in sickle cell anemia using the ultrasonic grey-scale technique. J Pediatr 96:1005–1008, 1980.
25. Brett M and Barker DJP: The world distribution of gallstones. Int J Epidemiol 5:335–341, 1976.
26. Malhotra SA: Epidemiological study of cholelithiasis among railroad workers in India with special reference to causation. Gut 9:290–295, 1968.
27. Nakayama F and Miyake H: Changing state of gallstone disease in Japan: Composition of the stones and treatment of the condition. Am J Surg 120:794–800, 1970.
28. Salen G and Tint GS: Nonsurgical treatment of gallstones. N Engl J Med 320:655–666, 1989.
29. Hay DW and Carey MC: Pathophysiology and pathogenesis of cholesterol gallstone formation. Semin Liver Dis 10:159–170, 1990.
30. Holan KR, Holzbach RT, Hermann RE, et al: Nucleation time: A key factor in the pathogenesis of cholesterol gallstone disease. Gastroenterology 77:611–617, 1979.
31. Carey MC and Lamont JT: Cholesterol gallstone formation. 1: Physical-chemistry of bile and biliary lipid secretion. Prog Liver Dis 10:139–163, 1992.
32. Lamont JT and Carey MC: Cholesterol gallstone formation. 2: Pathobiology and pathomechanics. Prog Liver Dis 10:165–191, 1992.
33. Carey MC and Cahalane MJ: The enterohepatic circulation. *In* Arias IM, Jakoby WB, Popper H, et al (eds): The Liver: Biology and Pathobiology, 2nd ed. New York, Raven Press, 1988, pp 573–616.
34. Kibe A, Holzbach RT, LaRusso NF, and Mao SJT: Inhibition of cholesterol crystal formation by apolipoproteins in supersaturated model bile. Science 225:514–516, 1984.
35. Holzbach RT, Kibe A, Thief E, et al: Biliary proteins: Unique inhibitors of cholesterol crystal nucleation in human gallbladder bile. J Clin Invest 73:35–45, 1984.
36. Burnstein MJ, Ilson RG, Petrunka CN, et al: Evidence for a potent nucleating factor in the gallbladder bile of patients with cholesterol gallstones. Gastroenterology 85:801–807, 1983.
37. Carey MC and Cahalane NJ: Whither biliary sludge? Gastroenterology 95:508–523, 1988.
38. Lee SP, LaMont JT, and Carey MC: Role of gallbladder mucus hypersecretion in the evolution of cholesterol gallstones: Studies in the prairie dog. J Clin Invest 67:1712–1723, 1981.
39. Lee SP, Carey MC, and LaMont JT: Aspirin prevention of gallstone formation in prairie dogs. Science 211:1429–1431, 1981.
40. Fridhandler TM, Davison JS, and Shaffer EA: Defective gallbladder contractility in the ground squirrel and prairie dog during the early stages of cholesterol gallstone formation. Gastroenterology 85:830–836, 1983.
41. Doty HE, Pitt HA, Kuchenbecker SL, and DenBesten L: Impaired gallbladder emptying before gallstone formation in the prairie dog. Gastroenterology 85:168–174, 1983.
42. Behar J, Lee KY, Thompson WR, and Biancani P: Gallbladder contraction in patients with pigment and cholesterol stones. Gastroenterology 97:1479–1484, 1989.
43. Bennion LJ, Knowler WC, Mott DM, et al: Development of lithogenic bile during puberty in Pima Indians. N Engl J Med 300:873–876, 1979.
44. Ruppin DC and Dowling RH: Is recurrence inevitable after gallstone dissolution by bile-acid treatment. Lancet 1:181–185, 1982.
45. O'Donnell LDJ and Heaton KW: Recurrence and re-recurrence of gallstones after medical dissolution: A long-term follow-up. Gut 29:655–658, 1988.
46. Apstein MD, George B, and Tchakarova B: The incidence of gallstones following spinal cord injury. Hepatology 16:154A, 1992.
47. Worobetz L, Inglis F, and Schaffer E: Ursodeoxycholic acid (UDCA) prevents gallstone formation during rapid weight loss (Abstract). *In* Falk Symposium No. 58: XI International Bile Acid Meeting: Bile acids as therapeutic agents. From basic science to clinical practice, 1990, p 97.
48. Cahalane MJ, Neubrand MW, and Carey MC: Physical-chemical pathogenesis of pigment gallstones. Semin Liver Dis 4:317–328, 1988.
49. Nakayama F: Quantitative microanalysis of gallstones. J Lab Clin Med 72:602–611, 1968.

50. Trotman BW, Ostrow JD, and Soloway RD: Pigment vs cholesterol cholelithiasis: Comparison of stone and bile composition. Am J Dig Dis 19:585–590, 1974.
51. Wosiewitz U: Limy bile and radiopaque, calcified gallstones: A combined analytical radiographic and micromorphologic investigation. Pathol Res Pract 167:273–286, 1980.
52. Donovan JM and Carey MC: Physical-chemical basis of gallstone formation. Gastroenterol Clin North Am 20:47–66, 1991.
53. Maki T: Pathogenesis of calcium bilirubinate gallstone. Ann Surg 164:90–100, 1966.
54. Sabiniski F and Wosiewitz U: The sugar spectrum of human cholesterol gallstones, mixed and pigment gallstones: Combined quantitative analysis of neutral sugars, *N*-acetylhexosamines, hexuronic and *N*-acetylnueraminic acids by capillary gas-liquid chromatography. J Clin Chem Clin Biochem 22:453–459, 1984.
55. Soloway RD, Trotman BW, and Ostrow JD: Pigment gallstones. Gastroenterology 72:167–182, 1977.
56. Kern F Jr, Erfling W, Simon FR, et al: Effect of estrogens on the liver. Gastroenterology 75:512–522, 1978.
57. Friedman GD, Kannel WB, and Dawber TR: The epidemiology of gallbladder disease: Observations in the Framingham study. J Chron Dis 19:273–292, 1966.
58. Honore LH: Cholesterol cholelithiasis in adolescent females: Its connection with obesity, parity, and oral contraceptive use—a retrospective study of 31 cases. Arch Surg 115:62–64, 1980.
59. Van der Linden W: Some biological traits in female gallstone disease patients: A study of body build, parity and serum cholesterol level with a discussion of some problems of selection in observational hospital data. Acta Chir Scand (Suppl) 269:1–94, 1961.
60. Maclure KM, Hayes KC, Colditz GA, et al: Weight, diet, and the risk of symptomatic gallstones in middle-aged women. N Engl J Med 321:563–569, 1989.
61. Bennion LJ and Grundy SM: Effects of obesity and caloric intake on biliary lipid metabolism in man. J Clin Invest 56:996–1011, 1975.
62. Jorgensen T: Gallstones in a Danish population: Relation to weight, physical activity, smoking, coffee consumption, and diabetes mellitus. Gut 30:528–534, 1989.
63. Sampliner RE, Bennett PH, Comess LJ, et al: Gallbladder disease in Pima Indians: Demonstration of high prevalence and early onset by cholecystography. N Engl J Med 283:1358–1364, 1970.
64. Braverman DZ, Johnson ML, and Kern F Jr: Effects of pregnancy and contraceptive steroids on gallbladder function. N Engl J Med 302:362–364, 1980.
65. Krejs GJ, Orci L, Conlon JM, et al: Somatostatinoma syndrome. N Engl J Med 301:285–292, 1979.
66. Buscail L, Tauber JP, Escourrou J, et al: Gallstone formation and occurrence of cholesterol monohydrate crystals in gallbladder bile of patients with long-term sandostatin treatment. Gastroenterology 96:A580, 1989.
67. Pomeranz IS and Shaffer EA: Abnormal gallbladder emptying in a subgroup of patients with gallstones. Gastroenterology 88:787–791, 1985.
68. Shaffer EA, McOrmond P, and Duggan H: Quantitative cholescintigraphy: Assessment of gallbladder filling and emptying and duodenogastric reflux. Gastroenterology 79:899–906, 1980.
69. The Coronary Drug Project Research Group: Gallbladder disease as a side effect of drugs influencing lipid metabolism: Experience in the Coronary Drug Project. N Engl J Med 296:1185–1190, 1977.
70. Logan GM and Duane WC: Lovastatin added to ursodeoxycholic acid further reduces biliary cholesterol saturation. Gastroenterology 98:1572–1576, 1990.
71. A Report from the Boston Collaborative Drug Surveillance Program: Oral contraceptives and venous thromboembolic disease, surgically confirmed gallbladder disease, and breast tumors. Lancet 1:1399–1404, 1973.
72. A Report from the Boston Collaborative Drug Surveillance Program: Surgically confirmed gallbladder disease, venous thromboembolism, and breast tumors in relation to postmenopausal estrogen therapy. N Engl J Med 290:15–18, 1974.
73. Honore LH: Increased incidence of symptomatic cholesterol cholelithiasis in perimenopausal women receiving estrogen replacement therapy: A retrospective study. J Reprod Med 25:187–190, 1980.
74. Eriksson M, Berglund L, Rudling M, et al: Effects of estrogen on low density lipoprotein metabolism in males: Short-term and long-term studies during hormonal treatment of prostatic carcinoma. J Clin Invest 84:802–810, 1989.
75. Thornton JR, Heaton KW, and MacFarlane DG: A relation between high-density-lipoprotein cholesterol and bile cholesterol saturation. BMJ 283:1352–1354, 1981.
76. Petitti DB, Friedman GD, and Klatsky AL: Association of a history of gallbladder disease with a reduced concentration of high-density-lipoprotein cholesterol. N Engl J Med 304:1396–1398, 1981.
77. Thijs C, Knipschild P, and Brombacher P: Serum lipids and gallstones: A case-control study. Gastroenterology 99:843–849, 1990.
78. Kadziolka R, Nilsson S, and Schersten T: Prevalence of hyperlipoproteinemia in men with gallstone disease. Scand J Gastroenterol 12:353–355, 1977.
79. Ahlberg J, Angelin B, Einarsson K, et al: Biliary lipid composition on normo- and hyperlipoproteinemia. Gastroenterology 79:90–94, 1980.
80. Sarles H, Chabert C, Pommeau Y, et al: Diet and cholesterol gallstones. Am J Dig Dis 14:531–537, 1969.
81. Attili AF and the GREPCO group: Dietary habits and cholelithiasis. *In* Capocaccia L, Ricci G, Angelico F, et al (eds): Epidemiology and prevention of gallstone disease. Boston, MTP Press, 1984, pp 175–181.
82. DenBesten L, Connor WE, and Bell S: The effect of dietary cholesterol on the composition of human bile. Surgery 73:266–273, 1973.
83. Sturdevant RAL, Pearce ML, and Dayton S: Increased prevalence of cholelithiasis in man ingesting a serum cholesterol lowering diet. N Engl J Med 288:24–27, 1973.
84. Pomare EW, Heaton KW, Low-Beer TS, and Espiner HJ: The effect of wheat bran upon bile salt metabolism and upon the lipid composition of bile in gallstone patients. Am J Dig Dis 21:521–526, 1976.
85. Scragg R, McMichael A, and Baghurst P: Diet, alcohol, and relative weight in gallstone disease: A case-control study. BMJ 288:1113–1119, 1984.
86. Fleming CR, Ludwig J, and Dickson ER: Asymptomatic primary biliary cirrhosis. Mayo Clin Proc 53:587–593, 1978.
87. Sherlock S: Primary biliary cirrhosis. *In* Bianchi L, Gerok W, and Sickinger K (eds): Liver and Bile. Falk Symposium No. 23. Lancaster, MTP Press, 1977, pp 319–340.
88. Van Berge Henegouwen GP, Brandt K-H, Ruben ATH, et al: High frequency of lithogenic bile in primary biliary cirrhosis. Neth J Med 25:89–93, 1982.
89. Bennion LJ and Grundy SM: Effects of diabetes mellitus on cholesterol metabolism in man. N Engl J Med 296:1365–1371, 1977.
90. Grodzki M, Mazurkiewicz-Rozynska E, and Czyzyk A: Diabetic cholecystopathy. Diabetologia 4:345–348, 1968.
91. Knowler WC, Carraher MJ, and Pettitt DJ: Diabetes mellitus, obesity and cholelithiasis. *In* Capocaccia L, Ricci G, Angelico F, et al (eds): Epidemiology and Prevention of Gallstone Disease. Lancaster, MTP Press, 1984, pp 85–91.
92. Lieber MM: The incidence of gallstones and their correlation with other diseases. Ann Surg 135:394–400, 1952.
93. Bates GC and Brown CH: Incidence of gallbladder disease in chronic hemolytic anemia (spherocytosis). Gastroenterology 21:104–109, 1952.
94. Dewey KW, Grossman H, and Canale VC: Cholelithiasis in thalassemia major. Radiology 96:385–388, 1970.
95. Merendino KA and Manhas DR: Man-made gallstones: A new entity following cardiac valve replacement. Ann Surg 177:694–704, 1973.
96. Tamalet E: La lithiase biliaire d'origine paludéene. J Med Fr 21:159–164, 1932.
97. Shull SD, Wagner CI, Trotman BW, and Soloway RD: Factors affecting bilirubin excretion in patients with cholesterol or pigment gallstones. Gastroenterology 72:625–629, 1977.

98. Bouchier IAD: Postmortem study of the frequency of gallstones in patients with cirrhosis of the liver. Gut 10:705–710, 1969.
99. Nicholas P, Rinaudo PA, and Conn HO: Increased incidence of cholelithiasis in Laennec's cirrhosis: A postmortem evaluation of pathogenesis. Gastroenterology 63:112–121, 1972.
100. Schwesinger WH, Kurtin WE, Levine BA, and Page CP: Cirrhosis and alcoholism as pathogenetic factors in pigment gallstone formation. Ann Surg 201:319–322, 1985.
101. Iber FL, Caruso G, Polepalle C, et al: Increasing prevalance of gallstones in male veterans with alcoholic cirrhosis. Am J Gastroenterol 85:1593–1596, 1990.
102. Acalovschi M, Badea R, Dumitrascu D, and Varga C: Prevalence of gallstones in liver cirrhosis: A sonographic survey. Am J Gastroenterol 83:954–956, 1988.
103. Blanckaert N, Kabra PM, Farina FA, et al: Measurement of bilirubin and its monoconjugates and diconjugates in human serum by alkaline methanolysis and high-performance liquid chromatography. J Lab Clin Med 96:198–212, 1980.
104. Di Padova C, Tritapepe R, DiPadova F, et al: Acute ethanol administration increases biliary concentrations of total and unconjugated bilirubin in rabbits. Dig Dis Sci 26:1095–1099, 1981.
105. Vlachevic Z, Yoshida T, Juttijudata P, et al: Bile acid metabolism in cirrhosis. III: Lipid secretion in patients with cirrhosis and its relevance to gallstone formation. Gastroenterology 64:298–303, 1973.
106. Trotman BW and Soloway RD: Pigment vs cholesterol cholelithiasis: Clinical and epidemiological aspects. Am J Dig Dis 20:735–740, 1975.
107. Heaton KW and Read AE: Gallstones in patients with disorders of the terminal ileum and disturbed bile salt metabolism. BMJ 3:494–496, 1969.
108. Cohen S, Kaplan M, Gottlieb L, and Patterson JF: Liver disease and gallstones in regional enteritis. Gastroenterology 60:237–245, 1971.
109. Whorwell PJ, Hawkins R, Dewbury K, and Wright R: Ultrasound survey of gallstones and other hepatobiliary disorders in patients with Crohn's disease. Dig Dis Sci 29:930–933, 1984.
110. Hill GL, Mair WSJ, and Goligher JC: Gallstones after ileostomy and ileal resection. Gut 16:932–936, 1975.
111. Sorenson TIA, Ingermann Jensen L, Klein HC, et al: Risk of gallstone formation after jejunoileal bypass increases more with a 1:3 than with a 3:1 jejunoileal ratio. Scand J Gastroenterol 15:979–984, 1980.
112. Magnuson TH, Lillemoe KD, and Pitt HA: The relationship of clinical risk factors to gallstone composition (Abstract). Hepatology 10:738, 1989.
113. Faloon WW, Rubulis A, Knipp J, et al: Fecal fat, bile acid, and sterol excretion and biliary lipid changes in jejunoileostomy patients. Am J Clin Nutr 30:21–31, 1977.
114. Nakayama F and Koga A: Hepatolithiasis: Present status. World J Surg 8:9–14, 1984.
115. Wosiewitz U, Schenk J, Sabinski F, and Schmack B: Investigations on common bile duct stones. Digestion 26:43–52, 1983.
116. Sauerbruch T, Stellaard F, Soehendra N, and Paumgartner G: Cholesteringehalt von gallengangssteinen. Dtsch Med Wochenschr 108:1099–1102, 1983.
117. Osnes M, Lotveit T, Larsen S, and Aune S: Duodenal diverticula and their relationship to age, sex and biliary calculi. Scand J Gastroenterol 16:103–107, 1981.
118. Lotveit T, Foss OP, and Osnes M: Biliary pigment and cholesterol calculi in patients with and without juxtapapillary duodenal diverticula. Scand J Gastroenterol 16:241–244, 1981.
119. Lotveit T: The composition of biliary calculi in patients with juxtapapillary duodenal diverticula. Scand J Gastroenterol 17:653–656, 1982.
120. Lotveit T, Osnes M, and Aune S: Bacteriological studies of common duct bile in patients with gallstone disease and juxta-papillary duodenal diverticula. Scand J Gastroenterol 13:93–95, 1978.
121. Messing B, Bories C, Kurstlinger F, and Bernier JJ: Does total parenteral nutrition induce gallbladder sludge formation and lithiasis. Gastroenterology 84:1012–1019, 1983.
122. Doty JE, Pitt HA, Porter-Fink V, and DenBesten L: Cholecystokinin prophylaxis of parenteral nutrition-induced gallbladder disease. Ann Surg 201:76–80, 1985.
123. Sitzmann JV, Pitt HA, Steinborn PA, et al: Cholecystokinin prevents parenteral nutrition induced biliary sludge in humans. Surg Gynecol Obstet 170:25–31, 1990.
124. Csendes A, Larach J, and Godoy M: Incidence of gallstones development after selective hepatic vagotomy. Acta Chir Scand 144:289–291, 1978.
125. Sapala MA, Sapala JA, Resto Soto AD, and Bouwman DL: Cholelithiasis following subtotal gastric resection with truncal vagotomy. Surg Gynecol Obstet 148:36–38, 1979.
126. Faberberg S, Grevsten S, Johansson H, and Krause U: Vagotomy and gallbladder function. Gut 11:789–793, 1970.
127. Stempel JM and Duane WC: Biliary lipids and bile acid pool size after vagotomy in man. Gastoenterology 75:608–611, 1978.
128. Shaffer EA: The effect of vagotomy on gallbladder function and bile composition in man. Ann Surg 195:413–418, 1982.
129. Nelson CP, Saik RP, Greenburg AG, et al: Truncal vagotomy causes biliary sludge formation. Curr Surg 39:30–33, 1982.
130. Baker HL and Hodgson JR: Further studies on the accuracy of oral cholecystography. Radiology 74:239–245, 1960.
131. Bartrum RJ, Crow HC, and Foote SR: Ultrasonic and radiographic cholecystography. N Engl J Med 296:538–541, 1977.
132. Conrad MR, Janes JO, and Dietchy J: Significance of low level echoes within the gallbladder. Am J Roentgenol 132:967–972, 1979.
133. Maringhini A, Ciambra M, Baccelliere P, et al: Sludge, stones, and pregnancy. Gastroenterology 95:1160–1161, 1988.
134. Lee SP, Maher K, and Nicholls JF: Origin and fate of biliary sludge. Gastroenterology 94:170–176, 1988.
135. Maringhini A, Marceno MP, Lanzarone F, et al: Sludge and stones in gallbladder after pregnancy: Prevalence and risk factors. J Hepatol 5:218–223, 1987.
136. Allen B, Bernhoft R, Blanckaert N, et al: Sludge is calcium bilirubinate associated with bile stasis. Am J Surg 141:51–56, 1981.
137. Roslyn JJ, Pitt HA, Mann L, et al: Parenteral nutrition-induced gallbladder disease: A reason for early cholecystectomy. Am J Surg 148:58–63, 1984.
138. Lee SP, Nicholls JF, and Park HZ: Biliary sludge as a cause of acute pancreatitis. N Engl J Med 326:589–593, 1992.
139. Ros E, Navarro S, Bru C, et al: Occult microlithiasis in "idiopathic" acute pancreatitis: Prevention of relapses by cholecystectomy or ursodeoxycholic acid therapy. Gastroenterology 101:1701–1709, 1991.
140. Lowenfels AB, Lindstrom CG, Conway MJ, and Hastings PR: Gallstones and risk of gallbladder cancer. J Natl Cancer Inst 75:77–80, 1985.
141. Comfort MW, Gray HK, and Wilson JM: The silent gallstone: A ten to twenty year follow-up study of 112 cases. Ann Surg 128:931–937, 1948.
142. Ralston DE and Smith LA: The natural history of cholelithiasis: A 15 to 30 year follow-up of 116 patients. Minn Med 48:327–332, 1965.
143. Newman HF, Northup JD, Rosenblum M, and Abrams H: Complications of cholelithiasis. Am J Gastroenterol 50:476–496, 1968.
144. Gracie WA and Ransohoff DF: The natural history of silent gallstones: The innocent gallstone is not a myth. N Engl J Med 307:798–800, 1982.
145. Sama C, Morselli-Labate AM, Venturoli N, et al: The natural history of asymptomatic and symptomatic gallstones: 10 year follow-up in the Sirmione study. Hepatology 16:87A, 1992.
146. Ransohoff DF, Gracie WA, Wolfensen LB, and Neuhauser D: Prophylactic cholecystectomy or expectant management for silent gallstones: A decision analysis to assess survival. Ann Intern Med 99:199–204, 1983.
147. Schein CJ: Acute cholecystitis in the diabetic. Am J Gastroenterol 51:511–515, 1969.
148. Turrill FL, McCarron MM, and Mikkelsen WP: Gallstones and diabetes: An ominous association. Am J Surg 102:184–190, 1961.
149. Turner RJ, Becker WF, Coleman WO, and Powell JL: Acute cholecystitis in the diabetic. South Med J 62:228–231, 1969.

150. Mundth ED: Cholecystitis and diabetes mellitus. N Engl J Med 267:642–646, 1962.
151. Hickman MS, Schwesinger WH, and Page CP: Acute cholecystitis in the diabetic: A case-control study of outcome. Arch Surg 123:409–411, 1988.
152. Walsh DB, Eckhauser FE, Ramsburgh SR, and Burney RB: Risk associated with diabetes mellitus in patients undergoing gallbladder surgery. Surgery 90:254–257, 1982.
153. Ransohoff DF, Miller GL, Forsythe SB, and Hermann RE: Outcome of acute cholecystitis in patients with diabetes mellitus. Ann Intern Med 106:829–832, 1987.
154. Sandler RS, Maule WF, and Baltus ME: Factors associated with postoperative complications in diabetics after biliary tract surgery. Gastroenterology 91:157–162, 1986.
155. Friedman LS, Roberts MS, Brett AS, and Marton KI: Management of asymptomatic gallstones in the diabetic patient. Ann Intern Med 109:913–919, 1988.
156. Diehl AK: Asymptomatic gallstones in diabetic patients. Ann Intern Med 110:1033–1034, 1989.
157. Weiss KM and Hanis CL: All "silent" gallstones are not silent. N Engl J Med 310:657–658, 1984.
158. Black WC, Key CR, Carmany TB, and Herman D: Carcinoma of the gallbladder in a population of southwestern American Indians. Cancer 39:1267–1279, 1977.
159. Carraher MJ, Wilson DL, and Knowler WC: Biliary carcinoma and mortality in Pima Indians: 15 year follow-up after an oral cholecystography survey (Abstract). Gastroenterology 86:1041, 1984.
160. Diehl AK: Gallstone size and the risk of gallbladder cancer. JAMA 250:2323–2326, 1983.
161. Berk RN, Armbuster TG, and Saltzstein SL: Carcinoma in the porcelain gallbladder. Radiology 106:29–31, 1973.
162. Koga A, Watanabe K, Fukuyama T, et al: Diagnosis and operative indications for polypoid lesions of the gallbladder. Arch Surg 123:26–29, 1988.
163. Kimura K, Ohto M, Saisho H, Unozawa T, et al: Association of gallbladder carcinoma and anomalous pancreaticobiliary ductal union. Gastroenterology 89:1258–1265, 1985.
164. Diehl AK: Epidemiology of gallbladder cancer: A synthesis of recent data. J Natl Cancer Inst 65:1209–1214, 1980.
165. Weiner PL and Lawson TL: Porcelain gallbladder. Am J Gastroenterol 64:224–227, 1975.
166. Cooke M: Limy bile. Proc R Soc Med 61:1110–1112, 1968.
167. Schwartz A and Feuchtwanger M: Radiographic demonstration of spontaneous disappearance of limy bile. Gastroenterology 40:809–812, 1961.
168. Festi D, Orsini M, DiBassi S, et al: Risk of gallstone formation during rapid weight loss: Protective role of gallbladder motility (Abstract). Third International Meeting, Pathochemistry, Pathophysiology and Pathomechanics of the Biliary System, Bologna, vol 26, 1992.
169. Rigas B, Torosis J, McDougall CJ, et al: The circadian rhythm of biliary colic. J Clin Gastroenterol 12:409–414, 1990.
170. Price WH: Gallbladder dyspepsia. BMJ (ii):138–141, 1973.
171. Koch JP and Donaldson RM Jr: A survey of food intolerances in hospitalized patients. N Engl J Med 271:657–660, 1964.
172. Thistle JL, Cleary PA, Lachin JM, et al: The natural history of cholelithiasis: The National Cooperative Gallstone Study. Ann Intern Med 101:171–175, 1984.
173. Kingston RD and Windsor CWO: Flatulent dyspepsia in patients with gallstones undergoing cholecystectomy. Br J Surg 62:231–233, 1975.
174. Ros E and Zambon D: Postcholecystectomy symptoms: A prospective study of gallstone patients before and two years after surgery. Gut 28:1500–1504, 1987.
175. Lund J: Surgical indications in cholelithiasis: Prophylactic cholecystectomy elucidated on the basis of long-term follow-up on 526 nonoperated cases. Ann Surg 151:153–162, 1960.
176. Wenckert A and Robertson B: The natural course of gallstone disease. Gastroenterology 50:376–381, 1966.
177. Friedman GD, Raviola CA, and Fireman B: Prognosis of gallstones with mild or no symptoms: 25 years of follow-up in a health maintenance organization. J Clin Epidemiol 42:127–136, 1989.
178. LaRusso NF, Hoffman NE, Hofmann AF, et al: Effect of primary bile acid ingestion on bile acid metabolism and biliary lipid secretion in gallstone patients. Gastroenterology 69:1301–1314, 1975.
179. Makino I, Shinozaki K, Yoshino K, and Nakagawa S: Dissolution of cholesterol gallstones by ursodeoxycholic acid. Jpn J Gastroenterol 72:690–702, 1975.
180. Angelin B, Ewerth S, and Einarsson K: Ursodeoxycholic acid treatment in cholesterol gallstone disease: Effects on hepatic 3-hydroxy-3-methylglutaryl coenzyme A reductase activity, biliary lipid composition, and plasma lipid levels. J Lipid Res 24:461–468, 1983.
181. Hardison WG and Grundy SM: Effect of ursodeoxycholate and its taurine conjugate on bile acid synthesis and cholesterol absorption. Gastroenterology 87:130–135, 1984.
182. Senior JR, Johnson MF, DeTurck DM, et al: In vivo kinetics of radiolucent gallstone dissolution by oral dihydroxy bile acids. Gastroenterology 99:243–251, 1990.
183. Fromm H and Malavolti M: Dissolving gallstones. Adv Intern Med 33:409–430, 1988.
184. Ell C, Schneider HT, Benninger J, et al: Significance of computed tomography for shock-wave therapy of radiolucent gallbladder stones. Gastroenterology 191:1409–1416, 1991.
185. Gleeson D, Ruppin DC, and the British Gallstone Study Group: Discrepancies between cholecystography and ultrasonography in the detection of recurrent gallstones. J Hepatol 1:597–607, 1985.
186. Iser JH, Murphy GM, and Dowling RH: Speed of change in biliary lipids and bile acids with chenodeoxycholic acid—is intermittent therapy feasible? Gut 18:7–15, 1977.
187. Thistle JL: Ursodeoxycholic acid treatment of gallstones. Semin Liver Dis 3:146–156, 1983.
188. Bachrach WH and Hofmann AF: Ursodeoxycholic acid in the treatment of cholesterol cholelithiasis, Parts 1 and 2. Dig Dis Sci 27:737–761 and 833–856, 1982.
189. Schoenfield L, Berci G, Carnovale R, et al: The effect of ursodiol on the efficacy and safety of extracorporeal shock-wave lithotripsy of gallstones: The Dornier National Biliary Lithotripsy Study. N Engl J Med 323:1239–1245, 1990.
190. Ertan A, Hernandez RE, Campeau RJ, et al: Extracorporeal shock-wave lithotripsy and ursodiol versus urosdiol alone in the treatment of gallstones. Gastroenterology 103:311–316, 1992.
191. Sackmann M, Pauletzki J, Sauerbruch T, et al: The Munich gallbladder lithotripsy study: Results of the first 5 years with 711 patients. Ann Intern Med 114:290–296, 1991.
192. Ell C, Kerzel W, Schneider HT, et al: Piezoelectric lithotripsy: Stone disintegration and follow-up results in patients with symptomatic gallbladder stones. Gastroenterology 99:1439–1444, 1990.
193. Gadacz TR and Crist DW: Anticipating the difficult cholecystectomy. Laparoscopic Surg 1:69–78, 1992.
194. Summary of the national Halothane study: Possible association between Halothane anesthesia and postoperative hepatic necrosis. JAMA 197:775–788, 1966.
195. NIH Consensus Development Panel on Gallstones and Laparoscopic Cholecystectomy: Gallstones and laparoscopic cholecystectomy. JAMA 269:1018–1024, 1993.
196. Southern Surgeons Club: A prospective analysis of 1518 laparoscopic cholecystectomies. N Engl J Med 324:1073–1078, 1991.
197. Gilliland TM and Traverso LW: Modern standards for comparison of cholecystectomy with alternative treatments for symptomatic cholelithiasis with emphasis on long term relief of symptoms. Surg Gynecol Obstet 170:39–44, 1990.
198. Gately JF and Thomas EJ: Acute cholecystitis occurring as a complication of other diseases. Arch Surg 118:1137–1141, 1983.
199. Svanvik J, Thornell E, and Zettergren L: Gallbladder function in experimental cholecystitis: Reversal of the inflammatory net fluid "secretion" into the gallbladder by indomethacin. Surgery 89:500–506, 1981.
200. Thornell E, Kral JG, Jansson R, and Svanvik J: Inhibition of prostaglandin synthesis as a treatment for biliary pain. Lancet 1:584, 1979.
201. Goldman L, Morgan JA, and Kay J: Acute cholecystitis: Correlation of bacteriology and mortality. Gastroenterology 11:318–325, 1948.

202. Dumont AE: Significance of hyperbilirubinemia in acute cholecystitis. Surg Gynecol Obstet 142:855–857, 1976.
203. Watkin DFL and Thomas GG: Jaundice in acute cholecystitis. Br J Surg 58:570–573, 1971.
204. Sanchez-Ubeda R, Rousselot LM, and Giannelli S: The significance of pancreatitis accompanying acute cholecystitis. Ann Surg 144:44–50, 1956.
205. Lesser PB and Warshaw AL: Differentiation of pancreatitis from common bile duct obstruction with hyperamylasemia. Gastroenterology 68:636–641, 1975.
206. Warshaw AL and Fuller AF Jr: Specificity of increased renal clearance of amylase in diagnosis of acute pancreatitis. N Engl J Med 292:325–328, 1975.
207. Laing FC, Federle MP, Jeffrey RB, and Brown TW: Ultrasonic evaluation of patients with acute right upper quadrant pain. Radiology 140:449–455, 1981.
208. Ralls PW, Colletti PM, Halls JM, and Siemsen JK: Prospective evaluation of 99m-Tc-IDA cholescintigraphy and grayscale ultrasound in the diagnosis of acute cholecystitis. Radiology 144:369–371, 1982.
209. Kane RA: Ultrasonographic diagnosis of gangrenous cholecystitis and empyema of the gallbladder. Radiology 134:191–194, 1980.
210. Handler SJ: Ultrasound of gallbladder wall thickening and its relation to cholecystitis. Am J Roentgenol 132:581–585, 1979.
211. Deitch EA: Utility and accuracy of ultrasonically measured gallbladder wall as a diagnostic criteria (sic) in biliary tract disease. Dig Dis Sci 26:686–693, 1981.
212. Freitas JE and Gulati RM: Rapid evaluation of acute abdominal pain by hepatobiliary scanning. JAMA 244:1585–1587, 1980.
213. Hall AW, Wisbey ML, Hutchinson F, et al: The place of hepatobiliary isotope scanning in the diagnosis of gallbladder disease. Br J Surg 68:85–90, 1981.
214. Mauro MA, McCartney WH, and Melmed JR: Hepatobiliary scanning with ^{99m}TC-PIPIDA in acute cholecystitis. Radiology 142:193–197, 1982.
215. Pedersen JH, Hancke S, Christensen B, et al: Ultrasonography, ^{99m}TC-DIDA cholescintigraphy, and infusion tomography in the diagnosis of acute cholecystitis. Scand J Gastroenterol 17:77–80, 1982.
216. Ram MD, Hagihara PF, Kim EE, et al: Evaluation of biliary disease by scintigraphy. Am J Surg 141:77–83, 1981.
217. Rosenthall L: An update on radionuclide imaging in hepatobiliary disease. JAMA 245:2065–2068, 1981.
218. Weissmann HS, Rosenblatt R, Sugarman LA, and Freeman LM: An update in radionuclide imaging in the diagnosis of cholecystitis. JAMA 246:1354–1357, 1981.
219. Weissmann HS, Berkowitz D, Fox MS, et al: The role of technetium-99m iminodiacetic acid (IDA) cholescintigraphy in acute acalculous cholecystitis. Radiology 146:177–180, 1983.
220. Shuman WP, Gibbs P, Rudd TG, and Mack LA: PIPIDA scintigraphy for cholecystitis: False positives in alcoholism and total parenteral nutrition. Am J Roentgenol 138:1–5, 1982.
221. Jarvinen HJ and Hastbacka J: Early cholecystectomy for acute cholecystitis: A prospective randomized study. Ann Surg 191:501–505, 1980.
222. Lahtinen J, Alhava EM, and Aukee S: Acute cholecystitis treated by early and delayed surgery: A controlled clinical trial. Scand J Gastroenterol 13:673–678, 1978.
223. McArthur P, Cuschieri A, Sells RA, and Shields R: Controlled clinical trial comparing early with interval cholecystectomy for acute cholecystitis. Br J Surg 62:850–852, 1975.
224. Van der Linden W and Sunzel H: Early versus delayed operation for acute cholecystitis: A controlled clinical trial. Am J Surg 120:7–13, 1970.
225. Van der Linden W and Edlund G: Early versus delayed cholecystectomy: The effect of a change in management. Br J Surg 68:753–757, 1981.
226. Fowkes FGR and Gunn AA: The management of acute cholecystitis and its hospital cost. Br J Surg 67:613–617, 1980.
227. Way LW: Pathogenesis and management of choledocholithiasis. *In* Fisher MM, Goresky CA, Shaffer EA, and Strasberg SM (eds): Gallstones. New York, Plenum Press, 1979. pp 411–427.
228. DenBesten L and Doty JE: Pathogenesis and management of choledocholithiasis. Surg Clin North Am 61:893–906, 1981.
229. Glenn F: Retained calculi with the biliary ductal system. Ann Surg 179:528–539, 1974.
230. Hermann RE: Common bile duct stones. *In* Moody FG (ed): Advances in Diagnosis and Surgical Treatment of Biliary Tract Disease. Chicago, Yearbook Publishers, 1983, pp 69–78.
231. Madden JL, Vanderheyden L, and Kandalaft S: The nature and surgical significance of common duct stones. Surg Gynecol Obstet 126:3–8, 1968.
232. Toouli J, Geenen JE, Hogan WJ, et al: Sphincter of Oddi motor activity: A comparison between patients with common bile duct stones and controls. Gastroenterology 82:111–117, 1982.
233. Glenn F and Beil AR: Choledocholithiasis demonstrated at 586 operations. Surg Gynecol Obstet 118:499–506, 1964.
234. Acosta JM and Ledesma CL: Gallstone migration as a cause of acute pancreatitis. N Engl J Med 290:484–487, 1974.
235. Kelly TR: Gallstone pancreatitis: Pathophysiology. Surgery 80:488–492, 1976.
236. Wolpers C: Relapses after spontaneous dissolution of gallstones. *In*: Back P and Gerok W (eds): Bile Acids in Human Diseases. Stuttgart-New York, FK Schattauer Verlag, 1972, pp 171–174.
237. Allen B, Shapiro H, and Way LW: Management of recurrent and residual common duct stones. Am J Surg 142:41–47, 1981.
238. Keighley MRB, Drysdale RB, Quoraishi AH, et al: Antibiotic treatment of biliary sepsis. Surg Clin North Am 55:1379–1390, 1975.
239. O'Connor MJ, Schwartz ML, McQuarrie DG, and Sumner HW: Cholangitis due to malignant obstruction of biliary outflow. Ann Surg 193:341–345, 1981.
240. O'Connor MJ, Schwartz ML, McQuarrie DG, and Sumner HW: Acute bacterial cholangitis. Arch Surg 117:437–441, 1982.
241. Boey JH and Way LW: Acute cholangitis. Ann Surg 191:264–270, 1982.
242. Berk JE: Choledocholithiasis. Am J Surg 55:96–101, 1941.
243. Pellegrini CA, Thomas MJ, and Way LW: Bilirubin and alkaline phosphatase values before and after surgery for biliary obstruction. Am J Surg 143:67–73, 1982.
244. Cameron JL: Acute cholangitis. *In* Moody FG (ed): Advances in Diagnosis and Surgical Treatment of Biliary Tract Disease. Chicago, Yearbook Publishers, 1983, pp 147–153.
245. Ausobsky JR and Polk HC Jr: Aspects of biliary sepsis. *In* Moody FG (ed): Advances in Diagnosis and Surgical Treatment of Biliary Tract Disease. Chicago, Yearbook Publishers, 1983, pp 133–146.
246. Ferrucci JT Jr: Imaging in obstructive jaundice. *In* Moody FG (ed): Advances in Diagnosis and Surgical Treatment of Biliary Tract Disease. Chicago, Yearbook Publishers, 1983, pp 57–68.
247. Beinart C, Efremidis S, Cohen B, and Mitty HA: Obstruction without dilation: Importance in evaluating jaundice. JAMA 245:353–356, 1981.
248. Vallon AG, Lees WR, and Cotton PB: Grey-scale ultrasonography in cholestatic jaundice. Gut 20:51–54, 1979.
249. Welch JP and Donaldson GA: The urgency of diagnosis and surgical treatment of acute suppurative cholangitis. Am J Surg 131:527–532, 1976.
250. Weissglas IS and Brown RA: Acute suppurative cholangitis secondary to malignant obstruction. Can J Surg 24:468–470, 1981.
251. Ikeda S, Tanaka M, Itoh H, et al: Emergency decompression of bile duct in acute obstructive suppurative cholangitis by duodenoscopic cannulation: A lifesaving procedure. World J Surg 5:587–593, 1981.
252. Kadir S, Baassiri A, Barth KH, et al: Percutaneous biliary drainage in the management of biliary sepsis. Am J Roentgenol 138:25–29, 1982.
253. Siegel JH, Safrany L, Ben-Zvi JS, et al: Duodenoscopic sphincterotomy in patients with gallbladders in situ: Report of a series of 1272 patients. Am J Gastroenterol 83:1255–1258, 1988.

254. Neoptolemos JP, Carr-Locke DL, Fraser I, et al: The management of common bile duct calculi by endoscopic sphincterotomy in patients with gallbladders "in situ." Br J Surg 71:69–71, 1984.
255. Davidson BR, Neoptolemos JP, and Carr-Locke DL: Endoscopic sphincterotomy for common bile duct calculi in patients with gallbladder in situ considered unfit for surgery. Gut 29:114–120, 1988.
256. Zimmon DS: Alternatives to cholecystectomy and common duct exploration (Editorial). Am J Gastroenterol 83:1272–1273, 1988.
257. Cotton PB: Endoscopic management of bile duct stone: Apples and oranges. Gut 25:587–597, 1984.
258. Berquist TH, May GR, Johnson CM, et al: Percutaneous biliary decompression: Internal and external drainage in 50 patients. Am J Roentgenol 136:901–906, 1981.
259. Perieras RV, Rheingold OJ, Hutson D, et al: Relief of malignant obstructive jaundice by percutaneous insertion of a permanent prosthesis in the biliary tree. Ann Intern Med 89:589–593, 1978.
260. Nakayama T, Ikeda A, and Okuda K: Percutaneous transhepatic drainage of the biliary tract. Gastroenterology 74:554–559, 1978.
261. Tylen U, Hoevels J, and Vang J: Percutaneous transhepatic cholangiography with external drainage of obstructive biliary lesions. Surg Gynecol Obstet 144:13–18, 1977.
262. Hoevels J, Lunderquist A, and Ihse I: Percutaneous transhepatic intubation of bile ducts for combined internal-external drainage in preoperative and palliative treatment of obstructive jaundice. Gastrointest Radiol 3:23–31, 1978.
263. Ferrucci JT, Mueller PR, and Harbin WP: Percutaneous transhepatic biliary drainage: Technique, results and applications. Radiology 135:1–13, 1980.
264. Schiff L: Jaundice: A clinical approach. *In* Schiff L and Schiff ER (eds): Diseases of the Liver, 6th ed. Philadelphia, JB Lippincott, 1987, pp 209–217.
265. Shaffer HA Jr, Buschi AJ, and Brenbridge NAG: Limitations of ultrasonography in evaluating patients with jaundice or cholecystectomy. South Med J 74:525–529, 1981.
266. Matzen P, Haubek A, Holst-Christensen J, et al: Accuracy of direct cholangiography by endoscopic or transhepatic route in jaundice—a prospective study. Gastroenterology 81:237–241, 1981.
267. Cotton PB: ERCP: Progress report. Gut 18:316–341, 1977.
268. Vennes JA: Management of calculi in the common duct. Semin Liver Dis 3:162–171, 1983.
269. Chuttani R, Bynum TE, and Apstein MD: A novel approach to papillotomy in patient with difficult Billroth II anastamosis. Gastroenterology 98:A575, 1990.
270. Pereiras R, Chiprut RO, Greenwald RA, and Schiff ER: Percutaneous transhepatic cholangiography with the "skinny" needle: A rapid, simple and accurate method in the diagnosis of cholestasis. Ann Intern Med 86:562–568, 1977.
271. Mueller PR, Harbin WP, Ferrucci JT Jr, et al: Fine-needle transhepatic cholangiography: Reflections after 450 cases. Am J Roentgenol 136:85–90, 1981.
272. Harbin WP, Mueller PR, and Ferrucci JT Jr: Transhepatic cholangiography: Complications and use patterns of the fine-needle technique: A multi-institutional survey. Radiology 135:15–22, 1980.
273. Soergel KH: Acute pancreatitis. *In* Sleisinger MH and Fordtran JS (eds): Gastrointestinal Disease: Pathophysiology, Diagnosis, Management, 4th ed. Philadelphia, WB Saunders, 1989, pp 1814–1842.
274. Howard JM and Ehrlich EW: Gallstone pancreatitis: A clinical entity. Surgery 51:177–184, 1962.
275. Block MA, Puig-LaCalle J, and Fallis LS: Acute pancreatitis associated with acute cholecystitis: The curative value of biliary tract surgery. Am J Surg 94:621–623, 1957.
276. Kelly TR and Swaney PE: Gallstone pancreatitis: The second time around. Surgery 92:571–575, 1982.
277. Acosta JM, Rossi R, and Ledesma CL: The usefulness of stool screening for diagnosing cholelithiasis in acute pancreatitis. Am J Dig Dis 22:168–172, 1977.
278. Ranson JHC: The timing of biliary surgery in acute pancreatitis. Ann Surg 189:654–663, 1979.
279. Medical Research Council Multicentre Trial of Glucagon and Aprotinin: Death from acute pancreatitis. Lancet 2:632, 1977.
280. Grendell JH and Cello JP: Chronic pancreatitis. *In* Sleisinger MH and Fordtran JS (eds): Gastrointestinal Disease: Pathophysiology, Diagnosis, Management, 4th ed. Philadelphia, WB Saunders, 1989, pp 1842–1872.
281. Neoptolemos JP, Carr-Locke DL, London N, et al: ERCP findings and the role of endoscopic sphincterotomy in acute gallstone pancreatitis. Br J Surg 75:954–960, 1988.
282. Littenberg G, Afroudakis A, and Kaplowitz N: Common bile duct stenosis from chronic pancreatitis: A clinical and pathologic spectrum. Medicine 58:385–412, 1979.
283. Paloyan D, Simonowitz D, and Skinner DB: The timing of biliary tract operations in patients with pancreatitis associated with gallstones. Surg Gynecol Obstet 141:737–739, 1975.
284. Burch JM, Feliciano DV, Mattox KL, and Jordon GL: Gallstone pancreatitis: The question of time. Arch Surg 125:853–860, 1990.
285. Kurtz RJ, Heimann TM, Beck AR, and Kurtz AB: Patterns of treatment of gallstone ileus over a 45-year period. Am J Gastroenterol 80:95–98, 1985.
286. Glenn F: Postcholecystectomy choledocholithiasis. Surg Gynecol Obstet 134:249–252, 1972.
287. Way LW, Admirand WH, and Dunphy JE: Management of choledocholithiasis. Ann Surg 176:347–359, 1972.
288. Safrany L and Neuhaus B: Intraduodenal manipulations of the common bile duct. Surg Ann 12:301–315, 1980.
289. Cotton PB and Vallon AG: British experience with duodenoscopic sphincterotomy for removal of bile duct stones. Br J Surg 68:373–375, 1981.
290. Salvioli G, Salati R, Lugli R, and Zanni C: Medical treatment of biliary duct stones: Effect of ursodeoxycholic acid administration. Gut 24:609–614, 1983.
291. Allen MJ, Borody TJ, Bugliosi TF, et al: Rapid dissolution of gallstones by methyl *tert*-butyl ether. N Engl J Med 312:217–220, 1985.
292. Mack E, Saito C, Goldfarb S, et al: Local toxicity of T-tube infused cholate in the rhesus monkey. Surg Forum 28:408–409, 1977.
293. Hofmann AF, Schmack B, Thistle JL, and Babayan VK: Clinical experience with monooctanoin for dissolution of bile duct stones: An uncontrolled multicenter trial. Dig Dis Sci 26:954–955, 1981.
294. Lillemoe KD, Gadacz TR, Weichbrod RH, and Harmon JW: Effect of monooctanoin (MO) on canine gastric mucosa. Surg Gynecol Obstet 155:13–16, 1982.
295. Way LW, Bernhoft RA, and Thomas MJ: Biliary stricture. Surg Clin North Am 61:963–972, 1981.
296. Thompson JE, Tompkins RK, and Longmire WP: Factors in management of acute cholangitis. Ann Surg 195:137–145, 1982.
297. Way LW: Biliary stricture. *In* Moody FG (ed): Advances in Diagnosis and Surgical Treatment of Biliary Tract Disease. Chicago, Yearbook Publishers, 1983, pp 133–146.
298. Pellegrini CA, Thomas MJ, and Way LW: Recurrent biliary stricture. Am J Surg 147:175–180, 1984.
299. Molnar W and Stockum AE: Transhepatic dilatation of choledochoenterostomy strictures. Radiology 129:59–64, 1978.
300. Bodvall B: The postcholecytectomy syndromes. Clin Gastroenterol 2:103–126, 1973.
301. Christiansen J and Schmidt A: The postcholecystectomy syndrome. Acta Chir Scand 137:789–793, 1971.
302. Toouli J: What is sphincter of Oddi dysfunction? Gut 30:753–761, 1989.
303. Tanaka M, Ikeda S, and Nakayama F: Change in bile duct pressure responses after cholecystectomy: Loss of gallbladder as a pressure reservoir. Gastroenterology 87:1154–1159, 1984.
304. Nebel OT: Manometric evaluation of the papilla of Vater. Gastrointest Endosc 21:126–128, 1975.
305. Geenen JE, Hogan WJ, Dodds WJ, et al: Intraluminal pressure recording from the human sphincter of Oddi. Gastroenterology 78:317–324, 1980.
306. Meshkinpour H, Mollot M, Eckerling GB, and Bookman L: Bile duct dyskinesia: Clinical and manometric study. Gastroenterology 87:759–762, 1984.

307. Hogan WJ, Geenen J, Vena R, et al: Abnormally rapid phasic contractions of the human sphincter of Oddi (tachyoddia) (Abstract). Gastroenterology 84:1189, 1983.
308. Hogan WJ, Geenen J, Dodds WJ, et al: Paradoxical motor response to cholecystokinin (CCK-OP) in patients with suspected sphincter of Oddi dysfunction (Abstract). Gastroenterology 82:1085, 1983.
309. Bar-Meir S, Geenen JE, Hogan WJ, et al: Biliary and pancreatic duct pressures measured by ERCP manometry in patients with suspected papillary stenosis. Dig Dis Sci 24:209–213, 1979.
310. Steinberg WM, Salvato RF, and Toskes PP: The morphine-prostigmin provocative test—is it useful for making clinical decisions? Gastroenterology 78:728–731, 1980.

26

Acute Diarrhea

JACQUELINE L. WOLF, MD

Diarrheal diseases are major causes of morbidity throughout the world and of significant mortality in underdeveloped areas of the world. In Asia, Africa, and Latin America, it is estimated that acute diarrhea causes 3 to 5 billion episodes of illness annually, resulting in 5 to 10 million deaths.[1] In the United States, there are an estimated 99 million acute cases of vomiting and/or diarrhea each year resulting in a minimum cost of $23 billion/yr in medical costs and lost productivity.[2]

The initial approach to a patient with diarrheal disease depends on whether the diarrhea has an acute onset or represents a recurrent or chronic condition. In this chapter, the assessment of patients with acute diarrhea is discussed.

Diarrhea is defined as an increase in daily stool weight (>200 g), stool liquidity, and usually stool frequency (>3 per day).[3] Acute diarrhea, or "gastroenteritis," is a common, generally self-limited problem that usually requires no specific treatment. Viruses, bacteria and their toxins, and parasites are the most frequent causes of the illness. The specific etiology need not be pursued unless the illness is prolonged more than 7 days, the patient has significant rectal bleeding or is extremely ill, or epidemiologic considerations are important. The sudden onset of lower abdominal cramping, watery diarrhea, nausea, and vomiting are characteristic. Because these manifestations are not unique to acute gastroenteritis, the examiner should be aware of the various other illnesses that may mimic gastroenteritis but have a more ominous portent (e.g., ischemic bowel disease, appendicitis, peritonitis, diverticulitis, pancreatitis, and inflammatory bowel disease). The bowel sounds in patients with gastroenteritis are usually normal or hyperactive, the temperature is normal or slightly elevated, and the white blood cell count is usually less than 9000 mm^3. Deviations from these generalizations should prompt suspicion of complicating factors.

It is helpful to classify acute diarrhea as *noninflammatory* or *inflammatory* (Table 26–1).[4] Noninflammatory diarrhea most commonly is caused by viruses, bacteria that produce toxins, or parasites. The proximal small intestine is the most common site of infection. Patients present with watery diarrhea that is usually devoid of fecal leukocytes.

Inflammatory diarrhea most commonly is caused by bacteria or parasites that invade the mucosa. The colon and ileum are the two areas most often infected. Patients most frequently present with dysentery, which is characterized by frequent small bowel movements with the stools often containing blood, pus, and mucus. Abdominal pain, tenesmus, and fever are common.

Although it is helpful to distinguish between the two patterns of diarrhea, in practice there is often overlap between the groups. *Aeromonas* and *Pleisomonas* cause both types of diarrhea. *Salmonella, Campylobacter,* and *Yersinia,* which usually cause inflammatory diarrhea, may only cause watery diarrhea.[4] In rotaviral infection, which usually causes noninfectious diarrhea, 6 to 31% of patients have fecal leukocytes and 50% of patients have mucus in their stools.[5–7]

TABLE 26–1. INFECTIOUS DIARRHEA SYNDROMES*

Features	Noninflammatory	Inflammatory
Pathogens	Rotavirus	*Shigella*
	Norwalk virus	*Salmonella*
	Enteric adenovirus	Invasive *Escherichia coli*
	Preformed toxin–induced diarrhea	*Yersinia enterocolitica*
	a. Staphylococcal	*Vibrio parahaemolyticus*
	b. *Clostridium perfringens*	*Entamoeba histolytica*
	c. *Bacillus cereus*	Gonococcal proctitis
	Vibrio cholerae	Herpes simplex
	Toxigenic *E. coli*	Chlamydial proctitis
	Enteropathogenic *E. coli*	*Clostridium difficile*
	Giardia lamblia	*Aeromonas*
	Cryptosporidium	*Plesiomonas*
		Enterohemorrhagic *E. coli*
Common site of localization	Proximal small intestine	Colon, ileum
Diarrhea	Watery	Dysentery
Fecal leukocytes	Usually absent	Often present

*Modified from Blacklow NR and Wolfson JS: Case records of the Massachusetts General Hospital: A six-year-old girl with diarrhea after exposure to animals. N Engl J Med 313:805, 1985, with permission from *The New England Journal of Medicine.*

NONINFLAMMATORY DIARRHEA

Viruses

Viruses account for most cases of noninflammatory diarrhea. There are three well-established groups of pathogens for viral gastroenteritis: Norwalk and Norwalk-like viruses, rotaviruses, and enteric adenoviruses. Other viruses that have been shown to cause gastroenteritis but are of lesser importance are the astroviruses, calciviruses, otofuke agent, and minireovirus.[7–9] The coronaviruses have not been shown conclusively to cause disease. Norwalk, an RNA-containing virus,[10] and Norwalk-like viruses are the typical viruses that cause epidemic gastroenteritis infecting predominantly older children and adults, accounting for approximately one third of these epidemics. Following experimental inoculation of volunteers with Norwalk virus, approximately 50% developed clinical illness and two thirds developed serologic evidence of infection following an incubation period of 18 to 48 hours.[7, 8, 9, 11] Typical symptoms last 24 to 48 hours and consist of diarrhea and vomiting associated frequently with low-grade fever, abdominal cramps, and myalgias.

Norwalk and Norwalk-like viruses affect the small intestine, producing a characteristic, albeit nonspecific, histologic lesion—the villi become shortened and the epithelial cells show vacuolization and shortening of the brush border. A lamina propria infiltrate of polymorphonuclear leukocytes and mononuclear cells occurs.[12] Malabsorption of D-xylose, fat, and lactose occurs and may persist for 1 week or longer.[9, 11] In the United States in volunteer studies immunity was short-lived, but following two exposures 6 months apart serum antibodies became associated with protection.[8, 13]

The human rotaviruses, segmented RNA–containing viruses, infect predominantly young children 6 months to 2 years of age.[7, 8] Rotaviral infection accounts for 40 to 60% of the cases of acute diarrhea occurring in the winter in hospitalized children of this age group. Adults are affected less severely than are children. In one large prospective family study, 32% of children and 17% of adults became infected in 1 year. Of those infected, 70% of children and 40% of adults were symptomatic.[14] The average incubation period is 1 to 3 days, with a mean duration of symptoms of 5 to 8 days. Vomiting, watery diarrhea, and low-grade fever are the most frequent initial symptoms. Symptoms of upper respiratory infection are also common. Spread is thought to be via a fecal-oral route but may be via a respiratory route.[7, 8] High levels of serum neutralizing antibody appear to be protective.[8, 15]

Enteric adenovirus infection usually occurs in children younger than 3 years of age (85%). The incubation period is 8 to 10 days. The illness is characterized by watery diarrhea lasting for an average of 9 days (5 to 12 days but may be prolonged) accompanied by only mild fever and vomiting.[8] It probably accounts for 4 to 10% of the diarrheal illness in these children.

Preformed Bacterial Toxins

Staphylococcus aureus, Clostridium perfringens, and *Bacillus cereus* contaminate food and produce toxin-mediated gastrointestinal symptoms. Staphylococcal and *B. cereus* toxins are preformed in the food, whereas the toxin of *C. perfringens* is elaborated in the intestine by vegetative spores.[16, 17] Of the bacterial food poisoning outbreaks in the United States from 1972 to 1976, 28% were identified as being due to *S. aureus,* 12% to *C. perfringens,* and 0.4% to *B. cereus.*

Staphylococcus aureus. The most common source of staphylococcal food poisoning is a protein-containing food such as ham or salami, but improperly refrigerated dairy products and pastries are also often implicated.[16] The illness begins abruptly with vomiting 1 to 7 hours after ingestion of contaminated food and is frequently associated with abdominal pain and watery diarrhea lasting 6 to 24 hours.[16, 17]

Clostridium perfringens. Beef, poultry, pork, and other meats are the most commonly implicated foods in *C. perfringens* food poisoning. Following an incubation period of 8 to 24 hours during which time the toxin(s) is (are) elicited, patients present with colicky abdominal pain, often in the upper abdomen, and diarrhea, usually without vomiting. The duration of illness is 1 to 2 days. *C. perfringens* usually produces an α-toxin that stimulates adenylate cyclase, but some strains may produce a β-toxin that causes a hemorrhagic necrotizing enteritis.[16]

Bacillus cereus. This agent is responsible for two distinct syndromes caused by different enterotoxins: (1) Disease is characterized by vomiting, with accompanying diarrhea in only one third of patients, occurring 1 to 5 hours after eating contaminated food and lasting 12 to 24 hours. This syndrome is due to a heat-stable toxin, and the disease mimics staphylococcal food poisoning. (2) Disease is characterized by abdominal pain and diarrhea, accompanied by vomiting in 23% of patients, occurring 6 to 20 hours after ingestion of contaminated food and lasting up to 36 hours. This syndrome is due to a heat-labile toxin that stimulates adenylate cyclase. The food most commonly implicated as the contaminated source for both syndromes is fried rice.[18]

Vibrio cholerae

Vibrio cholerae infection is the prototypic toxin-induced disease. Following an incubation period of a few hours to 6 days during which time the virbrios multiply in the small bowel,[19] the disease may have a gradual onset or a sudden onset with profuse watery diarrhea, vomiting, rapid dehydration, acidosis, muscular cramps, and circulatory collapse.[19] Treatment with an oral glucose-electrolyte solution or intravenous fluids can be lifesaving. Tetracycline can be useful for hastening the eradication of the vibrios from the stools.

The toxin of *V. cholerae* consists of a B-subunit with five identical units and an A-subunit made up of A_1 and A_2. The B-subunit binds to the GM-1 monosialoganglioside on the brush border of the intestinal absorptive cells. Following a conformational change in enterotoxin structure and a translocation of the receptor-toxin complex, subunit A_1 enters the cell, where it cleaves nicotinamide-adenine dinucleotide (NAD) to nicotinamide and adenasine diphosphate (ADP)-ribose. The ADP-ribose is transferred to the guanosine triphosphatase (GTP)–binding protein inhibiting the repression of adenylate cyclase by the GTP and thus promoting the formation of cAMP. Sodium chloride absorption from the lumen ceases, and active secretion from the crypt cells occurs.[19, 20]

Enterotoxigenic *Escherichia coli*

Many surveys of sporadic diarrhea in developed countries have shown that enterotoxigenic *Escherichia coli* (ETEC) are probably not important causes of diarrhea,[21, 22] but occasional outbreaks do occur.[23] On the other hand, ETEC diarrhea is of major importance to travelers in Mexico, Asia, Africa, and Latin America, where 35 to 70% of traveler's diarrhea is due to ETEC.[23, 24] (*Shigella,* 5 to 20%; *Campylobacter; Salmonella*; Rotavirus; Norwalk virus; *Giardia lamblia*; and *Entamoeba histolytica* account for most other diagnosed cases of traveler's diarrhea.) Following an incubation period of 8 to 96 hours, patients develop watery diarrhea lasting 24 to 36 hours. The ETEC produce a heat-labile enterotoxin (LT) that acts like the enterotoxin of *V. cholerae,* stimulating adenylate cyclase and/or a heat-stable enterotoxin (ST) that stimulates guanylate cyclase.

Enteropathogenic *Escherichia coli*

Enteropathogenic *E. coli* can cause diarrhea in adults, but most outbreaks are found in children. These organisms adhere to the brush border of the upper small intestine, do not produce the ST and LT enterotoxins, and cause diarrhea by an unknown mechanism.[21, 25]

Giardia lamblia

This organism causes the most frequently diagnosed intestinal protozoan infection in the United States.[26] It multiplies in the proximal small intestine and produces diarrhea by an unknown mechanism. It may produce diarrhea by invading the mucosa and eliciting a lesion with blunting of the villi and inflammation in the lamina propria, by physically blocking the epithelial surface with sheer numbers of *Giardia* organisms, or by inducing brush border enzyme deficiencies. Secondary bacterial overgrowth may contribute to diarrhea. The organism lives in contaminated tap water, well water, streams, and ponds and has become a cause of prolonged diarrhea in back-country hikers and in travelers.[27] It has become endemic and is currently a problem in day-care centers.[28] After an incubation period of 1 to 3 weeks, there is sudden onset of explosive, watery, often foul-smelling diarrhea, abdominal pain, flatulence, belching, and nausea. After a week or more, the acute illness may resolve or change into a low-grade chronic phase, with spontaneous remissions and exacerbations that may continue for months. This chronic phase may be associated with diarrhea, weight loss, and debility.[29] Malabsorption frequently occurs to a minor degree.

Cryptosporidium

These protozoan parasites infect the intestinal epithelial cells in immunocompetent and immunodeficient humans, as well as in a large variety of animals. Up to 4% of patients with diarrhea (particularly in summer) may be infected with *Cryptosporidium.*[4] The most common symptom is watery diarrhea accompanied by vomiting, anorexia, and abdominal pain lasting 5 to 10 days.[4, 30, 31] In immunocompromised patients, *Cryptosporidium* infection can cause a prolonged chronic diarrhea. To date, no effective treatment has been found.

INFLAMMATORY DIARRHEA

Inflammatory infectious diarrhea is caused by organisms that tend to localize in the ileum or colon, producing inflammation. In the United States, the most common etiologic organisms are *Shigella, Salmonella,* and *Campylobacter.* Dysentery is manifested by frequent small bowel movements, stools containing blood, mucus, or pus and is often accompanied by abdominal pain, tenesmus, and fever.

Shigella

Shigellosis is the most important cause of dysentery in the world. The organism is highly pathogenic so that the transfer of only 10 to 100 bacteria can lead to clinical infection. Because of the low infectious dose (ID_{50}), person-to-person spread is common, and low levels of contamination of food, milk, and water may be important. Children aged 6 months to 10 years are more susceptible to infection than are adults.[32, 33] The incubation period is 12 to 72 hours. Classically, the disease follows a biphasic course, beginning in the small bowel and followed 24 hours later by progression to the colon. Fever is usually the first symptom, followed by diarrhea and abdominal pain. Initially the patient passes watery, voluminous stools. These stools become more frequent and smaller in the second phase, at which time the patient may also have abdominal cramps and tenesmus. Gross blood is present in the stool of about 40% of patients in the second phase.

Respiratory symptoms are common and hyperpyrexic seizures and the hemolytic uremic syndrome occur in children. Symptoms usually last 4 to 7 days but may continue up to 14 days. Extraintestinal complications are rare, but some patients develop polyarthritis, conjunctivitis, and iritis, usually 10 to 14 days after the onset of dysentery. The colonic mucosa becomes ulcerated and inflamed, which may resemble the mucosa in patients with idiopathic ulcerative colitis when viewed with the sigmoidoscope. This illness can be fatal in children and in the elderly.

Salmonella

These are less pathogenic organisms, requiring approximately 10^5 bacteria to cause disease, making person-to-person spread less common than with *Shigella* infections. Infections are usually acquired from contaminated food or water, particularly from poultry products, eggs, unpasteurized milk, and shellfish. In fact, *Salmonella* is responsible for more cases of food poisoning than any other pathogen.[17] Dogs, cats, domestic livestock, and pet turtles, if infected, may also transmit the disease.[17, 32] In 1977, *S. typhimurium* accounted for 35% of the *Salmonella* isolates from human and nonhuman sources in the United States, but any species can be involved in individual cases. The incubation period is 6 to 48 hours, with symptoms usually lasting 1 to 7 days, but they can continue for up to 2 weeks. Watery diarrhea is common and may be accompanied by headache, chills, nausea, fever, and abdominal pain. Dysentery occurs much less frequently than nonbloody diarrhea. Acute symptoms usually abate after 48 hours but may be prolonged, lasting 1 week or longer. Decreased gastric acidity, malignancy, schistosomiasis, liver disease, alcoholism, immunosuppression, conditions associated with hemolysis, and chronic granulomatous disease of children predispose patients to salmonellosis and subsequent bacteremia.

Salmonella penetrate epithelial cells without causing marked mucosal ulceration, but instead produce an inflammatory response in the lamina propria. The diarrhea is caused in part by the inflammatory response and in part by the production of an enterotoxin. Fecal leukocytes are present in the stools of 36% of patients with *Salmonella* and 69% of patients with *Shigella* infections.[34]

Campylobacter

This organism is a common enteric pathogen in humans, accounting for up to 20% of cases of acute diarrhea during the peak season, which is during the summer in the United States.[32] As few as 500 *C. jejuni* bacteria can cause symptomatic disease.[35] Transmission is similar to that of *Salmonella,* as it may be transmitted directly from animals to humans by means of contaminated food or water or by person-to-person spread. Infected poultry and poultry products, shellfish, water, and unpasteurized milk are important vehicles for *Campylobacter* infection. There is a wide spectrum of severity of the disease, from asymptomatic or mild cases to life-threatening illness in the elderly or debilitated.[32] The incubation period is usually 3 to 5 days but may be as long as 10 days or as short as 1.5 days.[33] The duration of illness is usually 7 to 14 days, but 25% of patients have a relapse. In about half the patients, a febrile prodromal period of a few hours to days precedes the diarrhea. This is manifest by malaise, headache, dizziness, myalgias, backache, abdominal pain, or chills. Central abdominal pain lasts from a few hours to a few days, eventually becoming colicky, heralding the onset of diarrhea. Once the patient develops diarrhea, the stools rapidly become liquid and foul-smelling, and then watery. Visible blood appears in the stools of 30 to 50% of patients after a few days. Most stools contain polymorphonuclear leukocytes.[34] The organism persists in the stool for 2 to 5 weeks after an attack of *Campylobacter* enteritis if no antibiotics are administered. Antibiotics may reduce the relapse rate.

Invasive *Escherichia coli*

This organism produces a dysentery by invading the colonic mucosa. A large outbreak in 1971 was due to contaminated French cheese.[36] It is a less important cause of dysentery than is *Shigella, Salmonella,* or *Campylobacter.*

Enterohemorrhagic *Escherichia coli*

Since its first identification as a human pathogen in 1982 enterohemorrhagic *E. coli* has emerged as an important cause for outbreaks of bloody diarrhea in North America. In Washington state where *E. coli* 0157:H7, which is the most common cause of this syndrome, is reportable, but probably underdetected, the incidence in 1987 was 2.1 cases per 100,000 population compared with the 14.7 per 100,000 for *Salmonella,* 9.4 per 100,000 for *Campylobacter,* and 7.1 per 100,000 for *Shigella.*[37] After eating contaminated food the incubation period is 1 to 8 days (mean of 3.1 days).[38] Secondary spread occurs in households with a 3 to 8 day (mean of 4.8 days) incubation period. All ages can be infected, with the highest attack rate appearing to occur in children younger than 5 years of age with a second peak occurring in adults older than 60 years of age. Sixty percent of cases occur between June and September. The source of infection is usually contaminated ground beef, although raw milk or raw-milk products, poultry, or lamb or pork products may also be sources.[37, 38] The typical symptoms are bloody diarrhea with cramps lasting up to 11 days (mean of 3 to 7 days). Nausea and vomiting occur in about half the patients, and fever occurs in a third. The incidence of nonbloody diarrhea alone caused by this organism is unknown. In one outbreak in North Dakota, 93% had nonbloody diarrhea compared with 39% with bloody diarrhea.[39] Hemolytic-uremic syndrome and thrombotic thrombocytopenic purpura are serious complications, occurring in 12% of patients in one report.[37] The overall duration and severity of illness does not appear to be decreased by antibiotics.

When suspected, enterohemorrhagic *E. coli* should be cultured on Sorbitol-MacConkey medium for 24 hours for detection of non–sorbitol fermenting bacteria. It will not be detected on routine stool culture. After screening, all sorbitol-negative *E. coli* should be serotyped.

Aeromonas

Aeromonas hydrophila are gram-negative bacteria recently recognized as a cause of enteric infection. The clinical symptoms vary from voluminous watery diarrhea indistinguishable from cholera to dysentery.[40–43] *Aeromonas* produces heat-stable and heat-labile enterotoxins that are responsible for most of the symptoms.

Disease is usually mild and self-limited (1 to 7 days) but

may be severe and prolonged. In one study diarrhea persisted for over 2 weeks in approximately 40% of patients. Fecal leukocytes and heme-positive stools are present 50 to 60% of the time. Sepsis and extraintestinal infections occur. The disease course is shortened by treatment with antibiotics.

Plesiomonas

Plesiomonas shigelloides is a gram-negative bacteria of the same family as *Aeromonas* and *Vibrios. Plesiomonas* infection is strongly associated with eating uncooked shellfish within 48 hours of symptom onset and foreign travel.[44–46] Diarrhea with or without (50%) blood and abdominal cramps occur most commonly with vomiting in one third and fever in less than one quarter of patients. Symptoms may vary from watery diarrhea to severe dysentery. Stool polymorphonuclear leukocytes are common and abundant. Like *Aeromonas, Plesiomonas* enteritis is usually self-limited (average of 11 days) but may be prolonged. The organism is sensitive to trimethoprim/sulfamethoxazole and quinolones.

Yersinia enterocolitica

This gram-negative bacillus is carried by a wide range of animals. The modes of transmission to humans have not been clearly elucidated but include direct human contact, contaminated food (particularly raw milk), and contaminated water.[33, 47] The usual incubation period is 4 to 10 days, with the usual duration of illness being 2 weeks, but chronic infection that lasts for months is not uncommon.

The most common manifestation of disease is enterocolitis, occurring in one half to two thirds of patients. This syndrome is characterized by diarrhea associated frequently with abdominal pain and fever. Anorexia, weight loss, nausea, and fatigue are less common symptoms. Older children and adults may develop pseudoappendicitis with acute terminal ileitis or mesenteric adenitis. Some types of *Yersinia* induce polyarthritis and erythema nodosum. Occasionally, adults may present with an autoimmune-type disease manifested by meningitis, carditis, thyroiditis, hepatitis, and urethritis.

Diagnosis is difficult because culture of the organism is unreliable and requires 21 days of cold enrichment for optimal recovery. Serology may be diagnostic if antibodies in acute and convalescent serum are measured.

Vibrio parahaemolyticus

This organism is an uncommon cause of disease in the United States but accounts for up to 50% of the cases of acute gastroenteritis in Japan. It is widely distributed in the British coastal waters.[19, 48, 49] Illness occurs 2.5 hours to 4 days (usually 12 to 24 hours) following ingestion of contaminated seafood and usually lasts 2 to 3 days. An enterotoxin type of disease with diarrhea and abdominal cramps and commonly nausea, fever, headache, and vomiting occurs in 90% of cases; dysentery occurs in the minority of cases. Treatment is supportive.

Entamoeba histolytica

Within the United States, the most common mode of transmission for amebic colitis is person-to-person spread. Venereally transmitted outbreaks have been described, particularly among homosexuals.[50] A history of recent travel to Latin America, Africa, or Southeast Asia should also heighten suspicion. The disease is spread by the cyst form of *E. histolytica,* which is resistant to the usual municipal chlorination of water and to gastric acid. The motile trophozoite form encountered in the mucoid or bloody stools of symptomatic patients lyses at room temperature.

Most patients have asymptomatic infections. The onset of symptoms is usually gradual over several weeks and is manifested by abdominal discomfort and frequent, loose, watery stools containing variable amounts of blood and mucus with or without constitutional symptoms.[50, 51]

Gonorrheal Proctitis

Tenesmus and bloody stools can be caused by gonorrheal proctitis, a disease most frequently encountered in homosexuals. A history of rectal burning or pruritus preceding overt proctitis suggests this diagnosis. Inflammation with mucopurulent discharge is usually visible at the anal canal, and the diagnosis is suggested by a frankly purulent mucosal appearance at sigmoidoscopy. Gram stain of the exudate may reveal characteristic gram-negative intracellular diplococci. However, culture of the gonococcus directly onto a Thayer-Martin plate at the time of sigmoidoscopy should be performed in any patient with nonspecific proctitis in whom there is a suspicion of gonorrheal exposure.[52]

Chlamydia

Chlamydia have also been isolated from patients with proctitis or proctocolitis, especially homosexual men.[53] There are no specific clinical features that identify this agent except for lymphogranuloma venereum, but treatment for gonococcal proctitis is designed also to be sufficient for chlamydial infection.

Herpes Simplex

Herpes simplex type II may cause proctitis and has been found in 6 to 30% of homosexual patients with rectal symptoms.[53] Symptomatic disease is most common and presents as anorectal pain or burning, often exacerbated by bowel movements or anal intercourse, in about 95% of patients. Pruritus ani commonly occurs. Other frequent symptoms include constipation, mucoid or bloody discharge, and tenesmus. Sacral paraesthesias and difficulty in voiding, inguinal lymphadenopathy, and fever may also occur. In the normal host, the proctitis usually resolves within 3 weeks.

Pseudomembranous Colitis

The major risk factor for developing pseudomembranous colitis is treatment with antibiotics. Almost all antibiotics have been implicated. Ampicillin and the cephalosporins are the most commonly implicated antibiotics, although the incidence following clindamycin administration is probably the highest.[54]

The symptoms of antibiotic-associated colitis vary from mild diarrhea to pseudomembranous colitis. The reported incidence of diarrhea is 5 to 10% following ampicillin and 10 to 25% following clindamycin. Up to 10% of patients receiving clindamycin may develop pseudomembranous colitis.[55] The onset of symptoms typically occurs during the course of antibiotic therapy, usually 4 to 9 days after its initiation, but up to half the patients may have a delayed onset with symptoms beginning 2 to 6 weeks following discontinuation of the antibiotics.

Pseudomembranous colitis represents the most severe disease in the spectrum of antibiotic-associated colitis. It is typically manifested by fever, abdominal pains, abdominal tenderness, diarrhea, and a leukocytosis. Sigmoidoscopy may show characteristic 2- to 10-mm raised whitish or yellowish plaques on the mucosa, but the mucosa may be erythematous, edematous, or normal. Twenty-five to 70% of patients may have disease above the reach of the sigmoidoscope.[56, 57] The pseudomembranous colitis usually remits when antibiotics are stopped but frequently becomes more severe if antibiotics continue. If disease begins after cessation of antibiotics, specific antimicrobial therapy with metronidazole, vancomycin, or bacitracin may be necessary. Relapses occur in up to 24% of patients treated with antibiotics, and multiple relapses occur in 20 to 40% of patients with one relapse. Following antibiotic administration, there is a change in the colonic flora with an overgrowth of *Clostridia difficile. C. difficile*–produced toxins are etiologic agents for the gastrointestinal symptoms, but the presence of toxin is not the determining factor for deciding on treatment. A diagnosis is usually made by demonstration of toxin in the stool.

ENTERITIS OR DYSENTERY WITH SYSTEMIC INFECTIONS

In cases of dysentery, the offending organism invades the colonic mucosa, producing severe local inflammation with diarrhea and abdominal pain. Although the organism may gain transient access to the blood stream, bacteremia is usually of no consequence, and systemic infection does not occur.[58] Persistent fever sometimes occurs in patients with *Yersinia* infections.[47] By far, however, salmonellosis is the most common cause of systemic infection associated with enteritis.[17]

There are two syndromes associated with systemic salmonellosis: (1) spiking fevers with septicemia, and (2) constant fevers. *S. choleraesuis* is the organism associated most commonly with the spiking fever-septicemic syndrome.[59] In one series, 55% of patients with diarrhea caused by *S. choleraesuis* had a positive blood culture from a single, transient bacteremic episode.[60] Curiously, these patients often lack any gastrointestinal symptoms.

The second *Salmonella* syndrome is characterized by a continuous febrile course, as opposed to the episodic chills and fevers of the septicemic syndrome. Typhoid fever per se is rare; for example, there were only 95 isolations of *S. typhosa* from symptomatic patients in the United States in 1967, whereas one third of recent typhoid fever cases were associated with travel, chiefly to Mexico, Italy, and India.[61, 62] Thus, patients more often have a "typhoid-like" syndrome due to other species of *Salmonella* such as *S. paratyphi, S. schottmülleri,* and *S. hirschfeldii.*[17] These individuals are often thought to have infectious mononucleosis, because they may present with fever, lymphadenopathy, splenomegaly, and atypical lymphocytes in the peripheral blood stream.[60] Alternatively, the syndrome may consist only of fever and malaise lasting from 1 to 3 weeks. In this instance, the organism penetrates the intestinal epithelium with little or no damage and invades the blood stream. The pulse rate may be relatively slow, and the white blood cell count may be normal but with many immature forms. *S. schottmülleri* is the most common organism causing this syndrome in the United States, but any of the *Salmonella* species can produce it.[60] The diagnosis is established by obtaining a positive blood or stool culture.

The major problem for patients with *Salmonella* bacteremic syndromes is the development of focal infections. This complication occurs in 7% of patients with *Salmonella* sepsis and may include endocarditis or abscess of any organ developing as a result of transient bacteremia with or without gastroenteritis. Focal abscesses also may develop in previously asymptomatic *Salmonella* carriers, particularly those who are chronically debilitated, those who are taking corticosteroids, or those who have sickle cell anemia. Frequently, there is a suppurative complication in continuity with the gastrointestinal tract, such as appendiceal, psoas, or perineal abscesses or cholecystitis. An acute enteritis of the distal ileum, indistinguishable from acute appendicitis, can be the presenting manifestation of infection with *S. typhimurium.* Meningitis tends to occur in infants, and pneumonia occurs in very debilitated patients. Mycotic aneurysms of the aorta and osteomyelitis are particularly characteristic in adults. *Salmonella* osteomyelitis is usually an indolent infection, often multiply involving the ribs, spine, long bones, and shoulder joints.

MISCELLANEOUS CAUSES OF ACUTE DIARRHEA

Although most syndromes of acute gastroenteritis are infectious, there are other possible causes to consider (Table 26–2). Diarrhea may accompany therapy with broad-spectrum antibiotics, magnesium-containing antacids, quinidine, colchicine, cholestyramine, digoxin, and para-aminosalicylate. Drug-induced diarrhea is usually watery without cramping, nausea, or fever, and symptoms disappear with discontinuation of the medication.

Fecal impaction in the elderly or bedridden patient will produce an "overflow diarrhea." The rectal examination or abdominal radiograph is helpful in establishing this diagnosis.

Severe nausea and vomiting, if occurring within minutes to a few hours of ingestion of food or drink, should prompt

TABLE 26–2. MISCELLANEOUS CAUSES OF ACUTE GASTROINTESTINAL SYMPTOMS

Drug-related causes
Antibiotics
Magnesium-containing antacids
Quinidine
Colchicine
Para-aminosalicylic acid
Digitalis
Cathartics
Toxin-related causes
Heavy metals (e.g., lead, zinc, cadmium, copper)
Poisonous fish (e.g., ciguatoxin, scombrotoxin, pufferfish, shellfish)
Monosodium glutamate
Botulism
Mushroom poisoning (*Amanita phalloides* or *A. muscaria*)
Diarrhea associated with fecal impaction
Acute onset of a chronic or recurrent disorder
Diverticulitis
Inflammatory bowel disease
Villous adenoma
Malabsorption
Ischemic colitis or mesenteric artery thrombosis

suspicion of a chemical food poisoning. Heavy metal poisoning, for example, follows the imbibing of acidic or carbonated beverages that have been stored in metal containers lined with tin, copper, zinc, or cadmium. The patient may note a metallic taste, bloating (tin), or myalgias (cadmium, zinc). Acute nausea followed by burning in the mouth, circumoral and limb paresthesias, or urticaria is the pattern of food poisoning related to fish toxins. Scombrotoxin, which is elaborated by species in the tuna fish family, is the main cause of this poisoning in temperate zones, whereas in the tropics and in Hawaii, puffer fish and ciguatera poisoning are the most common. Ciguatera poisoning, which follows ingestion of affected fish in the red snapper group, produces paresthesias that may persist for months. A syndrome of gastrointestinal distress associated with the sensation of flushing or burning over the face, limbs, and chest is caused in some patients by eating excessive amounts of monosodium glutamate, the "Chinese restaurant" syndrome. In this instance, the symptoms are transient, lasting only a few hours.

Botulism is characterized by a descending motor paralysis, frequently with initial symptoms of dysphagia and diplopia after a latent period that averages 14 hours from ingestion of the toxin. Gastrointestinal disturbance may be minimal or altogether lacking in this type of food poisoning. Mushroom poisoning from the *Amanita* species produces severe nausea and vomiting, usually within 2 to 14 hours, often associated with altered mental status and visual disturbances. Renal and hepatic failure may complicate the illness.

DIAGNOSTIC STUDIES IN PATIENTS WITH ACUTE GASTROENTERITIS

Diagnostic studies in patients with acute gastroenteritis are usually not necessary, because most cases of gastroenteritis are short, self-limited, and not particularly severe. Diagnosis should be pursued in patients who have a prolonged illness for more than 7 days, severe symptoms, or significant bleeding or when epidemiologic considerations are important, such as in an outbreak of food poisoning.

The procedures that are most helpful in establishing the diagnosis in patients with acute gastroenteritis are (1) examination of the stool smear with methylene blue or Gram stain, (2) stool culture, (3) stool for *C. difficile* toxin, (4) stool examination for ova and parasites, and (5) sigmoidoscopy.

Stool Smear. A smear of rectal mucus or stool is prepared and stained, usually with Löffler's methylene blue dye, and examined under the microscope. Polymorphonuclear leukocytes will be present in the smear of most patients with the syndrome of dysentery and frequently in other cases of inflammatory diarrhea (see Table 26–1) when the colonic mucosa is invaded by bacteria. Note that blood in diarrheal stool is indicative of the inflammatory rather than noninflammatory etiologies. However, this finding is not specific since ischemia or other sources of bleeding present concurrently. Polymorphonuclear leukocytes will be absent in gastroenteritis produced by bacterial toxins (except for that of *C. difficile*) or by viruses when the infection involves the small bowel.[33] Occasionally, some viral infections will be associated with fecal leukocytes. Thus, *Shigella,* invasive *E. coli, Yersinia, C. fetus, Aeromonas, Pleisomonas* or *V. parahaemolyticus* is often associated with large numbers of fecal polymorphonuclear leukocytes. Some polymorphonuclear leukocytes appear in the stool in many *Salmonella* infections, although there is less surface mucosal inflammation. Unlike bacillary dysentery, amebic colitis often does not produce a fecal leukocytosis, an observation thought to be related to the lysis of white blood cells at sites of the amebic invasion.

Stool Culture. Culture of stool samples in appropriate media will establish the specific diagnosis in most cases of dysentery. *Salmonella* organisms generally are not difficult to grow, but three fresh stool specimens should be cultured for diagnosis. *Shigella* organisms are more difficult to isolate, because they are inhibited by the standard culture media almost as much as competing intestinal flora. Thus, if the index of suspicion is high for *Shigella,* three swabs of fresh stool should be cultured on *Salmonella-Shigella* (SS) or MacConkey agar. *Campylobacter* requires special media (Skirrow's or Butzler's) for culture.[32] Some laboratories routinely culture for *Salmonella, Shigella,* and *Campylobacter* if a stool culture is requested, but, for other laboratories, a *Campylobacter* culture must be requested. When there is a suspicion of *V. parahaemolyticus,* 1.5% NaCl must be added to the culture media to allow growth.[20] *Yersinia* grows on standard media but requires special techniques for identification. One should not neglect to culture suspected foods when it is necessary to investigate a common-source epidemic. Isolation of enterohemorrhagic *E. coli* is expedited by requesting isolation of *E. coli* not requiring sorbital for growth. D and H antigen typing is necessary for positive identification.

***Clostridia difficile* Toxin.** Diagnosis of *C. difficile* infection is usually made by detection of toxin from stool in a tissue culture cytotoxicity assay rather than by stool culture. Eighty-five to 100% of patients with pseudomembranous colitis and 15 to 27% of patients with antibiotic-associated diarrhea without pseudomembranes will have a positive stool toxin titer. *C. difficile* can be cultured from the stool in almost 100% of patients with toxin-positive antibiotic-associated diarrhea or colitis and in 15 to 30% of toxin-negative patients with antibiotic-associated diarrhea or colitis.[53]

Stool Examination for Ova and Parasites. The identification of *E. histolytica* is difficult. In acute cases, the examiner must seek the trophozoites. These will lyse or become unrecognizable on standing at room temperature, so that a warm, fresh stool should be examined within 1 hour of passage (or preserved by refrigeration at 4° C in polyvinyl alcohol). Identification is even more difficult when barium, laxatives, enemas, kaolin, or antibiotics are present. In fact, the stool may be negative for ova and parasites up to 3 weeks after a barium study. For identification of cyst forms in chronic carriers, one should stain stool with methylene blue in order to differentiate the nuclear detail of white blood cells from that of *E. histolytica* cysts. The serologic indirect hemagglutination test will reveal a positive titer in as many as 80 to 90% of patients with active amebic colitis and in no more than 2% of the general population.[50]

G. lamblia infection is diagnosed in 25 to 80% of patients by the presence of cysts in stools. Trophozoites are more difficult to identify. In patients passing mostly this form of the organism (i.e., those actively having diarrhea), definitive diagnosis may require duodenal aspiration or biopsy or both.

Sigmoidoscopy. The three major indications for sigmoidoscopy in patients with diarrhea of acute onset are (1) presence of blood, (2) occurrence during therapy with antibiotics, and (3) prolonged diarrhea. In patients with bloody diarrhea, sigmoidoscopy is not done to distinguish between dysentery and ulcerative colitis, which may produce a similar appearance in the rectum (although histology may differ), but to exclude other sources of bleeding. Sparing of the lower rectal mucosa in patients with bloody diarrhea may be caused by ischemic colitis, colon cancer, and some infections, including *Salmonella, Campylobacter,* and antibiotic-associated colitis. In addition to bacterial dysentery, amebiasis, syphilis, lymphogranuloma venereum, herpes simplex, *Chlamydia,* and radiation therapy may produce proctitis similar in appearance to ulcerative colitis.

On rectal biopsy, many patients with infectious diarrheal diseases have only a nonspecific, mild-to-severe mixed acute and chronic infiltrate of the superficial lamina propria, but, in some cases of bacterial dysentery (33% in one selected series), the histologic findings are identical to those of ulcerative colitis.[63]

Sigmoidoscopic findings may be more specific in patients with antibiotic-associated pseudomembranous colitis. Initially, there are minimally raised plaques 1 to 3 mm in diameter. The plaques become larger (4 to 8 mm) and more raised and may become confluent. Eventually, they appear as yellowish pseudomembranes superimposed on an erythematous, edematous mucosa with little friability or granularity.[54] The mucosal biopsy, which should include the margin of a plaque, shows an adherent pseudomembrane composed of polymorphonuclear leukocytes, fibrin, and epithelial debris. Patients taking antibiotics who have diarrhea without pseudomembranous colitis have an edematous, erythematous appearance of the mucosa without the plaque-like membranes or even a normal appearance.

CARE OF THE PATIENT WITH ACUTE DIARRHEA

Treatment of patients with acute diarrhea can be divided into four sections: (1) prevention of disease, (2) general measures of management of diarrhea, (3) indications for antibiotic therapy, and (4) management of antibiotic-associated diarrhea.

Prevention. Proper handling of food is most important for prevention of gastroenteritis. Improper refrigeration or inadequate cooking allows bacteria to multiply and produce toxin, which subsequently causes disease. Meats, rice, and vegetables should be adequately reheated prior to serving; this will destroy the heat-labile *B. cereus* toxin and many *C. perfringens* spores.

Viral gastroenteritis is spread from person to person and therefore is difficult to prevent. A major concern in cases that are not viral is to prevent epidemics by identifying cases and tracing a potential common source of infection. Shigellosis has a propensity to spread by person-to-person transmission under conditions of poor hygiene. Infection with *E. histolytica* in the absence of a history of traveling requires a serious effort to identify the source. *G. lamblia* can be acquired not only during travel but also commonly by ingestion of cysts from a contaminated water supply.

Asymptomatic carriage of *E. histolytica, G. lamblia,* and *Salmonella* is an important problem. The most frequent mode of transmission of *E. histolytica* within the United States is now sexual contact or close person-to-person contact with an asymptomatic cyst passer.[50] *G. lamblia* is carried by up to 33% of asymptomatic children in day-care centers.[28] In more than one half of all traceable outbreaks of *Salmonella* gastroenteritis, the source is an asymptomatic carrier employed as a food handler.[60] Only half of these carriers have a previous history of gastroenteritis, although the number of organisms excreted by asymptomatic carriers may equal the number found in patients with diarrhea. It is rare for the carrier state of *Salmonella* to last more than a couple of months postinfection except with *S. typhosa,* in which 3% of untreated patients become carriers and may excrete the bacteria for years. Of non-typhosa *Salmonella*–infected patients, it is estimated that about 0.2% become carriers.[60] About one third of the non-typhosa carriers have cholelithiasis, and two thirds are female.[64] Treatment with antibiotics is generally unsuccessful, and cholecystectomy is only successful in eradicating the carriage of the nontyphosa strain 50% of the time.

Traveler's diarrhea, or turista, is the syndrome of acute, watery diarrhea ubiquitous among travelers to certain underdeveloped nations; this is caused by a variety of pathogens, most frequently ETEC. Several studies have shown antibiotic prophylaxis to be beneficial in the prevention of traveler's diarrhea.[65–67] Treatment with a daily 100-mg dose of doxycycline decreased the rate of traveler's diarrhea in Peace Corps workers in Kenya from 60% in those treated with placebo to less than 10% in those treated with doxycycline.[66, 67] At present, most toxigenic *E. coli,* except in Far Eastern countries, are sensitive to doxycycline, which also has the advantage of being concentrated in the bowel lumen by the enterhepatic circulation. Trimethoprim/sulfamethoxazole has been shown to be effective in college students visiting Mexico, and erythromycin was effective in preventing traveler's diarrhea in a group of Americans attending a meeting in Mexico.[65] Unfortunately, there are many problems with the routine use of antibiotics for prophylaxis (i.e., sensitivity to the drugs; the potential risk that widespread prophylaxis may increase the numbers of R factor–mediated, multiply resistant strains of bacteria; change in the normal flora, which is important in protection against enteric pathogens; and the possibility that people taking prophylaxis will ignore sound preventive practices). Therefore, it is recommended that prophylactic antibiotics not be given for routine prevention of traveler's diarrhea. They should be limited only (1) to adults traveling for short periods of time to "high-risk" areas where it is not possible to obtain safe water and food, (2) to persons with decreased gastric acidity, a condition that predisposes to enteric infection, and (3) to those in whom electrolyte imbalance and fluid loss may be particularly hazardous.[65] For others, there is evidence supporting use of bismuth subsalicylate (Pepto-Bismol) as a means of preventing or treating diarrhea in travelers. In one study of travelers in Mexico, diarrhea developed in 23% of persons taking bismuth subsalicylate (60 ml four times daily for 21 days) compared with 61% of persons taking a placebo.[68] Vaccines may be helpful in the future for preventing traveler's diarrhea.

General Measures for Management and Control of Diarrhea. The main problems of patients with diarrhea are fluid and electrolyte imbalance and the possibility of systemic infection. Oral intake is the preferred route for fluid replacement, with hospitalization and intravenous hydration reserved for severely ill individuals. The oral liquids should be hypoosmolar and contain sodium and potassium (e.g., juices and fruit punch). Hyperosmolar fluids may exacerbate dehydration. Even in patients with severe diarrhea, oral rehydration is usually successful. For mild diarrhea, two bouillon cubes in water is an excellent source for salt repletion. Various commercially available electrolyte solutions, and Gatorade to a lesser degree, are good sources of electrolyte and sugar repletion. For moderate (3 to 10%) dehydration, an oral rehydration solution (ORS) is recommended. Solutions with a high-glucose concentration (>2.5%) may make the diarrhea worse because of an osmotic effect. Solutions should contain between 50 and 90 mEq/l of sodium, 20 to 30 mEq/l of potassium, and 2 to 2.5% glucose. The efficacy of this replacement program has been shown in infants and children. For moderate dehydration, infants should be given about 75 ml/kg in the first 8 hours and 75 ml/kg over the next 16 hours. For severe dehydration (>10%), severe vomiting, or severe gastric distention, parenteral fluid replacement is recommended.[69] More recently cereal and rice-based oral rehydration solutions have been shown to be superior to traditional glucose-based oral rehydration solutions. The cereal- and rice-based ORS[70] decrease stool volume by 20 to 60% and may shorten the duration of diarrhea in contrast to the glucose-based ORS that does neither. Some commonly available oral rehydration solutions are listed in Table 26–3. With the gradual reinstitution of a normal diet, the resumption of milk or milk products should be delayed because of a frequent lactose intolerance due to a lactase deficiency caused by mucosal damage, but there is no need to avoid fat, which is not osmotically active and provides needed calories.

To understand the general principles to be applied to the use of opiates, atropine, kaolinpectin, and other agents that diminish diarrhea, it should be recognized that diarrhea represents, in part, a normal defense mechanism that rids the bowel of an offending agent. Thus, to diminish diarrhea may prolong infection, and if one is dealing with a potentially invasive organism, such as *Shigella* or *Salmonella,* there is a risk of enhanced invasiveness and septicemia.[71] The more potent the agent used to diminish the diarrhea, the greater will be the potential for a problem with sepsis. In addition, it must be cautioned that excessive dosages of opiates or anticholinergics can produce paralytic ileus with potentially dire consequences. However, there is no contraindication to providing symptomatic relief in patients with uncomplicated acute gastroenteritis caused by the more usual agents—viruses or bacterial toxins. In these patients, bismuth subsalicylate, loperamide, or diphenoxylate can be used in small doses. Bismuth subsalicylate has been shown to reduce symptoms in students with toxigenic *E. coli* infection and volunteers with Norwalk infection.[72,73] It is given as 30 ml or 2 tablets every half hour for 4 hours, and after the first day, 30 ml or 2 tablets 4 times per day. In a trial comparing loperamide and bismuth subsalicylate in traveler's diarrhea, loperamide (8 mg/day) was superior in decreasing stool number.[74] The opiates should be used only in small doses for disabling diarrhea of the noninflammatory type.

Antibiotics. The use of antibiotics is restricted to patients who have bacterial dysentery, systemic infection, prolonged diarrhea caused by toxigenic *E. coli* infection of the small bowel, gonoccocal infections, *G. lamblia* infections, colitis due to *E. histolytica,* and perhaps *Vibrio* infections (Table 26–4).[76]

The duration of symptoms may be shortened by therapy with antibiotics in patients with diarrhea from toxigenic *E. coli, Shigella, Campylobacter fetus,* and invasive *E. coli.* The disadvantage of treating patients with *Shigella* infection is that the organisms rapidly acquire resistance. In uncomplicated *Salmonella* dysenteries, evidence is unequivocal that therapy with antibiotics may enhance the risk of developing a carrier state.[75]

Given these constraints, there are five practical indications for antibiotic use: (1) dysentery in infants, the very elderly, or the debilitated or in those with a particularly prolonged course due to *Shigella, Campylobacter,* or invasive *E. coli*; (2) patients with bacterial dysentery of any cause plus signs of septicemia, including repeated chills and fever in the setting of diarrhea, a typhoidal syndrome, or any manifestation of focal involvement beyond the intestinal lumen; (3) prolonged diarrhea due to toxigenic *E. coli*; (4) prolonged parasitic infection; and (5) gonococcal infection. Self-limited infection with *Campylobacter* need not be treated, but erythromycin (see Table 26–4) is usually given when diarrhea induced by this organism is prolonged in duration, severe, or multiply recurrent.

Prolonged diarrhea without a source, unless toxigenic *E. coli* is strongly suspected, should not be treated with antibiotics, but a search for the etiology should be made. This may include obtaining duodenal aspiration or biopsy to detect *G. lamblia* if stools are negative for ova and parasites (Fig. 26–1). Patients with septicemia or systemic manifestations should be treated initially with parenteral ampicillin, chloramphenicol, or a quinolone pending results of cultures. In patients with uncomplicated *Salmonella* or *Shigella* dysenteries, stool cultures should be repeated at 3 to 6 weeks, by which time most patients will have negative cultures, but antibiotic therapy is not recommended for the few patients who continue to excrete *Salmonella* up to 3 months after their illness.

TABLE 26–3. SOME ORAL REHYDRATION SOLUTIONS*

Solution	Na^+	K^+	Other Cations	Cl^-	Base	Other Anions	Carbohydrates	Cost/Quart†
HYDRA-LYTE—Jayco Powder (packet dilutes to 1 quart)	84	10	—	59	HCO_3 10 Citrate 20	—	Glucose plus sucrose: 2%	$1.23
INFALYTE—Pennwalt Powder (packet dilutes to 1 quart)	50	20	—	40	HCO_3 30	—	Glucose: 2%	$1.20
LYTREN—Mead Johnson Liquid (ready to use)	30	25	Ca Mg	25	Citrate 36	$SO_4$4 $PO_4$5	Glucose plus corn syrup: 7.7%	$2.73
ORAL ELECTROLYTE SOLUTION—Wyeth Liquid (ready to use)	30	20	Ca Mg	30	Citrate 23	$PO_4$5	Glucose: 7.5%	$1.20
PEDIALYTE—Ross Liquid (ready to use)	30	20	Ca Mg	30	Citrate 28	—	Glucose: 5%	$2.02
PEDIALYTE R.S.—Ross Liquid (ready to use)	60	20	—	50	Citrate 30	—	Glucose: 2.5%	$2.02
WHO Oral Rehydration Salts§ Powder (packet dilutes to 1 liter)	90	20	—	80	HCO_3 30	—	Glucose: 2%	$0.25‡

*From Travelers' diarrhea. Med Lett 25:29, 1983.

†Cost to the pharmacist, according to Drug Topics Red Book 1983 or the manufacturer.

‡Approximate cost per quart in the United States when purchased in lots of 5000 packets.

§Oral Rehydration Salts—Jianas Brothers Packaging, 2533 SW Blvd, Kansas City, MO; KBI, Berlin; ALLPACK, Waiblingen, West Germany; Geymont Sud, Anagni, Italy; others. Also available as Oralite—Beechman; Elotrans-Fresenius, Bad Homburg; Oral Rehydration Salts—Servipharm, Basel; Salvadora—LUSA, Lima.

TABLE 26–4. RECOMMENDED TREATMENT OF CAUSES OF ACUTE DIARRHEA

Organism	Symptom	Therapy (Adults)
Salmonella	Dysentery	Antibiotic not indicated
	Septicemia	Ampicillin, 1.0–3.0 g IV q 6 hr or quinoline, ceftriaxone, or cefotaxime
Shigella	Dysentery	Antibiotics may be indicated Tetracycline, 2.5 g po (single dose) in adults Ciprofloxacin, 500 mg po bid for 5 days Ampicillin, 500 mg po qid for 5 days or Trimethoprim/sulfamethoxazole, 160 mg/800 mg bid for 5 days
	Septicemia	Ampicillin, 1 g IV q 6 hr
Campylobacter		Antibiotic not usually indicated Erythromycin, 250–500 mg qid for 7 days Ciprofloxacin, 500 mg po bid for 5 days
Escherichia coli, Aeromonas, and *Plesiomonas*		Antibiotic not usually indicated Ciprofloxacin, 500 mg po bid for 5 days Trimethoprim, 160 mg/sulfamethoxazole, 800 mg bid for 5 days
Yersinia enterocolitica		Antibiotic not usually indicated Trimethoprim/sulfamethoxazole Ciprofloxacin, 500 mg po bid for 5 days
Vibrio parahaemolyticus		Fluid replacement only
Giardia lamblia		Metronidazole, 250 mg po qid for 7 days or Quinacrine, 100 mg po for 7 days Paromomycin, 500 mg tid for 10 days in pregnancy
Entamoeba histolytica	Dysentery	Metronidazole, 750 mg po tid for 7 days or Di-iodohydroxyquin, 650 mg tid for 20 days
	Asymptomatic cyst carrier	Dilonoxide furoate, 500 mg tid for 10 days
Pseudomembranous colitis		Antibiotic often not indicated Metronidazole, 250 mg po qid for 7 days or Vancomycin, 125 po qid for 7 days or Bacitracin, 20,000 U qid for 7 days

Antibiotic-Associated Diarrhea. The decision to treat this disease is not based simply on a toxin titer or the presence of pseudomembranes but has to be made after considering the clinical findings. Most patients who have the onset of disease while taking antibiotics, regardless of whether or not they have pseudomembranes, will improve with discontinuation of the antibiotic. Patients with mild disease or who are improving at the time of diagnosis can be watched without specific antimicrobial therapy.[54] Patients with more severe disease, those who will need to continue antibiotics, or those whose symptoms occur after discontinuation of antibiotics will need specific therapy. The efficacy of a 7-day course of metronidazole, 250 mg qid, vancomycin, 125 to 500 mg qid, and bacitracin, 20,000 units qid is the same.[54, 77] Metronidazole is the cheapest of the three drugs in the United States. Cholestyramine (4 g every 6 hours), which binds the toxin, may be an adjunct to therapy but should not be given at the same time as antimicrobial therapy because it may bind the medications. Relapses may be treated with the same drugs as the initial treatment or with an alternative drug.

SUMMARY: APPROACH TO THE PATIENT

The clinician first approaches a patient with acute diarrhea, nausea, and vomiting by considering both infectious and noninfectious etiologies for the acute illness. Drug or toxin ingestion or an acute abdominal process must be ruled out. Note is made of current medications, toxin exposure, travel history, animal exposure, and exposure to others with gastroenteritis. A careful physical examination is performed to exclude acute abdominal conditions such as appendicitis, salpingitis, or intestinal obstruction. It is particularly important to consider alternative diagnosis such as diverticulitis or intestinal ischemia in elderly patients with acute gastrointestinal symptoms. Sigmoidoscopic examination may be helpful if diarrhea has developed while the patient is taking antibiotics.

The initial approach to the patient with infectious diarrhea is determined by whether the clinical pattern is that of *acute noninflammatory* or *inflammatory* diarrhea (see Fig. 26–1).

Acute noninflammatory gastroenteritis is a mild illness that usually lasts less than 1 week and is usually due to infection of the small intestine. No diagnostic studies are needed unless there is an epidemic and a common source needs to be identified. Treatment is supportive with bismuth subsalicylate, loperamide, diphenoxylate or kaolin-pectin (opiates only if necessary), and fluids. The patient may eat anything tolerated, although generally it is recommended that one not ingest milk products. The diagnosis is most commonly a viral or bacterial toxin-induced gastroenteritis.

If the diarrhea is prolonged more than 1 week or if the patient has severely symptomatic diarrhea, stool cultures, a stool examination for polymorphonuclear leukocytes, and stool examinations for ova and parasites should be performed. If the test results are negative, further evaluation for *Giardia* or a chronic illness may be warranted (see Fig. 26–1).

Inflammatory diarrhea can vary from mild to severe, is usually associated with polymorphonuclear leukocytes and blood in the stool, and is due to inflammation of the terminal ileum or colon. Dysentery is the most severe form and is characterized by frequent small bowel movements, often

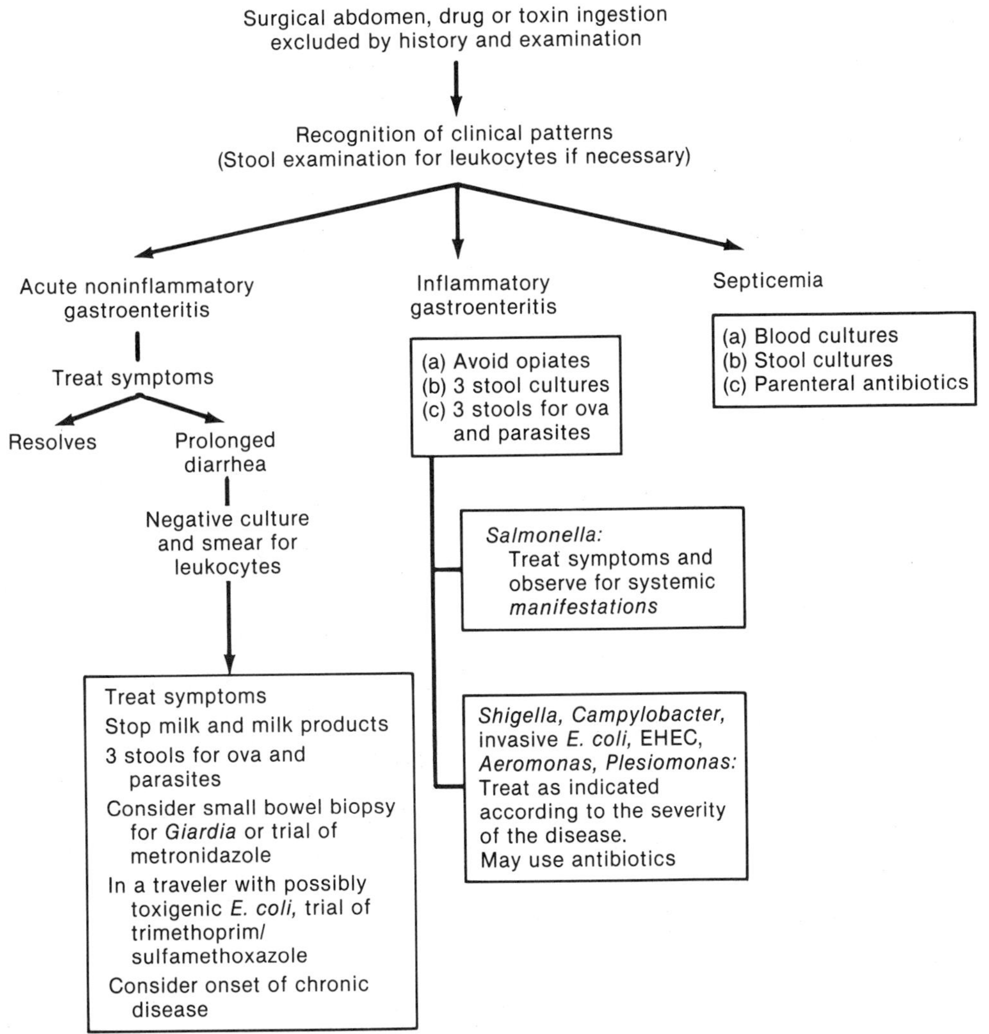

FIGURE 26–1. Approach to patients with acute diarrhea.

with blood, pus, and/or mucous-containing stools. It is treated according to the severity of the symptoms. Opiates and other antidiarrheal agents are withheld. Antibiotics, usually not indicated, may be given to selected patients, as discussed earlier and outlined in Table 26–4. Elderly or dehydrated patients require admission to the hospital. Most other patients do not require hospitalization. Three stool cultures for *Shigella, Salmonella,* and *Campylobacter* (and if suspected *Aeromonas, Plesiomonas,* or enterohemorrhagic *E. coli*) are obtained, if negative, three stools for ova and parasites are obtained (see Fig. 26–1). If negative, a sigmoidoscopic examination with direct culture of the mucosal exudate should be done, and the possibility of inflammatory bowel disease should be considered.

Diarrhea with signs of systemic infection manifested by recurrent chills or fever during or after a bout of dysentery requires therapy with a parenteral antibiotic.

ACKNOWLEDGMENTS

I acknowledge gratefully the contributions of Robert Smith, Jr., M.D., Z. Myron Falchuk, M.D., and William T. Branch, Jr., M.D., authors of the chapter on acute diarrhea in the first edition of this book.

REFERENCES

1. Kapikian AZ, Wyatt RG, Greenberg HB, et al: Approaches to immunization of infants and young children against gastroenteritis due to rotavirus. Rev Infect Dis 2:459, 1980.
2. Garthright WE, Archer DL, and Kvenberg JE: Estimates of incidence and costs of intestinal infectious diseases in the United States. Public Health Rep 103:107, 1988.
3. Krejs GJ and Fordtran JS: Diarrhea. *In* Sleisenger MH and Fordtran JS (eds): Gastrointestinal Disease: Pathophysiology, Diagnosis, Management, 3rd ed. Philadelphia, WB Saunders, 1983, p 257.
4. Blacklow NR and Wolfson JS: Case records of the Massachusetts General Hospital: A six-year-old girl with diarrhea after exposure to animals. N Engl J Med 313:805, 1985.
5. Hieber JP, Shelton S, Nelson JD, et al: Comparison of human rotavirus disease in tropical and temperate settings. Am J Dis Child 132:853, 1978.
6. Rodriquez WJ, Kim HW, Arrobio JO, et al: Clinical features of acute gastroenteritis associated with human reovirus-like agent in infants and young children. J Pediatr 91:188, 1977.
7. Wolf JL and Schreiber DS: Viral gastroenteritis. Med Clin North Am 66:575, 1982.
8. Blacklow NR and Greenberg HB: Viral gastroenteritis. N Engl J Med 325:252, 1991.
9. Dolin R, Treanor JJ, and Madore HP: Novel agents of viral enteritis in humans. J Infect Dis 155:365, 1987.
10. Jiang X, Graham DY, Wang K, and Estes MR: Norwalk virus genome cloning and characterization. Science 250:1580, 1990.

11. Blacklow NR, Dolin R, Fedson DS, et al: Acute infectious nonbacterial gastroenteritis: Etiology and pathogenesis. Ann Intern Med 76:993, 1972.
12. Schreiber DS, Blacklow NR, and Trier JS: The mucosal lesion of the proximal small intestine in acute infectious nonbacterial gastroenteritis. N Engl J Med 288:1318, 1973.
13. Parrino TA, Schreiber DS, Trier JS, et al: Clinical immunity in acute gastroenteritis caused by the Norwalk agent. N Engl J Med 297:86, 1977.
14. Wenman WM, Hinde D, Feltham S, et al: Rotavirus infections in adults: Results of a prospective family study. N Engl J Med 301:303, 1979.
15. Kapikian AZ, Wyatt RG, Levine MD, et al: Oral adminstration of human rotavirus to volunteers: Induction of illness and correlates of resistance. J Infect Dis 147:95, 1983.
16. Schneider J: Gastroenteritis due to *Staphylococcus aureus, Clostridium perfringens,* and *Bacillus cereus. In* Goodwin CS (ed): Microbes and Infections of the Gut. Melbourne, Blackwell Scientific, 1983, p 149.
17. Turnbull PCB: Food poisoning with special reference to *Salmonella*—Its epidemiology, pathogenesis, and control. Clin Gastroenterol 8:663, 1979.
18. Terranova W and Black PA: *Bacillus cereus* food poisoning. N Engl J Med 298:143, 1978.
19. Goodwin CS: Cholera and other vibrios, *Aeromonas* and *Plesiomonas. In* Goodwin CS (ed): Infections of the Gut. Melbourne, Blackwell Scientific, 1983, p 103.
20. Middlebrook JL and Dorland RB: Bacterial toxins: Cellular mechanisms of action. Microbiol Rev 48:199, 1984.
21. Gross RJ and Rowe B: *Escherichia coli* diarrhoea. *In* Goodwin CS (ed): Microbes and Infections of the Gut. Melbourne, Blackwell Scientific, 1984, p 79.
22. Dupont HL and Pickering LK: Infections of the Gastrointestinal Tract: Microbiology, Pathophysiology, and Clinical Features. New York, Plenum, 1980.
23. Rosenberg ML, Kaplan IP, Wachsmith K, et al: Epidemic diarrhea at Crater Lake from enterotoxigenic *E. coli.* Ann Intern Med 86:714, 1977.
24. Gorbach SL: Traveler's diarrhea. N Engl J Med 307:881, 1982.
25. Robins-Browne RM: Traditional enteropathogenic *Escherichia coli* of infantile diarrhea. Rev Infect Dis 9:28, 1987.
26. Wolfe MS: The treatment of intestinal protozoan infections. Med Clin North Am 66:707, 1982.
27. Barbour AG, Nichols CR, and Fukushima J: An outbreak of giardiasis in a group of campers. Am J Trop Med Hyg 25:384, 1976.
28. Pickering LK, Woodward WE, DuPont HL, et al: Occurrence of *Giardia lamblia* in children in day-care centers. J Pediatr 104:522, 1984.
29. Wolfe MS: Giardiasis. N Engl J Med 298:319, 1978.
30. Pitlik SD, Fainstein V, Garza D, et al: Human cryptosporidiosis: Spectrum of disease: Report of six cases and review of the literature. Arch Intern Med 143:2269, 1983.
31. Tzipori S: Cryptosporidiosis in animals and humans. Microbiol Rev 47:84, 1983.
32. Rowe B and Gross RJ: Salmonellosis, campylobacter enteritis, and shigella dysentery. *In* Goodwin CS (ed): Microbes and Infections of the Gut. Melbourne, Blackwell Scientific, 1984, p 47.
33. Wolf JL: Infectious diarrhea? What is the cause? Patient Care 17:79, 1977.
34. Pickering LK, DuPont HL, Olarte J, et al: Fecal leukocytes in enteric infection. Am J Clin Pathol 68:562, 1977.
35. Cover TL and Blaser MJ: The pathobiology of *Campylobacter* infections in humans. Annu Rev Med 40:269, 1989.
36. Marrier R, Wells TG, Swanson RC, et al: An outbreak of enteropathogenic *Escherichia coli* food-borne disease traced to imported French cheese. Lancet ii:1376, 1973.
37. Ostroff SM, Kobayashi JM, and Lewis JH: Infections with *Escherichia coli* 0157:H7 in Washington State: The first year of statewide disease surveillance. JAMA 262:355, 1989.
38. Ostroff SM, Griffin PM, Tauxe RV, et al: A statewide outbreak of *Escherichia coli* 0157:H7 infections in Washington State. Am J Epidemiol 132:239, 1990.
39. McDonough S, Heer F, and Shireley L: Foodborne outbreak of gastroenteritis caused by *Escherichia coli* 0157:H7—North Dakota, 1990. MMWR 40:265, 1991.
40. Freij BJ: *Aeromonas*: Biology of the organism and diseases in children. Pediatr Infect Dis 3:164, 1987.
41. Holmberg SD and Farmer JJ: *Aeromonas hydrophila* and *Plesiomonas shigelloides* as causes of intestinal infection. Rev Infect Dis 6:633, 1987.
42. Holmberg SD, Schell WL, Fanning GR, et al: *Aeromonas* intestinal infections in the United States. Ann Intern Med 105:683, 1986.
43. Challapalli M, Tess BR, Cunningham DF, et al: *Aeromonas*-associated diarrhea in children. Pediatr Infect Dis J 7:693, 1988.
44. Holmberg SD, Wachsmuth IK, Hickman-Brenner FW, et al: *Plesiomonas* enteric infections in the United States. Ann Intern Med 105:690, 1986.
45. Brenden RA, Miller MA, and Janda JM: Clinical disease spectrum and pathogenic factors associated with *Plesiomonas shigelloides* infections in humans. Rev Infect Dis 10:303, 1988.
46. Rain KC and Kelly MT: Clinical features, epidemiology, and treatment of *Plesiomonas shigelloides* diarrhea. J Clin Microbiol 27:998, 1989.
47. Goodwin CS: Yersinia infections, including mesenteric adenitis and gastrointestinal tuberculosis. *In* Goodwin CS (ed): Microbes and Infections of the Gut. Melbourne, Blackwell Scientific, 1984, p 241.
48. Bolen JL, Zamiska SA, and Greenough WB: Clinical features in enteritis due to *Vibrio parahaemolyticus.* Am J Med 57:638, 1974.
49. Rodrick GE, Hood MA, and Blake NJ: Human vibrio gastroenteritis. Med Clin North Am 66:665, 1982.
50. Krogstad DS, Spencer HJ, and Healy GR: Amebiasis. N Engl J Med 298:262, 1978.
51. Patterson M and Schoppe LE: The presentation of amoebiasis. Med Clin North Am 66:689, 1982.
52. Klein EJ, Fisher LS, Chow AW, et al: Anorectal gonococcal infection. Ann Intern Med 86:340, 1977.
53. Baker RW and Peppercorn MA: Gastrointestinal ailments of homosexual men. Medicine 61:390, 1982.
54. Bartlett JG: Antibiotic-associated colitis. Dis Mon 30:2, 1984.
55. Tedesco FJ, Barton RW, and Alpers DH: Clindamycin-associated colitis: A prospective study. Ann Intern Med 81:429, 1974.
56. Tedesco FJ, Corless JK, and Brownstein RE: Rectal sparing in antibiotic-associated pseudomembranous colitis: A prospective study. Gastroenterology 83:1259, 1982.
57. Seppälä K, Hjelt L, and Sipponen P: Colonoscopy in the diagnosis of antibiotic-associated colitis—a prospective study. Scand J Gastroenterol 16:465, 1981.
58. Grady GF and Keusch GT: Pathogenesis of bacterial diarrheas. N Engl J Med 285:831, 1976.
59. Saphra I and Winter J: Clinical manifestations of salmonellosis in man. N Engl J Med 256:1128, 1957.
60. Black PA, Junz LG, and Swartz MN: Salmonellosis—a review of some unusual aspects. N Engl J Med 262:811, 864, 921, 1960.
61. Aserkoff B, Schroeder SA, and Brachman PS: Salmonellosis in the United States—a five-year review. Am J Epidemiol 92:13, 1970.
62. Rice PA, Baire WB, and Gangarosa EJ: *Salmonella typhi* infections in the United States, 1967–1972: Increasing importance of international travelers. Am J Epidemiol 106:160, 1977.
63. Dickinson FJ, Gilmour HM, and McClelland BL: Rectal biopsies in patients presenting to an infectious disease unit with diarrheal disease. Gut 20:141, 1979.
64. Musher DM and Rubenstein AD: Permanent carriers of nontyphosa salmonellae. Arch Intern Med 132:869, 1973.
65. Merson MH: Prevention of traveler's diarrhea. Gastroenterology 84:424, 1983.
66. Sack DA, Kaminsky DC, Sack RB, et al: Prophylactic doxycycline for traveler's diarrhea. N Engl J Med 298:758, 1979.
67. Sack RB, Froehlich JL, Zulich AW, et al: Prophylactic doxycycline for traveler's diarrhea: results of a prospective double-blind study of Peace Corps volunteers in Morocco. Gastroenterology 76:1368, 1979.
68. Traveler's diarrhea. Med Lett 21:41, 1979.
69. Oral rehydration solution. Med Lett 25:19, 1985.
70. Khin-Maung U and Greenough WB: Cereal-based oral rehydration therapy. I: Clinical studies. J Pediatr 118:572, 1991.
71. DuPont HL and Hornick RB: Adverse effect of Lomotil therapy in shigellosis. JAMA 266:1525, 1973.

72. DuPont HL, Sullivan P, Pickering LK, et al: Symptomatic treatment of diarrhea with Bismuth subsalicylate among students attending a Mexican university. Gastroenterology 73:715, 1977.
73. Steinhoff MC, Douglas RG Jr, Greenberg HB, et al: Bismuth subsalicylate therapy of viral gastroenteritis. Gastroenterology 78:1495, 1980.
74. DuPont HL, Sanchez JF, and Ericsson CD: Comparative efficacy of loperamide hydrochloride and bismuth subsalicylate in the management of acute diarrhea. Am J Med 88(Suppl 6A):6A–15S, 1990.
75. Aserkoff B and Bennett JV: Effect of therapy in acute salmonellosis on salmonellae in feces. N Engl J Med 281:636, 1969.
76. Gorbach SL: Bacterial diarrhoea and its treatment. Lancet ii:1378, 1987.
77. Young GP, Ward PB, Bayley N, et al: Antibiotic-associated colitis due to *Clostridium difficile*: Double-blind comparison of vancomycin with bactitracin. Gastroenterology 89:1038, 1985.

27

Chronic Diarrhea

JERRY S. TRIER, MD

Chronic diarrheal disease may result from (1) diseases associated with *altered intestinal motility,* such as irritable bowel syndrome; (2) diseases that impair colonic fluid absorption due to a *colonic mucosal lesion,* such as ulcerative colitis; (3) disorders that result from intraluminal nonabsorbable substances, including laxatives, that *osmotically induce diarrhea*; (4) diseases in which there is *stimulation of intestinal secretion,* as with a tumor secreting humoral substances such as vasoactive intestinal peptide (VIP) or calcitonin; and (5) diseases that produce *intestinal malabsorption* either by interfering with intraluminal digestion as is seen in pancreatic insufficiency and obstructive jaundice or by resulting in impaired nutrient absorption due to a mucosal lesion of the small intestine, as occurs in celiac sprue. Diarrhea may also be functional, such as the irritable bowel syndrome. The evaluation of the patient should be directed toward defining the general category of diarrheal disease. Then, a specific disease can often be diagnosed, and appropriate therapy can be implemented.

APPROACH TO THE PATIENT

Obtaining a detailed history is crucial in the evaluation of a patient with chronic diarrhea. The frequency and volume of bowel movements must be estimated, and the presence or absence of associated features, such as weight loss, abdominal pain, or tenesmus, should be determined. Diarrhea means different things to different people, and an effort should be made to ascertain its features in each particular patient. There is no substitute for careful visual inspection of the patient's stools that he or she perceives as diarrheal. It should be determined whether there has been a change in stool frequency. Nocturnal diarrhea that wakes a patient from sleep is usually caused by a pathologic process, whereas diarrhea that disappears while a patient is sleeping may be either functional or organic in nature. Whether a stool floats or sinks is not characteristic of the presence or absence of steatorrhea; it is the gas content of the stool that determines its buoyancy.[1]

The typical daily diet contains approximately 2 liters of fluid; endogenous secretions, which include saliva, gastric juice, and biliary, pancreatic, and intestinal secretions, add an additional 7 liters. The absorptive capacity of the small intestine is so efficient that of the 9 liters of fluid, roughly 8 liters are normally absorbed by the time that the intestinal contents pass the ileocecal sphincter. Of the remaining fluid, the colon normally absorbs at least 0.8 liter; hence, normal stool contains less than 0.2 liter of fluid. In fact, the total mass of stool normally is 200 g or less per 24 hours.

Since stool mass in Western nations does not usually exceed 200 g/day, stool weight is a better index of diarrhea and malabsorption than is the number of bowel movements. Voluminous stools suggest disorders of the small intestine and proximal colon. They tend to be bulky and watery and may be foul-smelling. Pain from the small bowel and right colon is usually perceived by the patient in the periumbilical region or in the right lower quadrant.

Small quantities of loose stool suggest that the patient's problem is associated with left colonic or rectal dysfunction. The pain is usually referred to the left upper or lower quadrant. There may be tenesmus and urgency, or only mucus and flatus may be passed. The fecal matter may be bloody but is usually not foul-smelling.

Diarrhea alternating with constipation suggests the irritable bowel syndrome. The stool is often pebble-like in nature during the constipation phase. Constipation alternating with diarrhea can also be caused by obstructive lesions such as carcinoma of the colon.

A history of chronic ingestion of laxatives such as milk of magnesia or lactulose suggests the presence of *osmotic diarrhea,* although such a history may be difficult to obtain since laxative abuse is often surreptitious. Osmotic diarrhea occurs whenever the total tonicity of the intestinal contents is high, causing water to enter the lumen from the plasma and tissue spaces. In addition to laxative abuse, this occurs in patients with lactase and other disaccharidase deficiencies. It also occurs in any condition in which there is severe, generalized, malabsorption of dietary nutrients that remain in the gut lumen, adding to its osmolality.

The persistence of diarrhea when the patient is fasted indicates a *secretory* component. In this situation, even total abstinence from food will be associated with continued watery diarrhea. Such diarrhea is usually voluminous. The prototype of this group of illnesses is cholera, a disease that occurs in a unique clinical and geographic setting. However, chronic secretory diarrhea occurs in a number of other disorders such as the pancreatic cholera syndrome (watery diarrhea, hypokalemia, and acidosis caused by tumors of the pancreas that secrete VIP) and medullary carcinoma of the thyroid (calcitonin-mediated hypersecretion). In these conditions steatorrhea is generally absent.

Some diarrheas associated with a mucosal lesion and steatorrhea (e.g., celiac sprue) have a secretory component with net fluid secretion by the involved small intestine. Moreover, in steatorrhea, a secretory state can be produced in the colon by the interaction with the colonic mucosa of long-chain fatty acids, which, under normal circumstances, would be absorbed by the epithelium of the small intestine.[2] In contrast, short-chain fatty acids stimulate colonic ion absorption.[3] Bile salts, when present in excess, also induce a secretory diarrhea by interacting with colonic epithelial cells. Thus, patients with terminal ileal dysfunction or resection, as in Crohn's disease, may have this type of secretory diarrhea.[4, 5] In contrast to classical secretory diarrheas, the diarrhea associated with generalized malabsorption, ileal resection, and disaccharidase intolerance usually stops when the patient is fasting.

The physical examination often complements the history in the assessment of possible etiology. Extraintestinal manifestations can be prominent in a number of chronic diarrheal diseases. The nutritional state of the patient and the presence of peripheral edema, purpura, and tetany can provide clues suggesting malabsorption. Pallor may be associated with anemia caused by deficiency of vitamin B_{12}, folic acid, or iron due to their malabsorption.[6] Iron deficiency anemia may also reflect chronic intestinal blood loss associated with ulcerative colitis or Crohn's disease. Clubbing of the fingernails and a history of chronic pulmonary infection suggests cystic fibrosis. Evidence of chronic liver disease, especially jaundice, may suggest malabsorption due to inadequate delivery of bile salts required for normal intraluminal fat digestion. An abdominal mass in the right lower quadrant, fistula in the perineum, or perianal fissures suggest Crohn's disease.

Sigmoidoscopy should be an integral part of the physical examination in patients with chronic diarrhea. The mucosa in any chronic diarrheal disease may appear edematous, but bleeding with ulceration most often indicates the presence of an inflammatory condition such as ulcerative colitis, Crohn's colitis, or amebiasis. In the absence of gross bleeding, the stool must be tested for occult blood. At the time of sigmoidoscopy, stool or exudate should be smeared on the slide, stained with Wright's stain or methylene blue dye, and examined microscopically for the presence of polymorphonuclear leukocytes. These will be present in mucosal inflammatory disease such as ulcerative colitis, Crohn's colitis, amebiasis, and enteric infections caused by invasive microorganisms such as *Shigella* and *Salmonella.* They are absent in diarrhea caused by malabsorption, viral gastroenteritis, and irritable bowel syndrome.

Examination of wet mounts of mucus, exudate, or stool obtained at sigmoidoscopy for ova and parasites is often useful. If malabsorption is suspected, the stool should be examined microscopically for fat using Sudan stain. Unless the patient has taken unabsorbable lipids, such as castor oil or mineral oil, the presence of large amounts of oil droplets in the stool is highly suggestive of steatorrhea and, hence, malabsorption. An acid pH suggests carbohydrate malabsorption, as occurs in lactase deficiency. Additional diagnostic studies to be done depend on the clinical setting, the pattern of diarrhea, and the results of the initial evaluation and are described later.

DIAGNOSIS AND THERAPY

Irritable Bowel Syndrome

In the United States, irritable bowel syndrome is probably the most common cause of chronic diarrhea and lower abdominal discomfort.[7] Studies suggest that between 14 and 20% of population samples experience these symptoms with some regularity, but many do not seek medical aid.[8, 9] Symptoms may include nausea, flatulence, and abdominal distention, bloating, and pain, one or all of which may be present from time to time. Fever, gastrointestinal bleeding, or weight loss (unless the patient is severely depressed) are *not* part of the syndrome, and their presence should alert the physician to alternative diagnostic possibilities. The syndrome may affect a broad spectrum of individuals, ranging from children to older adults, but onset most commonly occurs in those between the ages of 20 and 35 years.[7] Onset of symptoms after the age of 60 years is possible but should stimulate a search for more specific underlying pathology.

Key features that help to distinguish irritable bowel syndrome from more ominous disease include (1) normal stool mass per 24 hours despite more frequent and loose stools, (2) disappearance of symptoms while the patient is asleep, and (3) a clear aggravation of symptoms with stress. A feeling of incomplete evacuation following a bowel movement is often present. Diarrhea alternating with constipation in cycles varying from 3 to 4 days to as much as 1 week is common. The constipated stool is often hard and in the form of either pellets or thin strings. Typically, stools are more frequent in the morning than later in the day. The initial stool, usually passed shortly after awakening, is often formed, whereas subsequent stools are looser and even watery. Urgency is common, often after meals. High pressures generated by the colon in its effort to empty may result in abdominal pain. In some patients, pain tends to localize to the left upper quadrant, giving rise to the so-called splenic flexure syndrome; more often, the pain is in the left lower quadrant, although pain may be located in any region of the abdomen, and its localization may vary from day to day. Patients frequently report the recurrent perceived need to defecate but with relatively scant stool excretion. The passage of mucus is prominent in some people but scant to absent in others. The passage of flatus or of a bowel movement frequently diminishes the patient's pain, at least transiently. During an episode of abdominal cramping, palpation may initially cause discomfort that often resolves when the examiner continues to apply gentle, steady pressure. A subgroup of patients with irritable bowel syndrome present with painless diarrhea without the typical cyclical diarrhea and constipation.

The cause of irritable bowel syndrome is unknown. To what extent some individuals who carry this diagnosis are affected by mild disaccharidase deficiency, carbohydrate intolerance, laxative abuse, or other unrecognized conditions is unknown. Abnormal intestinal motility has been documented; motility of the sigmoid colon was increased in patients with colic but was decreased in those with painless diarrhea.[10] Additionally, altered motility of the small intestine that correlates with cramping abdominal pain has been noted.[11–13] In many individuals, the periods of diarrhea occur under obviously stressful conditions (e.g., during final examinations or before interviews).[14] However, no single personality profile or psychiatric diagnosis has been consistently related to the irritable bowel syndrome.[7] Some patients show manifestations of depression or are experiencing a major personal loss. Others have been noted to be more anxious and obsessional than control populations.

Since functional bowel symptoms are highly prevalent, the likelihood that someone will request medical consultation for these symptoms may depend as much on his or her individual personality traits as on the severity of the symptoms. This may explain, at least in part, the reported high prevalence of psychiatric symptoms among patients with irritable bowel syndrome who seek medical care.[15]

Diagnostic Evaluation. Because there are no objective findings or specific diagnostic tests, this syndrome should be diagnosed only when one is reasonably certain that the patient has no other gastrointestinal disease. However, irritable bowel syndrome is sufficiently common in otherwise healthy young individuals that it becomes neither practical nor fruitful to perform extensive studies in each patient. If the patient is younger than 40 years of age and has a typical clinical pattern of episodic bowel dysfunction for several years or longer but no persistent pain or tenderness, weight loss, or other constitutional symptoms, evaluation can be attenuated and attention can be focused on management. In such individuals, the number of diagnostic studies may be limited to a careful history and physical examination, sigmoidoscopy, three stools tested for occult blood, a lactose tolerance test or breath test, or a trial of a milk-free diet together with such routine studies as a hematocrit, erythrocyte sedimentation rate, and serum potassium.[16]

Additional studies to be performed when symptoms are unusually severe or refractory include an upper gastrointestinal and small bowel barium contrast study, barium enema or colonoscopy with biopsy of the colonic mucosa, and examination of stools for fat, ova, and parasites. If dyspepsia is present, ultrasonography of the abdomen with attention to the gallbladder and pancreas may be indicated. In selected patients, this may be followed by a more extensive evaluation, for example, 72-hour collection of stool for weight or volume and fat, D-xylose tolerance test, and biopsy and/or duodenal aspiration for giardiasis if the findings in stools for ova and parasites are negative.

Management. The apparent prevalence of irritable bowel syndrome appears to be low in Africa where dietary fiber intake is much higher than in regions in which the population consumes the usual highly refined Western diet.[17] Hence, addition of fiber to the diet is widely used, although the evidence is conflicting,[18, 19] and truly definitive trials of potential treatment modalities for irritable bowel syndrome are not available.[20] Both unprocessed bran and psyllium colloid may be used, especially in patients with constipation or alternating constipation and diarrhea. Dosage varies from one patient to another, and several weeks or even months may be needed for a beneficial effect to be achieved. Up to 25% of patients have increased distention and flatus when a high-fiber diet is implemented, but in many patients, these symptoms improve with time and dosage adjustments. Three to 8 tablespoons of unprocessed, coarse bran and 1 to 3 tablespoons of psyllium colloid per day taken at meal time may be needed. One should begin with a low dose and instructions to increase the dose every 2 weeks until the stool achieves a soft and bulky consistency.

In a study of one extremely flatulent individual, flatus, as shown by its high hydrogen and CO_2 and low nitrogen content, was of intestinal origin and did not represent swallowed air. Milk, onions, beans, celery, carrots, raisins, wheat products, and Brussels sprouts were implicated in flatus production by a laborious process of elimination.[21] A simplified version of this approach using sequential elimination of milk, wheat products, and fermentable but nondigestable carbohydrates (legumes, cabbage) could be attempted in patients if flatus is a major complaint, especially if the patient's history suggests that these foodstuffs worsen symptoms. Excessive use of coffee, tea, sorbitol-containing gum, candy, or beverages or any other dietary aberration should also be identified and avoided. Glycerine suppositories may be used as needed for constipation, but laxatives should be avoided. Other medications, including anticholinergics and sedatives, may be added, but, in general, their effectiveness has not been documented.[20] If an antidiarrheal agent must be used, loperamide appears least addictive and has the longest duration of action.

Practicing physicians are aware of the frustrations, for both doctors and patients, engendered by continuous or recurrent symptoms, anxiety, and ensuing complaints of patients with the irritable bowel syndrome. Current recommendations are to consider treatment with antidepressants or psychiatric referral only when there are recognizable manifestations of depression or another psychiatric disorder in addition to the bowel symptoms.[16] Patients are helped by a continuous, supportive relationship with a physician. Hasty reassurance is to be avoided. The physician should attempt to educate the patient with regard to the nature of the condition and involve the patient in the management. The principal goal may be to enable patients to adjust to their chronic symptoms. In part, this requires giving the patient "permission" to be symptomatic. He or she should be reassured that complaints are legitimate. A common tactic is to place emphasis on forebearance in dealing with symptoms and challenge the patient to see how much can be accomplished in spite of the handicap.[22] Repeated diagnostic studies should be avoided unless there is a significant change in the pattern of symptoms. Fear of cancer by the patient should be suspected and dealt with by frank discussion. Follow-up is important, with the goal

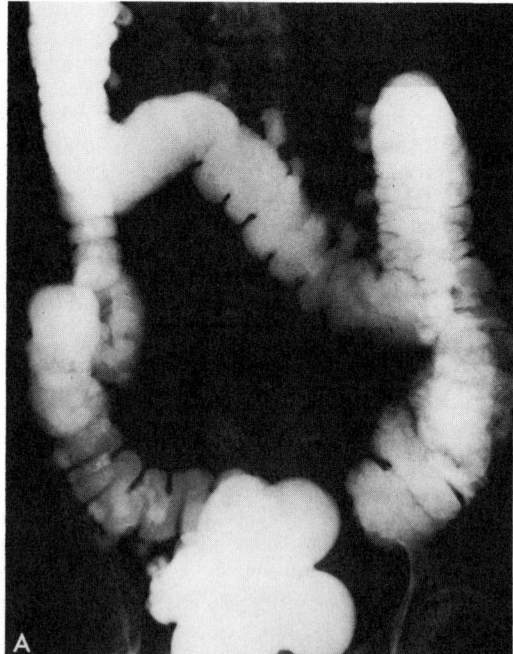

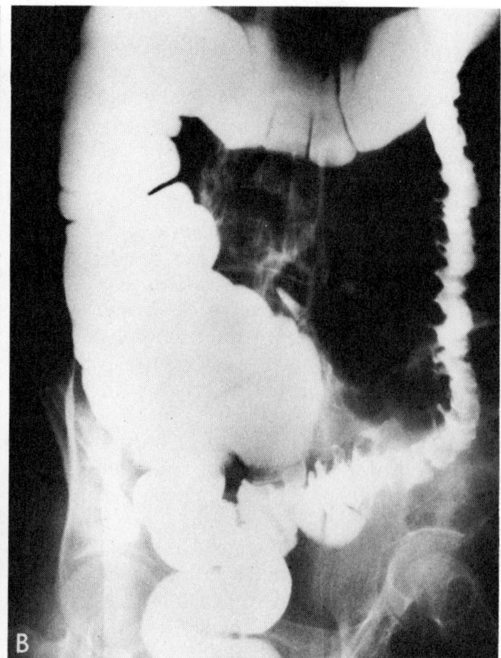

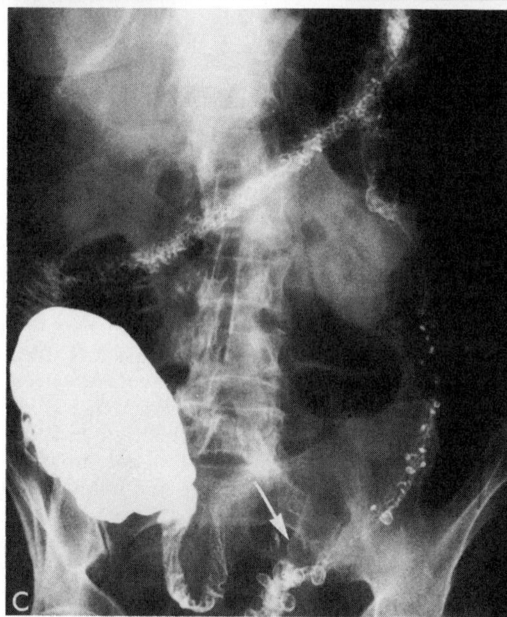

FIGURE 27–1. Radiologic features of diverticulosis and diverticulitis. Diverticuli may be asymptomatic or may be present in patients with symptoms identical to those of an irritable bowel syndrome. The barium enema can reveal a completely normal colon except for diverticula *(A)*. Patients with diverticulitis should be identified by the clinical findings of persistent pain, peritoneal irritation, fever, or leukocytosis. The barium enema may reveal spasm in a segment of colon with an irregular "saw-toothed" pattern *(B)*, which may be caused by colonic irritation but is an entirely nonspecific sign, since spasm for any reason produces it. The only specific radiographic sign of diverticulitis is barium outside a perforated diverticulum (as shown in the postevacuation film, *C*). This may represent the formation of walled-off microabscesses, or a gross perforation and abscess formation may be manifested by severe peritonitis, intestinal obstruction, or development of enteric fistulas. Computed tomography of the abdomen is a more sensitive and safer technique for detecting a pericolonic abscess. (Courtesy of Department of Radiology, Brigham and Women's Hospital, Harvard Medical School, Boston, Massachusetts.)

of gradually decreasing the frequency of office visits while maintaining a continuous relationship.

It has been suggested, though not proved, that *diverticulosis* may be a late consequence of the irritable bowel syndrome. Diverticula can be demonstrated by barium enema in 30% of people older than 60 years of age but are asymptomatic in most individuals.[23] The diverticula probably arise from herniations of colonic mucosa through weaknesses in the intestinal wall where blood vessels penetrate the muscularis propria. The intraluminal pressures required to cause these herniations are generated by the colons of some asymptomatic persons and of a substantial number of those with irritable bowel syndrome. Although a majority of those affected remain asymptomatic, some experience pain, flatulence, diarrhea, and constipation—symptoms indistinguishable from patients with irritable bowel syndrome without associated colonic diverticula. These diverticula may bleed when small blood vessels within them rupture. Many patients cease bleeding spontaneously with conservative therapy of bed rest, transfusion as needed, and a clear liquid diet. More persistent bleeding may stop with selective angiographic infusion of vasopressin (Pitressin) into the artery supplying the bleeding vessel or by embolization of the bleeding vessel at angiography. A few patients with refractory, life-threatening bleeding require surgical removal of the bleeding colonic segment. Diverticula may also become inflamed and produce diverticulitis characterized by fever, continuous as well as intermittent colicky pain, and/or signs of peritoneal inflammation, often localized to the left lower quadrant of the abdomen. Localized microabscesses are usually present, and abdominal CT scanning identifies the thickened inflamed colonic wall. Treatment with broad-spectrum antibiotics may be sufficient, but if frank rupture and abscess formation ensue (Fig. 27–1), surgical treatment with drainage and resection is usually required. Uncomplicated diverticulosis can be managed in the same manner as the irritable bowel syndrome.

PARASITIC AND INFECTIOUS CHRONIC DIARRHEA

Giardiasis can cause mild to severe chronic diarrhea.[24] If symptoms are severe, steatorrhea may often be present. Cysts in the stool establish the diagnosis but can be found in only approximately 60 to 70% of affected patients. Duodenal drainage and small intestinal biopsy usually reveal the trophozoites in the remaining 30 to 40% of patients. The treatment of choice is quinacrine hydrochloride, which is curative in 90 to 95% of patients. Metronidazole, although not approved for giardiasis in the United States, is also effective in 80 to 90% of patients.

Infections and parasitic infestations that normally produce acute, self-limiting diarrhea in immunocompetent individuals may produce chronic diarrheal disease with malabsorption in immunosuppressed patients. Indeed, chronic diarrhea occurs in up to 50% of North American patients with acquired immunodeficiency syndrome (AIDS).[25] For example, cryptosporidiosis produces a moderate self-limited diarrheal illness lasting 2 weeks or less in immunocompetent patients, but in patients with AIDS and other immunosuppressed populations, it produces chronic and often devastating diarrheal disease.[25, 26] Similarly, certain *Salmonella, Shigella,* and *Campylobacter* species cause self-limited diarrhea in most normal individuals but may produce chronic, relapsing diarrheal disease in patients with AIDS. The more common causes of chronic diarrhea and intestinal malabsorption in patients with AIDS are listed in Table 27–1.

Immunosuppressed patients with chronic diarrhea merit a thorough diagnostic evaluation since one or more causative specific pathogens can be identified in the majority.[25] Initially, the stool should be cultured thrice and assayed for *Clostridium difficile* toxin and examined for neutrophils and parasites using conventional and special (acid-fast, trichrome, iodine) preparations. If these studies are not conclusive, gastroduodenoscopy and colonoscopy should be considered to obtain biopsy specimens for histology and viral and mycobacterial culture. In addition, duodenal luminal contents should be examined for parasites. Electron microscopy of small intestinal and colonic biopsy samples may be required to establish the diagnosis in microsporidiosis and adenovirus infections, respectively.[25, 27] Patients in whom no causative agent can be identified may be suffering from infection or infestation with organisms that have not yet been recognized as potential pathogens. Whether or not infection of the intestine with the human immunodeficiency virus (HIV) itself causes viral disease is controversial.[28]

TABLE 27–1. CAUSES OF CHRONIC DIARRHEA IN AIDS

Parasitic	**Bacterial**
Cryptosporidia	*Salmonella*
Microsporidia	*Shigella*
Isospora belli	*Campylobacter*
Giardia lamblia	*Clostridium difficile*
	Mycobacterium avium–intercellulare
Viral	
Cytomegalovirus	**Fungal**
Adenovirus	*Histoplasma capsulatum*
Herpes simplex	
? HIV	

Upon isolation of a causative organism or organisms, appropriate treatment should be implemented. *Salmonella* and *Shigella* enterocolitis can be treated with ciprofloxacin, amoxicillin, or trimethoprim-sulfamethoxazole. *Campylobacter jejuni* infection can be treated with erythromycin or ciprofloxacin. *C. difficile* enterocolitis should be treated with metronidazole or vancomycin. *Isospora belli* infestation can be treated with trimethoprim-sulfamethoxazole or with pyrimethamine-sulfadoxine. Herpetic proctitis and cytomegalovirus colitis can be treated with acyclovir or ganciclovir, respectively. Unfortunately, there is no known effective therapy for adenovirus colitis or for *Cryptosporidium* or *Microsporidium* infestation. The efficacy of multiple drug regimens in the treatment of *Mycobacterium avium–intracellulare* in patients with AIDS is currently under study. There is some evidence that among patients with refractory AIDS-associated diarrhea, some will respond to administration of the somatostatin analog, octreotide.[29]

IDIOPATHIC INFLAMMATORY BOWEL DISEASE

Idiopathic inflammatory bowel diseases may develop in patients at any age, but the peak incidence of ulcerative colitis occurs between 19 and 49 years of age—that of Crohn's disease is between the ages of 10 and 30.[30–32] Ulcerative colitis occurs with about twice the frequency of Crohn's disease involving the small bowel and about four times that of Crohn's colitis.[30] These are chronic or recurrent illnesses that appear to be more prevalent in Jews of European extraction and that affect approximately one person per 1000 to 2000 people. The 10-fold increase in risk of developing these diseases among first-order relatives suggest that genetic factors are important in pathogenesis.[33]

Most patients with ulcerative colitis have an acute onset with bloody diarrhea followed by remissions and exacerbations. The clinical manifestations are mild during the initial episode in up to 50% of patients, and subsequent exacerbations tend to follow a similar pattern. The severity and character of diarrhea provides some insight into the extent of colonic involvement. Patients with disease involving one third or more of the colon may have severe diarrhea with many watery stools containing blood, mucus, and pus. In contrast, patients with disease confined to the rectosigmoid often have formed stools with several additional small-volume rectal discharges that contain blood, mucus, and pus. Of those patients with disease confined to the rectosigmoid at onset, only 5 to 15% ultimately progress to have involvement of a larger area of colon.[34]

Fever, weight loss, anemia, and constitutional symptoms are usually absent in individuals with disease limited to the rectum and distal sigmoid. Patients with extensive involvement of the colon often have manifestations of systemic illness, including fever, weight loss, fatigue, and anemia. Regardless of severity, the distal rectum is involved in virtually all patients with ulcerative colitis.[35]

The onset of Crohn's disease may be abrupt or insidious, but eventually, most patients develop either mild, moderate, or severe diarrhea. Hematochezia is uncommon in patients with disease limited to the small intestine, but stools are often positive for occult blood. In patients with colonic disease, hematochezia is more common. Gradual weight loss, low-grade fever, crampy abdominal pain, and anemia are common. Symptoms of intestinal obstruction may occur in those with small intestinal involvement. In some patients, severe diarrhea results from dysfunction of the terminal ileum, which allows bile salts to escape into the colon. In others, the presence of an ill-defined, tender mass in the ileocecal region or the presence of perianal disease, including fistulas or perirectal abscesses, suggest Crohn's disease.

Presence of an inflammatory process of some type can be confirmed if polymorphonuclear leukocytes can be identified on microscopic examination of the stool in patients with ulcerative colitis or Crohn's disease. Regardless of the severity, the patients may have extraintestinal manifestations, especially during exacerbations. These include acute synovitis, erythema nodosum, pyoderma gangrenosum, sclerosing cholangitis, episcleritis, and anterior uveitis.[31, 32, 36–38]

In some patients whose disease is confined to the colon, it may be impossible to differentiate between ulcerative colitis and Crohn's disease, although the presence of gross skip areas or focality of microscopic evidence of colonic mucosal inflammation suggests Crohn's disease. Extended follow-up of the patient ultimately often reveals the proper diagnosis (Table 27–2).

Diagnostic Evaluation. Active ulcerative colitis is almost always accompanied by an abnormal-appearing rectal mucosa at proctosigmoidoscopy. Early changes include mucosal edema resulting in decreased prominence of normal submucosal vessels, erythema, and a fine granular appearance of the mucosal surface. Friability is usually present. When the mucosa is traumatizied with a cotton swab or endoscope in patients with proctitis or colitis, petechiae appear and frank bleeding often results, whereas normal mucosa withstands this mild trauma. If the disease is more active, frank ulcers and bleeding are evident without wiping, and purulent exudate is prominent. Polymorphonuclear leukocytes are invariably seen if this exudate is examined microscopically.

Some patients with Crohn's colitis have mucosal changes visible at sigmoidoscopy that closely resemble those of ulcerative colitis, but many have normal-appearing rectal mucosa on sigmoidoscopy.[39] The appearance of the rectum can be characteristic, with fissures, fistulas, and/or a mucosa in which sharply demarcated ulcers are interspersed with normal-appearing areas.[40] It is crucial to rule out colitis caused by specific agents, especially in patients whose onset of symptoms is acute. Infectious bacterial colitis or proctitis and amebic colitis closely mimic the appearance and symptoms of idiopathic inflammatory bowel disease; hence, stool cultures, examination of stool for ova and parasites, and *Clostridium difficile* toxin determination are essential. Among patients who participate in receptive anal intercourse, gonococcal, herpetic, and syphilitic proctitis and lymphogranuloma venereum should be considered.

Rectal and colonic biopsies provide valuable confirmatory evidence in inflammatory bowel disease, although they are not in themselves diagnostic.[35, 41] In ulcerative colitis and proctitis, inflammation of the lamina propria, crypt abscesses, and a decrease in goblet cell mucus are characteristic but not specific findings, because they can also be seen in a variety of other inflammatory diseases, such as bacterial colitis. Alterations in glandular architecture with diminution of the number of glands and branching of glands are uncommon in acute bacterial colitis and suggest chronicity. Features suggesting Crohn's disease include focality of inflammation, the presence of granulomas, and inflammation of the deeper layers of the bowel wall (submucosa and muscularis propria), but biopsies in some patients with Crohn's colitis may appear indistinguishable from those seen in ulcerative colitis.[41] If, in Crohn's disease, the rectum appears grossly normal at sigmoidoscopy, the rectal biopsy is abnormal in about 10% of patients.[40]

Colonoscopy or barium enemas are indicated in patients with suspected inflammatory bowel disease when the diagnosis cannot be established at sigmoidoscopy or when the extent of disease is being determined. Colonoscopy and barium enemas are contraindicated in patients with ulcerative colitis or Crohn's colitis when there is severe or moderately severe acute disease or if the bowel is dilated and toxic megacolon is suspected. In this setting, the risk of serious complications such as perforation is increased. Preparation should be modified in patients with active disease and should consist of a clear liquid diet for 48 hours, followed by gentle tap-water enemas, only if necessary or administration of a polyethylene glycol electrolyte solution. Harsh laxatives are not needed and should be avoided; they can aggravate symptoms and induce complications.

Single-contrast barium studies may show shallow ulcerations along the edge of the bowel in ulcerative colitis and, with chronicity, loss of haustral markings and foreshortening of the colon. In Crohn's colitis, ulcerations interspersed with normal-appearing "skip areas" as well as ileal disease may be demonstrated. About 18% of patients with early ulcerative colitis have a normal single-contrast study.[42] Greater sensitivity is achieved by using air-contrast studies. A fine, diffusely granular appearance of the mucosa will be present in all except a few patients with active ulcerative colitis (Fig. 27–2).[42] Air-contrast studies show discrete, punched-out "aphthoid" ulcers within an otherwise normal mucosa in 40 to 50% of patients with early Crohn's colitis.[43]

Management. Ulcerative proctitis in which disease does not extend beyond the reach of the sigmoidoscope can generally be treated by corticosteroid enemas, sulfasalazine, 2 to 4 g/day, or both. If the disease is not responsive to local corticosteroids or if colonic involvement is more extensive, oral administration of corticosteroids (e.g., 40 to 60 mg/day of prednisone) may be required. This dosage is maintained until a remission is well established (usually 3 to 4 weeks) and then tapered gradually. Corticosteroids have not been shown to reduce the frequency of relapse.[44] In contrast, sulfasalazine, 2 g/day, has been shown to reduce the fre-

TABLE 27–2. FEATURES THAT HELP DISTINGUISH BETWEEN ULCERATIVE COLITIS AND CROHN'S COLITIS

	Ulcerative Colitis	Crohn's Colitis
Clinical features	Perianal abscesses, fistulas, and fissures rare Rectum involved	Perianal abscesses, fistulas, and fissures common Rectum may be spared
Radiology	Continuous involvement without skip areas No significant ileal involvement	Skip areas may be present Coexistent ileal disease may be present
Pathology	Diffuse, nonspecific mucosal inflammation Transmural inflammation uncommon	Inflammation may be focal or diffuse Granulomas present (~ 50%) Transmural inflammation common Deep fissures and ulcers common

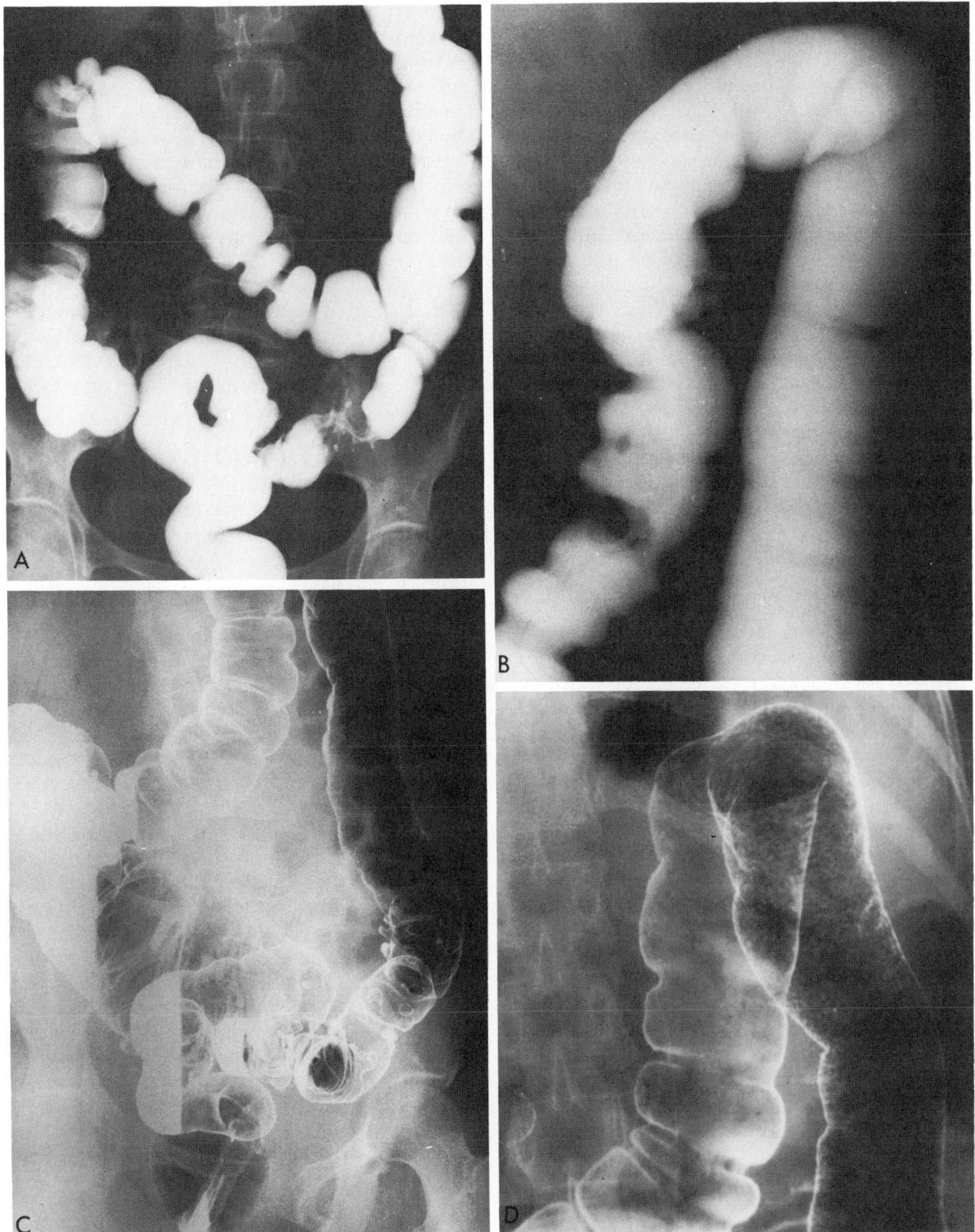

FIGURE 27–2. Radiologic features of ulcerative colitis. *A,* The single-contrast barium enema in this patient suggests a loss of haustral markings but otherwise is normal. *B,* No other findings, such as minute ulcerations at the edge of the lumen, can be identified. *C* and *D,* An air-contrast study of the same patient reveals the finely granular mucosal pattern, extending to the splenic flexure, that is typical of early or mild ulcerative colitis. (Courtesy of Department of Radiology, Brigham and Women's Hospital, Harvard Medical School, Boston, Massachusetts.)

quency of relapse in mild to moderate ulcerative colitis.[45] The active moiety in sulfasalazine is the aminosalicylic acid and newer preparations devoid of the sulfa moiety (mesalamine, olsalazine) are useful given orally to patients intolerant of sulfasalazine or as enemas (e.g., ROWASA rectal suspension enema) to patients who fail to respond to local corticosteroids.[46]

Patients with ulcerative colitis ultimately can be cured by total colectomy. The most frequent indications for surgery are life-threatening fulminant colitis with or without toxic megacolon, chronic debilitating disease that is refractory to medical therapy, and the risk of colon carcinoma. The risk of colon carcinoma depends on the extent and duration of disease and has been estimated to be 3 per cent or less during the first decade and up to 10% per decade thereafter in patients with ulcerative pancolitis.[47] The risk is only slight if disease is limited to proctosigmoiditis. It is recommended that careful surveillance in patients with extensive colonic involvement begin at the eighth to tenth year of disease, using colonoscopy.[48]

Crohn's disease responds less consistently to drug therapy and has a different natural history than ulcerative colitis. Acute exacerbations may respond to oral corticosteroids or to sulfasalazine, but there is no evidence that treatment with corticosteroids or sulfasalazine prolongs remissions or favorably influences the natural course of the disease.[49] In one study, sulfasalazine appeared most effective in patients with colonic involvement, whereas corticosteroids were most effective in patients with small bowel involvement.[49] Other possible effective agents in Crohn's disease include azathioprine[49] or its metabolite, 6-mercaptopurine,[50] and metronidazole.[51] Other drugs being evaluated include cyclosporine, methotrexate, chloroquine, and interferon,[46] but use of these agents should be limited to patients who are participating in controlled clinical trials until their efficacy has been documented. The role of surgery in Crohn's disease is limited to the treatment of complications, such as abscesses, enteric fistulas, strictures, and incapacitating medical intractability. As many as 75% of patients with Crohn's disease will eventually require surgery for complications.[52] However, surgery is not curative, and the high recurrence rate following resection of diseased bowel argues for limited resections and conservation of bowel, especially in patients with involvement of the small intestine.

OSMOTIC DIARRHEA

Lactose intolerance, a common cause of osmotic diarrhea, is highly prevalent, especially in blacks, American Indians, Asians, and Northern European Jews.[53] In primary lactose intolerance, there is an isolated acquired deficiency of lactase, a disaccharidase found in the brush border of intestinal absorptive cells with symptoms that are usually first manifest in adulthood. Secondary lactose intolerance may occur in any disease that causes extensive damage to the small intestinal mucosa, producing reduced mucosal lactase activity. Ingestion of lactose-containing dairy products results in abdominal cramps, bloating, and watery diarrhea. The diarrhea is induced by the osmotic effect of unabsorbed lactose and its breakdown products, which are produced by bacterial fermentation within the intestinal lumen. If stool electrolytes are measured during diarrhea, twice the sum of sodium and potassium is less than the stool osmolality, because the lactose and its breakdown products contribute to total osmolality. Unless the lactose load is unusually large, voluminous diarrhea is uncommon. Many but not all individuals with lactase deficiency recognize the association of their symptoms with ingestion of milk and other dairy products and spontaneously avoid these foods. Sensitivity to lactose varies among individuals, but diagnosis can usually be suspected if there is a sustained improvement during a therapeutic trial of a diet free of milk or other lactose-containing dairy products. The oral lactose tolerance test is of low specificity, but when necessary, diagnosis can be confirmed by small bowel biopsy, with assay of mucosa for lactase activity or by the measurement of hydrogen in the breath after oral administration of a lactose load (hydrogen breath test).[54]

Sucrose intolerance is associated with deficient activity of sucrase-isomaltase, another disaccharidase of the intestinal absorptive cell brush-border; malabsorption of glucose and galactose can result from congenitally defective active transport of these monosaccharides across the absorptive cell luminal membrane. These are rare disorders whose manifestations become apparent shortly after birth in affected individuals. In adults, a general intolerance for complex carbohydrates, in addition to steatorrhea, occurs in many diseases of the small bowel that are associated with generalized malabsorption.

Abuse of osmotic purgatives containing magnesium or sulfate produces a watery diarrhea of the osmotic type. Surreptitious laxative abuse can be extremely difficult to document; patients may deny using laxatives even when confronted with evidence and may switch from one type of laxative to another, which confuses the clinical state. If the stool contains more than 20 mM of magnesium per 24 hours or more than 4.5 mM of sulfate per liter, or if the sum of the sodium and potassium concentrations in liquid stool is less than the osmolality by more than 50 mM/l, the diagnosis of surreptitious laxative abuse should be considered.[55]

Diarrhea that accompanies generalized malabsorption is also associated with an osmotic component, because solubilized digestion products of unabsorbed foodstuffs and unabsorbed gastrointestinal secretions contribute to the oncotic pressure of the contents of the intestinal lumen.

SECRETORY DIARRHEA

Secretory diarrheas are characterized by large volumes of watery diarrhea that do not cease during 48 to 72 hours of fasting. Symptoms may be constant or may occur as intermittent attacks. Weight loss, dehydration, hypokalemia, nausea, vomiting, weakness, and crampy abdominal pain are features of the attacks. One form of the syndrome has been termed *pancreatic cholera,* or the watery diarrhea, hypokalemia, achlorhydria syndrome (WDHA). It is attributed, albeit not without controversy, to VIP secreted by noninsulin-producing tumors of the pancreas or, in 15 to 20% of patients, by ganglioneuromas or ganglioneuroblastomas.[56] Diarrhea in this syndrome is frequently accompanied by basal but not pentagastrin-fast achlorhydria, hypercalcemia, hyperglycemia, and dilatation of the gallbladder, all of which are probably induced by VIP or other putative humoral substances, such as prostaglandin E elaborated by the tumor. Determination of the plasma VIP level by radioimmunoassay is the only specific diagnostic test. Corticosteroids, octreoxide, indomethacin, lithium carbonate, or phenothiazines may reduce the diarrhea in some patients. However, responses may be transient, and efforts to localize the tumor and determine its extent and resectability by angiography and computed tomography should be carried out concurrently. Chemotherapy with streptozotocin and 5-fluorouracil has been helpful in most patients with unresectable tumors. A somatostatin analog, octreoxide, administered twice daily by subcutaneous injection was shown to produce long-term decreases in the volume of diarrhea and in release of VIP by the tumor.[57]

Clinical manifestations of a secretory type of diarrhea may also be present in Zollinger-Ellison syndrome, Addison's disease, carcinoid syndrome, medullary carcinoma of the thyroid, and villous adenoma. Most of these conditions can be recognized by their clinical features or laboratory tests (serum gastrin, calcitonin, urinary 5-hydroxyindoleacetic acid [HIAA]), and colonoscopy or barium enema. A most difficult clinical problem is distinguishing WDHA from surreptitious laxative or diuretic abuse, which probably occurs more commonly.[58] In secretory diarrheas, in contrast to osmotic diarrheas, twice the sum of stool sodium and potassium concentration is usually within 30 to 40 mM/l of equaling the stool osmolality. However, unlike osmotic cathartics, laxatives such as phenolphthalein, senna, and cascara produce a secretory diarrhea and may be continued surreptitiously while the patient is thought to be fasting. These purgatives can be detected in the stool by obtaining anthraquinone and phenolphthalein levels; they characteristically produce a dilated hypomotile colon which, after years, may have diminished haustral markings when seen on barium enema. With prolonged use, anthraquinones may produce melanosis coli of the rectum and distal colon, which can be recognized during proctosigmoidoscopy as brown to black mucosa pigmentation interrupted by pinhead-sized pale patches representing lymphoid follicles.

MALABSORPTION SYNDROME

Patients with malabsorption often excrete large volumes of diarrhea or stools. Not all patients have diarrhea, and some may even complain of constipation, but total stool mass is usually increased.[6] Diarrhea generally ceases or decreases markedly while the patient is fasting. Weight loss is common, often despite normal or even excessive caloric intake. Occasionally, patients present with osteopenic bone disease (bone pain or even pathologic fractures), with anemia caused by malabsorption of iron, folate, or even vitamin B_{12}, or with edema or ascites caused by hypoproteinemia secondary to exudation of serum proteins into the gut lumen.

The diseases that cause malabsorption can be divided into those that interfere primarily with the intraluminal phase of digestion and those that interfere primarily with the absorptive phase. Examples of the former include pancreatic exocrine insufficiency and hepatobiliary disease that may result in impaired delivery of bile into the lumen, whereas examples of the latter include a variety of mucosal diseases such as celiac sprue and Whipple's disease. The initial step in evaluation should be to document steatorrhea.[6] Staining of the stool for fat with Sudan 3 (Table 27–3) is a simple, rapid screening test that correlates remarkably well with quantitative stool fat analysis, the gold standard. Quantitative determination of stool fat requires that the patient be placed on a diet of known fat content, usually 80 to 100 g/day. After a 2- to 3-day equilibration period, stool is collected for 72 hours, and its fat content is determined chemically. Normal individuals excrete no more than 7 to 9 g/day of fat on this diet. Other less sensitive and less specific screening tests include the serum carotene and cholesterol, which are often low. Once steatorrhea has been documented, the D-xylose absorption test will usually show xylose malabsorption in patients in whom the mucosa is diffusely abnormal but not in those patients in whom only intraluminal digestion is impaired or in whom disease is confined to a small area of mucosa (e.g., pancreatic insufficiency, bile salt deficiency, and ileal dysfunction).[6] Radiographic studies of the small bowel are useful. If an abnormal mucosal pattern and/or dilatation are present, disease involving the intestinal mucosa is strongly suggested (Fig. 27–3).

In patients with malabsorption whose D-xylose absorption test is abnormal or in whom barium contrast studies suggest mucosal disease, a peroral small intestinal biopsy should be performed. There are a number of diffuse mucosal lesions (Whipple's disease and abetalipoproteinemia) and patchy mucosal lesions (lymphoma, eosinophilic enteritis, amyloidosis, and parasitic infestations) in which the pathology is specific and for which the biopsy may be diagnostic. The biopsy is abnormal but not diagnostic in, for example, celiac sprue, tropical sprue, and folate and vitamin B_{12} deficiency, because the histopathology is not specific. However, biopsy is valuable because it documents the presence of mucosal disease and the characteristic, if not specific, lesion. Precise diagnosis can then be established by other clinical information such as the patient's response to a gluten-free diet in suspected celiac-sprue, or geographic factors and the response to tetracycline and folate therapy in suspected tropical sprue. Normal small bowel biopsies are found in patients with postgastrectomy malabsorption, pancreatic exocrine insufficiency, and malabsorption due to hepatobiliary disease (Table 27–4). The diagnosis of celiac sprue can be established unequivocally only by a clinical and histologic response to a gluten-free diet.[59] The clinical response should be evident within a few weeks, although the mucosal abnormalities may require months or years to return to normal.[59]

TABLE 27–3. PERFORMING THE SUDAN STAIN

1. Place a small amount of stool (size of 1/2 of a "split pea") on a glass slide. If not liquid, add several drops water or saline and make a homogenate by using applicator stick as a pestle.
2. Add 2–3 drops of glacial acetic acid and 4–5 drops alcoholic solution of Sudan stain, mix, and add cover slip.
3. Heat with alcohol lamp or burner to boiling to facilitate hydrolysis of soaps to free fatty acids and to facilitate staining.
4. Examine under a microscope while slide is warm using low power to locate stained fat droplets and high power to examine droplets.
    - Normal: A few small droplets should be noticeable and represent normal fat excretion; these reassure the examiner that the slide has been prepared properly.
    - Abnormal: A much larger number and size of reddish-colored round droplets indicate steatorrhea.

Pitfalls: The skillful examiner gains experience by comparing an examination of stool from patients with steatorrhea with that from normal individuals. False-positive results may occur in patients receiving castor oil, mineral oil, and oil-based suppositories. False-negative results may result from barium diluting the stool. Failure to examine the slide while warm may result in conversion of the stained melted fat droplets to unstained needle-like fatty acid crystals. The slide should then be reheated and re-examined.

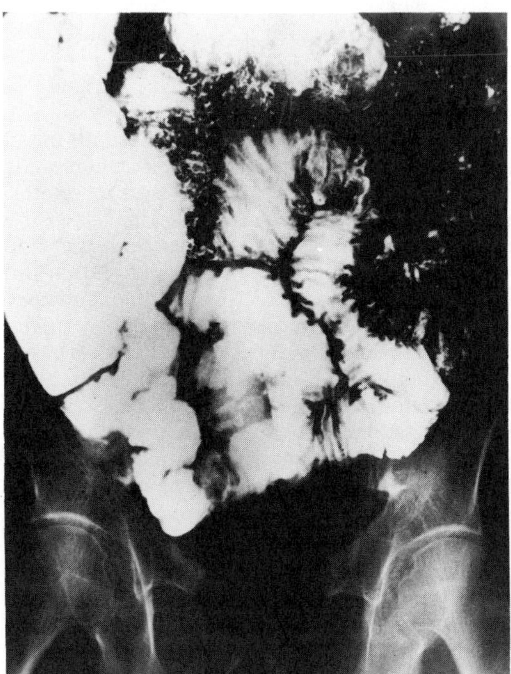

FIGURE 27–3. Radiologic features of the malabsorption syndrome caused by mucosal disease of the small bowel. The x-ray film shows dilatation and an abnormal mucosal pattern in addition to the nonspecific features of segmentation and fragmentation of barium.

TABLE 27–4. INFORMATION PROVIDED BY SMALL INTESTINAL BIOPSY

Disorders in Which Biopsy Is Diagnostic	
Diffuse Lesions	
Whipple's disease	Abetalipoproteinemia
Agammaglobulinemia	Giardiasis
Patchy Lesions	
Lymphoma	*Mycobacterium avium–intracellulare*
Lymphangiectasia	Cytomegalovirus
Eosinophilic enteritis	Coccidiosis
Systemic mastocytosis	Strongyloidiasis
Amyloidosis	Microsporidiosis
Crohn's disease	Cryptosporidiosis
Disorders in Which Biopsy Is Abnormal But Not Diagnostic	
Celiac sprue	Folate and B_{12} deficiency
Tropical sprue	Radiation enteritis
Unclassified sprue	Radiomimetic drugs
Infectious gastroenteritis	Malnutrition
Intraluminal bacterial overgrowth	Zollinger-Ellison syndrome
Disorders in Which Biopsy Is Normal	
Postgastrectomy malabsorption	Pancreatic exocrine insufficiency
Hepatic diseases	

Patients with malabsorption caused by chronic exocrine pancreatic insufficiency due to chronic pancreatitis, pancreatic carcinoma, or cystic fibrosis and patients with malabsorption caused by chronic hepatobiliary disease such as primary biliary cirrhosis, sclerosing cholangitis, or cholangiocarcinoma usually have normal xylose absorption and demonstrate a normal small intestinal mucosal pattern radiologically. Post-prandial or constant epigastric pain often radiating to the back are common features of chronic pancreatitis and pancreatic cancer. Abdominal ultrasound, abdominal computed tomography, and endoscopic retrograde cholangiopancreatography are helpful diagnostic maneuvers. Quantitation of sweat electrolyte secretion is of diagnostic value in suspected cystic fibrosis. Response to a therapeutic trial of oral pancreatic enzyme replacement may be helpful. Pancreatic exocrine function can be assessed by the secretin/cholecystokinin stimulation test or by the less cumbersome but less specific *N*-benzoyl-*L*-tyrosyl-*P*-aminobenzoic acid absorption test.

Overgrowth of bacteria in the proximal small intestine is associated with stasis, decreased acid secretion, and defective immunoglobulin production. Visceral scleroderma, multiple jejunal diverticula, small intestinal strictures, pernicious anemia, and acid-reducing gastric surgery are predisposing factors. Quantitative culture of jejunal fluid (including anaerobic and microaerophilic cultures) are diagnostic if properly done but require sophisticated bacteriologic methods. Abnormal vitamin B_{12} absorption, both with and without added intrinsic factor in the absence of ileal disease, has diagnostic value, because intraluminal bacteria bind this vitamin before it can be absorbed in the ileum. Treatment with ampicillin or tetracycline and metronidazole is useful as is surgical correction of stasis-producing lesions.

OTHER CAUSES OF DIARRHEA

Whenever the onset of diarrhea is acute, the possibility of drug-induced diarrhea must be considered. The patient's history may reveal the onset of diarrhea in concert with or shortly after the prescription of a new medication such as quinidine sulfate, colchicine, a magnesium-containing antacid, or an antibiotic. The diagnosis is confirmed if symptoms resolve when the suspected offending drug is discontinued.

Polyps and carcinoma of the colon may produce diarrhea associated with cramping and occult or gross bleeding into the stools. The diarrhea may be caused by overflow of liquid stool around a partially obstructing lesion. Villous adenomas, especially when located in the distal large bowel, may result in diarrhea characterized by copious mucus and hypokalemia, because the tumor secretes a protein- and potassium-rich fluid without producing luminal obstruction. All patients older than 40 years of age who present with a persistent change in bowel habits, crampy abdominal pain associated with diarrhea, or stools positive for occult blood should be evaluated with a colonoscopy or sigmoidoscopy and air-contrast barium enema.

REFERENCES

1. Levitt MD and Duane WC: Floating stools—flatus versus fat. N Engl J Med 286:973, 1972.
2. Poley JR and Hofmann AF: Role of fat maldigestion in pathogenesis of steatorrhea in ileal resection: Fat digestion after two sequential test meals without and with cholestyramine. Gastroenterology 71:38, 1976.
3. Binder HJ and Mehta P: Short-chain fatty acids stimulate active sodium and chloride absorption in vitro in the rat distal colon. Gastroenterology 96:989, 1989.
4. Hofmann AF and Poley JR: Role of bile acid malabsorption in pathogenesis of diarrhea and steatorrhea in patients with ileal resection. Gastroenterology 62:918, 1972.
5. Mekhjian HS, Phillips SF, and Hofmann AF: Colonic secretion of water and electrolytes induced by bile acids: Perfusion studies in man. J Clin Invest 50:1569, 1971.
6. Trier JS: Intestinal malabsorption: Differentiation of cause. Hosp Pract 23:195, 1988.
7. Drossman DA, Powell DW, and Sessions JT Jr: The irritable bowel syndrome. Gastroenterology 73:811, 1977.
8. Thompson WG and Heaton KW: Functional bowel disorders in apparently healthy people. Gastroenterology 79:283, 1980.
9. Drossman DA, Sandler RS, McKee DC, et al: Bowel patterns among subjects not seeking health care. Gastroenterology 83:529, 1982.
10. Powell DW: The irritable bowel syndrome. Intestinal motility. Gastroenterology 73:812, 1977.
11. Kellow JE and Phillips SF: Altered small bowel motility in irritable bowel syndrome is correlated with symptoms. Gastroenterology 92:1885, 1987.
12. Snape WJ, Wright SH, Battle WM, et al: The gastrocolic response: Evidence for a neural mechanism. Gastroenterology 77:1235, 1979.
13. Mitra R, Chura C, Rajendra GR, et al: Effect of progressive rectal distention in irritable bowel syndrome. Gastroenterology 66:770, 1974.
14. Mendeloff AI, Monk M, Siegel C, et al: Illness experience and life stresses in patients with the irritable colon syndrome and with ulcerative colitis. N Engl J Med 282:14, 1970.
15. Sandler RS, Drossman DA, Nathan HP, et al: Symptom complaints and health-care-seeking behavior in subjects with bowel dysfunction. Gastroenterology 87:314, 1984.
16. Sessions JT: The irritable bowel syndrome: Diagnosis, treatment, and prognosis. Gastroenterology 73:818, 1977.
17. Thompson WG: The irritable colon. Can Med Assoc J 111:1240, 1984.
18. Ritchie JA and Truelove SC: Treatment of irritable bowel syndrome with lorazepam, hyoscine, butylbromide, and ispaghula husk. Br J Med 1:376, 1979.
19. Longstretch GF, Fox D, Youkeles L, et al: Psyllium therapy in irritable bowel syndrome. Ann Intern Med 95:53, 1981.
20. Klein KB: Controlled treatment trials in the irritable bowel syndrome: A critique. Gastroenterology 95:232, 1988.
21. Sutalf LO and Levitt MD: Follow-up of a flatulent patient. Dig Dis Sci 24:652, 1979.

22. Whitehead WE and Schuster MM: Physiological management of the irritable bowel syndrome. Pract Gastroenterol 3:32, 1979.
23. Almy TP and Howell DA: Diverticular disease of the colon. N Engl J Med 302:324, 1980.
24. Chester AC, MacMurray FG, Restifo MD, et al: Giardiasis as a chronic disease. Dig Dis Sci 30:215, 1985.
25. Smith PD, Quinn TC, Strober W, et al: Gastrointestinal infections in AIDS. Ann Intern Med 116:63, 1992.
26. Current WL, Reese NC, Ernst JV, et al: Human cryptosporidiosis in immunocompetent and immunodeficient persons. N Engl J Med 308:1252, 1983.
27. Kotler DP, Francisco A, Clayton F, et al: Small intestinal injury and parasitic diseases in AIDS. Ann Intern Med 113:444, 1990.
28. Heise C, Dandekar S, Kumar P, et al: Human immunodeficiency virus infection of enterocytes and mononuclear cells in human jejunal mucosa. Gastroenterology 100:1521, 1991.
29. Cello JP, Grendell JH, Basuk P, et al: Effect of octreotide on refractory AIDS-associated diarrhea: A prospective, multicenter clinical trial. Ann Intern Med 115:705, 1991.
30. Monk M, Mendeloff AI, Siegel C, et al: An epidemiological study of ulcerative colitis and regional enteritis among adults in Baltimore: Social and demographic factors. Gastroenterology 56:847, 1969.
31. Cello JP and Schneiderman DJ: Ulcerative colitis. *In* Sleisenger MH and Fordtran JS (eds): Gastrointestinal Disease: Pathophysiology, Diagnosis, and Management, 4th ed. Philadelphia, WB Saunders, 1989, pp 1435–1476.
32. Donaldson RM, Jr: Crohn's disease. *In* Sleisenger MH and Fordtran JS (eds): Gastrointestinal Disease: Pathophysiology, Diagnosis, and Management, 4th ed. Philadelphia, WB Saunders, 1989, pp 1327–1358.
33. Orholm M, Munkholm P, Langholz E, et al: Familial occurrence of inflammatory bowel disease. N Engl J Med 324:84, 1991.
34. Sparberg M, Fennessy J, and Kirsner JB: Ulcerative proctitis and mild ulcerative colitis: A study of 220 patients. Medicine 45:391, 1966.
35. Flick AL, Voegtlin KF, and Rubin CE: Clinical experience with suction biopsy of the rectal mucosa. Gastroenterology 42:691, 1962.
36. Greenstein AJ, Janowitz HD, and Sachar DB: The extra-intestinal complications of Crohn's disease and ulcerative colitis. Medicine 55:401, 1976.
37. Lindor KD, Wiesner RH, MacCarty RL, et al: Advances in primary sclerosing cholangitis. Am J Med 89:73, 1990.
38. Dekker-Saeys BJ, Meuwissen SGM, Van Den Berg-Loonen EM, et al: II: Prevalence of peripheral arthritis, sacroiliitis, and ankylosing spondylitis in patients suffering from inflammatory bowel disease. Ann Rheum Dis 37:33, 1978.
39. Mekhjian HS, Switz DM, Melnyk CS, et al: National cooperative Crohn's disease study: Clinical features and natural history of Crohn's disease. Gastroenterology 77:898, 1979.
40. Hill RB, Kent TH, and Hansen RN: National cooperative Crohn's disease study: Clinical usefulness of rectal biopsy in Crohn's disease. Gastroenterology 77:938, 1979.
41. Goldman H and Antonioli DA: Mucosal biopsy of the rectum, colon, and distal ileum. Hum Pathol 13:981, 1982.
42. Bartram CI: Radiology in the current assessment of ulcerative colitis. Gastrointest Radiol 1:383, 1977.
43. Bull DM, Peppercorn MA, Glotzer DJ, et al: Crohn's disease of the colon. Gastroenterology 76:607, 1979.
44. Lennard-Jones JE, Misiewicz JJ, Connell AU, et al: Prednisone as maintenance treatment for ulcerative colitis in remission. Lancet 1:188, 1965.
45. Lennard-Jones JE, Connell AM, Barron JH, et al: Controlled trial of sulfasalazine in maintenance therapy for ulcerative colitis. Lancet 1:185, 1965.
46. Peppercorn MA: Advances in drug therapy for inflammatory bowel disease. Ann Intern Med 112:50, 1990.
47. Ekbom A, Helmick C, Zack M, et al: Ulcerative colitis and colorectal cancer: A population-based study. N Engl J Med 323:1228, 1990.
48. Ridell RH, Goldman H, Ransohoff DH, et al: Dysplasia in inflammatory bowel disease: Standardized classification with provisional clinical applications. Hum Pathol 14:931, 1983.
49. Summers RW, Switz DM, and Sessions JT Jr: National cooperative Crohn's disease study. Results of drug treatment. Gastroenterology 77:847, 1979.
50. O'Brien JJ, Bayless TM, and Bayless JA: Use of azathioprine or 6-mercaptopurine in the treatment of Crohn's disease. Gastroenterology 101:39, 1991.
51. Ursing B, Alm T, Barany F, et al: A comparative study of metronidazole and sulfasalazine for active Crohn's disease: The cooperative Crohn's disease study in Sweden. Gastroenterology 83:550, 1982.
52. Truelove SC and Pena AS: Course and prognosis of Crohn's disease. Gut 17:192, 1976.
53. Bayless TM: Recognition of lactose intolerance. Hosp Pract 11:97, 1976.
54. Bond JH and Levitt MD: Quantitative measurement of lactose absorption. Gastroenterology 70:1058, 1976.
55. Morris AI and Turnberg LA: Surreptitious laxative abuse. Gastroenterology 77:780, 1979.
56. Delvalle J and Yamada T: Secretory tumors of the pancreas. *In* Sleisenger MH and Fordtran JF (eds): Gastrointestinal Disease: Pathophysiology, Diagnosis, and Management, 4th ed. Philadelphia, WB Saunders, 1989, pp 1884–1900.
57. Gordon P, Comi RJ, Maton PN, et al: Somatostatin and somatostatin analogue (SMS 201-995) in treatment of hormone-secreting tumors of the pituitary and gastrointestinal tract and non-neoplastic diseases of the gut. Ann Intern Med 110:35, 1989.
58. Read NW, Krejs GJ, Read MG, et al: Chronic diarrhea of unknown origin. Gastroenterology 78:264, 1980.
59. Trier JS: Celiac sprue. N Engl J Med 325:1709, 1991.

28

Anorectal Disorders

ROGER L. CHRISTIAN, MD

Most Americans will be afflicted by one or more problems of the anorectal region during their lifetime. For many, the symptoms are minimal and may never require evaluation by a physician. For the individual who seeks medical attention, the clinician is faced with differentiating among several affictions of the anorectal region that are often interrelated.

EXAMINATION AND DIAGNOSTIC MEASURES

History

The physician should carefully elicit a description of symptoms and not be misled by the patient's usual self-diagnosis of hemorrhoids. The general health of the individual must be determined and consideration given to systemic disease that might produce abnormalities of the anorectum.

In addition, a careful history to discover upper or lower gastrointestinal dysfunction must be taken. The frequency of defecation, the character of the stool, and whether the patient is a "setter" or a "strainer" are important to learn. Finally, inquiries regarding the use of stool softeners, cathartics, and enemas must be made.

Symptoms associated with defecation should be sought. Inquiry should be made about pain with or following the bowel movement. The presence of blood (on the toilet paper or dripping into the toilet bowl), mucous or purulent drainage, the intermittent presence of a mass (or masses), and pruritus all should be considered.

Clinical Anatomy

To perform a meaningful examination, it is necessary to understand the anatomy of the anorectum. This region is approximately 4 cm in length (Fig. 28–1). The external boundary is at the anal verge, that is, the zone of change from normal skin of the buttocks to modified skin of the anal canal (without hair follicles or sweat glands). Midway through the anal canal is the junction between modified skin and cuboidal epithelium, most commonly known as the "dentate" or pectinate line. Deep to the modified skin at the dentate line are the anal crypts. At the base of each crypt, ducts to the anal glands open. These glands are usually in the submucosa, but many penetrate the internal sphincter and lie in the intersphincteric space.

An experienced examiner is often able to identify the dentate line by palpation. Skin tags are felt easily at this site. In the normal state, the junction can be identified readily by anoscopy. Modified skin has the appearance of a cloudy white membrane that abuts the purple-red mucosa of the rectum. Cutaneous sensory fibers accompany the modified skin to the dentate line.

Venous plexuses are deep to the skin and mucosa. The external hemorrhoidal veins are located external to the dentate line. As a result, they are invested with cutaneous sensory fibers. Just within the canal (and above the dentate line) are located the internal hemorrhoidal veins. These veins and overlying mucosa are not associated with cutaneous sensory fibers. This is the reason why inflamed internal hemorrhoids are usually heralded by painless bleeding.

Encircling the anal canal are two sets of muscles, the internal and external sphincters (see Fig. 28–1). The components of the external sphincter are under voluntary control. They maintain continence of stool and relax when defecation is initiated. The internal sphincter consists of smooth muscle and is, therefore, involuntary.

Physical Examination

Although examination primarily relates to the anal region, abdominal examination should not be neglected. In addition to searching for abdominal masses and tenderness, it should be determined whether the patient is constipated and has stool that one can palpate in the sigmoid colon or higher.

Anal examination begins with inspection of the perianal skin. Evidence of chronic irritation, scars, sinuses, or masses should be noted. The patient is asked to "bear down" as the examiner distracts the perianal tissues to see whether prolapse of hemorrhoids or mucosa or a fissure is present. Palpation around the anus may identify tender-

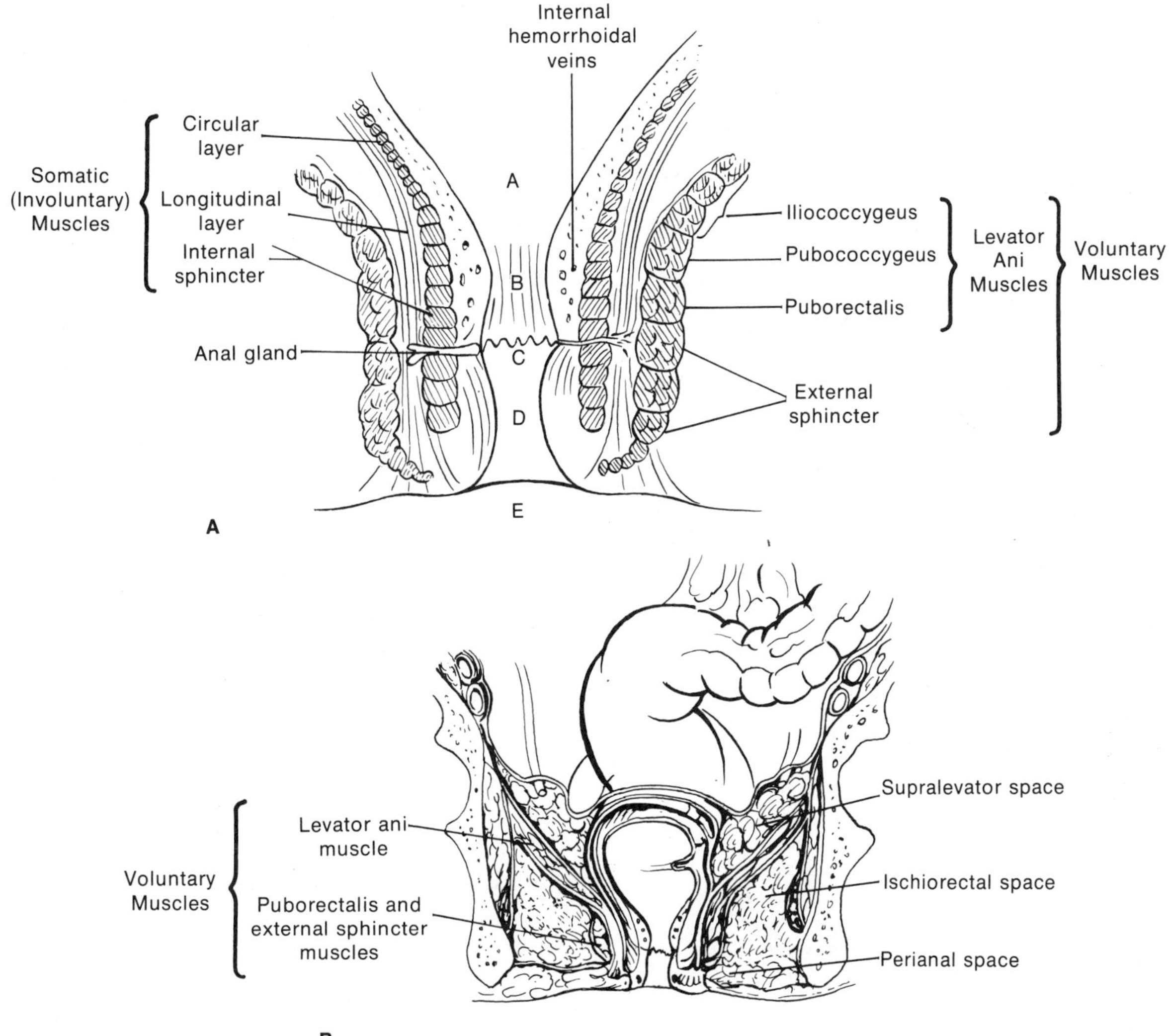

FIGURE 28–1. *A,* Clinical anatomy of anorectal region: (A) columnar epithelium; (B) cuboidal epithelium; (C) dentate line; (D) modified squamous epithelium; (E) normal skin beginning at the anal verge. *B,* Coronal section of anus, rectum, and pelvis. (Adapted from F. Netter, M.D.)

ness or induration at sites of inflammation, abscess, or fistula.

A well-lubricated finger then can be inserted into the anal canal. For the patient who has marked pain (and reflex spasm of the sphincter), insertion of the finger may be aided by having the patient bear down. As the Valsalva maneuver is performed and the anal canal descends, the sphincter relaxes. If the examining digit is held in position during this maneuver, the anus frequently will envelop the finger for a short distance. As the patient relaxes, the palpating finger follows the anal ring as it ascends to its normal position. After a moment of relaxation, the patient again strains "over" the fixed finger. By repeating the sequence several times, one is able to perform a limited examination. If one area is particularly sensitive, pressure can be applied against the opposite wall.

Abnormalities detected by palpation within the rectum include induration, abscess, fissure, or mass. If the patient has marked tenderness and the examination is thus limited, one must be certain that there is no internal abscess that is undetected. If complete examination is not possible, treatment should be started and the examination repeated in 1 to 3 days.

Anoscopy and Sigmoidoscopy

Two additional aids are used in evaluating disorders of the anorectal region. The anoscope is an instrument that should be used by all who practice primary care. Preparation for anoscopy is usually unnecessary. Positions that afford the best exposure are either the Sims' (lateral decubitus) or the knee-chest position.

The instrument is inserted only after digital examination has been performed to detect tenderness or a mass and to determine the axis of the anal canal. The instrument is lubricated and placed at the anal verge. As the patient bears down, it is advanced in a fashion similar to that described for digital examination. The anoscope is initially directed in line with the axis of the anal canal (for most patients, this means pointing the scope toward the umbilicus). Once beyond the level of the sphincter, the scope should be directed to follow the axis of the rectum along the curve of the sacrum. It is usually passed without difficulty to the shoulder of the instrument.

The anoscope is next stabilized, and the obturator is removed. Usually, the anterior wall of the rectum is seen. Frequently, a small area (1 cm^2) of ecchymosis is found where the obturator had rested. Normal mucosa is pink, smooth, and glistening. The instrument is angled so that the lumen of the rectum is seen. The scope is then withdrawn and moved in circular fashion so that the entire wall is inspected. As one approaches the sphincters, the presence of enlarged hemorrhoids may be demonstrated by asking the patient to bear down. Enlarged hemorrhoids will protrude into the lumen and will easily be seen.

If the patient has considerable discomfort during the terminal portion of the examination as the end of the anoscope runs over the area of sensitivity, reflex spasm of the anal sphincter will quickly expel the anoscope. For this reason, the examiner may be unable to obtain an adequate view and may initiate treatment on the basis of the symptoms and findings at palpation. Anoscopy can be repeated in several days, after the inflammation has subsided.

The rigid and flexible sigmoidoscopes also are used to evaluate the anorectum. Contrary to common belief, these instruments do not provide as good a view of the anal canal as the anoscope. This is particularly important to consider when seeking the source of hematochezia. Hemorrhoids that may be the site of blood loss can easily be overlooked. Finding a sinus opening is also more difficult with a sigmoidoscope. Disorders limited to the anal canal are best evaluated by anoscopy, except in the case of fissure.

COMMON SYMPTOM COMPLEXES

Bleeding

Multiple causes of hematochezia have been enumerated by Welch.[1] An adaptation of his classification lists the causes in order of approximate frequency (Table 28–1).

For bleeding that arises from the anorectum, the usual description is that of blood on the toilet paper. Occasionally the stool may be blood streaked, or the patient describes blood dripping into the toilet after defecation. The blood is usually "fresh" in that it is bright red in appearance (arterial in origin) and may be seen to clot.

Blood that arises from a site higher in the colon may be mixed with stool and darker in color. However, these alterations do not occur if the bleeding is brisk and the blood is evacuated quickly.

Rectal bleeding is usually painless. The complaint should be evaluated by inspection, digital examination, and anoscopy.

The extent of diagnostic work-up depends on symptoms, findings, and age of the patient. In a young patient whose bleeding is explained by a lesion visible on anorectal examination, one might proceed no further. For individuals above an arbitrary age of 35 or 40 years, or those with a family history of colonic cancer, sigmoidoscopy, barium enema, and/or colonoscopy are usually indicated to rule out other sites of blood loss.

The most common source of hematochezia is a hemorrhoid. Although the patient may describe considerable loss of blood each day, internal hemorrhoids may appear quiescent at the time of anoscopy. The bleeding may have occurred during the passage of a large and firm stool hours before. If there is easy prolapse of mucosa, which appears inflamed or bleeds with minimal abrasion, and the patient describes blood only on the toilet paper, the presumptive evidence is great that such is the source.

The second most frequent cause for bleeding is an anal fissure. The patient so afflicted usually has bleeding with defecation. Frequently a sharp or burning pain during and after a bowel movement is the primary symptom. It is common for the unaware physician and patient to assume "hemorrhoids" are the culprit. Anoscopy is usually precluded by marked discomfort. Treatment is based on a careful history and limited, but very specific, findings.

Whenever blood is mixed with stool or there is bloody diarrhea, one should suspect a disease process higher in the rectum or colon. Inflammatory conditions should be recognized easily by anoscopy or sigmoidoscopy. Several etiologies exist.

Ulcerative proctitis may present with tenesmus, a mucopurulent discharge, and either diarrhea or constipation. Findings at sigmoidoscopy include inflamed and friable mucosa, but the process is limited by a sharply defined border several centimeters above the dentate line.

Active ulcerative colitis is similar in appearance. If the mucosa appears intact, gentle wiping with a rectal swab may reveal an area of punctate hemorrhages representing ulcers. Barium enema or colonoscopy is usually necessary to define the extent of involvement. Since the disease may fluctuate, the mucosa can appear normal at times. Even then, a biopsy of the rectal mucosa often reveals atrophic changes.[2]

Crohn's disease of the colon may appear much like ulcerative colitis, but more characteristically there are perianal fistulas and inflammation out of proportion to the pain.

The gross and microscopic appearance of the mucosa in shigellosis, other acute dysenteries, or amebic colitis may mimic ulcerative colitis. The correct diagnosis is confirmed by appropriate microscopic and microbiologic studies of the stool.

Inflammatory changes may occur in rectal mucosa secondary to recurrent prolapse due to frequent straining, chronic use of cathartics, or enlarged hemorrhoids.[3]

Proctologic changes may also occur with nontraditional sexual practices. Anal receptive intercourse or sexual stimulation with foreign objects placed in the rectum can result in rectal ulcers and tears, prolapsed hemorrhoids, nonspecific proctitis, anal fissures, or perirectal abscesses. Coexistent also may be gonorrheal proctitis, with signs and symptoms that mimic idiopathic ulcerative colitis. Parasitic and other infectious causes of proctocolitis or proctitis also occur

TABLE 28–1. CAUSES OF HEMATOCHEZIA*

Most Common Causes
Hemorrhoids
Anal fissure
Less Common Causes
Cancer of the colorectum
Benign polypoid lesions of the colon
Inflammatory bowel diseases
Diverticulosis/diverticulitis
Unusual Causes
Anticoagulants and blood dyscrasias
Infectious disease (amebiasis, schistosomiasis, infectious diarrheas)
Meckel's diverticulum
Vascular lesions (ischemic colitis and mesenteric artery thrombosis)
Traumatic lesions (blunt or penetrating trauma)
Duodenal ulcer with extremely rapid bleeding
Intussusception
Small bowel tumors
Benign tumors of the colon
Unusual malignant tumors of the colorectum (leiomyomas, malignant lymphoma)
Arteriovenous malformations
Angiodysplasia of the colon

*Adapted from Welch CE: Colon hemorrhage. *In* Hardy JD (ed): Rhoads' Textbook of Surgery. Philadelphia, JB Lippincott, 1977, p 1196.

more commonly in homosexual men. By keeping these diagnoses in mind and performing appropriate cultures and smears, the physician will not overlook infectious diseases in patients with proctitis.[4]

Polyps, diverticula, arteriovenous malformations, and carcinoma usually bleed in a more erratic fashion. Depending on the site in the colon, local blood supply, and whether there is ulceration of the lesion, the hematochezia may assume different characteristics. Often the bleeding is very slow and only detected by testing for occult blood.

Pain

Another common symptom is pain. Table 28–2 lists several diagnoses in order of frequency.

The most prevalent conditions associated with pain are inflamed hemorrhoids, perianal abscess, and anal fissure. With the first two abnormalities, the discomfort is usually constant and aggravated by certain activities or postures. Remaining erect increases venous congestion and intensifies pain. Direct pressure while sitting also incites the discomfort.

Passage of stool may increase pain only slightly in the presence of inflamed hemorrhoids or abscess. In contrast, a fissure usually causes extreme discomfort during and after a bowel movement. An occasional patient with chronic fissure may experience little or no unpleasantness during defecation and find blood on the toilet paper as the only symptom.

Hemorrhoids become painful when inflammation or thrombosis develops. In an early stage, lax mucosa prolapses through the anal canal during defecation and spontaneously returns after the passage. Over time, there may be increased prolapse to the degree the patient must "tuck" the tissue above the sphincter to achieve comfort.

Increasing prolapse may suddenly get to the point at which the tissues no longer reduce, even with much pressure. Known as a "prolapsed and incarcerated internal hemorrhoid," this has the appearance of edematous tissue emanating through the anal canal. Since the external surface is rectal mucosa, it appears pink or "fleshy," with a mucous exudate. Several small clots may be seen, and areas of ulceration may be present. Pain is the primary complaint that brings the patient to the physician. The pain is constant and affected more by posture than by bowel actions. This process resolves over several days.

TABLE 28–2. CAUSES OF ANORECTAL PAIN

Most Common Causes
- Hemorrhoids
  - External anal thrombosis
  - Prolapsed thrombosed internal hemorrhoids
- Anal fissure
- Anorectal abscess
- Pilonidal abscess

Less Common Causes
- Inflammatory processes
  - Ulcerative proctitis
  - Ulcerative colitis
  - Granulomatous colitis
  - Bacterial and parasitic proctitis
  - Rectal prolapse
  - Traumatic proctitis
- Neoplastic processes
- Proctalgia fugax
- Coccygodynia

Thrombosis of an external hemorrhoidal vein is recognized as a purple mass covered with skin arising without the dentate line. During the early and most painful phase, the skin is taut and shiny. Direct pressure causes severe discomfort. As the process subsides, the overlying skin becomes wrinkled, and the mass diminishes in size. This condition is known variously as "external anal thrombosis" or "acute thrombosed hemorrhoid."

Anal fissure is the most misdiagnosed malady of the anal canal. Too frequently, a hasty history and cursory examination lead one to implicate "hemorrhoids." It is not unusual for a patient with a fissure to have been seen by several physicians and prescribed varying treatment regimens before the correct diagnosis is made.

An anal fissure is a linear ulceration in the modified skin just without the dentate line. The hallmark of this disorder is exquisite pain associated with passage of stool or examination. More than just an abrasion or tear in the epithelium, there is considerable inflammation that sensitizes the cutaneous pain fibers and causes marked discomfort. Typically, the fissure is situated in the posterior midline. Spreading the buttocks occasionally reveals the most external portion of the lesion as a small ulceration. A "sentinel pile" external to the fissure is frequently described but is not a constant finding. If present, it represents merely a fold of skin that may obscure or divert attention from the fissure.

When digital examination is permitted by the patient, the sphincter is found to be spastic. Induration surrounding the fissure is a subtle finding. The tender "trigger site" is barely within the anal verge and before the dentate line. If the patient permits anoscopy, the study is usually of little value, since the instrument is typically expelled by reflex contraction when the tender area is abraded.

Despite the marked discomfort, the physician should endeavor to palpate the rectum above the sphincter to be certain there is no occult abscess. If an abscess is considered likely, an examination under anesthesia may be necessary.

Abscess of the anorectal region becomes symptomatic according to its location. An abscess begins as infection in a perianal gland. If it does not resolve, the inflammatory process spreads in one of several directions, and the abscess develops in a distant location. As a result, symptoms and findings relate to the site of the infection. The variety of locations are depicted in Figure 28–2.

The most frequent site of abscess formation is the perianal region. In one report, anorectal abscesses were found to be perianal in 75% of cases; in 13%, abscesses were pelvirectal; and in 6%, they were ischiorectal. An additional small group was located near the anus but these were of uncharacteristic etiology (e.g., furuncles, sebaceous cysts, pilonidal abscesses, abscesses of Bartholin cysts, episiotomy abscesses, or hidradenitis suppurativa).[5]

Classification of abscesses is made on the basis of symptoms and location. Both perianal and ischiorectal abscesses are associated with severe localized pain. The perianal abscess is typically a well-demarcated swelling just without the anal verge. In contrast, the ischiorectal abscess is characterized by more diffuse induration and swelling over a larger region; it is deeper and does not have a tendency to "point." Owing to its deep location, the ischiorectal abscess frequently is not as promptly drained, since the diagnosis may not be certain or the physician may inordinately await the classic sign of fluctuance or softening.

Abscesses higher in the anal canal are more insidious, and symptoms are frequently more vague, usually associated with fever and systemic toxicity. Pain is usually expe-

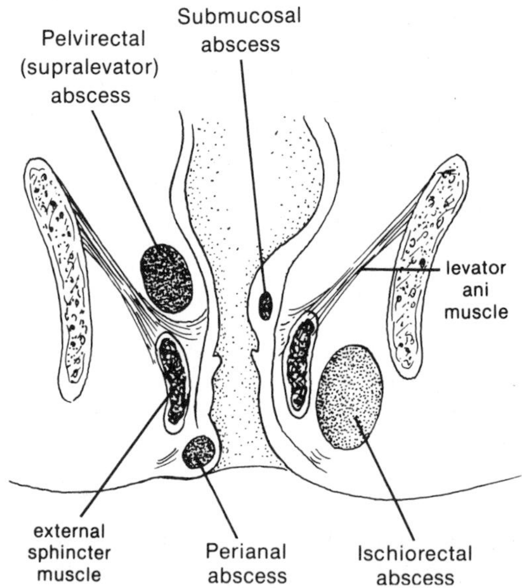

FIGURE 28–2. Common sites of anorectal abscesses.

rienced within the rectum or low pelvis. Palpation provides the diagnosis when a tender and boggy mass is discovered on rectal examination.

Early recognition and referral to a surgeon are of paramount importance in the care of the patient with an abscess. Delayed treatment may produce catastrophic sequelae. In their 10-year review of 184 patients admitted for perianal abscess, Bevans and colleagues reported nine patients who died of complications related to the anorectal process.[6] Thirty other patients had significant morbidity. The key factors in cases with complications were (1) delay in initial diagnosis and treatment, (2) inadequate initial therapy, and (3) associated systemic disease. Diabetes, blood dyscrasias, organic heart disease, chronic renal failure, and immunodeficient states were typical comorbid problems.

A frequent sequela of perianal abscess is fistula in ano. Following surgical or spontaneous drainage of an abscess, the process subsides, leaving a sinus opening in the skin that may persist or spontaneously close. When a new abscess forms in the same site, the likelihood of a fistula is great. Recurrent abscess formation or continuous drainage will persist until the internal opening is found and the tract unroofed.

When a fistula in ano develops, the clinician should consider the possibility of granulomatous disease. In one retrospective study, Scoma and colleagues found that of 232 patients with anal abscesses who were followed for more than 6 months, 154 developed fistulas, but in only 4% of these did it become apparent that the fistula was related to Crohn's disease.[5]

On the other hand, reviewing 500 patients with Crohn's disease, Homan and associates found that 28% developed an anal lesion, be it abscess, fistula, or fissure.[7] In 102 (20%), the anal disorder had preceded recognition of the granulomatous disease by 2 weeks to 12 years. Patients with granulomatous disease of the colon were twice as likely to develop an anal abnormality as those with small bowel disease alone.

Some patients complaining of anorectal pain have a pilonidal abscess. The discomfort in the low sacral area may not be discriminated from perianal discomfort. Inspection usually provides the diagnosis. Differentiating points include lack of anal tenderness or pain on defecation, absence of an anorectal mass, and absence of induration extending from the abscess to the anal canal.

Discomfort associated with proctitis or colitis is more vague and is usually described as tenesmus (spasm). This symptom may be variable and intermittent. Rectal pain coexistent with these disorders is likely to be caused by fissure, abscess formation, or inflammation related to hemorrhoids. In addition, the complaints usually include diarrhea.

With a bulky tumor of the rectosigmoid, tenesmus is a frequent complaint. However, if the lesion is low and invades the voluntary sphincter, or if the carcinoma is squamous in origin (anal carcinoma), pain may be more intense and constant and may mimic that of a fissure or prolapsed and incarcerated internal hemorrhoid.

Occasionally patients with coccygodynia or proctalgia fugax are seen. These are benign processes, but discomfort may prompt the patient to seek the opinion of a variety of specialists. Proctalgia fugax is a pain that seemingly arises in the rectum, recurs at irregular intervals, is usually of less than 10 weeks' duration, has no sequela, and is not associated with any identifiable anorectal lesion.[8] Coccygodynia, known by some as "television watchers' disease," is believed secondary to poor posture while sitting.[9] The levator ani, the coccygeus muscle groups, and the coccyx are found to be tender, probably owing to direct pressure and abnormal angulation. Relief is obtained by assuming correct posture while sitting. Body weight should be transferred from the lower spine to the ischial tuberosities and undersurfaces of the buttocks.

Those who engage in anal receptive intercourse are at risk of acquiring one of several painful proctologic lesions. In addition to lesions produced by trauma to the rectal tissue, proctitis and proctocolitis with infectious etiologies may occur. As a group, these are frequently referred to as "gay bowel syndromes," although they may also occur in women. Proctitis is manifested by anorectal pain, discharge, tenesmus, and hematochezia, with sigmoidoscopic findings limited to the distal 15 cm of bowel. Proctocolitis is manifested by blood- or pus-containing diarrhea, with sigmoidoscopic findings beyond 15 cm. Proctitis is most commonly associated with *Neisseria gonorrhoeae,* herpes simplex virus, *Chlamydia trachomatis* (non-LVG), and *Treponema pallidum.*[10] *Entamoeba histolytica* may produce proctitis or protocolitis, whereas *Campylobacter, Shigella, Chlamydia trachomatis* (LGV), and *Clostridium difficile* most often produce proctocolitis. Herpes simplex proctitis causes severe anorectal pain and tenesmus and may be associated with additional features of sacral paresthesias, difficulty in voiding, inguinal lymphadenopathy, and fever. Anorectal syphilitic chancres may be asymptomatic but are sometimes painful. The picture of diarrhea with normal sigmoidoscopic findings (enteritis) is commonly associated with *Giardia lamblia.* In almost one quarter of those with "gay bowel syndromes," more than one pathogen can be isolated by cultures and smears.[10]

Mass

Another complaint is a mass near or protruding through the anal canal. Frequently, the patient has little understanding of the problem and believes that a "hemorrhoid" is the cause. If associated symptoms are minimal, the patient may try several over-the-counter preparations before seeking advice from a physician.

An enlarged hemorrhoid or a skin tag is the most frequent cause for anal mass. An internal hemorrhoid that intermittently prolapses may be discovered only after the patient strains at stool. In early stages, it spontaneously retracts and may cause few symptoms. As the hemorrhoid enlarges with time, the patient may find it necessary to push the tissue back into the anal canal. Pain and bleeding may be variable at this stage.

A "skin tag" is a bit of floppy skin that may be the result of a thrombosed external hemorrhoid. It is usually painless, but it may bother the patient since the fleshy mass may make it difficult to maintain cleanliness.

A similar lesion is a hypertrophied anal papilla. Arising from modified skin at the dentate line, the mass is usually not discovered by the patient until it reaches a size when it may prolapse during defecation. Papillae appear as "fingers" of skin-covered tissue arising from the dentate line and pointing into the rectum. Size may vary from those barely noticeable to masses 1 cm or more in diameter and length.

Small isolated lesions of condyloma acuminatum present no difficulty in recognition. However, when a group of them obscure the anal canal, the diagnosis is more difficult. Closer inspection reveals the variegated surfaces of the warts. Spreading the buttocks may demonstrate less confluent areas. If digital examination is possible, small lesions may be detected in the anal canal.

As with any mass, consideration must always be given to possible carcinoma. Cancer presenting as an anal lesion is unusual, but skin carcinoma, melanoma, or anal carcinoma should be ruled out by biopsy. Malignancy may be masked by more conspicuous anorectal disease. Chronic or unusual problems should always arouse suspicion of possible malignancy.[11]

Pruritus Ani

This common and annoying symptom has several causes. In evaluating one with this complaint, the classification of Fromer should be considered (Table 28–3).[12] A certain number of patients have situations that are easily amenable to treatment. Once the anatomic and dermatologic situations have been ruled out, and once it is clear there is no systemic process that is playing a role, one is left with a large number of patients who fall into the idiopathic category.

TABLE 28–3. CLASSIFICATION OF PRURITUS ANI*

I. Anorectal abnormalities that cause local inflammation (25% of patients)
   - Papillitis and cryptitis
   - Prolapsed mucosa and hemorrhoids
   - Skin tags
   - Fissures and ulcers
   - Fistulas and draining sinuses
   - Neoplasms

II. Dermatologic abnormalities (~ 25% of patients)
   - Psoriasis
   - Seborrheic dermatitis
   - Contact dermatitis
   - Lichen sclerosis
   - Syphilis

III. Systemic or distant causes (~ 10% of patients)
   - Jaundice
   - Diabetes
   - Lymphomas
   - Allergy (hygienic pads, deodorants, douches, foods)
   - Parasites (especially pinworms)

IV. Idiopathic causes (~ 40% of patients)
   - Thought to represent low-grade inflammation, possibly aggravated by use of soaps

*Adapted from Fromer JL: Dermatologic concepts and management of pruritus ani. Am J Surg 90:805, 1955.

MANAGEMENT OF ANAL DISORDERS— ASCENDING LEVELS OF CARE

Basic Treatment: "Nostrums and Potions"

Most anorectal disorders occur in persons who have adopted the ways of Western civilization: a poorly balanced diet of highly refined foods, little exercise, and constant tension. For many patients, the judicious use of several medications and changes in personal habits may be the only measures needed for treatment.

The maintenance of bowel regularity with soft and bulky stools is of prime importance. A patient may believe that he or she is not constipated, but the physician may palpate stool in the sigmoid colon or cecum. After catharsis, large quantities of fiber and fluids should be added to the diet. Increasing fiber in the diet is the most logical approach. As yet, the Federal Drug Administration (FDA) has not established the recommended daily intake. Most dietitians suggest at least 5 g/day be consumed. This is best if spread over all three meals and reflecting several food groups.

For some people, a change in diet seems impossible. In such cases, the commonly used ground psyllium seed is helpful. Most people who need this agent require at least 1 tablespoon twice a day with meals.

Daily habits are also important. A pattern should be established that avoids an evening snack, includes a good breakfast to initiate the gastrocolic reflex, and then provides enough time for an unhurried bowel motion. Repeating this daily sequence and improving the diet will frequently alleviate chronic constipation.

Attention to hygiene is another element in the treatment of anorectal problems. The use of warm soaks (i.e., sitz baths), cleansing pads, or a perianal cleansing lotion helps to diminish inflammation. Too frequently, toilet paper irritates inflamed skin and mucosa. Gentle washing provides comfort and removes irritants. The witch hazel in cleansing pads acts as an astringent and seals the surfaces that may ooze. Each of these measures also improves the symptoms of nonspecific pruritus by reducing the associated inflammation, and witch hazel has a mild antipruritic effect.

One perineal lotion (Balneol) is a soothing emollient that contains oils and fatty acids to diminish irritation from toilet paper. Similar agents also are contained in several ointments and suppositories used to treat hemorrhoids (e.g., Anusol, Tronolane, and Preparation H). Most of these well advertised preparations were developed prior to the mandate of the FDA requiring that efficacy must be proved. Hence, production of these and similar compounds has continued. Despite therapeutic claims about Preparation H, there is no acceptable evidence that any of the ingredients within it are capable of reducing inflammation, shrinking hemorrhoids, or curing infection.[13]

Since inflammation is believed to aggravate hemorrhoids, topical corticosteroids are considered helpful in treatment by reducing edema. Suppositories are a commonly used vehicle to deliver this medication. However, appropriate distribution of the ingredients is not certain as the suppository melts. Better is the use of an aerosol foam to apply the hydrocortisone (Proctofoam-HC)[14] or one of several ointments (Anusol-HC or Corticaine). For most patients, these medications should be applied two times a day for 1 or 2 weeks.

When anorectal pain is the major symptom, over-the-counter ointments containing topical anesthetics may be beneficial. Applied every 4 hours and after each sitz bath and bowel movement, these medications usually provide significant relief when cutaneous nerve endings are exposed, as in ulcers and fissures.

If there is swelling and induration, the patient will also be more comfortable if he or she remains recumbent. This helps to diminish venous and lymphatic congestion and may promote healing. Ice packs applied to the anal area may provide additional comfort.

For the patient with a prolapsed and incarcerated internal hemorrhoid, prolonged rest in a recumbent position is a major element of treatment. Additional measures include alternating warm soaks (sitz baths) with ice packs, using topical anesthetics, and avoiding constipation. During the early phase, one might consider manual reduction with the placement of band ligatures cephalad to the area of prolapse.

Not to be confused with a prolapsed hemorrhoid is the external anal thrombosis (frequently called a thrombosed external hemorrhoid). This tender mass is covered by skin. By the time a patient seeks attention, the discomfort may be resolving and the clot may be well organized. At this phase, the skin may wrinkle over the thrombosis and there is much less tenderness. Treatment at this stage is symptomatic, similar to the prolapsed and incarcerated hemorrhoid. Topical ointments may be soothing and act as lubricant, but the anesthetic does not penetrate keratinized epithelium. If the patient arrives a few days after the thrombosis appears, drainage is the best option.

Hemorrhoids: Office Procedures

For the patient who has continuing problems with prolapsing hemorrhoids or bleeding, more aggressive intervention is required. Several modalities are available in the office setting that aim to destroy some of the excess tissue and fix the prolapsing mucosa high in the anorectum. The injection of an irritating chemical into the submucosa of the offending tissue has been used for many years. This procedure, which is simple and painless, may help to control bleeding but does little for prolapse.

For persistent bleeding and greater prolapse, the elastic ligature has found wide acceptance. The placement is simple to perform and requires only a forceps and simple applicator. The location and volume of tissue encompassed is easy to control. If placed far enough cephalad (1.5 to 2 cm above the dentate line), less than 10% of patients have pain sufficient to keep them out of work several days.[15]

There have been continuing reports of localized infection proceeding to systemic sepsis and occasional death following placement of a ligature. Although rare, these complications must be kept in mind for what some consider to be a simple procedure. Early suspicion of a problem followed by aggressive evaluation and treatment should favor a better outcome.[16]

Despite this, the long-term results from elastic bands seem excellent. In one study, almost 600 patients were followed 5 to 15 years. Although most patients required the placement of four or five ligatures, only 1.3% progressed to hemorrhoidectomy.[17]

Infrared photocoagulation is another modality that is gaining increased popularity. In several studies the results seem to be comparable with ligature when applied to smaller hemorrhoids. A major drawback is the initial cost and maintenance of complex equipment. Other authors report the use of bipolar electrocoagulation, direct current coagulation, and lasers. Although there are enthusiastic proponents, these techniques require expensive equipment and no long-term studies or cost comparisons have been made.[18]

Office-based treatment for an external anal thrombosis is incision and drainage. This is easily done after local anesthetic has been injected over the lesion. A simple incision allows the clot to extrude and relieves the marked discomfort. However, unless adequate overlying skin is excised, the thrombosis may reform in 24 hours and recreate the same process.[19]

Hemorrhoids: Hospital Procedures

When a patient has continued problems of pain, prolapse, or bleeding despite conservative management and use of the office procedures just described, operative hemorrhoidectomy remains the ultimate treatment. As a standard for success, the results of Ganchrow should be considered.[20] A retrospective study was performed 5 years following more than 2000 hemorrhoidectomy procedures. One half the patients responded to a questionnaire. Of these, 95% stated that their symptoms had been relieved. Only 28% of those operated on had residual minor rectal complaints. Itching was the most common of these but also mentioned were occasional complications including anal stenosis, perianal skin tags, persistent hemorrhoids, and soiling from partial incontinence.

Anal Fissure: Outpatient Therapies

For the initial phase of an anal fissure, stool softeners, topical anesthetics, and emollients are usually the only measures required. If these agents do not break the pain-spasm cycle, then an operative procedure is required. Lateral subcutaneous internal anal sphincterotomy is the operation of choice. This procedure involves transection of the thin ribbon of smooth muscle, the internal sphincter. The technique has been shown to promote healing more than 95% of the time.[21] Why this unusual procedure is successful is unclear. It may be that people who develop fissures have an abnormality of the internal anal sphincter with elevated resting pressure.[22]

Perianal Abscess: In- and Outpatient Therapies

For most perianal abscesses and in a selected number of ischiorectal abscesses, incision and drainage may be performed in the office setting. The procedure can be done with no more discomfort than accompanies the slow injection of anesthetic agent by a surgeon skilled in the use of local anesthesia. The risks are minimal in healthy, young individuals or in those with limited abscesses. However, in patients with compromised ability to deal with infection or in those with extensive phlegmon and cellulitis, careful exploration plus incision and adequate drainage in a more controlled environment is recommended. This is best done with the patient under general or regional anesthetic. Such patients should be hospitalized and closely observed to be certain that pelvic abscess, soft tissue phlegmon, or generalized sepsis does not occur.

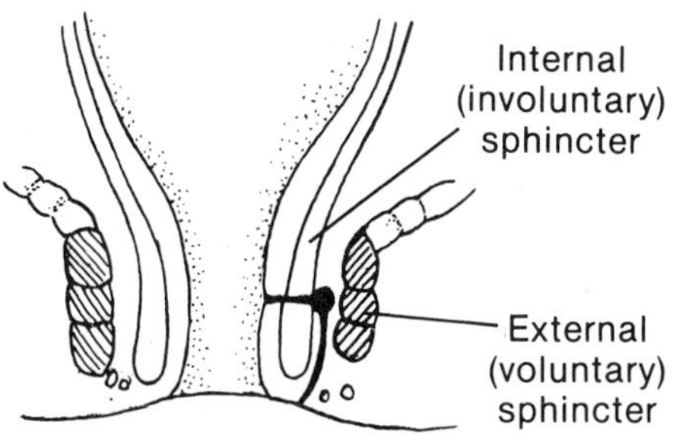

A. Intersphincteric, 45%

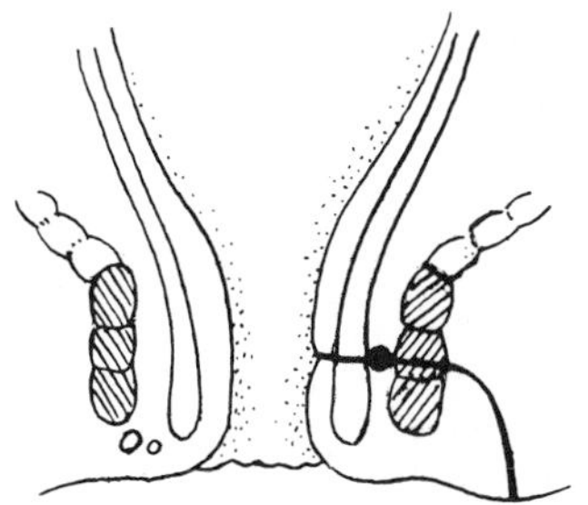

B. Transsphincteric, 30%

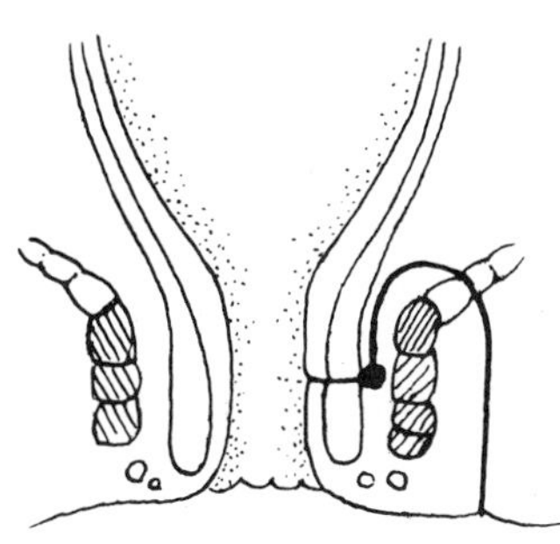

C. Suprasphincteric, 20%

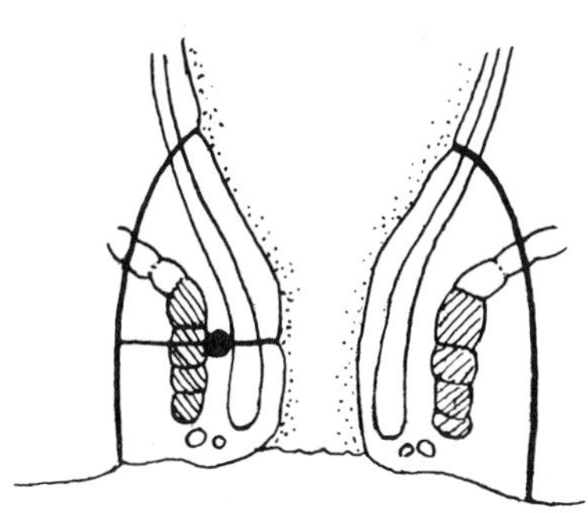

D. Extrasphincteric, 5%

FIGURE 28–3. Types of fistula in ano. The terms "trans-," "supra-," and "extra-" refer to the external (voluntary) sphincter. (Adapted from Parks AG, Gordon PH, Hardcastle JD: A classification of fistula in ano. Br J Surg 63:1, 1976.) Parks and associates analyzed 400 cases.

Following incision of a perianal abscess, the patient should be alerted that a subsequent fistula in ano may develop. For the patient who has recurrent abscess at the same site, anal exploration and fistulotomy are recommended.

Fistula In Ano: Operative Approaches

The treatment of fistula in ano is not urgent. Some patients refuse surgery and for many years accept persistent perianal drainage. Others experience a pattern of recurrent abscess formation, spontaneous drainage, slow resolution, and subsequent reformation of the abscess.

A fistula is a "tunnel" from the anal canal that penetrates the soft tissues and usually emanates outside the dentate line. The objectives of treatment are to uncover the fistula widely to allow healing from the deepest portion to the skin surface. Since the tract may pursue one of several directions (Fig. 28–3), the operation chosen relates to the tract and the sphincter. If the tract is superficial to the major voluntary (external) sphincter, the procedure is of little consequence. Only skin, mucosa, and perhaps some involuntary muscle are transected. However, if the tract has pursued a course through or around the external sphincter, then the operative procedure is more complex. Transection of this voluntary sphincter would cause incontinence of stool and flatus for months, and the patient might never regain full control. Alternative drainage procedures or the placement of a seton is used by the experienced colorectal surgeon.[23]

Pruritus Ani: Evaluation and Treatment

Once local anorectal, dermatologic, and systemic causes have been ruled out for this aggravating problem, one proceeds with a regimen to enhance anal cleanliness. This includes gentle cleansing, avoiding the use of anal preparations, and wearing loose cotton underwear to improve ventilation. In some patients, the elimination of certain dietary items and the regulation of bowel habits are also beneficial. Finally, the scratch-itch cycle is frequently broken by the topical use of hydrocortisone cream.[24]

REFERENCES

1. Welch CE: Colon hemorrhage. *In* Hardy JD (ed): Rhoads' Textbook of Surgery. Philadephia, JB Lippincott, 1977, p 1196.
2. Flick AL, Voegtlin KF, Rubin CE: Clinical experience with suction biopsy of the rectal mucosa. Gastroenterology 42:691, 1962.
3. Morson BC: Rectal biopsy in inflammatory bowel disease. N Engl J Med 287:1337, 1972.
4. Kilpatrick ZM: Gonorrheal proctitis. N Engl J Med 287:967, 1972.
5. Scoma JA: Incidence of fistulas subsequent to anal abscesses. Dis Col Rect 17:357, 1974.
6. Bevans DW Jr, Westbrook KC, Thompson BW, et al: Perirectal abscess: A potentially fatal illness. Am J Surg 126:765, 1973.
7. Homan WP, Tang C, Thorbjarnarson B: Anal lesions complicating Crohn's disease. Arch Surg 111:1333, 1976.
8. Peery WE: Proctalgia fugax: A clinical enigma. S Med J 81:621, 1988.
9. Thiele GH: Coccygodynia: Cause and treatment. Dis Col Rect 6:422, 1963.

10. Quinn TC, Stamm WE, Goodell SE, et al: Polymicrobial origin of intestinal infections in homosexual men. N Engl J Med 309:576, 1983.
11. Grodsky L: Unsuspected anal cancer discovered after minor anorectal surgery. Dis Col Rect 10:471, 1967.
12. Fromer JL: Dermatologic concepts and management of pruritus ani. Am J Surg 90:805, 1955.
13. Preparation H. Med Lett 18:108, 1976.
14. Proctofoam-HC for anorectal disorders. Med Lett 17:69, 1971.
15. Marsham D, Huber PJ Jr, Timmerman W, et al: Hemorrhoidal ligation—a review of efficacy. Dis Col Rect 32:369, 1989.
16. Quevedo-Bonilla G, Farkas AM, Abcarian H, et al: Septic complications of hemorrhoidal banding. Arch Surg 123:650, 1988.
17. Rothberg R, Rubin RJ, Eisenstat T, et al: Rubber band ligation hemorrhoidectomy—long-term results. Am Surg 49:167, 1983.
18. Smith LE: Hemorrhoidectomy with lasers and other contemporary modalities. Surg Clin North Am 72:665, 1992.
19. Oh C: Acute thrombosed external hemorrhoids. Mt Sinai J Med 56:30, 1989.
20. Ganchrow MI, Mazier WP, Friend WG, et al: Hemorrhoidectomy revisited—a computer analysis of 2,038 cases. Dis Col Rect 14:128, 1971.
21. Lewis TH, Corman ML, Prager ED, et al: Long-term results of open and closed sphincterotomy for anal fissure. Dis Col Rect 31:368, 1988.
22. McNamara MJ, Percy JP, Fielding IR: A manometric study of anal fissure treated by subcutaneous lateral internal sphincterotomy. Ann Surg 211:235, 1990.
23. Seow-Choen, Phillips RK: Insights gained from the management of problematical anal fistulae at St. Mark's Hospital 1984–88. Br J Surg 78:539, 1991.
24. Smith LE, Heinrichs D, McCullah RD: Prospective studies on the etiology and treatment of pruritus ani. Dis Col Rect 25:358, 1982.

29

Diseases of the Liver

DAVID NUNES, MB, MRCPI
J. THOMAS LAMONT, MD

The purpose of this chapter is to outline diagnostic and therapeutic approaches to patients with liver diseases likely to be encountered in a general medical or family practice, particularly (1) acute hepatitis, (2) chronic hepatitis, (3) alcoholic liver disease, (4) obstructive or cholestatic liver disease, and (5) infiltrative liver disease. These entities are generally quite simple to differentiate on the basis of the history, physical examination, and routine liver function studies.

VIRAL HEPATITIS

The physician in practice can manage the majority of hepatitis patients as outpatients. A working knowledge of the natural history and epidemiology is required in order to answer the patient's and the family's questions regarding duration of disease, risk of infection to others, and advisability of gamma globulin prophylaxis, vaccination, or interferon therapy.

Several new developments have significantly changed our approach to viral hepatitis. The description of hepatitis C and the availability of serologic tests for this virus have produced a more rational approach to what was previously called non-A, non-B (NANB) hepatitis. Interferon is allowing us to alter the natural history of these illnesses for the first time. Despite significant advances in these areas, new questions have arisen and much uncertainty regarding the best approach to the care of these patients remains. Human immunodeficiency virus (HIV) infection has added a new dimension to the management of these patients since viral hepatitis is frequently associated with HIV.

In this section we discuss the agents responsible for viral hepatitis in terms of their virology, epidemiology, natural history, and immune response, including discussion of the most appropriate use of diagnostic tests (Table 29–1). As the clinical presentations of the various types of acute and chronic hepatitis are similar, they are discussed together. Features specific to a hepatitis virus are discussed in the section on that virus.

TABLE 29–1. HEPATITIS VIRUSES

	Hepatitis A	Hepatitis B	Hepatitis C	Hepatitis D
Oral transmission	Yes	No	?(Unlikely)	No
Parenteral transmission	No	Yes	Yes	Yes
Incubation period	15–45 days	40–180 days	15–50 days	30–50 days
Mortality	0.1%	1–3%	1–2%	Up to 20%
Chronic infection	No	Yes (2–10%) Neonate 90%	Yes (50%)	Yes
Percent of seropositive US adults	25–50%	10%	0.5–1.5%	<1%

Clinical Features of Viral Hepatitis

Acute Viral Hepatitis. Most cases of viral hepatitis are asymptomatic and pass unnoticed as a nonspecific illness without jaundice. In the typical classical case with jaundice, the clinical course can be divided into three phases: prodromal, icteric, and recovery phases. The prodromal phase normally lasts for 1 to 2 weeks, during which time the patient complains of a loss of energy, muscle aches, nausea with loss of appetite, and right upper quadrant pain. Smokers characteristically lose their taste for cigarettes and reduce their intake or stop smoking. A low-grade fever is common, jaundice is absent, and the liver is frequently enlarged and tender.

After the prodromal phase the urine darkens, the stools lighten in color, and the patient becomes jaundiced. At this time the earlier constitutional symptoms start to abate, the patient feels better with resolution of fever, and a slow but definite improvement in energy and appetite. On examination the patient is jaundiced with scleral icterus and the liver is often palpable and tender. Splenomegaly may be present, particularly in children. Jaundice normally lasts for 1 to 4 weeks as the hepatitis gradually resolves. Resolution is often more rapid in children than in adults. Persistent lethargy and fatigue may be features for several weeks to months following the acute illness.

Patients with a slowly resolving or relapsing hepatitis pose several clinical problems. When relapsing hepatitis has developed on a background of hepatitis A, other causes of acute or chronic viral hepatitis should be excluded. In the absence of another cause for hepatitis, the patient can be reassured that there is no risk of chronic hepatitis. Patients with hepatitis B may progress to a chronic hepatitis and should be carefully followed. Superinfection with hepatitis D should be excluded, particularly when there has been a biphasic elevation in the transaminases.

Management. The management of acute viral hepatitis is purely supportive. In the early stages bed rest should be advised. Care should be taken concerning personal hygiene to limit spread of the virus. The patient should be meticulous about hand-washing and should use towels dedicated to his or her own use. As the constitutional symptoms resolve, a nutritious diet should be encouraged. Patients frequently find that meals high in carbohydrates and low in fats are better tolerated. Prolonged bed rest has no proven beneficial effects, but it seems prudent to advise patients to remain at home and maintain a low level of activity. If there is any deterioration in symptoms or signs, then bed rest may be warranted. Once the jaundice has resolved, the patient may gradually return to normal activities and should avoid alcohol for 6 months.

Laboratory Tests. The characteristic pattern of acute hepatitis is a marked elevation of the serum aspartate aminotransferase (AST) and alanine aminotransferase (ALT) to greater than ten times the upper limit of normal with only a mild increase in serum alkaline phosphatase and gamma-glutamyltranspeptidase (GGT). The level of transaminase is not a useful predictor of disease severity, as the levels may fall quickly as patients develop fulminant hepatitis. The transaminases may remain persistently abnormal for several months in normally recovering patients. The peak bilirubin level does, however, correlate with the duration of the illness. Severity of acute viral hepatitis is best indicated by abnormal prothrombin time (see later).

Fulminant Hepatitis. In fulminant hepatitis, features of hepatic failure develop within 8 weeks of onset of the clinical illness. In some cases the onset of liver failure may be so rapid that jaundice may not be present. Early features of impending hepatic failure include alteration in mentation and sleep pattern, and the development of fetor hepaticus and asterixis. Total anorexia, vomiting, and lethargy are common. By this time the prothrombin time is prolonged and the patient may have noticed easy bruising. Any of these features is an indication for the patient's admission to the hospital for supportive care.

The cause of acute fulminant hepatitis depends on the patient population and risk factors. In the United States NANB hepatitis is the most frequent cause, but current data would suggest that hepatitis C is rarely the cause, suggesting a role for other viruses or toxins in most cases. It is important to remember that patients who survive the acute illness will normally have a full recovery of liver function. Furthermore, liver transplantation has resulted in a significant improvement in long-term outcome in selected cases.[1] Therefore, early detection with aggressive supportive care is required, with early referral of the most seriously ill patients to a specialist unit with transplantation facilities.

Differential Diagnosis of Acute Viral Hepatitis. The differential diagnosis of acute viral hepatitis is strongly influenced by the personal risk factors. Careful attention to historical details will identify patients with definite risk factors for viral hepatitis, those with a significant history of contact with toxins, drugs, and other possibly infectious etiologies. During the prodromal phase it is frequently difficult to differentiate the illness from other acute viral infections, including acute infectious mononucleosis.

Hepatitis with severe right upper quadrant pain may be confused with gallbladder disease. Prominent vomiting and nausea may be misdiagnosed as acute gastroenteritis. During the icteric phase, causes of obstructive jaundice become part of the differential, though the marked elevation of serum transaminases usually distinguishes hepatitis from mechanical obstruction. Differentiation of viral hepatitis from a drug- or toxin-induced hepatitis requires a careful history and serologic tests.

Chronic Viral Hepatitis. With the advent of routine blood testing primary care physicians are seeing more asymptomatic patients with chronically abnormal liver blood tests, some of whom have chronic viral hepatitis. Patients with chronic active hepatitis may complain of malaise and easy fatigue but may deny a prior history of acute hepatitis. Those with chronic hepatitis B or C tend to have less florid symptoms and signs than patients with chronic autoimmune hepatitis and chronic hepatitis D.

If chronic viral hepatitis progresses to cirrhosis, the patient may present with the complications of portal hypertension: variceal bleeding, ascites, and spontaneous bacterial peritonitis. Hepatic failure may present with alteration in mentation, particularly daytime drowsiness and increased nocturnal activity with confusion. On examination these patients will have features of chronic liver failure:

palmar erythema, spider angiomata, asterixis, fetor hepaticus, and jaundice. An examination of the patient's mental state will reveal loss of recent memory, slowing of thought processes, and constructional apraxia. Ascites and peripheral edema are frequently present. Treatment is given as for any patient with liver failure, including the use of lactulose and oral antibiotics to reduce the level of encephalopathy and the judicious use of diuretics with or without abdominal paracentesis to treat ascites.

Hepatitis A. The hepatitis A virus (HAV) is a single, positively stranded RNA virus 27 to 28 nm in diameter and a member of the picornovirus family. The genome is approximately 7500 bases in length and codes for a viral polymerase, structural proteins, and a number of proteases. To date only one serotype has been recognized, although minor variations in the viral sequence have been documented.[2]

Epidemiology. Hepatitis A is spread by the fecal-oral route, resulting in a high rate of infection in developing nations where standards of personal hygiene and sanitation are low. In these communities the prevalence of IgG antibodies to HAV is as high as 90 to 95%, with the highest incidence of acute infection occurring in preschool-aged children. Hepatitis A is usually asymptomatic or associated with a nonspecific viral illness without jaundice. In more developed nations, the incidence of infection is lower and the seroprevalence of IgG antibodies is only 25 to 30%. Infection tends to occur at a later age, with a peak incidence between 5 and 14 years of age. Infection in adults is associated with a higher incidence of symptoms.

Infection in adults may occur after contact with infected children, and sporadic cases among the homosexual population have been reported. Outbreaks have also been reported in institutions for the mentally and physically disadvantaged and following consumption of clams and mussels harvested from beds contaminated by human sewage. People traveling from the developed world to areas with a high seroprevalence are also at increased risk of infection, and prophylactic measures are advised, especially for health-care workers (see later).

Hepatitis A has an incubation period of 15 to 50 days. The diagnosis is best made by measuring IgM antibodies to hepatitis A that are normally present by the onset of jaundice. IgM antibodies usually persist for 3 to 12 months and are replaced by permanent IgG antibody. Past exposure and immunity can be detected by measuring IgG antibodies. During the incubation period and for 1 to 2 weeks after the onset of jaundice the virus is excreted in the feces and patients should be considered infectious. Viremia is normally short-lived and occurs prior to the onset of jaundice. Because infection will not be clinically recognized for the majority of the infectious period, patient isolation is unlikely to alter the spread of disease.

Prognosis. Acute hepatitis A usually does not require any specific treatment, and laboratory monitoring of disease progress is normally all that is required. Hepatitis A accounts for less than 1% of all cases of fulminant hepatitis, and the mortality rate in large epidemics is less than 0.1%.

Occasionally, adult patients may experience a prolonged cholestatic illness with pruritus.[3] Such patients may benefit from a short course of prednisolone, tapering the dose from 30 mg over a 3-week period. Rarely, relapsing hepatitis occurs,[4] with an increase in liver enzymes and a reappearance of the virus in the stool. Chronic hepatitis A does not occur.

Prevention. Hepatitis A is best prevented by high standards of sanitation and personal hygiene, including meticulous washing of food and hands. Passive immunization with human immune serum globulin is recommended for nonimmune patients traveling to areas with a high incidence of infection and for close personal contacts of patients with hepatitis A. The recommended dosage is 0.02 ml/kg for pre-exposure prophylaxis and 0.02 ml/kg for postexposure prophylaxis. Such treatment confers protection for 2 to 3 months. Treatment of casual contacts and hospital personnel is not recommended.

Active immunization using live attenuated virus, inactivated virus, and recombinant proteins is presently undergoing development and clinical trials.[5, 6] When available it will become the vaccination method of choice for people traveling to high-prevalence areas, and possibly for children, homosexuals, and workers in contact with the virus.

Hepatitis B. The hepatitis B virus is a 42-nm particle known as the Dane particle. The outer envelope consists of a coat of surface proteins containing the hepatitis B surface antigen (HBsAg) and two other closely related proteins referred to as pre-S1 and pre-S2. Each of the three surface proteins is present in approximately equal quantities in the surface of the mature viral particle. Unlike HBsAg, the pre-S proteins are not excreted in a free form by infected hepatocytes. The pre-S1 protein is thought to be important in virus attachment and entry into hepatocytes.

Within the surface coat, the viral genome is contained within a core particle composed of a nucleocapsid core protein, the hepatitis B core antigen (HBcAg). A slightly smaller but related protein is actively secreted by hepatocytes containing replicating virus. This protein is referred to as the hepatitis B e antigen (HBeAg) and is a useful serologic marker of active viral replication.[7] Other more sophisticated markers of viral replication include measurement of HBV DNA and HBV DNA polymerase. These assays are becoming increasingly available for routine use to monitor response to therapy and as markers of infectivity.

The hepatitis B virus is noncytopathic; hence, the injury to the liver associated with infection results from the host's immune response. This has important implications in terms of the natural history and clinical manifestations of the disease.

Hepatitis B Serology. The hepatitis B surface antigen (HBsAg) appears in the blood of infected patients approximately 6 weeks after exposure, 1 to 2 weeks before the onset of any symptoms, and 4 to 6 weeks before the onset of jaundice (Table 29–2, Fig. 29–1). Shortly after the appearance of HBsAg, HBeAg is detectable, but usually at a lower titer. Approximately 2 weeks later, preceding both the onset of jaundice and a rise in liver enzymes, IgM antibodies to hepatitis B core antigen (anti-HBc) become detectable.[8] Measurements of HBsAg and anti-HBc IgM are the earliest and most reliable markers of acute hepatitis B infection and are best performed together.

In typical cases HBeAg disappears first, followed by the appearance of anti-HBe antibodies and the disappearance of HBsAg 4 to 6 weeks later. Persistence of HBeAg in serum for longer than 10 weeks is a reliable marker of chronic infection. Shortly after disappearance of HBsAg, antibodies to HBsAg will appear and are used as a serologic marker of long-term immunity. Anti-HBc IgM will persist for 3 to 12 months following an acute infection. Anti-HBc IgG antibodies are also a reliable marker of past natural infection but do not appear in those who have received recombinant HBsAg vaccination.

From a serologic viewpoint two types of chronic hepatitis B infection are recognized. In the replicative form, both HBeAg and HBsAg are present in the serum, indicating active viral replication. Mild to severe chronic active hepa-

TABLE 29–2. SEROLOGICAL MARKERS OF HEPATITIS B

Marker	Source	Antibody	Comment
HBsAg	Outer envelope protein	Anti-HBs	HBsAg found in acute and chronic infection. Antibody indicates prior infection or vaccination.
HBcAg	Nucleocapsid or "core" protein	Core antibody	IgM antibody indicates recent or active infection. IgG antibody is a marker of infection with natural virus both past and present.
HBeAg	Nonstructural protein	Anti-HBe	Marker of active viral replication and infectivity
HBV DNA	Viral DNA	None	Sensitive marker of active viral replication and infectivity
HBV DNA polymerase	Viral polymerase enzyme	None	Marker of virus in serum, replication, and infectivity

HBcAg = hepatitis B core antigen; HBeAg = hepatitis Be antigen; HBsAg = hepatitis B surface antigen; HBV = hepatitis B virus.

titis is found on liver biopsy, and serum of such patients is highly infectious. Loss of HBeAg may be heralded by an acute flare in the underlying hepatitis as the immune system clears replicating virus. In the nonreplicative form, HBsAg is present but HBeAg is absent. Such patients are frequently asymptomatic and have a low infectivity to others, and liver biopsy usually demonstrates only a chronic persistent hepatitis or a relatively normal appearance. Persistence of HBs antigenemia in the absence of HBeAg (the so-called carrier state) is thought to be due to integration of the virus into the host genome such that continuing expression of the HBsAg occurs without viral replication. Follow-up of carriers has demonstrated a low risk of cirrhosis.

In two clinical situations the normally measured serologic markers may be misleading. First, patients with severe acute hepatitis B may be HBsAg negative, probably as a result of an increased immune response leading to a loss of HBsAg. These patients will have raised anti-HBc IgM levels, underlining the importance of using both tests for the diagnosis of acute hepatitis. Second, a mutant form of hepatitis B has been described. This form fails to express HBeAg and is associated with a more severe illness.[9] This unusual "pre-core mutant" strain of the virus is found predominantly in the Mediterranean and Asia but does not appear to be a major problem in the United States at the present time.

Epidemiology. The hepatitis B virus is spread by percutaneous and permucous membrane exposure. In the developed world, infection occurs sporadically. Anti-HBc IgG is prevalent in intravenous drug abusers, homosexuals, sexually promiscuous groups, institutionalized patients, and health-care workers. As a result, either past or chronic infection is frequently found in patients with concomitant HIV disease. The carrier rate varies significantly worldwide with a seroprevalence of HBsAg of approximately 0.1% among healthy blood donors in the United States and Western Europe to as high as 15% in the Far East, where the disease is endemic and frequently contracted at childbirth. Between 5 and 10% of intravenous drug abusers and homosexuals are HBsAg positive.

Clinical Features. Hepatitis B infection is frequently an anicteric infection. Chronic hepatitis B carriers often give no history of an acute hepatitic illness. Indeed, patients who have an anicteric illness are probably at increased risk of becoming chronic carriers as this probably reflects an inadequate immune response to the primary infection.[10]

Acute hepatitis B tends to be more severe than acute hepatitis A or C, with a significantly higher incidence of acute fulminant hepatitis. However, in approximately 90% of cases, the disease runs a relatively benign self-limiting course. Persistent infection occurs in only 5 to 10% of acute cases. The rate of chronic infection is two to three times higher in males than in females and is significantly higher in immune suppressed groups such as those receiving chemotherapy or steroids, in neonatal infections, and in patients who have HIV-related immune suppression.[11] An acute serum sickness-type syndrome with arthralgia, an urticarial rash, fever, and proteinuria may be associated with acute hepatitis B.

The prognosis of chronic infection is related to the severity of the hepatitis. Patients with chronic persistent hepatitis on liver biopsy are at low risk of developing chronic active hepatitis and cirrhosis, while patients with chronic active hepatitis are at high risk of developing cirrhosis.[12] The long-term sequelae of chronic hepatitis B infection include the development of cirrhosis and hepatocellular carcinoma. In the Far East, where hepatitis B is endemic, up to 80% of all cases of hepatocellular carcinoma occur in HBsAg-positive individuals.

Treatment of Hepatitis B. In recent years a number of antiviral agents have been used in the treatment of chronic hepatitis B infection, including adenine arabinoside, acyclovir, and the interferons. At present α-interferon is the only recommended form of treatment, although combination therapies using other agents (including those already mentioned) are being assessed in an attempt to improve the overall response rate.

The type and extent of response to interferon may be divided into several categories. Patients considered to have a complete response (10%) clear the virus completely with loss of both HBsAg and HBeAg. Patients with a partial response (20 to 30%) clear HBeAg but remain HBsAg-positive. In both complete and partial responders, the extent and severity of liver damage as measured by liver histology and serum transaminases are reduced. Furthermore, data have demonstrated that longer term follow-up of these patients has shown that a significant number of patients who have cleared only HBeAg during the initial treatment regi-

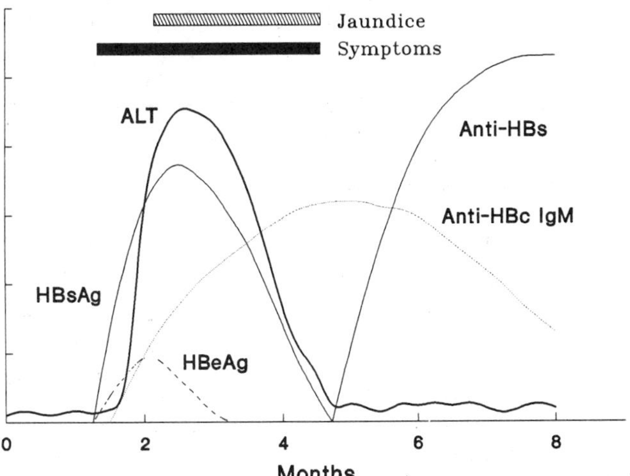

FIGURE 29–1. Time course for serologic markers in acute hepatitis B infection. (ALT = alanine aminotransferase.)

men will later clear HBsAg. Other patients (70%) demonstrate only a transitory improvement or show no improvement at all.[13]

A number of factors that may help to identify patients with hepatitis B who are most likely to respond to α-interferon have been determined.[14] Female patients with a recent onset of infection, normal immune system, high transaminase levels, and active hepatitis on liver biopsy are most likely to respond. Patients with long-standing disease, immune suppression, and only mildly abnormal liver transaminases are less likely to respond to α-interferon and thus are not good candidates for treatment. The poor response rate in patients of Far Eastern origin may in part be due to the early age of acquisition and the long duration of the illness at the time of commencing treatment, although genetic and other factors may be important. Some patients with early presymptomatic HIV disease have been treated successfully with interferon, and thus this is not an absolute contraindication to therapy. Patients receiving interferon for the treatment of hepatitis B frequently experience a rise in transaminase levels prior to seroconversion. This may result in a transient deterioration in liver function, and thus interferon should be used with great caution in patients with borderline liver function.

α-Interferon for hepatitis B infection is normally given in a dose of 5 to 10 million units subcutaneously three times weekly for 3 to 6 months. Unfortunately, side effects are experienced by most of those receiving α-interferon. Many patients have energy loss, muscle aches, fever, and other flu-like symptoms. These symptoms are usually worse immediately after injection and can be reduced by taking acetaminophen and advising that the drug be taken in the evening. Symptoms are usually worse during the first 2 to 3 weeks of therapy but may persist throughout the course of treatment. Diarrhea and thinning of the hair are reversible effects that usually occur later. Autoimmune conditions may be precipitated by the use of interferon, including hemolytic anemias, thrombocytopenias, thyroiditis, and a lupus-like syndrome. These are frequently asymptomatic and are noted by the appearance of auto antibodies. Therapy can be continued in the absence of clinical disease. Interferon may also induce a reversible thrombocytopenia and granulocytopenia. The aim is to maintain a platelet count of greater than 80–100 × 10^9/l and a total white blood cell count more than 1.5 × 10^9/l.

Interferon therapy should be monitored by weekly liver function tests and full blood cell count with platelet estimations during the first month and then every second week. Viral serology should be performed at four weekly intervals or if a response to therapy is indicated by a rise or sudden fall in transaminases. Patients who will respond to therapy will normally have done so after receiving treatment for 3 months. Patients who have shown no response by this time should have the treatment stopped.

Prevention and Immunization. Prevention of hepatitis B in the community requires a reduction of high-risk sexual behavior and a reduction in intravenous drug usage, such as for the prevention of HIV infection. A recombinant vaccine is now recommended for high-risk groups: intravenous drug abusers, prostitutes, homosexuals, and health-care workers (Table 29–3). Unfortunately, a significant proportion of these have already been exposed to the virus by the time they present for vaccination. Several countries, including the United States, are recommending hepatitis B vaccination in children. While protective antibody titers are achieved in 85 to 90% of young adults who receive the vaccine, the response rate is significantly lower in the elderly and in the immunosuppressed.[15] Furthermore, a

TABLE 29–3. HEPATITIS VACCINATION

Hepatitis	Situation	Individuals at Risk	Recommendation
Hepatitis A	Pre-exposure	Travelers to endemic areas	Hepatitis A immune serum globulin (0.02 ml/kg IM)
	Postexposure	Close personal contacts or children exposed in day-care centers or in institutions	0.06 ml/kg IM
Hepatitis B	Pre-exposure	Health care workers, hemodialysis staff, residents of mental and psychiatric institutions, promiscuous homosexuals, prostitutes, and travelers to endemic areas	Hepatitis B vaccine
	Postexposure	Infants of HBsAg-positive mothers, persons parenterally exposed to HBsAg: positive blood, sexual contacts of patients with acute hepatitis B	HBIG plus hepatitis B vaccine

HBIG = hepatitis B immune globulin; HBsAg = hepatitis B surface antigen; IM = intramuscularly.

rapid reduction in antibody titer occurs in a significant number of individuals who have shown an initial response. It is, therefore, recommended that all high-risk groups who have been vaccinated should have their antibody levels checked every 2 to 3 years to ensure continuing immunity.

Postexposure (needle-stick, sexual contact) prophylaxis can be achieved by the immediate administration of human immune globulin to hepatitis B. Nonimmune individuals with known parenteral, perinatal, or sexual exposure to hepatitis B should receive 0.06 ml/kg of the immune globulin followed by vaccination.

Hepatitis C Virus (HCV). The existence of a form of viral hepatitis unrelated to hepatitis A or B was first recognized in 1974.[16] Early attempts at characterizing the virus met with limited success. Electron microscopy, immunologic methods, and cell culture failed to identify the agent responsible for the disease. Only when modern molecular biology techniques were applied to the identification of this unknown agent was it reliably identified.[17] Since then there has been an explosion of new information regarding the genomic structure and epidemiology of the disease associated with the virus.[18]

Virology. The hepatitis C virus is a single, positively stranded RNA virus of approximately 10,000 bases,[19] which is thought to be related to the flavivirus (yellow fever virus) and pestivirus families.[20] The viral genome encodes for a single polypeptide that is subsequently cleaved into smaller proteins to produce the structural and nonstructural proteins necessary for viral replication.

Serology. First-generation serologic tests for hepatitis C depend on the detection of antibodies to recombinant viral proteins derived from the nonstructural region of the virus. Antibodies to this protein appear from 6 weeks to many months after exposure and may never be detected in a few patients.[21] False-positive test results are reported with many conditions associated with hypergammaglobulinemia, including autoimmune chronic active hepatitis and primary biliary cirrhosis.

Recently introduced second-generation tests incorporate the use of several viral proteins or methods of neutralization, thus reducing the number of false-positive results. Furthermore, the incorporation of structural proteins reduces the interval between exposure and seroconversion. By using several antigens impregnated on a paper strip, the recombinant immunoblot assay (RIBA) can be used to discern the pattern of antibody response and to confirm positive enzyme-linked immunosorbent assay (ELISA) results. At present no antigen detection system is available, making it difficult to distinguish past from present infection using serologic methods alone. HCV can be detected by amplification of viral RNA using the polymerase chain reaction (PCR), but this test is not available for routine clinical use.

Epidemiology. Testing for hepatitis C antibodies in routine blood donors has revealed a seroprevalence between 0.1 and 1%. Rates are higher in the minority groups in the United States and tend to be higher in Southern Europe than in Northern Europe.[22] There appears to be no sexual difference in positivity, but the rate rises progressively with age and then reaches a plateau at 40 to 50 years of age. In high-risk groups, such as hemophiliacs and intravenous drug abusers, the seroprevalence ranges from 50 to 80%.[23] Anti-HCV antibody testing in transfused patients has confirmed that the hepatitis C virus is the major cause of post-transfusion hepatitis, accounting for 90 to 95% of such cases.[24]

Household and sexual contacts of patients with hepatitis C have a slightly higher seroprevalence (2 to 8%) than does the general population. These data suggest that HCV may be transmitted sexually, but that this is a very inefficient method of transmission. Other reported modes of transmission include from a mother to her baby in the perinatal period and an anecdotal report of HCV infection following a human bite. More recently, transmission of HCV in patients receiving organ transplants has been reported.

Clinical Presentation. The presentation of hepatitis C is quite variable. A small proportion of patients present with jaundice following blood transfusion. This illness is usually mild and is rarely fatal.

Approximately 75% of patients who develop biochemical hepatitis following blood transfusion have no symptoms. A serum sickness-like illness with myalgia and arthralgia may occur but is less common than for hepatitis B infection. Hepatitis C is rarely associated with aplastic anemia.[21] This is of interest, because some flaviviruses are known to reproduce in the bone marrow. Both positively and negatively stranded HCV RNA have been demonstrated in mononuclear cells, suggesting active viral replication in these cells.

The clinical course of chronic hepatitis C is very variable. More than 50% of patients with acute post-transfusion hepatitis C will go on to develop chronic hepatitis, and of these approximately 25% will develop cirrhosis. Some patients with chronic hepatitis run a progressive clinical course with the development of cirrhosis and liver failure, whereas other patients may run a protracted course with minimal clinical disease. Factors that define the pathogenicity of infection remain poorly understood, but both genetic susceptibility and viral factors are probably important in defining disease expression.

Hepatitis C-related cirrhosis appears to run a benign course compared with alcoholic cirrhosis with a long interval to the development of complications. However, hepatocellular carcinoma may develop in patients with chronic HCV infection and cirrhosis. In Japan hepatitis C appears to be replacing hepatitis B as the major cause of hepatocellular carcinoma. Whether the virus has any direct oncogenic effect remains unclear.

Treatment. At present it is recommended that patients with known chronic hepatitis C should undergo liver biopsy and that patients with evidence of histologically progressive disease or disabling symptoms related to chronic hepatitis C infection should receive therapy. Patients with a mild histologic picture should be followed, and the need for treatment should be reassessed periodically. Treatment should be withdrawn or the dose reduced if severe side effects occur.

Selection of patients for interferon therapy remains a difficult problem. Long-term response rates are low with a significant incidence of treatment-related side effects and return of transaminase levels to pretreatment levels following treatment. Patients with established cirrhosis and secondary complications may have a lower response rate, and it may already be too late to expect any real clinical benefit. Young patients should be treated more aggressively than older patients. Loss of viral RNA and a fall in antibody titers appear to predict a good response to therapy with long-term remission. HCV antibody-negative patients with post-transfusion hepatitis respond with a rate similar to that seen in anti-HCV antibody-positive patients. The exact etiology in these antibody-negative cases needs further clarification, but the findings support the use of interferon in these patients.

The standard regimen for the treatment of hepatitis C is 3 to 5 million units of α-interferon three times weekly for 6 months. Treatment results in a 50% overall response rate in terms of normalization of transaminases during therapy, but up to 50% of these patients will have a biochemical relapse on discontinuation of therapy.[25] Biochemical response (normalization of transaminases) is associated with a reduction in the degree of hepatic inflammation on liver biopsy, but there is little information regarding its effect on the development of cirrhosis. However, a reduction in the incidence of cirrhosis would be expected if viral clearance is achieved.

α-Interferon treatment should be monitored as described in the section on hepatitis B. As with hepatitis B, lack of response after 3 to 4 months of therapy is normally an indication to stop interferon. Side effects are also as described in the section on hepatitis B, but are usually less marked, as the dose used is less. Patients with hepatitis C occasionally feel better when taking interferon, particularly when they have had marked constitutional symptoms before commencing the treatment. Those who demonstrate a partial or complete response are normally continued on therapy for 6 months.

Clear guidelines for patients who have a transitory or partial response, or who relapse on discontinuing treatment, are not available. It may be that longer courses or higher doses of α-interferon will result in a higher rate of viral clearance. Long-term use of a low maintenance dose of interferon has also been proposed, but little is known of the long-term toxicity of such treatment. The benefit of such therapy must be weighed against both the morbidity and cost of such a strategy, and such therapy should be limited to controlled studies.

Prevention. Early reports have suggested that screening donated blood for hepatitis C reduces the rate of post-transfusion hepatitis by approximately 75%. Inactivation of hepatitis C by heat and detergent treatment in pooled blood products such as factor VIII and IX is effective in preventing hepatitis C infection. The use of clean needles by drug addicts may also help to prevent the spread of infection. The cause of community acquired or sporadic hepatitis C is poorly understood. While the virus is probably spread by sexual contact, the rate of infection is low. It is probably prudent to recommend safe sexual practices in patients known to be actively infected, but whether safe sex will reduce the community rate of infection is unclear.

Hepatitis D. Hepatitis D, also referred to as delta hepatitis, is a very unusual virus first described in Italy in 1977.[26] It is a small, circularly stranded RNA virus whose surface coat is formed by the HBsAg. As a result, this virus requires coinfection with hepatitis B for the formation of new viral particles. Similar synergistic coinfection by viruses is found among some plant viruses. Hepatitis D infection may occur as coinfection, in which both hepatitis B and delta hepatitis are acquired together or as superinfection of patients with chronic hepatitis B infection who then develop hepatitis D. Distinction between these two forms of hepatitis D infection has important prognostic implications. Unlike hepatitis B, the hepatitis D virus is cytopathic and induces liver injury through direct hepatocyte damage.

Epidemiology. Hepatitis D occurs most frequently among intravenous drug abusers but may occur in any patient at risk of hepatitis B. It follows that the incidence of infection is high in HIV-positive groups, particularly intravenous drug abusers. Like hepatitis B, the virus is highly infectious with a high incidence of infection in nonimmune–exposed individuals. The prevalence of infection is highest in the equatorial regions of the world, with a higher seroprevalence in Southern Europe than Northern Europe and a high incidence in the Middle East, Southern India, and Africa.

Serology. The diagnosis of hepatitis D is normally made by measuring IgM antibodies to the virus. The presence of antihepatitis D IgM antibodies correlates with active infection and therefore persistence of these antibodies correlates with chronic infection. Persistent infection without anti-delta IgM antibodies may occur, and therefore absence of these antibodies does not always mean that infection has resolved. However, resolution of infection is normally heralded by a loss of IgM antibodies and the appearance of IgG antibodies. A window between the disappearance of IgM and the appearance of IgG antibodies sometimes occurs. Therefore serial testing may be necessary before an acute self-limiting infection can be ruled out.

Hepatitis D coinfection may be associated with failure to express the normal hepatitis B antigens, so that coinfection with hepatitis B is best detected by measuring anti-HBc IgM. In superinfection, hepatitis B viral synthesis is normally reduced and some patients may become seronegative for hepatitis B DNA, HBeAg, and occasionally HBsAg. Other more sophisticated tests for hepatitis D are also available; these tests include the detection of hepatitis D Ag by immunoblotting and HDV RNA by hybridization.

Clinical Presentation. The clinical presentation of hepatitis D depends in part on its relationship to hepatitis B infection. In general, hepatitis D adds to the morbidity and mortality of hepatitis B by increasing the incidence of fulminant hepatitis and the progression to cirrhosis. In acute coinfection with both viruses, complete resolution normally occurs as is seen in most patients infected with hepatitis B alone. However, the illness tends to be more severe, with many cases of fulminant hepatitis reported. Coinfection may be suggested by a biphasic rise in transaminases. In superinfection of hepatitis D on pre-existing hepatitis B, the patient often has a mild rise in transaminases but may have an acute hepatic illness that is occasionally fulminant. In this setting there is a higher incidence of progression to chronic hepatitis D, which is associated with a more rapidly progressive course to cirrhosis and liver failure than with hepatitis B infection alone.[27] Hepatocellular carcinoma is less frequently reported in these patients. This may, however, simply be a marker of the rapidly progressive liver disease in this group of patients, with many of them dying of the complications of cirrhosis and liver failure before the onset of hepatocellular carcinoma.

Prevention. The prevention of hepatitis D infection depends on preventing the spread of hepatitis B; therefore, all precautions recommended for the prevention of hepatitis B, including immunization, are effective at limiting the spread of hepatitis D. Treatment of hepatitis D with α-interferon has been disappointing, with almost universal relapse on discontinuation of treatment: It is thus not recommended at present.

ALCOHOLIC LIVER DISEASE

In no area of hepatology is preventive medicine more important than in alcoholic liver disease. The hepatologist sees patients with irreversible, end-stage alcoholic liver disease. In contrast, the generalist is in an excellent position to diagnose alcoholic liver disease in its earliest stages, when abstinence may allow complete healing. Considering the high cost and relative ineffectiveness of treatment of cirrhosis, "an ounce of prevention" is worth more than "a pound of cure" in the alcoholic patient.

Approximately 5% of the adult population in the United States are chronic alcoholics, and approximately one fifth of them will develop some form of liver disease. It is therefore not surprising that alcoholism is the commonest cause of liver disease in our society. The amount of ethanol consumed each day and the duration of that consumption, rather than the type of alcoholic beverage, are critical factors in the development of cirrhosis. As a rough guideline, the development of cirrhosis requires daily ingestion of at least six cans of beer, 6 oz of whiskey, or a quart of wine for at least 5 to 10 years. However, individuals vary considerably regarding their response to the effects of alcohol. For example, some individuals consume huge amounts of alcohol daily for many years without any deleterious effect, whereas others develop liver disease after several years of heavy drinking.

The pathogenesis of alcoholic liver disease is not known. Alcohol exerts a direct toxic effect on the liver both in humans and in experimental animals. For example, high doses of alcohol given to nonalcoholic human volunteers for several days causes mild fatty liver.[28] Similarly, baboons fed alcohol in large doses develop fatty liver that cannot be prevented by maintenance of adequate nutrition.[29] It should be noted that a causal relationship between fatty infiltration and subsequent cirrhosis has not been clearly established. A more likely precursor of cirrhosis is acute alcoholic hepatitis, characterized by hepatocellular necrosis as well as by severe inflammation of the hepatic parenchyma. Recurrent alcoholic hepatitis triggered by excessive alcohol intake may lead to nodular regeneration, fibrosis, and eventually cirrhosis. Early recognition of alcoholic liver disease is critically important, because cessation of drinking in patients with fatty liver or alcoholic hepatitis may prevent progression to cirrhosis. The early diagnosis of alcoholic liver disease is more likely to be made on an outpatient basis at a time when the patient is asymptomatic or only mildly symptomatic and the morphologic lesion is reversible. The patient with established cirrhosis with portal hypertension, ascites, and varices has a much poorer prognosis and may not benefit appreciably from abstinence.[30]

In office practice, the diagnosis of alcoholism may be difficult. The average alcoholic patient in this setting is fully employed and may have a stable social situation. Excessive drinking may be denied or not even recognized as excessive by the patient or family. The commonest cause for erroneous diagnosis in this situation is failure of the physician to ask the most useful questions for detecting alcoholism.

The patient should be asked especially about drinking at lunchtime or in the morning, missing work because of "hangovers," or any concern on the part of the family about drinking. It is worthwhile to inquire about the amount of alcohol required to produce inebriation, since the alcoholic is usually tolerant of relatively large amounts of alcohol. Special efforts to control drinking, such as "going on the wagon" sporadically, suggest that there may be a problem. Patients should be questioned about automobile accidents, drunk-driving violations, falls, sexual dysfunction, marital difficulties, and job changes that may be related to occult alcoholism. Occult alcoholism should also be suspected in patients with unexplained macrocytosis, gastritis, or peripheral neuropathy.

Alcoholic Fatty Liver

Fatty liver is the earliest and mildest form of alcoholic liver disease. The patient is usually asymptomatic or may have nonspecific symptoms such as malaise or aching in the right upper quadrant. The physical examination reveals an enlarged, smooth liver that is occasionally tender. Splenomegaly, spider angiomata, and gynecomastia are absent. Fatty liver may not produce any abnormality of liver function tests or may be accompanied by elevation of the gamma glutamyl transpeptidase. Minor elevations of the transaminases and alkaline phosphatase level may occur, but bilirubin, prothrombin time, and albumin values are normal. These abnormalities are often detected on screening blood tests in asymptomatic individuals. A similar clinical presentation can be observed in mild viral or drug hepatitis, severe obesity, and diabetes mellitus, which can usually be ruled out by appropriate historical or laboratory data. The diagnosis of alcoholic fatty liver can be confirmed by liver biopsy, which reveals fatty infiltration without significant necrosis, inflammation, or fibrosis. Liver biopsy is not necessary in all patients with suspected alcoholic liver disease. The diagnosis can often be confirmed by asking the patient to abstain entirely from alcohol for 2 or 3 months, during which time the liver should decrease in size and the transaminase levels return to normal. If abnormalities persist because of either failure to abstain (often denied) or the presence of other liver disease, then liver biopsy can establish the correct diagnosis. The procedure is invasive but may reinforce the necessity to stop all alcohol. This last point is particularly important in patients who do not realize that their drinking is excessive.

Acute Alcoholic Hepatitis

Acute alcoholic hepatitis reflects more intense damage to the liver and usually follows heavy binge drinking superimposed on years of chronic alcoholism. Fatty infiltration is accompanied by hepatic necrosis and inflammation of varying degrees, which can produce a spectrum of clinical signs and symptoms. In the classic case, the patient is moderately or severely ill and has right upper quadrant pain, jaundice, nausea, vomiting, and fever. Excessive drinking may be denied, especially if these symptoms have caused the patient to curtail drinking recently. Coexisting conditions such as alcoholic gastritis, peptic ulcer disease, pancreatitis, delerium tremens, and vitamin deficiencies are common. On physical examination, the liver is enlarged and tender, and localized direct and rebound tenderness and guarding in the right upper quadrant may be elicited. Jaundice, ascites, gynecomastia, spider angiomata, and palmar erythema are common, especially in patients with coexistent cirrhosis. Laboratory abnormalities include leukocytosis with a shift to the left, hyperbilirubinemia occasionally as high as 30 mg/dl, elevation of the transaminase levels up to 400 units/ml, and elevation of the alkaline phosphatase level to two or three times the normal value. Decreased serum albumin level and prolonged prothrombin time not corrected by administration of vitamin K are quite common.

Differential Diagnosis. Many variations on this "typical" pattern are encountered in practice, and diagnostic confusion is common. A small percentage of patients with acute alcoholic hepatitis develop a cholestatic pattern with marked elevation of bilirubin and alkaline phosphatase levels and little or no elevation of transaminase levels. These laboratory findings in a setting of fever, right upper quadrant pain, and tenderness can lead to an erroneous diagnosis of impacted common duct stone. Biliary obstruction may be suspected from an abnormal ultrasound study, which can detect gallstones or dilated bile ducts. In some patients, endoscopic retrograde cholangiopancreatography (ERCP) is required to establish the patency of the biliary tree. Differentiation of alcoholic hepatitis from biliary obstruction is extremely important because surgery in acute alcoholic hepatitis carries an extremely high morbidity and mortality. Diagnostic errors in this situation result from failure to obtain a history of alcohol abuse; inadequate physical examination with failure to appreciate spiders, gynecomastia, or other signs of chronic liver disease; and, perhaps most important, failure to realize that alcoholic hepatitis can mimic biliary tract disease.

Alcoholic hepatitis in its milder forms may mimic acute viral hepatitis. The patient may present with gradual onset of jaundice and anorexia with little or no pain or tenderness in the right upper quadrant. Laboratory findings include mild or moderate elevation of the bilirubin and elevation of the serum glutamic-oxaloacetic transaminase (SGOT) up to 400 units/ml.

Liver biopsy in alcoholic hepatitis reveals the pathognomonic features of fatty infiltration and alcoholic hyalin. Unfortunately, liver biopsy is frequently impossible because of prolonged prothrombin time or decreased platelets. In such patients, the diagnosis of acute alcoholic hepatitis is based on clinical features and the exclusion of biliary tract disease by ultrasonography or ERCP.

Management. The patient with suspected alcoholic hepatitis should be hospitalized because of the poor prognosis and need for intensive medical management. The prognosis of acute alcoholic hepatitis depends on the severity and duration of the inflammatory lesion and the presence of coexisting cirrhosis and its complications. A mortality of 25 to 50% can be expected in severely ill patients with prolonged prothrombin times, encephalopathy, bleeding, and ascites. The efficacy of corticosteroid therapy in this group of patients is still controversial, but recent reports appear to confirm a beneficial effect of corticosteroids in patients with hepatic encephalopathy.[31, 32] Patients with cholestatic acute alcoholic hepatitis appear to have a better prognosis, probably because synthetic function is preserved. Abstinence from alcohol, good nutrition, and treatment of infections, electrolyte abnormalities, and encephalopathy are the mainstays of therapy. The liver lesion heals slowly over a period of 6 weeks to 3 months. Failure of liver function tests to normalize after abstinence suggests underlying cirrhosis.

Alcoholic Cirrhosis

Cirrhosis is the great mimic among liver diseases because of the variability of its clinical manifestations. Many "compensated" cirrhotics are asymptomatic or have mild or nonspecific symptoms, particularly in those who have stopped drinking. Cirrhosis in this situation may be manifested by asymptomatic hepatosplenomegaly, mild ascites, or sexual dysfunction. In contrast, patients with "decompensated cirrhosis" have signs and symptoms of liver failure. A typical presentation is gradually increasing jaundice with moderate or severe impairment of synthetic function, as evidenced by hypoalbuminemia and hypoprothrombinemia. Portal hypertension, ascites, and esophageal varices are common in these patients and contribute to the significant morbidity and mortality.

Liver function abnormalities in cirrhosis cover a wide spectrum. Approximately 5% of patients with Laennec's cirrhosis present with normal liver function tests or with intermittent minor abnormalities. In the patient with decompensated cirrhosis, mild to moderate jaundice with bilirubin levels up to 10 to 15 mg/dl are common. The transaminase levels are usually less than 200 units/ml, except in the presence of alcoholic hepatitis. The serum albumin level is usually decreased, especially in the presence of ascites or edema. Severe jaundice and hypoprothrombinemia usually indicate end-stage cirrhosis or some additional cause of hepatocellular necrosis, such as alcoholic or viral hepatitis or heart failure.

The natural history of alcoholic cirrhosis is one of inexorable decline punctuated by episodes of hepatic decompensation accompanied by superimposed infection, bleeding, or encephalopathy. The major complications of cirrhosis are portal hypertension with esophageal varices, ascites, and hepatic encephalopathy.

Portal Hypertension and Bleeding Esophageal Varices. Nodular regeneration in the cirrhotic liver distorts the parenchyma and obstructs intrahepatic portal venous channels. Increased portal venous pressure leads to formation of collateral venous channels most prominent at the lower end of the esophagus (esophageal varices) and anus (hemorrhoids). Hemorrhage from varices is a severe complication of cirrhosis and carries a 1-month mortality of 50% in the severest form of cirrhosis (Child's C). The overall 5-year survival after an episode of bleeding varices is only 25%, with most deaths caused by recurrence of bleeding.

The acute medical management of bleeding esophageal varices is aimed at stopping hemorrhage as quickly as possible.[33] The current treatment of choice is endoscopic sclerotherapy or banding of varices with a small rubber band. Under direct vision through the fiberoptic endoscope the bleeding varix is identified and injected with a sclerosing solution or banded until bleeding stops. Repeat therapy may be required to control rebleeding. The procedure is relatively safe in skilled hands and provides temporary control in the majority of patients. Unfortunately, sclerotherapy exerts no effect on the underlying portal hypertension, and eventual rebleeding is quite common.[34] Studies have failed to confirm the usefulness of propranolol in preventing variceal hemorrhage. Patients with an acceptable surgical risk are usually referred for shunt surgery to provide permanent control of portal hypertension.

Portacaval shunts reduce the risk of variceal hemorrhage by decreasing portal pressure, but may also reduce blood flow to the liver and impair hepatic function. As a result there is only slight improvement in overall survival in shunted patients. The most important factor determining the outcome of shunt surgery is the severity of liver disease prior to operation. Child's classification of cirrhosis is a useful guide in assessing a patient for a portacaval shunt (Table 29–4).[35] The class A cirrhotic patient is clearly the optimal candidate for surgery and has an overall mortality of approximately 5%, class B 15 to 20%, and class C 50% or higher.

The patient who survives an episode of bleeding and who has relatively good liver function without intractable ascites is clearly the best operative candidate. But individuals with less serious hepatic impairment also fare better with nonoperative treatment. However, one or more episodes of life-threatening bleeding are usually considered a reasonable indication for shunt surgery, since the risk of another potentially fatal bleed is quite high. The decision to operate and the type of shunt are based in part on the urgency of the situation and the experience of the surgeon. In experienced hands, the distal splenorenal shunt developed by Warren appears to produce the least impairment of hepatic blood supply and the best preservation of hepatic function.

Ascites

Ascites, the accumulation of excessive fluid within the peritoneal cavity, is a complication of established cirrhosis and portal hypertension but may also occur in severe acute liver disease. Increased portal pressure, decreased serum albumin levels, and excessive retention of salt and water are responsible for fluid accumulation.[36] Urinary sodium excretion in patients with ascites is typically 10 mEq/day or less compared with a normal urinary sodium excretion of 40 to 80 mEq/day.

Clinical Features and Diagnosis. Ascites usually accumulates slowly over several or more months in the cirrhotic patient, in contrast to patients with viral or alcoholic hepatitis, who may accumulate ascites over a period of several weeks. The classic physical findings of ascites, shifting dullness and a fluid wave upon abdominal percussion, are present only when 1 liter or more of fluid is present. Small collections may be detected by pelvic ultrasound, since ascites accumulates first in the pelvis. In the presence of large effusions, the abdomen is tense, the umbilicus is everted, and the viscera cannot be palpated because of the intervening fluid.

The *differential diagnosis of ascites* in the cirrhotic patient includes (1) conditions other than ascites that cause abdominal distention and (2) causes of ascites other than cirrhosis. Abdominal distention can occur with excess abdominal fat, abdominal gas, bladder distention, pancreatic pseudocyst, or large intra-abdominal tumors, particularly of the ovary or uterus. It should also be remembered that patients with pre-existing cirrhosis can develop ascites for other reasons, such as spontaneous bacterial peritonitis or tuberculous peritonitis. The route of infection in spontaneous bacterial peritonitis is usually not obvious, but may

TABLE 29–4. CHILD'S CLASSIFICATION OF CIRRHOSIS

	Class A	Class B	Class C
Bilirubin	<2.0	2.0–3.0	>3.0
Albumin	>3.5	3.0–3.5	<3.0
Ascites	None	Easily controlled	Poorly controlled
Encephalopathy	None	Minimal	Advanced
Nutrition	Excellent	Good	Poor

*Adapted from Child CG and Turcotte JG: Surgery and portal hypertension. *In* Child CG (ed): The Liver and Portal Hypertension. Philadelphia, WB Saunders, 1969, p 50.

arise from small leaks in the bowel or from spontaneous bacteremia. The main symptoms are fever, abdominal pain, and signs of diffuse or localized peritonitis.

Diagnostic paracentesis is required to establish the diagnosis of cirrhotic ascites and rule out other conditions.[37] Approximately 20 ml of ascitic fluid is withdrawn from the flank via a narrow-gauge needle (22-gauge or smaller). The midline approach is avoided, except in tense ascites, because the air-filled bowel tends to float upward and prevents withdrawal of fluid. In typical, uncomplicated Laennec's cirrhosis, the ascitic fluid is clear and of a pale straw color and has a protein concentration of between 0.5 and 2.0 g/dl. The cell count is usually less than 300 cells/mm^3 and consists primarily of mononuclear and mesothelial cells. The presence of bacterial infection is indicated by an increase in the total white blood cell count above 300 cells/mm^3, of which more than 25% are polymorphonuclear leukocytes. The protein may be elevated to more than 3 g/dl. If spontaneous bacterial peritonitis is suspected, fluid should be examined carefully by Gram stain to confirm the presence of bacteria and should be sent for culture and sensitivity. Tuberculous peritonitis produces a mononuclear rather than a polymorphonuclear leukocytosis. The diagnosis may be confirmed by acid fast stain or culture of concentrated ascitic fluid or by the finding of caseating granulomata on peritoneal or liver biopsy. Tumors involving the peritoneum cause elevation of the red blood cell count and protein content of ascitic fluid. Cytology of spun fluid may confirm the diagnosis in up to 60% of cases.

Management of Ascites in the Cirrhotic Patient. The mainstays of therapy in ascitic patients are *salt* and *water restriction* and judicious use of *diuretics.* Since daily sodium excretion in the ascitic patient is usually less than 10 mEq, the cirrhotic patient retains a large proportion of dietary sodium and water. Dietary sodium should be restricted to a total daily intake of 20 mEq (~ 1.2 g of sodium chloride) by eliminating added table salt and avoidance of foods rich in sodium. Since cirrhotic patients with ascites have excessive urinary loss of potassium due to secondary hyperaldosteronism, it is necessary to supplement their diets with 25 to 50 mEq/day of potassium chloride to maintain a normal serum potassium level. The total daily intake of water should be limited to 1 l/day. Not surprisingly, this strict regimen is difficult to maintain and is not suitable for long-term outpatient management, except in the most compulsive patients. It should be initiated in the hospital and, if successful, continued in a modified form following discharge.

Edema fluid enters the intravascular space more rapidly than does ascitic fluid; therefore, in ascitic patients with significant peripheral edema, a maximum loss of 1 kg of body weight per day is appropriate. However, in those without peripheral edema, loss of 0.5 kg/day is safer, since greater losses may result in reduction of effective circulating plasma volume and further impairment of renal function.

Evidence suggests that use of diuretics for treatment of ascites may not be as hazardous as previously feared.[38] A reasonable initial approach is modified bedrest and salt and water restriction, as outlined previously, accompanied by aldactone (25 mg four times daily) and furosemide (40 mg/day or twice daily). Furosemide may be increased stepwise every third day to 80 or 120 mg/day if necessary, and aldactone may be increased to 50 mg four times daily. The patient should be carefully monitored for volume depletion as evidenced by weight loss of greater than 1 kg/day, hypotension, or oliguria, and replenished promptly with intravenously administered salt-poor albumin or plasma, as indicated. Approximately 5 to 10% of patients do not respond to a diuretic regimen and are considered refractory. These patients may be treated by large-volume paracentesis (5 to 10 liters) through a small-bore catheter. This procedure is generally safe, especially if accompanied by infusion of salt-poor albumin to maintain plasma volume.[39] Another approach is implantation of a plastic shunt (Leveen shunt) between the peritoneal cavity and the subclavian vein, which allows direct transfer of ascitic fluid into the vascular compartment. This procedure rapidly decreases ascites and, in selected patients, is a reasonable, safe, and convenient alternative to large-volume paracentesis.[40]

Hepatic Encephalopathy

Hepatic encephalopathy is an organic brain syndrome caused by accumulation in the blood of toxic metabolites, including ammonia, short-chain fatty acids, mercaptans, and skatoles, which normally are removed from portal blood by the liver. Hepatic encephalopathy may occur in severe acute liver diseases, such as fulminant viral hepatitis or halothane hepatitis in which the reduced number of functioning hepatic lobules is no longer capable of removing toxic compounds from blood. Hepatic encephalopathy also occurs in patients with chronic liver disease, particularly cirrhosis, and results from shunting of portal blood around the liver as well as a reduction in functioning hepatocyte mass.

Several mechanisms have been proposed to explain hepatic encephalopathy: (1) ammonia toxicity, and (2) endogenous substances that potentiate neuroinhibitor circuits in the brain. Ammonia is produced in the colon by the action of bacterial enzymes on proteins and urea and is then carried in portal blood to the liver, where it is converted to urea. In the presence of severe liver disease or portasystemic shunting, ammonia bypasses the liver and accumulates in various organs, including the brain, where it interferes with energy metabolism. Administration of ammonium chloride or amino acids (which are converted to ammonia) to patients with liver disease causes marked worsening of hepatic encephalopathy. Gastrointestinal bleeding, which increases the protein load delivered to the colon and thus enhances bacterial ammonia production, also precipitates or worsens hepatic encephalopathy. Recently, it has been suggested that increased neural inhibition in the brain, mediated by the gamma-aminobutyric acid (GABA)-benzodiazepine receptor complex, may be responsible for some of the manifestations of hepatic encephalopathy. According to this theory, increasing levels of endogenous compounds that occupy the receptor are capable of inhibiting neural transmission.[41]

Clinical Features. The clinical manifestations of hepatic encephalopathy include (1) a metabolic brain syndrome manifested by deterioration of intellectual function, personality changes, and an altered state of consciousness and (2) a neuromuscular disorder characterized by rigidity, flapping tremor (asterixis), and gait disturbance. These manifestations are not pathognomonic of hepatic encephalopathy and are seen in various forms in other organic brain syndromes. The diagnosis of hepatic encephalopathy is based on the occurrence of these features in a patient with liver disease and the exclusion of other conditions that may mimic hepatic encephalopathy.

In patients with fulminant hepatitis, encephalopathy develops rapidly, and deep coma may occur within several days of onset. In contrast, patients with cirrhosis or surgically created shunts may initially manifest only subtle personality changes or dulling of intellectual function. Asterixis, gait disturbance, and muscle rigidity are variable and may be unnoticed by the patient or family.

The diagnosis of hepatic encephalopathy is based on clinical criteria. Elevation of venous or arterial ammonia levels generally occurs in patients with hepatic encephalopathy. However, the serum ammonia level is occasionally elevated in patients without significant liver disease and in some patients with cirrhosis who do not have encephalopathy. A characteristic high-amplitude slow wave pattern is observed in the electroencephalogram (EEG) of patients with hepatic encephalopathy but is not specific for this condition. Fetor hepaticus is a peculiar musty, fruit-like odor on the breath of patients with hepatic encephalopathy. It is not present in all patients and is sometimes quite difficult to appreciate.

It is especially important to distinguish between hepatic encephalopathy and sedative or narcotic use, acute alcoholism, delerium tremens, bacterial meningitis, Korsakoff-Wernicke syndrome, and subdural hematoma or other head injuries because these conditions occur frequently in alcoholics and are easily confused with hepatic encephalopathy. Lumbar puncture, skull films, brain scan, computed tomography (CT) scan, or angiographic studies should be obtained as indicated to exclude these and other causes of neurologic signs and symptoms in the cirrhotic patient.

Treatment. Treatment of acute hepatic encephalopathy is aimed primarily at lowering the production of ammonia in the colon. The first step in the severely encephalopathic patient is to eliminate all protein intake in order to reduce ammonia production by colonic bacteria. If gastrointestinal bleeding has occurred, the blood remaining in the gut should be quickly removed with cathartics, and the source of blood loss should be treated aggressively. The nonabsorbable antibiotic neomycin is administered orally or by enemas at a dosage of 1 g every 6 hours. This drug reduces ammonia production by decreasing the number of ammonia-producing organisms in the intestine.

Lactulose is a synthetic, nonabsorbable disaccharide that is metabolized by colonic flora to organic acids and lowers the pH in the lumen. The acidic environment inhibits ammonia production by enteric bacteria and may also inhibit colonic uptake of ammonia. Lactulose usually produces a reduction of serum ammonia levels and improvement in hepatic encephalopathy within 24 to 48 hours. The drug is administered as a loading dose of 50 ml of syrup (65 g/dl of lactulose) every 2 hours until diarrhea occurs, then as a maintenance dose of 30 ml four times daily, adjusted as necessary to produce two or three loose stools per day.

The recently introduced benzodiazepine-GABA receptor antagonist, flumenazil, acts to block the actions of benzodiazepines in the brain. When administered to some patients with hepatic encephalopathy, this drug results in improvement in symptoms. Although not yet approved for treatment of hepatic encephalopathy, it is likely that this drug will be effective as a form of adjunct therapy.[42] The first therapeutic modality in outpatient treatment should be restriction of dietary protein, which, by itself, may allow the patient to return to a functional level. Protein intake should not be restricted to less than 40 g/day because of lack of palatability. In the event that protein restriction is unsuccessful, lactulose should be administered at the smallest dose that effectively controls symptoms.

CHOLESTASIS

The term "cholestasis" indicates stoppage or *stasis of bile.* In practice, the term refers to *obstructive jaundice* with elevation of bilirubin and alkaline phosphatase levels and only moderate elevation of transaminase levels. Most patients with cholestasis are diagnosed based on the history, physical examination, and liver function tests. However, in 10 to 20% of cases, the diagnosis will remain unclear after initial evaluation, and the patient will require hospitalization for further diagnostic tests.

Clinical Features

Patients with cholestasis describe gradual darkening of urine and skin and pale-colored stools, accompanied by gradually worsening pruritus. Patients with mechanical bile duct obstruction may describe symptoms of gallstone disease or pancreatic carcinoma. In chronic cholestasis, steatorrhea may result from deficiency of bile salts in the lumen of the small intestine. Because fat-soluble vitamins require bile salt micelles for optimal absorption, patients with cholestasis sometimes manifest osteomalacia (vitamin D) and hypoprothrombinemia (vitamin K). Another manifestation of chronic cholestasis, particularly in primary biliary cirrhosis, is hypercholesterolemia manifested clinically by waxy, yellowish, lipid deposits in the eyelids (xanthelasma) and over tendons (xanthomas).

Liver function tests reveal elevation of the bilirubin, usually to levels exceeding 10 mg/dl. The ratio of direct to indirect bilirubin is of little or no value in differentiating between intrahepatic and extrahepatic cholestasis. The alkaline phosphatase level is usually elevated to at least three times the normal value. Very high elevations of the alkaline phosphatase level ($>$ 5 to 10 times the normal value) may be seen in patients with primary biliary cirrhosis. The transaminase, lactic dehydrogenase, and albumin levels are usually only slightly affected. Hypoprothrombinemia is secondary to failure to absorb vitamin K from the intestine and can be corrected by injection of water-soluble vitamin K.

Differential Diagnosis

The clinical features of cholestasis just outlined are nonspecific and occur in either intra- or extrahepatic cholestasis. Additional findings sometimes suggest a specific etiologic diagnosis. *Extrahepatic biliary obstruction* due to stones or stricture frequently is accompanied by ascending cholangitis, with recurrent fever, chills, and acute onset of right upper quadrant pain in a jaundiced patient. *Pancreatic* or *biliary duct carcinomas* typically are not accompanied by ascending cholangitis but usually produce steadily deepening jaundice, constant, boring pain in the right upper quadrant or back, and weight loss. Chronic biliary tract obstruction for 6 months or longer can lead to *secondary biliary cirrhosis,* which may be difficult to distinguish from primary biliary cirrhosis (see further on).

It is now recognized that *viral hepatitis,* especially hepatitis A, can produce intense cholestasis that mimics common bile duct obstruction. Thus, a history of close personal contact or other exposure to viral hepatitis provides an important clue to the diagnosis of cholestatic hepatitis. *Drugs* most commonly associated with cholestasis are chlorpromazine and related compounds, methyltestosterone, gold, propylthiouracil, and chlorpropamide. A temporal relationship between starting the drug and the onset of jaundice is critical in establishing the diagnosis of drug cholestasis. *Pregnancy* and the taking of *oral contraceptive pills* are also associated with cholestatic jaundice. *Alcoholic hepatitis* may enter a cholestatic phase characterized by deep jaundice without significant elevation of transaminase levels. A history of alcohol abuse and the physical stigmata of Laennec's cirrhosis suggest this diagnosis.

Primary Biliary Cirrhosis. This is a chronic liver disease of unknown etiology characterized by progressive intrahepatic cholestasis culminating in cirrhosis. The disease occurs predominantly in women in the third to fifth decades. The classic presentation is the gradual onset of pruritis and low-grade jaundice with disproportionate elevation of alkaline phosphatase levels. Hypercholesterolemia, xanthelasma, and xanthoma may be prominent. Clinical features suggestive of an autoimmune disturbance, including Sjögren's syndrome and Raynaud's phenomenon, are found in some patients. The presence of mitochondrial antibody is highly suggestive of primary biliary cirrhosis, since it is found in approximately 95% of patients with primary biliary cirrhosis but in only a small percentage (< 5%) of other types of cholestasis.

Widespread use of multiphasic blood screening tests has uncovered many patients with *presymptomatic primary biliary cirrhosis.* These patients have isolated elevation of alkaline phosphatase levels, usually two to three times the normal value, with only slightly elevated or normal bilirubin and transaminase levels. Liver biopsy reveals chronic inflammation and destruction of intrahepatic bile ductules usually without cirrhosis. The disease may remain dormant for years before pruritus and jaundice develop.[44] Conversely, death from liver failure occurs in most symptomatic patients with primary biliary cirrhosis within 5 to 10 years after onset.

Postoperative Intrahepatic Cholestasis. This is a type of intrahepatic cholestasis seen in the immediate postoperative period, most commonly in patients who have undergone major operations complicated by extensive blood loss, infection, hypoxemia, and heart failure.[45] In the typical presentation, cholestasis appears 4 to 7 days after surgery and gradually worsens over several weeks. The bilirubin may reach levels of 10 to 30 mg/dl, is predominantly direct-reacting, and is accompanied by two- to five-fold elevation of alkaline phosphatase levels. Transaminase levels are usually normal or only slightly elevated. The pathophysiology of postoperative intrahepatic cholestasis is related to a combination of hypoxia, anesthesia, blood loss, infection, and heart failure, which impair the excretory function of the liver.

Diagnostic Studies. The major diagnostic problem is the identification of patients with jaundice who require surgery versus those with liver disease and a normal biliary tree. In many instances, this can be decided on clinical grounds—for example, a jaundiced patient recently started on chlorpromazine or one with a classic history of gallstones. In patients in whom the diagnosis is not clear, a more aggressive diagnostic approach is required.

The usual approach is to start with less invasive studies and proceed to more invasive ones. Abdominal ultrasonography is very useful for detecting gallstones, a mass in the head of the pancreas, or dilation of the common duct. Abdominal CT scanning also is helpful in the diagnosis of mass lesions in the pancreas or porta hepatis, but in the absence of obesity or excessive intestinal gas, CT scanning is not more sensitive than abdominal ultrasound.

ERCP provides precise information regarding the patency of the biliary tree and is the most sensitive and specific procedure in the diagnostic evaluation of patients with suspected extrahepatic obstruction or puzzling jaundice. ERCP involves placement of a plastic catheter in the papilla of Vater under endoscopic guidance and retrograde injection of dye into the pancreatic and biliary duct systems. ERCP is the procedure of choice in jaundiced patients with suspected pancreatic disease, as it is the only procedure that visualizes the pancreatic ductal system. ERCP may allow removal of stones, placement of stents or drains, and papillotomy. ERCP is somewhat safer than skinny-needle cholangiography, which involves blind puncture of the hepatic parenchyma and injection of dye.

Liver biopsy is the diagnostic procedure of choice in patients with suspected intrahepatic cholestasis who cannot be diagnosed by viral serology or a careful history of drug exposure. Liver biopsy involves increased risk and should not be done in jaundiced patients if there is evidence of bile duct obstruction by ultrasound, CT or ERCP, or in patients with abnormal clotting studies.

Liver biopsy provides a specific morphologic diagnosis in patients with primary biliary cirrhosis, alcoholic liver disease, viral hepatitis, and granulomatous hepatitis. The morphologic criteria for extrahepatic biliary obstruction are not absolute except in cases of longstanding high-grade block. Thus, liver biopsy cannot readily distinguish between intrahepatic and extrahepatic obstruction. In a significant proportion of patients (one fourth to one half), liver biopsy reveals cholestasis, but a specific etiology is not apparent. Idiopathic cholestasis may be caused in some patients by inapparent exposure to viruses, drugs, or toxins that damage the liver and cause an excretory defect.

INFILTRATIVE LIVER DISEASE

Infiltrative liver diseases include a diverse group of conditions characterized by (1) very mildly abnormal or normal liver function tests, (2) mild to moderate hepatomegaly, and (3) diffuse infiltration of the liver with fat, tumor cells, or granulomata. Probably the commonest type of infiltrative liver disease in practice is fatty infiltration secondary to obesity, diabetes, or alcoholism. Though less common, metastatic liver disease and granulomatous hepatitis are more serious diseases that may require specific therapy. The diagnosis of infiltrative liver disease can usually be made by liver biopsy, since the abnormal tissue is distributed throughout the entire substance of the liver. The typical liver function pattern in infiltrative disease includes predominant elevation of the alkaline phosphatase or gamma-glutamyl-transpeptidase level, minor elevation of transaminase levels, and normal bilirubin level and prothrombin time. The albumin level is often depressed in patients with cancer or tuberculosis or other infections. It is not uncommon to observe normal or near normal liver function tests even when widespread liver metastases or granulomata are present.

Hepatic Carcinoma

Hepatic metastases occur in approximately 30 to 50% of patients with carcinoma; the usual sites for the primary tumor are pancreas, colon, stomach, kidney, or breast. Tumor infiltration is widespread because the metastases are borne via portal vein or hepatic artery. In most patients, the site of the primary tumor is known, and spread to liver and other organs occurs late in the disease. However, in occasional patients, metastatic liver disease may be the initial symptom of malignancy. These may present with painful enlargement of the liver, fever of unknown origin, or signs of portal hypertension. Occasionally, tumor deposits may be so massive that normal liver tissue is replaced, and liver failure, including encephalopathy, occurs. In some patients with metastatic adenocarcinoma, the primary tumor cannot be found despite a rather exhaustive search.

The diagnosis of metastatic liver carcinoma is quite obvious in the typical patient previously treated for carcinoma who presents with weight loss; a large, nodular liver; and elevation of the alkaline phosphatase level. Although nonspecific, the finding of an elevated sedimentation rate or of carcinoembryonic antigen is suggestive of metastatic malignancy. Radionuclide liver scan or hepatic ultrasound are nonspecific but usually detect tumors greater than 2 cm in diameter. Blind percutaneous liver biopsy is positive in approximately 50 to 75% of patients with known metastases. The yield can be improved by obtaining two cores of tissue, by performing cytology on the fluid in the biopsy needle, and by aiming the needle at specific lesions using ultrasound. Hepatic metastases occasionally are quite vascular, and hemorrhage is a complication of liver biopsy in approximately 1 or 2% of patients.

Primary liver cancer or *hepatoma* is much less common than metastatic disease, comprising only 5% of all liver tumors. The majority of patients in the United States with hepatoma have pre-existing cirrhosis; thus, the tumor develops in a liver already distorted by fibrous bands and regenerative nodules. The symptoms are similar to those of metastatic cancer. Hepatomas are very vascular tumors and tend to bleed into the peritoneum. α_1-Fetoprotein, a fetal globulin that normally disappears from the serum at birth, appears in the serum of 60% of American patients with hepatoma. The presence of high levels of α_1-fetoprotein is relatively specific for hepatoma, occurring only rarely in other tumors involving the liver. The diagnosis is confirmed by liver biopsy. Hepatoma rarely may be localized to one lobe of the liver, particularly in younger individuals without preexisting liver disease. These tumors may be cured by hepatic resection; in contrast, hepatoma complicating cirrhosis is almost always multicentric and not amenable to surgical cure.

Granulomatous Liver Disease

Granulomata of the liver may be secondary to tuberculosis, sarcoidosis, lymphoma, ingestion of certain drugs, fungal infections, schistosomiasis, or brucellosis. Rarely, granulomatous hepatitis may be primary; that is, no underlying disease process can be found. The clinical features depend in large part on the underlying etiology. Patients with infectious granulomata, such as miliary tuberculosis, disseminated fungal infections, or brucellosis, are usually ill with fever, weight loss, and signs and symptoms of organ involvement elsewhere. In chronic conditions such as sarcoidosis, the evolution is more indolent, and signs and symptoms are less impressive. Liver function tests reveal an isolated elevation of alkaline phosphatase level to one or two times the normal value. In contrast to metastatic deposits in the liver, granulomata seldom exceed 1 or 2 mm in diameter; thus, ultrasound and liver scan results are seldom positive.

The most common causes of granulomatous liver disease are miliary tuberculosis, sarcoidosis, granulomatous hepatitis secondary to drugs, and idiopathic granulomatous hepatitis. Since these conditions involve the liver diffusely, needle biopsy generally provides the specific diagnosis.

Liver Transplantation. Hepatic transplantation has been improved to the point at which 1-year survivals of 75% are routine. Moreover, the quality of life of transplanted patients is excellent, making it a safe and effective alternative for many patients with end-stage liver disease. The generalist should be aware of the indications for liver transplant, and should be able to recognize when patients with acute fulminant liver disease should be referred to a liver transplant center.

Most transplant patients are younger than 50 years of age, but in recent years the age limit has increased, and successful transplants in 70 year olds have been achieved. The most urgent indication is fulminant drug or viral hepatitis in young adults or teenagers. The fatality rate of fulminant hepatitis without transplantation is approximately 75% in very ill patients; thus, transplantation is a reasonable alternative. Inherited metabolic diseases in children, including Wilson's disease, α_1-antitrypsin deficiency, congenital bile duct abnormalities and various storage diseases affecting the liver, may also benefit from liver transplantation. In adults, primary biliary cirrhosis, sclerosing cholangitis and cirrhosis from varying causes are the most frequent indications. The routine use of cyclosporine following liver transplantation has greatly improved 5-year survival, which in some centers has reached 80%.[46]

REFERENCES

1. Bismuth H and Samuel D: Liver transplantation in fulminant and subfulminant hepatitis. *In* Morris PJ and Tilney NL (eds): Transplantation Reviews 3. Philadelphia, WB Saunders, 1989, p 47.
2. Cohen JI: Hepatitis A virus: Insights from molecular biology. Hepatology 9:889, 1989.
3. Gordon SG, Reddy KR, Schiff L, et al: Prolonged intra-hepatic cholestasis secondary to acute hepatitis A. Ann Intern Med 101:635, 1984.
4. Glikson M, Galun E, Oren R, et al: Relapsing hepatitis A: Review of 14 cases and literature survey. Medicine 71:14, 1992.
5. Flehmig B, Heinricy U, and Pfisterer M: Immunogenicity of a killed hepatitis A vaccine in seronegative volunteers. Lancet i:1039, 1989.
6. Mao JS, Dong DX, Zhang HY, et al: Primary study of live attenuated hepatitis A vaccine (H2) strain in humans. J Infect Dis 159:621, 1989.
7. Hoofnagle JH and Di Bisceglie AM: Serological diagnosis of acute and chronic viral hepatitis. Semin Liver Dis 11:73, 1991.
8. Chau KH, Hargie MP, Decker RH, et al: Serodiagnosis of recent hepatitis B infection by IgM class anti-HBc. Hepatology 3:142, 1983.
9. Yoffe B and Noonan CA: Hepatitis B virus new and evolving issues. Digestive Dis Sci 37:1, 1992.
10. Dudley FJ, Fox RA, and Sherlock S: Cellular immunity and hepatitis associated (Australia) antigen liver disease. Lancet i:743, 1971.
11. Alexander G: Treatment of acute and chronic viral hepatitis. Ballière's Clinical Gastroenterology 3:1, 1989.
12. Lo KJ, Tong MG, Chien ML, et al: The natural history of chronic hepatitis B surface antigen positive liver disease in Taiwan. J Infect Dis 146:205, 1982.
13. Perrillo RP: Treatment of chronic hepatitis B with interferon: Experience in western countries. Semin Liver Dis 9:240, 1989.
14. Brook MG, Karayiannis P, and Thomas HC: Which patients with chronic hepatitis B virus infection will respond to α-interferon therapy? A statistical analysis of predictive factors. Hepatology 10:761, 1989.
15. Bruguera M, Cremades M, Salinas R, et al: Impaired response to recombinant hepatitis B vaccine in HIV-infected persons. J Clin Gastroenterol 14:27, 1992.
16. Feinstone SM, Kapikian AZ, Purcell RH, et al: Transfusion associated hepatitis not due to viral hepatitis A or B. N Engl J Med 292:769, 1975.
17. Choo Q-L, Kuo G, Weiner AJ, et al: Isolation of a cDNA clone derived from a blood borne non-A, non-B viral hepatitis genome. Science 359, 1989.

18. Alter HJ: Descartes before the Horse: I clone therefore I am: The hepatitis C virus in current perspective. Ann Intern Med 115:644, 1991.
19. Kato N, Hijikata M, Ootsuyama Y, et al: Molecular cloning of the human hepatitis C virus genome from Japanese patients with non-A, non-B hepatitis. Proc Nat Acad Sci USA 87:9524, 1990.
20. Feinstone SM: Hepatitis C virus. Eur J Gastroenterol Hepatol 3:572, 1991.
21. Alter HJ: The hepatitis C virus and its clinical relationship to the clinical spectrum of NANB hepatitis. J Gastroenterol Hepatol 1(Suppl):78, 1990.
22. Stevens CE, Taylor PE, and Pindyck J: Epidemiology of hepatitis C virus: A preliminary study in volunteer blood donors. JAMA 263:49, 1990.
23. Rumi MG, Colombo M, Gringeri A, et al: High prevalence of antibodies to hepatitis C virus in hemophiliacs treated with hepatitis C virus contaminated factor VIII concentrates. Ann Intern Med 112:379, 1990.
24. Alter HJ, Purcell RH, Shih JW, et al: Detection of antibody to hepatitis C virus in prospectively followed transfusion recipients with acute and chronic non-A, non-B hepatitis. N Engl J Med 321:1494, 1989.
25. Davis GL, Balart LA, Schiff ER, et al: Treatment of chronic hepatitis C with recombinant interferon α. N Engl J Med 321:1501, 1989.
26. Rizzetto M, Canese MG, Arico S, et al: Immunofluorescence detection of new antigen antibody system (delta/antidelta) associated to hepatitis B virus in the liver and serum of HBsAg carriers. Gut 18:997, 1977.
27. Saracco G, Rosina F, Brunnetto MR, et al: Rapidly progressive HBsAg positive hepatitis in Italy: The role of hepatitis delta virus infection. J Hepatol 5:274, 1987.
28. Rubin E and Lieber CS: Alcohol-induced hepatic injury in nonalcoholic volunteers. N Engl J Med 278:869, 1968.
29. Lieber CS and DeCarli LM: An experimental model of alcohol feeding and liver injury in the baboon. J Med Primatol 3:153, 1974.
30. Pande NV, Resnick RH, Yee W, et al: Cirrhotic portal hypertension: Morbidity of continued alcoholism. Gastroenterology 74:64, 1978.
31. Imperiale DF and McCullough AJ: Do corticosteroids reduce mortality from alcoholic hepatitis? A meta-analysis of randomized trials. Ann Intern Med 113:299, 1990.
32. Ramond M-J, Poynard T, Rueff B, et al: A randomized trial of prednisone in patients with severe alcoholic hepatitis. N Engl J Med 326:507, 1992.
33. Cello JP, Grendell JH, Crass RA, et al: Endoscopic sclerotherapy versus portacaval shunt in patients with severe cirrhosis and acute variceal hemorrhage. N Engl J Med 316:11, 1987.
34. The Copenhagen Varices Sclerotherapy Projects: Sclerotherapy after first variceal hemorrhage in cirrhosis. N Engl J Med 311:1589, 1984.
35. Child CG and Turcotte JG: Surgery and portal hypertension. *In* Child CG (ed): The Liver and Portal Hypertension. Philadelphia, WB Saunders, 1964, p 50.
36. Rocco VK and Ware AJ: Cirrhotic ascites: Pathophysiology, diagnosis and management. Ann Intern Med 105:573, 1986.
37. Hoefs JC: Diagnostic paracentesis: A potent clinical tool. Gastroenterology 98:230, 1990.
38. Gregory PB, Broekelschen PH, Hill MD, et al: Complications of diuresis in the alcoholic patient with ascites: A controlled trial. Gastroenterology 73:534, 1977.
39. Gines P, Arroyo V, Quintero E, et al: Comparison of paracentesis and diuretics in the treatment of cirrhotics with tense ascites: Results of a randomized study. Gastroenterology 93:234, 1987.
40. Stanley MM, Ochi S, Lee KK, et al: Peritoneovenous shunting as compared with medical treatment in patients with alcoholic cirrhosis and massive ascites. N Engl J Med 321:1632, 1989.
41. Jones EA, Skolnuck P, Gannal SH, et al: The gamma-aminobutyric acid A (GABA A) receptor complex and hepatic encephalopathy. Ann Intern Med 110:532, 1989.
42. Ferenci P, Grimm G, Meryn S, et al: Successful long-term treatment of portal-systemic encephalopathy by the benzodiazepine antagonist flumenazil. Gastroenterology 96:240, 1989.
43. Gordon SC, Reddy KR, Schiff L, et al: Prolonged intrahepatic cholestasis secondary to acute hepatitis A. Ann Intern Med 101:635, 1984.
44. Roll J, Boyer JL, Barry D, et al: The prognostic importance of clinical and histologic features in symptomatic and asymptomatic primary biliary cirrhosis. N Engl J Med 308:1, 1983.
45. Becker S and LaMont JT: Post-operative jaundice. Semin Liver Dis 8:2, 1988.
46. Iwatsuki S, Starzl TE, Todo S, et al: Experience in 1000 liver transplants under cyclosporine steroid therapy: A survival report. Transplant Proc 20(Suppl 1):945, 1988.

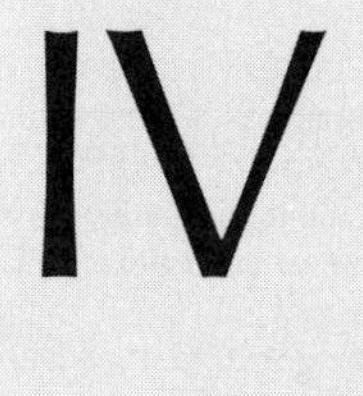

Genitourinary Problems

30 Abnormal Urinalysis

WILLIAM T. BRANCH, Jr., MD

An abnormal urinalysis, often obtained as a routine screening procedure, is commonly encountered in general medical practice. The approach always begins with a careful examination of the urine itself. The need for additional studies depends on the clinical setting as well as on findings in the urine.

Urinalysis

Albuminuria is detected by dipstick and abnormalities of the sediment by microscopic examination after centrifugation of 10 ml of urine for 5 to 10 minutes. In most cases in which proteinuria is detected by dipstick, the origin is from the glomerulus, and the proteinuria chiefly consists of albumin. The sensitivity of dipstick tests for albuminuria is variable; depending upon urinary concentration, it may record as little as 50 mg/day or miss as much as 300 mg/day.[1] Electrophoresis is necessary to identify Bence Jones or myeloma proteins and the proteins excreted in tubular diseases (α- and β-microglobulins and muramidase), since these are not detected by a dipstick. Albuminuria is also present in advanced interstitial nephritis, when the glomeruli are affected.

Dipstick examination may be used to screen the urine for red blood cells (RBC) and white blood cells (WBC). Dipsticks are reported to be positive in almost all urines containing 3 or more RBCs per high power field (RBC/hpf) but were positive in only 81 to 87% of those containing 1 to 3 RBC/hpf.[2] Dipsticks containing leukocyte esterase are reported to be positive in 97% of urines containing 1 to 3 or more WBC/hpf if read at 5 minutes but in only 90% if read at 1 minute.[2] The high sensitivity of the dipstick justifies using this method to prescreen and select urine for microscopic examination in low-risk populations.[2]

The sediment may contain RBCs, WBCs, epithelial cells, or casts. Normal limits are listed in Table 30–1.[3] The concentrated "button" of sediment in the test tube should be identified after centrifugation to avoid discarding it accidentally. After resuspending the button, one first examines

TABLE 30–1. NORMAL LIMITS FOR URINE SEDIMENT

Red blood cells	1–2/hpf
White blood cells	1–2/hpf (males) 1–5/hpf (females)
Epithelial cells	1–2/hpf (males) 1–5/hpf (females)
Hyaline or finely granular casts	1/10–20 hpf

under low power to identify casts before switching to high power for the cellular elements. The same normal limits for WBCs apply to epithelial cells, which arise from renal tubules or from transitional epithelium of the renal pelvis, ureters, and bladder, and to squamous epithelial cells from the vagina in female patients. In acute tubular necrosis, pyelonephritis, and glomerulonephritis, large numbers of tubular epithelial cells slough into the urine.

Hyaline or finely granular casts in urine sediment represent precipitated mucoproteins secreted by cells in the distal nephron. Cast formation of any type is promoted by increased proteinuria, stasis, acid urine, or agglutination of tubular cells, but casts containing RBCs or WBCs are always pathologic, since these cells normally are not found within tubules. Very broad casts arise from the larger collecting tubules, implying low flow as seen in chronic glomerulonephritis, and thus are called "renal failure casts." Any low-flow state, particularly acute tubular necrosis, can lead to a shower of hyaline or finely granular casts. WBC casts occur when there is inflammation within the glomeruli or tubules, although clumps of WBCs can arise from anywhere in the collecting system. If casts contain RBCs or if coarsely granular casts are heme-pigmented, there must be bleeding at the level of glomeruli or tubules. This would imply that a patient has glomerulonephritis, vasculitis, or, less commonly, acute interstitial nephritis or acute tubular necrosis.

Clinical Anatomy and Histopathology

The anatomy of the kidney and collecting system is illustrated in Figures 30–1 and 30–2. The clinician also should be familiar with the histopathology of glomerular lesions.

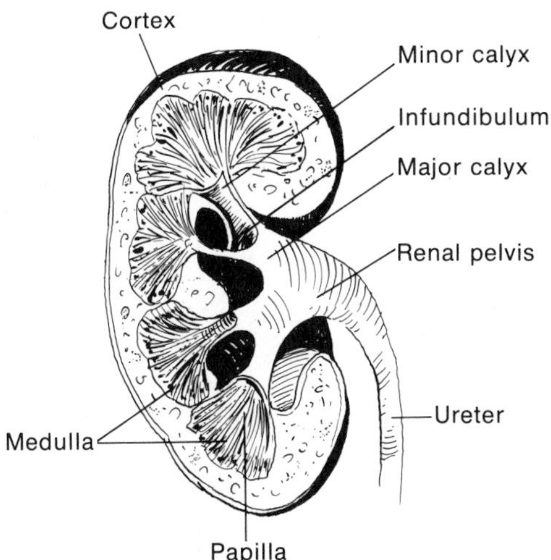

FIGURE 30–1. Clinical anatomy of the kidney. The renal pelvis divides into three major calyces; these each are connected by infundibula to groups of three or four minor calyces, into which drain the renal papillae.

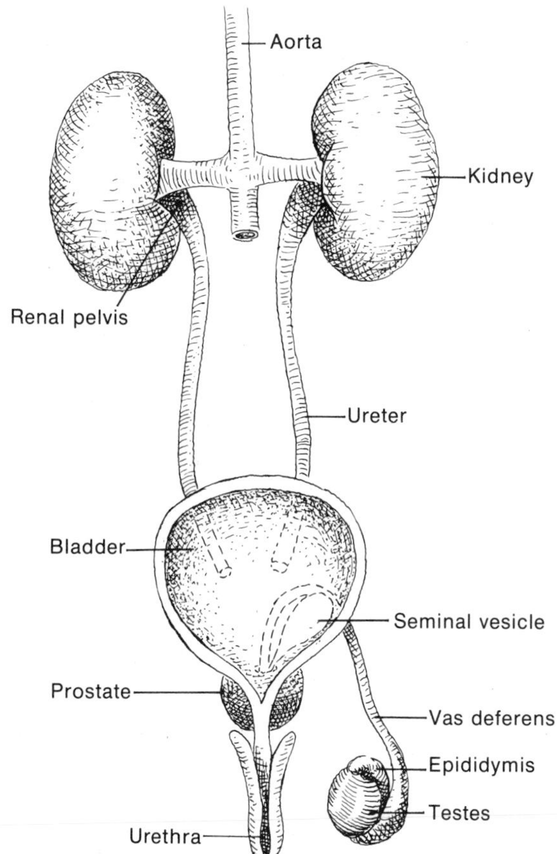

FIGURE 30–2. The kidneys and collecting systems.

One approach divides these into proliferative lesions and nonproliferative lesions by light microscopy. Proliferative lesions have increased cellularity within the glomerular mesangial matrix, either as an exudate consisting of polymorphonuclear leukocytes or as increased numbers of mesangial cells. The proliferative lesion is termed focal glomerulonephritis when only some parts of some glomeruli are involved; it is termed diffuse glomerulonephritis when all glomeruli are completely involved. Any of the proliferative glomerulonephritides may be accompanied by the finding of fibroepithelial crescents within glomeruli. These indicate an especially intense inflammatory response and are associated with the clinical syndrome of rapidly progressive glomerulonephritis.

In *minimal change* or *"nil" disease,* there are no light microscopic findings other than sometimes a slight mesangial prominence. Electron microscopy reveals nonspecific fusion of the epithelial cell foot processes of glomerular basement membranes in these patients. In *membranous glomerulonephritis,* there is a diffuse thickening of the capillary walls on light microscopy without mesangial proliferation. Electron micrographs show that this is due to deposits located on the epithelial side of the glomerular basement membrane. In *focal sclerosing glomerulonephritis,* there is focal and segmental shrinkage of glomerular tufts with capsular adhesions but no cellular proliferation. Heavy proteinuria may be associated with these nonproliferative lesions.

HEMATURIA

The incidence of microscopic hematuria in general medical patients is unknown, but in a survey of asymptomatic military recruits, 2 to 4 or more RBC/hpf were present in 5.2% of urinalyses performed and more than 8 RBC/hpf were present in 1%.[4] Gross hematuria occurs less frequently but was the chief complaint of 0.1% of emergency room patients.[5] The incidence of serious lesions is greater with gross hematuria than with microscopic hematuria. But whether hematuria is detected on routine examination or is the patient's complaint, the physician must plan an evaluation that is adequate to exclude serious causes but that spares expensive, invasive, and repeated studies as much as possible. If microhematuria is reported, its presence should be confirmed by repeat urinalysis. A culture is usually performed, even in asymptomatic patients, to identify those abnormalities that may be attributed to urinary tract infections. In female patients, routine urinalyses should not be collected during menses.

A positive dipstick (Hematest) result indicates that hematuria, hemoglobinuria, or myoglobinuria is present. If the test result is negative but the urine is discolored, another substance must account for red or brown urine. This can be bilirubin, porphyrin, or melanin (in metastatic melanoma). It also could be an ingested substance such as azodyes (Pyridium), nitrofurantoin, *para*-aminosalicylate, beets, and other drugs or substances.[6] Hemoglobinuria can be distinguished from myoglobinuria because in the latter the serum is clear when spun down. The approach to patients with red urine is outlined in Figure 30–3.

Sometimes the source of gross hematuria is apparent. The presence of clots usually indicates bleeding from the bladder. Initial hematuria comes from the urethra; terminal hematuria, which in women is sometimes present on toilet tissue, may be from the bladder neck, posterior urethra, or (in men) prostate. Blood appearing independently of micturition is from the distal urethra; unless the source is obviously trauma, a caruncle, or an ulcer, urethroscopy is necessary to exclude strictures or carcinomas. A brown or "smoky" color of hematuria reflects stasis in an acid urine, suggesting a renal origin. When RBC casts can be found, the source of bleeding almost certainly is within the renal parenchyma.

Dysuria plus hematuria usually, but not always, implies a urinary tract infection. Infection or another process producing inflammation is also likely whenever there is an excessive number of leukocytes in the urine. Painless midstream hematuria classically is associated with neoplasms and other structural abnormalities of the urinary tract.

Differential Diagnosis

Table 30–2 lists the findings to which hematuria was attributed in 1000 adult patients referred for gross hematuria,[7] together with findings in 500 asymptomatic adults with microscopic hematuria, all of whom had complete urologic evaluations.[8] Clearly, the incidence of various etiologies depends on how patients are selected as well as on findings in the urine. In a series largely drawn from an army recruiting center, 48% of subjects had calculous disease. Of patients referred to a nephrology group, 80% had lesions characterized as glomerulonephritis on renal biopsy.

Of greater importance to the clinician is knowing the probability of a serious or treatable disease when patients are found to have hematuria. About 5% of patients with asymptomatic microhematuria reported by Greene had lesions that represented a clear, immediate threat to their well-being or required major surgical intervention (Table 30–3).[8] Carcinoma of the bladder accounted for more than one third of the significant lesions. Notably, patients with fewer than 8 RBC/hpf were as likely to have a serious disease as those with more than 30. A more recent study of 200 patients with asymptomatic microhematuria yielded 11% with bladder carcinoma.[9] The increased number of bladder tumors in this series probably resulted from better recognition of carcinomas in situ but may also reflect the selection of patients by referral for urologic evaluation because their microhematuria was persistent. Sixty-two of the 64 patients with significant lesions in the two studies were older than 50 years of age. In younger patients with microhematuria, the odds favor benign or trivial causes. Of 1000 asymptomatic military recruits, 38.7% had 2 to 4 or more RBC/hpf on at least one urinalysis, done annually for 12 years, and only one of these 387 persons (who had 10 to 12 RBC/hpf) was eventually discovered to have bladder carcinoma.[4]

Gross hematuria, if not explained by cystitis, is more likely than microhematuria to be caused by a serious disease, as illustrated by the finding of carcinoma of the kidney or bladder in 18.4% of the 1000 patients referred for this reason for urologic examination.[7] It is also well known that serious lesions of the kidney or bladder may bleed only transiently.

The most common causes of hematuria are cystitis, urethritis, and bleeding from the prostate; the most serious are bladder and kidney carcinoma, calculous disease, and renal tuberculosis. In addition, glomerulonephritis is an important cause of hematuria, in which the question of whether or not to perform a renal biopsy may be raised.

Cystitis

Cystitis is the most common cause of gross hematuria, accounting for 22% of cases referred to urologists and 26% of those seen in an emergency room.[5,7] Most patients with cystitis have other symptoms, such as dysuria, frequency, fever, and suprapubic or flank pain,[5] but in the two series

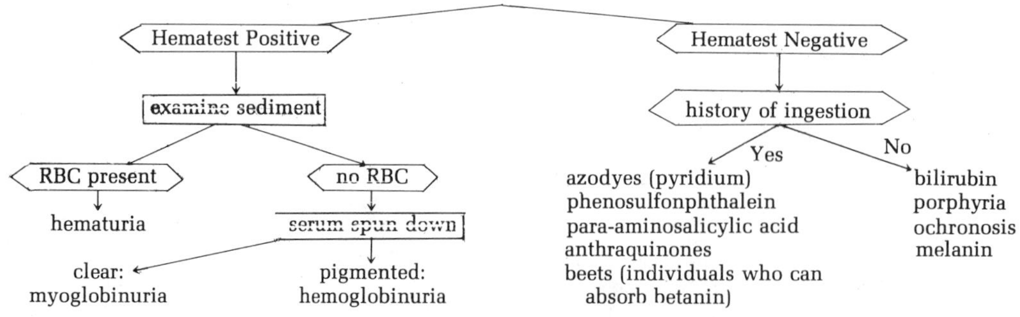

FIGURE 30–3. Approach to patients with red urine.

TABLE 30–2. FINAL DIAGNOSIS IN SELECTED PATIENTS WITH HEMATURIA*

	1000 Adults with Gross Hematuria (%)[7]	500 Adults with Asymptomatic Microhematuria (%)[8]
Bladder	**39.5**	**9.6**
Cystitis	22.0	3.4
Vesical neoplasm	15.0	1.8
Miscellaneous: trigonitis, diverticulum, varices, calculi, trauma, irradiation, chemical injury, foreign body	2.5	4.4
Prostate	**23.6**	**25.4**
Benign hyperplasia	12.5	23.6
Miscellaneous: varices, prostatitis, stricture, calculus, carcinoma	11.1	1.8
Kidney	**15.2**	**6.4**
Renal neoplasm	3.5	0.4
Glomerulonephritis	0.6	0†
Calculi	2.7	3.4
Pyelonephritis	3.0	0.2
Miscellaneous: renal cyst, hydronephrosis, horseshoe kidney, renal agenesis, trauma, polycystic kidneys, ptosis, infarct, nephrosclerosis, drug toxicity	4.4	2.4
Ureter	**6.5**	**2.2**
Calculus	5.3	0.4
Miscellaneous: tumor, stricture, ureteritis cystica, ureterocele	1.2	1.8
Urethra	**4.3**	**22.6**
Urethritis	1.3	21.2
Miscellaneous: stricture, calculus, tumor, foreign body, trauma, diverticulum, polyps	3.0	1.4
Other Causes	**2.4**	**0.8**
Tuberculosis	0.7	0
Miscellaneous: hemophilia, sickle cell disease, thrombocytopenia, sodium warfarin (Coumadin) overdose	1.7	0.8
Essential Hematuria	**8.5**	**34.4**

*Adapted from Kurdish GG: Determining the cause of hematuria. Postgrad Med *58*:118, 1975; and Greene LF, O'Shaughnessy EJ Jr, and Hendricks ED: Study of 500 patients with asymptomatic microhematuria. JAMA 161:610–613. Copyright 1956, American Medical Association.

†Excluded all with red blood cell casts or proteinuria.

of patients with asymptomatic microhematuria, cystitis was present in 3.4 to 10.5% despite the lack of symptoms.[8, 9] Generally, no further evaluation is necessary if the patient is a young woman with typical symptoms and a positive urine culture and if the symptoms resolve after treatment and the urine is clear on a repeat urinalysis.[10, 11] It is more puzzling if the result of the culture is negative in a patient complaining of dysuria. Transient hemorrhagic cystitis has been reported in adenovirus type 11 infection.[12] In other patients, sterile dysuria with or without pyuria or microhematuria can be noted in infections confined to the urethra. Whereas cystitis was common in patients with gross hematuria, the most common cause of unexplained microhematuria (22.6%[8]) was urethritis, often suggested by inflammation of the bladder trigone at cystoscopy (trigonitis).

TABLE 30–3. NATURE AND INCIDENCE OF SIGNIFICANT LESIONS IN 500 SELECTED PATIENTS WITH ASYMPTOMATIC MICROHEMATURIA*

Urologic Lesion	No. of Patients	%
Carcinoma of the bladder	9	1.8
Renal calculus	4	0.8
Renal cyst	4	0.8
Renal neoplasm	2	0.4
Ureteral calculus	2	0.4
Hydronephrosis	1	0.2
Occlusion of renal pedicle	1	0.2
Urethral stricture	1	0.2
		4.8

*Adapted from Greene LF, O'Shaughnessy EJ Jr, and Hendricks ED: Study of 500 patients with asymptomatic microhematuria. JAMA 161:610–616. Copyright 1956, American Medical Association.

Occasionally, patients with negative results on cultures have hematuria with frequency or dysuria that are chronic or recur frequently. Urinary tract tuberculosis and neurogenic bladder should be excluded. In postmenopausal women, chronic interstitial cystitis, a poorly understood idiopathic inflammatory process leading to fibrosis of the bladder, may cause these symptoms. In such cases, urgency or pain after voiding, progressive frequency of urination, and nocturia are indicative of a declining capacity for urine. Biopsy specimens may reveal fibrosis with round cell infiltration. The urine sediment may contain evidence of microscopic hematuria or pyuria. Similar clinical findings occur after cyclophosphamide therapy or several years after a course of radiation therapy. Of concern is to ensure that such patients do not have carcinoma of the bladder concurrently. In a series of 501 patients with symptoms of idiopathic, chronic interstitial cystitis, cystoscopies identified 15 patients (3%) who had bladder carcinoma.[13] Bladder carcinoma also has developed in patients after pelvic irradiation[14] and in patients thought to have interstitial cystitis due to long-term therapy with cyclophosphamide.[15] Interstitial cystitis is rare in men and creates a very high suspicion of malignancy.

Benign Prostatic Hypertrophy

The prostate is commonly the source of gross hematuria (23.6%[7]) and of microhematuria (25%[8]). The patient's history or examination may suggest chronic prostatitis or benign prostatic hypertrophy; however, even terminal hematuria can be caused by bladder neoplasia, so that one can never be certain that the prostate is the source of bleeding except by exclusion. Most commonly, a prostatic vein or varix ruptures, causing gross hematuria in patients with benign prostatic hyperplasia. Nevertheless, the prostate of any male patient with microscopic or gross hematuria should be examined carefully, since bleeding occurs in carcinoma of the prostate as well as in benign hypertrophy and chronic prostatitis. Many clinicians will also obtain a prostate specific antigen (PSA) level (see Chapter 34). Biopsies should be taken whenever there is induration or nodularity of the gland, elevated PSA, or any other features suggestive of malignancy.

Carcinoma of the Bladder

Bladder neoplasia is the major concern in patients with hematuria. Fifteen per cent with gross hematuria and 1.8 to 11% of patients with microhematuria had bladder tumors.[7–9] Age is an important feature in determining the likelihood of bladder carcinoma. Over the age of 65 years, the incidence reaches 1 case per 1000 population.[16] Below age 35 years, the lesion is unusual—about 1 case per 100,000 per year.[16] The tumor is associated with occupational exposure to dyes and organic solvents and with heavy cigarette smoking or analgesic nephropathy. Leather and rubber workers, textile workers, painters, hairdressers, shoemakers, and those exposed to coal, coke, asphalt, tar, or pitch may be at risk. Coffee, tea, and artificial sweeteners did not increase risk in several case-control studies, although the possibility of a small elevation of risk in subjects who reported very frequent use of artificial sweeteners was raised by one study.[17–19]

Intermittent, painless hematuria is the hallmark feature, although some patients present manifestations of cystitis (discussed previously) or bladder neck obstruction. Carcinoma of the bladder is staged according to the degree of invasion of the bladder wall. The most common lesions are confined to the submucosa (i.e., stage A) and have 70 to 80% 5-year survivals.[20, 21] In situ carcinoma (stage 0) is an anaplastic tumor sometimes associated with shorter survival, and 5-year survival is 50% or less in the more invasive stages (B, C, and D).[20, 21] It is important that patients with early-stage lesions treated by local resection have cystoscopy at regular intervals in anticipation of the very high (>60%) recurrence rate.

Carcinoma of the Kidney

Renal neoplasia was found in 3.5% of those with gross hematuria and 0.6% of those with microscopic hematuria.[7, 8] Ninety per cent of tumors in adults are renal cell carcinomas (hypernephromas). These are rare before the age of 40 years but increase in frequency, reaching death rates of 0.22 (men) and 0.12 (women) per 1000 in those older than 60 years of age.[22] Unfortunately, hematuria, which is present in 50 to 75% of cases, is often a late sign that indicates invasion of the vascular or collecting system. Other patients present flank pain, which may indicate obstruction, local extension, or, if continuous and aching in character, distention of the renal capsule. Because most tumors are discovered late in their course, as many as 40% of patients have palpable masses. A variety of systemic manifestations have been associated with these tumors: anemia, 41%; fever, 17%; elevated alkaline phosphatase level, 10%; hypercalcemia, 6%; erythrocytosis, 4%; myopathy, 3%; protein-losing enteropathy, rare; and possibly hypertension, 38%.[23] Alert clinicians can detect a few cases at early stages if these symptoms lead to an investigation of the urinary tract.

Seven to 8% of renal neoplasms are papillary tumors of the renal pelvis, usually transitional cell carcinomas.[24] These tumors characteristically present gross hematuria and less frequently flank pain or ureteral colic. In 30 to 40% of these lesions, there are additional malignant transitional cell tumors elsewhere in the ureters or bladder.

Calculous Disease

The prevalence of calculous disease in patients with hematuria varies from 3.8% in asymptomatic microhematuria[8] and 8% in symptomatic gross hematuria[7] to as high as 48% in a population with microhematuria selected from young, previously healthy army recruits.[4] Renal colic and hematuria are the presenting symptoms and signs in about 90% of men and 50% of women with calculous disease (the remaining female patients mostly have urinary infections). An identical colicky pain can be caused by clots, necrotic tumor fragments, necrotic papillae, or radiolucent calculi within the ureter. These must be considered whenever a radiopaque calculus cannot be identified in patients with hematuria and renal colic.

Glomerular Diseases

Glomerular abnormalities account for the majority of young patients with persistent asymptomatic microscopic hematuria or recurrent bouts of gross hematuria and no other findings in whom a structural abnormality of the urinary tract is not identified.[25] About 10% of patients with gross hematuria[7] and 20 to 34% of those with microhematuria[8, 9] are in this category. About two thirds of these patients have focal glomerulonephritis.[26] Various immunofluorescent patterns are associated with this histopathology, including diffusely distributed mesangial IgA, scattered deposits of complement, additional small deposits of IgM or IgG, and so on,[27] but patients whose only abnormality is hematuria most commonly have IgA deposition.[27] About one third of patients have mild but diffuse proliferative glomerulonephritis.[27] One might suspect benign familial hematuria if RBC and hemoglobin casts are also found in the urine of first-degree relatives with normal renal function.[28]

The presenting clinical sign is microhematuria found on routine urinalysis in about half the patients with focal glomerulonephritis; the others have recurrent bouts of gross hematuria, often following upper respiratory infections. Colicky pain can occur during the attacks, apparently caused by the passage of blood clots. Most episodes last a few days, although grossly bloody urine has persisted for as long as several months in occasional patients.[26]

The single most useful finding in the urine for identifying patients with hematuria due to glomerular disease is the presence of RBC or heme-pigmented granular casts. A meticulous search identified these in 94% of the 33 patients with focal glomerulonephritis in one series.[29] Only about half the patients with focal glomerulonephritis or mild diffuse proliferative glomerulonephritis have proteinuria, which is present in at least 90% of the patients with chronic glomerulonephritis.[26] Dysmorphic RBCs in the urine, identified by Wright's stain or phase contrast microscopy, are reported to indicate a glomerular source of bleeding, whereas crenated or "ghost" RBCs occur in hematuria of any etiology.[30, 31]

The short-term prognosis for patients with focal glomerulonephritis is often excellent. Hypertension or azotemia had not developed in 84 patients followed up to 10 years.[26, 29, 32] However, slowly progressive renal compromise is reported in some patients with IgA nephropathy and is common among those with marked proteinuria (> 1 g/24 hr).[27, 33] The short-term prognosis is good in patients with diffuse glomerulonephritis, although studies report signs of chronicity, usually hypertension or proteinuria, in 50% of adults who were followed for 2 to 15 years after apparent recovery from poststreptococcal glomerulonephritis.[34]

Findings in the urine can be limited to microscopic hematuria and a few RBC casts in many systemic illnesses associated with glomerulonephritis (see Table 30–9). In practice, a very careful history and examination should suffice to exclude systemic diseases if the only manifestation is microscopic hematuria.

Other Causes

RBCs appear in the urine in normal individuals after fever or prolonged heavy exercise. In one report of 47 long-distance runners, the urine specimen of 7 had more than 10 RBC/hpf, 18 had + or + + proteinuria, and some had RBC casts.[35] Hematuria following trauma may reflect urethral or bladder injury, requiring urethrography or cystography, or both; this injury should be suspected when urethral blood or pelvic fracture or hematoma is seen.[10] Blood may also reflect ureteral injury or renal contusion, which can be seen on intravenous pyelogram (IVP).[10] Acute thrombosis of the renal vein may present as hematuria accompanied by a tender, palpable kidney, to be followed later by proteinuria or the nephrotic syndrome. Emboli to the kidney may present flank pain and hematuria. In patients with medullary sponge kidneys, multiple small calculi form within the tubules and cause recurrent episodes of hematuria. Cases are identified by the characteristic brush-like medullary pyramidal blush and puddling of contrast seen in the renal collecting ducts on pyelography. Patients with unexplained clots or gross hematuria should also be checked for thrombocytopenia or clotting disorders. Conversely, patients with hematuria while on sodium warfarin (Coumadin) should have complete urologic evaluations, in case bleeding from an underlying lesion has been unmasked by anticoagulation therapy.

In addition to the ones just discussed, some urologic lesions in patients with hematuria include urethral stricture, renal cysts, hydronephrosis, polycystic kidneys, bladder calculi, and bladder diverticuli.[8] Sickle cell trait is found in many African-Americans with normal kidneys and otherwise unexplained microhematuria,[25] but these patients also require evaluation to exclude other sources of bleeding. Hematuria may accompany renal papillary necrosis or membranoproliferative glomerulonephritis in sickle cell anemia.[36] Papillary necrosis is also associated with diabetes and analgesic abuse. Renal tuberculosis is now uncommon, but hematuria, often accompanied by pyuria, is frequently the presenting complaint in patients who do have renal tuberculosis.[7, 37]

One patient with an arteriovenous malformation of the kidney was found in a series of 237 cases of hematuria.[25] Another investigator reported 17 young women with bouts of gross hematuria, flank pain, normal renal biopsies, and "subtle" renal angiographic abnormalities.[38] Even patients with persistent hematuria but normal light microscopy on renal biopsy need follow-up, since one study reported diffuse glomerular basement membrane thinning, which can lead to renal compromise.[39]

Diagnostic Studies and Approach to the Patient with Unexplained Hematuria

Renal ultrasonography or intravenous urogram, if not contraindicated, is usually the first procedure in patients whose hematuria remains unexplained by the history, physical examination, repeat urinalysis, and urine culture (Fig. 30–4). Some urologists now recommend ultrasonography as the procedure of choice because of its safety and lack of x-ray exposure, even though rarely ultrasonography might miss small nonobstructing renal pelvic or ureteral tumors.

Renal Mass Lesion

In one series, 6 to 10% of masses suggested by ultrasonography or intravenous urography were carcinomas; 70% were benign cysts; and the remainder consisted of pseudotumors (fetal lobulation or compensatory hypertrophy), hydronephroses, polycystic kidneys, renal abscesses, benign renal tumors, lymphomas, and hematomas (Table 30–4).[40] Undoubtedly, benign cysts account for an even larger proportion of patients when lesions are noted incidentally during ultrasonography or radiographs taken for other reasons, as opposed to those being evaluated for hematuria.

A noninvasive approach is justified whenever possible. Renal ultrasonography usually distinguishes pseudotumor and hypertrophy containing normal renal tissue from true renal masses. The first step in distinguishing benign cysts from renal cell carcinomas is to define the lesion as a simple cyst versus a solid or complex mass. Usually renal ultrasonography makes the distinction.[40–44] For lesions judged to be solid or complex on ultrasonography or intravenous urography, computed tomography (CT) scanning has become the next diagnostic test. A round lesion is judged to be benign by CT scanning if there is homogeneous attenuation, no enhancement using contrast, thin cyst-like walls, and a smooth interface with the renal parenchyma.[45] In one study, CT scanning accurately identified 56 consecutively encountered benign cysts.[45] Complex lesions by ultrasonography that appear entirely benign on CT scanning can be followed noninvasively by serial studies. If the lesion has indeterminate features, MRI may complement CT scanning in determining the need for surgical exploration. MRI can identify a thrombus in major vessels and can distinguish vessels from lymph nodes, but, without contrast, may fail to distinguish isodense renal neoplasms from surrounding parenchyma. Surgical exploration is generally indicated when CT scanning or magnetic resonance imaging (MRI) confirms the thick-walled, irregular, or solid appearance of a lesion that was previously thought to be suspicious.

Because of the accuracy of currently available imaging studies, diagnostic cyst puncture[46, 47] is done less frequently than in the past. It has a small complication rate of 0.75%,[48] and there is some concern that tumor seeding of renal carcinoma may result. In addition, even combining cystography, cyst fluid analysis, and cytology does not accurately identify all renal carcinomas. In one study, cyst puncture obtained fluid in 93% of 106 suspicious renal masses and identified six of seven patients with malignancies, but one patient later found to have a carcinoma had a totally negative cyst aspiration.[47] Because the doubling-time of renal cell carcinomas is reasonably fast, many urologists utilize serial studies with CT scanning or MRI to determine the need for surgery in somewhat suspicious masses.

Some benign lesions may require surgery but because the mortality rate of renal exploration is 0.72%,[44] surgery

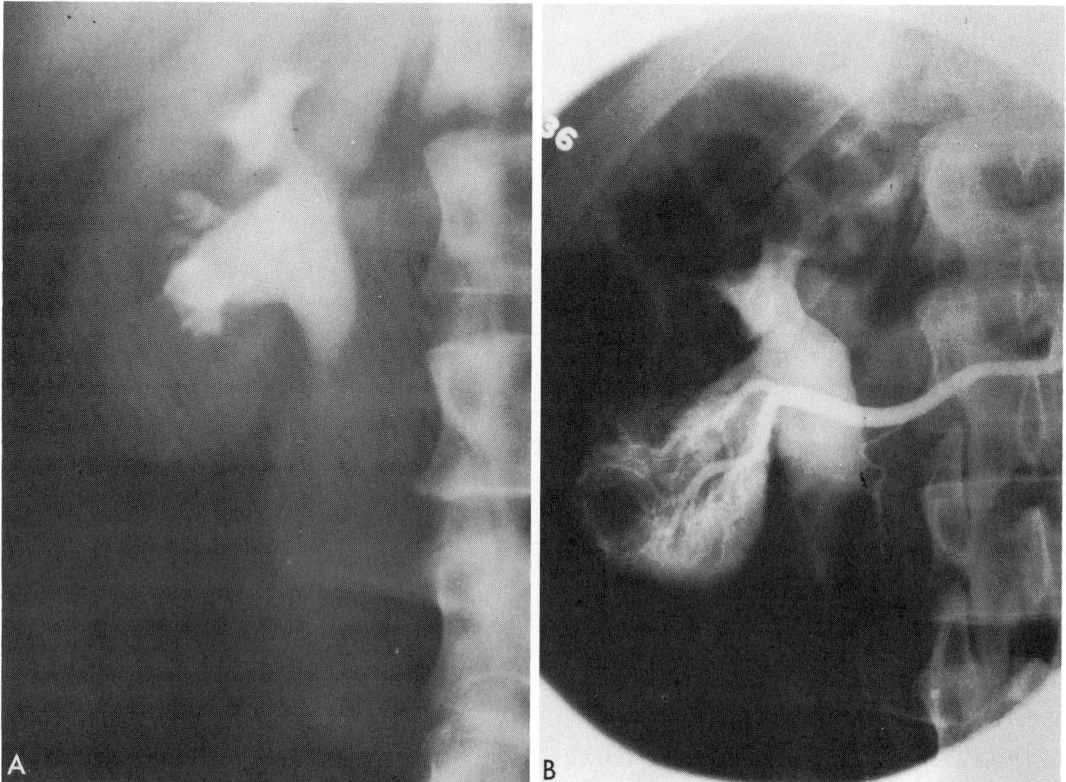

FIGURE 30–4. *A,* Results of urography in a previously asymptomatic middle-aged man who presented with flank pain and gross hematuria of several hours' duration. The urogram revealed no calculus (considered the most likely diagnosis by his physicians) but showed a slight dilatation of the renal pelvis on the right. A more subtle finding was the irregular lower medial aspect of the right renal cortex. In retrospect, this apparent irregularity or lobulation suggested a renal mass lesion to the radiologist. *B,* The patient whose urogram is shown in *A* had a cystic lesion, revealed by ultrasound; however, because of the suspicion of a thick wall on nephrotomography, an angiogram was performed. Tumor vessels were seen in one wall of the cyst, suggesting that necrosis within a hypernephroma had formed the cystic structure. (Courtesy of the Department of Radiology, Brigham and Women's Hospital, Harvard Medical School, Boston, Massachusetts.)

should be reserved for patients with thick or irregular walls or suspicious findings on cyst aspiration.

One should also consider performing cystoscopy to exclude concurrent carcinoma of the bladder in patients with hematuria and a benign renal cyst. Although hematuria is reported in about 15% of patients evaluated for benign cysts,[44] it may not be certain that the cyst causes the bleeding rather than being an incidental finding in a patient with another lesion.

Lesions of the Collecting Systems

More than half of renal calculi are within the ureter at presentation. They may best be seen by scrutinizing the plain abdominal film to detect radio-opaque calculi and may be missed on ultrasonography if not causing obstruction. Having the patient strain his or her urine through a piece of gauze may allow precise determination of the constituents of renal calculi, as well as identification of occasional tumor fragments and necrotic papillae, which appear grossly as a gray putty-like material.

Transitional cell carcinoma of the renal pelvis may cause hematuria and may be missed by ultrasonography unless it causes an obstruction. Intravenous urography also misses up to half of these lesions (Fig. 30–5),[24] and arteriography is not helpful, since there is no significant neovascularity in most transitional cell carcinomas.[49] Retrograde pyelography should be considered when there is suspicion of transitional cell carcinoma of the renal pelvis. The result of urinary cytology was positive in approximately 50% of patients who had this lesion in one series,[24] and its reliability can be enhanced if specimens are obtained by brush biopsy at the time of retrograde pyelography. In patients with an unexplained persistent radiolucent filling defect in the renal pelvis, who do not have known renal papillary necrosis or uric acid calculi, the etiology can be determined at times by detecting faint flecks of calcification within a partially radiolucent calculus or by characteristic acoustical and density differences between nonopaque calculi and renal pelvic tumors noted on ultrasonography or CT scanning.[50]

TABLE 30–4. FINAL DIAGNOSIS IN 206 PATIENTS REFERRED FOR RENAL MASS LESIONS*

Diagnosis	Number	%
Cysts	141	70
Pseudotumors	32	15
Tumors	13	6.5
Hydronephrosis	6	
Polycystic kidneys	5	
Abscess	4	
Hematoma	4	
Perirenal pseudocyst	1	
Total	206	

*Adapted from Pollack HM, Goldberg BB, Morales J, et al: A systematized approach to the differential diagnosis of renal masses. Radiology 113:153, 1974.

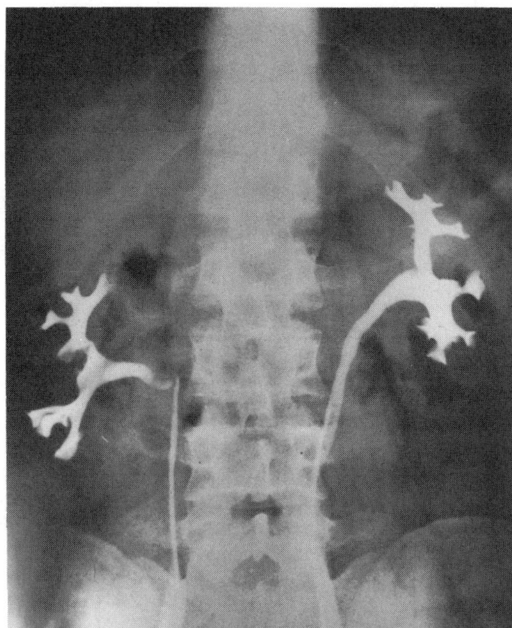

FIGURE 30–5. A 60-year-old woman was investigated for painless gross hematuria. The middle group of calyces on the right were not well visualized by intravenous urography; thus, retrograde pyelography was performed, confirming the finding that the infundibulum connecting the major to the minor calcyes has been occluded. Surgical exploration revealed a transitional cell carcinoma of the renal pelvis. (Courtesy of Department of Radiology, Brigham and Women's Hospital, Harvard Medical School, Boston, Massachusetts.)

Hematuria with Normal Upper Tracts

When the results of renal ultrasound or intravenous urogram are entirely normal, the chief consideration is carcinoma of the bladder. Less than half of these tumors are visible on cystograms.[51] Urinary cytology may be helpful, since most lesions that have clearly neoplastic cells will be detected. Unfortunately, some tumors that are invasive and thus behave malignantly are well differentiated, therefore negative urinary cytology does not rule out bladder cancer.[52] Cystoscopy should be performed. This procedure with biopsy of abnormally appearing areas is generally reliable. Cytology is useful as an adjunct, since of 262 patients developing bladder cancer in one study, 11 (4%) patients had initially negative cystoscopy results but positive urinary cytology results.[53]

One may raise the question of the need for cystoscopy in asymptomatic adults younger than 40 years of age with borderline (2 to 5 RBC/hpf) or transient microhematuria. Carcinoma of the bladder or kidney is rare in persons of this age in the absence of a history of exposure to bladder carcinogens or heavy cigarette smoking, whereas false-positive urinalyses containing 2 to 5 RBC/hpf are common.[41] In 1000 healthy recruits who had 12,227 routine urinalyses over 15 years, 38.7% had at least one urinalysis containing 2 to 4 or more RBC/hpf.[4]

Urologic evaluation including cystoscopy is recommended for persons older than 40 years of age[54] and those at increased risk of genitourinary cancer with reproducible asymptomatic microhematuria, and also for all persons with unexplained gross hematuria, even if transient.

No diagnosis was established by the urologic work-up in 20 to 34% of patients with persistent asymptomatic microhematuria[8, 9] and in 8.5% of those with gross hematuria.[7] Most probably have focal glomerulonephritis or other mild glomerular lesions. Follow-up of 191 patients for 10 to 20 years revealed no genitourinary malignancies in patients whose initial evaluation was negative.[41] Repeated cystoscopies and other studies were not recommended by these authors in the absence of gross hematuria, development of urinary tract infections, or changes in voiding characteristics.[41, 42] Patients with asymptomatic microhematuria and an initially negative urologic evaluation should have urine sediment, blood pressure, and renal function monitored during periodic health check-ups.

STERILE PYURIA

Most patients with pyuria have urinary tract infections, which can be diagnosed by the presence of typical symptoms—flank pain and fever in those with pyelonephritis, frequency and dysuria in those with lower urinary tract infections—together with positive urine cultures. The diagnosis is less evident in patients with sterile pyuria. Pyuria in the absence of a positive culture may denote prostatitis in male patients, may occur in patients of either sex in the setting of dysuria and other symptoms of urethritis, or may occur in asymptomatic patients.

Differential Diagnosis

Prostatitis

Culture-negative prostatitis occurs most frequently in young patients and is probably caused by *Chlamydia* or possibly by viruses or *Mycoplasma*. More commonly in older patients prostatitis represents persistent colonization of the gland by enteric pathogens. Generally at least a few colonies of gram-negative bacilli can be cultured from expressed prostatic secretions, and the clinical course is punctuated by bacterial urinary tract infections in addition to persistent, low-grade inflammation within the prostate. Prostatitis of these etiologies may be asymptomatic and often is detected by finding pyuria on routine urinalysis. There may be mild, intermittent dysuria, terminal dysuria or penile pain, and vague perineal discomfort.

Acute Urethritis

Except for the negative urine culture, the features of urethritis in women are similar to those of bacterial cystitis. The patient typically complains of frequency and dysuria intermittently present over several days. Pyuria (8 to 15 WBC/hpf) is typically present but not gross hematuria. About half the cases can be attributed to bacterial urethritis, which is generally a precursor of bladder infection. Often there is a history of recurrent urinary infections with positive cultures on previous occasions, and although the midstream urine may be sterile or contain a small number of organisms, culture of the first few drops of urine would detect larger numbers of gram-negative bacilli. Vaginitis must be excluded by history or examination. In a few cases, women with gonorrhea may complain of dysuria and have urethritis rather than salpingitis.

The remaining female patients probably have nongonococcal urethritis analogous to that occurring in men. In men, however, urethral discharge generally is present in addition to dysuria. Current evidence favors sexually acquired *Chlamydia* as the cause of most nongonococcal urethritis, with a small number of cases due to trauma, foreign bodies, and monilial or trichomonal infections.

Other Causes of Sterile Pyuria

When significant pyuria, especially if accompanied by hematuria, cannot be attributed to urethritis or prostatitis, the differential diagnosis includes renal mass lesions such as cysts or neoplasms, renal calculi, chronic interstitial cystitis, carcinoma of the bladder, glomerulonephritis, and urinary tract tuberculosis. Detailed discussion of the clinical findings in each of these is provided in the previous section (Hematuria) except for tuberculosis, which is now discussed.

Urinary Tract Tuberculosis

Genitourinary tuberculosis results from hematogenous seeding during a primary infection, leaving a focus for potential reactivation within the kidney. The initial lesion is a small granuloma in the parenchyma. In certain cases, the likelihood being unknown, spreading and coalescence eventually result in the rupture of caseous material into a minor calyx (Fig. 30–6*A*). From here, infection spreads into the calyceal system and renal pelvis, eventually seeding downward possibly to involve the ureter, bladder, prostate, seminal vesicles, and epididymis. The presenting symptoms may reflect localization at any of these sites. One third of patients with urinary tract tuberculosis have completely normal chest radiographs.[37, 55] Painless, gross hematuria is a common initial finding (~ 25%); many other patients first complain of fever and malaise (~ 20%), flank or back pain (~ 10%), epididymitis (~ 10%), or frequency and urgency of urination (~ 30%).[37, 55] It is not widely appreciated how often patients with urinary tuberculosis have symptoms of chronic cystitis, resulting from seeding of the bladder with infected urine. In some cases, bacterial cystitis or pyelonephritis has accompanied tuberculosis, so that even positive bacterial cultures do not exclude concurrent renal tuberculosis in patients whose symptoms are chronic or persistent. Generally, the tuberculin test is positive (88 to 95%).[37, 55]

The symptoms of tuberculous prostatitis, episodic dysuria and frequency, are the same as those of any chronic prostatitis accompanied by posterior urethritis (see Fig. 30–6*B*). However, the prostate gland typically is small and fibrotic in tuberculosis, whereas the gland is boggy and sometimes mildly tender in ordinary chronic prostatitis. Indurated seminal vesicles above the gland may also be palpable in tuberculosis. Concurrent involvement of the kidneys, ureters, and bladder is common; therefore, the midstream urine, which very often is clear in ordinary chronic prostatitis, should contain pus cells.

Diagnostic Studies and Approach to the Patient

If There Are Manifestations of Prostatitis

Whenever prostatitis is thought to be the source of pyuria, a three-glass urine test should be performed by collecting an initial, midstream, and terminal urine sediment. The terminal specimen is obtained by collecting the first 10 ml of urine following prostatic massage. The diagnosis of prostatitis is confirmed if the initial and midstream urine collections have few or no pus cells while the terminal specimen contains more than 15 WBC/hpf. Many cases of "unexplained" pyuria can be correctly attributed to prostatitis by using this test. The terminal urine specimen or expressed prostatic secretions should be cultured because management depends on making the distinction between abacterial and bacterial prostatitis.

Tuberculin testing is done in any patient with a history of exposure to tuberculosis or with sterile pyuria in the midstream urine. Continued suspicion or a positive tuberculin test result should lead to obtaining three or more cultures for tuberculosis and performing intravenous urography (see Fig. 30–6*B*).

If the Patient Has Dysuria

In women with abrupt or recent onset of dysuria, there is no practical way to distinguish between urethritis and cystitis while cultures are pending. In practice, the treatment is the same. Vaginitis must be excluded, usually by eliciting no history of a vaginal discharge. The symptoms usually resolve with appropriate treatment.

Another group of female patients have more chronic or intermittent symptoms of dysuria and urinary frequency but have negative cultures. Most patients with these symptoms are elderly women. Sometimes the explanation is atrophic vaginitis or a urethral caruncle, representing prolapsed urethral mucosa at the posterior aspect of the urethral meatus. In either case, the midstream urine, if carefully collected, is generally free of blood or pus. Initial treatment is usually topical estrogen.

There remain some women in whom the pelvic examination reveals no apparent cause for chronic, "sterile" dysuria. If the urine sediment is persistently abnormal, lesions of the kidneys and upper collecting tracts should be excluded by obtaining intravenous urography. Cystoscopy and cytologic study of the urine are also indicated to exclude the small possibility of bladder malignancy. Neurogenic dysfunction of the bladder can be excluded by cystometrography when frequency is a prominent manifestation. First morning urinary specimens for tuberculosis cultures as well as the tuberculin test should be obtained for those with persistent pyuria. When the result of the evaluation is otherwise negative, especially if pyuria accompanies urinary frequency, interstitial cystitis may be a possible diagnosis.

If symptoms are mild or intermittent, sitz baths may be helpful. Reassurance can be important, since some patients will have been subjected to repeated studies. Persistent frequency or nocturia can be alleviated partially in some patients by anticholinergic or smooth muscle-relaxing drugs such as propantheline bromide (Pro-Banthine) or imipramine.

In many young males with urethritis, the source is readily apparent because of penile discharge or documented by finding pus cells in only the initial specimen of a three-glass test. Therapy is determined by Gram staining and culturing the urethral exudate. Pending culture results, those with no history of exposure to gonococcus and with no gram-negative intracellular diplococci on the smear may be treated for nongonococcal urethritis. Additional studies are unnecessary unless the urine sediment remains abnormal. The urethral exudate of men with recurrent episodes of nongonococcal urethritis should also be examined for *Monilia* (KOH preparation) and for motile trichomonads (wet mount).

When dysuria cannot be attributed to urethritis in a man, the major considerations are cystitis and prostatitis. Examination and culture of midstream urine and urine obtained after prostatic massage generally localizes the source of symptoms to the bladder or prostate.

If There Is Asymptomatic Sterile Pyuria

Prostatitis and urethritis are excluded as causes of pyuria in male patients by using the three-glass test. Vaginal

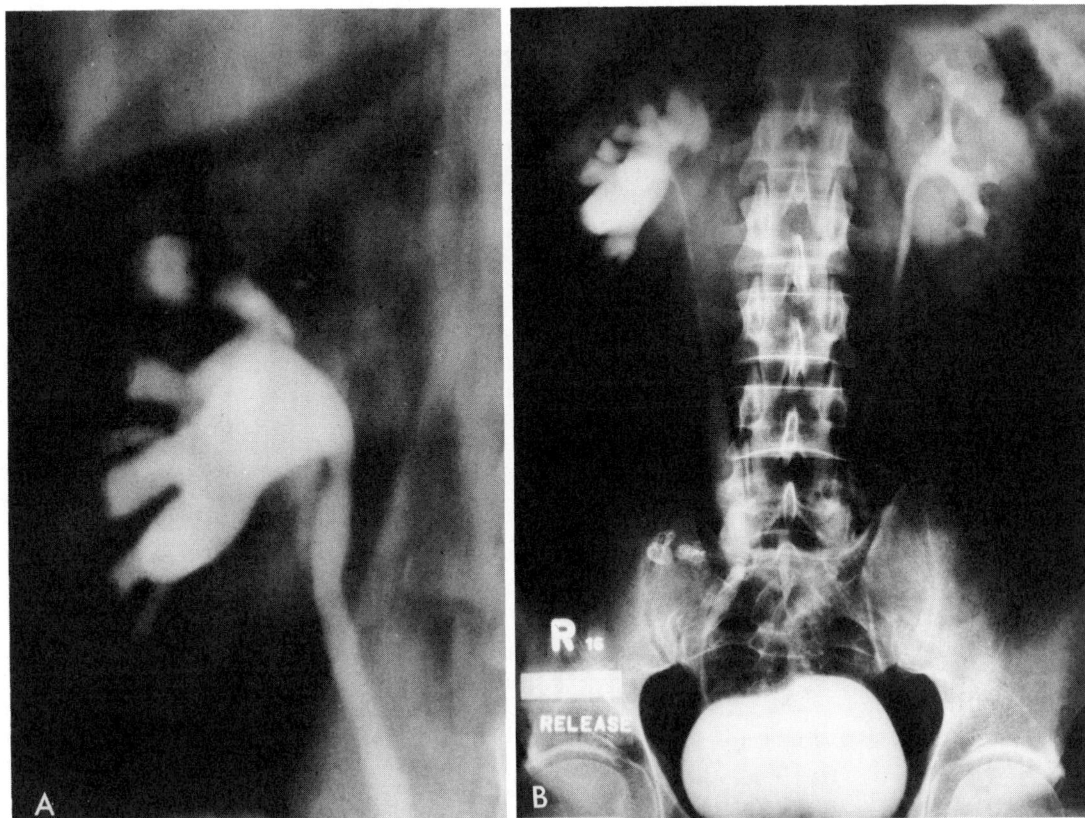

FIGURE 30–6. *A,* Renal tuberculosis. The pathogenesis of the lesion is illustrated by the cavitary lesion within the upper pole of the right kidney. This began as a granuloma caused by hematogenous spreading and has progressed to rupture into the upper pole calyces. From there, tuberculosis may disseminate downward within the urinary tract to involve the renal pelvis, ureter, seminal vesicles, prostate, epididymis, or bladder.

B, Intravenous urogram of a 39-year-old man with a 3-year history of episodic urinary frequency and dysuria. There was a family history of tuberculosis. The physical examination was entirely normal except for a small, firm, minimally tender prostate gland. An initial evaluation included a urinalysis showing 15 to 20 wbc/hpf, negative urine culture, and a positive tuberculin test result.

The urogram revealed thinning and narrowing of the right renal cortex with moderate ectasia of the intrarenal collecting system. The upper pole minor calyces show a marked irregularity and areas of excavation at the tips of the papilla. The lower pole minor calyces appear better preserved. A long stricture involves the proximal 3 cm of the right ureter from the UP junction. The result of the culture was positive for *Mycobacterium tuberculosis.* The patient received 2 years of therapy with isoniazid, pyridoxine, and ethambutol; it was also necessary to obtain repeat urograms to ascertain that progressive stricture with obstruction of the right kidney did not occur.

contamination in women is excluded by repeat urinalysis or, if necessary, by obtaining a specimen by catheterization. The work-up then begins with an intravenous urogram. If a mass lesion is suspected, the same diagnostic sequence may be followed, beginning with renal ultrasonography, as outlined in the Hematuria section. If there is no suspicion of a mass or obvious other lesion, such as a chronically obstructed or nonfunctioning kidney, one should examine the x-ray film carefully to exclude calculi or filling defects within the renal pelvis, or in the major or minor calyces. Urology work-up with cystoscopy is usually indicated when significant persistent, documented pyuria remains unexplained.

Tuberculosis is a consideration in patients with otherwise unexplained persistent pyuria. The radiograph may show a filling defect (abscess) within the kidney connected to the calyceal system. With progressive involvement there is scarring, distortion, and stricture formation in the adjacent collecting system and eventually in the ureter (see Fig. 30–6*A, B*). However, in one series, 25% of patients with genitourinary tuberculosis had normal or only mildly abnormal excretory urography.[55] Therefore, in cases in which suspicion is strong, a minimum of three first morning urine cultures should be done. Such cultures are positive in 90% of eventually proved cases; the 10% with false-negative cultures usually were found to have inadequately obtained specimens.[55]

PROTEINURIA

The upper limit of normal for proteinuria in adults is 150 mg/24 hr. In the absence of gross bleeding or inflammation within the collecting system, proteinuria comes from the renal glomerulus chiefly as albuminuria, from overloading the renal tubules with filtered protein such as myeloma proteins or lysozyme, or from tubular proteins lost because of interference with normal reabsorption by interstitial nephritis or other renal tubular disorders. In clinical practice, a 1 + reaction by dipstick provides a sensitive index of albuminuria at normal urine specific gravities. Proteinuria may be considered minimal in amounts of less than 0.5 g/24 hr, whereas more than 3 to 3.5 g/24 hr is often associated with the nephrotic syndrome. The clinical approach to a patient differs according to whether proteinuria is (1) associated with a systemic disease, (2) idiopathic, or (3) associated with the nephrotic syndrome.

TABLE 30–5. SYSTEMIC CONDITIONS AND OTHER CAUSES OF PERSISTENT PROTEINURIA

Common in clinical practice
- Congestive heart failure
- Hypertensive nephrosclerosis
- Diabetic benign nephrosclerosis
- Drug side effect, allergy, or toxicity: nonsteroidal anti-inflammatory agents, probenecid, captopril, D-penicillamine, mercury, gold, trimethadione, penicillins, aminoglycosides, etc.

Unusual causes, sometimes associated with the nephrotic syndrome
- Vesicoureteral reflux
- Diabetic intracapillary glomerulosclerosis (Kimmelstiel-Wilson disease)
- Amyloidosis
- Allergic reactions (bee stings, pollen, poison ivy, insect repellents)
- Heavy metal toxicity (mercury, bismuth, gold)
- Renal vein thrombosis
- Multiple myeloma and light chain nephropathy
- Hodgkin's disease and non-Hodgkin's lymphoma
- Solid tumors (renal cell, pancreatic, mesothelioma, colon, prostate)
- Systemic lupus erythematosus
- Chronic active hepatitis
- Secondary lues
- Quartan malaria
- Other chronic infections including shunt infections
- Hereditary nephritis (Alport's syndrome)
- Homograft rejection
- Myxedema
- Constrictive pericarditis
- Human immunodeficiency virus–associated nephropathy
- Other viral infections
- Heroin abuse nephropathy
- Sickle cell disease
- Renal allograph rejection
- Sarcoidosis
- Scleroderma
- Henoch-Schönlein purpura
- Goodpasture's syndrome
- Glycogen storage disease
- Massive obesity
- Analgesic abuse nephropathy
- Nephron ablation
- Resolving postinfectious glomerulonephritis

Differential Diagnosis

Proteinuria Associated with Systemic Diseases or Other Causes

Transient proteinuria may occur with fever or be associated with dehydration or gross hematuria. A variety of drugs including probenecid, fenprofen, gold, penicillamine, captopril, trimethadione, the penicillins, and aminoglycosides can produce proteinuria as a side effect or allergic or toxic reaction.[56] Vesicoureteral reflux and hydronephrosis produce proteinuria, and proteinuria also occurs in small amounts generally accompanied by RBCs or WBCs in the urine in some patients with pyelonephritis, nephrolithiasis, renal neoplasia, and renal tuberculosis. Moderate amounts of urinary protein characteristically are seen in congestive heart failure, benign diabetic nephrosclerosis, and hypertensive nephrosclerosis. Proteinuria as indicated by dipstick may be minimal or absent in patients with early interstitial nephritis, since the renal tubular α- and β-microglobulins and muramidase that appear early in the urine in the course of this syndrome are not detected by dipstick; these can be detected and quantified by electrophoresis of an aliquot of urine. In addition, any of the systemic diseases (to be discussed later) associated with the nephrotic syndrome or with nephritis can also present with only moderate amounts of protein in the urine (Table 30–5).

Idiopathic Proteinuria

Isolated proteinuria not associated with a systemic disorder is subdivided into several prognostically useful categories. The first distinction is to establish that the proteinuria has not occurred transiently (e.g., with exercise, fever, or dehydration). Proteinuria is then categorized as persistent (or constant)—that is, always present whether the patient is recumbent or upright—or as orthostatic: (1) either fixed and reproducible when the patient is upright or (2) transiently present (transient orthostatic proteinuria) on only 1 or 2 days each week.[57] Patients with orthostatic proteinuria of either type are usually found to have less than 1 g of urinary protein in 24 hours; have normal renal function, concentrating ability, and renal anatomy; and often cease to have proteinuria on follow-up.[56, 57] In one series, only 8% of patients with this pattern of proteinuria had definite morphologic evidence of renal disease. Twenty-year follow-up, possible in 36 of 43 patients, revealed no deterioration in renal function.[57] Histopathologic changes are noted more frequently (50 to 80%) in patients with persistent (or constant) proteinuria. The histologic alterations are quite heterogeneous (Table 30–6).[27] The short-term prognosis is also good, but in one series 50% of these patients developed hypertension after 5 years, and the risk of renal functional impairment was approximately 20% after 10 years.[56] Mild proteinuria has progressed to renal failure in a few patients who had partial nephrectomy of a solitary kidney.[58]

In patients whose only manifestation is isolated proteinuria, lesions present on renal biopsy could represent a healing phase. The urine sediment may help to select patients at higher risk: the presence of RBCs indicates a worse prognosis, RBC casts indicate glomerular disease, WBC casts indicate interstitial inflammation, granular or hyaline casts suggest renal origin of proteinuria, and lipid casts and oval fat bodies indicate nephrosis.[59]

Nephrotic Syndrome

The nephrotic syndrome develops when more than 3 to 3.5 g of urinary protein is excreted in 24 hours. The amount of proteinuria and diminution of serum albumin necessary to cause edema become less with increasing age. Clinical complications that frequently occur in patients with the nephrotic syndrome are listed in Table 30–7.[60]

Most adults with the nephrotic syndrome have minimal change disease, focal glomerular sclerosis, membranous glomerulonephritis, or mesangiocapillary (membranoprolif-

TABLE 30–6. HISTOPATHOLOGIC FINDINGS IN SELECTED CASES OF ISOLATED PROTEINURIA*

Diagnosis	No. of Patients	% of Patients
Normal or minimal change	32	49
Focal glomerulonephritis	17	25
Focal glomerular sclerosis	8	12
Membranous glomerulonephritis	6	9
Mesangiocapillary glomerulonephritis	2	
Total	65	

*Adapted from Morel-Maroger L, Leathan A, and Richet G: Glomerular abnormalities in nonsystemic diseases. Relationship between findings by light microscopy and immunofluorescence in 433 renal biopsy specimens. Am J Med 53:170, 1972.

TABLE 30–7. COMMON CLINICAL COMPLICATIONS OF THE NEPHROTIC SYNDROME*

	Complications
Hypovolemia	Postural hypotension Circulatory collapse Acute tubular necrosis
Diminished resistance to infection	Primary peritonitis Septicemia Cellulitis Urinary infections
Protein depletion	Osteoporosis Cutaneous striae Muscle wasting Apathy
Altered blood coagulability	Arterial thrombosis Venous thrombosis and pulmonary embolism
Reduced renal function	Uremia Hypertension
Miscellaneous	Secondary renal tubular disorders

*Adapted from Cameron JS: Nephrotic syndrome. BMJ 4:350, 1970.

erative) glomerulonephritis (MCGN)—although it should be appreciated that the nephrotic syndrome also occurs with other renal histopathologic lesions, as revealed by light microscopy (Table 30–8).[27] Minimal change disease shows minimal or no changes on light microscopy, but fusion of glomerular epithelial foot processes is visible on electron microscopy. Focal glomerular sclerosis has sclerosis of part or all of some glomeruli with associated tubular atrophy and interstitial fibrosis and is associated at times with vesicoureteral reflux.[61]

In membranous glomerulonephritis, soluble complexes of IgG and complement can be identified by immunofluorescence as a granular deposit on the epithelial side of the basement membrane.[27] In MCGN, the immunofluorescent deposits are on the endothelial side of the capillary basement membrane and are accompanied by mesangial proliferation.[27]

The nephrotic syndrome may be secondary to a systemic cause (see Table 30–5). Minimal change disease or membranous glomerulonephritis is noted on biopsy in many patients with these illnesses.[60] Patients with amyloidosis or diabetes mellitus have specific findings. Biopsies of patients with the nephrotic syndrome caused by allergy to fenoprofen and naproxen revealed acute interstitial nephritis accompanied by fusion of epithelial foot processes.[62] In 5% of elderly patients with persistently heavy proteinuria, abnormal monoclonal paraproteinuria was detected by immunoelectrophoresis.[63] Multiple myeloma was usually not present, but amyloidosis was noted by electron microscopy in some of these patients.

For adults with the nephrotic syndrome caused by primary renal disease, the short-term natural history can be estimated from outcomes of patients randomized to the untreated group in the British Medical Research Council Trial of Prednisone.[64] In minimal change disease, 25% of the group who received no treatment went into remission at 1 year and 60% by 2 years. Patients with membranous glomerulonephritis fared more poorly. After 2 years only 20% were free of proteinuria. Focal sclerosing glomerulonephritis was not specifically studied in that trial, but advanced renal failure occurs within 3 to 7 years after the onset in between a third and a half of patients with this lesion.[65–68] Renal function may remain normal for several years in MCGN but tends to decline rapidly during the final 1 to 2 years of illness.[69]

Diagnostic Studies and Approach to the Patient with Proteinuria

When idiopathic proteinuria is reported from the dipstick examination of a routine urinalysis, the first step is to question the patient and retest the urine to exclude transient proteinuria. Minor amounts of transient or intermittent proteinuria are commonly found in healthy young persons (0.4 to 14.8% of those tested routinely in some series[59]) and do not require extensive evaluation.[56] The systemic diseases and drug reactions associated with persistent proteinuria (see Table 30–5) generally have other manifestations that are recognizable from the history and physical examination. When persistent proteinuria is an isolated abnormality, the kidney is the source, so that the work-up usually includes definition of the renal anatomy with exclusion of vesicoureteral reflux or hydronephrosis by ultrasonography or intravenous urography. Such studies are usually normal. It seems reasonable also to obtain baseline creatinine clearance, quantitative 24-hour urinary protein, and urinary protein immunoelectrophoresis studies in patients with persistent proteinuria. Testing for antinuclear antibodies (ANA) or ASLO titer is recommended for those with clinical features of lupus or a history suggesting recent streptococcal infection.[56] Since there is no proved efficacy of treatment of glomerular lesions associated with only isolated proteinuria, a renal biopsy may not be indicated.[59] Clinical follow-up of the blood pressure, urinalysis, and serum creatinine or creatinine clearance is recommended on an annual basis for patients with persistent or constant proteinuria but can be done less often in those with only fixed or transient orthostatic proteinuria.[56]

Patients with a nephrotic syndrome should be evaluated for systemic diseases. Most of the causes listed in Table 30–5 are recognized clinically, but probably all patients should be tested for antinuclear antibodies, hypocomplementemia (C3 and C4 levels), monoclonal paraproteinuria, and glucose intolerance. Testing for viral infections may include hepatitis, Epstein-Barr, and cytomegaloviral serologies, blood and urine cultures for cytomegalovirus, and human immunodeficiency virus (HIV) testing. Fluorescein angiography establishes the presence of small vessel disease in diabetics with heavy proteinuria. Elderly patients who pre-

TABLE 30–8. BIOPSY FINDINGS IN SELECTED ADULTS WITH A NEPHROTIC SYNDROME[27]

Diagnosis	% of Patients
Minimal change disease	36
Focal glomerular sclerosis	10
Membranous glomerulonephritis	28
Mesangiocapillary glomerulonephritis	9
Mesangial proliferative glomerulonephritis	8
Diffuse exudative glomerulonephritis (acute poststreptococcal GN)	6
Focal and segmental proliferative glomerulonephritis	3
Total	100

*Adapted from More-Maroger L, Leathan A, and Richet G: Glomerular abnormalities in nonsystemic diseases. Relationship between findings by light microscopy and immunofluorescence in 433 renal biopsy specimens. Am J Med 53:170, 1972.

sent for the first time with otherwise unexplained nephrotic syndrome should be evaluated to exclude occult malignancy. A better prognosis is implied when there is a relatively small amount of proteinuria, highly selective proteinuria, and few red blood cells in the urine. Renal vein thrombosis can be detected in up to one half of patients with membranous glomerulonephritis if searched for angiographically.[70] Usually there are no complications, such as pulmonary embolism; the condition remains asymptomatic and is presumed to occur secondarily owing to the hypercoagulability associated with nephrosis. Patients with clinical evidence of pulmonary embolism or thrombophlebitis should have venography and, if the result of the study is positive, should receive treatment with anticoagulants.

Some underlying conditions may be treatable, so that renal biopsy is a consideration in patients with nephrosis. Primary care physicians should be generally familiar with the treatment options as they select patients for referral to a nephrologist. In the British Medical Research Council Trial of Prednisone, adults with minimal change disease showed no advantage after 2 years compared with the rate of spontaneous remissions.[64] The course of minimal change disease is variable, but steroids and immunosuppressants can induce remissions and be of palliative benefit in symptomatic adults.[3] Most patients with focal sclerosis on biopsy progressively worsen without responding to therapy, but some exhibit spontaneous remissions (10%) or possibly remissions induced by steroids (20%).[3] No treatment has been shown to be effective for MCGN, but low-dose alternate-day prednisone or combined therapy with aspirin and dipyramidole are tried in some patients.[3]

A randomized, double-blind trial used high doses of prednisone (125 mg) given on alternate days to adult patients with membranous glomerulonephritis.[71] Therapy was maintained until there was a response and then was tapered over a 10-week period but reinstituted if relapse occurred. After 3 years, progressive loss of renal function was slowed at little risk of toxicity in the treated group of these patients, all of whom were below the age of 65. More recent studies are conflicting.[72, 73] It was suggested to select adults for treatment with steroids or immunosuppressants who are in good health with recent onset of the nephrotic syndrome and a likelihood of progression to renal impairment as judged by heavy proteinuria (≥ 10 g/24 hr).[74] Because of the likelihood of spontaneous remission, corticosteroid therapy probably should not be offered to patients with minimal change disease unless they are symptomatic owing to protein wasting.

For patients who fail to respond and for elderly patients and others who are not candidates for steroid therapy, rest is helpful when the patient is in the edematous stage, but complete bedrest should be avoided because of the tendency for thrombosis.[60] Diet combines 100 g protein with moderate sodium intake. Diuretics are beneficial to control the edema in ambulatory patients, and potassium may be needed during this phase. Later, with onset of renal failure, there is less need for diuretics because of diminishing proteinuria. Albumin infusions are expensive and provide too transient a benefit to be useful, except in patients with acute hypovolemia or in those who otherwise are refractory and require initiation of diuresis. Antibiotics should be used therapeutically but not prophylactically, and good bacteriology studies are essential in every case, since the infecting organisms may be unusual.

Additional therapeutic modalities have been tried. Cytotoxic agents have been given to patients with proteinuria related to monoclonal paraproteinemia,[63] and colchicine to those with amyloidosis secondary to familial Mediterranean fever and possibly other causes.[75] Indomethacin may diminish proteinuria in the nephrotic syndrome but has no beneficial effect on renal function.[76] Worsening of renal function, attributed to impaired renal prostaglandin production, has been noted in some patients receiving indomethacin as well as other nonsteroidal anti-inflammatory drugs.[77]

GLOMERULONEPHRITIS

Patients with the syndrome of acute glomerulonephritis classically have proteinuria, some impairment of renal function, plus an active urine sediment containing RBCs, WBCs, increased casts, and heme-pigmented, coarsely granular, or RBC casts, and are frequently hypertensive. This syndrome is encountered less often than isolated hematuria, idiopathic proteinuria, and sterile pyuria. The short-term prognosis of glomerular diseases is generally good when the only manifestation is isolated hematuria or proteinuria; the prognosis is less certain in adult patients with clinical features suggesting glomerulonephritis. Additionally, in such patients, the renal manifestations are more likely to be part of a concurrent systemic illness. Hence, its potentially serious consequences mandate that this syndrome be considered in the differential diagnosis of patients with an abnormal urinalysis. Several subcategories of nephritis that may present with different clinical manifestations include poststreptococcal glomerulonephritis, systemic illnesses causing nephritis, MCGN, and rapidly progressive glomerulonephritis. It is necessary additionally to consider other causes of acute or progressive renal failure, such as acute tubular necrosis or acute interstitial nephritis, that also are manifested by an abnormal urinalysis plus renal compromise. Of patients with acute renal failure, the most common cause is acute tubular necrosis, which accounted for approximately 85% of cases in one series.[78] The remaining approximately 15% of patients, in whom renal biopsies were performed because of uncertainty about the diagnosis, had some form of glomerulonephritis (6.8%), atypical presentations of acute tubular or cortical necrosis (2.3%), acute interstitial nephritis (1.5%), hemolytic uremic syndrome or thrombotic thrombocytopenia purpura (1.5%), and a variety of other disorders including ischemic renal disease, myeloma kidney, amyloidosis, and diabetic nephropathy.[78]

Differential Diagnosis

Acute Poststreptococcal Glomerulonephritis

Acute poststreptococcal glomerulonephritis begins 1 to 2 weeks (occasionally 4 weeks) after an upper respiratory infection, pharyngitis, otitis media, or skin infection usually caused by types 1, 2, 41, or 49 β-hemolytic streptococci. In documented cases, glomerulonephritis occurred despite adequate penicillin therapy given shortly after the onset of impetigo or pharyngitis.[79] Nevertheless, patients should be treated in hopes that nephritis can sometimes be aborted; prophylaxis with benzathine pencillin may be necessary when an outbreak of infection with a nephritogenic strain of streptococci occurs within a closed community. Patients with nephritis typically complain of lethargy, malaise, and anorexia and have low-grade fevers. The three cardinal features are edema, oliguria, and hematuria. Edema is often periorbital and reflects fluid retention. There generally is mild to moderate hypertension (~ 150/100 mm Hg). Because the onset of hypertension is abrupt, the optic fundi may appear normal. The oliguria usually lasts no more than 4 days, although more prolonged cases occur and have a worse prognosis, with 1 to 2% of patients becoming uremic. Gross hematuria ("smoky" or "rust-colored" urine) is present initially in one third of the cases, whereas RBC casts are present invariably if sought carefully. In addition, the antistreptolysin O (ASO) titer should be elevated, and total hemolytic complement and particularly C3 levels are often diminished in serum; these levels typically return to normal within 1 month after the onset.

The clinical spectrum is broader than was previously suspected. Surveillance of the 3500 residents at Red Lake Indian Reservation during an epidemic of type 49 streptococcal infection detected 29 cases, all proved by biopsy, of which over half were entirely subclinical; the patients had no manifestations except abnormalities in the urine.[79]

The histopathologic findings in full-blown, acute cases consist of diffuse proliferative glomerulonephritis accompanied by a polymorphonuclear leukocytic exudate. As the syndrome resolves, light microscopy reveals diffuse mesangial proliferation.

It is estimated that 70% of adult patients with acute glomerulonephritis recover fully from the initial episode, but some patients follow a course of persistent proteinuria and microscopic hematuria or may develop renal insufficiency.[80] Some evidence of persistent renal involvement, chiefly trace to 1+ proteinuria or hypertension or both, was present in about half the adult patients in one series who were followed 15 years after apparently recovering from episodes of acute poststreptococcal glomerulonephritis.[34]

Eventually, some patients progress to a stage of chronic glomerulonephritis, characterized by slowly progressive azotemia, proteinuria, and hypertension. This syndrome is the most common cause of chronic renal failure and the most frequent indication for renal hemodialysis. In addition to poststreptococcal glomerulonephritis, any of the glomerulopathies discussed further on can lead to chronic glomerulonephritis.

Systemic Illnesses Causing Nephritis

Systemic illnesses reported to cause glomerulonephritis are listed in Table 30–9. Their etiology may be obvious, but occasionally the initial manifestation of a systemic disease can be the finding of RBCs, polymorphonuclear leukocytes, proteinuria, or casts in the urine.

Hypersensitivity angiitis is apparent from a typical purpuric skin rash over the lower extremities, often accompanied by arthralgias or symptoms of gastrointestinal purpura.

Many of the other conditions listed in Table 30–9—such as infected ventriculoatrial shunts, quartan malaria, leprosy, schistosomiasis, filariasis, and penicillamine or gold toxicity—occur only in special circumstances. However, specific diagnostic testing may be necessary to exclude HIV infection, subacute bacterial endocarditis, hepatitis B, systemic lupus erythematosus, cryoglobulinemia, and secondary lues in patients with unexplained glomerulonephritis.

Proteinuria and renal compromise associated with focal segmental sclerosis on biopsy may precede any manifestations of acquired immunodeficiency syndrome (AIDS) in HIV-associated nephropathy.[81]

Although in most systemic illnesses that present as nephritis light microscopy of renal biopsy specimens reveals nonspecific mesangial proliferative changes, special pathologic features that may be diagnostic in some cases include hematoxylin bodies and wire loops in systemic lupus erythematosus; necrotizing segmental arteritis and segmental necrosis of glomerular tufts in periarteritis nodosa (including hepatitis B-associated periarteritis); intimal thickening and concentric proliferation of intimal cells of the interlobular arteries in scleroderma; and necrotizing granulomas with vasculitis in Wegener's granulomatosis. A new test, the antineutrophilic cytoplasmic antibody (ANCA) test, has a positive result in Wegener's granulomatosis and other crescentic glomerulonephritides without immune glomerular deposits. Two conditions that mimic acute nephritis also have specific findings, intracapillary and arteriolar fibrin thrombi in the hemolytic uremic syndrome or postpartum renal failure, and "onion skin" lesions with fibrinoid arteriolar necrosis in malignant hypertensive nephrosclerosis. Cyclosporin A toxicity causes renal vasculitis. Many systemic conditions associated with nephritis demonstrate immunofluorescent deposits of complement and IgG within glomeruli, thought to originate as circulating immune complexes.[82] They are detectable in 70 to 80% of active cases.[83] Similar pathologic findings, even without clinical manifestations, have been noted in many patients who have a source of chronic antigenemia; for example, in 1.6% of solid tumor cases[84] and in many patients with leukemias or lymphomas.[85]

TABLE 30–9. SYSTEMIC DISEASES REPORTED TO BE ASSOCIATED WITH GLOMERULONEPHRITIS

Subacute bacterial endocarditis
Infected ventriculoatrial shunts
Hepatitis B
Quartan malarial nephrosis
Prolonged pneumococcal bacteremia
Other infections: leprosy, secondary syphilis, schistosomiasis, filariasis, infectious mononucleosis, varicella
Serum sickness
Systemic lupus erythematosus
HIV-associated nephropathy
Hypersensitivity angiitis (Henoch-Schönlein purpura)
Periarteritis nodosa
Wegener's granulomatosis
Scleroderma
Mixed connective tissue disease
Sjögren's syndrome
Relapsing polychondritis
Goodpasture's syndrome
Cryoglobulinemia
Waldenström's macroglobulinemia
Drugs: penicillamine, gold, heroin
Thyroiditis
Lymphoma, leukemia
Colonic carcinoma and other solid tumors
Intravenous cancer immunotherapy
Landry-Guillain-Barré syndrome
Subacute sclerosing panencephalitis

HIV = human immunodeficiency virus.

Mesangiocapillary Glomerulonephritis

This syndrome usually occurs in children and young adults and combines nephritic and nephrotic features. The initial manifestation may be an ordinary attack of nephritis followed by the onset of a nephrotic syndrome, or a patient may have the nephrotic syndrome plus hematuria.[69] Half the patients with MCGN show renal deterioration over a few years.[69] Almost all patients with MCGN have persistently low serum C3 levels with normal levels of C4, representing alternate pathway activation of complement. Sixty per cent of patients with MCGN (type II), and some patients with other types of acute proliferative glomerulonephritis, have C3 nephritic factor (C3Nef), an IgG autoantibody binding to an enzyme involved in alternate complement pathway activation in the serum.

Rapidly Progressive Glomerulonephritis

The hallmark of this syndrome is development of renal failure over a period of weeks. Symptoms include insidious onset of malaise, edema, and weight gain. The serum albumin is low, the patient is found to be anemic and to have oliguria and hematuria with RBC casts in the urine. Most patients with the idiopathic form remain normotensive and characteristically have normal serum complement levels.

Renal biopsy specimens show cellular proliferation and, most characteristically, fibroepithelial crescents within the majority of glomeruli. These crescents ultimately result in fibrosis. The prognosis is better if less than 40% of the glomeruli are involved by crescents.[86] In addition to sporadic idiopathic occurrences, rapidly progressive glomerulonephritis may be associated with many of the conditions listed in Table 30–9, including periarteritis nodosa, Wegener's granulomatosis, lupus erythematosus, hypersensitivity angiitis, essential mixed cryoglobulinemia, and Goodpasture's syndrome. The same syndrome may occur in very severe cases of poststreptococcal glomerulonephritis and MCGN. Recent studies of cases without associated systemic disease found many with a smooth, linear pattern of IgG deposition, suggesting antiglomerular basement membrane nephritis; a few with coarsely granular C3 and IgG, suggesting poststreptococcal nephritis; and several with negative immunofluorescent findings.[86] Some but not all of the patients with linear IgG deposition had pulmonary hemorrhages. Although fibrinogen is deposited within the glomeruli, there are no systemic clotting abnormalities and, unlike the hemolytic uremic syndrome, no microangiopathic hemolytic anemia. The absence of high-grade hypertensive retinopathy or of a grossly elevated blood pressure distinguishes this syndrome from malignant hypertension.

Other Causes of Acute Renal Failure

Oliguria with small amounts of reddish-brown urine is often the presenting manifestation in patients with acute tubular necrosis (ATN). The initial urinalysis usually reveals proteinuria, cylindruria, hematuria, and pyuria. "Dirty" brown granular casts and epithelial cell–containing casts are characteristically present, whereas RBC casts are noted infrequently in acute tubular necrosis. ATN is generally encountered in hospitalized patients with hypotension or sepsis. One condition that might present primarily as acute renal failure in a nonhospitalized, previously healthy individual is myoglobinuria caused by rhabdomyolysis. The urinalysis may reveal cellular elements and heme-pigmented casts because of the red myoglobin pigment. Most patients present with nausea and vomiting, myalgias, weakness, fever, and swollen, edematous limbs. The syndrome has been associated with heat, stress, and exercise in military recruits, and also with alcohol-induced coma and immobilization, convulsions, fever, hypothermia, cocaine toxicity, and treatment with mevacor.[87, 88] Sporadic cases have been reported in other apparently normal men who were thought to be stressed beyond their limit of muscular capacity. It is possible that these represent individuals with a genetic susceptibility, but in most cases, except for McArdle's syndrome, a biochemical abnormality has not been identified.[88]

Acute oliguric renal failure, usually but not always reversible, is also produced by high doses of radioiodinated contrast agents, including Renografin and Telepaque. In these cases, age and dehydration are factors, but the most important predisposing causes are diabetes and pre-existing renal disease.[89] The risk of renal compromise was 9% in diabetics who also had pre-existing renal insufficiency and received contrast material, but the risk was small for nondiabetics and for diabetics with normal renal function.[89]

Acute oliguric renal failure caused by allergic interstitial nephritis can develop in patients who are on cephalothin, methicillin, or other penicillin therapy.[90, 91] Fenoprofen, phenytoin, phenindione, cephalosporins, rifampin, allopurinol, thiazides, intravenous acyclovir, pentamidine, and sulfonamides are also reported to cause this reaction.[62, 92] Either gross or microscopic hematuria and usually proteinuria occur sometimes, but not always, accompanied by fever, skin rash, and arthralgias, and possibly blood eosinophilia and eosinophils in the urinary sediment.[93] Although RBC casts have been noted in the sediment of some cases, casts are described as being absent or few in the majority of instances.[62] Failure to recognize this syndrome, resulting in continuation of the offending agent, may lead to progressive and sometimes irreversible renal impairment.[62]

Nonsteroidal anti-inflammatory drugs may induce reversible renal compromise with a clear urine sediment, probably by the mechanism of prostaglandin inhibition, especially in elderly patients with underlying renal or cardiovascular disease.[94]

Other causes for renal failure include obstructive uropathy, massive uric acid overload, and direct tubular toxicity due to drugs such as the aminoglycosides, but most often there is little proteinuria or hematuria in these cases. Atheroembolic renal disease and other acute renovascular disease can occur spontaneously, in the presence of extensive atherosclerosis. Hematuria is minimal and RBC casts are rare in atheroembolic disease.[95] Multiple myeloma and bilateral renal artery occlusions may affect the kidneys without causing other obvious manifestations and should also be considered in patients with unexplained oliguria.

Patients with chronic interstitial nephritis have minimal proteinuria, and the urine sediment is generally clear. Most commonly the diagnosis is first suspected when an unexpected elevation of the blood urea nitrogen appears on routine testing. Specific symptoms, if present, consist of polyuria, renal tubular acidosis, salt wasting, or papillary necrosis. Most frequently, the syndrome results from regular abuse of analgesic drugs, most commonly combinations containing phenacetin. Often, the patient will have consulted the physician because of headache, backache, or another chronic symptom. Azotemia may have been discovered incidentally from a screening profile of blood chemistries. Information from the family may be necessary to help to confirm the analgesic use. Other etiologies include chronic potassium depletion, tophaceous gout involving the renal interstitium, renal ischemia, radiation-induced nephritis, hypercalcemia, medullary cystic kidneys, or hereditary nephritis.

Diagnostic Studies and Approach to the Patient

Hospitalization is required for most patients with oliguria and acute renal failure. The first step is to exclude obstructive uropathy, acute tubular necrosis, prerenal azotemia, underlying chronic renal disease, or another cause of renal failure instead of glomerulonephritis. It is important to determine if the patient has taken any drugs that may impair renal function. The next step in patients who are thought to have glomerulonephritis should be an evaluation for underlying systemic illness. Beyond this, the approach depends on the course of the patient's illness. Patients with acute poststreptococcal glomerulonephritis will usually recover after a brief interval with supportive management. Biopsy, tests for antiglomerular basement membrane antibody (ANTI-GBM) (present in 95%), and a trial of therapy with immunosuppressive agents or plasmapheresis is indicated in those following a course of rapidly progressive glomerulonephritis. In a few other patients, nephritis fails to resolve, a nephrotic syndrome ensues, or renal function gradually continues to deteriorate. In these, the major question is whether there are therapeutic measures that can affect long-term outcome.

The widespread availability of renal ultrasonography now makes it possible to identify dilatation of the ureter or hydronephrosis by noninvasive methods. The sensitivity of ultrasonography has been estimated at 98% for excluding obstructive uropathy,[42] although occasionally false-negative results are encountered in patients whose ureters are encased by tumor or fibrosis. In questionable cases, CT scanning should help.

Other ultrasonographically identifiable lesions include traumatic renal and perirenal hematomas, renal and perirenal abscesses, massive tumor replacement, and polycystic and multicystic kidneys.[42] The finding of bilaterally small, contracted kidneys is the hallmark of the syndrome of chronic as opposed to acute glomerulonephritis.

The urinalysis does not distinguish ATN, allergic interstitial nephritis, and sometimes other causes of acute renal failure from glomerulonephritis with certainty, unless myoglobinuria is also present. The finding of a clear urine sediment in a patient with oliguria may suggest urinary tract obstruction. In the absence of a preceding renal disease, patients retain tubular function early in the course of glomerulonephritis. Thus, the tubules continue extracting sodium, so that the sodium concentration in the urine of oliguric patients with acute glomerulonephritis (like those with prerenal azotemia), who are not on diuretics, is very low (mean of 22 mEq/l) compared with ATN (mean of 62 mEq/l) or obstructive uropathy (mean of 68 mEq/l).[96]* A correct diagnosis can be established in many difficult cases by using this test; however, a urinary sodium value in the range of 25 to 40 mEq/l is equivocal,[96] and the urine sodium and fractional excretion of sodium is low in hepatorenal syndrome and some nonoliguric types of ATN associated with radiocontrast agents, liver failure, burns, sepsis, and edematous states. Occasional patients with acute interstitial nephritis have been reported to have low urinary sodium concentrations, but the majority have high values.[62]

There are no findings in the urine to distinguish poststreptococcal glomerulonephritis from nephritis secondary to any of the systemic diseases listed in Table 30–9; thus, it is necessary to search in every case for any clinical feature that might suggest the diagnosis of a systemic illness. When there are no clinical findings outside the urinary tract in the face of documented, ongoing acute glomerulonephritis, one should consider obtaining ASO or ASO panel, blood cultures, HIV testing, antinuclear antibodies, hepatitis B–associated antigen, total hemolytic complement (CH50), C3 and C4 levels, cryoglobulin levels, rheumatoid factors, skin biopsy to detect IgA deposition, and a serologic test for syphilis.

Renal biopsy should be performed as early as possible when the clinical picture of rapidly progressive glomerulonephritis is recognized, since treatment may improve renal function in patients with crescentic glomerulonephritis, if begun prior to irreversible renal destruction.[97] Cyclophosphamide or chlorambucil plus high-dose methylprednisolone therapy given every other day is as effective as plasmapheresis and may entail fewer complications.[98, 99] In most cases the condition is not recurrent, so that therapy, when successful, may induce permanent remissions.

Studies have not shown immunosuppressive therapy to be beneficial in patients with slowly progressive, persistent idiopathic nephritis.[99] It is generally agreed as well that no therapy is beneficial for patients with MCGN.[69, 71, 99]

Although renal biopsy may yield prognostic information, there are few therapeutic implications of biopsy results in most patients with an episode of nephritis, unless a specific diagnosis of glomerulonephritis associated with rapidly progressive glomerulonephritis, lupus erythematosus, scleroderma, or Wegener's granulomatosis could be made. Complications of renal biopsy include gross hematuria in 5 to 7%, clinically important perirenal hematoma in 1.4%, failure to obtain renal tissue in 8%, acquired atrioventricular fistula especially in those hypertensive at the time of biopsy, and flare-up of infection in those infected at the time of biopsy.[100] There seems to be no need for biopsy in resolving or slowly progressive cases in which the renal function remains good, proteinuria is slight, serum complement is normal, and the initial attack was typical.[101] It is probably wise to obtain biopsies of patients with persistently active renal disease and severe hypertension or deteriorating renal function. Those with scleroderma may be improved by aggressive treatment of hypertension.[102] The "dense-deposit" variety of MCGN recurs so frequently after renal transplantation that biopsy information may be helpful in planning future management.[103] Focal glomerulosclerosis, immune complex-induced glomerulonephritis, and antiglomerular basement membrane glomerulonephritis may also recur, but not with great frequency, after transplantation.

*Oliguric patients with low urine sodium also have fractional excretion of sodium (FE_{Na}) <1%:

$$FE_{Na} = \frac{U_{Na} \times P_{cr}}{P_{Na} \times U_{cr}} \times 100$$

References

1. Pappes S: Asymptomatic proteinuria: Clinical significance. Postgrad Med 62:125, 1977.
2. Shaw ST, Poon SY, and Wong ET: "Routine urinalysis." Is the dipstick enough? JAMA 253:1596, 1985.
3. Brenner BM and Rector FC: The Kidney, 4th ed. Philadelphia, WB Saunders, 1991.
4. Froom P, Ribak J, and Benbassat J: Significance of microhematuria in young adults. BMJ 288:20, 1984.
5. Ingelfinger JR, Davis AE, and Grupe WE: Frequency and etiology of gross hematuria in a general pediatric setting. Pediatrics 59:557, 1977.
6. Abuelo JG: The diagnosis of hematuria. Arch Intern Med 143:967, 1983.
7. Kurdish GG: Determining the cause of hematuria. Postgrad Med 58:118, 1975.
8. Greene LF, O'Shaughnessy EJ Jr, and Hendricks ED: Study of 500 patients with asymptomatic microhematuria. JAMA 161:610, 1956.
9. Carson CC, Segura JW, and Greene LF: Clinical importance of microhematuria. JAMA 241:149, 1979.
10. Benson GS and Brewer ED: Hematuria-algorithms for diagnosis. II: Hematuria in the adult and hematuria secondary to trauma. JAMA 246:993, 1981.

11. Fair WR, McClennan BL, and Jost RG: Are excretory urograms necessary in evaluating women with urinary tract infections? J Urol 121:313, 1979.
12. Numazaki Y, Shigeta S, Kumasaka T, et al: Acute hemorrhagic cystitis in children: Isolation of adenovirus type II. N Engl J Med 278:700, 1968.
13. Utz DC and Zincke H: The masquerade of bladder cancer in situ as interstitial cystitis. J Urol 111:160, 1974.
14. Morrison AS and Cole P: Epidemiology of bladder cancer. Urol Clin North Am 3:13, 1976.
15. Wall RL and Clausen KP: Carcinoma of the urinary bladder in patients receiving cyclophosphamide. N Engl J Med 293:271, 1975.
16. Doll R, Payne P, and Waterhouse J (eds): International Union against Cancer: Cancer Incidence in Five Continents, Vol 1. New York, Springer-Verlag, 1966.
17. Morgan RW and Jain MG: Bladder cancer: Smoking, beverages and artificial sweeteners. Can Med Assoc J 111:1067, 1974.
18. Morrison AS and Buring JE: Artificial sweeteners and cancer of the lower urinary tract. N Engl J Med 302:537, 1980.
19. Hoover R, Strasser PH, Mason TJ, et al: Progress report to the Food and Drug Administration from the National Cancer Institute concerning the National Bladder Cancer Study. Bethesda, MD, National Cancer Institute, 1979.
20. Prout CR: Current concepts, bladder carcinoma. N Engl J Med 287:86, 1972.
21. Kolosseus RC, Fraley EE, and Blackard CE: Bladder cancer in man: An update. Minn Med 58:232, 1975.
22. Wynder EL, Mabuchi K, and Whitmore WF Jr: Epidemiology of adenocarcinoma of the kidney. J Natl Cancer Inst 53:1619, 1974.
23. Chisholm GD and Roy RR: The systemic effects of malignant renal tumors. Br J Urol 43:687, 1971.
24. Say CC and Hori JM: Transitional cell carcinoma of the renal pelvis: Experience from 1940 to 1972 and literature review. J Urol 112:438, 1974.
25. Burkholder GV, Dotin LN, Thomason WB, et al: Unexplained hematuria. JAMA 210:1729, 1969.
26. Hendler ED, Kashgarian M, and Hayslett JP: Clinicopathological correlations of primary hematuria. Lancet 1:458, 1972.
27. Morel-Maroger L, Leathan A, and Richet G: Glomerular abnormalities in nonsystemic diseases: Relationship between findings by light microscopy and immunofluorescence in 433 renal biopsy specimens. Am J Med 53:170, 1972.
28. Blumenthal SS, Fritsch C, and Lemann J Jr: Establishing the diagnosis of benign familial hematuria: The importance of examining the urine sediment in family members. JAMA 259:2263, 1988.
29. Rappaport A, Davidson DA, and Deveber GA, et al: Idiopathic focal proliferative nephritis associated with persistent hematuria and normal renal function. Ann Intern Med 73:921, 1970.
30. Fairley KF and Birch DF: Hematuria: A simple method for identifying glomerular bleeding. Kidney Int 21:105, 1982.
31. Chang BS: Red cell morphology as a diagnostic aid in hematuria. JAMA 252:1747, 1984.
32. Labovitz ED, Steinmuller SR, Henderson LW, et al: "Benign" hematuria with focal glomerulitis in adults. Ann Intern Med 77:723, 1972.
33. Kobayashi Y, Tateno S, Hikii Y, et al: IgA nephropathy: Prognostic significance of proteinuria and histologic alterations. Nephron 34:146, 1983.
34. Baldwin DS, Gluck MC, Schacht RG, et al: The long-term course of poststreptococcal glomerulonephritis. Ann Intern Med 80:342, 1974.
35. Castenfors J, Mossfeldt F, and Piscator M: Effect of prolonged heavy exercise on renal function and urinary protein excretion. Acta Physiol Scand 70:194, 1967.
36. Pollak VE and Ooi BS: Asymptomatic hematuria, diagnostic approach. Postgrad Med 62:115, 1977.
37. Christensen WI: Genitourinary tuberculosis: Review of 102 cases. Medicine 53:377, 1974.
38. Higgins PM and Aber GM: Renal pain and hematuria unexplained by complete urologic evaluation. Br J Urol 46:601, 1974.
39. Tiebosch AT, Frederik PM, van Breda Vriesman PJ, et al: Thin–basement-membrane nephropathy in adults with persistent hematuria. N Engl J Med 320:14, 1989.
40. Pollack HM, Goldberg BB, Morales J, et al: A systematized approach to the differential diagnosis of renal masses. Radiology 113:153, 1974.
41. Howard RS and Golin AL: Long-term follow up of asymptomatic microhematuria. J Urol 145:335, 1991.
42. Corwin HL and Silverstein MP: The diagnosis of neoplasia in patients with asymptomatic microscopic hematuria: A decision analysis. J Urol 139:1002, 1988.
43. Ferrucci JT Jr: Medical progress. Body ultrasonography (second of two parts). N Engl J Med 300:599, 1979.
44. Clayman RV, Williams RD, and Fraley EE: Current concepts in cancer: The pursuit of the renal mass. N Engl J Med 300:72, 1979.
45. McClennan BL, Stanley RJ, Melson GL, et al: CT of the renal cyst: Is cyst aspiration necessary? Am J Roentgenol 133:671, 1979.
46. Pearlstein AE: Hyperdense renal cysts. J Comput Assist Tomogr 7:1029, 1983.
47. Ekelund L and Karp W: Evaluation of solitary renal cystic lesions. Acta Radiol (Diagn) 19:321, 1978.
48. Lang EK: Renal cyst puncture and aspiration: A survey of complications. J Roentgenol 128:723, 1977.
49. Evans J: The accuracy of diagnostic radiology: Arteriography and nephrotomography. JAMA 204:131, 1968.
50. Brennan RE, Curtis JA, Kurtz AB, et al: Use of tomography and ultrasound in the diagnosis of nonopaque renal calculi. JAMA 244:594, 1980.
51. Lang EK: The roentgenographic assessment of bladder tumors: A comparison of diagnostic accuracy of roentgenographic techniques. Cancer 23:717, 1969.
52. Friedell GH, Soto EA, and Nagy GK: Cytologic and histopathologic study of bladder cancer patients. Urol Clin North Am 3:71, 1976.
53. Heney NM, Szyfelbein WM, Daly JJ, et al: Positive urinary cytology in patients without evident tumor. J Urol 117:223, 1977.
54. Messing EM, Young TB, Hunt VB, et al: The significance of asymptomatic microhematuria in men 50 or more years old: findings of a home screening study using urinary dipsticks. J Urol 49:237, 1987.
55. Simon HB, Weinstein AJ, Pasternak MS, et al: Genitourinary tuberculosis: Clinical features in a general hospital population. Am J Med 63:410, 1977.
56. Abuelo JG: Proteinuria: Diagnostic principles and procedures. Ann Intern Med 98:186, 1983.
57. Springberg PD, Garrett LE, Thompson AL, et al: Fixed and reproducible orthostatic proteinuria: Results of a 20 year followup study. Ann Intern Med 97:516, 1982.
58. Novick AC, Gephardt G, Guz B, et al: Long term follow-up after partial removal of a solitary kidney. N Engl J Med 325:1058, 1991.
59. Monin PAF: Urinary sediment in the interpretation of proteinuria. Ann Intern Med 98:254, 1983.
60. Cameron JS: Nephrotic syndrome. BMJ 4:350, 1970.
61. Torres VE, Vilosa JA, Holley KE, et al: The progression of vesicoureteral reflux neuropathy. Ann Intern Med 92:776, 1980.
62. Linton AL, Clark WF, Driedger AA, et al: Acute interstitial nephritis due to drugs: A review of the literature and report of nine cases. Ann Intern Med 93:735, 1980.
63. Mallick NP, Dosq S, Acheson EJ, et al: Detection, significance and treatment of paraprotein in patients presenting with "idiopathic" proteinuria without myeloma. Q J Med 47:145, 1978.
64. Black DAK, Rose G, and Brewer DB: Controlled trial of prednisone in adult patients with the nephrotic syndrome. BMJ 3:421, 1970.
65. Habib R: Focal glomerulosclerosis. Kidney Int 4:355, 1973.
66. Lim VS, Sibley R, and Spengo B: Adult lipoid nephrosis: Clinical and pathologic correlations. Ann Intern Med 81:314, 1974.
67. Jenis EH, Teichman S, Briggs WA, et al: Focal segmental glomerulosclerosis. Ann J Med 57:695, 1974.

68. Beaufils H, Alphonse JC, Guedon J, et al: Focal glomerulosclerosis: Natural history and treatment: A report of 70 cases. Nephron 21:75, 1978.
69. Cameron JS, Glasgow EF, Ogg CS, et al: Membranoproliferative glomerulonephritis and persistent hypocomplementemia. BMJ 4:7, 1970.
70. Wagoner RD, Stanson AW, Holley KE, et al: Renal vein thrombosis in idiopathic membranous glomerulopathy and nephrotic syndrome: Incidence and significance. Kidney Int 23:368, 1983.
71. Collaborative study of the adult idiopathic nephrotic syndrome: A controlled study of short-term prednisone treatment in adults with membranous nephropathy. N Engl J Med 301:1301, 1979.
72. Cattran DC, Delmore T, Roscoe J, et al: A randomized control trial of prednisone in patients with idiopathic membranous nephropathy. N Engl J Med 320:210, 1989.
73. Pontialli C, Zucchelli P, Passerini P, et al: A randomized trial of methylprednisolone and chlorambucil in idiopathic membranous nephropathy. N Engl J Med 320:8, 1989.
74. Danadio JV Jr, Torres VE, Velosa JA, et al: Idiopathic membranous nephropathy: The natural history of untreated patients. Kidney Int 33:708, 1988.
75. Ravid M, Robson M, and Kedar I: Prolonged colchicine treatment in four patients with amyloidosis. Ann Intern Med 87:568, 1977.
76. Shehadeh IH, Demers LM, Abt AB, et al: Indomethacin and the nephrotic syndrome. JAMA 241:1264, 1979.
77. Findling JW, Beckstrom D, Rawsthorne L, et al: Indomethacin-induced hyperkalemia in three patients with gouty arthritis. JAMA 244:1127, 1980.
78. Wilson DM, Turner DR, Cameron JS, et al: Value of renal biopsy in acute intrinsic renal failure. BMJ 2:459, 1976.
79. Kaplan EL, Anthony BF, Chapman SS, et al: Epidemic acute glomerulonephritis associated with type 49 streptococcal pyoderma. Am J Med 48:9, 1970.
80. Hinglais N, Garcia-Torres R, and Kleinknecht D: Long-term prognosis in acute glomerulonephritis. The predictive value of early clinical and pathologic features observed in 65 patients. Am J Med 56:52, 1974.
81. Bourgognier JJ, Meneses R, Ortiz C, et al: The clinical spectrum of renal disease associated with human immunodeficiency virus. Am J Kidney Dis 12:131, 1988.
82. Border WA: Immune complex detection in glomerulonephritis. Nephron 24:105, 1979.
83. Wilson CB and Dixon FJ: Diagnosis of immunopathologic renal disease. Kidney Int 5:379, 1974.
84. Sutherland JC, Vann Markhan R, and Mardiney MR: Subclinical immune complexes in glomeruli of kidneys postmortem. Am J Med 57:536, 1974.
85. Sutherland JC and Mardiney MR: Immune complex diseases in the kidneys of lympholeukemia patients: The presence of an oncornavirus-related antigen. J Natl Cancer Inst 50:633, 1973.
86. Spargo BH, Ofdonez NG, and Ringus JC: The differential diagnosis of crescentic glomerulonephritis: The pathology of specific lesions with prognostic implications. Hum Pathol 8:187, 1977.
87. Schrier RW, Henderson HS, Tisher CG, et al: Nephropathy associated with heat stress and exercise. Ann Intern Med 67:356, 1967.
88. Rowland LP and Penn AS: Myoglobinuria. Med Clin North Am 56:1233, 1972.
89. Purfrey PS, Griffiths SM, Barrett BJ, et al: Contrast material-induced renal failure in patients with diabetes mellitus, renal insufficiency, or both. N Engl J Med 320:143, 1989.
90. Burton JR, Lichtenstein NS, Colvin RB, et al: Acute renal failure during cephalothin therapy. JAMA 229:679, 1974.
91. Bennett WM, Plamp C, and Porter GA: Drug-related syndromes in clinical nephrology. Ann Intern Med 87:582, 1977.
92. Curt GA, Kaldany A, and Whitley LG: Reversible rapidly progressive renal failure with nephrotic syndrome due to fenoprofen calcium. Ann Intern Med 92:72, 1980.
93. Buysen JG, Houthoff HJ, Krediet RT, et al: Acute interstitial nephritis: A clinical and morphological study in 27 patients. Nephrol Dial Transplant J, 5:94, 1990.
94. Whetton A, Stout RL, and Spilman PS: Renal effects of ibuprofin, piroxicam, and sulindac in patients with asymptomatic renal failure. Ann Intern Med 112:508, 1990.
95. Kassirer JP: Atheroembolic renal disease. N Engl J Med 280:812, 1969.
96. Miller TR, Enderson RJ, Linas SL, et al: Urinary diagnostic indices in acute renal failure: A prospective study. Ann Intern Med 89:47, 1978.
97. Johnson JP, Whitman W, Briggs WA, et al: Plasmapheresis and immunosuppressive agents in antibasement membrane antibody-induced Goodpasture's syndrome. Am J Med 64:354, 1978.
98. Bruns FG, Fraley DS, Adler S, et al: Megadose methyl prednisolone versus plasmapheresis in the treatment of rapidly progressive glomerulonephritis (Abstract). Proc Am Soc Nephrology. 13th Annual Meeting, 1980, p 14A.
99. Cameron JS: The management of primary glomerulonephritis using immunosuppressive agents. Am J Nephrol 9(Suppl 1):33, 1989.
100. Wickre CG and Golper TA: Complications of percutaneous needle biopsy of the kidney. Am J Nephrol 2:173, 1982.
101. Cameron JS: Glomerulonephritis. BMJ 4:285, 1970.
102. Wagner C, Cooke CR, and Fries JF: Successful medical treatment of scleroderma in renal crisis. N Engl J Med 299:873, 1978.
103. Kassirer JP and McCluskey RT: Case records of the Massachusetts General Hospital. Recurrent nephrotic syndrome after a renal transplant. N Engl J Med 294:1108, 1976.

31

Sexually Transmitted Diseases

PART 1 ■ Salpingitis

RUTH TUOMALA, MD

Acute salpingitis and acute pelvic inflammatory disease (PID), used interchangeably in this chapter, refer to upper genital tract infection in women. PID actually represents a number of processes that occur when pathogenic organisms ascend from the vagina and cervix into the normally sterile uterus, fallopian tubes, and peritoneum, resulting in inflammation of these and nearby structures. Nontuberculous PID can be classified as primary or secondary. In primary PID, infection originates from a focus in the lower genital tract and may be exogenous; that is, venereal or iatrogenic (associated with an intrauterine device, dilatation and curettage, or hysterosalpingogram); or endogenous, the infecting organisms being part of the normal vaginal flora. Secondary PID, which is quite uncommon, arises from a focus outside the genital tract, such as in appendicitis or inflammatory bowel disease.

PUBLIC HEALTH IMPACT

It is difficult to overstate the importance of PID, both for the affected individual and for the society that bears the cumulative burden. Although PID is not reportable, estimates of its occurrence suggest that is accounts for 400,000 outpatient visits for a first diagnosis of PID and 5 to 20% of all gynecologic hospital admissions.[1] In 1990 the total direct and indirect costs of diagnosing and treating PID were estimated to be $4.2 billion.[2] Between 1979 and 1988, average annual hospital admissions were 181,700 for acute PID and 94,400 for chronic PID.[1] Less obvious but more important are the consequences of the sequelae of recurrent PID[3]: infertility, ectopic pregnancy, and chronic pelvic pain due to adhesions or persistent infection. The recurrent nature of salpingitis should prompt increased efforts at education, contact tracing, and long-term follow-up of women who have a first episode of illness. Rates of other sequelae increase with multiple episodes of acute infection as well as increasing duration of pain prior to treatment and severity of disease.[4] Approximately 20 to 30% of cases of infertility are thought to result from fallopian tube obstruction, most often as a consequence of PID. Data from prospective studies in Sweden suggest that tubal occlusion may result from a single clinical episode of PID 15 to 25% of the time. More than one half of women with a diagnosis of tuboovarian abscess (TOA) have reproductive difficulties. Ectopic pregnancy, which may result from salpingitis-associated tubal dysfunction, is seven to ten times more likely in women who have had PID than in those who have not. The reported number of ectopic pregnancies in the United States more than tripled between 1970 and 1983. Chronic pelvic pain occurs in approximately 18% of women who have had PID, some three times more often than in control subjects. These symptoms interfere with work and sexual functioning, may be associated with frequent visits to the physician, and often result in attempted palliative surgery, including hysterectomy. It is estimated that up to 90% of women with a diagnosis of chronic PID, which is often synonymous with chronic pain secondary to PID, eventually undergo surgery.[1] These long-term sequelae associated with PID are of increasing consequence to society and the health-care system when one considers that between 1987 and 1988 the highest hospitalization rates for PID were seen in teenaged girls.[1]

DIAGNOSIS

There are risk factors for the occurrence of PID that should be taken into account when taking a history from a woman who presents with pelvic pain. Most important, salpingitis is a disease of sexually active (in particular heterosexually active) women. Risk is increased by a history of sexually transmitted diseases, numbers of partners, frequency of intercourse, recent new partners, and age of first intercourse. A young age in itself increases risk of PID, with persons younger than 25 years of age being at greatest risk. The presence of an intrauterine device (IUD) increases the risk of PID; risk is decreased by use of barrier contraceptive methods and oral contraceptive pills. Studies have suggested that douching and smoking are risk factors for PID.[5–7]

The clinical diagnosis of salpingitis is made on the basis

of some combination of fever, lower abdominal pain and tenderness, adnexal tenderness with or without induration/masses, purulent cervical exudate, and peripheral leukocytosis or elevated sedimentation rate. However, there are serious problems with the accuracy of this diagnosis, as demonstrated by two laparoscopic studies and confirmed by multiple others from the United States, Canada, and Scandinavia. Jacobson and Westrom routinely performed laparoscopy on 814 patients with the clinical diagnosis of acute salpingitis and were able to confirm the diagnosis visually in only 532 cases (65%).[8] Ninety-eight patients (12%) were found to have other disorders, of which fully one half warranted immediate surgery, and 184 (23%) were "visually normal." The "visually normal" group were not treated for PID, although up to one quarter were treated for a variety of lower genital tract infections. A number of the women in this group were followed long-term and documented not to have the sequelae associated with PID. During the period of this study, an additional 91 cases of acute PID were detected during laparoscopy of patients with other preoperative diagnoses. Less than 60% of these 91 patients had abdominal pain and adnexal tenderness. Thus, the clinical diagnosis lacks both specificity and sensitivity.

Using more stringent clinical criteria, Sweet and coworkers,[9] in performing laparoscopy in 29 patients with acute salpingitis, found three misdiagnosed cases: one of acute appendicitis, one of ectopic pregnancy, and one of bowel obstruction. It is probable that when utilizing stringent criteria, milder or subclinical cases are frequently missed and that PID is even more frequent than is currently appreciated. Increased awareness of the potential subtlety of the diagnosis plus increased use of diagnostic laparoscopy may improve our awareness of the spectrum of disease.

The differential diagnosis of acute PID includes acute appendicitis, endometriosis, ectopic pregnancy, corpus luteum hemorrhage, pelvic adhesions, ovarian tumors, mesenteric lymphadenitis, and inflammatory bowel conditions. Acute PID should be considered in evaluating any sexually active woman who has abdominal pain or even less specific lower abdominal or genital complaints. There are no pathognomonic signs or symptoms of PID. Signs and symptoms that can be associated with a diagnosis of PID being present increase the accuracy of clinical diagnosis. Lower abdominal pain associated with PID is typically bilateral and is associated with tenderness; however either pain or tenderness may be worse on one side or unilateral. Vaginal discharge containing more than 10 polymorphonuclear leukocytes per high-power field (hpf) by wet mount is almost always present, though nonspecific; mucopus seen coming from the cervical os on pelvic examination provides additional evidence of PID. Dysuria, abnormal menstrual bleeding, anorexia, nausea and vomiting, and proctitis-type symptoms may occur with variable frequency in PID, although they are nonspecific findings. Peripheral leukocytosis occurs in less than half of the cases and is correlated with severity of presentation of clinical illness and fever. The sedimentation rate is usually elevated within a few days of onset of symptoms but is frequently normal early in the course of the episode. This is the only laboratory test found to have a significantly abnormal result in Westrom's series of women with PID, with the number being elevated in 75% of cases. It is, however, a nonspecific test. Noninvasive imaging studies such as ultrasound and a computed tomography (CT) scan can be helpful in diagnosing TOA in women with PID and can be used for following abscess resolution. However, imaging test findings suggestive of PID or TOA are nonspecific.

One wishes to treat all cases of PID in order to prevent sequelae. In more severe cases, in which lower abdominal pain and bilateral adnexal tenderness are accompanied by purulent cervical discharge or fever and other manifestations of pelvic infection, the clinical diagnosis may present little problem and may be reasonably secure. In such cases, initial laparoscopy is not warranted. However, when the diagnosis is uncertain, particularly in women at low risk, when there is need to exclude appendicitis or ectopic pregnancy or when the patient fails to respond to appropriate antimicrobial therapy, laparoscopic visualization is indicated (Table 31–1). In some cases, culdocentesis revealing an elevated white blood cell (WBC) count, with a normal count being 1500/ml, or endometrial biopsy diagnostic of endometritis can be helpful in establishing the diagnosis of inflammation of the upper genital tract. In general, it is appropriate to overdiagnose PID on an initial presentation of pelvic pain so as not to exclude those with mild disease from therapy. If long-term follow-up reveals repeated episodes of pain, laparoscopy should be liberally utilized to

TABLE 31–1. SPECIAL DIAGNOSTIC STUDIES TO CONSIDER FOR LOWER ABDOMINAL PAIN AND/OR VAGINAL BLEEDING IN WOMEN

	Indications	Findings
Radioimmunoassay for subunit of HCG	Possible ectopic pregnancy or intrauterine pregnancy	Highly sensitive and positive in low titer by the time of presentation in ectopic pregnancy; positive in high titer in the first trimester of intrauterine pregnancy
Culdocentesis	Suspected rupture of ectopic pregnancy or to confirm PID	Aspiration of blood from the pelvis that will not clot within a glass syringe More than 1500 WBC mm^3 suggests PID, appendicitis, or other causes of intra-abdominal inflammation
Endometrial aspiration biopsy (if pregnancy not desired)	Suspected spontaneous abortion	Chorionic villi obtained from uterus
Ultrasonography or CT scanning of the pelvis	Suspected ectopic pregnancy or ovarian cyst or abscess	Good sensitivity and specificity for detecting cysts, ectopic pregnancy, or masses but does not define the nature of a mass
Laparoscopy	Diagnosis uncertain or response to therapy incomplete	Will confirm or exclude diagnosis of salpingitis; will detect appendicitis, endometriosis, or ectopic pregnancy. Indicated when the diagnosis is in doubt, patient does not respond promptly to therapy, or surgery appears necessary

CT = computed tomography; PID = pelvic inflammatory disease; WBC = white blood cell establish a firm diagnosis. Laparoscopic grading systems may be useful for predicting duration of therapy and future sequelae.[10]

BACTERIOLOGY

The bacteriology of PID involves both sexually transmitted organisms and endogenous genital tract flora. Eschenbach and Holmes demonstrated that up to half of patients have polymicrobial, mixed aerobic-anaerobic peritoneal infections commonly involving the anaerobes *Peptostreptococcus, Peptococcus,* and *Bacteroides fragilis.*[11] Anaerobic and aerobic organisms isolated from these mixed infections are part of the usual vaginal flora and are similar to those found in other pelvic infections.[12] Some investigators have proposed that the presence of endogenous organisms represent superinfection following a process initiated by sexually transmitted organisms, mainly *Neisseria gonorrhoeae* and *Chlamydia trachomatis.*

Acute salpingitis can be generally classified as gonococcal, chlamydial, or nongonococcal-nonchlamydial on the basis of cervical culture results. Patients from whom *N. gonorrhoeae* is isolated are generally younger, are more acutely ill, and more often experience pain in the first 10 days of the menstrual cycle.[13] "Classic" chlamydial PID has an indolent course, with gradual onset of symptoms that tend to be more mild. Fever, peritoneal signs, and elevated WBC count occur less frequently, whereas intermenstrual bleeding and elevated sedimentation rates may be more common. Nongonococcal-nonchlamydial disease is more likely to present as an episode of recurrent disease with a subacute onset. Although less often are there peritoneal signs, masses may be more frequent. In particular, in the case of TOA, anaerobes are of primary concern. There is evidence that patients with gonococcal PID have a better prognosis with respect to response to therapy, duration of hospitalization, and subsequent risks of recurrence, infertility, and ectopic pregnancy, whereas women with chlamydial disease may have the worst prognosis with regard to fertility. All reasons for this are not understood, but persons who have gonococcal PID are probably likely to seek medical assistance earlier because of more acute onset of symptoms, whereas chlamydia may be associated with the greatest duration of inflammation prior to treatment. There is a great deal of overlap in both disease presentation and sequelae according to organisms present.

In 45 to 80% of patients with acute salpingitis, *N. gonorrhoeae* can be isolated from cultures of the cervix. The wide range of values is related to population variations in the prevalence of gonorrhea. *N. gonorrhoeae* can be isolated from the fallopian tube or from peritoneal fluid in 5 to 65% of patients whose cervical cultures yield the gonococcus. When the result of the smear is positive, a Gram stain of the cervical specimen is helpful, since the specificity is high if intracellular gram-negative diplococci are identified (>90%). However, the sensitivity of the Gram-stained smear, compared with cultures on selective medium, is only 48 to 71%.[13] Thus, a negative result of a smear does not reliably exclude *N. gonorrhoeae* as the cause in a patient with PID, and properly handled specimens should be taken for culture on selective media (e.g., Thayer-Martin). Cervical cultures are much more sensitive than Gram stains; their yield can be increased by 3 to 7% by simultaneously taking a culture from the rectum.[14]

Tissue culture for chlamydia, the "gold standard" for diagnosis, is costly, is time consuming, and requires transport at 4° C using special transport medium.[15] Direct aspiration of material from fallopian tubes and fimbrial biopsy for culture are the most specific ways to identify this pathogen in patients with salpingitis.[16] Rapid diagnostic tests for chlamydial infection of the cervix are now widely available. The direct-smear fluorescein-conjugated monoclonal antibody test is estimated to be approximately 90% sensitive and approximately 98% specific but requires an experienced microscopist using special equipment to interpret the results. The enzyme immunoassay (ELISA) test can be done more cheaply but has decreased sensitivity (67 to 90%) and specificity (92 to 97%). Both types of tests appear to be most specific when disease is suspected as opposed to when used as a screen. These tests may allow more rational choices of therapy for patients suspected of chlamydial infections and may also provide the imperative for contact tracing and long-term follow-up.

There is some evidence that *Mycoplasma* species may occasionally be pathogens in patients with salpingitis. Mardh and Westrom obtained specimens directly from fallopian tubes, isolating *M. hominis* from 4 of 50 women with salpingitis but from none of 50 control subjects.[17] Similar culture studies have documented *Ureaplasma urealyticum* to be present in some cases of infection. The contribution of such organisms to the overall problem of PID remains to be demonstrated.

TREATMENT

Compliant patients with a relatively clear-cut diagnosis and mild-to-moderate illness can generally be managed as outpatients. Guidelines published in 1993 by the Centers for Disease Control (CDC) for outpatient treatment of salpingitis are listed in Table 31–2. These guidelines are based on the need to cover for coexisting chlamydial infection as well as *N. gonorrhoeae.*[18] From 1985 to 1993 there was a change in the recommended outpatient therapy for gonorrhea because of increasing rates of penicillinase-producing *N. gonorrhoeae.* Ceftriaxone or cefoxitin or equivalent cephalosporin accompanied by probenecid are given immediately to treat for gonorrhea. Tetracycline—or doxycycline, which is more expensive but need be taken only twice daily—is then taken by mouth for 14 days to treat for *Chlamydia.* The same treatment is recommended for sexual partners of patients with gonorrhea, who should also

TABLE 31–2. CENTERS FOR DISEASE CONTROL RECOMMENDATIONS FOR OUTPATIENT TREATMENT OF PELVIC INFLAMMATORY DISEASE

Recommended Regimen A
Cefoxitin 2 g IM plus probenecid 1 g orally, or ceftriaxone 250 mg IM or an equivalent cephalosporin
plus
Doxycycline 100 mg orally 2 times a day for 14 days*
Recommended Regimen B (Nonpregnant)
Ofloxacin 400 mg orally 2 times a day for 14 days
plus
Clindamycin 450 mg orally 4 times a day,
or
Metronidazole 500 mg orally 2 times a day for 14 days

*Alternatives for patients who do not tolerate doxycycline: erythromycin base 500 mg orally 4 times a day for 14 days should be substituted for doxycycline/tetracycline in pregnant women. Uncomplicated chlamydial infections (urethritis, cervicitis) in pregnant women can be treated with erythromycin base 500 mg orally 4 times daily for 7 days or 250 mg orally 4 times daily for 14 days) or erythromycin ethylsuccinate (800 mg orally 4 times daily for 7 days or 400 mg orally 4 times daily for 14 days).[18]

IM = intramuscularly.

be examined and have specimens cultured. Patients who are allergic to or are unable to tolerate tetracyclines are given erythromycin for 14 days. Patients treated on an outpatient basis should be re-evaluated in a minimum of 72 hours. Pregnant women may be treated with a cephalosporin or spectinomycin in addition to erythromycin base or ethylsuccinate, but should not receive tetracyclines, erythromycin estolate, or quinolones (azithromycin, a single-dose alternative for uncomplicated chlamydial infections [urethritis, cervicitis], has not been shown to be safe in pregnancy).[18]

Hospitalization is indicated when the diagnosis is uncertain, when conditions such as appendicitis and ectopic pregnancy must be excluded, when a pelvic abscess is suspected, when the severity of the illness (which often means the presence of peritonitis) precludes use of oral antibiotics, or when the patient is pregnant, is an adolescent, is unable to follow an outpatient regimen, or fails to respond to outpatient therapy. The 1993 guidelines for treatment of hospitalized patients with PID are listed in Table 31–3.[18] The combination of doxycycline and cefoxitin or cefotetan contains a high risk of phlebitis if doxycycline is given by peripheral vein. If able to tolerate oral medications, oral doxycycline can be given because the drug achieves levels similar to those of the parenteral preparation. The combination of clindamycin and gentamicin may not provide optimal coverage for chlamydial infection, although comparative trials have suggested equal efficacy of the two suggested regimens in eradicating both *C. trachomatis* and *N. gonorrhoeae*.[19, 20] Cefoxitin, cefotetan, and clindamycin all cover penicillin-resistant *Bacteroides* species, but the clindamycin/aminoglycoside combination probably provides the best coverage when TOA or mixed anaerobic infection is suspected (e.g., in PID complicated by IUD). It has been suggested that the medical success rate in treating TOA is approximately 75%.[21]

The CDC guidelines are controversial because they are based on opinion rather than on data from carefully conducted clinical trials.[22] A few randomized trials have suggested that cure rates of the two regimens for hospitalized patients are equivalent. Other trials have suggested that outpatient treatment that employs more than one drug leads to better cure rates and fewer recurrences than does single-drug therapy. There is an opportunity for individualization of therapy, taking into account likely organisms involved, drug intolerances, cost, and prospects for long-term follow-up.

TABLE 31–3. CENTERS FOR DISEASE CONTROL RECOMMENDATIONS FOR INPATIENT TREATMENT OF PELVIC INFLAMMATORY DISEASE

Recommended Regimen A*
Cefoxitin 2 g IV every 6 hours
or
Cefotetan† 2 g IV every 12 hours
plus
Doxycycline 100 mg orally or IV every 12 hours (if not pregnant)
Recommended Regimen B‡
Clindamycin 900 mg IV every 8 hours
plus
Gentamicin 2 mg/kg IV or IM loading dose followed by 1.5 mg/kg every 8 hours

*Regimen A is given for at least 48 hours after the patient clinically improves. After discharge from the hospital, continue with doxycycline 100 mg orally twice daily for a total of 14 days.

†Other cephalosporins that provide adequate gonococcal, other facultative gram-negative aerobic, and anaerobic coverage may be used in appropriate doses.

‡Regimen B is given for at least 48 hours after the patient improves. After discharge from the hospital (if not pregnant), continue with doxycycline 100 mg orally twice daily for 14 days total. If chlamydia is strongly suspected, doxycycline may be started during hospitalization. Clindamycin 450 mg orally five times a day for 10–14 days may be considered as an alternative to doxycycline; however, it may provide less than optimal coverage against chlamydia.

IM = intramuscular; IV = intravenous.

It has been suggested that hospitalization for treatment of PID can also be utilized for intensive education of patients about the pathogenesis of PID, reducing risky behaviors, and recognition of early signs and symptoms of acute disease.[23] This may be particularly important in the successful long-term treatment of adolescents and in maximizing preservation of fertility.

A comprehensive approach to management of PID should also include evaluation of the patient for other sexually transmitted diseases (STDs) and contact tracing. Serosurveys of patients hospitalized with PID have suggested rates of HIV positivity of 6 to 16%.[24] Contact tracing of all male partners is necessary to prevent both reinfection and the further spread of disease. It is recognized that both gonorrhea and chlamydia can be asymptomatic in males. Cultures for both of these organisms or presumptive therapy should be minimum standards for partners.

PART 2 Penile Discharge and Urethritis

WILLIAM T BRANCH, Jr., MD

When a patient has penile discharge or dysuria, urethritis is generally present. Establishing the exact pathogen can be difficult, but in most cases proper therapy can be given if a differentiation between gonococcal and nongonococcal urethritis can be made. History and physical examination will not establish the diagnosis. Gram staining of the urethral discharge and, occasionally, culture, are required. Infections with multiple organisms may be the rule rather than the exception, and therapy must be planned accordingly.

Patient History

The symptoms of urethritis in male patients include vague penile discomfort, poorly localized penile itching, dysuria, and urethral discharge. The discharge can be colorless or frankly purulent. Further history should elicit:

1. Any previous history of STD, including syphilis, herpes simplex, gonorrhea, or nongonococcal urethritis
2. A recent exposure history, including male or female contacts, and symptoms of STD in these contacts
3. Any attempts at self-treatment (e.g., leftover antibiotics)
4. Allergies (especially penicillin)
5. Previous medical history (e.g., diabetes, urinary tract infection)

Physical Examination, Laboratory Examination, and Culture

A focused physical examination should include careful inspection for spontaneous or expressible urethral discharge, penile or other genital skin lesions, and inguinal lymphadenopathy.

Palpation for testicular or epididymal mass or tenderness, and rectal examination including an evaluation for prostatic and seminal vesicle tenderness, are important as well.

A sample of urethral discharge can be obtained by inserting a Calgiswab (calcium alginate swab) 2 cm into the distal urethra. This may result in useful specimens even in the absence of visible discharge. The swab is gently rolled against a clean glass slide, which is then air-dried for Gram staining. The same swab can be streaked onto a Thayer-Martin culture plate, using first a zigzag pattern and then cross-streaks. The culture plate should be at room temperature, and the plate must be promptly placed in a candle-jar after streaking. If the laboratory is at a distance, one can use culture media especially prepared for mailing.

Gram Stain. After air-drying, the slide should be *gently* flamed to fix the bacteria. Gram staining is performed as follows:

(1) Flood the slide for 5 seconds with gentian violet and rinse thoroughly with cold water; (2) flood the slide for 5 seconds with Gram's iodine and rinse thoroughly with cold water; (3) flood the slide for approximately 10 seconds with alcohol (95%) until the blue coloring begins to lift and then rinse thoroughly with cold water; (4) flood the slide for 5 seconds with fuscin and rinse thoroughly with cold water. Let the slide air-dry completely or gently pat it dry with a paper towel.

All Gram-stained smears should be examined under oil immersion microscopy.

GONOCOCCAL URETHRITIS

Incidence. Rates of gonorrhea declined overall in 1990 and 1991 but remain high for African-American adolescents and young adults.[25] The highest attack rates appear to be for men and women between the ages of 20 and 24 years, with ages 15 to 19 years being second.

Increasing gonococcal resistance to penicillin has been observed since the early 1970s. Chromosomally mediated, low-level resistance is likely due to mutations that alter the organism's surface permeability to penicillin.[25] Plasmid-mediated high-level resistance results from conjugation with gram-negative organisms carrying the resistance plasmid for penicillinase.[27] The penicillinase-producing *N. gonorrhoeae* (PPNG) were first found in the United States in 1976 among servicemen returning from Southeast Asia.

PPNG are common in Asia and have been increasingly common in the United States since 1980.[28–31] In 1991, 11% of gonorrhea isolates in a survey of STD clinics were PPNG, and, overall, 32.4% were resistant to penicillin, tetracycline, or both.[25] None demonstrated clinically significant resistance to currently recommended therapy (Table 31–4).[25]

Clinical Presentation. In men, gonorrhea develops in one fourth to one half of those exposed to a sexual partner with active infection.[32] The incubation period ranges from 2 to 14 days.[33] The true incidence of asymptomatic gonorrhea in men is not known, but probably it is unusual except for men with a history of STDs or recent exposure to multiple partners. The causative organism, *N. gonorrhoeae,* is a gram-negative diplococcus. The typical symptoms of *N. gonorrhoeae* infection are severe dysuria with a frankly purulent urethral discharge. Ascending infection can cause symptoms of epididymitis, including scrotal pain, swelling, tenderness, and fever. Some patients will be minimally symptomatic, with only slight dysuria or with asymptomatic mild discharge.

Findings on Gram Stain. If the Gram stain shows one or more polymorphonuclear leukocytes containing typical gram-negative diplococci within the cytoplasm, a diagnosis of gonorrhea can be made. In symptomatic men, the sensitivity of this test is over 93%, and the specificity is 98 to 100%.[34] The sensitivity of Gram stain in men probably exceeds that of culture, especially if transport times to the laboratory are long. Culture is optional when the Gram stain is clearly positive or clearly negative.[35]

Some Gram stains show only extracellular forms or atypical staining or morphology. Such stains should be regarded as indeterminate and a culture should be performed. Approximately half of such patients will have a positive culture.[32]

Treatment

Currently recommended treatment options for uncomplicated gonococcal infections in males are described in Table 31–4.[36] These protocols recognitize coexistent gonococcal and nongonococcal urethritis. The prevalence of coinfection with *Chlamydia* is approximately 20% of heterosexual men

TABLE 31–4. RECOMMENDED TREATMENT FOR URETHRITIS IN MALES*

Ceftriaxone 250 mg single IM dose plus doxycycline 100 mg orally twice daily for 7 days *or* tetracycline 500 mg orally four times a day for 7 days

Treatment Failures

Evaluate for reinfection or alternative diagnosis; if persistent NGU: erythromycin base or stearate 500 mg or ethylsuccinate 800 mg orally four times daily for 7 days *or* doxycycline 100 mg orally twice daily or tetracycline 500 mg orally four times daily for 7–21 days

Alternative Regimens

Cefixime 400 mg orally in a single dose, or ofloxacin 400 mg orally in a single dose, or ciprofloxacin 500 mg orally in a single dose

Spectinomycin 2 g IM in a single dose (plus doxycycline) if unable to tolerate cephalosporins or quinolones

*From MMWR 1993.

with gonorrhea.[37] Combined regimens provide single-dose coverage for *N. gonorrhoeae* plus additional days of doxycycline, to treat chlamydial infection. It is no longer considered sufficient to treat only for the gonococcus in heterosexual men.

Patients unable to tolerate cephalosporins may be treated with one of the alternative regimens. Ciprofloxacin has been used successfully in clinical trials and, like ofloxacin, has favorable pharmacokinetics.[36] No resistance to quinolones has been encountered in the US, but strains with decreased susceptibility are common in Asia.[36] Intramuscular spectinomycin is alternatively recommended, but is relatively ineffective against pharyngeal gonorrhea, and resistant strains are now reported in the US.[36] Even 7 days of doxycycline given alone does not suffice to treat resistant gonorrhea.

Patients with incubating syphilis (seronegative with no clinical signs of primary syphilis) are likely to be cured by the first regimen. However, serologic tests for syphilis are still indicated for patients being treated for gonorrhea, as the gonococcal treatment programs are inadequate for treating established syphilitic infection. Spectinomycin and the quinolones are not active against incubating syphilis, thus patients treated with these drugs should have the serologic test for syphilis in 1 month.[36, 37] All patients with gonorrhea should be offered confidential counseling and testing for HIV infection. Coexistent chlamydial infection is less common in homosexual men,[38] but CDC generally recommends treating all persons with gonorrhea simultaneously for presumptive chlamydial infection.

Follow-Up and Treatment of Contacts. Any patient presenting as a contact of an individual diagnosed as having gonorrhea should be examined, have specimens cultured, and then immediately be treated with one of the recommended regimens for gonococcal urethritis (described earlier). In treating female contacts, it is important to remember that tetracycline is contraindicated in pregnancy. Erythromycin can be used to treat coexistent chlamydial infection in pregnant women or in patients who are allergic to or intolerant of tetracycline.[36]

Treatment failure following combined ceftriaxone/doxycycline therapy is unusual. Follow-up cultures are not recommended, although repeat culture in 1 to 2 months will detect reinfection, along with any treatment failure.[36] Patients treated with alternative regimens not including ceftriaxone should have follow-up cultures done 4 to 7 days after completing therapy.[36]

The patient should abstain from sexual contact until he returns 1 week after completion of treatment for a repeat culture and for a confirmation of treatment of contacts. Although diagnosis and treatment are essential, the clinician must insist on proper epidemiologic follow-up and patient education. A busy clinician is advised to enlist existing resources to assist with this task. State epidemiologists or municipal public health agencies can be very helpful. The most effective epidemiologic intervention, however, will occur at the time of diagnosis. The clinician must educate the patient about the natural history of gonorrhea, the modes of transmission, and the reinfection rate. Explaining to the patient the possible consequences to his female contacts, especially the development of PID with secondary infertility and ectopic pregnancy risks, is a useful motivator. It is useful to put the burden of notifying contacts onto the patient, with the suggestion that contacts present themselves for culture and treatment. Prescribing medication for a patient unknown to the clinician is never a good practice.

NONGONOCOCCAL URETHRITIS

Etiology. Nongonococcal urethritis (NGU) may be caused by a variety of organisms, including *Candida albicans, Trichomonas vaginalis,* and herpes simplex virus, but the majority (~95%) of cases are due to infection with *Chlamydia trachomatis* (50% or more) or *Ureaplasma urealyticum* (20 to 40%).[36, 37] Evidence that *U. urealyticum* is a pathogen is confounded epidemiologically by the ubiquitous occurrence of the organism in many asymptomatic persons, but specific therapy for *U. urealyticum* has been effective in some symptomatic patients in whom urethral cultures were positive for this organism.[39, 40]

Incidence. The incidence of NGU (defined as urethritis from which *N. gonorrhoeae* is not cultured) is rapidly rising. In Great Britain, almost two thirds of cases of urethritis reported among men are nongonococcal.[41] NGU is at least as common as gonorrhea in men attending STD clinics in the United States and several times more common among men seen by private physicians.[37]

Clinical Presentation. Clinical assessment of the patient with NGU is the same as that for suspected gonorrhea. The symptoms are similar to those of gonorrhea but milder and less acute. The incubation period is longer (10 to 14 days). Patients should be asked the same questions regarding sexual history, previous STD, medications, and allergies. Dysuria is mild, and "itching" may be the predominant complaint. The urethral discharge may be scant and clear or mucoid.

Laboratory Assessment. In NGU, the Gram stain of the urethral discharge usually shows polymorphonuclear leukocytes (five or more leukocytes in three of five oil immersion fields) but no bacteria. A small number of pleomorphic bacterial forms may be seen, however. If no discharge is present, 15 or more polymorphonuclear leukocytes in one or more of five high-power fields in a centrifuged sediment of 10 ml of fresh first-voided urine indicates urethral inflammation.[42] Culture for gonorrhea and a serologic test for syphilis should be obtained. The diagnosis of NGU usually is made by exclusion of gonococcal disease (Fig. 31–1). Cultures for *C. trachomatis* and *U. urealyticum* are expensive and time-consuming. The new rapid methods for diagnosing *C. trachomatis* (discussed on page 360) are available, but since Gram staining provides a cheap, readily available, accurate test for gonococcal urethritis, and NGU can be diagnosed by exclusion, these methods have little applicability to male patients. The leukocyte esterase test may be used for screening urine of asymptomatic persons at high risk for STD, but a positive result should be confirmed by Gram stain.[36]

Treatment

NGU (without suspected gonorrhea) may be treated with doxycycline (100 mg orally 2 times daily for 7 days) or erythromycin base (500 mg orally 4 times daily for 7 days). Uncomplicated chlamydial infections also respond to azithromycin (1 g orally in a single dose).[36] Ofloxacin (300 mg orally 2 times daily for 7 days) is an alternative.[36] Ofloxacin is the only quinolone shown to be active against *Chlamydia.* Because *C. trachomatis* is an intracellular organism, an adequate period of antibiotic administration (usually 7 days) is needed, but single-dose azithromycin may be used for documented, uncomplicated *C. trachomatis* infection (i.e., contacts of patients, persons detected on screening).[36]

Persistent or progressive infection does occur, with resul-

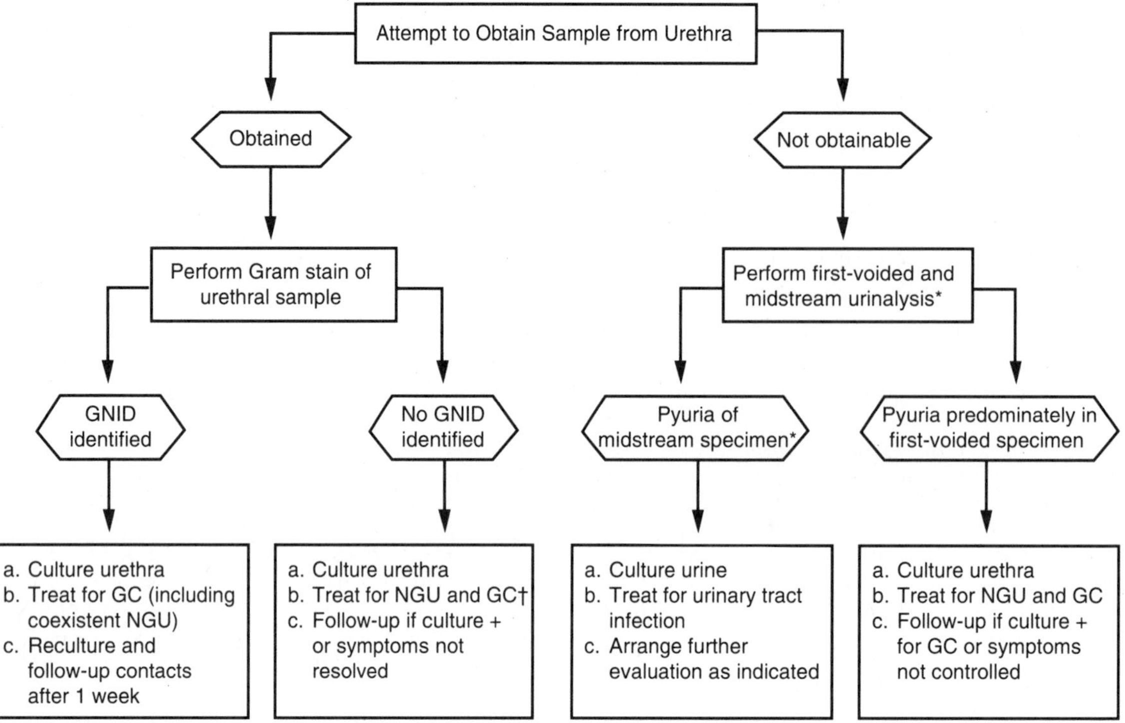

FIGURE 31–1. Approach to the male patient with penile discharge or burning.
*If significant pyuria is not identified in either specimen, a third-voided specimen following prostatic massage should also be examined.
†Combined NGU and GC treatment should be given (see Table 31–4) unless the diagnosis of NGU is unequivocal.

tant chronic urethritis, epididymitis, prostatitis, proctitis, and possibly Reiter's syndrome.[42] Patients in clinical studies in which cultures were done had a higher rate of relapse or persistence when the original chlamydial cultures were negative.[43] The etiology of persistent or recurrent NGU is not fully understood.[25, 44, 45] However, the regimen of ceftriaxone followed by doxycycline for 7 days is adequate treatment for gonococcal or chlamydial proctitis.[36] Chlamydial epididymitis should be treated with doxycycline for 10 days.

Sexual partners should be treated (within 30 days for symptomatic and 60 days for asymptomatic patients), even in the absence of symptoms. Seventy per cent of female contacts of men with chlamydial NGU have been reported to carry the organism; and the organism may be harbored for weeks or months in asymptomatic men and become the source of infection or reinfection of sexual contacts.[41] Barrier methods of contraception probably provide some protection against acquisition of chlamydial as well as gonococcal infections.

If the gonococcal culture and serologic test for syphilis are negative, and symptoms have resolved, no follow-up is required. If symptoms do not resolve, further evaluation or repeated treatment or both is required. Patients with dysuria in whom no discharge is obtainable by milking the urethra may have prostatitis or a disorder of the urinary tract instead of urethritis. A three-glass urine test should establish the source of symptoms in such cases (see Chapter 33). Tumors, foreign bodies, and strictures of the urethra should be considered in patients whose symptoms consist chiefly of a diminished urinary stream or difficulty in voiding; when necessary, these problems can be excluded by cystoscopy or urethrography. In patients with recurrent NGU, the discharge should be examined for *Candida* by KOH preparation (see p. 369) and for *Trichomonas* by a first-voided specimen of urine. The most likely causes of persistent or recurrent symptoms, however, are noncompliance with therapy, failure to treat the sexual partner, or acquisition of a new infection, either gonococcal or nongonococcal, from another sexual contact. Thus, the usual approach to the patient with continued symptoms will be to repeat the diagnostic studies and retreat the patient and his sexual partner with doxycycline or tetracycline for up to 3 weeks. If noncompliance was not the cause of failure to respond to adequate initial therapy, erythromycin (500 mg given orally, four times daily for 2 weeks[42]) should be substituted for doxycycline during the second course of therapy. Although tetracycline resistance has not been reported among *Chlamydia*, resistant strains of *U. urealyticum* are reported and usually are sensitive to erythromycin.[46]

ACKNOWLEDGMENT

The author acknowledges the contributions to this chapter of R. Kent Sargent, MD.

PART 3 ■ Genital Lesions

HARLEY A. HAYNES, MD

DIAGNOSIS AND MANAGEMENT

The presence of a genital lesion or lesions tends to evoke the specter of venereal disease in the minds of many patients and physicians. In fact, however, most genital lesions are not related to the classic venereal diseases such as syphilis, chancroid, lymphogranuloma venereum, and granuloma inguinale. If the spectrum of venereal disease is expanded to include 14 or 15 disorders known as STDs, the most common would be herpes simplex and condylomata acuminata. In many cases, a lesion is infectious but is not related to venereal disease. In other cases, a lesion of a noninfectious dermatologic disorder happens to be located on or near the anogenital region. A certain number of genital lesions are the result of trauma. For ease of classification, genital lesions may be grouped according to etiology, the major divisions being infectious and noninfectious (i.e., traumatic, secondary to a primary dermatologic disorder, and neoplastic). Although the classification given in Table 31–5 is too extensive for each entry to be discussed in detail in this chapter, it will provide the practitioner with an expanded differential diagnosis.

Patients, however, do not have etiologies; they have lesions and symptoms. Thus, descriptive morphology can be useful in classifying genital lesions, as shown in Table 31–6. Reference to a color atlas of sexually transmitted diseases may be very useful.[47] The most important of these lesions involve erosions or ulcerations; therein are found the major venereal disease presentations, at least in their early stages, as well as herpes simplex, trauma, carcinoma, and aphthous ulcers. This group of lesions—with erosion and/or ulceration—is most frequent, most demanding in terms of the differential diagnosis, and of greatest concern to the patient. While performing the physical examination of the anogenital area, the examiner should wear gloves.

Genital Erosions or Ulcers

The following conditions cause genital lesions manifested as erosions or ulcerations:

Erosions (±Crusts)	**Ulcerations**
Bullous diseases	Aphthous ulcers
Contact dermatitis	Bullous diseases
Ecthyma	Chancroid
Eczematous dermatitis	Erythema multiforme
Fixed drug eruption	Fungal infection (deep)
Herpes simplex	Foreign body reaction
Herpes zoster	Granuloma inguinale
Impetigo	Herpes simplex
Pediculosis pubis	Herpes zoster
Scabies	Hidradenitis suppurativa
Trauma	Human bite
	Laceration
	Pyoderma
	Squamous cell carcinoma
	Syphilis (primary)
	Trauma from zipper

The first step in evaluation is to determine the patient's history to find out whether *trauma* is the obvious cause of the genital lesion. For a traumatic etiology to be a possibility, the lesion should have some component of linearity and should have appeared promptly after the traumatic event, not several days or weeks later. A traumatic injury should have been noticeably painful at the time, and the lesion should be somewhat tender on examination. To be safe, a serologic test for syphilis should be obtained, even if trauma is suspected, and a darkfield examination should be performed if syphilis is a reasonable diagnostic possibility. The latent period for acquired herpes simplex or reactivation of herpes simplex seems to be quite short (~ 24 to 36 hours), thus this diagnosis must be considered even when the lesion appears to have been caused by trauma.

Erosions result after vesicles rupture, therefore one must inquire whether vesiculation occurred at the onset of lesions even if none is seen at the time of the examination. If the earliest manifestation is a vesicle, the lesion is most likely caused by *herpes simplex*. Either type 1 or type 2 may cause genital infection. A history of recurrent genital vesicular or erosive lesions makes recurrent herpes simplex a strong possibility. Vesicles may go unnoticed, however, and in most erosions and some ulcerations it is recommended that a Tzanck test be performed.

Tzanck Test. After any purulent exudate has been removed, a No. 15 scalpel blade can be used to scrape epithelial cells from the base of the lesion and to smear them onto a glass microscope slide for cytologic examination. The specimen should be air-dried, lightly heatfixed, and stained with Giemsa stain. A drop of immersion oil should be applied and a coverslip should be placed over the slide, permitting better optics when lower power lenses are used. Generally, low-power viewing is adequate to detect cells suspected to be multinuclear giant cells; one can then turn to a higher power for closer inspection of these cells.

The Tzanck test result is positive in about two thirds of patients with herpetic vesicles and in more than half of those with pustules but is often negative at the stage of crusting.[48] If the Tzanck test result is negative for vesicular or early erosive lesions, viral culture for herpes simplex virus can be done if there is compelling need to ascertain the diagnosis.

If neither trauma nor herpes simplex seems to be the etiology, one must next rule out *primary syphilis*. In addition, it is possible that a patient has both syphilis and herpes simplex simultaneously. The chancre of primary syphilis usually occurs 3 weeks after contact, never has a vesicular phase, and tends to be painless and nontender, or at least only minimally so. On physical examination, the lesions tend to look clean and nonpurulent and are characterized by palpable induration extending beyond the eroded or ulcerated central portion of the lesion by several millimeters. In the case of multiple chancres, each lesion tends to be smaller, less indurated, and somewhat more tender than the solitary lesion. The reasons for this are unknown.

TABLE 31–5. CLASSIFICATION OF GENITAL LESIONS BY ETIOLOGY CONTINUED

Infections
- *Viral*
  - Condylomata acuminata
  - Herpes simplex
  - Herpes zoster
  - Molluscum contagiosum
- *Bacterial*
  - Cellulitis
  - Chancroid
  - Ecthyma
  - Erythrasma
  - Folliculitis/carbuncle/abscess
  - Fusospirochetal (e.g., from human bite)
  - Granuloma inguinale
  - Impetigo
  - Secondary pyoderma
  - Syphilis
  - Trichomycosis axillaris
- *Chlamydial*
  - Lymphogranuloma venereum
- *Fungal/Yeast*
  - Candidiasis
  - Deep fungal (South American blastomycosis)
  - Tinea cruris
  - Tinea versicolor
- *Parasitic*
  - Pediculosis pubis
  - Scabies

Noninfectious
- *Traumatic*
  - Contact dermatitis
    - Allergic
    - Irritant
  - Foreign body/injection of drugs
  - Human bite or more superficial trauma by teeth
  - Laceration of vaginal or anal mucosa
  - Penile venereal edema
  - Suction edema, purpura, bullae, or erosions
  - Zipper laceration of penis
- *Secondary to a Dermatologic Disorder*
  - Aphthous ulcers
    - Simple
    - Severe (secondary to inflammatory bowel disease)
    - Behçet's disease
  - Balanitis xerotica obliterans (lichen sclerosus et atrophicus)
  - Bullous disorders
    - Epidermolysis bullosa
    - Erythema multiforme
    - Pemphigoid
    - Pemphigus vulgaris
  - Eczematous dermatitis
  - Epidermal inclusion cyst(s)
  - Fixed drug eruption
  - Hidradenitis suppurativa
  - Lichen planus
  - Penile lymphangitis
  - Pityriasis rosea
  - Plasma cell balanitis
  - Psoriasis
  - Sebaceous cyst(s)
  - Seborrheic dermatitis
- *Neoplastic*
  - Kaposi's sarcoma
  - Malignant melanoma
  - Squamous cell carcinoma in situ (erythroplasia of Queyrat)

When syphilis is suspected, a darkfield examination should be done.

By the time the examiner returns to the patient after the result of the Tzanck test has been found to be negative, a significant amount of clear serous fluid will have collected on the lesion. If necessary, the examiner, wearing gloves, squeezes the sides of the lesion gently but firmly to induce more serous transudation. This fluid is then collected with a clean scalpel blade or a clean cover slip, which is then placed on a scrupulously clean microscope slide. Ideally, enough fluid will be collected to fill the area beneath the cover slip. It is essential that the fluid specimen not be allowed to dry out, since the spirochetes, if present, will thus be killed and no longer visible. If additional fluid is needed, a normal saline solution containing no antibacterial additives may be added to the preparation immediately. It is suggested that two or three similar specimens be obtained, perhaps by a second individual, while the first slide is being examined under the darkfield microscope. If the result of the first preparation is negative, it is suggested that a total of three darkfield examinations be done at that sitting. If the lesion is strongly suggestive of primary syphilis, it may be desirable to have the patient return on a following day for additional darkfield examinations. It should be noted that antibiotic therapy with penicillin or tetracycline renders the darkfield result negative rather rapidly before cure has been ensured. In addition, this test may be rendered falsely negative by local antibiotic or germicidal applications or by the use of saline containing antibacterial agents. If typical spirochetes (i.e., *Treponema pallidum*) are found, assuring the diagnosis of primary syphilis, one should begin therapy promptly and register the patient with the Public Health Epidemiology Service, which will provide for interviews to determine all possible contacts of the patient who require examination and therapy. In early primary syphilis, serologic tests may still be nonreactive. Since the diagnosis can be confirmed only with the darkfield examination, it is desirable that the microscopy be performed by an experienced examiner. (See later discussion of Serologic Tests for Syphilis.)

If the Tzanck test and the darkfield examination results are negative, and the ulcer is somewhat painful and relatively soft, one must consider the diagnosis of *chancroid*. Chancroid is caused by a gram-negative coccobacillus, *Haemophilus ducreyi*. However, it is not generally possible to culture this in the routine bacteriology laboratory, because contaminants are likely to overgrow the specimen, and the bacterium is fastidious. Special medium for culturing the organism can be formulated by the laboratory after obtaining the recipe from the CDC in Atlanta. Since there is no serologic or skin test for chancroid, the diagnosis is generally made by means of clinical morphology and Gram stain of the lesion, which should show many polymorphonuclear leukocytes with gram-negative coccobacilli oriented like schools of fish swimming between them. According to the literature, approximately 15% of patients with chancroid also have syphilis, so that a darkfield examination for spirochetes should always be performed when a lesion is suspected of being chancroid.

If the diagnosis is still not made, and the lesion is somewhat exophytic and beefy in appearance, looking more like a tumor than a depressed ulceration, the diagnosis of *granuloma inguinale* should be considered. This disease, uncommon in the United States, is caused by a bacterium, *Calymmatobacterium granulomatis,* which produces inclusions in mononuclear cells known as Donovan bodies. These Donovan bodies are quite small, requiring an oil immersion lens for visualization on microscopy. Either an incisional punch or elliptical biopsy specimen may be sent for pathologic examination with special stains, or a piece of tissue from the lesion may be crushed and spread or touched on microscope slides to be stained by Giemsa stain. The advantage

TABLE 31–6. MORPHOLOGIC TERMS TO DESCRIBE GENITAL LESIONS

Atrophy or Scarring: Atrophy indicates a reduction in normal tissue elements. In the skin, there may be epidermal atropy with normal dermis, and normal skin markings are usually absent. In dermal atrophy, there is a decrease in dermal connective tissue, and the lesion is manifested as a depression in the skin. Scarring indicates a fibrotic reaction that may be atrophic or hypertrophic. Epidermis covering a scar is generally without normal skin markings and without appendages.

Edema: Swelling resulting from abnormal amounts of tissue fluid in the dermis. Edema may or may not be associated with other discrete lesions, including erythema.

Edema with Erythema: Edema combined with excessive redness of the skin and/or mucous membranes. Erythema is due to vasodilatation and therefore blanches with pressure from the examiner's finger or a transparent instrument. The presence of extravascular blood under the skin surface that does not blanch on pressure is termed purpura.

Erosion ± Crusts: A lesion in which part of the epidermis is removed but at least one cell layer of epidermis remains at the base is termed an erosion. Erosions allow tissue fluid to rise to the surface since the stratum corneum is absent, but bleeding does not occur because the dermis is exposed. When tissue fluid is mixed with numerous white blood cells, a seropurulent crust will form.

Erythema and Scaling ± Edema: In this sort of lesion, erythema of varying degrees of intensity is always seen, as well as the presence on the surface of the lesion of flaking of stratum corneum, called scaling. It is necessary to differentiate scaling from crusting.

Nodule: A nodule is a palpable, solid lesion located deeper than a papule, either in the dermis or in the subcutaneous tissue.

Papule: A papule is a solid, elevated, circumscribed lesion less than 1 cm in diameter, with most of the lesion above the plane of the surrounding skin rather than deep within it. The surface of the papule may be dome-shaped, flat-topped (as in lichen planus), or umbilicated (as in molluscum contagiosum). When papules become confluent and produce an elevation that occupies a relatively large surface area, the lesion is termed a plaque.

Pigmented Plaque or Nodule: This morphologic feature refers to raised lesions with increased pigmentation from melanin. At times an old ecchymosis with dark-colored purpura may simulate melanin pigmentation.

Pustule: A pustule is a circumscribed elevation of skin, usually less than 0.5 cm in diameter. It contains a purulent exudate that may be white, yellow, or greenish-yellow. Any condition capable of producing a vesicle can result in a pustule provided the vesicle is not promptly ruptured, and the fluid becomes turbid and relatively opaque owing to the presence of significant numbers of cells.

Ulceration: Ulcers are lesions in which the entire epidermis is missing, exposing the dermis. Very superficial ulcerations are difficult to distinguish from erosions and often have a similar diagnostic value.

Vesicle: A vesicle is simply a blister filled with reasonably clear fluid approximating serum. In a vesicle, either (1) part of the epidermis forms the roof and part the base, termed an intraepidermal vesicle, or (2) the entire epidermis forms the roof and the dermis forms the base. In herpes simplex and zoster, impetigo, and contact dermatitis, vesicles are intraepidermal. In the case of suction, fixed drug eruption, and many of the primary dermatologic blistering diseases, blisters are subepidermal.

of a biopsy is that one may check for the possible presence of squamous cell carcinoma.

Aphthous ulcers (often with concurrent oral lesions) and *recurrent erythema multiforme* (also often with oral lesions and possibly ocular and cutaneous lesions as well) represent differential diagnoses. *Fixed drug eruption,* usually having a characteristic violaceous, dusky color, may occur on the genitalia and may be recurrent. One would not expect lesions to be confined to the genitalia in other bullous diseases.

Squamous cell carcinoma of the genitalia tends to ulcerate or erode rather early and to be firm, relatively painless, and nontender. If a biopsy is going to be done, it will obviously take several days for a report to be available. When possible, it is desirable that therapy be withheld until the results of the biopsy are known. If this is not possible, but if the Tzanck test, darkfield examination, and Gram stain have all had negative results and serologic fluid samples have been drawn to be examined for syphilis, it is not unreasonable to treat for syphilis despite the negative darkfield examination if this diagnosis is likely. This should be done only when necessary, and it should be made clear that the diagnosis has not yet been confirmed.

Erosions of the Genital Area With Pruritus

In the case of rather severe pruritus with excoriations resulting in genital erosions, a parasitic infestation should be considered. The two most likely possibilities are *pediculosis pubis* and *scabies.*

A diagnosis of pediculosis pubis is rather easy if one inspects carefully for small, shiny, translucent nits attached to the pubic hair shaft. These nits are smaller than 1 mm in length. The adult lice tend to be attached to the skin or to hold onto a hair shaft and are about the color of a freckle or a café au lait spot, but on close inspection this "freckle" can be seen to be raised from the skin and to have legs on each side.

The diagnosis of scabies is more difficult. Generally lesions are also present in other than genital areas and particularly favor thin skin of the webs between the fingers, volar surfaces of the wrists, the axillae, breasts in women, the buttocks, and inguinal folds. One should look carefully to find nonexcoriated lesions in the hope of finding the scabetic burrow. The burrow is about as wide as a sewing needle and slightly irregular in direction, extending for several millimeters in length and terminating in a slightly larger portion, which has within it a gray dot, barely visible to the naked eye. This dot represents the adult female acarus. Microscopic diagnosis is made by placing a droplet of immersion oil on the skin and scraping away the overlying skin on top of the burrow until an erosion exists; the scraping is then examined under the microscope. A more thorough examination can be had if a shave biopsy is done of the burrow by taking a No. 15 or No. 10 scalpel blade and shaving off the skin of the top of the burrow, placing it on a microscope slide with a drop of potassium hydroxide or Swartz-Lamkin stain (without heating), applying a coverslip, and examining the specimen under low power. One looks for the adult acarus, for egg cases, and for fecal pellets, any one of which is diagnostic.

The approach to the problem of genital erosions or ulcerations has been outlined in Figure 31–2. This figure provides a summary only, and one should consult the text for details of the evaluation of patients.

Genital Lesions of Erythema and Scaling With or Without Edema

The etiologies of most genital lesions with primarily erythema and scaling are:

Candidiasis
Contact dermatitis
Eczematous dermatitis
Erythrasma

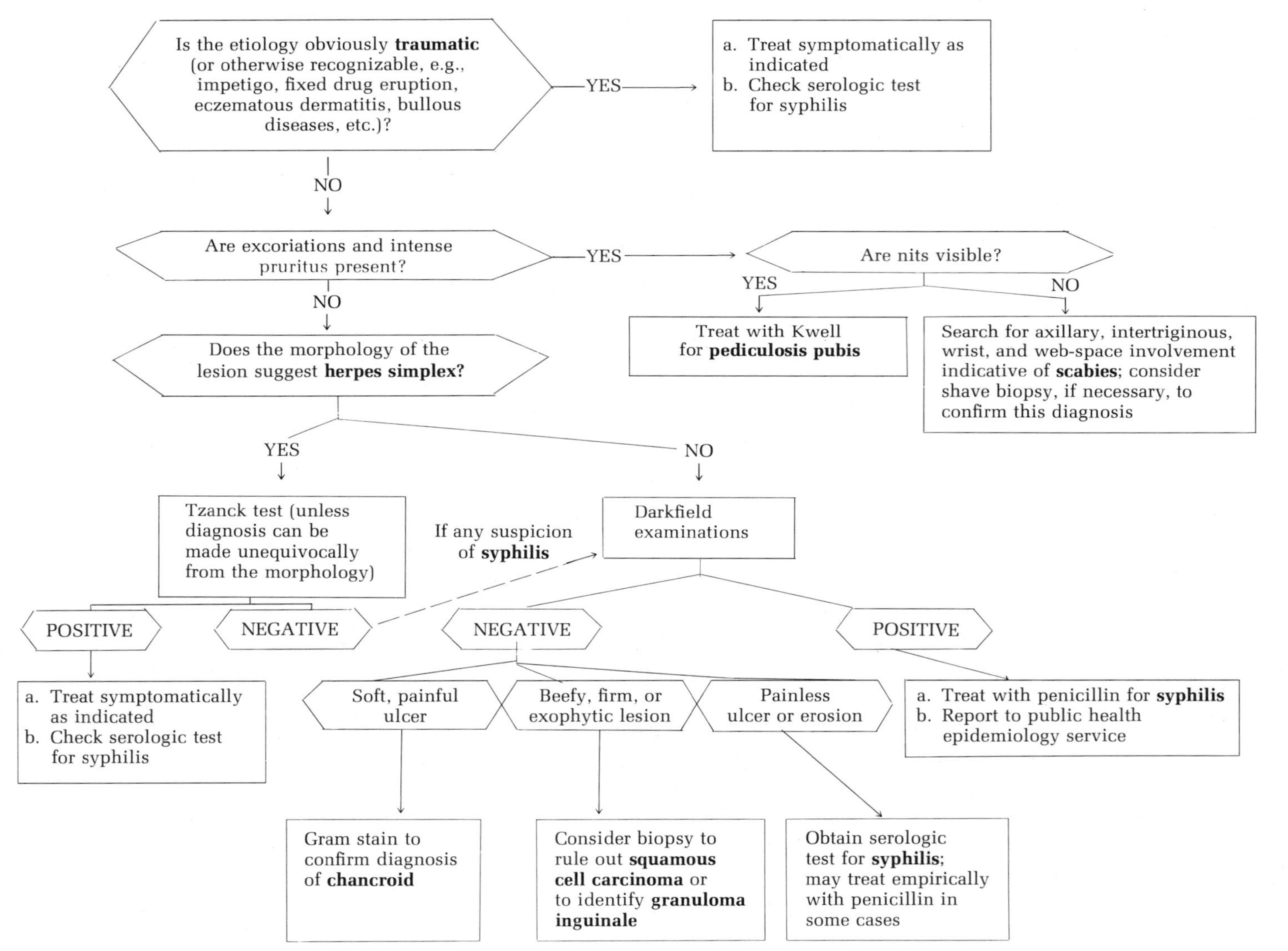

FIGURE 31–2. Approach to patients with genital erosions or ulcers.

Fixed drug eruption
Lichen planus
Pityriasis rosea
Psoriasis
Seborrheic dermatitis
Syphilis (secondary)
Tinea cruris
Tinea versicolor

Discrete lesions of erythema and scaling are termed *plaques*. The first step in evaluation of such plaques is to determine whether or not there are additional lesions over the cutaneous and mucocutaneous surface, or whether the lesions are confined to the genitalia. If lesions are widespread, other sites may provide a more characteristic morphology for diagnosis. Unless clinical inspection provides an almost certain diagnosis, the initial diagnostic maneuver in a patient with scaling plaques on the genitalia is usually to obtain a scraping of the scale for microscopic examination to detect fungi or yeast (Fig. 31–3). A small specimen can be obtained by using a No. 15 scalpel blade held perpendicular to the skin and stroked in a lateral fashion across the lesion. Scales are collected on a clean microscope slide, and a drop of potassium hydroxide (KOH) or Swartz-Lamkin stain is applied to the slide, which is then covered with a coverslip. The preparation is heated gently over a flame until tiny bubbles begin to form, at which point the slide is immediately placed on the counter to cool to prevent boiling. Once cooled, the slide is turned upside down onto a paper towel placed flat on the counter and is pressed firmly to squeeze out excess fluid and to thin out and flatten the specimen. The slide is then turned right side up and examined under the microscope using reduced illumination and a low-power lens, with a higher power employed as needed to evaluate suspicious areas.

All *fungal infections* and inflammatory *Candida infections* show septate branching hyphae. If in a relatively quiescent phase, *Candida* will show also budding yeast forms, and tinea versicolor will present a similar picture. If any of these features are found, the diagnosis becomes relatively simple. Currently it is no longer essential to differentiate between a tinea and a *Candida* infection, since therapeutic agents are effective against both. Clinically, the *tinea infection* tends to appear less acutely inflamed, to consist of an annular scaly plaque, and to spare the skinfolds proper. *Candida* infections, on the contrary, are likely to be most severe in the intertriginous folds and to be more inflammatory, with a tendency to produce satellite pustules at the edge of the plaque.

If the result of the scraping is negative for fungus or yeast, one must at least consider the possibility of *secondary syphilis*. Naturally, a history of a preceding chancre should be sought but the result may be negative, even in confirmed syphilis, since the lesion may escape notice. The lesions of secondary syphilis tend to be relatively asymptomatic, reddish-brown or copper in color rather than bright red, and characterized by minimal amounts of scale. In fact, the earliest lesions are only erythematous and slightly pal-

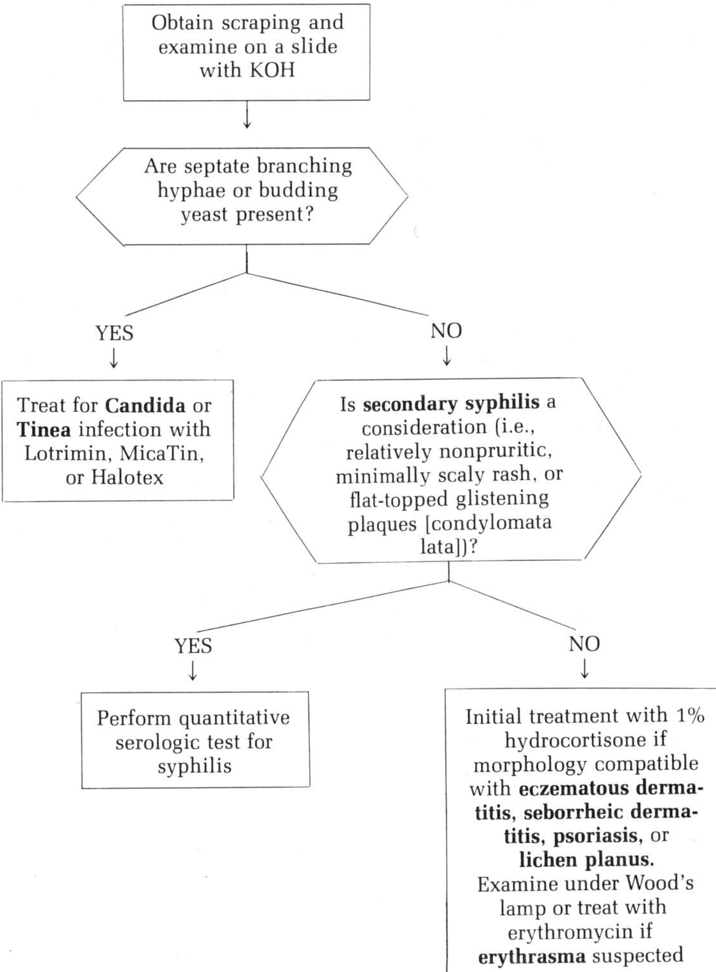

FIGURE 31–3. Approach to patients with scaling plaque confined to the genitalia.

pable, with no overlying alteration of the epidermis. Lesions tend to favor the genitalia, palms, and soles, although most patients with secondary syphilis have a truly generalized eruption that is often subtle and requires careful examination under excellent illumination. Generalized lymphadenopathy frequently occurs in secondary syphilis, as does a flu-like syndrome, and mucous membrane lesions consisting of white patches are sometimes seen. Secondary syphilis tends to occur about 6 weeks after the onset of the chancre and may overlap with a disappearing chancre. If untreated for several weeks, the lesions on hair-bearing areas tend to cause patchy alopecia, which is reversible with therapy.

Hypertrophic lesions in moist intertriginous areas, particularly the anogenital region, can occur in secondary syphilis and are called condylomata lata. In general, condylomata lata are flat-topped papules or plaques that glisten with a serous exudate, whereas condylomata acuminata are cauliflower-like, pointed papules that tend to be white and macerated. It is not unusual to be uncertain on examination about which lesion is present. Therefore, in all patients suspected of having condylomata acuminata, a complete examination for lesions of secondary syphilis as well as a serologic test for syphilis should be carried out. Serologic test results are positive in all cases of secondary syphilis, with the exception of the prozone reaction, described later in this chapter, which can be avoided by quantitative testing and does not influence the fluorescent treponemal antibody fluorescent (FTA-ABS) test.

Occasionally one sees *seborrheic dermatitis, eczematous dermatitis,* or *intertrigo* in the genital area. After obtaining a negative microscopic preparation for fungi and yeast, one can employ therapy of 1% hydrocortisone cream with or without 3% Vioform added to provide additional antimicrobial prophylaxis and some additional anti-inflammatory effect. This preparation is safe for long-term use and does not cause atrophy of the epidermis and dermis, as is seen with the more potent topical steroid preparations.

If slightly erythematous and somewhat pigmented plaques are present in the inguinal areas, and all the aforementioned test results are negative, the diagnosis of *erythrasma* should be considered. This is a bacterial infection by *Corynebacterium minutissimum,* a bacterium that produces a porphyrin, which allows a simple diagnosis by means of Wood's light inspection of the lesion after 24 hours without washing. If erythrasma is present, the skin lesion will fluoresce a dramatic coral-pink color. This lesion can be treated by oral or topical erythromycin.

Psoriasis and *lichen planus* may be limited to the genitalia, rendering the diagnosis much more difficult than would be the more typical case in which additional lesions occur elsewhere on the body. If one followed the preceding outline for evaluation and applied 1% hydrocortisone cream, one would do no harm and would benefit most patients. Biopsy of these lesions or referral to a dermatologist may be necessary for diagnosis.

Vesicular Genital Lesions

Bullous diseases
Contact dermatitis
Fixed drug eruption
Herpes simplex
Herpes zoster
Impetigo (bullous)
Suction bullae

The most important point to be made concerning intact vesicles found on the genitalia is that *vesicles are never caused by syphilis (except in the neonate).* Of course, this does not eliminate the possibility that a vesicular lesion could coexist with other lesions representing syphilis. After vesicles rupture, an erosion is present that may confuse the diagnosis. By and large, however, these patients will usually turn out to have *herpes simplex* and not one of the classic venereal diseases. The work-up should begin with a Tzanck test to examine cells from the base of a newly opened vesicle (Fig. 31–4). If this test result is positive, generally no further laboratory procedures are necessary, except for a test for syphilis to be obtained at this time and repeated in 1 month to ensure that subsequent lesions are not those of syphilis. If only vesicles are present, a darkfield examination is not indicated. If only vesicles are present and the Tzanck preparation is negative, one should repeat the Tzanck test, making sure that adequate numbers of epithelial cells have been collected from the base of the lesion. The next step is to aspirate fluid from an intact vesicle for Gram stain to investigate the possibility of *bullous impetigo,* which should show gram-positive cocci within polymorphonuclear leukocytes. *Contact dermatitis* should be quite pruritic and look like poison ivy dermatitis. *Bullae from suction* are generally larger than 1 or 2 mm, depending on what agent produced the suction. A *fixed drug eruption* tends to have a purplish or violaceous color and to be greater than 1 cm in diameter. Blistering diseases such as erythema multiforme, epidermolysis bullosa, bullous pemphigoid, and pemphigus vulgaris generally produce lesions elsewhere, such as in the mouth, eyes, or skin, to assist in the diagnosis.

Pustules

Genital lesions in which pustules are the prominent component include the following:

Bullous disorders
Candidiasis
Eczematous disorders
Folliculitis
Foreign body reaction
Herpes simplex
Herpes zoster
Hidradenitis suppurativa
Scabies

As mentioned previously, any disorder causing vesicles can result in pustules if the vesicles do not rupture before migration of significant numbers of cells into the vesicle fluid. Since the presence of pustules does not indicate de facto bacterial or viral infection, the examiner either recognizes the type of lesions and proceeds directly to the appropriate laboratory procedure or does not recognize them and must perform a Tzanck test, Gram stain on pustule contents, and KOH preparation of the epidermis scraped from the undersurface of the pustule roof as well as the pustule contents. If papules are found that are not yet pustular, scraping for *scabies* should be done. This will generally be futile when lesions already show pustulation. *Foreign body reactions* producing pustules may result from injection of foreign substances into the skin and are usually seen only in drug addicts and severely disturbed individuals. In patients with a history of *eczema,* this dermatitis may occur on the genitalia, and pustules can definitely occur in eczematous dermatitis. However, pustules do not

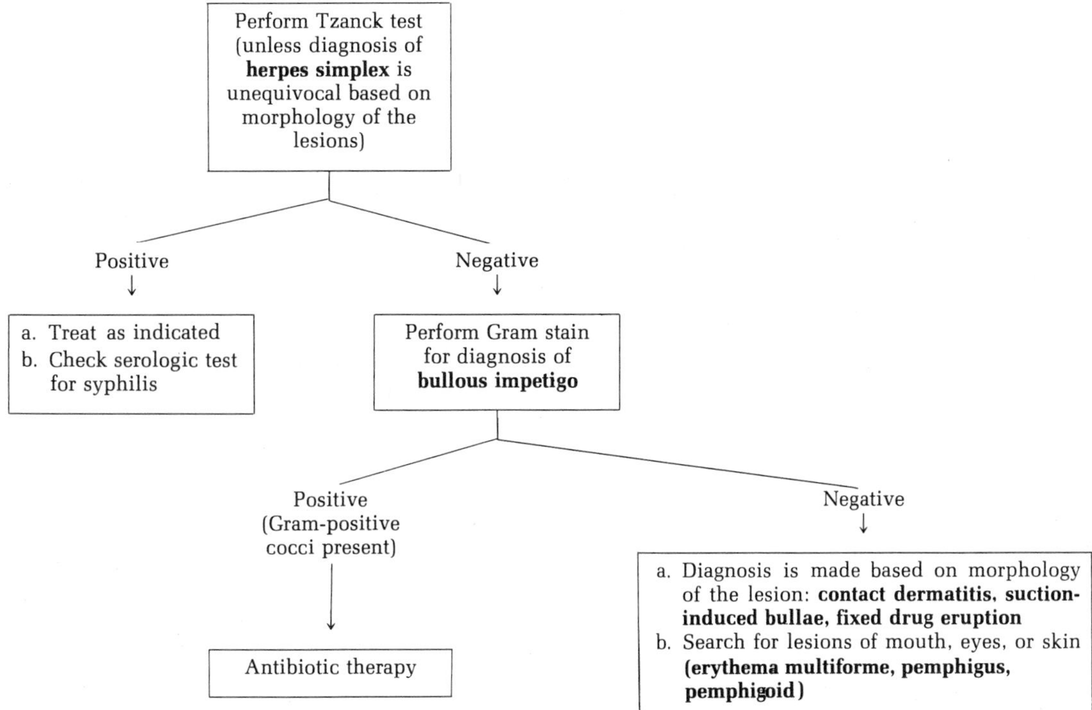

FIGURE 31–4. Approach to patients with vesicular genital lesions.

usually arise from normal skin but from areas showing erythema, scaling, and possibly excoriations. In folliculitis, hairs will be seen protruding from the midst of most pustules. Patients with *hidradenitis suppurativa* tend to have lesions in the pubis, groin, inner thighs, and axillae and often having scarring, clusters of comedones, and cystic nodules as well as more superficial pustules. Superficial pustules alone do not indicate this disorder.

Genital Papules

Condyloma acuminatum
Eczematous dermatitis
Lichen planus
Molluscum contagiosum
Psoriasis
Scabies
Syphilis (secondary)

Condylomata acuminata are the most common papular genital lesions. They are caused by one of the wart viruses and are spread by means of direct contact. The surface of the lesion is verrucous, containing multiple pointed papules packed tightly together. In moist intertriginous areas the lesions will become macerated and whitish-opaque. They occur on mucous membranes and modified mucous membranes as well as on the skin.

Molluscum contagiosum, another viral lesion, is less well known to most practitioners. It presents as a smooth, round papule, varying in size from barely visible to 3 or 4 mm in diameter. Characteristic papules are shiny and have the color of reasonably normal skin, but have a central depression or umbilication. Since these may become inflamed if traumatized, several inflammatory erythematous lesions, possibly with crusting, might be admixed with the noninflammatory lesions. If the diagnosis of molluscum contagiosum is suspected, the surface of the papule may be incised and the contents expressed onto a glass slide. The specimen is then flattened by a second glass slide and stained with Wright's or Giemsa stain. If the diagnosis is correct, large swollen epithelial cells filled with viral inclusions will be easily visualized.

Secondary syphilis, but not primary syphilis, may present papules or plaques in the genital area. The moist condylomata lata are often confined to the genital area, although they may also occur in the anal area. The result of the darkfield examination is positive and the serologic test for syphilis will always be positive if a sufficient sample is obtained. Unlike condylomata acuminata, the surfaces of condylomata lata are not verrucous; however, occasionally these two lesions cannot be well differentiated. Thus in any patient suspected of having condylomata acuminata, a serologic test should be performed to rule out secondary syphilis.

Scabies is quite pruritic—a very helpful clue to the diagnosis. Lesions commonly occur on the genitalia but are usually not confined to this area. They tend to extend to the thin skin of the pubis, inner thighs, volar surfaces of the wrists, webs between the fingers, axillae, buttocks, and breasts. Burrows should be sought and scraped for microscopic examination, as described earlier under erosions and pruritus (see p. 367).

Psoriasis and *lichen planus* are two primary dermatologic disorders that may present as genital papules or plaques. In men, both may cause lesions on the glans penis. The absence of lesions elsewhere on the skin may cause significant diagnostic confusion. Lichen planus tends to occur in the mouth as well as on the volar surfaces of the wrists and elsewhere. When papules in any of these locations are moistened with mineral oil, a characteristic white lacy pattern called Wickham's striae is revealed. This finding is diagnostic for lichen planus. In psoriasis, merely erythematous plaques with scaling will be seen. If no lesions are present at other sites, it may be necessary to confirm the diagnosis by biopsy.

Eczematous dermatitis produces a broad spectrum of skin lesions, including papules, erythema, scaling, crusting, excoriations, and so forth. In some patients, particularly blacks, papules alone may be present. Umbilication or significant erythema will be absent, although there may be some pigmentation. The surface of these lesions will be rather smooth. It is uncommon for genital lesions alone to occur in eczematous dermatitis, and the correct diagnosis is usually based on the finding of lesions elsewhere on the skin surface and a history of recurrent eczematous dermatitis.

Kaposi's sarcoma usually does not involve the genitalia, but when it does, it is seen as a purple-to-red papular lesion that blanches. When small, it may blanch completely; when larger, it may blanch partially to a brownish color.

Edema Without Erythema

Lymphogranuloma venereum (late)
Penile lymphangitis
Penile venereal edema
Suction

In both sexes the genitalia are subject to edema of striking degree from stimuli that would not cause this response elsewhere on the body. When only edema is seen, with no erythema or other kind of inflammatory lesions evident, the patient should be asked whether this condition is chronic or acute. If chronic, some form of lymphatic obstruction is likely, as in chronic *lymphogranuloma venereum,* lymphatic obstruction from lymphoma, hypoalbuminemia of many etiologies, or the presence of abdominal ascites. Acute genital edema is usually the result of trauma, such as *suction* or *friction,* the latter causing *penile venereal edema* after prolonged or repeated intercourse without adequate lubrication. In the case of *penile lymphangitis,* definite cord-like, firm, enlarged lymphatic vessels will be seen and should be palpated; it is unclear whether the etiology of this condition is traumatic or infectious, but the cords are nontender or only minimally tender. All these acute situations are self-limited and seem to require no therapy other than screening for possible STD, which might have been acquired during the encounter in question.

Edema with Erythema

Candidiasis
Cellulitis
Eczematous dermatitis
Fixed drug eruption
Plasma cell balanitis
Primary irritant dermatitis
Trauma

Genital *cellulitis* causing edema and erythema is associated with significant local pain and tenderness and often systemic reactions such as fever and malaise. *Candidiasis* may occasionally cause this morphologic reaction in both sexes and can be diagnosed by means of microscopic examination of vaginal secretions in women and of scrapings from epidermis on the glans or coronal sulcus in men. *Trauma* may be diagnosed on the basis of a peculiar configuration of the lesion and appropriate history. At times it may not be possible to distinguish trauma from cellulitis. If there is some question, therapy for the latter should probably be instituted. *Primary irritant dermatitis* usually results from chemical exposure to soap, douche preparations, fragrances, hygiene sprays, or contraceptive preparations. Occasionally, a history of an unusual chemical exposure will be elicited, such as some of the home remedies for real or feared pediculosis pubis. *Fixed drug eruption* may begin with a localized plaque of erythema and edema, usually greater than 1 cm in diameter, which rapidly assumes a violaceous color, may or may not blister, and tends to heal with hyperpigmentation. Localized areas of edema and erythema of a somewhat chronic nature on the glans penis may represent a peculiar kind of balanitis, histologically characterized by numerous plasma cells in the dermal infiltrate and termed *plasma cell balanitis.*

Atrophy or Scarring of the Genitalia

Balanitis xerotica obliterans
Bullous diseases
Foreign body reaction
Hidradenitis suppurativa
Lichen sclerosus et atrophicus
Trauma

The presence of atrophy or scarring of the genitalia does not indicate any acutely acquired STD. A chronic blistering problem will be revealed by the history. *Hidradenitis suppurativa* will be evident on physical examination of other areas, as mentioned earlier under Pustules. *Foreign body reactions* secondary to injection of drugs or other substances usually leave characteristic tracks and may have a positive history. Other kinds of *trauma* will generally appear to have resulted from an external injury, showing a geometric configuration, and may be confirmed by the history. A lesion of considerable importance, known as *lichen sclerosus et atrophicus* in both sexes and *balanitis xerotica obliterans* in men, is a disorder of unknown nature in which dermal edema and atrophy and epidermal atrophy often progress to a somewhat mutilating fibrosis. Minor trauma will cause purpura of the extremely fragile epidermis. These lesions may be quite pruritic and in men may result in urethral obstruction at the meatus, requiring surgical remedy. Such lesions have a characteristic appearance on skin biopsy.

Pigmented Genital Plaque or Nodule

Malignant melanoma
Nevus
Seborrheic keratosis
Squamous cell carcinoma (not usually pigmented)

The two most common pigmented lesions on the genitalia are *dermal nevi* and *seborrheic keratoses.* Pigmented nevi of the genitalia, as elsewhere on the body, generally show reasonably uniform tan pigmentation, with the epidermis intact, and are somewhat soft to palpation. Seborrheic keratoses are highly superficial vegetations that seem to be attached to the surface of the epidermis. The surface of the lesions consists of numerous tiny adjacent papules that tend to crumble off upon gentle scraping. Unlike genital warts, from which these lesions must be differentiated, seborrheic keratoses do not occur on the modified mucous membrane of the glans penis or prepuce or on the vulva or vagina. *Malignant melanomas* occur uncommonly in the genital area, including the vulva. As elsewhere, they generally present as a peculiar variegate pigmentation that is blue, brown, and black or sometimes red and white. The lesion also has a characteristic irregular outline. Pigmented lesions that are blue in color, if not readily explained by vascular structures, should be evaluated with the possibility of malignant melanoma in mind. In these cases, excisional biopsy by an appropriate specialist is often necessary. *Squamous cell carcinoma,* particularly the in situ plaques, may be pigmented in the genital area, although this is very unusual. In general, these lesions do not quite fit any of the preceding classifications, nor do they respond to topical steroid therapy or antifungal preparations, and thus often have to be diagnosed by biopsy.

Nodules

Abscess
Foreign body reaction
Hidradenitis suppurativa
Inclusion cysts
Penile lymphangitis
Sebaceous cysts

As can be seen from this list of etiologies for nodular genital lesions, the STDs do not appear as a customary manifestation. *Abscess* and *foreign body reaction* to injection should allow a reasonably straightforward diagnosis. *Sebaceous* or *epidermal cysts* may be numerous and are particularly frequent on the scrotum. *Hidradenitis suppurativa* was discussed earlier, under Pustules. *Penile lymphangitis* shows nodular, cord-like lesions in the subcutaneous tissue.

SEROLOGIC TESTS FOR SYPHILIS

In any genital lesions in which there is even a remote possibility of syphilis, serologic testing should be done. It should also be done if the patient might have been exposed to syphilis, whether or not lesions are present at the time, or might have some other STD.

Two types of tests detect syphilis: nontreponemal, measuring reaginic antibody, and treponemal, measuring antitreponemal antibody. Screening tests for syphilis employ some form of reaginic antibody test in which a nontreponemal antigen, prepared from cardiolipin-lecithin, reacts with reaginic antibodies in the patient's serum. Although most clinicians are familiar with the Hinton test and the Venereal Disease Research Laboratory (VDRL) test, today it is most likely that a rapid plasma reagin (RPR) test or an automated reagin test (ART) will be done. It is highly desirable that a quantitative serologic test be performed, since 1 to 2% of patients with early lesional syphilis may have a false-negative prozone phenomenon due to antibody excess interfering with the reaction. When present, a prozone phenomenon results in a nonreactive test on undiluted serum with a reactive test at some higher dilution. Specifying quantitative testing is not necessary with an ART, since this is done automatically. The RPR test has a lower incidence of prozone reactions than does the Hinton or VDRL test, but it is still desirable to have it quantitated. If this test is reactive, it should be repeated to exclude the possibility of laboratory error and to detect the rising titer that should be present in a recently acquired infection; a specific treponemal antibody test should also be performed.

The most common treponemal tests are the *microhemagglutination for T. pallidum (MHA-TP) test,* and the *FTA-ABS* test. The MHA-TP test is easier to do. False reactivity due to intercurrent viral or bacterial infections is detected by serum controls used to identify such heterophile antibody activity when it occurs in the MHA-TP test, permitting further evaluation with the FTA-ABS test.

The FTA-ABS test is the most sensitive and specific serologic test for syphilis readily available today. Results of the test are reported as nonreactive, borderline, 1+, 2+, 3+, and 4+. Three plus and 4+ reactions are significant positive results; nonreactive test results are negative. Borderline, 1+, and 2+ tests indicate indeterminate reactivity and should be repeated in the hope that the results will be significantly higher or lower, allowing a definite classification. Indeterminate results are difficult to interpret because they may represent antibodies to *T. pallidum* in low titers or antibodies to other treponemal organisms that are cross-reactive and not completely eliminated by absorption of the patient's serum. If the test result remains borderline or 1+, it is wise not to regard the test result as positive unless considerable clinical indications would contradict this. If the reading remains 2+, it may represent a significant positive test or may on occasion be a false-positive result. This is the most difficult test result to evaluate and requires considerable clinical judgment. If the treponemal test is nonreactive, a positive reaginic serologic test result does not indicate an infection with syphilis or any other treponemal disease but is likely caused by alteration of serum proteins due to recent immunization, viral disease, certain bacterial diseases, hepatitis, drug abuse, collagen vascular disease, pregnancy, dysproteinemia, or advanced age. It is also important to realize that, if the result was positive in the past owing to syphilis or other treponemal infection, the treponemal test result will remain positive after treatment and should not be used as a guide to the adequacy of therapy. In 95% of patients with a positive treponemal test result, the test result will remain positive for many years—possibly for the remainder of their lifetimes.

If a patient has a genital lesion that is strongly indicative of syphilis, it is desirable to perform both a quantitative reaginic test and a treponemal test simultaneously. If screening is to be done only as a routine procedure with no strong suspicion of syphilis, it is reasonable to perform only the reaginic test.

These serologic test results do not become positive immediately after infection. In fact, only about 25% of patients will have positive serologic test results during the first week of the chancre; each week thereafter, another 25% will develop a positive reaction, thus that at the end of 4 weeks one would anticipate a positive serologic test result in 100% of patients with lesional syphilis. Thus, a nonreactive test obtained 4 weeks after the onset of the lesion essentially rules out syphilis. The treponemal test result becomes positive slightly sooner than the reaginic test, so that a patient who has a positive reaginic test but a nonreactive treponemal test does not have syphilis. If early infectious syphilis is diagnosed and treated, it is desirable to perform the quantitative reaginic serologic test (RPR or ART) at monthly intervals to document the expected fall in titer. Patients with primary syphilis are expected to become nonreactive within 12 months of therapy and patients with secondary syphilis within 24 months, but the treponemal test remains positive.

THERAPY OF THE SEXUALLY TRANSMITTED DISEASES

It is strongly recommended that upon making the diagnosis of a major venereal disease, the clinician should contact the Department of Public Health (DPH). These diseases are all reportable, and such information is required for statistical purposes. In addition, the personnel at the DPH can assist the clinician regarding details of the diagnosis and current therapeutic guidelines. It is important that optimal therapy be instituted and that all sexual contacts of the patient be located and provided with appropriate therapy. This type of follow-up is generally the function of the epidemiology branch of the DPH but, of course, can be aided in many cases by the physician's explanation of its purpose and importance to the patient.

Syphilis. The CDC recommends a single dose of benzathine penicillin, 2.4 million units intramuscularly, for primary and secondary syphilis. In the Commonwealth of Massachusetts, it is recommended that a second, similar dose be administered 1 week later. The use of procaine penicillin requires injections daily or every other day for 10 days to 2 weeks and thus, from a logistic standpoint, is less feasible. Oral penicillin, while adequately therapeutic, does not ensure compliance; the entire recommended dose may not actually be taken, thus oral penicillin is not recommended. For patients allergic to penicillin, the alternative drug of choice is doxycycline, 100 mg orally two times daily for 14 days, or tetracycline, 500 mg four times daily for 14 days. The third-choice drug is erythromycin, given in the same dosage as tetracycline.

Syphilis of more than 1 year's duration (except neurosyphilis) should be treated with benzathine penicillin G, 2.4 million units intramuscularly once a week for 3 successive weeks. Alternatively, in the penicillin-sensitive patient (nonpregnant), treatment consists of tetracycline 500 mg four times daily or doxycycline 100 mg orally two times daily by mouth for 30 days.[49] For outpatient regimens, as opposed to hospitalization, the patient's compliance must be ensured. In patients with no neurologic signs or symptoms, the yield of cerebrospinal fluid examinations, the sensitivity of the CSF-VDRL test, and the likelihood of developing clinical neurosyphilis after treatment for late latent syphilis are all so low that this procedure is not routinely recommended,[50–52] but a positive HIV antibody test result is an indication for cerebrospinal fluid (CSF) examination. Some experts advise CSF examination and/or treatment for neurosyphilis for all patients coinfected with syphilis and human immunodeficiency virus (HIV), regardless of the clinical stage of syphilis.

CSF examination should be performed in all patients with clinical features of neurosyphilis, as well as prior to retreatment in patients who have relapsed after therapy, before treatment in patients receiving nonpenicillin regimens for syphilis, and in infants with congenital syphilis.[53] Currently recommended treatments for neurosyphilis include aqueous crystalline penicillin G, 12 to 24 million units intravenously per day, or procaine penicillin G, 2.4 million units intramuscularly per day, plus probenecid, 500 mg by mouth, each given for 10 days, followed by benzathine penicillin G, 2.4 million units intramuscularly weekly for three doses.[49]

Chancroid. The recommended regimens are azithromycin, 1 g orally in a single dose, or ceftriaxone, 250 mg intramuscularly in a single dose, or erythromycin, 500 mg by mouth 4 times daily for 7 days. Alternative regimens are amoxicillin, 500 mg, plus clavulanic acid, 125 mg orally 3 times daily for 7 days, or ciprofloxacin, 500 mg orally 2 times a day for 3 days.[49] Sexual partners should receive the same treatment. Susceptibility of *H. ducreyi* to antimicrobials varies geographically, and a clinical response to treatment should be ascertained. Lymph nodes resolve more slowly than the primary ulcer and, if fluctuant, may require aspiration by needle through healthy adjacent skin.

Granuloma Inguinale. Therapy for early lesions is similar to that for lymphogranuloma venereum. If resistance is encountered, ampicillin is the next choice.

Lymphogranuloma Venereum. Genital lesions cannot generally be seen in lymphogranuloma venereum, since the primary lesion is small and transient. The disease is caused by *Chlamydia trachomatis,* and the classic presentation is that of inguinal lymphadenopathy, with the typical lesions, including masses both above and below Poupart's ligament, giving rise to a so-called "groove" sign. Diagnosis is confirmed by complement-fixation testing on serum, since the Frei test is no longer available. The recommended therapy is doxycycline 100 mg orally two times daily for 21 days. Alternative regimens are tetracycline 500 mg, erythromycin 500 mg, or sulfisoxazole (or equivalent) 500 mg by mouth four times daily for 21 days.[49] Sexual partners should receive the same treatment.

Bubos should be aspirated, if necessary, rather than incised and drained, to prevent the formation of fistulas.

Condylomata Acuminata. These venereal warts can be extremely vexing to physician and patient alike. When a few lesions are present, they can be treated with the topical application of podophyllum resin, 20 or 25% in compound tincture of benzoin. This is to be applied sparingly *to the lesion only,* with the surrounding normal tissue protected by a coating of petrolatum if necessary. Dusting talcum powder over the application will help to reduce spread of the medication to adjacent tissue. The medication should be washed off with soap and water after 2 to 8 hours (or sooner if large amounts of podophyllum were needed). The longer this medication remains on the lesion, the more potent the reaction will be, resulting sometimes in painful erosions. A variation of this therapy designed for self-application by the patient is Condylox, applied to lesions twice daily for 3 consecutive days per week and repeated as required. Massive lesions should not be treated in this manner, since systemic toxicity may occur. Pregnant women also should probably not be treated with this agent. Electrofulguration, laser ablation, and cryosurgery with liquid nitrogen are alternative methods of treatment. In patients unresponsive to these measures, topical applications of 5-fluorouracil cream or intraurethral suppositories are more specialized therapeutic modalities. Great care must be taken when using this medication to avoid ulceration and erosion of sensitive tissue. This disorder is not a therapeutic indication for 5-fluorouracil topical therapy according to the packet insert approved by the Food and Drug Administration (FDA).

Molluscum Contagiosum. If only a small number of these lesions are present, they may be incised and expressed, removed by curettage, or removed by mild electrodesiccation. If untreated, these lesions may multiply or spread to sexual partners. When numerous lesions are present, the simplest way to treat them is by local liquid nitrogen therapy, either with a small-nozzle spray apparatus or by contact applications with a cotton applicator. Two 30-second applications should suffice to freeze the lesion, which will become necrotic and blister off without scarring. Repeat treatment might be necessary if any lesions remain or if the sexual contacts of the patient are not simultaneously treated. Again, cultures for gonococcal disease and serologic testing for syphilis are recommended in these patients.

Pediculosis Pubis. Treatment consists of either one or two applications to infested and adjacent areas of lindane (Kwell) (1%) lotion or cream washed off after 8 hours. An over-the-counter preparation of pyrethrins (RID), may be applied and washed off after 10 minutes; this is said to be equally effective. Sexual and other very intimate contacts should be treated as well.

Scabies. In general, lindane (Kwell) (1%) lotion is employed in the therapy of scabies. Kwell lotion may be applied thinly to the total skin surface from the neck down at bedtime and washed off the following morning. Soiled clothing and bedclothing should be laundered as soon as possible. All cohabitants and other intimate contacts should be treated similarly, and it is wise to repeat this therapy once, 1 week later. Excessive reapplications should be avoided because of possible neurotoxicity, and only the necessary volume for recommended therapy should be dispensed (i.e., 60 ml/person/application). A more recent therapy is 5% permethrin cream (Elimite) applied as indicated earlier. This preparation does not appear to cause neurotoxicity. Great care should be taken to include the distal subungual space under the fingernails in either treatment. Some patients develop a neurotic fear of parasites and tend to overtreat themselves. Since pruritus may persist for 2 weeks or so after therapy is effective, it is reasonable to prescribe an antihistamine such as chlorpheniramine maleate, 4 mg, one or two tablets every 4 to 6 hours as needed, as well as temporary application of a topical steroid of medium or low potency, such as triamcinolone 0.1% or hydrocortisone 1% cream. Treatment of young infants and pregnant women with lindane is not recommended because of some reports of neurotoxicity from overdosage. Alternative therapies include 5% permethrin (Elimite), 6% sulfur in petrolatum, which is highly effective but rather messy, and crotamiton lotion (Eurax).

***Candida* and Tinea Infections.** Therapeutic agents are now available that treat both tinea and *Candida* infections, thus a specific mycologic diagnosis is not always necessary. Examples of such agents are clotrimazole (Lotrimin), miconazole nitrate (Micatin), econazole (Spectazole), naftifine (Naftin), cyclopirox (Loprox), and ketoconazole (Nizoral). Usually it is not necessary to use a topical corticosteroid preparation as well. Combination agents containing triamcinolone, neomycin, gramicidin, and nystatin (e.g., Mycolog) are generally not recommended.

Herpes Simplex. Treatment with acyclovir, 200 mg by mouth, five times daily for 7 to 10 days, is now indicated if it is initiated within 6 days of the onset of a first or primary genital herpes simplex virus infection.[49] Acyclovir, 5 mg/kg of body weight intravenously every 8 hours for 5 to 7 days, may be administered to patients with severe symptoms or complications necessitating hospitalization.[49] Oral therapy may reduce systemic symptoms, and both oral and intravenous therapy are thought to reduce the duration of the eruptions by 3 to 5 and 7 days, respectively.[49] Oral therapy produces much lower blood levels but does not appear to cause the serious adverse effects, such as nephrotoxicity, that sometimes occur with intravenous acyclovir.[54] Topical acyclovir is not effective in reducing symptoms of primary genital herpes.[49]

Treatment of the primary infection does not influence the number or severity of subsequent recurrences. If a patient is known to have severely symptomatic recurrent genital herpes, oral therapy with acyclovir, 200 mg by mouth five times daily for 5 days, can be given if it is initiated within 2 days of the onset of the lesions, and this probably shortens the mean clinical course by about 1 day.[49]

The safety of acyclovir for treating pregnant patients is not established, and one should consult an obstetrician about possible prevention of neonatal herpes simplex virus infection. Continuous treatment with acyclovir is thought to reduce recurrent episodes of genital herpes by about 75% and this therapy can be considered for patients who do not plan to become pregnant and who have at least six such episodes per year.[49] An individualized dose of acyclovir, 200 mg by mouth, two to five times daily, should be given. Most people do well on 400 mg twice daily. Long-term safety has been established for as long as 5 years. After 1 year of continuous acyclovir administration, a break in therapy is recommended to permit assessment of the recurrence rate.[49, 54] Resistant strains of the virus may emerge during long-term therapy, but these appear to be less virulent than the sensitive strains.[54]

To avoid transmitting the disease to others, the patient should avoid sexual contact until the lesions have healed, even if taking acyclovir. Painful lesions may be treated as necessary with a topical anesthetic, such as viscous Xylocaine or Dyclone. It is reasonable to apply a germicidal agent such as Betadine ointment two or three times daily to reduce the likelihood of secondary bacterial infection, to act as a virucide for extracellular herpes virus contaminating the surface of the lesions, and to reduce its spread in patients not treated with acyclovir.

The patient must be warned that recurrence is possible without the need for reinfection from a partner. Failure to understand the pathogenesis of recurrent herpes simplex can lead to major conflicts between sexual partners. Most patients with recurrent herpes simplex will have fewer and milder cases over a period of several years. In some patients with recurrent lesions, a sensory syndrome of dysesthesia is present for a day or longer before lesions appear, and treatment may be started at this time. If mechanical trauma during intercourse seems to precipitate herpetic lesions, adequate lubrication (e.g., K-Y Jelly) should be ensured, if necessary, and use of a condom to provide some mechanical protection should be considered.

REFERENCES

Salpingitis

1. Rolfs RT, Galaid EI, and Zaidi AA: Pelvic inflammatory disease: trends in hospitalizations and office visits. Am J Obstet Gynecol 166:983–990, 1992.
2. Washington AE and Katz P: Cost of and payment source for pelvic inflammatory disease: Trends and projections, 1983 through 2000. JAMA 266:2565–2569, 1991.
3. Westrom L: Effect of acute pelvic inflammatory disease on fertility. Am J Obstet Gynecol 121:707, 1974.
4. Safrin S, Schachter J, Dahrouge D, and Sweet RL: Long-term sequelae of acute pelvic inflammatory disease: A retrospective cohort study. Am J Obstet Gynecol 166:1300–1305, 1992.
5. Marchbanks PA, Lee NC, and Peterson HB: Cigarette smoking as a risk factor for pelvic inflammatory disease. Am J Obstet Gynecol 162:639–644, 1990.
6. Aral SO, Mosher WD, and Cates W Jr: Self-reported pelvic inflammatory disease in the United States, 1988. JAMA 266:2570–2573, 1991.
7. Wolner-Hanssen P, Eschenbach DA, Paavonen J, et al: Association between vaginal douching and acute pelvic inflammatory disease. JAMA 263:1936–1941, 1990.
8. Jacobson L and Westrom L: Objectivized diagnosis of acute pelvic inflammatory disease: Diagnostic and prognostic value of routine laparoscopy. Am J Obstet Gynecol 105:1088, 1969.
9. Sweet RL, Mills J, Hadley KW, et al: Use of laparoscopy to

determine the microbiologic etiology of acute salpingitis. Am J Obstet Gynecol 134:68, 1979.
10. Soper DE: Diagnosis and laparoscopic grading of acute salpingitis. Am J Obstet Gynecol 164:1370–1376, 1991.
11. Eschenbach DA and Holmes KK: Acute pelvic inflammatory disease: Current concepts of pathogenesis, etiology and management. Clin Obstet Gynecol 18:35, 1975.
12. Sweet RL: Anaerobic infections of the female genital tract. Am J Obstet Gynecol 122:891, 1975.
13. Curran JW: Management of gonococcal pelvic inflammatory disease. Sex Trans Dis 6:174, 1979.
14. Riccardi NB and Felman YM: Laboratory diagnosis in the problem of suspected gonococcal infection. JAMA 242:2703, 1979.
15. Centers for Disease Control: *Chlamydia trachomatis* infections. MMWR 34 (Suppl 3):53S, 1985.
16. Mardh P-A, Ripa T, Svensson L, et al: *Chlamydia trachomatis* infection in patients with acute salpingitis. N Engl J Med 296:1277, 1977.
17. Mardh P-A and Westrom L: Tubal and cervical cultures in acute salpingitis with special reference to *Mycoplasma hominis* and T-strain mycoplasma. Br J Vener Dis 46:179, 1970.
18. Centers for Disease Control and Prevention: 1993 Sexually Transmitted Disease Treatment Guidelines. MMWR 42(RR-14):1–102, 1993.
19. Comparative evaluation of clindamycin/gentamicin and cefoxitin/doxycycline for treatment of pelvic inflammatory disease; a multi-center trial: The European Study Group. Acta Obstet Gynecol Scand 71:129–134, 1992.
20. Landers DV, Wolner-Hanssen P, Paavonen J, et al: Combination antimicrobial therapy in the treatment of acute pelvic inflammatory disease. Am J Obstet Gynecol 164:849–858, 1991.
21. Reed SD, Landers DV, and Sweet RL: Antibiotic treatment of tuboovarian abscess: Comparison of broad-spectrum beta-lactam agents versus clindamycin-containing regimens. Am J Obstet Gynecol 164:1556–1561, 1991.
22. Brunham RC: Therapy for acute pelvic inflammatory disease: A critique of recent treatment trials. Am J Obstet Gynecol 148:235, 1984.
23. Peterson HB, Walker CK, Kahn JG, et al: Pelvic inflammatory disease: Key treatment issues and options. JAMA 266:2605–2611, 1991.
24. Hoegsberg B, Abulafia O, Sedlis A, et al: Sexually transmitted diseases and human immunodeficiency virus infection among women with pelvic inflammatory disease. Am J Obstet Gynecol 163:1135–1139, 1990.

Penile Discharge and Urethritis

25. US Department of Health and Human Services, Public Health Service, Centers for Disease Control, National Center for Prevention Services, Division of STD/HIV Prevention, Surveillance and Information Systems Branch: Sexually transmitted disease surveillance 1991. Atlanta GA, US Department of Health and Human Services, 1991.
26. Sparling PR, Sarubbi FA Jr, and Blackman E: Inheritance of low-level resistance to penicillin, tetracycline, and chloramphenicol in *Neisseria gonorrhoeae*. J Bacteriol 124:740, 1975.
27. Eisenstein BI, Sox T, Biswamg G, et al: Conjugal transfer of the gonococcal penicillinase plasmid. Science 195:998, 1977.
28. US Department of Health and Human Services/Public Health Service: Global distribution of penicillinase-producing *Neisseria gonorrhoeae* (PPNG). MMWR 31:1, 1982.
29. Jaffe HW, Biddle JW, Johnston SR, et al: Infections due to penicillinase-producing *Neisseria gonorrhoeae* in the United States: 1976–1980. J Infect Dis 144:191, 1981.
30. Felman YM: Penicillinase-producing *Neisseria gonorrhoeae*—cases in New York City, 1979–81. NY State J Med 82:1556, 1982.
31. McCormack WM: Penicillinase-producing *Neisseria gonorrhoeae*—A retrospective. N Engl J Med 307:438, 1982.
32. Perez-Stable EJ: Urethritis in men. West J Med 138:426, 1983.
33. Schofield CBS: Some factors affecting the incubation period and duration of symptoms of urethritis in men. Br J Vener Dis 58:184, 1982.
34. Jacobs NF and Kraus SJ: Gonococcal and nongonococcal urethritis in men: Clinical and laboratory differentiation. Ann Intern Med 82:7, 1975.
35. Riccardi NB, and Felman YM: Laboratory diagnosis in the problem of suspected gonococcal infection. JAMA 242:2703, 1979.
36. Centers for Disease Control and Prevention: 1993 Sexually Transmitted Disease Treatment Guidelines. MMWR 42(RR-14):1–102, 1993.
37. Schacter J: *Chlamydia* infections. N Engl J Med 298:428, 1978.
38. Stamm WE, Koutsky L, Jourden J, et al: Prospective screening for urethral infection with *Chlamydia trachomatis* and *Neisseria gonorrhoeae* in men attending a clinic for sexually transmitted diseases. Clin Res 29:51A, 1981.
39. Brown MB, Cassell GH, Taylor-Robinson D, et al: Measurement of antibody to *Ureaplasma urealyticum* by an enzyme-linked immunosorbent assay and detection of antibody responses in patients with nongonococcal urethritis. J Clin Microbiol 17:288, 1983.
40. Taylor-Robinson D and McCormack WM: The genital mycoplasmas. N Engl J Med 302:1003, 1980.
41. Department of Health and Social Security: Sexually transmitted diseases: Extract from Annual Report of the Chief Medical Officer for the year 1972. Br J Vener Dis 50:73, 1974.
42. Felman YM and Nikitas JA: Nongonococcal urethritis: A clinical review. JAMA 245:381, 1981.
43. Hansfield HH, Alexander ER, Wang SP, et al: Differences in the therapeutic response of chlamydia-positive and chlamydia-negative forms of nongonococcal urethritis. J Am Vener Dis Assoc 2:5, 1976.
44. Toth A: Use of oral metronidazole HCI (Flagyl) for posturethritis syndrome. Urology 19:256, 1982.
45. Oriel JD and Ridgway GL: Comparison of tetracycline and minocycline in the treatment of non-gonococcal urethritis. Br J Vener Dis 59:245, 1983.
46. Treatment of sexually transmitted diseases. Med Lett 28:23, 1986.

Genital Lesions

47. Handsfield HH: Color Atlas and Synopsis of Sexually Transmitted Diseases. New York, McGraw-Hill, 1992.
48. Solomon AR, Rasmussen JE, Varani J, et al: The Tzanck smear in the diagnosis of cutaneous herpes simplex. JAMA 251:633, 1984.
49. Centers for Disease Control and Prevention: 1993 Sexually Transmitted Disease Treatment Guidelines. MMWR 42(RR-14):1–102, 1993.
50. Dans PE, Cafferty L, Otter SE, et al: Inappropriate use of the cerebrospinal fluid venereal disease research laboratory (VDRL) test to exclude neurosyphilis. Ann Intern Med 104:86, 1986.
51. Larsen SA, Hambie EA, Wobig GH, et al: Cerebrospinal fluid test for syphilis: Treponemal and nontreponemal tests. *In* Morisset R, et al (eds): Advances in Sexually Transmitted Diseases. Utrecht, The Netherlands, VNU Science Press, 1985, pp 157–162.
52. Wiesel J, Rose DN, Silver AL, et al: Lumbar puncture in asymptomatic late syphilis: An analysis of the benefit and risks. Arch Intern Med 145:65, 1985.
53. Hart G: Syphilis tests in diagnostic and therapeutic decision making. Ann Intern Med 104:368, 1986.
54. Goldberg LH, Kaufman R, Kurtz TO, et al: Long-term suppression of recurrent genital herpes with acyclovir: a 5-year benchmark. Arch Dermatol 129:582, 1993.

32

Urinary Tract Infections

WILLIAM T. BRANCH, Jr., MD

Most patients with infections of the urinary tract (UTIs) are seen initially by primary care physicians. The majority of these are women with acute dysuria, most often attributed to bacterial infection of the lower urinary tract (bladder and urethra) or to chlamydial infection of the urethra (the dysuria-pyuria syndrome).[1–3] Many cases represent sporadic infections in otherwise normal individuals. Occasionally, however, more difficult problems are encountered. An important subgroup of women with acute dysuria have subclinical pyelonephritis; these may require more prolonged treatment than do patients with bladder or urethral infection alone.[4] Other patients have fevers, chills, and flank pain in addition to dysuria, signifying acute pyelonephritis, and they often require hospitalization and parenteral antibiotic therapy. Others have frequent, recurrent infections, requiring consideration of long-term prophylaxis. Urinary tract infections in men also involve a different approach.

This chapter focuses on the problem of UTIs as seen from the perspective of the primary care physician. He or she generally must assume responsibility not only for initial treatment but also for the timing and extent of diagnostic evaluation, and for long-term follow-up of the patient.

NATURAL HISTORY

Pathogenesis

From 2 to 4% of women have positive results on midstream cultures (i.e., asymptomatic bacteriuria) in population surveys.[5–7] If women with asymptomatic bacteriuria are observed over a period of years, they tend to have recurrent, clinically manifested UTIs, particularly soon after marriage and during pregnancy. The most widely accepted hypothesis states that this is related to a tendency in some women for the gram-negative bacilli—especially strains exhibiting pathogenicity by adhering to mucosal cells—to colonize the vaginal introitus and bladder vestibule.[8] No anatomic defect can be identified. Episodes of lower tract infection in women are often associated with sexual intercourse, which has been shown to increase urine bacterial counts transiently tenfold in 30% of normal women.[27] Usually the bacteria that enter the bladder are vaginal flora, such as lactobacilli, diphtheroids, and α-hemolytic streptococci, which probably rarely produce infection.[4] Coliform organisms entering the bladder account for many episodes of sporadic cystitis, and for recurrent cystitis in women whose bladder vestibule is colonized by these organisms.[8]

Not all women with acute dysuria have UTIs. Some pain or discomfort on urination may be experienced by up to 21% of all women during the course of a year.[9] Of those seeking medical attention, one third to one half have negative results on cultures. Perhaps half of these patients have a low-grade bacterial urethritis and cystitis, with pyuria and gram-negative organisms on the first-voided specimen but low colony counts in midstream cultures.[1, 8, 10] Other patients, especially young women, suffer chlamydial urethritis, or possibly urethritis caused by *Mycoplasma*, viruses, or other organisms.[2, 11, 12] Dysuria without pyuria in women is also caused by vaginitis, mucosal atrophy, trauma, or other factors.

Most women with uncomplicated lower UTIs respond well to therapy and have few, if any, recurrences. In one study, 37.5% of previously asymptomatic women had a sporadic episode of bacteriuria during a 10-year prospective follow-up.[7] However, two studies of women who had been hospitalized for pyelonephritis reported that recurrent infections developed in 77 to 83% on long-term follow-up.[13, 14] It is also recognized generally that bacteriuria will recur within 1 year despite initially successful therapy in 80% of those who are subject to asymptomatic bacteriuria or previously had recurrent infections.[8] In some women, recurrent lower UTIs appear to follow the pattern of a cluster of several or more infections after an initial one. An interval of long-term freedom from infection may ensue if the urine can be sterilized for a sufficient time.[15]

Prognosis and Prognostic Factors

Intravenous urograms (IVPs) in patients selected because of either persistent asymptomatic bacteriuria (most have a history of at least several symptomatic episodes) or a hospitalization for pyelonephritis reveal caliectasis or renal cortical scarring or both in 10 to 20% of patients (Fig. 32–1).[5, 6, 14] However, when followed with serial studies, most adults with caliectasis do not develop new areas of scarring; furthermore, UTIs are rarely the cause of renal failure in adults, unless renal calculi or obstruction are also present. For example, among patients requiring dialysis, only 13% had pyelonephritis as the etiology of uremia, and only 3% were without stones or obstruction as an additional factor.[16] Nevertheless, a few adults with pyelonephritis do have adverse outcomes.[7, 14] Diabetics, in particular, are more subject to complications of UTIs, although they are no more likely than nondiabetics to develop bacteriuria.[17]

In children, it is thought that renal scarring is often related to infection in the presence of vesicoureteral reflux. Children, whose onset of UTIs occurs prior to the age of 5 years, more often develop scarring because the renal papillae have more open ducts in young children, which allows intrarenal as well as vesicoureteral reflux of infected urine.[17] High grades of vesicoureteral reflux produce more intrarenal reflux. In children, caliectasis and scarring increased from 25% in those with grade 1 reflux (a small amount partially filling the ureter) to 75% in those with grade 3, in which there is dilatation of the collecting system in addition to reflux reaching the renal pelvis (Fig. 32–2).[18] Children with recurrent urinary infections without vesicoureteral reflux had a low prevalence of renal scarring[19] and, as documented by ureteral cultures, a low incidence of upper UTIs.[20]

Fewer adults than young children have reflux associated with urinary infections, although one series of 158 patients referred for urologic evaluation of difficult infections included 30 (25%) with reflux.[25] In adults, about one third of cases of reflux are secondary to bladder carcinoma or to prostatic bladder outlet obstruction. Other adults with reflux have a relatively severe congenital anomaly with patulous ureteral openings or short intravesicular ureteral segments, or both. The relationship among reflux, progressive renal damage, and infection remains unclear in adults. Progressive renal scarring (in 15%), as well as death from advanced pyelonephritis (5%), has been associated with high-grade adult reflux.[26] Adults with sterile high-grade reflux are reported to develop progressive glomerulosclerosis in some cases.[52] In children, mild reflux may resolve after bladder dysfunction caused by recurrent cystitis is corrected by keeping the urine sterile,[53] but antimicrobial therapy is less successful in adults, with only 13% ceasing to reflux on medical therapy in one series.[25] Surgical ureteral reimplantation or endoscopic correction of high-grade reflux generally succeeds but warrants careful consideration and consultation with a urologist and nephrologist, because it may not alter prognosis if infections are controlled.[17, 26, 54]

Aside from reflux, the only urologic abnormality commonly found on urograms of women with complicated UTIs is renal calculi, found in 2 to 8%.[5, 6, 14] However, evidence of tissue infection, as opposed to mucosal involvement of the bladder, exists in about 30% of adult women whose clinical picture is only of lower UTIs. These patients have antibody-coated bacteria in the urine.[22] They may have subclinical pyelonephritis, presenting with dysuria and pyuria without the high fevers, chills, and flank pain of acute pyelonephritis. Nevertheless, most women with recurrent UTIs do not develop progressive renal scarring. The majority of those with antibody-coated bacteria respond to 10 days of therapy.[23, 24] Identification of the subgroup of women with persistent bacteriuria despite adequate therapy allows primary care physicians to focus their efforts related to urologic evaluation or more prolonged therapy on a small number of individuals. Recurrent uncomplicated UTIs in women after an interval of sterile urine—as opposed to persistent infections—chiefly present a problem in controlling symptoms and may not benefit from a work-up.

INITIAL ASSESSMENT AND THERAPY

Lower Urinary Tract Infections in Women

Most women with UTIs experience abrupt onset of frequency and dysuria but without flank pain, repetitive chills, or more than low-grade fever. These symptoms generally signal a lower UTI and are now subdivided into several categories.

Bacterial Lower UTIs. Bacteria colonizing the periurethral tissue may enter the urethra and produce infection by ascending into the bladder. In college women *Escherichia coli* accounted for 79% of positive urine cultures.[28] *Staphylococcus saprophyticus* caused 11%, and *Klebsiella* and *Proteus* accounted for 5%.[28]

Methods to confirm the diagnosis of bacterial lower tract infections have limitations. Pyuria (> 5 white blood cells [WBC]/hpf) in a woman is a nonspecific finding, sometimes present in vaginitis and other conditions. The presence of more than 10 white blood cells per high-power field plus 1+ bacteria in the centrifuged urine sediment was shown to differentiate urinary infection from vaginitis in most cases.[29]

Traditionally, urine cultures rely on a colony count of 10^5 or more to identify infection, but these criteria were derived from women with asymptomatic bacteriuria and from those with pyelonephritis.[8] Even so, the criterion of 10^5 or greater colonies per cubic millimeter has a false-negative rate of approximately 20% and a similar false-positive rate.[8] It is now recognized that women with bacterial lower UTIs, as opposed to those with asymptomatic bacteriuria or pyelonephritis, frequently have colony counts of less than 10^5 in midstream urine specimens, probably because in many infection is confined chiefly to the urethra with only early or low-grade bladder infection. Stamm and colleagues have proposed that the best diagnostic criterion for identifying symptomatic bacterial lower UTIs is 10^2 or greater colonies of urinary pathogens per cubic millimeter.[1]

Chlamydial Urethritis and the Dysuria-Pyuria Syndrome. It has been shown that in some populations one third to one half of women with dysuria have negative midstream cultures.[11, 12] Though some have bacterial urethritis, many have chlamydial urethritis.[2] Patients with urethritis caused by *Chlamydia* often have symptoms of several days as opposed to hours in duration and are less likely to have gross hematuria than patients with bacterial lower UTIs. Most are young women, and the history of a recent change in sexual partners is also elicited in many. However, *Chlamydia* are not present in about one third of women with dysuria, pyuria, and negative bacterial cultures.[2] Other organisms may cause this syndrome, including *Trichomonas vaginalis,* herpes simplex, and, especially in inner-city populations, *Neisseria gonorrhoeae*[4, 30, 31] and, rarely, tuberculosis, fungal infection, or an abscess located adjacent to the urinary tract.

Vaginitis and Other Causes of Dysuria without Pyuria. Vaginitis may cause the symptom of "burning urination" more often than UTIs. Usually the patient is also aware of having a vaginal discharge.[29] More than half of women with vaginitis can differentiate their symptom of burning on passage of urine through the labia from true

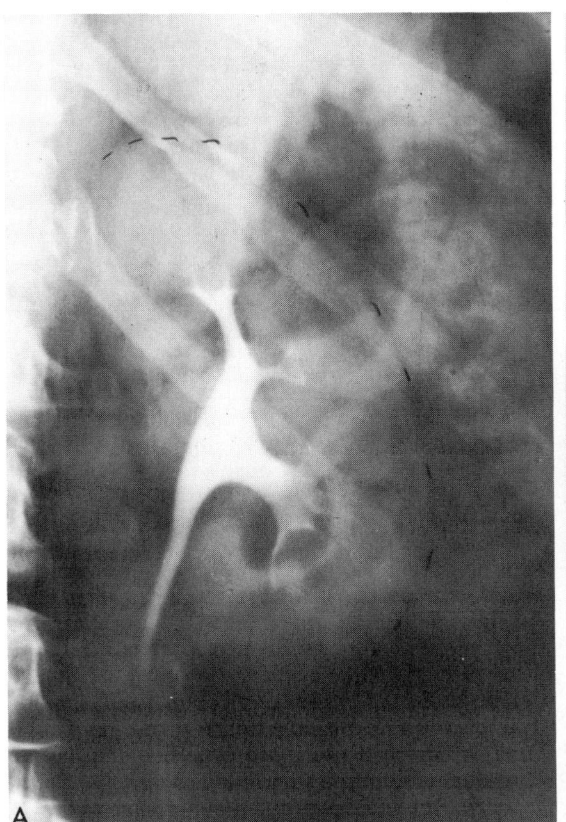

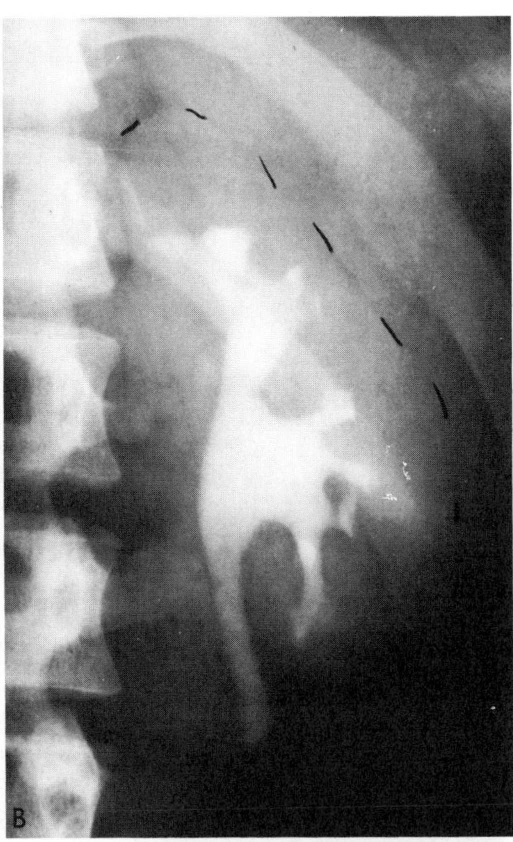

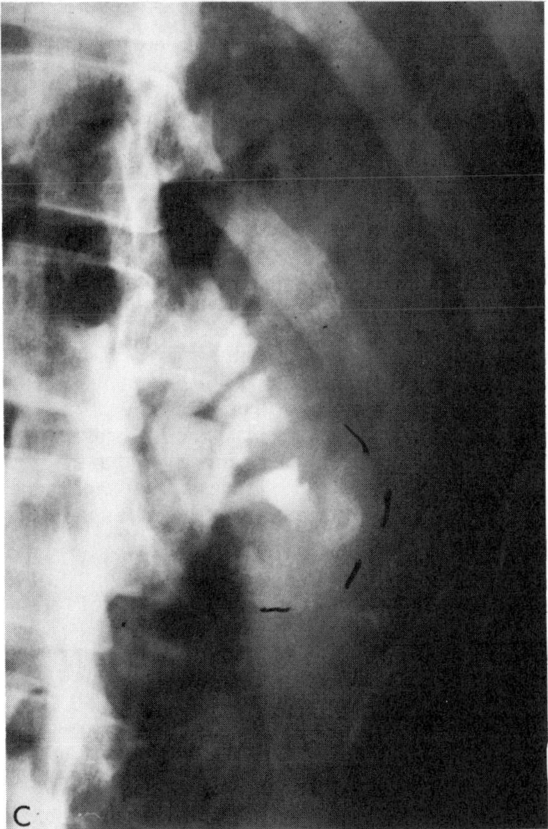

FIGURE 32–1. X-ray findings of pyelonephritis.

A, Normal excretory phase of intravenous urogram. The renal pelvis is divided into two or three major calyces, which are connected by infundibula to groups of minor calyces numbering 8 to 12, of which 2 to 4 are clustered in the upper, mid, and lower portions of the kidney, respectively. These normal calyces appear as small inverted cups showing the outline of each renal papilla, which is framed by a delicate, sharp fornix on either side. The renal cortex is smooth and uninterrupted by scarring or loss of parenchyma.

B, Calyceal blunting with an adjacent cortical scar. These changes are characteristic of pyelonephritis; dilatation of the minor calyes and loss of the delicate fornices cause calyces to appear blunted or clubbed. The focal parenchymal scar, which is adjacent to the calyceal damage, is also a hallmark of pyelonephritis.

C, Advanced pyelonephritis. Calyceal architecture is totally destroyed. The kidney is small and atrophic.

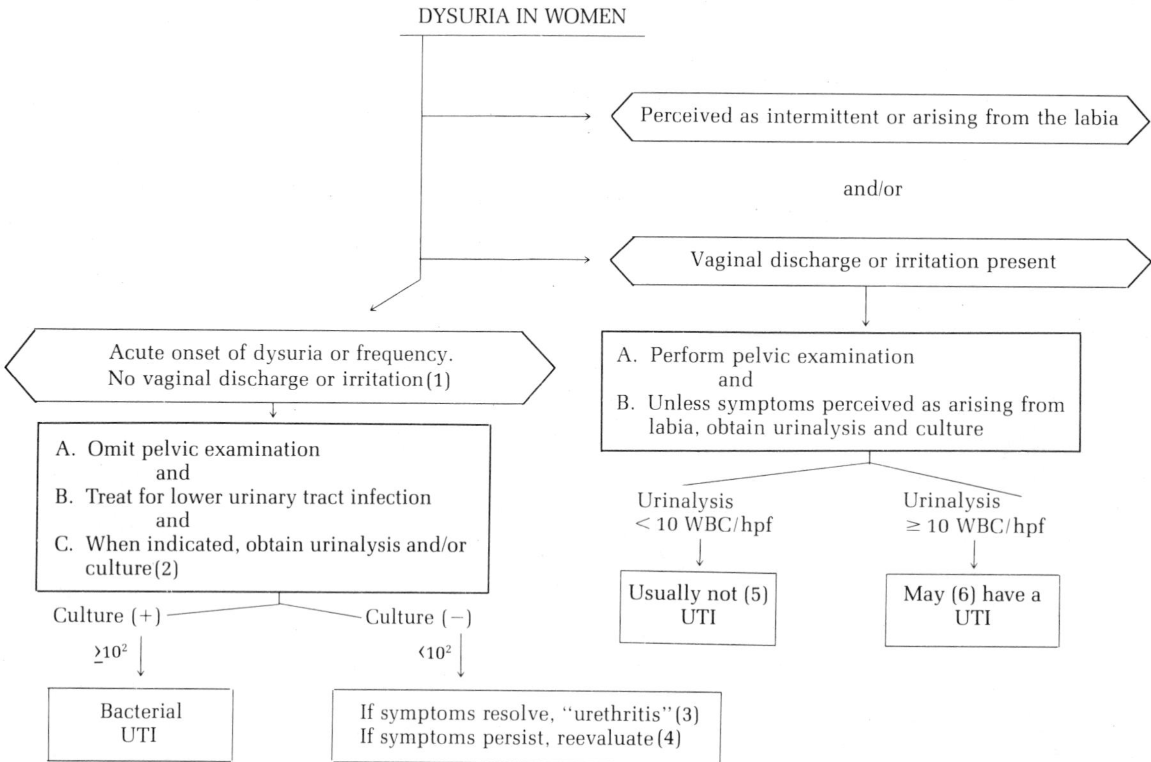

FIGURE 32–2. A strategy for evaluating women with acute dysuria or urinary frequency.

1. Although vaginitis occurs more commonly than urinary tract infections (UTIs), with no history of vaginal discharge or irritation the probability of vaginitis is 1% or less in women with dysuria.[29]
2. Because of the very high success rates of antimicrobial therapy, it may not be necessary in uncomplicated, sporadic cases to obtain urine culture unless symptoms persist or are recurrent.
3. The etiology of "urethritis" may be bacterial infection of the urethra (should be suspected when previous episodes of bacterial UTIs have been documented) or may be nonbacterial (presumably chlamydial). In either case, symptoms usually resolve after treatment for UTI.
4. The etiology of persistent or chronic dysuria in women may be inadequately treated cystitis or "urethritis," unrecognized vaginitis, trauma, urethral caruncle, interstitial cystitis, carcinoma of the bladder, tuberculosis of the bladder, and so on.
5. If vaginal discharge or irritation is present and there are < 10 white blood cells (WBC)/hpf, the probability of also having a UTI is 2% or less.[29]
6. Patients who have both acute dysuria and vaginal discharge or irritation and have 10 or more WBC/hpf have approximately a 24% probability of both vaginitis and UTI, a 24% probability of only vaginitis, a 19% probability of only UTI, and a 31% probability of other disorders;[29] other disorders include "urethritis," gonorrheal infections, herpes infections, and miscellaneous vaginal or pelvic abnormalities.

(internal) dysuria.[29, 32] Though herpetic, trichomonal, and gonorrheal vaginitis or cervicitis may induce a leukocyte response in vaginal fluid, candidal vaginitis does not, and the criterion of 10 WBCs or more per high-power field usually separates vaginitis from UTIs.[29]

In addition to vaginitis, there may be other causes of the acute urethral syndrome in women. Pyuria was not present in half of Stamm and colleagues' 32 patients with dysuria and negative bacterial cultures, and cultures of only one of them grew *Chlamydia*.[2] The other patients did not respond to antimicrobial treatment. Postulated causes of their symptoms include mucosal trauma and atrophy.[4]

Patients with persistent irritative bladder symptoms, with or without pyuria, as opposed to those with an acute but unexplained bout of dysuria, should be evaluated for possible neurogenic bladder, bladder carcinoma, tuberculous cystitis, or chronic interstitial cystitis.

Separating Lower UTIs from Subclinical Pyelonephritis. The clinician generally relies on the absence of repetitive chills or high fever and an absence of WBC casts in the sediment to distinguish a lower UTI from acute pyelonephritis. Flank or loin pain, unless associated with exquisite tenderness, does not reliably differentiate lower UTI from pyelonephritis. Furthermore, testing for antibody-coated bacteria suggests that in some populations approximately one third of patients with lower urinary tract symptoms actually have subclinical pyelonephritis.[22–24] The usefulness of this method is limited in clinical practice, however, because of poor standardization in different laboratories.[22]

The most practical means to identify patients with subclinical pyelonephritis who require further evaluation or treatment probably is detection of persistent bacteriuria on culture within 1 week following adequate therapy. For choosing initial therapy for patients suspected of having subclinical pyelonephritis, one must rely on the clinical and epidemiologic features. Women who fail to respond to single-dose or 3-day as opposed to 10-day therapy often have symptoms of longer duration and are from indigent populations with poorer access to medical care than women who responded to short-term therapy.[24] These criteria are imprecise. It seems best also to suspect subclinical pyelonephritis in women with lower tract symptoms whose histories include UTIs in childhood, previous multiple recurrent infections—especially three or more within the preceding year—hypertension, diabetes, known renal calculi or other urologic abnormalities, or symptoms, such as polyuria or nocturia, suggestive of tubulointerstitial disease.

Single-Dose Versus 7- to 10-Day Therapy. A number of reports demonstrate equally successful results using only a single dose or a 3-day course of an antimicrobial, compared with standard 7- to 10-day courses, in patients with uncomplicated lower tract infections.[23, 24, 33–38] A cure is generally defined as laboratory determination of a sterile urine 3 to 7 days after therapy. Later resumption of bacteriuria occurs commonly and is caused by *recurrence* or *reinfection,* in which the same or a different organism enters the bladder via the urethra, and not from *relapse* or *persistence* of organisms that failed to be eradicated by therapy. Using this criterion, single 320 mg/1600 mg doses of trimethoprim-sulfamethoxazole (2 Bactrim double-strength tablets) are estimated to be effective in 90% of patients, compared with 95% of patients given 7- to 10-day courses of the same antimicrobial.[37] The effectiveness of a single 3-g dose of amoxicillin was estimated to be 72%.[37] These antimicrobials, as well as nitrofurantoin, ampicillin, tetracycline, and many other agents, achieve high concentrations in urine and renal interstitium so that in vitro bacterial resistance does not always lead to failure of therapy.[21]

Women with subclinical pyelonephritis are less likely to respond to short-course (single-dose or 3-day) therapy than to 10-day therapy.[23] In one study, 15% of all women with lower tract symptoms relapsed shortly after receiving 3 Bactrim double-strength tablets, but only 3% relapsed after receiving 10 days of treatment.[39] Other studies confirm that most patients with antibody-coated bacteria in the urine respond to 10 days of treatment.[24] Thus, success using single-dose or 3-day treatment may depend on the selection of patients *unlikely* to have subclinical pyelonephritis. Patients whose urine is not sterile after adequate therapy, in the absence of bacterial resistance, are more likely to have evidence of caliectasis and scarring or other abnormalities on intravenous urograms.[23, 24, 33, 34] Although the numbers of patients reported to date are small, it appears that persistence of bacteriuria with the same organism within 1 week following therapy constitutes an indication to retreat for longer duration and raises the question of obtaining diagnostic studies (see further on).

Treatment Strategies

Vaginitis is excluded by the absence of a history of vaginal discharge, the presence of 10 or more WBC/hpf in the urine, and pelvic examination if necessary (see Fig. 32–2). Mucosal trauma, atrophy, and other causes of sterile dysuria without pyuria are excluded since these conditions do not produce pyuria. Thus, urinalysis should be performed at the time of presentation. Obtaining an initial urine culture is not necessarily correlated with successful treatment and is estimated to increase costs by about 40%,[37, 38] but it is believed to be standard practice by many clinicians and should be done when there is uncertainty about the diagnosis, suspicion of subclinical pyelonephritis, or the need to plan management for possible recurrent infections.

Single-dose trimethoprim-sulfamethoxazole (2 double-strength tablets) is probably the best choice of treatment for young, previously healthy, nonallergic women who present typical features within 1 to 2 days of onset and have no history of previous complicated infections.[37, 38] Women allergic to sulfa may receive single-dose therapy with amoxicillin (3 g po) or (if not pregnant) 3-day treatment with tetracycline, nitrofurantoin, or trimethoprim (200 mg/24 hr). Single-dose treatment produces fewer side effects—chiefly vaginitis, gastrointestinal symptoms, or rashes—which occur in only about 8% of patients compared with about 26% of patients who experience side effects during multiple-dose therapy.[37] However, failure to eradicate infection causes more prolonged morbidity, and added concern about persistent infection and the possible need for diagnostic studies. For this reason, 7 to 10 days of treatment probably represents a better choice for women from indigent or inner-city populations, with symptoms for more than several days or an unreliable history, or with any other aforementioned factor associated with subclinical pyelonephritis. Thus, single-dose or 3-day therapy is suited for reliable, healthy young women with *typical* symptoms and no complicating factors. Single doses or 3-day therapy may also be used for uncomplicated *recurrent* UTIs in women previously shown to respond to this treatment. Single-dose treatment has not been well studied in geriatric populations.

A follow-up urine culture is indicated within 1 week after completing therapy in women with persistent symptoms, and in those with any of the features previously listed associated with subclinical pyelonephritis. The patient with none of these factors whose response to treatment is complete may not benefit from a follow-up culture.[39, 40]

Before embarking on extensive evaluation or long-term treatment, one may wish to document persistent bacteriuria after a second trial of 7 to 10 days of adequate therapy. Patients with continuing symptoms but negative results on cultures after single-dose therapy may be suspected of having chlamydial urethritis. Such patients are generally young women or college students who are sexually active, have intermittent or stuttering dysuria, no hematuria, and no bacteria in the urine sediment. Some may respond to single-dose therapy with trimethoprim-sulfamethoxazole.[37] Effective regimens for nonpregnant patients failing to respond include doxycycline, 100 mg twice daily for 10 days,[3] tetracycline 500 mg four times daily for 7 days, or (if pregnant) erythromycin 500 mg four times daily for 7 days.[37]

Asymptomatic Bacteriuria in Women

Asymptomatic bacteriuria may be detected on follow-up of women who presented initially with symptomatic episodes or in evaluating those in whom pyuria was discovered on routine urinalyses. Given the benign natural history in most adults, screening programs for nonpregnant women generally have not been adopted. However, once detected, the problem is to what extent treatment or evaluation is indicated. Stamm suggests that the presence of pyuria distinguishes truly infected women from a somewhat larger number in whom the bacteriuria represents transient colonization.[10] One may choose to treat the former for 7 to 10 days and obtain a follow-up culture to exclude persistent infection. Although therapy usually eradicates bacteriuria transiently, a course of therapy has no discernible long-term influence on bacteriuria, owing to the very high recurrence rate in this population of patients.[6] Except in pregnancy, longer-term or repeated therapy does not appear to be justified in the absence of symptoms or a urinary tract abnormality.

Upper Tract Infections in Women

There is no evidence that most UTIs per se do not respond to oral therapy with an antibiotic.[21, 24, 33] However, when a patient has chills and fever clearly indicative of pyelonephritis, hospitalization generally is indicated, at least briefly, to achieve bactericidal blood and tissue levels sufficient for treating bacteremia. This consideration is particularly important in elderly individuals, those with underlying illnesses, or those infected following instrumentation of the genitourinary tract. Since adequate tissue and blood levels are not always obtained when antibiotics are given by the oral route, intravenous therapy is indicated in any patient with signs of septicemia. An aminoglycoside plus ampicillin or cefazolin is recommended until bacterial susceptibilities are known.[17] Most patients respond within 48 hours. If a septic course persists for longer than 72 hours, intravenous urography, which is somewhat better than renal ultrasonography,[41] should be done to rule out obstruction, which requires emergency urologic intervention, and to search for complications like perinephric abscess or renal carbuncle.

Patients with mild acute pyelonephritis have been treated successfully without hospitalization by some clinicians using well-absorbed oral agents such as the quinolones or trimethoprim-sulfamethoxazole given for 14 days.[42]

The question of whether some women with pyelonephritis, either *acute* or *subclinical,* require prolonged therapy for more than 10 days to eradicate the persistence within tissue foci of an inadequately treated infection is raised. Bacterial *persistence* in spite of therapy (i.e., relapse within 1 week with the same organism) may be caused by failure of single-dose or even 7- to 10-day therapy to eradicate pathogenic organisms from the vaginal and bladder vestibule with early reinfection of the bladder. It may also reflect (1) bacterial resistance or development of resistance to the antimicrobial; (2) struvite or giant staghorn calculi; or, rarely, (3) an atrophic kidney, bladder or urethral diverticulum, or other anatomic reservoir of infection in the urinary tract. Occasionally, infections that do not respond to several courses of conventional therapy given for 10 days in anatomically normal patients, may be eliminated by 6 weeks of therapy with a bactericidal agent administered orally in adequate doses.[36]

UROLOGIC EVALUATION

The purpose of the urologic evaluation in patients with UTIs is to exclude an abnormality of the urinary tract that is amenable to surgical correction or one that requires very careful follow-up or long-term efforts to keep the urine sterile. Studies generally are delayed for at least 6 weeks after an acute episode to allow transient vesicoureteral reflux to resolve. The diagnostic studies to be considered are IVP, cystoscopy, and voiding cystourethrography (VCUG) or radionuclide cystography. These studies are expensive and each carries a small risk, thus they should be reserved for selected patients. The risk of urography includes one to two cases of acute, usually reversible renal failure per 1000 patients, the majority of whom are diabetic, elderly, or dehydrated at the time of the examination, and about one death from anaphylaxis per 75,000 patients.[43, 44] Radiation exposure from the IVP or VCUG may entail a small risk of future malignancy for the patient[45] and if the patient is pregnant, especially in the first trimester, one must be concerned about the risk of future malignancy for the fetus.[46, 47] Cystoscopy, VCUG, and radionuclide cystography in women entail risk of introducing infection. Ultrasonography may be substituted for IVP in diabetics and patients with renal compromise if the purpose of the study is to rule out large stones, obstruction, or renal atrophy.

Although cystoscopy has a slightly higher yield of some abnormalities (i.e., urethral diverticuli), the abnormalities of most serious concern (i.e., infection stones or hydronephrosis) will be detected more often by urography. Data remain inadequate to give results of evaluations in adults with *persistent* infection suggesting a urologic abnormality, but the available data reveal a low yield in adults selected for other reasons. In schoolgirls and women with asymptomatic bacteriuria and recurrent infections, and in young women with acute pyelonephritis, the only frequently encountered abnormalities were caliectasis or renal cortical scarring, or both, in 10 to 20% and renal calculi in 2 to 8%.[5, 6, 14] Hydronephrosis, bladder outlet obstruction, and other abnormalities occurred in less than 1%.

Adult women in whom the only indication for diagnostic studies is *recurrent,* otherwise uncomplicated UTIs constitute the majority of those likely to be encountered by primary care physicians. These women rarely have correctable abnormalities.[48–50] Table 32–1 reveals that of 421 women who had urographic and other studies for this indication alone, the only abnormalities warranting surgical correction were three urethral diverticuli, one bladder diverticulum, and one colicovesical fistula.[17, 48, 50] Only seven of these 421 women with uncomplicated recurrences had caliectasis, renal scar, or a small kidney, and only five had signs of obstruction—none severe enough to require surgical correction.

Infection stones are encountered infrequently but are one abnormality that should not be overlooked. Infection with *Proteus mirabilis* or other urea-splitting bacteria is associated with formation of struvite (magnesium ammonium phosphate and apatite) calculi. Nephrotomography may be necessary to visualize flecks of calcium within these otherwise nonopaque stones. Once formed, the stones are a reservoir of persistent infection, virtually impossible to eradicate medically. Management generally involves a surgical approach, along with long-term antimicrobial prophylaxis. On the other hand, nonobstructing calcium oxalate and uric acid calculi may be only incidental findings in patients who also have UTIs.

Indications for Intravenous Urography. *Persistent* or *relapsing* bacteriuria with the same organism, which cannot be eradicated by several courses of 10 days or up to 6 weeks of adequate therapy, identifies a subgroup of patients more likely to have infection stones, pyonephrosis, ureteropelvic junctional obstruction, or other abnormalities. Some other clinical features that suggest the likelihood of a "complicated" infection requiring work-up include mixed or unusual organisms in the urine (e.g., *Pseudomonas, Proteus mirabilis*), pneumaturia (suggesting colicovesical fistula), severe hypertension, persistent hematuria, renal compromise, or a history suggesting recurrent infections in childhood, analgesic abuse, renal calculi, or obstructive symptoms. Severe pyelonephritis with sepsis requiring hospitalization may be an indication for urography. But a study of 67 hospitalized patients suggests that most lesions requiring surgical intervention, as opposed to abnormalities not altering treatment, are identified if IVPs are performed when patients remain febrile for more than 72 hours or have other complicating features.[41]

Voiding Cystourethrography or Radionuclide Cystography. Vesicoureteral reflux can be detected by VCUG or radionuclide cystography with ^{99m}Tc pertechnetate. The IVP cannot be relied on to show reflux, since even grade 3 reflux demonstrated by VCUG may not cause apparent dilatation of the ureters and renal pelves on routine IVP. Because VCUG and radionuclide cystography require catheterization of female patients, they should not be done unless the urine is sterile. The incidence of reflux is unknown in adults. Of 75 patients with uncomplicated recurrent infections, only one had transient reflux.[50] The yield of high grade reflux should be increased, however, if studies are

TABLE 32–1. RESULTS OF UROLOGIC EVALUATIONS IN 421 WOMEN WITH RECURRENT, OTHERWISE UNCOMPLICATED URINARY TRACT INFECTIONS

	Fowler, et al[50] (1981)	Engel, et al[48] (1980)	Fair, et al[49]* (1979)
Number of patients	104	153	164
Normal findings	83 (80%)	135 (88%)	145 (88%)
Incidental findings (duplications, other abnormalities of uncertain significance)	11 (11%)†	11 (7%)	12 (7%)
Renal scar or caliectasis	3	0	1
Renal calculi‡	2	1	1
Small or atrophic kidney	1	1	1
Ureteropelvic junctional obstruction	0	2§	0
Ureteral dilatation	0	0	3§
Ureteritis cystica	1	0	0
Bladder diverticulum	0	0	1
Colicovesical fistula	0	1	0
Urethral diverticuli	3	0	0

*Includes only intravenous urography; cystoscopy not done.

†Includes one renal cell carcinoma found at intravenous urogram (IVP) and one bladder carcinoma found at cystoscopy, both thought unrelated to urinary tract infections.

‡All small, nonobstructing calcium oxalate calculi, no infection stones.

§All mild, suggesting mild obstruction or reflux not requiring surgical correction; no cases with high-grade reflux were identified and only four cases with mild reflux.

Summary of abnormalities found:

—Possibly significant abnormalities found at IVP: 14 (3.5%) of 421 having IVP.

—Abnormalities found at IVP warranting surgical correction: 1 (<1%).

—Surgically correctable abnormalities found at cystoscopy: 4 (1.7%) of 227 having cystoscopy.

reserved for adults who have caliectasis and scarring on an IVP done to evaluate persistent bacteriuria, or recent severe pyelonephritis.

As mentioned, progression of caliectasis and scarring is uncommon in adults in the absence of reflux, calculi, or obstruction,[16, 19, 55, 56] leading one to postulate that most patients with negative VCUG findings but unexplained caliectasis probably had childhood reflux, which resolved when competency developed at the ureterovesical junction with growth of the bladder to adulthood. Presumably these patients are at low risk for developing progressive renal scarring in adulthood. Studies have demonstrated no differences in urethral diameters between women with recurrent infections and a control population.[57] Likewise, instrumental dilatations of the urethra had no influence on the number of recurrent infections in randomized trials.[58, 59] Thus, bladder outlet obstruction is rarely the cause of recurrent urinary tract infections in women.[17, 48, 50] When bladder outlet obstruction is suspected because of finding bladder trabeculations or postvoiding residual urine on urography, urethral calibration rather than VCUG is the best method of confirmation.

Cystoscopy. Cystoscopy may detect lesions not detected by IVP or VCUG, such as urethral diverticulum or ectopic ureterocele. Urethral diverticuli were reported in 1 to 2% of patients evaluated by cystoscopy for recurrent, uncomplicated UTIs in two series (see Table 32–1).[48, 50] In cases of reflux a more patulous appearance of the ureteral os at cystoscopy will help to estimate the likelihood that reflux will not resolve with medical management.

Physicians must weigh these advantages of cystoscopy against the potential for introduction of resistant organisms via instrumentation. For this reason, cystoscopy probably was employed too liberally in the past; however, in the absence of a radiologically demonstrable abnormality that explains the history, a single cystoscopic examination is indicated in patients with persistent or complicated infection. One may also consider cystoscopy in patients with multiply recurrent though otherwise uncomplicated UTIs.[4] One lesion that is unlikely to be identified without cystoscopy is carcinoma of the bladder. In elderly individuals, bladder cancers may show chronic or intermittent irritative symptoms that resemble UTIs or hematuria that may persist after treatment of apparent cystitis.

Urinary Tract Infections in Men

UTIs are uncommon in men younger than 50 years of age but achieve an incidence approaching that in women in men older than 70 years of age.[17] The pathogenesis of UTIs is different in men from that in women. Rather than recurrent bladder infestation via the urethra with organisms of fecal origin, many men are reinfected from organisms harbored within the prostate gland. Chronic prostatitis in these patients may be asymptomatic or manifested by mild frequency and urgency. The course is marked by recurrent episodes in which the urine becomes infected, uncommonly accompanied by acute epididymoorchitis and, rarely, acute prostatitis (see Chapter 33). Usually each episode responds promptly to therapy with antimicrobials; however, most antimicrobials to which gram-negative bacilli are sensitive do not achieve a sufficient level within the prostate to eradicate the source of infection, because of the high prostatic pH and need for lipid solubility. Thus, the source of reinfection persists following therapy. Recurrent infections can lead to prostatic fibrosis with contracture of the bladder neck and bladder outlet obstruction manifested by hesitancy, slowness of urinary stream, and frequency and urgency of urination.

In older men with UTIs, there may also be prostatic hypertrophy with postvoiding residual urine. This may allow bacteria to proliferate if organisms enter the bladder. This probably leads to bouts of infection once organisms are sequestered within the prostate.

Treatment of these conditions is discussed in the section on Long-Term Management and in Chapter 33.

Diagnostic Evaluation of Male Patients with Urinary Tract Infections. After an acute infection subsides, a three-glass urine test will confirm that chronic prostatitis is the source of infection (see Chapter 33). Microscopic examination should reveal 15 WBCs or more per hpf in the third (prostatic) specimen, whereas the first (urethral) and second (bladder) specimens show no, or significantly less, pyuria. Culture of the midstream specimen should be sterile if bacteriuria has been eradicated, whereas the prostatic specimen often contains small numbers of coliform organisms.

An IVP generally is indicated in male patients with urinary infection. If there is a relative contraindication to contrast, ultrasonography of the kidneys, upper tracts, and bladder could be performed in place of IVP. The work-up may possibly be deferred if the patient is a healthy man, with only one UTI, which is clearly related to prostatitis and which has not recurred on careful follow-up after adequate therapy. At IVP, a VCUG can also be obtained in men on voiding, thus visualizing the prostatic and membranous urethra sufficiently to detect obstructive dilatation. The postvoiding film following VCUG will detect gross reflux as well as allow an estimate of postvoiding residual urine. The estimation of residual urine is most important in men with UTIs, since the most likely factor contributing to recurrent infections, in addition to chronic prostatitis, is bladder outlet obstruction due to benign prostatic hypertrophy, stricture, or fibrotic scarring of the prostate. Cystoscopic examination is indicated if there is residual urine or obstructive voiding symptoms or if bladder tumor is suspected. Urethral strictures occurring distal to the prostatic urethra generally are manifested by symptoms such as a narrow urinary stream or inability to void, in addition to recurrent infections; however, if a stricture is clinically suspected in the penile or bulbous urethra (anterior urethra), a retrograde urethrogram should be obtained in addition to the VCUG.

LONG-TERM MANAGEMENT OF RECURRENT URINARY TRACT INFECTIONS

For practical purposes, one may subdivide patients with *recurrent* UTIs into three categories: (1) females with uncomplicated recurrent UTIs, (2) adult men without gross obstructive uropathy, and (3) men or women in whom infections are complicated by stones, obstruction, or other uropathy.

Women with Uncomplicated Recurrent Urinary Tract Infections

Compromise of renal function is not expected in the population of adult women who have recurrent UTIs but whose IVPs are normal. For the purposes of therapy, women whose only problem is recurrences of uncomplicated lower UTIs, insufficient to warrant obtaining an IVP, can also be assumed to be in this category. The goal of therapy is to minimize symptoms in these patients with the fewest side effects and least expense. Of course, one should revise the approach to treat more aggressively and obtain or repeat a work-up if such a patient develops persistent infection with urea-splitting or other unusual organisms, severe pyelonephritis, or any other complicating features.

Evidence suggests that several approaches effectively decrease the number of recurrent UTIs. Fifty milligrams of nitrofurantoin or 250 mg of penicillin G taken postcoitally usually prevents infection.[60] In a study of nitrofurantoin, 50 mg given as daily prophylaxis, only 15% of patients had recurrences of bacteriuria, as opposed to 80% of patients taking placebo.[61] An advantage of nitrofurantoin is low systemic concentrations and absorption by the small bowel, which minimize the likelihood of developing resistant colonic bacteria.[62] Using low doses and assuming normal renal function to excrete the drug, there are few dose-related side effects; however, multiple adverse effects, including chronic interstitial pneumonitis and allergic reactions, blood dyscrasias, neuropathies, and liver damage, are reported in patients taking long-term therapy.

Sulfisoxazole (Gantrisin) alters the fecal flora, possibly leading to a greater likelihood of infection with resistant organisms. Effective prophylaxis with less likelihood of colonization by resistant organisms is obtained with trimethoprim-sulfamethoxazole, 1 tablet taken at bedtime three times weekly.[63]

Self-administration of a single dose of trimethoprim-sulfamethoxazole (2 double-strength tablets) taken immediately at the onset of symptoms provides an alternative method for reducing morbidity in women with recurrent infections.[64] Although women in one study using this program experienced 2.2 infections per patient-year, as opposed to 0.2 episode per patient-year in women on daily trimethoprim-sulfamethoxazole prophylaxis, 30 of 35 such episodes responded to self-administered treatment.[64] No complications occurred in either group. Some increased numbers of trimethoprim-sulfamethoxazole–resistant *E. coli* were noted in women on daily prophylaxis.

Choice of a treatment strategy is probably best determined by the expected number of recurrent UTIs, as predicted from the patient's past experience. Self-administered single-dose treatment may be best for women with infrequent recurrences who have been shown to respond to this therapy. Postcoital prophylaxis may be best for women whose infections clearly recur in this setting. Those experiencing a cluster of recent infections can be treated by low-dose prophylaxis for several months, and those whose history indicates the likelihood of multiple recurrences within a single year may benefit from 6 months or more of low-dose prophylaxis.

Treatment of asymptomatic bacteriuria in otherwise normal women is not of long-term benefit,[6] with two exceptions. The first is pregnancy, in which there is a definite risk of pyelonephritis associated with bacteriuria,[65] in addition to concern that placental growth may be retarded in the presence of untreated bacteriuria.[66, 67] The second is when bacteriuria develops following use of an indwelling catheter, for example, postoperatively. This occurs in about one half of patients catheterized for more than 6 days and often does not resolve without a course of therapy, even after removal of the catheter.[68]

Chronic bacteriuria is common in aged persons of both sexes and may be associated with use of condom catheters in men.[76] Though these persons have a high mortality, this probably reflects their underlying debility and is not prevented by treatment of the bacteriuria.[77] One must be alert to the possibility of gram-negative sepsis caused by UTI, which may cause unexplained deterioration in an aged person without producing high fever, chills, dysuria, or other recognizable features; however, to date antimicrobial prophylaxis has not been shown to effectively sterilize the urine in incontinent nursing home residents and in other debilitated aged persons.[76]

Men with Recurrent Infections

Since organisms generally are harbored within the prostate rather than reinfecting the urine via the urethra, reinfection with new, resistant bacteria should occur less frequently in men; thus, it should be possible to prevent active infection by continuous use of any of a variety of agents to which an organism is sensitive. In the United States Public Health Service Study of prophylaxis with sulfamethizole, nitrofurantoin, or methenamine mandelate, the number of clinically manifested episodes was reduced by half.[69] Progressive renal failure was infrequent, occurring in only 5 of 249 men with recurrent or persistent bacteriuria who were followed for up to 10 years, three with complicating calculous disease or obstructive uropathy, and two with concomitant noninfectious renal problems that may have explained the outcomes.[69]

Trimethoprim-sulfamethoxazole, doxycycline, and the quinolones achieve effective concentrations within the prostate and are useful against gram-negative bacilli. Six to 12 weeks of therapy with one of these agents might prevent future infections by eradicating organisms from the prostate. However, relapse with the same organism has occurred in about half of patients treated for 12 weeks with trimethoprim-sulfamethoxazole.[70, 71] A reasonable strategy employs short-term therapy to treat sporadic infections, a trial of 6 to 12 weeks of treatment for those with recurrences, and longer-term prophylaxis plus consideration of surgery for those whose recurrences are associated with bladder outlet obstruction and post-voiding residual urine.

Patients with Complications

There is a potential for renal compromise when pyelonephritis occurs in the setting of calculi, obstruction, or high-grade vesicoureteral reflux. Such cases are difficult to treat with long-term prophylaxis because of the likelihood of selecting resistant organisms. In addition, when renal failure supervenes, antimicrobials are less concentrated in the urine, and drug toxicity (particularly with nitrofurantoin or methenamine mandelate) may result from cumulative doses of agents excreted chiefly in the urine. Thus, when the indications are clear, the first approach for patients with complications is correction of urologic abnormalities. Examples include struvite calculi, ureteropelvic junctional or other obstruction, bilateral high-grade reflux, or prostatic hypertrophy with a large volume of residual urine or dilated upper tracts.

In some patients, the indications for surgery are not so clear, particularly if only one kidney is involved and the other remains normal. Some examples include nonobstructing calcium oxalate calculi, mild reflux, and prostatism with small-to-moderate residual urine. Prophylaxis, using trimethoprim-sulfamethoxazole[62] or another agent, given for 6 months or longer, depending on the underlying condition, seems reasonable in these cases. Indications for surgery may be reconsidered if there is growth of a stone or progressive parenchymal damage on follow-up IVP.

In another group of patients, infections are complicated by anatomic or functional defects or massive residual urine volumes that are not reconstructable and prevent permanent eradication of infection. Examples include patients with neurogenic bladders or extensive radiation damage. In principle, one should avoid continuous antimicrobial prophylaxis in such patients to avoid selecting resistant organisms that pose a greater hazard to the patient. Treatment with bactericidal antibiotics can be reserved for symptomatic episodes.

Methenamine mandelate is sometimes useful in difficult cases. This drug decomposes to liberate formaldehyde and achieves bacteriostatic and bactericidal concentrations (> 10 μg/ml and > 28 μg/ml, respectively) at a urine pH of less than 6. Bacterial resistance is rare, and it is effective against gram-positive cocci and *Pseudomonas* species.[72] Methenamine mandelate may be most useful in patients with large residual urine volumes and less effective in those with indwelling Foley catheters,[72, 73] but unfortunately fails to prevent bacteriuria in half or more of patients with either problem.[72, 73] It should not be given in conjunction with sulfonamides and may produce metabolic acidosis in patients whose serum creatinine is more than 2 mg/dl.[72]

When the patient has an indwelling catheter, maintenance of sterile, closed drainage with nonobstructed, "downhill" flow rather than antimicrobial agents is emphasized.[68, 74] High infection rates are most closely correlated with disconnections of the catheter junctions but are not influenced, except adversely through selecting resistant organisms, by irrigations with antibiotics.[75] Infection of the catheter bag may be prevented by careful technique in the short term but almost always occurs in patients requiring chronic drainage; such patients may benefit from a program of intermittent self-catheterization when feasible.

REFERENCES

1. Stamm WE, Counts GW, Running KR, et al: Diagnosis of coliform infection in acutely dysuric women. N Engl J Med 307:463, 1982.
2. Stamm WE, Wagner KF, Ansel R, et al: Causes of acute urethritis syndrome in women. N Engl J Med 303:409, 1980.
3. Stamm WE, Running K, McKevitt M, et al: Treatment of the acute urethral syndrome. N Engl J Med 304:956, 1981.
4. Komaroff AL: Medical Progress: Acute dysuria in women. N Engl J Med 310:368, 1984.
5. Kunin CM: Asymptomatic bacteriuria. Annu Rev Med 17:383, 1966.
6. Asscher AW, Sussman M, Waters WE, et al: The clinical significance of asymptomatic bacteriuria in the non-pregnant woman. J Infect Dis 120:17, 1967.
7. Gillenwater JW, Harrison RB, and Kunin CM: Natural history of bacteriuria in school girls. N Engl J Med 301:396, 1979.
8. Stamey TA: Urinary Tract Infections. Baltimore, Williams & Wilkins, 1972.
9. Waters WE: Prevalence of symptoms of urinary tract infection in women. Br J Prev Soc Med 23:263, 1969.
10. Stamm WE: Measurement of pyuria and its relation to bacteriuria. Am J Med 75:53, 1983.
11. Gallagher DJA, Montgomerie JZ, and North JD: Acute infections of the urinary tract: The urethral syndrome in general practice. BMJ 1:622, 1965.
12. O'Grady FW, Charlton CAC, Fry IK, et al: *In* Bumfitt W and Asscher AW (eds): Urinary Tract Infections. New York, Oxford University Press, 1973, pp 81–91.
13. Little PJ and DeWardener HE: Acute pyelonephritis; Incidence of reinfection in 100 patients. Lancet 2:1277, 1966.
14. Parker J and Kunin CM: Pyelonephritis in young women. A 10–20 year follow-up. JAMA 224:585, 1973.
15. Kunin CM, Polyak F, and Postel E: Periurethral bacterial flora in women: Prolonged intermittent colonization with *Escherichia coli.* JAMA 243:134, 1980.
16. Schechter H, Leonard CD, and Scribner BH: Chronic pyelonephritis as a cause of renal failure in dialysis candidates. JAMA 216:514, 1971.
17. Rubin RH, Tolkoff-Rubin NE, and Cotran RS: Urinary tract infection, pyelonephritis, and reflux nephropathy. *In* Brenner BM and Rector FC (eds): The Kidney. Philadelphia, WB Saunders, 1991, pp 1369–1429.
18. Filly RA, Friedland GW Govan DE, et al: Urinary tract infections in children. II: Roentgenologic aspects. West J Med 121:374, 1974.
19. Fair WR, Govan DE, Friedland GW, et al: Urinary tract infec-

tions in children. I: Young girls with nonrefluxing ureters. West J Med 121:366, 1974.
20. Govan DE, Fair WR, Friedland GW, et al: Urinary tract infections in children. III: Treatment of ureterovesical reflux. West J Med 121:382, 1974.
21. Stamey TA, Govan DE, and Palmer JM: The localization and treatment of urinary tract infections: The role of bactericidal urine levels as opposed to serum levels. Medicine 44:1, 1965.
22. Mundt KA and Polk BF: Localizing urinary tract infections by detecting antibody-coated bacteria in urinary sediment. Lancet 4:1172, 1979.
23. Fang LST, Tolkoff-Rubin NE, and Rubin RH: Efficacy of single-dose and conventional amoxicillin therapy in urinary-tract infection localized by the antibody-coated bacteria technique. N Engl J Med 298:413, 1978.
24. Rubin RH, Fang LST, Jones SR, et al: Single-dose amoxicillin therapy for urinary tract infection: Multicenter trial using antibody-coated bacteria localization technique. JAMA 244:561, 1980
25. Senoh K, Iwatsubo E, Momos ES, et al: Nonobstructive vesicoureteral reflux in adults: Value of conservative treatment. J Urol 117:566, 1977.
26. Amar AD, Singer B, Lewis R, et al: Vesicoureteral reflux in adults: A twelve-year study of 122 patients. Urology 3:184, 1974.
27. Buckley RM Jr, McGuckin M, and MacGregor RR: Urine bacterial counts after sexual intercourse. N Engl J Med 298:321, 1978.
28. Latham RH, Running K, and Stamm WE: Urinary tract infections in young adult women caused by *Staphylococcus saprophyticus.* JAMA 250:3063, 1983.
29. Komaroff AL, Pass TM, McCue JD, et al: Management strategies for urinary and vaginal infections. Arch Intern Med 138:1069, 1978.
30. Curran JW: Gonorrhea and the uretheral syndrome. Sex Transm Dis 4:119, 1977.
31. Komaroff AL and Friedland G: The dysuria-pyuria syndrome. N Engl J Med 303:452, 1980.
32. Berg AO, Heidrich FE, and Finn SD: Establishing the cause of genitourinary symptoms in women in a family practice: Comparison of clinical examination and comprehensive microbiology. JAMA 251:620, 1984.
33. Bailey RR and Abbott GD: Treatment of urinary tract infection with a single dose of amoxicillin. Nephron 18:316, 1977.
34. Bailey RR and Abbott GD: Treatment of urinary tract infection with a single dose of trimethoprim-sulfamethoxazole. Can Med Assoc J 118:551, 1978.
35. Ronald AR, Boutros P, and Mourtada H: Bacteriuria localization and response to single-dose therapy in women. JAMA 235:1854, 1976.
36. Fang LS, Tolkoff-Rubin NE, and Rubin RH: Localization and antibiotic management of urinary tract infection. Annu Rev Med 30:225, 1979.
37. Carlson KJ and Mulley AG: Management of acute dysuria. A decision-analysis model of alternative strategies. Ann Intern Med 102:244, 1985.
38. Hooton TM, Running K, and Stamm WE: Single-dose therapy for cystitis in women. A comparison of trimethoprim-sulfamethoxazole, amoxicillin, and cyclacillin. JAMA 253:387, 1985.
39. Schultz HJ, McCaffrey LA, and Keys TF: Acute cystitis: A prospective study of laboratory tests and duration of therapy. Mayo Clin Proc 59:391, 1984.
40. Winickoff RN, Wilner SI, Gall G, et al: Urine culture after treatment of uncomplicated cystitis in women. South Med J 74:165, 1981.
41. Kanel KT, Kroboth FJ, Schwentker FN, et al: Role of intravenous urography in patients with acute pyelonephritis. Arch Intern Med 148:2144. 1988.
42. Tolkoff-Rubin NE and Rubin RH: Ciprofloxin in management of urinary infections. Urology 31:359, 1988.
43. Byrd L and Sherman RL: Radiocontrast-induced acute renal failure: A clinical and pathophysiologic review. Medicine 58:270, 1979.
44. Hartman GW, Hatery RR, and Witten DM: Mortality during excretory urography: Mayo Clinic experience. Am J Radiol 139:919, 1982.
45. Linos A, Gray J, Orvis A, et al: Low dose radiation and leukemia. N Engl J Med 302:1101, 1980.
46. Stewart A and Kneale GW: Radiation dose effects in relation to obstetric x-rays and childhood cancers. Lancet 1:1185, 1970.
47. Bross ID and Natarajan N: Genetic damage from diagnostic radiation. JAMA 237:2399, 1977.
48. Engel G, Schaeffer AJ, Grayhack JT, et al: The role of excretory urography and cystoscopy in the evaluation and management of women with recurrent urinary tract infections. J Urol 123:190, 1980.
49. Fair WR, McClennan BL, and Jost RG: Are excretory urograms necessary in evaluating women with urinary tract infections? J Urol 121:313, 1979.
50. Fowler JE Jr and Pulaski ET: Excretory urography, cystography and cystoscopy in the evaluation of women with urinary tract infection: A prospective study. N Engl J Med 304:462, 1981.
51. O'Hanley P, Low D, Romero I, et al: Gal-gel binding and hemolysin phenotypes and genotypes associated with uropathogenic *Escherichia coli.* N Engl J Med 313:414, 1985.
52. Torres VE, Velosa JA, Holley KE, et al: The progression of vesicoureteral reflux nephropathy. Ann Intern Med 92:776, 1980.
53. Edwards D, Normand CS, Prescod N, et al: Disappearance of vesicoureteric reflux during long-term prophylaxis of urinary tract infections in children. BMJ 2:285, 1977.
54. Scott JES: Management of ureteric reflux in children. Br J Urol 49:109, 1977.
55. Claessen I and Lindberg U: Asymptomatic bacteriuria in school girls. VII: Followup study of urinary tract in treated and untreated school girls with asymptomatic bacteriuria. Radiology 124:179, 1977.
56. Sanford JP: Urinary tract symptoms and infections. Annu Rev Med 26:485, 1975.
57. Graham JB, King LR, Kropp RA, et al: The significance of distal urethral narrowing in young girls. J Urol 97:1045, 1967.
58. Kaplan GW, Sammons TA, and King LR: A blind comparison of dilatation, urethrotomy and medication alone in the treatment of urinary tract infection in girls. J Urol 109:917, 1973.
59. Busch R, Huland H, Kollermann MW, et al: Does internal urethrotomy influence susceptibility to recurrent urinary tract infection? Urology 20:134, 1982.
60. Vosti KL: Recurrent urinary tract infections and prevention by prophylactic antibiotics after sexual intercourse. JAMA 231:934, 1975.
61. Bailey RR, Roberts AP, Gower PE, et al: Prevention of urinary tract infection with low dose nitrofurantoin. Lancet 2:1112, 1971.
62. Stamey TA, Condy M, and Mihara G: Prophylactic efficacy of nitrofurantoin macrocrystals and trimethoprim-sulfamethoxazole in urinary infections: Biologic effects on the vaginal and rectal flora. N Engl J Med 296:780, 1977.
63. Harding GKM, Buckwold FJ, Marrie TJ, et al: Prophylaxis of recurrent urinary tract infection in female patients: Efficacy of low-dose thrice weekly therapy with trimethoprim-sulfamethoxazole. JAMA 242:1975, 1979.
64. Wong ES, McKevitt M, Running K, et al: Management of recurrent urinary tract infections with patient-administered single-dose therapy. Ann Intern Med 102:302, 1985.
65. Whalley PJ: Bacteriuria of pregnancy. Am J Obstet Gynecol 97:723, 1967.
66. Naeye RL: Causes of the excessive rates of perinatal mortality and prematurity in pregnancies complicated by maternal urinary tract infections. N Engl J Med 300:819, 1979.
67. Zinner SH: Bacteriuria and babies revisited (Editorial). N Engl J Med 300:853, 1979.
68. Islam AKMS and Chapman J: Closed catheter drainage and urinary infection: Comparison of two methods of catheter drainage. Br J Urol 49:215, 1977.
69. Freeman RB, Smith WM, Richardson JA, et al: Long-term therapy for chronic bacteriuria in men: U. S. Public Health Service Cooperative Study. Ann Intern Med 83:133, 1975.
70. Meares EM: Prostatitis: A review. Urol Clin North Am 2:3, 1975.
71. Smith JW, Jones SR, Reed WP, et al: Recurrent urinary tract

infections in men: Characteristics and response to therapy. Ann Intern Med 91:544, 1979.
72. Kevorkicin CG, Merritt JL, and Ilstrup DM: Methenamine mandelate with acidification: An effective urinary antiseptic in patients with neurogenic bladder. Mayo Clin Proc 59:523, 1984.
73. Nilsson S: Long-term treatment with methenamine hippurate in recurrent urinary tract infection. Acta Med Scand 198:81, 1975.
74. Stamm WE: Guidelines for prevention of catheter-associated urinary tract infections. Ann Intern Med 82:386, 1975.
75. Warren JW, Platt R, Thomas RJ, et al: Antibiotic irrigation and catheter-associated urinary tract infections. N Engl J Med 299:570, 1978.
76. Freedman LR: Urinary-tract infection in the elderly (Editorial). N Engl J Med 309:1451, 1983.
77. Nicolle LE, Bjornson J, Harding GKM, et al: Bacteriuria in elderly institutionalized men. N Engl J Med 309:1420, 1983.

33

Prostatitis, Epididymitis, and Testicular Enlargement

KEVIN R. LOUGHLIN, MD
WILLET F. WHITMORE II, MD

Infection and inflammation of the prostate gland and epididymis are common disorders. Although easy to diagnose, they nevertheless represent some of the least understood and most difficult to treat of the nonmalignant urologic diseases. Despite considerable research data, establishing the precise etiology and instituting effective therapy are all too frequently a lesson in frustration for both the patient and the physician. The principles of successful treatment of these entities include isolation of the infectious organism when possible, treatment with the appropriate drug, and recognition of other disorders that may mimic these conditions.

PROSTATITIS

Prostatitis is an inflammatory process that involves the prostatic acini and surrounding stroma.[1, 2] It can occur either focally or diffusely within the gland, which accounts for some of the variety and variability of clinical symptoms. It presents as either a systemic febrile illness from prostatic sepsis or a localized inflammatory process without systemic manifestations. The less common acute form is invariably caused by bacterial invasion. Subacute or chronic prostatitis, although frequently the result of bacterial infection, includes many cases in which no agent is identified and the etiology remains obscure. Fungi, viruses, T strain *Mycoplasma, Chlamydia trachomatis, Ureaplasma urealyticum, Trichomonas vaginalis,* allergy, autoimmunity, and psychologic factors have all been implicated in the etiology of cases that clinically come under the heading of nonbacterial prostatitis.[3, 4] Age is no barrier to the development of any form of prostatitis, once puberty is reached.

Since the clinical presentation, treatment, and implications of acute and chronic prostatitis are quite different, they are discussed separately.

Acute Prostatitis

Acute prostatitis is a febrile illness that is accompanied by urinary tract infection and bacteremia. It is an uncommon disease and is usually associated with obstructing urethral abnormalities distal to the prostate. Acute prostatic infection may be hematogenous or may occur as a result of ascent of bacteria up the urethra. It infrequently progresses to chronic prostatitis but is often the result of an acute exacerbation of chronic bacterial prostatitis in the elderly patient. The diagnosis may not be made immediately because of the difficulty of distinguishing it from other forms of acute urinary tract infections. This is especially true in paraplegic patients. The treatment is aggressive medical management with urinary drainage, if appropriate. Antibiotics are the mainstay of treatment. The acutely inflamed prostate should be palpated gently in order to avoid inducing sepsis by excessive manipulation of the gland.

Most patients with acute prostatitis have symptoms and signs that clearly localize the process to the urinary tract. In the neurologically intact patient, the key diagnostic findings are exquisite prostatic tenderness accompanied by prostatic enlargement. Systematic gathering of appropriate data then dictates the subsequent steps to be taken in the diagnosis and management. The complete blood count (CBC) will show an elevated white blood cell count with a left shift. Electrolyte and blood urea nitrogen (BUN) values are usually normal, indicating that the urinary obstruction, if present, is acute. The urinalysis will show many white blood cells and bacteria. A Gram stain of the spun sediment usually, but not always, reveals the offending organism, allowing the clinician to differentiate between gram-positive and gram-negative infections. Then, after blood and urine cultures are obtained, broad-spectrum parenteral antibiotic coverage should be started immediately. If no organisms are seen, coverage for both gram-positive and gram-negative organisms should be maintained until culture results are available. It is important to begin parenteral antibiotics as soon as possible, since the poorly drained, edematous prostatic acini and ducts predispose their patients to bacteremia and septic shock. Hospitalization is indicated in most acute cases.

In patients with an obvious bladder outlet obstruction, as determined by history or physical examination, the bladder must be drained prior to further studies. This reduces hydrostatic pressure on the prostatic ducts and aids their drainage, as well as preventing ascending infection with pyelonephritis and its complications. If the bladder is not distended and the patient is voiding without difficulty, no manipulation is required. When a history of difficult voiding accompanies palpable bladder fullness, a urologist should be consulted regarding the preferred method of drainage. Placement of a urethral catheter, although it may be utilized in some of these patients, is not usually the best choice for bladder drainage, since passage of a catheter through an inflamed prostatic urethra and the presence of a foreign body may aggravate the inflammatory process. In most cases, a cystostomy tube should be placed, which usually can be done expeditiously by the percutaneous route using local anesthesia.

An intravenous urogram (IVP), which should be performed as an emergency in severely septic patients, is obtained eventually in most individuals suspected of having acute prostatitis. This confirms that the bladder and upper urinary tracts are not obstructed as well as eliminates any unsuspected abnormalities that could require surgical intervention. Prostatic massage is absolutely contraindicated in these patients, since septic shock can result. However, frequent gentle rectal examinations should be done to confirm gradual resolution of the tenderness and edema of the prostate.

In some cases, the prostate is obviously asymmetric, and the patient fails to improve clinically. In these cases, a prostatic abscess has developed and surgical drainage, either by transperineal needle aspiration or by transurethral incision of the abscess, is required. These procedures for prostatic abscess generally do not require consideration in patients who are improving clinically. A prostatic abscess is an uncommon complication.

The common organisms causing acute prostatitis reflect the bowel flora. Therefore, parenteral broad-spectrum antibiotics with good gram-negative coverage are usually instituted as initial treatment until the sensitivities from blood and urine cultures are available. A cephalosporin is the drug of choice in patients with impaired renal function, whereas an aminoglycoside is the drug of choice in patients with normal kidney function.

Once the patient is no longer febrile and the acute swelling and tenderness of the prostate have resolved, a thorough urologic evaluation is warranted. Acute prostatitis is often associated with anatomic abnormalities like urethral stricture or with neurogenic bladder disease that causes elevated voiding pressures. A retrograde urethrogram (to detect an anterior urethral stricture), a voiding cystourethrogram (to discover a posterior urethral stricture), a cystometrogram (to uncover neurogenic bladder disease in the absence of anatomic abnormality), and a cystoscopic evaluation are usually obtained following successful therapy. The patient can then be managed according to what results are found.

Chronic Prostatitis

Subacute or chronic prostatitis is second only to venereal urethritis as the most common urologic problem in adult men. Although the population incidence is unknown, cases occur at approximately equal rates through adulthood, and the percentage of cases with proved bacterial etiology increases gradually with age.[1] The patients may be asymptomatic or may have perineal and voiding discomfort.

Typically, the patient with chronic prostatitis has irritative voiding symptoms. However, obstructive symptoms may also be prominent. In the young patient, prostatitis is often preceded by venereal urethritis and can be precipitated by an acquired urethral stricture. In the older patient, or the patient with longstanding disease, chronic inflammation may cause scarring with secondary bladder neck contracture ("median bar"), or obstruction may result from edema and congestion of a gland that is already somewhat enlarged from benign prostatic hyperplasia (BPH). Less typical presentations include gross hematuria, and the septic complications of chronic bacterial prostatitis (*acute* pyelonephritis, cystitis, epididymitis, or prostatitis).

Current knowledge leads us to divide the disease into two subgroups: (1) bacterial prostatitis and (2) nonbacterial prostatitis. The treatment and prognosis are related to the etiology.

Bacterial prostatitis in the untreated patient is always accompanied by a urinary tract infection. The diagnosis is made by sequential urine collections (as is described) after infection has been cleared from the rest of the urinary tract with antibiotics. The organisms involved are gram-negative rods in more than 90% of cases.[2] Bacterial prostatitis responds clinically to appropriate antibiotic therapy in most cases, but usually the infection is not completely eradicated. Prolonged suppressive antibiotic therapy may be required to prevent recurrent symptoms and the complications of acute urinary tract infection.[2]

Nonbacterial prostatitis cannot be distinguished by history or physical examination from bacterial prostatitis. However, the result of the urine culture at initial presentation (before antibiotics have been taken) is negative. The

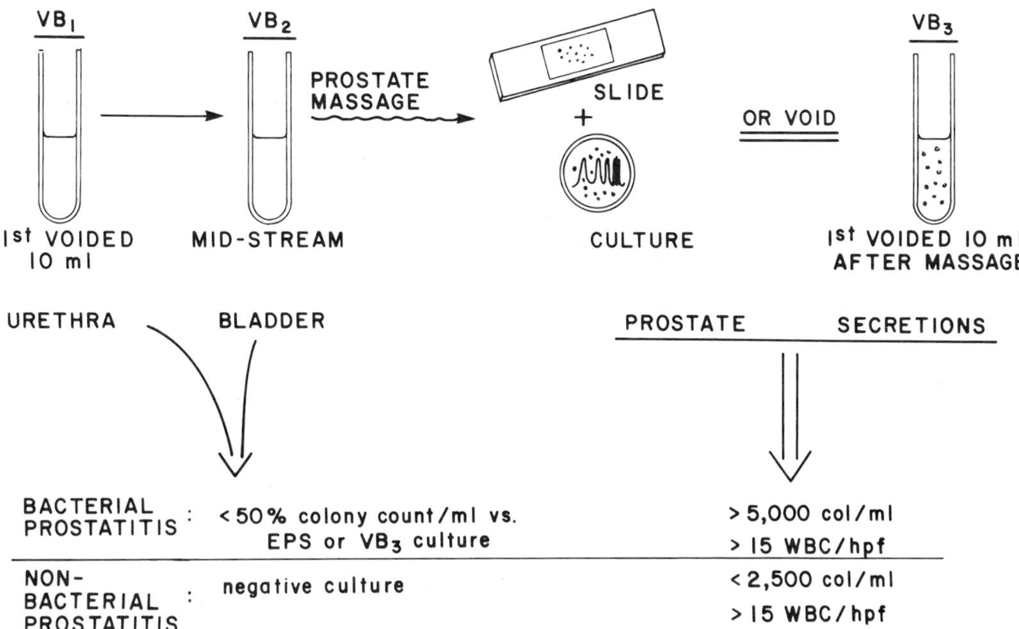

FIGURE 33–1. Diagnostic criteria for prostatitis. The diagnosis of prostatitis is made by showing pus cells in significant numbers in the secretions expressed by prostate massage. Culture of these secretions differentiates bacterial from nonbacterial prostatitis.

diagnosis is made by demonstrating increased numbers of white blood cells in the prostatic fraction of voided urine and by ascertaining the clinical history. The natural history, the incidence of recurrence following treatment, and the long-term sequelae of this disease have not been elucidated because of the lack of a precise definition and the apparent multiple and obscure etiologies. However, recent data on patients with so-called nonspecific urethritis have shown that about half of these patients actually have a *Chlamydia trachomatis* infection.[3] This information suggests that many cases of nonbacterial prostatitis are also probably caused by this difficult-to-culture agent. The usual clinical course of this disease, unless successfully treated with antibiotics or amebicides, is several months to years of remissions and exacerbations of symptoms, with subsequent complete recovery.

Any patient who has had recurrent episodes of prostatitis should be evaluated radiologically (e.g., by IVP and urethrogram) and cystoscopically to rule out any anatomic abnormalities. Other causes are also possible, including psychogenic and possibly "prostatodynia" due to disorders of innervation of the gland.[5] True prostatitis is usually accompanied by the presence of white blood cells in the prostatic secretions and by irritative voiding symptoms in addition to pelvic and perineal discomfort.

Diagnosis. The evaluation in every patient with prostatitis begins with a history, physical examination, microscopic analysis, and culture of the urine if it appears infected.

When the tentative diagnosis is urinary tract infection with chronic prostatitis, a culture of the urine should be obtained and the patient should be started on an antibiotic that will cover the common gram-negative enteric organisms that are usually responsible for urinary infections. The patient is told to return after at least 1 week of appropriate antimicrobial therapy for further evaluation. The most important point to be made regarding the initial evaluation of such a patient is that attempts to obtain prostatic secretions by prostate massage are deferred. If a urinalysis shows probable infection, prostatic massage without antibiotic coverage may result in septicemia. In addition, identifying the prostate as the source of the urinary infection can be done only when there is no active infection elsewhere in the urinary tract.

When the patient returns after a course of antibiotics and if the initial result of the culture was indeed positive, the urine specimens should be collected according to the techniques developed by Meares to localize the infectious process (Fig. 33–1).[2] If the result of the urine culture was negative or initial urinalysis was negative, prostatic secretions should also be examined to confirm the diagnosis.

The patient is instructed to prepare himself and to collect the first 10 ml of urine (VB_1) and then the usual midstream specimen (VB_2) (see Fig. 33–1). A rectal examination is then performed with prostatic massage. If enough prostatic secretions are expressed (EPS) to obtain culture and microscopic analysis, then this is sufficient. If minimal or no secretions are obtained, the patient is instructed to collect the first 10 ml of voided urine following massage (VB_3). This specimen has been shown to be an approximately 1/100 diluting of prostatic secretions.[2] If bacterial prostatitis is suspected, each specimen is sent promptly for culture, and the sediment is examined microscopically. If nonbacterial prostatitis is suspected, a culture is obtained only on EPS or VB_3 specimens.

The diagnosis of chronic prostatitis is made primarily on the basis of increased numbers of white blood cells (> 15 white blood cells per high-power field [hpf]) in the EPS or VB_3 specimens. Most normal persons have less than 2 white blood cells per hpf in prostatic secretions.[6] Irritative voiding symptoms or a tender prostate on rectal examination are nonspecific findings, although when all other causes of such findings have been excluded the diagnosis of prostatitis is usually invoked.

A specific organism is implicated as the causative agent if more than 5000 colonies/ml are found in the EPS or VB_c specimen and less than half that number in other specimens.[2] If the patient has bacterial urethritis, then the VB_1

specimen will yield the highest count. If all the counts are below 5000 colonies/ml, the examination should be repeated. In most cases, the organism will be gram-negative. *Escherichia coli* (in most cases), *Klebsiella, Proteus* species, and *Pseudomonas* are the usual organisms encountered. *Streptococcus faecalis* (enterococcus) and *Staphylococcus saprophyticus* are the only gram-positive organisms commonly found. Other gram-positive organisms can cause prostatitis, but their presence in low colony counts in normal individuals has implicated them as normal urethral flora in most cases.[2] Aggressive treatment for these organisms is indicated only if they are definitely localized to the prostate and are present in significant numbers.

When no organism is found and the white blood cell count is not greatest in the urethral or prostatic fluid, urinary tuberculosis and in situ carcinoma of the bladder or prostate should be considered in the differential diagnosis, especially in the older patient. These diseases commonly present irritative voiding symptoms because they stimulate an inflammatory submucosal reaction in the bladder. When the result of the tuberculin test is positive, tuberculous prostatitis or cystitis is best ruled out by serial urine cultures. Carcinoma in situ is most easily diagnosed by urine cytology. A PPD, urine cytology, IVP cystometrogram, and cystoscopy should be obtained in all patients who have irritative voiding symptoms that are inadequately explained by the clinical findings.

Bacterial invasion of the urinary tract in men, with the exception of gonococcal venereal urethritis, is uncommon at any age. Although statistics are not available, chronic bacterial prostatitis is thought to be the most common cause of relapsing urinary tract infection in adult men.[2] Because chronic bacterial prostatitis is a sufficient explanation for infection, patients with this diagnosis may be treated and followed without urologic evaluation unless persistent infection, frequent recurrences, or complications such as acute prostatitis epididymitis, or pyelonephritis develop. In men whose bacterial infection does not localize to the prostate, a significant urinary tract pathologic condition, such as a congenital abnormality causing urinary stasis or obstruction, stones, or tumor, must be ruled out. For this reason an IVP with voiding cystourethrogram and cystoscopy are indicated in these patients.

Treatment. The major therapeutic modalities for chronic prostatitis are: (1) specific antibiotic therapy, which is effective when a responsible organism is identified; (2) general symptomatic measures, which may be the only effective treatment for patients in whom a specific organism is not found; and (3) surgery, which should be offered to patients with extremely intractable symptoms or in whom prostatic obstruction is progressive.

Specific antibiotic therapy is initially directed at the acute cystitis and irritative symptoms that characterize the clinical presentation of bacterial prostatitis. When this acute infection has been controlled and the prostate has been shown to be the source of the infecting organism, a 4- to 6-week course of antibiotics may be sufficient to cure the patient.[2] However, most patients have a relapse within 12 months, and therefore the indefinite continuation of some form of suppressive therapy has been advocated.[1, 2] The chronically infected prostate has proved to be very resistant to sterilization because of the inability of most antibiotics to achieve therapeutic concentrations in the prostatic acini and ducts, where the organisms reside. Thus, the prostate serves as a reservoir of pathogenic bacteria. Experiments done in dogs and clinical experience in humans suggest that only antibiotics with lipid solubility reach therapeutic concentrations in prostatitic fluid.[2] Experimentally, only erythomycins, lipid-soluble tetracyclines (doxycycline), sulfa drugs, trimethroprim, and the quinolines fulfill these requirements.[1, 2] Of these compounds, the sulfa-trimethroprim combination provides good coverage of the gram-negative bacilli that are found in most cases of bacterial prostatitis and has been the standard therapy. When the organism involved is sensitive, the symptomatic response to therapy is gratifying in 80 to 90% of patients.[2] Preliminary results indicate that 15 to 25% will have the infection completely eradicated and that an additional 70% will be systematically improved.[2] The duration of therapy used in achieving these results varied from 2 to 12 weeks. In the 70 to 80% of patients whose organisms are not eradicated, a relapse of acute infection may be expected within 12 months.[2] Sulfa compounds, the sulfa-trimethoprim combination in suppressive doses, or urinary antiseptics such as methenamine mandelate or methenamine hippurate are used for long-term therapy for the prevention of recurrent acute infections in these patients. These agents are less likely to encourage the development of resistant organisms.

When no responsible agent is identified (nonbacterial prostatitis), it is current practice to prescribe a trial of therapy with tetracycline (500 mg four times daily) or doxycycline (100 mg twice daily) for 3 weeks. In these doses, tetracycline is effective against *Chlamydia trachomatis, Neisseria gonorrhoeae,* and T strain *Mycoplasma.* Such therapeutic trials are warranted in practice when special culture techniques for the isolation of these organisms are unavailable or unreliable.[3] If the patient has a good response to tetracycline and has a steady female partner, she should be treated as well because of the 70% incidence of cervical *Chlamydia* in patients with infected male partners.[3] An empiric course of metronidazole is also worth trying if antibiotics fail, since prostatitis cause by *Trichomonas* may be difficult to diagnose and some of these patients will have a good symptomatic response.

The fluoroquinolones have now also achieved wide application in the treatment of infections of the urinary tract, including prostatitis and epididymitis. The quinolones are excreted primarily by the kidneys, and laboratory studies have documented urinary levels of the quinolones that significantly exceed the minimal inhibitory concentrations (MICs) for sensitive or intermediate strains of gram-positive or gram-negative organisms.[7]

Animal studies, using a canine model, have also demonstrated relatively high prostate fluid/plasma concentrations for all the quinolones tested.[8–11] Because of this ability to achieve high prostatic fluid drug levels, quinolones are becoming increasingly popular for use in the treatment of bacterial prostatitis. In addition ofloxacin, norfloxacin, ciprofloxacin, and lomefloxacin have been shown to be efficacious in the treatment of *C. trachomatis* and *U. urealyticum.* Therefore, the quinolones have become an important option in the treatment of acute and chronic prostatitis as well as sexually transmitted diseases due to chlamydia or ureaplasma. The recommended doses for the treatment of prostatitis and other infections of the urinary tract are as follows: ofloxacin 200 to 400 mg twice daily, norfloxacin 400 mg twice daily, ciprofloxacin 250 to 500 mg twice daily, and lomefloxacin 400 mg once daily.

If antibiotic therapy fails, general symptomatic measures should be offered for relief. Avoiding the intake of substances that have produced prostatic irritation in the given patient is generally recommended. Sitz baths are most useful for the patient with nagging perineal discomfort or low back pain. An increase in sexual activity may add long-term benefit by providing physiologic prostatic drainage. Finally, oral antispasmodic agents such as imipramine, oxybutynin, propantheline bromide (Pro-banthine), flavoxate, hyoscyamine, and phenoxybenzamine can provide excellent relief from urinary frequency and urgency. Virtually all patients experience some measure of relief with minimal side effects if one or more of these agents are used appropriately.[1] It remains unproved whether prostatic massage accomplishes significant mechanical drainage of otherwise entrapped infected material in the prostatic ducts. In addition, frequent prostatic massage is a double-edged sword, since it itself produces prostatic inflammation.

Most patients with nonbacterial prostatitis experience transient symptomatic response to the antibiotics and symptomatic measures just described. Both the patient and the physician are frequently misled by spontaneous exacerbations and remissions of symptoms. In this setting, the patient often becomes dissatisfied with treatment and may go from one physician to another, only to have the treatment cycle repeated. The best way to manage these patients is to allow them to participate in the manipulation of therapy for symptomatic relief while assuring them that the syndrome is usually self-limited. Using a cooperative, aggressive approach enhances compliance and successful treatment of this frustrating disease.

Surgery is reserved for the rare patient who is truly crippled by his symptoms or when prostatic obstruction is the most prominent manifestation in elderly individuals with concomitant BPH or those with postinflammatory bladder neck contractures. The degree of obstruction in such cases can be documented by an IVP, uroflow test, and cystoscopy.

The choices of surgery are radical or simple prostatectomy. If the indication for surgery is refractory infection of the gland, one may perform radical prostatectomy, but this is a major operation and it produces impotence in many patients. For this reason, and because most patients respond to antimicrobials, radical prostatectomy is rarely employed for this indication. Simple prostatectomy with enucleation of the periurethral glands either by open surgery or by transurethral resection (TUR) is the operation usually performed. However, because this lesser procedure does not remove all the prostatic glands, potentially infected tissue is left behind.

In most cases, the indication for surgery is significant bladder outlet obstruction. A TUR is the procedure of choice for those who have a small prostate or inflammatory bladder neck contracture ("median bar"). Open prostatectomy is favored for patients who have a large gland (> 30g) with persistent obstruction from a swollen, infected prostate per se. This approach is advocated because the larger gland is more completely removed by using the open technique and because a TUR has the theoretical potential of sealing off pockets of infection in the remaining tissue.

Few studies are available reviewing the surgical treatment of patients operated on for irritative symptoms alone. In one well-studied but carefully selected series of 32 patients who had a TUR for this indication, 93% with prostatitis of either type were cured or improved.[12] Others have reported cure rates of about 30% with the remaining 70% having symptoms and persistent infection unchanged from the preoperative state,[1, 2]

In a few cases (< 5%), a patient's symptoms can be aggravated by surgery. The number of patients with irritative symptoms who ultimately do require surgery is unknown. However, the number is small, since most urologists adhere rather strictly to the criteria that the symptoms must remain uncontrolled after a maximal trial of conservative therapy and that patients under the age of 45 years must undergo a psychological evaluation preoperatively.

EPIDIDYMITIS

Epididymitis may be either acute or chronic. In most cases, epididymitis is thought to be secondary to the reflux of sterile or infected urine up the ejaculatory ducts and vas into the epididymis. The infection may also reach the epididymis through the perivasal lymphatics.

Acute Epididymitis

Epididymitis often occurs following strenuous physical activity, such as lifting heavy objects. It may also occur after considerable sexual excitement, urethral instrumentation, or prostatectomy.[13] The patient usually has onset of rather sudden pain in the scrotum that may radiate along the spermatic cord and even reach the flank. The pain is often quite severe, and the epididymis is exquisitely sensitive and may be swollen. The infection usually spreads from the lower to the upper pole of the epididymis. The patient may be afebrile; or, the temperature may reach 40° C (104° F). Irritative voiding symptoms and urethral discharge may also be present. The tunica vaginalis often secretes serous fluid, and a reactive inflammatory hydrocele may be present. The testis can become swollen from passive congestion but rarely becomes involved in the inflammation. The overlying scrotal skin may be erythematous but should be freely movable. Skin that appears to be fixed to the underlying epididymis suggests an abscess. Laboratory findings usually include a leukocytosis. Urinalysis may identify bacteria; pyuria is usually (but not always) present.

Differential Diagnosis. Torsion of the testicle, torsion of the appendages of the testis or epididymis, testicular tumor, testicular trauma, and mumps orchitis may also present as an acute scrotal mass or swelling.

Torsion of the testicle occurs in children; less commonly it may be seen in men. If the torsion is a 180-degree torsion of the testicle, the epididymis will be palpated anterior to the testis. The affected testis may also be noted to be riding somewhat high in the scrotum compared with its unaffected partner. In contrast to epididymitis, the testis itself is markedly tender, but pyuria is usually absent. Prehn's sign may be helpful in differentiation: if pain is relieved when the scrotum is elevated, the pain is due to epididymitis; if pain is not relieved or increased, then torsion of the testicle is the more likely diagnosis. A radioisotope scan or Doppler study of testicular blood flow will also distinguish epididymitis from testicular torsion. Normal or increased blood flow suggests epididymitis, whereas decreased blood flow signifies torsion. If torsion cannot be ruled out, the testis should be explored.

Torsion of the appendages of the testis or epididymis occurs virtually exclusively in prepuberal boys. The appendages may become twisted, causing scrotal pain and swelling. At times, the necrotic appendage can be seen through the scrotal wall as the so-called "blue-dot" sign. The epididymis is not tender.

Testicular tumor is usually painless. However, because of simple mass effect or because of internal hemorrhage, there may be sudden distention of the the tunica albuginea that will cause pain. The mass usually can be palpated as separate from the epididymis, and the urinalysis will be normal. If doubt exists, a scrotal ultrasound study is helpful in differentiating a tumor from epididymis. If a testicular tumor cannot be ruled out, orchiectomy through an inguinal incision should be performed.

Mumps orchitis results in a swollen scrotum, which is

often bilateral. There is usually parotitis and an absence of urinary symptoms, and the result of urinalysis is normal.

Treatment. Analgesics and antipyretics should be used to control pain and fever. Scrotal elevation and support provide symptomatic relief. Empiric antibiotic treatment should be instituted pending urine culture results. In patients younger than 50 years of age, tetracycline is the drug of choice since *Chlamydia* is the most common infecting organism. In patients older than 50 years of age, coliforms are the most common cause of infection, and a sulfa-trimethoprim combination is the drug of choice. Hospitalization is necessary if the patient is septic. The quinolones are an acceptable treatment alternative in patients who do not respond to first-line antibiotic therapy with either tetracycline or sulfa-trimethoprim.

Almost all episodes of acute epididymitis resolve spontaneously or after oral antibiotic treatment for 2 to 3 weeks. It usually takes much longer for the epididymis to return to its normal size. Sterility secondary to epididymitis is rare, although it may occur in cases of bilateral disease.

Chronic Epididymitis

Chronic epididymitis may occur after repeated frequent episodes of acute epididymitis, or it may appear insidiously. The epididymis is indurated and enlarged. Microscopically, the tissues are infiltrated with lymphocytes and plasma cells. The epididymis may or may not be tender but is always thickened. The urinalysis result is usually negative, unless an associated prostatitis is present. Tuberculosis may result in a chronic epididymitis that is associated with "beading of the vas" and sterile pyuria. Tumors of the epididymis are extremely rare, although ultrasound may aid in their diagnosis.

Antibiotic therapy is not as effective in treating chronic epididymitis as it is in treating acute epididymitis. Anti-inflammatory agents such as ibuprofen are used routinely when antibiotics have failed. Injections of local anesthetic agents into the spermatic cord also have been used for pain relief with some success. In severe, refractory cases, epididymectomy may become necessary.

PAINLESS SCROTAL MASSES

The scrotal mass is often a cause of anxiety for the patient and the physician. A scrotal mass or palpable induration of the testis in a young man should be considered a cancer of the testicle until proved otherwise. The most important decision to be made on physical examination is whether the scrotal mass or induration is inside or outside the testicle. Intratesticular masses or induration are usually tumors, although testicular abscess or hematoma must be considered if the history is appropriate.

At times, a hydrocele that surrounds the testicle will be difficult to distinguish from an intratesticular lesion. Transillumination of the scrotum with a flashlight in a completely dark room is a useful way of confirming the presence of a hydrocele. However, if the hydrocele is so large that the testis itself cannot be palpated, a scrotal ultrasound study should be performed to rule out a testis tumor. Most extratesticular scrotal masses lie superior to the testis in the scrotum. A scrotal hernia will transilluminate and can usually be reduced. Bowel sounds can be auscultated through the scrotal wall. A varicocele usually appears in the left scrotum because of the difference in venous drainage between the left and right gonadal vein. An epididymal cyst or spermatocele can usually be distinguished as a mass separate from the testicle by palpation. If it is large, a spermatocele may transilluminate. Some spermatoceles may be mildly tender. If a secure diagnosis of any scrotal mass cannot be made by physical examination, then a scrotal ultrasound study should be obtained to further delineate the pathology.

REFERENCES

1. Drach GW: Prostatitis: Man's hidden infection. Urol Clin North Am 2:499, 1979.
2. Meares M: Prostatitis. Urol Clin North Am 2:3, 1975.
3. Schacter J: Chlamydia infections. N Engl J Med 298:428, 1978.
4. Brenner H, Weidner W, and Schiefer HG: Studies on the role of *Ureaplasma urealyticum* and *Mycoplasma hominis* in prostatitis. J Infect Dis 147:807, 1983.
5. Barbalias GA, Meares EM Jr, and Sant R: Prostatodynia—clinical and urodynamic characteristics. J Urol 130:514, 1983.
6. Schaeffer AJ, Wendel EF, Dunn JK, et al: Prevalence and significance of prostatic inflammation. J Urol 125:215, 1981.
7. Naber KG: Use of quinolones in urinary tract infections and prostatitis. Rev Infect Dis 2: (Suppl 5):256–272, 1989.
8. Madsen PO, Baumueller A, and Hoyme U: Experimental models for determination of antimicrobials in prostatic tissue, interstitial fluid and secretion. Scand J Infect Dis 14(Suppl):145–150, 1978.
9. Dorflinger T, Larsen EH, Gusser TC, and Madsen PO: The concentration of various quinolone derivatives in the dog prostate. *In* Weidner W, Brunner H, Krause W, and Rothause CF (eds): Therapy of Prostatitis. Munich, W. Zuckschwerdt, 1986, pp 35–39.
10. Gasser TC, Graversen PH, and Madsen PO: Fleroxacin (RO23-6240) distribution in canine prostatic tissue and fluids. Antimicrob Agents Chemother 31:1010–1013, 1987.
11. Stein GE and Saravolatz LD: Randomized clinical study of ofloxacin and doxycycline in the treatment of urethritis and cervicitis. Rev Infect Dis 2(Suppl 5):236, 1989.
12. Smart GJ and Jenkins JD: The role of transurethral prostatectomy in chronic prostatitis. Br J Urol 45:654, 1973.
13. Tanagho EA: Nonspecific infections of the urinary tract. *In* Smith DR (ed): General Urology. Los Altos, CA, Lange Medical Publications, 1981, pp 153–198.

34

Benign and Malignant Enlargement of the Prostate

KEVIN R. LOUGHLIN, MD

Benign Prostatic Hypertrophy: Diagnosis and Treatment

As men age, the prostate gland enlarges (Fig. 34–1). It has been estimated that 5 to 10% of men at 40 years of age have prostatic enlargement, and 80% by 80 years of age have evidence of benign prostatic hypertrophy (BPH).[1, 2] Prostatic disease usually presents with symptoms that are very useful diagnostically. Decreased force of the urinary stream, hesitancy, straining to void, double voiding, and postvoid dribbling are encountered with prostatic enlargement and are referred to as obstructive symptoms. Urgency, dysuria, perineal discomfort, and pain at the head of the penis during or after voiding are frequently the consequence of prostatic inflammation and are referred to as irritative symptoms. Urinary frequency, nocturia, and hematuria are symptoms common to both irritative and obstructive disease.

Frequently, a patient will have a combination of irritative and obstructive symptoms. It then becomes a challenge to distinguish a progressive inflammatory problem, which has resulted in a stricture or edema, from a progressive obstructive problem causing secondary infection. A careful review of past symptoms often resolves this dilemma. Neurogenic bladder dysfunction usually shows these same symptoms and must be considered in the differential diagnosis. Incontinence, associated with urinary urgency in the absence of infection (spastic bladder) or resulting from overflow in a patient with urinary retention (flaccid bladder), is the most frequently encountered symptom of neurogenic bladder disease. The age of the patient is relevant to the diagnosis of prostatic diseases. In prepubertal youths (< 13 to 15 years old), the prostate is poorly developed, and prostatic disease is rare. Any prostatic mass in this age group should be considered malignant (sarcoma) until proven otherwise. Prostatitis can occur at any age following puberty. Clinical BPH and prostatic carcinoma are rare in patients younger than 45 years of age.

A basic knowledge of the anatomy of the prostate is essential for the interpretation of physical findings and for understanding the natural history of the diseases affecting it. For clinical purposes, the functional anatomy of the prostate may be considered to consist of four concentric layers (see Fig. 34–1*A*). The innermost layer is the transitional epithelium, which extends from the bladder to line the urethra. Surrounding this epithelium is a superficial bed of closely applied periurethral and submucosal glands whose ducts perforate the prostatic urethra at multiple points. These glands are most densely packed laterally and posteriorly and are the exclusive origin of benign prostatic hyperplasia. These glands are themselves encompassed by the so-called "true" prostatic exocrine glands that constitute the bulk of the prostate in the young adult. It is this portion of the gland in which prostatic carcinoma generally originates. The combined secretions of these glands form the seminal fluid. A fibrous sheath that encapsulates the entire prostate and seminal vesicles forms the outer layer.

The prostate is normally slightly larger than a golfball and encases that portion of the urethra that lies between the bladder neck and the urogenital diaphragm (prostatic urethra). Its base rests against the bladder neck, and the apex rests against the urogenital diaphragm. The function

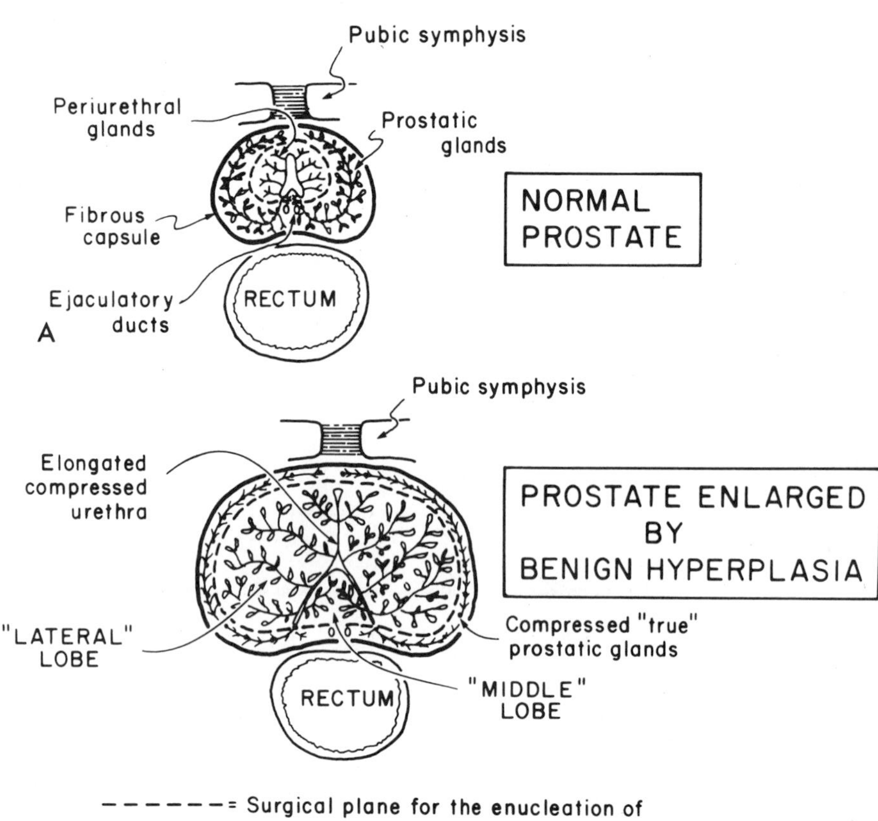

FIGURE 34–1. A diagrammatic transverse section of the prostate above the verumontanum. *A,* Clinical anatomy of the normal prostate showing the urethral lumen, the layers of prostatic glands, and the fibrous capsule. *B,* The natural history of prostatic hypertrophy. The periurethral glands, which are only a shallow submucosal layer in young men, become the bulk of the prostate in old age.

of the prostate along with the seminal vesicles is to furnish a nutrient fluid vehicle for the sperm during ejaculation.

The prostate is readily accessible to palpation. The size, consistency, symmetry, presence or absence of tenderness, and expressed secretions should be noted. The seminal vesicles are soft and are normally not distinguishable from the bladder wall on rectal examination (Table 34–1).

The size of the prostate is not really useful in diagnosis, since prostatic enlargement is only statistically related to the degree of obstruction. A normal-sized prostate may include a hypertrophied, nonpalpable, median lobe extending into the bladder. In addition, bladder neck contracture ("median bar") from chronic prostatitis can produce complete urethral obstruction without palpable enlargement of the prostate. Conversely, a very large gland may have no clinical significance other than being difficult to examine properly because of its bulk. The clinical usefulness of an estimate of size is in planning the operative approach in patients who require surgery. The convention among urologists is to estimate the size of the prostate by its weight in grams. The normal-sized gland (the size of a plum) is

TABLE 34–1. DIGITAL RECTAL EXAMINATION IN PROSTATIC DISEASE

	Prostatitis	BPH	Carcinoma
Size	Variable	Variable	Variable
Consistency	Boggy/irregular	Firm	Hard/irregular
Symmetry	Usually symmetric	Symmetric	Usually asymmetric
Tenderness	Often present	Absent	Absent
Secretions	Diagnostic	Not helpful	Not helpful to date

BPH = benign prostatic hypertrophy.

estimated as being about 20 g or less. A lemon-sized prostate weighs about 35 g, and a baseball-sized prostate weighs more than 60 g.

For diagnostic purposes, the consistency and symmetry of the prostate are its most important physical characteristics. With prostatitis, the gland may be either firm or boggy. Areas of acute inflammation are indurated and tender in comparison with uninvolved areas, and this may account for asymmetry. In addition, asymmetry can be caused by stones or rarely by abscess formation. Stones are visible radiologically, and an abscess is accompanied by fever and urinary tract infection. Benign hypertrophy is characterized by a firm, uniform consistency and symmetry. In men older than 45 years of age, prostate asymmetry is most commonly found in association with prostatic carcinoma, and therefore any patient in this age group with an unexplained asymmetric prostate should have a prostate ultrasound. The important diagnostic physical findings of carcinoma are areas of increased or asymmetric firmness, which can be very subtle. Discrete nodules and marked asymmetry constitute the more advanced form of the same lesion.

Prostate tenderness is a subjective finding and must be kept in perspective with the rest of the clinical picture. In patients with prostatitis, tenderness is roughly proportional to the extent and activity of the inflammatory process. Patients with BPH and carcinoma generally have little discomfort with palpation.

BPH is a nearly universal phenomenon of aging men. Before puberty, the prostate is immature in size and function; it reaches a fully functional state at puberty. It appears that BPH probably begins in men younger than 30 years of age,[3] although no clinical symptoms are seen in this age group. Autopsy series reveal that the percentage of men with pathologically identifiable BPH increases every year after the fourth decade.[3] Despite this finding, it has been estimated that there is only a 10% probability that a man who is 40 years old will require a prostatectomy for BPH if he lives to 80 years of age.[4] In men younger than 50 years of age, BPH is less common than prostatitis, urethral stricture, or neurogenic bladder disease as a cause of significant obstructive voiding problems. Thus, BPH is a diagnosis of exclusion in this younger age group.

Anatomically, BPH arises from the prostatic periurethral glands and stroma. As this tissue grows, forming an adenoma, the outer layers of prostatic glands are compressed, and the prostatic urethra becomes obstructed to a variable degree (see Fig. 34–1*B*). There are several important clinical implications of this anatomy. First, the individual growth pattern of the adenoma may be such that gross lateral lobe hypertrophy, which is present on physical examination, causes no significant obstruction. Conversely, minimal trilobar or median lobe hypertrophy, which feels insignificant when palpated, can result in urinary retention. Therefore, the size of the gland has only a statistical relationship to the degree of obstruction. Second, the compressed outer layers of prostatic tissue form a convenient capsule for the adenoma. This facilitates surgical removal with minimal risk of the loss of sexual function or continence. Finally, prostatic carcinoma usually arises from the so-called "true" prostatic glands, which, being compressed into this "capsule," are not removed surgically. Thus, the risk of developing prostatic cancer is unchanged by an operation for BPH.[5]

About half the patients present with straightforward obstructive voiding symptoms that have progressed over a period of years to the point of interfering with the patient's quality of life. The other half present with sequelae of BPH such as acute infection, gross hematuria, urinary retention, renal failure, and an overflow type of urinary incontinence. Of all voiding symptoms related to outlet obstruction, nocturia is the most objective and is considered the sine qua non for the diagnosis of significant BPH.

DIAGNOSIS

The evaluation of the patient with symptoms or signs of urinary tract obstruction includes history, physical examination, appropriate blood and serum studies, urinalysis, intravenous urogram (IVP), cystoscopy, uroflow, and measurement of postvoid residual urine.

After careful history and physical examination, a tentative diagnosis is made. Serum renal function tests and urinalysis confirm the absence of azotemia or infection that would delay definitive diagnostic evaluation and treatment. Prostate specific antigen (PSA) is a serine protease produced by both benign and malignant prostatic epithelium that can be measured in serum samples by immunoassay.[6] Although studies suggest that PSA may be useful in the early detection of prostate cancer,[7, 8] it is known that men with BPH or prostatitis can have elevated PSA levels and that men with prostate cancer can have normal PSA levels.[8–11] The interpretation of PSA levels can be confusing and is discussed more fully further on. An IVP or ultrasonic examination should be performed in all patients whose history, physical examination, or laboratory studies raise the suspicion of significant urinary tract abnormality. In BPH, the IVP can show changes consistent with bladder outlet obstruction (Fig. 34–2) and may serve to rule out other, unsuspected urinary tract abnormalities that are found in approximately one third of patients undergoing prostatectomy.[12] The uroflow test, which graphically demonstrates the time and rate of voiding, is valuable whenever there is doubt concerning the degree of obstruction in a patient who is able to void (Fig. 34–3).[13] The uroflow test is especially useful in determining the effects of therapy as well as the diagnosis. A cystometrogram should be performed whenever there is a question of neurologic disease as a contributing factor in patients with symptoms of voiding dysfunction. Some common examples of neurologic problems that affect bladder function are stroke, Parkinson's disease, diabetes mellitus, spinal injury, and demyelinating diseases. The cystometrogram enables the clinician to determine whether or not the patient's symptoms are due to neurogenic bladder dysfunction and to predict a favorable outcome for surgical or medical therapy, depending on the type of bladder found (Fig. 34–4).[14, 15] Cystoscopy should be performed in all patients who are to have a prostatectomy or who have hematuria. Faithful adherence to this rule prevents the potentially lethal complication of contaminating an open wound with an unsuspected transitional cell bladder cancer. In other patients, cystoscopy is indicated when there is a suspected lower urinary tract abnormality that is not clarified by other studies.

For the patient who has urinary retention, a catheter should be passed into the bladder. If the patient is difficult to catheterize, one should suspect a urethral stricture and a urologist should be consulted. Once the catheter is in place, about 200 ml of urine should be removed, and then the catheter should be briefly clamped. This allows the stretched mucosal vessels to refill slowly, thus avoiding the gross hematuria that sometimes is seen after rapid decompression of the bladder. The catheter may then be unclamped and the bladder allowed to drain freely. Next, the urine sediment is examined and should be normal. If the urine shows more than a few white blood cells, a culture is obtained, and antibiotics should be started immediately to curtail the likelihood of septicemia or parenchymal infection resulting from catheterization. Serum blood urea nitrogen (BUN) and creatinine values are needed to assess renal function. Patients with azotemia must be observed carefully after catheterization to prevent dehydration or hypokalemia from a postobstructive diuresis. In this regard, a urine creatinine to plasma creatinine ratio of 10 or greater is most indicative of iatrogenic rather than pathologic diuresis. The acid phosphatase level is usually normal in patients with retention due to BPH, but if not, the test should be repeated because a transient elevation may be caused by excessively vigorous prostatic examination or prostatic infarction. Twenty-four hours following the decompression, re-examination of the patient's prostate allows a much more accurate assessment of the true size and consistency. In the patient with urinary retention, the IVP should be obtained after he has stabilized on catheter drainage. If there is a history of urinary incontinence or neurologic disorder, a cystometrogram should be obtained. If the cystometrogram reveals a spastic type of neurogenic bladder, one should be very wary of performing prostate surgery, since severe incontinence or worsening of urinary frequency often results.

In the patient with a urinary tract infection, the infection should be cleared, and if symptoms persist or obstruction (as measured by IVP, uroflow, cystoscopy, and postvoiding residual urine volumes) plays an important role, prostatectomy is indicated. If the obstructive symptoms resolve with antibiotic therapy, the patient should be evaluated for

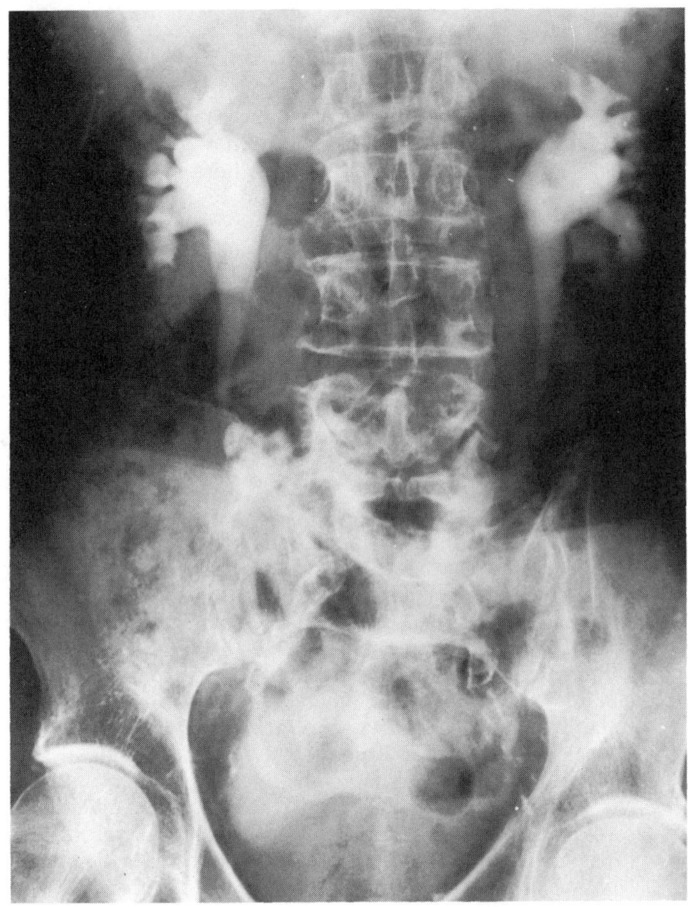

FIGURE 34–2. Intravenous urogram (IVP) of a patient with classic benign prostatic hypertrophy (BPH). Bladder outlet obstruction from BPH typically results in mild fullness of the upper collecting systems, distal ureteral J hooking, a trabeculated bladder (sometimes with secondary diverticula), and an elevated bladder floor from the enlarged prostate.

chronic bacterial prostatitis and should be treated accordingly (see Chapter 33).

TREATMENT

Transurethral resection of the prostate (TURP) has for several decades been the most common treatment alternative for treating bladder outlet obstruction. In 1991 more than 400,000 TURP procedures were performed at a cost exceeding 1 billion dollars.[12, 13] TURP is second only to cataract surgery as the most common surgical procedure performed on men older than 65 years of age in the United States. TURP has been associated with a mortality rate of approximately 0.2% and improvement in symptoms in more than 80% of patients.[14–16]

TURP is still the "gold standard" in terms of therapy. In a study by Nielson and associates,[17] urinary flow rates remained virtually unchanged from 1 to 7 years postoperatively. Fowler and associates reported on a group of more than 400 men who underwent TURP, and symptoms were improved in 93% of the patients with severe symptoms preoperatively and in 79% of patients with moderate symptoms preoperatively.[18] Therefore, since TURP is a highly effective modality in treating BPH, all new forms of therapy must be judged in comparison with TURP.

Despite this good track record, there are now many alternative therapies for the treatment of symptomatic BPH other than TURP. A primary care physician should be aware of the treatment alternatives and should be cognizant of the fact that the optimal treatment of prostatic obstruction varies from one patient to another. The common treatment alternatives that are currently available or under investigation are listed in Table 34–2.

MEDICAL THERAPY

There are two general approaches for the medical therapy of BPH. The first includes hormonal deprivation that will diminish the circulating levels of testosterone (T) or one of its metabolites (DHT). The second is the blockade of α-receptors that mediate the contractile properties of the bladder neck and prostate.

TABLE 34–2. TREATMENT ALTERNATIVES FOR BENIGN PROSTATIC HYPERTROPHY

Hormone Manipulation
LHRH analogs
Antiandrogens
5α-reductase inhibitors
α-Blockade
Invasive Therapy
Balloon dilatation
Transurethral incision of the prostate
Laser treatment
Stents
Hyperthermia

LHRH = luteinizing hormone–releasing hormone.

A. NORMAL

Flow rate cc/sec 30 20 10 0
10 20 30
TIME (sec)
Total vol. voided = 500

B. BLADDER OUTLET OBSTRUCTION (e.g. BPH)

Flow rate cc/sec 30 20 10 0
10 20 30
TIME (sec)
Total vol. voided = 300

Since flow rate is directly proportional to the volume voided, the following data obtained from UROFLOW studies of 300 normal men are required for interpretation.

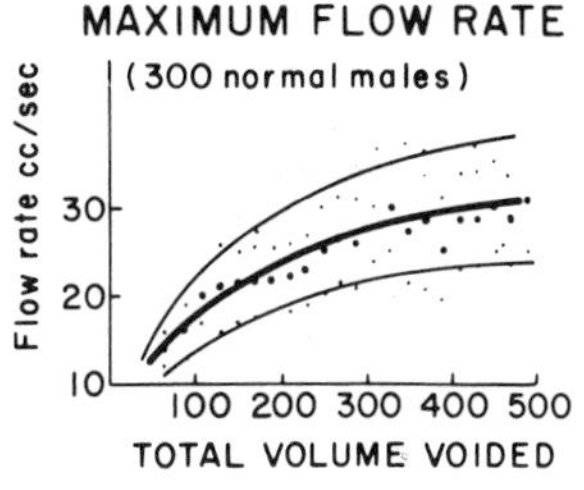

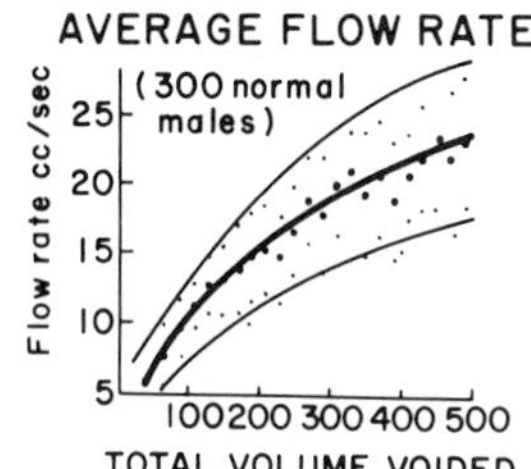

FIGURE 34–3. Typical uroflow curves. The patient (*A*) falls well within the range of normal, as seen on these graphs, whereas the patient with significant benign prostate hypertrophy (BPH) falls well below the minimum normal values for a 300-ml voided volume (*B*). For a given voided volume, a patient with significant urethral obstruction will have a flow rate below the lowermost line on both the maximum and average flow rate graphs.

A <u>Capacity</u>: Normal
<u>Proprioception</u> (sense of fullness and desire to void at normal volume): Intact
<u>Exteroception</u> (normal voiding sensation): Intact
<u>Motor Function</u>: Voluntary control of normal voiding contraction
<u>Post-Void Residual</u>: Negligible or increased in patients with true outlet obstruction (e.g. BPH)

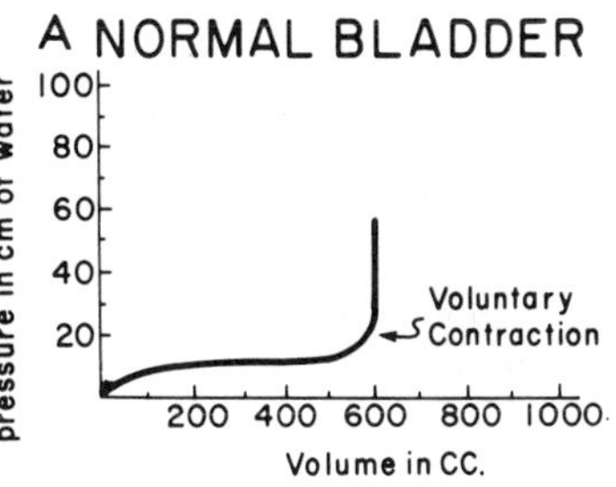

B <u>Capacity</u>: Reduced
<u>Proprioception</u>: Present or absent
<u>Exteroception</u>: Present or absent
<u>Motor Function</u>: absent voluntary control
<u>Post-Void Residual</u>: Variable

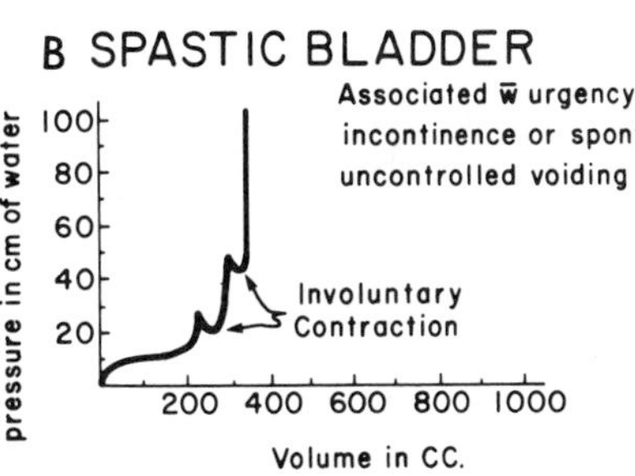

C <u>Capacity</u>: Increased except when catheter has been indwelling
<u>Proprioception</u>: Diminished or absent
<u>Exteroception</u>: Present or absent
<u>Motor Function</u>: Cannot initiate bladder contraction
<u>Post-Void Residual</u>: Large

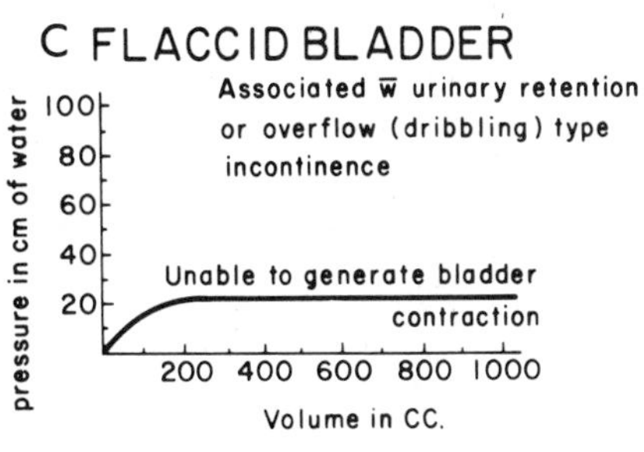

FIGURE 34–4. The three basic patterns of cystometrogram. Patients with benign prostate hypertrophy (BPH) who have pattern A may be expected to benefit from prostatectomy. A patient with pattern B deserves a more thorough urodynamic work-up before surgery for BPH is considered. Although these patients have symptoms that mimic prostatic obstruction, they are usually not obstructed, and surgery may aggravate their problem. Patients with pattern C may benefit from transurethral resection. Although the neurogenically induced flaccid bladder is not relieved by prostatectomy, the procedure reduces the resistance to emptying and, thus, may improve function.

The pathophysiology of BPH appears to be due at least in part to the stimulating effects of androgens on prostate tissue. Therefore, the pituitary gonadal axis plays an important role in prostatic growth. Neurons in the preoptic area of the hypothalamus secrete gonadotropin-releasing hormone (GnRH), also known as luteinizing hormone-releasing hormone (LHRH). LHRH is a small peptide that interacts with surface receptor sites on the plasma membrane of pituitary cells. LHRH stimulates the pituitary to release both luteinizing hormone (LH) and follicle-stimulating hormone (FSH). Secretion of LH causes the Leydig cells of the testicle to produce testosterone. Testosterone appears to have inhibiting effects on LHRH at the hypothalamic level and LH at the pituitary level.

The adrenals usually contribute only about 1% of circulating testosterone levels. The influence of adrenal androgens on prostatic cell growth is uncertain but appears to be minor.

Although testosterone is the major circulating androgen in men, the major tissue androgen is dihydrotestosterone (DHT). Testosterone diffuses into the prostatic cells, where it is converted to DHT by the enzyme 5α-reductase. Dihydrotestosterone then binds to steroid receptor complexes in the nucleus of the prostate, which ultimately causes cell growth. An understanding of this underlying physiology has led to the development of several clinical strategies to treat BPH with hormone deprivation.

LHRH Analogs

Peters and Walsh treated nine patients with bladder outlet obstruction secondary to BPH with nafarelin acetate, an LHRH analog, in a noncontrolled trial for 6 months.[19] Serum testosterone was reduced to castrate levels in all patients and this resulted in decreased libido and impotence. There was an average decrease of 24.2% in prostate size. Within 6 months after cessation of treatment, the prostates of all the men essentially returned to their pretreatment sizes. However, only three of the nine patients had significant clinical improvement as measured by symptom scores or peak uroflow. In similar studies, Garbilove and associates and Borsch and associates also demonstrated a decrease in prostate size after treatment with GnRH agonists.[20, 21]

Antiandrogens

Cyproterone acetate and flutamide are two antiandrogens that have been used clinically to treat BPH. Scott and Wade reported on the use of cyproterone acetate in an uncontrolled study of 13 men.[22] Urinary flow rates improved in nine men, and voiding symptoms improved in 11 men. Stone has reported on the use of flutamide in a randomized, double-blind study.[23] In his report, the men taking flutamide achieved a 41% decrease in prostate volume and a 46% increase in urinary flow rates. However, 53% of the men who were treated with flutamide developed breast pain and 11% developed diarrhea.

5α-Reductase Inhibitors

5α-reductase is the enzyme that converts testosterone to the intracellular androgen, DHT. It is known that DHT is the major intracellular androgen within the prostate and that it is necessary for the embryonic induction of the prostate.[24] Animal studies demonstrated that inhibitors of DHT were effective in the treatment of canine prostatic hyperplasia.[25, 26]

A highly effective 5α-reductase inhibitor with low toxicity has been synthesized (MK-906, finasteride, proscar) and is clinically available. This drug has low toxicity and has no significant side effects. Finasteride suppresses serum levels of DHT and reduces prostatic DHT content by approximately 90%.[27]

Early clinical experience with the drug has now been reported.[28] A double-blind study evaluated two doses of finasteride (1 mg and 5 mg) and placebo in a group of 895 men. Men treated with 5 mg of finasteride per day had a significant decrease in urinary symptoms ($P<.001$), an increase of 1.6 ml/sec (22%) in the peak urinary flow rate ($P<.001$) and a 19% decrease in prostatic volume after 1 year. The men treated with 1 mg of finasteride per day did not have a significant decrease in total urinary symptom scores.

α-Blockade

In the past 2 decades, researchers have noted that prostatic obstruction is related to dynamic and static components.[29] Caine and associates were the first to recognize that phenoxybenzamine, a nonselective α-blocker, was an effective form of therapy for males with obstructive urinary symptoms.[30] Since that time, 18 clinical trials for the treatment of BPH have been reported.[31] Sixteen of the 18 studies confirmed Caine's original observation that α-blockers are effective for the treatment of BPH. Terazosin and prazosin are two selective α-blockers that are presently being evaluated for the treatment of BPH.

Terazosin (Hytrin) is a long-acting selective α_1-adrenergic blocker that due to its long half-life can be administered as a once daily dose. Terazosin is presently approved by the Food and Drug Administration (FDA) as an antihypertensive drug. Lepor and associates reported on the use of terazosin in a group of 45 normotensive patients with symptomatic BPH.[32] The dose of terazosin was titrated to 5 mg per day providing significant side effects did not occur. The peak and mean urinary flow rates in the patients increased by 42% and 48%, respectively. The obstructive and irritative symptom scores improved by 63% and 35%, respectively. Side effects included erectile dysfunction, fatigue, lightheadedness, palpitations, nasal congestion, and asymptomatic hypotension. The most common dosage regimen used is 1 mg at bedtime for the first week, 2 mg at bedtime for the second week and 5 mg at bedtime for the third week. The 5 mg is the most common maintenance dose used, although some physicians increase the dose to 10 mg/day or 20 mg/day.

Prazosin (Minipress) is a selective α_1-adrenergic blocker that is used as an antihypertensive drug. Prazosin has a shorter half-life than terazosin, and the usual dose utilized is 1 mg twice daily.

Kirby and associates reported a randomized placebo-controlled study evaluating prazosin for the treatment of BPH.[33] The peak urinary flow rate improved by 59% and 6% in the prazosin- and placebo-treated groups, respectively.

INVASIVE THERAPY

Balloon Dilatation

Transurethral dilatation of the prostate (TUDP) is a procedure that appears particularly suited to younger patients with smaller prostates. Balloon dilatation involves dilating the prostatic urethra to between No. 75 and No. 90 French at high pressures (up to 110 psi).[34] Small prostates appear to give the best results with this procedure.[35, 36] As experience accrues, it appears that balloon dilatation may not achieve durable results. One report states that at 42 months after balloon dilatation, only 13% of patients still experienced significant symptomatic improvement.[37] Currently balloon dilatation appears to be best utilized in patients with mild obstructive symptoms who prefer less invasive therapy, but who are willing to accept the possibility of the need for subsequent treatment.

Transurethral Incision of the Prostate

Transurethral incision of the prostate (TUIP) was first popularized in the United States by Orandi.[38] The procedure requires a general or spinal anesthetic in most patients, although in selected patients it can be performed under local anesthesia.[39] The procedure requires a resectoscope equipped with a knife electrode. Incisions are made at the 5 and 7 o'clock positions from the ureteral orifice through the bladder neck and prostatic urethra to the verumontanum. The patients who are optional candidates for TUIP are patients with significant symptoms of bladder outlet obstruction secondary to BPH with a prostate gland of 30 g or less in size.[40]

Orandi has reported comparable results between TUIP and TURP in patients with relatively small prostates.[41] Those patients who underwent TUIP had a 79% improvement in peak uroflow compared with a 77% improvement in peak uroflow in the patients with TURP. Similar comparable results between TUIP and TURP have been demonstrated by other investigators.[42–45] Potential advantages of the TUIP appear to be decreased operating room time, shorter hospitalization, lower incidence of retrograde ejaculation, and less blood loss.

Laser Prostatectomy

Laser treatment of prostatic obstruction is presently still considered investigational by the FDA. Two approaches utilizing laser therapy for BPH are presently being examined. The first is a transurethral ultrasound-guided laser-induced prostatectomy (TULIP) in which prostatic tissue is compressed by an intraurethral balloon and neodymium:yttrium aluminum garnet (Nd:YAG) laser energy is directed at the compressed tissue. The laser energy penetrates the prostatic tissue and causes coagulation necrosis. The laser effect is monitored by ultrasound rather than by direct vision. Tissue sloughs off, and a channel is created in the prostatic urethra with minimal bleeding.[46] The TULIP procedure has several potential advantages over TURP. First, the TULIP procedure enables the patient to be discharged from the hospital in the morning after the procedure, compared with the 3- to 4-day hospitalization that is usually necessary after a TURP. Second, there is less bleeding associated with the TULIP technique, and therefore it is unlikely that a blood transfusion will be required. Finally, there appears to be less chance of retrograde ejaculation following TULIP compared with TURP.[47]

An alternative laser application for prostatic obstruction is the Visual Laser Ablation of the Prostate (V-LAP). In this procedure, an Nd:YAG laser beam passes through a No. 7.5 French probe, which is placed under direct vision through a No. 21 French cystoscope. The laser fiber is positioned under direct vision, and prostatic tissue is treated with 40 to 60 W of power. The laser fiber is moved to different areas of the prostatic urethra, and the tissue is treated with laser energy for 30 to 60 seconds.[48] Preliminary studies report improvement in symptom scores and mean uroflow rates, but follow-up is short.[49]

Prostatic Stents

The first use of a stent in the prostatic urethra was reported by Fabian in 1980.[50] This metallic stent was associated with encrustation, urinary tract infections, and stent migration. Over the ensuing decade several modifications have been made in prostatic stents that have reduced complications. There are currently two permanently implantable prostate stents available in the United States—the Urolume Wallstent (American Medical Systems, Minnetonka, MN) and the Intraprostatic Stent (Advanced Surgical Intervention, San Clemente, CA). Prostatic stents are not yet approved by the FDA and are still undergoing clinical trials.

The prostatic stents are finely woven tubular mesh made either of stainless steel (Urolume Wallstent) or titanium (Intraprostatic Stent). When fully expanded, the stents are 42F (Urolume Wallstat) or 39F (Intraprostatic Stent), respectively. Both stent models are positioned in the prostatic urethra by endoscopically controlled delivery systems under direct vision. The prostatic stent, when placed properly, extends from the bladder neck to the verumontanum, but not through the external sphincter. The stents can be placed under local anesthesia. Again, preliminary results with short follow-up suggest that the prostatic stents can achieve improvement in symptom scores and mean uroflow.[51]

Hyperthermia Treatment

The use of hyperthermia in the treatment of BPH is now being evaluated. The initial work reported by Servadio and associates used 915-Mz microwaves delivered through a transrectal probe in the 41 to 44° C range using the Prostathermer (Biodan Co, Rehovot, Israel).[52] Other machines have been developed that deliver the microwave energy through a transurethral probe and can achieve higher temperature (45 to 48° C) in the prostate.[53] The mechanism of action and effect of microwave therapy on the prostate is not yet fully understood.

The microwave treatments can be given under local anesthesia and require multiple treatments (generally 6 to 12 treatments, twice weekly) lasting 60 minutes. Complications that have been reported include small urethrorectal fistulas, which were not considered to be clinically significant, as well as hematuria and dysuria. The experience with microwave hyperthermia for treatment of BPH is still evolving. Its efficacy is still unproven, although the early experience looks promising.

SUMMARY

There is no single, optimal treatment for BPH, and the treatment must be individualized according to the patient's age, lifestyle requirements, and overall medical condition. Treatment is generally indicated when the patient's symptoms are sufficiently severe that he is willing to undergo the expenses and risk the side effects of intervention. Surgical treatment is usually mandatory for patients with obstruction, causing renal compromise (dilated upper tracts) or massive postvoiding residual urine, and should be considered in men with frequent urinary tract infections plus residual urine. For men seeking relief of symptoms, there is now the choice of medical or surgical therapy. Medical treatment is attractive in men who are either poor medical risks for anesthesia and surgery or for men who want to avoid potential side effects of surgery, such as retrograde ejaculation.

Balloon dilatation and prostatic stents seem to be best suited to men in whom palliation of symptoms is desired, but who are not considered to be good surgical candidates.

The utility and role of laser prostatectomy and microwave therapy is still evolving, but these therapies represent potential alternatives in the future.

TUIP is a reasonable consideration for a man with a relatively small gland (20 to 30 g). The efficacy of TUIP in the small prostate gland approaches that of TURP and has the benefit of decreased blood loss and a lower incidence of retrograde ejaculation.

The role of the physician treating a man with BPH is to explain to him the variety of treatment options that are now currently available. The physician's role should be to help the patient to make an informed decision and direct him to the therapy that is most appropriate for his circumstances.

Adenocarcinoma of the Prostate

Adenocarcinoma of the prostate is the most common internal cancer of men in the United States with 122,000 newly diagnosed cases in 1991.[54] The age-adjusted mortality rate from prostate cancer is 22.7 deaths per 100,000 men, and the incidence is 75 cases per 100,000 men.[55, 56] There appears to be racial differences in the incidence and mortality of prostate cancer. Native Japanese have an incidence of 5 per 100,000 men; however, when Japanese immigrate to the United States, their offspring demonstrate increases in clinical incidence and mortality that approximate United States Caucasians.[57] Black Americans have a mortality rate for prostate cancer that is two to three times the rate of Caucasians.[58]

DIAGNOSIS

The diagnosis of prostate cancer has undergone major changes in recent years. Central to these changes has been the use of prostate specific antigen (PSA) as a tumor marker. PSA is a serine protease that is an exocrine product of the human prostatic epithelium and serves a physiologic role in lysis of the seminal coagulum following ejaculation.[59] It should be recognized at the outset that PSA is produced by both benign and malignant prostate tissue and, therefore, cannot by itself serve as a screening test for prostate cancer. Catalona and associates have shown that the digital rectal examination and prostate specific antigen measurement together are the best screening test for prostate cancer.[60] Some experts now recommend that all men older than 50 years of age have an annual rectal examination and PSA level drawn. It is also advised that men with a family history of prostate cancer (first-degree relative) have annual rectal examinations and PSA levels starting at 40 years of age.

Although PSA alone is not a perfect screening test for prostate cancer, PSA levels do correlate with tumor grade, stage, and volume.[61] Patients with serum PSA values less than 10 ng/ml never had nodal metastases in the Stanford series.[61] Patients with serum PSA in the 10 to 25 ng/ml range had a 10% chance of pelvic nodal involvement, whereas in patients with PSA levels above 50 ng/ml almost two thirds were found to have nodal metastases. Although PSA levels correlate with tumor volume and stage, it should be emphasized that the correlations are gross enough that PSA alone cannot be used in an individual patient to define tumor volume or stage. Although there are conflicting reports in the literature, the preponderance of evidence supports the conclusion that a rectal examination performed by an experienced physician does not erroneously raise the serum PSA level.[62] Because of the increasing reliance on PSA, acid phosphatase is no longer used routinely as part of the screening process for prostate cancer. Acid phosphatase is not specific to the prostate, and elevations of acid phosphatase can be seen in gastric, pancreatic, lung, and breast cancer.

Early experience with transrectal ultrasound (TRUS) suggested that it might have a role as a screening modality for prostate cancer.[63] However, as experience accrued it became clear that TRUS was neither cost effective nor specific enough to serve as a screening device for prostate cancer.[64] TRUS has now found its niche as a tool for accurately directing the biopsies to the most suspicious areas of the prostate.[65]

The practical question, after the digital rectal examination (DRE) has been performed and the PSA has been returned, is which patients should have prostate biopsies performed? Cooner[66] has provided data that help to answer that question. Table 34–3 summarizes Cooner's data on almost 2700 men older than 50 years of age who were

TABLE 34–3. CANCER DETECTION RATE RELATED TO LEVELS OF SERUM PROSTATE SPECIFIC ANTIGEN AND DISTAL RECTAL EXAMINATION IN 2648 PATIENTS

Serum PSA	No. of Cancers/No. of Patients	
PSA (ng/ml)	DRE+	DRE−
≤4.0	46/446 = 10.3%	31/1265 = 2.5%
4.1–10.0	74/194 = 38.1%	19/343 = 5.5%
>10.0	168/256 = 65.6%	45/144 = 31.3%
Total	288/896 = 32%	95/1752 = 5.4%

DRE = digital rectal examination; PSA = prostate specific antigen.

evaluated for possible prostate cancer. Based on these data, we have advocated the following philosophy regarding which patients should undergo biopsy. All patients with a palpable prostatic nodule or suspicious induration, regardless of PSA level, should be advised to undergo biopsy. Patients with a normal rectal examination and normal PSA level should be followed annually.

Patients with a normal rectal examination and a PSA level above 10 ng/ml should be biopsied because the risk of an occult carcinoma is approximately 30%. The dilemma lies in the group with a normal rectal examination and a PSA level in the 4 to 10 ng/ml range. The approach to these patients must be individualized based on their age, size of their prostate gland, and overall health.

STAGE

Once the diagnosis is made, the next step is to determine the stage of the tumor. The system presently in use (Table 34–4) is reviewed under each subheading in the text.

The patient is staged by: (1) careful rectal examination; (2) PSA; (3) radioisotope bone scan; (4) abdominal computed tomography (CT) scan; or magnetic resonance imaging (MRI). Unfortunately, at the present time, no radiographic study can reliably determine the status of the pelvic lymph nodes. Because of this limitation of the radiologic studies, laparoscopic lymphadenectomy can be performed in patients with PSA levels of 30 ng/ml and above in patients in whom the knowledge of their nodal status would impact on their therapy.[67]

Stage A

The discovery of prostatic adenocarcinoma by the pathologist occurs in approximately 10% of patients who have a simple prostatectomy for benign disease. Detailed analysis of reported series of patients with stage A prostatic cancer has revealed two subgroups. The first group of patients has a small focus of differentiated tumor (stage A1), and the second group has multifocal, diffuse, or undifferentiated tumor (stage A2). Stage A1 prostatic cancer has a long natural history. The traditional dogma has been that there is no significant difference between the survival of these patients without treatment and that of age-matched controls. However, reports from Johns Hopkins Hospital and the Mayo Clinic suggest that not all stage A1 cancers are indolent.[68, 69] Epstein and associates reported 16% disease progression and 12% cancer deaths with stage A1 tumors.[68] Blute and associates[69] from the Mayo Clinic have reported a 27% disease progression, although no cancer deaths associated with stage A1 disease. These reports have led some urologists to treat stage A1 prostate cancer more aggressively (radical prostatectomy or external beam radiation), particularly in men in their 50s or early 60s.

Patients with stage A2 cancer statistically have a much more aggressive lesion, with reported 5- and 10-year survival rates of 32 to 50% and 14 to 31% respectively.[70, 71] Therefore, the clinical approach to patients with stage A tumors has been to evaluate carefully the prostatic tissue removed so that the patients can be placed into one of these two groups (Table 34–5).

Stage B

A nodule of adenocarcinoma, palpably confined within the prostate of an asymptomatic patient with a negative result on a bone scan, is a potentially curable cancer. Unfortunately, clinical stage B tumors constitute only about 10% of patients in representative series.[72, 73] The lack of a totally reliable screening test for this early cancer places much of the burden of detection on the examining finger of the patient's physician.

Treatment. The natural history and rate of progression of stage B disease is highly variable. Local extension or metastases may appear as early as 1 year or as late as 15 to 20 years after the initial diagnosis.[71, 74, 75] For this reason, uncertainties exist in choosing and evaluating therapy for these patients. However, eventual progression to metastatic disease and resultant death is the usual course in treatment failures and may be extrapolated to include untreated patients. The average patient with stage B disease is diagnosed at approximately 62 years of age, so that with otherwise good anticipated survival rates, the lethal potential of these tumors too often is realized. Using current knowledge, the anecdotal cases of so-called "latent" stage B cancer, allowing indefinite survival with a dormant tumor, cannot be separated from the majority with progressive disease. Accordingly, aggressive attempts at cure are justified for all patients, except for those of advanced age or those with concurrent illness that is expected to affect the 10-year survival rate. The traditional and arbitrary cut-off of patients older than 70 years of age for aggressive management has been based on an increased complication rate and diminishing returns in the survival of these patients

TABLE 34–4. STAGING OF PROSTATIC CARCINOMA

Stage A	Carcinoma within the prostate not detected clinically but found incidentally by the pathologist on tissue removed at prostatectomy for BPH. This is divided clinically into substages:
A1	Small focus of well-to-moderately differentiated carcinoma
A2	Diffuse, multifocal, or poorly differentiated carcinoma
Stage B	Disease palpably localized as a nodule in the prostate. This is subdivided into substages:
B1	Confined to one lobe or less than 1.5 cm in diameter
B2	Involving more than one lobe or greater than 1.5 cm in diameter
Stage C	Disease that is still confined locally but that invades surrounding structures
Stage D	Metastatic disease. This is clinically divided into substages:
D1	Small volume of tumor in lymph nodes adjacent to the prostate
D2	Distant metastases (usually lung or bone)

BPH = benign prostatic hypertrophy.

TABLE 34–5. SUMMARY TREATMENT PLAN FOR PROSTATIC CANCER

Stage	Patient Age (Years)	Tumor Volume and Grade	Treatment
A1	Any age	Focal and low-grade tumor	Observation or treatment (see text)
A2	<70	Diffuse or high-grade	Radiation or surgery
	>70	Diffuse or high-grade	Radiation or hormonal therapy
B1	<70	Nodule less than 1.5 cm, any grade	Radical surgery or radiation if negative or minimal nodal disease found at pelvic lymphadenectomy
	>70	Nodule less than 1.5 cm, any grade	Radiation or observation ± TUR, depending on age and underlying medical condition
B2	<70	Nodule greater than 1.5 cm, any grade	Radiation or radical surgery after evaluation of pelvic lymph nodes
	>70	Any size nodule, any grade	Observation, TUR
C	<70	Any size, any grade	Evaluation of pelvic lymph nodes and radical radiation therapy if nodes negative or minimal nodal disease
	>70	Any size, any grade	Observation until symptomatic, then palliation
D1	<70	Volume small by definition, any grade	Radiation therapy or observation until symptomatic
D2	Any age	Any size, any grade	Observation until symptomatic; hormonal therapy, palliative radiation; TUR, chemotherapy
or			
D1	>70		

TUR = transurethral resection.

with a tumor of uncertain malignant potential. A recent decision analysis concluded that treatment is unlikely to offer benefit to patients more than 75 years of age.[75a]

The clinician must choose from three accepted modes of therapy for aggressive management: (1) radical prostatectomy, (2) external supervoltage irradiation, and (3) interstitial irradiation with or without supplemental external irradiation. Similar 5- and 10-year survival rates have been demonstrated for patients selected for each of these treatment modalities, but randomized series are not available.

The selection of optimal treatment for patients with clinical stage B disease is facilitated by dividing them into stages B1 and B2. Stage B1 is a tumor confined to one lobe of the prostate or less than 1.5 cm in diameter on rectal examination. Stage B2 is any larger tumor that is still confined to the prostate (Fig. 34–5). This division has been based on the incidence of local lymph node metastasis found at pelvic lymphadenectomy (up to 50% for stage B2 versus less than 15% for stage B1) and the 15-year disease-free survival rates for patients who have had radical pros-

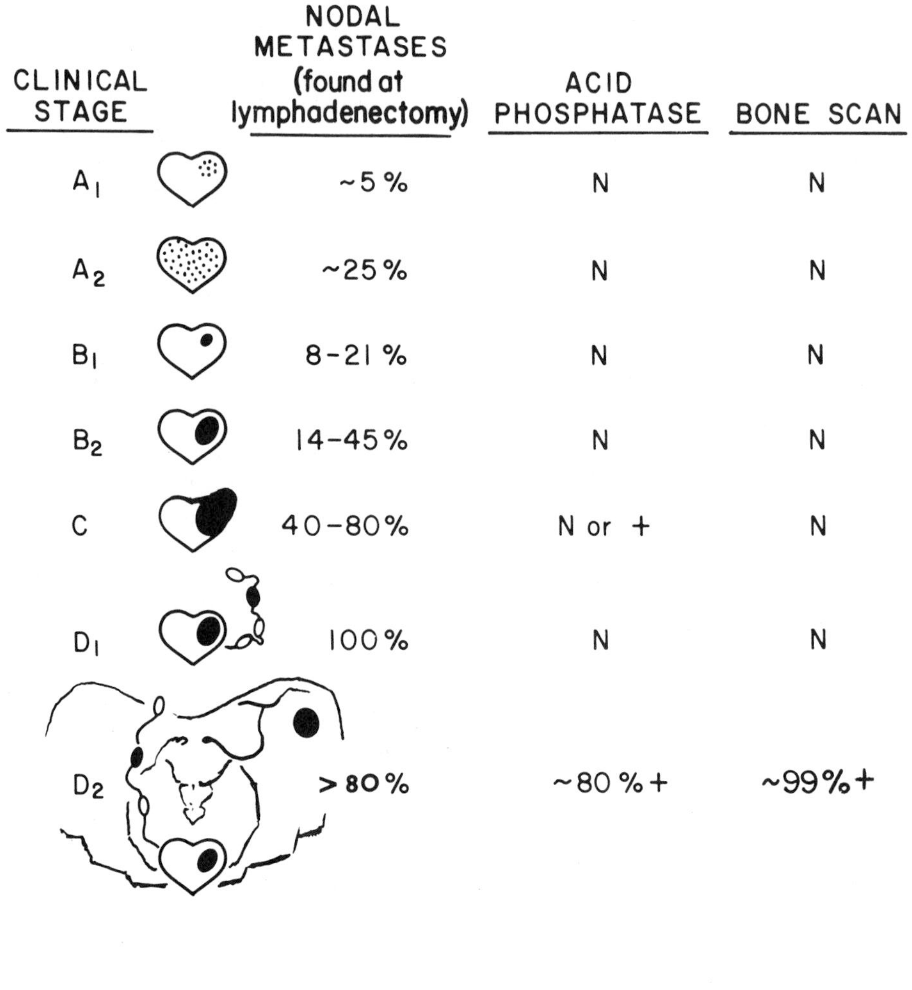

CLINICAL STAGE	NODAL METASTASES (found at lymphadenectomy)	ACID PHOSPHATASE	BONE SCAN
A_1	~5 %	N	N
A_2	~25 %	N	N
B_1	8–21 %	N	N
B_2	14–45 %	N	N
C	40–80 %	N or +	N
D_1	100 %	N	N
D_2	> 80 %	~80 % +	~99 % +

FIGURE 34–5. The clinical staging of prostate cancer is based on the digital palpation of the prostate, serum acid phosphatase level, and bone scan. The incidence of lymph node metastases generally increases with the clinical stage.

tatectomy without pelvic lymphadenectomy (18% for stage B2 versus 27% for stage B1) (Fig. 34–6).[76] Since removal of the cancer obviously results in cure if the tumor is truly localized, radical prostectomy appears at present to be the optimal treatment for the patient who has a true stage B1 cancer and an otherwise good life expectancy. For stage B2 lesions, a high incidence of nodal metastases and the likelihood of microscopic residual tumor (positive resection margins) following radical prostatectomy make surgery more controversial.[76] In these cases, radiation therapy, which has less immediate morbidity and mortality and a greater potential for eliminating microscopic locally invasive tumor, is a reasonable alternative therapy.

The advantages of a pelvic lymphadenectomy performed immediately prior to radical prostatectomy are debatable in patients with a stage B1 lesion. In those with B2 lesions, although data are not available to prove that survival is enhanced, the advantages of pelvic lymphadenectomy seem clear-cut because of the incidence of nodal metastases cited previously (see Fig. 34–5). Lymphadenectomy not only provides information regarding the true stage of the tumor but also spares the unfortunate patient with nodal metastases the morbidity of aggressive management that is likely to fail. The morbidity of pelvic lymphadenectomy is low, and the removal of microscopic nodal disease may improve survival. Careful histologic grading enables the surgeon to avoid pelvic lymphadenectomy in about a third of these patients. Patients with well-differentiated tumors with a Gleason histologic score of 2, 3, or 4 have a nearly zero incidence of lymph node involvement, whereas those with a histologic score of 8, 9, or 10 have a greater than 90% chance of lymph node spread.[74] Therefore, only the group with intermediate tumor differentiation requires surgical staging.

The presence of a small volume of metastatic tumor in pelvic lymph nodes discovered during lymphadenectomy has given rise to the subdivision of what is by definition a stage D tumor. Stage D1 is a clinical stage A, B, or C tumor with minimal nodal disease. Some of these patients have prolonged disease-free survival in combination with aggressive therapy to the prostate.[76]

Radiation therapy should be considered for patients with stage B2 tumors, for those with stage B1 tumors who are not surgical candidates by choice or because of age or medical contraindications, and/or those with minimal nodal disease at pelvic lymphadenectomy (stage D1). A dose of at least 6000 rads is required to eradicate the disease in most circumstances. Additional irradiation to the whole pelvis to a maximum tolerable dose of about 5000 rads has been advocated if pelvic lymphadenectomy is not performed.[77] This is designed to sterilize small amounts of metastatic disease that may be present in pelvic lymph nodes. However, the benefit of this additional treatment remains to be demonstrated, and the additional morbidity is high, so that most centers restrict the radiation fields.

In a large series of patients with unsegregated clinical stage B lesions given over 6000 rads in a small field to the prostate alone, the 5- and 10-year survival rates approximate those seen in similar patients having radical surgery (see Fig. 34–6). Improvement in these statistics is being sought by more aggressive staging techniques (pelvic lymphadenectomy) and by extending the irradiation field to encompass the surgically delineated tumor in selected patients.[77]

Interstitial irradiation has a theoretical advantage because of the extremely high doses of radiation that may be given. Doses of between 12,000 and 18,000 rads are readily achieved, with some apparent reduction in morbidity compared with the conventional doses (> 6000 rads) given by external irradiation.[78] Surgical exposure of the prostate through a lower abdominal incision is required for the careful placement of the radioactive seeds through hollow needles introduced into the prostatic substance under direct vision. This approach also allows simultaneous pelvic

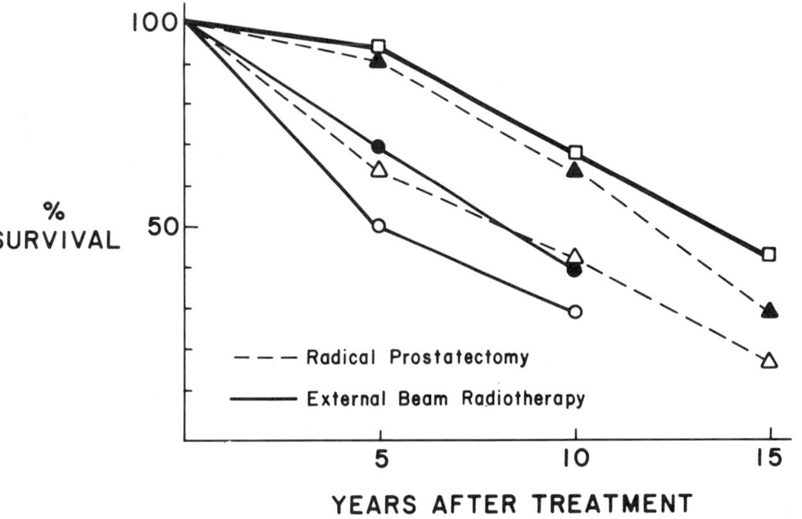

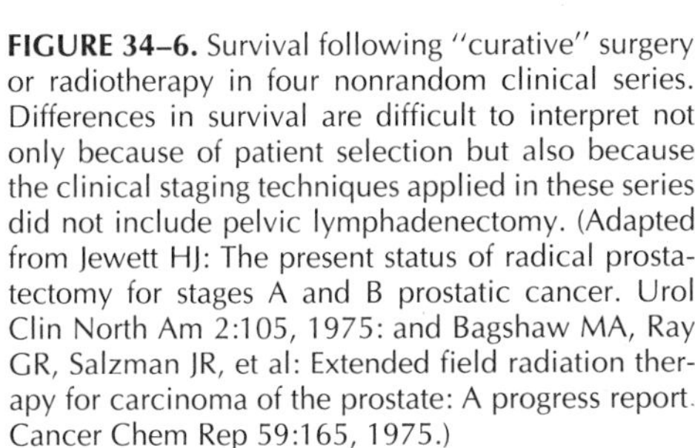
FIGURE 34–6. Survival following "curative" surgery or radiotherapy in four nonrandom clinical series. Differences in survival are difficult to interpret not only because of patient selection but also because the clinical staging techniques applied in these series did not include pelvic lymphadenectomy. (Adapted from Jewett HJ: The present status of radical prostatectomy for stages A and B prostatic cancer. Urol Clin North Am 2:105, 1975: and Bagshaw MA, Ray GR, Salzman JR, et al: Extended field radiation therapy for carcinoma of the prostate: A progress report. Cancer Chem Rep 59:165, 1975.)

lymphadenectomy. Unfortunately, there are some limiting practical disadvantages for this form of therapy. First, it is difficult to achieve an ideal placement of the radioactive seeds, which may result in erratic tumor dosage. Second, placement of the seeds is compromised by prior prostatic surgery or significant prostatic obstruction, which is present in most cases. Therefore, careful selection of patients is required. These obstacles have inspired programs of combined interstitial and external irradiation therapy that minimize these disadvantages.[80] The 5-year survival statistics with these newer techniques equal those of other therapies.[71] Because 15-year survival data are essential for the evaluation of therapy in early prostatic cancer (stages A and B), an attitude of healthy skepticism must still be maintained regarding these techniques.

Poor-risk patients generally include those who are older than 70 years of age and those who have major medical problems sufficient to reduce their 10-year life expectancy. The current approach to these patients is to give x-ray therapy to those judged to have a fair life expectancy but to advise only observation, with palliative treatment if or when the need arises, for those who are very aged or limited by medical illness.[79]

As with most aggressive approaches to malignancy, there are predictable complications with each form of therapy. Radical prostatectomy produces erectile impotence in more than 50% of patients and some degree of incontinence in 2 to 20%. Urethral stricture develops in less than 10%. The mortality of the procedure in well-selected patients is approximately 1%.[73] Curative radiation therapy produces impotence in approximately 50% of patients and, depending on field size and dosage, produces a permanent inflammatory cystitis or proctitis in approximately 10%.[75] Incontinence is uncommon. In general, a satisfactory outcome may be achieved for most complications using available medication and technology. For impotence, there are several very satisfactory prosthetic devices, as well as penile self-injection programs using prostaglandin E_1.

Stage C

Prostatic cancer with local extension into surrounding structures but without clinical evidence of metastases constitutes one third to one half of patients in representative series.[73] Usually, the patient presents symptoms typical of BPH or prostatitis. Less common presentations include hydronephrosis secondary to ureteral obstruction from subtrigonal tumor infiltration, constipation from gross prostatic enlargement, hematuria, hematospermia, lower extremity edema, and pelvic pain.

Diagnosis. The diagnosis and staging are based on the physical examination, which reveals palpable extension of tumor outside the prostate, together with a negative result on a bone scan and pelvic CT scan or MRI. Hydronephrosis from involvement of the ureter rather than from prostatic obstruction frequently is found with larger stage C tumors and may cause renal failure. Biopsy confirmation of the diagnosis is essential because this lesion may be mimicked by bladder carcinoma, renal carcinoma, or lymphoma involving the prostate, and the histologic grade is important for determining prognosis and treatment in some cases. If the patient has urinary retention in stage C disease, one may elect to perform a transurethral resection (TUR) of the prostate to relieve the severe bladder outlet obstruction as well as to obtain biopsy material for diagnosis. However, needle biopsy is preferred in patients who do not have outlet obstruction.

Treatment. Approximately 60% of these patients actually have subclinical metastases. Thus, the average reported survival rate of 3 to 4 years for this stage is skewed by a significant admixture of patients who really have stage D disease initially. The incidence of occult metastases is directly proportional to the size and grade of the primary tumor.[68–70] Radiation therapy has been the treatment of choice in most patients with stage C disease.[81]

The role of radical surgery in stage C disease is controversial. Several larger, uncontrolled series of selected patients with small tumors have indicated that some patients can be cured. However, there is solid evidence that the disease recurs locally in the majority of stage C patients treated surgically and that most of these patients have occult metastatic disease.[75] For these reasons, radical surgical procedures are being performed less frequently than radiation therapy in these patients.

Aggressive radiotherapy plays the central role in the treatment of stage C disease. It can provide good local control of the tumor in 85 to 90% of patients and may cure some patients.[72] Published survival statistics for external beam radiotherapy in selected patients at 5 and 10 years are 48% and 30%, respectively (see Fig. 34–6).[77] In comparing these results with the results from surgery (see Fig. 34–6), a strong bias in favor of good surgical results was created by selecting patients who had small tumors and favorable anatomy; the lack of proper staging by pelvic lymphadenectomy in the radiation therapy group must be recognized. In smaller stage C tumors, the anatomy is such that radioactive seeds can also be used, and lymphadenectomy can be done simultaneously.[80]

Follow-up of stage C patients after treatment requires determinations of serum creatinine and prostate specific antigen levels and a rectal examination every 6 months. An IVP should be performed if the serum creatinine level becomes elevated. A repeat bone scan should be done when symptoms of bone metastases develop. TURP is beneficial if bladder outlet obstruction is the only problem. Good local palliation can also be achieved with external beam radiotherapy.[69, 81] Temporary nephrostomy drainage may be required if the patient does not respond to radiation therapy. Permanent urinary diversion sometimes permits long-term survival.[82]

Stage D

Patients presenting with metastatic prostatic carcinoma (stage D) constitute about half of the patients in representative series. The presentation may be with local signs and symptoms of a pelvic tumor mass, such as are encountered with stage C cancer, but frequently metastatic carcinoma is the unfortunate finding on evaluation for arthritic pain or constitutional symptoms. Anemia, clotting abnormalities with gross hematuria, and symptoms of acute spinal cord compression are also common initial clinical events.

Diagnosis. The local cancer in these patients may be surprisingly subtle on physical examination, and local symptoms may be minimal. In these cases, the failure to make an early diagnosis by present techniques is not surprising. Confirmation should be obtained by needle biopsy of the prostate or by TUR.

Anemia, if present, is usually myelophthisic rather than nutritional. Microhematuria is common, but a few patients have gross hematuria. The prothrombin time and partial thromboplastin time in these patients may be markedly prolonged and the platelet count decreased. Although the mechanisms are not well defined, disseminated malignancy is a recognized cause of the diffuse intravascular coagulation syndrome, and also primary fibrinolysis occurs in patients with disseminated prostatic cancer. The bleeding that results can be life threatening. This may occur following TUR. The bone scan usually shows increased uptake of radioactive isotope in areas of pain from metastatic disease long before x-ray changes develop. Rarely, a lytic rather than a blastic metastatic lesion may fail to show on a bone scan but may be visible on an x-ray. A careful neurologic examination should be performed, especially if the patient has lower extremity weakness or paresthesias. Permanent parapelgia can result from spinal metastases unless this possibility is recognized and treated immediately.

Treatment. There is no true consensus regarding treatment of stage D prostate cancer. Although there have been reports advocating radical prostatectomy or radiation for stage D1 disease, most urologists consider that stage D1, D2, or D3 can only be palliated and not cured. Hormone therapy has emerged as the cornerstone of therapy for stage D disease. However, controversy continues whether early rather than late hormonal therapy is advantageous as well as whether total androgen blockade (testicular and adrenal androgens) is to be preferred over testicular androgen blockade alone.

Kramolwsky reported a retrospective study of 68 patients with surgically staged D1 disease.[83] Of the patients, 22 underwent immediate orchiectomy, 24 delayed orchiectomy, and 11 exogenous antiandrogen treatment (8 immediate and 3 delayed treatment), and 11 had no androgen deprivation. The patients were divided into two groups consisting of those who received immediate hormonal deprivation (30 patients) and those with delayed treatment (38 patients). The minimum follow-up was 60 months. The median time to progression to bone metastasis was 43 months in the delayed treatment group compared with 100 months in the immediate hormonal deprivation group (P = .0087). Likewise, the median time from diagnosis to death was 90 months in the delayed treatment group compared with 150 months in the immediate treatment group, which is not significant (P = .11).

There are three traditional methods of hormonal treatment: bilateral orchiectomy, daily oral estrogen therapy, and monthly injections with GnRH analogs. It should be recognized that these three treatment alternatives are therapeutically equivalent and that they all achieve the same endpoint—elimination of testicular androgens.

Seventy to 80% of prostate cancers are at least partially androgen dependent. The withdrawal of androgen provides a significant objective and subjective tumor response in these patients. Orchiectomy is advantageous in patients with a history of cardiovascular or thrombotic problems and in those who may have difficulty complying with a medical regimen.

Literally dozens of preparations are available to achieve suppression of androgen synthesis. The most popular is oral diethylstilbestrol, which is given in a standard dose of 3 mg/day to achieve maximum testosterone reduction in all men.[69] One mg per day of oral diethylstilbestrol reduces testosterone in many men and is effective clinically in these patients. Both 3 mg/day and 1 mg/day cause fewer cardiovascular complications than do 5-mg doses.[84] The treating physician should be aware that most men develop painful and aggravating gynecomastia with estrogen therapy unless they are given prophylactic breast irradiation (in the range of 700 to 900 rads given to each breast in a single dose prior to initiation of treatment).

Luteotropic Hormone-Releasing Hormone (LH-RH) Analogs. GnRH analogs are now available for the management of metastatic prostate cancer.[85] The mechanism of action is not completely understood, but with prolonged administration, the pituitary responsiveness to LH-RH is reduced, which results in a fall in serum testosterone, perhaps by decreasing LH receptors in the testis.[86,87] Thus, the agent achieves therapeutic results similar to those of estrogen without the cardiovascular risk in elderly men associated with taking estrogen. It also avoids the adverse psychological effects or orchiectomy. The Leuprolide Study Group reported that the objective response rate to leuprolide was similar to that of DES in 199 randomized patients with D2 prostate cancer followed for a median of 72 weeks.[85] Thirty-eight per cent of the patients had a partial or complete response, and 48% showed stabilization of disease. Side effects of leuprolide include hot flashes and decreased libido and impotence, but not gynecomastia. After initiation of this therapy, some patients develop a transient increase in serum testosterone, causing an acute "flare" of their disease. However, at 4 weeks after the start of therapy, the serum testosterone levels are in the castrate range, mimicking estrogen therapy.

A final unresolved question that remains in prostate cancer management is whether total androgen blockade (testicular and adrenal androgens) is superior to testicular blockade alone. A report by Crawford and associates suggests that total androgen blockade, which was achieved using a GnRH analog, leuprolide, and an antiandrogen, flutamide, which eliminated the effect of adrenal androgens, was superior to leuprolide alone.[88] They demonstrated a longer progression-free survival (16.5 versus 13.9 months; P = .039) and an increase in median length of survival (35.6 versus 28.3 months; P = .035). However, other groups have not been able to duplicate these results, and it remains unproven whether the addition of flutamide or other antiandrogens adds anything to traditional hormonal therapy.

Ketoconazole. Trachtenberg[89] reported on the use of ketoconazole, a nonestrogenic antifungal agent, in the treatment of 13 patients with stage D2 prostate cancer. Ketoconazole is administered in an oral dose of 400 mg every 8 hours and has been demonstrated to reduce rapidly both adrenal and testicular androgens. Trachtenberg noted a decrease in serum prostatic acid phosphatase levels and bone pain within 1 week of treatment. To date, the patients have been followed for 3 to 10 months without relapse. No feminizing or cardiovascular effects have been observed. Whether this drug will replace or augment standard hormonal therapies is not yet known.

Chemotherapy. 5-Fluorouracil and cyclophosphamide (Cytoxan) and estramustine phosphate and streptozotocin have each had an approximately 40% partial objective response rate in cross-over clinical trials.[90] These studies were done in patients who had failed or relapsed on hormonal therapy. The increased survival using these drugs is marginal, however (the 50% survival rate increased from 7 months to 12 months), and is counterbalanced by their morbidity. For these reasons, current general practice does not routinely include nonhormonal chemotherapy.

Palliation. Other therapy for stage D disease includes palliation of local symptoms. Radiotherapy, in addition to its use for relief for ureteral obstruction or chronic hematuria, plays an important role in the treatment of localized bone pain for metastatic lesions. Approximately 3000 to 3500 rads is the dose usually required for control of pain and treatment of impending pathologic fractures. Urinary diversion is occasionally necessary for patients who have bilateral distal ureteral obstruction from a tumor that does not respond to irradiation, but these patients rarely survive to leave the hospital postoperatively. The exception is the patient with renal failure as an isolated problem in whom the tumor otherwise is well tolerated and whose life expectancy, based on the minimal compromise of other vital organ systems, is good.

REFERENCES

1. Fowler FJ, Wennberg JE, Timothy RP, et al: Symptoms status and quality of life following prostatectomy. JAMA 259(20):3018, 1988.
2. McConnell JD: Antiandrogen therapy for benign prostatic hyperplasia. Monogr Urol 11(1):7, 1990.
3. Berry SJ, Coffey DS, Walsh PC, et al: The development of human benign prostatic hyperplasia with age. J Urol 132:474, 1984.
4. Grayhack JT and Sadlowski RW: Results of surgical treatment for benign prostatic hyperplasia. NIAMDD Workshop Proceedings, February, 1975. DHEW Publication No (NIH) 76-1113, pp 125–134.
5. Whitmore WF Jr: The natural history of prostatic cancer. Cancer 32:1104, 1973.
6. Wang MC, Valenzuela LA, Murphy GP, and Chu TM: Purification of a human prostate specific antigen. Invest Urol 17:159, 1979.
7. Cooner WH, Mosley BR, Rutherford CL, et al: Prostate cancer detection in a clinical urological practice by ultrasonography, digital rectal examination and prostate specific antigen. J Urol 143:1146, 1990.
8. Catalona WJ, Smith DS, Ratliff TL, et al: Measurement of prostate specific antigen in serum as a screening test for prostate cancer. N Engl J Med 324:1156, 1991.
9. Hudson MA, Bahnson RR, and Catalona WJ: Clinical use of prostate specific antigen in patients with prostate cancer. J Urol 142:1011, 1989.
10. Oesterling JE, Chan DW, Epstein JI, et al: Prostate specific antigen in the preoperative and postoperative evaluation of localized prostatic cancer treated with radical prostatectomy. J Urol 139:766, 1988.
11. Webster JP, Oesterling JE, Peters CA, et al: The influence of reversible androgen deprivation on serum prostate specific antigen levels in men with benign prostatic hyperplasia. J Urol 141:987, 1989.
12. Geller J: Benign prostatic hyperplasia: Pathogenesis and medical therapy. J Am Geriatr Soc 39:1208, 1991.
13. Oesterling J: Introduction and editorial comment. Urology 38 (Suppl):2, 1991.
14. Mebust WK, Holtgrewe HL, Cockett ATK, et al: Transurethral prostatectomy: Immediate and postoperative complications. A cooperative study of thirteen participating institutions evaluating 3885 patients. J Urol 141:243, 1989.
15. Lepor H and Rigvad G: The efficacy of transurethral resection of the prostate in men with moderate symptoms of prostatism. J Urol 143:533, 1990.
16. Bruskewitz RC, Larsen EH, Madsen PO, and Dorflinger T: Three year follow-up of urinary symptoms after transurethral resection of the prostate. J Urol 136:613, 1986.
17. Nielsen KT, Christensen MM, Madsen PO, and Bruskewitz RC: Symptom analysis and uroflowmetry 7 years after transurethral resection of the prostate. J Urol 192:1251, 1989.
18. Fowler FJ, Wennberg JE, Timothy RP, et al: Symptom status and quality of life following prostatectomy. JAMA 259:3018, 1988.
19. Peters CA and Walsh PC: The effect of nafarelin acetate, a luteinizing-hormone-releasing hormone agonist on benign prostatic hyperplasia. N Engl J Med 317:599, 1987.
20. Garbilove JL, Levine AC, Kirschenbaum A, and Droller M: Effect of a GnRH analogue (leuprolide) on benign prostatic hypertrophy. J Clin Endocrinol Metab 64:1331, 1987.
21. Borsch RW, Griffiths DJ, Blom JH, and Schroeder FH: Treatment of benign prostatic hyperplasia by androgen deprivation: Effects on prostate size and urodynamic parameters. J Urol 141:68, 1989.
22. Scott WW and Wade JC: Medical treatment of benign nodular prostatic hyperplasia with cyproterone acetate. J Urol 101:81, 1969.
23. Stone NN: Flutamide in treatment of benign prostatic hypertrophy. Urology 39:64, 1989.
24. Sitteri PK and Wilson JP: Testosterone formation and metabolism during male sexual differntiation in the human embryo. J Clin Endocrinol Metab 38:113, 1974.
25. Imperato-McGinley J, Guerrero L, Gautier T, and Peterson R: Steroid 5α-reductase deficiency in man: An inherited form of male pseudohermaphroditism. Science 186:1213, 1974.
26. Walsh PC, Madden JD, Harrock MJ, et al: Familial incomplete male pseudohermaphroditism, type 2: Decreased dihydrotestosterone formation in pseudovaginal perineoscrotal hypospadius. N Engl J Med 291:944, 1974.
27. Stoner E: The clinical development of a 5α-reductase inhibitor, finasteride. J Steroid Biochem 37:375, 1990.
28. Gormley GJ, Stoner E, Bruskewitz RC, et al: The effect of finasteride in men with benign prostatic hyperplasia. N Engl J Med 327:1185, 1992.
29. Gup DI, Shapiro E, Baumann M, and Lepor H: The contractile properties of human prostate adenomas: Insight into the development of intravesical obstruction. Prostate 15:105, 1989.
30. Caine M, Pfau A, and Perlberg S: The use of alpha adrenergic blockers in benign prostatic hyperplasia. Br J Urol 48:255, 1976.
31. Lepor H: Role of alpha adrenergic blockers in the treatment of benign prostatic hyperplasia. Prostate 3 (Suppl) 75, 1990.
32. Lepor H, Knapp-Maloney G, and Sunshine H: An open label dose titration study evaluating terazosin for the treatment of synmptomatic BPH. J Urol 144:1393, 1990.
33. Kirby RS, Coppinger SWC, Corcoran MO, et al: Prazosin in the treatment of prostatic obstruction: A placebo controlled study. Br J Urol 60:136, 1987.
34. Wozniak-Petrofsky J and Parra R: Diagnosis and treatment of benign prostatic hyperplasia. Hosp Med 28:117–124, 1992.
35. Marks LS: Value of balloon dilation in treatment of youthful patients with prostatism. Urology 39(1):31, 1992.
36. Creagh TA and Fitzpatrick JM: Nonmedical treatments for benign prostatic hyperplasia: balloons, stents, lasers and cryosurgery. Curr Opin Urol 2:8, 1992.
37. Oesterling JE: Introduction and editorial comment. Urology 38(Suppl) 2, 1991.
38. Orandi A: Transurethral incision of the prostate. J Urol 110:229, 1973.
39. Loughlin KR, Yalla SV, Belldegrun A, and Bernstein G: Transurethral incisions and resections under local anesthesia. Br J Urol 60:185, 1987.
40. Kletscher BA and Oesterling JE: Transurethral incision of the prostate: A viable alternative to transurethral resection. Semin Urol 10(4):265, 1992.
41. Orandi A: Transurethral incision of the prostate compared with transurethral resection of the prostate in 132 matching cases. J Urol 138:810, 1987.
42. Christiansen MM, Aagaard J, and Madsen PO: Transurethral resection versus transurethral incision of the prostate. Urol Clin North Am 17:621, 1990.
43. Dorflinger T, Osler M, and Larsen JF: Transurethral prostatectomy or incision of the prostate in the treatment of prostatism caused by small benign prostates. Scand J Urol Nephrol 104:77, 1987.
44. Larson EH, Dorflinger T, and Gassar TC: Transurethral incision versus transurethral resection of the prostate for the treatment of benign prostatic hypertrophy: A preliminary report. Scand J Urol Nephrol 104:83, 1987.
45. Hellstrom P, Lukkarinen O, and Kontturi M: Bladder neck incision of transurethral electroresection for the treatment of urinary obstruction caused by a small benign prostate: A randomized urodynamic study. Scand J Urol Nephrol 20:187, 1986.
46. Roth RA and Aretz HT: Transurethral ultrasound guided laser induced prostatectomy (TULIP procedure): A canine prostate feasibility study. J Urol 146:1128, 1991.
47. McCullough DL: This month in investigative urology: Transurethral laser treatment of benign prostatic hyperplasia. J Urol 146:1126, 1991.

48. Dixon CM and Lepor H: Laser ablation of the prostate. Semin Urol 10(4):273, 1992.
49. Costello AJ, Bowsher WG, and Bolton DM: Laser ablation of the prostate in patients with benign prostatic hypertrophy. Br J Urol 69:603, 1992.
50. Fabian KM: Der Intraprostatische "Partielle Katheter" (Urologische Spirale). Urology [A] 19:236, 1980.
51. Reddy PK, Evans R, and Eppel S: Prostatic stents in the treatment of benign prostatic hyperplasia. Semin Urol 10(4):260, 1992.
52. Servadio C, Leib Z, and Lev A: Local hyperthermia to canine prostate. Urology 35:156, 1990.
53. Servadio C: The use of hyperthermia for benign prostatic hyperplasia. Curr Opin Urol 2:12, 1992.
54. Boring CC, Squires TS, and Tong T: Cancer statistics, 1991. CA 41:19, 1991.
55. Devesa SS, Silverman DT, Young JL, et al: Cancer incidence and mortality trends among whites in the United States 1947–1984. J Natl Cancer Inst 79:701, 1987.
56. Carter HB, Piantadosi S, and Isaacs JT: Clinical evidence for and implications of the multistep development of prostate cancer. J Urol 143:742, 1990.
57. Akazaki K and Stemmerman GN: Comparative study of latent carcinoma of the prostate among Japanese in Japan and Hawaii. J Natl Cancer Inst 50:1137, 1973.
58. Ernster VL, Winkelstein W, Selvin S, et al: Race, socioeconomic status, and prostate cancer. Cancer Treat Rep 61:187, 1977.
59. Lilia H: A kallikrein like serine protease in prostatic fluid cleaves the predominant seminal vesicle protein. J Clin Invest 76:1899, 1985.
60. Catalona WJ, Smith DS, Ratliff TL, et al: Mesurement of prostate specific antigen in serum as a screening test for prostate cancer. N Engl J Med 324(17):1156, 1991.
61. Kabalin JN: Prostate specific antigen: Clinical use in the diagnosis and management of prostate cancer. Geriatrics 47(9):26, 1992.
62. Brawer MK, Schifman RB, Ahmann FR, et al: The effect of digital rectal examination on serum levels of prostate specific antigen. Arch Pathol Lab Med 112:1110, 1988.
63. Lee F, Littrup PJ, Torp-Pederson ST, et al: Prostate cancer: Comparison of transrectal ultrasound and digital rectal exam for screening. Radiology 168:389, 1988.
64. Chodak GW, Wald V, Parmer E, et al: Comparison of digital examination and transrectal ultrasonography for the diagnosis of prostate cancer. J Urol 135:951, 1986.
65. Hodge KK, McNeal JE, and Stamey TA: Ultrasound guided transrectal core biopsies of the palpably abnormal prostate. J Urol 142:66, 1989.
66. Cooner WH: Prostate-specific antigen, digital rectal examination and transrectal ultrasonic examination of the prostate detection. Monogr Urol 12:3, 1991.
67. Loughlin KR and Kavoussi LR: Laparoscopic pelvic node dissection in urologic malignancies. Contemp Urol 4(5):68, 1992.
68. Epstein JI, Paul G, Eggleston JC, and Walsh PC: Prognosis of untreated stages A-1 prostatic carcinoma: A study of 94 cases with extended follow up. J Urol 136:837, 1986.
69. Blute ML, Zincke H, and Farrow GM: Long-term follow up of young patients with stage A adenocarcinoma of the prostate. J Urol 136:840, 1986.
70. Grayhack JT and Sadlowski RW: Results of surgical treatment for benign prostatic hyperplasia. NIAMDD Workshop Proceedings, February, 1975. DHEW Publication No. (NIH) 76-1113, pp 125–134.
71. Boxer RJ: Adenocarcinoma of the prostate gland. Urol Surv 27:75, 1977.
72. Klein LA: Prostatic carcinoma. N Engl J Med 300:8324, 1979.
73. Catalona WJ and Scott WW: Carcinoma of the prostate: A review. J Urol 119:1, 1978.
74. Kramer SA, Spahr J, Brendler CB, et al: Experience with Gleason's histopathologic grading in prostatic cancer. J Urol 124:223, 1980.
75. Barzell W, Bean MA, Hilaris BS, et al: Prostatic adenocarcinoma: Relationship of grade and local extent to the pattern of metastases. J Urol 118:278, 1977.
75a. Fleming C, Wasson JH, Albertson PC, et al: A decision analysis of alternative treatment strategies for clinically localized prostate cancer. JAMA 269:2650, 1993.
76. Jewett HJ: The present status of radical prostatectomy for stages A and B prostatic cancer. Urol Clin North Am 2:105, 1975.
77. Bagshaw MA, Ray GR, Salzman JR, et al: Extended field radiation therapy for carcinoma of the prostate: A progress report. Cancer Chemother Res 59:165, 1975.
78. Whitmore WF Jr, Hilaris B, Grabstald H, et al: Implantation of ^{125}I in prostatic cancer. Surg Clin North Am 54:887, 1975.
79. Culp OS and Meyer JJ: Radical prostatectomy in the treatment of prostate cancer. Cancer 32:113, 1973.
80. Carlton CE, Hudgins PT, Guerriero WG, et al: Radiotherapy in the management of stage C carcinoma of the prostate. J Urol 116:206, 1976.
81. Gibbons RP, Mason JT, Correa RJ Jr, et al: Carcinoma of the prostate: Local control with external beam radiation therapy. J Urol 121:310, 1979.
82. Brin EN, Schiff M Jr, and Weiss RM: Palliative urinary diversion for pelvic malignancy. J Urol 113:619, 1975.
83. Kramolwsky EV: The valve of testosterone deprivation is stage D-1 carcinoma of the prostate. J Urol 139:1242, 1988.
84. Blackard CE, Byar DP, Jordan WP, et al: Orchiectomy for advanced prostatic carcinoma: A re-evaluation. Urology 1:553, 1973.
85. The Leuprolide Study Group: Leuprolide versus diethylstilbestrol for metastatic prostate cancer. N Engl J Med 311:1381, 1984.
86. Auclair C, Kelly P, Labrie F, et al: Inhibition of testicular luteinizing hormone receptor level by treatment with a potent luteinizing hormone agonist or human chorionic gonadotropin. Biochem Biophys Res Comm 76:855, 1977.
87. Schwarzstein L, Aparicio N, Turner D, et al: Luteinizing hormone (LH), follicle-stimulating hormone, and testosterone responses to consecutive injections of D-leucine-G-LH-releasing hormone ethylamide in normal men. Fertil Steril 28:451, 1977.
88. Crawford ED, Ersenberger MA, McLeod DG, et al: A controlled trial of leuprolide with and without flutamide in prostatic carcinoma. N Engl J Med 321:419, 1989.
89. Trachtenberg J: Ketoconazole therapy in advanced prostatic cancer. J Urol 132:61, 1984.
90. Murphy GP, Gibbons PR, Johnson DE, et al: A comparison of estramustine phosphate and streptozotocin in patients with advanced prostatic carcinoma who have had extensive irradiation. J Urol 118:288, 1977.

35

Urolithiasis

J. M. WITHERSPOON, MD

GENERAL FEATURES

Incidence and Prevalence

Almost 12% of Americans will have a kidney stone at some time in life. A systematic survey of hospital discharge data in 1952 revealed an average of 95 cases per 100,000, with wide regional variations.[1] A subsequent 25-year study noted a stable annual age-adjusted incidence rate for women of 36 per 100,000 per year, whereas the rate for men increased significantly from 78 to 124 per 100,000 per year during this period ($P < 0.02$).[2] By current estimates the nationwide incidence of urolithiasis is 164 per 100,000 per year. Unlike the developing countries of Asia, such as Turkey, India, and Thailand, where the attack rate of urate bladder stones is high in children and adolescents, in the industrialized countries of Europe and North America calcium stones of the upper urinary tract predominate in adults.

Prevalence data for a general population are more difficult to determine than are attack rates and the incidence of hospitalization, since stones remain silent in many untreated individuals. Screening ultrasound has discovered renal stones in 2% of urban adults[3]; a regional survey of 2000 adults detected a prevalence rate of calculi of 3.8%, using plain abdominal radiographs,[4] and stones have been identified in 5% of carefully studied postmortem specimens.[5]

A significant burden of illness can result, however. A Canadian study found symptomatic events in 30% of patients 3 years after incidental discovery of a urinary tract stone, and spontaneous passage occurred in only half of the cases.[6] The remaining patients required lithotripsy or other urologic intervention. Once the first episode has subsided, the natural cumulative recurrence rate appears to be 15% at 1 year, 35% at 5 years, and 50% at 10 years in the United States.[7] Urinary calcium predicts recurrences, as does the number of previous or asymptomatic stones. The lifetime recurrence rate is higher for men (65%) than for women (20%). Stone disease is uncommon in black patients and is usually secondary to chronic infection.

Active calcium stone–formers have 40 to 80 incidents per 100 patient-years. An average of every third or fourth incident requires hospitalization. Surgical procedures are performed at a rate of 10 to 30 per 100 stones. Prior to noninvasive lithotripsy, recurrent stone-formers often developed bilateral disease,[8] became chronically infected, and faced a risk of either partial or total nephrectomy that was approximately 30%.[9]

Although uncommon in American children, the pre-existing conditions and clinical presentation are similar to those found in adults,[10] except that gross hematuria associated with hypercalciuria in children may precede urolithiasis by several years.[11] Most of these children have a family history of stone disease. Their hypercalciuria may be very episodic on an unmodified diet, and both the very young and the elderly are susceptible to hidden variations in the vitamin D content of fortified milk, resulting in excessive calcium absorption and urolithiasis.[12]

Classification

Urolithiasis is not a single disorder but rather the clinical expression of a number of infectious, anatomic, and metabolic diseases. Time-honored classification schemes have relied on the predominant composition of stones by chemical analysis, infrared spectroscopy, x-ray diffraction photography, and polarization microscopy.[13] In routine practice, stone analysis predicts subsequent stone composition with nearly 90% accuracy, except when small calcium stones are followed by urinary tract infections and struvite urolithiasis.

In the United States and Europe, the majority of recovered stones consist of calcium oxalate that is relatively pure or admixed with varying amounts of calcium phosphate (Table 35–1). Pure and mixed calcium oxalate monohydrate (whewellite) or dihydrate (weddellite) accounts for 60 to 70% of stones; relatively pure calcium phosphate (apatite, hydroxyapatite, brushite) is found in only 6 to 8%; and magnesium ammonium phosphate hexahydrate (struvite) usually occurs with significant amounts of calcium phosphate and is found in 10 to 20%. Some calcium stones have a small uric acid nucleus. The underlying pathophysiology is more clinically relevant than is stone ultrastructure in most patients. Even trace amounts of phosphate in calcium oxalate stones are associated with high calcium

TABLE 35–1. CHEMICAL AND PHYSICAL CHARACTERISTICS OF URINARY STONES

Chemical Composition (Crystal Name)	Relative Frequency (%)	X-ray Opacity	Comments
Calcium oxalate monohydrate (whewellite) and dihydrate (weddellite)	30–35	Yes	Usually small, with a hempseed or mulberry shape, and brown or black color
Mixed calcium oxalate and calcium phosphate	30–35	Yes	
Calcium phosphate (apatite, hydroxyapatite, and brushite)	6–8	Yes	May have laminated staghorn configuration and light color. Associated with infection, stasis, and alkaline urine
Magnesium ammonium phosphate (struvite or "triple" phosphate)	10–20	Yes	
Uric acid	6–10	No	Ellipsoidal, tan or red-brown; associated with an acid urine
Cystine	2–3	Yes*	Multiple, faceted, and maple sugar in color
Others (see Table 35–2)	1–2	Maybe	Granular, often drug-induced

*Usually faint and granular.

excretion rates,[14] as well as high morbidity, but do not result from known abnormalities of phosphate metabolism.

Renal stones do not contain large amounts of both calcium and uric acid, but each may provide the unidentified nidus for crystal growth of the other component and respond to therapy. Uric acid stones without a calcium crystal at their center are encountered in 6 to 10% of all urinary calculi. Cystine and other metabolic stones are uncommon in the general practice setting. About 1% of analyzed stones are artifacts, such as pebbles, metallic shot, pencil graphite, fragments of bone or nail clippings, berries, and bird seed.[15] Recently, triamterene stones have been produced in patients receiving this potassium-sparing diuretic.[16]

Once the crystal composition is determined, clinical experience will dictate how a clinician perceives the association between urinary calculi and specific causal diseases. In a nationwide survey of urologists in 1955, individual estimates of the frequency of idiopathic stones ranged from 25 to 95%.[17] Specialists practicing in teaching hospitals encounter a number of patients with unusual, specific conditions such as primary and secondary hyperoxaluria, cystinuria, vitamin D and calcium excess, drug-induced kidney stones, renal tubular acidosis, and sarcoidosis, whereas in community practice, patients tend to have calculi secondary to infection, immobilization, or anatomic abnormalities of the genitourinary tract, with no underlying metabolic disease.[18]

A clinical classification of stone diseases is presented in Table 35–2. Patients with calcium or uric acid stones in whom no disorder can be found have been excluded. This group of truly idiopathic stone-formers constitutes 10 to 20% of the afflicted patients in a primary care practice. Approximately 30 to 40% of patients have hypercalciuria of some type, and 30 to 40% are hyperuricosuric. Classic causes of kidney stones such as primary hyperparathyroidism and gout are uncommon (5 to 10% each).

Pathogenesis

Several mechanisms are known to operate in stone formation, including urinary tract structural changes and physicochemical factors leading to precipitation of supersaturated crystalloids. In individuals with normal renal function, dehydration is an important consideration. For example, American troops stationed in desert areas during World War II had a high incidence of urolithiasis, as did immigrants to Israel whose low urine output was attributed to "European" drinking habits. In the United States there has been some evidence of a stone "season" during late summer. Strenuous exercise appears to further enhance the risks of calcium oxalate and uric acid stones. When combined with the effects of job-related fluid restrictions and a hot environment, kidney stones are occupational hazards for some outdoor workers, such as quarry drillers and postal deliverymen.[19] Seasonal peaks in calcium excretion between May and September noted in temperate zones may be due to enhanced vitamin D synthesis from increased sun exposure[20] and may result in an autumn or midwinter "harvest" of urinary stones. Finally, geographic variations and the alleged existence of a "stone-belt" in the southeastern United States may be inversely related to the hardness of drinking water,[21] although such a correlation is strongly influenced by diet, age, and family history. In rural Tennessee, for instance, white men with a positive family history and high urinary saturation with calcium oxalate have a lifetime risk of kidney stones approaching 90%.[22]

Clearly, supersaturation of uric acid, cystine, struvite (magnesium ammonium phosphate), and apatite (calcium phosphate) correlates strongly with the *formation frequency,* in which saturation is a function of concentration, ionic strength, and urine pH. A urine pH below 6.0 markedly diminishes uric acid solubility to less than 100 mg/l, whereas at pH levels above 6.5, urine is nearly always undersaturated with uric acid, approximating 1500 mg/l. The precipitation of cystine has a similar relationship to urine pH, but at higher levels of alkalinity; increasing urinary pH from 7.0 to 8.0 doubles cystine solubility from 400 to 800 mg/l. On the other hand, struvite precipitates in an alkaline urine with a pH above 7.2, which is often the case in urinary tract infections involving urea-splitting organisms. Elevated urine pH has a similar effect on calcium phosphate, which is highly insoluble at pH levels above 6.4, such as in infected urine, alkali abuse, or renal tubular acidosis. At pH levels above 7.4, calcium phosphate crystalluria is likely in all subjects unless urine calcium or phosphate concentrations are well below normal. Urine pH probably has little effect on calcium oxalate precipitation.

The nonlinear but strong effect of concentration on crystallization activity is important in hyperuricosuria, cystinuria, and hyperoxaluria, in which precipitation thresholds are easily exceeded at urinary uric acid excretion above 600 mg/day, cystine excretion above 300 mg/day, and oxalate excretion above 35 mg/day. Urine with an elevated calcium content ($>$ 300 mg/day) has only a slight tendency to reach threshold saturations for either calcium oxalate or calcium phosphate precipitation. For calcium stones to form, other promoting conditions usually exist, such as an inadequate

TABLE 35–2. CLINICAL CLASSIFICATION OF URINARY CALCULI

Disorder	Typical Stone Type
I. Calcium Stone Disease	
Hypercalciuric states	
Idiopathic hypercalciuria	Calcium oxalate
Primary hyperparathyroidism	Calcium phosphate
Dietary excess	Calcium oxalate
Sarcoidosis	Calcium oxalate
Hypervitaminosis D	Calcium oxalate
Renal tubular acidosis	Calcium phosphate
Hyperuricosuric states	Calcium oxalate
Hyperoxaluric states	Calcium oxalate
Primary hyperoxaluria	
Acquired gastrointestinal hyperabsorption	
Dietary indiscretion	
Vitamin C excess	
Ethylene glycol poisoning	
Secondary urolithiasis	
Infection stones	Calcium/triple phosphate
Obstructive urolithiasis	Calcium/triple phosphate
Medullary sponge kidney	Calcium oxalate
Polycystic kidney disease	Calcium phosphate
II. Uric Acid Stone Disease	Uric acid
Hyperuricosuric states	
Gout	
Myeloproliferative disorders	
Idiopathic hyperuricosuria	
Oliguria and acidosis (e.g., with chronic diarrhea, ileostomy)	
III. Cystinuria	Cystine
IV. Rare Metabolic Diseases	
Xanthinuria	Xanthine
APRTase deficiency	Uric acid
V. Drug-Induced Syndromes	Varied
(e.g., triamterene, phenazopyridine, furosemide, acetazolamide, phenylbutazone)	

inhibitory effect of normal urine on crystal precipitation or aggregation, seeding mechanisms for crystal nucleation and growth, or low urine volume. Of the inorganic inhibitors, the mean daily urinary citrate[23] and magnesium levels are frequently found to be low in several types of stone disease. Hypocitraturia occurs as an isolated finding in approximately 5 to 10% of patients and with other urinary abnormalities in up to 50%, but its level is only weakly related to the rate of stone recurrence.[24] Causes of hypocitraturia include a diet high in animal protein, hypokalemia, bowel disease, renal tubular acidosis, and thiazide diuretics. Although the value of routine citrate measurement is limited by its variability over time, levels tend to be normal in patients with a single stone episode.[25] Magnesium also forms soluble complexes with urinary calcium. Hypomagnesemia is usually dietary in origin or due to chronic alcohol ingestion. In calcium stone disease it is almost always accompanied by other urinary abnormalities, such as hypercalciuria, phosphate depletion, and hypocitraturia.

In the Western Hemisphere, where urinary calculi are almost always of renal origin, the characteristic microscopic architecture consists of concentric laminations, radial striations, and small spherules. A seed crystal may induce stone formation in urine supersaturated with another crystalline substance. Seeds of monosodium urate induce this form of nucleation by calcium salts. Electron-probe analysis has shown that some calcium oxalate stones have a calcium phosphate core of less than 40 μm in diameter. This finding has considerable significance, since the formation product threshold is much lower for calcium phosphate than for calcium oxalate. However, normal urine flow through the nephron into the collecting system usually is too rapid to allow even this amount of crystal aggregation.

In the absence of such lithogenic triggers as fixed particles or plaques in the collecting system, spontaneous nucleation followed by growth of free particles has not been convincingly demonstrated in vivo. Except for struvite, uric acid, and cystine calculi, for which extreme supersaturation may be both necessary and sufficient for crystal formation and growth, common calcium stones seem to require some additional binding or trapping mechanism, such as the mucoprotein matrix filaments found to constitute 2 to 10% of the weight of most stones.

There appears to be a cell-specific retention of calcium crystals by cultured renal epithelial cells that stimulates DNA synthesis and cellular proliferation.[26] This important initial step in stone disease is blocked by nephrocalcin, which is a glycoprotein found in normal human urine. Patients with active calcium nephrolithiasis produce an abnormal nephrocalcin lacking gamma-carboxyglutamic acid that fails to inhibit crystal formation.[27] Molecular abnormalities have been noted in another organic inhibitor, the Tamm-Horsfall protein, that contributes to crystal aggregation in severe recurrent calcium stone disease. Subtle morphologic characteristics of the pelvic-caliceal system may further predispose to stone growth.[28]

Anatomic abnormalities of the urinary tract and other causes of stasis are important factors modulating the clinical expression of urolithiasis. Clinically silent congenital defects such as hydronephrosis, a duplex or horseshoe kidney, medullary sponge kidney, and calyceal cysts are found in 5 to 20% of patients with calculi, depending on the diligence of radiologic evaluation. Unilateral ectopia and simple cysts per se probably do not increase the likelihood of stones but may predispose the patient to urinary infection and secondary stone formation. Renal calculi eventually occur in 15 to 20% of patients with polycystic kidney disease, even though their reduced concentration capacity may offer some protection against recurrent stone formation.

Clinical Manifestations and Differential Diagnosis

Since antiquity, the signs and symptoms of renal colic have been appreciated as a distinct and dreaded clinical syndrome. They were easily recognized by an experienced practitioner, such as John Tennent, who practiced in Williamsburg, Virginia, nearly 250 years ago:

Nevertheless some few of us be sitting too long at our Book, or our bottle, have, now and then, some Touches of the Gravel or Stones in the kidneys. This makes it self known, by a Pain across the Loins, by Urine ting'd with Blood, and mix'd with sand and jagged little stones. The stomach too is sometimes affected, and inclined to vomit.[29]

A typical attack begins suddenly as severe flank pain radiating toward the groin or genital area. Acute symptoms are due to stone movement, but their onset may occur at night or early in the morning. The pain is usually strong and spasmodic, lasting from minutes to hours, and is more severe than other symptoms, such as nausea and vomiting. Mild flank tenderness may be present, but peritoneal signs do not accompany an uncomplicated episode of urolithiasis. Frequency or urgency may be the primary symptom, especially if the stone is lodged at the ureterovesical junction. When there is associated urinary tract infection, the presentation may resemble acute pyelonephritis. Dysuria may result from secondary infection or movement of the stones into the bladder, and flank pain may persist for days after passage of the stone.

Most patients with calcium stones have their first episode between 20 and 40 years of age, but those receiving medical evaluation usually are 30 to 60 years old and have had several recurrences. Atypical patients with staghorn calculi may have chronic abdominal, flank, or back discomfort, sometimes evident for 1 year or more. An occasional patient will have symptoms simulating diseases of the gastrointestinal system, lumbar spine, or pelvic organs. Since urolithiasis is so uncommon in young women, hematuria and ureteral obstruction may be mistakenly attributed to endometriosis, pelvic cancer, or infection.[30]

In the absence of anatomic abnormalities, the right and left upper urinary tracts are equally likely to be involved in either solitary or recurrent stone formation. Up to 15% of patients have bilateral stones, but usually only one stone is symptomatic at the time of diagnosis. In North America, 60 to 80% of urinary calculi are ureteric, 20 to 30% are renal, and 5% are located in the bladder at the time of initial presentation.

Microscopic hematuria is a common finding, more often noted in the otherwise asymptomatic patient when quantitative techniques are used. Grossly hemorrhagic urine is less common; in one large series, urinary calculi accounted for 9% of the identified causes of gross hematuria, whereas infection (35%) and cancer (22%) were more frequent etiologies.[31] Hematuria without renal colic due to a stationary stone is similar to hematuria in autosomal dominant polycystic kidney disease. Strenuous activity is a frequently cited inciting event; bleeding may be intermittent and rarely lasts longer than 1 week; and it is usually self-limited, unless the patient has a coagulopathy. However, coumarin derivatives are thought to unmask silent stones and other urinary tract abnormalities with sufficient frequency to warrant periodic testing for blood in the urine in anticoagulated patients, so that major urinary bleeding can be avoided.

On plain films of the abdomen, occasional findings in acute renal colic include scoliosis with concavity toward the affected side and a stone in the path of the ureter at the ureteropelvic junction, the pelvic brim, or the ureterovesical junction, the site of most upper tract stones. When obstruction is present, the affected kidney will be enlarged. Plain abdominal x-rays alone usually add little to the clinical evaluation, due to their low sensitivity (60%) and specificity (70%).[32] Intravenous urography more reliably shows a delayed nephrogram and persistence of contrast in the collecting system even hours after stone passage. When backflow and pyelosinus rupture result from obstruction, the psoas margin will be obliterated by dye extravasated from the calyceal fornices and migrating into the lower abdomen.

The radiodensity of urinary calculi depends on their size, shape, and composition. In general, calcium-containing stones must be at least 2-mm thick to be seen. The only small stones likely to be seen on plain abdominal films are, in order of decreasing opacity, calcium phosphate (apatite), calcium oxalate, and magnesium ammonium phosphate (struvite). Cystine is partly radiodense but must be 4-mm thick or more to be visualized. Uric acid stones are radiolucent and are often difficult to find; even a large uric acid stone that nearly fills the renal pelvis may be missed by the untrained observer who does not perceive the slight reduction in pelvic opacification and localized edema in the ureteropelvic area.

Retrograde studies are indicated when excretory urography has failed to visualize the collecting system adequately, usually owing to poor renal function, or when the suspected stone cannot be identified. The differential diagnosis of opacities noted on x-ray includes calcified costal cartilage or blood vessels, phleboliths, gallstones, ingested tablets, and granulomas in the lung, lymph nodes, spleen, or pancreas. Radiolucent filling defects in the urinary tract may mimic stone disease, particularly in the renal pelvis, where tumors, blood clots, ectopic papillae, renal artery aneurysms, inclusion cysts, and cholesteatomas have been found.

Ultrasonography can detect stones 4 mm or larger in diameter, although actual stone size tends to be overestimated. It is the imaging technique of choice when iodinated contrast dye is contraindicated, to follow hydronephrosis, or in acute urolithiasis in children and pregnant women. The combination of ultrasonography and plain abdominal radiography has a diagnostic accuracy that is similar to that of intravenous urography.[33] In renal colic their sensitivity exceeds 80%, particularly when there has been time for dilatation of the collecting system to occur in the upper ureter.

The intravenous urogram remains the preferred imaging study to confirm the suspected stone's location, to assess renal function and collecting system anatomy, and to establish the presence of obstruction.[34] With oblique views or thin-section tomography it will usually distinguish renal parenchymal calcification from intrapelvic calculi. Diffuse deposition of calcium can be seen on histologic examination in many diseases, but when this is detectable radiographically, it constitutes nephrocalcinosis and usually involves the medullary portion of the kidneys.

Nephrocalcinosis is associated with the formation of renal stones in patients with idiopathic hypercalciuria, hyperparathyroidism, renal tubular acidosis, medullary sponge kidney, sarcoidosis, and hypervitaminosis D. Stones are not associated with the renal calcification of chronic glomerulonephritis, the hypergammaglobulinemic states, and chronic pyelonephritis unless renal tubular acidosis or chronic urinary tract infection is present. In the differential diagnosis of nephrocalcinosis, the intrarenal distribution of calcium may be helpful. Pinpoint stippling in the cortex is rare and suggests glomerulonephritis. Diffuse medullary calcium occurs in sarcoidosis and hypervitaminosis D. Fine streaks along the collecting ducts are seen in hyperparathyroidism. Round or oval deposits in the papillae suggest medullary sponge kidney disease, and when staghorn calculi accompany nephrocalcinosis, the likelihood of renal tubular acidosis or idiopathic hypercalciuria is great.

Renal calculi and cyst calcifications are difficult to distinguish in autosomal dominant polycystic kidney disease unless a computed tomography (CT) scan is done.[35] CT scanning with and without contrast provides three-dimensional localization of intrarenal stones and preoperative assessment of the thickness of overlying parenchyma. CT scanning is also useful in identifying uric acid and poorly mineralized matrix stones as small as 0.5 cm. Very small urinary calculi may be beyond the spatial resolution of CT scanning and other radiographic technologies.

Clinical Findings and Comorbid Conditions

Most patients tend to have recurrent disease when their relative risk is increased by a positive family history, dehydration, diet, obstruction, infection, and changes in urine pH. The hereditary factors in various types of urolithiasis are noted in Table 35–3, excluding the familial form of renal tubular acidosis, familial hyperparathyroidism, rare enzyme disorders, and the heterozygous form of cystinuria, which has been found in a few patients with calcium oxalate urolithiasis.

Age and sex are risk factors for urolithiasis. The ratio of men to women is 3:1 between 20 and 60 years of age when most stones first occur. Younger and older adults have little gender predominance, suggesting that estrogenic activity protects against stone formation. Urinary citrate levels also tend to be higher in premenopausal adult women than in men, providing some additional inhibitory protection.

There is an independent clinical association between urolithiasis and hypertension in regions with a high prevalence of calcium stones. Renal adenocarcinoma appears to be twice as likely in patients with a history of kidney stones as in controls.[36] Both of these associations seem to be linked by a diet high in animal protein.

Prolonged bed rest promotes stone disease, especially in young adults in whom immobilization results in bone resorption and marked elevation of urinary calcium. The effect can be rapid, and patients with spinal cord injury are most likely to develop renal stones within 3 months after injury.[37]

Ingestion of large quantities of vitamins D and A may lead to hypercalcemia and nephrolithiasis. Large doses of ascorbic acid also are associated with calcium stone disease. Doses at 2 g or less per day are presumed to have little effect, but since ascorbic acid is metabolized to oxalate, 4 g orally per day will increase urinary oxalate excretion by 20 mg/day and 8 g by 50 mg/day or more after 1 week of treatment.[38]

Antacid-induced hypophosphatemia, hypercalciuria, osteomalacia, and calcium nephrolithiasis have been noted after prolonged aluminum-magnesium hydroxide ingestion,[39] although the prevalence of kidney stones following iatrogenic phosphate depletion is unknown in the United States. Aluminum hydroxide, magnesium hydroxide, or aluminum carbonate gels bind dietary phosphates in the intestine. Chronic hypophosphatemia then leads to the increased production of 1,25-dihydroxylated vitamin D by the kidney, increased intestinal absorption of calcium, and increased urinary calcium. Iatrogenic oxaloprotein and aluminum-magnesium-urate stones have been noted in patients on chronic hemodialysis with a calcium oxalate core induced by vitamin D and calcium supplementation.[40]

Calcium Stones

Idiopathic Hypercalciuria

Most kidney stones are small (1 cm or less in diameter) and consist of calcium oxalate or a mixture of calcium oxalate and calcium phosphate. As first noted 50 years ago,[41] a number of the patients excrete high levels of urinary calcium but do not appear to have primary hyperparathyroidism or any other hypercalciuric disorder such as sarcoidosis or hyperthyroidism. Albright and associates[42] coined the phrase *idiopathic hypercalciuria* for this syndrome, which is found to occur in 60 to 70% of patients with stone disease and seems to be an inherited trait. Hypercalciuria is usually defined as urinary calcium excretion repeatedly exceeding 300 mg/day in men and 250 mg/day in women (or > 4 mg/kg/day in either sex), although there is considerable variability among ambulatory patients on ad lib diets. The overlap in urinary calcium between normal individuals and stone-forming patients is apparent in the observation that extreme hypercalciuria (> 600 mg/day) is rare in patients, and up to 30% of normal subjects are hypercalciuric on occasion.

Idiopathic hypercalciuria is associated with intestinal hyperabsorption of dietary calcium in one half of men and three quarters of women with calcium stones. Half of the adult relatives and children of these patients are hypercalciuric. Patients are normocalcemic; growth is normal; and there is no overt evidence of bone disease. Numerous isotopic studies of intestinal calcium transport have noted the range of absorption to be 30 to 50% of dietary intake for normal subjects and 40 to 80% for patients with idiopathic

TABLE 35–3. COMMON HEREDITARY FACTORS IN UROLITHIASIS

Disease	Mode of Inheritance	Typical Age of Diagnosis (Yr)
Idiopathic calcium stone disease	Polygenic or autosomal dominant	20–50
Primary gout with stones*	Polygenic	30–60
Cystinuria	Recessive	10–30
Primary hyperoxaluria	Recessive	5–10

**Note*: A hereditary predisposition to form uric acid stones has been noted in families without a history of clinical gout or hyperuricemia.

hypercalciuria. In comparison with stone-free controls, patients tend to have significantly higher levels of plasma 1,25-dihydroxyvitamin D, lower serum phosphorus levels (3.3 versus 3.8 mg/dl), increased renal phosphorus excretion, and higher urinary magnesium losses. Serum calcium is unchanged, indicating intact parathyroid regulation.

As calcium intake increases, normally there is a linear increment in urinary calcium excretion. In hypercalciuria, the incremental effect of dietary calcium is accentuated two- to threefold when other factors are carefully controlled. Dietary protein increases urinary calcium excretion proportional to the protein nitrogen, and urinary calcium increases modestly with increases in urinary sodium. Dietary phosphate varies from 500 to 2000 mg/day without much effect on urinary calcium excretion until phosphate deprivation is severe (~ 200 mg/day), enhancing 1,25-dihydroxyvitamin D synthesis by the kidney and increasing urinary calcium to 400 to 600 mg/day. This level of phosphate depletion is uncommon, except in patients with chronic alcoholism or malabsorption. Finally, urinary calcium increases transiently after carbohydrate administration, and some patients with calcium stone disease have been noted to have an exaggerated calciuric response to large amounts of glucose.

Sensitivity to dietary calcium can be used to identify a subgroup with intermittent *absorptive hypercalciuria* that occurs after meals owing to intestinal hyperabsorption. In such patients hypercalciuria can be corrected by dietary restriction or binding of intestinal calcium with cellulose phosphate, and the tubular reabsorption rate and renal threshold of calcium are normal. During low-calcium intake of 400 mg/day, 24-hour urinary calcium excretion falls to about 250 mg, and serum immunoreactive parathyroid hormone (iPTH) remains normal or low in these patients (< 25 μlEq/ml).[43, 44]

Absorptive hypercalciuria commonly affects well-nourished men in whom recurrent calcium urolithiasis occurs without apparent bone disease. After an oral load of 1 g of calcium, these individuals show an exaggerated increase in urinary calcium excretion, with calcium:creatinine ratios that are twice as high as those in normal controls (i.e., 0.20 to 0.35), or calcium/glomerular filtration rate increments that are abnormally high (i.e., > 0.20 Δ mg Ca/glomerular filtration rate [GFR]). After calcium loading, total and nephrogenous cyclic adenosine monophosphate (cAMP) excretion—a measure of parathormone (PTH) effect on the distal tubule—is reduced to the same degree as in normal individuals. These patients are mildly hypophosphatemic, possibly caused by a renal tubular "leak" of inorganic phosphate, and they have enhanced intestinal responsiveness to 1,25-dihydroxyvitamin D, which normally regulates transepithelial active transport of calcium and phosphorus. These findings suggest an association between disordered phosphate handling and uncontrolled 1,25-$(OH)_2D$ production in absorptive hypercalciuria, but they are not present in all patients with the disorder. However, the sequence of secondary events seems clear: a postprandial increase in the filtered load of urinary calcium and a significant postprandial suppression of parathyroid function result in hypercalciuria and increased risk of stone formation.

In contrast, a second major variant of idiopathic hypercalciuria exists in patients with increased fasting levels of urinary calcium (> 150 mg/day), subclinical evidence of negative calcium balance with bone mineral loss, and mildly elevated levels of circulating iPTH,[45] despite normocalcemia. In these patients, urinary cAMP is frequently elevated in the fasting state but is suppressed by oral calcium, and PTH increases appropriately in response to transient hypocalcemia[46]—observations that distinguish them from patients with primary hyperparathyroidism. This variant is called *renal hypercalciuria* and is thought to derive from a primary defect in proximal tubular resorption of fluid and electrolytes.[47] The relative proportions of renal and absorptive hypercalciuria are unknown in the general population, although adult patients with the latter variant are more numerous in selective, cross-sectional studies.

Measurement of urinary calcium, 1,25-$(OH)_2D$, PTH, and cAMP during calcium restriction and an overnight fast, followed by a metabolic diet containing 1000 mg of calcium, has been applied on a limited scale to outpatient populations.

A single, standardized protocol has not been established, however, and the primary benefit of controlled dietary conditions is identification of patients who appear to be hypercalciuric due to "calcium gluttony" or those at risk for excessive urinary calcium losses on a low-calcium diet.

Primary Hyperparathyroidism

Hypercalciuria with or without stone formation is found in 20 to 30% of patients with primary hyperparathyroidism, a disease that is found in 5 to 10% of all patients with nephrolithiasis and appears to increase the risk of symptomatic stone disease in young adults to 60 times that of the general population.

Since 1965, use of serum calcium measurements as an inexpensive screening test has increased the diagnosis of primary hyperparathyroidism. However, approximately 50% of all patients with hypercalcemia detected on routine testing have no symptoms, and the frequency with which urolithiasis leads to the recognition of hyperparathyroidism (5%) is much less than the frequency (50%) noted a decade ago.

Hypertension, emotional symptoms, osteopenia, osteitis fibrosa cystica, diminished renal function, and peptic ulcer disease are more commonly caused or aggravated by hyperparathyroidism than is calcium stone disease.

Urolithiasis due to hyperparathyroidism lacks specific clinical features. Occasionally, it may be marked by recurrence on therapy or rapid stone growth, by early involvement of both kidneys, by concomitant nephrocalcinosis, by a higher proportion of cases in women, or by an increased frequency of predominantly calcium phosphate (apatite) stones. However, patients with only two or three episodes of typical calcium oxalate stones during a 10- to 20-year period have been found to have parathyroid disease. Serum calcium is usually elevated, but not invariably so, and is seldom greater than 14 mg/dl.

Patients with renal stones usually do not have evidence of overt bone disease. However, cortical demineralization assessed by lumbar spine, forearm, and femoral neck absorptiometry occurs as frequently in patients with or without stone disease.[48] In general hypercalciuria also occurs as often (~ 30%) in either the "bone" or "stone" presentations of hyperparathyroidism. One study of selected patients identified a subgroup (not unlike the variant of idiopathic hypercalciuria) in whom plasma 1,25-$(OH)_2D$ was strikingly elevated, the calciuric response to oral calcium loading was increased, and the frequency of urolithiasis was four times that of the nonabsorptive group.[49] Hypercalcemic damage of the renal tubular epithelium followed by intracellular deposition of calcium salts may provide the nidus for stone formation.

The diagnosis of hyperparathyroidism in stone-formers requires the exclusion of other diseases associated with hypercalcemia and hypercalciuria, such as vitamin D intoxication, sarcoidosis, hyperthyroidism, myxedema, multiple myeloma, and the milk-alkali syndrome. Unsuspected hyperparathyroidism is a risk to patients treated for stones in whom long-term dietary calcium restriction may predispose to negative calcium balance and further bone loss or to patients who may become hypercalcemic on thiazide therapy. Surgical correction leads to slow dissolution of existing stones over years, a decrease of renal colic even though residual fragments are small and presumably mobile, and a virtual elimination of recurrences.[50] These results are the same for adenoma or primary hyperplasia but are less favorable when chronic infection has supervened.

Renal Tubular Acidosis

Urolithiasis is an uncommon but important complication of distal renal tubular acidosis (dRTA), whether it is the hereditary disorder or secondary to altered calcium metabolism and a variety of systemic, autoimmune, nephrotoxin, and tubulointerstitial diseases. Some of these diseases, such as hyperparathyroidism, medullary sponge kidney, hyperthyroidism, and chronic pyelonephritis, have additive lithogenic mechanisms. Hypercalciuria, hypocitraturia, and alkaline urine are the primary features of dRTA urolithiasis. Urinary phosphate wasting often occurs, and patients with metabolic acidosis are hyperchloremic and usually hypokalemic.[51]

Many of these patients have incomplete dRTA with normal serum chemistries, mean urinary pH during the day greater than 6.2, and failure to acidify the urine to less than 5.25 after ammonium chloride testing. Urinary citrate excretion may be very low (< 125 mg/day) with significant hypercalciuria and frequent recurrences of calcium oxalate or calcium phosphate stones. Up to one third of patients have been found to have this elusive but treatable form of dRTA.[52]

Hyperchloremic acidosis accompanied by a urine pH above 5.8 should lead to further evaluation of the patient for distal renal tubular acidosis. The proximal type II variant does not produce hypercalciuria and recurrent calcium stone disease. Whereas most forms of RTA in adults are secondary to systemic diseases or exposure to certain drugs and toxins like amphotericin B, lithium carbonate, and toluene, reports describe a small number of families with hypercalciuria, primary renal tubular acidosis, and early-onset calcium stone disease. Acidification defects of varying degrees of severity are especially prevalent when renal stones contain more than 20% calcium phosphate.

Hyperuricosuric Calcium Urolithiasis

Several relationships between calcium stone disease and disorders of uric acid excretion are well established. Patients with gout are at risk for both uric acid and calcium oxalate urolithiasis. Patients with primary hyperparathyroidism have an increased prevalence of both hyperuricemia and hyperuricosuria and may form mixed stones containing calcium and uric acid or may pass both calcium and uric acid calculi.

By far the most important interrelationship between uric acid abnormalities and stone disease exists in patients with idiopathic hyperuricosuria and recurrent calcium urolithiasis. In a survey of 460 patients who repeatedly formed calcium stones, about 25% were found to excrete more than 800 mg (men) or 750 mg (women) of uric acid in at least one 24-hour urine specimen.[53] The cause of calcium stone formation is unclear, but it may begin with heterogeneous nucleation of calcium oxalate by crystalline uric acid or monosodium urate, followed by epistaxial growth and facilitated by the absorption of inhibitors of calcium crystal aggregation by colloidal urate.

Early uncontrolled studies showing a dramatic fall in calcium stone recurrence after allopurinol treatment have been confirmed by a randomized trial of placebo-treated and allopurinol-treated patients.[54] Nearly 90% of the placebo group experienced stone recurrence, whereas only 20% of treated patients formed new stones during the 5-year study. For any single patient the effectiveness of allopurinol in reducing calcium-stone frequency is most clear when hyperuricosuria is marked or accompanied by hypercalciuria.

Uric Acid Stones

Uric acid nephrolithiasis accounts for up to 10% of recovered calculi in the United States, with an estimated prevalence of 0.01% of the adult population. Approximately 25% of patients with uric acid stones have gout or secondary hyperuricemia; the remainder usually are chronic protein overeaters and have acid urine. Even when nongouty patients have normal average daily uric acid excretion, they tend to show marked fluctuations with brief episodes of hyperuricosuria.

Several pathophysiologic factors are associated with uric acid stone formation: (1) hyperuricemia or hyperuricosuria; (2) decreased urine pH; and (3) decreased urine volume. Short-term risk of stone disease in asymptomatic hyperuricemia is low. In one large study of prepaid health plan members followed for 8 years, renal calculi were reported in 3% of those with asymptomatic hyperuricemia, in 1% of normouricemic controls, and in 15% of patients with gout.[55] Gender has a strong influence: at mildly elevated uric acid concentrations of 7 to 8 mg/dl, men have a greater lifetime risk of stones of any type (12.7%) than do women (7.1%) at the same serum level, who tend to be older and postmenopausal.[56] In untreated patients with gouty arthritis, the long-term incidence of urolithiasis was reported to be 22% in one series of 1228 patients.[57] Eighty-four per cent of these stones were found to be pure uric acid, whereas the remainder were either mixed calcium–uric acid stones, calcium oxalate alone, or calcium phosphate.

The mean age of onset for gouty stone formation is 44 years, 2 years later than the first attack of acute gouty arthritis, but stones precede arthritis in 40% of the patients. The risk of stone disease parallels the rate of urinary uric acid secretion, with stone formation rates of 10, 20, 35, and 50% at 24-hour excretion rates of less than 300, 300 to 700, 700 to 1100, and greater than 1100 mg, respectively. Since the average untreated patient with gout excretes only 70% as much uric acid as a normal individual at any plasma concentration of urate, the risk of gouty nephrolithiasis is greater in patients with secondary hyperuricemia than in individuals with primary gout at a comparable elevation of serum uric acid. Indeed, the reported prevalence of renal calculi in cancer patients receiving vigorous cytolytic therapy is 50%.[58] A third of patients with myeloproliferative disorders, such as polycythemia, leukemia, lymphoma, and multiple myeloma, will excrete more than 800 mg/day of urinary uric acid unless treated with allopurinol.

Normal adults on a regular diet have an average urinary uric acid concentration of 400 to 800 mg/day, depending on dietary purine intake, especially in men. At this level the urine is supersaturated with uric acid at a pH of 5.5, but not at 6.0. Since the average normal urine pH for a 24-hour period is about 6.2, the likelihood of spontaneous crystallization is low. The effect of urinary alkalinization is dramatic, increasing the solubility of uric acid tenfold between a pH of 6.0 and a pH of 7.0. In patients with uric acid calculi, urine pH typically is less than 6.0 in fasting morning specimens and has been found to be associated with a subnormal rise in urine pH in response to oral alkali administration, failing to simulate the "alkaline tide" that occurs postprandially in control subjects.[59]

Oliguria is an important factor in uric acid stone disease. Since sweat does not contain urate or uric acid, uncompensated loss of water through the skin during exposure to high environmental temperatures may contribute to the frequent clinical expression of stone disease in arid areas such as Israel. The combined effect of volume depletion and chronic acidosis is particularly apparent in patients with bowel resection or ileostomy for inflammatory bowel disease. Chronic diarrhea from any cause leads to bicarbonate loss in the stool, aciduria, and concentrated urine. Uric acid stones also can develop in individuals who frequently engage in strenuous exercise,[60] after prolonged fasting, following gastric or partial ileal bypass surgery, or on a high animal protein diet without adequate fluid intake.

Enzyme defects of purine metabolism, described in a small number of families, result in urate overproduction or urolithiasis. Most well-known of these disorders is the Lesch-Nyhan syndrome, in which extremely low levels of hypoxanthine-guanine phosphoribosyl transferase (HPRTase) are found in children who exhibit self-mutilation, choreoathetosis, spasticity, mental and growth retardation, and high levels of serum and urine uric acid levels. In this syndrome it is not unusual to find orange crystalline material in the diapers of neonatal patients, but the clinical manifestations of gout, including nephrolithiasis and gouty arthritis, are characteristic of older children who have less severe neurologic disturbances. Young adults with partial HPRTase deficiency may excrete more than 1000 mg/day of urinary uric acid and develop urolithiasis before age 30. Screening for reduced enzyme activity is advisable under these circumstances, particularly when family history suggests maternal inheritance.

Nephrolithiasis is only one of the renal manifestations of hyperuricemia. Gouty nephropathy, resulting from the crystallization of monosodium urate monohydrate in medullary interstitium and the papillae, was formerly common in patients with tophaceous gout. Its presence may reduce the likelihood of stone formation, since diminished concentrating capacity is an early pathophysiologic consequence of intramedullary urate deposition.[61] Acute intratubular crystallization of free uric acid is a well-recognized complication of chemotherapy in patients with myelo- or lymphoproliferative disease, made more likely by the acidosis and dehydration of chronic debilitation. Finally, the widespread use of phenylbutazone 30 years ago occasionally was associated with hyperuricosuria, uric acid stones, and bilateral ureteral obstruction, presumably because of direct inhibition of renal uric acid reabsorption.

Cystine Stones

Cystinuria is another cause of metabolic stone disease and seems to be a relatively common genetic disorder, with an autosomal recessive mode of inheritance. Membrane defects in the proximal tubule and small intestine result in excessive urinary cystine and the structurally related dibasic amino acids, lysine, arginine, and ornithine.

The intestinal defects have little clinical significance, since serum levels are usually normal, and cystine is derived from the essential amino acid methionine, the absorption of which is not impaired. Cystine, like other free amino acids, is readily filtered across the renal glomerulus and is reabsorbed by the proximal tubule.

The heterozygous genotype probably is not a cause of kidney stones.[62] The reported prevalence of homozygous cystinuria varies from country to country; however, based on newborn screening programs, overall worldwide prevalence is about 1 in 7000. The clinical expression of urolithiasis requires other factors, such as infection, low urine volume, and hyperuricosuria. Urinary excretion varies little from one day to another and normally is less than 21 mg/g of creatinine.

Cystine stones may occur at any age, but the initial presentation usually takes place in adolescence. The stones have a maple sugar appearance, are moderately radiopaque, and—like calcium oxalate, uric acid, and xanthine stones—contain little matrix protein. They vary in size from sand-like crystal aggregates to large staghorn calculi. The solubility threshold of urinary cystine is approximately 180 mg/g of creatinine; solubility is increased in a highly alkaline urine, nearly doubling above a pH of 7.8.[63] In cystinuria, decreased tubular reabsorption of cystine, the only naturally occurring amino acid sufficiently insoluble to precipitate and form stones, results in urine levels exceeding 250 to 300 mg/g of creatinine in homozygous stone-formers. Excretion rates increase from early childhood to midlife, but cystine urolithiasis is the only clinical manifestation of cystinuria.

Cystinuria contributes to about 2% of stones in adults and 8% in children. It affects both sexes equally, but recurrences are more frequent in men, who, if untreated, will die at an average age of 37 years.[64] More than 60% of men and women have their first stone by age 25. Most have had repeated episodes and bilateral disease before a diagnosis is made. Elevations in serum creatinine are common. Some patients develop chronic pyelonephritis and renal failure. A few have undergone kidney transplantation with normalization of urinary excretion of cystine and the other amino acids.[65]

Many patients with cystinuria have other lithogenic abnormalities, including hypocitraturia, hyperuricosuria, hypercalciuria, and defective renal acidification. Cystine mixed with calcium oxalate, calcium phosphate, and struvite in addition to noncystine calcium stones are common, in part due to chronic infection and therapeutic efforts to alkalinize the urine. Given the high morbidity, cystinuria should be considered in most patients with active urolithiasis. Cystine crystals found microscopically in the urinary sediment will make the diagnosis in some patients. The qualitative sodium cyanide nitroprusside test is highly sensitive to homozygous cystinuria, but false-positive results are common.[66] Patients who have a positive result on this screening test should have a quantitative urinary cystine determination, preferably on a 24-hour collection.

Calculi Secondary to Hyperoxaluria

Oxalic acid is an end-product of protein metabolism, important because of the insolubility of its calcium salt and because of its frequent occurrence in urinary calculi. It is found in a variety of foodstuffs, including leafy green vegetables, rhubarb, pepper, tea, and cocoa. Daily intake varies widely from 100 to 1000 mg, and normal urine is intermittently supersaturated with calcium oxalate. Intestinal absorption, which normally is only 3 to 5% of dietary intake, increases during calcium restriction due to binding in more soluble cationic salts and a decline in anaerobic bacteria that metabolize oxalic acid in the colon.[67]

Urinary excretion of oxalate varies from 10 to 40 mg/day (100 to 450 μmol/day), unrelated to age in adults but occasionally elevated in healthy young men. About 10% of urinary oxalate is derived from the diet, 30% results from ascorbate metabolism, and the largest fraction is the product of the oxidation of glyoxylate by lactic dehydrogenase and nicotinamide adenine dinucleotide.

Renal calculi related to secondary hyperoxaluria occur in only a few settings. Experimental vitamin B_6 deficiency has been noted to lead to hyperoxaluria in humans, but this deficiency state is rarely encountered. Oral intake of ascorbic acid must approach 5 g/day to have a major effect on the urinary excretion of oxalate. Ascorbic acid may interfere with some oxalate assay methods that overestimate its lithogenic potential at high dosages. Oxalic acid poisoning can occur from stain removers and ethylene glycol in antifreeze solutions, which are metabolized to oxalate; and prolonged exposure to methoxyflurane anesthesia, which is converted to oxalate in the liver, can result in massive hyperoxaluria, crystal formation within renal tubules, and oxalate nephritis leading to renal failure. Primary hyperoxaluria is a rare hereditary disorder, with two genetically and metabolically distinct types, characterized by recurrent calcium oxalate stones in a patient before 20 years of age.

The most common hyperoxaluric syndrome in adults is associated with ileal resection, inflammatory bowel disease, blind loop syndrome, and jejunoileal bypass surgery for morbid obesity. Hyperoxaluria in the range of 100 to 300 mg/day occurs in two thirds of these patients owing to a threefold increase in absorption of dietary oxalate.[68] Their fat malabsorption is strongly correlated with the level of hyperoxaluria and the risk of stone disease, since fatty acids form calcium and magnesium soaps and make oxalate available for absorption.

Urolithiasis can occur months or years following the onset of bowel disease or ileal surgery. Urinary oxalate typically exceeds 60 mg/day, but calcium excretion is low (< 100 mg/day) and serum calcium and phosphorus levels may be slightly below normal. Control of fat malabsorption by dietary substitution of medium-chain triglycerides, reduction of oxalate intake, or treatment with 2 to 4 g/day of oral calcium will decrease renal oxalate excretion in these patients. Since the colon is a major site of oxalate hyperabsorption, enteric hyperoxaluria does not occur when an ileostomy is performed. Cholestyramine also reduces urinary oxalate in these diseases, suggesting that bile salts may alter intestinal permeability to oxalate.

The lack of reliable methods to measure both urine and blood oxalate has given it a minor role in the pathogenesis of stone disease. Yet abnormal uptake and transport of oxalate may be an important cause of idiopathic calcium oxalate stones. Increased oxalate exchange in the erythrocytes of patients with active formation of these stones has supported the concept of a generalized cellular abnormality that is inherited and can be blocked by thiazides.[69] As a group these patients have increased intestinal oxalate absorption; however, since variations in dietary intake can be extreme, a single 24-hour urine sample of oxalate excretion will fail to distinguish stone formers from nonstoneformers.[70]

Infection Stones

Infection stones are one type of secondary urolithiasis that includes stones caused by obstruction at the ureteropelvic junction, ureteral strictures, horseshoe kidney, autosomal dominant polycystic kidney disease, medullary sponge kidney, urinary diversions, foreign bodies, and drugs that crystallize in the urinary tract. Infection stones may have a branched or staghorn configuration, filling the entire pelvic-caliceal system. They constitute 15 to 20% of analyzed urinary calculi in ambulatory patients and may occur at higher rates in chronically hospitalized patients, either as primary disease or as secondary laminar deposition on a pre-existing stone nidus. The risk factors include persistent or recurrent urinary tract infection, urinary alkalinity, and metabolic stone formation. Clinical history may reveal recent or remote exposure to broad-spectrum antibiotics and prior cystoscopic instrumentation.[1]

Infection stones consist of magnesium ammonium phosphate (struvite) frequently mixed with calcium phosphate (apatite) and called "triple phosphate." The stones result from chronic urinary infection with urease-producing bacteria, causing subsequent ureolysis and elevation of urinary alkaline, bicarbonate, and ammonia levels. Persistently increased urine pH above 7.2 is accompanied by calcium phosphate and magnesium ammonium phosphate precipitation. This process is aided by cellular debris and matrix proteins, which are commonly identified in infection stones and may account for the lithogenic properties of occasional organisms that do not split urea. Once initiated, a cycle of infection and stone formation ensues, with the calculi acting as a *locus minoris resistentiae* for bacteria beyond the reach of host defense mechanisms.[71]

Urologic instrumentation, surgical intervention for large stones, previous antimicrobial therapy, and progressive azotemia are associated with not only increased frequency of infection but also a shift in the bacteriologic pattern of stone washings or cultured fragments toward resistant, urease-producing organisms such as *Proteus* species (95% urease-positive), *Pseudomonas* (30% positive), *Klebsiella* (60% positive), *Serratia* (5 to 30% positive), and *Enterobacter* (3% positive).

E. coli, rarely associated with urease production, has been found to be the most frequent microorganism causing urinary infection in patients surgically treated for stone disease.[72] Consequently, bacterial cultures from removed calculi may not agree with previous or simultaneous midstream urine specimens, and multiple organisms may be present with differing antimicrobial sensitivity and virulence. These changes in the potential complexity of urinary tract infection resulting from urolithiasis occur more often in women than in men. The importance of unidentified infection is underscored by past observations that patients with untreated bilateral infection stones have a 25% mortality within 5 years and a 40% mortality within 10 years, confirming the gradual progression to end-stage renal disease in the absence of medical or surgical intervention. In addition to the chronic complications, acute bacteremia and septic shock from calculous pyelonephritis and obstruction can occur.[73]

In some patients recurrent calcium stone disease and urinary infection coexist without a causal relationship. Whereas more than 80% of removed struvite fragments have significant bacterial growth, perhaps 20% of calcium oxalate stones are also culture-positive. It may be that factors such as subtle urothelial injury, minor abnormalities in urine pH, osmolality, and glucose concentration, as well as coincidental stone formation, favor infection with common pathogens. A mild defect in renal acidification capacity, manifested as incomplete tubular reabsorption of bicarbonate, has been reported in persistent urinary infections associated with staghorn calculi.[74] An association has been noted between urinary stones and infection-prone conditions such as urethral diverticula in women and prostatic calculosis in men. Multiple confounding factors probably account for the variability of observed infection rates in stone disease. In a study of hospitalized patients with urolithiasis, only 8% of those with small calcium oxalate stones had a culture-proved urinary infection,[75] and a recent series documenting infection stones was dominated not by struvite but by calcium oxalate calculi.[76]

Upper tract calculi associated with infection occur in 30 to 50% of patients who have undergone ileal conduit and ureterosigmoidostomy diversion following pelvic surgery, but many of these patients have a history of ureteral dilatation or pyelonephritis prior to the urinary diversion procedure. Calculi consist of struvite, are frequently branched and bilateral, and are usually associated with urease-producing organisms. They may become clinically apparent more than 10 years after the procedure. In a study of 36 patients in whom calculi developed following ileal conduit diversion and who had frequent *Proteus* infections, high conduit residuals and hyperchloremic acidosis were important features that were not present in similar patients who did not form calculi.[77] Most of these stone-forming patients given an ammonium chloride load could not acidify the urine below pH 5.5 and may have had renal tubular acidosis associated with pyelonephritis and stone disease.

MANAGEMENT AND EVALUATION

Acute Renal Colic

Ureteral calculi frequently do not require surgical intervention or even minimally invasive fragmentation procedures, but presenting symptoms can be severe, unrelated to actual stone size, and patients plead for the most efficient use of time and diagnostic resources. After an appropriate history, physical examination, and urinalysis, either excretory urography or ultrasonography and plain abdominal x-ray should be obtained. Obstruction or fever as well as severe colic are indications for hospitalization and consultation with a urologic surgeon. However, in adults, most stones located in the ureters at the time of clinical presentation will be small enough to pass spontaneously at home. Patients should remain active and increase their fluid intake to approximately 3 l/day. They should be treated with analgesics, including opiates such as meperidine, and antibiotics may be necessary if bacteriuria is present. An attempt should be made to recover the stone. Children and adolescents with stone disease require specialized care because of the high probability of congenital abnormalities or infection. Further concern about radiation exposure, urethral injury after endourologic procedures, especially in small boys, and adverse effects of treatment on the developing kidney justify referral to a tertiary care facility. Similar complexities are confronted in the management of urinary stones in pregnancy, a rare event in the office practice of medicine. The physiologic hypercalciuria of pregnancy apparently is not associated with an increased risk of urolithiasis.[78]

Approximately 15% of ureteral calculi in adults measure 5 to 8 mm in diameter and lodge at the ureterovesical junction. They usually can be located by means of intravenous urography and can be removed by endoscopic manipulation; when this is unsuccessful (about 25% of first attempts), a second attempt at extraction can be deferred for several weeks. Ureteral stones that cannot be basket-captured can be pushed up into the renal pelvis "chamber" for extracorporeal shock-wave lithotripsy. Newer ureteroscopic maneuvers that utilize electrohydraulic or laser fragmentation are equally effective. Broad-spectrum antibiotics, such as ampicillin, cephalexin, or trimethoprim-sulfamethoxazole, should be administered for at least 2 weeks following ureteral manipulation. Some stones can be dissolved without surgery; nonobstructing uric acid stones dissolve with oral bicarbonate in as few as 6 days if the urinary pH is kept at 7; and cystine stones will dissolve with diuresis alone or combined with D-penicillamine. Symptomatic stones larger than 8 mm in diameter usually require specialized surgical procedures, many of which are now undertaken in an ambulatory setting.

Percutaneous nephrostomy and irrigation with alkaline solutions have been used to dissolve large uric acid and cystine stones obstructing the renal pelvis, either lodged in the proximal ureter or failing to respond to lithotripsy. Various solvents can enhance irrigation effectiveness. Percutaneous nephrolithotomy can also be used to manually fragment and extract calcium stones under limited or local anesthesia in patients who are poor surgical candidates or who are obstructed and have ureteral damage from prior stones. Significant bleeding, extravasation, and hypotension may occur. Large, branched calculi or imbedded, long-standing ureteral stones frequently require several treatment sessions.

The technologic transition from open to percutaneous manipulation has been achieved with considerable success at some medical centers at half the hospital costs. Only 1 to 2% of stone patients now require open surgery for stones of any size.[79] However, these endoscopic procedures require angiographic techniques, biplane fluoroscopy, balanced perfusion pressures to prevent pyelovenous backflow, and maintenance of sterile urine.

Extracorporeal shock-wave lithotripsy (ESWL), originally developed for noninvasive treatment of calcium stones, can now be applied to stones of widely varying composition.[80] Although technical skill is no longer a major consideration, successful fragmentation is dependent on stone size, location, crystalline structure, and certain patient factors such as extreme obesity. Early "first-generation" lithotriptors had patients immersed in water, with general anesthesia and two independent x-ray image conversion systems used to focus pulses of a spark discharge on the motionless stone. Discharges had to be electrocardiogram (ECG)-triggered to avoid cardiac arrhythmias. Newer equipment does not require underwater positioning or an anesthetic unless stents are placed, and ultrasound localization allows targeting of nonopaque calculi.

Ureteral, renal pelvic, and caliceal stones have been successfully fragmented by ESWL. Perhaps 70% of patients with urinary stones can be treated with this technique. Major complications are infrequent even with large, staghorn calculi. Renal colic from fragments is not uncommon, and ureteral obstruction can occur. Although well tolerated in the short term, hematuria, subcapsular hematomas, and elevated serum lactic dehydrogenase that may persist for several days are similar to the effects of blunt renal trauma.[81]

The risk of hypertension does not appear to be significantly increased in long-term follow-up after ESWL, and plasma renin activity or serum aldosterone are unchanged, as well as creatinine clearance. Effects on the growing kidney of children, the elderly with vascular disease, or ovarian function are uncertain. Retained fragments, often missed on plain abdominal films and tomograms,[82] may lead to subsequent stone formation. Post-lithotripsy fever is common, and patients frequently report the discomfort of the procedure to be much more severe than was anticipated.[83] Enthusiasm for this important technologic development is tempered by limited cost savings in most settings. Treatment periods may be prolonged; up to 60% of patients may require repeated ESWL sessions, depending on stone size. Ten per cent are discovered to have residual fragments after 2 months, if the stone is less than 1.5 to 2 cm in size. As the stone size increases, stone-free rates after ESWL drop precipitously.

Evaluation After the First Stone

Stone analysis, when available, can guide the initial evaluation. Uric acid, triple phosphate, and cystine composition direct attention to a diagnosis of gout, chronic infection or anatomic abnormalities, and cystinuria, respectively. Calcium phosphate stones suggest RTA, primary hyperparathyroidism, or infection. Calcium oxalate stones are usually idiopathic and require limited evaluation, except in the very young and in patients with a strong family history of urolithiasis.

After initial management, clinical assessment of patients with urolithiasis should focus on those aspects of the medical history, review of systems, and physical examination that may reveal associated diseases such as gout, urinary infection due to instrumentation, hyperparathyroidism, peptic ulcer disease, chronic bowel disease or surgery, malignancy, sarcoidosis, and thyrotoxicosis. Family history, dietary habits, and long-term use of medications, including over-the-counter mineral and vitamin supplements, should be carefully reviewed. A 1-week diary of diet, fluid intake, and several urinary pH measurements may be helpful. Laboratory tests should include routine urinalysis and a serum chemistry profile. The urine can be examined for cystine crystals, but triple phosphate, uric acid, and calcium oxalate crystalluria may be normal findings and are not indicative of active stone disease. If not done previously, intravenous pyelography (IVP) should be performed using bolus injection methods, since continuous infusion urography has been associated with urinary extravasation in stone disease. In children, voiding studies on IVP and cystography may be required to detect anatomic abnormalities. Attention should be paid to subtle details, such as mild nephrocalcinosis, small residual stones, and the existence of medullary sponge kidney that may coexist with either primary hyperparathyroidism or hypercalciuric urolithiasis.

Recently, the importance of medullary sponge kidney (MSK) in urolithiasis has been emphasized.[84] The diagnosis depends on careful review of high-quality IVPs for characteristic linear or spherical tubules in the renal papillae. The prevalence in stone-formers may approach 20% compared with 1% in patients without urolithiasis. One large study of 799 patients with "idiopathic" calcium stones found that women were more likely to have MSK, with high rates of stone recurrences and infection.[85] The latter complication had a significant association with prior cystoscopy. MSK does not appear to affect average urinary excretion of calcium or uric acid. Hypercalciuria is present in only a slightly higher fraction of patients than in controls, and prolonged urine transit time in ectatic ducts may be an important factor in stone formation.

A remote history of a single kidney stone elicited at a routine office visit or caliceal calcifications discovered as incidental findings should be approached circumspectly, especially in patients with vague complaints. One exception may be asymptomatic renal calculi found in women of childbearing age. These stones may be dislodged by the physiologic hydronephrosis of pregnancy, creating difficult management considerations. Women who are planning pregnancy should be offered metabolic and imaging studies leading to prophylactic ESWL treatment of their silent stone disease.

Evaluation of Recurrent Stone Formers

In most patients, the initial assessment will be normal. Those with a single episode of stone formation may be managed simply with increased fluid intake and periodic follow-up. Additional work-up is warranted for patients with one or more recurrences of renal calculi or for those with evidence of growth of residual calculi. Under these circumstances, the typical patient with calcium urolithiasis and an interval of 1 year or less between stone events is likely to have had three or more stone episodes, with at least a 60% probability of having some treatable metabolic disorder. The initial evaluation consists of a 24-hour urine collection to determine levels of calcium, uric acid, creatinine, oxalate, citrate, and magnesium, with the patient on a regular diet. Colorimetric screening tests for urinary cystine are appropriate in patients with active disease and are easy to perform. Measurement of serum iPTH is indicated in calcium stone disease, even when the serum calcium is normal.

Daily urine volume and early morning pH should be determined. A positive result on a qualitative test for cystine should be followed by 24-hour urine measurement. Homozygous cystinuria is defined as greater than 250 mg (1 mmol) cystine per g of creatinine. Reference values for other lithogenic states also have been established; however, given the multifactorial nature of stone formation, their clinical application may not be straightforward. Hyperoxaluria is generally considered to be greater than 45 mg/day (500 μmol/day); hypocitraturia at less than 320 mg/day (1.7 mmol/day); and hypomagnesiuria at less than 6 mEq/day (3 mmol/day or 7.3 mg/dl). In women, hypercalciuria is defined as greater than 250 mg/day (6.25 mmol/day) and hyperuricosuria as greater than 750 mg/day (4.4 mmol/day). Corresponding thresholds for men are 300 mg/day (7.5 mmol/day) of urinary calcium and 800 mg/day (4.7 mmol/day) of uric acid.

It is usually possible to base initial management on results of the 24-hour urine and iPTH level. Additional studies are considered for recurrent stone-formers in whom the cause of the metabolic defect remains unclear. It is often appropriate to repeat the 24-hour urine collection on a random diet, along with several measurements of serum calcium. When urinary calcium levels are very high (> 350 mg/day), the "renal" form of hypercalciuria can be confirmed by placing the patient on a restricted diet containing 400 mg of calcium, 800 mg of phosphorus, 1 g of protein per kg of body weight, and 70 to 100 mEq of sodium for several days, followed by an overnight fast and 2-hour urine collection. Persistently high calcium (> 15 mg/2 hr) excretion suggests renal hypercalciuria if there is no evidence of hyperparathyroidism. When fasting urinary calcium levels are normal, then the absorptive or "gastrointestinal" form of hypercalciuria can be pursued by drinking a synthetic meal (Calcitest) of 1 g of calcium, 200 mg of phosphorus, 25 mEq of sodium, and 400 calories, then obtaining a 4-hour urine collection after a 2-hour lag period to permit intestinal absorption. Patients with classical absorptive hypercalciuria have high urinary calcium excretion rates (> 60 mg/4 hr) under these loading conditions. Frequently, patient data do not simply fit either one of these categories, and some stone clinics no longer characterize hypercalciuria as absorptive or renal.[13] However, if strict dietary calcium restriction or intestinal binding with cellulose phosphate is begun without estimating the obligatory renal loss of calcium, patients will be exposed to long-term risks of bone demineralization.

There is considerable overlap between the subgroups of the absorptive variant, renal variant, and primary hyperparathyroidism. All stone-forming patients with hypercalciuria tend to have high rates of intestinal calcium absorption and elevated plasma 1,25-dihydroxyvitamin D synthesis. It has been suggested that alimentary hyperabsorption of calcium and disordered set-point control of 1,25-$(OH)_2D$ production after calcium loading,[86] with levels sufficient to produce some bone mineral loss during a low-calcium diet, may be findings of a continuous spectrum. At the extremes are (1) patients whose hyperabsorptive disorder is mimicked simply by giving 1,25-$(OH)_2D$ to normal controls, and (2) patients with less diet-dependent renal calcium excretion, more evidence of bone resorption, and an overriding coupling of increased PTH and 1,25-$(OH)_2D$ production. Many with the renal variant do not have evidence of parathyroid stimulation. Increased intestinal calcium absorption can occur independently of 1,25-$(OH)_2D$ in patients with the absorptive variant, and neither PTH nor phosphate levels safely exclude those who will not have persistent hypercalciuria on a low-calcium diet.

Preventive Therapy—General Measures

The first recommendation in the preventive treatment of all patients with recurrent urolithiasis is to increase fluid intake so that urine volume exceeds 2.5 l/day. Diuresis at this level increases urine flow rate, dilutes its constituents, and prevents stone recurrence in 60% of patients. Emphasis should be placed on increased water intake, regardless of stone type, to keep the urine dilute throughout the day and night, but even with encouragement some patients will not be able to sustain a significant increase in urine volume.[87] Patients with frequent calcium oxalate stones are advised to avoid drinking large amounts of beverages high in oxalate, such as tea, colas, beer, and fruit juice.

The inverse relationship between fluid intake and the risk of urolithiasis is possibly the single most important factor in the pathogenesis, natural history, and preventive treatment of all the stone diseases. In a classic demonstration of the effects of health education, Frank and DeVries reduced the prevalence of urolithiasis from 1.7 to 0.24% among European immigrants to Israel by stressing an adequate fluid intake and increasing urine output from an average of 0.8 to 1.1 l/day in the study group.[88] Many of these patients had uric acid stones and a diet rich in animal protein. Recently, 19% of patients attending an urban metabolic stone clinic were thought to have chronic dehydration. Most were men working in hot environments with dietary risk factors for urolithiasis.[89] Increasing urine volume from 1.7 to 2.5 l/day plus dietary advice led to a marked reduction of stone recurrences in a 5-year follow-up period.

When fluid intake is maintained, moderate activity may offer some protection against calcium stone formation. A number of surveys conducted in Europe have found the incidence greater among professional groups, such as physicians, and those with sedentary jobs, such as administrative and clerical workers, compared with farmers, forestry workers, and miners. These observations are confounded by the strong relationship between affluence and lithogenic diets. On the other hand, high levels of exercise (e.g., marathon running) appear to promote urinary calcium excretion, especially in white men.[90] It is clear that mechanical forces operating on the skeleton exert profound and varied influences on calcium metabolism.

In addition to maintaining a high urine volume, managing the patient's nutrition is important in preventing urolithiasis. In patients with idiopathic calcium stones or the hypercalciuria syndromes, there appears to be enhanced sensitivity to the calciuric effects of dietary protein,[91] as well as carbohydrate, sodium, and oxalate intake. The acidifying action of normal, high-protein diets reduces urinary citrate excretion that can be restored by modest vegetarianism. To prevent stone recurrences, the intake of animal protein should be limited to no more than five meals with meat, fish, or poultry per week, containing 1 g/kg/day of protein and less than 100 mEq/day of sodium.[92] An additional 10 to 20% reduction in urinary calcium can be achieved by dietary fiber (wheat, rice, or soy bran) in the range of 30 to 40 g/day. Bran has been shown to have this benefit in premenopausal women on a calcium-rich diet—a finding of considerable importance to the young female patient with a family history of osteoporosis.[93]

Calcium restriction to less than 100 mg/day is ill advised in most patients. For those with documented absorptive hypercalciuria dietary calcium can be reduced modestly to approximately 600 mg/day by eliminating milk, cheese, chocolate, fortified cereals, smoked fish, and canned meats. Such a limited calcium diet will be low in sodium, which will be of further benefit, but rigid calcium restriction is associated with 80% noncompliance and may produce bone demineralization. Osteopenia in patients with idiopathic stone disease occurs as frequently as in patients with primary hyperparathyroidism, and marked increases in bone turnover rates have been found in stone-forming patients on a low calcium diet.[94]

Chronic reduction of dietary calcium limits intestinal binding with oxalate, increases ^{14}C-oxalate absorption, and produces urinary oxalate levels that promote stone formation.[95] In some patients urinary oxalate excretion can reach 60 to 70 mg/day on a low calcium diet. This type of intermittent hyperoxaluria does not respond to dietary oxalate restriction, whereas patients with consistently elevated urinary oxalate have some benefit from elimination of such foods as spinach, collards, okra, rhubarb, sweet potatoes, nuts, tea, chocolate, pepper, wheat germ, cocoa, beets, swiss chard, soybean crackers, asparagus, and some berries. For similar reasons, calcium restriction is not recommended in enteric hyperoxaluric states, which are best managed by limiting oxalate-rich foods and by correcting the other nutritional problems secondary to malabsorption, such as dehydration, loss of bicarbonate, and steatorrhea. Reduction of dietary fat intake, its replacement by medium-chain triglycerides, and daily calcium or magnesium supplementation will lower renal oxalate excretion in most patients with ileal disease.

Patients with hyperuricosuric calcium urolithiasis may have normal urinary uric acid excretion on purine-restricted diets that contain approximately one third the normal daily purine consumption. Not only do these patients habitually consume meat, fish, poultry, and other foods rich in nucleoproteins—the main dietary source of purines—but also they excrete 10 to 15% more uric acid than do normal individuals at any level of dietary purine. Although controlled trials are lacking, one can reasonably conclude that the practical elimination of excessive amounts of purine-rich beverages (beer and wine) and foods will be helpful in some patients.

The effect of diet in gouty patients with uric acid stones is less straightforward, presumably because most of these patients are relative underexcretors of uric acid, and their risk of stone formation depends more on the total body urate pool than on dietary intake. In primary gout, proximal tubular secretion requires a higher plasma urate concentration than would suffice for the normal person to achieve an equivalent secretory rate. Since renal tubular reabsorption of urate is essentially a linear function of the filtered load, the total amount of excreted urinary uric acid will remain similar to that of nongouty subjects. Excessive uricosuria, when it does result from dietary intake, is seen more frequently in young age groups, occurring in 40% of patients 35 to 45 years of age but in less than 10% after 65 years of age. Hydration and alkalinization of the urine to a pH between 6.0 and 6.5 are usually effective preventive measures.

Once fluid intake and diet are addressed, the medication history may reveal iatrogenic factors that are important in stone disease. Vitamin D and vitamin A may lead to hypercalcemic nephrolithiasis. Large doses of ascorbic acid are also associated with calcium stone formation. Calcium phosphate stones may occur during acetazolamide treatment for glaucoma, owing to periodically alkaline urine. Triamterene, sulfonamides, and numerous other drugs may precipitate in the urinary tract.

Instrumentation of the urinary tract poses a considerable risk of iatrogenic infection and staghorn calculi formation in patients with renal stones. Although well-controlled studies are lacking, it is acceptable practice to use parenteral antibiotics, such as a cephalosporin or gentamicin, prior to and during invasive urologic procedures, followed by 2 weeks of oral antimicrobial therapy. Established or relapsing urinary tract infections in stone disease of all types require a prolonged course of antimicrobial drugs for several months. Prolonged therapy is also warranted following surgical removal of infection-induced struvite or calcium phosphate stones since persistent infection or stone recurrences can be expected in 40% of these cases, especially when residual fragments are refractory to dissolution.[96] Restriction of dietary phosphorus to less than 450 mg/day and reduction of intestinal phosphate absorption with aluminum carbonate (Basaljel) at 30 to 45 ml four times a day are supplemental measures that constitute the Shorr regimen for preventing growth or recurrence of infection stones. Whereas dietary phosphate reduction by the Shorr regimen is appropriate in infection-induced calculi, it may increase the risk of stone formation in calcium stone disease by stimulating the production of 1,25-$(OH)_2D$. This adverse effect of low phosphate intake is particularly important in patients with absorptive hypercalciuria or hyperparathyroidism.

The preventive approach to infection-induced stones includes acidifying the urine, antibiotic suppression of infection, and surgical correction of predisposing anatomic abnormalities. Preventing reflux and refraining from indwelling Foley catheters are particularly important in spinal cord–injured patients, reducing the risk of stones by one half to one third.[97] Long-term acidification of the urine after ESWL for infection stones, combined with culture-specific antibiotics, may reduce new stone formation and growth of residual stone fragments.

Renal colic can be a dramatic event, and many patients turn to nontraditional or home remedies with high expectation. In Chinese patients, acupuncture is as effective as intramuscular narcotic injections in relieving the colic of urolithiasis.[98] Hot baths or compresses and large doses of water and weak tea are popular and probably innocuous traditions in rural areas. Herbal medicine includes a number of substances meant to prevent stone recurrences, such as "Eisenberg's solution," which contains a large amount of citrate and has some scientific basis for its alleged effectiveness. *Rubia tinctorum* (common madder) is the essential ingredient in several kidney teas promoted for long-term prophylaxis of urolithiasis. Its red pigment, used to dye the trousers of French soldiers, also discolors the urine and obscures the presence of hematuria. Other anthraquinone glycosides in the plant are metabolized to highly genotoxic compounds and pose a significant carcinogenic risk.[99]

Preventive Therapy—Medications

Specific measures that are available to prevent a recurrence of calcium stones include thiazide diuretics, citrate preparations, allopurinol, phosphates, magnesium, and cellulose phosphate. Some of these medications still have not undergone controlled trials. The well-known observations that low-dose thiazide diuretics decrease urinary calcium and increase excretion of magnesium, zinc, and pyrophosphate, all of which inhibit calcium crystallization, have led to the increasing use of these drugs in calcium urolithiasis with or without hypercalciuria. The thiazides may decrease excessive intestinal calcium absorption, especially in patients with elevated 1,25-$(OH)_2D$ and PTH levels, but they seem particularly effective in renal hypercalciuria. The net effect on calcium balance appears to be positive, since thiazides provide some protection against loss of bone mineral content. Hydrochlorothiazide, 50 mg/day; trichlormethiazide, 4 mg/day; bendroflumethiazide, 5 mg/day; and chlorthalidone, 50 mg/day, can be used interchangeably to lower urinary calcium. In general, thiazides reduce recurrence rates to 50% of pretreatment levels in patients with frequent calcium oxalate stones, in randomized double-blind, placebo-controlled trials. The effect seems to be best with divided doses, prevention of hypokalemia, and control of dietary salt and protein intake. Since there seems to be an association among potassium deficiency, diminished excretion of citrate, and secondary hypercalciuria, potassium citrate is a preferred supplement for most patients. Excessive urinary sodium seems to attenuate the thiazide effect on calcium excretion, and dietary salt intake should be restricted to about 6 g/day.

In many medical centers, it is now the practice to begin therapy with low doses of thiazides in all patients with recurrent calcium urolithiasis who are shown to have hypercalciuria. Careful follow-up, including measurement of the serum calcium level, is necessary. Well-known side effects, like hypokalemia, hypercalcemia, hyperuricemia, glucose intolerance, and volume depletion necessitate discontinuation in 10 to 30% of patients on long-term thiazides for urolithiasis. Treatment failures are common when urinary citrate levels are low or when hyperuricosuria accompanies calcium stone formation, usually in hypercalciuric men. In these latter patients, the combined use of thiazides and allopurinol, at 100 mg twice daily, produces a tenfold reduction in stone production. Allopurinol may also decrease calcium stone recurrence in patients with no detectable metabolic disorder, other than mild hyperuricosuria. Three well-designed trials have demonstrated a significant benefit of allopurinol in these patients with calcium oxalate calculi.[100–102] Hydrochlorothiazide at 1 mg/kg/day is effective in childhood hypercalciuric stone disease and has few side effects.[103] At all ages serum calcium tends to rise, but iPTH falls and dystrophic calcification is not encountered during chronic therapy, unless the patient has unsuspected hyperparathyroidism.

The value of correcting hypocitraturia in urolithiasis has been known for 50 years. In 1985, the Food and Drug Administration (FDA) approved the use of potassium citrate in hypocitraturic calcium nephrolithiasis and in uric acid stone disease. It has been used successfully in patients with relapse on thiazides or allopurinol, in RTA, and in chronic diarrheal syndromes. Long-term therapy with 20 mEq three times daily in tablet form significantly reduces stone formation rates without the gastrointestinal distress seen with liquid preparations.[104] Shallow gastric erosions have been noted occasionally on endoscopy, usually without clinically significant bleeding. Typically, urinary pH increases to 6.5, but alkali-induced stones such as calcium phosphate do not occur because of the fall in urinary calcium levels. Citrate, either as Shohl's solution, equimolar mixtures of sodium and potassium citrate, or potassium citrate tablets is the treatment of choice for the calcium phosphate urolithiasis of distal RTA at 0.5 mEq/kg/day. In adults, the solutions are administered at 10 to 30 ml diluted with water, after meals and at bedtime; or two to four 5-mEq tablets are taken with a full glass of water with meals for all types of hypocitraturia.

Alkali ingestion is also effective in preventing metabolically active uric acid and cystine urolithiasis. Patients with uric acid stones can be treated with a variety of bicarbonate and citrate alkalinizers, to which acetazolamide can be added. Preparations containing sodium seem to have reduced effectiveness and a risk of calcium phosphate urolithiasis after long-term use. Total dosage depends on renal function, the amount of protein in the patient's diet, body weight, and the existence of medical complications such as congestive heart failure. Nocturnal urine pH should be checked periodically. In uric acid urolithiasis, a therapeutic urine pH of 6.5 can be achieved with 25 mEq of base at meals and bedtime, whereas patients with cystinuria will require twice this daily dosage to maintain the desired urine pH of 7.5. Uric acid stones, cystine stones, and calcium deposits within the kidney associated with RTA may disappear after treatment with absorbable alkali. In patients with RTA, urinary calcium excretion is reduced by 50%, and a 20-fold decline in stone recurrences has been noted.[105] The dosage of alkali required in cystinuria is poorly tolerated, and in cystinuric patients with mixed stones containing calcium it should be avoided in favor of achieving a urine volume of 3 l/day.

Patients at risk for uric acid stones should also maintain a high urine flow rate throughout the day. Such conservative management seems adequate for most patients with asymptomatic hyperuricemia. In those with clinical gout who are treated with uricosuric agents, alkalinization of the urine during the first 2 weeks of therapy, followed by long-term hydration, usually will prevent iatrogenic stone formation. Patients with metabolically active uric acid calculi and those with uric acid stones from myeloproliferative states or distal small bowel disease will benefit from allopurinol, 200 to 400 mg/day. The subgroup of patients with mixed calcium–uric acid urolithiasis may also require thiazides, once primary hyperparathyroidism has been excluded. Even patients with large, obstructing uric acid stones have had successful dissolution and salvage of renal function with the potent combination of liberal fluids, alkali therapy, and allopurinol.[106]

Asymptomatic relatives of patients with cystinuria need to maintain a high urine volume and periodic ultrasound surveillance throughout life. Those with crystalluria and urinary calculi who relapse on conservative therapy are candidates for D-penicillamine. This unique chelator reacts in vivo with cystine to form disulfide cysteine-penicillamine, which is 50 times more soluble in urine than is cystine. Supplemental pyridoxine, 50 to 100 mg/day, is recommended, since penicillamine combines with pyridoxal phosphate, the active metabolite of pyridoxine, to form a biochemically inactive compound. At dosages of 750 mg to 2 g/day existing stones shrink slowly after 6 to 12 months, provided that they are in pelvic-caliceal regions that are well perfused with urine. Active stone disease from cystinuria is an acceptable indication for penicillamine therapy, but adverse side effects are either common, including hypersensitivity rashes and fever, or potentially dangerous, such as proteinuria, bone marrow suppression, and epidermolysis bullosa. Cystine excretion is not sensitive to routine dietary manipulation. In all patients with cystinuria careful monitoring is important, since ESWL fragmentation can be accomplished readily with small, but not large cystine calculi.[107]

Calcium oxalate stones from the hyperoxaluria of ileal disease or small bowel resection can be prevented by dietary oxalate restriction, but compliance is low and the oxalate content of many prepared foods is not readily available. In a small number of these patients cholestyramine at 16 g/day has significantly reduced urinary oxalate excretion. Correction of hypocitraturia and hypomagnesuria may be helpful in many patients with urolithiasis complicating bowel disease. Magnesium oxide in dosages from 300 to 600 mg/day also may reduce idiopathic calcium stone recurrences in patients who cannot tolerate other therapy but is contraindicated in renal insufficiency or chronic urinary tract infection.

Orthophosphates, prepared as potassium acid phosphate, neutral mixtures (Neutra-Phos), or alkaline disodium and dipotassium phosphates have been used for decades to prevent recurrences of idiopathic calcium stones. The minimum effective dosage is 1500 mg/day, which increases the excretion of inorganic pyrophosphate, an inhibitor of stone formation, two- to threefold. Urinary calcium excretion falls in treated patients with hypercalciuria. The clinical response to chronic orthophosphate therapy, however, has been variable in unselected patients, and one double-blind, controlled study found that 25 patients receiving 1 g of acid phosphates daily showed no significant improvement in comparison with a placebo-treated group, 80% of whom remained stone-free during the 3-year follow-up period with hydration and a reduced calcium diet.[108] Side effects include diarrhea, abdominal discomfort, nausea, and soft tissue calcification. Phosphate therapy stimulates parathyroid activity in normal individuals but diminishes 1,25-$(OH)_2D$ and intestinal calcium absorption in patients with subtle hyperparathyroidism. Phosphates may be helpful in active stone-formers who are not candidates for parathyroid surgery or who have persistent hypercalciuria after removal of a parathyroid adenoma.[109] They are not indicated in MSK, infection stones, or renal insufficiency.

Sodium cellulose phosphate, a nonabsorbable ion-exchange resin with a high affinity for calcium, has been proposed for the treatment of active calcium stone formation, when absorptive hypercalciuria is carefully documented and bone disease is absent. Because of the potential for bone demineralization, cautious use in patients excreting more than 350 mg/day of urinary calcium or in thiazide resistent hypercalciuria is occasionally recommended. The dosage is 10 to 15 g/day, individualized according to urinary calcium excretion. Significant reduction in stone recurrence has been obtained in about 150 patients with very active calcium urolithiasis, reported in seven uncontrolled studies since 1974.[110] Hypomagnesemia, which may develop owing to resin binding, can be corrected by oral magnesium supplementation. Hyperoxaluria exceeding 50 mg/day is a troublesome side effect. Patients with renal hypercalciuria should not be treated with sodium cellulose phosphate because such therapy may induce secondary hyperparathyroidism and bone disease. Moreover, a significant sodium burden and the high cost (in excess of $4/day) preclude its widespread use. A few patients have developed acute joint pain on cellulose phosphate, possibly due to pyrophosphate synovitis.

Generally, patients with other uncommon causes of urolithiasis, such as hyperthyroidism, myxedema, and Cushing's disease, are best managed by specific therapy of the underlying disorder. For example, patients with sarcoidosis have increased fractional absorption of calcium, and hypercalcemia occurs when the compensatory ability of the kidneys is exceeded. Immunoreactive PTH is low, and nephrogenous cAMP may be undetectable. Plasma 1,25-dihydroxyvitamin D has been found to be markedly elevated in patients with normal renal function and in two anephric patients.[111] Additional in vitro evidence for extrarenal synthesis of 1,25-$(OH)_2D$ in sarcoidosis has been obtained from cultured pulmonary alveolar macrophages[112] and lymph node homogenates.[113] Prednisone reduces 1,25-$(OH)_2D$ to normal levels, corrects hypercalciuria, and provides preventive treatment for recurrent urolithiasis in sarcoidosis. One patient with silicone-induced granulomas, hypercalcemia, stone disease, hypercalciuria, and elevated plasma 1,25-$(OH)_2D$ has been described who also responded to glucocorticoid therapy.[114]

Finally, spurious foreign bodies are presented occasionally as evidence of stone disease by patients seeking narcotics or suffering from Münchausen's syndrome.[115] A suspicious history, an absence of microhematuria, and an alledged allergy to urogram dye might point to these complex psychiatric conditions, which are best managed by longitudinal care outside hospital emergency rooms.

REFERENCES

1. Boyce WH, Garvey FK, and Strawcutter HE: Incidence of urinary calculi among patients in general hospitals, 1948–1952. JAMA 161:1437, 1956.
2. Johnson CM, Wilson DM, O'Fallon WM, et al: Renal stone epidemiology: A 25-year study in Rochester, Minnesota. Kidney Int 16:624, 1979.
3. Oshibuchi M, Nishi F, Sato M, et al: Frequency of abnormalities detected by abdominal ultrasound among Japanese adults. J Gastroenterol Hepatol 6(2):165, 1991.
4. Scott R, Freeland R, Mowat W, et al: The prevalence of calcified upper urinary tract stone disease in a random population—Cumbernauld Health Survey. Br J Urol 49:589, 1977.
5. Rosenow EC: Renal calculi: Study of papillary calcification. J Urol 44:19, 1940.
6. Glowacki LS, Beecroft ML, Cook RJ, et al: The natural history of asymptomatic urolithiasis. J Urol 147(2):319, 1992.
7. Uribarri J, Oh MS, and Carroll HJ: The first kidney stone. Ann Intern Med 111(12):1006, 1989.
8. Williams RE: Long-term survey of 538 patients with upper urinary tract stone. Br J Urol 35:416, 1963.
9. Coe FL, Keck J, and Norton ER: The natural history of calcium urolithiasis. JAMA 238:1519, 1977.
10. Gearhart JP, Herzberg GZ, and Jeffs RD: Childhood urolithiasis: Experiences and advances. Pediatrics 87(4):445, 1991.
11. Garcia CD, Miller LA, and Stapleton FB: Natural history of hematuria associated with hypercalciuria in children. Am J Dis Child 145(10):1204, 1991.
12. Haddad JG: Vitamin D—Solar rays, the milky way, or both? N Engl J Med 326:1213, 1992.
13. Wilson DM: Clinical and laboratory evaluation of renal stone patients. Endocrinol Metab Clin North Am 19(4):973, 1990.
14. Ohman S, Larsson L, and Tiselius HG: Clinical significance of phosphate in calcium oxalate renal stones. Ann Clin Biochem 29(1):59, 1992.
15. Herring LC: Observations in the analysis of ten thousand urinary calculi. J Urol 88:545, 1962.
16. Ettinger B, Well E, Mandel MS, et al: Triamterene-induced nephrolithiasis. Ann Intern Med 91:745, 1979.
17. Buckland CE and Rosenberg M: Survey of urolithiasis in the United States. J Urol 73:198, 1955.
18. Williams RE: Long-term survey of 538 patients with upper urinary tract stone. Br J Urol 35:416, 1963.
19. Pin NT, Ling NY, and Siang LH: Dehydration from outdoor work and urinary stones in a tropical environment. Occup Med 42(1):30, 1992.
20. Transbøl I, Jørgensen FS, Lund B, et al: Seasonal variations in urinary excretion of calcium. BMJ 1:734, 1975.
21. Churchill D, Bryant D, Fodor G, et al: Drinking water hardness and urolithiasis. Ann Intern Med 88:513, 1978.
22. Thun MJ and Schober S: Urolithiasis in Tennessee: An occupational window into a regional problem. Am J Public Health 81(5):587, 1991.
23. Rudman D, Kutner M, Redel S, et al: Hypocitraturia in calcium nephrolithiasis. J Clin Endocrinol Metab 55:1052, 1982.
24. Hosking DH, Wilson DM, Liedtke RB, et al: Urinary citrate excretion in normal persons and patients with idiopathic calcium urolithiasis. J Lab Clin Med 106:682, 1983.
25. Hobarth K and Hofbauer J: Value of routine citrate analysis and calcium/citrate ratio in calcium urolithiasis. Eur Urol 19(2):165, 1991.
26. Lieske JC, Walsh-Reitz MM, and Toback FG: Calcium oxalate monohydrate crystals are endocytosed by renal epithelial cells and induce proliferation. Am J Physiol 262(4):F622, 1992.
27. Coe FL, Nakagawa Y, and Parks JH: Inhibitors within the nephron. Am J Kidney Dis 17(4):407, 1991.
28. Ishikawa Y, Kohri K, Iguchi M, et al: Influence of morphologic factors on calcium-containing stone formation. Urol Int 48(2):206, 1992.
29. Tennent J: Every Man His Own Doctor, or The Poor Planter's Physician. Facsimile of 1734 ed. Williamsburg, VA, Printing and Post Office, 1971.
30. Case 33-1992. N Engl J Med 327:481, 1992.
31. Koehler PR and Kyaw MM: Hematuria. Med Clin North Am 59:201, 1975.
32. Mutgi A, Williams JW, and Nettleman M: Renal colic: Utility of the plain abdominal roentgenogram. Arch Intern Med 151(8):1589, 1991.
33. Haddad MC, Sharif HS, Shahed MS, et al: Renal colic: Diagnosis and outcome. Radiology 184:83, 1992.
34. Cronan JJ: Contemporary concepts for imaging urinary tract obstruction. Urol Radiol 14:8, 1992.
35. Levine E and Grantham JJ: Calcified renal stones and cyst calcifications in autosomal dominant polycystic kidney disease: Clinical and CT study in 84 patients. Am J Roentgenol 159(1):77, 1992.
36. Maclure M and Willett W: A case-control study of diet and risk of renal adenocarcinoma. Epidemiology 1(6):430, 1990.
37. DeVivo MJ, Fine PR, Cutter GR, et al: The risk of renal calculi in spinal cord injury patients. J Urol 131:857, 1984.
38. Urivetzky M, Kessaris D, and Smith AD: Ascorbic acid overdosing: A risk factor for calcium oxalate nephrolithiasis. J Urol 147(5):1215, 1992.
39. Cooke N, Teitelbaum S, and Avioli LV: Antacid-induced osteomalacia and nephrolithiasis. Arch Intern Med 138:1007, 1978.
40. Daudon M, Lacour B, Jungers P, et al: Urolithiasis in patients with end stage renal failure. J Urol 147(4):977, 1992.
41. Flocks RH: Prophylaxis and medical management of calcium urolithiasis: The role of the quantity and precipitability of urinary calcium. J Urol 44:183, 1940.
42. Albright F, Henneman R, Benedict PH, et al: Idiopathic hypercalciuria (a preliminary report). Proc Roy Soc Med 46:1077, 1953.
43. Pak CYC, Ohata M, Lawrence EC, et al: The hypercalciurias:

Causes, parathyroid functions and diagnostic criteria. J Clin Invest 54:387, 1974.
44. Broadus AE, Insogna KL, Lang R, et al: Evidence for disordered control of 1,20-dihydroxyvitamin D production in absorptive hypercalciuria. N Engl J Med 311:73, 1984.
45. Coe FL, Canterbury JM, Firpo JJ, et al: Evidence of secondary hyperparathyroidism in idiopathic hypercalciuria. J Clin Invest 52:134, 1973.
46. Olmer M, Berland Y, and Argeni B: Absence of secondary hyperparathyroidism in most patients with renal hypercalciuria. Kidney Int 24(Suppl 16):S175, 1983.
47. Sutton RA and Walker VR: Responses to hydrochlorothiazide and acetazolamide in patients with calcium stones: Evidence suggesting a defect in renal tubular function. N Engl J Med 302:709, 1980.
48. Silverberg SJ, Shane E, Jacobs TP, et al: Nephrolithiasis and bone involvement in primary hyperparathyroidism. Am J Med 89:327, 1990.
49. Broadus AE, Horst RL, Lang R, et al: The importance of circulating 1,25-dihydroxy-vitamin D in the pathogenesis of hypercalciuria and renal-stone formation of primary hyperparathyroidism. N Engl J Med 302:421, 1980.
50. Jabbour N, Corvilain J, Fuss M, et al: The natural history of renal stone disease after parathyroidectomy for primary hyperparathyroidism. Surg Gynecol Obstet 172(1):25, 1991.
51. Rothstein M, Obialo C, and Hruska KA: Renal tubular acidosis. Endocrinol Metab Clin North Am 19(4):869, 1990.
52. Gault MH, Chafe LL, Morgan JM, et al: Comparison of patients with idiopathic calcium phosphate and calcium oxalate stones. Medicine (Baltimore) 70(6):345, 1991.
53. Coe FL and Kavalach AG: Hypercalciuria and hyperuricosuria in patients with calcium nephrolithiasis. N Engl J Med 291:1344, 1974.
54. Smith MJV and Boyce WH: Allopurinol and urolithiasis. J Urol 102:750, 1969.
55. Fessel WJ: Renal outcomes of gout and hyperuricemia. Am J Med 67:74, 1979.
56. Hall AP, Barry PE, Dawber TR, et al: Epidemiology of gout and hyperuricemia—a long-term population study. Am J Med 42:27, 1967.
57. Yü T-F and Gutman AB: Uric acid nephrolithiasis: Predisposing factors. Ann Intern Med 67:1133, 1967.
58. Riese RJ, Sakhaee K: Uric acid nephrolithiasis: Pathogenesis and treatment. J Urol 148:765, 1992.
59. Henneman PH, Wallach S, and Dempsey EF: The metabolic defect responsible for uric acid stone formation. J Clin Invest 41:537, 1962.
60. Sakhaee K, Nigam S, Snell P, et al: Assessment of the pathogenetic role of physical exercise in renal stone formation. J Clin Endocrinol Metab 65:974, 1987.
61. Klinenberg JR, Kippen I, and Bluestone R: Hyperuricemic nephropathy: Pathologic features and factors influencing urate deposition. Nephron 14:88, 1975.
62. Milliner DS: Cystinuria. Endocrinol Metab Clin North Am 19(4):889, 1990.
63. Dent CE and Senior B: Studies on the treatment of cystinuria. Br J Urol 27:317, 1955.
64. Watts RWE: Cystinuria and cystine stone disease. *In* Williams DI and Chisholm GD (eds): Scientific Foundations of Urology. London, Heinemann, 1976, p 320.
65. Krizek V, Erben J, Lazne M, et al: Disappearance of cystinuria after kidney transplantation. Br J Urol 55:575, 1983.
66. Pahira JJ: Management of the patient with cystinuria. Urol Clin North Am 14:339, 1987.
67. Allison MJ, Cook HM, Milne DB, et al: Oxalate degradation by gastrointestinal bacteria from humans. J Nutr 116:455, 1986.
68. Chadwick VS, Modha K, and Dowling RH: Mechanism for hyperoxaluria in patients with ileal dysfunction. N Engl J Med 289:172, 1973.
69. Baggio B, Gambaro G, Marchini F, et al: An inheritable anomaly of red-cell oxalate transport in "primary" calcium nephrolithiasis correctable with diuretics. N Engl J Med 314:599, 1986.
70. Wong SY, Slater SR, Evans RA, et al: Metabolic studies in kidney stone disease. QJ Med 82(299):247, 1992.
71. Rocha H and Santos LCS: Relapse of urinary tract infection in the presence of urinary tract calculi: The role of bacteria within the calculi. J Med Microbiol 2:372, 1969.
72. Holmgren K, Danielson BG, Fellstrom B, et al: The relation between urinary tract infections and stone composition in renal stone formers. Scand J Urol Nephrol 23(2):131, 1989.
73. Koga S, Arakaki Y, Matsuoka M, et al: Calculous pyelonephritis. Int Urol Nephrol 24(2):109, 1992.
74. Cochran M, Peacock M, Smith DA, et al: Renal tubular acidosis of pyelonephritis with renal stone disease. BMJ 2:721, 1968.
75. Cox, CE: Urinary tract infection and renal lithiasis. Urol Clin North Am 1:279, 1974.
76. Dajani AM and Shehabi AA: Bacteriology and composition of infected stones. Urology 21:351, 1983.
77. Dretler SP: The pathogenesis of urinary tract calculi after ileal conduit diversion. J Urol 109:204, 1973.
78. Kroovand RL: Stones in pregnancy and in children. J Urol 148:1076, 1992.
79. Segura JW: Surgical management of urinary calculi. Semin Nephrol 10(1):53, 1990.
80. Mulley AG Jr and Carlson KJ: Lithotripsy. Ann Intern Med 103:626, 1985.
81. Karlsen SJ and Berg KJ: Acute changes in kidney function following extracorporeal shock wave lithotripsy for renal stones. Br J Urol 67(3):241, 1991.
82. Jewett MA, Bombardier C, Caron D, et al: Potential for interobserver and intra-observer variability in X-ray review to establish stone-free rates after lithotripsy. J Urol 147(3):559, 1992.
83. Brown SM: Peri-operative anxiety in patients undergoing extracorporeal piezolithotripsy. J Adv Nurs 15(9):1078, 1990.
84. Ginalski JM, Portmann L, and Jaeger P: Does medullary sponge kidney cause nephrolithiasis? Am J Roentgenol 155(2):299, 1990.
85. Parks JH, Coe FL, and Strauss AL: Calcium nephrolithiasis and medullary sponge kidney in women. N Engl J Med 306:1088, 1982.
86. Coe FL: Treatment of hypercalciuria (Editorial). N Engl J Med 311:116, 1984.
87. Brickman AM, Ellison AF, Kliger AS, et al: Low urine volume in stone formers. Ann Intern Med 93:644, 1980.
88. Frank M and DeVries A: Prevention of urolithiasis. Arch Environ Health 13:625, 1966.
89. Embon OM, Rose GA, and Rosenbaum T: Chronic dehydration stone disease. Br J Urol 66(4):357, 1990.
90. Rodgers AL, Cox TA, Noakes TD, et al: Crystalluria in marathon runners. IV: Black subjects. Urol Res 20(1):27, 1992.
91. Wassertein AG, Stolley PO, Soper KA, et al: Case-control study of risk factors for idiopathic calcium nephrolithiasis. Miner Electrolyte Metab 13:85, 1987.
92. Goldfarb S: The role of diet in the pathogenesis and therapy of nephrolithiasis. Endocrinol Metab Clin North Am 19:805, 1990.
93. Jahnen A, Heynck H, Gertz A, et al: Dietary fibre: The effectiveness of a high bran intake in reducing renal calcium excretion. Urol Res 20:3, 1992.
94. Messa P, Mioni G, Franzon R, et al: Factors affecting fasting urinary calcium excretion in stone former patients on different dietary calcium intake. Scanning Microsc 6(1):239, 1992.
95. Smith LH: Diet and hyperoxaluria in the syndrome of idiopathic calcium oxalate urolithiasis. Am J Kidney Dis 17(4):370, 1991.
96. Silverman DE and Stamey TA: Management of infection stones: The Stanford experience. Medicine 62:44, 1983.
97. Hall SK, Hackler RH, Zampieri TA, et al: Renal calculi in spinal cord–injured patients: Association with reflux, bladder stones, and foley catheter drainage. Urology 34:126, 1989.
98. Lee YH, Lee WC, Chen MT, et al: Acupuncture in the treatment of renal colic. J Urol 147(1):16, 1992.
99. Blomeke B, Poginsky B, Schmutte C, et al: Formation of genotoxic metabolites from anthraquinone glycosides, present in Rubia tinctorum L. Mutat Res 265(2):263, 1992.
100. Smith MJV: Placebo versus allopurinol for renal calculi. J Urol 117:690, 1977.
101. Coe FL: Uric acid and calcium oxalate nephrolithiasis. Kidney Int 24:392, 1983.

102. Ettinger B, Tang A, Citron JT, et al: Randomized trial of allopurinol in the prevention of calcium oxalate calculi. N Engl J Med 315:1386, 1986.
103. Voskaki I, al Qadreh A, Mengrelic, et al: Effect of hydrochlorothiazide on renal hypercalciuria. Child Nephrol Urol 12(1):6, 1992.
104. Pak CYC, Fuller C, Sakhaee K, et al: Long-term treatment of calcium nephrolithiasis with potassium citrate. J Urol 134:11, 1985.
105. Coe FL and Parks JH: Stone disease in hereditary distal renal tubular acidosis. Ann Intern 93:60, 1980.
106. Sharma SK and Indudhara R: Chemodissolution of urinary uric acid stones by alkali therapy. Urol Int 48(1):81, 1992.
107. Katz G, Lencorsky A, Pide D, et al: Place of extracorporeal shock wave lithotripsy (ESWL) in management of cystine calculi. Urology 36:124, 1990.
108. Ettinger B: Recurrent nephrolithiasis: Natural history and effect of phosphate therapy: A double-blind controlled study. Am J Med 61:200, 1976.
109. Broadus AE, Magee JS, Mallette LE, et al: A detailed evaluation of oral phosphate therapy in selected patients with primary hyperparathyroidism. J Clin Endocrinol Metab 56:953, 1983.
110. Pak CYC: A cautious use of sodium cellulose phosphate in the management of calcium nephrolithiasis. Invest Urol 19:187, 1981.
111. Barbour GL, Coburn JW, Slatopolsky E, et al: Hypercalcemia in an anephric patient with sarcoidosis: Evidence for extrarenal generation of 1,25-dihydroxyvitamin D. N Engl J Med 305:440, 1981.
112. Adams JS, Stauma OP, Gacad MA, et al: Metabolism of 25-hydroxyvitamin D_2 by cultured pulmonary alveolar macrophages in sarcoidosis. J Clin Invest 72:1856, 1983.
113. Mason RS, Frankel T, Chan Y-L, et al: Vitamin D conversion by sarcoid lymph node homogenate. Ann Intern Med 100:59, 1984.
114. Kozeny GA, Bonbato AI, Bansal VK, et al: Hypercalciuria associated with silicone-induced granulomas. N Engl J Med 311:1103, 1984.
115. Atkinson RL and Earll JM: Munchausen syndrome with renal stones. JAMA 230:89, 1974.

36

Chronic Renal Failure

ROBERT C. MAY, MD
WILLIAM E. MITCH, MD

The major diseases leading to chronic renal failure (CRF) can be divided into those primarily affecting the glomeruli, those primarily affecting the tubules and renal interstitium, and inherited diseases that affect the glomeruli or interstitium or both (Table 36–1).[1, 2] Pathologic examination of the kidneys of patients with far-advanced CRF invariably reveals extensive glomerular and interstitial damage, regardless of the etiology of the initial disease. Thus, once CRF is established, clinical and metabolic manifestations of the disease are markedly similar because they are due mainly to an accumulation of unexcreted waste products.

The most frequent cause of progressive renal insufficiency is glomerulonephritis. This disorder is characterized by progressive damage to glomeruli that may result from a primary renal disease or from the secondary effects of a systemic disorder such as diabetes mellitus,[2] autoimmune disorders, allergic reactions, infections, and certain toxins. The next most frequent cause of progressive CRF is interstitial nephritis. Nonglomerular, progressive renal insufficiency was considered previously to be caused by chronic infection and was called pyelonephritis. It is now recognized that this is incorrect because in the absence of obstruction to urine flow, progressive CRF rarely, if ever, is caused by pyogenic infections.[3, 4] The more general term *interstitial nephritis* has replaced pyelonephritis. Interstitial nephritis may occur as a primary disease or secondary to drugs or other diseases such as hypertension, analgesic abuse, sickle cell disease, and gout.[5] The majority of patients with nonglomerular renal disease causing end-stage renal failure suffer from hypertensive glomerulosclerosis.[2] Somewhat surprisingly, antihypertensive therapy for pa-

TABLE 36–1. FREQUENCY OF DISEASES CAUSING END-STAGE RENAL FAILURE

Disease	% of Patients
Glomerulonephritis	35
Diabetes mellitus	25
Polycystic kidney disease	9
Interstitial diseases	31
Hypertensive nephrosclerosis; analgesic abuse; obstruction-infection; miscellaneous (uric acid sickle cell); undetermined	

*Data compiled from references 1 through 5 and 10.

tients with hypertensive nephrosclerosis has failed to prevent deterioration of renal function despite adequate blood pressure control.[6] Whether blood pressure measured in the physician's office is unrepresentative of mean blood pressure control or whether control by current standards is inadequate remains unclear. Black patients appear especially susceptible to developing CRF from hypertension.[7] This raises the possibility that factors not directly linked to blood pressure level, per se, may account for the progression of renal failure under these conditions.[8] Regardless, hypertensive nephrosclerosis is a major cause of end-stage renal failure in the United States.[9]

Hereditary diseases and in particular polycystic kidney disease (PCKD) are the third most common causes of progressive CRF. PCKD accounts for about 9% of patients in dialysis and transplant programs,[10] whereas other diseases such as medullary cystic disease or Alport's disease are considerably less frequent causes of end-stage renal failure. A detailed discussion of the pathologic processes and of the clinical manifestations of each disease process leading to CRF is beyond the scope of this chapter, although several points should be kept in mind when evaluating a patient with CRF.

First, an attempt should be made to determine whether damage is occurring primarily in the glomerulus or in the interstitium, because the course of certain diseases may be altered by therapy. For example, corticosteroids appear to decrease proteinuria in minimal change disease and may delay the progression of membranous glomerulonephritis to CRF.[11, 12] Corticosteroids and cytotoxic agents can diminish loss of renal function associated with lupus erythematosus, Wegener's granulomatosis, and certain types of arteritis,[13–15] and discontinuance of analgesics may interrupt the progressive course of analgesic nephropathy.[5] Suspicion of one of the collagen-vascular diseases is raised by multisystem symptoms and a more fulminant course. These patients rarely show CRF as the first manifestation of illness.

Glomerular damage should be suspected when a patient has gross or microscopic hematuria or more than 2 g/24 hr of albumin in the urine; finding a red blood cell cast in the setting of chronic renal involvement documents the presence of glomerulonephritis (Table 36–2). Patients with minimal change disease or membranous glomerulonephritis generally have more than 2 g/24 hr of albumin but few cells or casts in the urine. Renal damage associated with multiple myeloma is characterized by proteinuria caused by excretion of globulins or globulin fragments. These proteins may not be detected when urine is tested with albumin-specific test tapes but will cause an obvious precipitate when urine is mixed with an equal volume of 3 g/dl of sulfosalicylic acid. Thus, all patients with CRF from an undiagnosed illness should have urine tested for the presence of protein by both methods.

Interstitial disease is suggested by a predominance of white blood cells and renal tubular cells, white blood cell or tubular cell casts, and less than 2 g/24 hr of protein in the urine. In this situation, the possibility of analgesic-abuse nephropathy should be suspected and vigorously pursued. It is often difficult to obtain a history of prolonged analgesic use from these patients, but it is important to establish the diagnosis because discontinuing the analgesics may minimize renal damage. The presence of eosinophiluria has been cited as a useful marker of acute interstitial nephritis.[16] Nolan and associates examined eosinophiluria in unselected patients referred to a renal service for evaluation of an active urinary sediment and correlated the presence of eosinophiluria with the underlying diagnosis.[17] Eosinophiluria was noted in 10 of 11 patients with acute interstitial nephritis but was distinctly uncommon in acute tubular necrosis (0/30), acute pyelonephritis (0/10), and acute cystitis (1/15). It should be noted that eosinophiluria was not specific for acute interstitial nephritis since it was noted to be present in certain forms of glomerulonephritis, especially rapidly progressive glomerulonephritis (4/10), and in acute prostatitis (6/10). In this study, the investigators compared Hansen's stain with the more commonly employed Wright's stain to detect eosinophiluria in acute interstitial nephritis and found that Hansen's stain was much more sensitive (10/11 versus 2/11 with Wright's stain). Thus, the absence of eosinophiluria would be an argument against acute interstitial nephritis, but only if the more sensitive assay was used.

In addition to the urinalysis, information may be obtained from an abdominal radiograph. A finding of small kidneys bilaterally can result from diseases affecting either the glomeruli or interstitium. Large kidneys can be found in diabetic and amyloid nephropathy, myeloma of the kidney, and polycystic renal disease. Diagnosis of diabetic or amyloid nephropathy is usually obvious from extrarenal manifestations of the disease. PCKD is suggested by pain, hematuria, and enlarged kidneys. One study compared the presence of the mutant gene for autosomal dominant PCKD using genetic linkage analysis with sonographic findings of cystic disease in 17 families with autosomal dominant PCKD.[18] Forty of 48 members younger than 30 years of age had renal cysts, and all 27 who were older than 30 years of age had sonographic evidence of cysts. Few patients with PCKD are symptomatic until middle age; the median age for an elevation in serum creatinine was 38 years of age in men, and 39 years of age in women.[19] Thus, early sonography represents the most sensitive, practical test for the presence of PCKD. About 50% of patients with polycystic kidneys will have pain, whereas only 20 to 30% will have hematuria and palpably enlarged kidneys. The hematuria may be gross or microscopic and frequently is intermittent. Infection is a frequent complication of this illness.[10]

TABLE 36–2. CHARACTERISTICS OF URINALYSIS IN PATIENTS WITH CHRONIC RENAL FAILURE

	Urinalysis		
Primary Lesion	*Cells*	*Protein*	*Casts**
Glomerular	RBC, PMN, tubular	More than 2 g/day	RBC
Interstitial	PMN, tubular, occasional RBC	Less than 2 g/day	PMN or tubular cell

*A red blood cell (RBC) cast generally is diagnostic of a glomerular lesion, whereas a cast composed primarily of polymorphonuclear leukocytes (PMN) may be found in either glomerular or interstitial diseases.

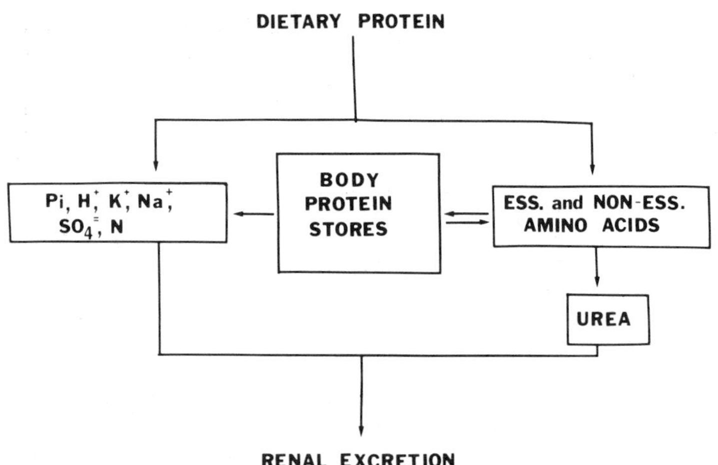

FIGURE 36–1. Digestion of dietary protein or catabolism of body protein enlarges the pool of essential and nonessential amino acids that can be used to synthesize body proteins. Amino acids can also be degraded, thus increasing urea production. Catabolism of endogenous or dietary protein also yields inorganic ions and other nitrogenous waste products that must be excreted. (From Mitch WE: Nutrition in renal disease. *In* Martinez-Maldonado M [ed]: Handbook of Renal Therapeutics. New York, Plenum, 1983, pp 349–373.)

Intravenous pyelography (IVP) can provide valuable information but may also cause further renal damage.[20] In the early stages of CRF, IVP can be useful for documenting that the patient has two kidneys of comparable size and has no evidence of obstruction from potentially remedied causes such as stones or strictures. IVP may also be useful in establishing the diagnosis of certain inherited cystic diseases such as PCKD or medullary cystic disease. In more advanced renal failure (serum creatinine value > 3 mg/dl), kidneys are poorly visualized unless a large dose of radiopaque contrast material is used. Unfortunately, large doses of iodinated contrast material can depress renal function profoundly, especially in those with diabetes and multiple myeloma.[20] The mechanism for renal damage is unknown but appears to be associated with or at least aggravated by dehydration. A report of the effects of prophylactic hydration of 100 patients who were undergoing angiography revealed no instances of acute renal failure nor of accelerated loss of renal function.[21] Although this report suggests a means of minimizing further renal injury, the value of the information to be gained from an IVP must be carefully weighed against the potential problems. This is especially true since the most important therapeutic information, the presence or absence of obstruction and kidney size, can be obtained by sonography.

The question of whether to obtain a renal biopsy is raised frequently during the evaluation of a patient with CRF. Discussion of the indications for a biopsy is not the purpose of this chapter.[22] A biopsy may be helpful in a patient with the nephrotic syndrome or in those suspected of having an autoimmune disease, because a treatable disease might be discovered. After the serum creatinine has reached a level higher than 5 mg/dl, the kidneys are usually shrunken unless the disease has progressed quite rapidly. A percutaneous renal biopsy when kidneys are small is rarely, if ever, advisable because unexpected injury could cause further loss of renal function. If therapeutic benefit is considered possible, then an open biopsy may be warranted, but this is unusual.

Goals of Therapy

The goals of therapy in managing patients with CRF include (1) lowering accumulated waste nitrogen and in particular urea nitrogen below the level that is associated with uremic symptoms, (2) maintenance of proper nutrition, (3) correction of mineral and electrolyte disorders, and (4) prevention of further progression of renal insufficiency. Meticulous medical management, as described further on, may delay the need for dialysis or renal transplantation for several years. Although dialysis and transplantation are frequently beneficial for patients with end-stage renal disease, they can be associated with considerable morbidity or even mortality. Therefore, delaying the need for dialysis or transplantation is viewed as an important and worthwhile goal by most patients with CRF.

WASTE NITROGEN ACCUMULATION

The signs and symptoms of uremia are directly related to the waste products that accumulate because of the loss of renal function. These waste products are derived from breakdown of dietary or endogenous protein stores. As indicated in Figure 36–1, metabolism of dietary protein or breakdown of body protein yields essential and nonessential amino acids and increases urea production because virtually all the nitrogen in amino acids is used to synthesize urea.[23] As shown in Figure 36–1, the breakdown of protein also increases the production of acid, potassium, phosphate, sulfate and other inorganic ions, as well as nitrogenous and non-nitrogen–containing organic waste products, including urea, ammonia, guanidino compounds, middle molecules, oxalic acid, phenols, and so on.[24] Subjects with normal kidneys excrete these products rapidly so that their concentrations in blood and body fluid are kept at a low level. In contrast, patients with renal disease may overproduce[25] and clear these compounds more slowly. The balance between production and elimination is achieved at the expense of high concentrations of a variety of toxic compounds in plasma and cells. It is not surprising, therefore, that increasing the dietary protein of patients with CRF increases their accumulation of these products and the symptoms of uremia. Thus, patients with CRF can be considered to have a type of progressive protein intolerance.

It is unknown which waste product(s) causes the symptoms of CRF. The possibility that the major uremic factor is urea has been studied extensively, but the data remain controversial. Infusion of urea into normal subjects does not produce uremic symptoms because the half-life of urea is only 6 to 8 hours, and more than 90% of the load is excreted after 1 day. In patients with CRF, the serum urea nitrogen (SUN) is maintained at a high level for a longer period of time; under these circumstances, uremic symptoms do develop. Johnson and colleagues added urea to the dialysis bath of patients undergoing regular hemodialysis treatment and raised the SUN to approximately

150 mg/dl.[26] After the SUN had been at this level for more than 1 week, the patients developed symptoms of uremia, including headache, lethargy, tremor, nausea, and gastrointestinal distress, even though the dialysis of other toxins was unchanged. Other studies have either failed to reproduce symptomatic uremia by infusing urea alone or have noted symptoms consistent with uremia, but only at extreme elevations in SUN.[27] Thus, it is more likely that SUN levels serve to indicate the accumulation of nitrogenous compounds, but urea, per se, is unlikely to be a major uremic toxin. Patients in the National Cooperative Dialysis Study with SUN above 100 had more symptoms and were hospitalized more frequently than were those whose SUN was maintained below 80 mg/dl.[28] These results indicate that the SUN is a useful index of uremic toxicity, but this is obvious from the relationships shown in Figure 36–1.

Simply stated, protein breakdown must increase the nitrogen available for urea synthesis and must increase the production of other waste products of protein catabolism. Based on these conclusions, an obvious way of reducing the symptoms of uremia would be to decrease dietary protein. The time to begin dietary protein restriction to treat the symptoms of uremia has not been settled, but it seems reasonable to begin altering the diet so as to maintain the SUN below 60 mg/dl. Dietary protein restriction should be started earlier in patients with persistent hyperphosphatemia or acidosis because a high-protein diet is invariably accompanied by increased accumulation of phosphate and acid (see Fig. 36–1).

The linear increase in urea production with dietary protein is useful because it can be used to estimate a steady-state SUN level that will result from a prescribed amount of dietary protein and the urea clearance of a patient. Calculation of the steady-state SUN (Table 36–3), in conjunction with the SUN-to-serum creatinine ratio, can be useful clinically as a rough measure of dietary compliance; a more accurate method is detailed in the section on Protein-Restricted Diets. The steady-state SUN and the ratio also may signal the presence of negative nitrogen balance or gastrointestinal bleeding. For example, the SUN-to-serum creatinine ratio of most patients with CRF is 10:1[29]; this ratio rises if the patient is eating an excessive amount of protein or if gastrointestinal bleeding, a further decline in renal function, or excessive catabolism of body tissues develops. The ratio can also rise in patients who develop dehydration. Conversely, the SUN-to-serum creatinine ratio is less than 10 in patients adhering to a low-protein diet.

TABLE 36–3. STEADY-STATE SUN RESULTING FROM DIFFERENT LEVELS OF DIETARY PROTEIN IN A PATIENT WITH CRF AND A CREATININE CLEARANCE OF 10 ML/MIN*

Diet		"Net" Urea Nitrogen (UuV)	Steady-State SUN (mg/dl)
Protein (g/day)	*Nitrogen (g/day)*		
100	16	13.5	156
60	9.6	7.1	82
40	6.4	3.9	45

*Dietary protein is assumed to be 16% nitrogen. If a patient with CRF is in nitrogen equilibrium and neither gaining nor losing body protein, then an average of 2.5 g/day of nonurea nitrogen (e.g., feces, urine creatinine, uric acid) results from metabolism. The difference between dietary nitrogen and this value is the quantity of "net" urea nitrogen that must be excreted each day to maintain the steady state. If creatinine clearance is 10 ml/min (on the average, urea clearance is 60% of creatinine clearance in patients with CRF), then urea clearance is 6 ml/min or 8.64 l/day. Rearrangement of the clearance formula, C = UV/P, and substitution of the daily quantity of urea to be excreted for UV permits calculation of P or the steady-state SUN resulting from a given protein intake. The answer in grams per liter is converted to milligrams per deciliter by multiplying it by 100.

It is emphasized that even a small amount of gastrointestinal bleeding will raise the SUN because the protein absorbed is broken down and converted to urea. Often, the bleeding is intermittent and requires several measurements of stool guaiac before it is detected.[30] A change in renal function alone should not affect the SUN-to-serum creatinine ratio; a rise in serum creatinine is accompanied by a proportional increase in SUN. These simple considerations are useful for determining when dietary compliance should be assessed more vigorously (see further on) and when the patient should be referred to the dietitian for dietary counseling.

MAINTENANCE OF NUTRITION

When treating patients with CRF with protein-restricted diets, the major concern is that they will develop negative nitrogen balance and protein wasting. This should not dissuade the physician, since body weight, serum proteins, and other indices of protein nutrition are well maintained with modern techniques of nutritional therapy.[31–34]

Normal adults require at least 0.6 g/kg/day of protein (~ 40 g of protein/day) to maintain neutral nitrogen balance.[35, 36] Early studies suggested that patients with CRF could achieve nitrogen balance with lower amounts of dietary protein; these "Giordano-Giovannetti–type" diets consisted of about 20 g/day of protein (~ 0.3/g/kg/day of protein). It was suggested that patients with CRF who had a large pool of urea nitrogen could utilize the nitrogen in urea to synthesize amino acids and, ultimately, protein.[37] More recent studies have shown that urea nitrogen is not utilized for protein synthesis to any significant extent by patients with CRF,[38–40] and this has prompted re-examination of the dietary protein requirements of these patients. It is now clear that their protein requirement is close to that of normal subjects; that is, they need at least 0.6 g/kg/day (~ 40 g/day of protein) to maintain neutral nitrogen balance and prevent protein wasting.[41] Most investigators increase the prescribed amount of dietary protein for patients with proteinuria. Although it is not firmly established that proteinuria does stimulate catabolism of body protein, it is customary to increase dietary protein by 1 to 1.5 g/day for each gram of protein lost in the urine.

It is insufficient to prescribe a diet consisting only of the minimum daily requirement of protein, because the diet may not contain an adequate supply of essential amino acids. To meet this requirement, 0.35 g/kg/day of the dietary protein should consist of the "high biologic value" type, which contains a high proportion of essential amino acids.

An example of a diet consisting of 40 g/day of protein is given in Table 36–4. This diet, as well as other diets used to treat patients with CRF, should always consider each patient's preferences for foods. Note that the diet provides approximately 35 kcal/kg/day and has a phosphorus content of less than 800 mg/day. The high-calorie content is prescribed to promote optimal utilization of the low-protein diet, whereas the low-phosphorus content can blunt the tendency toward hyperparathyroidism. Since it may be difficult to achieve the desired calorie intake while simultaneously restricting other foods, carbohydrate polymers are often prescribed. If these supplements are necessary, it is recommended that carbohydrates provide no more than 35% of the calories in order to limit the tendency of patients with CRF to develop hypertriglyceridemia. Another way to increase calories is to raise the polyunsaturated fat content of the diet (Table 36–5); raising the polyunsaturated-to-saturated fat ratio has been shown to reduce serum triglyc-

TABLE 36–4. LOW-PROTEIN (40 GRAMS), HIGH POLYUNSATURATED FAT DIET

Food Groups	Servings Daily	Suggested Foods	Foods to Avoid
Milk	½ cup	Skim, low-fat milk, buttermilk, low-fat yogurt, low-fat cheeses	Eggnog, milkshakes
Meat, fish, poultry	3 oz	Poultry, veal, fish, lean cuts of pork and beef	All others
Eggs	None	One egg or low-cholesterol egg product may be substituted for 1 oz of meat 2 to 3 times per week	
Breads and cereals	5 servings	One serving = 1 slice of bread; ½ cup cooked or ¾ cup dry cereal; 1 small potato; ½ cup rice, macaroni, or noodles	Any prepared with sauces containing additional milk, egg, or cheese
Vegetables	2 servings	Serving size varies with food selection	Lima beans, dried peas and beans, soybean products
Fruit	4 servings	Serving size varies with food selection	
Fat	As desired	Polyunsaturated oil and margarines, oil-based salad dressings, mayonnaise	Butter, saturated oils, cream, cream cheese, bacon, bleu cheese dressing
Beverages	As desired	Coffee, tea, fruit drinks, carbonated beverages, Kool-Aid	Any milk beverage in excess of allowed amount unless made with polyunsaturated, nondairy creamers. Fruit or vegetable juice in excess of allowed amount
Concentrated sweets	As desired	Jelly, jam, hard candy, syrup, honey, water or Italian ice, marshmallows, low-protein gelatin*	Regular gelatin, milk chocolate, creamy candies, desserts made with egg, milk, or flour above allowed amounts
Miscellaneous	As desired	All herbs and spices, lemon juice, flavoring extracts, vinegar, polyunsaturated nondairy creamers†	Nuts, coconut
Caloric supplements	If required to meet caloric needs	Glucose polymers	Protein supplements

*Dietary Specialties, Rochester, NY.
†Polyperx, Mitchell Foods, Fredonia, NY.

eride levels without raising the serum cholesterol of patients with CRF.[42]

In practice, a high-calorie intake is not forced on patients as long as they are not developing signs of malnutrition, such as weight loss or a decrease in serum albumin or transferrin. Obviously, the ongoing assistance of a skilled dietitian must be available to provide encouragement and counsel for patients being treated with protein-restricted diets.

There is evidence that certain vitamins may be insufficient with these diets. The major concern is that water-soluble vitamins such as pyridoxine, other B vitamins, and folic acid may be inadequate, and it is recommended that these patients with CRF receive a B vitamin complex containing 10 mg of pyridoxine and 1 mg of folic acid per day.[35, 43] In contrast, plasma levels of vitamin A are increased in patients with CRF; it has been suggested that this is associated with the development of uremic osteodystrophy and other uremic syndromes.[35] For this reason, multivitamin tablets containing vitamin A should not be prescribed for patients with CRF.

Other types of low-protein regimens have been extensively investigated in the treatment of patients with CRF. Generally, the diets have been more restrictive and have been studied in patients with moderately advanced CRF (serum creatinine > 5 mg/dl). Since restricting dietary protein below 0.6 g/kg/day of protein will cause negative nitrogen balance and protein wasting, the diets are always supplemented with a mixture of essential amino acids or ketoacids. Ketoacids are simply the carbon skeletons of essential amino acids, with the α-amino group replaced by a ketone group.[44] After ingestion, ketoacids are converted to the respective essential amino acid and can be used to synthesize body protein. In fact, ketoacids have been shown to substitute fully for essential amino acids in patients with CRF who were eating a protein-free diet and therefore had no other source of essential amino acids.[45] Ketoacid supplements are used widely in Europe and are being tested in the United States but are not commercially available at the present. A mixture of amino acids meeting the essential amino acid requirements is sold as Aminess tablets by Baxter Pharmaceuticals in the United States.

These more restricted diets have two potential advantages. First, the essential amino acid or ketoacid supplements provide the necessary essential amino acids so that dietary protein can be reduced to 0.3 g/kg/day of protein (~ 20 to 25 g/day of protein; Table 36–6) and consequently, the accumulation of waste products is reduced further. Second, it is unnecessary to restrict the type of protein eaten, thus the choice of foods is greater; this may explain why patients with CRF prefer the very low protein, supplemented-diet regimens.[46] When these regimens are used, a B vitamin complex–folic acid supplement and sufficient calcium to maintain calcium balance (see section on Calcium and Phosphate Homeostasis) are prescribed, just as with the diets providing 0.6 g/kg/day of protein.

Two important principles must be considered when using nutritional therapy. Compliance with the low-protein diet must be monitored, and signs of protein wasting must be detected early. Dietary compliance with the level of protein restriction can be assessed because urea production increases linearly with protein intake.[47, 48] In contrast, the excretion of nonurea nitrogen (the nitrogen contained in feces, urinary creatinine, uric acid, and unmeasured nitrogen) varies minimally with dietary protein and averages 31 mg/kg of body weight per day. This value does not depend on protein intake.[48]

The rate of urea production can be measured since it equals the rate of urea excretion plus the rate of change in the urea pool. The rate of urea excretion is the 24-hour urine urea nitrogen; the change in the urea pool can be calculated from changes in weight and SUN. Thus, as long as the SUN and weight are stable, the urea production rate (U) is equal to the 24-hour urine urea nitrogen, or $U_{UN}V$ in gN/day. Dietary compliance is assessed by assuming that nitrogen balance is zero. Then, intake of nitrogen (I_N) = U

TABLE 36–5. SAMPLE MEAL PATTERN OF 40-GRAM PROTEIN DIET

Breakfast
- Orange juice, 1/2 cup
- Cornflakes, 1 cup with 1/2 cup nonfat milk and 2 teaspoons sugar
- Toast, 1 slice with 2 teaspoons corn oil margarine and 1 tablespoon jelly
- Coffee with 3 tablespoons Polycose,* 1 oz Polyperx,† and 1 teaspoon sugar

Lunch
- Bread, 2 slices
- Lean roast beef, 1 oz
- Mayonnaise, 1 tablespoon
- Lettuce and tomato salad with 1 oz of oil and vinegar dressing
- Peaches, 2 medium
- Carbonated beverage 12 oz

Dinner
- Lamb chop, 2 ounces
- Small baked potato with 2 teaspoons margarine
- Small dinner roll with 1 teaspoon margarine
- Italian ice, 2/3 cup
- Coffee with 3 tablespoons Polycose,* 1 oz Polyperx,† and 1 teaspoon sugar

Between Meal Snacks
- Cranberry juice, 1 cup
- Lifesavers, 1 roll

Approximate Content:		*Kilocalories:*	
Protein	40 g	Protein	6%
Carbohydrate	407 g	Carbohydrate	65%
Fat	78 g	Fat	29%
Calories	2490	P:S	1.7:1
Phosphorus	620 g		
Sodium	1450 mg (63 mEq)		

*Polycose, a glucose polymer supplement (Ross Labs, Columbus, OH).
†Polyperx, a cream substitute composed predominantly of polyunsaturated fats (Mitchell Foods, Fredonia, NY).

+ 31 mg/kg/day of nitrogen. To convert the estimated nitrogen intake to grams of protein per day, I_N is multiplied by 6.25, since protein is 16% nitrogen.

Any patient who is in negative nitrogen balance must be identified as soon as possible so that measures can be taken to avoid further protein wasting. To accomplish this, each patient should maintain a daily record of weights, and serum albumin and transferrin levels should be measured periodically. If weight and serum protein levels remain stable, it can be concluded that the patient is in neutral nitrogen balance and maintaining body protein stores. On the other hand, if weight decreases or if serum albumin and transferrin gradually decline, the patient is probably in negative nitrogen balance and protein intake should be increased by 0.1 g/kg of body weight per day. The diet should also be carefully reviewed by the dietitian to ensure that there is an adequate calorie intake. If the patient continues to lose weight in spite of these adjustments, then dietary protein should be increased further and the patient should be fully evaluated for the presence of a catabolic illness.

ELECTROLYTE AND MINERAL DISORDERS—SALT AND WATER

Patients with CRF are able to maintain sodium balance even when creatinine clearance falls to 5 to 10 ml/min.[49] Several factors have been suggested to explain this adaptive phenomenon, including production of a natriuretic hormone and changes in physical factors regulating sodium reabsorption.[50, 51] An important therapeutic consequence of this adaptation is that sodium excretion is relatively fixed in these patients; patients with a creatinine clearance of 5 to 10 ml/min generally excrete 60 to 100 mEq of sodium per day (equivalent of 3.5 to 6 g of salt) and will continue to excrete this amount even when dietary salt intake is restricted. Although patients with mild CRF can excrete more sodium and can conserve sodium more easily than can those with more advanced CRF, even these patients have a relatively fixed rate of salt excretion.

The importance of this fact is that patients with CRF are susceptible to extracellular fluid (ECF) volume depletion whenever sodium intake is restricted to a level below the patient's obligatory sodium excretion. This may be particularly detrimental because autoregulation of renal blood flow is abnormal in CRF.[52] To ensure an adequate ECF volume, the diet should be designed to contain enough sodium so that the patient has a trace of pedal edema. To detect inadvertent ECF volume contraction early, patients should weigh themselves daily and alert the physician when weight loss exceeds 3 or 4% of body weight (~ 3 to 5 lb). Excessive contraction of ECF volume (> 6 lb weight loss) is generally accompanied by a 10 mm Hg or more decline in mean arterial blood pressure and an increase of 10 beats/min or more in heart rate upon rising from the supine position.

Some patients desire more salt in their diet because of prior eating habits rather than from any special requirement for salt or an inability to taste unsalted foods. Excessive dietary salt, like too little salt, can be detrimental, which emphasizes the important role of dietary education in establishing a proper salt intake. Fortunately, the taste perception for salt is not depressed by CRF, even though perception of sour and sweet tastes is occasionally impaired in such patients.[53] Because the serum sodium only gives the relationship between body sodium and body water, it alone should never be used as a guide for changing dietary salt.

The efficacy of furosemide in patients with CRF is shown

TABLE 36–6. SAMPLE MEAL PATTERN OF 25-GRAM PROTEIN DIET

Breakfast
- Rye toast, 2 slices with 2 teaspoons margarine and 1 tablespoon jelly
- Fruit cocktail, 1 cup
- Cranberry juice, 6 oz
- Coffee, 1 cup with Polyperx*

Midmorning Snack
- Coffee, 2 cups with Polyperx*

Lunch
- Large salad with lettuce, tomatoes, cucumbers, and radishes, 2 tablespoons French dressing
- Rye bread, 1 slice with 1 teaspoon margarine
- Large apple
- Cranberry juice, 6 oz
- Regular tomato juice, 6 oz

Dinner
- Lamb chop, 1 oz
- Rice, 1/2 cup with 1 teaspoon margarine
- Green beans, 2/3 cup with 1 teaspoon margarine
- Cranberry sauce, 1/2 cup
- Rye bread, 1 slice with 1 teaspoon margarine
- Diced fresh pear, 1 cup
- Cranberry juice, 6 oz
- Coffee, 1 cup with Polyperx*

Evening Snack
- Spearmint candy, 4 oz

Nutrient Breakdown:

Calories	2433
Carbohydrate	464 g
Protein	25 g
Fat	53 g
Sodium	1731 mg (75 mEq)
Potassium	2844 mg (73 mEq)
Phosphorus	430 mg

*Polyperx, a cream substitute composed predominantly of polyunsaturated fats (Mitchell Foods, Fredonia, NY).

by its ability to increase sodium excretion even in patients with almost no renal function.[54] In normal subjects, furosemide has a short duration of action, and after the drug is eliminated, an efficient compensatory response occurs, consisting of a sharp decrease in sodium excretion. This compensatory response leads to neutral sodium balance without any weight loss, unless the subject is eating a low-salt diet.[55] It is not known whether there is a compensatory response to furosemide in patients with CRF; there may not be one because the action of the drug is prolonged, and there is an "obligatory" sodium excretion that would act to blunt the compensatory response. Nevertheless, repetitive treatment with loop diuretics results in diminished natriuresis either in the short term or with prolonged therapy. This so-called braking effect may result from increased distal tubular sodium reabsorption.[56] Indeed, combination therapy using thiazide diuretics has been advocated for patients with diuretic resistance.[57,58] Moreover, not all loop diuretics have equal efficacy in patients with CRF. For example, a direct comparison of equally potent doses of bumetanide with furosemide in patients with CRF resulted in significantly greater natriuresis over 8 hours in patients receiving furosemide, despite no difference in the maximal fractional sodium excretion achieved.[59] The authors concluded that the difference was due to the greater nonrenal clearance for bumetanide. Thus, a number of considerations must be kept in mind when prescribing diuretic agents to patients with CRF.

Patients with CRF generally need large doses of furosemide because they accumulate organic anions that compete with furosemide for tubular secretion, thus decreasing the amount of drug reaching the active site of the kidney. Furosemide also has a "threshold" effect, meaning that there is little or no diuretic response until a sufficient amount of the drug reaches the loop of Henle. In practical terms, this means that a patient with CRF who responds to 80 or 120 mg of furosemide should not be given 40 mg twice daily, or little or no diuretic response will result.[51]

As long as an intact thirst mechanism exists and the patient has access to water, serum sodium is generally normal in patients with CRF. As with sodium, patients with CRF have a limited ability to respond either to a water load because their low glomerular filtration rate (GFR) limits free water excretion or to water deprivation because their concentrating capacity limits water conservation. Clinically important water intoxication in CRF may result from excessive intravenous administration of 5% dextrose in water or forcing fluids. If it becomes necessary to fast a patient with CRF, water should not be withheld. Just as with a normal subject, a patient with CRF adhering to a salt-restricted diet can develop serious hyponatremia during diuretic therapy. The physician is alerted to this complication by noting an excessive decline in body weight.

Correction of metabolic acidosis with sodium bicarbonate can lead to a dramatic improvement in symptoms of fatigue and weakness in CRF. Chronic metabolic acidosis has serious nutritional consequences, both on intermediary metabolism and on skeletal mineralization. In experimental animals with chronic acidosis, growth is stunted, nitrogen excretion is augmented,[60] and protein breakdown and oxidation of branched-chain amino acids are accelerated, both in the intact animal,[61] and in skeletal muscles incubated from animals with acidosis.[60] These results pertain to chronic uremia since the accelerated muscle protein breakdown and branched-chain amino acid catabolism are reversed by supplementing the animals with CRF with $NaHCO_3$.[62,63] These studies may be relevant to humans with CRF. For instance, Papadoyannakis and associates performed serial nitrogen balance studies on patients with CRF ingesting low-protein diets, either before or after correction of their accompanying acidosis, and noted an improvement in nitrogen balance when $NaHCO_3$ was given.[64] Likewise, Williams and associates examined nitrogen and 3-methylhistidine excretion (a marker for the breakdown of myofibrillar proteins in muscle) in patients with CRF receiving 0.6 g/kg protein diets before and after correction of their acidosis. Despite no change in dietary protein, nitrogen and 3-methylhistidine excretion were significantly reduced by correction of the acidosis.[65] Acidosis may likewise account for the lower branched-chain amino acid pools present in CRF.[66] Bergstrom and colleagues noted a striking linear relationship between predialysis bicarbonate concentrations and muscle valine concentrations in patients with CRF on maintenance hemodialysis.[66] These effects of metabolic acidosis are likely to have greater impact as the degree of protein restriction is increased. Metabolic acidosis may also affect carbohydrate metabolism since glucose intolerance and insulin resistance similar to the problems noted in patients with CRF were reproduced in normal subjects rendered acidotic.[67] Thus, it is imperative that metabolic acidosis is corrected in patients with CRF. To avoid all these problems, the serum bicarbonate should be kept above 20 mM. It is interesting that the sodium contained in sodium bicarbonate may be more easily excreted than an equimolar amount of sodium chloride,[68] thus the dietary sodium requirement may be underestimated slightly when calculated using the method in Table 36–7. This is detected by a gradual loss of weight. Occasional

TABLE 36–7. ESTABLISHING SALT REQUIREMENTS FOR PATIENTS WITH CHRONIC RENAL FAILURE

1. Determine daily average (2 to 3 days) of urine Na^+ excretion during period of stable renal function.
2. Determine quantity of sodium bicarbonate necessary to maintain serum total CO_2 at greater than 20 mM.
3. Calculate Na content of sodium bicarbonate and subtract from average daily Na^+ excretion to determine salt intake. One gram of sodium bicarbonate has 12 mEq of Na.
4. Maintain record of weight.

patients complain of belching when taking sodium bicarbonate; this can be alleviated by using sodium citrate (i.e., Shohl's solution, 1 mEq base/ml) since citrate is converted to bicarbonate. Note that some types of Shohl's solution contain a mixture of sodium and potassium citrate that could aggravate hyperkalemia. The use of citrate salts should be restricted to patients not receiving aluminum-containing compounds, since citrate will augment intestinal absorption of aluminum.[69]

Hypertension

Hypertension commonly accompanies CRF and may contribute to further progression of renal insufficiency. There is a heightened sensitivity of blood pressure to changes in sodium intake in CRF,[70] and when hypertension accompanies CRF, there is often hypersecretion of renin.[71] Initial therapy of hypertension is often directed at reducing total body sodium using furosemide or another "loop diuretic." Although thiazide diuretics may potentiate a loop diuretic, thiazides also will raise serum creatinine, presumably by lowering GFR.[72] Hence, combination therapy with thiazide and loop diuretics is usually restricted to hospitalized patients who, despite dietary sodium restriction and high-dose loop diuretic therapy, remain in positive sodium balance. Combined therapy requires close monitoring to prevent deterioration of renal function and the development of severe hypokalemia or hyponatremia. Changes in weight must be monitored carefully to avoid ECF volume depletion and worsening of renal insufficiency.

If diuretics alone do not control blood pressure, then centrally acting drugs or drugs affecting the peripheral nervous system or directly dilating vascular smooth muscle can be added.

The *centrally acting agents* clonidine, α-methyldopa, and reserpine are effective in patients with CRF, but with the development of drugs with fewer side effects, reserpine is rarely used. α-Methyldopa is often associated with sedation, partly due to an accumulation of sulfated metabolites, and it can cause impotence. The dose of α-methyldopa is 250 to 500 mg orally three to four times each day; if the serum creatinine level rises above 4 mg/dl, the interval between doses should be lengthened to two doses per day.

β-Blockers are often effective as antihypertensive agents; important differences exist among the commercially available drugs. For example, it has been reported that propranolol hastens the progression of CRF, at least in some patients.[73] In contrast, nadolol appears to be unique in apportioning a greater fraction of cardiac output to the kidney, thus preserving renal blood flow.[74] Until more definitive studies of the effects of β-blockers on the progression of CRF are available, these drugs should be reserved for patients with CRF who are unresponsive to other therapy or who require β-blockers to control the side effects of peripheral vasodilators like hydralazine or minoxidil. β-Blockers may be more efficacious than diuretics in patients with left ventricular hypertrophy or a prior history of myocardial infarction.[75, 76] When treatment with a β-blocker is necessary, nadolol seems to be a good choice. Since nadolol is excreted mainly by the kidney, its dose must be modified in patients with moderate renal insufficiency (serum creatinine > 5 mg/dl) to avoid toxicity.

Antihypertensive drugs dilating blood vessels either directly or by affecting the peripheral nervous system include α_1-antagonists (e.g., prazosin), calcium-channel blockers (e.g., nifedipine, verapamil), angiotensin-converting enzyme (ACE) inhibitors (e.g., captopril, enalapril), and miscellaneous agents such as minoxidil and hydralazine. *Hydralazine* is effective and does not depress renal blood flow or GFR.[77] It frequently causes a reflex increase in cardiac output and heart rate that is troublesome for patients with angina. As much as 100 mg of hydralazine can be given twice daily, but the total dose must not exceed 200 mg/day because the drug accumulates in patients with CRF and can cause a lupus-like syndrome. *Minoxidil,* like hydralazine, acts directly to vasodilate arterioles and has been shown to be effective in hypertensive patients with CRF who are unresponsive to other drugs. Although minoxidil does not depress renal blood flow or GRF, it has several serious side effects, including marked fluid retention, hirsutism, and rarely pericarditis and pericardial effusions during long-term therapy.[78] Because of these serious side effects, minoxidil should be reserved for patients with refractory hypertension. *Prazosin* causes peripheral vasodilatation by blocking α_1-receptors on nerves and vascular smooth muscle.[79] It does not depress renal blood flow or GFR and appears to be both safe and effective in patients with CRF. Unlike other direct-acting vasodilators, prazosin does not cause a reflex tachycardia and therefore does not require concomitant therapy with β-blockers.

Captopril blocks production of the potent endogenous vasoconstrictor angiotensin II, and, like minoxidil, it can lower the blood pressure in patients with CRF with refractory hypertension. Captopril has serious side effects, including acute renal failure, aplastic anemia, and hyperkalemia.[80–83] The daily dose should be reduced below 75 mg when creatinine clearance is less than 25 ml/min.[84, 85] Based largely on studies of experimental renal failure in rats, ACE inhibitors appear to arrest the progression of CRF. The protective effect of these agents is not due solely to lower systemic arterial pressures but is also due to the unique property of ACE inhibitors to dilate the efferent glomerular arteriole and lower intraglomerular capillary pressures.[86–88] Studies in humans have documented that ACE inhibitors may decrease proteinuria in diabetic nephropathy[89] and other types of chronic glomerulonephritis.[90] The patients who responded with a decreased proteinuria were those with higher peripheral renin activities; the degree to which proteinuria decreased was reversed if dietary sodium was reduced.[91] Whether ACE inhibitors are able to prevent renal failure in humans remains to be proved. Calcium channel blockers have also been shown to slow the rate of progression of CRF in rats; the protection did not correlate with the degree of blood pressure reduction.[92]

The use of ACE inhibitors in CRF requires meticulous follow-up. ACE inhibitors can decrease GFR in 20 to 30% of patients with CRF, although this adverse effect is usually reversible when the drug is stopped. Future studies are needed to clarify the role of ACE inhibitors in treating patients with CRF. Obviously, these potent drugs must be used with extreme caution in patients with CRF.

Guanethidine causes postural hypotension and depression of renal blood flow and GFR. For these reasons, it rarely is used in patients with CRF, though it may be effective when neither minoxidil nor captopril are tolerated.[93]

With the development of sustained-release preparations, *calcium channel blockers* are effective drugs for treating hypertension but can cause declines in GFR, rebound tachycardia, and progressive salt retention. Nifedipine, in high doses, has been shown to cause edema in 10 to 20% of patients.[94] The relationship between edema and salt retention is unclear in studies examining the pharmacodynamics of this agent.[95, 96] It remains unclear whether chronic renal failure will increase the incidence of edema, but the potency of these drugs makes them a valuable class of antihypertensives, both in patients with and without renal failure.

Potassium

Hyperkalemia is rarely a problem in patients with CRF, even when creatinine clearance falls below 10 ml/min, as long as the daily urine volume exceeds 1 liter. In fact, patients with CRF may have a deficit in total body potassium.[97] The ability to excrete potassium is maintained for at least three reasons: (1) There is a high rate of sodium and fluid delivery to the distal nephron; (2) there is increased aldosterone production; and (3) the postprandial increase in serum potassium directly promotes kaliuresis.[51] Virtually all potassium in the urine results from potassium secretion by the distal tubule. This secretory process depends on sodium delivery and aldosterone to maintain a favorable electrochemical gradient for potassium secretion.[98] Hence, hyperkalemia can develop in volume-depleted patients who experience a sharp decrease in urine volume. The importance of aldosterone is highlighted by the frequent development of hyperkalemia in patients with CRF who are given spironolactone.[99]

Besides the kidney, the gastrointestinal tract of patients with advanced CRF is important in excreting potassium.[100] The colon adapts to excrete potassium, and as with the kidney, the adaptation may be linked to higher levels of aldosterone or glucocorticoids.[101] This is important because chronic constipation may aggravate any tendency toward hyperkalemia. In treating constipation in CRF, magnesium salts must not be used because the patients excrete magnesium poorly and can develop magnesium intoxication.[99]

Most patients with CRF with moderate renal insufficiency (creatinine clearance of 20 to 30 ml/min) who are hyperkalemic are also diabetic and have low rates of renin and aldosterone production. This syndrome is called type IV renal tubular acidosis (RTA). The urine of some of these subjects can be acidified, but in most a limited ability to excrete an acid load is found;[99, 102] apparently, type IV RTA can be successfully treated with 0.1 to 0.3 mg/day of 9-fluorocortisone, although careful monitoring for signs of fluid overload is necessary.[103]

As renal function progressively declines, it may be necessary to restrict foods with a high potassium content, such as bananas, citrus fruits, and certain salt substitutes or salt-free soups. The serum bicarbonate of patients with CRF should be maintained above 20 mM (see earlier) because acidosis shifts potassium from the intracellular fluid to the ECF, thus aggravating any tendency toward hyperkalemia.[99]

Mild hyperkalemia is not associated with specific symptoms, although occasional patients complain of muscular weakness. A serum potassium level below 6 mEq/l is well tolerated by most patients with CRF, unless it has risen rapidly and has changed cardiac conduction.[99] Sequential electrocardiograms (ECGs) are useful in assessing the response to therapy.[104] The earliest ECG change is shortening of the QT interval; at higher levels (serum potassium > 6 mEg/l), the amplitude of T waves and the PR interval increase; subsequently, the QRS complex widens, and electrical activity of the atria disappears with the occasional appearance of bundle branch blocks.[105] In extreme hyperkalemia (serum potassium > 9 mEq/l), the QRS complex is replaced by a sine wave pattern, signaling impending cardiac standstill or ventricular fibrillation.[99, 106]

The treatment of hyperkalemia can be divided into acute and chronic phases, but all forms of therapy must reduce potassium stores and correct the abnormalities in cardiac conduction.[99] The most rapid method of reversing the cardiotoxic effects of potassium is to administer calcium intravenously. Calcium directly antagonizes the effect of hyperkalemia on cardiac conduction without changing serum potassium. A 10-g ampule of calcium chloride can be infused slowly during continuous ECG monitoring to avoid the cardiotoxic effects of calcium, including asystole. Intravenous calcium must never be administered simultaneously with sodium bicarbonate since calcium carbonate will precipitate. Extreme caution is necessary when intravenous calcium is given to a patient being treated with digitalis because of the danger of provoking arrhythmias. Moreover, intravenous calcium should not be given to patients with hyperphosphatemia because it will cause calcium deposition in tissues. Thus, it is unwise to treat hyperkalemia in patients with CRF with calcium intravenously, unless the patient is known not to have hyperphosphatemia.

Intravenous sodium bicarbonate is a rapid method for lowering serum potassium in normal subjects. It may be useful in acidotic patients with extreme hyperkalemia but without significant volume overload. Following injection of 1 to 2 ampules (44 to 88 mEq) of sodium bicarbonate, cardiac conduction rapidly improves owing to the rapid increase in serum sodium, which by itself improves cardiac conduction, and to a slower (30 to 60 minutes) effect attributable to redistribution of potassium into cells.[99] However, it should be noted that the use of intravenous $NaHCO_3$, whether administered as an isotonic or hypertonic solution, to patients with CRF has been shown to result in no drop in plasma potassium despite alkalinization of blood and an increase in plasma bicarbonate.[107] The use of β-adrenergic sympathomimetics has been used in patients with CRF with varied results. Blumberg infused epinephrine in hyperkalemic subjects with CRF and noted only a modest drop in serum K^+ (5.6 to 5.3 mEq/l); 5 of the 10 subjects had less than a 5% decline in plasma potassium. In contrast, the use of aerosolized albuterol resulted in a more significant response in patients with CRF, and it appears that its effect to lower plasma potassium may be additive to the effects of insulin.[108] Whether these discrepant results are caused by the type of drugs administered remains to be established. Nevertheless, it would not be wise to rely solely on sympathomimetics to treat hyperkalemia because of the lack of uniformity of response. Another method of reducing serum potassium is to infuse insulin, thus promoting cellular uptake of potassium within 30 to 60 minutes. Continuous infusion of 5 to 10 mU/kg/min of insulin will increase potassium disposal maximally[109]; glucose should be infused at approximately 10 mg/kg/min while serum glucose is monitored closely to avoid hypoglycemia. The efficacy of insulin has been tested in patients with CRF.[119] It produced a rapid, concentration-dependent decline in plasma potassium.[110] Thus, insulin remains the best-documented initial therapy for the treatment of hyperkalemia in the setting of CRF. With all these measures, there must be additional therapy directed at reducing potassium stores.

The two methods of reducing potassium stores are to use a cation exchange resin and dialysis. Cation exchange resins are negatively charged and equilibrated with sodium, although they have a higher affinity for potassium compared with sodium. Thus, after oral or rectal administration, potassium in the body is bound to the resin in exchange for sodium and eliminated through the gastrointestinal tract. To ensure elimination and to decrease transit time of the resin (Kayexalate), 50 g is mixed with an osmotic cathartic, such as 30 ml of a 10% sorbitol solution, and given orally. For patients who cannot be treated in this fashion, 50 g can be mixed with 200 ml of a 10% sorbitol solution and given as a retention enema for at least 1 hour; the efficiency of potassium removal by enema is much less than by oral administration.[111] For outpatients with hyperkalemia, 1 to 2 tablespoons/day of Kayexalate can be mixed in fruit juice and taken once or twice daily. Fortunately, sorbitol is rarely necessary in outpatients, but Kayexalate should not be taken concomitantly with aluminum hydroxide gels to avoid the formation of concretions in the gut or with other divalent cations because they will preferentially bind to the resin in place of potassium. Since the exchange of sodium for potassium is not 100%, only about 1 mEq of potassium is removed for every gram of Kayexalate taken orally.

The most efficient means of removing potassium from the body is hemodialysis; it is much more rapid and effective than peritoneal dialysis or Kayexalate. Indeed, with high-flux dialysis potassium clearance may exceed 90% of blood flow through the dialyzer. Serum potassium generally falls after 30 minutes of hemodialysis, but it takes at least 1 hour to initiate hemodialysis. For this reason, hemodialysis should never be relied on as sole therapy for severe hyperkalemia.[99] The average amount of potassium removed during hemodialysis often exceeds 1.5 mEq/kg, but this varies with the predialytic serum potassium, the duration of dialysis, the potassium concentration of the dialysis fluid,[112] and the clearance of small molecular weight solutes by the treatment as prescribed.

Calcium and Phosphate Homeostasis

A decline in renal function, regardless of etiology, is associated with abnormalities of the metabolism of calcium and phosphorus and of the hormones that regulate the concentrations of these minerals in body fluids. One of the first abnormalities in mineral metabolism in CRF is a rise in plasma immunoreactive parathyroid hormone (PTH), which can occur at a GFR of 30 to 50 ml/min (serum creatinine of 2 to 5 mg/dl).[113] The pathophysiology of the development of secondary hyperparathyroidism in CRF has been studied extensively and, at least in later stages of renal failure, appears to be closely linked to phosphate retention caused by a loss of renal function.[114] In the early stages of CRF, the relationship between phosphate retention and increased PTH secretion is more tenuous because phosphate is normal or somewhat reduced, although the plasma calcium level tends to be subnormal.

The hypothesis relating an increase in serum phosphate to the development of secondary hyperparathyroidism states that decreased phosphate elimination by the diseased kidney leads to an increase in postprandial plasma phosphate concentration even at relatively mild degrees of renal insufficiency. The risk in plasma phosphate subsequently leads to a decrease in serum ionized calcium, which stimulates PTH secretion. An increased plasma PTH level causes phosphaturia and lowers serum phosphate, thus permitting serum calcium to rise. In this scheme, the enhancement of phosphate excretion caused by PTH maintains the patient in neutral phosphate balance without hyperphosphatemia. To maintain a normal ionized calcium concentration, the rate of PTH secretion must be kept high, and this leads to reabsorption of bone calcium. However, studies of patients with early renal insufficiency have failed to reveal hyperphosphatemia.[115, 116] In vitro studies examining the solubility of calcium phosphate have cast doubt on the trade-off hypothesis. Adler and associates noted that an increase of 3.7 mg/dl in serum phosphate would be necessary in order to lower serum calcium to a level sufficient to stimulate PTH release.[117]

An alternative but closely linked hypothesis states that the primary abnormality leading to abnormal calcium and phosphorus metabolism in CRF is a decrease in conversion of 25-hydroxyvitamin D_3 to 1,25-dihydroxyvitamin D_3, the most active vitamin D metabolite. The impaired conversion is due partly to the decrease in renal mass, because the kidney is responsible for the 1-hydroxylation of 25-OH-cholecalciferol. However, changes in intracellular phosphate affect the activity of the enzyme; high-phosphate diets increase intracellular inorganic phosphate and depress hydroxylation, whereas low-phosphorus diets lower intracellular phosphate levels and augment the production of $1,25(OH)_2$-D_3, even in renal insufficiency.[118] These findings emphasize the importance of restricting dietary phosphate even early in the course of renal insufficiency. The lower concentration of the active form of vitamin D leads to impaired calcium absorption in the gastrointestinal tract, and this results in a lower level of serum ionized calcium, which in turn stimulates PTH secretion.[119]

Two other factors contribute to the increased level of PTH in CRF: resistance to the skeletal effects of PTH and decreased PTH degradation by the diseased kidney. Skeletal resistance to PTH may be due in part to decreased production of 1,25-dihydroxyvitamin D_3. The kidney is a major site of PTH degradation, and in CRF the rate of degradation is low.[120] The importance of PTH degradation in the pathogenesis of secondary hyperparathyroidism is not clear, but it does contribute to the high circulating levels of immunoreactive PTH. Immunoreactive PTH includes intact PTH; the amino terminal, active PTH fragment; and the inactive carboxy terminal fragment. Thus, some portion of measured PTH does not contribute to bone resorption but simply reflects decreased PTH degradation.[120]

Histologic evidence of renal osteodystrophy is a very common feature of CRF.[121] Secondary hyperparathyroidism leads to increased surface remodeling of bone with osteocytic and osteoclastic resorption, endosteal fibrosis, and increased numbers of osteoclasts.[121] Radiologically, hyperparathyroidism can be documented by finding subperiosteal resorption of bone in the phalanges of the hands, at the distal ends of the clavicles, and in the pelvis and teeth. In advanced secondary hyperparathyroidism, bone tumors filled with giant cells (brown tumors) can be seen growing from long bones primarily. A skull radiograph may show a finely mottled or "salt and pepper" appearance of bone, and "pseudofractures" of bones at sites where tendons insert may be seen owing to the concomitant presence of osteomalacia. X-ray studies also may reveal areas of increased bone density or osteosclerosis next to bones of decreased density. In the spine, these alterations in density appear as the "rugger jersey" sign.[122]

TABLE 36–8. DOSAGE AND ADVERSE EFFECTS OF ANTACIDS AND VITAMIN D PREPARATIONS

Drug	Usual Therapeutic Dose	Adverse Effects
Magnesium hydroxide Magnesium trisilicate (e.g., Maalox, Mylanta)		Should be avoided because they can produce symptomatic hypermagnesemia in patients with CRF
Aluminum hydroxide Aluminum carbonate (Amphojel, Basaljel, AlternaGEL, Nephrox)	30–60 ml or 3–4 capsules after meals, although more may be required	Constipation is frequent (less with AlternaGEL); nausea and anorexia can occur
Vitamin D	20,000–50,000 units/day	With vitamin D, hypercalcemia and an increased calcium × phosphorus product can occur. The initial dose should be small, and 2–4 weeks should elapse before a dose is increased. Avoid if serum phosphorus level is high
Dihydrotachysterol (Hytakerol)	0.2–0.5 mg/day	
1,25-Dihydroxycholecalciferol (Rocaltrol)	0.5–1 μg/day	

Many of the disabling features of CRF other than renal osteodystrophy may be caused in part by secondary hyperparathyroidism. These include peripheral neuropathy, impotence, pruritus, ischemic skin lesions, bone necrosis, anemia, lipid abnormalities, impaired insulin secretion,[123] and increased calcium content of the brain. In fact, PTH has been identified by some investigators as a "uremic toxin."[124] In addition, soft tissue calcification of vital organs in patients with CRF, including arteries, lung, and heart, is associated invariably with severe secondary hyperparathyroidism, and often the calcification can disappear following subtotal parathyroidectomy. Even more dramatic is the rapid healing of acral ischemic lesions in uremic patients with severe secondary hyperparathyroidism following subtotal parathyroidectomy.[125]

These considerations indicate why one of the most important goals in treating patients with CRF is the prevention of secondary hyperparathyroidism. Fortunately, this is possible because the rise in plasma phosphate appears to be the major determinant of the severity of secondary hyperparathyroidism. The concentration of this ion can be lowered by dietary manipulation and use of phosphate-binding gels.[126, 127]

In CRF, serum phosphorus should be kept between 3.5 and 4.2 mg/dl. Therapy directed at maintaining a normal serum phosphate level consists primarily of dietary phosphate restriction, but many patients also require phosphate-binding aluminum hydroxide gels or calcium salts to increase fecal phosphate excretion. Aluminum hydroxide binds phosphorus better after a meal, thus the binders should be given concomitantly with meals.[128] Due to the long-term effects of aluminum intoxication (dementia, anemia, and low-turnover bone disease with osteomalacia), limited phosphate adsorption can be accomplished using calcium carbonate. The lactate, citrate, and carbonate salts of calcium are equally potent when compared with each other, but their binding capacity is considerably less than aluminum hydroxide gels.[129, 130] Moreover, these agents have limited solubility in alkaline environments, thus their effectiveness may be lower in achlorhydric patients or in patients treated with H_2 blockers or blockers of gastric H-ATPase.[128] Nevertheless, control of hyperphosphatemia and suppression of secondary hyperparathyroidism have been accomplished with calcium salts. More soluble calcium salts that are unaffected by gastric pH, such as calcium acetate, have phosphate-binding capacities 2 times that of $CaCO_3$ and similar to aluminum hydroxide gels.[128] An effective dose is 2.4 to 5 g of calcium acetate, which also provides the 1500-mg daily calcium requirement for patients with CRF.

When a patient with a high serum phosphorus level begins therapy, response can be discouragingly slow for two reasons. First, the pool of accumulated phosphorus is very large in these patients, and even with a low-phosphorus diet and aluminum hydroxide or calcium salt use, phosphorus depletion occurs slowly. Thus, patience and perseverance are necessary to correct the high serum level. The other factor that can delay lowering of serum phosphate is a very high PTH level. This occurs because PTH-mediated dissolution of bone releases phosphorus, creating a constant endogenous phosphorus load.[125] Fortunately, hypersecretion of PTH to this degree rarely occurs.

Treatment of hyperphosphatemia consists of elimination of all foods high in phosphorus, such as dairy products (e.g., milk, cheese, cream) and excessive quantities of meat. Aluminum hydroxide gels (30 to 60 ml four times a day) or calcium salts (e.g., $CaCO_3$ 1.5 to 3 g four times a day) should also be prescribed. Compliance in taking binders is frequently poor because of the taste and because constipation develops. Basaljel and AlternaGEL or Nephrox may be alternated with Amphojel to provide a change in taste and improve compliance (Table 36–8); the liquid dosage form is preferred to capsules or tablets because it provides more efficient phosphate elimination.

Serum phosphorus is usually lowered after several weeks of adequate therapy. As phosphorus decreases, the serum calcium level almost always rises but may not reach normal levels. The reason for this is obscure but may be because of inadequate production of the active form of vitamin D, 1,25-dihydroxyvitamin D_3 or an inadequate intake of calcium, or both. Balance studies have indicated that the calcium requirement for patients with CRF is approximately 1500 mg/day,[131] which is greater than the requirement for subjects with normal renal function and suggests some abnormality in calcium absorption. Because protein restriction is accompanied by moderate calcium restriction, especially when dairy products are avoided, it will be necessary, after lowering the phosphate to normal, to give 1 to 1.5 g/day of elemental calcium, either as calcium salts (to bind the phosphorus) or calcium carbonate tablets (~ 40% calcium).

Neither calcium nor vitamin D should be given when the serum phosphorus level is high. If supplemental calcium does not raise the serum calcium to normal values, vitamin D may be added. Vitamin D can be given in several commercially available forms, including USP vitamin D, dihydrotachysterol, or 1,25-dihydroxyvitamin D_3 (see Table 36–8). Vitamin D (USP) must be converted to 25-hydroxyvitamin D_3 in the liver and then to the dihydroxy form in the kidney, thus the quantity needed in individual patients varies widely and can be more than 50,000 units daily. Dihydrotachysterol is considerably more potent because of a stereochemical similarity to 1,25-dihydroxyvitamin D_3. In general, patients require 0.2 to 0.5 mg/day to maintain the normal serum calcium level, but the initial dose should be 0.1 mg/day, and the dose should be increased only every 2 to 4 weeks to avoid vitamin D intoxication. 1,25-dihydroxy-vitamin D_3 has become commercially available (Rocaltrol), and patients can be given 0.25 μg/day of this drug initially, with the dose increased only every 2 to 4 weeks to avoid hypercalcemia. With any preparation of vitamin D, it is important to remember that hypercalcemia can lead to diminished renal function and can aggravate soft tissue deposition of calcium and phosphate. Rocaltrol has a short half-life, thus its biologic effects disappear relatively rapidly if hypercalcemia occurs.[132] The use of vitamin D in patients with CRF is controversial. Some investigators have noted that vitamin D caused a decline in renal function despite control of the serum calcium-phosphorus product.[133, 134] The explanation for the decline is obscure and has not been seen by others using similar treatment strategies.[135]

For at least two reasons, vitamin D should not be given when the serum phosphorus level is high. First, vitamin D promotes intestinal absorption of phosphorus as well as calcium.[136] Thus, the drug may appear to be relatively ineffective in increasing serum calcium because the increase in serum phosphorus blunts its calcium-raising effect (see previous discussion). Second, soft tissue deposition of calcium and phosphorus frequently occurs in patients with CRF and can be devastating. The tendency to deposit these elements increases as the product of calcium multiplied by phosphorus rises. Thus, at a product above 60 mg/dl^2, soft tissue accumulation of these minerals is certain to occur; it is advisable to keep the product below 40 mg/dl^2.

ENDOCRINE ABNORMALITIES

Multiple endocrine abnormalities can be seen in patients with CRF (Table 36–9).[137] Endocrine abnormalities are responsible in part for numerous uremic manifestations, including glucose intolerance (insulin), anemia (erythropoietin), osteodystrophy (PTH, vitamin D), hyperpigmentation (melanocyte-stimulating hormone [MSH]), gonadal and sexual dysfunction (follicle-stimulating hormone [FSH], luteinizing hormone [LH], prolactin, testosterone), and possibly salt wasting ("natriuretic hormone"). These can be caused by changes in one or more of the following: the circulating concentration of a hormone; the regulation of hormone secretion; the end-organ response to a hormone. When evaluating a patient with CRF for an endocrinopathy, it should be remembered that accumulation of a prohormone or an inactive metabolite of a hormone can substantially increase the plasma concentration of hormones measured by immunoassay because the antibodies used may not distinguish between the active hormone and these other molecules. Examples include accumulation of the precursors of insulin, glucagon, and the inactive C-terminal peptide fragment of PTH. This emphasizes the importance of knowing the specificity of antibodies in the hormone assay. Examples of abnormal regulation of hormone secretion include severe secondary hyperparathyroidism and prolactin. Abnormal end-organ response to PTH and insulin occurs in CRF.

TABLE 36–9. ENDOCRINE DYSFUNCTION IN CHRONIC RENAL FAILURE

Nature of Defect	Hormonal Defects
Diminished production of renal hormones	Decreased erythropoietin production Decreased conversion of 25-hydroxyvitamin D_3 to 1,25-dihydroxyvitamin D_3
Hormonal hypersecretion to re-establish homeostasis	Hyperparathyroidism Secretion of the "natriuretic hormone"
Decreased metabolic clearance of hormones	FSH, LH, prolactin, GH, MSH, gastrin
Blunted feedback response causing increased hormone secretion	LH, ACTH, prolactin
Defective tissue conversion of prohormone to hormone	T4 to T3 25-Hydroxyvitamin D_3 to 1,25-dihydroxyvitamin D_3
Decreased hormone production	Testosterone
End-organ unresponsiveness	Insulin PTH
Increased circulating inhibitors of hormones	Somatomedin inhibitory factor

Uremic patients frequently exhibit glucose intolerance, hyperinsulinemia, and hypertriglyceridemia.[138] Most studies indicate that uremia depresses insulin-stimulated glucose uptake by peripheral tissues and especially skeletal muscle.[139] This causes a higher blood glucose which, in turn, stimulates insulin secretion.[138] The peripheral resistance to insulin extends to activation of lipoprotein lipase, and this is partly responsible for the hypertriglyceridemia frequently seen in CRF.[140] The importance of hypertriglyceridemia in causing accelerated atherosclerosis in CRF is unsettled.[141] Fortunately, the insulin resistance of uremia is rarely severe enough to warrant treatment; plasma triglyceride levels can be lowered if dietary carbohydrates are restricted and a greater proportion of calories is supplied as unsaturated fat.[35, 42] Because the kidneys account for 20 to 30% of the metabolic clearance of insulin, diabetic patients frequently note that their insulin requirement falls as their renal function deteriorates.[142]

The anemia of uremia is largely a consequence of deficient erythropoietin production due to loss of kidney mass. Other factors that contribute to anemia include a blunted response to erythropoietin[143] and shortened red blood cell survival.[144] Recombinant erythropoietin (EPO) has been successfully employed in hemodialysis patients with a dose-dependent rate of correction of the anemia.[145] Studies of experimental uremia in rats raised the possibility that correction of the anemia of CRF with EPO might hasten the progression of renal failure.[146] Studies of EPO administration in predialysis patients with CRF have shown correction of anemia at doses similar to those employed in hemodialysis patients, indicating that dialyzable toxins do not contribute to the anemia of CRF in any important way.[147, 148] Patients receiving EPO experienced an improved sense of well-being, with less fatiguability, and increased libido (among male patients). EPO therapy did not result in any apparent acceleration in the rate of decline of creatinine clearance or in the reciprocal of serum creatinine concentration (SCr^{-1}) in the largest series reported to date.[149] Thus, it appears unlikely that EPO significantly accelerates the rate of decline of renal function, at least in short-term studies, but these studies do not give an answer as to whether treatment with EPO over a longer duration would hasten the decline of renal failure. Indeed, Watson and colleagues noted that three of the five patients whose GFR was being serially monitored experienced an abrupt decline in GFR; two of the patients were receiving EPO, the other patient received a placebo.[150] It should be noted that EPO was administered thrice weekly either intravenously or subcutaneously, the latter being a more efficient method of giving the agent.

Hypertension remains the most troublesome side effect of EPO therapy; the incidence of more severe hypertension increases as the rate of correction of the anemia increases. For this reason, all patients receiving EPO should be monitored carefully for accelerated hypertension. Generalized seizures have been also noted as a rare but dreaded complication. At present the Health Care Financing Administration (or Medicare) does not reimburse patients with CRF prior to the initiation of dialysis for EPO therapy; thus remuneration for EPO depends on other third-party insurers.

Anemia may be aggravated by gastrointestinal blood loss,[30] dysfunctional uterine bleeding, and folate or iron deficiency that can blunt the response to EPO; iron saturation less than 20% has been noted to be associated with EPO resistance.[151] However, patients with iron saturation above 20% can still be resistant until they are given iron supplements.[152] Thus, in patients with low values of saturation and resistance to EPO, a therapeutic challenge with iron is warranted. Iron deficiency and other treatable conditions should be sought whenever the degree of anemia changes or appears worse than expected for the degree of renal insufficiency; even patients with advanced CRF should have a hematocrit of approximately 25%. Serum iron is not a reliable index of deficient iron stores in patients with CRF who do not receive EPO; serum ferritin levels are more closely related to iron stores. As a general guideline, a ferritin level below 75 mg/l indicates iron deficiency.[153]

Evidence for gonadal dysfunction in CRF includes atrophic testes and diminished libido in men and amenorrhea or dysfunctional uterine bleeding and cystic ovaries in women.[154] Primary testicular dysfunction in men with CRF causes azoospermia and low testosterone levels. The intact hypothalamic and pituitary responses result in appropriately high plasma LH and FSH levels.[154] Successful transplantation corrects azoospermia and plasma testosterone, proving that uremia causes primary testicular failure.[155]

Less than 10% of premenopausal women with CRF have normal menstrual cycles; approximately 50% are amenorrheic; and about 40% have dysfunctional uterine bleeding. These changes are attributed to the absence of a midcycle LH surge caused by a defective hypothalamic response to the midcycle increase in estrogen production.[156] Dysfunctional uterine bleeding can be severe but generally responds to combined estrogen-progesterone preparations, indicating a normal uterine response to these hormones. Although infertility is the rule, conception can occur, but it is extremely unusual for women with advanced CRF (serum creatinine > 5 mg/dl) to carry a pregnancy to term. For this reason, sexually active women generally are advised to use contraceptive measures.

Hyperprolactinemia in CRF contributes to galactorrhea in women, and gynecomastia and perhaps sexual dysfunction in men. Hyperprolactinemia results in part from diminished clearance of prolactin because of decreased renal mass. Increased production of prolactin, which may be linked to secondary hyperparathyroidism, seems to be more important since long-term bromocriptine therapy can correct hyperprolactinemia.[157–159] This therapy may also improve male sexual dysfunction and occasionally, reinitiate cyclical changes in gonadotropins in women with CRF.[159,160] However, bromocriptine therapy is still considered experimental because long-term side effects have not been defined.

Several thyroid tests are abnormal in CRF; these include low-normal values of T4, decreased T3, and impaired peripheral conversion of T4 to T3.[161,162] These changes are not necessarily diagnostic of hypothyroidism; they can be seen in patients with other chronic illnesses. In fact, TSH levels tend to be normal in patients with CRF. The serum TSH level is the most important diagnostic test for identifying the rare patient with CRF who requires treatment with thyroid hormone.

Adrenal function is abnormal in CRF; 17-OH-corticosteroids accumulate in CRF and both free and total plasma cortisol levels are elevated, even though there is a normal diurnal secretory pattern.[163] The half-life of cortisol is prolonged in patients with CRF, suggesting impaired hepatic metabolism.[164] This alone cannot account for the twofold increase in plasma cortisol, since a higher plasma cortisol should reduce pituitary adrenocorticotropic hormone (ACTH) secretion. This suggests that there is an alteration in the set-point for feedback of the pituitary ACTH. Consistent with this interpretation, the dexamethasone suppression test in CRF shows a blunted suppression with a more rapid return of cortisol secretion. Indeed, overnight low-dose dexamethasone frequently fails to suppress cortisol secretion,[163] whereas chronic administration of higher doses of dexamethasone suppresses cortisol secretion.[165] The clinical implication of the mild hypercortisolism of CRF is unclear. In experimental animals, nitrogen utilization bears a complex relationship to glucocorticoid levels, and even mild increases may decrease nitrogen utilization.[166]

DRUG THERAPY

As outlined in Table 36–10, several factors must be considered when prescribing drugs for patients with CRF: abnormal clearance of the drug and its metabolites; changes in bioavailability; effects of drugs on renal function; and idiosyncratic reactions mimicking uremic symptoms. Many drugs are cleared from the body either by glomerular filtration or by active secretion of the drug into the proximal tubular lumen of the kidney, or both. Before prescribing for patients with CRF, it is necessary to consider whether the pharmacokinetics of the drug have been changed. For drugs excreted predominantly by the kidney, changes in drug clearance roughly parallel changes in the GRF. For patients with CRF, the dose intervals for commonly used drugs are given in Table 36–11. The dosing interval can also be calculated for drugs excreted by the kidney using a

TABLE 36–10. CHANGES IN DRUG METABOLISM AND ADVERSE DRUG EFFECTS IN CHRONIC RENAL FAILURE

Factors Causing Abnormal Drug Response	Examples
Altered bioavailability	
Change in first-pass metabolism	Propranolol, meperidine
Binding to aluminum gels	Digoxin
Altered protein binding	Weakly acidic drugs, phenytoin, warfarin
Decreased clearance	
Drug	Digoxin
Active metabolites	Sulfonamides, chlorpropramide, procainamide, normeperidine
Increased toxicity	
Effects on GFR	Calcium channel blockers, NSAIAs, propranolol
Idiosyncratic	Captopril, indomethacin
Dose-related	Aminoglycosides

TABLE 36–11. PRESCRIBING OF DRUGS FOR PATIENTS WITH CHRONIC RENAL FAILURE

Drug	Excreting Organ	Dosing in CRF: Serum Creatinine		Comments
		2 mg/dl	*10 mg/dl*	
Antibiotics				
Erythromycin	Liver	c (q 12 hr)	c (q 12 hr)	
Sulfamethoxazole Trimethoprim	Kidney	c (q 24 hr)	c (q 36 hr)	May increase serum creatinine by interfering with tubular secretion. Can achieve therapeutic levels in urine even in advanced CRF
Tetracycline	Kidney (Liver)	c (q 12 hr)	c (q 24 hr)	May increase BUN with high doses and ineffective for UTI at serum creatinine above 4 mg/dl. Doxycycline is preferred because it does not have these effects
Analgesics				
Aspirin	Kidney (Liver)	a (q 4–6 hr)	c (q 6–8 hr)	Avoid large doses because of GI irritation and possible depression of GFR
Acetaminophen	Liver	a (q 4–6 hr)	c (q 8 hr)	Avoid large doses, as metabolites can accumulate
Propoxyphene	Liver (Kidney)	a (q 4–6 hr)	a (q 4–6 hr)	
Codeine	Liver (Kidney)	a (q 4–6 hr)	a (q 4–6 hr)	
Pentazocine	Liver (Kidney)	a (q 4–6 hr)	a (q 4–6 hr)	
Psychoactive Agents				All these agents may cause excessive sedation
Phenobarbital	Liver (Kidney)	a (q 8 hr)	c (q 12 hr)	
Diazepam	Liver (Kidney)	a (q 8 hr)	a (q 8 hr)	
Flurazepam	Kidney	a (q 24 hr)	a (q 24 hr)	
Haloperidol	Liver (Kidney)	a (q 8 hr)	a (q 8 hr)	
Chlorpromazine	Liver	a (q 12 hr)	a (q 12 hr)	
Amitriptyline	Liver (Kidney)	a (q 8 hr)	a (q 8 hr)	
Cardiac Agents				
Procainamide	Kidney	c (q 4–6 hr)	c (q 8–12 hr)	Blood level advisable to prevent accumulation and toxicity such as lupus-like syndrome
Propranolol	Liver	a (q 6–8 hr)	b (50%)	There is a suggestion that the progression of renal insufficiency may be accelerated with this drug
Quinidine	Liver (Kidney)	a (q 6–8 hr)	a (q 6–8 hr)	Blood level advised to detect early toxicity
Hydralazine	Liver (Kidney)	c (q 24 hr)	c (q 36 hr)	Metabolites can accumulate and induce lupus-like syndrome. Total dose should be kept below 200 mg/dl
Methyldopa	Kidney (Liver)	a (q 6 hr)	c (q 8 hr)	May be associated with prolonged hypotension after beginning dialysis
Reserpine	Liver (Kidney)	a (q 24 hr)	a (q 24 hr)	May cause excessive sedation and GI distress or bleeding
Miscellaneous				
Warfarin	Nonrenal	a (q 24 hr)	a (q 24 hr)	Bleeding may be enhanced in CRF
Prednisone	Liver	a (q 8 hr)	a (q 8 hr)	Both prednisone and dexamethasone may augment catabolism and increase BUN.
Dexamethasone	Liver	a (q 6 hr)	a (q 6 hr)	They also may increase sodium retention

a = No change in dose or interval between doses. Normal interval indicated between parentheses.
b = Decrease dose by percentage indicated in parentheses without changing the interval.
c = Increase the interval between maintenance doses by the number of hours indicated in parentheses.
BUN = blood urea nitrogen; CRF = chronic renal failure; GFR = glomerular filtration rate; GI = gastrointestinal; UTI = urinary tract infection.

formula.* An alternative method for prescribing drugs is to use the normal dosing interval but to reduce the dose of the drug. Regardless of the method used, it is important to realize the considerable interindividual variability in drug elimination, so drug levels (especially for those drugs with a low therapeutic index) should be measured frequently to avoid drug toxicity.

Organic anions accumulate in uremic patients and tend to displace weakly acidic drugs (e.g., warfarin, diphenylhydantoin) from serum proteins. This generally is accompanied by an increase in the metabolism or excretion of the drug so that the steady-state, unbound drug concentration (the biologically important fraction) remains therapeutic. However, the measured drug concentration, which usually includes both the free and bound fractions, is subnormal, suggesting that the drug level is subtherapeutic. The best-studied example of this is phenytoin[169]; the total phenytoin level in patients with CRF treated with standard doses of the drug is low whereas the free or biologically active fraction remains in the therapeutic range. Raising the dosage of phenytoin in such patients would inappropriately increase the free drug level and could cause drug intoxication. Unfortunately, the degree to which uremia affects the measured and free concentration of most drugs is unknown, therefore it is imperative that patients be examined frequently for both clinical response and signs of drug toxicity.

Many drugs are converted to toxic or therapeutically active metabolites, which are eliminated by the kidney. For example, chlorpropamide is converted to an active hydroxymetabolite and procainamide is acetylated to form an active metabolite; both accumulate in patients with renal impairment.[170, 171] Meperidine (Demerol) is metabolized to normeperidine, which accumulates in patients with CRF.[172] Normeperidine is neuroexcitatory, and high plasma levels can cause seizures, thus this drug should be avoided in patients with CRF. Because it is difficult to predict which drugs will produce adverse reactions in CRF, drug therapy should be avoided unless it is clearly indicated and unless the potential therapeutic benefits considerably exceed any potential risks.

Drug therapy in CRF is also complicated by changes in the bioavailability of drugs. This may occur when intestinal absorption of the drug is impaired by concomitant administration of antacids. For example, digoxin absorption is markedly reduced when the drug is ingested with aluminum-containing, phosphate-binding gels.[173] Uremia also can change "first-pass" hepatic metabolism of drugs, thus changing the quantity of drug reaching the circulation. For example, both propranolol and lidocaine plasma levels may be excessive in patients with CRF given usual doses because their first-pass hepatic metabolism is reduced.[174]

Drug therapy can also be a major cause for unexplained deterioration of renal function in patients with CRF. For example, interstitial nephritis has been associated with many drugs, including furosemide, penicillinase-resistant penicillins, and all classes of nonsteroidal anti-inflammatory agents (NSAIAs).[175] If autoregulation of renal blood flow is impaired in CRF, excessive lowering of systemic blood pressure with antihypertensive drugs or contraction of the extracellular volume by overzealous use of diuretics can compromise the GFR. The renal circulation in patients with CRF appears to depend on calcium transport systems and local generation of vasoactive prostaglandins. Consequently, deterioration of the GFR can occur during treatment with calcium channel blockers[176] or inhibitors of prostaglandin synthesis (aspirin, NSAIAs).[175] Although sulindac was initially believed not to affect renal prostaglandin synthesis,[177] additional studies have not confirmed a renal-sparing effect.[178] Therefore, the use of any nonsteroidal anti-inflammatory drugs in patients with CRF should be limited to patients with a clear indication and only with careful monitoring for any decline in GFR. This rule may be especially true in patients with high-renin states, such as patients with proliferative glomerulopathies or those receiving therapy with either ACE inhibitors or diuretics.[179]

Finally, idiosyncratic reactions to drug can mimic an exacerbation of the underlying renal disease. As noted earlier, NSAIAs can induce an interstitial nephritis; they, as well as penicillamine, gold, probenecid, and captopril, can cause proteinuria and the nephrotic syndrome. The drug-induced nephrotic syndrome may become irreversible when proteinuria rises above 3 to 5 g/day, thus these agents should not be used unless absolutely necessary in patients with preexistent proteinuria.

Table 36–11 is a list of frequently prescribed drugs and changes in their dosing intervals for patients with CRF. Bennett and colleagues present an inclusive list of drugs and guidelines for their use in CRF.[180]

PROGRESSION OF CHRONIC RENAL INSUFFICIENCY

Once established, CRF progresses relentlessly to end-stage renal disease, even when the underlying disease that initiated kidney damage is no longer active. In patients with inherited diseases, such as PCKD, or metabolic diseases, such as diabetes mellitus, the progressive loss of renal function is undoubtedly linked to the primary disease process. No such explanation exists for the progression to end-stage renal disease of patients with poststreptococcal glomerulonephritis, previous renal cortical necrosis, or corrected vesicoureteral reflux. In these conditions, another process must be causing kidney damage after the initial renal disease becomes inactive.[181]

Until 1976, it was assumed that the clinical course of renal insufficiency in patients with CRF was unpredictable.[182] Difficulties with available methods of analyzing changes in renal function led to this conclusion. Repetitive measurement of inulin clearance or the clearance of radioactive substances by glomerular filtration was too cumbersome for routine clinical use. Measuring the SUN or urea clearance repetitively is not ideal for following the course of renal insufficiency, because the SUN is determined not only by the urea clearance but also by protein intake (see previous discussion) and urine flow. Because of the difficulties in obtaining accurate 24-hour urine collections, it was believed that repeated measurements of creatinine clearance in individual patients would be too imprecise to estimate the rate of loss of renal function. Finally, there is no simple method of analyzing the familiar hyperbolic relationship between serum creatinine and creatinine clear-

*New-dose interval in hours = dose interval for normal subjects in hours × 2.5 ÷ the creatinine clearance expressed in l/kg/day. The measured creatinine clearance in ml/min is converted to l/kg/day by multiplying by 1.44 and dividing by the patient's weight in kilograms. The creatinine clearance can be rapidly estimated from the serum creatinine (S) expressed in mg/l (multiply mg/dl by 10), using the following formulas based on age, sex, and weight of the patient:[167, 168]

For men, C_{Cr}(l/kg/day) = [28 − 0.2 age]S(mg/l)$^{-1}$ − 0.04

For women, C_{Cr}(l/kg/day) = [23.8 − 0.17 age]S(mg/l)$^{-1}$ − 0.04

These formulas predict creatinine clearance in patients with CRF with an error of less than 5%.

ance to determine the rate of loss of renal function of an individual patient.

These difficulties were circumvented when it was shown that the course of renal insufficiency could be described as a linear decrease in the reciprocal of serum creatinine concentration (S_{Cr}^{-1}) with time.[183] As shown in Figure 36–2, a plot of sequential values of S_{Cr}^{-1} of an individual patient with CRF is linear; the slope of this line, therefore, is an estimate of the rate of loss of renal function. In the first report of this relationship, more than 90% of the patients experienced a linear decline in S_{Cr}^{-1}, as their serum creatinine value increased from an average of 2.5 mg/dl to 14.5 mg/dl, regardless of the underlying disease. Subsequent studies have confirmed this relationship, though the frequency of patients demonstrating a linear decline in S_{Cr}^{-1} with time varies from 60 to 90%.[183–185]

The slope of the decline in S_{Cr}^{-1} with time can be calculated from an average of about seven measurements made over several months. Once the slope is determined, it can be used to predict when the patient will reach a serum creatinine concentration that usually is associated with the need to begin dialysis (i.e., ~ 10 mg/dl). Changes in the slope also can be used to determine whether the course of renal insufficiency has been altered by therapy (see subsequent discussion). Finally, an increase in the slope should alert the physician to evaluate the patient for other processes (e.g., infection, drug reaction) damaging the kidney.

In addition to the S_{Cr}^{-1} method, Rutherford and colleagues showed that the log of serum creatinine increased linearly and fitted the observed data better than changes in S_{Cr}^{-1}, at least in some patients.[184] In many cases, however, the slope of the logarithm function increased sharply late in the course of CRF, even though no associated clinical event or physiologic process could be identified. Thus, the use of the logarithmic method suffers because the future course of progression cannot be predicted from observations made early in the disease. Gretz and associates, for example, found that the prediction error for patients to progress from a serum creatinine of 5 to 10 averaged about 5 months using the S_{Cr}^{-1} method, but the error was about 20 months using the logarithmic method.[186]

The simplest pathophysiologic explanation for a linear decline of S_{Cr}^{-1} with time is that creatinine clearance decreases linearly with time and that glomerular function is lost at a constant rate.[187] This conclusion seems correct, since Barsotti and colleagues have reported that the creatinine clearance of patients with moderately advanced renal failure does decrease linearly with time regardless of the cause of CRF.[188] Moreover, in at least two diseases, GFR is lost at a constant rate; when GFR is reduced below approximately 85 ml/min, it declines at a constant rate in patients with diabetic nephropathy and in patients with PCKD.[187] Thus, a linear decline in S_{Cr}^{-1} with time is consistent with the constant rate of loss of GFR. The fact that both S_{Cr}^{-1} and creatinine clearance (or GFR) decline linearly with time suggests that creatinine excretion must remain constant throughout the course of renal failure. This is incorrect; creatinine excretion falls in patients with advanced CRF owing to increasing creatinine degradation.[168, 189] These apparently contradictory findings can be reconciled by taking into account the presence of a relatively constant rate of extrarenal creatinine clearance.

It is fortunate that changes in S_{Cr}^{-1} can be used to estimate the course of renal insufficiency since the day-to-day coefficient of variation of serum creatinine in patients with renal disease is only 6.5%, which is less than the variability of repetitive measurements of inulin or creatinine clearance.[187] It is emphasized that a single value of S_{Cr}^{-1} is a poor estimate of GFR, but that the change in S_{Cr}^{-1} with time reliably estimates changes in creatinine clearance and GFR. A single value of serum creatinine (or its reciprocal) is a poor estimate of GFR for the following reasons: Serum creatinine and creatinine excretion vary with meat intake; creatinine secretion contributes a significant amount to creatinine excretion as creatinine clearance declines; serum creatinine can remain within the normal range in patients with early CRF, even though they have had a decrease in GFR.[188]

The most important of these factors is the effect of dietary changes on serum creatinine. Cooking meat converts creatine to creatinine; normal subjects experienced a 52% increase in serum creatinine 1.5 to 3.5 hours after they ingested 225 g of boiled beef; 24 hours later, the serum creatinine had returned to control levels.[190] A patient with CRF who ate 225 g of boiled beef would also experience a rapid increase in serum creatinine, but it would not return to the basal value for a longer period, depending on the degree of renal insufficiency. Conversely, if meat were eliminated from the diet, serum creatinine and creatinine excretion would decrease, but the fall in creatinine excretion should be less than 15%, which is the average change observed in normal subjects eating a creatine-free diet.[188, 191]

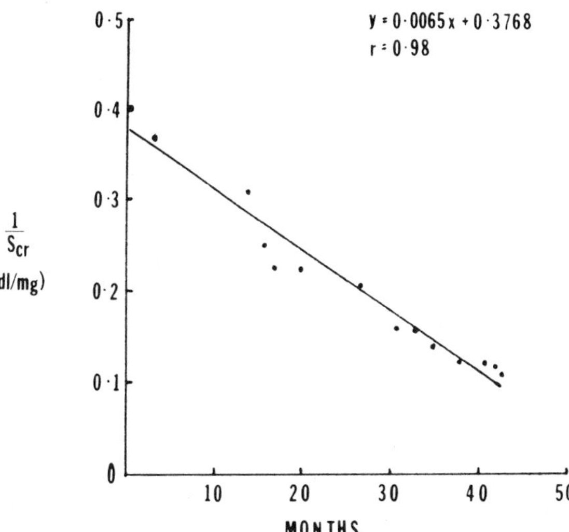

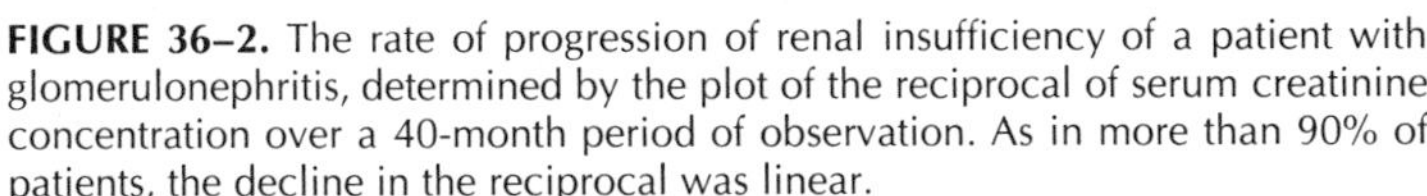
FIGURE 36–2. The rate of progression of renal insufficiency of a patient with glomerulonephritis, determined by the plot of the reciprocal of serum creatinine concentration over a 40-month period of observation. As in more than 90% of patients, the decline in the reciprocal was linear.

Thus, restricting dietary protein could lead to the false conclusion that the diet had changed the progression of renal insufficiency. Since the half-time to achieve a new steady state of creatinine excretion following a change in creatine intake is approximately 41 days,[168] an improvement in serum creatinine after beginning dietary protein restriction cannot be attributed to stabilization of renal function unless it persists for 4 months. If renal function continues to decline, serum creatinine must rise. Several other techniques have been devised to analyze the effects of therapy on progression of renal insufficiency.[34, 188, 192]

Mechanisms for the Progression of CRF

In the 1930s, it was reported that following subtotal nephrectomy rats develop a progressive rise in blood pressure and proteinuria, as well as increasing histologic damage to the kidney.[181, 193] Increasing dietary protein accelerated the loss of urea clearance. Brenner and associates provided persuasive evidence that the progression of renal insufficiency may be caused by an increase in both the pressure and flow of blood in the glomerulus occurring as an adaptation to loss of renal function.[194] They showed that this change in glomerular hemodynamics not only causes a "hyperfiltration response" but also is associated with glomerular capillary damage and glomerular sclerosis.

An alternative hypothesis invokes the alterations in calcium and phosphate metabolism caused by renal insufficiency.[195] Some portion of the beneficial effects of protein restriction might be due to dietary phosphate restriction. Laouari and associates re-examined this hypothesis and concluded that the beneficial effect of dietary phosphate restriction was more closely related to a decrease in protein and calorie intake than to phosphorus intake[196]; although this conclusion is controversial.[197]

A third hypothesis, that an accumulated nephrotoxin causes progressive renal insufficiency, is even more speculative because a specific nephrotoxin has not been identified, although dietary protein restriction does reduce serum oxalate levels and could limit the toxic effects of excessive oxalate accumulation in the damaged kidney.[198] In summary, studies indicate that dietary protein and phosphorus restriction can slow the loss of residual renal function in experimental CRF.

Investigation into the cause of progressive renal insufficiency in humans with CRF is understandably more limited because glomerular hemodynamics and the impact of calcium deposition on interstitial nephritis cannot be measured precisely with present techniques. However, a few studies address these potential mechanisms for progression of CRF in humans. For example, it is well established that chronic feeding of a low-protein diet reduces renal blood flow and GFR in normal subjects and that a high-protein meal raises renal blood flow and GFR. Bosch and colleagues confirmed this in normal subjects and showed that a large protein meal did not increase the creatinine clearance of patients with mild-to-moderate CRF.[199] They concluded that the glomeruli of the unresponsive patients already had a maximal hyperfiltration response and, therefore, GFR could not increase further in response to a high-protein meal. In examining the role of calcium and phosphorus in the progression of CRF in humans, Barsotti and colleagues measured the rate of loss of creatinine clearance and compared it with rates of phosphate excretion in two groups of patients fed the same low-protein diet but different amounts of phosphate.[200] Patients with a higher excretion rate of phosphate were losing renal function at a faster rate, and it was concluded that changes in mineral metabolism may contribute to the progression of renal insufficiency in humans. Clearly, further studies are needed to define the mechanisms contributing to progressive renal insufficiency.

Dietary Manipulation and Progression of CRF

Three dietary regimens have been used to slow progression of CRF. The variable in these diets is the amount of protein. They contain: (1) a conventional, low-protein diet of 0.6 g of protein/kg ideal body weight/day (primarily high-quality protein that provides essential amino acid requirements); (2) 0.3 g protein/kg/day of predominantly vegetable proteins supplemented with a mixture of essential amino acids (EAA); or (3) the same diet supplemented with a mixture of EAA and the nitrogen-free analogs of amino acids or ketoacids. These diets meet all nutritional requirements of patients with CRF (although after dialysis, the requirements increase) and reduce the symptoms of uremia.[201] Animal studies show that protein restriction slows the progression of CRF.

The protein requirement of normal subjects, approximately 0.6 g protein/kg of ideal body weight/day, is the same for patients with CRF.[201] However, nitrogen balance is possible only if the following conditions are met: (1) more than 60% of the protein must be of high biologic value (i.e., containing EAA); (2) caloric intake must be adequate (~ 35 kcal/kg/day)[202]; (3) B and C vitamins are supplemented; and (4) no coexisting catabolic condition is present (e.g., metabolic acidosis).[203] A skilled dietitian is needed to ensure that a nutritionally sufficient regimen is provided and that each patient's food preferences are included when recipes are planned. Compliance can be achieved with these diets during long-term therapy.[48, 201]

Dietary Protein Restriction and Progression of Renal Insufficiency

Maschio and associates reported an early trial of the effects of a low-protein diet on the progression of CRF.[31] Progression was assessed by evaluating changes in serum creatinine. The loss of renal function in treated patients with mild (serum creatinine 1.5 to 2.7 mg/dl) or moderate (serum creatinine 2.9 to 5.4 mg/dl) renal failure was much slower than in the controls group. Dietary compliance was not rigorously evaluated.

The Verona group updated the results of this regimen in 1989 by reporting on 390 patients treated with a low-protein diet for 54 ± 28 months.[204] Fifty-seven per cent of the patients had stable serum creatinine values; 11% had slower deterioration (defined as a decrease in the reciprocal of serum creatinine [Scr^{-1}] greater than -0.02 but less than -0.04 dl/mg/month); and 32% had rapid deterioration (> -0.04 dl/mg/month). Patients beginning the diet at an early stage of the disease seemed to have a more favorable course, as did patients with interstitial nephritis compared with those with chronic glomerulonephritis or PCKD. Initial values of serum creatinine, the degree of proteinuria, and systolic and diastolic blood pressures were found to be independent prognostic factors. With the low-protein diet, there were no adverse effects. Weight, anthropometric indices, and serum proteins were not compromised.[31] However, in the second 5 years, the concentration of protein in muscle biopsies decreased significantly as did serum albumin and transferrin (despite stable anthropometric measurements). These changes occurred only in a subgroup of eight patients who had lower values of energy intake (26 to 29 kcal/kg/day) than were prescribed. Thus, it is not clear that the problem was caused by inadequate dietary protein or by calories.

In a controlled evaluation of the influence of a low-protein diet, Rosman and coworkers reported the results of a prospective randomized trial involving 149 patients followed for at least 18 months (average of 24 months).[205] The amount of protein intake prescribed depended on the degree of renal insufficiency: Patients with a creatinine clearance between 30 and 60 ml/min were assigned to 0.6 g/kg/day of protein whereas those with a creatinine clearance between 10 and 30 ml/min were assigned to a diet containing 0.4 g/kg/day of high-quality protein. Progression was assessed from changes in serum creatinine and creatinine clearance. It was concluded that low-protein diets slow the loss of renal function and that patients younger than 40 years of age progressed more rapidly than did older subjects. The authors noted no adverse influence of protein restriction on nutritional status. Using the values of urea excretion reported by Rosman and associates, it can be calculated that protein intake must have been higher than was prescribed (Fig. 36–3).[48]

Results of a 4-year follow-up of 153 of the 248 patients who initially entered the study were reported by Rosman and coworkers.[206] The positive influence of the diet on progression was still noted, but it was most apparent in the group with more advanced renal insufficiency and glomerulonephritis. Any difference in rates of progression in patients with PCKD appeared to be related entirely to blood pressure control. In patients with other types of disease, blood pressure was not correlated with the preservation of renal function.

Both body weight and serum proteins were stable for 36 months. However, using data on urea excretion in the paper and the relationships described by Maroni and associates,[48] it can be estimated that the average intake was about 0.7 g of protein/kg body weight/day. A protein intake of 0.4 g/kg/day of protein would be well below the minimum daily protein requirement and cannot be recommended.[207]

Ihle and associates from Australia[208] conducted a prospective, randomized trial of a diet containing 0.4 g/kg/day of protein compared with unrestricted dietary protein in 64 subjects who were followed for 18 months. Results from patients who did not comply with the diet were excluded from the analysis. Changes in GFR were determined from the plasma disappearance of ^{51}Cr-EDTA. The groups were initially well matched for blood pressure, serum creatinine (range of 4 to 11 mg/dl), serum calcium, and phosphorus concentrations. End-stage renal failure developed in 9 of 33 patients (27%) who followed the unrestricted diets compared with only 2 of 31 (6%) who were thought to comply with the protein-restricted diet ($P < .05$). In addition, GFR decreased from approximately 15 to 6 ml/min in patients eating an unrestricted diet but did not change significantly in the protein-restricted group. Because patients who did not comply with the diet were excluded, the results assess the potential for benefit; they do not determine the influence of simply prescribing the diet. When the protein intake was calculated, the average was more than 0.7 g/kg/day (Fig. 36–4). Since the phosphorus content of the protein-restricted diet was approximately 30 to 40% less than that of the unrestricted diet, the relative importance of dietary protein versus phosphorus restriction on progression cannot be determined.

Regarding nutritional changes, serum albumin and anthropometric measurements remained stable during the 18 months of follow-up, but weight, serum transferrin, and total lymphocyte count all decreased significantly. These results could be due to an inadequate diet (although the average protein intake seemed to be above the minimum protein requirement). Since there are metabolic adaptations to a low-protein diet,[209] the alternative explanation is that advanced CRF prevented the patients from adapting to the diet. What is needed is a more complete understanding of the mechanisms of adaptation to these diets so that they can be used safely.

In contrast to these reports showing benefit, other prospective trials report that diet does not slow progression of CRF. Williams and associates randomly assigned 95 patients to one of three diets.[210] One diet contained 0.6 g/kg/day of protein, and the other had more than 0.8 g/kg/day of protein; a third group was given a diet containing 0.8 g/kg/day of protein and 800 mg/day of phosphorus (a low-phosphorus diet). The study design consisted of a 6-month stabilization period followed by observation of each group eating one of the specified diets for 19 ± 3 months. Dietary

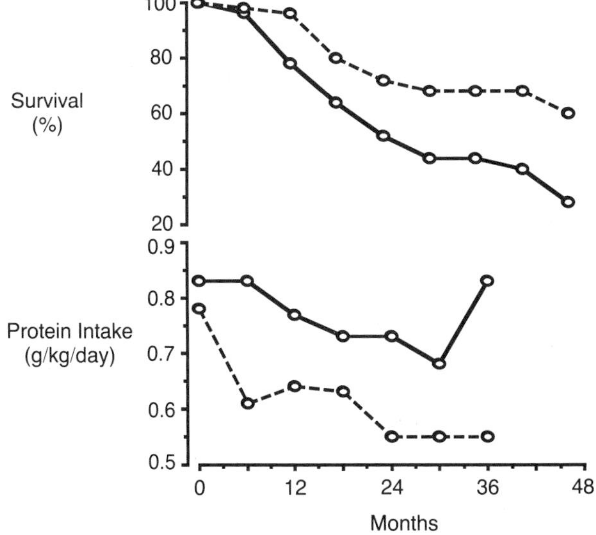

FIGURE 36–3. The survival to end-stage renal disease (persistent increase in serum creatinine) during treatment with a low-protein or a controlled diet is plotted as a percentage of enrolled patients surviving. Protein intake calculated from values of urea excretion during therapy is also shown. (From Maroni BJ, Steinman TI, and Mitch WE: A method for estimating nitrogen intake of patients with chronic renal failure. Kidney Int 27:58, 1985.) The results were calculated from the data of Rosman and associates (Rosman JB, ter Wee PM, Piers-Becht GP, et al: Prospective randomised trial of early dietary protein restriction in chronic renal failure. Lancet ii:1291, 1984, © The Lancet Ltd., 1984.) and show a significant ($P < .05$) effect of the low-protein diet.

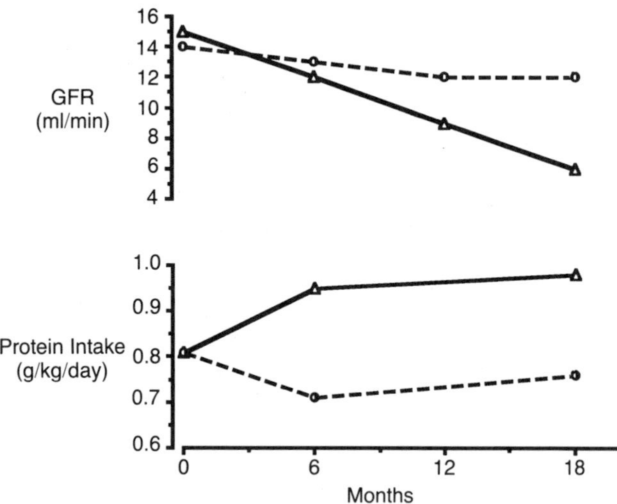

FIGURE 36–4. Changes in glomerular filtration rate (GFR) measured as the plasma clearance of iothalamate in patients prescribed a protein-restricted diet or an unrestricted diet. The calculated level of dietary protein as based on urea excretion is also shown (From Maroni BJ, Steinman TI, and Mitch WE: A method for estimating nitrogen intake of patients with chronic renal failure. Kidney Int 27:58, 1985. Used with permission of Kidney International.). The low-protein regimen significantly reduced the decline in GFR. (Drawn from the results of Ihle BU, Becker GJ, Whitworth JA, et al: The effect of protein restriction on the progression of renal insufficiency. N Engl J Med 321:1773, 1989; with permission from the New England Journal of Medicine.)

restriction did not slow the change in creatinine clearance (Fig. 36–5). However, as shown in Figure 36–3, the difference in protein intake was only 8 g/day on average. Regarding changes in nutritional status, the authors measured body weight, muscle mass (estimated from mid-arm muscle circumference and creatinine excretion), and serum transferrin and immunoglobulins. Body weight did not change significantly, although on average there was a slight decrease (1 to 2 kg) in groups fed the low-protein and low-phosphorus diets. Mid-arm muscle circumference as a measure of muscle mass was found to decline slightly (0.5 cm) but not significantly in the low-protein group. The other index of muscle mass, creatinine excretion, did not change, and serum transferrin and immunoglobulins did not fall in any of the groups. Thus, there was no evidence for an adverse nutritional effect of the diet, but there was no benefit on progression either.

The Northern Italian multicenter trial randomized 311 patients.[211] Since patients were stratified according to the degree of renal insufficiency, the number of patients in each group was not strikingly different from other trials.[208, 210] Progression was evaluated by analyzing the time for dialysis or doubling of serum creatinine ("renal survival"). The renal survival was slightly but not statistically better in patients who were prescribed the low-protein diet (27 versus 42 end-points in the control group). The authors suggested that the only factor that may have affected the rate of progression was the degree of proteinuria. The problem with this study is that the difference in protein intake was small. If it is assumed that the patients weighed 70 kg on average, the protein intake of the control group can be calculated from the urea excreted each day.[48] It was about 0.9 g/kg/day of protein for control patients; subjects fed the low-protein diet ate about 0.78 g/kg/day of protein. Regarding adverse effects on nutrition, the only factor measured was body weight, and no changes were found. Consequently, these results cannot be taken as evidence for nutritional efficacy.

The reason for the different conclusions reached in these trials is unclear. Possibilities are that dietary restriction does not change progression or that the difference in protein intake was too small to influence the loss of renal function. There is also the possibility that the inherent variability in repetitive measurements of creatinine clearance or serum creatinine may be too large to detect a difference,[212] although it is difficult to accept a conclusion that patients are improving or stable when their serum creatinine level is rising.

Fouque and associates performed a "meta-analysis" of published trials that permitted them to analyze a large number of patients.[213] A meta-analysis uses results from several studies in order to increase the number of patients. The critical issue in this type of analysis is to evaluate differences in frequency of a unique event in each trial, and Fouque and associates analyzed results from six studies of randomly assigned patients who were followed until they required dialysis or died. It was concluded that results from five of the six trials showed a reduction in the number of renal "deaths" (61 for low-protein diet groups versus 95 for control groups). These data permitted calculation of an odds ratio that estimates the likelihood of progressing to end-stage renal disease. The difference in the odds ratio was statistically significant ($P < .002$), which was consistent with the conclusion that dietary restriction preserves renal function. Although these results suggest a positive result, this type of analysis cannot prove the effectiveness of a low-protein diet.

Patients with progressive diabetic nephropathy can also respond to low-protein diets. This is important for two reasons: (1) a substantial proportion of patients with insulin-dependent diabetes develop renal failure and require dialysis; and (2) diabetes could complicate the nutritional responses to a protein-restricted diet. In a few reports, only changes in proteinuria with a low-protein diet were measured, and short-term protein restriction reduced proteinuria in diabetic patients with microalbuminuria.[214, 215] For-

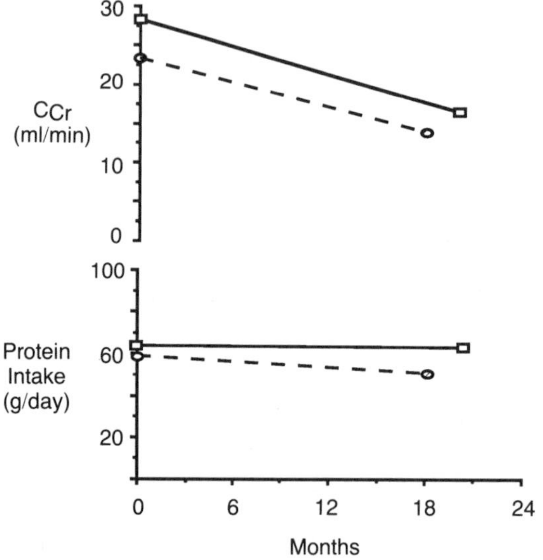

FIGURE 36–5. Changes in creatinine clearance during therapy with a low-protein and control diet in the trial conducted by Williams and associates (From Williams PS, Stevens ME, Fass G, et al: Failure of dietary protein and phosphate restriction to retard the rate of progression of chronic renal failure: A prospective, randomized, controlled trial. Q J Med 81:837, 1991, permission of Oxford University Press.). The protein intake was calculated from urea excretion. (From Maroni BJ, Steinman TI, and Mitch WE: A method for estimating nitrogen intake of patients with chronic renal failure. Kidney Int 27:58, 1985. Used with permission from Kidney International.) There was no effect on the progression of renal failure.

tunately, other than reducing proteinuria, low-protein diets can slow the rate of loss of GFR. A report from Guy's Hospital in London detailed the course of 19 insulin-dependent diabetic patients with persistent proteinuria who were eating an average of 1.13 g/kg/day of protein. When they were switched to a diet averaging 0.67 g/kg/day of protein, the rate of decline in GFR slowed significantly (from 0.61 to 0.14 ml/min/month); albuminuria also decreased.[215] This slowing of the rate of progression was significant, even when the results were adjusted for differences in blood pressure, energy intake, and glycosylated hemoglobin level. A more striking response was reported by Zeller and associates.[214] In their study, two groups of diabetic patients were randomly assigned to a diet containing 1 g/kg/day (35 patients) or to 0.6 g/kg/day of protein (33 patients). The investigators achieved reasonable compliance with the protein-restricted diet with no loss of body weight or muscle mass. The average decline in GFR and in creatinine clearance was significantly slowed by the protein-restricted diet. GFR decreased from a loss of 1.01 ml/min/month to only 0.36 ml/min/month; the loss of creatinine clearance declined from −0.81 to −0.33 ml/min/month. There was also slowing of the decline in Scr^{-1}, but the difference was not statistically significant. Some of the patients who had the unrestricted diet had stable values of GFR during the study. Although this makes their finding of a statistical difference more startling, it also indicates the difficulty in carrying out a trial in which progressive renal failure is being analyzed. Clearly, there is no good reason to study patients who do not have a measurable rate of progression. As in the report from London, other factors could not account for the apparent beneficial effect of the dietary regimen, including differences in blood pressure or glycemic control or the frequency of examinations. They concluded that the most likely explanation for slowing of the progression of CRF is the influence of dietary restriction.

Evidence that a more restricted diet (0.3 g/kg/day of protein) supplemented with a mixture of EAA slows progression of CRF is more tenuous. Alvestrand and Bergstrom studied 17 patients with well-defined rates of progression despite a conventional low-protein diet.[216] They found that an EAA-based regimen was effective in slowing the decline in Scr^{-1}. Only three of the 17 patients had no slowing of progression. However, an interim evaluation of the results from an ongoing prospective, randomized trial by the same group has cast doubt on whether the EAA-supplemented dietary regimen does slow progression of CRF.[217] In their view, any slowing of progression appeared to be most closely related to a small (2 mm Hg), but significant, reduction in diastolic blood pressure and possibly, more frequent examinations.

The effects of a ketoacid-based regimen on progression have also been studied. Barsotti and coworkers studied the rate of loss of creatinine clearance in 31 patients treated with a diet containing 0.5 g/kg/day of protein.[188] They observed that the decline in creatinine clearance was linear in patients with different types of disease. The pattern was interrupted in 11 of 12 patients who were changed to a regimen containing about 0.2 g/kg/day of protein plus supplements of calcium salts of ketoacids. Similar results were reported in a subsequent report of 48 patients: 27 of these patients were considered compliant and, on average, the loss of creatinine clearance in this group was halted; the loss of function was reversed from −0.65 to +0.15 ml/min/month ($P < .005$).[218] Other than calcium salts, basic amino acid salts of ketoacids have been tested. This ketoacid mixture was given as a supplement to a low-protein diet (only 0.3 g/kg/day of protein) and appeared to slow the loss of renal function. Among 17 patients with well-defined rates of progression (as assessed by changes in Scr^{-1}), 10 or 59% had a significantly slower rise in serum creatinine during long-term therapy (average of 20 months).[34] The effect was seen exclusively in patients who had not reached a stage of advanced renal failure (serum creatinine > 8 mg/dl).

The possibility that the response to an EAA-based regimen differs from that of a ketoacid-based treatment was tested by Walser and colleagues.[219] They evaluated changes in GFR while 12 patients (initial GFR of 13 ml/min) were treated with an EAA-based or ketoacid-based regimen before being crossed over to the other regimen. The ketoacid regimen appeared to slow progression more than the EAA regimen. Despite the small number of patients studied, the results are interesting because progression was blunted even though renal failure was advanced. Fortunately, there was no weight loss or decrease in normal values of serum albumin, even though dietary protein was greatly restricted.

In summary, it has not been proved that restricting dietary protein slows progression despite many provocative observations. One or more of the prospective, randomized multicenter trials now in progress may answer this question. On the other hand, it is hoped that this brief review will help readers when examining reports that evaluate the effects of dietary regimens on patients with CRF.

HEMODIALYSIS AND TRANSPLANTATION

In the United States nearly 15,000 patients per year develop end-stage renal failure, and currently nearly 150,000 patients are receiving kidney transplants or are maintained on hemodialysis.[220] Moreover, projections are that by the year 2000 approximately 240,000 patients will require treatment for end-stage renal failure. Until approximately 30 years ago, the majority of these patients died despite the most intensive medical management; with better techniques for dialysis and transplantation and with the greater availability of these therapies, many of these patients lead reasonably normal, productive lives for many years. Federal legislation has provided for funding of dialysis fees through the Medicare System for any patient who is enrolled in an approved dialysis program. Payment for the creation of the initial vascular access is the responsibility of the patient, but subsequent surgical fees related to dialysis are paid for by this federal program. Several dialytic therapies are now available, including home or center hemodialysis, continuous cycling peritoneal dialysis (CCPD), and continuous ambulatory peritoneal dialysis (CAPD). With these options, therapy can be individualized.

The hemodialysis machine has two major components: the dialyzer membrane, generally made from cellulose or plastic polymers, and the dialysate liquid. Blood from the patient passes through dialyzer tubing that is immersed in a bath containing a solution of ions in similar concentrations to that of plasma, but without any waste products. Dialyzer membranes are essentially impermeable to molecules with molecular weights greater than 5000 daltons, thus most waste products (but not proteins) can equilibrate with the bathing fluid. As a consequence of the concentration gradient between blood and dialysate fluid, waste products from the blood pass into the dialysis bath. This is oversimplified but does point out a major problem with dialysis—the nonselective nature of the process. In addition to waste products, amino, acids, vitamins, and other

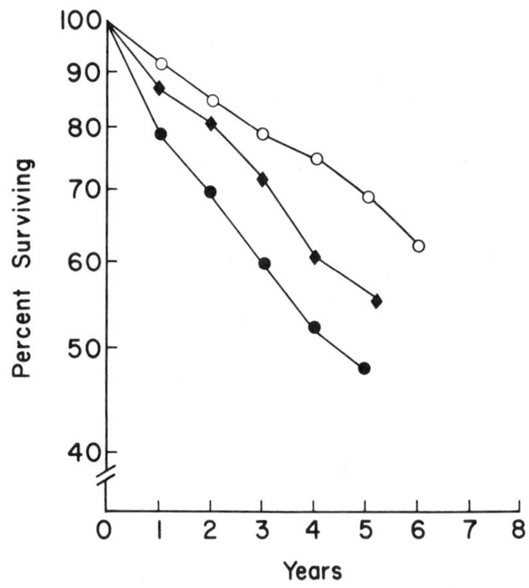

FIGURE 36–6. Survival of patients being treated by chronic hemodialysis. The graph shows that patients between 20 and 39 years of age (*open circles*) have an improved survival rate compared with patients older than 60 years (*solid circles*). After 6 years, about 50% of patients of all ages are surviving (*solid diamonds*).

nutrients are removed and must be replaced to prevent wasting of body protein stores. Excess fluid can also be removed, and electrolyte imbalances can be corrected.

Hemodialysis requires a reliable vascular access that permits blood to flow through the dialyzer. This was first accomplished with the Quinton-Scribner arteriovenous shunt consisting of Silastic tubing inserted into the cephalic vein and radial artery. The external shunt is still used occasionally for temporary vascular access, but its tendency to clot, the psychological problems of having tubes protruding from the arm, and the risk of infection have made internal arteriovenous fistulas the most common type of vascular access. Native fistulas are created near the wrist by anastomosing the radial artery to the cephalic vein. Alternatively, fistulas involving the brachial artery in the upper arm may be constructed in patients who have an unfavorable anatomy in the forearm. The higher pressure and flow of blood causes hypertrophy of superficial veins in the forearm, thus permitting repetitive venipuncture. The anastomosis is a relatively simple surgical procedure that need not require hospitalization, but usually 4 to 6 weeks are needed before the fistula can be used. Optimally, the fistula should be created before the patient becomes severely uremic; in general, fistulas are created when the serum creatinine is about 10 mg/dl, unless renal insufficiency is progressing rapidly. With the increasing age of patients entering dialysis, and the greater proportion of diabetics, vascular anatomy frequently precludes the construction of arteriovenous fistulas, and artificial grafts composed of either formalin-treated bovine carotid arteries or polytetrafluoroethylene have become the major type of vascular access used for hemodialysis. These grafts require approximately 2 weeks until they may be safely employed for dialysis. The useful life span of artificial grafts is shorter than that for native fistulas, due mainly to progressive intimal hyperplasia at the venous anastomotic site.[23] Moreover, they are more likely to become secondarily infected but demonstrate less signs of infection compared with native fistulas. A careful physical and ultrasonographic examination of grafts is needed in any hemodialysis patient who has a fever. In cases when graft placement is not feasible, permanent double-lumen Silastic catheters can be inserted and used immediately for dialysis. Unfortunately, they suffer from a greater infection rate, and their use should be restricted to patients with maturing native fistulas or to patients for whom no other graft can be placed.

Rates of survival of patients being treated by hemodialysis are shown in Figure 36–6; patients older than 60 years of age have a lower survival rate (75% 1-year survival) than do patients younger than 40 years of age (90% 1-year survival), and diabetic patients have the worst prognosis (65% 1-year survival). In the 1980s, the survival of patients on maintenance hemodialysis in the United States has declined, largely due to comorbid conditions associated with the increasing age of patients on hemodialysis. Indeed, as federal reimbursement schedules have decreased, there has been increasing pressure to reduce the dialysis time for patients and to resort to newer methods of high-flux hemodialysis to optimize small solute clearance. It remains unclear whether the shorter treatment times may be a factor in impaired survival or increased morbidity. Regrettably, if federal reimbursement continues to be limited, it is likely that these negative trends will continue or intensify.

Since the rehabilitation potential for patients receiving successful renal allograft transplants exceeds dialysis, there has been a growing trend toward renal transplantation. Transplants increased from 3200 in 1974 to almost 9000 in 1986, but the number of transplants has leveled off since then because of limitations in the supply of allografts.

The earliest renal transplants were performed at Peter Bent Brigham Hospital in Boston under the direction of Dr. John P. Merrill. Initially, only transplants between identical twins met with any great success; with prednisone and azathioprine therapy, renal transplantation in patients who are not genetically identical, including transplants from unrelated cadaver donors, are now possible.[222] Immunogenetic studies indicate that the probability of graft survival improves with the degree of identity of the major histocompatibility genes between recipients and living, related donors. It is unclear that histocompatibility antigen identity plays an important role in the survival of a renal transplant from an unrelated donor.[223] Improved use of immunosuppressive agents and antibiotics at surgery has increased patient survival markedly; infection is reduced to a 2% incidence, and operative mortality for all patients is now only 4% at the Brigham and Women's Hospital.[224] It has been reported that the 1-year survival rate of cadaveric renal allografts exceeds 80% when cyclosporin A is used.[223, 225] Cyclosporin A may permit the maintenance dosage of prednisone to be lowered. The ultimate role of cyclosporin A will require a more thorough characterization of its long-term toxicity.[225] Patients with poor allograft function or recurrent graft rejection during cyclosporin A therapy may have a dramatic improvement in renal function if the drug is stopped and azathioprine is used.[226]

It has become apparent that survival of kidneys transplanted from cadaver donors is enhanced if the patient has received at least 5 red blood cell transfusions.[227] Furthermore, prior blood transfusions from a related donor may enhance survival of a renal transplant from the same donor.[228] The mechanism for this effect of blood transfusion is poorly understood, but it does mean that a transfusion need not be withheld from patients with CRF.

This brief discussion addresses some of the essential aspects of treatment of patients with end-stage renal disease and should not be substituted for consultation with a nephrologist. Such consultation is especially important when renal function declines to a level indicating the need for placing an arteriovenous fistula.

COUNSELING THE PATIENT

Patients with CRF may seek assistance of the primary care physician in genetic counseling, in estimating the time before dialysis or transplantation will be required, or in the economic and practical aspects of dialysis therapy and renal transplantation. In responding to the patient, it can be emphasized with confidence that therapy for CRF is constantly improving and that further progress can be expected.

Regarding genetic counseling, several diseases culminate in CRF that may not become clinically apparent until after the primary child-bearing years of the third decade. These include polycystic and medullary cystic renal disease, both of which are inherited as an autosomal dominant trait with a high degree of penetrance of the gene.[229] Therefore, the chance that a child with an affected parent will have the disease approaches 50%. Prospective parents can be acquainted with these facts, and they or those who already have children may wish to know whether the disease is present in themselves or in the children. Frequently, but not always, the disease can be diagnosed by an IVP. However, in the case of children, it should be pointed out that there is no available therapy that will prevent the development of PCKD or medullary cystic disease. Thus, the psychological effects of knowing that a child has a chronic disease that may not have clinical manifestations for years may outweigh any diagnostic benefit. In other inherited diseases such as Alport's syndrome, CRF frequently becomes clinically manifest before the child-bearing years, and conception may not occur. Guidelines for advising relatives of these patients on the risk of developing these diseases are beyond the scope of this chapter and will require the assistance of a nephrologist.

The prognosis of a patient with CRF can be predicted reasonably accurately from calculation of the rate of change of the reciprocal of serum creatinine concentration with time (see previous discussion). However, this prognosis may be improved by nutritional therapy or by specific therapy for the underlying disease. Even if the course of the disease cannot be altered, mortality rates of patients being treated by dialysis or transplantation continue to decline, and a positive outlook can be conveyed to the patient.

Therapy of end-stage renal disease, including dialysis and transplantation, does impose a heavy burden on a patient and his or her family. The emotional and economic problems accompanying this aspect of CRF have been discussed in detail for physicians,[230] and they should not be dismissed lightly. Every attempt should be made to achieve the goals set forth in this chapter, including a vigorous attempt to preserve all residual renal function.

REFERENCES

1. Schechter H, Leonard CD, and Scribner BH: Chronic pyelonephritis as a cause of renal failure in dialysis candidates. JAMA 216:514, 1971.
2. Krakauer H, Grauman JS, McMillan MR, et al: The recent U.S. experience with treatment of end-stage renal disease by dialysis and transplantation. N Engl J Med 308:1558, 1983.
3. Gillenwater JY, Harrison RB, and Kunin CM: Natural history of bacteriuria in schoolgirls: A long-term case-control study. N Engl J Med 301:396, 1979.
4. Freeman RB, Smith WM, Richardson JA, et al: Long-term therapy for chronic bacteriuria in males. Ann Intern Med 83:133, 1975.
5. Murray T and Goldberg M: Chronic interstitial nephritis: Etiologic factors. Ann Intern Med 82:453, 1975.
6. Rostrand SG, Brown G, Kirk KA, et al: Renal insufficiency in treated essential hypertension. N Engl J Med 320:684, 1989.
7. Rostrand SG, Kirk KA, Rutsky EA, and Pate BA: Racial differences in the incidence of treatment for end-stage renal disease. N Engl J Med 306:1276, 1982.
8. Frohlich ED, Messerli FH, Dunn FG, et al: Greater renal vascular involvement in the black patient with essential hypertension: A comparison of systemic and renal hemodynamics in black and white patients. Miner Electrolyte Metab 10:173, 1984.
9. United States Renal DATA system 1991 Annual Data Report: III. Incidence and Causes of Treated ESRD. Am J Kidney Dis 18(Suppl. 2):30–37, 1991.
10. Danovitch GM: Clinical features and pathophysiology of polycystic kidney disease in man. *In* Gardner KD (ed): Cystic Diseases of the Kidney. New York, John Wiley, 1976, pp 125–150.
11. Jao W, Pollak VE, Norris SH, et al: Lipoid nephrosis: An approach to the clinicopathologic analysis and dismemberment of idiopathic nephrotic syndrome with minimal glomerular changes. Medicine 52:445, 1973.
12. Coggins CH (Collaborative Study of the Adult Idiopathic Nephrotic Syndrome): A controlled study of short-term prednisone treatment in adults with membranous nephropathy. N Engl J Med 301:1301, 1979.
13. Wagner L: Immunosuppressive agents in lupus nephritis: A critical analysis. Medicine 55:239, 1976.
14. Fauci AS and Wolff SM: Wegener's granulomatosis. Dis Mon April, pp 1–36, 1977.
15. Leib ES, Restivo C, and Paulus HE: Immunosuppressive and corticosteroid therapy of polyarteritis nodosa. Am J Med 67:941, 1979.
16. Corwin HL, Korbet SM, and Schwartz MM: Clinical correlates of eosinophiluria. Arch Intern Med 145:1097, 1985.
17. Nolan CR III, Anger MS, and Kelleher SP: Eosinophiluria—a new method of detection and definition of the clinical spectrum. N Engl J Med 315:1516, 1986.
18. Parfrey PS, Bear JC, Morgan J, et al: The diagnosis and prognosis of autosomal dominant polycystic kidney disease. N Engl J Med 323:1085, 1990.
19. Zeier M, Geberth S, Ritz E, et al: Adult dominant polycystic kidney disease—clinical problems. Nephron 49:177, 1988.
20. Carvallo A, Rakowski TA, Argy WP Jr, et al: Acute renal failure following drip infusion pyelography. Am J Med 65:38, 1978.
21. Eisenberg RL, Bank WO, and Hedgcock MW: Renal failure after major angiography. Am J Med 68:43, 1980.
22. Kassirer JP: Is renal biopsy necessary for optimal management of the idiopathic nephrotic syndrome? Kidney Int 24:561, 1983.
23. Mitch WE: Nutrition in renal disease. *In* Martinez-Maldonado M (ed): Handbook of Renal Therapeutics. New York, Plenum, 1983, pp 349–373.

24. Kelly RA and Mitch WE: Creatinine, uric acid, and other nitrogenous waste products: Clinical implication of the imbalance between their production and elimination in uremia. Semin Nephrol 3:286, 1983.
25. Ando A, Orita Y, Nakata K, et al: Effect of low-protein diet and surplus of essential amino acids on the serum concentration and the urinary excretion of methylguanidine and guanidinosuccinic acid in chronic renal failure. Nephron 24:161, 1979.
26. Johnson WJ, Hagge WH, Waggoner RD, et al: Effects of urea loading in patients with far-advanced renal failure. Mayo Clin Proc 47:21, 1972.
27. Merrill JP, Legrain M, and Hoigne R: Observations on the role of urea in uremia. Am J Med 14:519, 1953.
28. Lowrie EG, Laid NM, Parker TF, et al: The effect of hemodialysis prescription on patient morbidity: Report from the National Cooperative Dialysis Study. N Engl J Med 305:1176, 1981.
29. Dossetor JB: Creatininemia versus uremia: The relative significance of blood urea nitrogen and serum creatinine concentration in azotemia. Ann Intern Med 65:1287, 1966.
30. Rosenblatt SG, Drake S, Fadem S, et al: Gastrointestinal blood loss in patients with chronic renal failure. Am J Kidney Dis 1:232, 1982.
31. Maschio G, Oldrizzi L, Tessitore N, et al: Effects of dietary protein and phosphorus restriction on the progression of early renal failure. Kidney Int 22:371, 1982.
32. Alvestrand A, Ahlberg M, Furst P, et al: Clinical results of long-term treatment with a low protein diet and a new amino acid preparation in patients with chronic uremia. Clin Nephrol 19:67, 1983.
33. Mitch WE, Abras E, and Walser M: Long-term effects of a new ketoacid–amino acid supplement in patients with chronic renal failure. Kidney Int 22:48, 1982.
34. Mitch WE, Walser M, Steinman TI, et al: The effect of a ketoacid/amino acid supplement to a restricted diet on the progression of chronic renal failure. N Engl J Med 311:623, 1984.
35. Maroni BJ and Mitch WE: Nutrition in renal disease. *In* Klahr S and Massry S (eds): Contemporary Nephrology. New York, Plenum Press, 1985, p 599.
36. Scrimshaw NS: An analysis of past and present recommended dietary allowances for protein in health and disease. N Engl J Med 294:136, 1976.
37. Giordano C: Use of exogenous and endogenous urea for protein synthesis in normal and uremic subjects. J Lab Clin Med 62:231, 1963.
38. Mitch WE, Lietman P, and Walser M: Effect of oral neomycin and kanamycin in chronic uremic subjects. I: Urea metabolism. Kidney Int 11:116, 1977.
39. Mitch WE and Walser M: Effect of oral neomycin and kanamycin in chronic uremic subjects. II: Nitrogen balance. Kidney Int 11:122, 1977.
40. Varcoe R, Halliday D, Carson ER, et al: Efficiency of utilization of urea nitrogen for albumin synthesis by chronically uraemic and normal man. Clin Sci Mol Med 48:379, 1975.
41. Kopple JD and Coburn JW: Metabolic studies of low protein diets in uremia. I: Nitrogen and potassium. Medicine 52:583, 1973.
42. Sanfelippo ML, Swenson RS, and Reaven GM: Reduction of plasma triglycerides by diet in subjects with chronic renal failure. Kidney Int 11:54, 1977.
43. Kopple JD and Swendseid ME: Vitamin nutrition in patients undergoing maintenance hemodialysis. Kidney Int [Suppl] (2):79–84, 1975.
44. Walser M: Ketoacid therapy in chronic renal failure. Nephron 21:57, 1978.
45. Mitch WE and Walser M: Utilization of calcium L-phenyllactate as a substitute for phenylalanine by uremic subjects. Metabolism 26:1041, 1977.
46. Mitch WE, Collier VU, and Walser M: Treatment of chronic renal failure with branched-chain ketoacids plus the other essential amino acids or their nitrogen-free analogues. *In* Walser M and Williamson JR (eds): Metabolism and Clinical Implications of Branched-Chain Amino and Ketoacids. New York, Elsevier/North-Holland, 1981, p 631.
47. Cottini EP, Gallina DK, and Dominguez JM: Urea excretion in adult humans with varying degrees of kidney malfunction fed milk, egg, or an amino acid mixture: Assessment of nitrogen balance. J Nutr 103:11, 1973.
48. Maroni BJ, Steinman TI, and Mitch WE: A method for estimating nitrogen intake of patients with chronic renal failure. Kidney Int 27:58, 1985.
49. Coleman AJ, Avias M, Carter NW, et al: The mechanism of salt wastage in chronic renal disease. J Clin Invest 45:1116, 1966.
50. Bricker NS, Fine LG, Kaplan M, et al: The magnification phenomenon in chronic renal failure. N Engl J Med 299:1287, 1978.
51. Mitch WE and Wilcox CS: Disorders of body fluids, sodium and potassium in chronic renal failure. Am J Med 72:536, 1982.
52. Deen WM, Maddox DA, Robertson CR, et al: Dynamics of glomerular ultrafiltration in the rat. VII. Response to reduced renal mass. Am J Physiol 227:556, 1974.
53. Burge JC, Park HS, Whitlock CP, et al: Taste acuity in patients undergoing long-term dialysis. Kidney Int 15:49, 1979.
54. Allison MEM and Kennedy AC: Diuretics in chronic renal disease: A study of high dosage furosemide. Clin Sci 41:171, 1971.
55. Wilcox CS, Mitch WE, Kelly RA, et al: Response of the kidney to furosemide. I: Effects of salt intake and renal compensation. J Lab Clin Med 102:450, 1983.
56. Loon NR, Wilcox CS, and Unwin RJ: Mechanism of impaired natriuretic response to furosemide during prolonged therapy. Kidney Int 36:682, 1989.
57. Oster JR, Epstein M, and Smoler S: Combined therapy with thiazide-type and loop diuretic agents for resistant sodium retention. Ann Intern Med 99:405, 1983.
58. Ellison DH: The physiologic basis of diuretic synergism: Its role in treating diuretic resistance. Ann Intern Med 114:886, 1991.
59. Voelker JR, Cartwright-Brown D, Anderson S, et al: Comparison of loop diuretics in patients with chronic renal insufficiency. Kidney Int 32:572, 1987.
60. May RC, Kelly RA, and Mitch WE: Metabolic acidosis stimulates protein degradation in rat muscle by a glucocorticoid-dependent mechanism. J Clin Invest 77:614, 1986.
61. May RC, Masud T, Logue B, et al: Chronic metabolic acidosis accelerates whole body proteolysis and leucine oxidation in awake rats. Kidney Int 41:1535, 1992.
62. May RC, Kelly RA, and Mitch WE: Mechanisms for defects in muscle protein metabolism in rats with chronic uremia: The influence of metabolic acidosis. J Clin Invest 79:1099, 1987.
63. Hara Y, May RC, Kelly RA, and Mitch WE: Acidosis, not azotemia, stimulates branched-chain amino acid catabolism in uremic rats. Kidney Int 32:808, 1987.
64. Papadoyannakis NJ, Stefanidis CJ, and McGeown M: The effect of the correction of metabolic acidosis on nitrogen and potassium balance of patients with chronic renal failure. Am J Clin Nutr 40:623, 1984.
65. Williams B, Hattersley J, Layward E, and Walls J: Metabolic acidosis and skeletal muscle adaptation to low protein diets in chronic uremia. Kidney Int 40:779, 1991.
66. Bergstrom J, Alvestrand A, and Furst P: Plasma and muscle free amino acids in maintenance hemodialysis patients without protein malnutrition. Kidney Int 38:108, 1990.
67. DeFronzo RA and Beckles AD: Glucose intolerance following chronic acidosis in man. Am J Physiol 236:E328, 1979.
68. Hasted FC, Nolph KD, and Maher JF: $NaHCO_3$ and NaCl tolerance in chronic renal failure. J Clin Invest 56:414, 1975.
69. Molitoris BA, Froment DH, Mackenzie TA, et al: Citrate: A major factor in the toxicity of orally administered aluminum compounds. Kidney Int 36:949, 1989.
70. Koomans HA, Roos JC, Boer P, et al: Salt sensitivity of blood pressure in chronic renal failure. Hypertension 4:190, 1982.
71. Schalekamp MA, Beevers DG, Briggs JD, et al: Hypertension in chronic renal failure: An abnormal relation between sodium and the renin-angiotensin system. Am J Med 55:379, 1973.
72. Wollam GL, Tarazi RC, Bravo EL, et al: Diuretic potency of combined hydrochlorothiazides and furosemide therapy in patients with azotemia. Am J Med 72:929, 1982.

73. Bauer JH and Brooks LS: The long-term effect of propranolol therapy on renal function. Am J Med 66:405, 1979.
74. Textor SC, Fouad FM, Bravo EL, et al: Redistribution of cardiac output to the kidneys during oral nadolol administration. N Engl J Med 307:601, 1982.
75. Topol EJ, Traill TA, and Fortuin NJ: Hypertensive hypertrophic cardiomyopathy of the elderly. N Engl J Med 312:277, 1985.
76. Yusuf S, Peto R, Lewis J, et al: Beta blockade during and after myocardial infarction: an overview of the randomized trials. Prog Cardiovasc Dis 17:335, 1985.
77. Pierpont GL, Brown DC, Franciosa JA, et al: Effect of hydralazine on renal failure in patients with congestive heart failure. Circulation 61:323, 1980.
78. Drugs and Therapeutics: Minoxidil (Loniten). Med Lett 22:21, 1980.
79. Graham GR and Pettinger W: Prazocin. N Engl J Med 300:232, 1979.
80. Steinman TI and Silva P: Acute renal failure, skin rash, and eosinophilia associated with captopril therapy. Am J Med 75:154, 1983.
81. Hricik DE, Browning PJ, Kopelman R, et al: Captopril-induced functional renal insufficiency in patients with bilateral renal artery stenosis or renal artery stenosis in a solitary kidney. N Engl J Med 308:373, 1983.
82. Gavras I, Graff LG, Rose BD, et al: Fatal pancytopenia associated with the use of captopril. Ann Intern Med 94:58, 1981.
83. Textor SC, Bravo EL, Fouad FM, et al: Hyperkalemia in azotemic patients during angiotensin-converting enzyme inhibition and aldosterone reduction with captopril. Am J Med 73:719, 1982.
84. Kelly RA, Wilcox CS, Mitch WE, et al: Response of the kidney to furosemide. II: Effect of captopril on sodium balance. Kidney Int 24:233, 1983.
85. Romankiewicz JA, Brogden RN, Heel RC, et al: Captopril: An update review of its pharmacologic properties and therapeutic efficacy in congestive heart failure. Drugs 25:6, 1983.
86. Zatz R, Dunn BR, Meyer TW, et al: Prevention of diabetic glomerulopathy by pharmacological amelioration of glomerular capillary hypertension. J Clin Invest 77:1925, 1986.
87. Anderson S, Rennke HG, and Brenner BM: Therapeutic advantage of converting enzyme inhibitors in arresting progressive renal disease associated with systemic hypertension in the rat. J Clin Invest 77:1993, 1986.
88. Bauer JH, Reams GP, and Sunder ML: Renal protective effect of strict blood pressure control with enalapril therapy. Arch Intern Med 147:1397, 1987.
89. Taguma Y, Kitamoto Y, Futaki G, et al: Effect of captopril on heavy proteinuria in azotemic diabetes. N Engl J Med 313:1617, 1985.
90. Heeg JE, De Jong PE, Van der Hem GK, and De Zeeuw D: Reduction of proteinuria by angiotensin converting enzyme inhibition. Kidney Int 32:78, 1987.
91. Heeg JE, De Jong PE, Van der Hem GK, and De Zeeuw D: Efficacy and variability of the antiproteinuric effect of ACE inhibition by lisinopril. Kidney Int 36:272, 1989.
92. Dworkin LD, Levin RI, Bernstein JA, et al: Effects of nifedipine and enalapril on glomerular injury in rats with deoxycorticosterone-salt hypertension. Am J Physiol 259:F598, 1990.
93. Woosley RC and Nies AS: Guanethidine. N Engl J Med 295:1053, 1976.
94. Tuck ML, Bravo EL, Krakoff LR, et al: Endocrine and renal effects of nifedipine gastrointestinal therapeutic system in patients with essential hypertension. Am J Hypertension 3:333S, 1990.
95. Cappuccio FP, Markandu ND, Sagnella GA, et al: Acute and sustained changes in sodium balance during nifedipine treatment in essential hypertension. Am J Med 91:233, 1991.
96. MacGregor GA, Pevahouse JB, Cappuccio FP, and Markandu ND: Nifedipine, sodium intake, diuretics, and sodium balance. Am J Nephrol 7(Suppl 1):44, 1987.
97. Bilbrey GL, Carter NW, White MG, et al: Potassium deficiency in chronic renal failure. Kidney Int 4:423, 1973.
98. Good DW and Wright FS: Luminal influences on potassium secretion: Sodium concentration and fluid flow rate. Am J Physiol 236:F192, 1979.
99. May RC and Mitch WE: The treatment of hyperkalemia. *In* Whelton P and Whelton A (eds): Hyperkalemia and Potassium in Cardiovascular and Renal Medicine. New York, Marcel Dekker, 1986, p 453.
100. Hayes CP Jr, McLeod ME, and Robinson RR: An extrarenal mechanism for the maintenance of potassium balance in severe chronic renal failure. Trans Assoc Am Phys 80:207, 1967.
101. Hendler ED, Torretti J, Kupor L, et al: Effects of adrenalectomy and hormone replacement on NaK-AT-Pase in renal tissue. Am J Physiol 222:754, 1972.
102. DeFronzo RA: Hyperkalemia and hyporeninemic hypoaldosteronism. Kidney Int 17:118, 1980.
103. Sebastian A, Schambelan M, Lindenfeld S, et al: Amelioration of metabolic acidosis with fludrocortisone therapy in hyporeninemic hypoaldosteronism. N Engl J Med 297:576, 1977.
104. Ettinger PO, Regan TJ, and Oldewurtel HA: Hyperkalemia, cardiac conduction, and the electrocardiogram: A review. Am Heart J 88:360, 1974.
105. Bashour T, Hsu I, Gorfinkel HJ, et al: Atrioventricular and intraventricular conduction in hyperkalemia. Am J Cardiol 35:199, 1975.
106. Merrill JP, Levine HD, Somerville W, et al: Clinical recognition and treatment of acute potassium intoxication. Ann Intern Med 33:797, 1950.
107. Blumberg A, Weidmann P, Shaw S, and Gnadinger M: Effect of various therapeutic approaches on plasma potassium and major regulating factors in terminal renal failure. Am J Med 85:507, 1988.
108. Allon M and Copkney C: Albuterol and insulin for treatment of hyperkalemia in hemodialysis patients. Kidney Int 38:869, 1990.
109. DeFronzo RA, Felig P, Ferrannini E, et al: Effect of graded doses of insulin on splanchnic and peripheral potassium metabolism in man. Am J Physiol 238:E421, 1980.
110. Salem MM, Rosa RM, and Batlle DC: Extrarenal potassium tolerance in chronic renal failure: Implications for the treatment of acute hyperkalemia. Am J Kidney Dis 18:421, 1991.
111. Evans BM, Milne MD, Hughes Jones NC, et al: Ion-exchange resins in the treatment of anuria. Lancet 2:791, 1953.
112. Feig PH, Shook A, and Sterns RH: Effect of potassium removal during hemodialysis on the plasma potassium concentration. Nephron 27:25, 1981.
113. Reiss E and Canterbury JM: Genesis of hyperparathyroidism. Am J Med 50:679, 1971.
114. Slatopolsky E and Bricker NS: The role of phosphorus restriction in the prevention of secondary hyperparathyroidism in chronic renal disease. Kidney Int 4:141, 1973.
115. Prince RL, Hutchison BG, Kent JC, et al: Calcitriol deficiency with retained synthetic reserve in chronic renal failure. Kidney Int 33:722, 1988.
116. Wilson L, Felsenfeld A, Drezner MK, and Llach F: Alterered divalent ion metabolism in early renal failure: Role of $1,25(OH)_2D$. Kidney Int 27:565, 1985.
117. Adler AJ, Ferran N, and Berlyne GM: Effect of inorganic phosphate on serum ionized calcium concentration in vitro: A reassessment of the "trade-off hypothesis". Kidney Int 28:932, 1985.
118. Baxter LA and DeLuca HF: Stimulation of 25-hydroxyvitamin D_3-1 alpha hydroxylase by phosphate depletion. J Biol Chem 251:3158, 1976.
119. Massry SG and Ritz E: The pathogenesis of secondary hyperparathyroidism of renal failure: Is there a controversy? Arch Intern Med 138:853, 1978.
120. Freitag J, Martin KJ, Hruska K, et al: Impaired parathyroid hormone metabolism in patients with chronic renal failure. N Engl J Med 298:29, 1978.
121. Ritz E, Malluche HH, Krempien B, et al: Bone history in renal insufficiency. *In* David DS (ed): Calcium Metabolism in Renal Failure and Nephrolithiasis. New York, John Wiley, 1977.
122. Meema HE, Meindok H, and Oreopoulos DG: Radiology of renal osteodystrophy. *In* Brenner BM and Stein JH (eds): Contemporary Issues in Nephrology: Divalent Ion Homeostasis. New York, Churchill Livingstone, 1982, p 261.
123. Fadda GZ, Hajjar SM, Perna AF, et al: On the mechanism of

impaired insulin secretion in chronic renal failure. J Clin Invest 87:255, 1991.
124. Feinfeld DA: The role of parathyroid hormone as a uremic toxin: Current concepts. Sem Dialysis 5:48, 1992.
125. Collier VU and Mitch WE: Accelerated progression of chronic renal insufficiency after parathyroidectomy. JAMA 244:1215, 1980.
126. Kaplan MA, Canterbury JM, Bourgoignie JJ, et al: Reversal of hyperparathyroidism in response to dietary phosphate restriction in the dog. Kidney Int 15:43, 1979.
127. Slatopolsky E, Rutherford WE, Hruska K, et al: How important is phosphate in the pathogenesis of renal osteodystrophy? Arch Intern Med 138:848, 1978.
128. Sheikh MS, Maguire JA, Emmett M, et al: Reduction of dietary phosphorus absorption by phosphorus binders. J Clin Invest 83:66, 1989.
129. Slatopolsky E, Weerts C, Lopez-Hilker S, et al: Calcium carbonate as a phosphate binder in patients with chronic renal failure undergoing dialysis. N Engl J Med 315:157, 1986.
130. Cushner HM, Copley JB, Lindberg JS, and Foulks CJ: Calcium citrate, a nonaluminum-containing phosphate-binding agent for treatment of CRF. Kidney Int 33:95, 1988.
131. Kopple JD and Coburn JW: Metabolic studies of low protein diets in uremia. II: Calcium, phosphorus, and magnesium. Medicine 52:597, 1973.
132. Levine BS, Singer FR, Bryce GF, et al: Pharmacokinetics and biologic effects of calcitriol in normal humans. J Lab Clin Med 105:239, 1985.
133. Christiansen C, Rodbro P, Christiansen MS, et al: Deterioration of renal function during treatment of chronic renal failure with 1,25-dihydroxycholecalciferol. Lancet ii:700, 1978.
134. Christiansen C, Rodbro P, Christiansen MS, et al: Is 1,25-dihydroxycholecalciferol harmful to renal function in patients with chronic renal failure? Clin Endocrinol 15:229, 1981.
135. Baker LRI, Abrams SML, Roe CJ, et al: 1,25$(OH)_2D_3$ administration in moderate renal failure: A prospective double-blind trial. Kidney Int 35:661, 1989.
136. Brickman AS, Hartenbower DL, Norman AW, et al: Action of 1-hydroxyvitamin D_3 and 1,25-dihydroxyvitamin D_3 on mineral metabolism in man. I: Effects on net absorption of phosphorus. Am J Clin Nutr 30:1064, 1977.
137. Feldman HA and Singer I: Endocrinology and metabolism in uremia and dialysis: A clinical review. Medicine 54:345, 1974.
138. DeFronzo RA, Andres R, Edgar P, et al: Carbohydrate metabolism in uremia: A review. Medicine 53:469, 1973.
139. May RC, Clark AS, Goheer A, et al: Specific defects in insulin-mediated muscle metabolism in acute uremia. Kidney Int 28:490, 1985.
140. Bagdade JD, Porter P, and Bierman EL: Hypertriglyceridemia: A metabolic consequence of chronic renal failure. N Engl J Med 279:181, 1968.
141. Nestel PJ, Fidge NH, and Tan MH: Increased lipoprotein-remnant formation in chronic renal failure. N Engl J Med 307:329, 1982.
142. Rabkin R, Simon NS, Steiner S, et al: Effect of renal disease on renal uptake and excretion of insulin in man. N Engl J Med 282:182, 1970.
143. Wallner SF and Vantrin RM: Evidence that inhibition of erythropoiesis is important in the anemia of chronic renal failure. J Lab Clin Med 97:170, 1981.
144. Joske RA, McAlister JM, and Prankerd TAJ: Isotope investigations of red cell production and destruction in chronic renal disease. Clin Sci 15:511, 1956.
145. Eschbach JW, Egrie JC, Downing MR, et al: Correction of the anemia of end-stage renal disease with recombinant human erythropoietin: Results of a combined phase I and II clinical trial. N Engl J Med 316:73, 1987.
146. Garcia DL, Anderson S, Rennke HG, et al: Anemia lessens and its prevention with recombinant human erythropoietin worsens glomerular injury and hypertension in rats with reduced renal mass. Proc Natl Acad Sci 85:6142, 1988.
147. Eschbach JW, Kelly MR, Haley NR, et al: Treatment of the anemia of progressive renal failure with recombinant human erythropoietin. N Engl J Med 321:158, 1989.
148. Lim VS, DeGowin RL, Zavala D, et al: Recombinant human erythropoietin treatment in predialysis patients: A double-blind placebo-controlled trial. Ann Intern Med 110:108, 1989.
149. US Recombinant Human Erythropoietin Predialysis Study Group: Double-blind placebo-controlled study of the therapeutic use of recombinant human erythropoietin for anemia associated with chronic renal failure in predialysis patients. Am J Kidney Dis 18:50, 1991.
150. Watson AJ, Giminez LF, Cotton S, et al: Treatment of the anemia of chronic renal failure with subcutaneous recombinant human erythropoietin. Am J Med 89:432, 1990.
151. Van Wyck DB: Iron management during recombinant human erythropoietin therapy. Am J Kidney Dis 14:9, 1989.
152. Van Wyck DB, Stivelman JC, Ruiz J, et al: Iron status in patients receiving erythropoietin for dialysis-associated anemia. Kidney Int 35:712, 1989.
153. Van de Vyver FL, Vanhuele AA, Magelyne WM, et al: Serum ferritin as a guide for iron stores in chronic hemodialysis patients. Kidney Int 26:451, 1984.
154. Holdsworth S, Atkins RC, and Dekretser DM: The pituitary-testicular axis in man with chronic renal failure. N Engl J Med 296:1245, 1977.
155. Lim VS and Fang VS: Gonadal dysfunction in uremic man. Am J Med 58:655, 1975.
156. Lim VS, Henriguez C, Sievertsen G, et al: Ovarian function in chronic renal failure: Evidence suggesting hypothalamic anovulation. Ann Intern Med 93:21, 1980.
157. Sievertsen GD, Lim VS, Nakamatose C, et al: Metabolic clearance and secretion rates of human prolactin in normal subjects and in patients with chronic renal failure. J Clin Endocrinol Metab 50:846, 1980.
158. Raymond JP, Isaac R, Merceron RE, et al: Comparison between the plasma concentrations of prolactin and parathyroid hormone in normal subjects and in patients with hyperparathyroidism or hyperprolactinemia. J Clin Endocrinol Metab 55:1222, 1982.
159. Weizman R, Weizman A, Levi J, et al: Sexual dysfunction associated with hyperprolactinemia in males and females undergoing hemodialysis. Psychosom Med 45:259, 1983.
160. Gomez F, DeLacueva R, Wantes JP, et al: Endocrine abnormalities in patients undergoing long-term hemodialysis. The role of prolactin. Am J Med 68:522, 1980.
161. Lim VS, Fang VS, Katz AI, et al: Thyroid dysfunction in chronic renal failure: A study of the pituitary-thyroid axis and peripheral turnover kinetics of thyroxine and triiodothyramine. J Clin Invest 60:522, 1977.
162. Spector DA, Davis PJ, Helderman JH, et al: Thyroid function and metabolic state in chronic renal failure. Ann Intern Med 85:724, 1976.
163. Wallace EZ, Rosman P, Toshav N, et al: Pituitary-adrenocortical function in chronic renal failure: Studies of episodic secretion of cortisol and dexamethasone suppressibility. J Clin Endocrinol Metab 50:46, 1980.
164. Mishkin MS, Hsu T, Walker WQ, et al: Studies on the episodic secretion of cortisol in uremic patients on hemodialysis. Johns Hopkins Med J 131:160, 1972.
165. Workman RJ, Vaughn WK, and Stone WJ: Dexamethasone suppression testing in chronic renal failure: Parmacokinetics of dexamethasone and demonstration of a normal hypothalamic-pituitary-adrenal axis. J Clin Endocrinol Metab 63:741, 1986.
166. Quan ZY and Walser M: Effects of corticosterone administration on nitrogen excretion and nitrogen balance in adrenalectomized rats. Am J Clin Nutr 55:695, 1992.
167. Cockcroft DW and Gault MH: Prediction of creatinine clearance from serum creatinine. Nephron 16:31, 1975.
168. Mitch WE and Walser M: A proposed mechanism for reduced creatinine excretion in severe chronic renal failure. Nephron 21:248, 1978.
169. Reidenberg MM: The binding of drugs to plasma proteins and the interpretation of measurements of plasma concentrations of drugs in patients with poor renal function. Am J Med 62:466, 1977.
170. Stowers JM and Borthwick LJ: Oral hypoglycemic drugs: Clinical pharmacology and therapeutic use. Drugs 14:41, 1977.
171. Gilson TP, Lowenthal DT, Nilson HA, et al: Elimination of procainamide in end-stage renal failure. Clin Pharmacol Ther 17:321, 1975.

172. Szeto HH, Inturrisi CE, Houde R, et al: Accumulation of meperidine, and active metabolites of meperidine, in patients with renal failure or cancer. Ann Intern Med 86:738, 1977.
173. Brown DD and Juhl RP: Decreased bioavailability of digoxin due to antacids and kaolin-pectin. N Engl J Med 295:1034, 1976.
174. Lowenthal DT: Pharmacokinetics of propranolol, quinidine, procainamide, and lidocaine in chronic renal disease. Am J Med 62:532, 1977.
175. Clive DM and Stoff JR: Renal syndromes associated with nonsteroidal antiinflammatory drugs. N Engl J Med 310:563, 1984.
176. Diamond JR, Cheung JY, and Fang LST: Nifedipine-induced renal dysfunction. Am J Med 77:905, 1984.
177. Ciabattoni G, Cinotti GA, Pierucci A, et al: Effects of sulindac and ibuprofen in patients with chronic glomerular disease. N Engl J Med 310:279, 1984.
178. Brater DC, Anderson S, Baird B, and Campbell WB: Effects of ibuprofen, naproxen, and sulindac on prostaglandins in men. Kidney Int 27:66, 1985.
179. Garella S and Matarese RA: Renal effects of prostaglandins and clinical adverse effects of nonsteroidal anti-inflammatory agents. Medicine 63:165, 1984.
180. Bennett WH, Singer I, Golper T, et al: Guidelines for drug therapy in renal failure. Ann Intern Med 86:754, 1977.
181. Mitch WE: The influence of the diet on the progression of renal insufficiency. Annu Rev Med 35:249, 1984.
182. Maher JF, Nolph KD, and Bryan CW: Prognosis of advanced chronic renal failure: Unpredictability of survival and reversibility. Ann Intern Med 81:43, 1974.
183. Mitch WE, Walser M, Buffington GA, et al: A simple method of estimating progression of chronic renal failure. Lancet 2:1326, 1976.
184. Rutherford WE, Blondin J, Miller JP, et al: Chronic progressive renal disease: Rate of change of serum creatinine concentration. Kidney Int 11:62, 1977.
185. Oksa H, Pasternack A, Luomala M, et al: Progression of chronic renal failure. Nephron 35:31, 1983.
186. Gretz N, Manz F, and Strauch M: Predictability of the progression of chronic renal failure. Kidney Int 24:52, 1983.
187. Mitch WE: Measuring the rate of progression of renal insufficiency. *In* Mitch WE (ed): Contemporary Issues of Nephrology: The Progressive Nature of Chronic Renal Failure. New York, Churchill Livingstone, 1986, p 167.
188. Barsotti G, Guiducci A, Ciardella F, et al: Effects on renal function of a low-nitrogen diet supplemented with essential amino acids and ketoanalogues and of hemodialysis and free protein supply in patients with chronic renal failure. Nephron 27:113, 1981.
189. Mitch WE, Collier VU, and Walser M: Creatinine metabolism in chronic renal failure. Clin Sci 58:327, 1980.
190. Mayersohn M, Conrad KA, and Achari R: The influence of a cooked meal on creatinine plasma concentration and creatinine clearance. Br J Clin Pharm 15:227, 1983.
191. Heymsfield SB, Arteaga C, McManus C, et al: Measurement of muscle mass in humans: Validity of the 24-hour urinary creatinine method. Am J Clin Nutr 37:498, 1983.
192. Gretz N, Meisinger E, Getz T, et al: Low-protein diet supplemented by ketoacids in chronic renal failure: A prospective controlled study. Kidney Int 24(Suppl 16):S263, 1983.
193. Bischoff F: The influence of the diet on renal and blood vessel changes. J Nutr 5:431, 1932.
194. Brenner BM, Meyer TW, and Hostetter TH: Dietary protein intake and the progressive nature of kidney disease: The role of hemodynamically mediated glomerular injury in the pathogenesis of progressive glomerular sclerosis in aging, renal ablation, and intrinsic renal disease. N Engl J Med 307:652, 1982.
195. Donohue W, Spingarn C, and Pappenheimer AM: The calcium content of the kidney as related to parathyroid function. J Exp Med 66:697, 1937.
196. Laouari D, Kleinknecht C, Cournot-Witmer G, et al: Beneficial effect of low phosphorus diet in uremic rats: A reappraisal. Clin Sci 63:539, 1982.
197. Lumlertgul D, Burke TJ, Gillum DM, et al: Phosphate depletion arrests progression of chronic renal failure independent of protein intake. Kidney Int 29:658, 1986.
198. Barsotti G, Cristofano C, Morelli E, et al: Serum oxalic acid in uremia: Effect of a low-protein diet supplemented with essential amino acids and ketoanalogues. Nephron 38:54, 1984.
199. Bosch JP, Saccaggi A, Lauer A, et al: Renal functional reserve in humans: Effect of protein intake on glomerular filtration rate. Am J Med 75:943, 1983.
200. Barsotti G, Giannoni A, Morelli E, et al: The decline of renal function slowed by very low phosphorus intake in chronic renal patients following a low nitrogen diet. Clin Nephrol 21:54, 1984.
201. Maroni BJ: Requirements for protein, calories, and fat in the predialysis patient. *In* Mitch WE and Klahr S (eds): Nutrition and the Kidney. Boston, Little, Brown, 1993, p 185.
202. Kopple JD, Monteon FJ, and Shaib JK: Effect of energy intake on nitrogen metabolism in nondialyzed patients with chronic renal failure. Kidney Int 29:734, 1986.
203. Mitch WE: Uremia and the control of protein metabolism. Nephron 49:89, 1988.
204. Oldrizzi L, Rugiu C, and Maschio G: The Verona experience on the effect of diet on progression of renal failure. Kidney Int 36:S103, 1989.
205. Rosman JB, Meijer S, Sluiter WJ, et al: Prospective randomised trial of early dietary protein restriction in chronic renal failure. Lancet 2:1291, 1984.
206. Rosman JB, Langer K, Brandl M, et al: Protein-restricted diets in chronic renal failure: A four year follow-up shows limited indications. Kidney Int 36:S96, 1989.
207. FAO/WHO/UNU: Energy and Protein Requirements. (Technical Report Series 724.) Geneva, World Health Organization, 1985, p 1.
208. Ihle BU, Becker GJ, Whitworth JA, et al: The effect of protein restriction on the progression of renal insufficiency. N Engl J Med 321:1773, 1989.
209. Young VR: 1987 McCollum award lecture. Kinetics of human amino acid metabolism: Nutritional implications and some lessons. Am J Clin Nutr 46:709, 1987.
210. Williams PS, Stevens ME, Fass G, et al: Failure of dietary protein and phosphate restriction to retard the rate of progression of chronic renal failure: A prospective, randomized, controlled trial. Q J Med 81:837, 1991.
211. Locatelli F, Alberti D, Graziani G, et al: Prospective, randomized, multicentre trial of effect of protein restriction on progression of chronic renal insufficiency. Lancet 337:1299, 1991.
212. Mitch WE: Measuring the rate of progression of chronic renal insufficiency. *In* Mitch WE (ed): The Progressive Nature of Renal Disease. New York, Churchill Livingstone, 1992, pp 203–222.
213. Fouque D, Laville M, Boissel JP, et al: Controlled low protein diets in chronic renal insufficiency: Meta-analysis. BMJ 304:216, 1992.
214. Zeller KR, Whittaker E, Sullivan L, et al: Effect of restricting dietary protein on the progression of renal failure in patients with insulin-dependent diabetes mellitus. N Engl J Med 324:78, 1991.
215. Walker JD, Dodds RA, Murrells TJ, et al: Restriction of dietary protein and progression of renal failure in diabetic nephropathy. Lancet 2:1411, 1989.
216. Alvestrand A and Bergstrom J: Amino-acid supplements and the course of chronic renal disease. *In* Mitch WE (ed): The Progressive Nature of Renal Disease. New York, Churchill-Livingstone, 1986, p 219.
217. Bergstrom J, Alvestrand A, Bucht H, and Gutierrez A: Progression of chronic renal failure in man is retarded with more frequent clinical follow-ups and better blood pressure control. Clin Nephrol 25:1, 1986.
218. Barsotti G, Morelli E, and Guiducci A: Three years' experience with a very low nitrogen diet supplemented with essential amino acids and keto-analogues in the treatment of chronic uremia. Proc Eur Dial Transplant Assoc 19:773, 1982.
219. Walser M, Hill S, and Ward L: Progression of chronic renal failure on substituting a ketoacid supplement for an amino acid supplement. J Am Soc Nephrol 2:1178, 1992.
220. Levinsky NG and Rettig RA: The medicare end-stage renal disease program: A report from the Institute of Medicine. N Engl J Med 324:1143, 1991.

221. Chervu A and Moore WS: An overview of intimal hyperplasia. Surg Gynecol Obstet 171:433, 1990.
222. Guttmann R: Renal transplantation. N Engl J Med 301:975, 1979.
223. Strom TB: The improving utility of renal transplantation in the management of end-stage renal disease. Am J Med 73:105, 1982.
224. Tilney NL, Strom TB, Vineyard GC, et al: Factors contributing to declining mortality rate in renal transplantation. N Engl J Med 299:1321, 1978.
225. Merion RM, White D, Thiru S, et al: Cyclosporine: Five years' experience in cadaveric renal transplantation. N Engl J Med 310:148, 1984.
226. Rocher LL, Milford EL, Kirkman RL, et al: Conversion from cyclosporine to azathioprine in renal allograft recipients. Transplantation 38:669, 1984.
227. Opelz G, Grover B, and Terasaki P: Induction of high kidney graft survival rate for multiple transfusions. Lancet 1:1223, 1981.
228. Cochrum K, Hanes D, Potter D, et al: Improved graft survival following donor specific blood transfusions. Transplant Proc 13:190, 1981.
229. Schemki RN: Genetics in cystic kidney disease. *In* Gardner KD (ed): Cystic Diseases of the Kidney. New York, John Wiley, 1976, p 83.
230. Campbell JD and Campbell AR: The social and economic costs of end-stage renal disease. N Engl J Med 299:386, 1978.

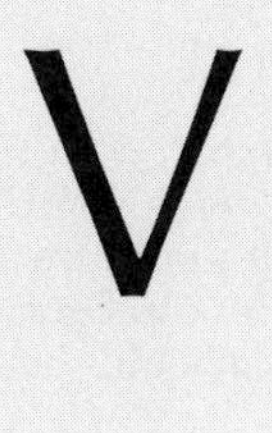

Gynecologic Problems

37

Vaginitis and Cervicitis

BEVERLY WOO, MD

Vaginitis

Vaginitis is a common and often perplexing problem for women. It may cause considerable discomfort and may be a source of embarrassment. Symptoms include vaginal discharge, severe itching or burning of the vaginal area, urinary frequency or burning, and/or dyspareunia. Some patients are hesitant even to mention an annoying discharge to their physician, thus the problem may not be detected except by the physical examination. In one gynecologist's practice, 72% of the young, sexually active females consecutively seen had one or more of the vulvovaginitides.[1]

Evaluation of the Patient

The history begins with the patient's description of the amount, color, consistency, and odor of the vaginal discharge; possible itching, burning, or pain in the vaginal area; abdominal, pelvic, or back pain; and urinary frequency, urgency, or burning. Information about the duration of various symptoms and attempts at self-treatment as well as a complete gynecologic and sexual history should be obtained; one should record (1) the menstrual history, including the date of the last menstrual period; (2) previous pregnancies and abortions; (3) method(s) of contraception; (4) previous vaginal infection(s) and treatment(s), a history of sexually transmitted disease, or possible exposures; and (5) personal hygiene habits such as douching or the use of sprays or deodorants. Finally, inquiry should be made about the presence of systemic illnesses, such as diabetes mellitus, and the patient's use of any medications. The physical examination should include observation of vaginal secretions or discharge, and the appearance of the vaginal mucosa, cervix, urethra, Skene's glands, and Bartholin's glands.

Normal and Abnormal Vaginal Secretions

Physiologic variations in vaginal secretions are known. Many women experience an increasing amount of vaginal secretion up to the time of ovulation, with a subsequent decline until menses. Pregnancy, stress, and sexual excitement may also cause changes in the amount or quality of vaginal secretion.

The normal vaginal secretion is colorless and odorless, with an acidic pH between 3.8 and 4.2. Examination of normal vaginal secretion shows a predominance of a long, thick, nonmotile, gram-positive bacillus, which is the anaerobic Döderlein bacillus. This organism probably protects the vagina from infection with more pathogenic organisms by acting upon the glycogen present in vaginal epithelial cells to produce lactic acid and create an acidic pH that is unfavorable for the growth of other bacteria. A change in the vaginal environment caused by a change in pH, as in pregnancy, or a change in the bacterial flora, as from systemic antibiotics, facilitates the development of vaginal infection.

In patients with vaginitis, the amount of vaginal secretion can be greatly increased. The color may become white, yellow, green, or gray. The consistency of the discharge may be thick or bubbly, depending on the degree of infection and the relative amounts of mucus and leukocytes.

Laboratory Methods

The microscopic examination is the most important step in the analysis of vaginal secretions. A drop of vaginal fluid is placed on one microscope slide with a single drop of warm saline solution and a coverslip. A similar slide should be prepared with a drop of vaginal fluid mixed with a drop of potassium hydroxide (KOH) of 10 to 20% concentration. The patient's use of a douche or the contamination of the vaginal secretion with lubricating jelly during the pelvic examination interferes with the usefulness of this procedure. The vaginal fluid mixed with saline should be examined first. In the presence of significant infection, the Döderlein bacillus is no longer present. Instead, one may see stippled epithelial cells, the so-called "clue" cells characteristic of bacterial vaginosis. One may also identify the motile protozoan *Trichomonas vaginalis.* In atrophic vaginitis, only small, round, basal epithelial cells are seen because there is insufficient estrogen to produce the large, flat, superficial type of vaginal epithelial cells. Polymorphonuclear leukocytes are seen in trichomonal and herpetic infections as well as in mucopurulent cervicitis and gonococcal cervicitis, but not in bacterial vaginosis. In rare cases, the presence of crenated red blood cells in a purulent discharge may alert the examiner to the presence of pyohematometrium. On the second slide, the KOH solution will dissolve most of the cellular material present and facilitate the search for the long, thin, septate hyphae and small, oval, budding yeast forms of *Candida albicans* (Fig. 37–1).

Nickerson's or Sabouraud's medium can be used to culture *C. albicans*. Cultures for *T. vaginalis* and *Gardneralla vaginalis* generally are not indicated in routine office practice. If gonorrhea is suspected as the cause of a purulent discharge, an appropriate culture should be done (see later).

Differential Diagnosis

The major etiologies of vaginitis are (1) *T. vaginalis* infection, (2) *Candida* infection, (3) Bacterial vaginosis (formerly *G. vaginalis* infection), and (4) atrophic vaginitis (Table 37–1). Less common infectious causes of vaginitis include *mobiluncus* species, *chlamydia trachomatis*, herpes simplex virus, human papillomavirus, *Enterobius vermicularis* (pinworm), and *Giardia lamblia.*[2] Urinary tract infections must be excluded when "burning" on urination is a prominent symptom. *Neisseria gonorrhoeae* and mucopurulent or other types of cervicitis may also be encountered in patients with vaginal symptoms. Less common causes are irritation from contraceptive creams and jellies, condoms, tampons, douches, or vaginal deodorants; malignant lesions of the cervix, endometrium, or vagina; and pyometrium due to benign cervical stenosis or associated with carcinoma of the uterine fundus or cervix. Rarely, women may have chronic or recurrent vaginal irritation due to allergic reactions to semen. Use of condoms or precoital antihistamines are used in these cases.[3]

Trichomonas vaginalis INFECTION

In the United States, there has been a 40% decrease in the incidence of *Trichomonas* vaginitis during the past 15 years.[2] This may be due to effective treatment with metronidazole for women with vaginitis and their sexual partners, as well as decreased sexual partners and increased use of condoms resulting from concern about human immunodeficiency virus (HIV) infection.[2] Some women may be asymptomatic carriers of the organism,[4] and it may proliferate and cause symptoms when the vaginal pH is high, (usually >5.0), such as during pregnancy or the last half of the menstrual cycle, when there are excessive secretions or blood in the vagina, or when there is bacterial overgrowth. There is strong evidence for its sexual transmission, but the organism has also been demonstrated in women who are not sexually active. The organism may be carried asymptomatically in the male urethra and prostrate and has a clear predilection for survival in the female Skene's and Bartholin's glands. Hence, topical agents generally are not sufficient to eradicate *Trichomonas* in female patients, and reinfection may occur from the male consort. Although *Trichomonas* vaginitis is generally considered to be an annoying source of discomfort rather than a serious medical problem, possibly it may contribute to infertility by altering the vaginal milieu.[5] *Trichomonas* also is statistically more likely to be present in patients with carcinoma in situ of the cervix, but this association is not thought to be causal; the inflammatory changes (class II Papanicolaou smears) often induced by trichomonal cervicitis have not been found to progress to dysplasia.[6]

The most common symptoms of a patient with *Trichomonas* vaginitis are a profuse, foul-smelling discharge and

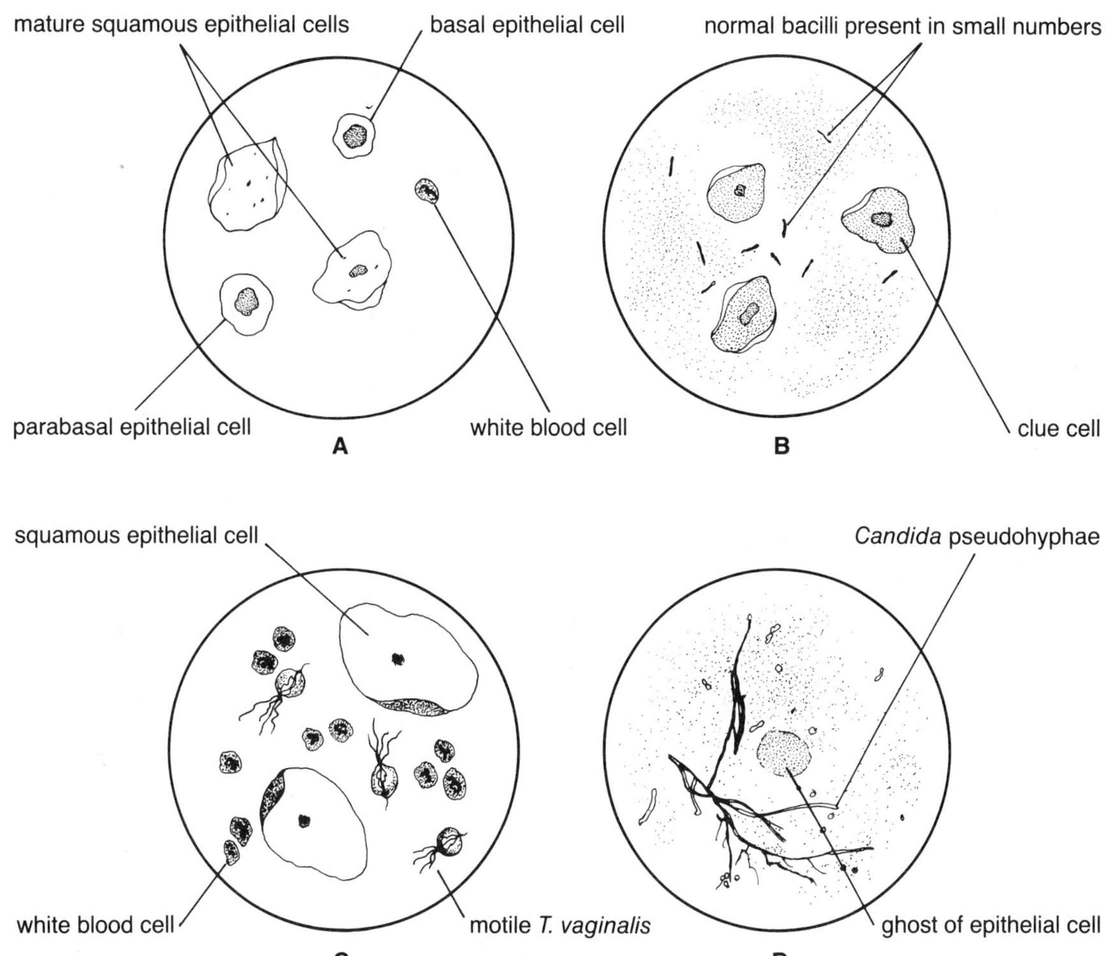

FIGURE 37–1. Normal and abnormal findings on vaginal wet and KOH preparations. *A*, Normal cells seen in vaginal wet preparation (under high dry). *B*, Clue cells seen on wet preparation (under high dry). *C*, *Trichomonas vaginalis* seen on wet preparation using saline. Recognition is greatly enhanced by motility of the organism (under high dry). *D*, *Candida* pseudohyphae in KOH preparation (under low power). (Adapted from Fischer PM, Addison LA, Curtis P, et al: The Office Laboratory. East Norwalk, CT, Appleton-Century-Crofts, 1983.)

burning and itching of the introitus. Symptoms may develop acutely but are more likely to develop gradually and to have been present for 1 week longer in trichomonal than in candidal vaginitis.[7] Urethritis with typical burning on urination may be present.[7] The discharge itself is usually thin, yellow or yellow-green, bubbly or frothy, and malodorous but is almost never curd-like.[7] On physical examination, the introitus is usually bathed in the abnormal discharge. The vulva and urethra as well as the vaginal mucosa may appear inflamed. The examiner occasionally sees "strawberry spots," which are red granular areas on the cervix and the upper fornix of the vagina. In patients with chronic or asymptomatic infection with *Trichomonas*, varying amounts of a discharge may be found without evidence of inflamed mucosa.

TABLE 37–1. DIAGNOSES IN 821 EPISODES OF WOMEN WITH GENITOURINARY COMPLAINTS*

	%
Vulvovaginitis	70
Candida albicans (49%)	
Trichomonas vaginalis (12%)	
Nonspecific vaginitis (36%)	
Combined *C. albicans* and *Trichomonas* (2%)	
Urinary tract infections	12
Combination of urinary tract infection and vulvovaginitis	2
Herpes progenitalis, asymptomatic carriers of *N. gonorrhoeae*, cervicitis, atrophic vaginitis, and miscellaneous disorders	14
Normal examination despite complaints	1

*Adapted from McCue JD, Komaroff AL, Pass TL, et al: Strategies for diagnosing vaginitis. J Fam Pract 9:395, 1979.

Only 1% of the patients in this study were older than 45 years of age.

The diagnosis is made most expeditiously by examining a drop of the vaginal fluid mixed with a drop of warm saline solution on a microscope slide and covered with a glass coverslip. Tap water is not a suitable substitute, but optionally, the vaginal fluid may be mixed with a 1% solution of cresyl blue and isotonic saline solution to stain the epithelial cells violet but leave trichomonal organisms colorless. This "wet prep" should be examined immediately because the organisms become immobile if the sample is allowed to become chilled or dry. On microscopic examination, *T. vaginalis* is a round or oval organism with flagella that appears to be slightly larger than a leukocyte and much smaller than the epithelial cells. One can usually see organisms moving about vigorously in a whirling or jerking motion. Probably most symptomatic patients are identified by this examination, although positive cultures or Papanicolaou smears with negative microscopic examination are reported in some cases.[7–13] For example, in one study, the result of the wet preparation was positive in only 50.4% of patients with positive cultures, but only about half these patients were complaining of an abnormal discharge at the time of the evaluation.[9] The sensitivity of the wet preparation was correlated with the amount of discharge noted on examination;[9] thus, it seems likely that organisms will be identified in 80 to 90% of symptomatic patients but in a smaller number of asymptomatic carriers or those with a very minimal discharge. Since *Trichomonas* is the only flagellate found in the female genital tract, positive wet preparations are highly specific.

The most effective treatment for *Trichomonas* is oral metronidazole (Flagyl), which may be given as 250 mg three times daily for 7 to 10 days or as a single dose of 2 g.[14, 15] A single dose of 1 or 1.5 g is effective in some patients, but the 2-g dose is superior, especially in women with greater body weight.[16] In most men, *Trichomonas* will clear from the urinary tract spontaneously within a short time, thus reinfection can be avoided by having the male partner use a condom for a total of 3 weeks.[17] In apparent treatment failures, however, both the patient and her partner should receive courses of metronidazole. In women, metronidazole in a 500-mg vaginal suppository can be added once daily for refractory cases. Reinfection is the most common cause of recurrences, but treatment failures have also been noted from metronidazole resistance,[18] drug malabsorption,[19] and inactivation of metronidazole by vaginal bacteria.[20]

Metronidazole sometimes produces an unpleasant metallic taste in the mouth. Patients may also experience an "Antabuse" effect if they drink alcohol while taking metronidazole and should be cautioned to abstain during the period of medication. Its use is contraindicated in the presence of hepatic disease, blood dyscrasias, or diseases of the central nervous system. Since metronidazole has been shown to potentiate the effects of sodium warfarin (Coumadin) by lengthening the prothrombin time,[21] it seems reasonable to recommend the single-dose method of treatment for patients taking warfarin.

Although teratogenic effects of metronidazole have not been clearly substantiated, most physicians refrain from prescribing it if the patient is pregnant. Metronidazole is a carcinogen for animals, but two human studies revealed no excess occurrence of cancer in patients treated with metronidazole.[22, 23] The numbers of patients in these studies were only sufficient to exclude a large excess risk of cancer within about 10 years of exposure to the drug.[15]

I recommend that treatment of trichomonal infection with metronidazole be confined to patients with symptoms. Treatment of asymptomatic *Trichomonas* infection is not warranted because of the potential toxicity of the medication. The Papanicolaou smear is not a practical method for making the diagnosis of trichomonal vaginitis, but women with cellular changes indistinguishable from dysplasia, together with *Trichomonas* on the Papanicolaou smear, should receive a trial of therapy followed by a repeat smear. If the cytologic changes are due to the infection, the Papanicolaou smear should become normal in a few weeks after eradication of the organism.

When metronidazole cannot be used, topical clotrimazole, 100 mg/day for 7 days, or povidone-iodine for 7 to 28 days is an alternative treatment, with cures expected in one half to two thirds of patients.[24, 25]

Candida INFECTION

The incidence of *Candida* vaginitis has doubled between 1980 and 1990. Although *C. albicans* is the most common etiologic agent, infection with other *Candida* species or *Torulopsis glabrata* can cause vaginitis with similar features. *Candida* vaginitis occurs almost exclusively in women between puberty and the menopause, suggesting a role for hormonal influences. The source of *C. albicans* may be the gastrointestinal tract, where the organism is a common inhabitant. Infection also seems to be transmissible by sexual intercourse. Certain factors may predispose an individual to candidal vaginitis. The most common of these is the use of systemic antibiotics. *Candida* vaginitis occurs frequently in women with diabetes mellitus or during pregnancy. Both these conditions alter the vaginal fluid by increasing the content of glycogen and thus may create a more favorable medium for candidal growth. The use of some types of oral contraceptives may also predispose an individual to the development of *Candida* vaginitis, although this remains a controversial area.

The patient with *Candida* vaginitis usually complains of a thick, white vaginal discharge accompanied by severe itching, as well as burning, local pain, and irritation. Urinary burning and frequency as well as dyspareunia due to lack of normal lubrication are also frequently reported symptoms. Many women can distinguish between this "external" dysuria, produced by passage of the stream of urine across inflamed labia, and truly "internal" dysuria, which is associated with cystitis or urethritis.[7]

On examination, the discharge usually appears thick and white, with a cottage cheese–like or "curd-like" appearance, adhering to the intensely inflamed vaginal mucosa. The character of the discharge is often of diagnostic value; in one study, a curd-like discharge was noted in 77% of women with candidal infection but in only 14% of those with other types of vaginitis.[7] Characteristically, bleeding may be induced by efforts to dislodge the white discharge. An abrupt onset of symptoms, intense pruritus, and inflammation of the vulva with satellite lesions also favor the diagnosis of yeast infection. In one study, absence of odor on provider examination was the most valuable predictive sign for *Candida* infection.[26]

To establish the diagnosis, a sample of the vaginal discharge should be mixed with 1 to 2 drops of 10 to 20% KOH solution and examined under the microscope. With the cellular material dissolved by the KOH solution, one can more easily identify the small, oval, budding yeast cells and long, thin, septate hyphae of *C. albicans*. One can also plate a culture of the discharge on Nickerson's or Sabouraud's medium and look for growth, appearing after 4 to 5 days. Cultures are somewhat more diagnostically sensitive (80 to 90%) than are microscopic examinations (60 to 80%) but are less specific for clinical infection, since 10 to 20% of asymptomatic women harbor yeast in the vagina.[7, 8, 27, 28] Generally, the microscopic examination, together with the history and physical examination, is adequate for making the diagnosis.

Treatment consists of a topical antifungal agent such as nystatin (Mycostatin), miconazole (Monistat), clotrimazole (Gyne-Lotrimin), or teconazole (Terazol) in a cream or suppository form daily for 3 or 7 days. Seven-day treatment packs of clotrimazole and miconazole have become available "over-the-counter" at generally lower prices than when purchased with a prescription. At this time, the 3-day formulations, which contain a higher dose of medication per day, are only available with a prescription. Use of any of these drugs has an initial cure rate of about 90%. Treatment may be continued through a menstrual period, and a pad rather than a tampon should be employed to absorb the flow. An important part of treatment is to remove any predisposing factors when possible.

Bluestein and associates studied a group of women without vaginitis who received antibiotics for an acute respiratory, urinary, or skin infection.[29] One third of the women developed candidal vaginitis, whereas 5% developed nonyeast vaginitis. Pruritus or discharge was highly correlated with *Candida* vaginitis. Women who develop these symptoms in the setting of antibiotic therapy can reasonably be treated without an examination.

At least 5% of patients with initial resolution of symptoms and signs of candidal vaginitis after treatment develop recurrent symptoms within 4 weeks. In women with recurrent candidal vaginitis, clotrimazole used for days 5 through 11 of four consecutive menstrual cycles reduced the number of symptomatic episodes to 1 in 18 patients, compared with 10 episodes in 19 patients on placebo. Symptoms recurred, however, in one third of the clotrimazole-treated patients within 6 months of stopping prophylactic treatment.[30] Some gynecologists advise continued treatment for 1 week prior to each menstrual period in recurrent cases or use of a condom by the sexual partner.[31] Oral antifungal therapy can be prescribed for patients with unusually difficult cases of recurrent or chronic vaginitis. Among women with recurrent candidal vulvovaginitis, daily ingestion of 8 ounces of yogurt containing *Lactobacillus acidophilus* was associated with decreased vaginal colonization by *Candida* species and episodes of infection. Direct application of lactobacilli to the vagina using yogurt or tablets has also been suggested.[32]

BACTERIAL VAGINOSIS (NONSPECIFIC VAGINITIS, *Gardnerella vaginalis* INFECTION)

Bacterial vaginosis is probably the leading cause of vaginitis in the United States, associated with more than one third of all cases. In 1955, Gardner and Dukes described an association between "nonspecific bacterial vaginitis" and a small, gram-negative bacillus called *Haemophilus vaginalis*, then *Corynebacterium vaginale* and now *Gardnerella vaginalis*.[33] Bacterial vaginosis is characterized by lack of lactobacilli and overgrowth of aerobic and anaerobic bacteria, including *G. vaginalis, Mycoplasma hominis, Bacteroides bivius* and other *Bacteroides* species, and the recently named species *Mobiluncus mulieris* and *M. curtisii*.[34] Because this infection occurs in women between puberty and menopause and in postmenopausal women treated with estrogens, it appears that an estrogenic effect on vaginal epithelium is necessary for its vigorous growth. Coexisting infection with *T. vaginalis* has been described frequently and is attributed to the increased vaginal pH associated with bacterial vaginosis.[35] Organisms associated with bacterial vaginosis may also cause pelvic inflammatory disease.[34]

Patients with bacterial vaginosis have a variable amount of thin, homogeneous, gray vaginal discharge. The most characteristic and often the only manifestation of infection is a strongly disagreeable odor, often described as "fishy" or "rotten." Many patients are too embarrassed to complain of the odor; others become conditioned to it and find it no longer noticeable. In a few cases, the major manifestation is a persistent discharge or "wetness," which may prompt the patient to wear a pad or tampon. Patients generally experience less severe vaginal burning and itching than do those with trichomonal or candidal infections, because bacterial vaginosis causes very little tissue invasion and inflammation.

The physical examination is notable for mild or absent inflammation of the vulva and vagina. The discharge is characteristically smooth, with a tendency to coat the vaginal epithelium. The pH is typically higher than 4.5. Addition of a few drops of 10% potassium hydroxide solution to the vaginal fluid results in the release of a fishy odor.

Microscopic examination of the vaginal discharge mixed with normal saline classically shows few if any leukocytes but a large number of epithelial cells that appear stippled or granulated owing to adherence of bacilli on the cell surfaces. These cells, called "clue cells" by Gardner and Dukes,[33] are highly suggestive of bacterial vaginosis. In fact, "clue cells" are often very difficult to identify. From a practical point of view, the presence of the clinical features just described with no evidence of *T. vaginalis* or *C. albicans* infection should suggest the diagnosis of bacterial vaginosis in a woman who is premenopausal or who is postmenopausal but receiving estrogen therapy.

Treatment for this condition often proves difficult. In the past, sulfanilamide vaginal creams or suppositories have been used, as well as systemic tetracycline and ampicillin. However, *G. vaginalis* generally is resistant to sulfonamides and tetracycline in vitro. In fact, sulfa-containing vaginal creams have been shown to provide no more relief from symptoms than does a bland cream or base alone,[36] and use of sulfa carries the risk of sensitization. Ampicillin has excellent in vitro activity against *G. vaginalis*, but reports of its clinical efficacy vary from over 90% in two studies[37, 38] to about 33% in another well-designed, randomized trial.[39] Pheifer and associates achieved excellent results in treatment using oral metronidazole (Flagyl) but poor results using sulfa-containing vaginal cream and oral doxycycline as well as oral ampicillin.[39] Oral metronidazole is the most effective treatment. A recently published meta-analysis concluded that there was no significant difference in the cure rate (85 to 87%) with four treatment regimens of different durations: (1) a single dose of 2 g; (2) 2 days of treatment with 2 g/day; (3) 5 days of treatment with 400 mg two or three times daily; and (4) 7 days of treatment with 500 mg twice daily.[40] Some studies have shown that the 1- or 2-day treatment regimens are associated with a lower incidence of candidal vaginitis than are longer courses of therapy.[41–43] Although the currently recommended treatment is 7 days of 500 mg twice daily, the single dose therapy may be preferable because it appears to be equally effective and may be associated with decreased side effects and increased compliance. Metronidazole should not be used during pregnancy. An alternative treatment regimen is ampicillin, 500 mg four times daily for 7 days. Treatment of the sexual partner is not generally associated with a decreased risk of recurrent infection but may be reasonable if the patient experiences early recurrences. Metronidazole, 2 g orally every month on the third day of menses, may decrease recurrences in difficult cases.[43]

ATROPHIC VAGINITIS

Atrophic vaginitis may cause an abnormal vaginal discharge in women who have low estrogen levels due to any cause, including natural menopause or surgical or radiation castration. The vaginal epithelium becomes thin and atrophic when deprived of estrogen. Normal superficial vaginal epithelial cells are lost, leaving only the basal cell layer, which is susceptible to infection and inflammation even with little or no trauma. Typical symptoms are an abnormal vaginal discharge, often accompanied by vaginal and vulvar burning, soreness, or pruritus. There may also be urinary burning, frequency, and urgency; vague lower abdominal discomfort; and sometimes vaginal bleeding. The physical examination and microscopic examination of the vaginal discharge should always be carried out to rule out other causes of vaginitis. On physical examination, the vaginal epithelium appears pale pink and very dry rather than bluish-red and moist. A urethral caruncle, representing prolapsed urethral epithelium, may be present. Constricting fibrosis may partially close off the upper part of the vagina, while the skin of the vulvar area is thin, having a parchment-like appearance.

Treatment for the condition is local estrogen in the form of a vaginal cream or suppositories. Treatment converts the vaginal mucosa from an atrophic to a cornified state.[44] Daily applications of conjugated estrogens (Premarin) or estradiol to the vagina do produce stable serum estrogen levels equivalent to the normal follicular phase levels in ovulating women.[44] Most women can lengthen the interval between doses to weekly or monthly applications of the cream or suppository after about 1 month of daily therapy.

Neisseria gonorrhoeae INFECTION

Because the stratified squamous vaginal epithelium in the normal adult protects against infection by the gonococcus, gonorrheal vaginitis (as opposed to salpingitis or cervicitis) is extremely rare except in children, pregnant women, and postmenopausal women. During pregnancy, the vaginal epithelium is altered, and in postmenopausal women the thin, parchment-like vaginal epithelium may be fragile; in these cases, the gonococcus may cause vaginitis. However, gonorrhea can be carried in the cervix of premenopausal women without detectable symptoms or might present as increased discharge or urinary frequency and burning.

The physical examination in children, pregnant women, or postmenopausal females with gonorrheal vaginitis reveals an intense inflammatory response that causes the vaginal canal to be extremely red, swollen, and edematous. Examination may be exquisitely painful, and there may be a profuse quantity of pus. There is often involvement of the vulva and painful involvement of the urethra and of Skene's and Bartholin's glands. In premenopausal women, the gonococcus sometimes involves only the endocervical epithelium without producing salpingitis; in such cases, the cervical os will be filled with pus, while the cervix may appear edematous and soft. There can be an inflamed cervical erosion or small abscesses in nabothian cysts. Very few adult females with symptoms of vaginitis will have a gonococcal etiology, however. In one study of 478 symptomatic females, 29 (4%) had positive cultures for *N. gonorrhoeae*, but all were felt to be asymptomatic carriers with vaginitis of a different cause.[7] In the asymptomatic carrier, there often are no findings on pelvic examination or merely an abnormal but scanty discharge. Diagnostic tests for and treatment of gonococcal infection are described in Chapter 31.

FOREIGN BODIES

An abnormal vaginal discharge can be caused by irritation from any object placed in the vagina. The most common foreign body is a retained vaginal tampon that has been forgotten at the time of the last menses. Other objects may be a forgotten contraceptive diaphragm, a pessary, or some other item inserted into the vagina.

SUMMARY, APPROACH TO PATIENTS WITH VAGINITIS

It is most important in all cases of vaginitis to make every effort to identify a specific cause. A small number of patients (~ 2%) have mixed infections (see Table 37–1). The saline wet mount and KOH preparation will be negative for *Trichomonas* and *Candida* in more than half of the patients encountered in a general medical practice, and many of these patients probably have bacterial vaginosis. However, the finding of many leukocytes on microscopic examination suggests that the source of the discharge may be cervicitis. In addition, in symptomatic patients the false-negative rate of wet and KOH preparations for both *Trichomonas* and *Candida* is probably 10 to 20%. If the clinical picture is highly suggestive of candidal vaginitis, because the onset is abrupt, a rash with satellite lesions is present, pruritus is prominent, and/or the discharge is curd-like, but the KOH preparation fails to reveal yeast, one could culture the discharge on Nickerson's medium in hope of confirming the diagnosis and prescribe a trial of anticandidal therapy rather than treating for bacterial vaginosis. Postmenopausal women with symptomatic vaginitis generally should be treated with topical estrogen.

When therapy fails or symptoms are recurrent despite the approach just outlined, the patient should be instructed to discontinue treatment for several days and not to douche prior to the examination. Then a very careful, complete examination, with repeat saline and KOH preparations, should be performed. At that time, one should also consider whether the diagnosis may actually be cervicitis, allergy to a foreign substance, or allergy to the previously prescribed treatment. In the absence of these factors, the patient should be treated with specific therapy for the most likely etiology based on a review of the history and clinical and microscopic findings. If the recurrence has followed shortly after apparently successful initial therapy, one should also consider simultaneously treating the patient's sexual partner.

All patients with vaginitis should be instructed to avoid the use of constricting undergarments or perineal napkins, excessive or overly concentrated douches (one half cup of vinegar to 2 quarts of warm water is sufficient), or irritating agents, including repeated bathing and exposure to soap. If no abnormalities can be identified on the physical examination of a woman whose complaint is vaginal discharge, one should review with the patient information concerning the normal amounts and quality of vaginal discharge.

Cervicitis

The endocervix, lined with columnar epithelial cells, is susceptible to infection by *N. gonorrhoeae, C. trachomatis*, and herpes simplex virus. Cervicitis caused by these sexually transmitted pathogens can have important clinical consequences for both pregnant and non-pregnant women. In particular, cervicitis from *N. gonorrhoeae* and *C. trachomatis* may be associated with infection of the uterus or fallopian tubes leading to increased risks of ectopic pregnancy and infertility, and *N. gonorrhoeae* may cause widespread infection via hematogenous dissemination. Chlamydial infection during pregnancy greatly increases the risk of inclusion conjunctivitis and pneumonia in newborns.

Women with cervicitis may be asymptomatic, or they may be aware of an abnormal discharge indistinguishable from symptomatic vaginitis. On examination, the cervix may appear red, congested, and friable, with bleeding easily induced by a cotton-tipped swab. Additional findings on examination include yellow mucopus originating in the endocervical canal and ectocervical ulcerations.

It may be difficult to differentiate infectious cervicitis from cervical ectopy (normal ectopic columnar epithelium) by physical examination. Columnar epithelium appears "redder" than the usual appearance of cervical epithelium and may be associated with cloudy-appearing mucus. Distinguishing ectopy from cervicitis is best done by noting yellow mucopus in cervicitis and by examination and cultures of endocervical secretions. A cotton swab should be inserted gently into the endocervix, with care to avoid contamination by vaginal secretions. The swab should be rolled onto a glass slide and be Gram stained. Large numbers of squamous cells and vaginal flora in the specimen suggest that contamination by vaginal secretions has occurred. Otherwise, the uncontaminated endocervical specimen should be examined to determine the number of polymorphonuclear leukocytes per high-power field (hpf) and to identify intracellular gram-negative diplococci. Culture of the endocervix should be done for *N. gonorrhoeae* and also for *C. trachomatis* in some circumstances (see Chapter 31).

Brunham et al suggested that the term *mucopurulent cervicitis* be used to describe cervicitis associated with an endocervical exudate, defined as the presence of either visible yellow mucopus or 10 or more leukocytes per hpf in a specimen of endocervical mucus.[45] In 100 randomly selected nonmenstruating women seen at a sexually transmitted diseases clinic, cervical infection with *N. gonorrhoeae, C. trachomatis*, or herpes simplex virus was associated with these findings. *C. trachomatis* was isolated from the cervixes of 20 of the 40 women who met criteria for mucopurulent cervicitis and from only 2 of 60 women without mucopurulent cervicitis. Isolation of herpes simplex virus was associated with ectocervical ulcers on examination.

Women with mucopurulent cervicitis should generally be treated for *N. gonorrhoeae, C. trachomatis*, or herpes simplex virus. Treatment for *C. trachomatis* is recommended for women with endocervical mucopus or increased polymorphonuclear leukocytes with or without gonococcal infection, since the two frequently coexist. Women who are sexual contacts of men with nongonococcal urethritis should also receive treatment for *C. trachomatis* infection. Treatment consists of doxycycline, 100 mg twice daily, or tetracycline, 500 mg four times daily, for 7 days.[46] During pregnancy or when tetracyclines cannot be given, erythromycin, 500 mg four times daily for 7 days, should be prescribed. A single dose of 1 g of azithromycin has been shown to be as effective as 7 days of doxycycline for uncomplicated chlamydial urethritis and cervicitis.[47] Treatment is generally not necessary for patients with cervical ectopy without cervicitis.

Post-treatment cultures are obtained in women with gonococcal cervicitis. Women with confirmed or suspected chlamydial cervicitis are followed with examinations to be certain that abnormalities resolve after treatment.

REFERENCES

1. Gardner HL: Vulvovaginitis: Prevalence and diagnosis. Med Times 106:22, 1978.
2. Kent HL: Epidemiology of vaginitis. Am J Obstet Gynecol 165:1168, 1991.
3. Jones WR: Allergy to coitus. Aust N Z J Obstet Gynecol 31:137, 1991.
4. Dunkelberg WE, Skeggs R, Kellogg DS, et al: Relative incidence of *Corynebacterium vaginale (Haemophilus vaginalis), Neisseria gonorrhoeae*, and *Trichomonas* spp. among women attending a venereal disease clinic. Br J Ven Dis 46:187, 1970.
5. Green TH: Gynecology: Essentials of Clinical Practice. Boston, Little, Brown, 1977, p 376.
6. Koss LG and Wolinska WH: *Trichomonas vaginalis* cervicitis and its relationship to cervical cancer. A histocytological study. Cancer 12:1171, 1959.
7. McCue JD, Komaroff AL, Pass TL, et al: Strategies for diagnosing vaginitis. J Fam Pract 9:395, 1979.
8. McLennan MD, Smith JM, and McLennan CE: Diagnosis of vaginal mycosis and trichomoniasis: Reliability of cytological smear, wet smear and culture. Obstet Gynecol 40:231, 1972.
9. Fouts AC and Kraus SJ: *Trichomonas vaginalis*: Reevaluation of its clinical presentation and laboratory diagnosis. J Infect Dis 141:137, 1980.
10. Burch TA, Rees CW, and Kayhoe DE: Laboratory and clinical studies on vaginal trichomoniasis. Am J Obstet Gynecol 76:658, 1958.
11. Rothenberg RB, Simon R, Chipperfield E, et al: Efficacy of selected diagnostic tests for sexually transmitted diseases. JAMA 235:49, 1976.
12. McCann JS: Comparison of direct microscopy and culture in the diagnosis of trichomoniasis. Br J Ven Dis 50:450, 1974.
13. Perl G: Errors in the diagnosis of *Trichomonas vaginalis* infection. Obstet Gynecol 39:7, 1972.
14. Fleury FJ, VanBergen WS, Prentice RI, et al: Single dose of 2 grams of metronidazole for *Trichomonas vaginalis* infection. Am J Obstet Gynecol 128:320, 1977.
15. Goldman P: Metronidazole. N Engl J Med 303:1212, 1980.
16. Pattison CM: Metronidazole in a single dose for the treatment of trichomoniasis. Br J Ven Dis 58:121, 1982.
17. Hildebrandt RJ: Trichomoniasis: Always with us—but controllable. Med Times 106:44, 1978.
18. Mullerm M, Merngassner JG, Miller WA, et al: Three metronidazole-resistant strains of *Trichomonas vaginalis* from the United States. Am J Obstet Gynecol 138:808, 1980.

19. Roe FJC: Metronidazole: Review of its uses and toxicity. J Antimicrob Chemother 3:285, 1977.
20. Ralph ED and Clarke DA: Inactivation of metronidazole by anaerobic and aerobic bacteria. Antimicrob Agents Chemother 14:377, 1978.
21. Kazmier FJ: A significant interaction between metronidazole and warfarin. Mayo Clin Proc 5:782, 1976.
22. Beard CM, Noller KL, O'Fallon WM, et al: Lack of evidence for cancer due to use of metronidazole. N Engl J Med 301:519, 1979.
23. Friedman GD: Cancer after metronidazole. N Engl J Med 302:519, 1980.
24. Schnell JD: The incidence of vaginal *Candida* and *Trichomonas* infections and treatment of *Trichomonas vaginitis* with clotrimazole. Postgrad Med J 50(Suppl):79, 1974.
25. Henderson JN and Tait IB: The use of povidone-iodine (Betadine) pessaries in the treatment of candidal and trichomonal vaginitis. Curr Med Res Opin 3:157, 1975.
26. Schaaf VM, Perez-Stable E, and Borchardt K: The limited value of symptoms and signs in the diagnosis of vaginal infections. Arch Intern Med 150:1929, 1990.
27. Burgess SG, Mancuso PG, Kalish PE, et al: Clinical and laboratory study of vaginitis: Evaluation of diagnostic methods and results of treatment. N Y State J Med 70:2086, 1970.
28. Davis DA: Vaginal moniliasis in private practice. Obstet Gynecol 34:40, 1969.
29. Bluestein D, Rutledge C, and Lumsden L: Predicting the occurrence of antibiotic-induced *Candida vaginitis* (AICV). Fam Pract Res J 11:319, 1991.
30. Davidson F and Mould RF: Recurrent genital candidosis in women and the effect of intermittent prophylactic treatment. Br J Ven Dis 54:176, 1978.
31. Meeker CI: Candidiasis—an obstinate problem. Med Times 106:26, 1978.
32. Hilton EH, Isenberg HD, Alperstein P, et al: Ingestion of yogurt containing *Lactobacillus acidophilus* as prophylaxis for candidal vaginitis. Ann Intern Med 116:353, 1992.
33. Gardner HC and Dukes CD: *Haemophilus vaginalis* vaginitis: A newly defined specific infection previously classified "nonspecific" vaginitis. Am J Obstet Gynecol 69:962, 1955.
34. Mardh P: The vaginal ecosystem. Am J Obstet Gynecol 165:1163, 1991.
35. Fleury FJ: Is there a "nonspecific" vaginitis? Med Times 106:37, 1978.
36. Sulfa vaginal creams. FDA Drug Bull 10:6, 1980.
37. Lee L and Schmale JD: Ampicillin therapy for *Corynebacterium vaginale (Haemophilus vaginalis)* vaginitis. Am J Obstet Gynecol 115:786, 1972.
38. Rodgers HA, Hesse FE, Pulley HC, et al: *Haemophilus vaginalis (Corynebacterium vaginale)* vaginitis in women attending public health clinics: Response to treatment with ampicillin. Sex Trans Dis 5:18, 1978.
39. Pheifer TA, Forsyth PS, Durfee MA, et al: Nonspecific vaginitis: Role of *Haemophilus vaginalis* and treatment with metronidazole. N Engl J Med 26:1429, 1978.
40. Lugo-Miro VI, Green, M, and Mazur L: Comparison of different metronidazole therapeutic regimens for bacterial vaginosis: A meta-analysis. JAMA 268:92, 1992.
41. Jerve F, Berdal TB, Bohman P, et al: Metronidazole in the treatment of non-specific vaginitis (NSV). Br J Ven Dis 60:171, 1984.
42. Perdon A, Hanna JH, Morse PL, et al: An evaluation of single-dose metronidazole treatment for *Gardnerella vaginalis* vaginitis. Obstet Gynecol 64:271, 1984.
43. Baldson MD: *Gardnerella vaginalis* and its clinical syndrome. Eur J Clin Micr 1:288, 1982.
44. Martin PL, Yen SSC, Burnier AM, et al: Systemic absorption and sustained effects of vaginal estrogen creams. JAMA 242:2699, 1979.
45. Brunham RC, Paavonen J, Stevens CE, et al: Mucopurulent cervicitis—the ignored counterpart in women of urethritis in men. N Engl J Med 311:1, 1984.
46. Centers for Disease Control and Prevention: 1993 STD Treatment Guidelines. MMWR (SS-14)1–102, 1993.
47. Martin DH, Mroczkowski TF, Dalu ZA, et al: A controlled trial of a single dose of azithromycin for the treatment of chlamydial urethritis and cervicitis. N Engl J Med 327:921, 1992.

38

Common Gynecologic Problems: Pelvic Mass, Chronic Pelvic Pain, Endometriosis, Premenstrual Syndrome, and Menopause

PHILLIP G. STUBBLEFIELD, MD

The assessment of gynecologic problems generally begins with an adequate pelvic examination. The patient must consent to and be adequately prepared for the examination in advance. During the examination, the examiner should inform the patient before touching her and before each phase of the examination. It is helpful to maintain verbal communication as the examination proceeds. A female assistant should be present. The examining room should contain a firm examination table with stirrups or knee holders, a good light, an assortment of specula, swabs, an Ayres spatula, Cytobrush, glass slides and fixative for cytology, small bottles of saline solution, small bottles of 10% potassium hydroxide for the examination of fresh secretions, media for vaginal and gonorrheal cultures, and tests for chlamydia. Most important is privacy. Many women find the standard Graves' bivalve speculum and its plastic copies to be uncomfortable; a better alternative is the medium Pedersen speculum, because it is narrow but long. The small, pediatric Pedersen is especially useful for adolescent and elderly women.

PELVIC EXAMINATION

With the patient in the lithotomy position, the vulva is inspected for any white areas, condylomata, or other lesions and is then gently palpated for subcutaneous tumors or cysts. In elderly women, areas of pruritus deserve special attention and probably a biopsy to rule out vulvar carcinoma in situ. Pigmented lesions here, as on other skin surfaces, deserve scrutiny; they may be melanomas. The labia are gently separated by the examiner's thumb and a finger so that the introitus can be inspected. Disorders of pelvic support are evaluated by asking the patient to bear down as if straining at stool. Descensus of the anterior wall represents cystocele and, if the posterior wall is involved, rectocele. Descent of the cervix toward the uterus is prolapse. These abnormalities are graded as first degree if present, second degree if the introitus is reached, or third degree if there is protrusion beyond the introitus.

Speculum Examination. A metal specula must be warmed to body temperature. The examiner spreads the labia and gently introduces the speculum to its full length and opens it to visualize the cervix. If the cervix cannot be easily located, one should not continue probing at the expense of patient discomfort, but instead, should remove the speculum, insert a finger to locate the cervix by palpation, and then reintroduce the speculum in the proper direction. The cervix is inspected, and any lesions are noted. Particular attention is paid to the squamocolumnar junction, where the somewhat erythematous columnar endocervical epithelium changes to the light pink, squamous epithelium of the vagina. At this junction, a white lesion that does not wipe away with a swab is likely to be either a condyloma acuminatum, dysplasia, or carcinoma in situ and will require a biopsy. A fungating, vascular lesion is likely to be actual carcinoma. A benign endocervical polyp may be seen as a smooth, red protuberance from the cervical canal. As the speculum is removed, the vaginal walls are inspected. (Screening for cervical carcinoma is discussed in Chapter 72; see page 935 for a description of the technique of obtaining specimens for cytology.)

Bimanual Examination. A bimanual examination is performed by introducing one finger through the introitus; if this finger goes in easily, a second finger is introduced beside it. If the introitus only admits one finger comfortably or if the patient seems unable to relax, it is best to proceed with a one-finger examination. To insist on using two fingers increases the patient's discomfort and reduces her ability to relax. Throughout the pelvic examination, the patient's cooperation is important, but the bimanual examination is impossible without it. If the abdominal wall is tensed, the examiner may feel masses that are not there or fail to appreciate true tumors that are present. Tenderness of the pelvic organs is an important finding, but the examiner must be gentle; otherwise, the examination of normal organs will produce pain and mislead the examiner. If the patient has trouble relaxing, it will help if the examiner introduces his fingers into the vagina and then waits with the other hand resting gently on the abdomen while encouraging the patient to think of relaxing her abdominal muscles.

As the examination begins, the upper vagina is palpated for nodules that could represent adenosis or metastatic cancer. The cervix is palpated and then grasped by placing a finger on either side of it in the lateral fornices. From this position, with one third of the uterus between the examiner's fingers, it is usually easy to palpate the uterine corpus between the hand in the vagina and the hand on the abdomen. Uterine size and contour are noted. Is the uterus symmetric, or is one side distorted by a fibroid tumor? Is the uterine corpus in anterior, mid, or posterior position with reference to the axis of the cervix? One should attempt to record the size of the corpus in centimeters, as for example $7 \times 5 \times 4$, the dimensions of the normal uterus. Women taking oral contraceptives and elderly women usually have smaller than average uteruses, affording a frequently available opportunity for the inexperienced examiner to prove that he or she can detect such differences.

Adnexal Examination. The examiner's vaginal fingers are both repositioned in one lateral fornix, and the abdominal hand is swept from the uterus over to the side to palpate the ovary. This motion is repeated to examine the opposite ovary. The ovaries are normally sensitive to compression, as the male physician can readily demonstrate to himself by self-examination of the testes. Normal ovaries are readily palpable in slender women during the reproductive years but may be hard to find because of their smaller size in women taking oral contraceptives. The ovaries are hard to identify in obese women, and the examiner frequently must be content with the rationalization that failure to feel an ovary is synonymous with the absence of any pathologic enlargement. Often the left adnexa is more easily examined if the right-handed examiner moves to the patient's side rather than standing at the end of the table. The size of any adnexal mass is described three-dimensionally in centimeters. The shape, consistency (cystic or solid), degree of fixation to other structures, and tenderness of all adnexal masses should be noted. The size of the ovary can be compared with an immediately available reference, the uterine corpus, in most women. The ovaries should be less than half the size of the normal corpus. Palpation of an ovary of apparently normal size in a postmenopausal woman is pathologic, because the ovaries normally regress to a small size in women in this age group. In one study, 20 postmenopausal women with an asymptomatic palpable ovary had surgical exploration. Thirteen had ovarian neoplasms, and of these, three were malignant.[2] Hence, the presence of a palpable ovary in a woman several years postmenopause is reason to obtain a pelvic ultrasound study, a serum CA 125 assay, and ask for repeat examination by a gynecologic specialist. Masses other than the ovary can be palpated in the adnexae (e.g., an ectopic pregnancy, a paraovarian cyst, or a pedunculated fibroid).

Rectovaginal-Abdominal Examination. The examiner's index finger is gently introduced into the rectum, allowing time for the sphincter to relax. The first finger is then reintroduced into the vagina, and the pelvic organs are again palpated between the examiner's two hands. This maneuver is often very illuminating. What may have been thought to be a moderately enlarged uterus on vaginal examination may now be appreciated as a solid ovarian tumor lying behind a normal-sized uterus. Nodules between the uterus and the rectum are an important finding, indicating either endometriosis of the uterosacral ligaments or metastatic tumor. One simple procedure to help differentiate an enlarged uterus from an adnexal mass is to replace the vaginal speculum and insert a uterine sound through the cervical canal to the top of the uterine cavity to demonstrate its size, shape, and direction.

After the rectal examination has been completed, stool is routinely checked for occult blood.

PELVIC MASS

Some of the more common conditions producing pelvic masses in women are listed in Table 38–1. Diagnosis is aided by a thorough examination with a careful description of the findings. Where is the mass located: midline, right or left side, posterior to the uterus? How large is the mass? Is the mass the bladder? Is it in fact the uterus? Does it arise from the uterus or is it separate? Is it firm or cystic, and what is its shape? Is it mobile or fixed? Is it tender to gentle palpation?

An enlarged uterus in a woman of reproductive years must always be considered a pregnancy until this can be ruled out. The next most common diagnosis is uterine leiomyoma(s). A mass arising from the uterus that is firm, irregular in contour, and nontender is almost always a fibroid, *but* it could also be an ovarian tumor adherent to the uterus. Fibroids of modest dimension, not yet large enough to fill the pelvis, if not producing symptoms of pain or hemorrhagic menses can be followed for years and may never require surgery unless they start to enlarge or become otherwise symptomatic. However, such a plan of management for an ovarian cancer is ill advised. In the postmenopausal woman, enlarging fibroids are of much greater concern, because the possibility of leiomyosarcoma is greater.

Ultrasound examination (abdominal and vaginal) is helpful in determining whether a mass is truly arising from the uterus or is ovarian in origin. If the ultrasound picture is also consistent with fibroids, if the ovaries can be seen as normal and separate from the mass, and if there is no evident hydronephrosis by ultrasound, periodic examination is sufficient management for the premenopausal woman.

Adnexal masses are usually ovarian in origin. The most common ovarian masses in women during the reproductive years are benign retention cysts. If the mass is 5 cm in diameter or less and feels cystic, standard practice is to follow the patient for 1 or 2 months, waiting for the cyst to regress spontaneously. During the waiting period, the patient is cautioned against any vigorous activity that might result in torsion of the adnexa containing the cystic ovary. If there is any possibility of pregnancy, a sensitive assay for β-human chorionic gonadotropin (HCG) should be performed to rule out ectopic pregnancy. Masses larger than 5 cm may still regress spontaneously, but the larger the mass, the less likely it is to be only an ovarian retention cyst. Although malignant ovarian tumors can be found in women of any age, the older the woman, the greater is the risk.

Ultrasound examination is helpful in differentiating uni-

TABLE 38–1. SOME CONDITIONS PRESENTING AS A PELVIC MASS

Female Internal Genitalia
Vagina
Adenosis
Inclusion cyst
Cyst of Gartner's duct
Carcinoma
Imperforate hymen
Cervix
Carcinoma*
Uterus
Pregnancy, normal and abnormal*
Uterine anomaly
Leiomyoma(s)* and leiomyosarcoma
Adenomyosis
Carcinoma of the endometrium or cervix*
Ovary
Physiologic cyst (follicular or corpus luteum)*
Ovarian pregnancy
Retention cyst*
Benign tumor* (e.g., endometrioma, dermoid teratoma, cystoma, cystadenoma, fibroma)
Malignant tumor* (e.g., carcinoma, stromal tumors, germ cell tumors)
Parovarian or broad ligament
Parovarian tumor
Fallopian tube
Tubal pregnancy*
Hydrosalpinx or pyosalpinx*
Tubo-ovarian abscess*
Carcinoma of fallopian tube
Other Organs
Urinary tract
Normal bladder (urinary retention)
Carcinoma of the bladder
Pelvic kidney
Gastrointestinal tract
Diverticulitis with abscess*
Appendiceal abscess
Carcinoma*
Carcinoid tumor
Volvulus
Peritoneum
Endometriosis with adhesions*
Inflammatory pseudocyst
Mesothelioma
Retroperitoneum
Teratoma
Sarcoma

*Most common conditions.

locular, thin-walled cysts, which are likely to regress, from structurally more complex masses, which will probably require intervention. Endovaginal ultrasonography is especially useful in evaluating adnexal masses. However, ultrasonography is not yet totally reliable for this determination. Gynecologic referral is indicated when a small mass persists for more than a month or two, for masses larger than 5 cm, or for a mass of any size in the postmenopausal woman.

Laparoscopy, which is a surgical procedure, is the next step. A small incision is made in the fold at the lower edge of the umbilicus, a needle is inserted into the abdominal cavity to establish a pneumoperitoneum with CO_2 gas, and a trocar 6 to 8 mm in diameter is then thrust into the abdominal cavity. A telescope carrying a fiberoptic light source is inserted through the trocar sheath to visualize the abdominal viscera. Laparoscopy is an invasive procedure, and serious complications, although rare, have occurred. For the most part, such complications reflect poor surgical technique; however, if there is an adhesion of intestine to the abdominal wall underlying the umbilicus, intestinal perforation may occur with introduction of the trocar. To prevent this, a variation of technique, termed *open laparoscopy*, is used when the patient has a history of generalized peritonitis or of multiple surgical procedures. In younger women, an apparent thin-walled simple cyst may be needle-aspirated under laparoscopic guidance, with the fluid sent for cytologic examination, and the cyst wall biopsied. Recent advances in laparoscopic instrumentation now allow the experienced gynecologic surgeon to perform complete removal of ovarian cysts and total oophorectomy without laparotomy.[3] However, proper management of an ovarian cancer requires laparotomy, complete removal of the mass without spill, a thorough staging examination of the entire abdominal content with multiple biopsies of peritoneal surfaces, and in most cases, complete hysterectomy with bilateral salpingo-oophorectomy.

The tubo-ovarian complex of chronic pelvic inflammatory disease can also present as a pelvic mass; however, the patient most often would also have chronic pelvic pain.

CHRONIC PELVIC PAIN

The symptom of chronic lower abdominal pain must be taken seriously. In the past, if results of the pelvic examination were negative, this problem was often considered to be psychosomatic. With the availability of laparoscopy, we now realize that a physical basis for the pain can be found in many cases.[4] However, there is a substantial minority of patients in whom the cause of the pain remains obscure, even after laparoscopy, or in whom pain persists despite definitive therapy for a specific condition.[5]

The sensory innervation of the pelvic organs is complex. Visceral somatic pain fibers travel with the sympathetic nerves in the hypogastric plexus through the dorsal root ganglia to enter the spinal cord at segments T-10 to S-2. There is some segmental localization, with T-10 the primary cord segment for the ovary, T-12 for the uterus, and L-1 for the bladder and vagina.[6] In addition, there are sacral visceral sensory nerves for the same organs, which are carried in the sacral parasympathetic nerves, along the pudendal nerve, to enter the spinal cord at S-2 to S-4. With this dual sensory innervation, different sensations from the same organ may travel different routes to the spinal cord, as, for example, stretch sensations from bladder and vagina are said to travel with the sacral visceral afferents whereas inflammatory pain is said to travel with the thoracolumbar afferents. Pain from pelvic organs can be referred to skin supplied from nerves of the same spinal segment—hence, to the corresponding dermatomes of the anterior abdominal wall, to the skin over the sacrum, and to the anterior aspects of the thighs. Pain from the ovary may be felt in the lower quadrant of the abdomen over the affected ovary, but it also can be referred to the T-10 dermatome around the umbilicus.

Evaluation of the Patient. A thorough history of the patient is taken and integrated with the findings of the pelvic examination. The pain should be characterized as to when it occurs, and its relationship to the menstrual cycle should be determined. Primary dysmenorrhea is present for only a few hours before the menstrual flow begins; then it resolves. In primary dysmenorrhea, by definition, there is no identifiable pathology. However, the physical basis for the pain is now fairly well understood. Most women with dysmenorrhea can be shown to produce higher than normal levels of prostaglandins in the uterus just prior to menstruation, and, as a result, the force of the uterine contractions that proceed the menstrual flow is measurably greater than in women who do not experience pain.[7] Pain that is present for as long as 2 or 3 days before menstruation or that persists for 2 or 3 days after the flow has started suggests demonstrable pathology such as endometriosis. One should determine its relationship to intercourse, bowel movements, and urination, as well as its location.

Pain in one lower quadrant or both lower quadrants suggests adnexal pain, as from chronic tubal inflammation or adhesions. Pain felt in the lower midline and radiating to the low back and front of the thighs suggests uterine pain. A generalized distribution, shifting location, and rushes of cramping pain suggest intestinal origin. Confusion of pain from the female internal genitalia with pain from the intestine is very common. If the history is suggestive of intestinal origin, especially in patients in whom there is a history of constipation or constipation alternating with diarrhea, one should suspect the spastic colon syndrome.

The physician should inquire about a history of sexually transmitted disease, use of an intrauterine contraceptive device, previous abdominal surgery, previous tubal pregnancy, or unexplained infertility. Much of chronic pelvic pain is explained by previous pelvic inflammatory disease (PID) with adhesions. The association with a known episode of PID or of appendicitis suggests that chronic tubal inflammation or pelvic adhesions will be found; however, the absence of this history does not rule out chronic PID. For many patients, the first episode is not recognized. This is especially the case with chlamydial salpingitis. A history of more insidious onset and of painful menstruation that has become progressively more severe, with the pain now lasting for several days around the time of menstruation, suggests endometriosis. One should inquire as to whether the patient has pain with intercourse and, if so, when. Pain around the introitus with penetration suggests inadequate lubrication from inhibited sexual response or vaginitis, but the symptom of pain felt only with deep thrusting suggests that significant pelvic pathology will be found, most commonly endometriosis or adhesions.

The physical finding of an enlarged uterus is significant. A symmetrically moderately enlarged, tender uterus and the history of severe pain only at the time of menstruation is suggestive of adenomyosis, or so-called internal endometriosis. In this condition, endometrial glands are found deep within the wall of the uterus. An irregular, enlarged uterus is likely to contain fibroid tumors, although as previously noted, these tumors can be confused with ovarian masses. Large fibroid tumors may produce a sensation of pressure and of fullness, but they do not usually produce severe pain unless degeneration of the fibroid is occurring. In general, it is best to search for other sources before attributing severe pain to a fibroid. An adnexal mass may be found. Cystic tumors may produce pain from stretching of the ovarian capsule if they grow rapidly. If endometriosis exists or if the ovary is confined by adhesions, pain is more likely. Unfortunately, most ovarian malignancies do not seem to produce pain until they are far advanced, and, even then, the pain is mild, diffuse, associated with nausea, and often mistakenly attributed to a gastrointestinal origin. A nondistinct fullness of one or both adnexae, associated with tenderness and some fixation of the uterine corpus, is suggestive of pelvic adhesions from previous PID.

Uterine prolapse or a large cystocele may produce discomfort that is characteristically described as a pulling sensation, rather than sharp pain or cramping, and is usually associated with the symptom that "everything is falling out."

An interesting approach to chronic pelvic pain has been proposed by Slocum. He states that many women with pelvic pain exhibit "trigger points," small areas of skin or fascia that are hyperesthetic.[8] Pressure on a trigger point is said to reproduce the patient's symptom. He advises that the "trigger points" be injected with local anesthetic. (This work requires validation by others.)

Psychological Assessment. As part of the initial evaluation concerning chronic pelvic pain, one should inquire about the patient's major life events since childhood. What is the present family constellation? What is the patient's level of physical and emotional functioning? Is she disabled by the pain, or is she able to work in spite of it? Is there a history of recurring, poorly documented physical complaints? A history of physical abuse as a child can be elicited in a substantial minority of these patients.[9]

Diagnostic Studies. The white blood cell count and differential determination are obtained, although these will usually be normal in patients with chronic pelvic pain. The erythrocyte sedimentation rate (ESR) is more useful. An elevated ESR may be the only laboratory finding in chronic PID. Urinalysis and culture may be helpful. An ultrasound examination of the pelvis with vaginal and abdominal probes is most useful. A normal ultrasound study does not rule out disease, and positive ultrasound findings require other confirmation, but the findings can be helpful. A 1-cm ovarian cyst is a normal finding, but a 2- to 3-cm complex cyst, which is too small to be palpated, may represent an endometrioma or an area of adhesion of intestine to the ovary.

For some conditions, a therapeutic trial of medical management may also be diagnostic and should precede invasive studies. Pain primarily felt only in the days around menstruation should be treated by antiprostaglandin medications. Adequate doses must be used: for example, ibuprofen, 800 mg to start, followed by 400 to 600 mg every 6 hours. Another approach is a trial of oral contraceptives to suppress ovulation. Prior to such therapy, however, one must consider the patient's age and other risk factors for vascular disease. Another approach to be strongly considered in the management of chronic pain is complete suppression of ovarian function with gonadotropin-releasing hormone (GNRH) analogs. If spastic colon is suspected, a few weeks' trial of a high-fiber diet or bulk-inducing laxatives is advised.

The finding of tender adnexae and moderate elevation of the ESR or a history suggestive of PID suggests chronic PID. A course of oral antibiotics combined with an antiprostaglandin is indicated. One such regimen is doxycycline, 100 mg twice a day (see Table 31–2), and ibuprofen, 400 mg four times a day, for 10 days. If these maneuvers fail or are not appropriate, the next step in evaluation is diagnostic laparoscopy.

Pelvic pain can be psychogenic in origin, and psychological factors tend to assume a role in any pain of long duration. However, unless the patient has flagrant psychopathology, she merits diagnostic laparoscopy. Even if obvious psychopathology is present, the patient should probably still have laparoscopy, but only after an initial psychiatric evaluation. Patients with multiple somatic complaints are the most difficult to manage. A borderline personality does not prevent the development of endometriosis nor protect one from sexually transmitted disease, but it makes it difficult to interpret symptoms and clinical findings. Often, even in this context, a diagnostic laparoscopy is appropriate and serves to reassure the patient as to what is *not* wrong.

Findings at Laparoscopy. The results of one laparoscopy series are detailed in Table 38–2.[10] This series includes only patients whose pain had persisted in the same location for longer than 6 months; it does not include patients whose worsening symptoms had required earlier intervention. A control group is included, which is composed of women who had no symptoms identified preoperatively but had requested laparoscopic tubal sterilization. Most of the patients with pain had positive findings at laparoscopy, even though most of them had negative findings at preoperative pelvic examinations. Pelvic abnormalities were sometimes found in the asymptomatic group. However, there were differences. For example, when adhesions were found in the women with pain, the adhesions were more likely to envelop, confine, or bind an organ, whereas in the women without pain, the adhesions were more often loose. In the pain group, the finding of adhesions was usually associated with a history of previous PID or of prior surgery. Endometriosis was also found in the group without pain, but when these women were questioned again after surgery, they usually reported the presence of recurring discomfort but had not thought it severe enough for complaint. Interestingly, the large pelvic veins seen at laparoscopy that are sometimes taken as evidence of "pelvic congestion syndrome" were seen more often in the control group than in the pain group and could not be related to pain. The finding of retrograde menstruation in the pain group may not be particularly significant, because other investigators have reported that if examined in the perimenstrual days, 90% of cycling women will exhibit blood in the peritoneal fluid.[11] Other laparoscopy series have not consistently found as high a percentage of patients with positive findings as that illustrated in Table 38–2; however, the criteria for inclusion in other studies have not been as stringent.

Management. Treatment subsequent to laparoscopy depends on the illness. Prolonged antibiotic therapy may produce a remission for the patient with chronic PID, especially if the ESR is elevated. The course of chronic PID is that of remission and relapse. Cultures of infected fallopian tubes yield a variety of organisms, predominantly anaerobic. Hence, prolonged treatment with a synthetic tetracycline is the first choice for outpatient management, but no one agent is effective against all the likely pathogens. Clindamycin or the combination of metronidazole with ampicillin may produce remission when tetracycline has failed. Whether or not chronic PID without abscess involves actual infection is not yet clear, but, in practice, antibiotic therapy often seems to work (see Tables 31–2 and 31–3).

Surgery for chronic PID is reserved for cases resistant to medical therapy or when there have been repeated recurrences. The few cases in which the findings are predominantly unilateral hold the most hope. Unilateral salpingo-oophorectomy may have dramatic results. When the disease is bilateral, conservative surgery with lysis of adhesions may be beneficial, but relapse is very common. The best course is to persist in attempts at medical management as long as feasible, then plan surgical removal of uterus, tubes, and both ovaries. The availability of in vitro fertilization makes an in-between step of bilateral salpingectomy or even bilateral salpingo-oophorectomy worth considering, but the efficacy of such an approach in treatment of pain is unknown.

TABLE 38–2. FINDINGS AT LAPAROSCOPY IN 100 PATIENTS WITH PELVIC PAIN PRESENT FOR MORE THAN 6 MONTHS IN THE SAME LOCATION COMPARED WITH 50 PATIENTS REQUESTING STERILIZATION*

	Patients With Pelvic Pain	Sterilization Patients
Number of women	100	50
Age range	18–55	23–47
Median age	29	35
Pathologic findings (%)	83	29
Endometriosis	32	15
Pelvic adhesion of reproductive organs	38	12
Bowel adhesions	10	2
Liver adhesions	3	0
Nonpathologic findings (%)	17	71
Retrograde menstruation	5	0
Large pelvic veins	3	15
Normal pelvis	9	56

*From Kresch AJ, Seifer DB, Sachs LB, et al: Laparoscopy in 100 women with chronic pelvic pain. Obstet Gynecol 64:672, 1984. Reprinted with permission from the American College of Obstetricians and Gynecologists.

ENDOMETRIOSIS

Endometriosis is a condition of unknown cause in which tissue that is almost identical to normal endometrium is found in abnormal places. The most common sites for endometriosis are the surface of the ovaries and the peritoneum adjacent to the uterus, tubes, and ovaries, especially that of the cul-de-sac behind the uterus, the area where gravity would produce pooling of fluid dripping from the fallopian tubes. Endometriosis has also been described in such remote locations as the umbilicus, the knee, and the lung, where it may produce monthly episodes of hemoptysis. Major theories of causation include retrograde menstruation through the fallopian tubes into the abdominal cavity, with implantation of endometrial cells on peritoneal surfaces,[12] metaplasia of tissue of embryonic origin, lymphatic or vascular metastasis, direct implantation into surgical scars, and combinations of the aforementioned, with metaplasia of peritoneal tissue stimulated by menstrual fluid.[13] Studies in monkeys that develop spontaneous endometriosis have demonstrated altered cellular immune response with diminished rejection of autografts, suggesting a possible immune deficiency etiology for human endometriosis as well.[14] Delayed childbearing and regular ovulation without interruption for pregnancy are thought to play a role. There is a weak familial tendency, with sisters and mothers of affected women more often having endometriosis than do mothers-in-law or sisters-in-law.[15] Obstructive abnormalities of the genital tract confer strong risk for the condition. Women who have endometriosis had earlier menarche and report shorter menstrual cycles but more prolonged menstruation and heavier flow than controls, suggesting that a greater opportunity for peritoneal contamination with menstrual blood increases risk.[15]

Endometriosis may present in a variety of ways. Clinically, one may suspect endometriosis from a history of primary dysmenorrhea of increasing severity and poor response to antiprostaglandin medication. Endometriosis is a common finding when laparoscopy is done to evaluate unexplained infertility. The mechanism for pain or for infertility in association with endometriosis is not clear; however, the peritoneal fluid of women with endometriosis contains high levels of prostaglandin metabolites. Fluid from women with pain of chronic PID or adhesions does not differ from normal in prostaglandin content.[16] Endometriotic implants are presumed to synthesize prostaglandins, as does normal endometrium. Endometriosis may present as a mass lesion, an endometrioma, of one or both ovaries. Although endometriomas are often unexpected findings at routine pelvic examination, they may leak or rupture and present as an acute abdominal catastrophe with peritoneal signs and a low-grade fever. Rarely, endometriomas become secondarily infected and present as acute PID.

Diagnosis. The pelvic examination is frequently abnormal in women with endometriosis, with tenderness behind the uterus, a mass in the ovary, nodules on the uterosacral ligaments, or, rarely, blue spots visible on the cervix. Definitive diagnosis, however, requires laparoscopy. Laparoscopic findings range from minimal, with a few small blue implants on the surface of an ovary or over the uterosacral ligaments, to severe, with bilateral endometriomas and major adhesions obliterating the fallopian tubes. Laparoscopy findings may be quite subtle. Typical findings are small blue nodules and surrounding areas of brown discoloration; however, it has been appreciated that peritoneal folds, white plaques, and so forth, often prove to be endometriosis when biopsies are examined histologically. Characteristically, the patient whose only symptom is disabling dysmenorrhea will be found to have endometriosis involving only the peritoneum of the uterosacral ligament; however, because this structure carries important afferent sensory nerves, the anatomic finding does correlate with the symptoms.

Management. Management of endometriosis is determined by the severity of the disease, the symptoms, and the patient's wishes, that is, pain relief or improvement in fertility. Depending on the location of the implants, minimal endometriosis can be treated with electrocautery or laser under laparoscopic guidance or by hormonal therapy. Extensive endometriosis responds somewhat to hormonal therapy, but surgical resection of large implants is usually also required. Endometriomas respond poorly to hormonal therapy and almost always need to be resected.

Estrogens alone, androgens, progestins, and combination oral contraceptives containing both estrogen and a progestin have been used in the past, but current therapy favors danazol or GNRH analogs. Danazol is a very weak androgen; its mechanism of action is complex. At therapeutic doses, it blocks the midcycle surge of gonadotropins and, hence, prevents ovulation and produces amenorrhea. In addition, danazol inhibits many of the enzymes necessary for steroidogenesis.[17] Its efficacy has been demonstrated in controlled trials of women followed by laparoscopy.[18] Women treated with danazol usually begin to experience relief soon after therapy is begun, in contradistinction to estrogen-progestin therapy, in which symptoms may become worse before they begin to improve. A dose of 800 mg/day is standard, but 400 mg will produce amenorrhea and stop pain and is adequate treatment for most women. Mild androgenic side effects, such as oily skin and increased acne, weight gain, and reduction in breast size, are common. At the higher dose, a few women may develop hirsutism or even deepening of the voice. Emotional changes, moodiness, and depression are encountered by some women. Treatment is continued for 6 to 9 months.

Two forms of GNRH analog are presently available. Nafarelin is administered daily by absorption across the nasal mucosa. Leuprolide acetate is available as a once-a-month injection of the depot form, Depot Lupron. The GNRH agonists have been found highly effective.[19] Whether or not they are superior to danazol is not clear, though there is a widespread clinical impression that relief of pain from endometriosis lasts longer after GNRH analog therapy than after therapy with danazol. As would be expected from an androgen, danazol has an adverse effect on lipids, producing significant reduction of high-density lipoprotein during therapy. GNRH agonists have little effect on lipids when given in 6-month courses, but the marked hypoestrogenic state produced is associated with menopausal symptoms of hot flashes and vaginal dryness and results in a reduction in bone density.[20] Unfortunately, hormonal treatment rarely produces long-lasting cure of endometriosis, and symptoms frequently recur a few months or years after completion of therapy. Surgical resection appears to produce longer-lasting remission, although no randomized trial has been reported. Depending on the extent of the endometriosis and the patient's wishes, a recurrence may be managed with another course of hormonal therapy or with surgery. Definitive treatment of the disease requires removal of all visible endometriosis, the uterus, tubes, and both ovaries. This dramatic step should be delayed as long as possible by courses of hormonal therapy and by conservative surgery.

PREMENSTRUAL SYNDROME

Physical and emotional symptoms occur in many women in the luteal phase of the menstrual cycle and are relieved when menstrual flow begins. Formerly called *premenstrual tension,* in recent years this condition has been labeled the *premenstrual syndrome* (PMS).[21] Thirty to 40% of menstruating women are said to be affected by PMS to some extent. It appears that there is no one "syndrome" but at least three kinds of illness, similar only in being related to the menstrual cycle. Some women suffer from specific illness such as seizures, recurrent dermatitis, migraine headaches, or asthma, which are seemingly triggered by the menstrual cycle and occur at the same time each month. There are also women who have major psychiatric illnesses that appear to be exacerbated during the premenstrual phase. The more common problem, distinguished by some as "primary PMS,"[22] consists of a cluster of symptoms that vary in severity among women and from cycle to cycle, that appear only in the luteal phase, that begin to diminish after the onset of menstruation, and that appear when criteria for other psychiatric diagnoses are lacking. Common physical symptoms are weight gain, edema, a bloated sensation, breast-swelling and tenderness, headache, fatigue, and lethargy. Common emotional symptoms are extreme irritability, emotional lability, crying spells, depression, anxiety, and cravings for salty foods and sweets. The most severe form of PMS has been called the late luteal phase dysphoric disorder (LLPDD) and is proposed as a specific psychiatric diagnostic category in the DSM system for the classification of mental disorders.[23] The diagnosis of LLPDD is applied only when the symptoms are severe, have occurred during most menstrual cycles in the past year, and disappear within a few days of onset of the follicular phase.[23]

Secondary premenstrual syndromes are those conditions with symptoms that increase premenstrually but in which there are also sufficient other symptoms to enable diagnosis of another psychiatric illness.[22]

The causes of PMS are unknown. Women with PMS do not differ from controls in terms of daily follicle-stimulating hormone, luteinizing hormone, estradiol, progesterone, or androgens.[24] According to Reid and Yen,[25] the sex steroids estrogen and progesterone influence neuronal activity in many areas of the brain. Yen's group has proposed that the symptoms have to do with effects of the cycling sex steroids on serotonergic and noradrenergic receptors and on endorphins, oxytocin, and vasopressin.[25, 26] Normally, β-endorphins, the endogenous opioids, increase in peripheral blood during the luteal phase. Women with PMS have lower β-endorphin blood levels, and the current concept is that they suffer from symptoms of withdrawal to their own opioids.[24]

Diagnosis. A general history and physical examination of the patient are helpful in diagnosing PMS. Women presenting with the complaint of "PMS" may have a variety of other conditions ranging from hypothyroidism to major affective illness to menopause. The patient is then asked to keep an inventory of her symptoms, rating each on a simple scale of 0 (not present) to 3 (severe) at the end of each day and also noting the onset of menstruation. There is no laboratory test for this condition. If symptoms fit the pattern just described, clearing completely for at least 1 week after the onset of menstruation, primary PMS is diagnosed. An atypical symptom pattern suggests a different etiology, frequently psychiatric.

Management. For many years it was thought that PMS was caused by inadequate production of ovarian progesterone in the luteal phase. Treatment with vaginal progesterone suppositories was common.[21] However, even high-dose vaginal progesterone is no more effective than a placebo.[27] Pyridoxine (vitamin B_6) has also been widely prescribed, and some randomized trials have shown benefit.[28] Others have found this agent ineffective, and there is considerable risk of serious neurotoxicity if more than modest doses are used.[24] The first scientifically proven effective therapy was ovulation suppression with a GNRH analog.[26] Symptoms return when treatment is stopped, and the drug is very expensive. Because estrogen production is severely reduced with GNRH analog therapy, symptoms and side effects of menopause are produced. GNRH analogs can be combined with estrogen and progestin, so-called "give back" treatment, and continued indefinitely, but the problem of high cost remains.[29] Permanent relief is provided by surgical bilateral oophorectomy and estrogen replacement.[30, 31]

Less dramatic alternatives exist. These include calcium supplementation, 1000 mg/day,[32] and the prostaglandin synthetase inhibitors.[33] Low-dose danazol (200 mg/day, taken continuously) has consistently been found effective, although benefit may be limited to those who become anovulatory.[34] Women who continue to ovulate on danazol must use contraception, because masculinization of a female fetus could follow if pregnancy occurred. Various psychoactive agents appear promising. The benzodiazepine alprazolam is effective but is potentially addictive, thus treatment must be carefully supervised.[35] Doses of 0.25 mg are given two or three times a day during the luteal phase and then tapered for 2 to 3 days with the onset of menses.

Buspirone, a new anxiolytic drug unrelated to benzodiazepines or barbiturates and thought to have low addictive potential, has also been found useful in controlled trials.[36] The dose is 10 mg twice a day during the luteal phase. The antidepressant fluoxetine was found effective in a small, controlled trial with continuous therapy of 20 mg/day.[37]

A reasoned approach to the problem is to ask the patient to track her symptoms for a minimum of 2 months to make the diagnosis. During this time dietary alterations are advised: Avoid red meat, caffeine, chocolate, and salty foods; add 1000 mg/day of calcium. Regular aerobic exercise is frequently prescribed. Often the identification and recognition of the problem and these lifestyle changes are sufficient. If the problem persists, minimal pharmacologic intervention is offered at first. The diuretics spironolactone or triamterene are prescribed for luteal phase fluid retention, and prostaglandin synthetase inhibitors are used for headache and dysmenorrhea.[33] If emotional symptoms are significant and persist after these minimal interventions, one of the psychoactive drugs (alprazolam or buspirone) is added under close supervision. For further relief an ovulation suppression regime is chosen, such as danazol, 400 mg/day, or a GNRH analog. Women who have severe symptoms and who desire permanent sterilization can be considered for oophorectomy, or hysterectomy-oophorectomy after a thorough evaluation and initial less intrusive medical management.

Women who have cycle-triggered illnesses may benefit from hormonal suppression of the menstrual cycle with oral contraceptives if this is medically appropriate or by progestin therapy alone. Affective disorders that are exacerbated by the menstrual cycle are best managed by a psychiatrist.

MENOPAUSE

Menopause is the cessation of menstruation and occurs on the average at 51 years of age in the United States. Natural menopause is the result of a gradual process of ovarian failure that takes place over several years. Fewer and fewer ovarian follicles remain that will respond to pituitary stimulation, and, during these years, baseline levels of the gonadotropins, follicle-stimulating hormone (FSH), and luteotropic hormone (LH) gradually rise. Eventually, there are no more ovarian follicles that will respond, and the menses cease. As part of this gradual process, the menstrual cycles become less regular. There are skips and delays. There may also be anovulation in some cycles, when prolonged estrogen production without progesterone produces dysfunctional uterine bleeding and, not infrequently, endometrial hyperplasia (see Chapter 39).

Ovarian follicles are the main source of the most potent natural estrogen, estradiol, and, as the follicles are used up, estradiol falls to very low levels. After menopause, alternative pathways for estrogen production become more important. The ovaries continue to produce androgens, androstenedione, and testosterone.[38] The prehormone androstenedione, produced in the ovarian stroma and by the adrenal glands, is converted to the weak estrogen estrone,[38] and this serves as a precursor for production of estradiol.[39] The main site of conversion of androstenedione to estrone is in adipose tissue; hence, women who are relatively fat tend to produce more estrogen after menopause than do slender women.[38] This fact appears to explain the clinical observation that obese women are at greater risk for endometrial cancer[38] and at less risk for osteoporosis than are slender women.

A number of symptoms occur in association with the progressive ovarian failure of the premenopausal years and become worse after menopause. These include somatic alterations such as hot flashes, vaginal dryness, headaches, breast pain, and weight gain. Psychological alterations such as fatigue, irritability, lability of mood, anxiety, crying spells, and insomnia have also been described. In the past, these symptoms were thought to be of psychoneurotic origin. Our current concept is that many of these symptoms are signs of estrogen withdrawal and continued estrogen deficiency.

The classic menopausal symptom is the hot flush or flash. Subjectively, the woman feels suddenly unbearably hot, and the skin becomes flushed. During the hot flash, skin temperature actually increases a degree or more, and body core temperature falls temporarily. Estrogen deficiency appears to induce a disorder of central thermoregulatory hypothalamic α-adrenergic mechanisms. In menopausal women, heating provokes hot flashes and cooling reduces them. The α_2-agonist clonidine inhibits α-adrenergic receptors and reduces hot flashes. The α_2-inhibitor yohimbine provokes hot flashes in menopausal women.[40]

A sleep disorder is frequently associated with hot flashes, that is, more time is required to fall asleep, and there are frequent awakenings that occur at the time of hot flashes. Erlik, Meldrum, and Judd have clearly demonstrated that women who suffer most from hot flashes produce lower levels of estrogens than do women who are not symptomatic and that symptomatic women have significantly lower body weight for height.[38] Placebo-controlled trials have demonstrated the efficacy of estrogen replacement to reduce the frequency of hot flashes and improve sleep. Estrogens do not abolish all hot flashes for all women; some women continue to suffer, even when on adequate estrogen replacement therapy. Clonidine therapy often helps them.

Genital atrophy as a result of estrogen deficiency produces another constellation of symptoms: failure of sexual lubrication, vaginal dryness and pain with intercourse, urinary frequency, and dysuria. These symptoms usually respond dramatically to estrogen replacement.

Emotional lability, depression, anxiety attacks, loss of energy, and other psychological symptoms have been much more difficult to study. They are not as clearly related to estrogen deficiency as are hot flashes. They do not respond as well or as consistently to estrogen replacement therapy. However, placebo-controlled crossover trials have demonstrated reduction in irritability, anxiety, depression, and headaches with estrogen therapy.

Research has begun to establish a role for ovarian androgens in preventing some of these symptoms. Women subjected to surgical menopause lose their main source of estradiol but also lose much of their androstenedione and testosterone. Women given androgens or androgen-estrogen combinations after surgical menopause experienced fewer symptoms and a greater sense of well-being than did women treated with estrogens alone.

The role of estrogen in the prevention of osteoporosis is well established. The benefits of estrogens in preventing osteoporosis and in its treatment have been documented in controlled trials. This topic is discussed in detail in Chapter 54.

Cardiovascular disease is also a concern of the menopausal years. The incidence of cardiovascular disease increases steadily with age. The age-specific incidence for women lags about 10 years behind that for men.[41] Women who undergo premature menopause have accelerated cardiovascular disease unless they are given estrogen replacement.[42] After menopause, circulating lipoproteins change in a way that would be predictive of increased cardiovascular risk: high-density lipoprotein (HDL) cholesterol decreases and low-density lipoprotein (LDL) cholesterol increases.[43] Estrogen replacement therapy more than compensates for these adverse changes.

Many studies have demonstrated a potentially beneficial change in the lipids with estrogen therapy: LDL decreases and HDL increases.[41] In a randomized, blinded, cross-over study, Walsh and colleagues demonstrated that daily doses of 0.625 mg or 1.25 mg conjugated estrogens decreased mean LDL by 15% and 19%, respectively.[44] The same doses increased HDL by 16% and 18%, respectively. Several studies document an apparent 40 to 50% reduction in risk of heart attack for estrogen-treated women.[41] This reduction in risk is physiologically plausible, given the lipid effects. There may be additional direct beneficial effects of estrogen on the vessel wall. On the other hand, critics note that the benefit of estrogen could be an artifact of patient selection, that physicians may have prescribed estrogens preferentially for healthy women and withheld them from women with cardiovascular risk factors. A very large randomized trial will be required to determine the truth.

Hormonal replacement therapy has real and theoretical risks. One of the known risks is endometrial cancer (see Chapter 39). This risk appears to be totally preventable provided that (1) estrogens are administered in combination with progestins[45] and (2) the patients are periodically subjected to endometrial biopsy. Another known risk is a modest increase in gallbladder disease, with an estimated incidence of 131 per 100,000 persons attributed to estrogen therapy.[46]

Patients with abnormally elevated triglycerides are at risk for marked hypertriglyceridemia with resultant fulminant pancreatitis if they are treated with systemic estrogens. Because thrombosis has been associated with oral contraceptives, risk has been imputed to menopausal estrogen replacement, even though the doses used are much lower.[46, 47]

Gordon and colleagues studied several of the coagulation factors in menopausal women on different doses of ethinyl estradiol.[48] They found no changes in prothrombin time, factor X, fibrinogen, factor VII, or fibrinopeptide A; however, a mild shortening of the thromboplastin time and elevation of factor XII were found. Antithrombin III was reduced in women given 20 μg/day of ethinyl estradiol but not in those given 5 or 10 μg. A 0.625- to 1.25-mg dose of conjugated estrogens, the drug most often used for menopausal estrogen replacement in the United States, would be comparable to 5 to 10 μg of ethinyl estradiol, whereas the dose used in oral contraceptives has ranged from 30 μg to 100 μg, three to 20 times greater.[49] There is probably a threshold dose for significant procoagulant effect. Our usual postmenopausal doses are probably below the threshold. Indeed, a review concluded that there is no association between menopausal estrogens and thrombosis.[50]

The possibility that estrogen replacement may increase the risk for breast cancer continues to create great concern. The larger doses of hormones used for oral contraceptives have no overall effect on breast cancer risk.[51, 52] However, there may be a low level of risk for a subset of young women with prolonged exposure to oral contraceptives.[51, 52] Several large studies have found use of postmenopausal estrogens unrelated to breast cancer.[53] Others have found a low level of risk with long-term use, 10 to 15 years or more.[54] A very large recent case control study found no increase in breast cancer risk from unopposed conjugated estrogens, even after long periods of use.[55] A meta-analysis by Khoo and Chick of 16 hormone replacement studies found no significant risk among hormone replacement users, overall or in relation to duration of use or interval since first use.[53] They found that the addition of progestin was possibly protective. A meta-analysis by another group concluded that there is risk.[56] The controversy is far from resolved, but I find the evidence on balance reassuring. Even if the worst scenario is true, prolonged use of estrogens could at most increase breast cancer by a relative risk of 1.2 to 1.4 (20 to 40% increase). On the other hand, the evidence is even stronger that menopausal estrogens reduce heart attack risk by approximately 50%, and since cardiovascular disease is a more common cause of death for women than is breast cancer, the net effect of hormone therapy would be one of benefit.[41]

Clinical Management. Whether all menopausal women should receive hormonal therapy is not yet clear. Certainly, women who have premature menopause, either spontaneously or after oophorectomy, should have estrogen replacement at least until age 51 years, the time of average natural menopause. There are two reasonable approaches for women who have menopause at the normal age: Treat all menopausal women unless they have a contraindication, or treat based on an assessment of the individual woman's symptoms, risk for osteoporosis, and lipid profile. Presently, we favor the latter approach and encourage the patient to decide, based on her individual circumstances. We offer estrogen replacement therapy to menopausal women who have symptoms of estrogen deficiency: hot flashes, the associated sleep disorder, and urogenital atrophy. We also attempt therapy of psychological symptoms such as irritability, lability of mood, anxiety, and depression, provided that these symptoms are not isolated but are accompanied by clear-cut estrogen deficiency symptoms such as hot flashes. If women are not symptomatic, I do not offer estrogens routinely but rather advise measurement of bone density and a fasting lipoprotein profile. A bone density that is close to the fracture threshold suggests this woman would benefit from estrogens. Similarly, elevated LDL or low HDL would argue for estrogen therapy to reduce heart disease risk, unless the triglyceride level is very high as well.

Choice of Regimens for Hormonal Replacement. Most of our knowledge of the long-term effects of hormone replacement therapy comes from studies of women treated with estrogen only, unopposed by progestational hormone. Unopposed estrogen, even taken cyclically with a drug-free period each month, produced endometrial hyperplasia at 1 year in 30% of patients treated with 0.625 mg/day of conjugated estrogens and in 57% of those taking 1.25 mg/day and has been associated with a several-fold increase in risk for endometrial cancer.[57] Use of progestin for 11 days or more each month markedly reduces the occurrence of hyperplasia and is thought to prevent endometrial cancer as well.[45]

Conventionally, women have been advised to take estrogens cyclically. There is no proved benefit for this plan and no physiologic rationale. Bothersome hot flashes frequently return during the time that one is not taking hormones. Equilin, the potent equine estrogen in conjugated estrogen, lasts for weeks in the body after the last dose, so that 1 week off medication accomplishes little. Presently, there are three acceptable regimens for the administration of hormone replacement therapy for menopausal women: (1) continuous or cyclic low-dose estrogen without progestin, but with an annual endometrial biopsy to detect hyperplasia; (2) continuous or cyclic low-dose estrogen with a progestin added for 13 to 14 days each month; and (3) continuous low-dose estrogen plus continuous low-dose progestin, with both taken every day.

A daily estrogen dose of conjugated estrogens (Premarin), 0.625 mg, is sufficient to prevent loss of bone density and provides significant improvement in circulating lipoproteins.[44, 58] Choice of specific progestin and dose must be done with care because the progestin may partly reverse the beneficial effect of the estrogen on lipids if too high a dose is used.[59] Typically, daily doses of 10 mg of medroxyprogesterone acetate (Provera) have been used, but this is now known to be too much to maintain ideal lipid effects and frequently causes side effects of abdominal cramping, bloating, and premenstrual-like symptoms.[60] We suggest a dose of 5 mg/day for 13 to 14 days each month when cyclic progestin therapy is chosen or 2.5 mg/day for continuous progestin therapy.[61] Irregular spotting and bleeding are common initially, but women who persevere and reach 6 months on therapy usually develop endometrial atrophy and experience amenorrhea thereafter.[61] For some this may be preferable to the monthly bleeding pattern that occurs when progestins are taken cyclically.

Estrogens can also be administered transdermally. Transdermal estrogens are effective in relieving estrogen deficiency symptoms but do not have the beneficial effects on lipids demonstrated with oral estrogen. This may be a benefit for the patient with severe hypertriglyceridemia who otherwise could not be given estrogens safely, but other women would unnecessarily give up a known benefit of therapy. Progestin therapy is as necessary with transdermal as with oral estrogen to protect the patient from endometrial hyperplasia. In our practice, we use estrogens alone for women who have had a hysterectomy. In women without a hysterectomy, whether or not to perform an endometrial biopsy before starting estrogen therapy and subsequently during therapy is unclear; the prevailing opinion is that biopsies are unnecessary. One group demonstrated that women who received 12 days of progestin each month and who bled after day 10 of therapy invariably had secretory endometrium on biopsy. Women who bled before day 10 often had proliferative endometrium on biopsy, which was a signal that a larger dose of progestin was needed.[62] Thus, women on cyclic estrogen-progestin therapy may be adequately protected if a biopsy is done whenever there is bleeding other than at the expected time. Women on the continuous regimen, estrogen and progestin every day, would have a biopsy if they bleed after the initial 6 months. My preference is for a Pipelle biopsy (see Chapter 39) done before therapy is started and at intervals of 2 to 3 years. I believe that this is justified by series such as that of Koss, who found endometrial cancers in 6.96/1000 supposedly asymptomatic women screened in New York,[63] by Leather's report of endometrial cancer developing in women on continuous estrogen/progestin therapy,[64] and because of Gelfand's report that a small percentage of patients given cyclic estrogen plus Provera had hyperplasia on biopsy after 1 year.[57] The ideal length for therapy is not known. Accordingly, we encourage a discussion of benefits and risk on an annual basis with each patient.

Women who have few complaints after menopause are producing relatively more estrogen[38] and, hence, are probably at increased risk for endometrial cancer. Such women should be considered for screening in order to detect this disease, if present (see Chapter 39).

REFERENCES

1. Barber HRK: Cancer of the ovary. *In* van Nagell JR Jr and Barber HRK (eds): Modern Concepts of Gynecologic Oncology. Boston, John Wright-PSG, 1982, pp 252–253.
2. Miller RC, Nash JD, Weiser EB, and Hoskins WJ: The postmenopausal palpable ovary syndrome: A retrospective review with histopathologic correlates. J Reprod Med 36:568, 1991.
3. Nezhat F, Nezhat C, and Silfen SL: Videolaseroscopy for oophorectomy. Am J Obstet Gynecol 165:1323, 1991.
4. Roseff SJ and Murphy AA: Laparoscopy in the diagnosis and therapy of chronic pelvic pain. Clin Obstet Gynecol 33:137, 1990.
5. Steege JF: The evaluation and treatment of women with pelvic pain. *In* Sciarra JJ, McElin TW, and Droegemueller W (eds): Gynecology and Obstetrics, Vol 6. Philadelphia, Harper & Row, 1984.
6. Carpenter MB and Sutin J: Human Neuroanatomy, 8th ed. Baltimore, Williams & Wilkins, 1983.
7. Dawood MY: Dysmenorrhea. Clin Obstet Gynecol 33:168, 1990.
8. Slocum JC: Chronic somatic, myofascial, and neurogenic abdominal pelvic pain. Clin Obstet Gynecol 33:145, 1990.
9. Rapkin AJ, Kames LD, Darke LL, et al: History of physical and sexual abuse in women with chronic pelvic pain. Obstet Gynecol 76:92, 1990.

10. Kresch AJ, Seifer DB, Sachs LB, et al: Laparoscopy in 100 women with chronic pelvic pain. Obstet Gynecol 64:672, 1984.
11. Halme J, Hammond MG, Hulka JF, et al: Retrograde menstruation in healthy women and in patients with endometriosis. Obstet Gynecol 64:151, 1984.
12. Sampson JA: Peritoneal endometriosis due to the menstrual dissemination of endometrial tissue into the peritoneal cavity. Am J Obstet Gynecol 14:422, 1927.
13. Kitchin JD III: Endometriosis. *In* Sciarra JJ, McElin TW, and Droegemueller W (eds): Gynecology and Obstetrics, Vol 1. Philadelphia, Harper & Row, 1984.
14. Dmowski WP, Steele RW, and Baker GF: Deficient cellular immunity in endometriosis. Am J Obstet Gynecol 141:377, 1981.
15. Goldman MB and Cramer DW: The epidemiology of endometriosis. Prog Clin Biol Res 323:15, 1990.
16. Dawood MY, Khan-Dawood FS, and Wilson L: Peritoneal fluid prostaglandins and prostanoids in women with endometriosis, chronic pelvic inflammatory disease, and pelvic pain. Am J Obstet Gynecol 148:391, 1984.
17. Barbieri RL and Ryan KJ: Danazol: Endocrine pharmacology and therapeutic applications. Am J Obstet Gynecol 141:453, 1981.
18. Noble AD and Letchworth AT: Medical treatment of endometriosis: A comparative trial. Postgrad Med J 55(Suppl 5):37, 1979.
19. Dlugi AM, Miller JD, and Knittle J: Lupron depot (leuprolide acetate for depot suspension) in the treatment of endometriosis: A randomized, placebo-controlled, double-blind study. Fertil Steril 54:419, 1990.
20. Dawood MY, Lewis V, and Ramon J: Cortical and trabecular bone mineral content in women with endometriosis: Effect of gonadotropin releasing hormone agonist and danazol. Fertil Steril 52:21, 1989.
21. Dalton K: The Premenstrual Syndrome and Progesterone Therapy. Chicago, Year Book Medical Publishers, 1977.
22. Steiner M, Haskett RF, and Carroll BJ: Premenstrual tension syndrome: The development of research diagnostic criteria and new rating scales. Acta Psychiatr Scand 62:177, 1980.
23. American Psychiatric Association: Diagnostic and Statistical Manual of Mental Disorders, 3rd Rev. ed. Washington, DC, American Psychiatric Association, 1987, pp 367–369.
24. Cihal HJ: Premenstrual syndrome: An update for the clinician. Obstet Gynecol Clin North Am 17:457, 1990.
25. Reid RL and Yen SSC: Premenstrual syndrome. Am J Obstet Gynecol 140:874, 1981.
26. Muse KE, Cetel NS, Futterman LA, et al: The premenstrual syndrome: Effects of "medical ovariectomy." N Engl J Med 311:1345, 1984.
27. Freeman E, Rickels K, Sondheimer SJ, and Polansky M: Ineffectiveness of progesterone suppository treatment for premenstrual syndrome. JAMA 264:349, 1990.
28. Doll H, Brown S, Thurston A, and Vessey M: Pyridoxine (vitamin B_6) and the premenstrual syndrome: A randomized, crossover trial. J R Coll Gen Pract 39:364, 1989.
29. Mortola JF, Girton L, and Fisher U: Successful treatment of severe premenstrual syndrome by combined use of gonadotropin-releasing hormone agonist and estrogen/progestin. J Clin Endocrinol Metab 72:252A, 1991.
30. Casper RF and Hearn MT: The effect of hysterectomy and bilateral oophorectomy in women with severe premenstrual syndrome. Am J Obstet Gynecol 162:105, 1990.
31. Casson P, Hahn PM, Van Vugt DA, and Reid RL: Lasting response to ovariectomy in severe intractable premenstrual syndrome. Am J Obstet Gynecol 162:99, 1990.
32. Thys-Jacobs S, Ceccarelli S, Bierman A, et al: Calcium supplementation in premenstrual syndrome: A randomized crossover trial. J Gen Intern Med 4:183, 1989.
33. Johnson SR: Premenstrual syndrome and dysmenorrhea. *In* Rayburn WF and Zuspan FP (eds): Drug Therapy in Obstetrics and Gynecology, 3rd ed. St Louis, MO, Mosby Year Book, 1992, pp 355–374.
34. Halbreich U, Rojansky N, and Palter S: Elimination of ovulation and menstrual cyclicity with danazol improves dysphoric premenstrual syndromes. Fertil Steril 56:1066, 1991.
35. Harrison WM, Endocott J, and Nee J: Treatment of premenstrual dysphoria with alprazolam: A controlled study. Arch Gen Psych 47:270, 1990.
36. Rickels K, Freeman EW, Sondheimer S, et al: Buspirone in the treatment of premenstrual syndrome. Lancet 1:777, 1989.
37. Stone SB, Pearlstein TB, and Brown WA: Fluoxetine in the treatment of late luteal phase dysphoric disorder. J Clin Psychol 52:290, 1991.
38. Erlik Y, Meldrum DR, and Judd HL: Estrogen levels in postmenopausal women with hot flashes. Obstet Gynecol 59:403, 1982.
39. Judd HL, Shamonki IM, Frumar AM, et al: Origin of serum estradiol in postmenopausal women. Obstet Gynecol 59:680, 1982.
40. Freedman RR, Woodward S, and Sabharwal SC: Alpha-2 adrenergic mechanism in menopausal hot flushes. Obstet Gynecol 76:573, 1990.
41. Barrett-Connor E and Bush TL: Estrogen and coronary heart disease in women. JAMA 265:1861, 1991.
42. Gambrell RD: The menopause: Benefits and risks of estrogen-progestogen replacement therapy. Fertil Steril 37:457, 1982.
43. Egeland GM, Kuller LH, Matthews KA, et al: Hormone replacement therapy and lipoprotein changes during early menopause. Obstet Gynecol 76:776, 1990.
44. Walsh BW, Schiff I, Rosner B, et al: Effects of postmenopausal estrogen replacement on the concentrations and metabolism of plasma lipoproteins. N Engl J Med 325:1196, 1991.
45. Voigt LF, Weiss NS, Chu J, et al: Progestogen supplementation of exogenous oestrogens and risk of endometrial cancer. Lancet 338:274, 1991.
46. Boston Collaborative Drug Surveillance Program: Surgically confirmed gallbladder disease, venous thromboembolism, and breast tumors in relation to postmenopausal estrogen therapy. N Engl J Med 290:15, 1974.
47. Petitti DB, Wingerd J, Pelligrin R, et al: Risks of vascular disease in women. JAMA 242:1150, 1979.
48. Gordon EM, Williams SR, Frenchek B, et al: Dose dependent effects of postmenopausal estrogen and progestin on antithrombin III and factor XII. J Lab Clin Med 111:52, 1988.
49. Mandel FP, Geola FL, Ju JKH, et al: Biologic effects of various doses of ethinyl estradiol in postmenopausal women. Obstet Gynecol 59:673, 1982.
50. Young RL, Goepfert AR, and Goldzieher HW: Estrogen replacement therapy is not conducive of venous thromboembolism. Maturitas 13:189, 1991.
51. Schlesselman JJ: Cancer of the breast and reproductive tract in relation to use of oral contraceptives. Contraception 40:1, 1989.
52. Stadel BV, Rubin GL, Webster LA, et al: Oral contraceptives and breast cancer in young women. Lancet 2:970, 1985.
53. Khoo SK and Chick P: Sex steroid hormones and breast cancer: Is there a link with oral contraceptives and hormone replacement therapy? Med J Aust 156:124, 1992.
54. Steinberg K: A meta-analysis of the effect of estrogen replacement therapy on the risk of breast cancer. JAMA 265:1985, 1991.
55. Kaufman DW, Plamer JR, de Mouzon J, et al: Estrogen replacement therapy and the risk of breast cancer: Results from the case-control surveillance study. Am J Epidemiol 134:1375, 1991.
56. Sillero-Arenas M, Delgado-Rodriguez M, Rodrigues-Canteras R, et al: Menopausal hormone replacement therapy and breast cancer: A meta-analysis. Obstet Gynecol 79:286, 1992.
57. Gelfand MM and Ferenczy A: A prospective 1-year study of estrogen and progestin in postmenopausal women: effect on the endometrium. Obstet Gynecol 74:398, 1989.
58. Genant HK, Cann CE, Ettinger B, et al: Quantitative computed tomography of vertebral spongiosa: A sensitive method for detecting early bone loss after oophorectomy. Ann Intern Med 97:699, 1982.
59. Hirvonen E, Malkonen M, and Manninen V: Effects of different progestogens on lipoproteins during postmenopausal replacement therapy. N Engl J Med 304:560, 1981.
60. Clisham PR, deZiegler D, Lozano K, et al: Comparison of continuous versus sequential estrogen and progestin therapy in postmenopausal women. Obstet Gynecol 77:241, 1991.
61. Weinstein L, Bewtra C, and Gallagher JC: Evaluation of a

continuous combined low-dose regimen of estrogen-progestin for treatment of the menopausal patient. Am J Obstet Gynecol 162:1534, 1990.

62. Padwick MI, Pryse-Davis J, and Whitehead MI: A simple method for determining the optimal dosage of progestin in postmenopausal women receiving estrogens. N Engl J Med 315:930, 1986.
63. Koss LG, Schreiber K, Oberlander SG, et al: Detection of endometrial carcinoma and hyperplasia in asymptomatic women. Obstet Gynecol 64:1, 1984.
64. Leather AT, Savvas M, and Studd JWW: Endometrial histology and bleeding patterns after 8 years of continuous combined estrogen and progestogen therapy in postmenopausal women. Obstet Gynecol 78:1008, 1990.

39

Abnormal Uterine Bleeding

PHILLIP G. STUBBLEFIELD, MD

From menarche to menopause, with the exception of pregnancy, women normally experience periodic vaginal bleeding at intervals of 3 to 5 weeks, with each episode lasting 5 to 7 days and associated with characteristic symptoms that precede the onset of bleeding. Normal vaginal bleeding is determined by cyclic release of the sex steroids estrogen and progesterone from the ovaries in response to gonadotropins released by the brain. In the normal menstrual cycle, even as menstruation is occurring, an ovarian follicle is already beginning to mature and to release estrogen. Under the influence of the ovarian estrogen, the lining of the uterus changes from a menstrual to a proliferative pattern. Through positive feedback interactions between the ovaries and the hypothalamus and pituitary, a midcycle surge of the luteinizing hormone is triggered by rising levels of ovarian estrogen. This luteinizing hormone surge, in turn, triggers ovulation, and after that event, the ovarian follicle transforms itself into the corpus luteum, which produces both estrogen and progesterone. Under the influence of progesterone, the proliferative endometrium is transformed into the secretory pattern, and then with the death of the corpus luteum and the fall in the levels of the two steroid hormones, the next menstrual period begins, and the superficial lining of the uterus is shed once again. In ovulatory cycles, the late secretory endometrium also manufactures prostaglandins, which are involved in the mechanism of menstruation and which account for many of the associated symptoms.

Bleeding that occurs at shorter or longer intervals than anticipated or that differs from the customary amount is perceived as abnormal by the patient and may signal any of several abnormalities.

Bleeding that occurs at the normally expected time but that is heavier than normal is described as *menorrhagia* or alternatively as *hypermenorrhea.* Symptoms that suggest an abnormally excessive amount of bleeding are the passage of clots for more than a few hours during a menstrual cycle and "flooding" (i.e., the menstrual blood soaks through a tampon or pad and then onto the woman's clothing). There is a wide variety in the absorbency of the different sizes of tampons or pads presently on the market. However, if a patient reports soaking through a pad or tampon every hour for several hours, this is an abnormally excessive amount of bleeding.

Bleeding that occurs between menstrual periods is referred to by the patient as spotting. The commonly used medical terms for this are *metrorrhagia* or *intermenstrual flow. Polymenorrhea* refers to episodes of bleeding at shorter than normal intervals, i.e., less than 21 days apart, rather than to an excessive amount of flow. *Oligomenorrhea* refers to episodes of bleeding at intervals longer than 35 days, and *amenorrhea* refers to the absence of bleeding. Another pattern of abnormal bleeding is *postcoital bleeding*. Women who have vaginal bleeding more than 1 year after menopause are described as having *postmenopausal bleeding.*

Abnormal uterine bleeding generally has one of five causes: (1) abnormal pregnancy, (2) dysfunctional uterine bleeding, (3) benign organic lesions, (4) malignant lesions of the cervix or uterus, and (5) coagulopathy.[1–3] In many cases, the patient's detailed history of her bleeding pattern will allow the clinician to suspect which of the five possible etiologies is the correct one. Thus, bleeding in association with *pregnancy*, in most cases will follow a period of amenorrhea, and the patient will have the associated symptoms of prolonged breast tenderness, urinary frequency, and morning nausea that frequently characterize pregnancy. These comments notwithstanding, patients with early spontaneous miscarriage or ectopic pregnancy may not have characteristic pregnancy symptoms and may not have a period of recognizable amenorrhea.

Dysfunctional uterine bleeding implies the absence of any detectable organic lesion or pregnancy. It is usually anovulatory and is distinguished by an erratic pattern rather than by normal cyclicity and, in most cases, by the absence of menstrual discomfort, unless the amount of blood clots passed is so great that the patient experiences pain just from the cervical dilatation that accompanies the passage of large clots.

Benign organic lesions of the uterus, such as leiomyomata, are usually associated with excessively heavy menstruation that occurs at the normally expected time and is associated with the usual menstrual symptoms, including cramping discomfort that begins a few hours before the episode of bleeding.

Polyps of the cervix and other benign cervical lesions are frequently associated with *postcoital bleeding*. However, postcoital bleeding is also one of the characteristic signs of invasive cancer of the uterine cervix, as is other intermenstrual bleeding. Bleeding in the perimenopausal period and especially *postmenopausal bleeding* have a high association with cancer of the uterine corpus, that is, endometrial carcinoma. Generalized coagulopathy as a cause of excessive and prolonged menstrual bleeding is rare. However, a significant percentage of patients who develop systemic coagulopathy may have excessive menstrual flow as an early sign of their illness.

SPECIFIC CAUSES OF ABNORMAL UTERINE BLEEDING

Pregnancy

When women in the reproductive years have abnormal uterine bleeding, three questions must be answered. (1) Is the patient pregnant? (2) If so, is the pregnancy intrauterine or extrauterine (ectopic)? (3) If intrauterine, is the pregnancy normal or abnormal? When bleeding is associated with second and third trimester pregnancy, the diagnosis is generally obvious because of the uterine size. However, the most common time for bleeding during pregnancy is in the first trimester, when the uterus may be only minimally enlarged and when differentiating between a pregnant and a nonpregnant state is not possible on clinical grounds alone. Pregnancy tests used in previous years were relatively insensitive. Early gestations and abnormal pregnancies often yielded negative test results. Present pregnancy tests are specific for the β moiety of the human chorionic gonadotropin molecule (β-HCG) and are extremely sensitive. Serum β-HCG assays that will detect as little as 5 to 10 mIU/ml are commonly available, and there are several excellent urine pregnancy tests that will detect 25 to 50 mIU/ml. Consequently, if performed and reported correctly, a negative test result is proof that pregnancy does not exist.

Generally, spontaneous abortion of an intrauterine pregnancy is associated with a history of amenorrhea and symptoms of pregnancy and then with the fairly sudden onset of heavy vaginal bleeding with clots and low abdominal cramping pain. On pelvic examination, the uterus will be found soft and moderately enlarged, the cervix will be partially dilated, and placental tissue will be in the process of being extruded. In such a circumstance, the diagnosis is obvious and the treatment equally obvious—a uterine curettage procedure—unless it appears that the patient has already passed the conceptus in toto and the bleeding has now subsided. Bleeding without cramping and without associated cervical dilatation is considered a threatened abortion; although many such patients will ultimately go on to lose the pregnancy, this is not true in all cases. Five to 10% of women who ultimately deliver a normal baby at term will report some first-trimester vaginal bleeding. Ultrasound examination, especially if performed with a vaginal probe, may help determine whether the conceptus is normal at the time, and therefore whether pregnancy may continue, or whether it is abnormal and very likely will go on to miscarriage.

In the most obvious case of *ectopic pregnancy*, the uterus is minimally enlarged, and there is marked tenderness of one uterine adnexa and possibly a palpable mass. However, the early symptoms of ectopic pregnancy may be minimal, as may be the physical findings. Ectopic pregnancy is very common, occurring in one or more of 100 pregnancies. Therefore, any woman of reproductive age with abnormal vaginal bleeding and pelvic pain merits a sensitive β-HCG–specific pregnancy test.

Dysfunctional Uterine Bleeding

For the most part, dysfunctional uterine bleeding is associated with anovulation and involves bleeding from a proliferative endometrium. Anovulation is commonly seen in the young woman immediately after menarche and in the premenopausal woman. Anovulation can also be seen in the intervening years, especially in association with obesity or with the Stein-Leventhal syndrome and related disorders or major systemic illness.[2–5] With a failure of ovulation, the ovarian follicle may produce excessive amounts of estrogen, with resultant continued stimulation of the endometrium, and ultimately, irregular and excessive bleeding occurs. In the young adolescent, the patient's age and the physical examination are sufficient to suggest a diagnosis of anovulation. After pregnancy is excluded, it is reasonable to proceed directly to hormonal therapy. Unless contraindicated, first choice of therapy would be one of the higher-dose oral contraceptives, which combine estrogen and a progestin. Either norethindrone acetate, 2.5 mg, with 0.05 mg ethinyl estradiol (Norlestrin 2.5/50), or norgestrel, 0.5 mg, and 0.05 mg of ethinyl estradiol (Ovral) is given twice a day for 10 days. This will terminate the current episode of bleeding and produce endometrial atrophy, so that the withdrawal bleeding that occurs at the end of treatment will be minimal. When estrogens are considered contraindicated, hormonal management can be by progestins alone, for example, medroxyprogesterone acetate (Provera), 10 mg twice a day for 10 days. Profuse anovulatory bleeding that persists despite treatment with oral agents can be controlled by curettage (see later) or with high-dose estrogen therapy (conjugated estrogens, 25 mg, given intravenously every 4 hours until bleeding stops).[5] An oral progestin, such as medroxyprogesterone acetate, must be given after estrogen administration in order to avoid recurrent heavy bleeding. The cessation of hormonal therapy will be associated in each case with a new episode of withdrawal bleeding, but this bleeding should be of a lesser magnitude than that which resulted in the need for therapy.

Beyond adolescence, anovulation and the production of ovarian estrogen unopposed by progesterone may have already produced a hyperplasia of the lining of the uterus. An endometrial biopsy is advised, and then hormonal therapy should be begun immediately. Biopsy can be accomplished by various instruments. We use the Pipelle instrument, which is described subsequently. An alternative that is both diagnostic and therapeutic for the present episode is full curettage performed as an office procedure without dilatation or anesthesia by means of one of the small-diameter vacuum cannula systems.

Women with anovulatory bleeding very likely will continue to have anovulatory cycles in the future. Consideration must be given to their long-range therapy, which may involve the use of progestational agents or estrogen and a progestational agent in combination, or the induction of ovulation (see Chapter 41).

Uncommonly, dysfunctional uterine bleeding in the form of prolonged menstruation may occur in an *ovulatory* cycle in association with inadequate function of the corpus luteum or because of a corpus luteum that persists an abnormally long time. In these cases, endometrial biopsy taken during the bleeding episode will show a secretory endometrium but with an unusual pattern described as irregular shedding. Persistent bleeding caused by irregular shedding can be controlled with estrogen and progestin; if persistent corpus luteum is the etiology, suppression of ovulation for several months with oral contraceptive pills is advisable.[5]

Finally, even though synthetic estrogens and progestins are often used in the therapy of dysfunctional uterine bleeding, sex hormone therapy can also produce an abnormal bleeding pattern. Women taking oral contraceptives frequently experience intermenstrual bleeding—a symptom that, if persistent, may require selection of a different oral contraceptive with an increased dose of either the progestin or estrogen component (see discussion in Chapter 40).

Organic Disease of the Uterus or Cervix

Benign organic disease of the uterus or cervix is suggested by a regular pattern of bleeding and normal menstrual symptoms, which have a very high correlation with the presence of ovulatory cycles. Uterine leiomyomata may be suspected if the pelvic examination shows an irregularly enlarged, firm uterus. However, leiomyomata of small size not detectable by pelvic examination can also cause menstrual hemorrhage when they are close to the lining of the uterus (submucosal). Polyps of the endometrium can also produce excessively heavy, but regular, menstrual bleeding.

One of the fairly common organic causes of abnormal bleeding is chronic endometritis, an inflammation of the lining of the uterus. The bleeding pattern is that of excessive and prolonged menstrual periods, with intermenstrual bleeding as well. Chronic endometritis can follow spontaneous or induced abortion or childbirth, is a common occurrence with *Chlamydia trachomatis* infection of the upper genital tract, and it is also seen in association with the wearing of intrauterine contraceptive devices. The same pattern of abnormal bleeding can be associated with intrauterine device use even without any histologic evidence of chronic endometritis and will usually resolve when the device is removed.

In the premenopausal years, endocervical epithelium frequently is found extending well onto the exocervix, where it may become inflamed, producing chronic cervicitis. Mucopurulent cervicitis is often gonorrheal or chlamydial in etiology, and its presence requires the specific tests for these conditions (see Chapter 31); it can be treated with cefoxitin IM plus oral tetracycline. Cervical ectropion, even without mucopurulent cervicitis, may be a cause of intermenstrual bleeding and postcoital bleeding. Polyps of the endocervical epithelium protruding through the cervix can produce the same symptoms. The diagnosis is suspected because the exocervix bleeds during pelvic examination when wiped with a cotton swab, and it appears raw and friable. Ectropion and chronic cervicitis as causes of bleeding can be managed quite effectively by cervical cautery or cryosurgery. However, before this is carried out, cervical cytology should be performed, and biopsy specimens should be taken of the cervix to rule out malignancy. The cervical polyp is dealt with by twisting it off at its base with an instrument such as a Kelly clamp. The base is then cauterized with a silver nitrate applicator. The polyp, of course, is sent for histologic examination.

After excluding pregnancy, the next step in evaluation of the woman with abnormal uterine bleeding is a properly timed endometrial biopsy performed as an office procedure. If the biopsy is performed during the luteal phase of the cycle or at the beginning of menstruation, the biopsy should show secretory or menstrual endometrium, respectively. This finding excludes anovulation as a cause of the bleeding. Both leiomyomata and anovulation commonly occur in perimenopausal women, so the finding of a proliferative rather than a secretory endometrium does not exclude the presence of leiomyomata but does suggest that the abnormal bleeding is caused by anovulation rather than the fibroid.

If abnormal bleeding persists after an office biopsy that showed normal secretory menstrual endometrium, further evaluation is needed. Vaginal-probe ultrasound is advised to look for uterine fibroids, and hysteroscopy will probably be necessary. Hysteroscopy is the direct examination of the uterine cavity with a small telescope passed through the cervical canal. Polyps and small fibroids can be removed hysteroscopically without major surgery. Currently, there is great interest in the treatment of chronic menorrhagia with hysteroscopically guided ablation of the endometrium using either radio frequency electric current or neodymium: yttrium-aluminum-garnet laser.[6]

Malignant Organic Lesions

Estrogen-secreting *ovarian neoplasms*, the most commonly encountered of which are granulosa-theca cell tumors, may produce periods of amenorrhea followed by heavy, irregular uterine bleeding clinically indistinguishable from dysfunctional uterine bleeding; thus, a careful pelvic examination with palpation of the ovaries is an essential component in the evaluation of every woman with abnormal uterine bleeding. Abnormal vaginal bleeding from *carcinoma of the cervix* is, unfortunately, a late symptom. Generally, the pattern is that of intermenstrual bleeding and postcoital bleeding. By the time cervical carcinoma produces bleeding, the diagnosis generally is obvious on pelvic examination by the presence of a fungating mass arising in the cervix. *Endometrial* cancer is, for the most part, a disease of the postmenopausal woman, and its characteristic symptom is irregular vaginal bleeding and spotting. However, endometrial carcinoma will be found in a few women (<2%)[7] who have excessive uterine bleeding in the perimenopausal years and, although rare, will occasionally be found in premenopausal women with excessive bleeding. Hence, sampling the endometrium is recommended for all perimenopausal women with this complaint. For adults in the premenopausal years, a single episode of dysfunctional bleeding can be treated with hormones, but, as mentioned previously, recurrent episodes or bleeding not controlled by hormones warrants endometrial sampling. Techniques for sampling the endometrium are described further on in this chapter.

Coagulopathy

Generally, coagulopathy as a cause of abnormal vaginal bleeding is infrequent, and, therefore, we do not routinely perform coagulation studies. However, if heavy menstrual periods persist after the diagnoses of abnormal pregnancy, dysfunctional uterine bleeding, and benign or malignant organic lesions have been excluded, then a complete investigation of the patient's coagulation system is indicated. Menstrual hemorrhage is a common problem in women with acquired coagulopathy, such as that associated with acute leukemia and von Willebrand's syndrome.

POSTMENOPAUSAL BLEEDING AND ENDOMETRIAL CANCER

The risk of malignancy is substantial among women with symptoms of postmenopausal bleeding. In two series, malignancies were present in 24% and 13%, respectively, of all patients with postmenopausal bleeding.[8, 9] The probability was nearly as great in those with only contact bleeding (21%) or spotting (19%) as in those with frank bleeding (27%); although older patients were at higher risk, malignancies were present in 14% of those between the ages of 45 and 54.[8] Benign conditions commonly associated with postmenopausal bleeding included estrogen administration (13%), atrophic endometrium (12%), senile vaginitis (9%), ulceration of the cervix associated with prolapse (7.5%), cervical polyps (7%), and endometrial polyps (4%).[8, 9] Because any of these benign conditions could be present concurrently in patients with bleeding caused by malignancies, all patients with postmenopausal bleeding require complete diagnostic evaluation.

The incidence of endometrial carcinoma increases markedly with age, to about one case per 10,000 women at age 40 years, but nearly one case per 1000 women between the ages of 55 and 65 years.[10] From the point of view of the epidemiologist, risk factors associated with endometrial cancer are (1) variations of normal anatomy or physiology (obesity, nulliparity, and menopause after age 50 years); (2) the presence of certain abnormalities or diseases (diabetes mellitus, high blood pressure, Stein-Leventhal syndrome); and (3) exposure to known external causes of the disease (history of pelvic irradiation and exposure to exogenous estrogen).[11] These predisposing factors are primarily hormonal, and have in common the exposure either to endogenous or to exogenous estrogens over a long period of time unopposed by progesterone, as occurs in anovulatory states in premenopausal women and in postmenopausal women. The use of unopposed estrogen in the treatment of postmenopausal symptoms increases the risk of endometrial carcinoma. Estimates of the relative risks for estrogen-treated women obtained from eight independent case-controlled studies vary from risk ratios of 3.0 to 8.0.[12] The risk is probably greatest with high doses of estrogen (e.g., conjugated estrogens [Premarin], 1.25 mg/day) and with longer durations of therapy (e.g., 7 years or longer); lower estrogen doses or shorter durations of therapy probably increase the risk also but to a lesser extent. Although conjugated estrogens have been most commonly used in the United States and are, therefore, most often implicated as a cause of endometrial cancer, any other exogenous estrogen would be expected to carry the same risk.

Our current concept is that unopposed estrogen, whether endogenous or exogenous, is associated with the development of endometrial hyperplasia. The endometrial hyperplasias have been classified as either simple or atypical, based on the presence of cytologic atypia on biopsy. Each group is further subdivided, based on the degree of glandular complexity and crowding on histologic examination. Progression of simple hyperplasia to endometrial cancer appears uncommon. In Kurman and associates' series, one of 93 (1%) patients with this pattern developed cancer during follow-up. On the other hand, patients whose lesions had both cellular atypia and a high degree of complexity progressed to cancer in 10 of 35 cases (29%).[13]

The step-by-step progression from mild to severe premalignant lesions that occurs with squamous carcinoma of the cervix has not been as clearly demonstrated for endometrial cancer. Indeed, the large screening program reported by Koss and colleagues found endometrial hyperplasias to be no more prevalent than frank carcinomas, which led those investigators to conclude that in older women, adenocarcinoma may occur with no preceding hyperplasia.[14]

Techniques for Detection of Endometrial Carcinoma or Its Precursor Hyperplasias

The standard Papanicolaou smear taken as a scrape of the exocervix detects approximately 50% of endometrial carcinomas and is therefore not adequate to rule out endometrial cancer. Aspiration of the endocervix using a cytology pipette and rubber bulb was initially reported to increase detection,[15] but a large study was not able to confirm this.[14] Endocervical sampling with a Cytobrush may well improve detection of endometrial lesions, but this effect has not yet been demonstrated. The sensitivity of endocervical cytology is increased if the cytologist reports as suspicious any normal-appearing endometrial cells seen in the postmenopausal woman or endometrial cells seen during the luteal phase of the menstruating woman.

The standard means for diagnosing endometrial lesions has been surgical dilatation and curettage. This was usually performed under general anesthesia in a hospital. In this procedure, tapered metal rods are used to stretch the cervical canal to a diameter of 9 to 10 mm so that a good-sized curette can be inserted into the uterine cavity to scrape the walls. Over the years, the use of small curettes inserted without the need for dilatation has developed. Among these small curettes are the Duncan, Kervorkian, and Novak instruments. More recently, small-bore, flexible plastic cannulas (the Vabra and the Karman) have been introduced for vacuum curettage of the endometrium. These small steel curettes and vacuum curettes obtain actual pieces of endometrium that can be fixed, sectioned, and studied by conventional histology.

The value of the small steel curette has been demonstrated by Ferenczy and colleagues.[16] They evaluated 400 patients whose endometrial biopsies were performed in the office with the Kervorkian curette. Endometrial biopsy specimens obtained with the Kervorkian curette were as good as or better than those obtained by conventional surgical dilatation and curettage. Ferenczy and colleagues obtained adequate tissue for diagnosis in 91.8% of cases. When compared with surgical dilatation and curettage or hysterectomy, diagnostic accuracy was 96.2%. All seven endometrial cancers were correctly diagnosed. Seventy-three per cent of the patients required no further surgical procedure.[16]

The Pipelle device (Pipelle, Unimar Inc., Wilton, CT) developed in France has been widely adopted as the method of choice for endometrial biopsy. The Pipelle is a flexible, small-bore plastic catheter of 2.5 mm external diameter. Its lumen contains a semi-rigid plastic stylet with a small gasket near its tip. The stylet serves to stiffen the instrument for ease of insertion through the cervical canal, and when the stylet is rapidly withdrawn, a vacuum is created that is sufficient to obtain a generous suction biopsy of the endometrium. Several studies have compared the Pipelle device to other means for endometrial sampling. Compared with the Novak suction curette, the Pipelle was as effective in obtaining adequate tissue and was less painful.[17, 18] In a study of patients with known endometrial cancer who had endometrial biopsies with the Pipelle in the doctor's office without anesthesia, the Pipelle biopsy correctly diagnosed cancer in 39 of 40 specimens (97.5% sensitivity).[19] In one case, the Pipelle biopsy showed atypical endometrial hyperplasia, the preceding dilatation and curettage specimen was read as grade 1 adenocarcinoma, while the hysterectomy specimen was interpreted as adenocarcinoma in situ.

Ultrasound offers considerable promise as a way to determine which patients need endometrial biopsy. In the small series reported to date, if the endometrium was no thicker than 4 mm on examination with vaginal-probe ultrasound, biopsy always showed either an inactive or low-estrogen–stimulation histologic pattern. Endometrium measured as more than 4 mm could be a normal proliferative pattern but could also be hyperplasia or cancer.[20] There are no cost savings to using ultrasound rather than endometrial biopsy, and patients with endometrial thickness greater than 4 mm will still need a biopsy. However, ultrasound is less invasive than a biopsy, is painless, and can be performed by a technician.

Error is possible in endometrial biopsy. One may sample only the lower uterine segment and not the fundus. A well-trained gynecologic pathologist will suspect this on examination of the tissue and will so indicate. Another source of error is that some patients with endometrial cancer will show only necrotic tissue and fibrin on endometrial biopsy.[21] Such findings mandate surgical dilatation and curettage. Complications are possible with any of the techniques for sampling of the endometrium. Some patients experience strong vagal reactions and syncope, and it is possible to perforate the uterus by insertion of any instrument into the uterine cavity. Nonetheless, occurrence of complications in large series with endometrial sampling has been rare.

Technique for Endometrial Biopsy with the Pipelle

A pelvic examination is performed to confirm the position and size of the uterus. The cervix is exposed with a speculum and cleansed with an antiseptic solution. We advise injecting 1 to 2 ml of 1% plain lidocaine into the anterior lip of the cervix before placement of a tenaculum. Next, the Pipelle is introduced through the cervical canal into the uterine cavity. With practice, the operator learns to sense when the internal os has been traversed. If the Pipelle cannot be inserted without force, the attempt should be abandoned and gynecologic consultation obtained. In about 3% of postmenopausal women, the cervix is too stenotic for endometrial biopsy without dilatation. Dilatation in these cases requires special small dilators and considerable skill.

Once the Pipelle is in the uterine cavity, the stylet is withdrawn to the stop, creating a vacuum. The Pipelle is then gently rotated, advanced, and retracted, taking care not to withdraw the tip from the endometrial cavity until the plastic pipette is filled with endometrial tissue. The Pipelle is then withdrawn and evacuated onto a piece of absorbent paper to create a block of tissue that is then placed in formalin, with the paper included, for fixation. In the patient who is actively bleeding, the first pass with the Pipelle may obtain only blood clot. In this case, the Pipelle should be reintroduced and the procedure repeated so that actual endometrium is obtained. There is no need to cut the end off the Pipelle to evacuate the tissue.

Full surgical dilatation and curettage and hysteroscopy with the patient under anesthesia is indicated for further diagnosis if the endometrial biopsy specimen shows any of the following: inadequate tissue or only lower uterine segment, fibrin and necrosis, or any of the *atypical* endometrial hyperplasia patterns. It should also be performed if postmenopausal bleeding persists after endometrial biopsy.

Great caution is required if any kind of hyperplasia is diagnosed from an endometrial biopsy. In the premenopausal woman, simple hyperplasias can be presumed, at least initially, to be the result of temporary unopposed estrogen associated with anovulation, and treatment would be prescribed with a progestational agent, such as medroxyprogesterone acetate, 5 to 10 mg/day, started on day 14 of the cycle, continued for 14 days, and repeated each cycle. Subsequently, endometrial biopsy would be repeated after 3 months to confirm that hyperplasia did not persist. Postmenopausal women on unopposed estrogen need to have progestin therapy added for at least 14 days each month, and then need to be rebiopsied to prove that the hyperplasia is gone. Atypical hyperplasia is of much greater concern, because it may coexist with endometrial carcinoma and has a high probability of progression. The young woman who wishes to have children requires complete evaluation with hysteroscopy, surgical dilatation and curettage, prolonged progestin therapy, repeat curettage to rule out persistent hyperplasia, and regular biopsies thereafter. The postmenopausal patient not on hormone therapy and the younger woman who does not desire further pregnancies are probably best served with hysterectomy if they have atypical hyperplasia.

Screening Asymptomatic Women for Endometrial Cancer: Should It Be Done?

Whether or not asymptomatic women who are not receiving estrogens should have periodic endometrial sampling is not yet clear. There are no risk factors sufficiently powerful to identify a group of women who can be excluded from screening.[11] Although obesity, nulliparity, age greater than 50 years at menopause, and exogenous estrogen therapy are risk factors in endometrial cancer, Richardson has observed that of women with endometrial cancer, 78% were *not* obese, 58% were *not* nulliparous, 22% were *younger* than 49 when they ceased menstruating, and 43 to 89% had received *no* hormone replacement.[22] Cramer has suggested that at a minimum women who are followed-up for 15 years beginning at age 50 years have a cumulative risk of 1% of developing endometrial carcinoma if they are not receiving estrogens and up to 7% if they are receiving estrogens.[10] Twenty per cent of women with endometrial cancer report no symptoms of abnormal bleeding. Whitehead and colleagues have reported that of women with no abnormal bleeding requesting estrogen therapy for menopausal symptoms, 2% already had endometrial carcinoma present on biopsy before estrogen therapy was started, and 7% had one of the hyperplasia patterns present.[23] Koss's group found endometrial carcinoma at the rate of 6.96 per 1000 when 2586 asymptomatic women aged 45 or more years were screened in New York City.[14] Ferenczy and Gelfand have suggested that all women have endometrial sampling once they reach 50 years of age, and that high-risk women, regardless of age, have this procedure performed. They suggested that as a minimum there should be an initial endometrial biopsy; if the biopsy result is negative and satisfactory, the biopsy could be repeated at intervals of 2 to 3 years.[24] Screening with vaginal-probe ultrasound as described earlier may offer yet another alternative.

Gambrell has proposed a different approach to the detection of endometrial hyperplasia or cancer in asymptomatic women: the progesterone-challenge test.[25] If postmenopausal women bleed in response to progesterone, they may have sufficient endogenous estrogen production to place them at risk for endometrial cancer. A small-scale test of this idea was reported by Hanna and colleagues. Twenty-five menopausal women who did not bleed when given a progestin had normal endometrial biopsy specimens, but three of the five women who bled after receiving the progestin had endometrial hyperplasia on biopsy.[26] In a separate study, 30 asymptomatic postmenopausal women and 10 women with biopsy-proven adenomatous hyperplasia were given the progestin. The progesterone challenge test had a sensitivity of 100% and a specificity of 92%.[27]

None of these approaches has as yet been widely accepted, and no prospective study of their cost-effectiveness in a large, randomly selected population has been performed. Nevertheless, in view of the facts that early endometrial carcinoma is highly curable and that the techniques are readily available, screening with ultrasound, progesterone-challenge test, or endometrial biopsy deserves serious consideration.

Recommendations for Assessment and Follow-up of Postmenopausal Women

1. *Postmenopausal bleeding.* Any woman with postmenopausal bleeding of any degree should be promptly evaluated with an endometrial sampling by the small curette or with a vacuum Pipelle curettage performed in the doctor's office. If the symptoms of postmenopausal bleeding persist after a normal biopsy, then hysteroscopy and full surgical dilatation and curettage should be performed.
2. *Other indications for biopsy.* Other clear-cut indications for endometrial biopsy are a cervical Papanicolaou smear that shows endometrial cells during the luteal phase of the cycle in the perimenopausal woman, a smear that shows any endometrial cells at all in the postmenopausal woman, bleeding after the administration of a progesterone-challenge test, or endometrial thickness greater than 4 mm on vaginal-probe ultrasound measurement.

REFERENCES

1. Schnatz PT: Bleeding and amenorrhea. *In* Romney SL, Gray MT, Little AB, et al (eds): Gynecology and Obstetrics: The Health Care for Women. New York, McGraw-Hill, 1975, pp 179–197.
2. Cowan BD and Morrison JC: Management of abnormal genital bleeding in girls and women. N Engl J Med 324:1715, 1991.

2a. Goldfarb JM and Little AB: Abnormal vaginal bleeding. N Engl J Med 302:666, 1980.

3. Long CA and Gast MJ: Menorrhagia. Obstet Gynecol Clin North Am 17:343, 1990.
4. Yen SSC and Jaffe RB: Reproductive Endocrinology. Philadelphia, WB Saunders, 1978.
5. Speroff L, Glass RH, and Kase NG: Clinical Gynecological Endocrinology and Infertility, 4th ed. Baltimore, Williams & Wilkins, 1989, p 265.
6. Goldrath MH, Fuller TA, and Segal S: Laser photovaporization of endometrium for the treatment of menorrhagia. Am J Obstet Gynecol 140:14, 1981.
7. Ferenczy A, Guralnick M, and Gelfand MM: Out-patient diagnostic techniques for endometrial carcinoma. Comp Ther 4:27, 1978.
8. Keirse MJNC: Clinical review. Aetiology of postmenopausal bleeding. Postgrad Med J 49:344, 1973.
9. Inglis RN, Weir JH, and Shayka A: An improved device for office endometrial biopsies. Contemp Obstet Gynecol 13:61, 1979.
10. Cramer DW: Epidemiology of the gynecologic cancers. Comp Ther 4:9, 1978.
11. MacMahon B: Risk factors for endometrial cancer. Gynecol Oncol 2:122, 1974.
12. Weinstein MC: Estrogen use in postmenopausal women—costs, risks, and benefits. N Engl J Med 303:308, 1980.
13. Kurman RJ, Kaminski PF, and Norris HJ: The behavior of endometrial hyperplasia: A long term study of "untreated" hyperplasia in 170 patients. Cancer 56:403, 1985.
14. Koss LG, Schreiber K, Oberlander SG, et al: Detection of endometrial carcinoma and hyperplasia in asymptomatic women. Obstet Gynecol 64:1, 1984.
15. Richart RM: The debate over screening for endometrial cancer. Contemp Obstet Gynecol 14:100, 1979.
16. Ferenczy A, Shore M, Guralnick M, et al: The Kervorkian curette: An appraisal of its effectiveness in endometrial evaluation. Obstet Gynecol 54:262, 1979.
17. Stoval TG, Ling FW, and Morgan PL: A prospective, randomized comparison of the Pipelle endometrial sampling device with the Novak curette. Am J Obstet Gynecol 165:1287, 1991.
18. Silver MM, Miles P, and Rosa C: Comparison of Novak and Pipelle endometrial biopsy instruments. Obstet Gynecol 78:828, 1991.
19. Stovall TG, Photopulos GJ, Poston WM, et al: Pipelle endometrial sampling in patients with known endometrial carcinoma. Obstet Gynecol 77:954, 1991.
20. Varner ER, Sparks JM, Cameron CD, et al: Transvaginal sonography of the endometrium in postmenopausal women. Obstet Gynecol 78:195, 1991.
21. Steiner GJ and Craig JM: Endometrial biopsy: A valuable adjunct in diagnosis and management of adenocarcinoma of the uterine corpus. Obstet Gynecol 24:389, 1964.
22. Richardson GS: Rationale for the format of the workshop and summary of non-endocrine aspects of endometrial carcinoma. *In* Richardson GS and MacLaughlin DT (eds): Hormonal Biology of Endometrial Cancer, Vol 42. International Union Against Cancer. Geneva, 1978, p 3.
23. Whitehead MI, McQueen J, Beard RJ, et al: The effect of cyclical estrogen therapy and sequential estrogen-progestogen therapy on the endometrium of postmenopausal women. Acta Obstet Gynecol Scand 65(Suppl):91, 1977.
24. Ferenczy A and Gelfand MM: Appraisal of techniques for the office diagnosis of corpus carcinoma and its precursors. J Diagn Gynecol Obstet 1:49, 1979.
25. Gambrell ED: The menopause: Benefits and risks of estrogen-progestogen replacement therapy. Fertil Steril 37:457, 1982.
26. Hanna JH, Brady WK, Hill JM, et al: Detection of postmenopausal women at risk for endometrial carcinoma by a progesterone challenge test. Am J Obstet Gynecol 147:872, 1983.
27. Toppozada MK, Ismail AA, Hamed KS, et al: Progesterone challenge test and estrogen assays in menopausal women with endometrial adenomatous hyperplasia. Int J Gynaecol Obstet 26:115, 1988.

40

Contraception

MITCHELL D. CREININ, MD
PHILIP D. DARNEY, MD, MSc

The primary health care of women often involves helping them avoid or time pregnancies. The purpose of this chapter is to present a historical perspective of fertility control methods in medical care, a framework for evaluating and prescribing the most commonly used contraceptive methods, and a discussion of the risks and benefits of each.

Effective and safe contraception involves the knowledgeable and responsible participation of both partners. In choosing a method of contraception, both partners must decide what they want from contraception. For example, if protection against sexually transmitted disease (STD) is of primary importance, then a barrier method is the best choice. If high efficacy is more important, then hormonal contraception, like oral contraceptives or levonorgestrel implants (Norplant) may be a better choice. If high efficacy without the need for user compliance (e.g., to remember to take a pill) is important, then an intrauterine device (IUD) or an implant may be a good selection. Once a couple decides on the features that are most important, it is easier to help them select a method, or combination of methods, to best provide them with safe and effective contraception.

Modern methods of birth planning—hormonal and intrauterine conception—have been available only since the late 1950s. These methods have made contraception less burdensome and have made birth planning possible for anyone. Birth prevention has not, however, always depended on the contraceptive methods that are discussed in this chapter; long before industrial technology and social morality permitted the distribution of contraceptives, families found other means by which to limit their size.[1] The advent of the "family planning movement" in Britain and the United States preceded by many years significant medical responsibility for birth control. The development of modern contraception resulted from a timely interaction of social, technologic, and medical events in the early 1950s.[2] Clinical trials and widespread availability of modern contraceptive methods followed by the early 1960s. Statistical and epidemiologic methods developed especially for the evaluation of contraceptives have, over the past 30 years, created a vast literature about the safety, side effects, and effectiveness of birth control.

CONTRACEPTIVE EFFECTIVENESS, SAFETY, AND ACCEPTABILITY

The effectiveness of any method of contraception in preventing unwanted pregnancy is dependent on the inherent properties of the method as well as the person using the method. "Theoretical effectiveness" refers to the maximal effectiveness of a contraceptive when it is used precisely as prescribed or recommended by the manufacturer. "Use effectiveness," on the other hand, refers to the success a sample of persons using a particular method has in preventing pregnancy; it reflects compliance and the conditions of use. Table 40–1 shows the theoretical and use effectiveness of the most common methods of contraception in use today.

Use effectiveness approaches theoretical effectiveness with methods that are not coitus related and do not depend on user compliance. Thus, methods such as sterilization, IUDs, intramuscular medroxyprogesterone acetate (Depo-Provera), and levonorgestrel implants (Norplant) have very similar theoretical and use-effectiveness rates. In addition, the efficacy for a given method is dependent on the population in which the method is studied. For example, the effectiveness of a contraceptive method varies by age group (Fig. 40–1) and tends to increase with each continuous year of use. For patients requesting advice, use effectiveness is probably a more helpful guide in choosing a method.

Effectiveness of a contraceptive technique was initially measured by the *Pearl Index:* the number of pregnancies per 100 woman-years of use. This method has several deficiencies that the newer life-table methods take into account by calculating "net" rates of discontinuation. These net rates eliminate all but one reason for discontinuation. Using *multiple-decrement life-table* discontinuation rates, a clinician can describe the probability of discontinuation for various reasons (e.g., pregnancy, side effects, or dissatisfaction) after a particular number of months of use. As with the *Pearl Index,* the life-table–based rates of contraceptive continuation depend on the features of the population studied. It is important, therefore, that the life-table continuation rates the clinician uses to assist a prospective user of contraception be derived from an appropriate population.

TABLE 40–1. FAILURE RATES DURING THE FIRST YEAR OF USE IN THE UNITED STATES*

	% of Women with Pregnancy	
Method	*Theoretical Effectiveness (%)*	*Use Effectiveness (%)*
No method	85.0	85.0
Vasectomy	0.1	0.15
Levonorgestrel implants	0.2	0.2
Depo-Provera	0.3	0.3
Tubal ligation	0.2	0.4
Combination pill	0.1	3.0
Minipill	0.5	3.0
Intrauterine device		3.0
TCu380A	0.8	<1.0
Progestasert or Progesterone T	2.0	2.0
Condom	2.0	12.0
Cervical cap	6.0	18.0
Diaphragm	6.0	18.0
Sponge		
Parous women	9.0	28.0
Nulliparous women	6.0	18.0
Withdrawal	4.0	18.0
Periodic abstinence		20.0
Calendar	9.0	
Ovulation	3.0	
Symptothermal	2.0	
Postovulation	1.0	
Spermicide	3.0	21.0

*Adapted from Trussell J, Hatcher RA, Cates W, Jr, et al: Contraceptive failure in the United States: An update. Stud Fam Plann 21:51, 1990.

In addition to effectiveness, safety and acceptability have traditionally been considered important characteristics of contraceptive methods. Evaluation of contraceptive safety has depended not so much on special methodology, as has the study of effectiveness, but rather on extensive application of standard epidemiologic and statistical methods for measuring drug-related complications. Contraceptive acceptability is the extent to which individuals or populations find a particular contraceptive method to be practical. Acceptability is obviously important because it has great influence on the use effectiveness of contraception and on personal sexual satisfaction.

ORAL CONTRACEPTION

Following clinical trials in 1956 and Federal Drug Administration (FDA) approval in 1960, use of oral contraceptives in the United States accelerated rapidly until initial enthusiasm was tempered by evidence of toxicity. Initial formulations contained relatively large doses of synthetic estrogens and progestogens, providing a very high level of efficacy but also undesirable clinical and metabolic effects. Use declined, then accelerated, so that by 1976, nearly one third of all American women aged 15 to 44 years relied on oral contraception.[3] Their popularity decreased again in the late 1970s, after reports of their association with arterial disease—principally myocardial infarction—in women older than 40 years of age.[4, 5] In 1978, the World Health Organization recommended using oral contraceptives containing the lowest possible estrogen and progestin doses to maintain efficacy but minimize side effects.[6] Improvements initially focused on dose reductions of the original formulations, followed by variation of the steroid dosing through the cycle in biphasic and triphasic regimens. With lower-dose formulations, popularity again surged, and by 1988, nearly 20% of American women aged 15 to 44 years used oral contraception.[3]

Formulations and Mechanism of Action

A clinician reviewing the more than 60 different trade names of oral contraceptives marketed around the world might conclude that they present an impossible prescribing dilemma; these products are derived from two types of synthetic estrogen and nine types of synthetic progestins. Although the list of oral contraceptives is long, low-dose pills with 20 to 35 μg of ethinyl estradiol combined with 0.15 to 1.0 mg of a progestogen are appropriate for the majority of prescribing situations. The progestins commonly used vary considerably in their progestogenic, estrogenic, and androgenic potencies, thereby leading to varying side effects. Until recently, the estrogen component was the focus of the epidemiologist's criticism and the clinician's attention, resulting in a gradual decrease from 150 μg to the doses presently available. Recently, more attention has been given to the progestin component, leading to the development of new synthetic progestins (e.g., norgestimate, gestodene, and desogestrel) with better cycle control and a lower incidence of side effects because they have little androgenic and estrogenic activity.

Both the estrogen and the progestogen components act on the hypothalamus to inhibit gonadotropin secretion so that ovulation is inhibited. The hypothalamus is "fooled" into thinking that the woman is pregnant, with the high levels of estrogen suppressing follicle-stimulating hormone secretion and progestogen suppressing luteinizing hormone secretion. Progestin-only pills ("minipills") will suppress ovulation in some, but not all, cycles by inhibiting the luteinizing hormone surge; however, because of the lack of estrogen, endometrial instability occurs, resulting in irregular endometrial shedding.

Although the estrogen component is important in maintaining a stable endometrial lining, the progestogen component exerts a dominant influence on the character of the lining, resulting in a hypotrophic endometrium unsuitable for ovum implantation. In addition, the progestogen promotes secretion of a thick cervical mucus, which retards sperm penetration. Progestogens may also alter oviductal transport of both sperm and egg. These supplementary contraceptive effects are important adjuvants, especially when a pill is missed and ovulation may occur, or with progestin-only pills, which do not reliably inhibit ovulation.

Effectiveness

A safe and acceptable contraceptive method is not likely to please many users if it is also not reasonably effective. Oral contraceptives are theoretically so effective that a clinician can assure the patient that if she takes the pills as directed, she will not become pregnant. Method failures usually are related to a delay in the initiation of the following cycle when the patient extends the 7-day pill-free interval; this extension allows the ovary to escape suppression. Thus, the 28-day package, with seven placebo pills, improves patient compliance. Typical failure rates during the first year of use are 3.0%, but with very motivated subjects, an annual failure rate of 0.1% is achievable.[7] Efficacy decreases significantly without estrogen, as in the progestin-only "minipill."

Oral Contraceptives and Cardiovascular Disease

A major problem encountered by clinicians when discussing the side effects of birth control pills is that the data

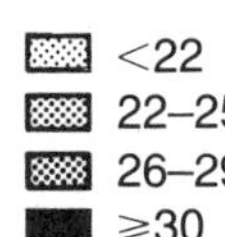

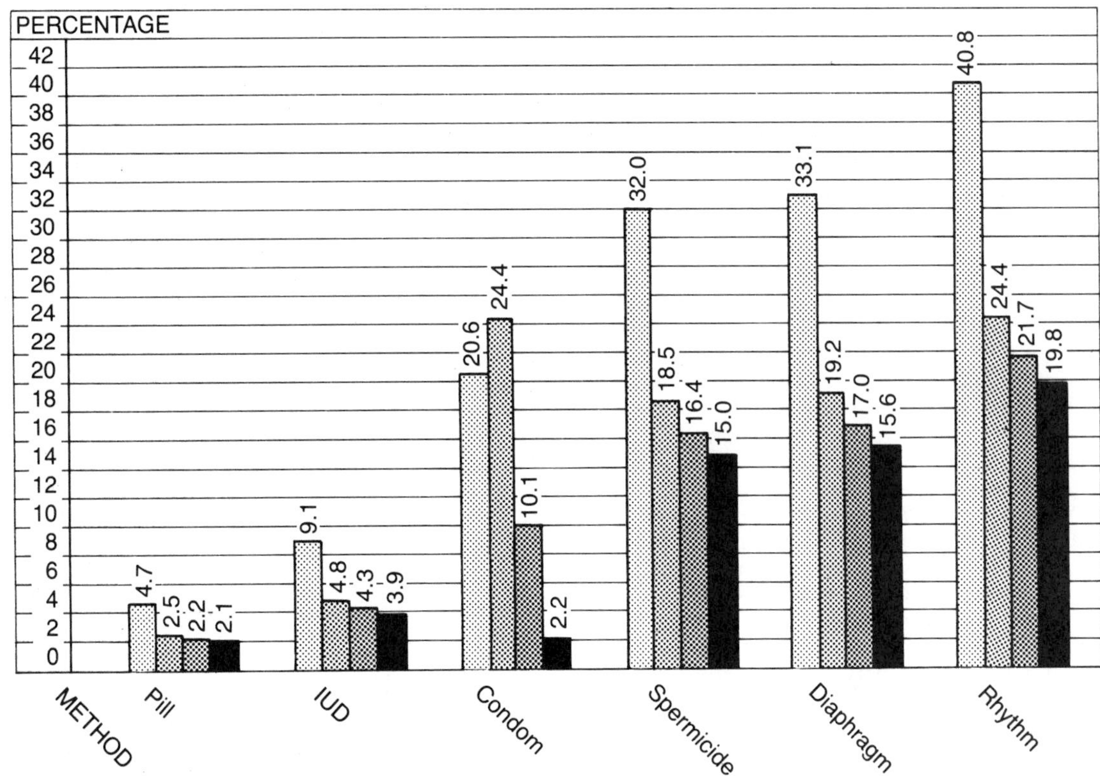

FIGURE 40–1. Estimated percentage of currently married women who become pregnant within the first year of contraceptive use, by type of methods used, according to age-group of women, 1970 to 1976. (From Ory HW, Forrest JD, and Lincoln R: Making Choices: Evaluating the Health Risks and Benefits of Birth Control Methods. New York, Alan Guttmacher Institute, 1983.)

often presented to patients are derived from older pills of higher dosage, whereas clinicians presently use low-dose pills and new formulations.

The birth control pill was first implicated as a causative agent of thromboembolic disease in young women as a result of the studies of Vessey and Doll in Britain.[8] This early evidence found support in other retrospective evaluations, but long-term prospective studies by the Royal College of General Practitioners,[4, 9] the Oxford/Family Planning Association,[5, 10] the Kaiser Walnut Creek study,[11] the Nurses Health Study,[12] and the Puget Sound study[13–15] have found much lower levels of mortality than predicted by the retrospective analyses. Much was learned from these studies about what types of patients develop cardiovascular disease when they use oral contraceptives. These studies indicated that the risk of myocardial infarction with pill use was increased only in women over the age of 35 who also smoked cigarettes. In addition, the British data implicated a relationship between progestin dose and cardiovascular disease, but only in doses that are no longer used in currently available pills. The majority of the conclusions derived from these older studies implicated pill doses greater than those available today or involved pill use in patients who would not be prescribed birth control pills today because of underlying risk factors for cardiovascular disease. More recent studies of low-dose formulations in healthy women show no increased incidence of stroke or cardiovascular deaths.[15–18]

Metabolic Effects

In addition to their contraceptive effects, oral contraceptives cause metabolic changes that may cause major and minor side effects and, hence, affect their safety and acceptability. For example, the estrogen component alters blood coagulability by increasing fibrin formulation and platelet aggregation and decreasing antithrombin III activity. These effects, however, have been found only with pills containing ≥ 50 μg of ethinyl estradiol. Studies of the blood coagulation system and the use of low-dose pills show no overall change in blood coagulability, with slight increases in thrombin formation offset by increased fibrinolytic activity. The progestogen component can rarely cause a slight increase in blood pressure in users of low-dose pills, a slight decrease in glucose tolerance, and a decrease in ratios of high- to low-density serum lipoproteins. Oral contraceptives also affect bile solubility, resulting in concern for women with impaired liver function or those who have a propensity to form gallstones. This factor does not appear to be important for women who have normal liver function.

When considering these effects, clinicians should discriminate between statistical significance and clinical significance. The clinical significance of changes in serum lipoproteins, carbohydrate metabolism, and blood pressure with low-dose oral contraceptives (<50 μg of ethinyl estradiol), are usually negligible.

Oral Contraceptives and Cancer

Ever since birth control pills were first prescribed, women and their physicians have been concerned about the possibility that their long-term use might increase the risk of cancer. Reassuring evidence shows that oral contraceptives decrease the risk of developing endometrial and ovarian cancer by one half.[19, 20] In the 1980s, approximately 2000 cases of endometrial cancer and 1700 cases of ovarian cancer were averted annually in the United States by past and current use of oral contraceptives. Whether oral contraceptives increase the incidence of premalignant and malignant changes of the cervix is still unclear; because results of studies disagree, the risk is assumed to be small.[21, 22] An apparent cervical cancer increase may be due to increased surveillance because pill users have more frequent Papanicolaou smears.[21] Also, confounding factors related to number of partners and lack of barrier contraception (risk factors for the development of cervical cancer) are difficult to control for in these studies.

Likewise, multiple conflicting studies have been published regarding the risk of breast cancer, and the cumulative experience results in no increased risk; oral contraceptives may promote earlier development of breast cancers and not new cancer. The Centers for Disease Control[23] conducted the largest case-control study on the subject and showed an increased risk of early breast cancer only in young women with early menarche who used oral contraceptives for a long time before their first birth. Duration of use, long-term use, or specific type of estrogen or progestin did not affect the overall risk of breast cancer. Women using birth control pills are somewhat less likely to develop breast cancer at an older age, a finding that suggests that breast cancer may be diagnosed earlier in pill users. In addition, no increased risk was found in women with risk factors for breast cancer, specifically benign breast disease or a family history of breast cancer. The incidence of benign breast disease is also decreased by the use of oral contraceptives.

Benign hepatocellular adenoma was once considered to be more common in birth control pill users. However, the incidence is related to the duration of use and steroid dosage. No cases of these tumors have been reported with low-dose oral contraceptive use. Similarly, there is no evidence linking oral contraceptive use to melanoma,[24] hepatocellular carcinoma,[25] gall bladder cancer, colon cancer, renal carcinoma, or pituitary tumors.[26]

Interactions with Other Drugs

The two classes of drugs that have been reported to alter oral contraceptive effectiveness are antibiotics and anticonvulsants. Several antibiotics interfere with enterohepatic circulation of oral estrogens, and there are several dozen case reports of women who have become pregnant while taking antibiotics with their contraceptive steroid preparations. However, antibiotics implicated in reducing the bioavailability of oral contraceptives (e.g., ampicillin, tetracycline, erythromycin, and nitrofurantoin) do not change plasma levels of the contraceptive steroids and have not been found in a large database review to result in method failure.[27]

Several reports have confirmed the occasional failure of oral contraceptives in patients receiving anticonvulsants. Phenytoin, carbamazepine, primidone, and phenobarbital are known to stimulate the hydroxylation of steroids, thereby affecting the duration and intensity of their action. They may also increase the concentration of sex-hormone binding globulin and thereby reduce the biologic effectiveness of contraceptive steroids. Likewise, the antituberculosis agent rifampin is a potent enzyme-inducing agent that enhances the metabolism of both the estrogenic and progestogenic components of oral contraceptives. Still, oral contraceptives provide a very effective method of birth control for women taking these medications and do not affect the seizure threshold or the effectiveness of the anticonvulsants themselves. If a patient on medications that affect liver metabolism cannot use another form of contraception, then an oral contraceptive with 50 μg of ethinyl estradiol taken at the same time every day is an acceptable alternative.

Beneficial Effects

The noncontraceptive benefits of birth control pills include regular menses with decreased flow, less dysmenorrhea, less anemia, decreased incidence of endometrial and ovarian cancers and benign breast disease and pelvic inflammatory disease (PID). Women who use birth control pills for more than 12 months have one third the incidence of symptomatic PID found in nonusers.[28] In addition, there are fewer ectopic pregnancies, benign ovarian cysts, and uterine leiomyomata, and improvement of rheumatoid arthritis.

The risk of death from cardiovascular disease among nonsmoking women using oral contraceptives under 35 years of age is extremely small—approximately one or two deaths per 100,000 users per year.[29] When the reduced risks of PID, ectopic pregnancy, and endometrial and ovarian cancer are also considered, the low-dose birth control pill has a positive effect on women's health and provides a substantial cost savings for the health care system (Table 40–2).

Oral contraceptives are also used frequently to manage disorders unrelated to fertility control, including dysfunctional uterine bleeding, dysmenorrhea, menorrhagia-related anemia, endometriosis, acne, and hirsutism. Also, they act as a simple means to provide hormone replacement for the young woman with hypothalamic amenorrhea and to regulate cycles in the oligo-ovulatory woman.

Other Effects

Because oral contraceptives are often prescribed to younger women who have not begun or not completed childbearing, their effects on subsequent fertility are of great importance. Early reports from the Royal College of General Practitioners[30] and the Oxford Family Planning Association[31, 32] noted a delay in conception in former pill users. The Royal College of General Practitioners study found that 85% of nulliparous and 93% of parous women were pregnant by the end of 2 years after cessation of pill use. The Oxford Family Planning Association study also confirmed a slight delay, but more recent analysis has shown this delay to be concentrated in nulliparous women 30 to 34 years old. Overall, at the end of 2 years, 82% of former pill users had given birth, compared with 89% of women who had used other methods. This delay is explained by an apparent "slow start" during the first 3

TABLE 40–2. HOSPITALIZATIONS PREVENTED ANNUALLY BY USE OF ORAL CONTRACEPTIVES*†

Disease	No. of Hospitalizations Prevented Annually Per 100,000 Pill Users	No. of Hospitalizations Prevented Annually†
Benign breast disease	235	25,100
Benign ovarian cysts	35	3700
Iron-deficiency anemia‡	320	34,200
Pelvic inflammatory disease		
Total episodes with	600	64,200
hospitalization‡	156	16,700
Ectopic pregnancy	117	12,500
Rheumatoid arthritis‡	32	3400
Endometrial cancer§	5	2000
Ovarian cancer§	4	1700

*Adapted from Mosher WD and Pratt WF: Use of family planning services in the United States: 1982 and 1988, Advance data from vital and health statistics; No. 184. National Center for Health Statistics, Hyattsville, MD, 1990; and Ory HW: The noncontraceptive health benefits from oral contraceptive use. Fam Plann Perspect 14:182, 1982.

†Except where noted, based on 10.7 million current users of oral contraceptives in the United States.

‡Episodes prevented regardless of whether hospitalization occurred.

§Based on an estimated 39 million American women who have ever used oral contraceptives (as of 1982).

months after cessation of oral contraceptives as compared with other methods (Table 40–3).[33] From 3 to 12 months, the conception rates are approximately the same. After 12 months, the pregnancy rate among former pill users increases such that by 24 months, 90% of these women had conceived.

In view of these data, the clinician can confidently explain to a woman who has not yet borne children that use of oral contraceptives is not a threat to future childbearing. There is no increase in the incidence of spontaneous abortion after stopping oral contraception. Also, there is no evidence that periodic cessation (a "pill holiday") is warranted; sometimes, it only results in unintended pregnancy.

The use of oral contraceptives increases the incidence of some conditions—migraine headache, hay fever, ocular dryness, and gallbladder disease in women who are known to have cholelithiasis. Oral contraception should be used with caution in these patients. There is no evidence that the use of oral contraceptives in the pubertal woman who has menstruated impairs growth or development.

Contraindications

The epidemiologic studies described previously point out the principal medical contraindications to oral contraceptive use. Women with deep-vein thrombophlebitis, a past history of thromboembolic disorders, severe hypertension, atherosclerotic disease, or impaired liver function should not use oral contraceptives. Women with known or suspected breast cancer or other estrogen-dependent cancers likewise should not use estrogen-containing oral contraceptives. Women with undiagnosed abnormal genital bleeding should not receive birth control pills without a full evaluation, including a pregnancy test. Ideally, women who are known or suspected to be pregnant should not take oral contraceptives; however, two initial reports on the teratogenicity of oral contraceptives have been disproven by 10 times as many reports refuting any such effects.

The greatly increased risk of death due to myocardial infarction or other thromboembolic disease among women over the age of 35 who are also heavy smokers is clear. In the past, it was recommended that women over the age of 40 not use oral contraceptives because of a higher risk of myocardial infarction. However, re-evaluation of the data on which these recommendations were based revealed that this risk existed only in women with other risk factors for cardiovascular disease, e.g., cigarette smoking and uncontrolled hypertension (Table 40–4). More recent studies suggest that oral contraceptive use in women older than 40 years of age is relatively safe in the absence of smoking, hypercholesterolemia, hypertension, or other causes of vascular disease.[12] Thus, women older than 35 years of age without risk factors for cardiovascular disease can safely use oral contraceptives but should have their blood pressure, serum cholesterol, and fasting blood sugar evaluated annually.

Selection and Use

The choice of a particular oral contraceptive preparation depends on assessment of the risk factors described previously as well as cost, preference for certain packaging and instructions, and the woman's and her clinician's experience with various preparations (Table 40–5). In most situations, the preparation of choice is the one containing the lowest dose of estrogen and progestogen consistent with an acceptable menstrual pattern. Only under unusual circumstances is the dose >35 μg of ethinyl estradiol and, for some women, it is as low as 20 μg. A history of intolerable minor side effects with previous use of low-dose combinations may alter this plan, but the best course is to try a different low-dose preparation.

Breakthrough bleeding commonly occurs during the first 2 or 3 months of oral contraceptive use. Its incidence depends on the dose of synthetic estrogen (increased with preparations containing <30 μg) and type of progestogen (decreased with the newer progestogens, even with estrogen doses <30 μg). It is important that women be informed that this harmless but annoying symptom generally disap-

TABLE 40–3. CONCEPTION RATES ACCORDING TO PRIOR METHOD OF CONTRACEPTION*

	Conception Rates (%)			
Months to Conception	*Pill (n = 1086)*	*IUD† (n = 451)*	*Diaphragm (n = 903)*	*All Other (n = 774)*
1–3	38.9	54.1	65.4	58.3
4–6	18.3	18.6	15.3	16.9
7–9	11.2	10.0	7.0	8.9
10–12	6.8	4.9	3.8	4.0
≥13	24.8	12.4	8.5	11.9

*From Linn S, Schoenbaum SC, Monson RR, et al: Delay in conception for former "pill" users. JAMA 247:629, 1982. Copyright 1982, American Medical Association.

†IUD = intrauterine device.

TABLE 40–4. Annual Deaths/100,000 Women by Age Group*

Age	<20	20–24	25–29	30–34	35–39	40–44
No method	—	7.4	9.1	14.8	25.7	28.2
Pill/nonsmoker	—	0.7	1.1	2.1	14.1	32.0
Pill/smoker	—	3.6	6.8	13.7	51.4	117.6
Maternal mortality†	7.2	6.5	7.7	11.8	23.0	55.9

*Adapted from Cramer DW and Cann CI: Risks and benefits of oral contraceptive use in women over 35. Maturitas 1:99, 1988.

†Deaths/100,000 live births in the United States from 1979 to 1988.

pears after 3 pill cycles and can be controlled, if necessary, with a slightly higher dose of estrogen. If breakthrough bleeding persists beyond the third cycle or becomes disturbingly heavy, the best approach is to administer 20 μg of ethinyl estradiol for 7 days when the breakthrough bleeding is persistent or heavy. Usually, this treatment is necessary for only two or three cycles, after which better cycle control is commonly achieved.

Amenorrhea resulting from inadequate estrogen stimulation of the endometrium is not generally as troubling to patients as is breakthrough bleeding. With each cycle, the oral contraceptive user has as much as a 13% chance of failing to have a withdrawal bleed, depending on the formulation.[34, 35] Women who are aware that their menses will almost certainly be 2 to 3 days shorter and, rarely, may disappear altogether when they use oral contraceptives are unlikely to be alarmed at the occurrence of these symptoms. Some women will, for personal or cultural reasons, be distressed by failure to have a "normal" menses. This concern is best alleviated by selecting a new oral contraceptive with slightly more synthetic estrogen or a different progestogen. In addition, if a woman is amenorrheic while using an oral contraceptive and has been sexually active during that cycle, a highly sensitive urine or serum pregnancy test should be performed. If a woman continues to be amenorrheic in following cycles and is taking the pills correctly, repeated pregnancy tests are not necessary.

Among the less serious but bothersome effects of estrogen are cyclic weight gain (due to fluid retention), breast fullness and tenderness, and nausea. These symptoms occur rarely with low-estrogen formulations and, when they do occur, are likely to subside after the first 3 months of use. Uncommon effects of estrogen that can become worse with prolonged use include darkening of breast and facial skin (chloasma) and photodermatitis. The complaint of pill-related weight gain has been disproven in multiple studies of low-dose preparations that showed no major differences among the various products. Approximately as many women gain weight as lose weight with oral contraceptives. If weight gain is a problem, the clinician should reassure the patient about the lack of association and direct her to evaluate her diet and level of exercise. If weight gain persists or the patient desires to change preparations because of weight gain, then a pill with a less androgenic effect should be used. Side effects due to an excess of progestogen are rarely seen with the doses used in pills today and may be absent altogether with the newer progestogens.

Despite its high effectiveness, use of oral contraception

TABLE 40–5. CURRENT ORAL CONTRACEPTIVES IN THE UNITED STATES

	Progestin	Dose (mg)	Estrogen	Dose (μg)
Multiphase Preparations				
Ortho-Novum 7/7/7 (Ortho)	Norethindrone (7)	0.5	Ethinyl estradiol	35
	Norethindrone (7)	0.75		35
	Norethindrone (7)	1.0		35
Tri-Norinyl (Syntex)	Norethindrone (7)	0.5	Ethinyl estradiol	35
	Norethindrone (9)	1.0		35
	Norethindrone (5)	0.5		35
Triphasil (Wyeth-Ayerst)				
Tri-Levlen (Berlex)	Levonorgestrel (6)	0.05	Ethinyl estradiol	30
	Levonorgestrel (5)	0.075		40
	Levonorgestrel (10)	0.125		30
Jenest (Organon)	Norethindrone (7)	0.5	Ethinyl estradiol	35
	Norethindrone (14)	1.0		35
Low-Dose Preparations				
Ovcon-35 (Mead-Johnson)	Norethindrone	0.4	Ethinyl estradiol	35
Brevicon (Syntex)	Norethindrone	0.5	Ethinyl estradiol	35
Modicon (Ortho)	Norethindrone	0.5	Ethinyl estradiol	35
Ortho-Novum 1/35 (Ortho)	Norethindrone	1.0	Ethinyl estradiol	35
Norinyl 1/35 (Syntex)	Norethindrone	1.0	Ethinyl estradiol	35
Loestrin 1/20 (Parke-Davis)	Norethindrone acetate	1.0	Ethinyl estradiol	20
Loestrin 1.5/30 (Parke-Davis)	Norethindrone acetate	1.5	Ethinyl estradiol	30
Nordette (Wyeth-Ayerst)	Levonorgestrel	0.15	Ethinyl estradiol	30
Lo-Ovral (Wyeth-Ayerst)	Norgestrel	0.3	Ethinyl estradiol	30
Demulen 1/35 (Searle)	Ethynodiol diacetate	1.0	Ethinyl estradiol	35
High-Dose Preparations				
Ovcon-50 (Mead-Johnson)	Norethindrone	1.0	Ethinyl estradiol	50
Ortho-Novum 1/50 (Ortho)	Norethindrone	1.0	Mestranol	50
Norinyl 1/50 (Syntex)	Norethindrone	1.0	Mestranol	50
Norlestrin 1/50 (Parke-Davis)	Norethindrone acetate	1.0	Ethinyl estradiol	50
Ovral (Wyeth-Ayerst)	Norgestrel	0.5	Ethinyl estradiol	50
Progesterone Only ("Minipill")				
Micronor (Ortho)	Norethindrone	0.35		
Nor-Q.D. (Syntex)	Norethindrone	0.35		
Ovrette (Wyeth-Ayerst)	Norgestrel	0.075		

still results in hundreds of thousands of unintended pregnancies due to poor patient compliance each year. Compliance requires a melding of personal behavior, an understanding of the potential side effects, and a strong desire to avoid pregnancy. Noncompliance with oral contraceptive use often stems from a lack of knowledge; the majority of women, when faced with questions regarding the safety and side effects of oral contraceptives, turn to their friends or newspapers and, rarely, to their physicians. It is important for the clinician, when initially prescribing an oral contraceptive, to take the time to explain the facts and myths of oral contraception. The clinician should review:

1. How oral contraception works;
2. The risks and benefits of oral contraception with an emphasis on safety and noncontraceptive benefits;
3. How and when to take the pills;
4. The side effects that can affect compliance and what to do should one or more occur;
5. The warning signs of dangerous but rare and unlikely side effects (e.g., leg swelling).

Because most women who stop using oral contraception do so without consulting a physician, it is important to establish an open line of communication and to emphasize that the patient should call or return for any problems or concerns before she stops taking the pills. In addition, she should return after the first 3 months of use to review the above points and to address any questions, concerns, or other problems. If a clinician takes the time at the initiation of oral contraceptive therapy to discuss these issues with the patient, many problems, including unwanted pregnancy, can be avoided.

Postcoital Contraception

High doses of oral estrogen or estrogen containing oral contraceptives can be used to prevent implantation after fertilization has occurred. If therapy is begun within 72 hours of midcycle intercourse, pregnancy results in approximately 1% of cases, as compared with 15 to 20% of untreated patients.[32] The use of these hormones early in gestation has not been shown to cause problems should the treatment fail; use immediately after fertilization has either an "all-or-none" effect on the pregnancy. Diethylstilbestrol, 25 mg twice daily for 5 days, is very effective as a postcoital contraceptive but causes nausea and breast tenderness. A more acceptable alternative is administration of high-dose ethinyl estradiol and norgestrel, two tablets taken immediately, followed by two more tablets 12 hours later. This regimen has the advantages of a shorter treatment course and less nausea. Copper-releasing intrauterine devices have also been proven to be effective postcoital contraceptives when placed in the uterine cavity within 5 days of intercourse.[36] Should treatment fail to prevent pregnancy, the patient should be offered a therapeutic abortion.

LONG-ACTING HORMONAL CONTRACEPTION

Levonorgestrel Implants (the Norplant System)

Subdermal implants containing synthetic progestins were approved for use in the United States in December 1990 and are the first new contraceptive in the past 30 years. They have been used throughout the world by over 2 million women and have an impressive record of effectiveness and safety. The Norplant System consists of six silastic capsules, each filled with 36 mg of levonorgestrel. The capsules are implanted under the skin and removed at the patient's request or at the end of 5 years, when the hormone levels are no longer adequate to provide contraception. Placement and removal require a minor surgical procedure using local anesthesia.

Mechanism of Action

Norplant works by releasing a low, steady dose of levonorgestrel. Plasma concentrations are sufficient to prevent conception within 24 hours of insertion. The amount of levonorgestrel released per day during the first year of use is 25 to 50% that of combination levonorgestrel–containing oral contraceptives.[37] After the first year, the rate of release decreases gradually so that by the end of 5 years, plasma levels are insufficient to reliably prevent conception.

As with oral contraceptives, the Norplant System has several mechanisms by which pregnancy is prevented. Levonorgestrel acts centrally to inhibit the luteinizing hormone surge, resulting in suppression of ovulation in approximately two thirds of menstrual cycles over 5 years. Should ovulation occur, fertilization is prevented by the thick, scant cervical mucous caused by the continual presence of progestogen. Additionally, the constant low levels of levonorgestrel suppress the estradiol-induced cyclic maturation of the endometrium, resulting in an atrophic lining unsuitable for implantation.

Effectiveness

The Norplant System pregnancy rate in the first year of use is 0.2/100 woman-years.[38] All of these pregnancies except one were present at the time of insertion, therefore, the corrected first-year pregnancy rate is 0.01/100 woman-years. The pregnancy rate gradually increases over the 5 years, with a cumulative pregnancy rate of 2.9/100 woman-years. This 5-year cumulative rate is approximately the same as with oral contraceptives or an intrauterine device in the first year alone (Table 40–6).

Ectopic pregnancy is rare with the Norplant System, occurring at a rate of 0.28/1000 woman-years.[38] In comparison, the overall ectopic pregnancy rate in the United States is 1.7/1000 women aged 15 to 44.[39] Ectopic pregnancies account for approximately 14% of pregnancies that occur with the use of the Norplant System. Thus, for women reporting amenorrhea, especially after a period of regular

TABLE 40–6. USE-FAILURE AND CONTINUATION RATES OF SELECTED CONTRACEPTIVE METHODS

	Use-Failure Rate		
Year	*Levonorgestrel Implants (%)*	*OCP (%)**	*IUD (%)†*
1	0.2	3	3
2	0.2	—	—
3	0.9	—	—
4	0.5	—	—
5	1.1	—	—
	Continuation Rate		
	~90	50–75	~75

*OCP = oral contraceptive.
†IUD = intrauterine device.

bleeding, pregnancy should be ruled out by a sensitive urine or serum pregnancy test.

Advantages and Disadvantages

Levonorgestrel implants are a safe, highly effective method of continuous contraception that requires little user compliance or motivation and is rapidly reversible. Because the implants do not contain estrogen, they can be used in women with contraindications for estrogen-containing contraceptives (e.g., a history of thrombosis or estrogen-dependent cancer). Sustained release avoids the high initial dose of injectables and the daily hormone surge seen with oral contraceptives. These surges, along with "first-pass" hepatic metabolism, are thought to account for the changes in lipids and coagulation sometimes seen with oral contraceptive use. Additionally, use is not coitus related; thus, use effectiveness closely approximates theoretical effectiveness.

As with any contraceptive, there are also disadvantages:

1. Irregular bleeding occurs in 80% of users, primarily during the first year. Many women and their partners find this change unacceptable. The endometrium is unstable because of variable suppression of endogenous estrogen production and a lack of cycling of the progestin, resulting in unpredictable shedding.
2. The initiation and discontinuation of levonorgestrel implants require a simple surgical procedure, limiting the ability of the user to start and stop use without a clinician.
3. Initiation and discontinuation costs are high because of the cost of the implants and because a surgical procedure is required for implantation and removal.
4. The implants may be visible under the skin, although this does not seem to bother most women.
5. The implants do not protect against STDs.

Levonorgestrel implants are absolutely contraindicated in only five circumstances: unexplained vaginal bleeding, acute liver disease, benign or malignant liver tumors, active thromboembolic disease, and breast cancer. In addition, because levonorgestrel is metabolized in the liver, the effectiveness is decreased in women who are using medications that induce hepatic microsomal enzymes, such as phenytoin, carbamazepine, phenobarbital, and rifampin.

Side Effects

Menstrual Effects. Menstrual irregularities are the single most common problem associated with Norplant System use. In the first year, roughly 60% of women will experience some alteration of their menstrual cycles, most commonly spacing of bleeding episodes, changes in duration and volume of flow, and spotting (Table 40–7).[40] Oligomenorrhea or amenorrhea also occurs, but less frequently. After the first year, approximately 60% of women have regular cycles.[41] Should amenorrhea occur after a period of regular menses, a sensitive urine or serum pregnancy test should be obtained. Women who are amenorrheic throughout their use of levonorgestrel implants are unlikely to become pregnant. Thus, once negative results on a pregnancy test are obtained, serial tests are not necessary.

Despite the increased number of spotting and bleeding days, hemoglobin values increase in anemic women, and no change or a slight improvement is found in women with normal blood counts.[42] When very heavy bleeding occurs with the Norplant System, small decreases in hemoglobin have been noted. If the bleeding is intolerable or worrisome, the patient may benefit from a short course of estrogen, usually 0.2 mg of ethinyl estradiol daily for 21 days.

Metabolic Effects. The sustained, low serum concentrations of levonorgestrel cause no significant metabolic changes. Multiple studies of varied populations have shown no appreciable change in carbohydrate metabolism, liver function, blood coagulation, immunoglobulin levels, serum cortisol levels, blood chemistries, and serum lipoproteins.[43–50]

General Effects. In addition to menstrual changes, multiple other effects have been reported: headache, mastalgia, hyperpigmentation over the implants, hirsutism, depression, mood changes, anxiety, nervousness, ovarian cyst formation, and galactorrhea. Many of these effects are similar to problems with oral contraceptives, and some may not be due to levonorgestrel. Reassurance is adequate therapy for many complaints, and other symptoms respond to simple therapies. Most patients will find these side effects tolerable after an explanation as to their cause and reassurance that they pose no serious health risk.

The most common side effect after menstrual irregularities is headache. Headaches vary from mild bitemporal to migraines, with onset of symptoms usually related to the insertion of the implants. For patients who do not obtain relief with acetaminophen or prostaglandin synthetase inhibitors, removal is common. Among women who discontinue the Norplant System, approximately 20% do so because of headaches.[38]

Women will experience both weight gain and weight loss. These changes may be related to diet and exercise as well as to the androgenic activity of levonorgestrel.

Mastalgia usually occurs premenstrually and is associated with fluid retention. These symptoms usually decrease with duration of use and respond to local treatment, like a tight-fitting bra. Women rarely request removal of the implants because of mastalgia.

Galactorrhea occurs and is more common if the implants are inserted near the end of lactation, especially if the patient continues to receive nipple stimulation. It is important not to ignore the discharge and to rule out pathologic disease with a breast exam, pregnancy test, and a prolactin level assessment. If the discharge is bloody or discolored, it should also be sent for cytologic examination. Decreasing the amount of breast and nipple stimulation will usually resolve this problem.

Acne is more common if the patient had cyclic acne in the

TABLE 40–7. MENSTRUAL PATTERNS OF NORPLANT USERS*

Menstrual Pattern	First Year	Second Year	Third Year
8 or more days bleeding	44%	27%	24%
15 or more days bleeding	15%	4%	7%
70 or more days without bleeding	37%	30%	22%
90 or more days without bleeding	26%	19%	15%
Bleeding days	54 days	48 days	48 days

*Adapted from Sivin I, Alvarez-Sanchez F, Diaz S, et al: Three-year experience with Norplant subdermal contraception. Fertil Steril 39:799–808, 1983. Reproduced with permission of the publisher, The American Fertility Society.

past or a problem with acne when taking oral contraceptives. The acne is a result of the androgenic activity of levonorgestrel in combination with a decrease in sex hormone–binding globulin levels, resulting in increased free androgens. Treatment involves good hygiene with a skin cleanser and topical antibiotics (1% erythromycin or 1% clindamycin solution).

Ovarian cysts occur because the low serum level of levonorgestrel does not suppress follicle-stimulating hormone enough to arrest ovarian follicle growth. However, the luteinizing hormone surge is usually inhibited so that ovulation does not occur. Some of these follicles continue to grow and can, on occasion, cause pain or be palpated during a pelvic exam. Because these are simple cysts, further evaluation is not indicated unless the cysts become large and painful or fail to regress over 2 to 3 months.

Genital herpes outbreaks have been reported to be more common after implant insertion in patients with a past history of genital herpes. These outbreaks usually occur during episodes of prolonged bleeding or spotting when pad use is increased and, therefore, may be due to the increased local irritation. Use of tampons instead of pads and acyclovir suppression have been successful in treating this problem.

Patient Selection and Use

If a patient desires levonorgestrel implants, a detailed description of the effectiveness, advantages, disadvantages, side effects, risks and benefits, and insertion and removal techniques should be provided. This counseling is important because it will help prospective users decide if they can tolerate the menstrual changes and other side effects, and thereby prevent dissatisfaction and discontinuation.

Implant insertion can be performed at any time of the menstrual cycle, provided pregnancy is ruled out. Various subcutaneous sites have been used in clinical trials, and the greatest satisfaction and ease of insertion has been found to be in the upper inner portion of the nondominant arm. Insertion is performed under local anesthesia by a specially trained practitioner. Potential complications of insertion include infection, hematoma formation, local irritation, and expulsion of capsules. The majority of these problems occur during the first few weeks after implantation and in fewer than 1% of patients.[52]

Removal is a more difficult procedure that also requires special training and takes from a few minutes to 1 hour, depending on how carefully the capsules were inserted and the experience of the clinician. In women who discontinue using the implants to become pregnant, world-wide life-table pregnancy rates are approximately the same as with women who have not used any contraception. After removal of the implants, levonorgestrel levels are unmeasurable within 48 hours, and most women have normal ovulatory cycles during the first month.

Counseling

The most common reason women request levonorgestrel implants is because of failure or dissatisfaction with other methods of contraception. It is important to counsel patients about the similarities and differences between this approach to contraception and the methods the patient may have used in the past. Because a surgical procedure is required for insertion and removal, and because of the expense of levonorgestrel implants, their use is indicated only when long-term birth control is desired.

Women at risk of acquiring STDs, including human immunodeficiency syndrome, must consider that levonorgestrel implants provide no protection against these diseases. A woman at risk of STDs may still wish to use the implants to prevent pregnancy because of its high efficacy and convenience. However, she should also be counseled about the importance of using barrier methods to protect against the transmission of STDs.

Finally, because menstrual irregularities are common, all prospective users must understand the range of possible changes and that it is not possible to predict what effect levonorgestrel will have on each individual's menses. Stressing that these changes are expected and do not represent illness increases patient comfort with the implants. In addition, the patient should be reminded that most women revert to normal menstrual cycles with increasing duration of use. Without reassurance prior to insertion, women are more likely to terminate use before time can improve unacceptable bleeding. If during the course of reviewing all of the potential side effects it becomes obvious that the menstrual changes would be unacceptable to the patient or to her partner, the clinician should encourage the patient to consider other methods of contraception.

Depo-Provera

Like levonorgestrel implants, a depot intramuscular injection of medroxyprogesterone acetate (Depo-Provera) is a progestin-only contraceptive providing long-term, highly efficacious contraception. Injection of 150 mg every 3 months is nearly as effective as levonorgestrel implants. The side effects are similar: menstrual irregularities, mastalgia, weight change, and depression. The incidence of irregular bleeding is 30% in the first year and approximately 10% thereafter; most women become amenorrheic after several injections. After discontinuing therapy, it takes 6 to 8 months for the drug to completely clear the body. Return of normal menses and ovulatory function is delayed, but even after long-term use, the risk of permanent infertility is not increased.

Norethindrone enanthate in a dose of 200 mg intramuscularly every 2 months is equally as effective as Depo-Provera.[53] The side effects are similar, except that there is 50% less amenorrhea after 1 year of use and 33% less amenorrhea after 2 years of norethindrone enanthate use.

INTRAUTERINE DEVICE

The history of the development, trial, and application of the IUD parallels that of the oral contraceptive. The availability of modern plastics and recognition of the need for improved contraception in a crowded world encouraged Margulies and Lippes in the late 1950s to design and evaluate IUDs that resumed their shape after their insertion into the uterine cavity. The medical community was then won over by the extensive evaluative efforts of the Population Council, and IUDs were widely promoted in family planning programs in developing countries. Enthusiasm for IUDs was high because they offered contraceptive protection that was at once highly effective, long-lasting, inexpensive, independent of coitus, and completely reversible. Disillusionment followed, spurred on by problems from the Dalkon Shield. Introduced in 1970, the Dalkon Shield was associated with a high rate of pelvic infection, and its production was discontinued in 1975. Unfortunately, American women and their clinicians applied this experience to all IUDs, and interest in their use declined. Distribution within the United States was discontinued, and the economic burden of legal costs related to the IUD dissuaded further production. The number of women using IUDs in the United States declined from 2.2 to 0.7 million between 1981 and 1988.[3]

Worldwide development and use of the IUD proceeded. Progesterone-containing IUDs continued to be distributed in the United States from their time of FDA approval in 1976. Copper IUDs were improved through the 1980s, building on the knowledge gained from IUDs of the past. Currently, two IUDs are available in the United States, the TCu-380A (ParaGard, GynoPharma Corp.) and the progesterone T (Progestasert, Alza Corp.). Both provide effective and safe contraception. Information about the risk factors for IUD-associated pelvic infection and infertility (multiple sexual partners, young age at first intercourse, and failure to use a barrier method) has allowed more intelligent selection of candidates for IUD use.

Mechanism of Action

The exact mechanism of action of IUDs is not fully understood. It is most commonly hypothesized that the primary contraceptive effect of IUDs results from stimulating the proliferation of inflammatory cells within the endometrium, creating an environment hostile to sperm and unfavorable to implantation. Recent studies have shown the effects of the IUD to extend to the fallopian tubes, inhibiting fertilization or tubal function related to fertilization.[54] In addition, progesterone-containing IUDs cause a decidualization of the endometrium, leading to atrophy of the glands and a thickening of the cervical mucus, creating a barrier to sperm penetration.

Effectiveness

The TCu-380A has been approved for use in the United States for 8 years. The progesterone-releasing IUD must be replaced every year because the progesterone is depleted in 12 to 18 months. The nonmedicated IUDs (e.g., Lippes' Loop) never have to be replaced unless problems occur. IUDs with greater amounts of copper have consistently lower failure rates than do other types. With the TCu-380A, the pregnancy rate in the first year is less than 1%, the expulsion rate, 6%; and the removal rate, 12%, mainly for bleeding and pain.[55] The continuation rate at 1 year is approximately 82/100 women and decreases by 15 to 20% per year thereafter.

Complications

Infection is the most serious complication associated with IUDs. Infections that are truly related to the IUD occur within the first 3 months of use and are felt to be due to contamination of the uterine cavity at the time of insertion with organisms from the vaginal flora.[56] Infections that occur later are likely to be sexually transmitted. Because sexual behavior is an important factor in the pathogenesis of PID, women who are at low risk are unlikely to experience upper-tract infection while using an IUD. Women who have culture results positive for gonorrhea or chlamydia without evidence of upper-tract infection should be treated appropriately but do not require IUD removal. These patients, however, should be thoroughly counseled that the high-risk sexual behavior that led to the sexually transmitted disease could result in PID, possibly leading to infertility and chronic pelvic pain. Should any signs of upper-tract disease be present, the IUD should be removed and appropriate antibiotic therapy instituted.

Pregnancy with an IUD in place should prompt suspicion of ectopic pregnancy. About 3 to 4% of IUD pregnancies are extrauterine (Table 40–8). Copper-releasing IUDs have a much lower ectopic pregnancy rate than progesterone-releasing IUDs. In fact, the ectopic pregnancy rate with progesterone-releasing IUDs is more than twice that of women not using contraception. The protection against ectopic pregnancy afforded by the copper-releasing IUDs makes their use acceptable in women with a prior ectopic pregnancy and no risk factors for PID.

Spontaneous abortion is a more likely complication of pregnancy with IUD use than is ectopic pregnancy. The spontaneous abortion rate for women wearing IUDs is approximately 50%, as compared with approximately 15% for all pregnant women.[57] Pregnancies that occur despite the device or that were conceived before IUD insertion are more likely than other pregnancies to result in septic abortion, especially in the second trimester, or preterm delivery in the third trimester. Because of the high risk for spontaneous and septic abortion, IUDs should be removed if pregnancy is diagnosed and the string is visible. After removal of an IUD with visible strings, the spontaneous abortion rate is about 30%.[58] If the device cannot be easily removed, the woman should be offered therapeutic abortion. If a woman pregnant with an IUD in place shows evidence of uterine infection, therapeutic abortion and removal of the device should be undertaken after initiation of antibiotic therapy (e.g., gentamicin and clindamycin, or cefoxitin or cefotetan and doxycycline).

Although infection and spontaneous abortion are the cause of most serious IUD complications, bleeding and pain are the symptoms most often responsible for IUD discontinuation. Five to 15% of women discontinue IUD use within 1 year because of these symptoms.[59] Because IUDs can alter menstrual patterns, the clinician must take a careful menstrual history before discussing with a woman whether an IUD is appropriate. Women who experience heavy and prolonged menses or dysmenorrhea may not tolerate copper

TABLE 40–8. ECTOPIC PREGNANCY RATES FOR VARIOUS CONTRACEPTIVE METHODS OVER 1 YEAR*

	% Risk of Ectopic Pregnancy	Ectopic Pregnancy/ 10,000 Users
No method	0.2	17.0
Combination OCP‡	0.2	0.6
Minipill	2–4†	6–8
Intrauterine device	3–4	9.0
TCu-380A		2.0
Progesterone T		68.0
Vasectomy	0.2	0.03
Tubal ligation	16.0	6.4
Levonorgestrel implant	14.0	2.8
Depo-Provera	13.0	4.0
Periodic abstinence	0.3	0.6
Withdrawal	0.2	0.4
Spermicide	0.3	0.6
Sponge	0.2	0.4
Cervical cap	0.2	0.4
Diaphragm	0.2	0.4
Condom	0.2	0.2

*Adapted from Kost K, Forrest D, and Harlap S: Comparing the health risks and benefits of contraceptive choices. Fam Plann Perspect 23:54, 1991.

†From Graham S and Fraser IS: The progestogen-only mini-pill. Contraception 26:373, 1982. Used with permission of Butterworth-Heinemann.

‡OCP = oral contraceptive.

IUDs but may benefit from progesterone-releasing IUDs, which actually decrease menstrual blood loss. Cramping pain is generally limited to the first few months of IUD use, and treatment with prostaglandin synthetase inhibitors is usually helpful.

Patient Selection and Use

Women who have borne children, who do not have prolonged menstrual periods marked by excessive pain or bleeding, who are at low risk of STDs, and who desire highly effective contraception without personal inconvenience are ideal candidates for the IUD. The most important determinant in the selection of patients is not age or parity, but, rather, risk factors for STDs. In addition, women with uterine anomalies may not accommodate an IUD, and a uterus that is too small or too large will result in compromised effectiveness. Women with an allergy to copper or Wilson's disease should not use copper IUDs; immunocompromised patients and women at risk for endocarditis should not use IUDs.

Cervical culture for gonorrhea and chlamydia should be done for women who are considering an IUD. A positive culture result in an otherwise asymptomatic woman should receive routine treatment and prompt questioning as to whether an IUD is a good choice. If the patient has not had a recent Papanicolaou smear, one should be obtained during the examination. The uterus should be sounded; for successful IUD use, the uterus should sound between 6 and 10 cm, inclusive of the cervical canal. A bimanual examination should then be performed, with particular attention paid to the uterine position, size, and mobility. If the clinician finds the pelvic organs to be abnormal or there is excessive tenderness to uterine or cervical manipulation, IUD insertion should be postponed until further investigation assures the absence of infection.

Each IUD package contains a full explanation of the risks and benefits of the IUD and the insertion and removal procedures; the clinician and patient should review this form together. The patient should always be shown her IUD prior to insertion and should receive an explanation of the insertion procedure. The IUD can be safely inserted at any time during the menstrual cycle but can also be delayed until menses if pregnancy is a possibility. Immediately prior to insertion, the IUD should be loaded into its plastic inserter according to the directions provided with the package. This should be accomplished using a no-touch technique, preserving sterility and negating the need for hand-scrubbing, draping, or gowning. The cervix is swabbed with an antiseptic solution and the anterior lip grasped with a tenaculum after local anesthetic is injected at the tenaculum site. A paracervical block using 1% chloroprocaine hydrochloride (Nesacaine) is injected; inclusion of atropine, 0.4 mg, with the anesthetic will decrease the incidence of vasovagal reaction with insertion. Steady traction is exerted on the tenaculum to straighten the cervical canal, and the inserter is advanced through the cervical os into the uterine cavity. The directions should then be followed to place the IUD high in the fundus. The strings are cut to a length of about 4 cm from the external os. If they are cut too short initially, they will be difficult for the inexperienced user to feel. The strings can always be cut shorter later if they protrude from the introitus. Because most women experience uterine cramping during and immediately after insertion, prostaglandin synthetase inhibitors should be administered prior to insertion and during the 24 hours thereafter. Doxycycline, 200 mg, administered orally 1 hour prior to insertion, will provide protection against insertion-related infection but probably is of little benefit to the woman at low risk for STDs.

Following insertion and after uterine cramping has abated, the woman should examine herself vaginally to palpate the strings. It is often helpful to use a mirror so that she can actually see the cervix and protruding strings prior to feeling them. She should then be instructed to palpate the strings prior to each act of intercourse until she returns for a follow-up examination after her next menses. Thereafter, self-examination following each menses is probably adequate to assure that her IUD is in place. She should also be instructed to use another contraceptive and return for evaluation if she fails to feel the IUD strings.

Complications of IUD insertion include perforation, bleeding from the tenaculum site, and vasovagal reaction from acute cervical dilation. Among experienced inserters of IUDs, perforation occurs with approximately 0.1% of procedures. Frequent causes are failure to properly assess the uterine position and inaccurate definition of the cervical canal. Rarely do such perforations cause injury to the pelvic or abdominal contents. Often, they go undetected until the device is noted to be absent on a subsequent examination. Unless there is excessive bleeding, suggesting laceration of a uterine vessel, removal of the perforated IUD is not an emergency.

Follow-up Care and Removal

The follow-up visit after the menses following insertion should include the patient's account of her experience with the IUD, including her ability to feel the string and changes in her menses, as well as a pelvic examination to determine the intrauterine position of the IUD and the absence of signs of pelvic infection. A common problem at IUD follow-up visits is an inability to visualize the string in the cervical canal, especially if the string was cut too short. The patient should be assured that inability to feel or see the string usually means that it has retracted and not that the IUD has perforated the uterus or has been expelled. The strings can often be identified by gently rotating a cytologic brush within the cervical canal. If this maneuver fails, a uterine sound can be introduced into the intrauterine cavity and carefully withdrawn so as to rub across the device. Should this fail to detect the IUD, the clinician must suspect either undetected perforation at the time of insertion or undetected expulsion. The position of the IUD is then best determined by ultrasound or, lacking that, with anterior-posterior, lateral, and oblique films of the pelvis with a radio-opaque marker (i.e., a uterine sound) in the uterine cavity. If the IUD is found to be in the uterine cavity, the patient and clinician can be reassured. If the device is perforating the myometrium or is in the abdominal cavity, removal is necessary, usually by laparoscopy.

At the time of routine Papanicolaou smear, the cytologist may report presence of *Actinomyces*-like organisms. The frequency of such reports ranges from 1 to 25% of IUD users, depending mainly on how hard the cytologist looks for the organisms, the type of IUD (higher with inert, plastic-only devices and lower with copper-containing devices), and the duration of use.[60–62] Although unusual, occurrence of intra-abdominal *Actinomyces* infections in association with IUD use has been reported. The most cautious course, therefore, is to remove the IUD and treat with penicillin G, 500 mg orally four times daily for 1 month. If the patient then wishes to resume use of an IUD, a copper-containing one should be inserted.

Removal is easily accomplished by grasping the string with any appropriate clamp and pulling with firm traction.

If the string cannot be visualized, the steps as mentioned above can be used to localize the device. If the IUD is then found to be intrauterine, it can be removed with a Facit ureteral stone forceps directed to the area where the device was localized. If the IUD cannot be grasped using the forceps, then removal with sonographic guidance or via hysteroscopy is necessary. If the patient wishes to continue using an IUD, a new device can be placed at the time of removal as long as infection is not present.

Fertility returns promptly after removal. Pregnancy rates in women who have IUDs removed because of a desire to become pregnant are similar to those in women who discontinued use of other methods of contraception (see Table 40–3).[63] In women with monogamous relationships, there is no evidence of an increased risk of infertility after IUD use.

BARRIER METHODS

Renewed concern over the transmission of STDs, especially the human immunodeficiency virus, has reawakened interest in condoms and other barrier methods of contraception. Barrier contraceptives also reduce the incidence of cervical cancer by half. When used correctly, the condom, diaphragm, and cervical cap can be highly effective. Chemical barriers, however, are far less effective than hormonal or intrauterine contraception.

Diaphragm

The diaphragm is a dome-shaped latex cup with a rim made of flexible steel. Rim diameters range from 50 to 105 mm in increments of 5 mm, the most commonly used sizes being 70 to 80 mm. There are three types of steel rims: a flat spring that bends only in the lateral plane, a coil spring flexible in all directions, and an arching spring ("all flex") that is also flexible in all directions but assumes an arch shape when flexed laterally.

When properly fitted, a diaphragm provides comfortable and safe protection at low cost. Improper fitting or prolonged retention can cause vaginal irritation. Rarely, women or their partners may be allergic to the latex or the spermicide used with the diaphragm. Urinary tract infections are twice as common in women using diaphragms as in women using oral contraceptives.[64] For these women, consider refitting with a smaller diaphragm; also, voiding after intercourse is helpful and, if necessary, a postcoital prophylactic antibiotic (e.g., nitrofurantoin, 100 mg) can be prescribed. The principal contraindication to diaphragm use is inability to insert and remove the diaphragm properly; most commonly, this problem results from the reluctance of the woman to touch (or have her partner touch) her genitalia.

The typical use-failure rate for diaphragms is 15 to 20% after 1 year of use. Older, well-educated married women with longer use achieve efficacy rates greater than 95%, but young women can also achieve similar results if properly counseled and highly motivated. Whether diaphragms can be effective without spermicide has not been determined.

Fitting the Diaphragm. The diaphragm must fit with the posterior portion of the rim in the posterior fornix and the anterior portion under the pubic symphysis. The most important point in selecting the correct diaphragm is to choose the kind of spring the patient can use most easily and the largest size comfortably accommodated. Most women find the arching spring easiest to insert properly because the curve tends to guide the diaphragm posteriorly under the cervix. The first step in fitting a diaphragm is a routine bimanual examination, with special attention to the mobility of the uterus, the position and size of the cervix, and the shape of the anterior and posterior vaginal walls. The presence of a rectocele or cystourethrocele make diaphragm use more difficult. For these patients, the flat-spring diaphragm, which does not permit bending from back to front, may be useful.

The diaphragm size for fitting is chosen by the examiner at the time of the pelvic examination. The middle finger is placed in the posterior fornix, and the point at which the index finger hits the pubic symphysis is marked with the thumb. This distance is measured, and the corresponding fitting ring or diaphragm is inserted. The final size is determined by noting if the diaphragm is pressed too snugly behind the pubic symphysis or if it comes out with bearing down. The diaphragm is removed by hooking a finger under the anterior rim and pulling outward. After finding the appropriate size, the patient should demonstrate that she can place and remove the diaphragm correctly and feel her cervix behind the diaphragm to assure proper placement.

During or after fitting of the diaphragm, the user should be instructed in the use of spermicide and the timing of insertion and removal. Prior to insertion, spermicide should be placed around the rim, and a teaspoonful should be placed in the central portion. Because the spermicide is active for approximately 6 hours, women can insert the diaphragm up to 6 hours prior to intercourse. The diaphragm must be left in place for at least 6 hours after coitus. If additional acts of intercourse occur before the 6 hours pass, additional spermicide should be applied in the vagina in front of the diaphragm using a vaginal applicator. For intercourse that occurs more than 6 hours after insertion, the diaphragm should be removed and the spermicide reapplied.

After removal, the diaphragm should be washed with soap and water and dried. Periodically, the diaphragm should be filled with water to check for leaks. The fit should be assessed yearly and with a weight change of 10 pounds or more or following pregnancy or pelvic surgery. If cleaned regularly, stored dry, and kept away from powders and oil-based lubricants, diaphragms should last for several years.

Cervical Cap

The cervical cap has been used in Europe nearly as long as the diaphragm. There are several designs, the best of which is the thimble-shaped cavity rim latex ("Prentif") cap, the only one approved for use in the United States (Cervical Cap, Los Gatos, CA). US trials have shown the cap to be as effective as the diaphragm, although somewhat more difficult to fit (they come in only 4 diameters: 22, 25, 28, and 31 mm) and more difficult to situate properly over the cervix. Proper fit of one of the four sizes cannot be accomplished in up to 10% of women.[65]

Like the diaphragm, the cervical cap must be left in place at least 6 hours after sexual intercourse, but may be left for several days with no known risk for toxic shock syndrome. It need not be used with a spermicide; however, a teaspoonful of spermicide is usually placed in the cap before application. The spermicide is reported to decrease the incidence of foul-smelling discharge, a common complaint when the cap is left in place longer than 24 hours. The most common cause of failure is dislodgement during intercourse; users must check the fit of the cap over the cervix after insertion and again after each act of intercourse.

Condoms

Condoms are usually made from thin latex rubber, although 1% are still made from the less efficacious lamb's intestine ("natural skin"). They come in various shapes, colors, textures, and with or without spermicide. Condoms fit over the erect penis to act as a barrier to the transmission of sperm as well as the organisms responsible for STDs and human immunodeficiency syndrome. Like the diaphragm, they do not have serious side effects but may reduce penile sensation and, thus, sexual satisfaction. The major advantages besides protection from STDs are low cost and ready availability.

High effectiveness rates have been achieved in older, married couples experienced in using condoms. The lower use effectiveness rate of 80 to 85% is found in younger, unmarried couples with little contraceptive experience. Effectiveness of the condom increases with correct and consistent use. If lubricants are used, they must be water based because oil-based lubricants or vaginal creams can weaken the latex. After intercourse, the man must withdraw his penis while it is still erect, holding the condom at the base to prevent spillage. Because condoms break up to 2% of the time[66, 67] and fall off up to 13% of the time,[66] couples should remember that concomitant use of vaginal spermicide greatly decreases the risk of pregnancy and disease transmission in these cases. If there is any spillage or if the condom breaks, spermicide, if not already present, should be applied in the vagina immediately.

Female condoms ("Reality," Wisconsin Pharmaceutical Co., Jackson, WI), recently approved for use in the United States, are pouches made of polyurethane or latex. Like the "male" condom, they should provide an effective barrier to STDs and pregnancy.

Spermicides

Spermicidal foams, jellies, creams, films, and suppositories have a wide range of reported efficacy. Efficacy seems more dependent on the population studied than the agent used, with typical failure rates of approximately 20%/yr. With ideal use, as with other barrier methods, a pregnancy rate of approximately 3%/yr can be achieved with spermicides. Spermicides used in conjunction with a diaphragm or condom are most effective.

All spermicidal preparations consist of two components, an inert base and a spermicide (nonoxynol 9, octoxynol 9 or menfegol). These preparations act by damaging the cell membranes of sperm as well as bacteria responsible for STDs. Spermicide must be applied 10 to 30 minutes prior to intercourse and most remain effective for up to 8 hours after application. Tablets and suppositories are effective for less than 1 hour after insertion. Reapplication of any type of spermicide is needed for each coital episode.

Like condoms, spermicides are inexpensive, readily available, and have virtually no side effects. One or the other partner is rarely (1 to 5%) allergic to the propellant or spermicide, and this problem is usually easily solved by changing products.

Contraceptive Sponge

The vaginal contraceptive sponge ("Today," Whitehall Labs, NY) is a soft, dome-shaped sustained-release system for nonoxynol 9. Release of the spermicide is initiated by soaking the sponge with water prior to insertion. A central dimple helps the user place it over the cervix, and a braided cord assists with its removal. The sponge may be inserted immediately before intercourse or up to 24 hours beforehand. Like the diaphragm, it should remain in place at least 6 hours after coitus before removal.

The major advantage of the contraceptive sponge is that it provides continuous protection for up to 24 hours, regardless of frequency of intercourse. Side effects are uncommon; fewer than 10% of users complain of vaginal irritation, and allergic reactions occur in approximately 4%.[68] Because the sponge comes in only one size, proper fit may be difficult, especially in parous women. Accordingly, the first-year failure rate for parous women (28%) is double that of nulliparous women (14%) in the United States.[69]

NATURAL FAMILY PLANNING

Concern over chemical and mechanical interference with natural bodily processes like reproduction has encouraged some couples to control conception by periodic abstinence. Approximately 1% of reproductive-age women practiced some form of fertility timing in 1988, a dramatic decline since the 1960s. To make this method more reliable than the 30 to 40 pregnancies per 100 woman-years of use resulting from menstrual timing alone, techniques for detecting ovulation have been developed. Whatever approach to timing is used, natural family planning requires commitment from both partners. Techniques are based on following basal body temperature or the consistency of cervical mucus, as well as the length of the menstrual cycle. Counselors who are especially devoted to, and familiar with, ovulation timing are probably best qualified to teach this method to interested couples. Efficacy is increased by the use of barrier methods if intercourse occurs during the 2 weeks around ovulation.

STERILIZATION

Sterilization is the most common method of family planning used by couples in both developed and developing countries. Since 1970, approximately 1 million sterilization procedures have been performed annually in the United States.[70] Prior to 1973, vasectomies were more common than fallopian tube interruption. In 1988, 24% of couples used sterilization for contraception, 17% female and 7% male.[3, 71]

The popularity of surgical contraceptive sterilization is due to its high effectiveness, low incidence of side effects, and ease of use. Vasectomy is safer, simpler, and less costly than female sterilization. Both are equally effective, and both are intended to be permanent. Failure rates vary by method, but all are less than 1% in the first year.

Male sterilization is easily performed as an outpatient procedure using local anesthesia. The most common complications of vasectomy are hematoma, surgical site infection, and epididymitis, all occurring in approximately 1.5% of procedures.[72] Granuloma formation from leakage of sperm is a rare and, most often, self-limiting complication, occurring in 0.3% of procedures.[72] Complication rates vary according to the operator's experience and the type of procedure. The only reported long-term complication is a slightly increased rate of prostate cancer. Mortality is rare (0.3/100,000 procedures).

Female sterilization is increasingly performed as an out-

TABLE 40–9. DEATH-TO-CASE RATE FOR LEGAL ABORTIONS BY TYPE OF PROCEDURE AND WEEKS OF GESTATION, UNITED STATES, 1972 TO 1980*†

	Weeks of Gestation						
Type of Procedure	*≤8*	*9–10*	*11–12*	*13–15*	*16–20*	*≥21*	*Total*
Curettage	0.4	1.2	2.1	0.0	0.0	0.0	0.9
Dilatation and evacuation	0.0	0.0	0.0	3.6	10.7	15.0	5.5
Instillation	0.0	0.0	0.0	6.1	13.0	15.4	10.6
(Saline)	(0.0)	(0.0)	(0.0)	(1.9)	(16.2)	(15.1)	(12.6)
(Prostaglandin and other agents‡)	(0.0)	(0.0)	(0.0)	(14.1)	(6.6)	(16.0)	(7.1)
Hysterotomy/hysterectomy	0.0	51.4	35.3	65.6	64.6	135.0	44.6
Total§	0.5	1.3	2.2	5.4	13.6	17.7	1.9

*From Centers for Disease Control: Abortion Surveillance, 1979–80, issued May, 1983.
†Deaths per 100,000 abortions, based on distributions of abortions for which type of procedure and weeks of gestation are known.
‡Denominators for rates include abortions reported as "other" type of procedure (1% of all abortions with procedure known).
§Includes four deaths for which type of procedure was classified as "other" and two for which type of procedure was unknown.

patient procedure via laparoscopy or minilaparotomy using general, regional, or local anesthesia. Approximately 40 to 50% of procedures are performed in the immediate postpartum period via minilaparotomy at the level of the umbilicus,[73] and the remainder are performed as interval procedures. The incidence of complications is <1% and is dependent on the level of surgical skill. Most laparoscopic injuries are related to the trocar or other surgical instruments. Mortality (1.5/100,000 procedures) is slightly higher than that of vasectomy and is most commonly a result of an anesthetic complication.[74] In comparison, maternal mortality rates are 9.1/100,000 live births.[75] Under experiment are hysteroscopic techniques to inject occlusive materials into the fallopian tubes.

Pregnancy that occurs in women who have had tubal occlusion is more likely to be ectopic than in women using no method; however, the overall risk of an ectopic pregnancy after sterilization is lower than if the procedure had not been performed (see Table 40–8). Bipolar tubal occlusion is more likely to result in ectopic pregnancy than is mechanical occlusion. In the first year after sterilization, about 6% of pregnancies will be ectopic, whereas the majority of pregnancies that occur thereafter will be ectopic.[76] The cause of the increase is that the rate of intrauterine pregnancies decreases over time, whereas the ectopic pregnancy rate remains constant.

Physicians counseling their patients about sterilization should inform them that it is intended, but not guaranteed, to be a permanent procedure and should be confined to persons who are certain that there is no possibility of ever desiring to have more children. Informed consent is very important. To this end, some state governments and, for indigent patients, the federal government, require special consent procedures stipulating age limits, mental capacity requirements, and waiting periods between signing the consent forms and undergoing the procedure. Although sterilization is a safe procedure, patients must be informed of the hazards of infection, bleeding, and bowel injury at surgery. In addition, they should be informed about the minor side effects, such as diaphragmatic and shoulder pain resulting from gas infused into the abdomen during laparoscopy. Women and men alike can be assured that sterilization has few, if any, long-term ill effects on health, although some women experience menstrual changes.[77, 78]

ABORTION

Surgical Abortion

The availability of safe, legal abortion has had the greatest impact on maternal health since the introduction of antibiotics, which prevented maternal deaths from sepsis, and blood banking, which prevented maternal deaths from hemorrhage. Legalization has made abortion available to nearly all women and has dramatically reduced abortion complications. Still, because abortion is a surgical procedure with greater risks than other forms of fertility control, it should be used as a back-up for a method failure and not as a primary means of contraception. Legal abortion services provide health planners with an excellent example of economic, acceptable delivery of needed health services that have had a measurable, positive impact on health status. An accelerated decline in abortion-related mortality occurred after the legalization of abortion (as early as 1968 in some states and throughout the United States after January 1973).[79]

Abortion is a safe surgical procedure with a mortality rate of 0.5/100,000 procedures if performed before 12 weeks' gestation.[79] In the United States, approximately 88% of abortions are performed in the first trimester.[80] After the twelfth week of gestation, the death-to-case rate increases by approximately 50% with each additional week. Abortions performed after 20 weeks' gestation have a death-to-case rate of more than 20 times that of abortions performed at less than 9 weeks' gestation. The risk of death also varies independently with the type of procedure performed, shown in Table 40–9. A disproportionate percentage of the mortality has recently been shown to be due to complications of general anesthesia.

As with mortality rates, morbidity rates vary primarily with the duration of the pregnancy and the method of abortion. Table 40–10 shows rates of common complications of first-trimester procedures. During the first trimester, 99% or more of procedures are performed by suction evacuation with or without sharp curettage.[80] Abortions in the second trimester are usually achieved by cervical dilation and uterine evacuation. Procedures using intra-amniotic hypertonic saline or intra-amniotic or intracervical prostaglandins account for fewer than 15% of second-trimester terminations; these types of procedures have decreased in incidence over the past 15 years because of a higher rate of associated complications than occur in dilation and uterine evacuation.[80] Clinicians who perform or refer patients for abortion must counsel patients that (1) early abortion, preferably before 9 weeks' gestation, is safer than late abortion, and (2) that evacuation is safer, simpler, and less expensive than instillation of hypertonic saline or prostaglandins for late abortions.

Multiple studies have repeatedly shown that early abortion has no adverse effects on future fertility. Conditions such as secondary infertility, cervical incompetence, spontaneous abortion, prematurity, and abnormalities of pla-

TABLE 40–10. COMPLICATIONS OF FIRST-TRIMESTER ABORTION*

Major Complications (Hospitalization Required)	Incidence	%
Retained tissue	1:3617	0.0277
Sepsis	1:4722	0.0212
Uterine perforation	1:10,625	0.0094
Hemorrhage	1:14,166	0.0071
Inability to complete	1:28,333	0.0035
Tubal pregnancy	1:42,500	0.0024
Minor Complications (Managed as Outpatient)	*Incidence*	*%*
Mild infection	1:216	0.4630
Reaspiration, same day	1:553	0.1808
Reaspiration, later	1:596	0.1678
Cervical stenosis	1:6071	0.0165
Cervical laceration	1:9444	0.0106
Underestimated gestational age	1:15,454	0.0065
Convulsion	1:25,086	0.0040

*Adapted from Hakim-Elahi E, Tovell HM, and Burnhill MS: Complications of first trimester abortion: A report of 170,000 cases. Obstet Gynecol 76:929, 1990.

centation and labor have all been investigated. Repeated abortions, especially in the second trimester, may be associated with a slightly increased risk of cervical incompetence or late spontaneous abortion, but conclusive evidence is lacking.[81]

Currently, the safest abortion procedure available in the United States is minimal cervical dilation and rapid uterine evacuation by suction curettage. This procedure is usually performed with a paracervical block and accompanying systemic (oral or parenteral) analgesia, sedation, or both. Cervical dilation can be accomplished mechanically using rigid dilators. However, placement of hydrophilic dilators in the cervical canal 4 to 24 hours prior to the abortion is safer and decreases the risk of uterine perforation below that achieved with mechanical dilation. Women who test Rh negative, D^u negative should be treated with Rh immune globulin following the procedure.

Serious psychological reactions to abortion occur infrequently. Emotional problems can occur when patients have a history of mental illness, immature interpersonal relationships, unstable relationships full of conflict with their partners, or negative relationships with their mothers. Ambivalence about the abortion or evidence of coercion to obtain the abortion by the partner or the patient's parents also helps predict increased frequency of emotional problems. The physician or other counselor must, therefore, help the patient make her own decision about the abortion and then guide her to the medically safest procedure.

Abortion procedures are best performed by medical personnel who perform them voluntarily and who have thorough training in the technical, social, political, and psychological aspects of abortion and contraception.

Mifepristone (RU-486)

In France, mifepristone (RU-486) has been used in combination with a prostaglandin analog as a medical alternative for early pregnancy termination. Mifepristone is an antiprogesterone that was first used as an abortifacient in humans in 1982. Since its introduction, mifepristone has been studied extensively in France, China, Scandinavia, and the United Kingdom, which have provided considerable data on its efficacy and safety. When used alone in a single 600-mg oral dose, mifepristone causes abortion in 80% of users within 49 days or less of amenorrhea[82]; addition of a prostaglandin analog increases the efficacy to 94 to 99%.[82–84] The course of treatment consists of mifepristone, 600 mg orally, followed 36 to 48 hours later by intravaginal gemeprost (prostaglandin E_1 analog), intramuscular sulprostone (prostaglandin E_2 analog), or oral misoprostol (prostaglandin E_2 analog). Failure of this treatment regimen is very rare at 42 days or less of amenorrhea, and there is a 6 to 7% failure rate between 43 and 69 days of amenorrhea.[82, 83] The vast majority of pregnancies are expelled within 24 hours after administration of the prostaglandin analog.

The two major problems associated with this treatment are pain and bleeding. Most women reported abdominal pain during the first 4 hours after receiving the prostaglandin analog, and the percentage requiring narcotic analgesia depended on the amount and type of analog used. The studies from the United Kingdom reported that three times as many nulliparous women as multiparous women will require narcotic analgesia.[83]

Virtually all women experience bleeding after receiving mifepristone and a prostaglandin analog, regardless of the treatment outcome. Subjectively, blood loss in the United Kingdom studies seemed severe in 16% of users by 2 days after treatment, but fewer than 1% felt so after 9 days.[83] Changes in hemoglobin before and 7 days after treatment, however, showed a significant decrease in fewer than 1% of patients. Likewise, in the French studies, fewer than 1% of women required a surgical abortion because of hemorrhage and 0.05% or fewer of women required a blood transfusion.[84]

Overall, medical treatment for early pregnancy termination avoids a surgical procedure and its associated risks in approximately 95% of patients. The risks and side effects of this medical treatment are fewer than or equal to those of surgical abortion, with the additional benefit of lower cost. Also, mifepristone has been shown to decrease the interval to delivery in prostaglandin-induced second-trimester terminations[85, 86] and to be effective in cervical priming before induction for intrauterine fetal demise.[82] It has potential uses as a luteal-phase abortifacient and for labor induction at term, but these uses are limited by the lack of information on the effects of mifepristone on the developing fetus and neonate.[82] Mifepristone use in the United States is presently limited by the political debate over the legality of abortion as well as by the lack of availability of the prostaglandin analogs used in Europe.

REFERENCES

1. Wrigley EA: Population and History. London, World University Library, 1969.
2. Goldzieher VW and Rudel MW: How the oral contraceptives came to be developed. JAMA 230:421, 1974.
3. Mosher WD and Pratt WF: Contraceptive use in the United States: 1973–88, Advance data from vital and health statistics; No. 182. Hyattsville, MD, National Center for Health Statistics, 1990.
4. Beral V and Kay CR: Mortality among oral contraceptive users. Lancet ii:727, 1977.
5. Vessey MP, Doll R, Peto R, et al: A long-term follow-up study of women using different methods of contraception—an interim report. J Biosoc Sci 8:373, 1976.
6. World Health Organization: Steroid contraception and risk of neoplasia. WHO Tech Rep Ser 1978, #619.
7. Trussell J, Hatcher RA, Cates W Jr.: Contraceptive failure in the United States: An update. Stud Fam Plann 21:51, 1990.
8. Vessey MP and Doll R: Investigation of relation between use

of oral contraceptives and thromboembolic disease. BMJ 2:199, 1968.
9. Kay CR: Oral contraception and health: The Royal College of General Practitioners study. Am J Epidemiol 102:458, 1975.
10. Vessey MP, McPherson K, and Johnson B: Mortality among women participating in the Oxford/Family Planning Association Contraceptive Study. Lancet ii:731, 1977.
11. Ramcharm S, Pellegrin FA, Ray RM, et al: The Walnut Creek Contraceptive Drug Study: A prospective study of the side effects of oral contraceptives. J Reprod Med 25:346, 1980.
12. Stampfer MJ, Willett WC, Colditz GA, et al: A prospective study of past use of oral contraceptive agents and risk of cardiovascular diseases. N Engl J Med 319:1313, 1987.
13. Porter JB, Hunter JR, Danielson DA, et al: Oral contraceptives and nonfatal vascular disease—recent experience. Obstet Gynecol 59:299, 1982.
14. Porter JB, Hunter JR, Jick H, et al: Oral contraceptives and nonfatal vascular disease. Obstet Gynecol 66:1, 1985.
15. Porter LB, Hershel J, and Walker AM: Mortality among oral contraceptive users. Obstet Gynecol 70:29, 1987.
16. Royal College of General Practitioners Oral Contraceptive Study: Further analyses of mortality in oral contraceptive users. Lancet i:541, 1981.
17. Vessey MP, McPherson K, and Yeates D: Mortality in oral contraceptive users. Lancet i:549, 1981.
18. Vessey MP, Villard-Mackintosh L, McPherson K, et al: Mortality among oral contraceptive users: 20 year follow-up of women in a cohort study. BMJ 299:1487, 1989.
19. The Cancer and Steroid Hormone Study of the CDC and NICHD: Combination oral contraceptive use and the risk of endometrial cancer. JAMA 257:796, 1987.
20. The Cancer and Steroid Hormone Study of the CDC and NICHD: The reduction in risk of ovarian cancer associated with oral-contraceptive use. N Engl J Med 316:650, 1987.
21. Irwin KL, Rosero-Bixby L, Oberle MW, et al: Oral contraceptives and cervical cancer risks in Costa Rica: Detection bias or causal association? JAMA 259:59, 1988.
22. Brinton LA, Reeves WC, Brenes MM, et al: Oral contraceptive use and risk of invasive cervical cancer. Int J Epidemiol 19:4, 1990.
23. The Cancer and Steroid Hormone Study of the CDC and NICHD: Oral contraceptive use and the risk of breast cancer. N Engl J Med 315:405, 1986.
24. Hannaford PC, Villard-Mackintosh L, Vessey MP, et al: Oral contraceptives and malignant melanoma. Br J Cancer 63:430, 1991.
25. WHO Collaborative Study of Neoplasia and Steroid Contraceptives: Combined oral contraceptives and liver cancer. Int J Cancer 43:254, 1989.
26. Milne R and Vessey M: The association of oral contraception with kidney cancer, colon cancer, gallbladder cancer (including extrahepatic bile duct cancer) and pituitary tumors. Contraception 43:667, 1991.
27. Szoka PR and Edgren RA: Drug interactions with oral contraceptives: Compilation and analysis of an adverse experience report database. Fertil Steril 49(Suppl):31S, 1988.
28. Rubin GL, Ory HW, and Layde PM: Oral contraceptives and pelvic inflammatory disease. Am J Obstet Gynecol 144:630, 1982.
29. Kost K, Forrest JD, and Harlap S: Comparing the health risks and benefits of contraceptive choices. Fam Plann Perspect 23:54, 1991.
30. Royal College of General Practitioners: The outcome of pregnancy in former oral contraceptive users. Br J Obstet Gynaecol 83:608, 1976.
31. Vessey MP, Wright NH, McPherson K, et al: Fertility after stopping different methods of contraception. BMJ 276:265, 1978.
32. Vessey MP, Smith MA, and Yates D: Return of fertility after discontinuation of oral contraceptives: Influence of age and parity. Br J Fam Plann 11:120, 1986.
33. Linn S, Schoenbaum SC, Monson RR, et al: Delay in conception for former "pill" users. JAMA 247:629, 1982.
34. Reiter SL and Baer LJ: Initial selection of oral contraceptives. J Reprod Med 35:547, 1990.
35. Percival-Smith RKL, Yuzpe AA, Desrosiers JA, et al: Cycle-control on low-dose oral contraceptives: A comparative trial. Contraception 42:253, 1990.
36. Fasoli M, Parazzini F, Cecchetti G, et al: Post-coital contraception: An overview of published studies. Contraception 39:459, 1989.
37. Darney PD, Klaisle CM, Tanner S, et al: Sustained-release contraceptives. Curr Probl Obstet Gynecol Fertil 13:89, 1990.
38. Sivin I: International experience with Norplant and Norplant-2 contraceptives. Stud Fam Plann 19:81, 1988.
39. Centers for Disease Control: Ectopic pregnancy surveillance, 1970–1987. CDC surveillance summaries, December, 1990. MMWR 39:9, 1990.
40. Sivin I, Alvarez-Sanchez F, Diaz S, et al: Three-year experience with Norplant subdermal contraception. Fertil Steril 39:799, 1983.
41. Shoupe D, Mishell DR, Bopp BL, et al: The significance of bleeding patterns in Norplant implant users. Obstet Gynecol 77:256, 1991.
42. Fakeye O and Balogh S: Effect of Norplant contraceptive use on hemoglobin, packed cell volume, and menstrual bleeding patterns. Contraception 39:265, 1989.
43. Croxatto HB, Diaz S, Robertson DN, et al: Clinical chemistries in women treated with levonorgestrel implant (Norplant) or a TCu200 IUD. Contraception 27:281, 1983.
44. Konje JC, Otolorin EO, and Ladipo OA: Changes in carbohydrate metabolism during 30 months on Norplant. Contraception 44:163, 1991.
45. Shaaban MM, Elwan SI, El-Sharkawy MM, et al: Effect of subdermal levonorgestrel contraceptive implants, Norplant, on liver functions. Contraception 30:407, 1984.
46. Singh K, Viegas OAC, Liew D, et al: Two-year follow-up of changes in clinical chemistry in Singaporean Norplant acceptors: Metabolic changes. Contraception 39:129, 1989.
47. Shaaban MM, Elwan SI, El-Kabsh MY, et al: Effect of levonorgestrel contraceptive implants, Norplant, on bleeding and coagulation. Contraception 30:421, 1984.
48. Abdulla K, Elwan SI, Salem HS, et al: Effects of early postpartum use of the contraceptive implants, Norplant, on the serum levels of immunoglobulin of mothers and their breastfed infants. Contraception 32:261, 1985.
49. Bayad M, Ibrahim I, et al: Serum cortisol in women users of subdermal levonorgestrel implants. Contracept Deliv Syst 4:133, 1983.
50. Shaaban MM, Elwan SI, et al: Effect of subdermal levonorgestrel contraceptive implants, Norplant, on serum lipids. Contraception 30:413, 1984.
51. Roy S, Mishell DR Jr., Robertson DN, et al: Long-term reversible contraception with levonorgestrel-releasing Silastic rods. Am J Obstet Gynecol 148:1006, 1984.
52. Klavon SL and Grubb GS: Insertion site complications during the first year of Norplant use. Contraception 41:27, 1990.
53. World Health Organization: Multinational comparative clinical evaluation of two long-acting injectable contraceptive steroids: Norethisterone enanthate and medroxyprogesterone acetate. Final report. Contraception 28:1, 1983.
54. Alvarez F, Brache V, Fernandez E, et al: New insights on the mode of action of intrauterine contraceptive devices in women. Fertil Steril 49:768, 1988.
55. Sivin I, El Mahgoub S, McCarthy T, et al: Long-term contraception with the levonorgestrel 20 mcg/day (LNg 20) and the Copper T 380Ag intrauterine devices: A five-year randomized study. Contraception 42:361, 1990.
56. Lee NC, Rubin GL, and Borucki R: The intrauterine device and pelvic inflammatory disease revisited: New results from the Women's Health Study. Obstet Gynecol 72:1, 1988.
57. Foreman H, Stadel BV, and Schlesselman S: Intrauterine device usage and fetal loss. Obstet Gynecol 58:669, 1981.
58. Tatum HJ, Schmidt FS, and Jain AK: Management and outcome of accidental pregnancies associated with copper T intrauterine devices. Am J Obstet Gynecol 145:596, 1983.
59. IUDs: An appropriate contraceptive for many women. Population Reports, Population Information Program, The Johns Hopkins University, Series B, Number 4. July 1982.
60. Chapin DS and Sullinger JC: A 43-year old woman with left buttock pain and a presacral mass. N Engl J Med 323:183, 1990.

61. Keebler C, Chatwani A, and Schwartz R: Actinomycosis infection associated with intrauterine contraceptive devices. Am J Obstet Gynecol 145:596, 1983.
61A. Duguid HLD: Actinomycosis and IUDs. Int Plann Parenthood Fed Med Bull 17:3, 1983.
62. Petitti DB, Yamammoto D, and Morgenstern N: Factors associated with actinomyces-like organisms on Papanicolaou smears in users of IUDs. Am J Obstet Gynecol 145:338, 1983.
63. Rioux JE, Cloutier D, Dupont P, et al: Pregnancy after IUD use. Adv Contracept 2:185, 1986.
64. Fihn SD, Latham RH, Roberts MS, et al: Association between diaphragm use and urinary tract infection. JAMA 254:240, 1985.
65. Richwald GA, Greenland S, Gerber MM, et al: Effectiveness of the cavity-rim cervical cap: Results of a large clinical study. Obstet Gynecol 74:143, 1989.
66. Trussell J, Warner DL, and Hatcher RA: Condom slippage and breakage rates. Fam Plann Perspect 24:20, 1992.
67. Albert AE, Hatch RA, and Graves W: Condom use and breakage among women in a municipal hospital family planning clinic. Contraception 43:167, 1991.
68. Edelman DA, McIntyre SL, and Harper J: A comparative trial of the Today contraceptive sponge and diaphragm. Am J Obstet Gynecol 150:869, 1984.
69. McIntyre SL and Higgins JE: Parity and use-effectiveness with the contraceptive sponge. Am J Obstet Gynecol 155:796, 1986.
70. Association for Voluntary Sterilization: Estimate of US sterilizations, 1984. New York, Association for Voluntary Sterilization, 1985.
71. Mosher WD and Pratt WF: Use of family planning services in the United States: 1982 and 1988, Advance data from vital and health statistics; No. 184. National Center for Health Statistics, Hyattsville, MD, 1990.
72. Wortman J: Vasectomy—what are the problems? Popul Rep D(2):25, 1975.
73. Centers for Disease Control: Surgical sterilization surveillance: Tubal sterilization and hysterectomy in women aged 15–44 years, 1979–1980. CDC surveillance summaries, September, 1983. MMWR 32:1, 1983.
74. Escobedo LG, Peterson HB, Grubb GS, et al: Case fatality rates for tubal sterilization in US hospitals. Am J Obstet Gynecol 160:147, 1989.
75. Centers for Disease Control: Maternal mortality surveillance, 1979–1986. CDC surveillance summaries, July, 1991. MMWR 40:1, 1991.
76. Chi IC, Laufe LE, and Atwed R: Ectopic pregnancy following female sterilization procedures. Adv Plann Parenthood 16:52, 1981.
77. Peterson HB, Huber DH, and Belker AM: Vasectomy: An appraisal for the obstetrician-gynecologist. Obstet Gynecol 76:568, 1990.
78. Rulin MC, Davidson AR, Philliber SG, et al: Changes in menstrual symptoms among sterilized and comparison women: A prospective study. Obstet Gynecol 79:749, 1989.
79. Centers for Disease Control: Abortion surveillance, United States, 1984–1985. CDC surveillance summaries, September, 1989. MMWR 38:11, 1989.
80. Centers for Disease Control: Abortion surveillance, United States, 1988. CDC surveillance summaries, July, 1991. MMWR 40:15, 1991.
81. Hogue CJ: Impact of abortion on subsequent fecundity. Clin Obstet Gynecol 13:951, 1986.
82. Ulmann A and Dubois C: Clinical trials with RU 486 (mifepristone): An update. Acta Obstet Gynecol Scand Suppl 149:9, 1989.
83. UK Multicentre Trial: The efficacy and tolerance of mifepristone and prostaglandin in first trimester termination of pregnancy. Br J Obstet Gynaecol 97:480, 1990.
84. Silvestre L, Dubois C, Renault M, et al: Voluntary interruption of pregnancy with mifepristone (RU 486) and a prostaglandin analogue: A large-scale French experience. N Engl J Med 322:645, 1990.
85. Hill NCW, Selinger M, Ferguson J, et al: The physiological and clinical effects of progesterone inhibition with mifepristone (RU 486) in the second trimester. Br J Obstet Gynaecol 97:487, 1990.
86. Urquhart DR, Bahzad C, and Templeton AA: Efficacy of the antiprogestin mifepristone (RU 486) prior to prostaglandin termination of pregnancy. Hum Reprod 4:202, 1989.

41

Amenorrhea Syndromes

ROBERT G. DLUHY, MD

Amenorrhea for at least 3 months in a patient with previous menstruation is the generally accepted definition of secondary amenorrhea. Secondary amenorrhea may be seen under certain physiologic circumstances (postmenopausally and following pregnancy). A diagnosis of primary amenorrhea is usually made in a patient who has never menstruated. Patients with primary amenorrhea have a high incidence of gonadal (e.g., ovarian dysgenesis) or embryologic abnormalities (e.g., uterine agenesis), suggesting that primary amenorrhea results from genetic diseases. However, there are clear-cut examples of patients with gonadal dysgenesis who began to menstruate at puberty, only to have their cycles cease secondarily. Thus, amenorrhea should be viewed from a pathophysiologic viewpoint to define whether the absence of menstruation is secondary to (1) anatomic diseases or end-organ abnormalities, (2) gonadal failure, or (3) abnormalities of the central nervous system-hypothalamic-pituitary regulation of gonadotropin secretion. Numerous hormonal factors, such as prolactin, have been found to modify gonadal steroid and pituitary gonadotropin secretion, potentially implicating these factors in abnormalities of menstruation.

PHYSIOLOGY OF THE NORMAL MENSTRUAL CYCLE

The median menstrual cycle length is 28 days, but prolonged intermenstrual intervals are commonly seen in association with anovulatory cycles (especially in adolescence and in the transition to the menopause). In the absence of ovarian function, follicle-stimulating hormone (FSH) levels are higher than levels of luteinizing hormone (LH), resulting in a greater FSH:LH ratio than observed during the reproductive years of the normal woman. Thus, high FSH:LH ratios are observed in prepubertal and postmenopausal women. In the prepubertal girl, gonadotropin secretion is low, owing to immaturity of hypothalamic gonadotropin-releasing hormone (GnRH), whereas in the postmenopausal woman, gonadotropin secretion is increased, owing to the failure of the ovary and the subsequent decline in ovarian negative-feedback inhibition.

The normal menstrual cycle can be divided into follicular, ovulatory, and luteal phases (Fig. 41–1).[1] In the early follicular phase, FSH and LH gradually rise while estrogen and androgen levels remain constant; in the late follicular phase, ovarian estradiol secretion begins to rise gradually and then rapidly and is accompanied by a decline in FSH and a steady rise in LH levels. The midcycle ovulatory phase is characterized by a rapid and sharp rise in LH level (the so-called LH peak or surge); follicular rupture occurs approximately 16 to 24 hours after the LH peak. The rise in serum estradiol, which triggers the LH peak, reaches its peak approximately 1 day before the LH surge.

Following ovulation, a corpus luteum is formed, with a

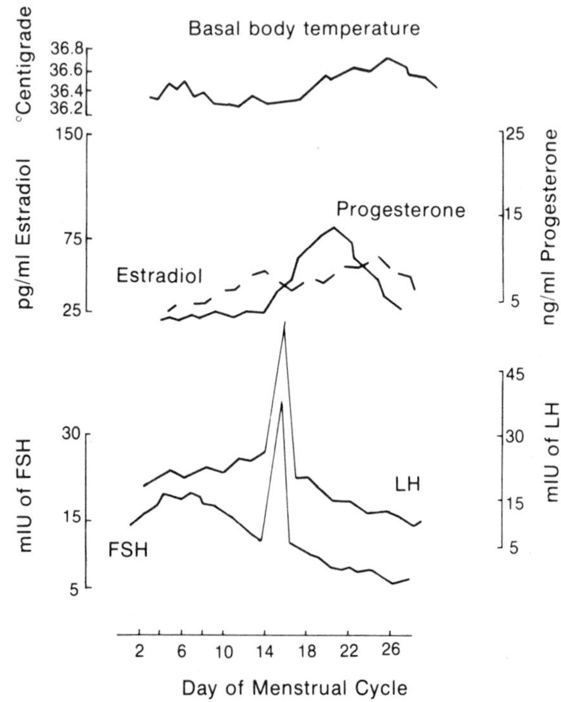

FIGURE 41–1. Mean daily basal body temperature, plasma estradiol, progesterone, and follicle-stimulating hormone and luteinizing hormone levels during normal menstrual cycles. (Adapted from Scommegna A and Dmowski WP: Dysfunctional uterine bleeding. Clin Obstet Gynecol 10:221, 1973.)

subsequent marked increase in progesterone secretion and a smaller rise in estrogen levels. The marked rise in progesterone levels centrally produces the elevation of basal body temperature. The elevated progesterone and estrogen levels in the luteal phase are subsequently accompanied by declines in FSH and LH levels. Unless pregnancy occurs, estrogen and progesterone levels decline in the late luteal phase and are accompanied by vasospasm of endometrial vessels, endometrial necrosis, and withdrawal menstrual bleeding. FSH begins to rise in the late luteal phase to initiate follicular growth for the next menstrual cycle. The regulation of this complex cyclic pattern of hormone release involves inherent cyclic activities as well as feedback regulation of the hypothalamic-pituitary-ovarian axis. Some aspects of the cyclic behavior of human menstruation, such as folliculogenesis, reside in the ovary and are gonadotropin independent.

Gonadotropin secretion by the pituitary gland depends on and is regulated by hypothalamic GnRH. The regulation of GnRH is complex and includes the hypothalamic content of biogenic amines and prostaglandins; the major control is the feedback loop provided by ovarian steroid output. This negative feedback regulation of GnRH is primarily by estradiol and explains the rise in gonadotropin output in the postmenopausal woman. Moreover, estradiol acts to augment pituitary LH reserve (i.e., the synthesis and storage of LH) and modulates the sensitivity of the pituitary gonadotropins to GnRH. Although the feedback of estradiol on GnRH release is primarily negative, there is also evidence for positive midcycle regulation of GnRH. Thus, as estrogen levels rise over time during the follicular phase, a positive action on GnRH is ultimately achieved, culminating in the midcycle LH surge.

The endometrium reflects the cyclic nature of ovarian steroid secretion.[2] The follicular phase is characterized by a proliferative endometrium with abundant mitoses; the increased progesterone levels that occur after ovulation convert the proliferative to a secretory endometrium. Failure of implantation of a fertilized ovum leads to a prostaglandin-induced vasoconstriction and subsequent shedding of the endometrial tissue, or menstruation. It should be evident that estrogen deficiency is associated with atrophy of the endometrium. Anovulatory cycles associated with inappropriate estrogen levels, abnormal estrogen-to-progesterone ratios, or both would be associated with a proliferative endometrium, leading to an irregular shedding, or episodes of amenorrhea.

The vaginal epithelium and cervical mucus also can be viewed as sensitive indices of hormonal secretion at each period of life and during the course of each menstrual cycle. The vaginal epithelium shows a progressive increase in numbers of cornified cells prior to ovulation, in parallel with the increasing levels of estrogen. In the postmenopausal woman who is estrogen deficient, the vaginal epithelium will be atrophic. In the prepubertal or postpubertal amenorrheic young woman, an estrogenic smear makes a diagnosis of hormonal deficiency highly unlikely. Therefore, the vaginal smear serves as a biologic assay of the degree of ovarian function. The cervical mucus also reflects estrogen activity; arborization (or ferning) and increased elasticity (ability to withdraw the mucus into a long thread, or spinnbarkeit) reflect estrogen stimulation and are maximally apparent at midcycle, just prior to ovulation.[3] Thus, the presence of cervical mucus can also be used in an amenorrheic patient as a bioassay of endogenous estrogen production.

Evaluation of gonadal disorders often requires the determination of genetic sex. A simple technique is to sample the buccal mucosa for a chromatin mass near the nuclear membrane (Barr's or sex chromatin body). These bodies are nonfunctioning X chromosomes and are observed in 30% or more of cell nuclei from normal women. In patients with gonadal dysgenesis syndromes, something is wrong with the second sex chromosome in at least some of the patient's cells. Most of these patients will have a low proportion of sex chromatin-positive cells; they lack a second X chromosome and have 45 rather than 46 chromosomes. However, numerous gonadal dysgenesis variants exist, including mosaicism (absent X chromosome only in some cell lines), as well as structural abnormalities of the second sex chromosome. The karyotype obtained from tissue grown in culture, usually of human leukocytes, allows precise characterization of the individual chromosomes and is the preferred chromosome analysis test, if available. The Y chromosome can also be specifically identified by fluorescent staining with quinacrine; the H-Y cell surface antigen is an alternative test to detect Y chromosomal material.

PRIMARY AMENORRHEA

The diagnosis of primary amenorrhea, or failure to initiate menstruation, is made when the clinician is most likely not dealing with delayed menarche. Because menarche occurs between the ages of 9 and 16 years, a diagnosis of delayed menarche should still be considered as long as the patient is in the 9-to-16–year range. It is important in such patients to determine whether normal secondary sex characteristics are present or absent.[4] Because growth of breasts and the appearance of axillary and pubic hair usually precede the first menses, the presence of these signs in an amenorrheal patient as old as 16 years suggests a diagnosis of delayed menarche. In many of these patients, there also may be a family history of delayed menarche. On the other hand, absence of normal secondary sex characteristics in patients 16 years of age or older points to the diagnosis of primary amenorrhea.

The evaluation of patients with a working diagnosis of primary amenorrhea should then focus on the two major etiologic possibilities: gonadal and extragonadal abnormalities[5, 6] (Table 41–1). Gonadal abnormalities include ovarian diseases, such as gonadal dysgenesis, polycystic ovarian disease, or genetic maleness; extragonadal etiologies include dysgenesis of the müllerian ducts and hypogonadotropic states (panhypopituitarism or isolated hypogo-

TABLE 41–1. CAUSES OF PRIMARY AMENORRHEA

Delayed menarche
Gonadal abnormalities
Gonadal dysgenesis (Turner's syndrome, XO, and variants)
Polycystic ovarian disease
Genetic males (testicular feminization)
Hermaphroditism (XX/XY)
Physical damage (e.g., chemotherapy or irradiation)
Immune etiologies (isolated or in association with other autoimmune diseases)
Enzyme defects
Galactosemia
17 α-Hydroxylase deficiency
Extragonadal etiologies
Dysgenesis of the müllerian ducts
Vaginal atresia or aplasia
Hypothalamic-pituitary dysfunction, including isolated hypogonadotropism
Onset in adolescence of other causes of amenorrhea (see Table 41–2)—especially anorexia nervosa and exercise-induced amenorrhea

nadotropism). It is also important to remember that a phenotypic female does not necessarily reflect the genetic sex of the patient because male gonadal failure or resistance to the action of androgen in the male fetus will lead to phenotypically normal female external genitalia.

History and Physical Examination

The family history may help exclude certain rare familial syndromes (e.g., pure gonadal dysgenesis). Lymphedema during the neonatal period is also commonly seen in a chromatin-negative gonadal dysgenesis. Sexual immaturity strongly suggests the diagnosis of a gonadal basis for the amenorrhea, implying deficient ovarian and adrenal output of sex steroids. These patients also will have eunuchoid proportions, owing to failure of epiphyseal fusion of their long bones (arm span is greater than height; crown-pubis less than symphysis pubis-floor measurements). On the other hand, the presence of breast development and sexual hair in a female patient with primary amenorrhea is consistent with either delayed menarche or end-organ uterine or vaginal abnormalities (vaginal septum, vaginal atresia, imperforate hymen, absence of the uterus, or endometrial diseases, such as tuberculosis).

The general physical examination also may reveal findings characteristic of gonadal dysgenesis (Turner's syndrome).[7] These patients are characteristically of short stature (less than 58 inches) and may exhibit webbing of the neck, short metacarpals, increased carrying angles at the elbows (cubitus valgus), low hairline, high-arched palate, and numerous café au lait spots and black freckles. Genetic men with testes (male pseudohermaphroditism) have variable phenotypes ranging from a truly feminine appearance to incomplete masculinization. They have varying degrees of peripheral resistance to androgen action (5α-reductase deficiency, or a receptor disorder, testicular feminization), or abnormalities in androgen synthesis.[8] An important clue on physical examination in the testicular feminization syndrome is a phenotypically normal female with primary amenorrhea with absent or scant axillary and pubic hair, despite normal breast development.

Genital Examination

Female patients with ambiguous external genitalia are most commonly evaluated before puberty, usually in the neonatal period. Determination of the nuclear sex of these individuals is the first test to rule out a diagnosis of female pseudohermaphroditism (genetic female with adrenogenital syndrome).

In female patients with primary amenorrhea whose external genitalia are phenotypically normal, an important first step is to determine whether the vagina is present or absent; an absent or nonpatent vagina is seen in patients with vaginal atresia or aplasia (Fig. 41–2). If a vagina is present, it is then necessary to determine whether the cervix is present or absent. Absence of a cervix is most commonly encountered in genetic males with testicular feminization syndrome. Presence of the male gonad is associated with regression of müllerian structures (upper vagina and uterus) so that a short vagina ends in a blind pouch. This diagnosis is further supported by normal breast development and sparse or absent sexual hair. Testes may be palpable in the inguinal canals, and the buccal mucosal smear reveals a chromatin-negative sex. Karyotyping (demonstrating a Y chromosome by special techniques) and measurement of testosterone levels confirm the diagnosis. A positive family history is obtained in two thirds of patients with this syndrome.

If the physical examination reveals a vagina and a cervix, the next step is to determine the nuclear sex of the patient (see Fig. 41–2). If the patient tests chromatin negative, additional karyotyping should be performed to determine whether a Y chromosome is present. Absence of a Y chromosome points to a diagnosis of gonadal dysgenesis; presence of a Y chromosome suggests a diagnosis of true hermaphroditism, testicular feminization, or mixed gonadal dysgenesis. Identifying patients with primary gonadal abnormalities with a Y chromosome is important because these patients are at high risk for developing gonadal tumors; accordingly, the gonadal tissue in these patients should be excised.[9] An important finding that confirms the diagnosis of primary gonadal failure (i.e., gonadal dysgenesis) is elevated gonadotropin levels; in such cases, gonadotropins are elevated after puberty, and a characteristically high FSH:LH ratio will be found.

Possible diagnoses in the patient with primary amenorrhea, who tests chromatin positive by buccal smear or XX by karyotyping, and who has a patent vagina and a cervix include delayed puberty, pituitary insufficiency, chronic anovulation, and chromatin-positive gonadal dysgenesis. If gonadotropin levels are elevated, a diagnosis of gonadal dysgenesis is likely, although an additional possibility is the resistant ovary syndrome. Normal or low levels of pituitary gonadotropins are consistent with delayed puberty or a number of hypothalamic-pituitary diseases, including isolated hypogonadotropic hypogonadism, chronic anovulation, and pituitary and suprasellar neoplasms. In addition to radiographic imaging of the pituitary gland, administering progesterone and estrogen-progesterone combinations is often indicated to assess uterine responsiveness and the degree of estrogenization. These tests will be discussed subsequently in the section on secondary amenorrhea.

SECONDARY AMENORRHEA

Secondary amenorrhea is usually defined as the absence of menses for at least 3 months in a patient with previously established normal menstrual function. As opposed to genetic diseases, acquired diseases of the pituitary-ovarian axis are the most common causes of secondary amenorrhea. However, it is again emphasized that patients with genetic diseases, who ordinarily present with primary amenorrhea, may initiate menses for varied periods of time; pregnancies also have been reported. Thus, the definition of primary versus secondary amenorrhea should be viewed as arbitrary, and the pathophysiology of acquired amenorrhea should always be sought.

At the outset, the differential diagnosis of secondary amenorrhea includes possible pregnancy and menopause. Age and history of sexual activity with or without the use of contraceptives may be helpful, but a pregnancy test should always be obtained before a diagnostic evaluation is initiated (Fig. 41–3). Prior use of oral contraceptive therapy also should be questioned because transient failure to resume spontaneous menses after discontinuation of contraceptive steroids occurs in a significant fraction of treated patients. Although the diagnostic possibilities include many organic etiologies, a large group of patients in the early and midreproductive years will be encountered in whom secondary amenorrhea will be temporarily related to weight loss, exercise, or psychogenic factors, with no organic pathology emerging over time.[10] These patients have

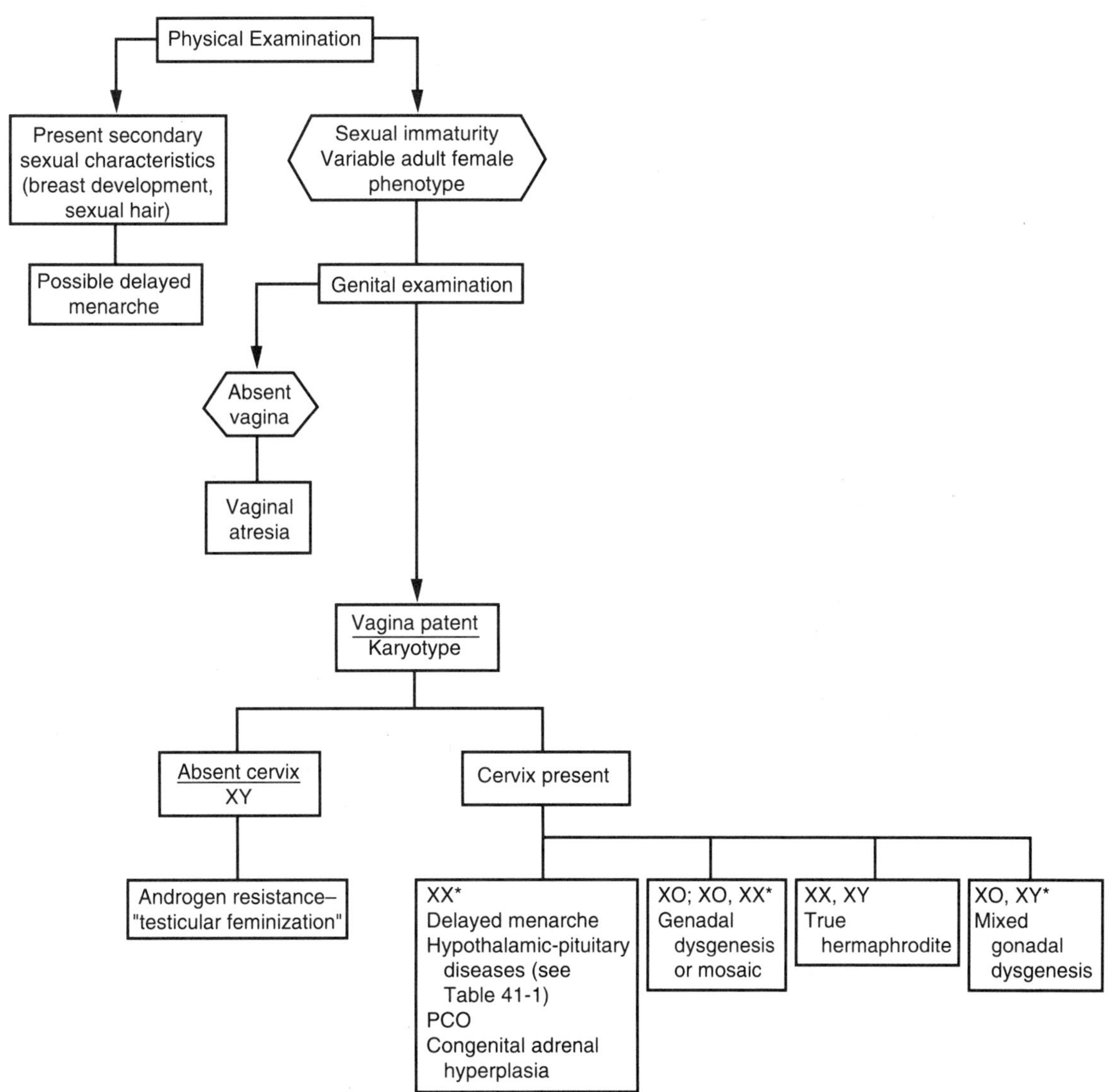

FIGURE 41–2. Evaluation of the patient with primary amenorrhea and female external genitalia. *-Elevated levels of FSH, LH. †-Normal or low levels of follicle-stimulating hormone and luteinizing hormone.

chronic anovulation syndrome. Their FSH and LH levels are similar to those observed in menstruating women in the early follicular phase of their cycles. Anovulation occurs secondary to acyclic gonadotropin secretion, probably related to endogenous opioid inhibition of GnRh release. The functional nature of this disorder is evidenced by the resumption of menses over time or following psychological counseling in some of these patients. On the other hand, an orderly approach to the patient with secondary amenorrhea is required to exclude diseases with specific therapies, such as pituitary tumors, anorexia nervosa, or uterine abnormalities (Table 41–2).

Because cyclic menstrual bleeding requires a normally functioning uterus and a patent cervix and vagina, diseases of these end-organs should be considered early in the differential diagnosis of secondary amenorrhea. Carcinoma and stenosis of the cervix can be ruled out by the physical examination. Intrauterine synechiae (Asherman's syndrome) also should be excluded.[11] A history of endometritis, either postpartum or postabortal following dilatation and curettage, should be sought. The diagnosis of uterine stenosis can be confirmed by hysteroscopy or a hysterosalpingogram; the treatment is lysis of the adhesions.

Ovarian Causes

The causes of secondary amenorrhea in which the ovary is the primary abnormality range from failure of ovarian function to hyperplastic or neoplastic ovarian diseases that hypersecrete androgens, estrogens, or both and secondarily lead to alterations in the rhythmic release of FSH and LH (see Table 41–2).

The mean age at which menopause (or cessation of ovarian function) occurs is approximately 50 years, with about half of women reaching menopause between 45 and 50 years of age. However, menopause may occur prematurely and has been reported in each decade following menarche. In general, premature ovarian failure is defined by cessation of menses following spontaneous sexual maturation before the age of 35 years. The diagnosis is clinically suggested by vasomotor instability (vasodilatation leading to warmth or hot flushes, followed by sweating). Physical examination may reveal signs of estrogen deficiency (diminution in breast size, vaginal atrophy with decreased mucus production, and dyspareunia). The diagnosis of premature ovarian failure is confirmed by finding elevated levels of pituitary gonadotropins with the characteristically high

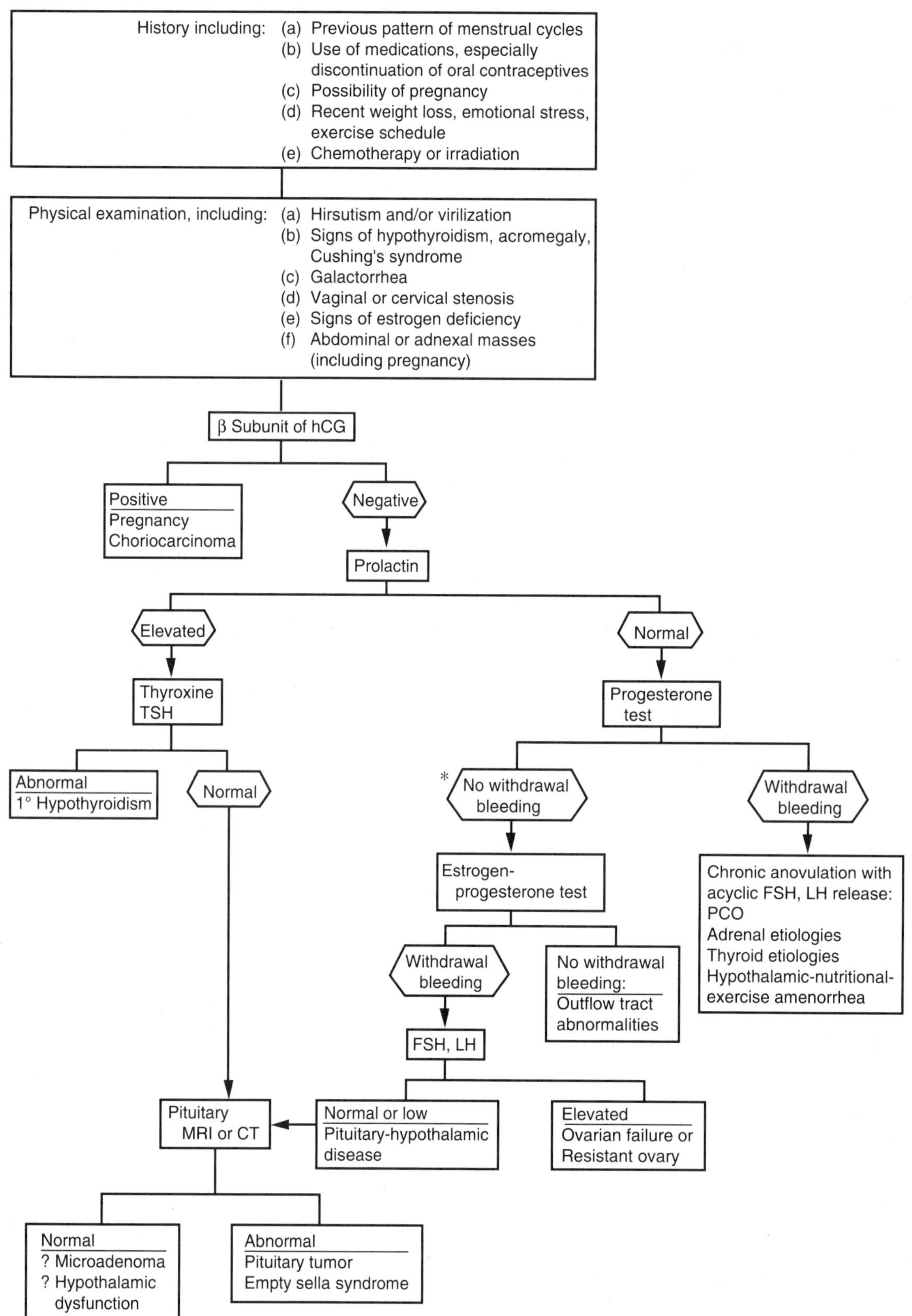

FIGURE 41–3. An initial approach to the patient with secondary amenorrhea. *-A negative test result does not provide definitive evidence for an abnormality in this axis. Failure of the patient to comply or poor gastrointestinal absorption is a common cause for a false-negative progesterone withdrawal test. Poor absorption of progesterone after intramuscular injection may also be seen, especially in the obese individual. Finally, the estrogen-progesterone ratio achieved at the uterus may not be physiologic, and withdrawal bleeding may fail to occur.

TABLE 41–2. CAUSES OF SECONDARY AMENORRHEA

Pregnancy
Chronic anovulation (hypothalamic) syndrome of functional, nutritional, or psychogenic etiology
  Following stressful life events
  Anorexia nervosa
  Associated with chronic illness
  Exercise-induced
End-organ abnormalities
  Carcinoma of the cervix
  Cevical stenosis
  Intrauterine synechiae (Asherman's syndrome)
  Uterine stenosis
Ovarian causes
  Menopause or premature ovarian failure
  Ovarian neoplasia
    Granulosa-theca cell tumors (feminizing)
    Arrhenoblastomas (virilizing)
    Adrenal rest, lipoid cell tumors, hilar cell tumors, or dysgerminomas
  Polycystic ovarian disease
Adrenal etiologies
  Cushing's syndrome due to hyperplasia, neoplasia, or ectopic ACTH* production
  Adrenogenital syndromes
Hypothalamic-pituitary causes
  Primary anterior pituitary insufficiency (idiopathic or postpartum pituitary necrosis—Sheehan's syndrome)
  Pituitary tumors
    Chromophobe adenomas
    Functioning pituitary tumors (e.g., causing acromegaly)
  Hyperprolactinemic states (see Table 41–3)
  Amenorrhea following discontinuation of oral contraceptive steroids (may unmask other hypothalamic-pituitary axis abnormalities)
Thyroid disease
  Hyperthyroidism
  Primary hypothyroidism with or without hyperprolactinemia

*ACTH = adrenocorticotropic hormone.

FSH:LH ratio. Premature ovarian failure may be idiopathic, or it may occur in the course of a syndrome of multiple endocrine end-organ failures (Addison's disease, Hashimoto's thyroiditis, pernicious anemia).[12] Autoimmune destruction probably underlies the pathogenesis of the failure of these endocrine target organs, as evidenced by the high prevalence of antibody titers directed at thyroid, adrenal, and ovarian tissues in these patients.[13] An additional amenorrhea syndrome with high gonadotropin levels is the resistant ovary due to antibodies directed at the ovarian gonadotropin receptors. In this situation, potentially functioning ovarian follicles may respond to the exogenous administration of large amounts of gonadotropins.

Ovarian tumors producing elevated estrogen levels, androgen levels, or both commonly produce chronic anovulation and secondary amenorrhea syndromes. As the result of inappropriate sex hormone feedback signals, pituitary gonadotropin secretion becomes acyclic. The resultant FSH and LH levels are either low or normal.

The most common functioning ovarian neoplasm is the granulosa-theca cell tumor.[14] Heavy and irregular menstrual bleeding, alternating with periods of amenorrhea, is the commonest complaint in premenopausal women. Sexual precosity in prepubertal girls or genital bleeding in postmenopausal women also suggests the diagnosis of granulosa cell tumor. These neoplasms range in size from 1 to 30 cm and are palpable by bimanual abdominal pelvic examination in approximately 80% of patients. Although anovulation and amenorrhea are secondary to elevated estrogen levels, signs of androgen excess may additionally be found if the tumor also contains luteinizing stromal cells.

Ovarian tumors producing androgens commonly produce virilizing syndromes in premenopausal and postmenopausal women.[15] Progressive and severe hirsutism is variably associated with signs of virilization (deepening of the voice, male habitus, and clitoromegaly), depending on the magnitude and duration of the testosterone elevation. The most common virilizing ovarian neoplasm is arrhenoblastoma. The majority of these neoplasms occur in women less than 40 years of age and are commonly palpable on physical examination. Amenorrhea is the commonest abnormality found in association with these tumors. Secondary amenorrhea is probably secondary to abnormal feedback regulation of gonadotropin secretion by elevated estrogen levels, which result from extraglandular conversion of androgenic compounds produced by the ovarian neoplasm. Other androgen-producing ovarian neoplasms include adrenal rest or lipoid cell tumors, hilar cell tumors, and dysgerminomas.

Polycystic Ovarian Disease. An important disease category consistently associated with anovulation, infertility, and menstrual abnormalities ranging from oligomenorrhea to secondary amenorrhea is the polycystic ovarian syndrome. This syndrome of chronic anovulation includes a group of heterogeneous disorders that have as a common basis varying degrees of androgenization and acyclic secretion of estrogens (usually estrone) and pituitary gonadotropins. The acyclic estrogen levels provide abnormal feedback signals for the regulation of pituitary gonadotropins, leading to suppressed FSH and tonically elevated LH levels. Numerous specific disorders (e.g., Cushing's syndrome, androgen-producing ovarian neoplasms, and congenital adrenal hyperplasia) can produce this characteristic hormonal pattern secondary to extraglandular peripheral conversion of androgenic precursors to estrogens. However, most often these specific disorders are not in evidence, and the primary abnormality is diagnosed.

As a group, patients with the polycystic ovarian syndrome usually share many common clinical features that often commence at or about the time of menarche: varying degrees of hirsutism (in some instances, true virilization), progressive menstrual irregularity and oligomenorrhea (sometimes progressing to secondary amenorrhea), and infertility.[16,17] Thus, the appearance of symptoms and signs over a prolonged period is useful in making the diagnosis of polycystic ovarian syndrome. This prolonged period is in contrast to the more abrupt onset of signs and symptoms in patients with ovarian or adrenal neoplasms.

Studies of androgen levels in patients with polycystic ovarian syndrome reveal elevated levels of androgenic steroids, including testosterone, androstenedione, and sometimes the adrenal androgen (dehydroepiandrosterone sulfate)[16,18,19] In other instances, increased levels of free androgenic steroids are found in the presence of normal plasma steroid levels because of decreased levels of sex hormone–binding globulin. Many studies point to the ovary as the major site for increased androgen production, but numerous additional studies suggest a combined ovarian-adrenal source. Some patients (20%) with longstanding polycystic ovarian syndrome may become severely hirsute and virilized. Therefore, this disease should be included in the differential diagnosis of virilizing syndromes in women, along with adrenal and ovarian neoplasms. An additional subset of patients with the disease has been identified with signs of androgen excess, acanthosis nigricans, and insulin-resistant diabetes mellitus. Insulin resistance in polycystic ovarian syndrome independent of the degree of obesity is also well established.[20] The insulin-resistant state and associated hyperinsulinemia have been linked to a number of other abnormalities commonly observed in polycystic ovarian syndrome, such as hyperlipidemia and hypertension.

The characteristic pituitary gonadotropin hormonal profile of patients with polycystic ovarian syndrome is a low or normal FSH level, with the LH level tonically elevated to levels often observed in normal menstruating women at the time of the midcycle ovulatory surge. It has been proposed that elevated acyclic estrogen (mainly estrone) levels result from extraovarian peripheral conversion of ovarian androgens (especially androstenedione); these levels of estrogen probably suppress FSH secretion while enhancing GnRH stimulation of LH secretion. A vicious circle becomes established because the elevated LH levels, in turn, tonically stimulate the ovary to produce excessive quantities of androgens. Chronic anovulation results from failure of follicular maturation, in part related to the suppressed FSH levels. Although in the established syndrome the ovarian changes are apparently secondary to altered gonadotropin levels, it is not clear whether the primary hormonal abnormality that initiates these changes originates in the ovary, the adrenal gland, or the pituitary-hypothalamic regulation of gonadotropin release. Familial polycystic ovarian syndromes are consistent with genetic etiologies,[21] whereas others have suggested abnormal modulation of neuroendocrine mechanisms regulating GnRH release.[22]

The differential diagnosis of menstrual irregularity, obesity, and hirsutism should include ovarian and adrenal etiologies. Symptoms and signs of concomitant cortisol excess point toward an adrenal lesion. The diagnosis of polycystic ovarian syndrome is best established by the history of signs and symptoms dating to the pubertal period, along with the characteristic FSH:LH ratio. Bilaterally enlarged ovaries may be palpable by bimanual abdominal-pelvic examination; ultrasonography also may reveal bilaterally enlarged cystic ovaries. Transvaginal transduction is recommended for ovarian visualization in the obese patient. Testosterone production is variable, but the levels are generally lower than those seen in patients with androgen-producing ovarian tumors. In virilized patients, polycystic ovarian disease may be difficult to differentiate from an ovarian neoplasm. If physical and ultrasonographic examinations are not adequate, venous catheterization may localize the androgen elevations and provide a definitive diagnosis.

Hypothalamic-pituitary Causes

Failure of a hypothalamic-pituitary unit may occur secondary to functional or structural defects arising in either locus or to abnormal higher CNS interactions with the hypothalamus. Patients may have incomplete or complete pituitary insufficiency (panhypopituitarism); if pituitary insufficiency is partial, gonadotropin secretion and growth hormone secretion are characteristically the first to be lost. Clinically, panhypopituitary patients appear chronically ill and suffer from severe malaise and fatigue. The physical examination often reflects signs of multiple hormone deficiencies. Dry, thin, wrinkled skin and loss of axillary and pubic hair reflect combined deficiencies of growth hormone, adrenal androgen, and thyroid hormones.

Primary Anterior Pituitary Failure. Primary pituitary insufficiency may be idiopathic or may result from vascular infarction, pituitary tumors, or infiltrative disorders (granulomas, metastatic tumors, and hemochromatosis). Vascular infarction of the pituitary gland may be seen in nonpregnant women or male patients who have diseases of the microvasculature (diabetes mellitus or sickle cell disease). More commonly, vascular infarction occurs in the immediate postpartum period in patients who become acutely hypotensive following hemorrhage at the time of delivery (Sheehan's syndrome).[23] It appears that the enlarged pituitary gland of pregnancy is at risk because of the precarious nature of its blood supply. Failure to lactate and then spontaneously resume menses is an important clue for the early diagnosis of postpartum pituitary failure.

Pituitary tumors are an important consideration in the differential diagnosis of secondary amenorrhea. The tumor may destroy normal gonadotropin-producing cells, compress the pituitary stalk, or involve the hypothalamus because of suprasellar extension. In addition to producing anterior pituitary failure, the tumor tissue itself may be nonfunctional or hormonally productive (functional). Functioning pituitary tumors may produce prolactin (amenorrhea-galactorrhea syndromes), growth hormone (acromegaly), adrenocorticotropic hormone (Cushing's syndrome), or rarely, thyroid-stimulating hormone (hyperthyroidism). An important recent advance has been the detection of small, functioning pituitary tumors or microadenomata less than 10 mm in diameter, which are best diagnosed by magnetic resonance imaging of the pituitary gland aided by the administration of the contrast agent gadolinium. Prolactin-producing pituitary microadenomata are particularly important because they are being diagnosed with increasing frequency in patients with secondary amenorrhea, galactorrhea, or both.

Hyperprolactinemia. Elevated prolactin levels are known to produce chronic anovulation as well as the amenorrhea-galactorrhea syndrome.[24] The elevated prolactin levels lead to acyclic gonadotropin release and decreased pulsatile LH secretion due to suppression of hypothalamic GnRH release.[25] The etiologies of the amenorrhea-galactorrhea syndrome include hyperplastic and neoplastic transformation of the pituitary lactotropes. Persistent galactorrhea following pregnancy with resumption of menses is not uncommon (Chiari-Frommel syndrome). Many patients with hyperprolactinemia have ultimately been found to have small microadenomata by magnetic resonance imaging (MRI) of the pituitary gland. The natural history of pituitary microadenomas is not known, but the overwhelming majority do not progress to become macroadenomas.[26]

Pituitary prolactin secretion is under tonic hypothalamic suppression by the prolactin inhibitory factor dopamine.[27, 28] Further, dopamine receptors have been identified on prolactin-secreting pituitary lactotropes. Therefore, prolactin secretion may be elevated by primary pituitary pathology, or prolactin levels may rise secondarily when the hypothalamic dopaminergic inhibitory influence is interrupted. Thus, destructive lesions of the hypothalamus (e.g., craniopharyngioma, granulomatous diseases, and metastatic tumors), interruption of the pituitary stalk (from head trauma or surgery), and depletion of the dopamine content of the hypothalamus or blocking of dopaminergic pituitary lactotroph receptors by pharmacologic agents will all lead to elevated prolactin levels. The absolute prolactin level is a helpful diagnostic point, because levels in excess of 150 to 200 ng/ml (normal is <15 to 20 ng/ml) are almost always associated with demonstrable pituitary adenomas by high-resolution computed tomography or MRI.[24] Moreover, the height of the prolactin level generally correlates with the size of pituitary adenomas.[29]

Primary hypothyroidism can be associated with variable elevations in prolactin levels, as well as with enlargement of the sella turcica.[24, 30] Thus, a prolactin-secreting tumor can be erroneously diagnosed if primary hypothyroidism is not recognized. Treatment with replacement doses of thyroid hormone corrects all of the endocrine abnormalities. Hyperprolactinemia has also been seen in patients with polycystic ovarian disease and following discontinuation of oral contraceptive steroids. In the latter patients, a primary underlying abnormality of the hypothalamic-pituitary axis, such as a pituitary microadenoma, may have been masked by the oral contraceptive steroids and is revealed when they are discontinued.

Table 41–3 summarizes the physiologic, pathologic, and pharmacologic causes of hyperprolactinemia.

Galactorrhea (milky discharge from the breasts in men and nonpuerperal women) is generally, but not invariably, associated with hyperprolactinemia. Galactorrhea may be accompanied by amenorrhea and anovulation, or menses may remain regular. The latter circumstance often occurs postpartum, and normal prolactin levels are usually encountered. In women with secondary amenorrhea but without galactorrhea, hyperprolactinemia will be found in 15 to 20% of patients.[31] However, the likelihood of finding elevated prolactin levels in a patient population with secondary amenorrhea increases greatly if concomitant galactorrhea is present. Patients with hyperprolactinemia and oligoamenorrhea may develop signs of estrogen deficiency, possibly including decreased bone density.[32, 33] Hirsutism is sometimes seen in hyperprolactinemic patients.

Treatment of patients with amenorrhea-galactorrhea syndromes logically should be directed at the specific etiology of the elevated prolactin levels (e.g., thyroid replacement in hypothyroidism). In patients with hyperprolactinemia that is idiopathic or secondary to a pituitary microadenoma or macroadenoma, the dopamine agonist bromocriptine suppresses the elevated prolactin levels regardless of etiology in approximately 85% of patients. Bromocriptine also reduces the size of macroprolactinomas in over 50% of patients because of a reduction in cell volume. Transsphenoidal surgery may be needed in some patients with macroadenomas who do not respond to bromocriptine treatment, especially subjects with optic chiasm compression.

Disordered Regulation of Gonadotropin Secretion (Psychogenic, Nutritional, and Exercise-related Causes)

Secondary amenorrhea may be seen in association with emotional upsets or serious psychiatric illness (severe depression, psychosis, and anorexia nervosa). Both ends of this spectrum illustrate that stress and the central nervous system can influence endocrine gland function. Psychogenic or hypothalamic amenorrhea in young women following stressful life events is a common cause of secondary amenorrhea. In these patients, higher centers in the central nervous system probably produce secondary amenorrhea by altering the hypothalamus, leading to acyclic gonadotropin release. Gonadotropin levels are usually in the follicular phase range. Appropriate therapy and counseling often reverse the secondary amenorrhea, illustrating the functional nature of the hypothalamic abnormality.

Secondary amenorrhea is also seen in athletes, such as long-distance runners, who exercise vigorously.[34] Weight loss and a decrease in the percentage of body weight as fat correlate with menstrual abnormalities. Reversal of this syndrome occurs with reduction of physical activity and with weight gain of as little as 3 to 5 lb, with a corresponding increase in the percentage of body weight as fat.

In contrast to hypothalamic amenorrhea, anorexia nervosa is a serious psychiatric disorder (seen almost exclusively in adolescent girls) that is characterized by excessive dieting, distortion of body image, and repulsion of food, leading to severe weight loss and malnutrition.[35] Secondary amenorrhea is an important feature of this syndrome and may be coincident with or precede the loss of weight. Gonadotropin levels are low and show a reduced and delayed response to GnRH, suggesting acquired hypothalamic dysfunction. Additional support for hypothalamic dysfunction includes abnormalities of temperature regulation and mild diabetes insipidus in a substantial number of patients with anorexia nervosa.[36] Adrenal and thyroid function test results are also altered. As in chronic starvation, serum T_4, and to a greater extent, T_3, levels are reduced, but thyroid-stimulating–hormone secretion is not elevated. The low T_3 levels, which reflect decreased peripheral conversion from T_4, may have physiologic consequences that lead to decreased metabolism of both testosterone and cortisol. Elevated cortisol levels in the blood have been found and reflect a decreased metabolic clearance of cortisol in association with the preservation of an inappropriately normal cortisol secretory rate.[37] The functional nature of all of these endocrine abnormalities is illustrated by their reversal following successful weight gain and psychotherapy.

Other chronic diseases associated with severe malnutrition (e.g., tuberculosis, cirrhosis, uremia, and AIDS) may also lead to secondary amenorrhea. These patients with an acquired form of hypothalamic hypogonadotropic hypogonadism further illustrate the relationship between body weight and reproductive function.

Amenorrhea (with or without hyperprolactinemia) is also seen in a small percentage of women who discontinue treatment with oral contraceptives (so-called postpill amenorrhea). Unless menses resumes spontaneously within 6 months, these patients should be investigated as are other women with secondary amenorrhea to rule out lesions (e.g., a pituitary adenoma) that prompted or appeared coincident with oral contraceptive use.

TABLE 41–3. ETIOLOGIES OF HYPERPROLACTINEMIA

Physiologic	Pathologic	Pharmacologic
Pregnancy	Prolactin-secreting pituitary tumor	Thyrotropin-releasing hormone
Postpartum	Hypothalamic disorders:	Medications
(Nonnursing mothers, days 1–7)	Functional: Chiari-Frommel syndrome	Estrogen
(Nursing mothers after suckling)	Organic: e.g., craniopharyngioma, metastatic disease, sarcoid	Antihypertensives—methyldopa, reserpine
Stress		Phenothiazines
Exercise	Pituitary stalk section	Tricyclics (amitriptyline, imipramine)
Sleep	Primary hypothyroidism	Dopamine receptor blockers (metaclopramide)
Hypoglycemia	Polycystic ovarian disease	Butyrophenones (haloperidol)
	Renal failure	
	Cirrhosis	
	Empty-sella syndrome	

Endocrine Diseases Associated with Secondary Amenorrhea

Hyperthyroidism and Hypothyroidism. Hyperthyroidism is commonly associated with oligomenorrhea, which may progress to cessation of menses; menstrual flow is usually scant. In this disorder, the increased concentration of thyroxine is associated with increased levels of testosterone-estradiol-binding globulin, with a resultant decrease in the metabolic clearance rate of these hormones. There also is an associated increased peripheral conversion of androgens to estrogens in the thyrotoxic state.[38] The resulting acyclic elevations of estrogen levels lead to anovulation and tonically elevated LH levels. Hypothyroidism also is associated with failure of ovulation and infertility or abortion. Menstrual bleeding is usually irregular and often excessive (menorrhagia), but secondary amenorrhea may also be seen. In some patients, the menstrual irregularity and anovulation are associated with galactorrhea and elevations in circulating levels of prolactin.[39] In contrast to the hyperthyroid state, hypothyroidism is associated with decreased circulating levels of sex hormone-binding globulin and an increase in metabolic clearance of testosterone and estrogen. These alterations, plus accompanying abnormalities in the peripheral conversion of androgens to estrogens, lead to disturbances in the feedback regulation of gonadotropin release, with resultant anovulation, dysfunctional bleeding, or both. Normal menstrual function is usually restored when the euthyroid state is reestablished.

Diseases of the Adrenal Cortex. Secondary amenorrhea may be seen in primary adrenocortical insufficiency. This may result from coincidental premature ovarian failure (with elevated gonadotropin levels),[12] or hypothalamic hypogonadotropic hypogonadism may result if cachexia and malnutrition are severe.

Chronic anovulation and amenorrhea also occur in patients with Cushing's syndrome. Possible explanations include alteration in central nervous system rhythms and acyclic estrogen levels derived peripherally from androgenic precursors, which secondarily alter gonadotropin release. Finally, in Cushing's syndrome, chronic anovulation may secondarily lead to abnormalities in ovarian androgen production, resulting in formation of polycystic ovaries.

Clinical and Laboratory Testing

Diagnostic Trial of Progesterone (Progesterone Test). A practical test of the integrity of the hypothalamic-pituitary-ovarian-uterine axis is the progesterone withdrawal bleeding test[40] (see Fig. 41–3). Medroxyprogesterone acetate (Provera) is the oral preparation of choice (10 mg once or twice daily for 5 to 10 days), because it has a greater and more prolonged effect on the endometrium than does progesterone. The progesterone test may also be performed by giving the patient 100 mg of progesterone intramuscularly. Vaginal bleeding within 1 week following the administration of a progestational agent indicates that (1) the pituitary gland secretes gonadotropins, (2) the ovary is responding to the gonadotropins with sufficient output of estrogen to cause endometrial proliferation, and (3) the uterus is capable of responding to both estrogen and progesterone.

Thus, withdrawal flow in a patient with amenorrhea provides *indirect* evidence for the integrity of the hypothalamic-pituitary-ovarian-uterine axis. Accordingly, amenorrheic patients with chronic anovulation syndromes (e.g., hypothalamic amenorrhea, polycystic ovarian disease, hyperprolactinemia syndromes, and thyroid and adrenal diseases) will often respond to progesterone administration with withdrawal bleeding. On the other hand, patients who are estrogen deficient (e.g., ovarian failure or pituitary insufficiency) would be expected to have a negative response. However, a negative test result does not provide definitive evidence for an abnormality in this axis. Failure of the patient to comply and poor gastrointestinal absorption are common causes for a false-negative progesterone withdrawal test result. Poor absorption of progesterone after intramuscular injection may also be seen, especially in the obese individual.

Finally, the estrogen-progesterone ratio achieved at the uterus may not be physiologic, and withdrawal bleeding may fail to occur. Nevertheless, in patients with a negative progesterone test result, additional studies are required to determine the locus of the abnormality. In patients with primary amenorrhea, the first diagnosis to rule out is agenesis of the uterus and vagina. Beyond the physical examination, this possibility is excluded if withdrawal bleeding occurs within a week after the oral administration of combined estrogen-progesterone treatment (1.25 mg/day of conjugated estrogen for 20 days with medroxyprogesterone acetate, 10 mg/day for the last 10 to 14 days). Thereafter, studies should aim to examine the integrity of each locus in the axis in an attempt to define whether the amenorrhea is dysfunctional (e.g., chronic anovulation syndromes) or is due to ovarian or pituitary failure.

Blood Follicle-stimulating and Luteinizing Hormone Levels. Basal serum gonadotropin (FSH and LH) levels are often not diagnostic in hypothalamic-pituitary disorders because low versus normal values are not distinguishable in assay systems.

On the other hand, basal levels of gonadotropins are diagnostic if the levels are clearly elevated, as in gonadal failure or resistant ovary syndrome. Thus, in patients with primary or secondary amenorrhea, three- to fivefold increases of FSH and LH above normal (with an increased FSH:LH ratio) are diagnostic of a hypergonadotropic form of amenorrhea (see Table 41–1). Tonically elevated LH levels in association with normal FSH levels strongly point to polycystic ovarian disease.[19] A single elevated LH level, however, may not be diagnostic in an oligomenorrheal patient, as it may represent an ovulatory surge. Low serum FSH and LH levels in the amenorrheic woman are expected in hypothalamic or pituitary diseases (e.g., pituitary tumors, and anorexia nervosa), but the levels may be indistinguishable from early follicular phase levels in menstruating women. Thus, further workup may be indicated if the levels are low or normal, especially if withdrawal bleeding cannot be provoked by the progesterone test (see Fig. 41–3) in a patient with secondary amenorrhea. Responsiveness of FSH and LH to GnRH stimulation has not proved useful in differentiating hypothalamic from pituitary causes of secondary amenorrhea. Pituitary imaging may be indicated if a clinical diagnosis is not apparent (such as in severe weight loss).

Prolactin. The normal level of prolactin in women in most assay systems is less than 20 ng/ml, with no significant differences noted during the menstrual cycle. Prolactin levels rise physiologically in response to stress, during pregnancy and sleep, and in postpartum nursing and nonnursing mothers (see Table 41–3). Accordingly, in any patient with secondary amenorrhea, pregnancy should first be ruled out by a β-subunit of human chorionic gonadotropin determination before additional diagnostic studies are obtained. Prolactin levels also are not interpretable in severely stressed or hypothyroid patients or in patients taking antidopaminergic, some antihypertensive, or psychotropic drugs because prolactin levels are secondarily elevated in these situations (see Table 41–3). Several repeat samples should be taken to estimate the basal secretion of prolactin.

The demonstration of hyperprolactinemia does not distinguish patients with idiopathic or disordered regulation of secretion from patients with prolactin-secreting pituitary neoplasms. Therefore, the diagnosis of an adenoma requires radiographic confirmation. Many also believe that most patients with idiopathic hyperprolactinemia have micro-adenomas that escape visualization with even the most advanced radiographic techniques. However, a level greater than 150 to 200 ng/ml correlates strongly with the demonstration of a pituitary adenoma by high-resolution computed tomography or MRI.[24] Prolactin-stimulation tests (e.g., thyrotropin-releasing hormone and chlorpromazine) are not useful in differentiating disorders of prolactin regulation from prolactin-secreting pituitary tumors.

Summary of the Approach to the Patient with Secondary Amenorrhea

The pattern of previous menstrual cycles should be carefully documented to determine whether longstanding menstrual irregularity may have resulted from a progressive syndrome, such as polycystic ovarian syndrome, or whether abrupt cessation of menses in a woman previously cycling normally suggests an acquired lesion affecting the pituitary-hypothalamic-ovarian axis. A β-subunit of human chorionic gonadotropin should be obtained at the outset to exclude pregnancy.

The *history* should include information on recent weight change, emotional upset, exercise schedule, and use of medications (including recent withdrawal from oral contraceptive pills). Symptoms of multiple hormonal deficiencies, visual symptoms, or headaches point toward a hypothalamic-pituitary etiology. A history of long-term or recently progressive hirsutism suggests increased production of adrenal or ovarian androgens or both. The presence of galactorrhea suggests hyperprolactinemia. Symptoms of hyperthyroidism or hypothyroidism should also be sought.

The *physical examination* should include a search for (1) hirsutism or virilization (male habitus, temporal recession, clitoromegaly), (2) hypothyroidism, (3) endocrine hyperfunction syndromes (acromegaly, Cushing's syndrome, hyperthyroidism), (4) galactorrhea, (5) vaginal or cervical stenosis, (6) estrogen deficiency (breast and vaginal mucosal atrophy), and (7) adnexal or abdominal masses (including enlargement of the pregnant uterus). The history or the physical examination will strongly suggest a diagnosis that can be confirmed by a specific laboratory test (e.g., thyroid indices or thyroid-stimulating hormone levels) in many cases. Hirsutism and virilization should lead to the measurement of serum testosterone and adrenal androgen (dehydroepiandrosterone sulfate) levels.

Even in the absence of galactorrhea, a serum prolactin level should be obtained in women with persistent amenorrhea. If the prolactin level is elevated, it should be repeated, thyroid indices should be obtained, and, if the latter are normal, the patient should be evaluated for a possible macroadenoma or microadenoma of the pituitary (see later discussion).

If the history, physical examination, β-subunit of human chorionic gonadotropin, and prolactin level do not suggest a specific diagnosis, the next step might be administration of a progestational agent (see Fig. 41–3). Withdrawal flow within 7 to 10 days implies integrity of the hypothalamic-pituitary-ovarian-uterine axis, proving adequate estrogen production and uterine responsiveness. Thus, evidence of withdrawal flow suggests a diagnosis of chronic anovulation with acyclic gonadotropin release (as in hypothalamic amenorrhea or polycystic ovarian syndrome). Moreover, withdrawal flow excludes a diagnosis of pregnancy as well as states of significant estrogen deficiency—such as premature menopause or pituitary gonadotropin insufficiency. Usually, in addition to the clinical assessment, LH levels are obtained in patients with amenorrhea who bleed after receiving progesterone. A low or normal level suggests hypothalamic amenorrhea. Tonically elevated LH levels and normal FSH levels strongly suggest the diagnosis of polycystic ovarian syndrome in the absence of thyroid or adrenal disease, especially if the patient is obese and hirsute and has a longstanding history of oligomenorrhea since adolescence. As with prolactin, single measurements of LH may be misleading. Pooled sampling has been suggested for LH:FSH when clinically indicated.[41]

A patient who fails to have withdrawal flow after receiving progesterone might also represent a false-negative response. Failure to comply with an oral medication schedule or, rarely, the possibility of poor gastrointestinal absorption should lead to the administration of progesterone parenterally. Patients with failure to bleed because of inadequate estrogen will usually have low plasma levels of estradiol. If this is not the case, one should reconsider the possibility of chronic anovulation caused by hyperprolactinemia, thyroid disease, excess adrenal corticosteroids, or adrenal or ovarian androgens. In patients with low plasma levels of estradiol, the estrogen-progesterone test should produce withdrawal flow; lack of withdrawal bleeding after this test may identify subjects with outflow tract abnormalities.

If the patient fails to bleed after progesterone administration, has a low plasma estradiol level, and bleeds after administration of estrogen plus progesterone, or if there is any suggestion by physical examination of inadequate estrogenization (vaginal mucosal or breast atrophy), FSH and LH levels should be obtained. If these are elevated, the patient has ovarian failure or resistant ovary syndrome. If the FSH and LH levels are low or normal, the differential diagnosis includes pituitary-hypothalamic diseases, such as anorexia nervosa, pituitary insufficiency, or pituitary tumor. Radiographic imaging of the pituitary gland is usually in order. Reference values for pituitary gonadotropin and steroid hormone levels in normal menstruating adult women are provided in Table 41–4.

Evaluation of Hyperprolactinemia. The patient with hyperprolactinemia and galactorrhea-amenorrhea should have a careful radiologic evaluation of the pituitary gland by MRI aided by the administration of the contrast agent gadolinium.[42] As previously discussed, the size of prolactin-secreting pituitary tumors correlates well with the height of the prolactin elevation; in general, levels exceeding 150 to 200 ng/ml (normal: $<$ 20 ng/ml) strongly correlate with the diagnosis of a pituitary neoplasm. When a pituitary macroadenoma is diagnosed, formal visual field testing should also be performed. Prolactin levels above the normal range but not greatly elevated (20 to 150 ng/ml) should be viewed as indeterminate; they do not distinguish disorders of prolactin regulation from small pituitary tumors of less than 10 mm in size (microadenomata). The diagnosis of a microadenoma ultimately depends on its demonstration by MRI, generally as a radiolucent defect within the pituitary gland following administration of the contrast agent gado-

TABLE 41–4. REPRESENTATIVE REFERENCE VALUES FOR PITUITARY PEPTIDE AND STEROID HORMONE LEVELS IN NORMAL MENSTRUATING WOMEN

Hormone	Value
Prolactin	5–20 ng/ml
FSH*—Follicular phase	5–30 mIU/ml
Midcycle peak	2 × baseline
Postmenopausal	40–250 mIU/ml
LH†—Follicular phase	5–30 mIU/ml
Midcycle peak	3–5 × baseline
Postmenopausal	>30 mIU/ml
Plasma progesterone	
Follicular phase	<150 ng/dl
Luteal phase	>500 ng/dl
Plasma estradiol (varies over entire menstrual cycle)	
Days 1–10	25–75 pg/ml
Days 20–30	75–150 pg/ml
Plasma testosterone	30–100 ng/dl
Plasma androstenedione	0.5–3 ng/ml

*FSH = follicle-stimulating hormone.
†LH = luteinizing hormone.

linium. Unless fertility is desired (see subsequent discussion) and when the radiologic findings are equivocal, patients with modest prolactin elevations should be followed for evidence of an increase in the size of a possible pituitary neoplasm by means of annual serial prolactin levels. Imaging of the pituitary gland by MRI on a periodic basis (every 2 to 3 years) should be considered additionally, especially if symptoms appear (such as headaches) or if prolactin levels are rising.

MANAGEMENT ISSUES

Management of Hyperprolactinemia

The clinical presentation of patients with hyperprolactinemia is a broad spectrum ranging from galactorrhea with preservation of menses to anovulation or oligoamenorrhea syndromes. Moreover, the etiologies of hyperprolactinemia include pituitary neoplasms (microadenomas or macroadenomas) as well as disorders of prolactin regulation. Thus, the decision to treat depends on the issues raised by the particular patient.

When a prolactin-secreting pituitary tumor is diagnosed and treatment is elected to lower prolactin levels, therapeutic alternatives include transsphenoidal resection, external irradiation, and the use of dopamine agonists.[42] External irradiation is usually reserved for following surgical decompression, where medical treatment with bromocriptine has also been shown to fail.

The overall success rate in lowering prolactin levels into the normal range, with resumption of menses, following the transsphenoidal microdissection of a pituitary microadenoma, is approximately 85% in centers that routinely perform this procedure. Surgery may also be indicated to decompress large tumors with suprasellar extension that causes visual field impairment (see later discussion). Transsphenoidal surgery is associated with low rates of morbidity, but sepsis, the development of diabetes insipidus, and pituitary insufficiency have all been reported.

Because dopamine physiologically lowers prolactin secretion, it is not surprising that up to 85% of patients with hyperprolactinemia (including neoplasms) respond to the dopamine agonist bromocriptine with suppression of prolactin levels into the normal range.[42] This medication is administered in increasing doses, beginning with 1.25 to 2.5 mg at bed time (with a snack) to 2.5 mg twice or three times a day (with meals). The dose is increased until prolactin levels are suppressed into the normal range. Side effects are minor and include nausea and vomiting. Postural hypotension may transiently occur after the initiation of bromocriptine therapy, but this effect can be ameliorated if the medication is taken at bedtime. Menses and ovulatory cycles resume in approximately 75% of patients. If the goal is resumption of menses for purposes of fertility, the drug should be discontinued as soon as pregnancy is diagnosed.

A potential danger to such a bromocriptine-treated patient, who has not received prior primary treatment of a known pituitary macroadenoma, is that the trophic effect of high levels of estrogen during the latter half of pregnancy will produce enlargement of the tumor.[43] This circumstance may lead to visual field impairment or a neurosurgical emergency. Thus, the size of the pituitary neoplasm should be assessed by MRI before bromocriptine therapy is begun in patients desirous of pregnancy. Visual field examination should also be performed in all such patients. The patient with a pituitary macroadenoma should receive primary tumor therapy, usually transsphenoidal surgery, before induction of ovulation is attempted. Patients with hyperprolactinemia secondary to a pituitary microadenoma (<10 mm in size) are not at great risk from ovulation induction by bromocriptine without prior primary pituitary therapy.[43]

A difficult management issue is a young woman with an elevated prolactin level and amenorrhea who does not desire pregnancy. Studies indicate that such patients are probably at increased risk for developing osteopenia because the mineral content of the skeleton (as assessed by photon densitometry) is reduced in such patients, compared with that of age-matched cycling females.[32, 33] Because the majority of these patients have a microadenoma, transsphenoidal surgery has been recommended to "cure" them. Although long-term follow-up of such patients whose prolactin levels were surgically reduced into the normal range is limited, a recurrence rate of up to 50% has been reported over a 5-year follow-up, and there is a reappearance of amenorrhea.[44] Such patients may be candidates for long-term bromocriptine therapy, but it is recommended that therapy be periodically interrupted and the status of the patient reassessed.

In general, prolactin levels rise when bromocriptine therapy is discontinued, indicating the necessity for chronic continuous therapy. In this situation, the choice is between the risk and benefits of chronic chemotherapy versus those of the secondary amenorrheic state. Finally, bromocriptine reduces tumor size as well as prolactin levels in up to 50% of patients. As a result some have advocated its use as primary therapy for prolactin-secreting macroadenomas.[45] This is a reversible involution of the tumor mass by reducing cell volume.[46] Because cell loss secondary to necrosis does not occur, the tumor re-expands within weeks after discontinuation of therapy. However, life-long therapy with bromocriptine, tapered to a low dose, appears to be indicated, especially for tumors that extend into surrounding neural structures. This therapy may shrink the tumor mass for years, even in patients with extensive tumors.[47]

Induction of Ovulation by Other Agents

Clomiphene Citrate. Treatment with clomiphene citrate (50 to 100 mg daily for 5 days) may be used to induce ovulation in nonhyperprolactinemic, anovulatory patients who desire to become pregnant. Clomiphene citrate is felt to act as a competitive inhibitor of estradiol at the level of the hypothalamus or pituitary, leading to an ovulatory surge in gonadotropins approximately 7 days after completion of the 5-day course.[48] Because the action of clomiphene fundamentally depends on its antiestrogenic properties, this agent is unlikely to produce an increase in gonadotropins and an ovulatory surge in an estrogen-deficient patient. It is frequently used in patients with the polycystic ovarian syndrome but obviously will be of no use in patients with pituitary or ovarian failure.

Gonadotropin levels should be measured on the last day of clomiphene administration to document pituitary responsiveness. A diagnosis of presumed ovulation can be confirmed by the finding of a luteal phase level of progesterone (greater than 500 ng/dl) approximately 2 weeks after the last day of clomiphene administration.

Gonadotropin Administration. Parenteral administration of human menopausal gonadotropin (FSH) (Pergonal) in conjunction with LH (human chorionic gonadotropin) may be used to induce ovulation in patients with functional gonadal tissue (e.g., hypopituitary patients and many patients with oligoamenorrhea syndromes, such as polycystic ovarian disease). Therapy is difficult and expensive and should be performed only by an experienced infertility expert. Multiple births and excessive ovarian stimulation with ovarian enlargement are potential problems with this therapy.

Gonadotropin-Releasing Hormone Administration. Pulsatile GnRH has been used successfully to induce ovulation in patients with primary and secondary hypothalamic amenorrhea. As with gonadotropin administration, this therapy is expensive and should be performed by an infertility expert.

Suppressive Therapy

A major issue in patients with polycystic ovarian disease is the management of hirsutism. Suppressive therapy with oral contraceptive steroids has been shown to reduce androgen levels in patients with polycystic ovarian disease. The decline in the production of testosterone also correlates with the suppression of elevated levels of LH. Induction of regular endometrial shedding using oral contraceptives may also protect against the future development of endometrial hyperplasia or carcinoma in these patients. Improvement in hirsutism frequently occurs but the basic defect is not corrected because discontinuation of oral contraceptive steroids leads to the return of abnormal hormonal patterns. In some patients with polycystic ovarian disease, adrenal androgen overproduction has been demonstrated to be the primary abnormality (e.g., congenital adrenal hyperplasia syndrome). Under this circumstance, adrenal suppression with glucocorticoids would be a logical first choice of therapy. In refractory patients with progressive, severe hirsutism, combined treatment with the antiandrogen spironolactone and ovarian suppression may be indicated.

Replacement Therapies

Patients with primary hypogonadism are usually treated by hormonal replacement at approximately 12 years of age to promote growth as well as the development of secondary sex characteristics. Oral contraceptives can be used; alternatively, sequential estrogen-progesterone therapy may be employed in these patients as well as in postmenopausal subjects. A schedule that has been used commonly in postmenopausal patients includes the oral administration of 0.625 to 1.25 mg/day of conjugated estrogens (or 0.01 to 0.02 mg/day of ethinyl estradiol) for 3 weeks of each month, with 5.0 to 10 mg of medroxyprogesterone acetate daily for the last 10 to 14 days of estrogen therapy. The addition of progestational agents has eliminated the risk of endometrial carcinoma in such patients. However, patients on this schedule should be followed regularly and indefinitely; in some instances, periodic endometrial biopsy may be indicated. Patients treated with sequential estrogen-progesterone or oral contraceptive therapies should be followed up for possible side effects, such as alterations in lipid and carbohydrate metabolism. In postmenopausal women who do not wish to re-experience withdrawal bleeding, daily combined estrogen and progesterone therapy may also be used for replacement therapy.

Progestins. If the problem is dysfunctional uterine bleeding (presence of irregular, excessive, out-of-phase uterine shedding in association with anovulatory cycles), treatment with cyclically administered progestational agents (e.g., medroxyprogesterone acetate, 10 mg/day for 5 to 10 days monthly or bimonthly)[49] may control the bleeding. Use of medroxyprogesterone acetate (e.g., 5.0 to 10 mg/day taken orally for the last 10 to 14 days of each month) may reduce the risk of endometrial carcinoma in patients with the chronic dysfunctional uterine bleeding of polycystic ovarian disease. An alternative treatment schedule would be oral contraceptive replacement therapy. Large doses of intramuscular medroxyprogesterone acetate (150 mg every 90 days) will produce prolonged anovulation and amenorrhea. This therapeutic schedule has been used when one wishes to suppress ovulation but estrogens are contraindicated, as in patients with bleeding disorders and endometriosis.

REFERENCES

1. Yen SSC: The human menstrual cycle. *In* Yen SSC, Jaffe RB (eds): Reproductive Endocrinology: Physiology, Pathophysiology, and Clinical Management. Philadelphia, WB Saunders, 1978, pp 126–151.
2. Rakoff AE: Hormonal cytology in gynecology. Clin Obstet Gynecol 4:1045, 1961.
3. Moghissi KS: Ovulation detection. Endocrinol Metab Clin North Am 21:39, 1992.
4. Rebar RW and Connolly HV: Clinical features of young women with hypergonadotropic amenorrhea. Fertil Steril 53:804, 1990.
5. Rebar RW and Cedars MI: Hypergonadotropic forms of amenorrhea in young women. Endocrinol Metab Clin North Am 21:173, 1992.
6. Philip J, Sele V, Trolle D: Primary amenorrhea. A study of 101 cases. Fertil Steril 16:795, 1965.
7. Turner HH: A syndrome of infantilism, congenital webbed neck, and cubitus valgus. Endocrinology 23:566, 1938.
8. Griffin JE: The androgen resistance syndromes: 5α-reductase deficiency and related disorders. *In* Scriver et al (eds): The Metabolic Basis of Inherited Disease, 6th ed. New York, McGraw-Hill, 1989, pp 1919–1944.
9. Scully RE: Gonadoblastoma: A review of 74 cases. Cancer 25:1340, 1970.
10. Nelson MA, Dyment PG, Goldberg B, et al: Amenorrhea in adolescent athletes. Pediatrics 84:394, 1989.
11. Asherman JG: Amenorrhea traumatica (atretica). J Obstet Gynaecol Br Emp 55:23, 1948.
12. Neufeld M, MacLaren N, and Blizzard R: Autoimmune polyglandular syndrome. Pediatr Ann 9:154, 1980.

13. Rabinowe SL, Raunikar VA, Dib SA, et al: Premature menopause: Monoclonal antibody defined T lymphocyte abnormalities and antiovarian antibodies. Fertil Steril 51:450, 1989.
14. Hodgson JE, Dockerty MB, Mussey RD: Granulosa cell tumor of the ovary: A clinical and pathological review of 62 cases. Surg Gynecol Obstet 81:631, 1945.
15. Malkasian GD Jr, Dockerty MB, Mussey RD: Functioning tumors of the ovary in women under 40. Obstet Gynecol 26:669, 1965.
16. Young RL and Goldzieher JW: Clinical manifestations of polycystic ovarian disease. Endocrinol Metab Clin North Am 17:621, 1988.
17. Morris DV: Hirsutism. Clin Obstet Gynecol 12:649, 1985.
18. Judd HL: Endocrinology of polycystic ovary disease. Clin Obstet Gynecol 21:99, 1978.
19. Yen SSC: The polycystic ovarian syndrome. Clin Endocrinol 12:177, 1980.
20. Pasquali R, Venturoli S, Paradisi R, et al: Insulin and C-peptide levels in obese patients with polycystic ovaries. Horm Metab Res 14:284, 1982.
21. Givens JR: Familial polycystic ovarian disease. Endocrinol Metab Clin North Am 17:771, 1988.
22. Quigley ME, Rakoff JS, and Yen SSC: Increased luteinizing hormone sensitivity to dopamine inhibition in polycystic ovary syndrome. J Clin Endocrinol Metab 52:231, 1981.
23. Sheehan HL and Murdoch R: Postpartum necrosis of the anterior pituitary: Pathological and clinical aspects. J Obstet Gynaecol Br Emp 45:456, 1938.
24. Kleinberg DL, Noel GL, and Frantz AG: Galactorrhea: A study of 235 cases, including 48 with pituitary tumors. N Engl J Med 296:589, 1977.
25. Sauder SE, Frager M, Case GD, et al: Abnormal patterns of pulsatile luteinizing hormone secretion in woman with hyperprolactinemia and amenorrhea: Responses to bromocriptine. J Clin Endocrinol Metab 59:941, 1984.
26. Koppelman MCS, Jaffe MJ, Rieth KG, et al: Hyperprolactinemia, amenorrhea and galactorrhea: A retrospective review of twenty-five cases. Ann Intern Med 100:115, 1984.
27. Leblanc H, Lachelin G, Abu-Fadil S, et al: Effects of dopamine infusion on pituitary hormone secretion in humans. J Clin Endocrinol Metab 43:669, 1976.
28. MacLeod RH, Kimura H, and Login I: Inhibition of prolactin secretion by dopamine and piribedil (ET-495). *In* Pecile A, Muller EE (eds): Growth Hormone and Related Peptides. New York, Elsevier, 1976, pp 443–453.
29. Child DF, Nader S, Mashiter K, et al: Prolactin studies in "functionless" pituitary tumors. BMJ 1:604, 1975.
30. Edwards CR, Forsyth IA, and Besser GM: Amenorrhea, galactorrhea, and primary hypothyroidism with high circulating levels of prolactin. BMJ 3:462, 1971.
31. Franks S, Murray MAG, Jecquier AM, et al: Incidence and significance of hyperprolactinemia in women with amenorrhea. Clin Endocrinol 4:597, 1975.
32. Schlechte J, Walkner L, and Kathol M: A longitudinal analysis of premenopausal bone loss in healthy women and women with hyperprolactinemia. J Clin Endocrinol Metab 75:698, 1992.
33. Biller BMK, Baum HBA, Rosenthal DI, et al: Progressive trabecular osteopenia in women with hyperprolactinemic amenorrhea. J Clin Endocrinol Metab 75:692, 1992.
34. Bullen BA, Skrinar GS, Beitins IZ, et al: Induction of menstrual disorders by strenuous exercise in untrained women. N Engl J Med 312:1349, 1985.
35. Katz JL: Psychoendocrine considerations in anorexia nervosa. *In* Sachar EJ (ed): Topics in Psychoendocrinology. New York, Grune and Stratton, 1975, pp 121–133.
36. Mecklenburg RS, Loriaux DL, Thompson RH, et al: Hypothalamic dysfunction in patients with anorexia nervosa. Medicine 53:147, 1974.
37. Boyar RM, Hellman LD, Roffwarg H, et al: Cortisol secretion and metabolism in anorexia nervosa. N Engl J Med 296:190, 1977.
38. Southern A, Olivo J, Gordon GG, et al: The conversion of androgens to estrogens in hyperthyroidism. J Clin Endocrinol Metab 38:207, 1974.
39. Honbo KS, Van Herle AJ, and Kellett KA: Serum prolactin level in untreated hypothyroidism. Am J Med 65:782, 1978.
40. Kletzky OA, Davajan V, Nakamura RM, et al: Clinical categorization of patients with secondary amenorrhea using progesterone-induced uterine bleeding and measurement of serum gonadotropin levels. Am J Obstet Gynecol 121:695, 1975.
41. Goldzieher JW, Ozier TS, Smith KD, et al: Improving the diagnostic reliability of fluctuating hormone levels by optimized multiple-sampling techniques. J Clin Endocrinol Metab 43:824, 1976.
42. Klibanski A and Zervas NT: Diagnosis and management of hormone-secreting pituitary adenomas. N Engl J Med 324:811, 1991.
43. Molitch ME: Pregnancy and the hyperprolactinemic woman. N Engl J Med 312:1364, 1985.
44. Serri O, Rasio E, Beauregard H, et al: Recurrence of hyperprolactinemia after selective transsphenoidal adenomectomy in women with prolactinoma. N Engl J Med 309:280, 1983.
45. Molitch ME, Elton RL, Blackwell RE, et al: Bromocriptine as primary therapy for prolactin-secreting macroadenomas. Results of a prospective multicenter study. J Clin Endocrinol Metab 60:698, 1985.
46. Nissim M, Ambrosi B, Bernasconi V, et al: Bromocriptine treatment of prolactinomas: Studies on the time course of tumor shrinkage and morphology. J Endocrinol Invest 5:409, 1982.
47. Liuzzi A, Dallabonzana D, Oppizzi G, et al: Low doses of dopamine agonists in the long-term treatment of macroprolactinomas. N Engl J Med 313:656, 1985.
48. Igarashi M, Ibuki Y, Ubo HK, et al: Mode and site of action of clomiphene. Am J Obstet Gynecol 97:120, 1968.
49. Goldfarb JM and Little AB: Abnormal vaginal bleeding. N Engl J Med 302:666, 1980.

42

Hirsutism

GORDON H. WILLIAMS, MD

Hirsutism is commonly defined as an excess of body hair in a woman in a more or less male pattern of distribution. Although this is a common problem, the exact incidence is unclear because it is dependent on not only hormonal but also genetic and social factors. For example, Western European and North American women are more hirsute than Asians but are less hirsute than Near Eastern women. Conversely, in a relatively homogeneous racial group, there may be a discrepancy between what is perceived to be excess body hair and what can be objectively measured as such. McKnight, in a study of 400 white Welsh university students reported that nearly 10% of them felt that they had an excess of body hair.[1] However, in this group, the frequency of hirsutism as just defined may actually have been higher (Table 42–1). In general, normal women do not have hair on the upper back or upper abdomen and seldom on the chin (10%) or sternum (3%). Thus, incidence figures can be properly interpreted only by knowing both the racial composition of the population studied and whether subjective or objective methods were used. In white North American women, some degree of hirsutism may be present in as many as 10%.[2–4]

Hirsutism may result from androgen excess syndromes or drug ingestion, or it may be familial or idiopathic (Table 42–2). The frequency of excess androgen secretion as a cause of hirsutism is probably quite small in the absence of other signs of increased androgen production. Indeed, some investigators have suggested that as low as 1% of patients with simple hirsutism have an endocrine abnormality.[2–4] On the other hand, if other signs or symptoms of androgen excess are present (Table 42–3), particularly if signs of virilization are noted, the probability that androgen production is increased is quite high.

REGULATION OF HAIR GROWTH

Alterations in hair growth may be secondary to a change either in the hair-growth cycle or in the pattern of distribution of the various types of hair. Hormones, particularly androgens, can alter either of these aspects.

The mature hair consists of the hair shaft, which is the visualizable cylinder; the hair follicle, which is the epidermal pocket of cells that holds the hair; and the hair bulb at the base of the hair, which contains the actively proliferating epidermal cells.[5, 6] Within the hair bulb is the papilla, where the hair shaft is formed.

There are three general types of human hair, one prenatal and two postnatal. *Lanugo* hairs are a dense, fine growth over the entire skin surface of the embryo and are usually lost during fetal life. *Vellus* hairs are finely textured, unpigmented hairs present on apparently hairless areas of the human skin. They are usually only 2 to 3 mm in length. *Terminal* hairs are longer, coarser, and pigmented, imparting a hairy appearance to a particular area of the body (Fig. 42–1).

The total number of hair follicles in an adult is approximately 5 million, with nearly 20% found on the scalp. No new hair follicles appear after birth, and indeed with time there is a gradual decrease in the number of follicles; nearly 50% are lost between the fourth and the ninth or tenth decade of life.[7]

It is likely that all terminal hair arises from vellus hair. After conversion of a vellus into a terminal follicle, one or more terminal hair growth cycles occur, and then the follicle either dies or reverts to a vellus follicle. The terminal follicle has three distinct phases to its growth cycle. The active, growing phase is the *anagen* stage, whereas the resting phase is called the *telogen* stage. A transition phase from the one to the other is called the *catagen* phase.[8] Anatomically, specific differences exist between a hair follicle in the anagen phase and one in the telogen phase. The hair bulb and papilla retract toward the skin during the

TABLE 42–1. MALE HAIR PATTERNS DETECTED IN 400 WELSH WOMEN*†

Area	% of Women
Upper lip	26
Periareola	17
Linea alba	35
Upper pubic triangle	10
Lumbar sacral region	16
Arms and legs (coarse hair)	84

*Data from McKnight E: The prevalence of "hirsutism" in young women. Lancet i:410, 1964.
†The women were between the ages of 18 and 24 years.

TABLE 42–2. CAUSES OF HIRSUTISM

Familial
Idiopathic
Drugs: Minoxidil, diazoxide, phenothiazines, hexachlorobenzene, phenytoin, androgens, ACTH,* glucocorticoids
Androgen overproduction
  Ovarian
    Hyperplasia: Polycystic ovaries, hilus cell hyperplasia
    Tumor: Arrhenoblastoma, hilus cell, adrenal rest, granulosa cell, Brenner
  Adrenal
    Hyperplasia
      Cushing's syndrome
      Congenital adrenal hyperplasia
    Tumor: Virilizing adrenal carcinoma or adenoma

*ACTH = adrenocorticotropic hormone.

telogen phase, and the hair is often termed a "club hair" (see Fig. 42–1).

The rate of hair growth is approximately the same in various parts of the body, around 0.35 mm per day. Although in men the rate of growth of scalp and facial hair may be somewhat faster and the growth rate on the extremities somewhat slower, generally the length that a terminal hair reaches is determined not so much by its rate of growth as by its duration of growth. Scalp and facial hair have anagen stages lasting several years, whereas body hair grows for only 3 or 4 months. Thus, the density of hair in a given area is in part related to the per cent of hair follicles in a growing rather than a resting phase. Usually, at any one time, 80% scalp hair follicles are in the growing or telogen stage.

CLASSIFICATION OF TERMINAL HAIR

Two types of terminal hair can be distinguished: *asexual* hair—that is, terminal hair whose growth is not dependent on androgens; and *sexual* hair. Sexual hair may be divided into two subgroups: *ambosexual* hair, whose growth is modified by a low concentration of androgen, as present in women, and *male sexual,* controlled by levels of androgen in men.[9, 10] Terminal hair found on the scalp, eyebrows, and, to a lesser extent, the forearms and legs in both sexes and at all ages is asexual. Its development appears to be intrinsic and only minimally under the influence of hormonal secretion. The conversion of vellus into terminal follicles on the face, chest, shoulders, back, and abdomen requires levels of androgen as found in men. On the other hand, the formation of axillary terminal hairs requires only the level of androgen found in women. It is therefore ambosexual. Pubic hair is divided into an upper and lower triangle; the lower triangle is ambosexual, whereas the upper triangle is sexual. Extremity hair is of mixed control. The most significant factors are probably intrinsic or hereditary. However, the formation of terminal follicles is in part influenced by the level of androgens.

Other hormones may also affect hair growth. *Glucocorticoids* seem to prolong the telogen stage and may shorten the active, growing stage. On the other hand, *thyroid* hormone favors the anagen stage. Estrogen does not have a consistent effect on hair growth, although in pregnancy the anagen stage is prolonged. Growth hormone may contribute to the growth of eyebrow or eyelash hair and hair on the extremities.

DIFFERENTIAL DIAGNOSIS

The causes of hirsutism can be divided into four broad categories: familial, idiopathic, androgen excess, and drugs (see Table 42–2).[2–4, 11] In general, the first two conditions are not associated with other signs of androgen excess, that is, oligomenorrhea, significant acne, or virilization. Likewise, drug-induced hirsutism is usually not associated with other signs and symptoms of androgen excess, unless the drug is an androgen. The other drugs that produce an increase in body hair include phenothiazines, minoxidil, and anticonvulsants, such as phenytoin. Each of these drugs, particularly minoxidil, produces a generalized increase in hair growth not just in androgen target areas.[12–14] The underlying mechanism is not clear but may be related to the ability of these drugs to convert vellus into terminal follicles.

If drugs are excluded, the only known causes of hirsutism amenable to treatment are those secondary to excess production of androgens by either the adrenal gland or the ovary.

Characteristics of the Androgen Excess Syndromes

Clinically, it is important to distinguish between simple hirsutism and hirsutism associated with virilization. In most cases of simple hirsutism, there is no known cause for the increased hair growth. On the other hand, if the patient is virilized as well as hirsute, increased levels of androgens will usually be found.[2–4, 15] The signs and symptoms of androgen excess can be divided into four areas (see Table 42–3). Besides hirsutism, there may be oligomenorrhea, acne, or virilization. The four components of virilization are temporal balding, change in body habitus from a female to a male pattern (i.e., loss of pelvic fat and increase in upper torso muscular development), clitoral enlargement, and deepening of the voice. In general, the degree of virilization is a reflection of both the duration and the degree of excess androgen secretion, although significant virilization can be present with minimal changes in testosterone production, and a significant increase in testosterone production may be associated with minimal signs of virilization (Fig. 42–2).[16, 17] Finally, the occurrence of oligomenorrhea in a hirsute patient increases the probability that an excess secretion of androgen will be found. Thus, the evaluation of the hirsute patient should include a careful history of the onset of menarche, past and present menstrual history, and reproductive capacity as well as a careful physical evaluation for signs and symptoms of androgen excess.

Adrenal Virilization

Adrenal virilizing syndromes result from excess production of adrenal androgens, such as dehydroepiandrosterone

TABLE 42–3. SIGNS AND SYMPTOMS ASSOCIATED WITH INCREASED ANDROGEN PRODUCTION IN WOMEN

Hirsutism
Oligomenorrhea
Acne
Virilization
  Temporal balding
  Enlarging of clitoris
  Deepening of voice
  Change of body habitus

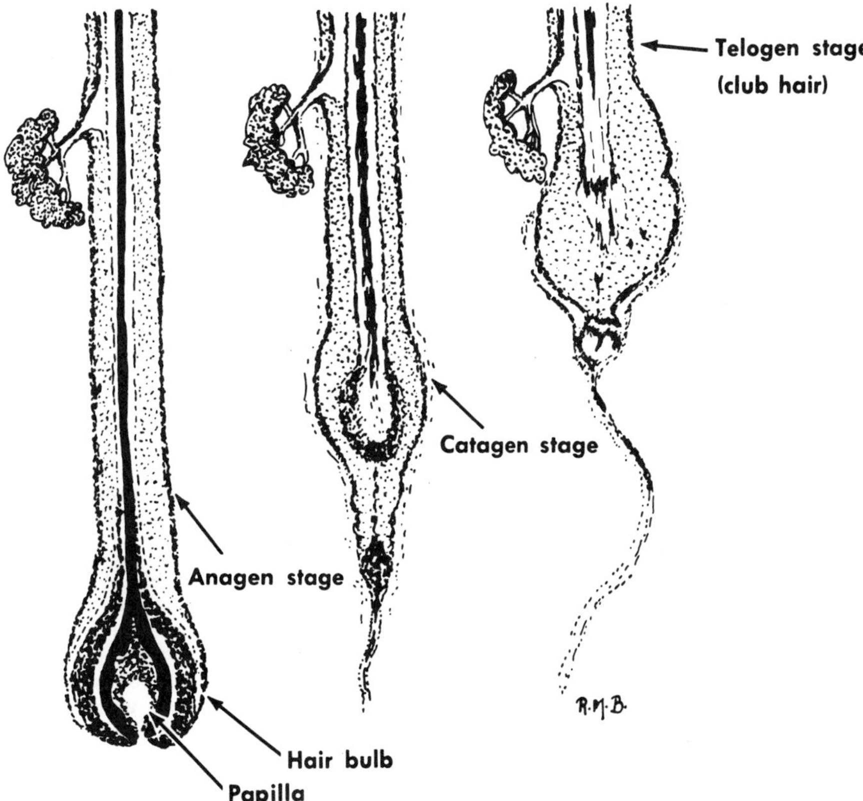

FIGURE 42–1. Growth cycle of a terminal hair. Anagen is the active growing phase, catagen a short transitional stage, and telogen a resting stage. Note the change in the hair bulb and papilla to a club shape in the telogen stage. (From Stewart WD, Danto JL, and Maddin S: Dermatology: Diagnosis and Treatment of Cutaneous Disorders. St. Louis, CV Mosby, 1974, p 10.)

and Δ-4-androstenedione, which can be converted into testosterone in peripheral tissue, with the elevated testosterone levels producing most of the virilization.[18,19] As in other states of adrenocortical hyperfunction, the syndrome may result from hyperplasia of both adrenal glands or an adenoma or carcinoma of one. It also may arise in a congenital form, congenital adrenal hyperplasia, secondary to a 21- or an 11-hydroxylase or a 3β-hydroxy-Δ^5-steroid dehydrogenase enzyme deficiency. In some cases, this form of excess androgen production may not be manifest in childhood but only after menarche (the so-called late-onset or nonclassical congenital adrenal hyperplasia).[20–22]

The adrenal virilizing syndromes may be associated with secretion of greater or smaller amounts of other adrenal hormones, and they may therefore present as "pure" syndromes of virilization or as "mixed" syndromes associated with excess production of glucocorticoids, for example, Cushing's syndrome. For convenience, it is appropriate to

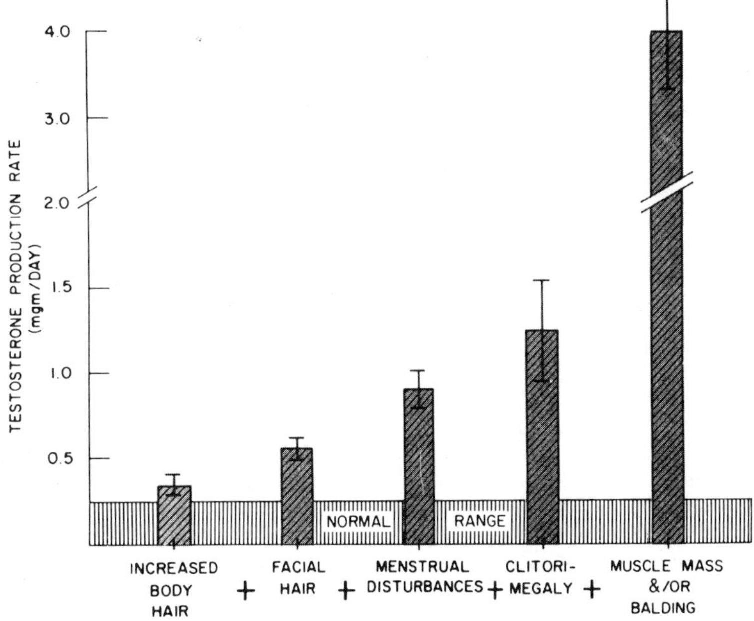

FIGURE 42–2. Correlation of testosterone production rates with the development of virilization. (Adapted with permission from Kirschner MA: Hirsutism and virilization. *Resident & Staff Physician* 25:118, 1979. © (May 1979) by Romaine Pierson Publishers, Inc.)

divide the adrenal causes of androgen overproduction into *tumors* and *hyperplasia*.

Adrenal Tumors. Adrenal *adenomas* and *carcinomas* may cause a pure or mixed virilizing syndrome.[18] Because adrenal androgens are weak compared with gonadal androgens, adrenal virilization is usually characterized by *large increments* in urinary 17-ketosteroid excretion and plasma dehydroepiandrosterone (DHEA) sulfate levels, and often with less impressive clinical signs of virilization. Virilizing adrenal adenomas are rare. On the other hand, adrenal carcinomas are the most common adrenal tumor causing virilization. They usually are associated with high urinary 17-ketosteroid excretion and plasma DHEA sulfate levels, and a moderate increase in 17-hydroxycorticoid excretion—often disproportionately so when compared with cortisol excretion. They characteristically show no increase in steroid excretion when stimulated with adrenocorticotropic hormone (ACTH) and also fail to suppress with dexamethasone administration. They are often associated with marked virilization of sudden onset.[18]

Adrenal Hyperplasia. Adrenal hyperplasia can be of two types. Both types are secondary to increased secretion of ACTH, but the mechanisms underlying the increased secretion are different. In *Cushing's syndrome,* the increased ACTH is the result of a functional or anatomic derangement in its secretion, that is, a pituitary or extrapituitary ACTH-producing tumor or a dysfunction in the hypothalamic-pituitary axis.[18] In addition to signs and symptoms of excess androgen production, these patients also show evidence of glucocorticoid hypersecretion, for example, glucose intolerance, striae, ability to bruise easily, central adiposity, osteoporosis, and hypertension.

A second form of hyperplasia is due to a defect in a steroid enzymatic step (usually either the C-21- or C-11-hydroxylase but also the 3β-hydroxy-Δ^5-steroid dehydrogenase) required for the formation of cortisol.[20–23] As a result of this defect, cortisol production falls, resulting in activation of the hypothalamic-pituitary-adrenal axis and increased ACTH release to overcome the block. This process results in a buildup of precursors behind the block, which then spill over into the adrenal androgen pathway—for example, Δ-4-androstenedione and DHEA sulfate. Because this defect is inherited, it is often observed in infants. Virilization in the female neonate is associated with ambiguous external genitalia (female pseudohermaphroditism). In patients with significant enzyme deficiency, hirsutism without other signs of virilization is uncommon.

The most common adrenal defect associated with hirsutism is a partial enzyme deficiency. This has been termed *late-onset* or *nonclassical* congenital adrenal hyperplasia.[20–23] Its prevalence among hirsute women has been estimated to be between two and 35%, depending on the population.[24–25] Its frequency increases if menstrual irregularities are also present. As with the classical form, the nonclassical form can be produced by partial deficiencies in the C-21- or C-11-hydroxylase or the 3β-hydroxy-Δ5-steroid dehydrogenase enzymes. Although 21-hydroxylase deficiency dominates the nonclassical like it does the classical forms of congenital adrenal hyperplasia, the relative frequency of a partial deficiency in the other two enzymes is somewhat greater.[22] In all cases, the defect is inherited as a recessive trait. Deficiency of 21-hydroxylase is closely linked to the human leukocyte antigen loci. Thus, human leukocyte antigen major histocompatibility typing has been used to determine the frequency of this enzyme deficiency in the general population.[26] Such surveys for the most part also determine the general frequency of nonclassical congenital adrenal hyperplasia. In the general white population, an estimated 0.2 to 0.3% of women have this defect. This number increases to nearly 4% in Jews originating in Eastern Europe.[27]

Some investigators have reported that a minority of patients with nonclassical congenital adrenal hyperplasia may have two enzyme deficiencies, that is, C-21- and C-11-hydroxylase.[28] However, it is more likely that the abnormal steroid patterns suggestive of this dual enzyme deficiency is caused by excess adrenal androgen production rather than a second enzyme deficiency. Confirmation of this possibility awaits specific genotyping in these patients.

Finally, some patients with hirsutism may have increased responsiveness of their adrenal gland to ACTH, even though classic Cushing's syndrome or an enzyme deficiency is not apparent.[29] Thus, more subtle abnormalities in adrenal function may also be present.

Ovarian Virilization

Ovarian causes of excess androgen production can also be divided into tumorous and hyperplastic conditions. The most common ovarian tumor causing hirsutism and virilization is the arrhenoblastoma, but other ovarian tumors, such as adrenal rest tumors, granulosa cell tumors, hilar cell tumors, and Brenner's tumors, have also been associated with virilization.[30–32] Virilization due to ovarian tumors is characterized by normal or only moderate elevations of urinary 17-ketosteroids because the neoplasm usually secretes the potent androgen testosterone.[15] Thus, with the exception of adrenal rest tumors, baseline 17-ketosteroid excretion in excess of 20 mg/day or increased plasma DHEA sulfate levels are unusual. As with adrenal neoplasms, steroid secretion by ovarian tumors is usually not acutely suppressed by dexamethasone administration. With the exception of adrenal rest tumors, they are also largely independent of ACTH stimulation.

By far, the most common ovarian cause of excess androgen production is ovarian hyperplasia or polycystic ovaries. This syndrome, first described by Stein and Leventhal in 1935, consists of various characteristics that fall into three general areas.[33] First, the most consistent feature is anovulation with amenorrhea or oligomenorrhea and episodes of menorrhagia. Second, production of estrogens is uninterrupted. Thus, there is a proliferative endometrium with the development of adenomatous hyperplasia in some cases. Finally, there is evidence of androgen overproduction. As opposed to tumors, whether of ovarian or adrenal origin, virilization is less common with polycystic ovaries, whereas hirsutism is quite frequent. In most cases, the 17-ketosteroid excretion rate is greater than normal. Although the 17-ketosteroid excretion is reduced by dexamethasone, the residual level is often greater than in normal subjects. Plasma levels of androstenedione and, to a lesser extent, testosterone are usually increased, as are their production rates.[34]

Several studies have documented that the polycystic ovary produces increased amounts of androstenedione but decreased amounts of estradiol. Thus, the increased estrogen levels found in patients with polycystic ovaries are not the result of increased ovarian production rates but rather an increased peripheral conversion of androstenedione into estrone. The serum levels of follicle-stimulating hormone (FSH) and luteinizing hormone (LH) are variable.[34–36] Often they are normal; however, the FSH is frequently lower than normal, whereas the LH is higher and characteristically shows frequent peaks of low magnitude. Further, LH response to LH-releasing hormone is usually enhanced, suggesting that the increased LH levels may be due to an increased sensitivity of the pituitary to the releasing hormone. This may be secondary to the increased estrogen levels,[36] decreased dopaminergic activity,[37] or both.

In some women with polycystic ovaries, hyperinsulinism also occurs.[38, 39] In some of these subjects, acanthosis nigricans is a third component of the syndrome. The pathophysiologic link between hyperinsulinism and increased androgen production or polycystic ovary syndrome is unclear. However, currently available data suggest that these processes may be independent. For example, there is no correlation between the presence or absence of polycystic ovaries, the degree of hirsutism, or the levels of androgens and the degree of insulin resistance in women with hirsutism.[38, 39]

Pathologically, the ovaries are usually enlarged to several times the normal size. Typically, beneath a thickened capsule are many small follicular cysts, thus giving the name polycystic ovaries. Often, the follicular cysts are in various stages of atresia, with luteal cells that are hyperplastic, luteinized, or both, but seldom are mature follicles seen.

Several theories have been developed to account for the altered steroid output by these ovaries. It has been amply documented that increased androgen production from any source may produce this syndrome. For example, patients with Cushing's syndrome or congenital adrenal hyperplasia have been shown to have anatomic and biochemical changes in their ovaries similar to those found in patients with idiopathic polycystic ovaries.[40] Thus, the ovarian lesion may not be a primary process. However, in at least some women with polycystic ovaries, long-term adrenal suppression does not modify testosterone or androstenedione levels.[41] A second hypothesis is that there is a deficiency in the conversion of androstenedione into estrone by the ovary. Although some in vitro data favor this hypothesis, data from other studies do not.[19] Furthermore, this hypothesis does not explain the amelioration of the symptoms of this syndrome by wedge resection of the ovary or by administration of clomiphene or gonadotropin or both.

Third, primarily on the basis of data derived from studies in the rat, the pathogenesis of the polycystic ovary syndrome has been reported to be secondary to a derangement in the relationship between the ovary and the hypothalamic pituitary axis. Finally, the most recently proposed mechanism is hyperinsulinemia, which is known to exist in some patients with polycystic ovary syndrome. As noted earlier, however, there is minimal correlation between the level of insulin and the level of androgens or the presence or absence of polycystic ovaries in hirsute women.[38, 39] Hence, the specific cause of this syndrome still remains in doubt.[42]

SPECIAL DIAGNOSTIC PROCEDURES

The evaluation of the hirsute woman begins with a careful history and physical examination. If drugs are excluded, the next step is to determine whether other evidence for excess androgen production is present and whether there are signs and symptoms of ovarian or adrenal pathology. Specifically, it is important to assess any evidence for Cushing's syndrome and whether the patient's menstrual cycles are normal. Most patients with Cushing's syndrome, if examined carefully, will have findings suggestive of increased glucocorticoid secretion and, therefore, can be distinguished from patients with other causes of excess androgen production.

Normal menstrual cycles are distinctly uncommon if the hirsutism is secondary to ovarian pathology and unusual if secondary to adrenal disease.[42] Thus, hirsutism without virilization, beginning after puberty and accompanied by oligomenorrhea, is more likely to be of ovarian than of adrenal origin. However, oligomenorrhea still occurs frequently with adrenal disease. On the other hand, nonvirilized patients with hirsutism and regular menses are most likely to have idiopathic or familial hirsutism.

A *sudden onset* of *progressive hirsutism* and *virilization* suggests an adrenal or ovarian neoplasm. Because adrenal tumors secrete weak androgens (e.g., DHEA), virilizing adrenal neoplasms are characterized by high urinary 17-ketosteroid excretion rates, usually in excess of 30 to 40 mg/24 hours or by increased plasma DHEA sulfate levels, in excess of 3.5 μg/ml. However, the occasional patient will have only an increase in 17-ketosteroid excretion rate. Failure to reduce 17-ketosteroid or DHEA sulfate levels to normal following dexamethasone suppression (0.5 mg orally every 6 hours for 2 days) supports a diagnosis of virilizing adrenal tumor and excludes congenital adrenal hyperplasia. On the other hand, virilization due to ovarian tumors is characterized by normal or only modest or no elevations in urinary 17-ketosteroids or plasma DHEA sulfate levels and significant elevations in plasma testosterone levels.[42, 43]

Thus, measurements of baseline urinary 17-ketosteroids and plasma DHEA sulfate are the best screening tests for ruling out adrenal tumors in patients with hirsutism.[42, 43] Urine 17-ketosteroid levels of less than 15 mg/24 hours or plasma DHEA sulfate levels of less than 3.5 μg/ml are extremely rare when hirsutism is secondary to an adrenal tumor. Urine steroid values should be interpreted with caution, however, because undercollection is a common problem. The completeness of the urine collection can be assessed by measuring the creatinine level. Usually, 1 g of creatinine is excreted per 50 kg of body weight per 24 hours. Plasma DHEA sulfate levels do not suffer from this drawback but because of periodic fluctuations and variations in sulfatase activity, they may not be as precise. Plasma DHEA levels are particularly vulnerable to this criticism because of its short half-life. Although a normal 17-ketosteroid excretion rate and DHEA sulfate level virtually eliminates an adrenal tumor as the cause of hirsutism, the other causes of excess androgen production may be associated with either normal or elevated levels of these steroids. Slightly increased levels are of limited benefit in the differential diagnosis, except in excluding idiopathic hirsutism.

Determining the plasma testosterone level is also useful in evaluating patients with hirsutism. Again, its specificity lies in its ability to rule out a particular cause of androgen excess, not in its ability to discriminate among the various types. It is extremely unlikely that patients with hirsutism and normal plasma testosterone levels have an ovarian neoplasm.[1–4, 42, 43] On the other hand, an elevated level is not useful in differentiating the various forms of androgen excess from each other.

A particularly heated debate has raged concerning the value of total versus "free" testosterone as a diagnostic tool. In some patients with hirsutism (particularly those with oligomenorrhea), the circulating levels of testosterone-estradiol–binding globulin are low. Therefore, the total testosterone may be normal and yet the free testosterone (that not bound to testosterone-estradiol–binding globulin and therefore biologically active) may be elevated. Thus, most textbooks suggests that free testosterone levels should be obtained.[42, 43] Several investigators, however, question the wisdom of this approach and its inherently greater costs.[44, 45] One of these concluded that "the indirect estimation of AFT (apparent free testosterone) in addition to [testosterone] is time-consuming, costly, without practical value in selecting the proper treatment, and therefore, not mandatory in the routine evaluation of androgenized women."[44]

Patients with Cushing's syndrome can be readily differentiated from other patients with hirsutism by measuring a 24-hour cortisol-excretion rate (normal is < 100 μg) or by their response to the overnight dexamethasone suppression test. This test is highly reliable and specific. False-negative results are almost unheard of. The test is performed by giving the patient 1 mg of dexamethasone at bedtime and obtaining a plasma cortisol level between 7 and 10 AM the following morning. The plasma cortisol level should be less than 5 μg/dl in most laboratories. A value less than that virtually excludes Cushing's syndrome as the cause of hirsutism. On the other hand, an elevated value does not necessarily mean that the patient has Cushing's syndrome because the false-positive rate of this test is 10 to 15%.[18] If a patient has an elevated plasma cortisol level in response to the overnight dexamethasone suppression test, a standard low-dose dexamethasone suppression test should then be performed by giving 0.5 mg of dexamethasone every 6 hours for 48 hours. Either a 24-hour urine specimen is obtained on the second day of the dexamethasone administration or a plasma cortisol level is obtained after completion of the 48 hours, or both are obtained. The plasma cortisol level should again be less than 5 μg/dl. In the 24-hour urine specimen, the cortisol level should be less than 30 μg, and 17-hydroxysteroids, less than 3 mg. Again, creatinine should be measured in the urine collections to verify completeness of the collection.

Thus, a normal 17-ketosteroid excretion rate, DHEA sulfate plasma level, plasma testosterone level, and overnight dexamethasone suppression test would exclude adrenal or ovarian tumors and Cushing's syndrome as causes for the hirsutism (Table 42–4). One is then left with differentiating between congenital adrenal hyperplasia, polycystic ovaries, and idiopathic hirsutism. Often patients with congenital adrenal hyperplasia will have elevated 17-ketosteroid or DHEA sulfate levels and precursors behind the enzyme blocks, that is, 11-deoxycortisol for 11-hydroxylase deficiencies, 17-hydroxyprogesterone for 21-hydroxylase deficiencies, and an increased ratio of 17-hydroxypregnenolone to 17-hydroxyprogesterone for 3β-hydroxy-Δ^5-steroid dehydrogenase deficiencies. It has now been reported, though, that as many as 30% of patients with hirsutism, oligomenorrhea, and normal basal 17-ketosteroid levels, although usually elevated DHEA sulfate plasma levels, may have partial adrenal enzyme deficiencies.[20–23, 28, 29] This conclusion was based on the finding of a buildup of precursors behind the block when the entire enzyme system was stressed by administering pharmacologic doses of ACTH (Fig. 42–3). In normal subjects, the adrenal enzyme system is particularly efficient, and there is little buildup of cortisol precursors. On the other hand, in an early study, 13 of 31 patients with hirsutism and oligomenorrhea showed a buildup of precursors when ACTH was administered.[28] Similar results have been obtained with measurement of blood levels of these precursor steroids.[20–23, 29]

Thus, these individuals can be screened with plasma DHEA sulfate levels. However, even a normal value does not exclude the possibility of a mild form of congenital adrenal hyperplasia. Therefore, if the index of suspicion is high, an ACTH stimulation test should be performed.[22, 46–49] The most convenient approach is to administer synthetic ACTH (cosyntropin) in a dose of 0.25 mg intramuscularly or intravenously over 1 to 2 minutes. Plasma levels of the precursor steroids (17-hydroxyprogesterone, 17-hydroxypregnenolone, and 11-deoxycortisol) should be measured before and 1 hour after the ACTH is administered.

Some investigators have suggested that a 1-hour stimulation test is not sufficient to distinguish all patients with congenital adrenal hyperplasia from normal.[28] They would administer ACTH continuously intravenously for 4 to 24 hours. If administered for 24 hours, 0.5 mg of cosyntropin is administered in 1000 ml of 5% dextrose in water. One advantage of the 24-hour infusion is the ability to measure the levels of urinary metabolites of the precursor hormones, specifically pregnanetriol (a metabolite of 17-hydroxyprogesterone) and tetrahydro-11-deoxycortisol (a metabolite of 11-deoxycortisol). Yet, in studies of families with 21-hydroxylase deficiency, 60- and 360-minute infusions yielded similar results.[20] There have been no comparative studies in patients with hirsutism to verify the reliability of the short versus the long infusion tests. However, because of its convenience, most investigators have adopted the rapid cosyntropin stimulation test and measure steroids 1 hour

TABLE 42–4. LABORATORY EVALUATION OF HIRSUTISM-VIRILIZING SYNDROMES

	Ovarian		Adrenal			
	*PCO**	*Ovarian Tumor*	*CAH†*	*Adrenal Neoplasm*	*Cushing's Syndrome*	**Idiopathic**
Urinary 17-ketosteroids or plasma DHEA‡ sulfate	N↑	N	N↑	↑↑↑	N↑	N
Plasma testosterone	N↑	↑↑	N↑	N↑	N↑	N
Serial LH§ levels	N↑	N	N	N	N	N
Precursor of cortisol biosynthesis						
Basally	N	N	N↑	N↑	N	N
Following ACTH‖ infusion	N	N	↑↑	N↑	N	N
Cortisol levels following overnight dexamethasone suppression test	N	N	N	↑	↑	N

*PCO = polycystic ovarian syndrome.
†CAH = congenital adrenal hyperplasia.
‡DHEA = dehydroepiandrosterone.
§LH = luteinizing hormone.
‖ACTH = adrenocorticotropic hormone.

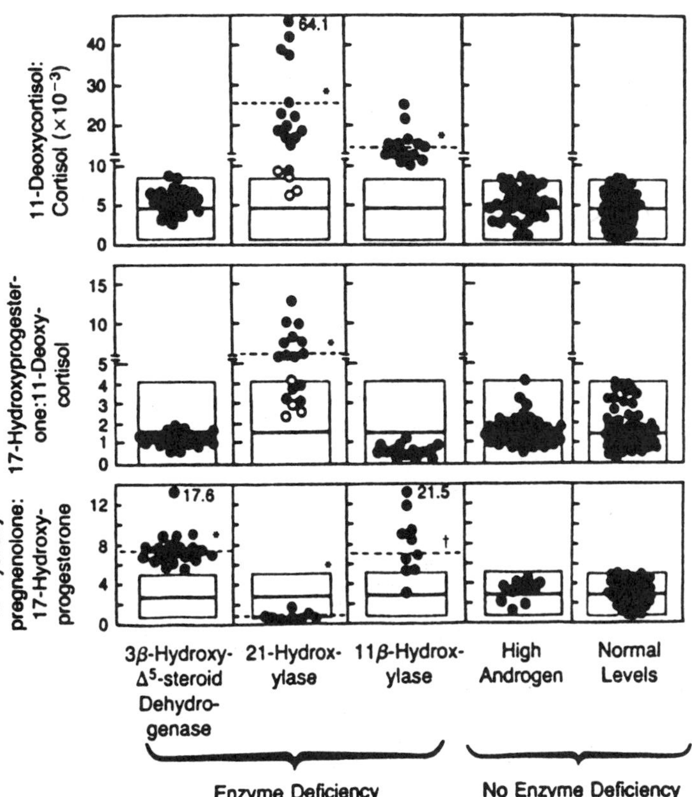

FIGURE 42–3. Plasma steroid precursor-to-product ratios 60 minutes after ACTH stimulation in women with nonclassical congenital adrenal hyperplasia due to deficiency of 3β-hydroxy-Δ^5-steroid dehydrogenase, 21-hydroxylase, or 11β-hydroxylase and in 118 woman with no adrenal biosynthetic defect. Boxed values are the mean ± 2D ratios for 26 normal women. Solid circles denote affected women, and open circles denote obligate carriers. Asterisks ($P < .005$) and the dagger ($P < .05$) indicate significant differences from normal values. Dashed lines indicate the mean values for the affected women. (From Eldar-Geva T, Hurwitz A, Vecsei P, et al: Secondary biosynthetic defects in women with late-onset congenital adrenal hyperplasia. N Engl J Med 323:866, 1990. Reprinted with permission of the New England Journal of Medicine.)

later. Of importance in menstruating patients, the test should be performed in the follicular phase of their cycle.[48] Thus, finding a normal plasma level of steroid precursors or their metabolites in the urine in response to ACTH administration effectively rules out an adrenal enzyme deficiency (see Table 42–4).

Some investigators have suggested that hirsute women who do not have evidence of congenital adrenal hyperplasia or polycystic ovarian syndrome are hirsute because of an abnormality in peripheral androgen metabolism. Specifically, they suggest that peripheral 5α-reductase activity is increased in these individuals, producing a more androgenic peripheral steroid pattern that results in the hirsutism. Evidence supporting this claim are increased levels of 3α-androstanediol and its glucuronide and sulfate conjugates.[50–52] If correct, then measurement of this steroid may be useful to determine if abnormal peripheral androgen metabolism is present. Other studies, however, report that the level of this steroid or its conjugates does not provide any information beyond that obtained by measuring plasma testosterone.[53–55] Indeed, in one study, serum androstanediol glucuronide not only paralleled the levels of commonly measured androgens but also did not correlate with the degree of facial hirsutism.[54]

The only definitive way of determining whether *polycystic ovaries* are present is by visual inspection. Commonly this is done by laparoscopy. In some cases, an elevation of the plasma LH level will provide circumstantial evidence for the presence of polycystic ovaries.[34–36, 43] However, many patients with polycystic ovaries do not have elevated LH levels. Thus, the finding of a normal level is not helpful. Finally, abdominal computed tomography holds great promise in evaluating the adrenal area, whereas ultrasonography has been particularly useful for examining the ovaries.

SUMMARY OF THE APPROACH TO THE PATIENT

Evaluation of Simple Hirsutism

A patient with simple hirsutism without oligomenorrhea, virilization, or signs of Cushing's syndrome has better than a 95% chance of having idiopathic hirsutism. The primary conditions to be excluded are ovarian or adrenal tumors. Thus, a complete history and physical examination with a careful search for signs and symptoms of Cushing's syndrome or virilization in conjunction with a baseline 24-hour 17-ketosteroid excretion rate, plasma DHEA sulfate level, and a plasma testosterone determination to rule out adrenal and ovarian tumors would suffice. If oligomenorrhea is also present, then the probability that an adrenal or ovarian lesion will be found increases by as much as 10-fold. In addition to these procedures, it would be appropriate to perform an overnight dexamethasone suppression test for Cushing's syndrome, to obtain a plasma LH level to assess the probability of polycystic ovaries, and in some cases (i.e., those with an elevated plasma DHEA sulfate level or severe enough manifestations to warrant consideration of prednisone therapy) to perform a cosyntropin infusion test to rule out an adrenal enzyme deficiency. Measurement of steroid precursors for all three potential enzyme deficiencies is important. The value of also measuring the level of androstanediol or its glucuronide or sulfate conjugates is unclear. Obviously, an abnormal result from any of the tests listed earlier requires further evaluation. If the patient is not interested in having children, making a definitive diagnosis of polycystic ovaries (i.e., hospitalization with laparoscopy) may not be warranted because treatment of the hirsutism is only marginally successful.[43]

Evaluation of Virilization

In patients who have signs and symptoms of virilization, as opposed to just hirsutism, there is a very high probability that a specific abnormality of ovarian or adrenal hormonal secretion will be found. Therefore, a careful and thorough evaluation to establish the proper diagnosis and initiate the correct treatment is warranted. Not only should these individuals have the previously mentioned tests, but also if the diagnosis remains undetermined, further studies should be performed, including adrenal computed tomographic scan, ultrasonography of the pelvis, and, if necessary, laparoscopy.

MANAGEMENT OF HIRSUTISM

Treatment of patients with virilizing syndromes due to adrenal or ovarian tumors requires surgical removal of the lesion, if at all possible (Table 42–5). In some cases this is not feasible, and therefore, appropriate chemotherapy may be necessary. In patients with Cushing's syndrome, various therapeutic approaches may be warranted. If a discrete, ACTH-producing lesion is present, then surgical removal of that tumor should be attempted. If pituitary-hypothalamic dysfunction is the cause, however, often bilateral adrenalectomy is the treatment of choice.

In patients with partial *adrenal enzyme deficiencies,* because the excess androgen production is secondary to increased ACTH secretion, treatment is directed at suppressing ACTH release with exogenous glucocorticoids (see Table 42–5). The preferred agent is prednisone. Some investigators use dexamethasone because it is a longer-acting steroid. However, this advantage in suppressing adrenal function increases the probability of developing steroid-induced side effects, even when dexamethasone is administered in relatively low doses (0.25 to 0.5 mg/day). Several parameters can be used to monitor the response to therapy. The two biochemical parameters usually followed initially at monthly intervals and later at 3-month intervals are plasma DHEA sulfate levels and urinary 17-ketosteroid excretion rates. Usually the most sensitive biologic indicator of a change in androgen levels is the sebum content of the skin.[10] This can be evaluated qualitatively by asking the patient how frequently she washes her hair, or the sebum production can actually be quantified. Changes in sebum content usually occur within days after a reduction in androgen production. In contrast, it may take several months for the menses to become regular and a year or more for a significant change in facial hair growth to occur.

TABLE 42–5. TREATMENT OF HIRSUTISM

Surgery
Ovarian or adrenal tumors
Cushing's syndrome
Wedge resection of polycystic ovary (infrequent)
Prednisone: congenital adrenal hyperplasia
Estrogen-progesterone combination: polycystic ovaries
GnRH agonist: polycystic ovaries
Mechanical treatment of hair
Electrolysis
Depilatories
Plucking, waxing
Shaving
Bleaching
Nonspecific drug therapy
Spironolactone
Cyproterone acetate ± ethinyl estradiol
Flutamide

The usual program is to administer prednisone, 5 mg orally every 12 hours, until the biochemical parameters and sebum production have been suppressed for 3 months. Then the prednisone can be reduced to 2.5 mg every 8 hours. If after 3 more months of therapy both clinical and biochemical responses have been sustained, then a further reduction of prednisone to 2.5 mg twice daily may be tried. The goal should be to reduce the prednisone to the lowest dose possible and still suppress urine or plasma androgen levels and maintain normal menstrual cycles. In some patients with mild enzyme deficiencies, a single 2.5-mg dose of prednisone at bedtime to reduce the normally occurring morning peak in ACTH secretion may be sufficient to maintain normal cycles and reduce hair growth.[18]

It is unclear how long prednisone is needed. Some patients with documented enzyme deficiencies and good clinical responses to prednisone have been symptom-free for 2 to 3 years after prednisone was stopped. On the other hand, some patients require a daily dose of prednisone of 10 mg to maintain normal levels of 17-ketosteroid excretion, or plasma DHEA sulfate, menstrual cycles, and hair growth. If this level of prednisone is necessary, then the patient should be made aware of the potential side effects of long-term administration of pharmacologic doses of glucocorticoids so that an appropriate risk-benefit analysis can be made.

The management of the patient with polycystic ovaries depends in part on whether she wishes to become pregnant (see Table 42–5). If ovulation is the primary goal of therapy, then clomiphene or a combination of follicle-stimulating hormone (Pergonal) and human chorionic gonadotropin may be useful.[42, 43] This form of therapy should be instituted only after a definitive diagnosis has been established, which may include laparoscopy, and then only by a physician skilled in the use of these agents because significant side effects may occur if they are used improperly. If a patient is not interested in achieving fertility, then suppression of ovarian function with estrogens or estrogen-progesterone combinations, such as low-dose estrogen birth control pills or a gonadotropin-releasing hormone agonist (e.g., leuprolide), may be tried.[39, 43, 56, 57] Again, as with adrenal lesions, the most sensitive index of androgen suppression is a change in sebum production. Excess hair growth takes a long time to regress. If estrogen therapy is used, menstrual periods will be regularized because of the hormonal therapy and therefore cannot be used as an index of suppression of androgen production. Because the basic abnormality in this syndrome is likely to be in the hypothalamic-pituitary axis, estrogen suppressive therapy probably does not alter the basic pathophysiology but simply modifies its expression. Whether this is true for agonist therapy is uncertain, although as with estrogen therapy, the regularity of menses no longer can be used as an index of effective therapy because the gonadotropin-releasing hormone agonist will likely induce amenorrhea. Thus, the efficacy of ovarian suppressive therapy in reducing hair growth and other androgen effects is less than the efficacy of the treatments used for ovarian and adrenal tumors or adrenal hyperplasia.[43, 56, 57]

Several experimental procedures have also been used to treat patients with polycystic ovaries. One approach was to administer high-dose depo-medroxyprogesterone acetate intramuscularly every 15 days.[58] The rationale behind this approach was to suppress LH release. After 5 months of therapy, a significant decrease in the rate of hair growth was noted. However, amenorrhea also occurred, and whether other long-term side effects may occur is still unclear.

Idiopathic Hirsutism

As noted earlier, the majority of patients will have no definable cause for simple hirsutism. Even in some patients in whom the cause is known, treatment of the primary lesion may not be feasible; therefore, measures directed at mechanically removing the excess hair may be necessary.[59, 60] Five techniques have been used (see Table 42–5). The most effective, but also the most costly, is *electrolysis*. A galvanic (direct) current destroys the hair follicle itself. Needles are attached to the electrolysis machine and are placed into the hair follicles. The procedure is effective but time-consuming. Because there are more than 1400 follicles/square inch of body surface, a significant number of treatments are necessary to produce a discernible change in the growth of hair. With earlier machines, there was a high probability of scarring and pain; both occur infrequently with currently used equipment. However, the investment of time and money remains considerable. Twice-weekly sessions for several years are necessary to produce a significant change in most cases. A related procedure is *diathermy*. However, it is only infrequently used because of the relatively high risk of scarring.

Depilatories consist of commercially available creams that contain barium or calcium sulfide or calcium thiosulfate. These agents work by breaking the disulfide bonds in the hair shaft. They do not alter the hair follicle and therefore do not alter the rate of hair growth. They may, however, be locally irritating and therefore produce a dermatitis, in some cases, requiring the use of topical steroids. The mechanical removal of hair, plucking, is also effective in eliminating the hair but usually does not alter the hair follicle. Therefore, the growth of new hair continues. Waxing is a related method in which large numbers of hair can be removed simultaneously by placing wax or tape and glue depilatories on the face and then suddenly pulling them off while they are still pliable. Plucking and waxing may irritate the hair follicle, and thus cause it to grow more rapidly, or produce an infection in the hair follicle itself. The simplest and safest way to remove hair is by *shaving*. Shaving, however, is the technique used least by hirsute females. The primary objection is the belief that shaving increases the rate or thickness of subsequent hair growth. However, no objective data support this belief.

Bleaching of the hair provides another method. The hair is depigmented and therefore rendered less conspicuous. Bleaching is often used to treat hair on the upper lip and the sideburn area. A solution of hydrogen peroxide and ammonia is the most commonly used agent and is readily available from commercial sources.

Numerous nonspecific pharmacologic approaches also have been used. All have approached the problem by attempting to lower the effective concentration of androgens at the hair follicle, by inhibiting androgen production, accelerating its degradation, blocking its transport, or inhibiting its binding to cytosolic binding sites. The agents include cyproterone acetate, flutamide, spironolactone, cimetidine, and bromocriptine. Both cyproterone acetate and spironolactone act at two sites—blocking binding to receptor sites and inhibiting production.[61] In most studies, cyproterone acetate (50 to 100 mg) was given in combination with ethinyl estradiol. Both were given cyclically. The success rate was usually 50 to 70%, with minimal side effects. However, long-term follow-ups have not been reported.[61–63] Some clinical trials have used as little as 2 mg of cyproterone acetate.[63] Although suppression of hair growth is not as great as with higher doses, the difference may not be significant when contrasted with the decrease in side effects. Spironolactone is usually given either continuously at doses of 100 to 200 mg/day or cyclically. It appeared effective both clinically and biochemically in 75 to 90% of cases.[61, 64, 65] Indeed, it may be effective even when no changes in androgen levels are observed. Its potential side effects include activation of the renin-angiotensin system, natriuresis, and hyperkalemia. However, in two studies of 69 patients followed for 1 year, none of these symptoms was observed. Results with cimetidine and bromocriptine have been mixed.[61, 66] Flutamide is a new antiandrogen that is presently undergoing clinical testing. In one report, a significant reduction in hair growth was observed after 3 months of therapy.[67] However, no long-term studies or assessments of potential side effects have been published. Finally, 5α-reductase inhibitors may produce an overall favorable reduction in peripheral androgen activity in women with hirsutism.[68] However, no studies have been reported using these agents. It is important to stress that none of these drugs have been approved by the FDA for treatment of hirsutism, and the long-term consequences are still unknown.

REFERENCES

1. McKnight E: The prevalence of "hirsutism" in young women. Lancet i:410, 1964.
2. Erkkola R and Ruutiainen K: Hirsutism: Definitions and etiology. Ann Med 22:99, 1990.
3. Forber AP: Hirsutism. *In* Fitzpatrick TB, Arndt KA, et al (eds): Dermatology in General Medicine. New York, McGraw-Hill, 1971.
4. Breckwoldt M, Zahradnik HP, and Wieacker P: Hirsutism: Its pathogenesis. Hum Reprod 4:601, 1989.
5. Stewart WD, Danto JL, and Maddin S: Dermatology: Diagnosis and Treatment of Cutaneous Disorders. St. Louis, CV Mosby, 1974, p 10.
6. Ferriman D: Human Hair Growth in Health and Disease. Springfield, IL, Charles C Thomas, 1971.
7. Montagna W and Dobson RL: Hair Growth. New York, Pergamon Press, 1969.
8. Kligman AM: The human hair cycle. J Invest Dermatol 33:307, 1959.
9. Rook A: Endocrine influences on hair growth. BMJ 1:609, 1965.
10. Strauss JS and Pochi PE: Recent advances in androgen metabolism and their relation to the skin. Arch Dermatol 100:621, 1969.
11. Wieland RG, Vorys N, Folk RL, et al: Studies of female hirsutism. Am J Med 41:927, 1966.
12. Livingston S, Petersen DC, Boks LL et al.: Hypertrichosis occurring in association with Dilantin therapy. J Pediatr 47:351, 1955.
13. Baker L, Kaye R, Root AW, et al: Diazoxide treatment of idiopathic hypoglycemia of infancy. J Pediatr 71:494, 1967.
14. Dormois JC, Young JL, and Nies AS: Minoxidil in severe hypertension: Value when conventional drugs have failed. Am Heart J 90:360, 1975.
15. Preedy JRK: Endocrine investigation in hirsutes. *In* Brown AC (ed): The First Human Hair Symposium. New York, Medcom Press, 1974, p 97.
16. Kirschner MA and Bardin CW: Androgen production and metabolism in normal and virilized women. Metabolism 21:667, 1972.
17. Kirschner MA: Hirsutism and virilization. Res Staff Phys 25:118, 1979.
18. Williams GH and Dluhy RG: Diseases of the adrenal cortex. *In* Wilson J, Braunwald E, Isselbacher K, et al (eds): Harrison's

Principles of Internal Medicine, 12th ed. New York, McGraw-Hill, 1991, p 1713.
19. Givens JR: Hirsutism and hyperandrogenism. Adv Intern Med 21:221, 1976.
20. New MI and Levine LS: Recent advances in 21-hydroxylase deficiency. Annu Rev Med 35:649, 1984.
21. Speiser PW, Dupont J, Zhu D, et al: Disease expression and molecular genotype in congenital adrenal hyperplasia due to 21-hydroxylase deficiency. J Clin Invest 90:584, 1992.
22. Eldar-Geva T, Hurwitz A, Vecsei P, et al: Secondary biosynthetic defects in women with late-onset congenital adrenal hyperplasia. N Engl J Med 323:855, 1990.
23. Chrousos GP, Loriaux L, Mann DL, et al: Late-onset 21-hydroxylase deficiency mimicking idiopathic hirsutism or polycystic ovarian disease. Ann Intern Med 96:143, 1982.
24. Killeen AA, Hanson NQ, Eklund R, et al: Prevalence of nonclassical congenital adrenal hyperplasia among women self-referred for electrolytic treatment of hirsutism. Am J Med Genet 42(2):197, 1992.
25. Akinci A, Yordam N, Ersoy F, et al: The incidence of nonclassical 21-hydroxylase deficiency in hirsute adolescent girls. Gynecol Endocrinol 6:99, 1992.
26. Balsamo A, Revelli A, Borelli I, et al: Hormonal profiles in Italian late-onset adrenal hyperplasia correlate with HLA class III polymorphisms. Gynecol Endocrinol 6:91, 1992.
27. Speiser PW, Dupont B, Rubinstein P, et al: High frequency of nonclassical steroid 21-hydroxylase deficiency. Am J Hum Genet 37:650, 1985.
28. Newmark S, Dluhy RG, Williams GH, et al: Partial 11- and 21-hydroxylase deficiencies in hirsute women. Am J Obstet Gynecol 127:594, 1977.
29. Meikle AW, Worley RJ, and West CD: Adrenal corticoid hyperresponsiveness in hirsute women. Fertil Steril 41:575, 1984.
30. Boivin Y and Richard RM: Hilus cell tumors of the ovary. A review with a report of 3 new cases. Cancer 18:231, 1965.
31. Norris HJ and Taylor HB: Virilization associated with cystic granulosa tumors. Obstet Gynecol 34:629, 1969.
32. Pedowitz P and Pomerance W: Adrenal-like tumors of the ovary. Review of the literature and report of two new cases. Obstet Gynecol 19:183, 1962.
33. Goldzieher JW: Polycystic ovarian disease. Fertil Steril 35:371, 1981.
34. DeVane GW, Czekala NM, Judd HL, et al: Circulating gonadotropins, estrogen and androgens in polycystic ovarian disease. Am J Obstet Gynecol 121:496, 1975.
35. Berger MJ, Taymor ML, and Patton WC: Baseline gonadotropin levels and secretory patterns in patients with typical and atypical polycystic ovarian disease. Fertil Steril 26:619, 1975.
36. Rebar R, Judd HL, Yen SSC, et al: Characterization of the inappropriate gonadotropin secretion in polycystic ovary syndrome. J Clin Invest 57:1320, 1976.
37. Quigley ME, Rakoff JS, and Yen SS: Increased luteinizing hormone sensitivity to dopamine inhibition in polycystic ovary syndrome. J Clin Endocrinol Metab 52:231, 1981.
38. Toscano V, Bianchi P, Balducci R, et al: Lack of linear relationship between hyperinsulinemia and hyperandrogenism. Clin Endocrinol 36:197, 1992.
39. Wild RA, Alaupovic P, and Parker IJ: Lipid and apolipoprotein abnormalities in hirsute women. The association with insulin resistance. Am J Obstet Gynecol 167:575, 1992.
40. Kirschner MA and Jacobs JB: Combined ovarian and adrenal vein catheterization to determine the site(s) of androgen overproduction in hirsute women. J Clin Endocrinol 33:199, 1971.
41. Laghelin GC, Judd HL, Swanson SC, et al: Long-term effects of nightly dexamethasone administration in patients with polycystic ovarian disease. J Clin Endocrinol Metab 55:768, 1982.
42. McLachlan RI, Healy DL, and Burger HG: The ovary. *In* Felig P, Baxter J, Broadus J, et al (eds): Endocrinology and Metabolism, 2nd ed. New York, McGraw-Hill, 1987, p 951.
43. Hatch R, Rosenfield RL, Kim MH, et al: Hirsutism: Implications, etiology, and management. Am J Obstet Gynecol 140:815, 1981.
44. Schwartz U, Moltz L, Brotherton J, et al: The diagnostic value of plasma free testosterone in non-tumorous and tumorous hyperandrogenism. Fertil Steril 40:66, 1983.
45. Carlstrom K, Gershagen S, and Rannevik G: Free testosterone/SHBG index in hirsute women: A comparison of diagnostic accuracy. Gynecol Obstet Invest 24:256, 1987.
46. Bates GW, French GM, Humphries BB, and Blackhurst DW: Outcome of corticotropin stimulation testing in women with androgen excess and ovulatory dysfunction. Am J Obstet Gynecol 167:308, 1992.
47. Hawkins LA, Chasalow FI, and Blethen SL: The role of adrenocorticotropin testing in evaluating girls with premature adrenarche and hirsutism/oligomenorrhea. J Clin Endocrinol Metab 74:248, 1992.
48. Harracksingh C, Benjamin F, Deutsch S, and Seltzer VL: Comparison of the adrenocorticotropic hormone stimulation test in the follicular and luteal phases of the menstrual cycle. Int J Fertil 37:123, 1992.
49. Siegel SF, Finegold DN, Lanes R, and Lee PA: ACTH stimulation tests and plasma dehydroepiandrosterone sulfate levels in women with hirsutism. N Engl J Med 323:849, 1990.
50. Kirschner MA, Samojlik E, and Szmal E: Clinical usefulness of plasma androstanediol glucuronide measurements in women with idiopathic hirsutism. J Clin Endocrinol Metab 65:597, 1987.
51. Greep N, Hoopes M, and Horton R: Androstanediol glucuronide plasma clearance and production rates in normal and hirsute women. J Clin Endocrinol Metab 62:22, 1986.
52. Whorwood CB, Ueshiba H, and delBlazo P: Plasma levels of C19 steroid glucuronides in premenopausal women with nonclassical congenital adrenal hyperplasia. J Steroid Biochem Mol Biol 42:211, 1992.
53. Vogt C, Dericks-Tan JS, Kuhl H, and Taubert HD: Is 3α-, 17β-androstanediol-glucuronide a diagnostic marker in women with androgenic manifestations? Gynecol Endocrinol 6:85, 1992.
54. Salman K, Spielvogel RL, Shulman LH, et al: Serum androstanediol glucuronide in women with facial hirsutism. J Am Acad Dermatol 26:411, 1992.
55. Pang S, Wang M, Jeffries S, et al: Normal and elevated 3α-androstanediol glucuronide concentrations in women with various causes of hirsutism and its correlation with degree of hirsutism and androgen levels. J Clin Endocrinol Metab 75:243, 1992.
56. Wild RA, Demers LM, Applebaum-Bowden D, and Lenker R: Hirsutism: Metabolic effects of two commonly used oral contraceptives and spironolactone. Contraception 44:113, 1991.
57. Loy R and Seibel MM: Evaluation and therapy of polycystic ovarian syndrome. Endocrinol Metab Clin North Am 17:785, 1988.
58. Correa de Oliveira RF, Novaes LP, Lima MB, et al: A new treatment for hirsutism. Ann Intern Med 83:817, 1975.
59. Wagner RF Jr: Physical methods for the management of hirsutism. Cutis 45:319, 1990.
60. Richards RN, Uy M, and Meharg G: Temporary hair removal in patients with hirsutism: A clinical study. Cutis 45:199, 1990.
61. Hammerstein J, Moltz L, and Schwartz U: Antiandrogens in the treatment of acne and hirsutism. J Steroid Biochem Mol Biol 19:591, 1983.
62. Chapman MG, Jeffcoate SL, and Dewhurst CJ: Effect of cyproterone acetate-ethinyloestradiol treatment on adrenal function in hirsute women. Clin Endocrinol 17:577, 1982.
63. Belisle S and Love EJ: Clinical efficacy and safety of cyproterone acetate in severe hirsutism: Results of a multicentered Canadian study. Fertil Steril 46:1015, 1986.
64. Cumming DC, Yang JC, Rebar RW, et al: Treatment of hirsutism with spironolactone. JAMA 247:1295, 1982.
65. Carmina E and Lobo RA: Peripheral androgen blockade versus glandular androgen suppression in the treatment of hirsutism. Obstet Gynecol 78:845, 1991.
66. Grandesso R, Spandri P, Gangemi M, et al: Hormonal changes and hair growth during treatment of hirsutism with cimetidine. Clin Exp Obstet Gynecol 11:105, 1984.
67. Marcondes JA, Minnani SL, Luthold WW, et al: Treatment of hirsutism in women with flutamide. Fertil Steril 57:543, 1992.
68. Brooks JR: Treatment of hirsutism with 5α-reductase inhibitors. Clin Endocrinol Metab 15:391, 1986.

43

The Infertile Couple

BRUCE H. ALBRECHT, MD
ISAAC SCHIFF, MD

Management of involuntary infertility has changed dramatically over the past decade: new treatments based on scientific analyses of fertility factors are rapidly replacing the empiric remedies of the past. These changes increase the need for general practitioners to become familiar with the biologic foundations of fertility, for only with this knowledge can the rationale for today's more effective therapies be understood. In its allotted length, this chapter cannot hope to present a comprehensive, detailed account of the evaluation and treatment of infertility; for such coverage, other sources are available.[1–8] It can, however, present the basic problems general physicians are likely to encounter in examining an infertile couple and describe the circumstances in which it would be worthwhile to refer the couple to a specialist for further consultation and evaluation.

The American Fertility Society defines *infertility* as the failure of a couple to achieve conception after engaging in one or more years of regular sexual intercourse without practicing any contraceptive measures. The definition is extended by some researchers to include couples in which the woman becomes pregnant but fails to deliver a viable infant. *Primary infertility* refers to couples who have never produced previous pregnancies or children; *secondary infertility* refers to couples who have previously produced children but have failed to achieve a pregnancy after one or more years of trying. *Recurrent pregnancy loss* refers to a woman who has had three or more spontaneous abortions.

The definition of (involuntary) infertility is not an arbitrary one but rather is derived from observation of the cumulative pregnancy rate of normally fertile couples (Fig. 43–1). Normal couples, who have an estimated 15 to 20% chance of pregnancy during each month of exposure, show a 50% chance of pregnancy by the third to fourth month, and a 76% chance by the sixth to eighth month. After one year, 85 to 95% of healthy couples will have achieved a pregnancy. Thus, in general, if a couple has not achieved a pregnancy after less than 1 year of trying, they should be reassured. It is appropriate, though, to initiate an evaluation after just 6 months in couples older than 30 to 35 years of age, and even earlier in couples in whom a cause of infertility may be obvious—for example, when amenorrhea or previous pelvic infections are seen, or when the man has small testicles.

It has been estimated that in the United States about 10 to 15% of couples experience involuntary infertility, and the number of cases may be rising. Possible reasons for this increase include the recent steady rise in the number of

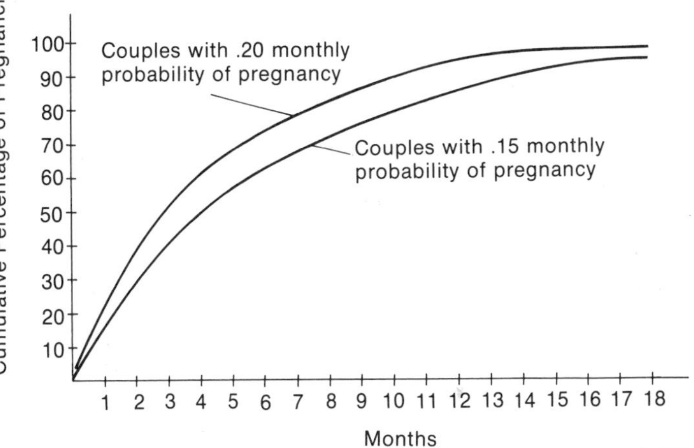

FIGURE 43–1. The cumulative percentage of pregnancies occurring during the first 18 months of unprotected coitus in normal couples with a monthly probability of pregnancy of 0.15 to 0.20. (From Cramer DW, Walker AM, and Schiff I: Statistical methods in evaluating the outcome of infertility therapy. Fertil Steril 1979; 32:80–86. Reproduced with permission of publisher, The American Fertility Society.)

cases of sexually transmitted diseases, resulting in an increase in pelvic inflammatory disease; the probable increased exposure of American couples to environmental toxins; and the recent trend in delaying child bearing to the later reproductive years, all of which can lead to decreased pregnancy rates. An inherent age-related decline in female fertility seems to begin after age 30 years.[9] The possible biologic explanations for this decline include hypothalamic aging, increased luteal or other ovulatory defects, reduced ovum viability, and increased pregnancy wastage.

Present figures show that about 75% of infertile couples will eventually seek medical help. This high figure is partly due to the unavailability of babies for adoption that has occurred because of the widespread use of therapeutic abortion for unwanted pregnancies and the changed attitude toward the single mother. The process of adopting a child often calls for 3 to 5 years of waiting, and adoption of a second child is usually impossible. Thus, there is strong public demand for the expansion of research into the causes and treatment of infertility. In 1974, the American College of Obstetricians and Gynecologists responded to this demand by establishing a subspecialty certification board in Reproductive Endocrinology.

APPROACH TO THE INFERTILE COUPLE

When working with an infertile couple, it must be emphasized at the outset that infertility is a problem of the couple, not just the female partner. Couples must be evaluated as a unit, and motivation for the evaluation should come from *both* partners. An infertility investigation tends to place emotional stresses on a couple, who may already be under a great deal of stress from the pressures of infertility and its accompanying issues of sexual identity and compatibility.[10]

It is estimated that approximately 40 to 50% of infertile couples will have male factors, 60 to 70% will have female factors, and 10 to 20% will have no identifiable cause for their infertility. This total is greater than 100 because in 25 to 30% of couples the infertility is of multiple etiology.

The fertility of a couple depends on the culmination and normal interaction of numerous factors. The man must produce an adequate number of healthy, motile sperm, which must traverse the male reproductive tract and be ejaculated into a normal female reproductive tract. Here, the sperm must penetrate the cervical mucus and ascend through the uterus and fallopian tubes to the ampulla, where fertilization takes place. Obviously, this must occur simultaneously with ovulation in the female, which is a response to the proper stimulation of the ovarian follicles by an intact hypothalamic-pituitary mechanism. The released ovum must be "picked up" by the freely mobile, healthy fallopian tube, where fertilization and division to the blastocyst stage occur during the week following ovulation. Implantation of the blastocyst then occurs on the endometrial bed, which has been prepared over the preceding 3 weeks (since the last menstruation) in response to the hormonal products of the ovary, from which the ovum was produced. Continued hormonal and nutritional support of the conceptus is necessary over the next 260 days.

It is obvious that many more basic events and factors can be defective in a woman. On the other hand, because an expensive and prolonged investigation of the woman serves no useful purpose if the man is infertile, an adequate evaluation of the man should be performed very early in the evaluation of a couple.

Four basic areas need to be covered in an infertility evaluation (Table 43–1). These tests are designed to evaluate the anatomy, physiology, and sexual compatibility of the couple. Additional areas requiring evaluation will be discussed in the following sections.

EVALUATION OF THE MAN

History and Physical Examination

The evaluation should begin with a general medical history and physical examination, with special attention to certain pertinent factors. Although the age-related reproductive decline in men is not as marked as in women, the sperm count and motility do gradually decrease. Occupation is a significant factor because exposure of the scrotum to excessive heat (e.g., as may be common in cross-country truck drivers, bakers and cooks, and foundry workers), radiation, lead, and organic chemicals, particularly pesticides, may be detrimental to spermatogenesis. In addition, current use of common ingestants such as nicotine, alcohol, and marijuana should be noted, as they have been implicated as being detrimental to normal spermatogenesis.

Numerous complicating factors should be looked for during the complete medical history. Diabetes and neurologic diseases may be associated with retrograde ejaculation and impotence. Infectious diseases, such as postpubertal mumps orchitis, or tuberculous or gonococcal epididymitis, may affect fertility. Medications that should be particularly noted include sex hormones, antihypertensive medications, spironolactone, nitrofurantoin, cimetidine, and chemotherapeutic agents. Damage to the testes may have occurred due to trauma, cryptorchidism, or previous repairs for cryptorchidism or hernias during which the spermatic artery or ductus deferens may have been inadvertently tied off.

The physical examination should concentrate on the secondary sex characteristics and the genitalia. If the patient appears to be inadequately virilized, the diagnosis of delayed pubertal maturation should be considered. The location of the urethral meatus should be assessed, as a hypospadias can result in failure of the ejaculate being deposited in the vagina. Testicular consistency is probably more important than size: a soft, rubbery testicle, regardless of it size, is generally associated with severe oligospermia or azoospermia. The testes of Klinefelter's syndrome are typically small (< 2 cm) but may be firm. Epididymal induration or irregularities can be due to old infection and may indicate an obstruction. Vascular engorgement of the venous plexus in the scrotum indicates a varicocele, which can be related to abnormalities of gonadal function. Unilateral testicular atrophy of varying degrees is fairly common with a varicocele; therefore, disproportionate testicular size (differential > 0.5 cm) should alert the examiner to this possibility. A varicocele is best diagnosed by having the patient stand erect and perform a Valsalva maneuver while the examiner palpates both right and left spermatic cord regions. This method accentuates the dilated varicosities. Studies on the diagnosis of varicoceles by scrotal examination with Doppler probes, thermograms, ultrasounds, and venograms show a high rate of abnormal test results in

TABLE 43–1. BASIC INFERTILITY EVALUATION

1. Semen analysis
2. Documentation of normal ovulatory function
3. Postcoital examination
4. Patency of fallopian tubes

fertile men with normal semen analyses. Therefore, the physical examination remains the mainstay of diagnosis.

Causes of Male Infertility

Table 43–2 lists causes of male infertility. The genetic causes of infertility are rare and can usually be suspected on the basis of the physical examination.

Klinefelter's syndrome (XXY chromosomal pattern) affects 1:600 male births. Most patients with this syndrome have elevated gonadotropin values and low androgen levels; consequently, masculine characteristics are absent or underdeveloped and, on examination, the patients have a eunuchoidal habitus, gynecomastia, and small, firm testes. Semen analysis usually shows azoospermia, and testicular biopsy reveals hyalinization.

XYY syndrome occurs in 1:1000 male births. These patients are usually tall, and they may have a tendency to manifest increased aggressiveness and criminal behavior. Although impaired spermatogenesis is usually seen, normal fertility has been documented.

Reifenstein's syndrome, another genetic abnormality related to infertility, is characterized by eunuchoidal habitus, gynecomastia, hypospadias, Leydig's cell hypoplasia, and azoospermia. Patients have a normal 46,XY chromosomal pattern but reduced levels of testosterone and dihydrotestosterone.

Primary testicular diseases are more common causes of male infertility. Cryptorchidism is the most common disorder of sexual differentiation in men. Approximately 1% of full-term infants have an undescended testis at 1 year of age, and 10% of these have a bilateral defect. Unilaterally, cryptorchid patients undergoing orchidopexy prior to puberty have a 62% fertility rate, versus 46% if corrected after puberty. A similar trend is seen in patients with bilateral cryptorchidism (30% fertility rate versus 13%). These data suggest an inherent defect in the undescended testis despite surgical correction, in addition to a secondary insult that occurs in the testicle exposed to the higher temperature of the extrascrotal location. Further evidence attesting to the inherent testicular defect in this condition comes from histologic studies that show bilateral testicular abnormalities in unilateral cryptorchidism, and the increased malignant potential of both the ectopic and the eutopic testis of the unilaterally cryptorchid patient.

TABLE 43–2. CAUSES OF MALE INFERTILITY

Genetic
Klinefelter's syndrome
XYY syndrome
Reifenstein's syndrome
Primary testicular disorders
Cryptorchidism
Sertoli-cell–only syndrome (germinal cell aplasia)
Mumps orchitis
Chemicals and drugs
Irradiation
Endocrine problems
Kallmann's syndrome (hypogonadism and anosmia)
Panhypopituitarism
Hyperprolactinemia
Male adrenogenital syndrome
Partial androgen resistance
Ductal obstruction
Epididymal
Congenital absence of the ductus deferens
Ejaculatory duct
Previous ligation of the ductus deferens
Infection
Ejaculatory disorders
Retrograde ejaculation
Impotence
Varicocele

Sertoli-cell–only syndrome, or germinal cell aplasia, is a primary testicular disease diagnosed only by testicular biopsy, which shows small seminiferous tubules, complete absence of germinal epithelium, and the presence of Sertoli's cells and normal-appearing Leydig's cells. On examination, patients with this syndrome have small, soft testicles and an elevated follicle-stimulating hormone (FSH) level, probably resulting from the lack of inhibin production because there are no germinal cells. Testosterone and luteinizing hormone (LH) values are normal because the Leydig cells are present and functional.

Mumps orchitis is a rare complication of mumps in prepubertal boys, but 30% of postpubertal men develop orchitis when mumps parotitis occurs. Mumps orchitis is bilateral in up to 33% of individuals and causes testicular damage in 75% of patients, resulting in subsequent presentation with severe oligospermia or azoospermia and atrophy of the testicle or testicles.

The list of exogenous chemicals and drugs that may directly or indirectly affect testicular function continues to expand. Direct-acting compounds, including flutamide, cyproterone acetate, spironolactone, cimetidine, colchicine, sulfasalazine, and nitrofurantoin in high doses, are toxic to spermatogenesis. Indirect-acting compounds, such as the androgens, progestins, and estrogens, can inhibit spermatogenesis by suppressing the hypothalamic-pituitary axis. A growing number of infertile males are arising from the widespread use of alkylating agents and antimetabolites in the treatment of malignancies and immunologically mediated diseases. These patients usually have permanent sterility following the discontinuance of the medications, but occasionally spermatogenesis may recover over a period of months to many years. Occupational exposure of chemical plant workers and field workers to 1,2-dibromo-3-chloropropane, the active ingredient in a soil fumigant, has been shown to impair testicular function. Commonly used drugs like ethanol, tetrahydrocannabinol, and cocaine have been shown to reduce spermatogenesis and testicular size and affect sperm count. Cigarette smoking is associated with sperm abnormalities, especially when a varicocele is also present.[11] Calcium channel blockers have recently been shown to reversibly render normal sperm incapable of fertilization.[11a] Low-grade and unrecognized exposure to toxic agents may contribute to the impairment seen in men with so-called idiopathic subfertility.

With greater survival rates of childhood and adult cancer patients, the number having received gonadal irradiation is also increasing. Spermatogonia are very radiosensitive, whereas Leydig's and Sertoli's cells appear to be much more resistant. There may be an age-related effect, with the prepubertal testicle more prone to damage. The effect is dosage dependent. No significant effects occur following a single exposure of the testicle to 200 rads, but azoospermia is observed in men who receive more than 700 rads. Recovery of spermatogenesis may occur up to 4 to 5 years after radiation exposure of as much as 600 rads.

The most common endocrine disorders that cause infertility are the result of impaired production of gonadotropins. Kallmann's syndrome, a rare disorder characterized by hypogonadism and anosmia, is thought to be caused by a defect in the hypothalamus. Patients with this syndrome, as well as those hypogonadotropic hypogonadal patients with an intact sense of smell, do not undergo normal puberty and thus have a eunuchoidal appearance. Panhypopituitarism is a treatable disorder that generally is acquired but can be congenital and obviously is associated not only with infertility but also with the signs of thyroid and adrenal insufficiency, as well as with dwarfism, if congenital. Men with hyperprolactinemia frequently have low gonadotropin and testosterone levels and may show infertility caused by oligospermia, loss of libido, impotence, and gynecomastia. Congenital or adult-onset adrenogenital syndrome can be difficult to recognize in men, as opposed to women, because men may have only oligospermia. The diagnosis can be confirmed by observing elevated urinary serum dehydroepiandrosterone sulfate (DHEA-S) and 17-OH progesterone levels.

Men with ductal obstruction present with azoospermia. The most common congenital abnormality of the male ductal system is atresia of the cauda epididymis or the proximal part of the vas deferens. Absence of the vas deferens may occur unilaterally or bilaterally. Although the cause of most congenital obstructions is unknown, intrauterine exposure to diethylstilbestrol may result in obstructive epididymal lesions. Small testes, epididymal cysts, and poor semen quality have also been observed in diethylstilbestrol-exposed men.[12] Recently, ejaculatory duct obstruction has been recognized as a new cause of obstructive azoospermia and oligospermia (associated with very low ejaculate volumes) by transrectal ultrasound demonstration of mild seminal vesicle or ampullary dilation. Transurethral resection of the ejaculatory ducts leads to a dramatic improvement in semen quality.[7] In the preantibiotic era, the most common cause of obstructive azoospermia was gonorrheal infection of the cauda epididymis. Tuberculosis can involve the epididymis and vas, but treatment with chemotherapeutic agents can result in spontaneous recanalization. Today, the most common cause of ductal obstruction is vasectomy for voluntary sterilization. Unintentional iatrogenic injury to the vas has also been observed in inguinal operations, such as herniorrhaphy and orchiopexy, particularly when performed in children, and varicocelectomy.

Asymptomatic infections of the male reproductive tract are uncommon, and few data support the contention that this is a common cause of male infertility; however, it should be looked for by a good history and genital examination. Men with convincing clinical or microscopic evidence of urethritis, prostatitis, or epididymitis should have cultures taken, but even without bacteriologic proof of genital infection, they should be treated with doxycycline. In the absence of concurrent symptoms, *Chlamydia* organisms are rarely isolated from normal men, and in studies of asymptomatic men with unexplained infertility, *Chlamydia* organisms have not been cultured.

Retrograde ejaculation is produced by any factor that disrupts the action of the internal sphincter. This may occur in patients who during childhood had operative correction of their bladder neck concurrent with ureteral reimplantation. It is also seen in patients with a functional sympathectomy resulting from diabetes mellitus or a disrupted sympathetic innervation due to a spinal cord injury or a retroperitoneal lymph node dissection, as for testicular cancer. Similar dysfunction of the sympathetic nervous system may result from pharmacologic treatment with antihypertensives (phenoxybenzamine, guanethidine, L-methyldopa, prazosin, and thiazides), antidepressants (amitriptyline, imipramine, and phenelzine sulfate), and antipsychotics (thioridazine, haloperidol, chlorpromazine, perphenazine, and trifluoperazine).[7] Retrograde ejaculation should be suspected whenever the semen volumes are low or negligible. The diagnosis can be made by examining a urine specimen obtained after orgasm for high numbers of sperm.

Impotency may be a result of infertility or can be the cause of infertility. Antihypertensive drugs, such as reserpine and guanethidine, can cause impotency and should be discontinued in favor of other medications. The diagnosis of hyperprolactinemia should be considered in the man with both impotency and oligospermia. Psychotherapy or behavior modification may help those with psychogenic impotence. Electroejaculation has been used successfully in patients with spinal cord injury and in those who cannot ejaculate following retroperitoneal lymph node dissection for cancer.

A varicocele may be found in 10 to 20% of normal men, but if semen abnormalities are found, this number approaches 40%. As such, it is perhaps the major correctable cause of male infertility. Approximately 90% of varicoceles are on the left side, as anatomic considerations of the left internal spermatic vein are distinctively different from the right. The left internal spermatic vein enters the left renal vein, whereas the right internal spermatic vein drains directly into the inferior vena cava. The left renal vein is squeezed between the superior mesenteric artery and the aorta, causing proximal venous distention in a significant percentage of men. The effect of a varicocele seems to be related to its mere presence and not necessarily to its size. Even in men with unilateral varicoceles, microscopic examination has shown abnormalities of spermatogenesis in both testicles. On semen analysis, these patients characteristically have abnormal morphology, consisting of tapered and immature forms (present in 95% of patients), decreased motility (in 90% of patients), and lower sperm counts (in about 70%). Current research on the pathophysiologic mechanism by which the varicocele alters testicular function favors the hypothesis that in response to the elevated left testicular venous pressure, bilaterally elevated testicular arterial flow occurs, elevating the testicular temperature, which in turn is detrimental to spermatogenesis.

In 25 to 30% of men with oligospermia, thorough investigation will fail to identify a specific etiology. The probability of these men impregnating their partners is low but variably reported as 1 to 35%. In our experience, when the sperm count is below 20 million/ml, the pregnancy rate is less than 15%, and when it is below 10 million ml, pregnancy is rare.

Semen Analysis

Semen analysis, the most important part of the male evaluation, provides information about sperm motility and morphology as well as the absolute number of sperm present. If it is normal, further investigation can be temporarily halted. The semen analysis can be performed at any time, but optimally there should be a 36- to 72-hour abstinence from ejaculation because frequent ejaculation may depress the sperm number, whereas prolonged abstinence may decrease the motility. Because some plastic jars may affect the sperm motility, glass containers are preferred. Collection of semen by means of a condom also results in a loss of motility owing to spermaticidal agents in the condom. If masturbation is not possible, for religious or psychological reasons, then special semen collection condoms may be used. Withdrawal techniques should not be used because the first portion of the semen, which is sperm-enriched, may be lost. Obviously, analysis is best performed at any time during the menstrual cycle other than ovulation.

What constitutes a normal semen analysis is difficult to define.[8] The count should be at least 20 million sperm/ml but preferably more than 40 million sperm/ml. The volume is 1.5 to 4 ml, and after the specimen has been allowed to sit for 15 to 30 minutes, it should liquefy and have a watery rather than a gelatinous consistency. The motility of the sperm should be greater than 60% at 2 hours from collection, with good forward progression of the sperm. The role of sperm morphology in fertility is less clear, and its main importance may be diagnostic. A high percentage of tapering and immature forms is often a clue to the presence of a varicocele.

Increased use of computer-assisted semen analysis will enable more objective evaluation of sperm concentration and in addition provides the opportunity to more accurately estimate the motility characteristics of the sperm. Of all the parameters measured in a typical semen analysis, motility has been considered the most important for predicting fertility[13]; however, subjective and imprecise measurement of sperm motion is inherent in visual estimation of motility by the human eye as performed in a manual semen analysis. Computer-assisted sperm analysis can rapidly and objectively determine the sperm concentration, per cent motility, velocity, linearity, and an array of sophisticated sperm motion parameters. Studies of sperm from fertile men suggest that the lower limit of normal sperm velocity is 30 μm/sec.[14] In addition, the sperm from fertile men appear to have a greater lateral head displacement.[15] It is possible that the measurement of computer-assisted sperm analysis parameters may be able to substitute for other more expensive and difficult sperm function tests.

It needs to be emphasized that the "normal" sperm count does not describe the number of sperm necessary for initiating pregnancy. It has been demonstrated by in vitro fertilization that only a minimum density (10,000 to 50,000/ml) of quality sperm need to be present for sperm penetration of the ovum. A study of women undergoing hysterectomy who had artificial insemination 15 to 45 minutes prior to surgery showed that only one of every 14 million sperm placed in the vagina reached the oviduct, whereas one of every 5000 sperm in the cervical mucus reached the oviduct.[16] Although this study does not suggest the minimum number of sperm needed, it does point out the fact that many barriers exist between the vaginal seminal pool and the site of fertilization of the ovum. Certainly as the sperm number and the percentage of normal and motile forms decrease, the ability to impregnate decreases. Unfortunately, in oligospermic men, even the motile sperm do not fertilize as well as equal numbers of sperm from normospermic men.[17] The chance of a pregnancy is remote if the semen analysis reveals fewer than 10 million sperm/ml and fewer than 40% active sperm at 2 hours.

If the first semen analysis result is completely normal, it may not be necessary to repeat the test. If the findings are abnormal, however, repeat analyses should be performed. Normally fertile men can have transient abnormalities in their semen analysis owing to stress, infection, or environmental factors. Any generalized illness, particularly when associated with a high fever, can cause impaired testicular function, and because spermatogenesis takes approximately 74 to 78 days from its initiation until the appearance of mature spermatozoa in the ejaculate, any illness within the 3 months prior to a semen analysis could potentially affect semen quality. For this reason, a patient with an abnormal analysis result should have it repeated at monthly intervals for 2 to 3 months. If repeated analyses reveal abnormalities, the investigation should continue.

Sperm Function Tests

Motile sperm are not necessarily capable of fertilization. Sperm must undergo capacitation and acrosome reaction, penetrate the zona pellucida, and fuse with the oolemma for the sperm to be capable of ovum penetration.

The zona-free hamster egg sperm penetration assay tests the ability of the sperm to capacitate, undergo acrosome reaction, and enter the ooplasm.[8] In a large study of known fertile and infertile men, the percentage of penetration in the fertile group ranged from 14 to 100%, with a mean of 56.3% and, in the infertile group, less than 10%. When the male partner of an infertile couple is found to have a sperm penetration of less than 10%, we find the fertilization rate with in vitro fertilization to be reduced, but even with a sperm penetration assay of zero we have seen fertilization and pregnancies. Another biologic assay is the hemizona assay, which uses the zona pellucida from human eggs to measure the ability of sperm to bind to the zona pellucida, which is the first step in the fertilization process.[8] Both of these assays are costly, difficult to perform, and often have poor reproducibility; therefore, their role in the evaluation of the infertile male remains controversial.

Assays that are easier to perform and have excellent reproducibility include the acrosin assay and the hypo-osmotic swelling test.[8] A normally functioning sperm membrane is required for successful union of the gametes; therefore, a test of membrane function might be correlated with the likelihood of sperm fertilizing an egg. This assay assesses ability of the sperm to transport fluids across its membrane under hypo-osmolar conditions, indicating membrane integrity and normal function. Correlation of the in vitro fertilizing capacity of the sperm with the hypo-osmotic swelling test shows that the majority of semen samples that fertilize oocytes have greater than 60% swelling in the hypo-osmotic swelling test, and when the value is less than 50%, most of the specimens were infertile. The acrosin assay measures the content of the acrosin enzyme, which is an important acrosomal enzyme involved in the acrosome reaction and sperm binding to, and penetration of, the zona pellucida. It may also indicate the integrity of the acrosomal cap in that after the acrosome reaction has occurred, the measurement of the acrosin content will be low. A low measurement of acrosin will be measured if the acrosome reaction has occurred prematurely or if the acrosin content of the sperm is initially low. The acrosin content can also be used as a measure of damage sustained by cryopreservation. The freeze-thaw procedures damage the acrosomal membrane so that acrosin is released. The measurement of the acrosin content before and after cryopreservation may be useful as an indicator of successful cryopreservation of the sperm. Comparison of in vitro fertilization rates and acrosin content shows that when the content is less than 14 uIU/10^6 sperm, fertilization is unlikely to occur, but nearly all men with an acrosin content of greater than 25 uIU/10^6 sperm fertilized at least some of their partner's eggs.

All of these assays correlate with the results of in vitro fertilization attempts and aid particularly in the evaluation of the subfertile male partner, but none of them can allow the clinician to conclusively tell a couple that the man's sperm are capable or incapable of fertilizing his partner's eggs. Only in vitro fertilization can answer this question.

Endocrinologic Evaluation of the Infertile Man

The testes have two distinct but related roles, consisting of endocrine functions (Leydig and Sertoli cells) and reproductive functions (germ cells). LH is primarily responsible for stimulating testosterone secretion by the Leydig cells, whereas FSH acts on the Sertoli cells. For spermatogenesis to occur, FSH must be available to initiate the functioning of the seminiferous tubules, and LH is necessary to stimulate testosterone production so that spermatogenesis can be both initiated and maintained. Normal spermatogenesis occurs only when the Sertoli cells and the seminiferous epithelium are bathed in an appropriate androgen milieu. Because Leydig cells produce most of the body's circulating testosterone, measurement of serum testosterone provides an indirect indication of intratesticular testosterone concentration. Because LH secretion is regulated by the inhibitory feedback of circulating testosterone, the serum LH level reflects the adequacy of Leydig cell function. Serum FSH secretion is controlled by the negative feedback from not only testosterone but also inhibin, which seems to be produced by the spermatogenic components, and FSH is therefore of great value in assessing the state of the seminiferous epithelium.

The endocrinologic evaluation of infertile men yields abnormal results in fewer than 10%, but because it can contribute to the diagnosis and prognosis of the patient's infertility problem, an evaluation (Table 43–3) is routinely performed for men with severe oligospermia and azoospermia or evidence of impaired sexual function. A normal level of FSH in an azoospermic man indicates spermatogenic capability. In men with azoospermia due to severe destruction of the germinal epithelium, serum FSH levels are usually elevated, and further testing and therapy are for naught. Combined elevations of FSH and LH levels are seen with severe testicular damage, reflecting a decline in both the spermatogenic and androgenic functional components of the testes. When the FSH, LH, and testosterone levels are low, the prolactin level should be evaluated. If the prolactin level is high, an evaluation for a pituitary tumor is performed. If the prolactin level is not elevated, one must be concerned about pituitary failure; testing for deficiencies of other pituitary hormones (thyroid-stimulating hormone, adrenocorticotropic hormone, and, possibly, growth hormone) should be performed. If the other pituitary hormones are normal, hypogonadotropic hypogonadism on a congenital basis (in the absence of pubertal development) or an acquired basis (in the presence of normal sexual development) can be diagnosed. When the diagnosis of congenital or adult-onset adrenogenital syndrome is present, adrenal suppression with replacement doses of glucocorticoids will correct the endocrine abnormality and often result in an improved semen analysis.

TREATMENT OF MALE INFERTILITY

All physicians who evaluate the male members of infertile couples will frequently be confronted with oligospermia (sperm count of less than 20 million/ml) or asthenospermia (sperm motility of less than 50%). Unfortunately, because of the limited understanding of the pathophysiology of male reproduction, many therapeutic alternatives have unproved efficacy.

Surgical therapy of a varicocele should be carried out in the patient who has oligospermia or asthenospermia. In addition, because studies of adolescents with asymptomatic varicoceles have shown that progressive deterioration of gonadal function and testicular histology occurs as they age,[18] surgery should be recommended to these young patients, especially those with ipsilateral testicular growth retardation. Therapy consists of left spermatic vein ligation. Heretofore, this has been accomplished by an inguinal approach, but more recently a less invasive laparoscopic technique has been described.[19] Although little improvement in sperm morphology is often seen following surgery, sperm counts and motility improve postoperatively in 40 to 70% of patients. A beneficial effect of surgery on testicular histology can also be seen. Successes with respect to the parameters on semen analysis, as well as on subsequent pregnancy rates of their partners, are greater in men whose presurgery sperm counts are higher than 10 to 20 million sperm/ml. In some series, as many as 50% of patients undergoing surgery are able to impregnate their partners within a year of therapy. The value of hormonal therapy, either alone or in combination with a varicocelectomy, is

TABLE 43–3. ENDOCRINE EVALUATION FOR ABNORMAL SEMEN ANALYSIS

Level	Elevated	Normal	Low
FSH*	Primary testicular problem of germinal epithelium	Some functioning germinal epithelium present Nonendocrine problem	Hypogonadotropic hypogonadism Panhypopituitarism Pituitary failure
LH†	Poor Leydig cell function (usually associated with a low testosterone level) Partial androgen resistance (usually associated with high testosterone and normal FSH levels)	Normal testosterone levels	As above Also excessive testosterone production, particularly from adrenal or exogenous intake
Testosterone	Exogenous intake Adrenal or testicular tumor Partial androgen resistance		Hypogonadotropic hypogonadism Panhypopituitarism Pituitary failure Leydig cell failure
Prolactin	Functional hyperprolactinemia Pituitary adenoma Usually associated with low testosterone, LH, and FSH levels Also associated with impotence		
DHEA‡-sulfate	Adrenal tumor Cushing's syndrome Congenital or adult-onset adrenogenital syndrome (usually associated with an elevated 17-OH progesterone level)		

*FSH = follicle-stimulating hormone.
†LH = luteinizing hormone.
‡DHEA = dehydroepiandrosterone.

unclear. In patients with counts of less than 10 million/ml, either human chorionic gonadotropin (hCG) or clomiphene citrate combined with surgery may result in a greater improvement in semen quality and a higher pregnancy rate than surgery alone.

The approach to azoospermia is summarized in Figure 43–2. First, the patient's FSH level should be determined. If the FSH level is elevated, primary testicular failure is diagnosed, and the couple should be offered donor artificial insemination. The finding of low FSH and testosterone levels indicates hypogonadotropic hypogonadism, which can be treated as outlined below in this section. When the FSH level is normal, the patient should be questioned about the volume of ejaculate. Low volumes are seen with congenital absence of the ductus deferens, and because of the usual concurrent absence of the seminal vesicles, the ejaculate will not contain fructose. In patients with azoospermia and positive seminal fructose but no evidence for retrograde ejaculation, transrectal ultrasound is performed. Recently, ejaculatory duct obstruction has been recognized as a new cause of obstructive azoospermia and oligospermia associated with very low ejaculate volumes and demonstration of mild seminal vesicle or ampullary dilation by transrectal ultrasound.[7] Transurethral resection of the ejaculatory ducts can lead to a dramatic improvement in semen quality. Scrotal exploration and vasography can pinpoint obstruction elsewhere along the ejaculatory tract. Direct observation of the epididymis can usually locate an obstruction in this structure. Prior to a surgical repair for obstruction, an endocrine evaluation is mandatory, and a testicular biopsy should be obtained. The presence of an elevated FSH level or an abnormal testicular biopsy result

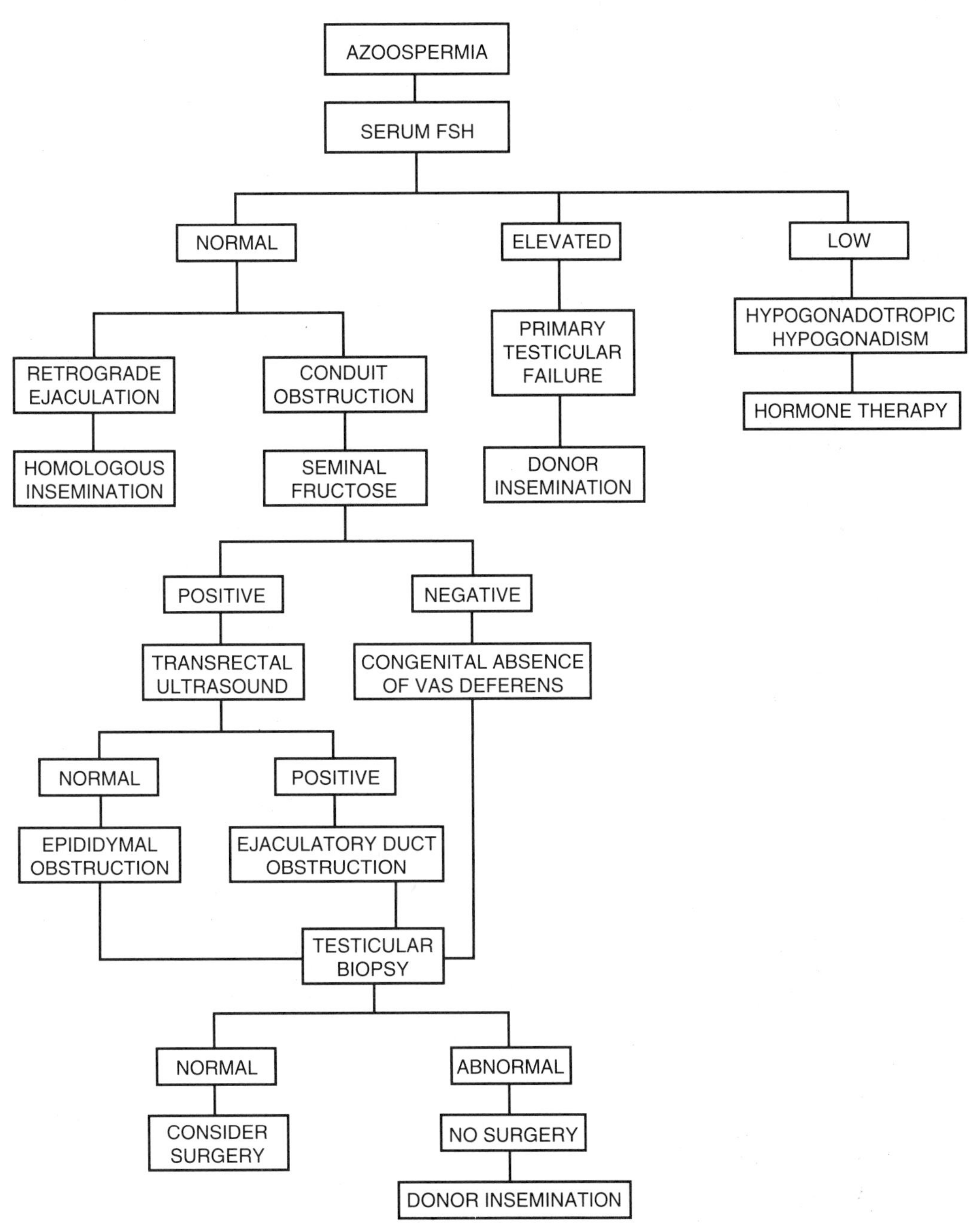

FIGURE 43–2. Approach to azoospermia.

is a contraindication to surgery. Surgical reanastomosis of the ligated ductus deferens leads to a pregnancy rate of approximately 40 to 50%, but surgical repair of the other causes of obstruction is successful in fewer than 10% of cases.

Treatment of retrograde ejaculation entails artificial insemination or the administration of drugs that enhance sympathetic stimulation.[7] Agents such as pseudoephedrine (60 mg, four times a day), ephedrine (50 mg, four times a day), or phenylpropanolamine (75 mg, twice a day) may be used in an effort to close the bladder neck at the time of ejaculation. Pharmacologic treatment has a chance to work only if the retrograde ejaculation is of neuropathic etiology; it does not seem helpful if it is secondary to bladder neck surgery. When medical treatment fails, semen must be retrieved from the bladder to perform artificial insemination. The patient is instructed to empty his bladder prior to masturbation or coitus, and then a postorgasmic urine specimen, alkalinized by oral administration of sodium bicarbonate, is collected. Alternatively, an appropriate buffer solution can be instilled into the bladder prior to ejaculation. The diluted semen specimen is centrifuged at 300 rpm for 10 minutes. The sperm pellet thus obtained is used for homologous intrauterine insemination.

Gonadotropin deficiency or hypogonadotropic hypogonadism, when congenital, is usually secondary to a hypothalamic deficiency of gonadotropin-releasing hormone (GnRH). Low-dose, chronic, pulsatile administration of GnRH can be used to initiate testicular function and puberty.[20] Most patients with acquired gonadotropin deficiency have matured sexually and have pituitary failure. Exogenous gonadotropin therapy is very successful in stimulating spermatogenesis.[7] hCG, which has LH-like activity, is administered at 1500 to 2500 IU intramuscularly three times a week. When the testosterone levels are elevated into the normal range or after approximately 2 to 3 months, human menopausal gonadotropin (hMG), which has an equal ratio of FSH and LH activity, is also administered (37.5 to 150 IU). In some men, hCG alone can maintain spermatogenesis once it is established. Gonadotropin secretion may also be suppressed by hyperprolactinemia, which is usually due to a pituitary tumor. Surgical treatment of the pituitary tumor, if one is present, or treatment with bromocriptine, to lower the prolactin levels, can restore sperm counts and testosterone levels to normal.

In cases of oligospermia in which no etiologic factor is determined, testosterone rebound therapy, GnRH, hMG/hCG, tamoxifen citrate and clomiphene citrate have been used empirically.[7, 21] Unfortunately, the results of these treatments have been inconsistent and, in the few controlled studies, often disappointing. We use clomiphene citrate, 25 mg per day, in patients with normal pretreatment FSH levels. Based on several reports, it appears that about 50% of patients treated with clomiphene have at least some increase in sperm counts, and 25 to 30% may achieve conception in their partners. Semen analyses are monitored at monthly intervals, beginning at 8 weeks after therapy is initiated; if a response is not seen by 4 months, the therapy is abandoned. Much experimental evidence suggests that prostaglandins have an inhibitory influence on reproductive function, and controlled studies using indomethacin and ketoprofen have shown a significant increase in both sperm count and motility and a pregnancy rate of 20 to 35% (compared with 8% in the control groups).[22] It has been recognized for many years that increased testicular temperatures could result in a decreased rate of sperm production. Efforts at cooling the testicles have included ice packs and the application of the testicular hypothermia device. Unfortunately, compliance with the treatments seems to be a major problem, but in one study a 66% improvement in seminal parameters was seen in the treatment group after 4 months of application, and the pregnancy rate in that group was 27%, far superior to that of the control group.[23] Attempts to freeze and subsequently thaw and pool specimens for artificial insemination have not been particularly successful because the motility of thawed sperm from oligospermic men is usually very poor. (Artificial insemination by the male partner is covered in the next section.)

There are no specific treatments for asthenospermia, and when a varicocele has been excluded, patients with poor motility have a poor prognosis. The asthenospermic patient who has a varicocele should be advised to have surgery. Drugs that impair semen motility should be avoided if possible. Azulfidine used to treat ulcerative colitis, heroin, and methadone, as well as tetrahydrocannabinol, the principal metabolite of marijuana, have been observed to impair sperm motility. Coital lubricants, such as Vaseline, K-Y jelly, Lubafax, and Surgilube, should be avoided because they may be spermicidal. If a lubricant is needed, the use of Replens (Columbia Labs) has been shown not to interfere with the sperm motility seen on postcoital examination. In a double-blind study of the oral administration of kallikrein (600 kU/day) to 90 oligoasthenospermic men, sperm density and motility were improved, and conception rates were 38 and 16% for the kallikrein and the placebo-treated groups, respectively.[24] Some investigators have used hCG injections, which can sometimes cause a severe decline in the sperm count. Some studies have shown an association of decreased sperm motility in men colonized with T-strain mycoplasma. The eradication of the infection from the semen of infertile men following doxycycline therapy improves sperm motility, but the link between such colonization and male infertility is speculative. Oral vitamin C administration has been observed to improve the sperm motility and pregnancy rate.

When the seminal volume is very low, and particularly if the postcoital examination shows very few sperm, patients may benefit from homologous artificial insemination. When seminal volumes are elevated, and particularly if the sperm count and motility are somewhat decreased, insemination can be performed using either a split ejaculate or a washed and concentrated specimen. In general, the first portion of the ejaculate has a marked increase in the concentration and motility of the sperm. Split ejaculates can also be used when semen shows increased viscosity and failure to liquefy because the first portion of the ejaculate tends to be much less viscous.

Homologous Artificial Insemination

The use of artificial insemination with the male partner's semen—that is, homologous artificial insemination (AIH)—is not new and was actually used more than a century before donor artificial insemination. Table 43–4 gives several indications for its use. AIH for the category related to problems of sexual intercourse is highly successful. For the other indications, AIH remains more controversial and is the topic of the rest of this section.

The use of intravaginal or intracervial AIH has not proved efficacious except in cases related to problems of sexual intercourse. The pregnancy results of intrauterine insemination using washed and concentrated sperm (AIH-IUI) may be improved, but these results are uncertain because most studies thus far have lacked proper controls.[25]

The sperm-washing and concentrating procedure is a

TABLE 43–4. INDICATIONS FOR HOMOLOGOUS ARTIFICIAL INSEMINATION

Problems related to sexual intercourse
Impotency and refractory premature ejaculation
Frigidity and vaginismus
Inadequate coital activity
Hypospadias and penile curvature
Procidentia, anterior cervix, and vaginal stenosis or septum
Semen abnormalities
Oligospermia
Asthenospermia
Oligoasthenospermia
Increased viscosity
Low semen volumes
High semen volumes with low sperm density
Abnormal sperm–cervical mucus interaction
Abnormal cervical mucus
Prior endocervical trauma and absent cervical mucus
Normal mucus and semen analysis with abnormal interaction

very simple technique that removes the prostaglandins from the seminal fluid and reduces the volume such that all the sperm in an ejaculate can be deposited into the uterine cavity. On the day of insemination, a fresh masturbatory semen specimen is collected and allowed to liquefy (10 to 20 minutes). When a problem of liquefaction is known, a split ejaculate specimen is collected. The semen specimen is placed in a centrifuge tube and diluted with phosphate-buffered solution to a final volume of about 12 ml. After centrifugation at 300 rpm for 10 minutes, the fluid is separated from the sperm pellet. Buffer solution is added to increase the pellet to 0.2 to 0.3 ml, and it is then ready for insemination directly into the uterine cavity. Daily blood or urine samples are obtained from the woman to monitor for the LH surge, and intrauterine inseminations are performed on the 2 days following the LH surge.

The results of AIH-IUI are variable, depending on the indications, but in most studies the conception rate is low. Because the spontaneous pregnancy rate in a similar control group has been measured in only one study, the therapeutic value of AIH-IUI has remained uncertain. In a preliminary report using natural intercourse as the control, the pregnancy rate per cycle of therapy in couples with abnormal semen was 30.5%, and for natural intercourse, 1.4%.[26] Couples with an abnormal sperm-cervical mucus interaction but normal cervical mucus and semen analysis may have up to a 60% chance of achieving a pregnancy through AIH-IUI. Unfortunately, because the majority of couples receiving AIH-IUI have abnormal semen, the overall success rate of AIH-IUI is discouragingly low. Currently, because most of our pregnancies appear to occur in the first 6 to 8 months, we stop AIH after that time and consider superovulation and AIH-IUI (see section on Assisted Reproductive Technologies) or donor artificial insemination.

Donor Artificial Insemination

Because many forms of male infertility cannot be treated or respond poorly to therapy, donor artificial insemination (DAI) using a donor semen specimen may be considered. The moral and legal questions of the procedure have not been fully answered at the present time, and for some couples, there are religious considerations as well. The couple should be counseled on all aspects of donor insemination prior to beginning this treatment. Pre-DAI counseling should include a consultation with a psychiatrist or social worker experienced in this subject.

Technically, the DAI procedure has become more complicated than just obtaining fresh semen specimens from anonymous donors who match the male partner's physical characteristics. Careful screening of the donor is important not only for an excellent semen analysis but also for general health, intelligence, and the absence of known genetic abnormalities and sexually transmissible diseases. In 1990, a consensus committee of the American Fertility Society issued "New Guidelines For The Use Of Semen Donor Insemination: 1990" (Fertil Steril 53[Supple 1], 1990) specifically addressing the issues of selection and screening of donors and the use of frozen semen specimens that have been quarantined for at least 180 days, after which the donor is retested for sexually transmissible diseases to maximize the safety of DAI.

Unless obvious fertility problems are determined at the time of the medical history and physical examination, our evaluation of the woman undergoing DAI is minimal and consists only of proof of ovulation and a normal hysterosalpingogram. Timing of DAI is accomplished as already described for AIH-IUI. Pregnancy is achieved within 6 months in 75% of normally fertile women.[9] If pregnancy has not occurred by that time, the evaluation of the woman is completed. Our couples are told at the outset that very few pregnancies occur after a year of inseminations and that inseminations will be discontinued at that time.

EVALUATION AND TREATMENT OF THE WOMAN

History and Physical Examination

The evaluation of the female partner should begin simultaneously with that of the man. Again, a thorough medical history and physical examination are important. The gynecologic history should include an assessment of the menstrual pattern, including age of menarche, cycle interval and duration, and quality of flow. Symptoms of ovulation should be noted. These include mittelschmerz (midcycle ovulatory pain), increased midcycle discharge, molimina (premenstrual symptoms, such as breast tenderness, bloating, acne, and mood changes), and dysmenorrhea. Previous pregnancies (including spontaneous and therapeutic abortions) and the interval of coitus without contraceptive measures should be noted, and the male partner at the time of those conceptions should be established. If there have been previous pregnancies, possible intervening etiologic events of infertility must be identified. These may include a new sexual partner, problems with the use of an intrauterine device, pelvic inflammatory disease, intra-abdominal operations, and onset of symptoms suggestive of endometriosis. A history of pelvic inflammatory disease is very important because a single bout of infection renders the patient infertile in 12 to 15% of cases; with recurrent episodes, a doubling of the likelihood of infertility occurs with each infection. Prior surgery, especially operations directed toward the pelvic organs or the appendix, is a common cause of infertility. Prior surgery for an ectopic pregnancy suggests the possibility that the remaining tube also has abnormalities. The chance of a normal pregnancy after an ectopic one is in the range of only 25%, and the likelihood of another ectopic pregnancy is markedly increased over normal.

Initially, questions about intercourse should be limited simply to the use of artificial lubricants or postcoital douching and the presence of dyspareunia. Care should be taken to interfere as little as possible with the couple's usual coital habits, to avoid unnecessary stress on the relationship. If semen analysis results are normal but the postcoital examination reveals no sperm, then questions about coital techniques and positions should be explored. Some of the most common sexual problems encountered in this patient population are either too frequent or too infrequent intercourse. Often, neither partner understands when the fertile time of the woman's menstrual cycle, and thus the optimal time for intercourse, occurs. The importance of adequate coital exposure is suggested by the fact that coitus four or more times a week is twice as effective in achieving pregnancy as coitus twice or fewer times a week.[27] Using urinary LH surge testing, couples can be counseled to abstain from the midfollicular phase until the day of the LH surge and the following day. Based on the fact that survival of normal sperm in normal cervical mucus is approximately 1 to 2 days, this recommendation should ensure the presence of viable sperm during the 12 to 24 hours that the ovum is capable of being fertilized, without depleting the "sperm reserve."

During the physical examination, special attention should be paid to endocrine and reproductive features. Thyroid examination should include not only palpation of the gland, but also examination for exophthalmos, lid lag, tremor, and deep tendon reflexes. The breasts should be checked for expressible galactorrhea. The hair distribution should be noted, especially the presence of facial hair and a male escutcheon. These features, as well as an enlarged clitoris, are signs of hyperandrogenicity. Bimanual examination should search for evidence of congenital anomalies, tumors of the uterus and other pelvic organs, and endometriosis. In addition, a Papanicolaou smear and other routine laboratory tests should be performed at this time.

With the preliminary histories and physical examinations completed, the physician should proceed to the testing of the four basic areas, as previously outlined (see Table 43–1). The semen analysis has already been discussed. The remaining three areas primarily involve the woman.

Documentation of Normal Ovulatory Function

Documentation of ovulation should precede any other testing in the woman. The great majority of women with regular monthly menstrual cycles are ovulating, particularly if moliminal symptoms and dysmenorrhea occur; nevertheless, the fertility of the menstrual cycle needs to be evaluated.

The simplest technique for documenting ovulation is the basal body temperature. This is best done with a basal body thermometer each morning on awakening and prior to any physical activity. The temperature in women in the proliferative phase of the menstrual cycle is usually below 36.7° C (98° F). As ovulation approaches, a drop in the temperature may be observed. When ovulation occurs, the corpus luteum begins to produce progesterone, which has a thermogenic effect on the hypothalamus, causing a 0.3 to 0.6° C (0.5 to 1° F) rise in the basal temperature for the next 14 days. Temperature elevated for 10 days or less is suggestive of a luteal phase defect. Although the temperature chart is useful in determining whether a woman is ovulating, it is not useful to couples in timing coitus because the fertile period precedes the rise in temperature. For this reason, we ask patients to take temperatures for specific purposes, such as initial conformation of ovulation in a new patient and initial evaluation in anovulatory patients of their response to ovulation induction with clomiphene citrate.

The most precise prediction of the timing of ovulation is by LH monitoring. Daily serial blood samples, beginning several days prior to expected ovulation, will show an increase in the concentration of this hormone from approximately 5 to 10 mIU/ml to over 20 mIU/ml at the time of the preovulatory LH surge. Ovulation usually occurs on the day after the surge, as evidenced by collapse of the follicle on ultrasound monitoring. This method is practical only if your hormone laboratory can provide same-day service and if your patients are willing to expend the necessary effort, time, and money. We generally recommend the use of urine LH testing when it is necessary to know the precise day of ovulation.[28] This is important for timing periovulatory ultrasounds, the postcoital examination, and artificial inseminations.

Technically, ovulation can be defined as the release of an ovum from the graafian follicle. In the past, ovulation was assumed to occur when the indirect evaluation criteria (biphasic basal temperature chart, elevated serum progesterone level, and a biopsy specimen with secretory endometrium) were present. A transvaginal ultrasound performed the morning after the LH surge allows the observation of the preovulatory follicle cyst. During spontaneous ovulatory cycles, the ultrasound image of the follicle cyst should demonstrate crisp margins and measure 18 to 22 mm in average diameter on the day after the LH surge. On the following day, ultrasound should confirm collapse of the ovarian follicle, which suggests release of the ovum from the follicle cyst. The follicle can go through the normal stages of development without ovum release; this is termed the *luteinized unruptured follicle syndrome* (LUF). The diagnosis can be suspected when ultrasound examination fails to document disappearance of the preovulatory follicle 48 hours after the LH surge, or when laparoscopy in the early luteal phase fails to document the ovulation stigma on the corpus hemorrhagicum. Luteinized unruptured follicle syndrome probably occurs in as many as 10% of menstrual cycles in normal women, but because it is rarely a repetitive problem, it is an infrequent cause of infertility. If the syndrome is documented in subsequent menstrual cycles, treatment with clomiphene citrate or human menopausal gonadotropins can be attempted; when this fails, the gamete intrafallopian transfer (GIFT) procedure can be used.

The ultrasound can also be used to evaluate the endometrial development during the menstrual cycle and the likelihood of a subsequent pregnancy. An endometrial thickness, measured in the longitudinal view across the uterine fundus, of greater than 9 mm is associated with a high likelihood of subsequent implantation. The appearance of peripheral echogenicity with a central dark area of reduced echogenicity divided by the highly echogenic endometrial surface (the so-called halo pattern) is associated with a significantly higher pregnancy rate than an endometrium characterized by the presence of a homogeneous echo-dense pattern. When the thickness is greater than 9 mm and a halo pattern is present, the pregnancy rate/embryo transfer was 33%, compared with only 7% when the echo-dense pattern, a thickness of less than 9 mm, or both were seen.[29]

Eight days after the midcycle LH surge is observed, a plasma progesterone level is obtained. A value of greater than 3 ng/ml suggests that ovulation has occurred, and a midluteal progesterone level of greater than 15 ng/ml is generally associated with a normal luteal phase.[30] An endometrial biopsy, which is an invasive procedure, should not

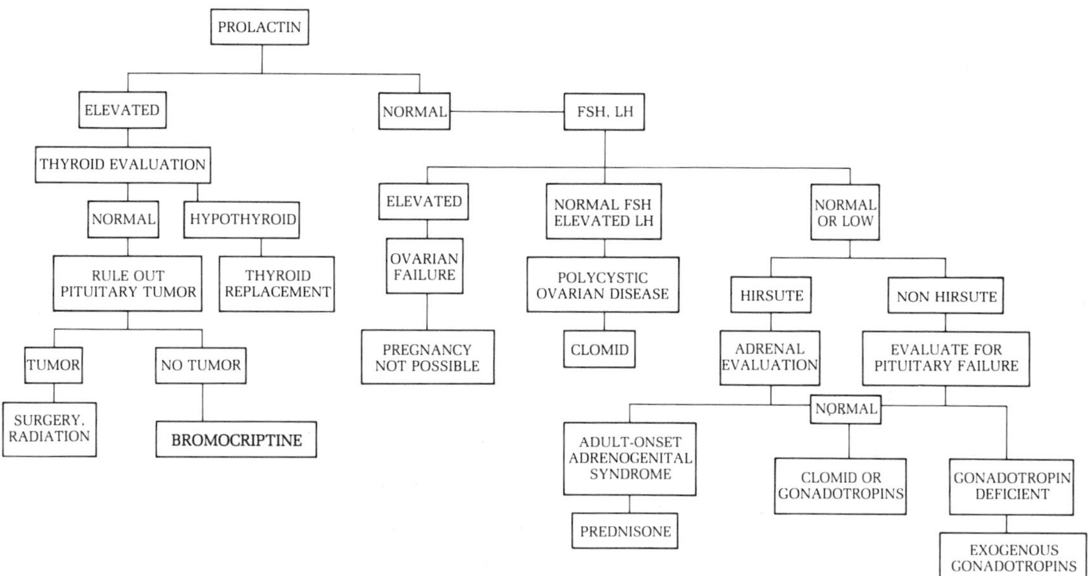

FIGURE 43–3. Endocrine evaluation for anovulation.

be performed just to confirm ovulation. If a luteal phase defect is suspected by a short-duration temperature rise (< 11 days) or a serum progesterone in the midluteal phase of less than 15 ng/ml, an endometrial biopsy is performed approximately 11 days after LH surge. Patient discomfort during this procedure varies greatly; thus, we usually administer a paracervical block with 10 ml of 1% chloroprocaine hydrochloride, which eliminates most of the pain. If the histologic dating of the endometrial tissue lags 3 days or more behind that expected by counting forward from the day of the LH surge or backward from the onset of the subsequent menstrual period, then a diagnosis of luteal phase defect is possible. Because luteal phase defect can be an isolated rather than a recurrent event, two abnormal biopsy results are required to make the diagnosis. Because of the discomfort and expense associated with endometrial biopsy, some investigators use direct measurements of serum progesterone levels as a means of diagnosing the adequacy of the luteal phase. Although the exact values of progesterone that are needed to rule out an inadequate luteal phase are in dispute, it is our feeling that when a series of progesterone measurements drawn 5, 8, and 11 days after the LH surge are greater than 8, 15, and 8 ng/ml, respectively, we do not find an abnormal timed endometrial biopsy. Treatment with clomiphene citrate, hCG injections, vaginal progesterone suppositories, and bromocriptine have all been used with varying success.[31–34] Adequacy of therapy should be assessed by repeating the endometrial biopsy or series of progesterone measurements on the medication. When the biopsy reflects a normal endometrial histology, the pregnancy rate becomes that of the normal population.[35]

Although fecundity declines with advancing maternal age, this decline is probably more closely related to ovarian status than to chronological age per se. The fact that menopause occurs at different ages in different women suggests that the age-related reduction in fecundity may also occur at different rates in different women. One indicator of ovarian function is the basal FSH level on day 3 of the menstrual cycle. The serum level of FSH increases as ovarian function declines.[36] Although each hormone laboratory needs to establish its normal range for FSH, we find that an FSH over 30 mIU/ml indicates menopause; when the FSH is between 20 and 30 mIU/ml, no live pregnancies have been produced; between 16 and 20 mIU/ml, a reduction in pregnancy rate, and an increase in abortions are seen; and when the FSH is less than 16 mIU/ml, the chances for pregnancy seem to be good. Because of the grave implications of an elevated FSH level, repeated observation should be obtained before advising a woman to forego fertility treatments or to pursue donor ova (see the section on Donor Ova). In women who have fluctuating FSH values, we have observed a higher pregnancy rate during cycles in which the FSH on day 3 of the cycle is below 16 mIU/ml; therefore, we initiate treatment only during cycles associated with a low FSH, and if an FSH of over 16 mIU/ml repeatedly returns, we recommend discontinuing fertility treatment.

If a woman is amenorrheic or is having anovulatory bleeding, an endocrine evaluation should be performed, as outlined in Figure 43–3. In addition, women with menstrual abnormalities should have a careful nutritional and eating-disorder history taken. In one study, 16.7% of infertility patients with menstrual dysfunction were found to have an eating disorder.[37] If an eating disorder or a correctable endocrinopathy is found, the patient should be treated appropriately prior to consideration of pregnancy.

In all women with amenorrhea, and particularly those with galactorrhea, a plasma prolactin determination is essential. If the prolactin level is elevated, a pituitary tumor must be excluded by magnetic resonance imaging or computed tomographic scanning of the sella turcica. In the majority of cases, a very small tumor of less than 1 cm in size, termed a *microadenoma,* is found. In approximately 5 to 10% of patients with hyperprolactinemia, hypothyroidism is also present. The postulated mechanism is that the elevation of both prolactin and thyroid-stimulating hormone is secondary to increased thyrotropin-releasing hormone. To substantiate a diagnosis of hypothyroidism, measurement of thyroid-stimulating hormone is more sensitive than simple screening for thyroxine and tri-iodothyronine uptake.

The presence of estrogenic cervical mucus is helpful in predicting which women will respond to 10 mg of medroxyprogesterone acetate orally for 5 days or 100 mg of progesterone-in-oil intramuscularly by having withdrawal menses, and to clomiphene citrate with ovulation. Women with hypothalamic, pituitary, or ovarian failure usually have estrogen deficiency and therefore do not have estrogenic mucus and will not have withdrawal bleeding in response to progestogens, nor will they ovulate while taking clomiphene citrate. The women with ovarian failure will be distinguished from the others by menopausal levels of serum FSH and LH. Differentiation of hypothalamic and pituitary disease may be difficult. Most patients with pituitary failure will also demonstrate adrenal and thyroid deficiencies. Hypothalamic disease is essentially a deficiency of GnRH.

Withdrawal bleeding in response to progestogens occurs when endogenous estrogen is present and usually indicates ovarian dysfunction, as seen with polycystic ovarian disease and other hyperandrogenic states. Polycystic ovarian disease, which is associated with an increase in androgen production, with 70% of the affected women complaining of hirsutism, almost invariably begins at puberty; later onset of symptoms arouses suspicion of some other hyperandrogenic state. In hirsute or virilized women, serum testosterone, androstenedione, and DHEA-S determinations are helpful in assessing whether the source is the ovary or the adrenal glands and whether a tumor is likely to be present. When the DHEA-S level is elevated, a component of adrenal hyperandrogenism is present, and when the level is greater than 350 μg/ml, Cushing's disease and adrenal tumors must be ruled out. When the DHEA-S level is greater than 200 μg/ml, partial adrenal suppression using 5 mg of prednisone at bedtime rarely initiates spontaneous menses but can enhance the patient's responsiveness to clomiphene citrate.

Four major therapeutic regimens are available for ovulation induction. For complete details, see the reference list at the end of this chapter.[1–4, 30, 38–40] Because some of these techniques require expert knowledge and sophisticated laboratory testing, they generally are best performed by a fertility specialist. In brief, the four regimens are as follows: (1) clomiphene citrate with and without hCG, (2) human menopausal gonadotropins and hCG, (3) bromocriptine, and (4) GnRH. Clomiphene citrate is administered initially at 50 mg/day, days 5 through 9 of the menstrual cycle, but if ineffective, the dose is raised by increments of 50 mg/day up to 150 mg/day for 5 days. If still unsuccessful, a regimen of clomiphene followed by an injection of hCG can be tried when a 20- to 24-mm follicular cyst is visualized on an ovarian sonogram (approximately 5 to 7 days following the last clomiphene tablet).[40] If treatment is still unsuccessful, hMG and hCG are used to stimulate the ovary to ovulate. Of course, in women with pituitary failure or hypophysectomy, a trial of clomiphene can be eliminated, and hMG therapy should immediately follow. For the subgroup of patients with hyperprolactinemia in whom a pituitary tumor has been ruled out (see Fig. 43–3), one may use bromocriptine to lower the prolactin level and initiate the resumption of ovulatory menstrual cycles.[39] If these patients become pregnant, they should immediately discontinue taking the bromocriptine, although it appears to be safe in pregnancy. Patients with hypothalamic failure have been shown to respond to intravenous or subcutaneous pulsatile administration of low doses of GnRH with ovulation and pregnancy.[38]

In general, the results of ovulation induction are very good. Except for those with ovarian failure, nearly all anovulatory patients can be made ovulatory with some form of treatment, and 60 to 80% are able to conceive. However, ovulation induction should be performed only by those well trained in its proper management, because complications of ovarian hyperstimulation and multiple pregnancy are fairly frequent.

Sperm–Cervical Mucus Interaction

After ovulation has been established, the patient is scheduled for postcoital examination (Sims-Huhner Test) 1 or 2 days prior to the expected date of ovulation as predicted by a review of the patient's recent basal body temperature charts. Alternatively, patients using urine LH monitoring are scheduled for postcoital examination the morning after the LH surge. The couple is asked to have sexual intercourse, and examination 6 to 16 hours later consists of evaluating the cervical mucus and the number and motility of sperm present in the mucus. As ovulation approaches, the amount of mucus is greatly increased, and its water content rises significantly, producing a clear, acellular mucus with increased elasticity (spinnbarkeit) and decreased viscosity. In addition, the ferning capacity (formation of crystals in a fern-shaped pattern) is enhanced as ovulation approaches because of increased levels of salts in the mucus. All these factors help increase sperm survival in the cervical mucus within the female genital tract. Live, motile sperm have been identified in good cervical mucus typically for 48 hours but as long as 5 days after the last coitus. Constant "insemination" of the upper genital tract from this sperm reservoir occurs over a prolonged interval. Within 24 to 48 hours after ovulation, the rising progesterone levels cause a marked decrease in the quantity of mucus and an increase in mucus viscosity and cellularity, which present a barrier to sperm penetration.

At the time of the examination, mucus from the internal os is aspirated using a tuberculin syringe fitted with a 16-gauge plastic intravenous catheter. The volume of mucus can be observed, and a portion of the mucus can be placed on a microscope slide and stretched to assess the spinnbarkeit. A cover slip is placed over the majority of the mucus for microscopic evaluation, and the remainder is allowed to dry for assessment of the ferning pattern. If the quality of the mucus is not optimum (i.e., spinnbarkeit greater than 6 cm, ferning maximal or 3 on a scale of 0 to 3, moderate to copious in quantity, and relatively acellular when examined microscopically), then no definitive statements can be made regarding the quality of the sperm–cervical mucus interaction. If the patient is still preovulatory, she is asked to return every 48 hours for repeat examinations until ovulation. If ovulation has already occurred, as indicated by a temperature rise on the basal temperature chart, the examination is repeated during the next menstrual cycle. LH monitoring can ensure precise timing for the postcoital examination. Patients are asked to have coitus the night of the LH surge and to come to the office the following morning for the postcoital examination.

When good mucus is present, five or more sperm/high-power field, with good motility and linear progression, is considered an adequate result. However, what constitutes a normal examination and its prognostic significance are matters of dispute. When both the semen analysis and the cervical mucus are normal, there does seem to be an excellent correlation between quality of postcoital examination and prognosis for conception. The findings are: if two tests show no sperm present, no pregnancy is seen within 2 years; if only nonmotile sperm are seen, a 25% pregnancy rate is seen within 2 years; if a fair test is obtained, there is a 50% pregnancy rate; with a good test, approximately 70%; and with an excellent test, approximately a 90% pregnancy rate within 2 years.[41] Although the postcoital examination cannot replace the semen analysis as the only step in evaluation of men, it may be useful in assessing the functional significance of a semen analysis with low concentration, low motility, or low volume. For example, in men with sperm counts of less than 20 million sperm/ml, a postcoital test showing one or more progressively motile sperm resulted in a pregnancy rate of 41%, as opposed to a 17% pregnancy rate when no sperm or no progressively motile sperm were seen.[42]

If the preovulatory timing is good and the mucus quality is poor, then cervicitis should be ruled out. Cervical cultures for gonorrhea, *Ureaplasma urealyticum* (T-strain mycoplasma), and *Chlamydia trachomatis* should be performed, and both the man and the woman are treated if the culture results are positive. Even in the absence of positive cultures, mucopurulent mucus with microscopic evidence of abundant leukocytes should be treated empirically with doxycycline or erythromycin. Some patients with an inadequate amount of mucus respond to the administration of low doses of estrogen, 0.02 mg of ethinyl estradiol or 0.3 mg of conjugated estrogens, for the 5 to 7 days preceding the expected time of ovulation. If the patient has had prior cervical conization or cautery, the endocervical glands may have been destroyed and will no longer respond to estrogen stimulation. Occasionally, patients with very thick, tenacious cervical mucus will respond to the oral administration of guaifenesin (200 mg four times daily), a bronchial mucolytic agent.

If results are normal on a semen analysis and the postcoital examination reveals excellent cervical mucus but no sperm, an extremely low number of sperm, or sperm with low motility, a repeat postcoital examination should be scheduled. In addition, coital technique should be carefully assessed. If repeated examinations consistently reveal no sperm or only immobilized sperm or sperm with shaking tails but no progressive motility, sperm antibody testing should be performed.[43]

The antigenicity of spermatozoa and seminal plasma components has been recognized since the turn of the century. When sperm antibodies are present in a woman, sperm may be unable to penetrate the cervical mucus, or, once in the mucus, their motility is retarded. Men can also produce autoantibodies against their own sperm, which can cause the sperm to fail to migrate through the female genital tract. Other antifertility mechanisms of sperm antibodies may be the inactivation of acrosomal enzymes or inhibition of sperm attachment to, or penetration of, the zona pellucida.

Many tests for antibodies have been developed; some have a very high incidence of positive results in infertile couples (40 to 80%) and a large number of false-positive results (10 to 40%). Currently, the most widely accepted test for sperm antibodies is the immunobead binding test.[43] It has a relatively low frequency of positive test results in infertile couples (only 9% positives in couples with otherwise negative infertility evaluations) and almost no false-positive results in fertile couples. In one study, only 15.3% of untreated males with greater than 50% of their sperm antibody bound achieved a pregnancy, compared with 66.7% of men with fewer than 50% of their sperm bound.[44] In a study of the role of sperm antibodies in in vitro fertilization, women who have IgG sperm antibodies directed toward the sperm tail have lower fertilization rates in vitro when their sera are used in the culture media, and men who have IgA antibodies that are tail directed have a reduced ability to fertilize eggs.[45]

The best treatment for immunologic infertility has yet to be demonstrated. Most studies have not had appropriate controls, and therefore proper interpretation has been impossible. High doses of methylprednisolone on a continuous or interrupted schedule seem to have a therapeutic effect in some studies.[46] AIH-IUI has a comparable pregnancy rate without the risk of high-dose steroids (including aseptic necrosis of the femoral head), but the spontaneous abortion rate approaches 50%.[47]

In summary, abnormal sperm–cervical mucus interaction is determined by evaluation of the postcoital examination. Abnormal postcoital examinations can be categorized into five etiologies: (1) abnormal sperm, (2) abnormal cervical mucus quality or quantity, (3) cervicitis, (4) sperm antibodies, and (5) the unexplained abnormal postcoital examination in the absence of all the above factors. Except for cervicitis, which should be treated with antibiotics, all of the other causes of an abnormal postcoital examination results can be treated by AIH-IUI (see the section on Homologous Artificial Insemination). It should be noted, however, that although AIH-IUI enhances the chances of pregnancy when the postcoital examination results are abnormal, empiric use of AIH-IUI does not seem to be of value, and therefore the greatest importance of the postcoital examination is perhaps to determine therapy.[48]

Tests of Tubal Patency

If the woman is ovulating, her partner has a normal semen analysis, and the postcoital test results are normal, the next step is to rule out tubal disorders, which may be responsible for 30% of infertility. Even though some physicians prefer at this point to have the patient try to achieve pregnancy for an additional 6 months, we proceed immediately with tests of tubal patency because as many as half the patients who have pelvic adhesions have no antecedent history of pelvic inflammatory disease, septic abortion, abdominal or pelvic surgery, or use of an intrauterine device.[49]

The standard test for tubal patency for many years was Rubin's test, or tubal insufflation with carbon dioxide, but because of limited information and a high incidence of false-positive results, it is rarely used today. Currently, the conventional test is the hysterosalpingogram, which not only provides information about tubal patency but also reveals distortion of the endometrial cavity from uterine anomalies, fibromyomas, endometrial polyps, and intrauterine synechiae.[5] In addition, if dye remains confined to the areas adjacent to the ends of the tubes, peritubal pelvic adhesions may be suspected. Although the hysterosalpingogram can be performed with routine radiographs, the amount of information gained by the experienced observer is greatly increased when the hysterosalpingogram is performed with slow, controlled injection of contrast media with fluoroscopic observation. The test is performed in the midfollicular phase of the cycle to avoid interference with, or irradiation of, an early pregnancy. Incidentally, hysterosalpingography (especially with oil-based contrast media) may also have a therapeutic effect by mechanically dislodging mucus plugs from the tubes or by breaking adhesions and thus helping achieve tubal patency and pregnancy.[50]

The hysterosalpingogram has the disadvantage of not diagnosing a significant number of patients with pelvic adhesions or endometriosis because tubal problems sufficient to show on radiographs are not present.[49] In addition, hypersensitivity to the iodine-containing dye is rarely encountered, but probably the most serious complication of hysterosalpingography is the occurrence of severe pelvic infection. This probably happens only extremely rarely in patients with normal pelvic structures but may occur in 10% of patients with pelvic adhesions or obstruction.[51] Patients with a strong history of prior pelvic inflammatory disease or radiographic evidence for pelvic disease should be treated prophylactically with a broad-spectrum antibiotic, such as doxycycline.[51]

Laparoscopy can be used to directly examine the pelvic organs for disease; however, it does have the disadvantages of needing to be performed in the hospital, carrying the risks of general anesthesia and surgery, and yielding no information about the configuration of the uterine cavity. For these reasons, laparoscopy alone does not replace hysterosalpingography but rather complements it. If the patient has not already had a hysterosalpingograph, we perform a hysteroscopy to directly observe the uterine cavity for synechiae, polyps, submucous myomata, and abnormalities in configuration. Many infertility surgeries, such as lysis of adhesions, excision and destruction of endometriosis, fimbrioplasties, and neosalpingostomies, can be performed through the laparoscope by pelviscopic techniques. Laparoscopy also has the advantage of allowing us to confirm pelvic adhesions or tubal blockage and to avoid a major operation if the observed pelvic and tubal disease is so extensive that the chances for successful surgical repair are exceedingly small. These patients should be offered in vitro fertilization.

We offer laparoscopy to patients with normal results on infertility investigations, in an attempt to exclude all anatomic possibilities for their infertility; however, currently when a patient has normal hysterosalpingographic and pelvic examination results and a history that does not suggest the possibility of pelvic adhesions or endometriosis, we generally recommend performing an assisted reproductive technology procedure such as GIFT or zygote intrafallopian transfer (ZIFT) at the same time as the diagnostic laparoscopy (see the section on Assisted Reproductive Technologies).

Surgical conditions of the fallopian tube can be categorized as obstruction at multiple sites, distal occlusion at the fimbria, proximal obstruction at the uterotubal junction, and peritubo-ovarian adhesions that do not obstruct the tube. The last, which is the most amenable to surgery—particularly if the adhesions are filmy—may have a prognosis for pregnancy of 50 to 70%. The pregnancy rate following operations attempting to correct multiple sites of obstruction is so poor that we consider this to be a contraindication to surgery. Operation for a distal obstruction has a pregnancy rate of 5 to 50%, depending on whether the obstruction is associated with a hydrosalpinx and the degree of tubal mucosal destruction. Major surgical repair of proximal obstruction gives a success rate of 30 to 45%. Fluoroscopically guided transcervical fallopian tube catheterization achieves a similar pregnancy rate in proximal obstruction and is a much less invasive procedure.[52] All attempts to repair obstruction in tubes damaged by an inflammatory process are in contrast to the 75 to 85% pregnancy rates following microsurgical repair of tubal sterilizations. Certainly the restoration of tubal patency following inflammatory disease is more successful than the resulting pregnancy rate. This discrepancy is due to the fact that the fallopian tube is much more than a conduit from the ovary to the uterus, and damage to the tubal mucosa is irreversible and certainly not repaired by surgery.

Prior to operation, the patient should be advised that in general her chances of failure may be as great as or greater than her chances of success. The success of operation depends on the location of the obstruction, the etiology for the pathologic abnormalities, the type of surgical procedure to be performed, and the expertise of the surgeon. We certainly feel that infertility surgery should be undertaken only by a gynecologist trained in and regularly performing infertility surgery. Further details on surgical techniques appear in the reference list.[1-3, 6]

The future holds promise in several areas. Research is ongoing in the use of postsurgical adjuncts to decrease the likelihood for adhesion reformation. Laser surgery has captured the imagination of the lay public, but with today's equipment no substantial improvement in pregnancy rates has been demonstrated. New laparoscopic instrumentation and the techniques to use them are rapidly changing the field of infertility from a major surgical endeavor to ambulatory, minimally invasive surgery. The list of surgical procedures that have been performed by pelviscopy seems to grow almost weekly; however, the safety and efficacy of pelviscopic procedures have yet to be established. As pregnancy rates with in vitro fertilization and embryo transfer increase, many patients with a poor prognosis for pregnancy following surgery will elect not to have reconstruction by major surgery. Nevertheless, if a minimally invasive surgical procedure can be performed at the same time as the diagnosis, then the use of pelviscopic infertility surgery will continue to expand.

Endometriosis

The incidence of endometriosis in the normal population is unknown but is estimated to be 5 to 20%. In an infertile population, the incidence of endometriosis appears to be higher, quoted in various studies at 10 to 40%. Patient complaints of dysmenorrhea, particularly if it is not well controlled by the nonsteroidal anti-inflammatory agents, may be due to endometriosis. The occurrence of deep pelvic pain with intercourse is a cardinal sign of endometriosis. On pelvic examination, tender nodularity of the uterosacral ligaments can sometimes be identified. Nevertheless, the diagnosis of endometriosis is usually not obvious and cannot be made with certainty without laparoscopy.

The etiology of infertility associated with endometriosis is difficult to explain. When tubo-ovarian adhesions are present, the cause of the infertility is obvious, but frequently the endometriosis is present only on the peritoneum in the cul-de-sac and on the uterosacral ligaments. Thus, the relationship between infertility and endometriosis is frequently unknown. Even more obscure is the relationship between treatment, either surgical or medical, and prognosis for pregnancy.[53-55]

Surgical treatment is generally advised when adhesions or endometriomas are present. Lysis of adhesions and excision of endometriomas can be performed by pelviscopic techniques. Pregnancy rates of 30 to 50% can be expected. In mild disease, the controversy is much greater. Pregnancy rates from 30 to 75% have been quoted by different investigators, but in one study of conservative surgery versus expectant management of mild endometriosis, no significant difference was seen. Nevertheless, because the diagnosis can be made only at the time of a laparoscopy, this procedure provides the opportunity for pelviscopic treatment by excision or ablation of the endometriotic lesions by laser or cautery.

Nonsurgical treatment of mild endometriosis with the testosterone derivative danazol has been shown to be very effective at relieving the symptoms of dysmenorrhea and pelvic pain associated with endometriosis. Some early studies showed pregnancy rates in infertile patients with mild endometriosis of 50 to 70%. More recently, several investigators, including us,[54] have questioned the efficacy of danazol for the treatment of infertility associated with mild endometriosis. In one randomized study, the pregnancy rate was not different in the treated and untreated groups.[55] The newest treatment modality is medical hypophysectomy using GnRH analogs (leuprolide acetate [Lupron] and nafarelin acetate [Synarel]). Analog therapy may be even more effective at relieving the pain symptoms of endometriosis, but there is no evidence that it can increase a patient's chances of becoming pregnant. The likely reason for the failure of medical therapies to enhance pregnancy rates is that these medications are effective only at suppressing endometriosis, and once the therapy is discontinued, there is regrowth and reactivation of the endometriosis.

NORMAL INFERTILE COUPLE: UNEXPLAINED INFERTILITY

After thorough evaluation, 10 to 20% of infertile couples will be left with no definitive cause for their infertility. This probably reflects our lack of knowledge regarding the etiology and treatment of infertility. The fertility potential of a specific couple is a complex interaction of the fertility potentials of each member of the couple. Either member of an infertile couple may no longer be infertile when paired with a different, more fertile partner.

Traditionally, the semen analysis has been used as the sole evaluation of male fertility. Recently it has been shown that the motile sperm count (sperm count × per cent motility) is related more closely to pregnancy rates than either the sperm count or the per cent motility alone.[56] In couples whose male partners had a motile sperm count of more than 60 million/ml, an almost 90% pregnancy rate occurred in an average time to conception of 6 months. When the motile sperm count was less than 30 million/ml, only 50% conceived, in an average of 10 months. Nevertheless, this modification of the traditional semen analysis is still only a descriptive evaluation of the semen.

In a small study of in vitro fertilization of human oocytes obtained at diagnostic laparoscopy from patients with unexplained infertility, a high rate of fertilization failure was noted.[57] This information has prompted some investigators to use in vitro fertilization as a diagnostic procedure to determine whether abnormalities of gametes or their transport are causing infertility. Multiple oocytes are recovered from a patient and exposed to sperm from the male partner and a matched fertile donor. Fertilization by the donor sperm but not with the male partner's indicates an abnormality of the latter's sperm. Fertilization by both specimens suggests some barrier in vivo to normal sperm transport or function or to normal ovum release or pick-up by the fallopian tube. Fertilization by neither specimen indicates an abnormality with the oocyte. If fertilization occurs with the male partner's sperm, the patients can be encouraged to have additional assisted reproductive technology procedures. In the case of oocyte defects, donor ova can be offered (see the section on Assisted Reproductive Technologies). In the case of sperm defects, the couple can be advised to proceed with donor artificial insemination.

The postcoital examination evaluates the sperm and cervical mucus interaction, which consists only of sperm entry into, and survival within, the cervix. Laparoscopic recovery of sperm from the pelvic cavity enables assessment of the adequacy of sperm transport into the upper genital tract.[58] The spontaneous pregnancy rate in the positive sperm recovery group was nearly 50%; in the negative group, only 10%. Of particular note is the fact that the results of the postcoital tests and the laparoscopic sperm recovery showed poor correlation. This fact is probably part of the explanation for the high pregnancy rate of patients undergoing the GIFT procedure.

Ovulation, defined as the release of an ovum from the graafian follicle, is assumed to occur when the indirect evaluation criteria (biphasic basal temperature chart, elevated serum progesterone, secretory endometrium, and conformation by ultrasound examination) are present. The follicle can go through the normal stages of development, and an ultrasound examination can document disappearance of the preovulatory follicle, but ovum release may not occur; this is termed the *trapped ovum syndrome*. Although this diagnosis has been documented histologically by finding the trapped ovum in the hemorrhagic corpus luteum, there is no practical clinical means of making this diagnosis. However, this diagnosis can be suspected to be another partial explanation of why the pregnancy rate is so high with the GIFT procedure in unexplained infertility.

Several clinical studies have suggested that *Ureaplasma urealyticum* (T strain mycoplasma) may be associated with reproductive failure. In general, the frequency of *U. urealyticum* in the cervical mucus of women and the semen of men increases from fertile control subjects to explained infertile control subjects to couples with unexplained infertility. In one study, T-mycoplasma was recovered from the semen in 19% of normal men, in 47% of men with infertility of known etiology, and in 76% of men with unexplained infertility.[59] In most randomized studies of couples with positive *U. urealyticum* genital colonization, antibiotic treatment has not been effective at improving conception rates when compared with placebo; however, in a study of couples with unexplained infertility, in which a higher incidence of cervical and endometrial T mycoplasma was seen, treatment resulted in improvement in fertility only in the cases with the positive endometrial culture results.[60]

ASSISTED REPRODUCTIVE TECHNOLOGIES

An increasingly popular treatment for infertile couples is the ever-increasing list of assisted reproductive technologies. In vitro fertilization was the first of these technologies, but the GIFT and ZIFT procedures have surpassed in vitro fertilization as more common clinical techniques in most infertility clinics. In addition, superovulation and AIH-IUI has become a commonly used assisted reproductive technology procedure. The use of donor ova is relatively new but rapidly expanding. All of the procedures, which are done in special centers with expertise in these techniques, are now increasingly considered for couples who have unexplained infertility or have not responded to other more conventional treatments.

Superovulation and AIH-IUI

In women with normal ovulatory function, superovulation with clomiphene citrate or human menopausal gonadotropins[61] is used to enhance timing of insemination and to provide more than one egg for fertilization. Although this treatment or variations thereof are widely use for male infertility, the major use is for unexplained infertility. The cycle fecundity achieved with superovulation and AIH-IUI in women with minimal endometriosis, cervical factor, or unexplained infertility is close to that achieved by women without fertility problems. Comparing AIH-IUI alone, superovulation alone, and superovulation combined with AIH-IUI in the treatment of unexplained infertility, the pregnancy rate/cycle was 2.2, 6.1, and 26.4%, respectively.

However, the success must be balanced against the risk of multiple births with this approach.

In Vitro Fertilization

During the dozen or so years since the birth of the first baby conceived by in vitro fertilization, the indications for this technique have changed from irreparable tubal factor to any fertility problem not responsive to conventional fertility treatments back to irreparable tubal factor. The current success rate of in vitro fertilization ranges from 10 to 30%, and because the chance for pregnancy in successive attempts does not change appreciably in the first four to six cycles of treatment, the cumulative pregnancy rates reported for six cycles of treatment are not significantly different from the pregnancy rate for fertile couples. Unfortunately, most couples find the emotional, physical, and financial consequences of in vitro fertilization treatment so burdensome that going beyond a single attempt can be difficult. Although no major breakthroughs have emerged recently to significantly change the success rates, the procedure itself has become easier for the patients to endure. Since 1986, the majority of ovum retrievals have been accomplished by ultrasound-guided transvaginal-needle aspirations, thereby avoiding laparoscopy and the attendant general anesthesia.

Gamete Intrafallopian Transfer

Insights into the etiology of unexplained infertility can be gained from the observation that the GIFT procedure is highly successful when applied to this group of patients. In our experience, the success rate of GIFT is approximately 40%. In essence, the GIFT procedure assures the simultaneous presence of sperm and ova in the ampullary portion of the fallopian tubes. It has been used for the treatment of unexplained infertility and infertility unresponsive to conventional treatments when the woman has patent fallopian tubes. It can even be used to overcome impairment of ovum pick-up due to tubo-ovarian adhesion, as long as the tube is open and accessible for catheterization at the time of a laparoscopy. The advantage of the GIFT procedure when compared with in vitro fertilization is that the pregnancy rate is approximately twice as high. The disadvantages include the risks of laparoscopy and general anesthesia, a higher frequency of ectopic pregnancies, and no knowledge about the sperm and egg interaction unless pregnancy occurs.

Zygote Intrafallopian Transfer

The zygote intrafallopian transfer (ZIFT) procedure is a hybrid of GIFT and in vitro fertilization, combining the best of both procedures but at the price of an increased financial cost. Ovum retrieval is accomplished by ultrasound guidance, thus avoiding laparoscopy and general anesthesia; fertilization of the ova is confirmed by in vitro techniques, and then any fertilized eggs (zygotes) are returned to the patient's fallopian tubes via laparoscopy, yielding an improved pregnancy rate. Current data suggest that the pregnancy rates for comparable patients are identical for GIFT and ZIFT; therefore, the only advantage of ZIFT is to confirm normal gamete interaction (i.e., fertilization). For this reason, ZIFT is especially valuable in the treatment and evaluation of male infertility.

Donor Oocytes

Oocyte donation has become a viable medical alternative for the treatment of infertility in women with the inability to produce normal oocytes—for example, women with premature ovarian failure or basal FSH levels greater than 16 mIU/ml and inheritable genetic diseases. Somewhat ironically, both the implantation and pregnancy rates in women receiving donated oocytes appear to be significantly higher than the rates attained by patients using their own gametes. This is probably because of the endometrial abnormalities related to the ovarian hyperstimulation in women using their own oocytes, a situation avoided by using the natural hormonal cycle in the oocyte recipients.[62]

The questions surrounding the appropriate application of the assisted reproductive technologies remain unanswered. These concerns are hotly debated and no consensus exists, nor is likely to exist, but The Ethics Committee of the American Fertility Society has attempted to address the issues in its report "Ethical Considerations of the New Reproductive Technologies" (Fertil Steril 53[Suppl 2], 1990).

Currently, we recommend in vitro fertilization for patients with severely damaged fallopian tubes; ZIFT, for patients with open tubes and male factors; and GIFT, for patients with open tubes and unexplained infertility or non–male factor infertility unresponsive to conventional treatments. Because these techniques are rapidly evolving, interested couples for whom an assisted reproductive technology may be applicable should discuss the possibilities with a reproductive specialist.

PROGNOSIS FOR THE INFERTILE COUPLE

According to most reports, the eventual fertility rate for most initially infertile couples, irrespective of etiology, is about 50 to 60% (Table 43–5). The longer a couple has been infertile, the lower the likelihood is for achieving a pregnancy. The diagnosis also affects the chances for a success-

TABLE 43–5. CUMULATIVE PREGNANCY RATES AT 36 MONTHS AFTER INITIATING INFERTILITY EVALUATION*

	No. of Patients	Cumulative 36-Month Pregnancy Rate (%)
Duration of Infertility		
12–23 months	399	63
24–35 months	288	54
36–47 months	161	38
48–71 months	156	27
> 72 months	141	37
Primary Clinical Diagnosis		
Ovulation defect	349	66
Idiopathic infertility	154	61
Seminal factor	351	44
Cervical factor	59	44
Endometriosis	49	29
Tubal factor	183	27
Prior Fertility		
This partnership	202	63
Previous relationship	133	41
None	810	48
Overall	1145	51

*Adapted from Collins JA, Wrixon W, James LB, et al: Treatment-independent pregnancy among infertile couples. Reprinted by permission from the New England Journal of Medicine 309:1201, 1983.

ful outcome. Couples with secondary infertility are more likely to attain conception than those with primary infertility.[63]

The efficacy of treatment for any particular diagnosis is difficult to assess because few well-controlled studies exist. Several studies suggest that treatment-independent pregnancies account for at least one third of the conceptions among infertile couples.[63]

To couples with unexplained infertility, the physician might explain that the chances for conception are low if the infertility has lasted more than 4 years; however, occasional patients may become pregnant after many years of trying. Couples in this situation should not be exposed to unnecessary therapeutic regimens and prolonged, expensive follow-ups; nevertheless, if the couple has not been evaluated by a reproductive endocrinologist, the physician should make such a referral, if the couple so desires.

In previously infertile women who do eventually become pregnant, the pregnancy wastage is greater than that seen in the normal pregnant population. The incidence of ectopic pregnancy is about five times the normal rate, spontaneous abortion is increased, and the perinatal mortality rate is doubled. Therefore, the infertile patient who is fortunate enough to conceive should not be treated in the ordinary manner but should be followed carefully throughout her pregnancy.

The anxiety and stress indirectly caused by the infertility may lead to marital discord and divorce of couples. The marital partners often experience a sense of emotional isolation and feelings of inadequacy because of their inability to accomplish what is for others the natural act of procreation. Husbands blame wives, and wives blame husbands. Thus, infertility should be seen not merely as an inconvenience but as a major life crisis. Above all, the emotional aspects of infertility must not be overlooked. The partners should be encouraged by their physician to discuss their problems openly with each other as well as with the attendant medical staff. Calling on the assistance of a group such as Resolve (Resolve, 1310 Broadway, Somerville, MA 02144–1731), a national nonprofit organization that specializes in counseling, educating, and furnishing emotional support for the infertile couple, should also be considered.

REFERENCES

1. Speroff L, Glass RH, and Kase NG: Clinical Gynecologic Endocrinology and Infertility, 3rd ed. Baltimore, Williams & Wilkins, 1989.
2. Yen SSC and Jaffe RB (eds): Reproductive Endocrinology: Physiology, Pathophysiology, and Clinical Management, 3rd ed. Philadelphia, WB Saunders, 1991.
3. Garcia C-R, Mastroianni L, Amelar RD, and Dubin L (eds): Current Therapy of Infertility, 3rd ed. Philadelphia, BC Decker, 1988.
4. Yee B (ed): Ovulation Induction. Infertil Reprod Med Clin North Am 1:1, 1990.
5. Hunt RB and Siegler AM: Hysterosalpingography: Techniques and Interpretation. Chicago, Year Book Medical Publishers, 1990.
6. Semm K: Operative Manual for Endoscopic Abdominal Surgery. Chicago, Year Book Medical Publishers, 1987.
7. Lipschultz LI and Howards SS (eds): Infertility in the Male, 2nd ed. St. Louis, Mosby–Year Book, 1991.
8. Acosta AA, Swanson RJ, Ackerman SB, et al (eds): Human Spermatozoa in Assisted Reproduction. Baltimore, Williams & Wilkins, 1990.
9. Albrecht BH, Cramer DW, and Schiff I: Factors influencing the success of artificial insemination. Fertil Steril 37:792, 1982.
10. Menning BE: Infertility: A Guide for the Childless Couple. Englewood Cliffs, NJ, Prentice-Hall, 1988.
11. Klaiber EL, Broverman DM, Pokoly TB, et al: Interrelationships of cigarette smoking, testicular varicoceles and seminal fluid indexes. Fertil Steril 47:481, 1987.

11a. Benoff S, Cooper GW, Hurley I, et al: The effect of calcium ion channel blockers on sperm fertilization potential. Proceedings of the American Fertility Society, Montréal, Abstract No. 2, 1993.

12. Gill WB, Schumacher GFB, and Bibbo M: Structural and functional abnormalities in the sex organs of male offspring of mothers treated with diethylstilbestrol (DES). J Reprod Med 16:147, 1976.
13. Aitken RJ, Best FSM, Richardson DW, et al: An analysis of sperm function in cases of unexplained infertility: Conventional criteria, movement characteristics and fertilizing capacity. Fertil Steril 38:212, 1982.
14. Holt WV, Moore HDM, and Hillier SG: Computer-assisted measurement of sperm swimming speed in human semen: Correlation of results with in vitro fertilization assays. Fertil Steril 44:112, 1985.
15. Feneux D, Serres C, and Jouannet P: Sliding spermatozoa: A dyskinesia responsible for human infertility? Fertil Steril 44:508, 1985.
16. Settladge DSF, Motoshima M, and Treadway DR: Sperm transport from the external cervical os to the fallopian tubes in women: A time and quantitation study. Fertil Steril 24:655, 1973.
17. Matson PL, Turner SR, and Yovich JM: Oligospermic infertility treated by in vitro fertilization. Aust N Z J Obstet Gynaecol 26:84, 1986.
18. Okuyama A, Koide T, Itatani H, et al: Pituitary-gonadal function in schoolboys with varicocele and indications of varicocelectomy. Eur J Urol 7:92, 1981.
19. Aaberg RA, Vancaillie TG, and Schuessler WW: Laparoscopic varicocele ligation: A new technique. Fertil Steril 56:776, 1991.
20. Coelingh-Bennink HJT, Dogterom AA, Lappohn RE, et al: Pulsatile GnRH, 1985: Proceedings of the 3rd Ferring Symposium. Haarlem, the Netherlands, A Ferring Publication, 1986.
21. Wang C, Chan C-W, Wong K-K, et al: Comparison of the effectiveness of placebo, clomiphene citrate, mesterolone, pentoxifylline, and testosterone rebound therapy for the treatment of idiopathic oligospermia. Fertil Steril 40:358, 1983.
22. Barkay J, Harpaz-Kerpel S, Ben-Ezra S, et al: The prostaglandin inhibitory effect of antiinflammatory drugs in the therapy of male infertility. Fertil Steril 42:406, 1984.
23. Zorgniotti AW, Cohen MS, and Sealfon AI: Chronic scrotal hypothermia: Results in 90 infertile couples. J Urol 135:944, 1986.
24. Schill WB: Treatment of idiopathic oligozoospermia by kallikrein: Results of a double-blind study. Arch Androl 2:163, 1979.
25. Allen NC, Herbert CM, Maxson WS, et al: Intrauterine insemination: A critical review. Fertil Steril 44:569, 1985.
26. Kerin JFP, Kirby C, Peek J, et al: Improved conception rate after intrauterine insemination of washed spermatozoa from men with poor quality semen. Lancet i:533, 1984.
27. MacLeod J and Gold RA: Semen quality in relation to age and sexual activity. Fertil Steril 4:194, 1953.
28. Corsan GH, Ghazi D, and Kemmann E: Home urinary luteinizing hormone immunoassays: Clinical applications. Fertil Steril 53:591, 1990.
29. Sher G, Herbert C, Maassarani G, and Jacobs MH: Assessment of the late proliferative phase endometrium by ultrasonography in patients undergoing in-vitro fertilization and embryo transfer (IVF/ET). Hum Reprod 6:232, 1991.
30. Hammond MG and Talbert LM: Clomiphene citrate therapy of infertile women with low luteal phase progesterone levels. Obstet Gynecol 59:275, 1982.
31. Cline DL: Unsuspected subclinical pregnancies in patients with luteal phase defect. Am J Obstet Gynecol 134:438, 1979.
32. Jones GS: The luteal phase defect. Fertil Steril 27:351, 1976.
33. Soules MR, Wiebe RH, Aksel S, et al: The diagnosis and therapy of luteal phase deficiency. Fertil Steril 28:1033, 1977.
34. Seppala M, Hirvonen E, and Ranta T: Hyperprolactinaemia and luteal insufficiency. Lancet i:229, 1976.

35. Daly DC, Walters CA, Soto-Albors CE, et al: Endometrial biopsy during treatment of luteal phase defects is predictive of therapeutic outcome. Fertil Steril 40:305, 1983.
36. Toner JP, Philput CB, Jones GS, and Muasher SJ: Basal follicle-stimulating hormone level is a better predictor of in vitro fertilization performance than age. Fertil Steril 55:784, 1991.
37. Stewart DE, Robinson E, Goldbloom DS, and Wright C: Infertility and eating disorders. Am J Obstet Gynecol 163:1196, 1990.
38. Miller DS, Reid RR, Cetel NS, et al: Pulsatile administration of low-dose gonadotropin-releasing hormone: Ovulation and pregnancy in women with hypothalamic amenorrhea. JAMA 250:2937, 1983.
39. Mornex R, Orgiazzi J, Hugues B, et al: Normal pregnancies after treatment of hyperprolactinemia with bromoergocryptine, despite suspected pituitary tumors. J Clin Endocrinol Metab 47:290, 1978.
40. O'Herlihy C, Pepperell RJ, and Robinson HP: Ultrasound timing of human chorionic gonadotropin administration in clomiphene-stimulated cycles. Obstet Gynecol 59:40, 982.
41. Hull MGR, Savage PE, and Bromham DR: Prognostic value of the postcoital test: Prospective study based on time-specific conception rates. Br J Obstet Gynaecol 89:299, 1982.
42. Kroeks MVAM and Kremer J: The role of cervical factors in infertility. *In* Pepperell RJ, Hudson B, and Wood C (eds): The Infertile Couple. New York, Churchill-Livingstone, 1980, p 122.
43. Bronson RA, Cooper GW, and Rosenfeld DL: Autoimmunity to spermatozoa: Effect on sperm penetration of cervical mucus as reflected by postcoital testing. Fertil Steril 41:609, 1984.
44. Ayvaliotis B, Bronson R, Rosenfeld D, and Cooper G: Conception rates in couples where autoimmunity to sperm is detected. Fertil Steril 43:739, 1986.
45. Witkin SS, Viti D, David SS, et al: Relation between antisperm antibodies and the rate of fertilization of human oocytes in vitro. J Assist Reprod 9:9, 1992.
46. Mathur S, Baker ER, Williamson HO, et al: Clinical significance of sperm antibodies in infertility. Fertil Steril 36:486, 1981.
47. Albrecht BH, Saunders DT, Betz G, et al: Efficacy of intrauterine homologous artificial inseminations. Abstract No. 29, American College of Obstetricians and Gynecologists, District VIII, Denver, 1989.
48. Quagliarello J and Arny M: Intracervical versus intrauterine insemination: Correlation of outcome with antecedent postcoital testing. Fertil Steril 46:870, 1986.
49. Maathius JB, Horbach JGM, and Van Hall EV: A comparison of the results of hysterosalpingography and laparoscopy in the diagnosis of tube dysfunction. Fertil Steril 23:428, 1972.
50. Schwabe MG, Shapiro SS, and Haning RV: Hysterosalpingography with oil contrast medium enhances fertility in patients with infertility of unknown etiology. Fertil Steril 40:604, 1983.
51. Pittaway DE, Winfield AC, Maxon W, et al: Prevention of acute pelvic inflammatory disease following hysterosalpingography: Efficacy of doxycycline prophylaxis. Presented at the Society for Gynecologic Investigation, 30th Annual Meeting. 1983 (Abstract No. 399).
52. Kumpe DA, Zwerdlinger SC, Rothbarth LJ, et al: Proximal fallopian tube occlusion: Diagnosis and treatment with transcervical fallopian tube catheterization. Radiology 177:183, 1990.
53. Schenken RS and Malinak LR: Conservative surgery versus expectant management for the infertile patient with mild endometriosis. Fertil Steril 37:183, 1982.
54. Butler L, Wilson E, Belisle S, et al: Collaborative study of pregnancy rates following danazol therapy of stage I endometriosis. Fertil Steril 41:373, 1984.
55. Seibel MM, Berger MJ, Weinstein FG, et al: The effectiveness of danazol on subsequent fertility in minimal endometriosis. Fertil Steril 38:534, 1982.
56. Steinberger E and Rodriguez-Rigau LJ: The infertile couple. J Androl 4:111, 1983.
57. Trounson AO, Leeton JF, Wood C, et al: The investigation of idiopathic infertility by in vitro fertilization. Fertil Steril 34:431, 1980.
58. Templeton AA and Mortimer D: The development of a clinical test of sperm migration to the site of fertilization. Fertil Steril 37:410, 1982.
59. Friberg J and Gnarpe H: Mycoplasmas in semen from fertile and infertile men. Andrologia 6:45, 1974.
60. Stray-Pedersen B, Eng J, and Reikvan TM: Uterine T-mycoplasma colonization in reproductive failure. Am J Obstet Gynecol 130:307, 1978.
61. Hurst BS and Wallach EE: Superovulation with intrauterine insemination: Empiric therapy for infertile couples. Postgrad Obstet Gynecol 10:6, 1990.
62. Sauer MV, Paulson RJ, and Lobo RA: Reversing the natural decline in human fertility: An extended clinical trial of oocyte donation to women of advanced reproductive age. JAMA 268:1275, 1992.
63. Collins JA, Wrixon W, Janes LB, et al: Treatment-independent pregnancy among infertile couples. N Engl J Med 309:1201, 1983.

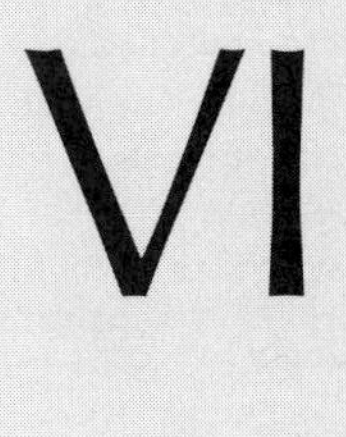

VI

Endocrine Problems

44

Thyroid Diseases

P. REED LARSEN, MD

Thyroid diseases are commonly encountered and usually can be managed in the office setting. The actual prevalence of thyroid abnormalities in the population is unknown but must be very great. For example, in one series of 821 patients autopsied at the Mayo Clinic in whom there was no clinical suspicion of thyroid disease prior to death, 50% were found to have thyroid abnormalities.[1] Many of these were revealed only on histologic section. Most were benign, and a large portion were follicular adenomas. It is difficult to say what fraction of these physical abnormalities might be recognized clinically, but a fair estimate would be that about 5% of the population has a palpable abnormality of the thyroid gland.

In addition to these anatomic abnormalities, thyroid dysfunction, either hypothyroidism or hyperthyroidism, is also common. Screening studies of a single community in England, for example, revealed a prevalence of hypothyroidism and hyperthyroidism of about 1%.[2] Screening programs have been able to detect congenital hypothyroidism at a frequency of about 1 in 4000 births.[3]

APPROACH TO THE PATIENT

History

The changes in the secretion rate of the thyroid gland are gradual; therefore, the changes in the patient's symptomatology are also gradual. Often, the patient does not recognize the degree of impairment of a normal state of health until after resolution of the symptoms of either hyperthyroidism or hypothyroidism. Therefore, it is incumbent on the physician taking the history to seek evidence for any change in well-being.

For as yet unknown reasons, thyroid diseases are considerably more common in women than in men. The ratio of women to men is generally five to 10 to one for all forms of thyroid disease; thus, this possibility should be considered especially strongly in women with nonspecific symptomatology.

Symptoms of Hypothyroidism. The complaints of the patient with hypothyroidism are often nonspecific. These may include generalized fatigue, cold intolerance, weight gain, constipation, coarsening of the skin, dryness of the hair and skin, lethargy, and slow speech, all of which should alert the physician to the possibility that the patient is hypothyroid. The weight gain in hypothyroidism is usually not great—only five to 10 lb on the average. Obese patients who are found to be hypothyroid should be cautioned that they will probably not alleviate this problem merely by appropriate therapy of the hypothyroidism.

Symptoms of Hyperthyroidism and Graves' Exophthalmos. The symptomatology suggesting hyperthyroidism is usually obvious in the younger patient but may be extremely subtle in the elderly. The elderly patient may present with depression, weight loss associated with anorexia, and congestive heart failure associated with atrial fibrillation.[4] In fact, the symptoms of congestive heart failure often are so much more dramatic than those of the other metabolic effects of excess thyroid hormone in the elderly that the presence of unexplained cardiac decompensation or atrial fibrillation should lead the physician to consider the diagnosis of hyperthyroidism.

The involvement of the eyes in patients with the form of hyperthyroidism known as Graves' disease has been well described. Patients may seek the physician's attention for this problem initially and may not be aware of the symptoms of hyperthyroidism, which often accompany this disease. In addition, elucidation of the symptomatology of eye disease will often allow the physician to make the clinical diagnosis of Graves' disease, as opposed to toxic nodular goiter or subacute thyroiditis, solely on a clinical basis. The symptoms of eye disease that should be reviewed with the patient include photophobia, wind sensitivity, frequent tearing, periorbital swelling, edema, a foreign body or sandy sensation in the eyes, and, more significantly, diplopia, particularly in distance vision. A change in visual acuity may be an important symptom of optic nerve involvement.

Previous Radiation Exposure to the Head, Neck, or Chest. One additional factor of extreme importance in the general medical evaluation of any patient is whether a history of exposure to thyroidal irradiation exists. In the recent past, radiation was used to treat many forms of disease of the head and neck, including chronic tonsillitis, eustachian tube dysfunction, acne, hemangiomas of the face or neck, and ringworm, as well as status thymicolymphaticus. Five to 10% of patients with a history of significant exposure to radiation will develop papillary thyroid carcinoma within 20 years of exposure.[5] Likewise, the presence of a thyroid nodule on physical examination should lead to thorough questioning of the patient (and the patient's parents, if possible) regarding the possibility of radiation exposure of the thyroid.

Physical Examination

The physical examination of the patient with thyroid disease may reveal suggestive evidence of pathology but is often inconclusive. An exception is resting tachycardia, which in the younger patient is virtually a sine qua non for establishing the diagnosis of hyperthyroidism. Only rarely have I observed a young patient with thyrotoxicosis of a significant degree whose resting pulse did not exceed 90 beats per minute in the outpatient setting. In addition to this finding, patients with moderate-to-severe hyperthyroidism will have all the peripheral and dramatic manifestations of thyroid hormone excess and present no difficulty in recognition. Particular attention needs to be given to examining the eyes for the presence or absence of chemosis, conjunctival irritation, conjunctival injection, and impairment of extraocular movements. These are important in confirming the diagnosis of Graves' disease.

Dry, coarse skin and hair, periorbital puffiness, slight swelling of hands and fingers, and change in ring size should suggest the possibility of myxedema. The most useful physical correlate of this condition in a clinical setting is the delay in the relaxation phase of the deep tendon reflexes. Like tachycardia, the sign is not specific because in other circumstances (peripheral neuropathy, malnutrition, and hypothermia) the relaxation phase of the deep tendon reflexes is prolonged.

Examination of the Thyroid

The first step in the examination is to observe the patient while he or she is swallowing with the neck slightly extended. By this simple maneuver, one can usually appreciate the size of the thyroid gland, the normal gland often being just visible. From inspection, the physician can often determine whether the thyroid gland is enlarged and, if so, whether this enlargement is nodular or diffuse and whether nodularity is limited to a single area of the thyroid or is bilateral. Following inspection of the lower neck during swallowing, the position of the trachea is ascertained by palpation of the sternal notch, and any deviation is noted. Such deviation is extremely common in older patients with large, nontoxic nodular goiters and may not be visible on inspection.

The next step is to locate the thyroid isthmus, generally found just below the cricoid cartilage. I prefer the anterior approach to the thyroid gland, particularly for appreciation of the presence or absence of nodular lesions. Palpation of each lobe of the thyroid gland is performed using the thumb of the hand corresponding to the side of the thyroid gland to be evaluated. The left thumb is used to compress the left lobe against the trachea. During the swallowing maneuver, it moves up and down underneath the thumb, allowing ready recognition of small irregularities or nodules. In addition to appreciation of the presence or absence of nodularity, the consistency of the thyroid gland can also be evaluated. Increased consistency is characteristically noted in patients with Hashimoto's thyroiditis and sometimes in those with Graves' disease. Another aspect of the thyroid examination that is more subtle is determination of the size of the pyramidal lobe, which is generally palpable in any patient with diffuse thyroid disease. It often presents as a small, cylindric mass extending superiorly from the isthmus, often to as high as the superior border of the thyroid cartilage. It is enlarged in patients with diffuse thyrotoxicosis due to Graves' disease and in any other condition that leads to generalized enlargement of the thyroid. Specific tenderness of the thyroid gland is usually limited to acute inflammatory diseases caused by either acute bacterial or, more commonly, subacute, presumably viral, thyroiditis. Rarely, patients with Hashimoto's thyroiditis have thyroid tenderness.

The physician should then determine whether the thyroid gland extends below the sternum and also evaluate the adequacy of the thoracic inlet by having the patient extend the arms over the head, observing for evidence of

TABLE 44–1. RESULTS OF SERUM T4,* THBR,† FREE T4 INDEX, TSH,‡ and T3§ MEASUREMENTS IN VARIOUS CLINICAL CIRCUMSTANCES

	Anticipated Results				
Diagnostic Category	*T4 RIA‖ (μg/dl)*	*THBR*	*Free T4 Index*	*T3 RIA (ng/dl)*	*TSH (μU/ml)*
Euthyroid					
Normal TBG¶	5–10.2	0.85–1.10	5–10	60–180	0.5–5.0
Elevated TBG	7.5–18.0	0.50–0.90	5–11	90–300	0.5–5.0
Reduced TBG	1.0–6.0	1.05–2.00	3–8	10–70	0.5–5.0
FDH**	12–20	0.85–1.10	12–20	60–180	0.5–5.0
Hypothyroid					
Normal TBG	0–5.0	0.50–0.90	0–4	0–130	>5.0
Hyperthyroid					
Normal TBG	8.0–50.0	1.05–1.70	10–80	180–1000	<0.5

*T4 = thyroxine.
†THBR = thyroid hormone binding ratio.
‡TSH = thyroid-stimulating hormone.
§T3 = triiodothyronine.
‖RIA = radioimmunoassay.
¶TBG = thyroxine-binding globulin.
**FDH = familial dysalbuminemic hyperthyroxinemia.

jugular venous distention during the maneuver. In addition, the neck is examined for the presence of enlarged lymph nodes, particularly when a solitary nodule has been found. In older patients, kyphosis sometimes alters the tracheal position so that the thyroid cartilage is found at the level of the sternal notch, which obviates palpation of the thyroid gland.

After completing the history and physical examination, the physician should have an excellent idea of whether the patient has significant thyroid disease. If the thyroid gland is enlarged, the physician should be reasonably confident that this enlargement is causing hyperthyroidism or is a result of hypothyroidism. If the patient has symptoms suggesting hyperthyroidism, it should be apparent whether it is associated with diffuse or nodular thyroid enlargement.

Laboratory Evaluation

Sensitive thyroid-stimulating hormone (TSH) assays have become so useful and precise that in the outpatient setting, a strong argument can be made that simple measurement of TSH will suffice to categorize patients into one of three groups[6]: euthyroid (serum TSH concentrations are between 0.5 and 5 μU/ml); hyperthyroid (serum TSH concentrations <0.5 μU/ml or the lower limit of normal for that particular assay); or hypothyroid. In the last case, if the cause of hypothyroidism is thyroid failure (as is the case in over 99% of such patients) the serum TSH is always greater than 5 μU/ml and in most symptomatic patients, greater than 15 μU/ml. In the hyperthyroid group, it is often possible to correlate the level of TSH with the clinical severity of the hyperthyroidism. In patients with obvious clinical hyperthyroidism, serum TSH is virtually always less than 0.2 μU/ml or undetectable, depending on the lower limits of the TSH assay. In patients in whom autonomous thyroid function is present (toxic nodule or mild Graves' disease), serum TSH concentrations will usually be found between 0.2 and 0.4 μU/ml. The major important exception to exclusive dependence on measurements of serum TSH as a biochemical approach to assessing thyroid status is that in patients with hypothalamic or pituitary hypothyroidism (secondary or tertiary hypothyroidism), serum TSH concentrations are often normal or even slightly elevated even when serum thyroid hormone concentrations are low. In such patients, the TSH is thought to be biologically ineffective. As a practical strategy, if the suspicion of thyroid disease is low but sufficient to justify testing, then the assay of serum TSH alone is adequate for screening purposes. On the other hand, if the clinician's index of suspicion of thyroid dysfunction is high, both an estimate of serum thyroid hormone concentration and its free fraction as well as a serum TSH should be quantitated.

If the clinician does not have access to a laboratory in which a reliable sensitive TSH assay is available, then the best screening test for thyroid dysfunction is the combination of a serum thyroxine (T4) accompanied by an index of the fraction of thyroid hormones that are free. The latter estimate can be determined in several ways, but the recent recommendations of the American Thyroid Association[8] are that such estimates be referred to as a thyroid hormone binding ratio (THBR) (Table 44–1). In many laboratories, the estimates of the free fractions of thyroid hormones are achieved by a resin or charcoal triiodothyronine (T3) uptake test. In essence, this test estimates the unoccupied binding sites available on circulating thyroxine-binding globulin (TBG). The resin or charcoal uptake of the isotope deviates from normal in the same direction as does the free fraction of circulating thyroid hormones. Thus, in a pregnant patient in whom serum T4 and TBG are both elevated, the resin T3 uptake is subnormal, indicating that the fraction of the total hormone that is free is subnormal. The free T4 can be estimated by normalizing the uptake (dividing the patient's uptake by the midnormal uptake percentage for that laboratory, i.e., calculating the THBR) and multiplying this value by the serum total T4 or T3. The product is termed the free T4 (or T3) index. In this way, a total T4 measurement can be corrected for the plasma TBG concentration (see Table 44–1).

Common causes of elevation or reduction of serum TBG are listed in Table 44–2. The most common cause of an elevation in serum TBG is an increase in estrogen production either due to pregnancy, oral contraceptive agents, or postmenopausal estrogen therapy. The increase in TBG is now thought to be due to estrogen-induced alterations in the glycosylation pattern of TBG such that its clearance by the liver is reduced.[9] The reduction in clearance leads to a doubling or trebling of TBG during pregnancy. Because the central feedback inhibition of TSH secretion reflects the free hormone, not the total, the total serum T4 is elevated when the free fraction is reduced. In conditions in which TBG concentrations are low, serum T4 is proportionately reduced but the free fraction is elevated. Thus again, the product of the total T4 and the THBR (the free T4 [T3]

TABLE 44–2. COMMON CLINICAL CIRCUMSTANCES IN WHICH THE CONCENTRATION OF CIRCULATING THYROXINE-BINDING GLOBULIN IS ALTERED

TBG* increased
Pregnancy
Estrogen therapy in excess of replacement
Oral contraceptive administration
Newborn infants
In certain families (X-linked)
TBG decreased
Chronic protein malnutrition
Hepatic failure
Nephrotic syndrome
Androgen therapy in excess of replacement
In certain families (X-linked)
After L-asparaginase

*TBG = thyroxine-binding globulin.

index) is in the normal range. At both extremes of TBG concentration, however, this simple correction is not effective, and apparent deviations from normal occur. A definitive assessment of the patient's thyroid status under these circumstances can be confirmed by measurement of serum TSH.

The utility of this approach to estimating free hormone concentrations is more obvious when the effect of increases or decreases in thyroid function on these two tests is evaluated (see Table 44–1). Because in hyperthyroidism serum T4 production is increased but TBG remains constant, unoccupied sites on TBG are reduced, and the T3 uptake or THBR is increased. The opposite occurs in hypothyroidism. Thus, under these circumstances, a combination of an elevated T4 and THBR leads to an amplification of the deviation of the T4 from normal. The opposite occurs in hypothyroidism. From a simplistic point of view, if both the serum hormone concentration and the THBR deviate from normal in the same direction, the problem can usually be attributed to an alteration in thyroid hormone production rates. On the other hand, if the deviations of total serum hormone and THBR are in opposite directions, the problem is usually an abnormality in binding protein. Of course, combinations of altered TBG and thyroid hormone production can occur, and in these situations the quantitation of serum TSH is especially useful.

When the free T4 index is used to assign a thyroid functional status, the clinician should keep in mind several situations in which an elevated result does not indicate the presence of hyperthyroidism. This phenomenon can occur in patients who are ill, particularly with acute psychosis or hyperemesis gravidarum, or who have received oral contrast agents for evaluation of the function of the gallbladder or are taking amiodarone.[10–12] In these conditions, the conversion of serum T4 to T3, a step that activates thyroxine, is impaired. In the case of the sick patient, the reason for the impairment of conversion is not yet well understood. In the case of patients receiving the iodinated drugs, it has been hypothesized that there is inhibition of T4 to T3 conversion by the drug.[13] As a result, the pituitary gland is activated to release thyroid-stimulating hormone (TSH). T4 production is stimulated, and serum T4 levels increase above the upper limits of normal. Such patients appear to have biochemical hyperthyroidism. However, the history usually does not suggest the presence of this disease, and the tests may even have been requested because of a suspicion of hypothyroidism. Under these circumstances—that is, when blood tests suggest hyperfunction and the clinical data do not—serum TSH and T3 determinations should be obtained. In patients with an elevated serum T4 level due to impairment of conversion, serum T3 concentrations are reduced, and serum TSH levels may be detectable or even increased, which is not the case in patients with bona fide hyperthyroidism. This distinction should allow separation of most sick patients from those who have hyperthyroidism.

A rarer cause of similar findings is the presence of excess quantities of an albumin in the serum that binds T4 but not T3 more strongly than does the bulk of serum albumin.[14] Such patients have an elevated free T4 index, as estimated from the total T4 and T3 resin uptake. Total serum T3 and TSH levels are normal in this disorder, which is transmitted as an autosomal dominant.

It follows from this discussion that if a patient with true hyperthyroidism should become ill enough to require hospitalization, then serum T4 and T3 resin uptake may well be increased, but owing to the impairment of T4 to T3 conversion, serum T3 levels may have fallen into either the high or midnormal range. In such patients, the normal serum T3 level is misleading, and the patients are still hyperthyroid in spite of the impaired conversion. In this uncommon situation, the serum TSH level will be reduced. Such diagnostic problems usually arise in the severely ill patient who is hospitalized, not in the ambulatory setting.

Interpretation of Serum TSH Concentrations. As mentioned, the exquisite sensitivity of the pituitary thyroid feedback loop to alterations in thyroid hormone production rates makes the accurate estimation of serum TSH the most clinically useful test of thyroid dysfunction. Table 44–3 shows conditions in ambulatory patients that can be associated with abnormal serum TSH concentrations. By and large, all individuals living in an iodine-sufficient country who have an elevated serum TSH will have primary hypothyroidism or a failing thyroid gland usually resulting from autoimmune thyroid disease. The other causes are much rarer and are included only for completeness. The commonest causes of a reduction in serum TSH are autonomous thyroid function or over-replacement with thyroid hormone. It is important to recognize that from 10 to 30% of patients may have a subnormal TSH level during the first trimester of normal pregnancy. This is especially true in hyperemesis gravidarum. Women with hydatidiform mole may even develop mild clinical hyperthyroidism. In these conditions, it is thought that human chorionic gonadotropin, a weak stimulator of the thyroid, is causing excessive T4 release, suppressing pituitary TSH.[15] Occasionally, in patients with acute psychosis or depression, serum TSH may also be transiently reduced.[10] This can sometimes make a clinical therapeutic decision difficult, but the condition resolves spontaneously when the acute problem subsides.

Quantitation of Circulating Antithyroglobulin and Thyroid Microsomal Antibodies. In certain forms of thyroid disease (Graves' disease and Hashimoto's thyroiditis) that appear to have an immunologic basis, antibodies to human thyroglobulin or thyroid microsomes may be found in the serum. The microsomal antigen is now recognized to be thyroid peroxidase.[16] The presence of these antibodies may provide useful information about the etiology of the thyroid disease. Test results for these antibodies are reported as the greatest dilution of the unknown serum that gives a positive response or as units in the case of the thyroid microsomal antibody. In Hashimoto's disease, over 90% of patients will have an elevated titer of thyroid microsomal antibody, whereas only 50 to 60% of such patients will have antithyroglobulin antibodies. In Graves' disease, roughly half the patients will have positive thyroid microsomal antibody results, and about 20 to 30% will have a

TABLE 44–3. CONDITIONS IN AMBULATORY PATIENTS THAT MAY BE ASSOCIATED WTIH ABNORMAL SERUM TSH* CONCENTRATIONS

	Expected TSH (μU/ml)	Thyroid Status	Free T4† Index
TSH Elevated			
Primary hypothyroidism	6–500	↓	↓
Iodine deficiency	6–150	N‡, ↓	↓
Thyroid hormone resistance			
"Thyrotroph" alone	5–15	↑	↑
Generalized	5–50	N, ↓	↑, ↑↑
Thyrotroph tumor	5–15	↑	↑
Hypothalamic-pituitary dysfunction	1–20	↓	↓
Psychiatric illness	0.4–10	N	N
Test artifact (endogenous antimouse γ globulin antibodies)	10–500	N	N
TSH Reduced			
Hyperthyroidism	<0.1	↑	↑, T3↑§
Euthyroid Graves' disease	0.2–0.5	N(↑)	N(?T3↑)
Autonomous nodules	0.2–0.5	N(↑)	N(?T3↑)
Excess thyroid hormone treatment	0.1–0.5	N, ↑	N, ↑
First-trimester pregnancy	0.2–0.5	N(↑)	N(↑)
Hyperemesis gravidarum	0.2–0.5	N(↑)	↑(N)
Hydatidiform mole	0.1–0.4	↑	↑
Acute psychosis or depression (rare)	0.4–10	N	N(↑)
Elderly (small fraction)	0.2–0.5	N	N

*TSH = thyroid-stimulating hormone.
†T4 = thyroxine.
‡N = normal.
§T3 = triiodothyronine.

positive antithyroglobulin determination. About 15% of the population without known thyroid disease will have a positive response to either test. Therefore, both are useful in establishing a high degree of suspicion regarding the presence of autoimmune thyroid disease. In some patients in whom thyroid tissue has been totally destroyed, even if this has occurred via an immunologic mechanism, the thyroid microsomal antibody may be present in very low titer. In most patients with Hashimoto's disease, there is a rough correlation between the extent of thyroid involvement and the antibody titer.

Radioisotope Procedures

The radioactive iodine uptake is becoming considerably less important as an index of thyroid function for two reasons. First, the specific tests for serum thyroid hormones and TSH now available have limited its utility. The uptake result will generally add very little to what is already known about thyroid status on the basis of these tests. Second, the uptake may be spuriously reduced, owing to the presence of iodinated contrast material or increased iodine in the diet. Its major uses are to identify the thyroid gland as the source of elevated serum thyroid hormone levels when this is in question and to differentiate hyperthyroidism due to Graves' disease from that associated with subacute thyroiditis. The "normal" result for the 24-hour radioactive iodine uptake is from 0 (in a patient ingesting iodide) to as high as 30%. The reason for the absence of a lower limit is the frequency with which excess iodine is now encountered in the population.

The most common reason for performing a thyroid scintiscan is to ascertain whether nodular enlargement of the thyroid represents a functioning or nonfunctioning lesion. The nodule should be outlined by palpation prior to scanning because the scan cannot delineate the extent of a nodule at the periphery or near the isthmus of the thyroid. The choice of scanning technique and agent usually is a function of the current practice in the local nuclear medicine department. The most sensitive technique for evaluation of the possibility of a cold thyroid nodule is the pertechnetate scan using the gamma camera with pinhole collimator. This technique has the advantages of low radiation dose to the thyroid and resolution sufficient to allow recognition of small lesions (as small as 5 mm in diameter under ideal circumstances). The major disadvantage is that an occasional malignant nodule will concentrate pertechnetate but not iodine isotope (see further on).

In the patient with Graves' disease in whom there is an easily palpable, diffusely enlarged thyroid gland, the scan adds nothing to what is already known and is a needless expense. On the other hand, in the presence of hyperthyroidism in a patient in whom, for various reasons, palpation of the thyroid gland is not possible, localization of the increased uptake to a normally shaped thyroid gland in the neck provides worthwhile information.

Ultrasound

Ultrasonography of the thyroid is most useful in the patient with an apparently solitary nodule, in whom one can determine whether the nodule is solid, mixed (multiloculated), or cystic. Simple cystic lesions are the minority of thyroid nodules but can be treated by aspiration and often will not recur, thus saving the patient the risk and expense of a potential surgical procedure. In addition, the ultrasound may be used to document with precision the size of the thyroid lesion, so that its change with time and treatment can be reliably evaluated. A multiloculated cyst of the thyroid gland appears to have the same significance as a solid lesion; that is, it may be a malignant tumor. Ultrasound may also be used to guide needle placement during fine-needle aspirations.

Nonspecific Biochemical Abnormalities

In patients with hypothyroidism, the concentration of cholesterol and triglycerides may be elevated. In addition, the patient with severe hypothyroidism may have elevation in some circulating serum enzymes, including creatinine phosphokinase, lactic dehydrogenase, and serum glutamic-oxaloacetic transaminase. With therapy of hypothyroidism, these enzymatic abnormalities return rapidly to normal.

About 10% of patients with hyperthyroidism may have modest elevations in serum calcium levels. This appears to be associated with an elevation in unbound calcium and is presumably a function of elevated bone turnover. Similarly, a rise in alkaline phosphatase level is common and may be derived from either increased bone turnover or hepatic abnormalities. The concentration of direct bilirubin may also be slightly elevated in the severely thyrotoxic patient.

Mild anemia may occur in prolonged hypothyroidism or hyperthyroidism and is usually corrected with treatment of the thyroid. Hyponatremia is a rare manifestation of severe hypothyroidism, and hypothyroidism may be associated with the so-called serum-inappropriate antidiuretic hormone syndrome.

DIAGNOSIS AND TREATMENT

On the basis of the clinical examination and the measurements of thyroid function, it should be possible to group patients into one of several distinct categories. These categories are defined in terms of both the type of thyroid abnormality and the functional thyroid status. Table 44–4 depicts the general classification of patients with thyroid disease that will be used in this discussion. As is apparent from this table, any type of thyroid physical abnormality can be associated with any level of thyroid function. In fact, significant thyroid dysfunction may occur without any palpable thyroid abnormality. Although the classification in Table 44–4 is arbitrary, it provides a useful scheme for assessing ambulatory patients.

Abnormalities of Thyroid Size or Shape

Diffuse Goiter. The physician will often be able, on the basis of the clinical history, to suspect one category of thyroid dysfunction (Table 44–5). However, even if a clear distinction cannot be made, the presence of diffuse thyroid enlargement is indication for the basic studies of thyroid function. These tests should include a sensitive serum TSH as well as a serum T4 and THBR determination. Interpretation of the sensitive TSH results should be done with the clinician mindful of causes of a suppressed TSH presented in Table 43–3. If serum TSH is suppressed and the serum free T4 index is not elevated, then the patient may well have T3 thyrotoxicosis, and a serum T3 level should be determined as well. However, this determination is not usually necessary if the patient's diet has sufficient iodine. On the basis of these tests, a functional category can be assigned.

TABLE 44–4. CLASSIFICATION OF THYROID DISORDERS

I. Abnormalities in the size or shape of the thyroid gland
  A. Diffuse goiter
  B. Multinodular goiter
  C. Solitary or dominant nodule
    Patients with each of the above are further subdivided according to the level of thyroid function
II. Thyroid dysfunction without palpable thyroid abnormalities
  A. Hyperthyroidism
  B. Hypothyroidism
III. Evaluation of patients with a history of thyroidal radiation exposure

Diffuse Goiter with Hyperthyroidism (Graves' Disease). The clinical suspicion of hyperthyroidism is confirmed by finding an elevated estimated serum free T4 or T3. Over 95% of hyperthyroid patients with diffuse goiter have Graves' disease. The other major diagnosis that should be considered in such individuals is that of "painless" thyroiditis (subacute lymphocytic thyroiditis).[17] The latter should be suspected if hyperthyroidism is less than 2 months in duration and of abrupt onset. The thyroid may be minimally enlarged (or even normal) and either tender or painless. Occasionally, patients with Hashimoto's thyroiditis may present a similar picture, especially in the postpartum period.[18] The presence of these conditions can be confirmed by finding a low thyroidal ^{123}I uptake in association with elevated serum thyroid hormone concentrations. The hyperthyroidism of subacute thyroiditis is selflimited, requiring only symptomatic therapy with anti-inflammatory agents (salicylates or prednisone) and, rarely, β-adrenergic blockade.

Therapy of the patient with Graves' disease will depend on the severity of the symptoms. If the patient is severely ill, then immediate institution of treatment with antithyroid drugs is indicated. My choice of therapeutic agent in severely ill patients is propylthiouracil given at a dosage of from 450 to 750 mg/day, depending on the clinical severity of the patient's disease. This dosage is recommended because of its capacity to inhibit T4 to T3 conversion when given at high doses.[19, 20] The propylthiouracil is given in three doses, and a white blood count and differential determination are obtained at the start of therapy as a baseline. This is important because a rare patient (approximately 5/1000) will develop agranulocytosis, and it is important to know the basal neutrophil count, which may be slightly reduced in untreated Graves' disease. The patient is cautioned about the symptoms of agranulocytosis (infections), and no routine white blood count is obtained subsequently. The patient is seen 2 to 4 weeks after initiation of therapy, again depending on the clinical severity of the syndrome. Most patients will experience symptomatic relief within the first 2 weeks of the onset of effective antithyroid drug therapy.

The antithyroid drug methimazole (Tapazole) may also be used for initiation of treatment, and its dosage will vary from 15 to 60 mg, in divided dosages. This drug at this dosage is as effective as propylthiouracil in inhibiting thyroid hormone synthesis, but it does not inhibit peripheral conversion of T4 to T3 as does propylthiouracil.[19, 20]

In my experience, β-adrenergic blocking agents are not routinely necessary in the treatment of patients with hyperthyroidism. In addition to their potential for reducing cardiac output, their effect on pulse rate may confuse the clinician as to whether adequate inhibition of thyroid hormone synthesis has been achieved.

The effectiveness of antithyroid drug therapy is monitored both by the clinical symptomatology of the patient and by the serial T4 and T3 uptake tests. In general, an improvement in symptomatology is preceded by an appropriate decrease in the level of serum thyroid hormones. Most patients can be tapered to less than 450 mg/day of propylthiouracil after 2 to 3 months of therapy.

Once control of the acute symptoms of hyperthyroidism has been achieved, a decision must be made about what the long-term approach to treatment will be. The three major options are chronic antithyroid drug therapy, surgery, and radioactive ^{131}I therapy. The use of chronic anti-

TABLE 44–5. CHARACTERISTICS OF DIFFUSE GOITER

Clinical evaluation	Hypermetabolic	Normal	Hypometabolic
Results of:			
Total serum T4*	↑	N†	↓
T3 resin uptake	↑	N	↓
Estimated free T4 index	↑	N	↓
Total serum T3‡	(↑)	N	NI§
TSH	↓	N	↑
Thyroid functional status	Hyperthyroid	Euthyroid	Hypothyroid
Further diagnostic studies:			
TMA‖ (or ATA¶)	N or ↑	N or ↑	↑ (or N)
24-hr radioactive iodine uptake	↑ or ↓**	NI	NI
Thyroid scan	NI	NI	NI
Therapy	Antithyroid drugs: definitive therapy with ^{131}I or surgery	Observe (with or without T4 therapy) depending on TSH††	T4 therapy

*T4 = thyroxine.
†N = normal.
‡T3 = triiodothyronine.
§NI = not indicated.
‖TMA = thyroid microsomal (peroxidase) antibody.
¶ATA = antithyroglobulin antibody.
**Useful primarily when the question of subacute thyroiditis has been raised.
††TSH = thyroid-stimulating hormone.

thyroid drug therapy in patients with Graves' disease is based on previous studies of the natural history of this disease, which indicate that a certain proportion of patients with Graves' disease will undergo spontaneous remission within 6 to 18 months after initiation of antithyroid drug therapy. As far as is known, the antithyroid drug therapy itself does not influence the development of a remission but keeps the patient asymptomatic until a remission might occur. Studies in the last decade have suggested that in the United States the anticipated remission rate is somewhat lower than was observed 30 years ago.[21] These results suggest the possibility that only 10 to 15% of patients with Graves' disease will undergo spontaneous remission. Many thyroidologists are opting for earlier definitive therapy with radioactive iodine or surgery in such patients, particularly in the older age group. A recent study from Japan, however, raises the possibility that a therapeutic strategy combining methimazole and T4 for a period of 1 to 2 years, followed by sufficient T4 to suppress TSH, may lead to a higher fraction of remissions than occurs if TSH is allowed to return to its normal level.[22] The mechanism by which this result is obtained is not clear, and the study is being repeated in several clinics in the United States as of this writing. The only potential complication of continuing T4 in a patient with Graves' disease in remission is that if hyperthyroidism recurs, it may be more severe.

During the early long-term antithyroid drug therapy treatment period, the patient is seen every 4 to 8 weeks, and the clinical and biochemical thyroid status is monitored as outlined previously. In most patients receiving antithyroid drug therapy, monitoring the serum free T4 index is satisfactory. However, as treatment progresses, serum TSH should also be monitored. An index of satisfactory control of thyroid hormone production is an increase of serum TSH into the low-normal range. In most patients receiving antithyroid drug therapy, there is progressive depletion in thyroidal iodine, resulting in an increase of the ratio of T3 to T4 in thyroid gland secretion. As a result, a reduction of serum T4 to subnormal levels may be required before serum TSH returns to normal. In such patients, serum T3 should also be monitored. If the combination of antithyroid drug and T4 mentioned above is to be employed, the T4 should not be added until serum TSH becomes detectable. At this point, a replacement dose of T4 is added (see later discussion) and the combination of medications continued for a year's time, at which point the antithyroid drug is discontinued. If this approach is not taken, then it is reasonable to monitor serum TSH and adjust the antithyroid drug dose to maintain TSH in the normal range of 0.5 to 5 μU/ml. This therapy is continued at least 6 months or sometimes for 1 year, after which the patient may be evaluated for the presence of a spontaneous remission. Signs suggesting remission are a reduction in the requirement for antithyroid drug to extremely low levels or a decrease in the size of the thyroid gland.

When antithyroid drugs are discontinued, the patient should have thyroid tests repeated after approximately 4 weeks. In the patient who is not receiving T4, TSH can be monitored because a recurrence of hyperthyroidism will be preceded by a suppression of TSH. In the early phases of a relapse, serum T3 may become elevated while serum T4 is still normal because of the previous induction of intrathyroidal iodine deficiency by antithyroid drug therapy. If a relapse does not occur within the first few months of treatment, the patient may be followed at 3- to 6-month intervals. Usually, relapses will appear within the first 6 months after discontinuation of antithyroid drugs. Patients should be cautioned that the reappearance of symptoms indicates a need for reinstitution of treatment. If a relapse occurs, then a decision must be made as to whether radioactive iodine, surgery, or a second trial of antithyroid drugs is in order.

Thyroid Ablation. Two forms of ablative therapy are available, radioactive iodine (^{131}I) and surgery. Radioactive iodine has been in use since the late 1940s, and the only complication associated with this approach has been the high prevalence of hypothyroidism supervening at some time after therapy. Although this may occur in only 10 to 15% of patients in the first year following radioactive iodine therapy, as many as 80 to 90% will develop hypothyroidism by 20 years after treatment. In discussing treatment alternatives, this probability should be emphasized to the patient. Surgical treatment has the advantage of producing more rapid results and probably a lower incidence of hypothyroidism in the long-term follow-up. However, there are no extensive studies that establish this conclusively. Of course, the complications of recurrent laryngeal nerve injury and hypoparathyroidism, as well as the morbidity and rare surgical mortality, must be considered. The cost of surgical therapy is roughly 10 to 20 times that of radioactive iodine therapy.

In the female who anticipates pregnancy at some time in the future the potential for ovarian radiation needs to be considered because much of the administered radioiodine is excreted by the kidney. Recent estimates of the ovarian dose are approximately 3 rads/10 mCi administered dose, that is, about twice that received during radiographic contrast studies performed during an evaluation for infertility.[23] Unfortunately, we are not likely to have definitive answers to the possible genetic risk of the use of therapeutic ^{131}I in the near future, if ever. Therefore, the decision must be based on the incomplete data at hand. In my opinion, radioactive iodine is a safe and effective therapy for all nonpregnant patients over the age of 21. One stipulation is that the patients are advised to avoid pregnancy within 6 months of ^{131}I treatment to allow dissipation of any possible short-lived radiation effects.

Surgery is recommended for patients younger than 21 years in whom a remission does not appear within a year of onset of therapy or who are dissatisfied with, or unable to maintain, a chronic antithyroid drug program. Surgical therapy should be preceded by rendering the patient euthyroid, along with 10 days of iodide treatment (1 drop saturated solution of potassium iodide [SSKI] twice a day) to reduce the size of the thyroid gland further. The patient should have no symptoms of hyperthyroidism when surgery is undertaken. Following surgery, it is important to evaluate the patient both clinically and biochemically for the development of hypothyroidism, which can occur at any time after therapy.

Thyroid Storm. A patient in whom hyperthyroidism is accompanied by severe tachycardia, fever, abdominal pain, and disorientation, or in whom acute bacterial infection accompanies hyperthyroidism, may be said to have the clinical condition designated *thyroid storm.* Such patients should be hospitalized and treated vigorously with a combination of antithyroid drugs, iodides to inhibit release of thyroid hormones from the gland, and agents to block peripheral conversion of T4 to T3.[24] Because the oral cholecystographic agents iopanoic acid (Telepaque) and ipodate (Oragrafin) block conversion of T4 to T3 in humans, they may even be superior to propylthiouracil as inhibitors of peripheral conversion as well as providing a source of iodide.[25, 26] General supportive measures, such as cooling, steroid therapy, and reduction of fever with nonsalicylate, antipyretic agents, should be instituted. Salicylates should not be used because they displace T4 and T3 from TBG, thus raising free thyroid hormone levels even higher. β-adrenergic blocking agents are also indicated in most patients.

Pregnancy. Pregnancy is a common complicating condition in the hyperthyroid patient because both conditions have their peak incidence in young women. The principle of therapy of the pregnant hyperthyroid patient is to reduce antithyroid drug dosage to its absolute minimum. This reduction is necessary because the antithyroid drugs cross the placenta and may inhibit thyroid hormone synthesis in the fetus.[27] Accordingly, overdosage may be accompanied by the development of fetal goiter, which may, in turn, cause tracheal obstruction at the time of delivery. In addition, the possibility of fetal hypothyroidism needs to be considered.

In the management of pregnant patients, it is important that monthly visits and biochemical monitoring be maintained. Serum T4 and THBR as well as TSH should be monitored. The natural history of Graves' disease appears to be influenced by pregnancy. In the first trimester, thyroid stimulation by circulating immunoglobulin is highest. As pregnancy progresses, the intensity of this stimulation is reduced in the typical patient. Following delivery, there is often a rebound increase in circulating thyroid immunostimulators and an exacerbation of hyperthyroidism. Thus, a patient may require relatively larger doses of propylthiouracil in the first trimester, lower doses during the second, and may be able to discontinue the medication altogether in the third trimester. However, following delivery, the antithyroid drug will often need to be reinstituted if the patient is not nursing.

Propylthiouracil is used in preference to methimazole in pregnant patients because the latter drug crosses the placenta more readily. Iodide should never be given as long-term therapy to the pregnant hyperthyroid patient because the fetal thyroid is sometimes not able to adapt to high levels of plasma iodide, and a goiter in the fetus from iodine-induced inhibition of hormone synthesis may supervene.[28] A total propylthiouracil dosage of up to 400 mg/day is usually safe with respect to fetal thyroid function, but even this low dosage has been associated with the development of fetal goiter in a few patients.[27] If hyperthyroidism during pregnancy cannot be controlled with small amounts of propylthiouracil, then surgery is performed, usually in the second trimester. Preparation for surgery may include short-term (7–10 days) administration of iodides to decrease the vascularity of the thyroid gland. Such therapy offers no danger to the fetus and will facilitate the performance of the surgery.

In the medical treatment of pregnant hyperthyroid patients, I do not favor the combination of antithyroid drugs and T4 (or T3) supplementation. Maternal thyroid hormones do not cross the placenta in quantities adequate to supplant fetal thyroid function,[29] but administration of exogenous T4 to the mother may obscure the fact that the antithyroid drug dose is excessive. It is usually best to manage patients by monitoring maternal serum TSH levels, maintaining them in the slightly subnormal (0.2 to 0.5 μU/ml) range, but being especially cognizant of the progress of the pregnancy itself. Although desirable to achieve a completely euthyroid state, the goal of therapy during pregnancy is to minimize the risk of intrauterine hypothyroidism to the fetus. Therefore, the pulse, rate of weight gain, and fetal growth should be monitored in collaboration with an obstetrician. If both physicians are satisfied with the clinical progress of the pregnancy, then a small degree of chemical hyperthyroidism can be tolerated. Because TBG is elevated, the normal range for serum T4 and T3 is significantly higher during pregnancy.

Therapy of Exophthalmos with Graves' Disease. Fortunately, severe eye disease associated with Graves' disease is rare.[30] When exophthalmos does occur, it is often mild and self-limiting, not requiring aggressive therapy. However, patients with progressive exophthalmos should be evaluated and followed in conjunction with a thyroidologist and ophthalmologist because an increase in retro-orbital pressure can, on occasion, lead to optic atrophy and blindness. In general it is best not to attempt surgery for diplopia until such time as the orbital inflammation has stabilized or remitted for 3 years. Symptomatic treatment of periorbital swelling, which may occur during sleep, may be achieved by administration of a diuretic at bedtime and elevation of the head of the bed.

Diffuse Goiter Associated with the Euthyroid State. The presence of a diffuse goiter without functional abnormality usually indicates that the patient is in a presymptomatic phase of hyperthyroidism or hypothyroidism. The patient who is in the early phases of Graves' disease will usually have slight thyroid enlargement, high normal serum thyroid hormone concentrations, and a subnormal serum TSH level. A thyroid microsomal (peroxidase) antibody determination may be positive. If TSH concentrations are significantly reduced, then treatment for hyperthyroidism with low doses of antithyroid drugs should be instituted. A patient whose TSH is still in the normal range does not require treatment but should be followed up for the development of hyperthyroidism in the future. On the other hand, if thyroid hormone levels are in the low-normal range, the possibility of early Hashimoto's disease may be suspected, especially in the adolescent or young adult. In these situations, serum TSH levels may be found to be elevated, even though the serum T4 level is still within the normal range. Such patients should be treated with T4 as though they were hypothyroid, in anticipation of the development of frank hypothyroidism and possible further thyroid enlargement.

Diffuse Goiter in Association with Thyroid Hypofunction. Patients in this category usually have Hashimoto's disease, as evidenced by an elevated circulating titer of antimicrosomal or antithyroglobulin antibodies. The hypothyroidism may first become apparent in the postpartum period when it may be only transient.[18] Usually, however, Hashimoto's disease progresses inexorably to hypothyroidism at a variable rate.

Any patient with a low serum T4 not explained on the basis of TBG deficiency, phenytoin, or salicylates who does not also have an elevated TSH should be suspected of having pituitary or hypothalamic disease and evaluated accordingly. Measurement of the serum T3 level is not indicated in the hypothyroid patient because it is a poor discriminator between patients with normal thyroid function and those with compensated but clinically significant thyroid dysfunction.[26]

Treatment of the Hypothyroid Patient. In the past, hypothyroidism has been adequately treated with thyroid extract, with combinations of T4 and T3, and with T4 alone. Because the last is probably more physiologic in light of our present knowledge, it is my preference. Recent studies using sensitive TSH assays have indicated that an appropriate dose of T4 in most patients is approximately 0.7 μg/lb ideal body weight. Overdosage should be avoided because of the potential for accelerating bone turnover, leading to osteopenia.[31] This is especially important in women who will undergo lifelong therapy. The institution of therapy may begin with complete or with a subreplacement dosage. In elderly patients, those in whom there is any suspicion of coronary artery disease and those who have had longstanding, severe hypothyroidism, the initial dose should be 25 μg of T4 (see later discussion). After a period of 4 to 6 weeks, the dose can be doubled (assuming no adverse symptoms have appeared), with further adjustments made until TSH returns to normal and clinical euthyroidism has supervened. In the young, healthy patient, a complete replacement dose may be initiated immediately because even under these circumstances, serum T4 will not become normal for 4 to 6 weeks.

Serum T4 concentration should be in appropriate range for the serum TBG level. This is particularly important in pregnant patients or in those receiving oral contraceptives or estrogen. Furthermore, recent studies have established that during pregnancy there is usually an increased T4 requirement.[32] This need may appear as early as 6 to 8 weeks' gestation or not until the third trimester. For this reason, patients with hypothyroidism should be cautioned to notify their physician when they become pregnant so that monitoring of TSH can be instituted. The increase in the required dose is only about 50%, although it may be greater in some individuals. Following delivery, the T4 dosage should be returned to the prepregnancy level.

Patients receiving T4 should be monitored on an annual basis once a replacement dosage is determined. The T4 requirements are remarkably stable, with the exception of pregnant patients, as mentioned above, and in patients entering their eighth decade, in whom the dose should be reduced by about 25%. Thyroid replacement requirements in children are higher per pound of ideal body weight than adults, a fact that should be kept in mind in the adolescent patient.[3] The institution of therapy with carbamazepine (Tegretol) will increase thyroid hormone requirements because of an acceleration of T4 degradation. Amiodarone, which blocks the activation of T4 to T3, may have a similar effect. Rifampicin treatment has also been associated with an increase in thyroid hormone requirements. Cholestyramine and colestipol will block T4 absorption. The development of sprue or diabetic diarrhea can also impair T4 absorption. Any of these events occurring in the hypothyroid patient should lead to more careful and frequent monitoring of serum TSH to ensure that appropriate adjustments are made.

As mentioned, institution of therapy in the hypothyroid patient with coexistent coronary artery disease should be performed quite judiciously. Retrospective studies have suggested that hypothyroid patients with angina should be evaluated for surgically remediable coronary artery lesions before institution of treatment for hypothyroidism.[33] The reason for this is that some patients do not have sufficient myocardial blood flow to sustain the increases in cardiac output required in the euthyroid state. Other studies have shown that even in patients with moderately severe hypothyroidism, no unusual complications occur during surgery. Thus, therapeutic decisions in patients presenting with this constellation of symptoms should involve both cardiologic and endocrinologic consultation to weigh the risks and benefits of either approach.

Subclinical Hypothyroidism. In some patients, slight thyroid enlargement associated with a low-normal T4 and THBR levels but modest TSH elevation (5 to 10 μU/ml) is present. Carefully controlled studies show that treatment of such patients generally produces no clinical benefits.[34, 35] Nevertheless, the slight thyroid enlargement per se may be an indication for T4 replacement. In my experience, there are no clinical manifestations of hypothyroidism in patients in whom TSH concentrations are less than 10 μU/ml. If thyroid peroxidase antibodies are present, therapy should be instituted in anticipation that further deterioration of thyroid function will occur.

The Patient with Multinodular Goiter

Hyperthyroidism Due to Toxic Nodular Goiter. Multinodular goiter (Table 44–6) is the commonest thyroid abnormality and is usually associated with normal levels of thyroid function. However, occasionally hyperfunction supervenes in a patient with longstanding multinodular goiter (Plummer's disease), and special aspects of this form of hyperthyroidism need to be emphasized. The diagnosis of hyperthyroidism in such patients is made by measuring serum T4, THBR, and TSH levels. It is particularly important to remember that patients with this disease may have subtle manifestations of hyperthyroidism, or "apathetic or masked hyperthyroidism." If the free T4 index is normal and TSH is suppressed, serum T3 should be measured to establish the diagnosis because there is an increased inci-

TABLE 44–6. CHARACTERISTICS OF MULTINODULAR GOITER

Clinical evaluation	Hypermetabolic	Normal	Hypometabolic
Results of:			
Total serum T4*	↑	N†	↓
T3 resin uptake	↑	N	↓
Estimated free T4 index	↑	N	↓
Total serum T3‡	(↑)	N	NI§
TSH	↓	N or ↑	↑
Thyroid functional status	Hyperthyroid	Euthyroid	Hypothyroid
Further diagnostic studies:			
TMA‖ (or ATA¶)	N or ↑	N or ↑	N or ↑
24-hr radioactive iodine uptake	NI	NI	NI
Thyroid scan	Uptake by one or more nodules (occasionally diffuse uptake)	Uptake by one or more nodules (occasionally diffuse uptake)	NI
Therapy	Antithyroid drugs: ^{131}I or surgery	Observe with or without T4 therapy; surgery—if indicated from local symptoms and no response to T4	T4 therapy

*T4 = thyroxine.
†N = normal.
‡T3 = triiodothyronine.
§NI = not indicated.
‖TMA = thyroid microsomal (peroxidase) antibody.
¶ATA = antithyroglobulin antibody.

dence of suppressed TSH in elderly patients who have apparently normal thyroid function.[36] A thyroid scan should be obtained to document the cause of the hyperthyroidism if this is present. Patients should then be treated with antithyroid drugs to achieve a euthyroid state followed by definitive therapy with radioiodine. It is important that patients be rendered euthyroid prior to radioiodine therapy to avoid the rare circumstance of radioiodine inducing a release of thyroid hormone, which can exacerbate cardiac or other symptoms of hyperthyroidism. The dose of radioiodine required for such patients is usually about twice that needed for patients with Graves' disease because the distribution of radioisotope in the nodular thyroid gland is often heterogeneous. Such patients should then be followed regularly after treatment to detect the development of hypothyroidism. Surgical treatment for the patient with toxic nodular goiter is indicated if there is physical obstruction to breathing or swallowing or if the thyroid gland is so enlarged that it causes a severe cosmetic abnormality.

Multinodular Goiter in the Euthyroid Patient. This is a relatively common condition, particularly in women over the age of 60 years. Its etiology is still unknown, but many studies have suggested that the presence of mild abnormalities in thyroid hormone synthesis leads to chronic low-grade TSH hyperstimulation.[37] With prolonged low-grade TSH stimulation, thyroid nodules become autonomous, and the patient develops a fixed (autonomous) but normal level of thyroid function. As with the other forms of thyroid enlargement, serum T4, THBR, and TSH will dictate the proper course of therapy. If TSH is suppressed, radioiodine treatment is usually given. On the other hand, low-normal thyroid function test results may indicate the presence of hypothyroidism, which is sometimes associated with Hashimoto's thyroiditis. In such patients, assuming thyroid function is not autonomous, prophylactic T4 replacement is indicated to reduce TSH to normal and prevent further thyroid enlargement. During treatment, patients should be monitored with yearly serum T4 and TSH determinations to ascertain that thyroid autonomy has not developed during suppressive treatment. Iodide should not be administered to patients with nontoxic nodular goiters because it may induce clinical hyperthyroidism. If the thyroid gland is sufficiently enlarged as to cause physical symptoms or tracheal compromise, surgical therapy may be indicated. This should be followed by permanent T4 replacement.

Multinodular Goiter with Hypothyroidism. This condition is uncommon but may supervene in patients with combined multinodular goiter and Hashimoto's thyroiditis. The latter is usually revealed by the presence of antimicrosomal antibodies, and treatment of the hypothyroidism is the same as has been previously described. Some decrease in thyroid size may be anticipated, and thyroid replacement should be employed before resorting to surgery for an enlarged thyroid gland.

Patient with a Solitary or Dominant Thyroid Nodule

Solitary Nodule Associated with Hyperthyroidism. Most solitary thyroid nodules are follicular adenomas (Table 44–7). These have usually lost the capacity to transport iodide and therefore are nonfunctional in terms of their ability to synthesize thyroid hormone, despite the presence of other biochemical characteristics that are typical of normal thyroid tissue. However, if the nodule does retain its ability to trap iodine, hyperthyroidism may occur. The size of the thyroid nodule may be of some value in determining whether hyperthyroidism is likely. If the nodule is greater than 4 cm in diameter and is functional, hyperthyroidism is often present. Hyperthyroidism also is more often present if the patient is over the age of 60 years. When present, hyperthyroidism frequently is due to "T3 thyrotoxicosis," as was the case in 16 (25%) of 62 patients with toxic autonomously functioning thyroid nodules in one series.[38] Antithyroid drugs may be necessary to render the patient euthyroid before definitive therapy is undertaken.

Radioactive iodine is usually the treatment of choice in the older patient with a solitary toxic thyroid nodule. This is an ideal disease to treat with this agent because the radioactivity and consequent destruction are concentrated in the area of hyperfunction. On the other hand, in the

TABLE 44–7. CHARACTERISTICS OF SOLITARY OR DOMINANT THYROID NODULE

<table>
<tr><td>Clinical evaluation</td><td>Hypermetabolic</td><td>Normal</td><td>Hypometabolic</td></tr>
<tr><td>Radiation history</td><td>+* or −†</td><td>+ or −</td><td>+ or −</td></tr>
<tr><td>Results of:</td><td></td><td></td><td></td></tr>
<tr><td>Total serum T4‡</td><td>↑</td><td>N§</td><td>↓</td></tr>
<tr><td>T3|| resin uptake</td><td>↑</td><td>N</td><td>↓</td></tr>
<tr><td>Estimated free T4 index</td><td>↑</td><td>N</td><td>↓</td></tr>
<tr><td>Total serum T3</td><td>(↑)</td><td>N</td><td>NI¶</td></tr>
<tr><td>TSH**</td><td>↓</td><td>N</td><td>↑</td></tr>
<tr><td>Thyroid functional status</td><td>Hyperthyroid</td><td>Euthyroid</td><td>Hypothyroid</td></tr>
<tr><td>Further diagnostic studies:</td><td></td><td></td><td></td></tr>
<tr><td>TMA†† (or ATA‡‡)</td><td>N or ↑</td><td>N or ↑</td><td>N or ↑</td></tr>
<tr><td>24-hr radioactive iodine uptake</td><td>NI</td><td>NI</td><td>NI</td></tr>
<tr><td>Thyroid scan</td><td>Nodule is F§§</td><td>Nodule is
F ↓ or NF|||| (solid or cystic)</td><td>Nodule is
F ↓ or NF (solid or cystic)</td></tr>
<tr><td>Ultrasound</td><td>NI</td><td>F: NI
NF: solid or cystic</td><td>F: NI
NF: solid or cystic</td></tr>
<tr><td>Needle aspiration or biopsy</td><td>NI</td><td>F: NI
NF: solid +, cystic +</td><td>F: NI
NF: solid +, cystic ±</td></tr>
<tr><td>Therapy</td><td>Antithyroid drugs; surgery or radioactive iodine</td><td>Individualized therapy</td><td>T4 therapy</td></tr>
</table>

*+ = yes.
†− = no.
‡T4 = thyroxine.
§N = normal.
||T3 = triiodothyronine.
¶NI = not indicated.
**TSH = thyroid-stimulating hormone.
††TMA = thyroid microsomal (peroxidase) antibody.
‡‡ATA = antithyroglobulin antibody.
§§F = functioning.
||||NF = not functioning.

younger patient whose thyroid nodule is particularly large, this is a disadvantage because irradiation of the extranodular tissue may reach levels that are associated with the propensity for future malignancy. In patients under 21 years of age, such nodules should be excised surgically after rendering the patient euthyroid.

Normal thyroid function may follow therapy owing to the re-establishment of function in the previously suppressed area of the thyroid gland. If this does not occur, then T4 replacement therapy is required. In the young patient undergoing surgery, inspection of the remainder of the thyroid gland should be performed at the time of surgery. If inspection shows normal tissue and only a portion of a thyroid lobe has been removed, then T4 therapy is usually not necessary. On the other hand, if there is a suggestion of additional underlying thyroid disease or the presence of Hashimoto's disease, then T4 should be administered.

Solitary or Dominant Nodule in a Euthyroid Patient. If a patient with a solitary or dominant nodule proves to have a normal free T4 index and TSH level, then an evaluation for the possibility of thyroid malignancy must be performed. Malignancy may be present in anywhere from 5 to 8% of such patients. Historical factors pointing to an increased risk of malignancy are a family history of thyroid tumors, particularly medullary carcinoma, a history of prior exposure of the thyroid to irradiation in infancy or childhood, or a rapid change in the size of the thyroid nodule. In patients with a family history of medullary carcinoma, the diagnosis of multiple–endocrine neoplasia type IIA or B should be considered and a serum calcitonin measurement obtained. If this is elevated, the patient should be evaluated for the presence of hyperparathyroidism (see Chapter 45) or pheochromocytoma (see Chapter 10). Subsequent referral to a surgeon for definitive therapy follows.

In patients with a thyroid nodule and a history of external neck irradiation in childhood, the risk of thyroid malignancy is sufficiently high (on the order of 10 to 30%, depending on the dose of x-ray) that referral to a surgeon is also indicated.[5] Rapid enlargement of a thyroid nodule, particularly in an elderly patient, suggests the possibility of anaplastic carcinoma, which requires immediate intervention in hopes of obtaining a surgical cure. The development of a firm nodular lesion in a patient with pre-existing Hashimoto's thyroiditis suggests the possibility of lymphoma, and appropriate evaluation of the patient with eventual tissue confirmation of the diagnosis should be performed.[39]

The most cost-effective first test for the evaluation of a euthyroid patient with a solitary nodule is the fine-needle aspiration of the thyroid. Because this technique requires considerable skill both in performance and evaluation, such patients should be referred to a physician specializing in this procedure who has the advice of an experienced cytopathologist. About 5% of such nodules will be cystic and may not recur after needle aspiration. However, a cystic lesion does not eliminate the possibility of malignancy, and the clinician should not be falsely reassured by this finding. About 5 to 10% of thyroid needle aspirates will be found to be highly suggestive of malignancy, with the most common diagnosis that of papillary carcinoma. Surgical therapy is indicated for such individuals. In another 30%, the findings will suggest a follicular lesion, and no determination will be possible as to whether the lesion represents an adenoma or carcinoma. In general, the next step in such patients is to perform a thyroid scan using ^{123}I. If the nodule proves to be functional with respect to radioiodine, then the risk of a malignancy is virtually eliminated. Such patients may be followed up with radioiodine therapy if the nodule grows and particularly if the patient develops hyperthyroidism. If the nodule is not functioning, the patient should be referred for surgery for definitive diagnosis. A preoperative chest radiograph should be performed.

About 60% of thyroid aspirates are judged to be benign, colloid, or hyperplastic. These patients should have thyroid imaging. If the nodule is not functioning, a trial of TSH suppressive therapy is appropriate, and sufficient T4 should be administered to reduce the TSH level to between 0.2 and 0.4 μU/ml. Such patients are followed at 4-month intervals, with the option of repeating the fine-needle aspiration or excision if the nodule enlarges or fails to decrease in size. It should be recognized that fine-needle aspiration cytology can never completely eliminate the question of malignancy in a thyroid nodule. However, a benign cytologic result may, together with the rest of the clinical picture, reduce the statistical chance that malignancy is present to a level sufficiently low that surgery is not indicated. However, the patient should be advised of the remote possibility of malignancy so that his or her final decision regarding the therapeutic options is fully informed.

In centers lacking expertise in the evaluation of cytologic material obtained by fine-needle aspiration, a decision for surgery may be made in solid, nonfunctioning nodules, as judged by thyroid scintigraphy and ultrasonography, that do not become smaller during thyroid therapy to suppress TSH secretion. This approach leads to surgery in about 60 to 70% of patients with solitary nodules, as opposed to 40 to 50% using the fine-needle aspiration technique as a screening tool.

Solitary or Dominant Nodule in a Hypothyroid Patient. The presence of a thyroid nodule in a hypothyroid patient does not have the serious connotation that it does in a patient who is euthyroid. The hypothyroid patient obviously has thyroid disease. Often, the nodule is the only residual functioning thyroid tissue remaining, having hypertrophied in response to TSH. In such patients, serum T4 levels may be only modestly decreased, and the thyroid scan shows evidence of function only in the area corresponding to the thyroid nodule. With suppression of TSH, some decrease in the size of the nodule can be anticipated.

The nonfunctioning nodule in the patient with hypothyroidism may be somewhat difficult to evaluate because uptake in the thyroid will usually be very low under these circumstances. Therefore, the connotation of lack of function is not nearly what it is in the patient who is otherwise euthyroid. More anatomic information can be achieved by ultrasound. If this shows a cystic lesion and the patient has diffuse thyroid disease sufficient to cause hypothyroidism, no further diagnostic evaluation is indicated. If the nodule is solid, then a trial of T4 therapy is indicated. Because TSH is elevated, which could have stimulated growth of the nodule, this therapeutic trial is even more important than it is in the euthyroid subject. As with euthyroid patients, if the patient has a history of thyroid exposure to radiation, then the nodule should be treated as though it has a 30% chance of malignancy. Hypothyroidism does not protect against the development of thyroid malignancy under these circumstances.

Thyroid Dysfunction Without Palpable Thyroid Abnormalities

Hyperthyroidism. Rarely, the physician will encounter a patient who has symptoms and biochemical test results indicating the presence of thyroid hyperfunction but does not have a palpably abnormal thyroid. Four possibilities are to be considered in this situation: (1) Graves' disease with no thyroid enlargement, (2) subacute painless thyroiditis, (3) factitious exogenous thyroid hormone ingestion, and (4) ectopic hyperthyroidism, such as occurs in struma ovarii. Certainly the last possibility is most remote, and the reader is referred to more specialized texts for a discussion of this and other rare causes of hyperthyroidism.[24]

To differentiate between the remaining three possibilities, the most useful diagnostic test is a 24-hour radioactive iodine uptake with a thyroid scan. With hyperthyroidism due to Graves' disease, the uptake will be normal or elevated, and the gland will be normally situated in the neck. In the patient who has painless subacute thyroiditis with hyperthyroidism, thyroid uptake will be reduced, and no gland will be visible in the neck. A scan need not be performed in the postpartum patient, but she can be observed, as clinical hyperthyroidism will resolve with time.[18] In the patient who is taking exogenous thyroid hormone surreptitiously, the gland is small and the iodine uptake also is suppressed. To differentiate between painless thyroiditis and surreptitious exogenous thyroid hormone ingestion, serum thyroglobulin may be measured. If the patient is ingesting thyroid hormone, serum thyroglobulin is generally low. In subacute thyroiditis, serum thyroglobulin is elevated.

Antithyroid drug therapy is of no use in hyperthyroidism resulting from subacute thyroiditis, though β-adrenergic blocking agents can be used to alleviate symptoms; agents that block T4 to T3 conversion (see previous discussion) may be of use in the severely toxic patient; and salicylates or corticosteroids can relieve local pain.

Hypothyroidism. Patients commonly present with symptoms and biochemical tests suggesting hypothyroidism and have no palpable thyroid gland. This is especially common in older people, in whom Hashimoto's thyroiditis has progressed to complete destruction of the thyroid. Such patients should have confirmation of the diagnosis by measurement of serum TSH levels. Antimicrosomal and antithyroglobulin antibodies may be present, but not necessarily because their levels may decline after the thyroid tissue has been destroyed. Hypothyroidism without palpable thyroid tissue may also occur in the neonate and in postpartum women.

Patient with a History of Thyroidal Radiation Exposure

Because of the previously widespread use of irradiation to the face and neck in the treatment of various lesions, the physician occasionally is consulted by a patient who has been informed that as a child he or she had exposure of the thyroid gland to radiation. Such patients should have ultrasonography to determine if nodules are present. If one or more nodules greater than a 0.5 cm are detected, especially if not documented previously, then referral for surgery should be strongly considered. If no significant nodularity is present, then the patient should be followed. There is disagreement as to whether these patients should also receive TSH suppressive therapy.[40, 41] There is ample evidence in experimental models that the irradiated thyroid requires TSH to develop thyroid malignancies. It is also known that thyroid carcinoma cells contain TSH receptors and respond biochemically to TSH.[42] Therefore, it makes good theoretical sense to suppress TSH in patients who have a history of childhood thyroid irradiation, but no data have accumulated to show benefit from this approach. My current strategy is to inform the patient of the controversy regarding the issue and to recommend annual follow-up without TSH suppression using ultrasound to evaluate questionable lesions.

REFERENCES

1. Mortenson JD, Woolner LB, and Bennett WA: Gross and microscopic findings in clinically normal thyroid glands. J Clin Endocrinol Metab 15:1270, 1955.
2. Tunbridge WMG, Evered DC, Hall R, et al: The spectrum of thyroid disease in a community: The Whickham survey. Clin Endocrinol 7:481, 1977.
3. Fisher DA: Management of congenital hypothyroidism. J Clin Endocrinol Metab 72:523, 1991.
4. Davis PJ and Davis FB: Hyperthyroidism in patients over the age of 60 years. Clinical features in 85 patients. Medicine 53:161, 1974.
5. DeGroot LJ: Diagnostic approach and management of patients exposed to irradiation to the thyroid. J Clin Endocrinol Metab 69:925, 1989.
6. Klee GG and Hay ID: Assessment of sensitive thyrotropin assays for an expanded role in thyroid function testing: Proposed criteria for analytic performance and clinical utility. J Clin Endocrinol Metab 64:461, 1987.
7. Surks MI, Chopra IJ, Mariash CN, et al: American Thyroid Association guidelines for use of laboratory tests in thyroid disorders. JAMA 263:1529, 1990.
8. Larsen PR, Alexander NM, Chopra IJ, et al: Revised nomenclature for tests of thyroid hormones and thyroid-related proteins in serum. J Clin Endocrinol Metab 64:1089, 1987.
9. Ain KB, Mori Y, and Refetoff S: Reduced clearance rate of thyroxine-binding globulin (TBG) with increased sialylation: A mechanism for estrogen-induced elevation of serum TBG concentration. J Clin Endocrinol Metab 65:689, 1987.
10. Spratt DI, Pont A, Miller MB, et al: Hyperthyroxinemia in patients with acute psychiatric disorders. Am J Med 73:41, 1982.
11. Bouillon R, Naesens M, Van Assche FA, et al: Thyroid function in patients with hyperemesis gravidarum. Am J Obstet Gynecol 143:922, 1982.
12. Wiersinga WM, Endert E, Trip MD, and Verhaest-de Jong N: Immunoradiometric assay of thyrotropin in plasma: Its value in predicting response to thyroliberin stimulation and assessing thyroid function in amiodarone-treated patients. Clin Chem 32:433, 1986.
13. Larsen PR: Thyroid-pituitary interaction: Feedback regulation of thyrotropin secretion of thyroid hormones. N Engl J Med 306:23, 1982.
14. Docter R, Bos G, Krenning EP, et al: Inherited thyroxine excess: A serum abnormality due to an increased affinity for modified albumin. Clin Endocrinol 15:363, 1981.
15. Glinoer D, De Nayer P, Bourdoux P, et al: Regulation of maternal thyroid during pregnancy. J Clin Endocrinol Metab 71:276, 1990.
16. Portmann L, Fitch FW, Havran W, et al: Characterization of the thyroid microsomal antigen, and its relationship to thyroid peroxidase, using monoclonal antibodies. J Clin Invest 81:1217, 1988.
17. Woolf PD: Transient painless thyroiditis with hyperthyroidism: A variant of lymphocytic thyroiditis? Endocrine Rev 1:411, 1980.
18. Amino N, Mori H, Iwatani Y, et al: High prevalence of transient post-partum thyrotoxicosis and hypothyroidism. N Engl J Med 306:849, 1982.
19. Abuid J and Larsen PR: Triiodothyronine and thyroxine in hyperthyroidism: Comparison of the acute changes during therapy with antithyroid agents. J Clin Invest 54:201, 1974.
20. Laurberg P, Torring J, and Weeke J: A comparison of the effects of propylthiouracil and methimazole on circulating thyroid hormones and various measures of peripheral thyroid hormone effects in thyrotoxic patients. Acta Endocrinol 108:51, 1985.
21. Wartofsky L: Low remission after therapy for Graves' disease. Possible relation of dietary iodine with anti-thyroid therapy results. JAMA 226:1083, 1973.
22. Hashizume K, Ighikawa K, Sakurai A, et al: Administration of thyroxine in treated Graves' disease. N Engl J Med 324:947, 1991.
23. Robertson JS and Gorman CA: Gonadal radiation dose and its genetic significance in radioiodine therapy of hyperthyroidism. J Nucl Med 17:826, 1976.
24. Larsen PR and Ingbar SH: The thyroid gland. *In* Wilson JD, and Foster DW (eds): Williams Textbook of Endocrinology, 8th ed. Philadelphia, WB Saunders, 1992, pp 357–487.
25. Wu SY, Shyh TP, Chopra IJ, et al: Comparison of sodium ipodate (oragrafin) and propylthiouracil in early treatment of hyperthyroidism. J Clin Endocrinol Metab 54:630, 1982.
26. Larsen PR, Silva JE, and Kaplan MM: Relationships between circulating and intracellular thyroid hormones: Physiological and clinical implications. Endocrine Rev 2:87, 1981.
27. Cheron RG, Kaplan MM, Larsen PR, et al: Neonatal thyroid function after propylthiouracil therapy for maternal Graves' disease. N Engl J Med 304:525, 1981.
28. Fradkin JE, Wolff J: Iodide-induced thyrotoxicosis. Medicine 62:1, 1983.
29. Vulsma T, Gons MH, and de Vijlder JJM: Maternal-fetal transfer of thyroxine in congenital hypothyroidism due to a total organification defect or thyroid agenesis. N Engl J Med 321:13, 1989.
30. Jacobson DH and Gorman CA: Endocrine ophthalmopathy: Current ideas concerning etiology, pathogenesis and treatment. Endocrine Rev 5:200, 1984.
31. Stall GM, Harris S, Sokoll LJ, and Dawson-Hughes B: Accelerated bone loss in hypothyroid patients overtreated with L-thyroxine. Ann Intern Med 113:265, 1990.
32. Mandel SJ, Larsen PR, Seely EW, and Brent GA: Increased need for thyroxine during pregnancy in women with primary hypothyroidism. N Engl J Med 323:91, 1990.
33. Hay ID, Duick DS, Vlietstra RE, et al: Thyroxine therapy in hypothyroid patients undergoing coronary revascularization: A retrospective analysis. Ann Intern Med 95:456, 1981.
34. Nystrom E, Caidahl K, Fager G, et al: A double-blind crossover 12-month study of L-thyroxine treatment of women with "subclinical" hypothyroidism. Clin Endocrinol 29:63, 1988.
35. Cooper DS, Halpern R, Wood LC, et al: Thyroxine therapy in subclinical hypothyroidism. A double-blind, placebo-controlled trial. Ann Intern Med 101:18, 1984.
36. Sawin CT, Geller A, Kaplan MM, et al: Low serum thyrotropin (thyroid stimulating hormone) in older persons without hyperthyroidism. Arch Intern Med 151:165, 1991.
37. Peter HJ, Studer H, Forster R, et al: The pathogenesis of "hot" and "cold" follicles in multinodular goiters. J Clin Endocrinol Metab 55:941, 1982.
38. Hamburger JI: Evolution of toxicity in solitary nontoxic autonomously functioning thyroid nodules. J Clin Endocrinol Metab 50:1089, 1980.
39. Larsen PR: Thyroid lymphoma. Case records of the Massachusetts General Hospital. N Engl J Med 316:931, 1987.
40. Stockwell RM, Barry M, and Davidoff F: Managing thyroid abnormalities in adults exposed to upper body irradiation in childhood: A decision analysis. Should patients without palpable nodules be scanned and those with scan defects be subjected to subtotal thyroidectomy? J Clin Endocrinol Metab 58:804, 1984.
41. DeGroot LJ, Reilly M, Pinnameneni K, et al: Retrospective and prospective study of radiation-induced thyroid disease. Am J Med 74:852, 1983.
42. Field JB, Boom G, Chou MCY, et al: Effects of thyroid-stimulating hormone on human thyroid carcinoma and adjacent thyroid tissue. J Clin Endocrinol Metab 47:1052, 1978.

45

Hypercalcemia

THOMAS J. MOORE, MD
EDWARD M. BROWN, MD

In recent years, hypercalcemia has been recognized as a much more common problem than was previously suspected.[1, 2] The major factor contributing to our increased awareness has been the development of multichannel autoanalyzers that measure calcium levels as part of routine blood screening. The signs and symptoms of hypercalcemia are generally vague and nonspecific, and the differential diagnosis of this condition is broad and complex. Fortunately, because of the development of more discriminating laboratory methods, we are now able to assess the significance of an elevated calcium level and to diagnose and treat the underlying disorder in most patients.

Calcium Homeostasis

Calcium not only is important for skeletal integrity but also is vital for normal plasma membrane activity, nerve conduction, muscle contraction, enzymatic activity, coagulation, and hormone secretion.[3] As a result, mammals have developed a carefully controlled system of maintaining the total and ionized serum calcium levels within the narrow ranges of 8.5 to 10.5 mg/dl (2.1 to 2.6 mM) and 4.5 to 5.5 mg/dl (1.1 to 1.4 mM), respectively.

The normal human body contains approximately 1 to 2 kg of calcium, of which over 99% is stored in bone.[3] The average American diet provides 0.5 to 1 g/day of calcium. The percentage of ingested calcium actually absorbed into the circulation ranges from 25 to 75% and is regulated by vitamin D. Calcium losses occur through the kidneys and through secretion of calcium back into the gut lumen. The balance between calcium absorption, storage, and loss is regulated by parathyroid hormone, vitamin D, and calcitonin.[3]

Parathyroid Hormone

Like many peptide hormones, parathyroid hormone (PTH) is synthesized as a longer peptide (prepro-PTH) and is then shortened to an 84 amino acid peptide that is recognized as the major stored and secreted form of hormone.[4] The physiologic purpose of PTH is to maintain the circulating level of calcium, and the secretion of PTH is regulated by the serum calcium level: Low calcium stimulates and high calcium suppresses PTH secretion.[3] PTH affects the calcium level through direct and indirect actions on bone, kidney, and intestine. In bone, it increases mineral resorption by increasing the number and activity of osteoclastic cells, and inhibiting the bone-forming osteoblasts. This mobilizes calcium out of bone stores and into the circulation. In the kidney, PTH increases the distal tubular reabsorption of filtered calcium, decreasing calcium excretion. Finally, PTH indirectly promotes calcium absorption in the intestine by activating vitamin D (see further on). The actions of PTH on bone and kidney are mediated by intracellular second messengers, including 3′,5′ cyclic adenosine monophosphate (cAMP) and products of the hydrolysis of inositol phospholipids.

Vitamin D

Our current understanding of vitamin D suggests that this vitamin could also be called a hormone, since it is converted to a more active form by the body and this activation is under feedback control.[5] The vitamin D precursor, 7-dehydrocholesterol, is stored in the skin and can be converted by sunlight to vitamin D_3 (cholecalciferol).[6] Another form of vitamin D, D_2 or calciferol (formed by irradiation of yeast), is added to many milk and cereal products. In the body, both these vitamin D precursors are activated by a series of two hydroxylations (Fig. 45–1). The first step is 25-hydroxylation, which takes place in the liver. The extent of this conversion seems related to the amount of substrate available and is not under tight feedback control. The 25-hydroxy-vitamin D (25-OHD) is then 1-hydroxylated in the kidney to $1,25(OH)_2D$. It is now known that this is the active vitamin D metabolite. The 1-hydroxylation step is tightly controlled: PTH, low serum calcium and phosphate, and low $1,25(OH)_2D$ levels all stimulate 1-hydroxylation.[5] Sensitive and specific assays have been developed for both 25-OHD and $1,25(OH)_2D$. The 25-OHD, which circulates bound to an α-globulin vitamin D-binding protein, is the predominant form of vitamin D in the blood, and its levels fluctuate seasonally, being highest in late summer. The

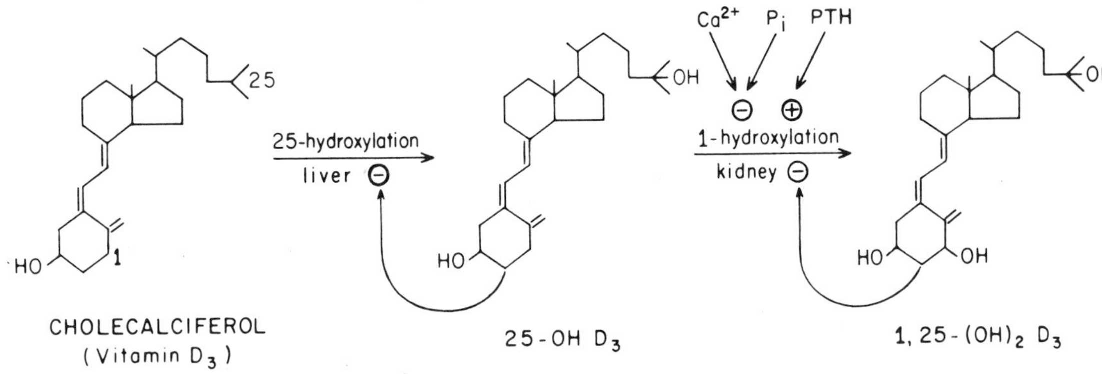

Ca2+ Pi PTH
25-hydroxylation
liver ⊖
1-hydroxylation
kidney ⊖
CHOLECALCIFEROL (Vitamin D_3)
25-OH D_3
1, 25-$(OH)_2$ D_3

FIGURE 45–1. Steps in the activation of the "hormone" vitamin D.

normal range is 10 to 55 ng/ml in the serum. The $1,25(OH)_2D$ assays remain technically difficult but are now available through several commercial laboratories. Normal levels are 20 to 60 pg/ml and do not vary seasonally. For clinical purposes, a 25-OHD determination gives an excellent indication of vitamin D deficiency or excess.[5, 7]

The physiologic function of vitamin D is to elevate serum calcium and phosphate levels. The main mechanism for this is through $1,25(OH)_2D$-mediated stimulation of intestinal calcium and phosphate absorption.[5] Although $1,25(OH)_2$ vitamin D does enhance the synthesis of the osteoblast-specific protein, osteocalcin, suggesting the possibility of direct regulation of bone formation, vitamin D, either alone or in concert with PTH, promotes calcium resorption from bone.[5] However, since the mineralization of bone matrix depends ultimately on circulating calcium and phosphate concentrations, the predominant effect of the intestinal and bone-resorbing actions of vitamin D is to contribute indirectly to bone formation by maintaining adequate circulating concentrations of these ions. Vitamin D also promotes calcium and phosphate reabsorption from the renal tubular filtrate, but the physiologic importance of this action is uncertain.

Calcitonin

Calcitonin is a 34 amino acid peptide produced by the parafollicular or C cells of the thyroid gland.[8] It is a potent hypocalcemic agent in some species (e.g., the rat) that acts by reducing bone resorption and by increasing renal calcium excretion, but its actions in normal adult humans are modest at best. For example, in states of calcitonin excess (medullary thyroid carcinoma) or deficiency (total thyroidectomy), calcium and bone homeostasis remain essentially normal. Currently, the principal clinical use of calcitonin is to decrease osteoclastic activity in states of increased bone turnover, including Paget's disease, hypercalcemia, and some forms of osteoporosis.[8]

HYPERCALCEMIA

Hypercalcemia results from excessive movement of calcium into the extracellular fluid from bone and intestine for which there is not adequate compensation by renal calcium excretion. Most causes of hypercalcemia mobilize calcium from bone, while excessive ingestion of calcium as well as the various forms of vitamin D excess (both endogenous and exogenous) increase gastrointestinal absorption of calcium. A few causes of hypercalcemia enhance renal tubular reabsorption of calcium *directly* (e.g., primary hyperparathyroidism, familial hypocalciuric hypercalcemia, thiazides, or therapy with lithium), whereas in most causes, dehydration and the effects of hypercalcemia per se on glomerular filtration rate and renal tubular function limit calcium excretion.

The finding of an elevated calcium level, therefore, may signal underlying disease, but several factors can cause false elevations of the serum calcium level and should be ruled out. Most laboratories define the normal range for an assay as the mean value ± 2 standard deviations for a group of subjects without known disease (the 95% confidence limits). Thus, by definition, 2.5% of subjects are expected to have calcium levels above the normal range. Many such subjects will have calcium levels within the accepted normal range if determinations of their levels are repeated. In addition, when these normal subjects do have elevated calcium levels, they are minimal elevations (usually less than 0.4 mg/dl outside the normal range), so that the farther above the normal range, the more likely it becomes that a pathologic cause for the hypercalcemia exists.

Serum protein levels must also be considered in evaluating the serum calcium level. Calcium in the blood is present in both bound and unbound form. Half of the total circulating calcium is bound to albumin and to a lesser extent globulins; a very small percentage is bound to anions (citrate and phosphate). The other half circulates unbound as ionized calcium. It is this ionized fraction that is available for the metabolic and other needs of cells and is carefully monitored and regulated by the factors involved in calcium homeostasis. Routine serum calcium assays measure both bound and unbound forms of calcium. As a result, elevated albumin or globulin concentrations may raise the total serum calcium level while the ionized fraction remains normal. In rare individuals with multiple myeloma, a calcium-binding immunoglobulin is produced that elevates total but not ionized calcium levels. In addition, prolonged tourniquet-induced venous stasis can cause hemoconcentration and increase plasma protein concentrations with consequent elevated calcium levels. Conversely, a truly elevated calcium level can be falsely lowered into the normal range in states of hypoproteinemia. Measurement of the actual ionized serum calcium level would clarify these problems, but ionized calcium assays are not routinely available. A rough correction of the calcium level for abnormalities in albumin can be calculated by allowing 0.8 mg/dl of calcium for every 1.0 g abnormality in albumin level. However, hypoalbuminemia is much more common than elevated albumin levels and thus, on this basis, spurious "hypocalcemia" is much more common than "hypercalcemia."

TABLE 45–1. MANIFESTATIONS OF HYPERCALCEMIA

Central Nervous System: Lassitude, easy fatigability, poor memory, depression, obtundation, coma
Ophthalmic: Band keratopathy
Cardiovascular: Hypertension
Digestive: Anorexia, nausea, vomiting, constipation, ulcers, pancreatitis
Genitourinary: Renal stones, nephrocalcinosis, decreased urine-concentrating capacity, renal insufficiency
Muscular: Weakness (especially proximal)
Skeletal: Osteoporosis, fractures, bone pain, brown tumors, bone cysts
Joints: Pseudogout

Manifestations

Making a clinical diagnosis of hypercalcemia is often difficult because of the vague, nonspecific nature of the symptoms and the lack of findings on physical examination. The traditional triad of "bones, stones, and groans" is seldom seen now that most patients are diagnosed early in the course of their disease. However, even with early hypercalcemia there are several common symptoms (Table 45–1), and the diagnosis can frequently be suspected if several of these symptoms occur together.

The most frequent complaints of the hypercalcemic patient are weakness and easy fatigability.[9–11] Usually these are subjective symptoms, but occasionally objective proximal muscle weakness can be demonstrated. Mental changes are also common and are particularly evident in older individuals. The changes in part depend on the serum calcium level (especially common if above 13 mg/dl) and range from memory loss and difficulty in concentrating to depression and even to frank obtundation. Gastrointestinal symptoms are also frequent and include anorexia—frequently with weight loss (suggestive of underlying malignancy)—vomiting, constipation, and symptoms of pancreatitis. Ulcer disease may be more prevalent in hypercalcemic patients, perhaps because of hypercalcemia-induced gastrin release and increased gastric acid output. The mechanism causing the pancreatitis is not clear. Renal stones are related to the amount of hypercalciuria and occur in 30 to 40% of patients with hyperparathyroidism in some series.[9–11] Polyuria and nocturia may be seen because hypercalcemia impairs maximum urinary concentration. Bone pain, gout, and pseudogout have also been associated with hypercalcemia (especially hyperparathyroidism).

On physical examination, the only finding directly related to hypercalcemia is corneal band keratopathy, seen as gray or white calcium deposits in the superficial layers of the cornea that are usually first observed near the limbus at 3 and 9 o'clock and, when severe, extend linearly across the cornea (Fig. 45–2). Band keratopathy, when grossly visible, is a late finding; more commonly it is seen only by slit-lamp examination. Hypertension seems to occur with increased frequency, either from hypercalcemia-related renal damage or from a direct action of calcium on vascular smooth muscle or perhaps other cells.

Differential Diagnosis

When hypercalcemia has been confirmed in the laboratory, several possible diagnoses must be considered (Table 45–2). The relative frequencies with which various disorders are encountered depends on how patients are selected. Among medical inpatients, malignant disease is the most common cause of hypercalcemia; in asymptomatic patients detected by outpatient screening, hyperparathyroidism accounts for over 90% of the pathology, and malignant disease for only 3 to 4%.[12]

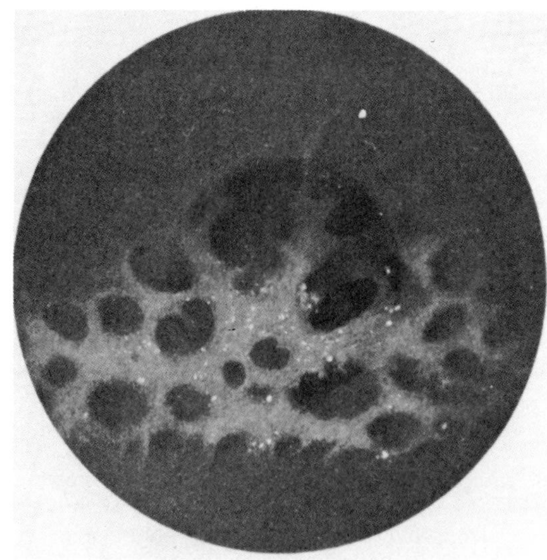

FIGURE 45–2. Unusually far-advanced hypercalcemic band keratopathy.

Hyperparathyroidism. In primary hyperparathyroidism, hypercalcemia is the result of excessive PTH secretion by one or more abnormal, enlarged parathyroid glands. The latter are generally less sensitive than normal to the suppressive effects of hypercalcemia on parathyroid function. A single parathyroid adenoma is present in 80 to 85% of cases, with hyperplasia involving all parathyroid glands in

TABLE 45–2. DIFFERENTIAL DIAGNOSIS OF HYPERCALCEMIA

- Hyperparathyroidism
  - Parathyroid adenoma (85%)
  - Parathyroid hyperplasia (15%)
  - Parathyroid carcinoma (<1%)
- Familial hypocalciuric hypercalcemia (FHH)
- Malignant diseases
  - Direct bone involvement
    - Localized (metastases)
    - Diffuse (multiple myeloma)
  - Production of humoral factors
    - PTH-related peptide (HHM)
    - Prostaglandin E_2
    - Cytokines
    - Ectopic PTH
- Thiazide diuretics
- Vitamin D excess
  - Exogenous
  - Endogenous
    - Sarcoidosis and other granulomatous diseases
    - Some lymphomas (especially adult T cell)
- Adrenal insufficiency
- Thyrotoxicosis
- Paget's disease and immobilization
- Milk-alkali syndrome
- Miscellaneous possible causes
  - Acromegaly
  - Hypothyroidism
  - Vitamin A intoxication
  - Pheochromocytoma
  - Lithium therapy
  - Postrenal transplant
- Theophylline administration

approximately 15% and parathyroid carcinoma in less than 1%. Occasional patients may have two or even three adenomas. Parathyroid hyperplasia is seen most commonly in families with multiple endocrine neoplasia (MEN) syndromes but may also be seen as isolated familial parathyroid hyperplasia or sporadically in individual patients. Most affected members of families with MEN I develop primary hyperparathyroidism, whereas a smaller fraction develop islet cell tumors of the pancreas (about a third) or pituitary tumors (15%). Families with MEN II syndrome have medullary carcinoma of the thyroid, pheochromocytomas, and parathyroid hyperplasia. In some cases, the parathyroid hyperplasia may be markedly asymmetric, and the possibility of MEN should be considered in any patient with primary hyperparathyroidism. If a diagnosis of MEN II is made, provocative testing to evaluate for the possible presence of medullary carcinoma of the thyroid should be carried out using infusion of pentagastrin as described in standard texts.[10, 11]

Most enlarged parathyroid glands, including those in MEN I, are probably monoclonal (i.e., arising from a single abnormal cell), due to mutations in one or more genes involved in the control of parathyroid cellular function.[13, 14] About two thirds of parathyroid tumors from MEN I and one quarter of parathyroid adenomas show allelic losses from regions of chromosome 11 that may encode a growth suppressor gene. An additional small fraction of adenomas (<10%) have a separate chromosomal rearrangement involving chromosome 11, which involves a gene (prad 1) likely involved in cell cycle control.[15]

The use of multichannel autoanalyzers in the outpatient setting has dramatically increased the apparent prevalence of primary hyperparathyroidism.[2] Rather than being a rare condition with severe hypercalcemia and far advanced clinical sequellae, such as recurrent nephrolithiasis and severe hyperparathyroid bone disease, primary hyperparathyroidism in the modern day is a much milder condition with a prevalence of 1:1000 in most series and as high as 4:1000 in Sweden. Like most endocrine diseases, primary hyperparathyroidism is more common in women than in men (2:1). It usually appears between the fourth and sixth decades and is rarely seen in childhood, except in affected members of MEN kindreds.

Only 10 to 20% of hyperparathyroid individuals have nephrolithiasis or classical parathyroid bone disease (osteitis fibrosa cystica). Some patients also have signs, symptoms, or complications regarded as specifically related to hyperparathyroidism or hypercalcemia in general, including peptic ulcer disease, pancreatitis, gout, pseudogout, or diminished renal function. The frequency of these conditions is relatively low in modern series, however, and not necessarily clearly higher than that in the general population. Most patients with primary hyperparathyroidism have no symptoms or less specific manifestations such as fatigue, muscular weakness, constipation, nocturia, depression, or other psychiatric symptoms. Whereas the latter are common in the population at risk for primary hyperparathyroidism, these symptoms do improve following surgery in a variable number of patients, suggesting a causal link to the disease in at least some patients. Studies have also focused on possible cardiovascular complications of primary hyperparathyroidism. Hypertension is present with an increased prevalence (as high as 50%) in many (although not all) series. This elevated blood pressure may normalize following successful parathyroidectomy but often does not. Studies from Sweden have raised the possibility of an excessive cardiovascular mortality in hyperparathyroid individuals, perhaps caused by hypertension or other cardiovascular complications of chronically elevated levels of serum calcium or PTH.[16] Even asymptomatic patients with primary hyperparathyroidism may have undergone excessive loss of bone mass, generally cortical in excess of trabecular bone, which potentially puts them at risk of fracture.[17] Studies suggest that in patients with mild primary hyperparathyroidism, particularly postmenopausal women, spinal bone density is reduced by 5 to 10% and cortical bone density by 10 to 20% relative to age-matched controls. The extent to which the prevalence of fracture is increased in this population is not known with certainty, but there is probably a modest increase in fracture risk in hyperparathyroid patients in the United States. Following successful parathyroidectomy, bone density improves but does not normalize.[18]

Laboratory findings in most patients with primary hyperparathyroidism reflect the mild clinical presentation of the disorder.[2, 9–11] Hypercalcemia is mild (often 1 mg/dl above the upper limit of normal for total calcium). In patients with very mild or intermittent hypercalcemia, the measurement of serum ionized calcium may permit a diagnosis to be made with greater confidence, but determination of total calcium generally suffices. Serum phosphorus is usually in the lower half of the normal range, and frank hypophosphatemia is uncommon. An elevation in alkaline phosphatase of skeletal origin is unusual but may be seen in the occasional patient with overt osteitis fibrosa cystica. The measurement of the osteoblast-specific protein, osteocalcin, is another marker of the increase in skeletal turnover, which is nearly universal in patients with primary hyperparathyroidism but is not clinically indicated in most cases. Electrolytes and renal function are generally normal, and most patients do not show a clearcut reduction in serum chloride concentration.

Bone radiographs may show the classic changes of subperiosteal bone resorption in the occasional patient with overt hyperparathyroid bone disease, but in most cases they are normal or may show diffuse osteopenia (Fig. 45–3). The determination of bone mineral density has become an important part of the evaluation and therapy of the

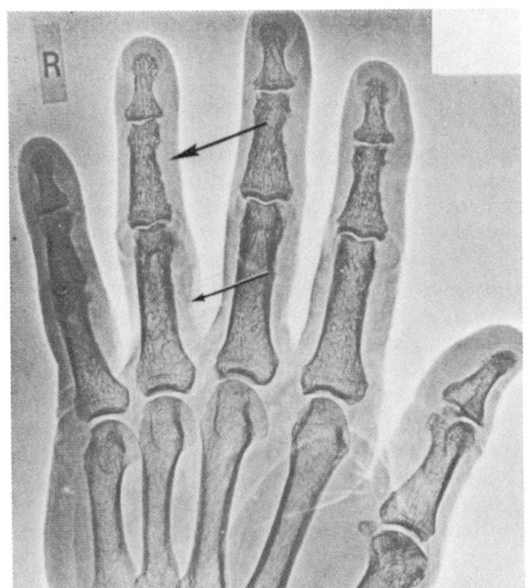

FIGURE 45–3. Subperiosteal bone resorption in the hand of a patient with hyperparathyroidism. The large arrow indicates the characteristic, irregular cortical margin; the small arrow indicates the normal cortical appearance for comparison.

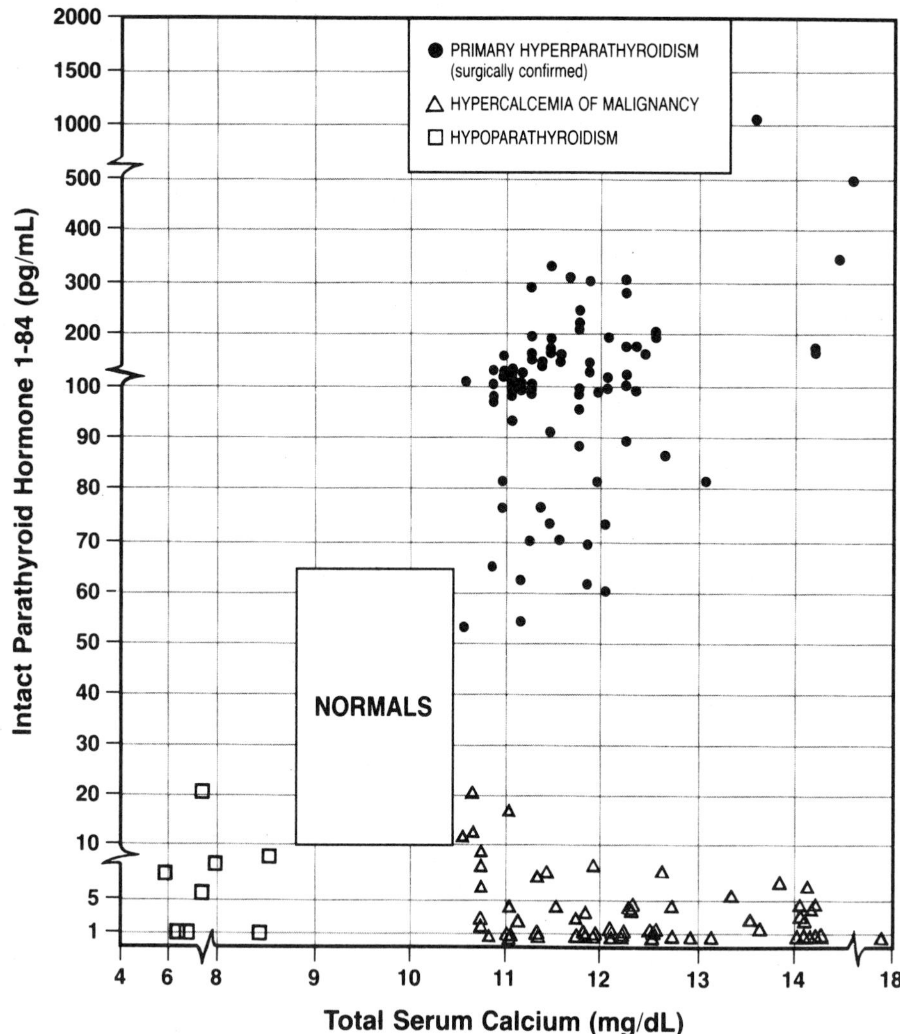

FIGURE 45–4. Nomogram showing the relationship between total serum calcium concentration and serum intact parathormone (PTH) measured using an immunoradiometric assay. Note the excellent separation between the levels of intact PTH in patients with primary hyperparathyroidism and those with hypercalcemia of malignancy. In addition, most patients with idiopathic hypoparathyroidism have frankly low values of intact PTH that in many cases are within the sensitivity range of the assay (>1 pg/ml). (Courtesy of Nichols Institute Diagnostics.)

hyperparathyroid patient.[17] This is particularly true in individuals at risk for bone loss for other reasons, such as postmenopausal women. Although the optimal skeletal site for determining bone density is controversial, a site(s) rich in cortical bone is preferred (e.g., the radius or proximal femur). Because of the significant morbidity and even mortality associated with hip fracture, the measurement of the latter may provide information that is important in the management of older hyperparathyroid individuals.

The development of highly sensitive and specific immunoradiometric and immunochemiluminescent "sandwich" assays for PTH has greatly simplified the assessment of parathyroid activity in primary hyperparathyroidism and other hypercalcemic conditions.[19] Such assays detect only intact, largely bioactive PTH by virtue of utilizing two different antibodies directed at the two ends of the molecule. In one such assay,[19] an antiserum directed at the carboxy terminal half of the molecule is attached to a plastic bead, while a second iodinated antiserum that binds to the amino terminus is in a soluble form. Only the intact PTH molecule will crosslink the labelled, soluble antiserum to the bead. Such assays, for the first time, readily measure a wide range of values for PTH from grossly elevated ones (1500 pg/ml) to the lower limit of the normal range for PTH (10 to 65 pg/ml) and even into the range of PTH values seen in overtly hypoparathyroid individuals (e.g., 1 to 10 pg/ml) (Fig. 45–4).[19] More than 90% of patients with primary hyperparathyroidism have frankly elevated levels, whereas individuals with essentially all other forms of hypercalcemia except familial hypocalciuric hypercalcemia (FHH) (see later) and the rare hypercalcemia of malignancy due to ectopic production of authentic intact PTH have frankly suppressed PTH levels (<10 pg/ml).[20] Not surprisingly, these improved assays have largely replaced not only all of the indirect measures of parathyroid function (e.g., tubular reabsorption of phosphate, serum chloride) but also more specific indices such as urinary cAMP excretion and the other less specific, single antibody assays employed previously for diagnosing hyperparathyrodism (e.g., C-, N-, and midmolecule PTH assays). A major advantage of the intact assays over the older C- and midmolecule assays is the relatively minor effect of renal dysfunction on the clearance of intact PTH. Thus, elevated levels of intact PTH in the presence of chronic renal insufficiency generally reflect true secondary hyperparathyroidism.

Much has been written about so-called "normocalcemic" hyperparathyroidism. This condition, characterized by a normal serum calcium value and an elevated PTH level, is probably quite rare. In most instances, if the calcium is measured often enough, several definitely elevated values will be found. In some patients, associated conditions that tend to lower the serum calcium (e.g., hypoalbuminemia, vitamin D deficiency, hypothyroidism, or the use of calciuric diuretics) may keep the calcium in the normal range. The diagnosis should be suspected when hyperparathyroid-related problems, such as renal stones and osteoporosis, are seen in a normocalcemic patient. Normocalcemic hyperparathyroidism, which is a primary disorder of the parathyroid glands, should not be confused with secondary hyperparathyroidism (such as is seen in chronic renal insufficiency), in which the increase in PTH secretion is an attempt to raise a low serum calcium level into the normal range. In normocalcemic hyperparathyroidism, the serum calcium level is almost always at the upper limit of normal, and the level of serum ionized calcium may be frankly elevated.

Familial Hypocalciuric Hypercalcemia. FHH is transmitted as an autosomal dominant condition.[21] The clinical presentation resembles that of hyperparathyroidism in that the hypercalcemia is often mild and longstanding and associated with normal or slightly elevated PTH levels. The parathyroid glands from affected subjects generally show histologic evidence of only mild hyperplasia.[21] These subjects rarely develop renal stones, bone disease, or other complications of their hypercalcemia. Even removal of three and a half parathyroid glands (the usual surgical procedure for parathyroid hyperplasia) rarely corrects the hypercalcemia. The cause of this unusual syndrome ($<1\%$ as common as hyperparathyroidism) remains unclear, but the abnormal gene has been localized to chromosome 3.[22]

The diagnostic hallmarks of the disorder are mild to moderate hypercalcemia and relative *hypocalciuria* in the setting of autosomal dominantly inherited hypercalcemia in other affected family members. Urinary calcium excretion in these patients, despite their hypercalcemia, is very low (usually <100 mg/24 h) with the ratio of the clearance of calcium to that of creatinine being less than 0.01.[21] Because of the benign course of FHH and its poor response to parathyroidectomy, we recommend measuring 24-hour urinary calcium excretion in hypercalcemic patients who have a family history of hypercalcemia or in whom previous subtotal parathyroidectomy has failed to correct the hypercalcemia. If urinary calcium excretion and the urinary calcium to creatinine clearance ratio are low, FHH should be considered and family members screened for hypercalcemia, but most patients require no intervention to treat their hypercalcemia.

Malignant Disease. Currently, malignant disease is the second most common cause of hypercalcemia. The serum calcium level in malignant disease may be extremely high—levels of 15 to 20 mg/dl are not uncommon, whereas such levels are distinctly unusual in primary hyperparathyroidism. Two possible mechanisms are involved.[23] First, tumors can directly invade bone, releasing calcium into the circulation as bone is destroyed. This bone resorption may be mediated by local production of humoral factors such as prostaglandins or osteoclast-activating factor, produced either by the tumor cells or by lymphocytes and monocytes in the metastasis.[23] Breast cancer is the most common cause of hypercalcemia of this type. Hypercalcemia occurs in more than 30% of patients with advanced breast cancer and accounts for over 50% of all cases of malignancy-related hypercalcemia.

Hematologic malignancies (myeloma, lymphoma, and some leukemias) are also common causes of hypercalcemia. Myeloma cells and activated T and B lymphocytes release lymphokines, such as interleukins 1 α and β, interleukin-6, tumor necrosis factors α and β, and transforming growth factor α, that have osteoclast-activating activity.[24] Prostaglandins, especially PGE_2, can also stimulate bone resorption and have been implicated as causes of hypercalcemia in certain circumstances.[25] Some lymphomas, including adult T cell leukemia/lymphoma, are associated with hypercalcemia that is mediated by $1,25(OH)_2$ vitamin D[26] or PTH-related peptide (see later).

The second way that tumors can cause hypercalcemia is indirect, by producing a humoral factor that stimulates bone resorption without actual bone metastases, a syndrome now called humoral hypercalcemia of malignancy (HHM).[27, 28] It should be pointed out that the presence of skeletal metastases does not rule out this form of hypercalcemia. Many patients with solid tumors metastatic to bone have hypercalcemia in which a humoral mediator plays a dominant role, and HHM is now thought to be the most common mechanism underlying hypercalcemia in patients with solid tumors.

The most important humoral mediator of HHM is the so-called PTH-related peptide or PTHrP,[28] which is a particularly common mediator of the hypercalcemia produced by squamous cell cancers of the lung, head and neck, esophagus, and female genital tract, as well as renal cell carcinomas.[27] This tumor-derived peptide has predicted isoforms varying from 139 to 173 amino acids, arising from alternative splicing at the carboxy terminus, but it is not yet known which form(s) of the molecule are secreted by tumors. The similarity of PTHrP to PTH is limited to identity in eight of the first 13 amino acids at the N-terminus (Fig. 45–5). Nevertheless, the two peptides interact with classical PTH receptors in kidney and bone with remarkably similar potency. Circulating levels of PTHrP are low in normal subjects,[29] and the peptide is not thought to contribute to systemic calcium homeostasis under normal circumstances. Hypercalcemia results when production of PTHrP by a tumor raises the circulating levels of the peptide sufficiently to produce hypercalcemia, presumably mediated through PTH receptors. This produces a hypercalcemic syndrome characterized by elevated PTHrP levels, suppressed intact PTH, elevated urinary cAMP, and low or normal $1,25(OH)_2$ vitamin D levels.[27] It is quite possible that additional factors produced by the tumor contribute to the hypercalcemia and other features of this syndrome. For example, another tumor-derived factor inhibiting the 1-hydroxylation of vitamin D has been suggested as a possible cause of the generally low levels of $1,25(OH)_2$ vitamin D in this syndrome, despite the high circulating levels of PTH-like bioactivity. PTHrP is also produced by a number of normal tissues, including skin, pancreatic islets, stomach, adrenal glands, and lactating breast, but its role in normal physiology is poorly understood.[28]

Thiazide Diuretics. Thiazides decrease renal calcium excretion and may also increase bone resorption. Because of these effects, thiazides are being used to treat patients with idiopathic hypercalciuria as well as those with hypoparathyroidism (in an effort to raise serum calcium levels). When thiazides are given to a normal person, the decrease in renal calcium excretion may cause a transient elevation in the serum calcium level (rarely greater than 11.5 mg/dl). The serum calcium level usually returns to normal within 7 to 10 days[30] as the homeostatic controls of the serum calcium level adapt to the decreased calcium excretion. Thus, thiazides should be considered as a cause of hypercalcemia only when they have been recently started. However, if a patient for some reason has an increased bone turnover rate (e.g., Paget's disease, unsuspected bone me-

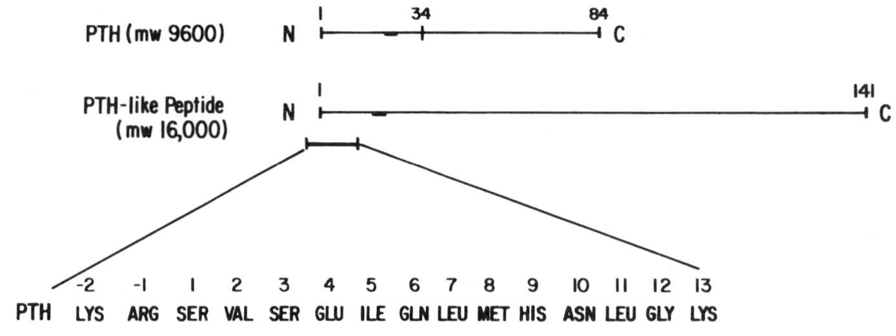

FIGURE 45–5. A schematic comparison of selected structural features of human parathormone (PTH) and PTHrP. The expanded areas show the only regions of aminio acid homology between the two proteins—identity in eight of 13 amino acids at the amino termini of both proteins (note that amino acids -1 and -2 are also identical but are cleaved off during processing of the mature proteins). (From Broadus AE, et al: Humoral hypercalcemia of cancer. Identification of a novel parathyroid hormone–like peptide. Published by permission from the New England Journal of Medicine 319:556, 1988.)

tastases), then thiazides may cause persistent hypercalcemia. Any patient with hypercalcemia who is on long-term thiazides should be evaluated for other causes of increased skeletal turnover.

Vitamin D Excess. Vitamin D excess may arise from either endogenous or exogenous sources. *Exogenous* vitamin D excess is most commonly encountered in hypocalcemic patients who are taking pharmacologic doses of vitamin D to maintain a normal serum calcium level (usually 50,000 to 100,000 units/day). The vitamin D metabolite causing hypercalcemia in this setting is likely to be 25-OHD, because 25-OHD serum levels are greatly elevated (often 5-fold or more), whereas the $1,25(OH)_2D$ levels range from low to slightly elevated. In addition, there have been clusters of cases of vitamin D excess in England in the 1950s and in Boston in 1991 due to excessive vitamin D fortification of milk.[31, 32] A hypercalcemic patient with a high serum vitamin D level but no obvious source of vitamin D should be evaluated by taking a careful dietary history and even analyzing the vitamin D content of any fortified nutrients. Since vitamin D is extensively stored in fat and has a slow turnover rate, hypercalcemia may persist for 1 to 2 months or even longer after vitamin D is discontinued.

Endogenous causes of vitamin D excess have only recently been recognized. This clinical situation was first recognized in patients with sarcoidosis who develop hypercalcemia with elevated $1,25(OH)_2D$ levels. This pattern has been observed in anephric patients with sarcoidosis, suggesting a nonrenal site for 1-α-hydroxylation of vitamin D. It is now known that macrophages, derived from granulomatous tissue or pulmonary alveoli, are capable of 1-hydroxylating 25-OHD.[33–35] The regulation of this enzyme is not the same as in the kidney: PTH does not stimulate macrophage 1-hydroxylation. The macrophage enzyme is also not regulated by phosphate but, unlike the enzyme in the kidney, is markedly inhibited by glucocorticoids. It is likely that macrophage activation of vitamin D is also responsible for hypercalcemia in other granulomatous disorders (e.g., coccioidomycosis, berylliosis).

Adrenal Insufficiency. Hypercalcemia may be seen in acute adrenal insufficiency, especially in children. The mechanism of this finding is unclear. Pharmacologic doses of glucocorticoids block intestinal calcium absorption via a direct effect on the mucosa in the proximal small bowel, and also reduce renal calcium reabsorption.[36] It has been speculated that the hypercalcemia of adrenal insufficiency is related to the absence of these glucocorticoid effects. In many cases, however, volume contraction also plays an important role, elevating total calcium concentration out of proportion to ionized calcium, which may be normal.

Thyrotoxicosis. Hypercalcemia may be seen in up to 25% of patients with hyperthyroidism; the prevalence may be as high as 50% if ionized calcium levels are measured.[37, 38] Hyperthyroidism increases bone turnover with osteoclastic activity outweighing osteoblastic activity. PTH levels are low. Hypercalciuria is common, resulting primarily from increased bone resorption. Renal phosphate reabsorption is increased in thyrotoxicosis with a tendency toward hyperphosphatemia. Hypercalcemia in this setting is usually mild but may occasionally reach levels of 15 mg/dl or greater.

Paget's Disease and Immobilization. Paget's disease is a combined osteoclastic-osteoblastic overactivity that is not usually associated with hypercalcemia. However, when a patient with active Paget's disease is immobilized (frequently because of some unrelated illness), hypercalcemia may develop. This is related to the decrease in osteoblastic activity, which occurs concomitantly with the decrease in physical activity. The net result is that osteoclastic activity becomes predominant and serum calcium levels increase. Immobilization-related hypercalcemia may also be seen without Paget's disease in conditions characterized by increased bone turnover, such as mild hyperparathyroidism, or in growing children.

Milk-Alkali Syndrome. In this syndrome, hypercalcemia develops in patients treated with large amounts of milk and absorbable antacids for peptic ulcer disease.[39] Characteristically, the serum calcium level rises within 1 week after therapy is begun, and patients complain of headache, nausea, and vomiting. If therapy is discontinued early, the serum calcium level usually returns promptly to normal, and renal function is preserved, but if therapy is prolonged, metastatic calcification, with nephrocalcinosis, renal insufficiency, and alkalosis, may result. The pathogenesis of the disorder is not clear, but the major factor is probably the massive calcium intake associated with the older ulcer treatment schedules. In addition to the milk, the antacids used in these patients contained calcium carbonate and daily calcium intake could reach 10 to 20 g/day. The associated alkalosis contributes to increased renal tubular calcium reabsorption as well as the development of nephrocalcinosis. This syndrome is rarely seen now that most antacids no longer contain calcium. A few antacids containing calcium carbonate are still in use, however (e.g., Tums, Alka-2, and Titralac) and calcium carbonate is also commonly used as a calcium suplement (e.g., to reduce bone loss), although seldom in high enough doses to produce hypercalcemia.

In addition, calcium carbonate is sometimes used as a phosphate binder in patients with renal insufficiency. These patients often have alterations in calcium metabolism (e.g., secondary hyperparathyroidism and variable 1-hydroxylation of vitamin D). Some of these patients become hypercalcemic when given calcium carbonate,[40] and serum calcium should be routinely monitored in this setting.

Other Causes of Hypercalcemia. Acromegaly, hypothyroidism, vitamin A intoxication, treatment with theophylline, pheochromocytoma, and the watery diarrhea, hypokalemia, achlorhydria (WDHA) syndrome have been reported to be associated at times with hypercalcemia. Pheochromocytoma can be associated with the MEN II syndrome but also possibly causes hypercalcemia in the absence of this syndrome. Hypercalcemia associated with lithium therapy has also been reported in 10 to 15% of patients receiving the drug. Lithium administration reduces urinary calcium excretion.[41] In vitro, lithium reduces the sensitivity of parathyroid cells to calcium, demanding a higher calcium level to suppress PTH secretion.[42] Thus, patients taking lithium may resemble those with mild hyperparathyroidism: hypercalcemia and high-normal PTH levels. The calcium level may normalize if lithium is discontinued in some patients, but others may, in fact, harbor a parathyroid adenoma. Mild hypercalcemia that slowly resolves has been described in postrenal transplant patients and is thought to be related to pre-existing parathyroid hyperplasia caused by uremia.

Approach to the Hypercalcemic Patient

Hypercalcemia is frequently discovered during routine blood screening in nonhospitalized patients, and the evaluation of these patients can be largely accomplished in an outpatient setting (Table 45–3). The degree of hypercalcemia is an important clue to the significance of the underlying problem. As has been mentioned earlier, minimal elevations in serum calcium (e.g., 10.5 to 10.9 mg/dl) may be seen in as many as 2.5% of normal subjects. The first step in evaluating these minimal calcium elevations is usually to repeat the level. Many normal subjects whose calcium levels fall at the upper end of the normal distribution will be found to have normal values when the test is repeated. The presence of hypercalcemia on repeated samples, even though the levels are only slightly elevated, suggests underlying pathology and requires further evaluation.

The work-up of hypercalcemia includes a careful history and physical examination to evaluate such possibilities as thiazide or lithium use, vitamin D or A abuse, thyrotoxicosis, adrenal insufficiency, the milk-alkali syndrome, or malignancy. Although hypercalcemia causes few demonstrable physical findings per se, careful examination may supply clues to an underlying malignancy, thyrotoxicosis, adrenal insufficiency, or sarcoidosis.

In addition to the history and physical examination, routine laboratory tests are sometimes helpful in the differential diagnosis. A low serum phosphate level suggests disorders in which there is an excess of a phosphaturic substance—either hyperparathyroidism, ectopic PTH, or PTHrP production by a tumor. An elevated bone-derived alkaline phosphatase level (heat labile) is seen in hyperparathyroidism, some malignancies, Paget's disease, and thyrotoxicosis, whereas an increased liver-derived alkaline phosphatase (heat stable) and other liver enzymes are more suggestive of malignancy or sarcoidosis. Although low-grade anemia may be seen with any cause of hypercalcemia, particularly with impaired renal function, a hematocrit of less than 30% in the absence of renal insufficiency or gastrointestinal bleeding suggests malignancy.

TABLE 45–3. APPROACH TO THE HYPERCALCEMIC PATIENT

A. History and physical examination
   1. History of thiazide use, vitamin D use, or milk-alkali syndrome
   2. Weakness, anorexia, weight loss, or other manifestations of malignancy, thyrotoxicosis, or adrenal insufficiency
   3. Physical findings suggesting sarcoidosis, thyrotoxicosis, adrenal insufficiency, or malignancy
B. Exclude false-positive calcium value (when calcium is only slightly elevated)
   1. Repeat calcium level—consistent elevation suggests pathology
   2. Serum albumin value, 0.8 mg/dl calcium for every 1 g abnormality in albumin level
C. Review of routine laboratory tests
   1. Low serum phosphate (suggests PTH excess)
   2. Increased bone-derived alkaline phosphatase (hyperparathyroidism, malignancy, Paget's disease)
   3. Abnormal liver function tests (malignancy, sarcoidosis)
   4. Anemia (obtain serum and urine protein electrophoresis to exclude multiple myeloma; evaluate for underlying malignancy)
   5. Chest film, screening for malignancy
D. PTH assay
   1. Low normal or undetectable—suggests nonparathyroid etiology
   2. High normal or elevated—hyperparathyroidism, familial hypocalciuric hypercalcemia, or ectopic PTH production
   3. Midnormal—clinical follow-up and repeat PTH assay in 2–3 months

PTH = parathyroid hormone.

The most important laboratory distinction to make in the initial evaluation of the hypercalcemic patient is the differentiation of PTH versus non–PTH-dependent forms of hypercalcemia. This distinction has been greatly simplified by the newer PTH assays described earlier.[19] A high-normal or elevated intact PTH level in the setting of overt hypercalcemia is virtually diagnostic of primary hyperparathyroidism but can also be seen in the rare patient with ectopic hyperparathyroidism as well as occasional patients with FHH. Mild to moderate elevations in PTH and serum calcium levels are seen in most hyperparathyroid subjects. Much more severe elevations, particularly when accompanied by overt systemic manifestations (e.g., weakness, anorexia, and weight loss) increase the probability that the patient has either parathyroid carcinoma or ectopic hyperparathyroidism. Most patients with FHH and rare individuals with primary hyperparathyroidism have mid-normal levels of intact PTH. A low-normal or, more commonly, a frankly suppressed intact PTH level in the face of hypercalcemia indicates a non–PTH-dependent form of hypercalcemia.[10,11] In such cases, if a malignancy is present it is often clinically obvious. The role for PTHrP assays in the evaluation and management of patients with malignancy-associated hypercalcemia is not yet clear. In patients with hypercalcemia of uncertain etiology, such assays may be useful in uncovering the presence of the occasional occult tumor producing hypercalcemia. It is also possible that the measurement of PTHrP may be useful as a tumor marker in monitoring responses to therapy, although this has not yet been shown to be the case.

The basis for other nonparathyroid hormone–dependent

hypercalcemias may also be apparent from the history and physical examination, but in some such cases as well as in some malignancies additional laboratory evaluation may be needed to uncover the cause. Such testing might include blood tests such as thyroid function tests, adrenal function testing, vitamin D—25(OH) vitamin D or $1,25(OH)_2$ vitamin D—or vitamin A levels, and serum (and, if necessary, urinary) protein electrophoresis, as well as radiologic or biopsy evaluation of tissues potentially involved by sarcoidosis, malignancy, or other infiltrative processes. It should be emphasized, however, that hyperparathyroidism and clinically apparent malignancies comprise about 90% of hypercalcemic individuals; more detailed laboratory testing for less common causes only need be undertaken in a few patients in whom the diagnosis is inapparent after initial routine laboratory tests as well as a PTH determination.

Occasionally, a patient may be seen with borderline hypercalcemia and a normal level of PTH, results that do not permit definitive differentiation of mild hyperparathyroidism from other causes of hypercalcemia. If there is no evidence of malignancy on initial testing and the calcium level remains abnormal on repeat testing, the best approach may be to follow the patient carefully and repeat the calcium and PTH levels in 2 to 3 months. Repeat evaluation such as this usually permits the distinction between mild, but biochemically more apparent hyperparathyroidism and the progression of other causes of hypercalcemia.

TREATMENT

The treatment of hypercalcemia ultimately depends on the treatment of the underlying disease. In some cases, the solution is obvious (e.g., discontinue thiazides or vitamin D); in others, it is extremely complex (e.g., metastatic malignancy). Rather than discuss treatment of the various disorders that can cause hypercalcemia, this section deals with the special problems of treating hyperparathyroidism and then discusses the medical methods available to treat hypercalcemia of whatever cause.

Hyperparathyroidism

In hyperparathyroidism, several therapeutic approaches have been suggested. There is general agreement that surgical removal of the abnormal parathyroid gland or glands is the treatment of choice in patients with a serum calcium level of 12 mg/dl or greater or in those with recurrent renal stones, hypercalcemic nephropathy, neuromyopathy, or progressive metabolic bone disease, regardless of the calcium level.[10, 11] However, there is less agreement about how to treat asymptomatic patients with less severe hypercalcemia because it is uncertain whether all these patients ultimately progress to more severe disease.

In one prospective study, 142 patients with so-called "biochemical" (e.g., mild, largely asymptomatic) hyperparathyroidism were given no specific therapy and were followed for 10 years to assess the natural course of their disease.[43] Nineteen subjects failed to participate in ongoing follow-up, reducing the number of patients who were evaluated to 123. Of these, 33 (27%) underwent parathyroid surgery during the 10 years, for various reasons (worsening renal failure or hypercalcemia, renal stones, bone disease, or simply discomfort with the knowledge that they harbored a parathyroid tumor, albeit benign). Most of the patients did not progress to severe hypercalcemia or significant complications of their hyperparathyroidism during the 10 years of their follow-up. Subsequent studies have confirmed these general results, and this subject was reviewed in detail at a National Institutes of Health Consensus Conference.[44]

However, before this watchful waiting approach to therapy is widely applied, two notes of caution should be emphasized. First, asymptomatic patients (and their physicians) may lose sight of the potential seriousness of their condition and be lost to follow-up, allowing their disease to progress without adequate medical attention. Second, mild hyperparathyroidism may exert its metabolic effects so slowly that a longer period of follow-up than is presently available may be needed before we can be certain of the full consequences of the "no treatment" approach. This hazard may be particularly relevant for metabolic bone disease. None of the currently available studies has adequately assessed the potential progression of PTH-induced osteopenia, especially in young women, in whom 15 or 20 years of untreated hyperparathyroidism could conceivably result in clinically significant, irreversible osteoporosis. Until the results of a careful prospective study of the progression of metabolic bone disease in these patients becomes available, we recommend parathyroid exploration in all patients who have hyperparathyroidism with serum calcium levels above 12 mg/dl, with symptomatic hypercalcemia, or with active renal stone or bone disease, and in asymptomatic patients if they are younger than 60 years of age. "Watchful waiting" seems most appropriate in older, asymptomatic patients in whom the appearance of osteoporosis, if it develops slowly, would be less problematic. Finally, the financial cost of long-term surveillance may also be a factor. The cost of medical follow-up currently exceeds that of a surgical approach after 5 to 6 years.[2]

Regarding the surgical approach to hyperparathyroidism, optimal treatment for parathyroid adenoma and carcinoma is resection of the tumor. For parathyroid hyperplasia, the current recommendation is removal of three and one half glands, leaving behind a portion of one gland with its blood supply intact. Usually this remnant is sufficient to prevent postoperative hypoparathyroidism.

There are several pitfalls in parathyroid surgery. It is not always easy to locate all parathyroid glands because of variability in size, number, and position (glands are sometimes found in the thymus, thyroid, or mediastinum). In addition, parathyroid hyperplasia may be markedly asymmetric with one or more nearly normal-sized glands on gross appearance. Furthermore, it may be very difficult, if not impossible, to distinguish adenoma from hyperplasia on frozen section histology. The decision of how many glands to remove often depends on the surgeon's judgment of the gross appearance of the glands combined with input from frozen section analysis at the time of surgery. The most important factor determining the success of parathyroidectomy is the skill and experience of the surgeon. An experienced surgeon can locate and remove the offending gland(s) at least 90 to 95% of the time during the first neck exploration.

Operative mortality is very rare—usually related to some preoperative illness increasing the patient's risk—and morbidity (e.g., vocal cord paralysis, hemorrhage, and pneumonia) is 1 to 2%. Persistent hyperparathyroidism after surgery occurs in 3 to 5% of cases and is generally a result of missing an adenoma. Recurrent hyperparathyroidism (i.e., that developing after a variable period of normocalcemia) is rare with adenomas but more common in parathyroid hyperplasia, particularly with MEN I in which it may occur in 50% or more of cases followed for 5 to 10 years postoperatively. Permanent hypoparathyroidism requiring oral vitamin D or calcium supplements occurs in another 3 to

5% of cases. Transient hypocalcemia after parathyroidectomy is seen fairly commonly (20 to 30%), especially in patients with metabolic bone disease and elevated alkaline phosphatase levels. This hypocalcemia is probably a result of rapid deposition of calcium in bone (so-called "hungry bone" syndrome). These patients, if asymptomatic, may require calcium supplements but seldom for more than 1 month. The administration of estrogen replacement to postmenopausal women with hyperparathyroidism or inorganic phosphate can be an effective method of reducing serum and urine calcium levels in patients who refuse surgery, are unacceptable surgical risks, or in whom parathyroidectomy was unsuccessful (see next section).

Specialized techniques to localize parathyroid tissue preoperatively are available in many centers.[44] Ultrasonography, scintigraphy, magnetic resonance imaging, or computed tomography scanning can localize 60 to 80% of abnormal parathyroid glands. A higher success rate can be achieved by using selective arteriography and selective venous blood sampling of the cervical (particularly the thyroidal) veins with PTH immunoassays of the samples. Absolute identification of a lesion identified by one of these techniques as parathyroid tissue can be accomplished by needle aspiration followed by performing a PTH assay on the diluted aspirate. Experienced surgeons are generally successful in defining a parathyroid abnormality in most cases operated on for the first time without the use of such tests. Therefore, specialized parathyroid localization tests are reserved for patients who have had previous unsuccessful neck explorations, because abnormal glands are notoriously difficult to locate after the cervical anatomy has been distorted. The localization and removal of abnormal parathyroid glands is most frequently successful when performed in a center where a team approach is employed involving highly experienced and dedicated radiologists and surgeons.

Medical Therapy of Hypercalcemia

Successful therapy of hypercalcemia involves reversing factors that initiated it (i.e., increased bone resorption, enhanced gastrointestinal absorption of calcium [if present], and inadequate renal calcium excretion).[10, 11] Advances in the development of potent, nontoxic inhibitors of bone resorption have modified the traditional approach to the therapy of hypercalcemia during the past several years.[45] Previously, vigorous hydration with saline (6 liters or more/day) combined with the use of potent loop diuretics to enhance renal calcium excretion were a major focus of therapy and were combined with inhibitors of bone resorption as necessary. The latter included agents such as plicamycin (formerly known as mithramycin), calcitonin, and, in some cases, glucocorticoids, phosphates, or cyclooxygenase inhibitors (e.g., indomethacin).[10, 11] The advent of the potent intravenous bisphosphonates, particularly APD,[46] and gallium nitrate,[47] has simplified the acute as well as the chronic therapy of the hypercalcemic patient considerably (details follow).

Acute Therapy of Severe Hypercalcemia

Acute, vigorous medical therapy should be initiated in any patient with severe hypercalcemia (e.g., of the order of 14 mg/dl or greater) (Table 45–4). Such patients usually have symptoms clearly related to the electrolyte disturbance, including nausea, vomiting, polyuria, polydipsia, or significant mental disturbances (i.e., lethargy, stupor, or coma). Some patients have symptoms at lower levels of calcium (particularly older individuals and those in whom hypercalcemia is of rapid onset) and may also warrant such therapy. All such patients are dehydrated and should receive sufficient intravenous saline (generally 0.9%) to restore a normal state of hydration. In patients with modest prerenal azotemia (a creatinine of 2 mg/dl or less) and a clear sensorium, rehydration can usually be achieved with 2 to 3 liters during the first 12 to 24 hours. In some cases, it may be necessary to administer potassium and magnesium salts in sufficient quantities to correct hypokalemia and hypomagnesemia. Only in patients in whom volume overload becomes a problem, such as those with severely impaired cardiac or renal function, is the use of loop diuretics required, because the addition of these agents greatly increases the need for intensive monitoring with measurements of central venous pressure as well as the risk of iatrogenic fluid and electrolyte imbalance.

TABLE 45–4. TREATMENT OF SEVERE HYPERCALCEMIA

1. Establish adequate hydration (e.g., 2–3 liters normal saline in 24 hours)
2. Administer inhibitors of bone resorption
   a. APD (Pamidronate), 30–90 mg IV over 4–24 hours; may repeat after 7 days

   or

   b. Gallium nitrate, 200 mg/m^2/day IV continuous infusion for 5 days
3. Glucocorticoids for steroid-responsive tumors or for vitamin D excess (e.g., prednisone 40–60 mg/day)

Unless there is a dramatic response to hydration alone during the first 12 to 24 hours, a potent inhibitor of bone resorption, such as a bisphosphonate or gallium nitrate (see later), should be added to the therapeutic regimen.[45] Because these agents may have some risk for nephrotoxicity in dehydrated patients, they are generally withheld until adequate hydration has been achieved. In occasional patients in whom hypercalcemia is life-threatening at presentation (e.g., those with very severe hypercalcemia, arrhythmias, severe dehydration, and/or stupor or coma), rehydration should be carried out more aggressively during the first few hours so that a bisphosphonate or gallium nitrate can be administered earlier. In addition, it may be necessary to use additional, more rapidly acting agents, such as calcitonin or, in rare cases, peritoneal or hemodialysis, during the first 12 to 24 hours of therapy. Although calcitonin is an inhibitor of bone resorption, studies have indicated that its hypocalcemic actions during the first 24 to 48 hours result to a significant extent from its calciuric actions.

Bisphosphonates (formerly called diphosphonates) are effective inhibitors of bone resorption that have been evaluated and used extensively during the past 5 to 10 years. In the United States, clinical studies have shown etidronate to be an ineffective agent for treating hypercalcemia when administered orally but modestly effective when administered intravenously at a dose of 7.5 mg/kg/day for 3 to 5 days. The actions of this agent when administered in the latter fashion are relatively short-lived (generally < 1 week), and repeated courses of intravenous administration are required to control hypercalcemia. Much more potent is aminohydroxypropilidine diphosphonate (APD or Pamidronate), which has recently received FDA approval for intravenous therapy of hypercalcemia of malignancy with or without bone metastases.[46, 48] A single intravenous dose of 30 to 90 mg of this agent for 4 to 24 hours produces normocalcemia within 2 to 4 days in 70 to 90% of individuals with all varieties of hypercalcemia. The calcium-lowering effect persists for 1 to 3 weeks. This dose may be repeated after a minimum of 7 days as needed to control hypercalcemia with very limited toxicity except for transient low-grade fever and lymphopenia, which seldom require cessation of therapy.

Gallium nitrate (Ganite) has also received FDA approval for intravenous use in treatment of hypercalcemia of malignancy. It is administered at a dose of 200 mg/m^2/day for 5 days as a continuous intravenous infusion and produces normocalcemia in about 70% of hypercalcemic patients with an onset of action of 3 to 6 days and a duration of 10 to 12 days following cessation of therapy.[47] Gallium nitrate produces some nephrotoxicity at the higher doses used for cancer chemotherapy (300 mg/m^2/day), and there is probably a small risk of this type of toxicity in the dose used to treat hypercalcemia. The drug may be administered repeatedly as required to control chronic hypercalcemia. There has been a wider experience with the use of APD than with gallium nitrate, and the former appears to induce normocalcemia in a somewhat higher fraction of patients. Both cost the pharmacy $300 to $400 for a single course of therapy, and oral formulations of both agents are in the process of being developed. Specific therapy for the underlying malignancy should, of course, be initiated as soon as is feasible.

As noted earlier, the combination of intravenous hydration and antiresorptive therapy controls hypercalcemia in most symptomatic patients with a sufficiently severe electrolyte abnormality to warrant hospitalization. In selected patients with hypercalcemia, alternative forms of therapy may be appropriate. In some malignancies, hypercalcemia is very responsive to administration of glucocorticoids (e.g., prednisone, 40 to 60 mg/day). This is particularly true for those in whom hypercalcemia is mediated by excessive production of 1,25$(OH)_2$ vitamin D as well as in granulomatous disorders in which hypercalcemia has a similar pathophysiology (and, of course, Addison's disease).[26] In the first two cases, glucorticoids inhibit both the production of 1,25$(OH)_2$ vitamin D as well as its action on gastrointestinal calcium absorption.[26, 36] Ketoconazole as well as chloroquine and hydroxychloroquine have also lowered the levels of 1,25$(OH)_2$ vitamin D in this setting in scattered case reports,[49, 50] but there is insufficient experience to recommend their routine use for this purpose at this time.

Chronic Therapy of Hypercalcemia

The chronic medical therapy of hypercalcemia has also been simplified by the advent of potent antiresorptive agents. Many such patients will have an underlying malignancy, and specific treatment for the tumor or any other chronic causes of hypercalcemia is a cornerstone of the successful chronic therapy of hypercalcemia. These patients should also remain well hydrated with a liberal intake of salt and 3 to 4 l/day of fluids. If needed, repeated courses of APD or gallium nitrate may be administered at the time of recurrence of hypercalcemia. In the case of APD, it may be administered as a single 4- to 6-hour intravenous infusion of 30 to 60 mg in the outpatient setting. Clearly, it is always important that the patient be aware of the symptoms of early hypercalcemia so that more intensive therapy may be initiated before the development of severe hypercalcemia.

In several types of hypercalcemia, specific forms of chronic therapy may be appropriate that differ from those just described. In postmenopausal women with symptomatic primary hyperparathyroidism who refuse or are not candidates for surgery, administration of 0.625 to 2.5 mg/day premarin (or conjugated equine estrogen) reduces bone turnover and urinary calcium excretion and may lower serum calcium concentration to near normal levels.[51] Doses of premarin of 1.25 mg/day or more are higher than those generally used to treat the symptoms and complications of the menopause, and a full consideration should be given to the relevant risk:benefit issues as described in Chapter 54. The newer bisphosphonates (e.g., pamidronate) are also effective in lowering the serum calcium concentration in primary hyperparathyroidism but raise the level of PTH concurrently and have the theoretical, long-term risk of stimulating further growth of the abnormal parathyroid gland(s). Oral administration of phosphate (e.g., Neutra-phos) in four daily doses of 250 to 500 mg may also be useful in this setting,[52] although this form of therapy also raises PTH levels. Patients treated with oral phosphate must also be monitored regularly for evidence of metastatic calcification and decline in renal function. Rare patients whose hypercalcemia is known to be mediated by excessive production of prostaglandins by a tumor may respond well to administration of indomethacin.

REFERENCES

1. Boonstra CE and Jackson CE: Hyperparathyroidism detected by routine serum calcium analysis. Ann Intern Med 63:468, 1965.
2. Heath H, Hodgson SF, and Kennedy MA: Primary hyperparathyroidism: Incidence, morbidity, and potential economic impact in a community. N Engl J Med 302:189, 1980.
3. Brown EM: Extracellular Ca^{2+}-sensing, regulation of parathyroid cell function, and the role of Ca^{2+} and other ions as extracellular (first) messengers. Physiol Rev 71:371, 1991.
4. Habener JF, Rosenblatt M, and Potts JT: Parathyroid hormone: Biochemical aspects of biosynthesis, secretion, action, and metabolism. Physiol Rev 64:985, 1984.
5. Haussler MR and McCain TA: Basic and clinical concepts related to vitamin D metabolism and action. N Engl J Med 297:974, 1977.
6. Holick MF: The cutaneous photosynthesis of pre-vitamin D_3: A unique photoendocrine system. J Invest Dermatol 76:512, 1981.
7. Hughes MR, Baylink DJ, Jones PG, et al: Radioligand receptor assay for 25-hydroxyvitamin D_2D_3 and 1,25-dihydroxyvitamin D_2D_3: Application to hypervitaminosis D. J Clin Invest 58:61, 1976.
8. Austin LA and Heath H: Calcitonin: Physiology and pathophysiology. N Engl J Med 304:269, 1981.
9. Mallette LE, Bilizekian JP, Heath DA, et al: Primary hyperparathyroidism: Clinical and biochemical features. Medicine 53:127, 1974.
10. Aurbach GD, Marx SJ, and Spiegel AM: Parathyroid hormone, calcitonin, and the calciferols. *In* Wilson JD and Foster DW (eds): Textbook of Endocrinology, 7th ed. Philadelphia, PA, WB Saunders, 1985, p 1137.
11. Stewart AF and Broadus AE: Mineral Metabolism. *In* Felig P, Baxter JD, Broadus AE, and Frohman LA (eds): Endocrinology and Metabolism, 2nd ed. New York, McGraw-Hill, 1987, p 1317.
12. Lee DBN, Zawada ET, and Kleeman CR: The pathophysiology and clinical aspects of hypercalcemic disorders. West J Med 129:278, 1978.
13. Arnold A, Staunton CE, Kim HG, et al: Monoclonality and abnormal parathyroid hormone genes in parathyroid adenomas. N Engl J Med 318:658, 1988.
14. Friedman E, Sakaguchi K, Bale AE, et al: Clonality of parathyroid tumors in familial endocrine neoplasia type 1. N Engl J Med 321:213, 1989.

15. Motokura T, Bloom T, Kim HG, et al: A novel cyclin encoded by a bcll-linked candidate oncogene. Nature 350:512, 1991.
16. Palmer M, Adami H-O, Bergstrom R, et al: Survival and renal function in persons with untreated hypercalcemia: A population-based cohort study with 13 years of follow-up. Lancet i:59, 1987.
17. Silverberg SJ, Shane E, De La Cruz, et al: Bone disease in primary hyperparathyroidism. J Bone Miner Res 4:283, 1989.
18. Martin P, Bergmann P, Gillet C, et al: Partially reversible osteopenia after surgery for primary hyperparathyroidism. Arch Intern Med 146:689, 1986.
19. Nussbaum SR, Zahradnik R, Lavigne J, et al: Highly sensitive two-site immunoradiometric assay for parathyrin and its clinical utility in evaluating patients with hypercalcemia. Clin Chem 33:1364, 1987.
20. Yoshimoto K, Yamasaki R, Sakai H, et al: Ectopic production of PTH by small cell lung cancer in a patient with hypercalcemia. J Clin Endocrinol Metab 68:976, 1989.
21. Marx SJ, Attie MF, Levine MA, et al: The hypocalciuric or benign variant of familial hypercalcemia: Clinical and biochemical features in fifteen kindreds. Medicine 60:397, 1981.
22. Chou YH, Brown EM, Levi T, et al: The gene responsible for familial hypocalciuric hypercalcemia maps to chromosome 3 in four unrelated families. Nature Genetics 1:295, 1992.
23. Mundy GR: Hypercalcemia of malignancy revisited. J Clin Invest 82:1, 1988.
24. Mundy GR: Hypercalcemic factors other than parathyroid hormone-related protein. Endocrinol Metab Clin North Am 18:795, 1989.
25. Seyberth HW, Segre GV, Morgan JL, et al: Prostaglandins as mediators of hypercalcemia associated with certain types of cancer. N Engl J Med 293:1278, 1975.
26. Adams JS: Vitamin D metabolite-mediated hypercalcemia. Endocrinol Metab Clin North Am 18:765, 1989.
27. Stewart AF, Horst R, Deftos LJ, et al: Biochemical evaluation of patients with cancer-associated hypercalcemia: Evidence for humoral and nonhumoral groups. N Engl J Med 303:1377, 1980.
28. Strewler GJ and Nissenson RA: Hypercalcemia in malignancy. West J Med 153:635, 1990.
29. Budayr AA, Nissenson RA, Klein RF, et al: Increased serum levels of a parathyroid hormone-like protein in malignancy-associated hypercalcemia. Ann Intern Med 111:807, 1989.
30. Middler S, Pak CYC, Murad F, et al: Thiazide diuretics and calcium metabolism. Metabolism 22:139, 1973.
31. British Pediatric Association: Hypercalcemia in infants and vitamin D. BMJ 2:149, 1956.
32. Jacobus CH, Holick MF, Shao Q, et al: Hypervitaminosis D associated with drinking milk. N Engl J Med 326:1173, 1992.
33. Mason RS, Frankel T, Chan Y, et al: Vitamin D conversion by sarcoid lymph node homogenate. Ann Intern Med 100:59, 1984.
34. Reichel H, Koeffler HP, and Norman AW: Production of 1 alpha, 25-dihydroxyvitamin D_3 by hematopoietic cells. Prog Clin Biol Res 332:81, 1990.
35. Adams JS, Sharma OP, Diz MM, and Endres DB: Ketoconazole decreases the serum 1,25-dihydroxyvitamin D and calcium concentration in sarcoidosis-associated hypercalcemia. J Clin Endocrinol Metab 70(4):1090, 1990.
36. Hahn TJ, Halstead LR, and Baran DT: Effects of short term glucocorticoid administration on intestinal calcium absorption and circulating vitamin D metabolite concentrations in man. J Clin Endocrinol Metab 52:111, 1981.
37. Baxter JD and Bondy PK: Hypercalcemia of thyrotoxicosis. Ann Intern Med 65:429, 1966.
38. Burman KD, Monchik JM, Earll JM, and Wartofsky L: Ionized and total serum calcium and parathyroid hormone in hyperthyroidism. Ann Intern Med 84:668, 1976.
39. McMillan DE and Freeman RB: The milk-alkali syndrome: A study of the acute disorder with comments on the development of the chronic condition. Medicine 44:485, 1965.
40. Meric F, Yap P, and Bia MJ: Etiology of hypercalcemia in hemodialysis patients on calcium carbonate therapy. Am J Kidney Dis 16(5):459, 1990.
41. Miller PD, Dubovsky SL, McDonald KM, et al: Hypocalciuric effect of lithium in man. Miner Electrolyte Metab 1:3, 1978.
42. Brown EM: Lithium induces abnormal calcium-regulated PTH release in dispersed bovine parathyroid cells. J Clin Endocrinol Metab 52:1046, 1981.
43. Sholz DA and Purnell DC: Asymptomatic primary hyperparathyroidism: 10 year prospective study. Mayo Clin Proc 56:473, 1981.
44. Potts JT Jr: Proceedings of the NIH consensus development conference on diagnosis and management of asymptomatic primary hyperparathyroidism. Bone Mineral Res 7(Suppl 2): S1, 1991.
45. Treating cancer-associated hypercalcemia. Drug Ther Bull 28:85, 1990.
46. Pamidronate. Med Lett 34:1, 1992.
47. Warrell RP, Israel R, Frisone M, et al: Gallium nitrate for acute treatment of cancer-related hypercalcemia: A randomized, double-blind comparison to calcitonin. Ann Intern Med 108:669, 1988.
48. Ralston SH, Dryburgh FJ, Cowan RA, et al: Comparison of aminohydroxypropylidene disphosphonate, mithramycin, and corticosteroid/calcitonin in treatment of cancer-associated hypercalcemia. Lancet i:907, 1985.
49. Glass AR, Cerletty JM, Elliott W, et al: Ketoconazole reduces elevated serum levels of 1,25-dihydroxyvitamin D in hypercalcemic sarcoidosis. J Endocrinol Invest 13(5):407, 1990.
50. Bia MJ and Insogna K: Treatment of sarcoidosis-associated hypercalcemia with ketoconazole. Am J Kidney Dis 18(6):702, 1991.
51. Marcus R, Madvig P, Crim M, et al: Conjugated estrogens in the treatment of postmenopausal women with hyperparathyroidism. Ann Intern Med 100:633, 1984.
52. Broadus AE, Magee JS, Mallette LE, et al: A detailed evaluation of oral phosphate therapy in selected patients with primary hyperparathyroidism. J Clin Endocrinol Metab 56:953, 1983.

46

Diabetes Mellitus

ALDO A. ROSSINI, MD
JOHN P. MORDES, MD

DIABETES MELLITUS: A CHRONIC DISEASE EPIDEMIC

Diabetes mellitus describes a class of disorders characterized by hyperglycemia. An ancient disease described in Pharaonic and Vedic texts, diabetes has grown increasingly prevalent among young and old, among men and women, and in both developed and developing nations. Diabetes afflicts nearly one in 20 persons in Western society. Most persons with diabetes are 40 years of age or older, but some were afflicted before 5 years of age. In the United States about 500,000 cases are diagnosed annually. In 1990, 7 million people knew that they had diabetes, but an equal number with the disease remained undiagnosed. Among certain Americans the disease has epidemic proportions.[1] It afflicts women and blacks about twice as frequently as white males. The prevalence among Hispanics may be one in five. The cost of caring for diabetes and its complications in the United States in 1987 exceeded $20 billion.[2] It is impossible to avoid diabetes in the office practice of medicine.

Diabetes is not only a common and costly disorder but also a chronic one that can be refractory to treatment. Physicians who take care of patients with diabetes encounter recurrent frustration. Demanding diseases of this kind enervate caregivers. It can be difficult to generate enthusiasm for treating diabetes despite its domination of the lives and long-term health prospects of those affected. But diabetes *is* treatable, and the rewards of good treatment are great. Good diabetes care is important for many reasons.

- Diabetes can be rapidly fatal. Diabetic ketoacidosis, hyperosmolar hyperglycemic nonketotic coma, alcoholic ketoacidosis, and hypoglycemia are medical emergencies. More often than not, they can be prevented.
- Chronic hyperglycemia causes debilitating symptoms. The polydipsia, polyuria, and nocturia of diabetes can make the patient's life miserable. Wide excursions of glycemia affect vision. Uncontrolled diabetes induces fatigue, weakens surgical scars, and predisposes the patient to infections that range from intertrigo to mucormycosis.
- Diabetes can devastate pregnancy, increasing the risk of congenital malformations, neonatal complications, and maternal morbidity and mortality.
- Finally, chronic diabetes leads almost inevitably to secondary complications. More than 2 million Americans are hospitalized each year because of these related disorders.[3] Compared with the general population, persons with diabetes are 25 times more likely to become blind, 17 times more susceptible to renal failure, five times more likely to suffer a gangrenous extremity, and twice as susceptible to heart disease. It appears increasingly likely that appropriate treatment of diabetes may retard if not prevent some of these complications.

Perhaps because the sequelae of diabetes are so grave, we normally regulate glycemia with extraordinary precision. Plasma glucose concentration varies only between approximately 60 and 120 mg/dl (3.3 to 6.7 mM) despite extremes of activity and food intake. The American Diabetes Association has defined normal plasma glucose concentrations; values for adults are given in Table 46–1. An understanding of how this remarkable control is achieved is the key to understanding its derangements. It is here that diabetes management is grounded.

PATHOPHYSIOLOGY

Insulinization: The Key to Glucose Homeostasis

Control of plasma glucose concentration is achieved by precise regulation of the "insulinization" of body tissues.

TABLE 46–1. NORMAL PLASMA GLUCOSE CONCENTRATIONS FOR NONPREGNANT ADULTS*

Fasting plasma glucose ≤115 mg/dl (≤6.4 mM)
2-hour postprandial glucose <140 mg/dl (<7.8 mM)

*These values have been established by the American Diabetes Association: Clinical practice recommendations 1990–1991. Diab Care 14(Suppl 2):1, 1991.

Insulinization is a function of the concentration of circulating insulin and the sensitivity of tissues to that insulin. Figure 46–1 outlines the basic interactions.

After we eat, plasma glucose concentration rises but is held within the normal range by insulin secreted from pancreatic β cells. Insulin promotes the transport of glucose into cells where it is either metabolized to generate energy, stored for later use as glycogen, or metabolized to lipid and kept as a long-term energy reserve.

When we fast, plasma glucose concentration falls but again remains in the normal range, this time as the result of decreased insulin secretion. The decline in insulin concentration leads to hepatic glycogenolysis and the release of glucose into the circulation.

Fasting longer than 12 to 16 hours initiates a second tier of adaptive mechanisms. Peripheral tissues like muscle begin to use free fatty acids for fuel instead of glucose. The concentration of free fatty acids is regulated by residual circulating insulin through its control of lipolysis as well as glycemia. Gluconeogenesis continues to supply glucose for the central nervous system, but at the price of muscle breakdown to provide amino acids, since glucose cannot be synthesized from lipid.

Fasting longer than 72 hours initiates a third tier of adaptive processes. Now even the brain uses an alternative fuel, the ketone bodies. As less glucose is consumed, gluconeogenesis declines, muscle is spared, and everything that can be done metabolically to survive famine is in place.

At all times and under all conditions, such as gourmandizing or starving, insulin regulates plasma glucose concentration. In the fed state, abundant insulin secretion precludes hyperglycemia. In the fasted state, low levels of insulin adjust rates of lipolysis, glucose transport, and gluconeogenesis. Normally we are always "insulinized" to just the appropriate degree.

Diabetes Mellitus: Disorders of Insulinization

Diabetes occurs when deficient insulinization disrupts normal metabolic regulation. This can in turn result from many different pathologic processes. Diabetes is not one disease but consists of a family of syndromes that share only two things in common—hyperglycemia and some abnormality of insulinization. There are two principal routes to abnormal insulinization.

The first route is absolute insulin deficiency. The archetype of this condition is type I or "juvenile" diabetes. Pancreatectomy, pancreatic carcinoma, pancreatitis, and several toxins can also reduce circulating insulin concentrations to near zero.

The second route to abnormal insulinization is *relative* insulin deficiency due to insulin insensitivity (or "resistance"). The commonest form of this disorder is obesity-related type II or "maturity onset" diabetes. Patients with corticosteroid dependence, uremia, coronary ischemia, and many other conditions can also develop hyperglycemia despite normal or moderately elevated levels of circulating insulin. They are mildly insulin insensitive and "relatively" insulin deficient. Their hyperglycemia may not be permanent or severe. More extreme are cases of lipoatrophic diabetes and cases of insulin resistance associated with virilization and acanthosis nigricans, in both of which hyperglycemia occurs in the presence of extremely high insulin concentrations.[4]

Other diabetogenic mechanisms include synthesis of abnormal ("mutant") insulin molecules, circulating antagonists to insulin or its receptors, and molecular defects in insulin receptors.[5] There are probably dozens of routes to both insulin deficiency and resistance, and the list of abnor-

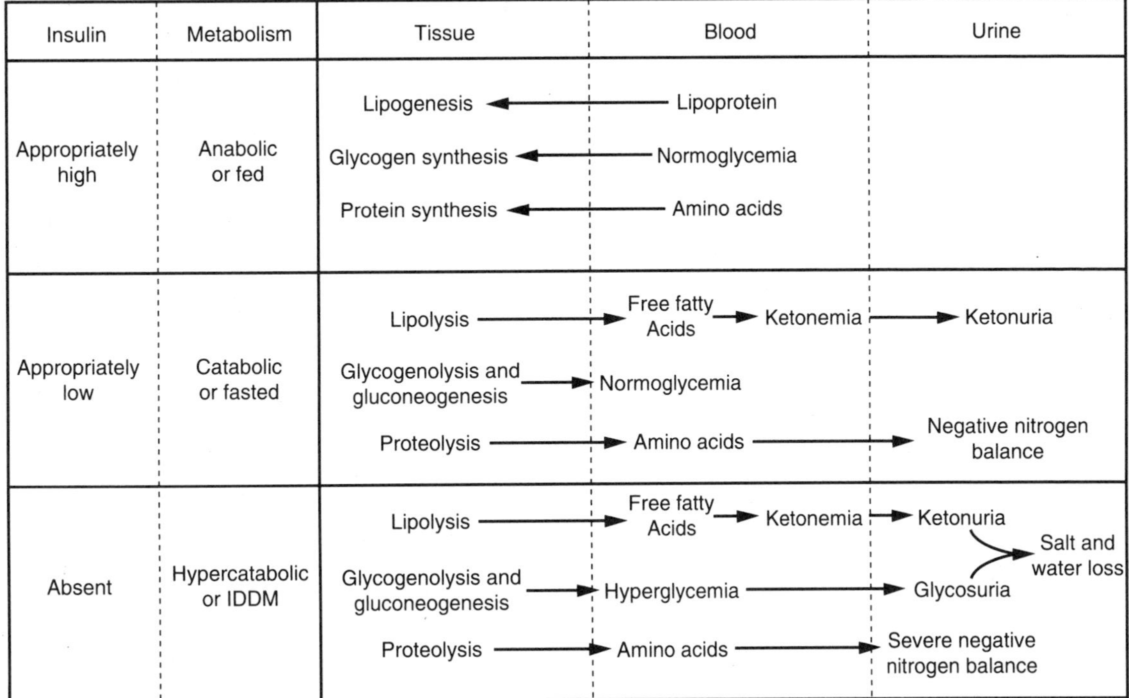

FIGURE 46–1. General overview of the key metabolic processes that are regulated by insulin. IDDM = Insulin-dependent diabetes mellitus.

malities that can cause diabetes is certain to expand. Few of these abnormalities are understood in detail, but the principle of insulinization unifies them all and provides the key to clinical management.

CLASSIFICATION

Rationale and Limitations

To bring order to the numerous diabetic syndromes, a classification system has been devised and is given in Table 46–2.[6] An important principle to note is that age of onset (i.e., "maturity-onset" versus "juvenile-onset") does not classify diabetes. Ketosis-resistant diabetes can occur in overweight children. Ketosis-prone diabetes with insulin deficiency may develop in lean adults. Even "ketosis-resistant" and "ketosis-prone" are imprecise classifiers. Obese patients with type II diabetes can become ketoacidotic, especially during surgery, trauma, or infection.

The distinction between "insulin-dependent" and "non–insulin-dependent" is important, but the terms are easily misused. The distinction is biologic, not therapeutic or semantic. All patients with type II non–insulin-dependent diabetes (NIDDM) in the basal (unstressed) state retain the capacity to secrete insulin; for them exogenous insulin injections are supplemental, not essential, for life. Persons with type I, insulin-dependent diabetes mellitus (IDDM) cannot survive without exogenous insulin.

The classification gives caregivers important guidance. The goals, strategies, and tactics of therapy for lean patients who produce no insulin are very different from those appropriate for obese patients who produce insulin, but not enough to compensate for insensitivity. Misclassification of diabetes also interferes with epidemiologic and clinical research.

Most people with hyperglycemia suffer from idiopathic diabetes mellitus (see Table 46–2). Approximately 80 to 90% of them have type II NIDDM; 5 to 10% have type I IDDM. NIDDM includes a subgroup of nonobese but ketosis-resistant individuals. Table 46–3 summarizes important features that distinguish IDDM and NIDDM. The other forms of diabetes mellitus are much less common.

Insulin-Dependent (Type I) Diabetes Mellitus

IDDM results from the destruction of pancreatic β cells by an autoimmune process.[7,8] Those affected circulate little or no insulin. IDDM, often referred to as juvenile diabetes, develops abruptly in children and adolescents of normal body weight but can occur at any age. Untreated IDDM progresses to ketoacidosis as gluconeogenesis and lipolysis proceed without restraint in the absence of insulin.

TABLE 46–2. CLASSIFICATION OF HYPERGLYCEMIC STATES*

Diabetes Mellitus
1. Type I: Insulin-dependent type (IDDM); susceptible to ketosis
2. Type II: Non–insulin-dependent type (NIDDM); resistant to ketosis
3. Diabetes associated with certain conditions or syndromes (see Tables 46–4 and 46–5)

Impaired Glucose Tolerance (IGT)
Abnormality in glucose levels intermediate between normal and overt diabetes

Gestational Diabetes Mellitus (GDM)
Glucose intolerance with onset during pregnancy

*From the National Diabetes Data Group: Classification and diagnosis of diabetes mellitus and other categories of glucose intolerance. Diabetes 28:1039, 1979.

Non–Insulin-Dependent (Type II) Diabetes Mellitus

Formerly called maturity or adult onset diabetes, NIDDM results from insensitivity to insulin. The disease develops insidiously and can appear at any time between adolescence and old age. "Maturity onset diabetes of the young" (MODY) is an autosomal dominant, heritable variant of the disorder.[9] Concentrations of circulating insulin are relatively low but are not absent in NIDDM; those affected are underinsulinized but are not uninsulinized. In general, there is enough insulin to control lipid mobilization and prevent ketosis. An intercurrent stress can precipitate extreme hyperglycemia, hyperosmolality, coma, and lactic acidosis in patients with NIDDM.

The cause of the disease at the cellular level is not yet known. At least two defects appear to be required, a peripheral defect in insulin action *and* a defect in insulin production. The latter may be caused by inadequate numbers of β cells or by some other defect in the secretory process.

More than 80% of patients with NIDDM are obese, and, interestingly, most of them belong to the subset of overweight individuals* who carry their excess adiposity around the waist.[10] The disorder can often be managed with diet, exercise, and oral hypoglycemic drugs, and almost all obese persons with diabetes respond to weight reduction alone. Some obese patients need exogenous insulin to control hyperglycemia and its symptoms. Lean patients with NIDDM tend more often to require insulin therapy and may have a different pathogenetic process.

Impaired Glucose Tolerance

Impaired glucose tolerance (IGT) is a metabolic abnormality characterized by mildly elevated fasting plasma glucose concentration or by a glucose tolerance test that is borderline abnormal. Affected individuals progress to overt diabetes at the rate of 1 to 5%/y. Others may remain glucose intolerant or revert to normal.

Patients with IGT often become frankly diabetic when stressed. Their risk of atherosclerotic cardiovascular disease and neuropathy is greater than that of the general population, but they tend to remain free of microangiopathic retinal and renal disease. IGT is not innocuous and should never be trivialized as a "touch of sugar" or the like.

Gestational Diabetes

Gestational diabetes (GDM) appears during the later stages of pregnancy in women not known to have diabe-

*Obese individuals can be classified according to the primary site of accumulation of fat. It is generally either around the waist ("android" or "abdominal" obesity) or in the hips and thighs ("gynoid" or "gluteofemoral" obesity). Obesity occurring around the waist carries significant risk of morbidity and mortality, whereas obesity around the hips does not. The distinction can be quantified by computing the waist:hip circumference ratio (WHR). In both men and women, the WHR predicts heart disease, diabetes, stroke, and death independent of total body fat mass. In men, the risk of these diseases increases markedly when the WHR is greater than 1.0; in women, the risk increases when the ratio is greater than 0.8.

TABLE 46–3. CHARACTERISTICS OF IDIOPATHIC DIABETES MELLITUS

Characteristics	IDDM	NIDDM
Epidemiology		
Prevalence	1.3/1000	~20/1000
Per cent of all diabetes	5 to 10%	90 to 95%
Diabetic:nondiabetic death rate ratio	4–11:1	2–4:1
Prevalence by sex	Approximately equal	F>M
Age at onset	<20 years	>40 years
Peak age for onset	12–14 years	45–64 years
Family history of diabetes	Frequent	More frequent
Clinical Manifestations		
Islets:		
Acute	Insulitis	Unknown
Chronic	Severe reduction of β cell mass with α and δ cells spared	Mild reduction of β cell mass
Insulin secretion	Absolute deficiency	Relative deficiency
Insulin resistance	Often present but not severe	Common
Immunogenetics	HLA-B8, B15, B18, DR3, DR4, DQβ3.1	None
Islet cell antibodies	Present	Infrequent
Association with other autoimmune disease	Yes	No
Clinical onset	Rapid	Insidious
Therapy		
Caloric intake	Maintenance	Usually requires reduction
Insulin	Always	Almost never the initial therapy
Oral hypoglycemic agents	Almost never useful	Frequently useful
Exercise	Balanced against food intake and insulin	To increase caloric utilization

IDDM = Insulin-dependent diabetes mellitus; NIDDM = Non–insulin-dependent diabetes mellitus.

tes.[11] It occurs in women whose insulin secretory capability is inadequate to meet the amplified metabolic demands of pregnancy. Untreated maternal hyperglycemia causes big babies that are harder to deliver and more likely to experience neonatal complications including hypoglycemia. GDM requires insulin therapy for the duration of the pregnancy. Only 2% of women with GDM remain hyperglycemic after delivery, but 40% eventually develop overt diabetes within 15 years. Most have NIDDM, but IDDM is occasionally observed.

Other Types of Diabetes Mellitus

"Secondary" diabetes mellitus is precipitated by many diseases and drugs, some of which are listed in Tables 46–4

TABLE 46–4. GLUCOSE INTOLERANCE ASSOCIATED WITH CERTAIN CONDITIONS AND SYNDROMES*

Hypoinsulinemic States	Hyperinsulinemic States	Other Syndromes, Genetic and Congenital
Pancreatic disease	Hormonal antagonism	Chromosomal abnormalities
Pancreatectomy	Glucocorticoid excess	Down's syndrome
Pancreatic carcinoma	Cushing's syndrome	Turner's syndrome
Pancreatitis	Exogenous steroids	Klinefelter's syndrome
Hemochromatosis	Growth hormone excess	Inborn errors of metabolism
Retroperitoneal fibrosis	Acromegaly	Glycogen storage disease type I
β Cell cytotoxins	Glucagon excess	Familial hyperlipidemia, type IV
Streptozotocin	Glucagonoma	Acute intermittent porphyria
Alloxan	Estrogen excess	Hyperglycerolemia
L-Asparaginase	Oral contraceptives	Neuromuscular syndromes
Vacor (rodenticide)	Pregnancy	Ataxia telangiectasia
Inhibition of insulin synthesis or release	Prolactin excess?	Myotonic dystrophy
Hypokalemia	Insulin receptor abnormalities	Huntington's chorea
Hyperaldosteronism	Defect in insulin receptors	Friedreich's ataxia
Diuretic therapy	Congenital lipodystrophy	Laurence-Moon-Biedl syndrome
Hypochloremic alkalosis	Associated with acanthosis nigricans and virilization	Prader-Willi syndrome
Hypocalcemia	Antibodies to insulin receptors	
Catecholamine excess	Abnormal insulins	
Stress, burns, trauma	"Mutant" insulins	
Infection	C-peptide defects	
Pheochromocytoma		
Sympathomimetic drugs		
Other pharmacologic agents (see Table 46–5)		
Malnutrition		

*From National Diabetes Group: Classification and diagnosis of diabetes mellitus and other categories of glucose intolerance. Diabetes 28:1039, 1979.

TABLE 46–5. SOME DRUGS THAT CAUSE HYPERGLYCEMIA AND INTERFERE WITH DIABETES CONTROL*

β Cell Toxins and Drugs that Interfere with Insulin Synthesis or Secretion	Drugs that Interfere with Insulin Action	Uncertain Mechanism of Action	Counterregulatory Drugs
β-Adrenergic blockers	Prednisone	Nicotinic acid (niacin)	Catecholamines
Calcium channel blockers	Dexamethasone	Oral contraceptives	Dopamine
Clonidine		Opioids	Dobutamine
Diazoxide		Naloxone	
Diuretics (thiazides; furosemide)		Phenothiazines	
Lithium		Benzodiazepines	
Levodopa		Tricyclics	
Phenytoin		Indomethacin	
L-Asparaginase		Amiodarone	
Pentamidine†		Cimetidine	
Streptozotocin		Salmon calcitonin	
Alloxan			

*From O'Byrne S and Feely J: Effects of drugs on glucose tolerance in non–insulin-dependent diabetics. Part I in Drugs 40:6, 1990 and Part II in Drugs 40:203, 1990.
†Initially causes hypoglycemia; later causes β cell loss.[70, 71]

and 46–5. The pathophysiology varies with the particular association and is often complex and poorly understood. Use of listed drugs or the diagnosis of an associated illness suggest the possibility of hyperglycemia.

Malnutrition-related diabetes mellitus (MRDM) is a common disorder in the Third World. Patients are usually young adults.[12] The pathophysiology is not clear. A painful fibrocalculous variant is associated with pancreatic stones, fibrosis, and endocrine atrophy. Low concentrations of insulin are present in MRDM, and ketosis is rare.

Statistical Risk Classes

Previous abnormality of glucose tolerance describes patients with normal glucose tolerance but a history of overt diabetes or impaired glucose tolerance. That abnormality may have been spontaneous or associated with illness or pregnancy. With stress, glucose intolerance often recurs in these individuals. This category keeps individuals who are currently well from being labeled as diabetic. That in turn is beneficial to patients both psychologically and when seeking insurance or employment.

Potential abnormality of glucose tolerance refers to individuals whose risk of diabetes is greater than that of the general population. It is a category whose importance will grow as methods of diabetes prevention are perfected. It replaces the terms "prediabetes" and "latent diabetes." Those with a higher than average diabetes risk include children and siblings of persons with diabetes, the obese (NIDDM), and individuals who circulate certain autoantibodies (e.g., islet cell antibodies [ICA], islet cell surface antibodies [ICSA], glutamic acid decarboxylase [GAD], and insulin autoantibodies [IAA]) or who express certain major histocompatibility complex antigens (IDDM). Those with potential risk of IDDM often have loss of the first phase of insulin secretion that is normally observed during *intravenous* glucose tolerance testing. Autoantibodies, HLA antigens, and intravenous glucose challenge are research tools that are not germane to clinical practice at present.[13, 14]

DIAGNOSIS

When To Be Suspicious

The onset of diabetes can be insidious or fulminant depending on the extent of underinsulinization and intercurrent stress. The prevalence of diabetes warrants its consideration in nearly every patient, but certain circumstances warrant exceptional suspicion. Individuals with previous abnormalities of glucose tolerance or any of the conditions listed in Table 46–4 are at risk. More than 60% of obese individuals eventually develop diabetes; anyone more than 20% above ideal body weight should be evaluated.* All women who have had frank gestational diabetes or a large infant (>9 lb or ~4.5 kg) are at risk for NIDDM. Finally, because glucose tolerance declines with age, it is reasonable to measure a fasting plasma glucose concentration in the elderly.

Family history is a useful guide to physicians when assessing risk for diabetes. In the case of IDDM, a parent with diabetes confers a 2 to 4% risk of the disorder in a child. Identical twins have a 50% shared risk. In the case of NIDDM, heritability is more pronounced. The presence of NIDDM in any first-degree relative should prompt an evaluation of the disease. The genetics of diabetes are discussed in more detail below (Table 46–6).

Diagnosis of IDDM

Subclinical IDDM probably smolders for years, autoimmune β cell destruction being an indolent process. Progressive loss of glucose tolerance can be detected weeks to years before the onset of symptoms of hyperglycemia. Paradoxically, some patients in the prodromal phase of IDDM have symptoms of hypoglycemia, perhaps due to the release of insulin from dying β cells.

---

*Practicing physicians can readily diagnose obesity by calculating a patient's **relative weight.**

$$\text{Relative weight} = \frac{\text{Actual body weight}}{\text{Ideal body weight}}$$

Relative weight >1.2 (20% "excess") is a practical definition of obesity.

This definition is useful clinically because it defines the threshold of trouble. Life table analyses show an increase in both morbidity (e.g., diabetes) and mortality once an individual is 20% or more overweight. This epidemiologic association is the rationale for this definition of obesity, both qualitatively and quantitatively. Ideal body weight for use in the equation can be obtained from reference tables but is also easy to estimate:

Females: 100 lb + 5 lb per inch of height above 5 ft.
Males: 106 lb + 6 lb per inch of height above 5 ft.
The ideal weight range is ± 10% of the calculated value.

TABLE 46–6. HERITABILITY OF DIABETES*

	IDDM	NIDDM
Overall U.S. population risk	~0.3%	~6%
Both parents with the same disorder	~30%	~30% Frank NIDDM >50% Impaired glucose tolerance
One parent with the disorder	2–4%†	10–20%
A monozygotic twin with the disorder	~50%	~100%
A sibling with the disorder	5–17% depending on HLA type ‡	~25%

*From Eisenbarth ES: Type I Diabetes Mellitus: A Chronic and Predictable Autoimmune Disease. Kalamazoo, Upjohn Corporation, 1989 and Soeldner JS: The etiology of diabetes. In Kozak GP (ed): Clinical Diabetes Mellitus. Philadelphia, WB Saunders, 1982, pp 21–31.

The estimates are probabilities of the *same type* of diabetes occurring in a relative of an individual with diabetes.

†IDDM occurs somewhat more often when the affected parent is the father.

‡IDDM is more common when the affected sibling is HLA identical.

Before untreated IDDM progresses to diabetic ketoacidosis (DKA), patients often note a subtle prodrome and can pinpoint when it began. Episodically increased plasma glucose concentrations lead progressively to polyuria, polydipsia, weight loss, fatigue, polyphagia, nocturia, and irritability. All the symptoms are amplified by intercurrent infection or other stress, and, if undiagnosed, progress until DKA ensues. IDDM has been detected incidentally after routine blood or urine testing, but this is uncommon.

DKA may be the first indication of IDDM. Symptoms and signs include tachypnea, tachycardia, dehydration, orthostatic hypotension, abdominal pain, nausea, vomiting, and confusion.[15] Abdominal pain may mimic appendicitis; lipemic serum and hyperamylasemia may suggest acute pancreatitis. In addition to the classic prodromal symptoms, there may be an antecedent history of viral illness, trauma, or emotional stress.

Diagnosis of NIDDM

DKA almost never signals the onset of NIDDM, because insulinization in that disorder can almost always suppress lipolysis. DKA in patients with NIDDM generally occurs in the context of extreme stress (e.g., sepsis, stroke, or myocardial infarction). Elderly patients with new onset of diabetes and DKA should be evaluated for cancer of the pancreas, which occurs in 10 to 15% of such cases. The mechanism is unknown.

NIDDM is occasionally diagnosed for the first time in patients with hyperosmolar hyperglycemic nonketotic coma (HHNKC). Such patients are usually elderly, are uniformly azotemic, and have some form of impaired response to thirst in addition to underinsulinization.[15] Intercurrent illness is also common, as is historical evidence of impaired or previously abnormal glucose tolerance. The plasma glucose concentration in HHNKC may be very high (1000 to 2000 mg/dl, 55 to 110 mM), due to dehydration.

Much more typically, the onset of NIDDM is indolent. Often it is discovered serendipitously when blood or urine glucose testing is performed for other reasons. Most patients voice only nonspecific complaints. Retrospectively, almost all patients will recall fatigue and weakness that progressed during the months before the detection of hyperglycemia. Family members may have noted increased irritability and lethargy. Weight gain often precedes the laboratory diagnosis of NIDDM.

The "polys." As blood glucose concentrations periodically exceed the renal threshold for reabsorption ($T_M \approx 180$ mg/dl,10 mM), polyuria and nocturia occur intermittently. The increase in the frequency of these symptoms is often so gradual that they are attributed to "getting old." If patients are known to have other diseases, they and their physicians may attribute the increase in urination to congestive heart failure, diuretic use, prostatic hypertrophy, or chronic venous insufficiency. Increased thirst and dry mouth are also common symptoms of NIDDM that result from the osmotic diuresis of glucose. An old clinical maxim holds that nocturia followed by a drink of water indicates the presence of diabetes, whereas nocturia without one is more likely to be due to some other disorder.

Vision. Blurred vision is common among patients with undiagnosed diabetes. It occurs because hyperglycemia induces changes in lens chemistry that in turn induce osmotically driven distortion of lens geometry. Frequent revision of eyeglass prescription is a common harbinger of diabetes. Paradoxically, some elderly patients notice improved visual acuity in the months before the diagnosis of NIDDM due to a favorable distortion of the lens.

Itch. Pruritus frequently vexes persons with untreated and uncontrolled diabetes. Often attributed to dry skin, it generally has other causes. Recurrent monilial vaginitis is common in women with diabetes, and uncircumcised males are susceptible to balanitis. Inframammary and inguinal dermatophytoses occur more readily in the setting of hyperglycemia, and are particularly common among obese persons with diabetes. Diabetes should also be suspected in patients with recurrent, severe carbuncles and furuncles. A summary of common symptoms of hyperglycemia is given in Table 46–7.

Complications of Diabetes Can Occur Before the Disease Is Diagnosed

NIDDM may worsen so indolently that the disease remains undiagnosed until a complication of the disorder occurs. Retrospectively, mild hyperglycemia may have been charted but regarded as inconsequential. Hyperglycemia is never innocuous. Ophthalmologists occasionally diagnose diabetes. Both background and proliferative diabetic retinopathy can occur after years of chronic moderate hyperglycemia. The initial manifestation of NIDDM can also be an unexplained neuropathy. Symptoms typically include leg pain, cramps, or paresthesias that are easily misattributed to vascular insufficiency, venous stasis disease, or arthritis. Less commonly, cranial nerves are affected. Finally, the detection of any form of premature vascular disease should raise the possibility of diabetes. A description of the complications of diabetes follows.

TABLE 46–7. SYMPTOMS OF HYPERGLYCEMIA

Polyuria, polydipsia, nocturia
Polyphagia
Weakness, fatigue, lethargy
Weight change
Pruritus
Blurry vision
Irritability
Nocturnal leg cramps
Nocturnal paresthesias of the toes

Laboratory Confirmation of Diagnosis

We have emphasized that diabetes mellitus is not simply hyperglycemia, but when it comes to diagnosis there is only one pathognomonic clinical criterion—inappropriately elevated plasma glucose concentration. Diabetes can almost always be diagnosed just by measuring fasting or postprandial plasma glucose concentrations. The oral glucose tolerance test (OGTT) is rarely necessary to diagnose diabetes in adults. OGTTs are essential only in the diagnosis of impaired glucose tolerance and gestational diabetes; occasionally, they are useful in the diagnosis or exclusion of diabetes in children. Plasma glucose concentrations that establish the presence of diabetes, IGT, and GDM have been defined by the American Diabetes Association and are summarized in Table 46–8.[14] Glycohemoglobin assays are not sensitive enough to use for diagnosing diabetes.

Individual laboratories may adjust the "normal" and "diagnostic" values to account for variation in the method of analysis and the type of specimen. Venous blood, capillary blood, whole blood, and serum also give slightly different results. In general, 120% of the laboratory's upper limit of normal for fasting glucose concentration is the threshold for diagnosing diabetes. Maximum 2-hour postprandial glucose concentration should not exceed 140% of maximum fasting levels.

Clinicians have greater diagnostic leeway than do clinical investigators. The rigid definitions required for research protocols should not define clinical practice. Clinicians must, however, exclude human and laboratory error, and testing for diabetes should be performed at least twice before considering the diagnosis firm.

The extent to which an individual patient is evaluated should be tempered by clinical judgment. A fasting plasma glucose concentration of 120 mg/dl (6.7 mM) in a young, obese, hyperlipidemic individual could represent IGT, but an OGTT is unnecessary. The patient needs vigorous efforts at weight reduction, irrespective of any further test results. A fasting value of 140 mg/dl (7.8 mM) probably does not require intervention in an 80 year old; in a thin child it is a portent that demands additional study. As a cliché states, treat the patient, not the laboratory.

TABLE 46–8. LABORATORY DIAGNOSIS OF DIABETES*

Diagnosis of Diabetes in Nonpregnant Adults

A. Plasma glucose concentration ≥200 mg/dl in the context of classic symptoms of diabetes
B. Fasting plasma glucose concentrations ≥140 mg/dl on two occasions
C. Fasting plasma glucose concentration is <140 mg/dl, but two oral glucose tolerance tests demonstrate a 2-hour plasma glucose concentration *and* one additional intervening value both ≥200 mg/dl after a 75-g glucose challenge

Impaired Glucose Tolerance

Fasting plasma glucose concentration is <140 mg/dl, but during a 75-g oral glucose tolerance test the 2-hour value is ≥140 mg/dl but <200 mg/dl *and* at least one additional intervening value is >200 mg/dl

Gestational Diabetes Mellitus

An oral glucose tolerance test performed wtih a 100-g glucose challenge showing at least two of the following:
Fasting plasma glucose concentration >105 mg/dl
1-hour value >190 mg/dl
2-hour value >165 mg/dl
3-hour value >145 mg/dl

Diabetes Mellitus in Children

A. A random plasma glucose concentration >200 mg/dl plus classic symptoms of diabetes
B. Fasting plasma glucose concentration ≥140 mg/dl on two occasions, and two oral glucose tolerance tests (using a 1.75 g/kg challenge) demonstrate a 2-hour value ≥200 mg/dl

*Criteria established by the American Diabetes Association: Clinical practice recommendations 1990–1991. Diab Care 14(Suppl 2): 1, 1991.

Glucose Tolerance Tests

Indications. Nonpregnant patients rarely require the 3-hour OGTT to diagnose or exclude diabetes. The 5-hour OGTT is *never* necessary to diagnose diabetes. The OGTT is necessary only to establish gestational diabetes or IGT and in a few other circumstances.[14]

For example, a patient with one of the complications of diabetes, perhaps a cranial nerve palsy, is suspected to have diabetes but has normal fasting and postprandial plasma glucose concentrations. In this circumstance, an OGTT may provide useful information. Whatever the outcome, other causes of the index disorder (e.g., tumor or multiple sclerosis) still have to be excluded.

Another indication for OGTT testing is to adjudicate the diagnosis in patients whose fasting and postprandial results are equivocal or inconsistent or whose diagnosis of diabetes is based on an OGTT that may have been performed incorrectly. The diagnosis of diabetes carries important legal and economic consequences; the 3-hour OGTT, if performed correctly, approximates a diagnostic gold standard for distinguishing diabetes from IGT and normal glucose tolerance. The OGTT is the only standard for establishing the diagnosis of gestational diabetes. Note that the glucose challenge used for GDM is 100 g, not the 75 g used in nonpregnant adults.[14]

The only other indication for the OGTT is to evaluate patients for possible reactive hypoglycemia.[16] In such cases the test is carried out for 5 or even 6 hours. Symptomatic hypoglycemia fulfilling Whipple's triad* several hours after the oral glucose load is the diagnostic criterion.

Correct Performance. The OGTT must be performed under strictly standardized conditions or the results may be invalid.[14] The commonest problem is incorrect preparation. Patients sometimes starve themselves before the test in the mistaken belief that this maneuver enhances carbohydrate tolerance. It actually has the opposite effect by causing a temporary decline in insulin's synthetic and secretory capability. Subjects must ingest a minimum of 150 g of carbohydrate (the equivalent of ~½ lb of dry pasta or ~5 cups of cooked pasta) daily for 3 days before the test. Patients must also be ambulatory, free from intercurrent illnesses, and not receiving drugs that impair carbohydrate tolerance (see Table 46–5). During the test the patient should be seated and should not smoke.

EVALUATION OF DISORDERS ASSOCIATED WITH DIABETES

After a diagnosis of diabetes mellitus has been confirmed, clinicians must evaluate all except the youngest patients with IDDM for the complications of diabetes. These complications are described later in detail. In addition, all patients should be evaluated for disorders that are either unusually prevalent among those with diabetes or that con-

*Whipple's triad: Criteria for the diagnosis of hypoglycemia include (1) plasma glucose concentration less than 50 mg/dl (2.8 mM); (2) symptoms of hypoglycemia; and (3) resolution of symptoms with administration of glucose.

tribute to the development of hyperglycemia. Nonendocrine conditions that exacerbate hyperglycemia include burns, trauma, myocardial infarction, sepsis, and treatment with drugs that impair insulin secretion or interfere with the action of insulin. These conditions are listed in Table 46–4.

Endocrine Hyperfunction

Disturbances that lead to the production of counterregulatory hormones induce hyperglycemia. These hormones include catecholamines, cortisol, growth hormone, and glucagon. Each is normally released into the circulation to meet sudden energy need or to counteract hypoglycemia. Corresponding endocrine diseases that cause diabetes include pheochromocytoma, Cushing's syndrome, acromegaly, and glucagonoma. Hyperthyroidism, hyperaldosteronism, and somatostatinoma may also be associated with worsening glucose tolerance. These disorders can often be excluded by history and physical examination. Laboratory testing should be reserved for patients with symptoms or signs of endocrinopathy.

Autoimmune Diseases Associated with IDDM

IDDM is autoimmune in origin, and other immune disorders are common in patients with this type of diabetes. The prevalence of autoimmune thyroid disease is about 30 times higher among patients with IDDM than in the general population.[17] Addison's disease, hypergonadotrophic hypogonadism, idiopathic hypoparathyroidism, pernicious anemia, vitiligo, relapsing polychondritis, and alopecia areata are also more prevalent in persons with type I diabetes.[8] The same may also be true of nontropical sprue and rheumatoid arthritis, but the data are equivocal.

Rare Forms of Diabetes

Listed in Table 46–4 are some very rare causes of hyperglycemia that are associated in ways that are poorly understood with other disorders. Lipoatrophic diabetes mellitus is associated with extreme insulin resistance and the absence of subcutaneous and visceral fat. Diabetes is also associated with the syndrome of acanthosis nigricans, virilization, and severe insulin resistance. Finally, Friedreich's ataxia, Huntington's chorea, stiff man syndrome, and myotonic dystrophy are neurologic disorders associated with diabetes.

APPROACH TO PATIENTS KNOWN TO HAVE DIABETES

Duration of Hyperglycemia

Having diagnosed diabetes, it is very important to determine its duration. Secondary complications of diabetes appear 10 to 15 years after the onset of the disease, not after its detection. The duration of disease in part guides the orientation of care. An old clinical maxim states that the "physiologic age" of a patient with uncontrolled diabetes is the sum of the chronologic age and the number of years of hyperglycemia. Awareness of duration and "physiologic age" has obvious implications. Care of recent onset diabetes should focus on control and on the prevention of complications. The longer that diabetes has been present, the more emphasis must be given to the detection and treatment of complications.

In the case of new onset IDDM, duration is seldom an issue. Because of its insidious onset, NIDDM may be present but may be undetected for years. Some patients have been told that they have a "touch of sugar" or "mild diabetes," but in the absence of treatment, they remain unaware that a serious disease condition is present. A careful history can give excellent clues to duration. In the case of women with diabetes, pregnancy history can disclose antecedent GDM. Because glucose determinations are a part of nearly every chemistry profile, both hospital records and notes of previous caregivers can give clues to the duration of IGT.

Assessment of Past and Current Control of Diabetes

The next question to consider is glycemic control since the onset of diabetes. Assessment of control can exploit many sources of information.[14]

The first is the record of blood glucose determinations. In contemporary practice, most patients with diabetes now have access to "fingerstick" self-monitored blood glucose (SMBG) determinations both at home and in the physician's office. The collated record of glucose determinations can provide an excellent index of glycemic control. Unfortunately, not all patient logs are accurate.[18]

The second source of information is provided by measures of glycosylation. These include total glycosylated hemoglobin and hemoglobin A_{1c} determinations. These tests provide indices of average glycemic control during the preceding 2 to 3 months and are exceptionally useful in cases when blood glucose determinations are unavailable or of suspect reliability. A more complete discussion of these tests follows.

The third source of information is the clinical history. Polyuria, polydipsia, and nocturia bespeak poor control. Fatigue, irritability, and disturbance of vision suggest wide excursions in glycemia. Weight gain also suggests poor control, as does a history of vaginitis, furunculosis, or intertrigo.

The fourth source of information is the history of treatment. Progression from unsuccessful diet treatment to a series of oral agent failures and perhaps finally to insulin indicates periods of refractory control.

Status of Complications and Other Relevant Conditions

In all except recent onset cases, clinicians must assess relevant organ systems for complications of diabetes. As noted earlier, detection of a complication sometimes even predates the diagnosis of diabetes. Symptoms, signs, previous evaluation, treatments, and current status of complications should be documented. The individual complications are discussed in the final section of the chapter; what follows are guidelines for nonspecialist practitioners evaluating a patient with diabetes who is not well known to them.

Eyes. What is the patient's subjective evaluation of his or her sight? Have there been frequent changes in prescription? Has the patient ever had an ophthalmologic evaluation? If so, when?

Nervous System. Does the patient have paresthesias or dysesthesias? Is there evidence of autonomic dysfunction in the form of impotence or postural hypotension?

Kidneys. Is proteinuria known to be present? Is there a history of abnormal renal function?

Vascular System. Is there a history of angina, heart failure, claudication, stroke, or foot ulcer? Have any of these conditions been investigated previously?

Intercurrent Risk Factors. Diabetes amplifies other risk factors for cardiovascular disease. Patients with diabetes are particularly in need of counseling and evaluation with regard to serum lipid concentration, hypertension, smoking, and physical fitness.

Drugs. The modern pharmacopeia is too large to know in detail, but many agents in common use do affect glycemia and control of diabetes. The tendency of medical practice to be fragmented, with many providers prescribing drugs to the same patient, enhances the risk of adverse consequences for persons with diabetes. The evaluation of a patient with diabetes should include not just a list of current medications but also an annotation of those that affect glycemia and those whose effects on diabetes are not familiar to the physician. An excellent example of common medications that affect diabetes is the thiazide class of diuretics. Prescribed for diuresis, hypertension, and other conditions, thiazides inhibit insulin secretion directly, increase serum lipid concentrations, and lower serum potassium concentrations, impairing insulin secretion. Some drugs that can affect glycemia are listed in Table 46–5.

PHYSICAL EXAMINATION OF PATIENTS WITH DIABETES

All patients with diabetes require careful physical examination on a regular basis. Diabetes is a chronic disorder that inevitably affects and changes its host. There are few patients in medicine who pose such a challenge to the examiner.

No single physical finding is pathognomonic of diabetes. Many findings are specific (e.g., proliferative retinopathy and necrobiosis lipoidica diabeticorum), but none establishes or excludes the diagnosis. Many signs characteristic of diabetes are caused by complications; some are associated with only rare forms (e.g., acanthosis nigricans); still others are associated with diseases that are common in patients with diabetes (e.g., vitiligo, psoriasis, and herpes zoster).

Necrobiosis lipoidica diabeticorum occurs in approximately 2% of persons with diabetes, four times more frequently in women, and it precedes the onset of impaired carbohydrate intolerance in 20% of affected individuals. Lesions are typically pretibial. They begin as slightly red maculopapules but progress to form purplish plaques with sharply defined elevated borders, glistening surfaces, and slight scaling. The final stage is that of sclerodermoid, atrophic lesions that eventually ulcerate and can become secondarily infected.

Diabetic dermopathy is the term applied to brown skin spots that usually occur in patients with IDDM of long duration. Rarely it may be an early finding. The lesions are multiple, deeply pigmented, well circumscribed, round, small, finely scaled, and atrophic. Bullosis diabeticorum, consisting of multiple tense blisters on the fingers or toes, is seen with diabetic peripheral neuropathy.

Less specific skin and connective tissue findings in persons with diabetes are listed in Table 46–9. *Vitiligo* is more common in both patients with IDDM and NIDDM than in the general population for unknown reasons. *Acanthosis nigricans* is a rare finding that is associated with insulin resistance and elevated insulin levels. The lesion is characterized by the distinctive sandpaper-like hyperpigmented areas on the neck, axillae, and other areas of flexion. Among patients older than 50 years of age with herpes zoster, as many as 17% have coexisting diabetes.

TABLE 46–9. INTEGUMENTARY MANIFESTATIONS OF DIABETES

Necrobiosis lipoidica diabeticorum
Diabetic dermopathy
Linear excoriative dermatitis
Bacterial and fungal skin infections
Multiple noduli cutanei
Multiple large hyperpigmented skin tags, especially in males
Eruptive xanthomas secondary to severe hypertriglyceridemia
Xanthochromia, secondary to elevated levels of serum carotene, especially in patients with poor nutrition or inadequate insulin therapy
Dupuytren's contractures
Atrophic changes, including loss of hair and decreased skin temperature in distal extremities
Psoriasis
Mucormycosis
Acanthosis nigricans
Porphyria cutanea tarda

Unexplained organomegaly is occasionally detected in patients with diabetes. Hepatomegaly accompanied by right upper quadrant pain is usually associated with uncontrolled type I diabetes and is caused by a lipid accumulation within hepatocytes. Hepatomegaly also occurs in the context of obese type II diabetes, but in addition to fatty infiltration, pericentric fibrosis, intracellular hyalinization, and perihepatocyte collagen deposition are found. In both instances, circulating liver enzyme concentrations tend to be elevated, but bilirubin remains normal. Parotid gland enlargement is sometimes also observed in NIDDM.

Eye findings include "snowflake" cataracts in IDDM, premature senile cataracts in any patient with longstanding diabetes, and Adie's pupil—one that responds slowly or not at all to light. Background diabetic retinopathy can often be detected by the nonophthalmologist even in the undilated eye. There are now good data to suggest that physicians who regularly examine eyes ophthalmoscopically become skillful in the detection of early changes that then warrant in-depth investigation by a specialist.[19] Microaneurysms, flame hemorrhages, and cotton wool spots are not difficult to detect. More advanced diabetic changes including neoproliferative disease and vitreous hemorrhage are obvious and require immediate referral. Office practitioners have an important role to play in the early detection of diabetic eye disease.

Neurologic findings include loss of pain and temperature sensation, especially in a "stocking-glove" distribution. Proximal muscle weakness affects mostly the legs. Cranial nerve palsies most often present as third cranial nerve lesions with sparing of the pupillary light reflex. Bell's palsy and femoral palsy are also common. Autonomic neuropathy may be detected in the form of orthostatic hypotension, anhidrosis, facial hyperhidrosis, or resting tachycardia.

LABORATORY INVESTIGATION OF PATIENTS WITH DIABETES

Prudent care of uncomplicated diabetes often requires laboratory investigation beyond that required to establish

TABLE 46–10. INDICES OF METABOLIC CONTROL

	Normal	Acceptable	Poor
Fasting plasma glucose	115 mg/dl (6.4 mM)	140 mg/dl (7.8 mM)	>200 mg/dl (11.1 mM)
2-Hour postprandial Plasma glucose	140 mg/dl (7.8 mM)	200 mg/dl (11.1 mM)	>235 mg/dl (13.1 mM)
Total glycosylated Hemoglobin	8%	10%	>12%
Hemoglobin A_{1c}	6%	8%	>10%

Note: Mean plasma glucose was 155 mg/dl with glycosylated hemoglobin (A_{1c}), about 7.0% in the DCCT,[20] values somewhat below those that have been acceptable when currently available treatment means and personnel are used.

the diagnosis (see Table 46–8) and assess control (Table 46–10). The American Diabetes Association recommends the diagnostic and surveillance studies shown in Table 46–11 for defining associated complications and risk factors.[14] Obviously, patients with diabetes should undergo other laboratory studies relevant to other conditions revealed by history and physical examination. The tests specifically relevant to the assessment of diabetes control are discussed more fully later in the section on good control.

TREATMENT OVERVIEW

Goals, Strategies, and Tactics

Goals. The long-term goals of diabetes therapy are (1) normal life span; (2) minimization of disabling complications; (3) normalization of daily life; and (4) freedom to pursue any reasonable educational, occupational, recreational, and social activity.

Current treatment makes it possible, but not easy, to achieve these four goals that sometimes verge on being mutually exclusive. Strategies and tactics that might prolong life and reduce disability can interfere with normal daily living and restrict the activities accessible to patients with diabetes. The suitability and relative priority of each goal must be adapted to each patient's clinical and personal circumstances.

Strategies. Therapeutic strategies include (1) control of hyperglycemia without frequent or severe hypoglycemia; (2) reduction of associated cardiovascular risk factors; (3) adaptation of therapy to each patient's clinical, educational, occupational, and economic circumstances; (4) provision for patient education at the time of diagnosis and at intervals throughout the course of therapy; and (5) prompt treatment of complications of diabetes when they occur.

Control of Blood Sugar. No clinician would argue the benefit of reducing glycemia to levels that prevent polyuria, nocturia, and chronic fatigue, perhaps 180 mg/dl (10 mM), but this "loose" form of control does not restore normoglycemia. Data now demonstrate that "tight" control using three or more daily insulin injections or an insulin pump to achieve mean glucose levels of about 155 ± 30 mg/dl (8.6 ± 1.7 mM) and glycosylated hemoglobin values of about 7% prevents or slows the development of the microangiopathic complications of IDDM.[20] Supportive data come from studies of intensive insulin therapy,[21] pancreas transplantation,[22] and the basic science study of advanced glycosylation end-products, the carbohydrate "rust" of tissues that is created by nonenzymatic linkage of glucose to protein.[23] Additional convincing data come from studies of diabetic pregnancy.[24, 25]

Restoration of normoglycemia resolves many metabolic and physiologic abnormalities that predispose to complications.[26] These include derangements in carbohydrate (e.g., sorbitol), protein, lipoprotein, phospholipid, and cholesterol metabolism; nerve conduction velocity; leukocyte and platelet dysfunction; and nonenzymatic glycosylation of hemoglobin and other tissues.

"Tight" control in patients with IDDM, however, failed to reach the target glycosylated hemoglobin value of 6.05%, despite the use of a team of experienced diabetologists, nurses, and nutritionists, and despite the occurrence of hypoglycemic reactions in many patients.[20] Nevertheless, to the extent practical, we advocate giving high priority to the control of hyperglycemia in young patients with diabetes for whom the prevention of complications is now a key goal. The Diabetes Control and Complications Trial (DCCT) showed decreases in background retinopathy (after an initial increase possibly attributable to increased insulin), in microalbuminuria and albuminuria, and in neuropathy.[20] "Tight" control benefited patients with IDDM who had not yet developed complications (primary prevention) and those with early complications (secondary prevention).[20] Although results of studies of "tight" control in patients with NIDDM are not available at the time of this writing, these patients develop similar complications, albeit at a later age, since the disease starts later in life. A prudent approach for NIDDM would stress weight loss and exercise to keep plasma glucose as low as possible.

Tactics. Therapeutic tactics include diet, exercise, exogenous insulin, oral hypoglycemic agents, medications for associated or complicating disorders, and specific educational programs.

What Is Good Diabetes Control?

The plasma glucose concentration that defines satisfactory control is not the same for all patients with diabetes. For the elderly, those with advanced complications of diabetes, and patients without glucose counterregulatory mechanisms, "tight" control is probably inappropriate. The elderly and infirm require control adequate only to prevent the symptoms of hyperglycemia: polydipsia, polyuria, nocturia, and polyphagia.

For the newly diagnosed patient with NIDDM, every effort should be made to achieve constant normoglycemia by means of diet, weight reduction, and increased physical activity. For active, growing children with IDDM, plasma glucose concentrations between 80 and 160 mg/dl (4.5 to 9.0 mM) are acceptable. The pregnant woman with diabetes, on the other hand, requires meticulous control, with fasting plasma glucose concentrations less than 105 mg/dl (5.8 mM) and 2-hour postprandial values less than 120 to 140 mg/dl (6.7 to 7.8 mM).[14] Plasma glucose levels and glycosylated hemoglobin values approaching those of the

TABLE 46–11. LABORATORY EVALUATION OF DIABETES*

Fasting plasma glucose concentration
Glycosylated hemoglobin
Fasting lipid profile
Serum creatinine in adults, or if proteinuria is present
Urinalysis: Urinary protein excretion should be measured by a microalbuminuria method if available
A test of thyroid function, preferably a thyroid-stimulating hormone, by sensitive assay
Electrocardiogram in adults

*Recommendations of the American Diabetes Association: Clinical practice recommendations 1990–1991. Diab Care 14 (Suppl 2): 1, 1991.

DCCT should be sought in most young adults with IDDM, but this approach may be tempered at times by the means of the practitioner and his or her team to educate the individual patient and avoid severe hypoglycemia.

How to Assess Diabetes Control

The best way to assess control is to combine fingerstick *self-monitoring of capillary blood glucose (SMBG) concentrations* with periodic determinations of glycosylated hemoglobin. Measurement of fasting plasma glucose concentration during outpatient visits has much less value because it is seldom representative of average glycemia. Guidelines for control in nonpregnant adults have been established by the American Diabetes Association and are shown in Table 46–11.[14]

In the era of self-monitoring of blood glucose, *urine testing* is clearly an inferior index of glycemic control and is not recommended.[14] Variability in renal resorption of glucose, patient compliance, and drug interference have always limited the utility of this measure. We advocate it only as "better than nothing" for patients who cannot or will not measure capillary glucose concentrations.

Glycohemoglobin, either total glycosylated hemoglobin or hemoglobin A_{1c}, is the best single method for periodic assessment of control of diabetes.[27, 28] The steady nonenzymatic glycosylation of tissue proteins yields an excellent index of average glycemia; the biochemical reactions detected by the test may actually play a major role in the pathogenesis of complications of diabetes. The glycosylated hemoglobin gives an index of control for the 3 months preceding the test (during which time erythrocyte mass will have turned over). Contemporary assays for glycohemoglobin are reliable and reproducible, but anemia, hemoglobinopathies, uremia, and certain medications may cause factitious values. There are several different glycohemoglobin methods (e.g., chromatographic, colorimetric, HPLC), and each has its tradeoffs in cost and sensitivity to the confounding factors just listed. It is important for the office practitioner to be aware of a laboratory's assay method and to be familiar with its specific limitations, if any.

Total glycosylated serum protein *(fructosamine)* provides information analogous to that provided by the glycohemoglobin.[29] Determination of fructosamine provides an index of glycemic control over a shorter period (1 to 3 weeks) than does a glycohemoglobin measurement (2 to 3 months). The fructosamine determination is not in wide use at this time.

Reduction of Cardiovascular Risk Factors

Cardiovascular disease deserves a special place in treatment because it kills many more persons with diabetes than do DKA, HHNKC, and renal failure combined. Every patient with diabetes must be evaluated for cardiovascular risk factors and counselled in their reduction. Treatable risk factors include cigarette smoking, hypertension, and hypercholesterolemia. When caring for obese, hypertensive, hypercholesterolemic, sedentary patients with diabetes who smoke, attention to blood glucose alone is unlikely to influence long-term morbidity and life expectancy, although there was a trend toward fewer macrovascular complications with "tight" control in the DCCT.[20]

NUTRITION

Goals and Strategies

Nutrition is essential to good diabetes therapy. The goal of dietary management is maintenance of ideal body weight using a healthy diet tailored to an individual's lifestyle and food preferences (Table 46–12). It is a goal that in the past has been difficult to achieve but has now become more easily realized as national awareness of the importance of diet increases.

Strategies for achieving dietary compliance begin with nutrition consultation. Physicians seldom acquire, maintain, or have the time to provide the information needed to manage diet. Comprehensive nutrition counseling by either a registered dietitian or a diabetes nurse educator can have a significant beneficial effect on diabetes management. We advise reliance on these resources in the nutritional management of all patients with diabetes.

General Nutritional Principles

Rational dietary prescriptions for patients with IDDM and NIDDM must include (1) total calories; (2) percentage and type of carbohydrates; (3) percentage and types of fats; (4) proteins; (5) meal spacing; and (6) modifications for exercise and complicating disorders.

The number of calories prescribed varies with age, body habitus, and activity level. About 10 cal/lb are needed for homeostasis in the absence of activity; another 3 cal/lb (for an office worker) to 10 cal/lb (for a laborer) are needed to supply energy needed for activity. The principles behind caloric prescriptions are given later. The actual composition of the diet should conform to the guidelines now widely espoused by both the American Heart and American Diabetes Associations.[14] These guidelines focus on the provision of a nutritious, palatable diet that minimizes the risk of atherosclerotic heart disease.

This diet provides more than half of its calories as carbohydrate and reduces fat to 30% or less of total energy intake. The physician must teach the patient with diabetes that this emphasis on carbohydrate is an emphasis on complex sugars, fruits, rice, breads, and starches. Concentrated sweets obviously impair diabetes control, but carbohydrate restriction per se has no role in diabetes management. When ingested singly, different carbohydrates differ with respect to subsequent postprandial glucose concentrations; they are said to have different "glycemic potential." However, when these different carbohydrates are eaten as part of a normal meal, effects on postprandial glucose are less

TABLE 46–12. DIETARY MANAGEMENT OF DIABETES

Goal:	Ideal body weight manufactured by a varied diet conforming to the recommendations of the American Heart Association and American Diabetes Association
	• <30% of calories from fat
	• 55–60% of calories from carbohydrate, principally complex forms
	• 15–20% of calories from protein (0.8 g/kg)
	• Avoidance of excessive sodium intake (<3000 mg/day)
Tactics:	Counselling by a dietitian or diabetes nurse educator
	• Regularization of dietary habits
	• Three meals a day
	• Snacks only for patients treated with insulin
	Behavior modification for refractory obesity

evident. Consumption of modest amounts of sucrose is acceptable if control of diabetes is maintained. The use of approved artificial sweeteners in reasonable quantities is sanctioned by the American Diabetes Association.[14] Reduction of sodium, cholesterol, and saturated fat intake is prudent for everyone, but particularly so for patients with diabetes whose risk of heart disease is particularly great.

Limited quantities of alcohol, a glass of wine nightly, for example, are an acceptable part of the diet of any adult with diabetes and may even exert a beneficial effect on plasma lipid composition.[30, 31] In the patient with IDDM, excessive ethanol ingestion may lead to wide fluctuations in plasma glucose concentration, with hyperglycemia at the time of ingestion, and potentially severe hypoglycemia 6 to 12 hours thereafter. The caloric content of alcoholic beverages must also be included in the estimates of daily consumption.

Nutritional Tactics in IDDM

For the patient with IDDM, nutritional therapy aims to minimize oscillations in plasma glucose concentration caused by meals and exercise. Nutritional prescriptions for children with diabetes must also allow for normal growth and development. Adequate calories, protein, and trace nutrients must be supplied in the framework of appropriate injections of exogenous insulin. As the child grows, dietary prescriptions must be modified. Measurements of height and weight should be made at regular intervals, and the information should be plotted on standard growth charts. Deviations from the predicted growth curves in the absence of other illnesses suggest inadequacy of diet and insulin therapy.

Minimizing oscillations in plasma glucose requires consistency in composition and spacing of food intake. Most patients with IDDM need one or more snacks in addition to three meals daily. Depending on the patient's activity pattern, the initial dietary prescription might include a bedtime snack and perhaps an afternoon snack. Midmorning snacks may be added if the interval between breakfast and lunch is prolonged or if the individual experiences frequent midmorning hypoglycemic reactions.

Various formulas have been suggested for distribution of calories during the day; no one is clearly superior. We advocate simply dividing total calories into sixths (or twelfths), with one sixth for breakfast, two sixths for lunch, two sixths for supper, and one twelfth for each of two snacks. Whatever formula is used, the patient must be consistent on a daily basis.

In the patient with IDDM, food also prevents and treats hypoglycemic reactions. In this regard, any biases against giving "sugar" to persons with diabetes should be identified and overcome. Patients and their families must feel free to use any form of readily absorbable glucose to treat hypoglycemia. If the hypoglycemic reaction is not due to missing a meal or unanticipated physical activity, the patient should reduce insulin dosage on the following day.

There is general consensus that a program of instruction in the equivalence of portions of various foods ("exchanges") can facilitate control of diabetes in patients treated with insulin. A knowledge of exchanges enables an individual to anticipate mismatches between insulin and food intake and to take appropriate action. Instruction in these food exchanges is a valuable component of diabetes education programs. In reality, however, few individuals with diabetes adhere closely to exchange based diets over the long term. Those unable or unwilling to focus this degree of attention on each meal can, in fact, often achieve the same result by frequent self-monitoring of glucose combined with intensive insulin therapy. These shortcomings notwithstanding, we advocate instructing patients with IDDM in both the general strategy of prudent diet and the specific advantages that a knowledge of exchanges can provide to the motivated individual.

Nutritional Tactics in NIDDM

When treating obesity-related NIDDM, it is realistic to focus on short-term goals that, although not ideal, may enhance insulin sensitivity sufficiently to restore glucose tolerance to normal. It is better to achieve modest success than to discourage all efforts at weight reduction because of rigid insistence on unattainable goals.

The rate of success using diet alone to achieve weight loss is very low. Only approximately 25% of people enrolling in diet clinics lose 20 lb, and less than 5% lose 40 lb.[32] The number that maintain weight loss for more than 1 year is even less. What success can be achieved requires individualization of the degree of caloric restriction. In general, daily deficits between 250 and 500 calories are advisable. Deficits of this magnitude result in the loss of 0.5 to 1 lb of adipose tissue (at ~3600 cal/lb) per week. Rates of weight loss in this range may be more easily maintained in the long term.

Adequate intake of vitamins and minerals is difficult to achieve if caloric intake is <1200 cal/day. Severely restricted diets require multivitamin supplementation. Diets for patients with NIDDM should be hypocaloric until ideal body weight or acceptable glycemic control is achieved. Meal spacing is important only to the extent that it enhances weight reduction. Patients with the "night eating syndrome" should not skip breakfast or lunch. Snacks and bedtime feedings are not necessary.

Diets that provide up to 65% of total calories as complex carbohydrates may improve OGTT responses in some patients. In contrast, popular low-carbohydrate, high-protein diets are often successful in achieving short-term weight reduction but have poor long-term records and may eventually impair insulin secretion.

Behavior Modification

The majority of obese persons who are able to lose weight gain it back within 2 years. Until effective anorectic agents become available for long-term use, the only supplemental intervention that can be recommended for weight reduction is behavior modification. Not every obese patient is a candidate; patients who became obese during adulthood achieve greater success than do patients whose obesity developed during childhood. The latter group may experience disturbing psychological symptoms if they attempt to reduce to "ideal" weight. Patients with serious psychiatric disturbances are also poor candidates for behavior modification. These programs should be organized by psychologists trained in behavioral theory and methodology.

EXERCISE

Exercise is essential for optimal control of all types of diabetes.[14] A sedentary lifestyle predisposes to obesity and exacerbates other medical problems. Exercise lessens the likelihood of obesity and enhances insulin sensitivity in all individuals regardless of body habitus. It also improves lipid profiles and lessens cardiovascular risk.

Physicians must first educate patients with diabetes with regard to the value of exercise and fitness. This is a critical responsibility. Too often patients consider exercise as less important than medication. In particular, physicians need to point out that substantial benefits can accrue from small investments in activity.

Physicians must of course assess the relative risk of exercise for each patient, but some physical activity should be advocated for all except the bedridden. Individuals who are clearly out of shape and those with diabetes of long duration obviously require thoughtful counseling as to the appropriate level of exercise with which to begin (Table 46–13).

Regular exercise has three notable benefits in NIDDM. First, it increases daily caloric deficits without compromising intake of essential nutrients. Second, it enhances glucose uptake by muscle. Finally, it may actually reduce appetite, thus facilitating adherence to a hypocaloric diet.

Physicians can define realistic and achievable goals for their patients and help them integrate an exercise program into their lifestyle. It is essential that the program be planned, regular, and gradually progressive. Sporadic, excessively stenuous exercise carries definite risks and offers few long-term benefits. Insisting that a patient, or better yet, the family take a 20- to 30-minute walk each day is often an appropriate starting point and can be as important as insisting on compliance with medication. By gradually increasing the pace, the patient can increase the distance walked each day without increasing the time allotted to this activity.

A number of special caveats related to exercise must be taught to patients who depend on insulin. The risk of hypoglycemia is enhanced as a result of increased glucose consumption by muscle during strenuous activity. Patients need to perform self-monitoring of blood glucose both before and after exercise. A low blood glucose concentration before exercise requires prophylactic carbohydrate supplementation, but hyperglycemia after strenuous exercise should *not* be treated with additional insulin. In the latter case, hyperglycemia is probably due to the catecholamine surge associated with the exercise. As it dissipates, glucose concentration falls quickly; supplemental insulin can induce severe hypoglycemia. Finally, because exercise enhances insulin sensitivity, it should be anticipated that progressive, consistent exercise may lower a patient's overall insulin requirement. The same general caveats apply to patients treated with oral agents, but exercise-induced hypoglycemia is an uncommon problem in such cases.

TABLE 46–13. EXERCISE AND DIABETES

Educate patients as to benefits
Determine the cardiovascular risk
Set realistic goals
Suggest methods to integrate the program into patients' lifestyles
Counsel patients on the glycemic implications of exercise
1. Increased need for self-monitored blood glucose determinations for evaluation before and after exercise
2. Increased need for carbohydrate before exercise
3. Reduction in insulin requirements with increasing fitness
4. Avoidance of inappropriate insulin treatment of postexercise hyperglycemia

Obtain the counsel of experts (e.g., diabetes nurse educator, exercise physiologists, cardiologists) as needed

INSULIN THERAPY

Goals and Strategies of Insulin Treatment in Type I Diabetes

Patients with IDDM require insulin for the prevention of ketoacidosis and survival. Even when fasting, they require exogenous insulin to maintain control over hepatic gluconeogenesis, ketogenesis, glycemia, and lipolysis. Almost all patients with type I diabetes require multiple injections of insulin to achieve adequate control throughout the day. In the absence of endogenous insulin, it is impossible to supply appropriately high concentrations of insulin at mealtime and appropriately low concentrations at other times with a single injection. The required injections may take many forms, including (1) multiple injections of intermediate and regular insulin; (2) a single injection of long-acting insulin plus multiple injections of regular insulin with meals; and (3) continuous infusions of regular insulin by pump supplemented with boluses at mealtimes. These alternatives are discussed more fully later.

Goals and Strategies of Insulin Treatment in Type II Diabetes

Patients with NIDDM not adequately controlled by diet and exercise require exogenous insulin to *supplement* endogenous production. Such patients need to reduce fasting hyperglycemia, allowing repletion of pancreatic β cell insulin reserves and fostering endogenous secretion of insulin in response to meals. Because even insulin-treated patients with NIDDM still have endogenous insulin reserves, they retain some capacity for autoregulation of carbohydrate metabolism. They can often be managed with a single injection of intermediate-acting insulin each morning. Some patients require two injections, but more complicated programs usually do little to enhance control in refractory patients.

Insulin Kinetics and Preparations

All practitioners must know something about the onset, peak, and duration of action associated with available insulin preparations. Table 46–14 lists the kinetic properties of commonly used insulin preparations. In the past, most insulins were beef, pork, or beef/pork combination products that contained traces of other proteins like proinsulin. These have largely been replaced by highly purified beef and pork insulins and by human insulin produced by recombinant DNA technology. Table 46–15 provides information on specific beef, pork, and recombinant human insulin products on the market to date.

Most patients can be treated with an intermediate-acting insulin (NPH or Lente), with or without the addition of regular insulin (crystalline zinc insulin). Long-acting insulin (Ultralente) is used in conjunction with multiple injections of regular insulin before meals in intensive insulin treatment regimens.* Continuous subcutaneous insulin infusions by pump require special buffered formulations of regular insulin to prevent precipitation. Semilente insulin has a slightly longer onset, peak, and duration of action than does regular insulin.

For the rapid insulinization needed to treat diabetic ke-

*The manufacture of long-acting protamine zinc insulin in the United States was discontinued at the end of 1991.

TABLE 46–14. INSULIN KINETICS

Type of Insulin	Onset of Action (hr)	Peak of Action (hr)	Duration of Action (hr)
Short-Acting			
Regular beef/pork	0.5–1	2–4	6–8
Regular beef	0.5–1	2–4	6–8
Regular pork	0.5–1	2–4	6–8
Regular human	0.5	1–4	6–8
Semilente beef/pork	1–2	3–8	10–16
Semilente beef	1.5–2	5–7	12–16
Intermediate-Acting			
NPH beef/pork	1–2	6–12	18–26
NPH beef	1–2	6–12	18–26
NPH pork	1–2	6–12	18–26
NPH human	1–2	6–12	18–24
Lente beef/pork	1–3	6–12	18–26
Lente beef	1–3	8–12	20–24
Lente pork	1–3	8–12	18–22
Lente human	1–3	6–10	18–22
*Prolonged-Acting**			
Ultralente beef/pork	4–6	14–24	28–36
Ultralente beef	4–6	16–24	28–36
Ultralente pork	4–6	8–20	24–28

*Long-acting protamine zinc and beef Ultralente insulins are no longer being manufactured.

toacidosis, hyperosmolar coma, and (with glucose) life-threatening hyperkalemia, only regular insulins should be used. These may be given intravenously (for immediate effect), intramuscularly (with onset in 5 to 30 minutes), or subcutaneously. Intermediate and long-acting insulins can be given only subcutaneously.

Most insulin used today is U-100, containing 100 units (~3.6 mg/ml). U-500 insulin is used principally in the treatment of severe insulin-resistant states. The manufacture of U-40 insulins was discontinued in 1991. The administration of small doses of insulin to young children who might formerly have received U-40 preparations can be facilitated by the use of newer, more accurate 0.25 and 0.3 ml syringes that measure insulin doses in $\frac{1}{2}$ unit increments.

Mixing Insulins

Regular insulin may be mixed in a syringe with NPH. The mixture retains characteristics of both the regular and the NPH; there is rapid onset and both an early peak (1 to 2 hours) and an intermediate peak (8 to 14 hours). It is now recommended that regular not be mixed with Lente,[14] but patients controlled using such a mixture need not change. Mixtures of Semilente, Lente, and Ultralente insulin yield preparations that, according to Eli Lilly, Inc., produce a clinical response from the mixture that is the same as that expected from these insulins administered separately.

Fixed Ratio Combination Insulins

As a convenience to patients, premixed combinations of 30% regular and 70% NPH insulin are available in the United States. Other ratios are available in Europe. We recommend these fixed ratio insulins primarily for patients with NIDDM. Because they have residual endogenous insulin secretion, they can compensate for a mismatch between meal size and the relative amounts of NPH and regular insulin. Patients with IDDM with no capacity for internal adjustment must retain the ability to adjust the composition of each insulin injection.

Human Insulin

Human insulins may have a slightly faster onset and a shorter duration of action when compared with conventional purified animal insulin preparations (see Table 46–14). They also produce lower titers of circulating insulin antibodies than do beef and pork insulin. For this reason, human insulins are recommended in the treatment of patients with allergy to animal insulin. Some authorities recommend that human insulins be used in all patients who are starting insulin for the first time, both because of antibody production and because economic forces are likely to make this the most readily available form of insulin in the future. There is no need to switch patients who are successfully managed on animal insulins to human insulins in the absence of a specific indication. It has been suggested that

TABLE 46–15. INSULIN PREPARATIONS AVAILABLE IN THE UNITED STATES

Product	Manufacturer	Form	Strength
Rapid-Acting (onset ½–4 hours)			
Humulin Regular	Lilly	Human	U-100
Humulin BR (for pumps only)	Lilly	Human	U-100
Novolin R (Regular)	Novo Nordisk	Human	U-100
Novolin R Penfill (Regular)	Novo Nordisk	Human	U-100
Velosulin Human (Regular)	Novo Nordisk	Human	U-100
Velosulin Pork (Regular)	Novo Nordisk	Pork	U-100
Iletin I Regular	Lilly	Beef/Pork	U-100
Iletin I Semilente	Lilly	Beef/Pork	U-100
Iletin II Regular	Lilly	Beef	U-100
Iletin II Regular	Lilly	Pork	U-100, U-500
Purified Pork R (Regular)	Novo Nordisk	Pork	U-100
Standard Regular	Novo Nordisk	Pork	U-100
Standard Semilente	Novo Nordisk	Beef	U-100
Intermediate-Acting (onset 2–4 hours)			
Humulin L (Lente)	Lilly	Human	U-100
Humulin N (NPH)	Lilly	Human	U-100
Insulatard Human NPH	Novo Nordisk	Human	U-100
Novolin L (Lente)	Novo Nordisk	Human	U-100
Novolin N (NPH)	Novo Nordisk	Human	U-100
Novolin N Penfill (NPH)	Novo Nordisk	Human	U-100
Iletin I Lente	Lilly	Beef/Pork	U-100
Iletin I NPH	Lilly	Beef/Pork	U-100
Iletin II Lente	Lilly	Beef	U-100
Iletin II NPH	Lilly	Beef	U-100
Iletin II Lente	Lilly	Pork	U-100
Iletin II NPH	Lilly	Pork	U-100
Insulatard NPH	Novo Nordisk	Pork	U-100
Purified Pork (Lente)	Novo Nordisk	Pork	U-100
Purified Pork N (NPH)	Novo Nordisk	Pork	U-100
Standard NPH	Novo Nordisk	Beef	U-100
Long-Acting (onset 4–6 hours)			
Humulin U (Ultralente)	Lilly	Human	U-100
Iletin I Ultralente	Lilly	Beef/Pork	U-100
Standard Ultralente	Novo Nordisk	Beef	U-100
Mixtures (All are 70% NPH, 30% Regular Insulin)			
Mixtard 70/30	Novo Nordisk	Pork	U-100
Mixtard Human 70/30	Novo Nordisk	Human	U-100
Novolin 70/30	Novo Nordisk	Human	U-100
Novolin 70/30 Penfill	Novo Nordisk	Human	U-100
Humulin 70/30	Lilly	Human	U-100

TABLE 46–16. SCHEDULES FOR INSULIN ADMINISTRATION

Prebreakfast	Prelunch	Presupper	Bedtime	Comments
N	—	—	—	Rarely suitable for IDDM
N + R	—	—	—	Regular covers breakfast
N	—	N	—	Usual starting regimen for IDDM
N + R	—	N + R	—	Treatment for IDDM providing coverage of meals and sleep
N + R	—	R	N	Variant on previous regimen
N + R	R	R	N	Intensive control regimen providing greater mimicry of normal insulin secretory patterns
R	R	U + R	—	Alternative intensive control regimen with one less injection

N = NPH or Lente insulin; R = regular insulin; U = Ultralente insulin. Additional strategies might include:
1. Ultralente (70%) and Lente (30%) mix at bedtime plus regular insulin before meals.
2. Continuous subcutaneous insulin infusion by pump.

some patients using human insulin are more susceptible to hypoglycemia unawareness (see later) than are patients using animal insulins, but this remains a subject of controversy and is not a contraindication to the use of human insulin.

Tactics of Insulin Administration

Insulin regimens are designed to mimic normal insulin responses to feedings. In patients with NIDDM, physicians provide exogenous insulin supplementation to enhance *endogenous* β cell response to meals. Patients with IDDM have no endogenous reserves, and insulin administration in the patient with IDDM must make allowance for each meal.

In the nonpregnant adult with IDDM, the easiest and least disruptive program is two daily insulin injections. Increasing the number of injections enhances a patient's ability to tailor insulin to meals and exercise but demands more injections and self-monitoring of blood glucose. Complex strategies can become increasingly disruptive of normal living and may enhance the risk of hypoglycemia. Insulin infusion pumps allow the most fastidious control over plasma glucose concentration but pose the risks of both severe hypoglycemia (if the pump keeps running during stupor or coma) and DKA (if the pump malfunctions). The pump is discussed later in the section on intensive therapies.

The patient and the physician must decide together on the best insulin administration strategy. That choice varies with age, education, insight, duration of diabetes, ability to respond to hypoglycemia, and the presence of complications.

The *split mix* is the simplest method for IDDM and is the best one for newly diagnosed patients. The patient on a split mix administers a mixture of regular and intermediate insulin, 20 to 30 minutes before breakfast, and a second injection of a mixture of regular and intermediate insulin, 20 to 30 minutes before supper. The morning regular insulin modulates the plasma glucose concentration after breakfast; the morning intermediate insulin is maximally effective after lunch and during the afternoon; the evening regular insulin covers supper; the evening intermediate provides insulinization during the night. Dosage and scheduling are modified according to the results of self-monitoring of blood glucose.

The most generally useful recommendation is to inject two thirds of the total requirement in the morning and one third in the evening. The intermediate:regular insulin ratio is usually approximately 2:1. It is important to teach the patient to adjust only one component of the mix at a time. In general, the intermediate-acting insulin should receive priority when the dose is adjusted; changes in short-acting insulins can be thought of as "fine tuning" the regimen in response to individual diet and exercise habits. It is also essential that the patient learn to expect insulin requirements, and thus insulin doses, to vary over time.

Patients ideally choose the dose of both morning and evening insulin based on self-monitoring of blood glucose and experience with hypoglycemia over the previous 1 to 2 days. Once doses are chosen, they should not, if possible, be altered for 1 to 2 days so that the pattern of glycemic control associated with the regimen can be evaluated by SMBG.

Adjustments of the basic split mix regimen are generally straightforward. Hyperglycemia at noon should prompt an increase in the next morning's regular insulin dosage; hyperglycemia at supper should be followed by an increase in the morning intermediate; hyperglycemia at bedtime should be treated with increasing evening regular; and hyperglycemia before breakfast necessitates increasing the evening intermediate. Hypoglycemic symptoms or self-monitored blood glucose determinations below the target range before lunch should result in a reduction of the next morning's regular insulin. Symptoms of low glucose concentrations during the afternoon should prompt a reduction in the morning intermediate, and so on.

Other Schedules. Many minor and major alterations of the basic split mix insulin schedule can be used. Some are listed in Table 46–16. Selection of the appropriate schedule depends on factors including age, type of diabetes, target blood glucose concentration, diet, patient compliance, and the results of self-monitoring of blood glucose. When attempting to determine which pattern to employ, a measurement of blood glucose concentration before each meal and at bedtime is desirable. Other schedules may be devised as needed to compensate for unusual work, exercise, or travel needs.

Adjusting Insulin Dosage

Whatever the schedule, both physician and patient must understand the rationale for adjustments in dosages. Adjustments must be deliberate and made according to a predetermined plan. On a daily basis, decisions regarding adjustments must be made by the patient, and there is no text or computer program that can provide the correct adjustment advice for an individual. The physician's role is primarily to see that the patient is properly educated. Specific adjustments of the split mix regimen have been discussed earlier. Table 46–17 and the following section list some general guidelines that can be used by both the physician and the patient for adjusting most insulin regimens.

TABLE 46–17. SAMPLE GUIDELINES FOR ADJUSTMENT OF INSULIN DOSE BASED ON THE PATTERN OF PREMEAL AND BEDTIME BLOOD GLUCOSE MEASUREMENTS

Pattern	Prebreakfast	Prelunch	Presupper	Bedtime	Adjustment
1: Patient on 1 dose of NPH in the morning	P	P	P	P	↑ Intermediate insulin 10%
2: Patient on 1 dose of NPH in the morning	A	P	A	A	Add regular insulin
3: Patient on 1 dose of NPH plus regular in the morning	P	A	A	A	Split ⅔–⅓
4: Patient on split mix	A	A	P	A	↓ Afternoon snack
5: Patient on split mix	A	A	A	P	↓ Bedtime snack
6: Patient on split mix	P	P	A	A	↑ Evening intermediate

P = poor control (hyperglycemia); A = adequate control. Alternative approaches if these adjustments are not adequate might include those outlined in Table 46–14.

The magnitude of daily adjustments should be agreed on in advance. A reasonable rule of thumb is to adjust the total insulin dosage by no more than 10%/day. A frequent cause of unstable diabetes is adjustment by increments that are excessive. Patients with unstable diabetes may need to adjust their dose daily (see later). More stable diabetes may require no changes for days or weeks. For many patients with diabetes, adjustments every 2 to 4 days are appropriate.

The physician and the patient must agree on desirable glycemic control. For individuals with labile diabetes, self-monitored blood glucose concentrations of 100 to 180 mg/dl (5.6 to 10 mM) may be the optimum achievable. The target for patients with more stable diabetes is 80 to 140 mg/dl (4.4 to 7.8 mM). Because insulin requirements vary constantly, regular adjustments are essential for optimal control. It is not adequate to have the patient examined every 3 months by a physician who then makes a specific recommendation for insulin adjustment. Most patients can and must be guided to a level of understanding that permits them to regulate their insulin appropriately on a daily basis. The physician in this setting is the navigator, not the helmsman.

Sick Day Rules

During illness, insulin requirements for patients with type I diabetes generally increase as a result of increased insulin resistance. With SMBG and intelligent adjustment of insulin doses, DKA can usually be prevented. If, however, a patient cannot maintain control after 48 hours of acute illness, he or she should contact the physician for help whether or not ketonuria is present. During illness, supplemental injections of regular insulin are often required temporarily. Guidelines for these adjustments, the classical "sick day rules," are outlined in Figure 46–2.

Basically, patients should check self-monitored capillary blood sugars every 4 hours and, if hyperglycemia is present, urine should be checked for ketonuria. Supplemental regular insulin is taken every 4 hours until ketonuria clears and normoglycemia is restored. If ketonuria and hyperglycemia (≥300 mg/dl) are not controlled within 24 hours, the patient should be examined by a physician. Arterial pH of less than approximately 7.2 or serum bicarbonate level of less than approximately 15 mEq/l are indications for the patient to be hospitalized.

The most common "sick day" error is made by patients who are unable to eat because of nausea and vomiting; they may take no insulin in a mistaken effort to avoid hypoglycemia. But decreasing their insulinization is, of course, the quickest route to DKA. Combined with the insulin resistance and predisposition to dehydration associated with infectious gastrointestinal illness, DKA can occur with lethal celerity. If a patient with diabetes cannot keep liquids down for more than 8 to 12 hours and has persistent hyperglycemia and ketonuria, the risk of worsening ketoacidosis is very high, and the individual should be seen in the emergency department.

Starting Insulin Treatment

It is not necessary to hospitalize most patients to begin insulin therapy. Of course, patients with ketoacidosis should be hospitalized for prompt treatment. In addition,

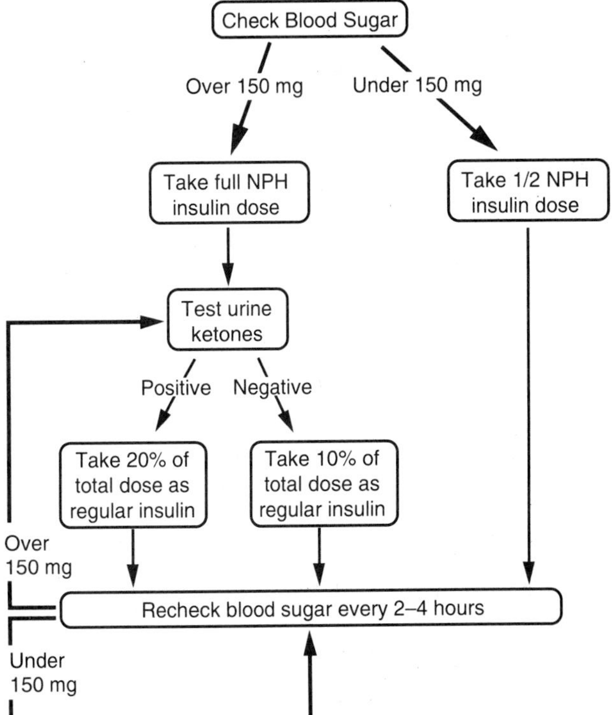

FIGURE 46–2. General outline for self-care by the patient with insulin-dependent diabetes when the patient is ill. These guidelines must, of course, be individualized according to the age, insight, and self-care capabilities of the patient.

patients of any age with unusual handicaps or with extreme fear of self-injection may prudently be hospitalized to institute therapy. The average patient with NIDDM who requires insulin to control hyperglycemia may be started on therapy as an outpatient. It is reasonable to begin with 15 to 20 units of intermediate insulin each morning and expect to have to increase the dosage gradually until adequate control is achieved. Again, the objective of insulin therapy in the patient with NIDDM is to supplement endogenous production, not to supply exogenously the total requirement for insulin.

Intensive Insulin Therapies

Intensive injection therapy and continuous subcutaneous infusions of insulin by pump (CSII) are alternative strategies for achieving tight control of diabetes. Intensive therapy generally consists of a single daily injection of intermediate or long-acting insulin plus three or more additional injections of regular insulin before meals. The pump provides analogous treatment, a continuous basal infusion of regular insulin that is supplemented by three to five additional premeal boluses. Neither form of intensive therapy can be offered to patients unwilling or unable to devote substantial time and attention to its use. To be successful, both regimens demand 4 to 8 SMBG glucose determinations daily and the intellectual ability to translate the results into appropriate modifications of each bolus or injection of insulin. When appropriately selected, motivated patients can achieve the same excellent results using either method. Multiple injections are more cumbersome, but pumps are very expensive. Being mechanical devices, it is also possible that pumps might malfunction, leading to either DKA or severe hypoglycemia, but reports of such problems are rare. Newer pumps contain internal self-test systems and alarms. The American Diabetes Association recommends that intensive treatment with insulin pumps be prescribed only at medical facilities that have a professional team skilled in their use.[14]

Notes About Injections

The traditional teaching about rotation of injection sites has changed. It is now recommended that one area (e.g., the abdomen or arm) be used for several weeks, with the injection site rotating within that area. The recommendation reflects the discovery of variability in insulin absorption from one region to another and is intended to provide longer periods of relative absorptive consistency. Technique should be assessed whenever a new patient is enrolled into a physician's practice. Patients should be counseled not to inject into the leg or arm before exercise involving these extremities. In the interest of saving money, the limited reuse of syringes has been shown to be generally safe, but in the absence of severe financial constraint, the American Diabetes Association discourages the practice.[14] To reduce the discomfort of injection to a minimum, we recommend the use of insulin syringes that feature newer 29-gauge lubricated needles.

Various devices intended to enhance compliance and control are also available to patients. Infusion pumps have been mentioned earlier. Insulin injection "pens" are cartridge-like devices designed to make it more convenient to administer multiple injections. Each cartridge holds at least 1 day's supply of insulin. The patient dials in the dose and pushes a button to administer it. The pens do not provide continuous insulin but facilitate compliance with intensive treatment regimens. Much more popular in Europe than in the United States, they require special insulin refills and skilled instruction in their use. Jet injectors administer insulin transcutaneously without a needle by using high pressure. Devices similar in principle are used in mass vaccination programs. Insulin jet injectors offer no proven biologic advantage over conventional insulin injections. They are expensive and require maintenance, but many patients prefer them to needles. Finally, many devices (e.g., magnifiers) are available that make injecting insulin more convenient or more precise for certain patients. Such patients can conveniently be apprised of these devices by their diabetes nurse educator.

Sensitivity to Regular Insulin

Sensitivity to regular insulin is a poorly understood and inadequately appreciated problem that afflicts many patients with long-term diabetes, generally those with IDDM. After many years of diabetes, the frequency of hypoglycemic reactions begins to increase, and diabetes control appears to become "brittle" in the absence of intercurrent illness, renal failure, or adrenal insufficiency. In such patients the problem often appears to be enhanced sensitivity to even very small doses of regular insulin. One strategy for restoring normoglycemia in longstanding diabetes that is out of control is to reduce greatly the regular insulin in the regimen. A final uncommon cause of sensitivity to insulin is the Houssay phenomenon: sensitivity to insulin in the context of pituitary insufficiency due to either a tumor or ablation.

COMPLICATIONS OF INSULIN THERAPY

Hypoglycemia

A major side effect of therapy with insulin and, to a lesser extent, the oral agents is hypoglycemia. Patients and families should be taught how to recognize hypoglycemia and how to deal with it (Table 46–18). Hypoglycemia in the patient with IDDM often results from delays in meals or irregular patterns of exercise. If hypoglycemia occurs for either of these reasons, the insulin dose on the following

TABLE 46–18. HYPOGLYCEMIA

Signs and Symptoms	
Hunger	Diaphoresis
Pallor	Headache
Dizziness	Nervousness or trembling
Blurred vision	Irritability
Crying	Confusion
Inability to concentrate	Drowsiness or fatigue
Poor coordination	Abdominal pain or nausea
Inappropriate actions/responses	

Treatment

At the first sign of any of the aforementioned warnings, give sugar immediately. Any one of the following forms is acceptable

Sugar: 5 small cubes, 2 packets, or 2 teaspoons

Fruit juice: $\frac{1}{2}$ to $\frac{2}{3}$ cup

Carbonated beverage (not diet or sugarless soda): 6 oz

Candy: $\frac{1}{4}$ to $\frac{1}{3}$ candy bar

Concentrated carbohydrates (e.g., Insta-Glucose Tubes; Glucose Squeeze Bottles, B-D Glucose Tablets, Insulin Reaction Gel Foil Packets, or Dextrosol Tablets)

day should not be reduced. Rather, every attempt should be made to return eating and exercise patterns to normal. Hypoglycemic reactions occurring for reasons that cannot be identified should be followed by a decrease in the appropriate insulin the following day, as outlined earlier. There are, of course, many other causes of hypoglycemia in addition to exogenous insulin. These causes are beyond the scope of this chapter. We have discussed them in detail elsewhere.[33]

Treating Hypoglycemia Orally and with Glucagon

Most hypoglycemic reactions can be treated with sugar by mouth. Orange juice, soft drinks, candy, and glucose products designed for individuals with diabetes to carry with them are equally effective. If the person with diabetes does not respond and is unable to swallow, intramuscular glucagon (1 mg) should be given immediately and the patient brought to an emergency room for evaluation. If the patient has not responded within 5 minutes, a second injection of glucagon should be given en route to the hospital. After a severe insulin-induced hypoglycemic reaction, the patient should be observed for several hours to ensure that hypoglycemia does not recur. A determination of the type of insulin responsible for a reaction, whether short, intermediate, or long-acting, may be helpful in determining how long a period of observation is needed. Any person known to have diabetes who is unconscious should be presumed to be hypoglycemic and should be treated with glucose intravenously. This should be done immediately or immediately after obtaining blood for later glucose determination, but only if the blood sampling can be done without delay.

Hypoglycemia Unawareness

It has been estimated that 25% of patients with IDDM experience hypoglycemia unawareness.[34] The factors involved include duration of diabetes, chronicity of hypoglycemic episodes, and loss of counterregulatory capability due to autonomic neuropathy. As noted earlier, this may be more common among users of human insulin. Hypoglycemia unawareness is also more frequent in patients receiving β-adrenergic blockers.

Insulin Allergies

Some patients develop a local reaction after insulin injections. This consists of erythema, pruritus, and mild induration. It is most common when insulin injections are first started and is less common with human insulins. These localized skin reactions usually subside without further treatment.

True insulin allergy, mediated by IgE antibodies, is rare. In almost all cases, the patient has received intermittent insulin injections in the past. When urticaria or anaphylaxis occurs after a subcutaneous insulin injection, the patient nearly always has received insulin previously without untoward effect. Other allergic reactions to insulin are in fact allergies to some component of the solution in which the insulin is suspended. These include protamine and preservatives like methylparaben. Substitution of an equivalent insulin, Lente for NPH, for example, may solve the problem.

Patients with type I diabetes and true insulin allergy need to be desensitized by a specialist. They are injected with a very small amount of human insulin, and the dose is increased as rapidly as tolerated. Insulin-allergic patients with NIDDM can also be desensitized, but the patient may wish to reconsider alternative methods of treatment, particularly diet and exercise.

Antibody-Mediated Insulin Resistance

Local and systemic insulin allergies must be distinguished from IgG-mediated insulin resistance. "Insulin resistance" is present in patients who require more than 200 units of insulin daily for 2 days or more in the absence of DKA, infection, or endocrinopathy. Most patients with insulin resistance in the absence of intercurrent illness have IgG anti-insulin antibodies. Insulin resistance associated with acanthosis nigricans, lipoatrophy, or enhanced subcutaneous proteolysis is rare.

All patients receiving insulin develop low titers of anti-insulin antibodies, but only rare patients with high titers become resistant. Treatment can be difficult. Patients taking beef or pork insulin should be switched to human insulin, but cross-reactivity may frustrate this tactic. If a resistant patient has IDDM, very large insulin doses (up to several thousand units daily) may be required. One may also attempt to inhibit antibody production by giving corticosteroids. This should be attempted only in the hospital because, if the treatment is successful, a precipitous fall in plasma glucose may occur, and intravenous glucose may be needed. Fortunately, IgG-mediated insulin resistance is usually self-limiting, rarely lasts for more than 1 year, and tends not to recur.

Lipoatrophy and Lipohypertrophy

Some patients develop localized areas of lipoatrophy or lipohypertrophy in response to subcutaneous insulin. Such patients should have their injection insulin techniques reviewed to ensure that they are preparing and administering the insulin correctly. Pockets of lipoatrophy can be treated with small injections of insulin into the margins of the atrophied areas. Human or highly purified pork insulin should be used, and subsequent rotation of insulin sites may help. Lipohypertrophy does not usually respond to this technique.

Syndrome X

Studying normal weight populations, several investigators have observed that up to 20% may be to some degree insulin resistant. These have been called "metabolically obese, normal-weight" individuals, or persons with "syndrome X." They are remarkable not merely because of insulin resistance, but also because they appear to have the same vascular complications that afflict the patients with insulin-resistant diabetes. Some investigators studying these associations have speculated that chronically high concentrations of circulating insulin may have adverse effects on plasma lipids and blood pressure and thus induce vascular disease. This theoretical toxicity of hyperinsulinemia is a controversial subject under active study.[35]

If there are risks associated with chronic hyperinsulinemia, this would call into question the wisdom of treating obese, insulin-resistant patients with large

(>100 units/day) doses of insulin. This issue, too, is controversial and unresolved.[36, 37] For the practitioner, it is only important to realize that even if syndrome X proves to be real, that fact should not alter treatment of NIDDM. Rather, it should only reinforce established principles. Diet, exercise, and weight loss (not insulin) are the definitive, first-line therapies in NIDDM.

UNSTABLE IDDM

The term "brittle diabetes" should be avoided. Uncontrolled diabetes is common, but uncontrollable diabetes is rare. Factors contributing to fluctuations in control of diabetes are variability in food intake and exercise, errors in self-testing and insulin techniques, intercurrent illnesses, emotional stress, and the use of interfering medications. Some common causes of changing diabetes control are listed in Table 46–19.

Increased Insulin Resistance

Stress, particularly infection, is the most important factor to consider when control is lost, particularly in patients with longstanding diabetes who were previously stable. The stressor need not be an obvious one. Malignancy, major infection, unplanned pregnancy, and new onset coronary ischemia are only a few of the common problems whose presence may be heralded by loss of diabetes control. In addition, there are six occult infections that should not be overlooked. These are dental abscesses, gingivitis, sinusitis, osteomyelitis, cholecystitis, and chronic pyelonephritis. The causes of insulin resistance described earlier are quite rare in comparison.

Abnormal Glucose Counterregulation

Abnormalities in counterregulatory systems, particularly glucagon and epinephrine, can also contribute to unstable diabetes control.[38] A mild degree of counterregulatory impairment is common in all patients with diabetes after the disease has been present for several years. More severe impairment is less common and much more difficult to treat. Unless a primary care physician is experienced in the treatment of unstable diabetes with impaired counterregulation, such patients should probably be referred to a diabetologist.

Exercise

Exercise can have a major impact on control. Vigorous exercise can increase absorption of insulin injected into an active extremity but have little effect on injections in the abdomen. In well-controlled patients with IDDM, exercise also enhances glucose uptake by muscle and can result in hypoglycemia. In the poorly controlled patient with IDDM, exercise can increase hepatic glycogenolysis, gluconeogenesis, and ketogenesis; exacerbate hyperglycemia; and lead to ketoacidosis.

Insulinization

Both underinsulinization and overinsulinization can result from errors in injection, the prescription of new medications, gradual change in body weight, intercurrent illness, and change in level of physical activity. Most commonly the real problem is the reluctance of the patient to adjust the insulin dose or to call for advice regarding the dose, following a change in the circumstances just described. Patient education is the key to solving this problem. Finally, whenever *declining* insulin requirements are observed in longstanding diabetes, changes in thyroid, adrenal, and renal function should be excluded.

Causes of Hyperglycemia in the Morning

The *Somogyi phenomenon* effect describes posthypoglycemic, rebound hyperglycemia due to secretion of counterregulatory hormones.[39] It is seen occasionally in patients with IDDM who experience hypoglycemia during the night. They may not awaken during the reaction, but in the morning, they complain of fatigue, headaches, sweats, or bizarre dreams. Hyperglycemia and ketonuria are present before breakfast. Misguided attempts to prevent *rebound* morning hyperglycemia by increasing the dose of insulin lead to more frequent and more severe nocturnal hypoglycemic episodes and more rebound hyperglycemia during the following morning. Diagnosis of nocturnal hypoglycemia can be made by obtaining a self-monitored fingerstick blood glu-

TABLE 46–19. POSSIBLE CAUSES FOR CHANGES IN DIABETES CONTROL

Increasing Insulin Requirement	Decreasing Insulin Requirement
1. Increased food intake	1. Decreased food intake
2. Decreased level of exercise	2. Increased exercise
3. Increased insulin resistance	3. Increased insulin sensitivity
a. Obvious infections	a. Regular insulin sensitivity with long duration of diabetes
• Viral infections	b. Impaired renal function
• Bacterial (urinary, foot)	c. Endocrine disease (e.g., adrenal insufficiency, hyperthyroidism)
b. Occult infections Osteomyelitis; sinusitis; dental abscess; gallbladder disease; pyelonephritis	d. Liver disease
c. Malignancy	e. Medications (e.g., alcohol, β-blockers)
d. Vascular disease (e.g., myocardial ischemia)	4. Insulin injection errors
e. Medications (e.g., corticosteroids)	
f. Stress	
g. Endocrine diseases (e.g., Cushing's syndrome)	
h. Rebound after hypoglycemia	
i. Pregnancy/menstruation	
4. Insulin injection errors	

TABLE 46–20. ORAL HYPOGLYCEMIC AGENTS AVAILABLE IN THE UNITED STATES

Generic Name	Trade Name	Manufacturer	Dosage Range (mg/day)	Approximate Biologic Half-Life (hr)
Tolbutamide	Orinase	Upjohn	500–3000	4
Chlorpropamide	Diabinese	Pfizer	100–750	36–72
Acetohexamide	Dymelor	Lilly	500–1500	5
Tolazamide	Tolinase	Upjohn	100–750	7
Glyburide	Diabeta	Hoechst	1.25–20	24
	Micronase	Upjohn	1.25–20	24
Glipizide	Glucotrol	Roerig	5–40	24

cose concentration at 2 or 3 AM. Appropriate treatment is either a reduction in total insulin dosage or modified spacing of insulin and meals.

Use caution when attributing poor control of diabetes to the Somogyi phenomenon. If reducing the dose of insulin does not improve control, other explanations must be sought and different modifications in therapy tried.

The *dawn phenomenon* refers to a rise in plasma glucose concentration that occurs in everyone beginning about 5 AM.[40] It is due to increasing concentrations of circulating counterregulatory hormones that are under circadian control. Unlike the Somogyi phenomenon, which tends to occur around 3 AM, the modest increase in glycemia due to the dawn phenomenon responds to increased insulinization.

The *previous night's meal* exerts a major influence on fasting glycemia. Alterations in the quantity or timing or either supper or snack are common causes of loss of control.

TREATMENT OF DIABETES WITH ORAL HYPOGLYCEMIC AGENTS

Classes and Mechanisms of Action

Table 46–20 lists the oral hypoglycemic agents (OHA) available in the United States. All are sulfonylurea compounds. The newer second-generation drugs, glyburide and glipizide, are more potent than the older agents and may be effective in some patients refractory to first generation agents. Some studies suggest that the newer agents may have fewer side effects.[41]

The sulfonylureas useful in the treatment of diabetes are thought to work via several mechanisms. They enhance release of insulin from pancreatic β cells. In addition they appear to reduce insulin resistance and block hepatic gluconeogenesis. Other oral agents that act by different mechanisms are under development. These agents include biguanides such as metformin and other compounds that may have entirely different mechanisms of action. These are not available in the United States at this writing.

Indications

The pharmacology of sulfonylureas indicates their suitability for treating NIDDM but not IDDM. Therapy with oral hypoglycemic agents is limited to type II patients whose diabetes has proved refractory to diet and exercise. Because of concerns about possible teratogenicity, the drugs are contraindicated in gestational diabetes. Basic information on the use of oral hypoglycemic agents is summarized in Table 46–21; our algorithmic approach to their use is shown in Figure 46–3.

Like the insulins, sulfonylureas are available as short, intermediate, and long-acting compounds. Tolbutamide has the shortest duration of action; it is metabolized in the liver to *inactive* metabolites that are excreted by the kidney. Tolazamide, acetohexamide, glyburide, and glipizide are metabolized to other *active* compounds by the liver. Their duration of action is classified as intermediate and lasts 18 to 24 hours. They can be given once daily. The long-acting compound chlorpropamide is minimally metabolized and has a duration of action of 36 to 72 hours. It is excreted almost entirely by the kidneys.

Patients with liver disease should not receive tolbutamide; patients with renal disease should not be given chlorpropamide. In both cases, excretory failure may lead to severe hypoglycemia. Elderly patients and others at particular risk from hypoglycemia may best be treated with the agents that have a shorter half-life.

Side Effects

The major side effect of these drugs is hypoglycemia. The most important clinical point is that oral agent–induced hypoglycemia is very long in duration and can recur after initial treatment with glucose. Any patient with hypoglycemia due to an oral agent should be hospitalized, monitored closely, and given a continuous infusion of glucose until the oral agent has been completely metabolized.

Minor side effects include rashes and gastrointestinal complaints. Acetohexamide has uricosuric effects. Glyburide and glipizide increase free water clearance. Chlorpropamide can cause the syndrome of inappropriate antidiuretic hormone secretion (SIADH), posing the risk of both hyponatremia and hypoglycemia in elderly patients with renal impairment. Uncommon severe side effects of sulfonylurea compounds include hepatotoxicity, generalized hy-

TABLE 46–21. GUIDELINES FOR THE USE OF ORAL HYPOGLYCEMIC AGENTS

1. First-line treatment of NIDDM is diet and exercise. If these two measures do not normalize glycemia, then oral hypoglycemic agents should be *added* to this regimen
2. Characteristics of patients most likely to respond to oral agents:
   - Onset of diabetes after 40 years of age
   - Duration of diabetes <5 years
   - Normal weight or obese
   - No previous use of insulin, or diabetes controlled with <40 units/day of insulin
3. Absolute contraindications
   - Allergy to sulfonylurea compounds
   - Insulin dependent (type I) diabetes mellitus
   - Pregnancy
4. Relative contraindications
   - Intercurrent illness (e.g., infection, trauma, ischemic heart disease)
   - Liver or renal disease
   - Known allergy to sulfur-containing antibiotics and diuretics

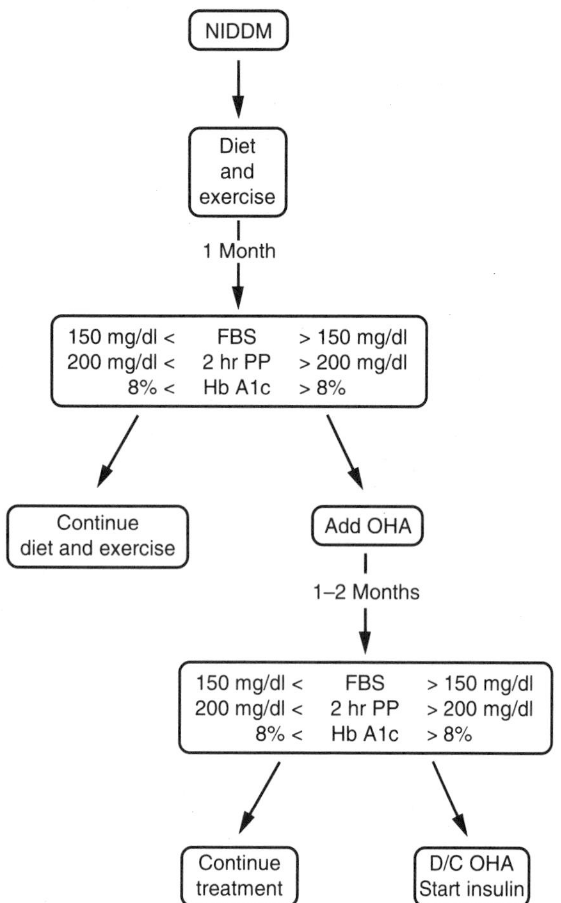

FIGURE 46–3. General approach to the treatment of patients who are candidates for treatment with oral hypoglycemic agent. Each case must, of course, be individualized.

persensitivity reactions, and agranulocytosis. Patients allergic to sulfur-containing antibiotics and diuretics (e.g., furosemide) may also be allergic to sulfonylureas, but such cross-reactivity is rare. The use of oral hypoglycemic agents in sulfa allergic patients is discouraged. If it cannot be avoided, the oral agent should be started under close supervision.

All sulfonylurea drugs occasionally produce disulfiram (Antabuse)-like reactions in patients who also ingest alcohol. Glyburide and glipizide are probably less problematic in this regard. They are also less likely to be displaced from albumin and potentiated by drugs like aspirin, phenylbutazone, and warfarin. Drug interactions with oral agents are listed in Table 46–22.

As noted earlier, all sulfonylureas can produce severe hypoglycemia. This may occur inadvertently in patients with worsening excretory function, as a result of overdosage, and occasionally as a result of dispensing errors due to similarities among the names of many of the drugs, as shown in Table 46–23.

Treatment Failure

Primary treatment failure refers to patients who never achieve satisfactory control in response to oral agents. *Secondary treatment failure* refers to patients who initially respond satisfactorily, but whose glycemic control later deteriorates. The rates of failure are hard to estimate; perhaps 40% of suitable candidates fail primarily, and another 10 to 30%/yr fail secondarily. Patient selection is important. The older the patient and the shorter the duration of the diabetes, the greater is the likelihood of success. Patients with normal or above-normal weight also fare better than do patients who are underweight. If a patient remains inadequately controlled after 3 months of treatment, there is little point in continuing sulfonylurea therapy; instead, renew efforts at dietary management or begin insulin injections.

The second-generation agents, although more potent, are probably not more effective therapeutically than chlorpropamide. Patients who fail secondarily on an older agent may respond to one of the newer drugs.

Some patients controlled on oral agents remain in satisfactory control on a suitable diet if the drug is discontinued. For this reason, it is reasonable to reduce the dosage and, occasionally, to stop the drug entirely to determine if therapy is still warranted. An algorithm for the use of OHA is given in Figure 46–3.

TABLE 46–22. DRUG INTERACTIONS THAT AFFECT ORAL HYPOGLYCEMIC AGENTS

Potentiators	Antagonists
Acute ethanol ingestion	Chronic alcoholism
Anabolic steroids	Corticosteroids
Phenylbutazone	Phenytoin
Clofibrate	Diazoxide
Chloramphenicol	Phenothiazines
Cyclophosphamide	Rifampin
Guanethidine	Thiazides
Oral anticoagulants (warfarin)	
Monoamine oxidase inhibitors	
Propranolol	
Salicylates	
Methysergide (Sansert)	
Sulfonamides	
Tetracyclines	

Combining Insulin and Oral Agents

Because oral agents decrease insulin resistance and block hepatic gluconeogenesis, it is reasonable to believe that they could be useful in *potentiating* the effects not only of residual endogenous insulin secretion but injected insulin as well. In theory, administration of both drugs should enhance control while reducing the dose of exogenous insulin. Although an attractive concept in principle, the practice of combining oral agents with insulin injections has not proved useful in IDDM and may have only limited use in NIDDM.[42] The recommended strategy is to use an intermediate or long-acting insulin at bedtime and the oral

TABLE 46–23. MEDICATION-DISPENSING ERRORS THAT CAN CAUSE HYPOGLYCEMIA

Prescribed Medication	Dispensed Medication
Acetazolamide (Diamox)	Acetohexamide (Dymelor)
Dyazide	Dymelor
Dialume ($A1(OH)_3$)	Diabinese
Tolectin	Tolinase
Diamox	Diabinese
Chlorpromazine	Chlorpropamide

agent in the morning, but treatment must be individualized and efficacy evaluated critically in each patient.

PATIENT EDUCATION

Every competent person with diabetes must assume some responsibility for management of the disease. Diabetes requires daily, sometimes hourly decision making that no caregiver can provide. Effective diabetes care requires effective patient education.

At the time of diagnosis, psychological factors may impair a patient's receptiveness to learning. Nearly everyone has acquired misinformation from the media and fears diabetes and its complications. Deal with these fears at the outset. Only then can effective learning take place.

Patients should learn what type of diabetes is present; the goals, strategies, and tactics of therapy; and the rationale for each. The information can be made as simple or as sophisticated as circumstances dictate. All patients should know about complications in a general way but need specific instruction in the signs and symptoms of certain complications, particularly ketoacidosis and hyperosmolar nonketotic coma. Patients should understand how to respond to changes in the control of their diabetes and when to obtain medical advice promptly. With understanding, the patient is in a better position to regulate therapy on the basis of rational self-interest and self-motivation.

Topics of Instruction

Dietary instruction should be provided by a registered dietitian or other trained health educator. The dietitian can provide specific recommendations, adapted to the patient's educational, economic, and cultural circumstances. In some cases, major changes in eating behavior may be desirable, but the smaller the alterations, the greater is the chance for success. Dietary fads should be dealt with openly but sympathetically; a "frontal attack" is the least effective way to diminish their attractiveness. Provision must be made for follow-up, evaluation, and modification of dietary prescriptions. Obviously, reinforcement of the role of nutrition by the physician is helpful.

Self-monitoring of blood glucose is now standard practice. In the absence of physical or intellectual handicaps, all patients with diabetes should learn self-monitoring techniques. The desirable frequency of monitoring varies with the individual patient. In general, patients with IDDM should obtain a minimum of two values daily; three to four determinations are preferable if at all possible. All methods require the patient to obtain capillary blood by pricking the finger with a small lancet attached to a spring-loaded device. Because of the risk of transmitting infection, the lancets should not be reused, nor should the devices be shared with anyone. All currently available glucose monitoring systems require both a drop of capillary blood and a disposable test strip. Specific manufacturer's instructions for each glucose meter must be followed exactly. The technology is constantly advancing. Consultation with a specialist in diabetes management or a diabetes nurse educator is necessary to stay abreast of developments.

The blood sugar can be estimated by comparing the color on some strips with a standardized color chart, but this method is susceptible to error. A meter is preferred and will be paid for by many insurance carriers. The results should be recorded in a diary or logbook.

Diaries for recording self-monitored blood glucose results are very valuable. Meter manufacturers often provide logbooks to record measurement data. Simple sheets of paper with six columns are preferable (Fig. 46–4). In the first column, the patient records the day's insulin dose. In the next four columns, values obtained before each meal and at bedtime are recorded as needed. The last column is used for comments, including a log of reactions and notes concerning meals and exercise. Patients must be educated with regard to the need for accurate data and should be discouraged from making up numbers to please the caregiver. Even a few accurate values can be useful. The patient should bring the diary when visiting the physician or nurse educator.

Urine testing for glucose should be used only when patients cannot or will not perform SMBG.[14] In those cases, second-voided specimens four times daily are required for patients with IDDM; less frequent determinations suffice for patients with NIDDM. In either case, the patient should understand why the test is necessary and how to interpret the semiquantitative grading of glycosuria. The major use of urine testing is for the detection of ketones by insulin-treated patients during illness. Detection of ketonuria is a major component of the "sick day rules."

Learning correct insulin injection techniques is a critical need for all IDDM and insulin-treated NIDDM patients. Cleaning of the stopper and injection of air should precede withdrawal from the vial. When two kinds of insulin (usually regular and NPH) are drawn into the same syringe, it is recommended that the regular insulin be drawn up first.

For subcutaneous injections, the patient picks up a fold of skin, holds the fold between the thumb and index finger, and injects into the fat layer. Injection sites should be rotated within a given area as described earlier in the section on injection techniques. Injections into exactly the same site should occur no more often than once a month. Inconsistencies in injection techniques may lead to variation in the dose injected and its absorption.

Instruction on the recognition and treatment of *hypoglycemia* is obviously crucial not only for all patients with IDDM but also for patients taking oral hypoglycemic agents. Patients on insulin or OHA must be counseled on the importance of carrying some form of carbohydrate with them at all times. They must also be encouraged to wear a bracelet or necklace (e.g., Medic-Alert) that can alert caregivers to the presence of diabetes in the event of loss of consciousness from any cause.

The counterregulatory hormone *glucagon* is available as a therapeutic agent for the treatment of hypoglycemia. It is given *intramuscularly*, not subcutaneously, for the treatment of severe hypoglycemic reactions. The technique for using the drug has been described earlier in the section on insulin and hypoglycemia. The technique should be taught to family members likely to care for the hypoglycemic person with diabetes.

With regard to *foot care*, individuals with longstanding diabetes should trim their own nails only with great care. Feet should be inspected daily, washed gently, and dried carefully. Patients should not use chemicals like mercurochrome or full-strength povidone-iodine on their feet. They should wear soft cotton or wool socks and shoes that have been carefully fitted and broken in. Going barefoot, wearing open sandals, wearing thongs, and using hot soaks are high-risk activities for persons with longstanding diabetes and should be forbidden. Lanolin is useful for dry skin, and lamb's wool will prevent maceration between the toes. No lotion should be placed between the toes. As needed, a podiatrist should be consulted to cut nails, care for calluses, and assist in the proper fitting of shoes. All patients with

Date	Insulin	Blood Tests Before Eating				NOTES (Record changes in diet, stress, exercise reactions, illness, urine tests, etc.)
		Break-fast	Noon Meal	Evening Meal	Bedtime Snack	

FIGURE 46–4. Example of a simple sheet of paper suitable for use as a self-monitored blood glucose log.

diabetic neuropathy must exercise caution to avoid not only abrasion, pressure, and impact injuries but also thermal injury. Bath water temperature must always be tested with the hand; feet must never be placed next to a radiator or space heater. The basic rules of foot care are summarized in Table 46–24.

Genetic Counseling

Physicians should speak frankly about genetics when appropriate. There are many misconceptions about the heritability of diabetes. NIDDM poses a greater genetic risk to offspring and relatives than does IDDM. If one identical twin has NIDDM, the concordance in the second twin is almost 100%. In contrast, if one identical twin has IDDM, the concordance for diabetes is only about 50%. The prevalence of diabetes among the offspring of two parents with IDDM is only about 2 to 4%. Some key reference figures on heritability are shown in Table 46–6.[43, 44]

TABLE 46–24. BASIC RULES OF FOOT CARE FOR PATIENTS WITH DIABETES

Avoid going barefoot
Avoid open-toed shoes and sandals
Wear only comfortable shoes, even if unstylish
Break in new shoes gradually
Always wear stockings
Use lanolin-containing moisturizers regularly
Cut nails with utmost care; trim them straight across
Treat corns and calluses promptly; use a pumice stone
Report *any* foot infection immediately and have it treated

Organization of Patient Education

The organization of patient education depends on the type of practice and on the resources available. In most cases, it is most effective and efficient to have a trained nurse educator provide the instruction. The physician should reinforce educational efforts and be available to answer additional questions. Never assume that patients who have had diabetes for many years understand management principles adequately. It has been reported that 30 to 60% of patients taking insulin make medication errors, and the problem is more common in those with long-term diabetes than in newly diagnosed patients.

Evaluation of the Effectiveness of Patient Education

Physicians must judge the success of diabetes education for each patient with respect to both comprehensiveness and assimilation of the information. Sick day rules are easy to forget. Refresher sessions are needed for patients whose retention of essential information is inadequate.

Failure to understand basic differences between IDDM and NIDDM has led to confusion and inappropriate, ineffective patient education. For example, instruction in meal spacing, snacks, and the treatment of hypoglycemia is essential for patients with IDDM, whereas the patient with NIDDM needs to focus on weight loss through diet and exercise. The degree of independence that each patient should and can assume will vary according to insight and maturity, but the goal is always to encourage as much responsibility as possible.

Psychosocial Support

Diabetes disrupts people's lives in many ways. It causes needless embarrassment and fear in both adults and children. There are also direct and indirect financial implications. Medications and supplies are costly, but more troublesome is the discrimination against individuals with diabetes by vendors of health, disability, and life insurance. Diabetes also carries with it the potential for discrimination in employment despite the fact that affected individuals, with rare exceptions, are legally entitled to, and medically fit for, any position for which they are otherwise qualified. A successful education program will provide persons with diabetes with the assistance needed to overcome these hurdles. The American Diabetes Association and the Juvenile Diabetes Foundation provide a wide range of educational materials, and regional affiliates of both national organizations are often helpful in providing information regarding local resources for patient education.

SPECIAL PROBLEMS IN THE MANAGEMENT OF DIABETES

Diabetes in Children

About 1 in 600 children in the United States has IDDM. This amounts to about 150,000 cases at any given time. The impact of IDDM on the young is initially devastating, but with special attention, the lives of affected children can quickly and successfully be returned to normal.[45, 46] It is crucial for the child that the physician develop a strong alliance with the parents. Parents require help and should be put in contact with local support organizations mentioned earlier. Peer acceptance is one of the biggest problems. We encourage attendance at summer camps for children with diabetes. At camp, the children can learn about their disease among their peers, learn that they are not alone, and learn that they can do anything a child without diabetes can do. It is difficult for a child to live with IDDM, but it can be done. Some goals, strategies, and tactics for the care of IDDM in children are outlined in Table 46–25.

TABLE 46–25. CARE OF DIABETES IN CHILDREN

Goals:	1. Overall good health
	2. Normal growth and development
	3. As normal a lifestyle as possible
	4. Emotional well-being
	5. Positive attitude on the part of caregivers
Strategies:	1. Diabetes education
	2. Growth and development assessment
	3. Glucose control to minimize future diabetic complications
	4. Minimize hypoglycemic episodes
	5. Consult with health professionals (e.g., child psychologists, diabetes nurse educators) as needed
Tactics:	1. Frequent blood sugar monitoring
	2. Appropriate nutrition and exercise plan
	3. Use of growth and development charts
	4. Use of combination insulin regimen (split mix)
	5. Insulin dosage adjustments
	6. Sick day rules
	7. Awareness of the symptoms of hypoglycemia
	8. Participation in support groups (e.g., camps, organizations like the American Diabetes Association and Juvenile Diabetes Foundation)

Diabetes in Adolescence

Adolescence is synonymous with turmoil. The psychological and hormonal maturation that always troubles teenagers is doubly difficult for those with a disorder that renders them different. Their control inevitably tends to suffer as they change in size, activity, and physiology.[46] Adolescents with IDDM are the patients most likely to ignore their illness, fabricate self-monitored glucose results, commit dietary indiscretions, and forget the snacks that must precede exercise. They are also the group most likely to use their disease for secondary gain, typically by omitting insulin and courting DKA. Physicians must realize that adolescents do not always hear as they listen. The most important thing that health care providers can give to adolescents with IDDM is the knowledge that they will always be available for them when asked to be of help.

Diabetes in the Elderly

The proportion of Americans who are 70, 80, and 90 years of age is growing rapidly, and the prevalence of diabetes in these age groups is also rising. Factors that contribute to the frequency of diabetes in older persons include the "normal" reduction in glucose tolerance that accompanies aging, intercurrent illness, and medications. Diabetes in both established and newly diagnosed elderly patients requires thoughtful consideration of goals and risks.[47]

Target glucose concentration for elderly patients with diabetes must be carefully individualized. As more 60- and 70-year-old persons live to be 80 and 90 years of age, a degree of control suitable for minimizing long-term complications may appear appropriate for certain patients. It must always be remembered, however, that the elderly are more frail than the young, and management of hyperglycemia must take this into account. The consequences of hypoglycemia in the very elderly can be grave. Hypoglycemia that a child could shrug off can induce stroke, myocardial infarction, or, if consciousness is lost, a hip fracture, in an elderly patient unable to recognize or respond to it.

In particular, it must be remembered that the elderly are likely to be receiving many other prescription medications. Four pharmacologic issues need to be considered with respect to diabetes in the elderly: (1) Drugs (e.g., thiazides) can unmask latent glucose intolerance. Changing the drug can restore glucose tolerance. (2) In patients with known diabetes, drugs can worsen control either directly (e.g., steroid injections into arthritic joints) or indirectly (e.g., warfarin) by interfering with oral hypoglycemic agents. (3) Some drugs like diisopyramide and enalapril can enhance the likelihood of hypoglycemia, and β-adrenergic blocking agents can mask the symptoms of hypoglycemia. (4) Finally, liver disease and impairment of renal function can alter the metabolism of any drug in the elderly. Diabetes-related medication errors compound all these problems. It has been estimated, for example, that insulin dosage errors of up to 20% are common in elderly patients with any degree of visual impairment.[47]

It is worth pointing out that the frailness of the elderly is not only physical but also psychological. The latter can result from the death of spouse or peers, financial constraints, age-related forgetfulness, and medications. Just as with children, physicians must establish an alliance with the elderly that maintains their sense of worth and hence their sense of purpose in caring for diabetes. Table 46–26 summarizes key issues in the care of diabetes in the elderly.

Diabetes and Pregnancy

Gestational Diabetes. About 1 to 3% of pregnancies are complicated by diabetes.[11] Of these, 90% are cases of gestational diabetes. Screening for hyperglycemia is essential in all pregnant women, particularly those with previous abnormalities of glucose tolerance, obesity, a history of recurrent spontaneous abortion, or a previous high birth weight infant (>9 lb or 4.5 kg).

All pregnant women should be screened for diabetes between weeks 24 and 28 of gestation.[48] The standard procedure consists of a 50-g oral glucose load given without regard to time of day or time of last meal. Venous plasma glucose is drawn 1 hour later. Values of 140 mg/dl (7.8 mM) or greater should be followed by a full diagnostic OGTT performed as described earlier. Formal diagnostic criteria for GDM are in Table 46–8. Alternative, somewhat simpler threshold criteria for the initiation of insulin therapy in diabetes include a fasting plasma glucose concentration greater than 105 mg/dl (5.8 mM) and a 2-hour postprandial glucose concentration greater than 120 mg/dl (6.7 mM) on two separate occasions within 2 weeks.

TABLE 46–26. CARE OF DIABETES IN THE ELDERLY

Goals:	1. Individualize target glycemia according to age and self-care capabilities
	2. Seek to minimize short-term versus long-term complications as appropriate to age and overall health
	3. Minimize interference with lifestyle. Prevent both hyperglycemic symptoms and hypoglycemic events
Strategies:	1. Diet and exercise suitable to overall health and lifestyle
	2. Evaluation of potential drug interactions
	3. Consider alterations of drug metabolism induced by organ failure or by other medications
	4. Integration of diabetes care into care of other medical problems
	5. Address psychosocial aspects of care Loneliness Finances
Tactics:	1. Adjust frequency of self-blood sugar monitoring according to target glycemic control
	2. Key the nutrition and exercise health plans to individual needs
	3. Preferentially use oral agents or a single morning insulin injection
	4. Make appropriate medication adjustments
	5. Teach sick day rules
	6. Teach awareness of hypoglycemia symptoms
	7. Encourage support group participation

Gestational diabetes is always treated with insulin. Human insulin is preferred to minimize development of maternal antibodies to insulin that cross the placenta. The teratogenic potential of oral agents is unknown, and they are contraindicated in pregnancy. Diet is an important component of GDM management but is keyed to the evolution of the pregnancy and not to the treatment of diabetes. Starvation-induced ketosis may be harmful to the developing fetus.[49] For this reason dietary management of GDM must emphasize carbohydrate intake, and weight loss must be avoided. Current recommendations call for a total weight gain of 22 to 26.5 lb (8.8 to 10.6 kg) during the course of pregnancy. The presence of GDM classifies a pregnancy as high risk. Treatment should be undertaken as a joint intervention by an experienced obstetrician and a physician skilled in diabetes management.

Insulin treatment regimens for GDM are similar to those used for NIDDM. A single morning dose of intermediate-acting human insulin is often sufficient to maintain normal fasting blood levels and to allow for appropriate endogenous insulin secretion following meals.

As noted earlier, gestational diabetes almost always resolves after delivery, but women who have been affected with the condition are at risk for subsequent permanent diabetes. The official recommendation of the American Diabetes Association is to evaluate them on the first postpartum visit with a 2-hour OGTT using a 75-g glucose load.[14]

Pregnancy and Pre-existing Diabetes. Most women with diabetes who become pregnant have IDDM. Uncontrolled IDDM puts both the mother and the fetus at risk. The risk of congenital malformations in women with uncontrolled IDDM is greatly increased, but that risk can be reduced to the average population risk if diabetes is brought under control before conception.[24, 25] The teratogenic effects of hyperglycemia and ketosis appear to be maximal during the first few weeks of gestation. The most important thing an office practitioner can accomplish for a young woman with IDDM who desires pregnancy is to educate her as to the need for glycemic control *before* trying to conceive.

The normal upper limits of fasting and postprandial glycemia are different in pregnant women. During a normal pregnancy, fasting plasma glucose concentrations do not exceed 60 mg/dl (3.3 mM), although postprandial glucose concentration may rise to 165 mg/dl (9.2 mM). During diabetic pregnancy, target fasting blood sugar values are 60 to 100 mg/dl (3.3 to 5.6 mM). The postprandial target value is less than 120 to 140 mg/dl (<6.7 to 7.8 mM).

The method of choice for managing the pregnant woman with diabetes is an insulin pump coupled with frequent SMBG measurements.[50] Because renal threshold for glucose is reduced in pregnancy, urine testing can be misleading and its use is discouraged. The preferred approach minimizes the risks associated with diabetic pregnancy.[25] If continuous infusion of insulin is not possible, regular insulin before each meal combined with long-acting insulin once daily can provide the same degree of control and needed flexibility. Mixtures of regular and intermediate-acting insulins given twice daily constitute the minimal acceptable regimen.

Metabolic status constantly changes during pregnancy, and frequent adjustment of insulin therapy is required. The general trend is for insulin requirements to remain stable or fall slightly during the first trimester, then to increase substantially. Maximum insulin dose may be two or three times the prepregnancy requirement.

Delivery. In the last weeks of pregancy, there may be a slight decline in insulin requirements. Substantial declines (>50% of the maximum dose) indicate fetal distress. Frequent hypoglycemic reactions in the third trimester of pregnancy should prompt assessment of fetal and placental viability.

Insulin requirements usually fall dramatically after delivery. On the day of delivery, the insulin dosage should be reduced to 50% or less of the *prepregnancy* dose in all patients, and glucose should be given intravenously. Most patients with GDM will no longer require insulin after delivery. A reasonable rule after delivery is to withhold insulin until the plasma glucose level reaches at least 200 mg/dl (11.1 mM). Subsequent doses can be estimated from those used before pregnancy or by taking one third of the maximum dosage during pregnancy and adjusting according to the results of blood testing.

The importance of reducing insulin at the time of delivery cannot be overemphasized. Permanent neurologic deficits have occurred in patients who developed severe hypoglycemia because of failure to appreciate the precipitous fall in insulin requirements after delivery.

The timing of delivery can be optimized by the use of sophisticated methods for monitoring the maturation and health of the fetus and placenta. Delivery between 36 and 38 weeks of gestation has generally been counselled. The longer a woman has had diabetes, the earlier the delivery should be performed, but it should not usually take place before week 36. Mothers with GDM may be delivered as late as week 39. The decision rests with the obstetrician.

Maternal Risk. Pregnancy poses special risks to women with diabetes, particularly those with longstanding IDDM. Pregnancy may precipitate diabetic retinopathy, and ophthalmoscopic examinations should be performed frequently until delivery. In the patient with pre-existing retinopathy, neovascular proliferation may progress rapidly and require photocoagulation.

Pre-existing diabetic nephropathy may worsen during pregnancy. A rapid decline in renal function is an ominous development. Pregnant women with diabetes but without pre-existing nephropathy generally do not become azotemic during pregnancy.

Pregnant women are susceptible to urinary tract infection, and diabetes amplifies the risk. Pregnant women with diabetes should have regular urinalyses to exclude pyuria. When pyuria or bacteriuria is documented, appropriate cultures should be obtained and therapy instituted.

Diabetic Comas

Treatment of the DKA and HHNKC is beyond the scope of this book. In the section that follows, we focus on the issues of recognition and initial approach. Our strategies for the treatment of diabetic coma have been presented elsewhere.[15, 51]

Diabetic Ketoacidosis. The clinical presentation of DKA has been described earlier. When ketoacidosis is the presenting manifestation of new onset IDDM, the patient should be hospitalized. Development of DKA may be more subtle in patients already receiving insulin. It is usually associated with some precipitating factor. In addition to febrile illnesses, alcohol abuse and severe emotional stress can lead to ketoacidosis. Emotional instability contributes to errors in insulin dosage, self-testing for control, misrepresentation of the results of testing, and disregard for the severity of symptoms. Emotionally immature individuals sometimes precipitate DKA by omitting insulin.

Fluids, electrolyte replacement, insulin, and careful monitoring are the keys to therapy. Most cases deserve admission to an intensive care unit (ICU). The preferred method of treatment, after the institution of fluid and electrolyte therapy, is continuous insulin infusion. Each patient must be evaluated for intercurrent illness. Patients who die of DKA usually have some underlying complication like myocardial infarction or sepsis.

Prevention is the best treatment, and the keys to prevention are careful attention to education, stressing sick day rules and the response to ketonuria. The key to successful education is a good working alliance with the patient.

Hyperosmolar Hyperglycemic Nonketotic Coma (HHNKC). All persons with diabetes are susceptible to the syndrome of hyperglycemic hyperosmolar nonketotic coma, but the disorder can also occur in glucose-intolerant patients not previously diagnosed with hyperglycemia. The usual presentation is in the middle-aged or elderly patient with mild NIDDM treated with diet alone or with diet and oral agents. Most patients experience a prodromal phase of several days to several weeks, during which they have progressive polyuria and polydipsia. Cerebral function becomes impaired, and confusion, stupor, and coma follow. Nursing home patients are particularly at risk because they may depend on others for things to drink, and their somnolence is easily overlooked.

Associated illnesses are common. Some degree of azotemia is invariable, and cardiovascular impairment is extremely frequent. Infections, myocardial or cerebral infarction, hemorrhage, trauma, and burns may all precipitate the syndrome. Dialysis, hyperalimentation, and various drugs are among the iatrogenic precipitants (see Table 46–5). Whatever the precipitating cause, the patient develops hyperglycemia, glycosuria, and an osmotic diuresis. If thirst fails to compensate for urinary fluid loss, severe dehydration ensues.

Laboratory diagnosis of HHNKC is straightforward. Urinalysis shows glycosuria but minimal ketonuria. Plasma glucose concentrations usually exceed 600 mg/dl (33 mM) and may exceed 2000 mg/dl (111 mM). Serum acetone is minimal or absent. Serum osmolality usually exceeds 350 mOsm/kg. Any patient suspected of having HHNKC should be admitted to hospital for emergency fluid, electrolyte, and insulin therapy.

Diabetes and Surgery

Patients with diabetes who need elective surgery should be evaluated preoperatively to assess control and to search for complications like nephropathy that could complicate the procedure. The normotensive patient who requires a procedure should be sent to the operating room with an infusion of 5% dextrose in 0.45% saline. Scheduling the procedure as a first case greatly simplifies management.

If an insulin-treated patient is well controlled, it is our practice to use subcutaneous intermediate-acting insulin (NPH or Lente) in a total dose calculated from previous requirements. The simple calculation is made as follows. The total amount of intermediate-acting insulin plus half the total regular insulin used on the day prior to surgery are added together. One half of this total dose of insulin is administered as intermediate-acting insulin early on the morning of surgery; the other half is given in the recovery room, again as intermediate-acting insulin. For example, a patient taking 32 units of NPH insulin and 8 units of regular insulin each morning would receive 18 units of NPH on the morning of surgery and 18 units of NPH in the recovery room. This method precludes intraoperative hypoglycemia yet also provides enough insulin to counter the stress of the procedure.

Frequent monitoring of blood glucose intraoperatively is mandatory. Patients who are poorly perfused after surgery require either frequent boluses of intravenous regular insulin or continuous infusion pump therapy together with frequent blood glucose determinations.

Patients with NIDDM controlled by diet alone generally require little special attention preoperatively but may require insulin postoperatively. In the case of patients with NIDDM treated with oral agents, the drug should be withheld on the day of surgery. Postoperatively, insulin may be used until metabolic stability is achieved, if necessary.

Hypoglycemia in the postoperative patient is more dangerous than mild hyperglycemia. Postoperative insulin should be titrated to achieve a "surgical range" plasma glucose concentration of 200 to 250 mg/dl (11.2 to 13.9 mM). Attempting to treat hyperglycemia with subcutaneous regular insulin alone often leads to wide fluctuations in plasma glucose levels. Postoperative diabetes control in an ICU is best achieved by continuous infusion of insulin. Patients who are stable should receive intermediate-acting insulin twice daily. Once the patient is stable, efforts to achieve better glycemic control are justified for many reasons; hyperglycemia interferes with immune system function and weakens the strength of surgical wounds.[52] Our approach to the care of diabetes during emergency surgery, ICU management, and postsurgical periods is outlined in detail elsewhere.[53]

Pancreatectomy and Diabetes

Diabetes in patients who have undergone pancreatectomy for cancer or pseudocyst removal, and in some individuals with severe pancreatitis, is difficult to manage. These patients are susceptible to wide swings in glycemic control due in large measure to the loss of glucagon-mediated counterregulation. Unlike patients with IDDM who lose only β cells, pancreatectomized individuals lose all the cellular components of the islet, including the glucagon-secreting α cells.

The prudent target for glycemic control in pancreatectomized patients is generally higher than it would be in patients with IDDM. Treatment obviously requires insulin and should emphasize the close coordination of meals with therapy. Six small daily feedings together with a split mix is a reasonable initial strategy. The dose of insulin needed is usually relatively small.

COMPLICATIONS

In the penicillin era, Osler's dictum (regarding lues) might well be modified to state: "To know diabetes is to know medicine." Complications of diabetes can directly or indirectly affect essentially all body systems. In addition to vascular, eye, nerve, and kidney complications, diabetic skin, bone, leukocytes, and platelets can be adversely affected by the disease. Immune responses and surgical wound strength are also impaired. Not least, diabetes can precipitate severe psychosocial and economic disruptions.

The issue of control and complications has been addressed earlier. Complications affect IDDM and NIDDM patients with the same frequency after diabetes has been present for 15 to 20 years. Complications of IDDM are frequent in young adults in the prime of life, and for this reason they sometimes seem more devastating than the complications of NIDDM. There is, however, no difference in the severity of complications that occur in longstanding IDDM and NIDDM. Once major complications have occurred, tight control of diabetes, even by pancreas transplantation, seems to have little benefit. Tight control does diminish complications, however, if instituted prior to or early in their development.[20] Early recognition of complications allows early treatment.

Anterior Eye Disorders

Acute refractory changes in persons with diabetes can be due to osmotic shifts of water into the lens. As plasma glucose concentration rises and falls, the eye becomes myopic and hyperopic, respectively. Individuals with newly diagnosed or poorly controlled diabetes should not purchase new glasses until stable and acceptable glycemia is achieved.

Cataract formation may be related to similar osmotic disturbances, perhaps involving sorbitol. Persons with diabetes develop cataracts earlier than do those without the disease, and their opacities progress more rapidly. Patients with poorly controlled diabetes may also develop subcapsular "snowflake" cataracts. Cataract surgery in patients with diabetes is usually successful.

Glaucoma occurs three times more frequently in persons with diabetes than in individuals of the same age who are not hyperglycemic. Early detection and treatment prevent nerve damage and usually preserve vision.

Rubeosis iritis is characterized by new blood vessel growth on the anterior iris. A severe form of glaucoma may ensue when these vessels involve the anterior chamber angle. This can cause pain and rapidly lead to blindness. Referral to an ophthalmologist is mandatory.

Posterior Eye Disorders: Diabetic Retinopathy

Diabetic retinal disease is a complex problem.[54] There are two categories: (1) background or nonproliferative retinopathy and (2) proliferative retinopathy. Background retinopathy is characterized by capillary dilatation, capillary closure, microaneurysms, venous dilatation, venous beading, and loop formation. There are also extravascular lesions including cotton wool spots, hard exudates, and small hemorrhages. Proliferative retinopathy implies neovascularization; this new vessel formation is both intraretinal and preretinal. At its extreme, proliferative retinopathy results in fibrosis retinitis proliferans with contractures and eventual retinal detachment.

Estimates of the prevalence of diabetic retinopathy vary. In general, some retinopathy exists in nearly all patients who have had diabetes for more than 20 years, but this does not necessarily imply impairment of vision. Only about 2% of patients with diabetes progress to legal blindness with visual acuity poorer than 20/200.

Background retinopathy is the earliest change in the retina of patients with diabetes. It reflects breakdown of the blood-retina barrier, with serious leakage that can be demonstrated by fluorescein angiography. More sensitive methods (vitreous fluorophotometry) have shown alterations in the blood-retina barrier even in persons with newly diagnosed diabetes. These changes are quantitatively correlated with both the duration of diabetes and degree of control. Evidence supports the view that good glycemic control is of benefit in preventing or delaying the onset of background retinopathy.

Microaneurysms appear as small red dots and represent dilatation of retinal capillaries at their venous end. They are the earliest ophthalmoscopic sign of background retinopathy. Microaneurysms are abnormally permeable and allow transudation of intravascular fluid that forms hard exudates. These are sharply defined, yellow-white, lipoprotein-containing deposits in the middle layers of the retina; products of neuronal cell degeneration may also be embedded in them. Both microaneurysms and hard exudates can undergo spontaneous resolution and reformation. Unless the center of the macula is involved, these lesions rarely cause significant visual disturbances.

Diffuse retinal edema can reduce vision if it involves the macula. Unfortunately, retinal edema is difficult to detect with the ophthalmoscope. Fluorescein angiography will usually reveal the characteristic picture known as cystoid macular edema.

Soft exudates or cotton wool spots are infarctions in the nerve fiber layer of the retina. These lesions are similar to those seen in patients with hypertension. They are indicative of axonal swelling of the nerve fiber layer, secondary to ischemia.

Intraretinal microvascular abnormalities (IRMA) are a more advanced form of background retinopathy. IRMA consist of shunt vessels, pre-existing capillaries, and intraretinal neovascularization, usually adjacent to areas of occluded capillaries. IRMA are intermediate in severity between background and proliferative diabetic retinopathy.

Tight control appears to increase retinopathy somewhat in the first year. The DCCT showed decreased background retinopathy by about 50%, however, after 3 or more years of tight control.[20]

Proliferative retinopathy refers to the development of new blood vessels in the retina. These vessels typically occur on or near the optic disk but may occur elsewhere. Such vessels form fans or fronds tangential to the plane of the retina. With proliferation of the fibrous-glial supporting tissue, adhesions to the vitreous humor become prominent. Thickening and shortening of the fibrous tissue elevates vessels off the retina into the vitreous.

Rupture of new vessels leading to vitreous hemorrhage can occur suddenly. The patient may experience a shower of "floaters" or complete loss of vision depending on the extent of the hemorrhage. Tractional retinal detachments also occur. Eventually, some patients reach an "involutional" stage. No further hemorrhage or detachment occurs, but the patient is left with an ischemic retina and impaired vision. In many cases, proliferative retinopathy becomes more malignant. About 20% of eyes with untreated proliferative retinopathy progress to visual acuity poorer than 5/200 within 2 years.

Photocoagulation is the mainstay of treatment. High-energy laser light causes thermal injury in the retinal pigmented epithelium, destroying neovascular tissue. The procedure is thought to eliminate critical areas of ischemia or hypoxia, the postulated source of factors thought to stimulate neovascularization. Because photocoagulation requires good visualization of the fundus, it cannot be performed on patients who have extensive hemorrhage.

Vitrectomy is used to treat hemorrhages that do not clear spontaneously. The surgeon removes the blood from the vitreous cavity and injects a clear salt solution in its place. If the patient has not suffered irreversible retinal damage, vitrectomy can restore vision. Electroretinography and ultrasonography have been used to evaluate the status of the retina preoperatively, excluding cases unlikely to benefit from vitrectomy.

Screening procedures are obviously the purview of trained specialists. The responsibility of primary care physicians is to identify patients with diabetes who are in need of referral. Patients with newly diagnosed diabetes should be examined ophthalmoscopically to determine whether retinopathy is present. Annual funduscopic examinations are a reasonable minimum. Identification of background retinopathy should prompt referral to an ophthalmologist. Once retinopathy is present, the primary care physician must see to it that ophthalmologic follow-up care is maintained. Middle-aged and elderly patients should have ocular pressures measured to exclude glaucoma regularly.

Renal Complications

Renal failure occurs in nearly half of patients with IDDM within 25 years of the diagnosis of diabetes. Patients with NIDDM also develop diabetic nephropathy. All patients with diabetes should have a urinalysis yearly, and serum creatinine concentration should be measured if proteinuria is detected. Diabetic nephropathy is defined as the presence of a persistently positive urinary dipstick test for albumin in a person with diabetes, or a urinary albumin excretion rate of >0.3 g/day (albuminuria) or of >0.03 g/day (microalbuminuria, as defined by some authorities), in the absence of other renal diseases.[55]

Microalbuminuria not detectable by dipstick urinalysis is the first clinical manifestation of diabetic nephropathy and generally antedates changes in serum creatinine concentration.[56] Defined as the excretion of 0.03 to 0.3 g of protein per day, its quantification requires special methodology. The detection of microalbuminuria theoretically allows the earliest possible institution of appropriate therapies, and this test is regarded by some as the test of choice for the protein component of urinalysis. At this writing, however, it remains to be established that the detection of microalbuminuria will lead to meaningful clinical benefits.

When *proteinuria* is detected, creatinine clearance and measurement of 24-hour urinary protein excretion should be obtained. Massive proteinuria may be associated with hypoalbuminemia, edema, hyperlipidemia, and other features of the nephrotic syndrome. Diabetic nephropathy often parallels the development of diabetic retinopathy. If proteinuria exists in the absence of retinopathy, especially if the proteinuria is associated with azotemia, one should suspect other causes of renal insufficiency.

Microscopic hematuria and casts are also associated with early diabetic nephropathy, but other causes of microscopic hematuria or casts obviously must not be overlooked. *Pyuria* is observed frequently, urinary tract infections probably being more common in those with diabetes than in those without it. Persons with diabetes are particularly susceptible to the acute complications of urinary tract infection, including papillary necrosis, pyelitis, and perinephric abscess. Asymptomatic bacteriuria in patients with diabetes should be treated.

Hypertension is a common problem in patients with diabetes; those with obesity and hyperinsulinemia appear particularly susceptible. When present, it accelerates the progression of diabetic nephropathy, initiating a vicious circle that leads to worsening hypertension. Blood pressure should be recorded at every visit, and even mild hyperten-

TABLE 46–27. CLASSIFICATION AND EVALUATION OF DIABETIC NEUROPATHY

Disorder	Symptoms	Clinical Assessment
Polyneuropathy	Pain, paresthesia, or anesthesia intensified at night, starting in lower extremities	Loss of pinprick and vibratory sensation, stocking-glove distribution; absent ankle reflexes
Mononeuropathies		
Mixed spinal nerves	Pain and weakness in distribution of spinal nerves	Loss of muscle strength, reflexes, and pinprick and vibratory sensation in spinal nerve distribution
Cranial nerves	Sudden weakness of nerve distribution; diplopia if cranial nerve III, IV, or VI involved; pain may be present	Muscle paresis or paralysis; cranial nerve III involved, preservation of pupillary light reflex
Radiculopathy	Pain in dermatome distribution	Loss of pinprick and vibratory sensation over dermatome
Amyotrophy	Weakness on getting up from a chair, weight loss, myalgia, and painful paresthesias	Muscle wasting and weakness, usually in pelvic girdle, fasciculation, loss of pinprick sensation
Autonomic Neuropathies		
Gastroparesis	Fullness and regurgitation of food postprandially	Gastric distention; decreased peristalsis; gastric barium retention
Diarrhea	Nocturnal diarrhea Unpredictable diarrhea	Normal jejunal biopsy Steatorrhea
Bladder	Hesitancy; incomplete emptying of bladder; small urine volume	Residual urine after voiding
Impotence	Inability to achieve or maintain erection	No erection under any circumstances; associated autonomic neuropathy
Postural hypotension	Light-headedness when walking or from supine to standing position	Postural hypotension without vagal or sympathetic compensation (e.g., tachycardia following hypotension; bradycardia following Valsalva maneuver)

sion should be treated promptly. Drugs of choice for treating hypertension in diabetes are the angiotensin-converting enzyme (ACE) inhibitors.[57] These potent drugs* have minimal effects on control of diabetes, but they have occasionally been associated with hypoglycemia,[58, 59] may cause hyperkalemia in patients with even mild diabetic renal insufficiency, and are contraindicated in pregnancy. Calcium channel blockers are also effective. Although they can impair insulin secretion, they, like the ACE inhibitors, are generally free of significant adverse consequences on control of diabetes and lipid metabolism.[60] Drugs in both of these classes are vasoactive and ACE inhibitors, and diltiazem may diminish proteinuria in patients with diabetic nephropathy. β-Adrenergic blockers and diuretics should be avoided because of their adverse effects on diabetes control.

Renal biopsy is rarely necessary to diagnose diabetic nephropathy. When performed to exclude other renal disorders, it shows characteristic lesions including nodular glomerulosclerosis (described by Kimmelstiel and Wilson) and, more commonly, diffuse glomerulosclerosis. Exudative glomerular lesions and sclerosis of afferent and efferent arterioles may also be seen. In patients with poorly controlled diabetes, glycogen and lipid deposition can occur in renal tubules; such lesions are probably reversible with good control of diabetes.

Any of these lesions, alone or in combination, may lead to progressive renal insufficiency. If the serum creatinine level exceeds 2 mg/dl, the creatinine clearance should be measured, and the patient generally should be referred to a nephrologist for further evaluation and treatment. It is uncommon for diabetic nephropathy, once detected, to stabilize. The time from detection to dialysis may range from months to years.

The *risk of angiography in patients with both diabetes and nephropathy* deserves comment. Nephropathy has commonly been thought to render patients with longstanding diabetes particularly susceptible to acute renal failure after angiographic procedures are performed. With the advent of modern reagents and techniques, however, the risk of angiography may not be any higher than it is in patients without diabetes.[61] A prudent course of action for attending physicians should be to alert radiologists to the presence of diabetes, to hydrate such patients before study, and to minimize dye loads during the procedure.

Treatment of diabetic nephropathy focuses principally on efforts to prevent it by strict glycemic control, aggressive treatment of hypertension, and treatment of a neurogenic bladder if one develops. Tight control has been shown to reduce the occurrence of microalbuminuria and albuminuria,[20] although longer follow-up would be needed to demonstrate decreased renal failure, a "harder" endpdoint. There is also evidence that ACE inhibitors reduce microalbuminuria and may retard the progression of renal failure, even in normotensive diabetics.[62] After proteinuria has appeared, some authorities advocate a low-protein diet. This is said to reduce renal hyperfiltration, delaying the progression of nephropathy.

End-stage diabetic nephropathy can be treated by hemodialysis, chronic ambulatory peritoneal dialysis (CAPD), and renal transplantation. In general, patients with diabetes tolerate dialysis well, but they often experience accelerated proliferative retinopathy and myocardial infarction. Some centers have reported more favorable responses to peritoneal dialysis. In view of the complications experienced during dialysis, some authorities recommend renal transplantation as early as possible after the onset of renal failure. Transplantation has proved remarkably successful in many patients with diabetes. Cotransplantation of the pancreas is now performed in several medical centers, and, when successful, the reversal of diabetes is associated with retardation (but not reversal) of diabetic retinopathy and neuropathy and also with enhanced survival of the renal graft.[22]

Diabetic Neuropathy

Diabetic neuropathy takes many forms; one classification system is shown in Table 46–27. The pathophysiology is

*Among these are benazepril, captopril, enalapril, fosinopril, lisinopril, quinapril, and ramipril.

not well understood. Acute mononeuropathies are probably ischemic. The sorbitol pathway may be involved in reversible nerve conduction disturbances. Evidence now suggests that tight control prevents or retards the progression of diabetic neuropathy.[20]

Polyneuropathies are very common and consist of bilateral symmetric sensory disturbances. They usually involve the lower extremities more than the upper extremities. Gradually progressive hypesthesia and anesthesia lead to neuropathic foot ulcers and neuropathic arthropathy (Charcot joints). The latter most often affects tarsal, tarsometatarsal, and metatarsophalangeal joints. Night cramps and burning paresthesias are particularly discomforting. Severe loss of vibratory sense and proprioception may mimic vitamin B_{12} deficiency or syphilis, both of which should therefore be excluded. Multiple tense blisters on the fingers or toes (bullosis diabeticorum) may rarely accompany neuropathy.

Better control of diabetes may help alleviate painful neuropathic symptoms, but the effects are unpredictable and may depend on the extent of irreversible damage. Many medications have been used to relieve pain and paresthesias. Tricyclic antidepressants, trifluoperazine, clonazepam, mexiletine, phenytoin, thiamine, and vitamins B_6 and B_{12} have all been used successfully in some patients, but none yields predictable benefit. The tricyclics are, in our experience, the most effective agents, but the painful symptoms often subside after several months, and analgesic therapy may be all that is needed.

Our approach is to begin with analgesia, for example acetaminophen or propoxyphene. Our second line of treatment consists of amitriptyline (50 to 150 mg qhs), clonazepam (0.5 to 3 mg/day), or mexiletine ($\leq$10 mg/kg/day). These are potent drugs with significant neurologic and cardiovascular side effects to which patients with diabetes may be particularly susceptible. The clinician treating painful diabetic neuropathy with these agents must be thoroughly familiar with their pharmacology.

Another alternative is the topical, transcutaneous administration of capsaicin as a cream.[63] This agent, the chemical that gives pepper its taste, interferes with the action of substance P, which is a neurochemical mediator of pain. After a brief initial period of burning sensations associated with the application of the cream, many patients achieve good control of pain. Again, the effect on any given patient cannot be predicted, and many patients find the need for multiple daily applications unacceptable.

Mononeuropathy and mononeuropathy multiplex usually occur suddenly. Thought to be ischemic in origin, these neuropathies carry an excellent prognosis with resolution within several months. They involve, respectively, a single nerve, or two or more nonadjacent nerves, with accompanying muscle weakness, wasting, or pain. Most commonly involved are the femoral, obturator, and sciatic nerves in the legs; the median and ulnar nerves in the arms; and cranial nerves III, IV, and VI with extraocular muscle palsy. Bell's palsy is also common in diabetes.

Other causes of mononeuropathy must be excluded. If doubt exists, a neurologist should be consulted. One subtle finding indicative of the diabetic origin of cranial neuropathy is the preservation of pupillary light reflexes in the presence of a third cranial nerve palsy. This constellation suggests preservation of parasympathetic fibers located in the periphery of the third cranial nerve and an ischemic, diabetic pathogenesis involving the vasa nervorum.

Diabetic amyotrophy or asymmetric motor neuropathy typically involves proximal muscles of the lower extremities, especially in older men with mild diabetes. Recovery may take up to 2 years. Apart from maintaining glucose control, no specific therapy is available. Occasionally, affected patients may benefit from tricyclic antidepressant therapy. *Mixed sensory-motor polyneuropathies* are particularly troublesome. Again, therapy consists of close attention to control of diabetes, analgesia, and protective devices. *Diabetic autonomic neuropathies* affect cardiovascular, gastrointestinal, and genitourinary function.

Signs of *cardiovascular autonomic neuropathy* include postural hypotension, vasomotor instability, and fixed-rate, resting tachycardia. Cardiac autonomic dysfunction can be detected by simple office observations: absence of bradycardia in response to the Valsalva maneuver, absence of sinus arrhythmia in response to deep breathing, and absence of cardioacceleration in response to standing. Fixed, resting tachycardia may increase the risk of arrhythmia, especially after myocardial infarction. Orthostatic hypotension can be treated effectively with fludrocortisone (Florinef) and elastic support stockings.

Gastrointestinal complaints in longstanding diabetes that are not of gallbladder origin are usually associated with *gastrointestinal autonomic neuropathy.* Affected patients tend also to have peripheral neuropathy, areflexia, and signs of cardiac autonomic dysfunction. Several different esophageal disorders can produce dysphagia in patients with diabetes. Difficulty occurs principally when swallowing solids. Diabetic dysphagia may cause retrosternal pain that can be severe enough to lead to food avoidance, undernutrition, and weight loss. *Esophageal candidiasis* is another, often overlooked, component of dysphagia in patients with diabetes. Diagnosis requires esophagoscopy. Dyspepsia can also be due to a reduction in the force of esophageal peristalsis. This can eventually lead to symptoms and signs of reflux esophagitis. Esophageal manometry establishes the diagnosis.

Gastroparesis diabeticorum describes a syndrome of postprandial fullness, nausea, bloating, epigastric pain, regurgitation, and vomiting. Regurgitation of undigested food 1 to 2 hours after eating is the commonest history. The diagnosis can be established by barium studies, by endoscopy, and by radionuclide transit measurements.

Constipation can be a problem in diabetes of even brief duration and is related to poor dietary habits and dehydration. In longstanding diabetes, patients may develop constipation due to depressed myotonic contractility of the colon. Intermittent *diarrhea* may also be present. This is generally watery, voluminous, and easily mistaken for a malabsorption syndrome. Fecal incontinence may result from the loss of both sensory and motor function at the anal sphincter.

Therapy of diabetic gastrointestinal autonomic dysfunction can be as simple as dietary modification emphasizing bulking agents. For patients with gastroparesis, frequent small feedings of puréed food can be effective. Raising the head of the bed and asking the patient to ambulate after meals can also provide substantial relief. Occasionally gastrointestinal prokinetic agents like metoclopramide (Reglan) are effective in the relief of gastroparesis diabeticorum; they are less useful in the treatment of other diabetic enteropathies. The investigational drug cisapride has similar effects, and cholinergic agonists like bethanechol (Urecholine) provide another alternative. Preliminary data indicate that erythromycin may also benefit certain patients with gastroparesis.[64] About half of patients with "diabetic diarrhea" respond to broad-spectrum antibiotics like tetracycline.

Autonomic neuropathy affecting the genitourinary tract induces neurogenic bladder dysfunction, retrograde ejaculation, and impotence. Detection of the neurogenic bladder is of particular importance because urinary stasis predisposes to infection and ureteral reflux can lead to hydronephrosis and the induction or acceleration of renal failure. Patients with autonomic bladder dysfunction should be taught to void on a regular schedule and to enhance emptying by manual application of suprapubic pressure. Cholinergic drugs like bethanechol (Urecholine) are sometimes helpful. The diagnosis is readily established by ultrasonography.

No treatment is available or required for retrograde ejaculation. Physicians must be reassuring because the condition, although benign, frequently leads to anxiety in the patient or his partner. Impotence in men with diabetes can be the consequence of psychological disturbances, chronic hyperglycemia alone, medication side effects, and vascular disease in addition to autonomic neuropathy. The office practitioner can intervene by improving control of diabetes, eliminating potential offending medications, and listening for evidence of psychological problems. Refractory organic impotence is best managed by referral to a specialist skilled in the diagnosis and treatment of this difficult problem. Impotence that is due to diabetic neuropathy with or without vascular insufficiency can be treated by penile prostheses or intermittent injections. Androgen therapy is of little or no benefit in such patients. The most important responsibility of the office practitioner is to inquire about these problems. Too often they are ignored, with significant adverse consequences on quality of life.

Cardiovascular Complications

Arteriosclerotic coronary, cerebral, and peripheral vascular disease leading to myocardial infarction, stroke, intermittent claudication, and foot ulcer is exceptionally common in patients with diabetes. The mechanisms are not well understood, although the hyperlipoproteinemia associated with chronic uncontrolled diabetes is likely to play a role. Longstanding diabetes is sometimes associated with extensive vascular calcification. The dietary and lifestyle recommendations of the American Heart Association, together with control of diabetes or IGT, offer the only reasonable route to prevention.

Patients with diabetes do suffer "silent" myocardial ischemia, although the relative frequency of the problem in comparison with the general population is not clear.[65] A baseline electrocardiogram should be performed on all patients with diabetes older than 40 years of age and at a younger age if there is a family history of heart disease.

Persons with diabetes occasionally develop cardiomyopathy in the absence of coronary artery insufficiency, hypertension, or valvular disease. Impaired left ventricular function in such patients leads to severe, often refractory, congestive heart failure. Its pathophysiology is not well understood but may be related to disease of small vessels within the heart.

Infections in Patients with Diabetes

Poorly controlled diabetes (mean glucose ≥250 mg/dl, 14 mM) is associated with alterations of leukocyte function that impair migration, phagocytosis, and bacteriostatic activity. Lymphocyte function is also depressed.

Cholelithiasis is strongly associated with hyperlipoproteinemia, obesity, and multiparity; cholecystitis is consequently common among individuals with diabetes. The presence of asymptomatic gallstones in a patient with diabetes should not be considered an absolute indication for surgery,[66] but rather a cause for vigilance. Clinicians must be aware that gallstones in patients with diabetes can be associated with *occult* cholecystitis. The typical case involves an unexplained fever, increased insulin resistance, and nausea. Ascending cholangitis complicating cholecystitis in patients with coexisting diabetes can be fatal.

Vaginal and cutaneous candidiasis is especially common in obese individuals with diabetes. Other infections seen more commonly than in the general population include aspergillosis, blastomycosis, tuberculosis, gas gangrene, and cryptococcal meningitis. Mucormycosis, a very uncommon fungal infection of the nasopharynx, tends to occur in *acidotic* patients with diabetes.

In addition to appropriate antibiotic and antifungal therapy, reinstitution of good diabetes control is imperative. Hospitalization is often necessary to effect such measures.

FUTURE DEVELOPMENTS

In the era of molecular technology, the promise of significant advances in the prevention, treatment, and cure of diabetes has grown steadily brighter. Unfortunately, promises still take years or decades to translate into medical reality. As of this writing, there are neither cures nor miracle therapies just around the corner. What follows is a brief summary of some promises that are further in the future.

Treatments

A major unmet need in diabetes treatment is for an implantable glucose sensor that will match exogenous insulin administration to metabolic need. All current insulin treatments, including external pumps and internally implanted reservoir systems, are "open loop." They can only approximate metabolic need. A transcutaneous glucose sensor is likely to appear before an implantable one, and this will assist patients willing to use it frequently to adjust their insulin pump or injection schedule. Evidence that tight control benefits patients may hasten such advances.

Transcutaneous and nasally administered insulin formulations have not yet achieved consistent therapeutic success and will probably not be available soon. Adjunctive treatments with insulin-like growth factors and proinsulin are also unlikely to make a major impact on diabetes care soon, but these agents and others continue to be actively investigated.

A completely different aspect of diabetes care involves agents intended to prevent or ameliorate complications. Several aldose reductase inhibitors for treatment of neuropathy remain under development and may be available relatively soon. Even more exciting is the prospect of agents that prevent the synthesis of "advanced glycosylation endproducts" (AGEs), the purported biochemical detritus of chronic hyperglycemia that may lead to vascular disease.[23, 67] The first such agent, aminoguanidine, is currently under study.[68]

Cures

Normal pancreatic β cells constitute the best glucose-monitoring and insulin delivery system. Successful pancreatic transplantation is now a reality for patients with

IDDM with end-stage renal disease. Cotransplantation of both a kidney and a pancreas enhances renal allograft survival and quality of life. In this setting, the risk of chronic immunosuppression is acceptable. Pancreatic transplantation into younger persons with diabetes is controversial. The obvious benefits cannot easily be weighed against the potential risk of decades of chronic immunosuppression. For better or worse, the unavailability of donor organs has tended to make the issue moot. Most authorities agree that pancreas transplantation will at best serve only a minor fraction of the population with diabetes. Transplantation of isolated human pancreatic islets would be preferable, but suffers from the limitations, as does whole pancreas transplantation. Transplantation of xenogeneic islet grafts, perhaps from pigs, would solve the issue of availability, but methods for preventing rejection remain to be perfected. Transgenic human tissues engineered to express the insulin gene and secrete insulin in response to glucose have begun to be developed.

An alternative to ordinary transplantation is the sequestration of histoincompatible or even xenogeneic insulin-secreting cells. The strategy is to enclose the tissues within a semipermeable barrier that permits the diffusion of glucose, insulin, and nutrients but prevents access to the cells of the immune system. Two implementations of the sequestration strategy are under development. One coats the islets with a polymer gel, forming small spherules that can then be implanted. The other, the "biohybrid pancreas," puts islets in chambers that are nourished by blood that circulates through semipermeable hollow fibers obtained from a surgical arteriovenous connection. These devices have proved successful in short-term animal trials.[69] The time frame for clinical availability is not known.

Somatostatin inhibits the insulin-antagonistic hormones glucagon and growth hormones; it also inhibits the secretion of other polypeptide hormones. Efforts are being made to develop analogs of somatostatin that are specific for glucagon inhibition and that have prolonged durations of action. Whether such analogs will prove clinically effective remains to be seen.

Prevention

It is now possible to prevent IDDM-like autoimmune diabetes in several animal models. Prevention strategies include immunosuppression, immune system modification by transfusion of lymphocytes, prophylactic administration of exogenous insulin, and several more radical pharmaceutical and surgical (e.g., thymectomy) strategies. Only immunosuppressive drugs like cyclosporine and azathioprine have been tested in humans. Cyclosporine clearly can reverse IDDM in children if given early, but it must be taken chronically or the disease reappears immediately. Trials of immunosuppression continue on a restricted research basis only. Investigations of other strategies are even earlier stages. The fact that limited success has already been achieved, however, makes us confident that additional research will devise clinically useful methods in the foreseeable future.

Because there are currently no safe and accepted methods for preventing IDDM, there is little justification for ordering HLA typing or evaluating for the presence of autoantibodies, as some commercial firms suggest. Patients at risk for IDDM because they are close relatives of patients can best be followed by periodic monitoring of fasting and postprandial glucose concentrations.

In regard to NIDDM, the key to prevention is the prevention of obesity. A large trial is underway to determine whether tight control retards the progression of complications in NIDDM.

CONCLUSION

In the end, we are left with daily responsibility for early and accurate diagnosis of diabetes, for institution of appropriate therapy, and for provision of effective patient education programs. Even within the limitations of current therapeutics, it remains possible to treat the disease well, ameliorate many of its complications, and enable patients to achieve a quality of life that need be second to none.

REFERENCES

1. Kovar MG, Harris ML, and Hadden WC: The scope of diabetes in the United States. Am J Public Health 77:1549, 1987.
2. Bransome ED Jr: Financing the care of diabetes mellitus in the U.S. Diabetes Care 15(Suppl.1):1, 1992.
3. National Diabetes Data Group: Diabetes in America: Diabetes Data Compiled in 1984. Bethesda, U.S. Department of Health and Human Services, 1985.
4. Moller DE and Flier JS: Insulin resistance: Mechanisms, syndromes, and implications. N Engl J Med 325:938, 1991.
5. Taylor SI, Cama A, Accili D, et al: Genetic basis of endocrine disease. 1: Molecular genetics of insulin resistant diabetes mellitus. J Clin Endocrinol Metab 73:1158, 1991.
6. National Diabetes Data Group: Classification and diagnosis of diabetes mellitus and other categories of glucose intolerance. Diabetes 28:1039, 1979.
7. Eisenbarth GS: Type I diabetes mellitus: A chronic autoimmune disease. N Engl J Med 314:1360, 1986.
8. Rossini AA, Handler ES, Greiner DL, et al: Insulin dependent diabetes mellitus. Hypothesis of autoimmunity. Autoimmunity 8:221, 1991.
9. Bowden DW, Gravius TC, Akots G, et al: Identification of genetic markers flanking the locus for maturity-onset diabetes of the young on human chromosome 20. Diabetes 41:88, 1992.
10. Kissebah AH and Peiris AN: Biology of regional body fat distribution: Relationship to non-insulin-dependent diabetes mellitus. Diabetes/Metab Rev 5:83, 1989.
11. Barss VA: Diabetes and pregnancy. Med Clin North Am 73:685, 1989.
12. Viswanathan M: Pancreatic diabetes in India: An overview. *In* Pololsky S and Viswanathan M (eds): Secondary Diabetes: The Spectrum of the Diabetic Syndromes. New York, Raven Press, 1980, pp 105–116.
13. Ziegler AG, Ziegler R, Vardi P, et al: Life-table analysis of progression to diabetes of anti-insulin autoantibody-positive relatives of individuals with type I diabetes. Diabetes 38:1320, 1989.
14. American Diabetes Association: Clinical practice recommendations 1990–1991. Diabetes Care 14 (Suppl 2):1, 1991.
15. Rossini AA and Mordes JP: The diabetic comas. *In* Rippe JM, Irwin RS, Alpert JS, et al (eds): Intensive Care Medicine, 2nd ed. Boston, Little, Brown, 1991, pp 963–975.
16. Hofeldt FD: Reactive hypoglycemia. Endocrinol Metab Clin North Am 18:185, 1989.
17. Payami H, Joe S, and Thomson G: Autoimmune thyroid disease in type I diabetic families. Genet Epidemiol 6:137, 1989.
18. Mazze RS, Shamoon H, Pasmantier R, et al: Reliability of blood glucose monitoring by patients with diabetes mellitus. Am J Med 77:211, 1984.
19. Nathan DM, Fogel HA, Godine JE, et al: Role of diabetologist in evaluating diabetic retinopathy. Diabetes Care 14:26, 1991.
20. The Diabetes Control and Complications Research Group: The effect of intensive treatment of diabetes on the development and progression of long-term complications in insulin-dependent diabetes mellitus. N Engl J Med 329:977, 1993.
21. Dahl-Jorgensen K: Near-normoglycemia and late diabetic com-

plications: The Oslo study. Acta Endocrinol 115 (Suppl 284):4, 1986.
22. Robertson RP: Pancreas transplantation in humans with diabetes mellitus. Diabetes 40:1085, 1991.
23. Brownlee M: Glycosylation of proteins and microangiopathy. Hosp Pract 27 (Suppl 1):46, 1992.
24. Miller E, Hare JW, Cloherty JP, et al: Elevated maternal hemoglobin A_{1c} in early pregnancy and major congenital anomalies in infants of diabetic mothers. N Engl J Med 304:1331, 1981.
25. Jovanovic L, Druzin M, and Peterson CM: Effect of euglycemia on the outcome of pregnancy in insulin-dependent diabetic women as compared with normal control subjects. Am J Med 71:921, 1981.
26. DCCT Research Group: Epidemiology of severe hypoglycemia in the diabetes control and complications trial. Am J Med 90:450, 1991.
27. Larsen ML, Horder M, and Mogensen EF: Effect of long-term monitoring of glycosylated hemoglobin levels in insulin-dependent diabetes mellitus. N Engl J Med 323:1021, 1990.
28. Service FJ, O'Brien PC, and Rizza RA: Measurements of glucose control. Diabetes Care 10:225, 1987.
29. Smart LM, Howie AF, Young RJ, et al: Comparison of fructosamine with glycosylated hemoglobin and plasma proteins as measures of glycemic control. Diabetes Care 11:433, 1988.
30. Scott J: Lipoprotein(a). BMJ 303:663, 1991.
31. Moore RD, Smith CR, Kwiterovich PO, et al: Effect of low-dose alcohol use versus abstention on apolipoproteins A-I and B. Am J Med 84:884, 1988.
32. Bray GA: Treatment for obesity. *In* Brodoff BN and Bleicher SJ (eds): Diabetes Mellitus and Obesity. Baltimore/London, Williams & Wilkins, 1982, pp 322–332.
33. Desemone J, Mordes JP, and Rossini AA: Hypoglycemia. *In* Rippe JM, Irwin RS, Alpert JS, et al (eds): Intensive Care Medicine, 2nd ed. Boston, Little, Brown, 1991, pp 1000–1009.
34. Gerich JE, Mokan M, Veneman T, et al: Hypoglycemia unawareness. Endocr Rev 12:356, 1991.
35. Reaven GM: Banting lecture 1988: Role of insulin resistance in human disease. Diabetes 37:1595, 1988.
36. Reaven GM: Insulin resistance and compensatory hyperinsulinemia: Role in hypertension, dyslipidemia, and coronary heart disease. Am Heart J 121(Suppl):1283, 1991.
37. Stern MP and Mark AL: "Syndrome X": Is it a significant cause of hypertension? Hosp Pract 27(Suppl 1):37, 1992.
38. Kleinbaum J and Shamoon H: Impaired counterregulation of hypoglycemia in insulin-dependent diabetes mellitus. Diabetes 32:493, 1983.
39. Shalwitz RA, Farkas-Hirsch R, White NH, et al: Prevalence and consequences of nocturnal hypoglycemia among conventionally treated children with diabetes mellitus. J Pediatr 116:685, 1990.
40. Perriello G, De Feo P, Torlone E, et al: The dawn phenomenon in type 1 (insulin-dependent) diabetes mellitus: Magnitude, frequency, variability, and dependency on glucose counterregulation and insulin sensitivity. Diabetologia 34:21, 1991.
41. Gerich JE: Oral hypoglycemic agents. N Engl J Med 321:1231, 1989.
42. Peters AL and Davidson MB: Insulin plus a sulfonylurea agent for treating type 2 diabetes: Metabolic effects of combination glipizide and human proinsulin treatment in NIDDM combination insulin-sulfonylurea therapy. Ann Intern Med 115:45, 1991.
43. Eisenbarth GS: Type I Diabetes Mellitus: A Chronic and Predictable Autoimmune Disease. Kalamazoo, Upjohn Corporation, 1989.
44. Soeldner JS: The etiology of diabetes. *In* Kozak GP (ed): Clinical Diabetes Mellitus. Philadelphia, WB Saunders, 1982, pp 21–31.
45. Lorenz RA and Wysocki T: The family and childhood diabetes. Diabetes Spectrum 4:262, 1991.
46. Siminerio L and Betschart J: Children with Diabetes. Alexandria, VA, American Diabetes Association, 1986.
47. Morley JE and Kaiser FE: Unique aspects of diabetes mellitus in the elderly. Clin Geriatr Med 6:693, 1990.
48. Cousins L, Baxi L, Chez R, et al: Screening recommendations for gestational diabetes mellitus. Am J Obstet Gynecol 165:493, 1991.
49. Rizzo T, Metzger BE, Burns WJ, et al: Correlations between antepartum maternal metabolism and intelligence of offspring. N Engl J Med 325:911, 1991.
50. Jovanovic L, Peterson CM, Saxena BB, et al: Feasibility of maintaining normal glucose profiles in insulin-dependent pregnant diabetic women. Am J Med 68:105, 1980.
51. Mordes JP, Tranquada RE, and Rossini AA: Lactic acidosis. *In* Rippe JM, Irwin RS, Alpert JS, et al (eds): Intensive Care Medicine, 2nd ed. Boston, Little, Brown, 1991, pp 994–1000.
52. Yue DK, McLennan S, Marsh M, et al: Effects of experimental diabetes, uremia, and malnutrition on wound healing. Diabetes 36:295, 1987.
53. Mordes JP and Rossini AA: Management of diabetes in the critically ill patient. *In* Rippe JM, Irwin RS, Alpert JS, et al (eds): Intensive Care Medicine, 2nd ed. Boston, Little, Brown, 1991, pp 955–962.
54. Frank RN: On the pathogenesis of diabetic retinopathy: A 1990 update. Ophthalmology 98:586, 1991.
55. Selby JV, FitzSimmons SC, Newman JM, et al: The natural history and epidemiology of diabetic nephropathy: Implications for prevention and control. JAMA 263:1954, 1990.
56. Arieff AI: Proteinuria and microalbuminuria as predictors of nephropathy. Hosp Pract 27 (Suppl 1):51, 1992.
57. Marre M, Leblanc H, Suarez L, et al: Converting enzyme inhibition and kidney function in normotensive diabetic patients with persistent microalbuminuria. BMJ 294:1448, 1987.
58. Arauz-Pacheco C, Ramirez LC, Rios JM, et al: Hypoglycemia induced by angiotensin-converting enzyme inhibitors in patients with non–insulin-dependent diabetes receiving sulfonylurea therapy. Am J Med 89:811, 1990.
59. Buller GK and Perazella M: ACE inhibitor-induced hypoglycemia. Am J Med 91:104, 1991.
60. Ferrier C, Ferrari P, Weidmann P, et al: Antihypertensive therapy with Ca^{2+} antagonist verapamil and/or ACE inhibitor enalapril in NIDDM patients. Diabetes Care 14:911, 1991.
61. Parfrey PS, Griffiths SM, Barrett BJ, et al: Contrast material-induced renal failure in patients with diabetes mellitus, renal insufficiency, or both: A prospective controlled study. N Engl J Med 320:143, 1989.
62. Ravid M, Savin H, Jurin I, et al: Long-term stabilizing effect of angiotensin-converting enzyme inhibition on plasma creatinine and on proteinemia in normotensive type II diabetic patients. Ann Intern Med 118:577, 1993.
63. Capsaicin Study Group: Effect of treatment with capsaicin on daily activities of patients with painful diabetic neuropathy. Diabetes Care 15:159, 1992.
64. Janssens J, Peeters TL, Vantrappen G, et al: Improvement of gastric emptying in diabetic gastroparesis by erythromycin: Preliminary studies. N Engl J Med 322:1028, 1990.
65. Alpert JS, Chipkin SR, and Aronin N: Diabetes mellitus and silent myocardial ischemia. Adv Cardiol 37:297, 1990.
66. Pickleman J and González RP: The improving results of cholecystectomy. Arch Surg 121:930, 1986.
67. Brownlee M, Cerami A, and Vlassara H: Advanced glycosylation end products in tissue and the biochemical basis of diabetic complications. N Engl J Med 318:1315, 1988.
68. Hammes H-P, Martin S, Federlin K, et al: Aminoguanidine treatment inhibits the development of experimental diabetic retinopathy. Proc Natl Acad Sci (USA) 88:11555, 1991.
69. Sullivan SJ, Maki T, Borland KM, et al: Biohybrid artificial pancreas: Long-term implantation studies in diabetic, pancreatectomized dogs. Science 252:718, 1991.
70. O'Byrne S and Feely J: Effects of drugs on glucose tolerance in non–insulin-dependent diabetics (Part I). Drugs 40:6, 1990.
71. O'Byrne S and Feely J: Effects of drugs on glucose tolerance in non-insulin-dependent diabetics (Part II). Drugs 40:203, 1990.

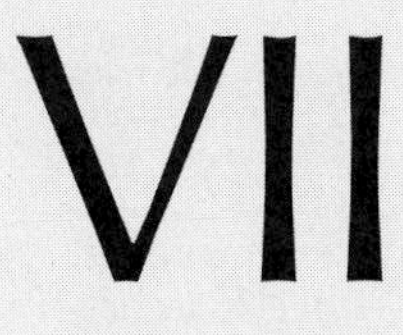

Hematologic Problems

47

Evaluation of an Abnormal Blood Count

A. JACQUELINE MITUS, MD
DAVID S. ROSENTHAL, MD

Routine automated blood counting often reveals unanticipated hematologic abnormalities, the preliminary evaluation of which falls to the internist. This chapter focuses on the integration of the history, physical examination, and ancillary laboratory studies in the work-up of various hematologic derangements. "Cytopenias" (e.g., anemia, thrombocytopenia, and leukopenia) and "cytoses" (e.g., erythrocytosis, thrombocytosis, and leukocytosis) are addressed.

ANEMIA

Anemia is generally defined by a hemoglobin count of less than 14g/dl (hematocrit <40%) in the male or a hemoglobin count of less than 12 g/dl (hematocrit < 36%) in the female. The prevalence of anemia varies between sexes and age groups, being highest among infants (5.7%) and young women (5.8%).[1] In the aged population, overall, 12% of individuals are anemic, and males are affected more commonly than females (17.7% versus 8.4%).[2]

General Approach

The evaluation of anemia is facilitated by a framework from which to approach the problem. The history and physical examination are critical and often suggest the underlying pathophysiologic process. An acute drop in hemoglobin and hematocrit (bleeding, hemolysis) causes orthostatic

TABLE 47–1. EVALUATION OF ANEMIA

Reticulocyte Count	
Decreased (production abnormality) (normocytic except where noted)	*Elevated (bleeding and increased destruction) (generally macrocytic)*
I. Ingredient deficiency	I. Blood loss (normocytic)
Iron deficiency (microcytic)	II. Intrinsic red blood cell abnormality
Folate deficiency (macrocytic)	Membrane defect
Vitamin B_{12} deficiency (macrocytic)	Enzymopathy
Low erythropoietin-renal failure	Hemoglobinopathy* (microcytic)
II. Bone marrow suppression	III. Extrinsic red blood cell defect
Inflammation-anemia of chronic disease (normocytic and microcytic)	Autoantibody
Infection	Infectious organism
Toxin	"Environmental" abnormality
III. Myelophthisic process	
Fibrosis	
Metastatic cancer	
Granuloma	
IV. Primary bone marrow defect (stem cell disorder)	
Aplastic anemia (macrocytic or normocytic)	
Myelodysplasia (macrocytic or normocytic)	
Acute leukemia	

*Certain hemoglobinopathies (e.g., thalassemia) are considered to be problems of production (ineffective erythropoiesis) and destruction. See text.

symptoms, palpitations, shortness of breath and, in the elderly, may precipitate myocardial ischemia, congestive heart failure, or confusional states. By contrast, when anemia develops slowly allowing for compensatory mechanisms, the patient may become acclimated to extremely low counts (hemoglobin < 6 to 7 g), noting only mild dyspnea or fatigue. Specific complaints and findings can suggest the origin of anemia; pica and koilonychia are associated with iron deficiency, glossitis, and neuropathy with pernicious anemia. The social, occupational, and family history can be equally informative (see later).

As with all cytopenias, anemia can be considered a problem of decreased production or excessive destruction (Table 47–1). The reticulocyte count plays a critical role in differentiating between these two pathophysiologic processes. When reduced, a defect in red blood cell synthesis is presumed, whereas reticulocytosis implies abnormal loss of red blood cells, either due to bleeding or hemolysis. It is important to remember that the reticulocyte count is reported as a percentage of total red blood cells. This value must be corrected in the anemic patient to account for the decrease in the absolute number of cells [$retic_{corrected} = retic_{observed} \times$ (observed hematocrit/normal hematocrit)]. Without this adjustment, the reticulocyte count may be misinterpreted as elevated when, in fact, it is inappropriately low for the degree of anemia.

Causes of diminished red blood cell production may be thought of as arising from defects in the developmental pathway of the erythrocyte. Commonly, there are deficiencies in the fundamental ingredients necessary for red blood cell production and differentiation (e.g., iron, folate, vitamin B_{12}, and erythropoietin). Normal erythropoiesis may be hindered by environmental factors (e.g., infections, toxins) and extraneous processes impinging on the marrow (e.g., fibrosis, metastatic cancer). Finally, primary defects in the hematopoietic progenitor (e.g., aplastic anemia, myelodysplasia, leukemia) also give rise to hypoproliferative anemia (see Table 47–1).

Increased destruction of red blood cells, hemolysis, is incited by intrinsic red blood cell defects (e.g., hemoglobinopathy, enzymopathy, or membrane abnormalities) and by extrinsic causes (e.g., antibodies, infectious organisms, or "environmental" irregularities) (see Table 47–1).

The red blood cell indices can further aid in the evaluation of anemia. The mean corpuscular volume (MCV) is calculated by dividing the hematocrit by the red blood cell number. Small, microcytic cells are defined by an MCV of less than 80 fl, whereas macrocytosis is present when the MCV exceeds 100 fl. Reviewing the peripheral smear, a normal red blood cell should approximate the size of a lymphocyte nucleus (the "micro-yardstick" of hematology[3]). The mean corpuscular hemoglobin (MCH = hemoglobin/red blood cell count) and mean corpuscular hemoglobin concentration (MCHC = hemoglobin/hematocrit) serve as markers of red blood cell protein synthesis and categorize anemia as hypochromic (decreased hemoglobinization), normochromic, or hyperchromic.

Decreased Production (Hypoproliferative Anemia)

Microcytic (Iron Deficiency, Anemia of Chronic Disease, Sideroblastic Anemia, Thalassemia)

Normal adult hemoglobin consists of a heme moiety (tetrapyrrole ring surrounding a single ferrous ion) and four interlocking globin chains (two α–β-globin dimers) (Fig. 47–1). Abnormalities of any of these factors will give rise to an anemia that is characterized by microcytosis and hypochromia. Iron deficiency is the most common cause encountered by the internist. Ordinarily, 1 mg of elemental iron meets daily requirements, but in pregnancy and infancy, this need may increase three- to fourfold. Although iron depletion through blood loss is the most important cause, increased demand (pregnancy), malnutrition, and malabsorption are also causes. Pica, angular cheilosis, koilonychia (spooned, ridged, brittle nails), and dysphagia from esophageal webs (Plummer-Vinson syndrome) are associated with severe longstanding depletion. Chronic inflammation, due to indolent infections or autoimmune processes, gives rise to inappropriate utilization of iron and a picture easily confused with iron deficiency. Through mechanisms not completely elucidated, in anemia of chronic disease (ACD), iron is retained in the reticuloendothelial system and is thus inaccessible for incorporation into hemoglobin. The hematocrit is in general only mildly depressed (low 30s), although more severe anemia (hematocrit of 25%) can be

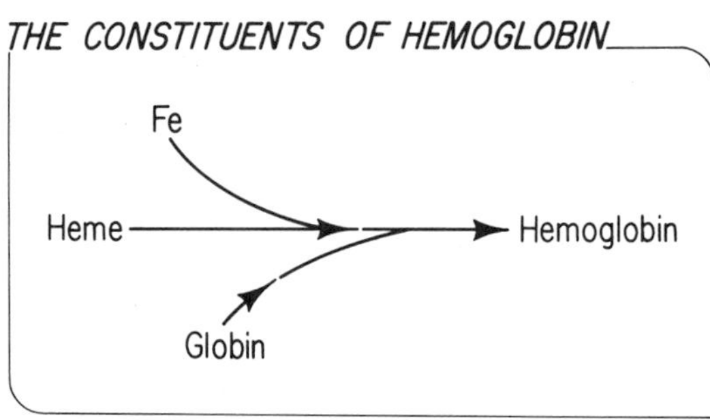

FIGURE 47–1. The three components of hemoglobin.

seen. In most cases, indices reveal a normocytic normochromic process, but in one fourth of cases, microcytosis dominates.[4] The term ACD continues to confuse internists and hematologists alike. It has been suggested that "anemia of inflammation" or anemia of "defective iron reutilization" is more accurate.[4,5] Although it is critical to distinguish ACD from iron deficiency, this differentiation is not always straightforward. In both cases, serum iron is depressed. The total iron-binding capacity (TIBC; transferrin), is helpful; elevated in iron deficiency; and low in chronic disease. Ferritin is the best measure of total body iron stores. Consequently it is depressed in iron deficiency; however, because it acts as an acute phase reactant, it is typically high in inflammatory or infectious states (Fig. 47–2). The most difficult scenario is the iron-deficient patient with ongoing inflammation. Here, it has been suggested that a ferritin level greater than 50 μg/l renders the possibility of iron deficiency unlikely.[4]

Aberration of any of the numerous synthetic steps involved in heme synthesis gives rise to a refractory anemia marked by inappropriate accumulation of iron in the mitochondria of red blood cells. These iron-laden mitochondria ally themselves in a perinuclear ring in nucleated red blood cells, a pathologic configuration called ringed sideroblast. The hallmark of sideroblastic anemia, ringed sideroblasts are easily distinguished from normal siderocytes in which only occasional iron particles are scattered in the cytoplasm. Sideroblastic anemia may be congenital or acquired, and in most cases, the cause is poorly understood. Secondary causes include vitamin B_6 (pyridoxine) deficiency and toxin exposure (e.g., alcohol, lead, isoniazid, or chloramphenicol). Idiopathic acquired sideroblastic anemia is believed to represent a primary hematopoietic stem cell disorder and is categorized as a myelodysplastic syndrome (refractory anemia with ringed sideroblasts).

The final component essential to the manufacture of hemoglobin is adequate and balanced synthesis of globin chains. The thalassemias are a group of congenital diseases arising from absent or reduced production of the normal adult classes of globins, α or β (α-thalassemia and β-thalassemia, respectively). α-Thalassemia is prevalent in those of black African and Asian descent, whereas β-thalassemia is found in individuals heralding from the Mediterranean basin. Imbalance of the two chains leads to decreased hemoglobinization, shortened survival, and premature death of red blood cell precursors within the marrow, a process referred to as ineffective erythropoiesis. Excesses of unmatched α or β chains precipitate and deform the normally pliable erythrocyte, leading to cell injury and lysis. This process occurs both in the marrow and in the peripheral circulation; therefore, decreased or ineffective production and increased destruction are both operative in thalassemia. Clinically, the anemia can vary from mild to severe and is markedly hypochromic and microcytic. The peripheral smear is often striking, revealing a myriad of red blood cell abnormalities including teardrops, target cells, schistocytes (fragmented red blood cells), and nucleated red blood cells (Fig. 47–3).

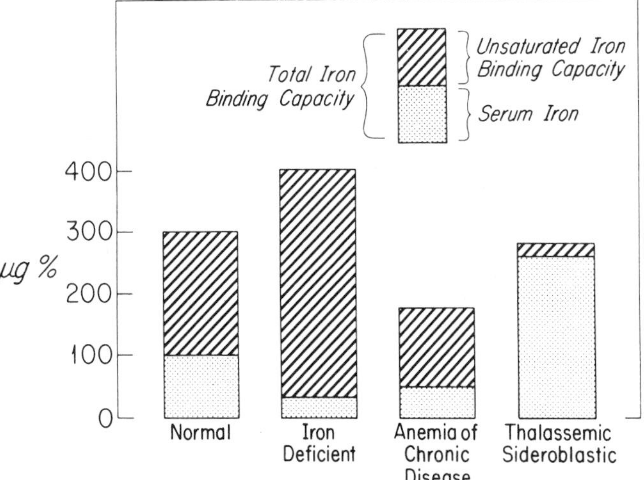

FIGURE 47–2. Serum iron level and total iron-binding capacity in the diagnosis of iron deficiency and other anemias.

Macrocytic (Megaloblastic Anemia, Liver Disease, Aplastic Anemia, Myelodysplasia, Alcoholism, Hypothyroidism)

Cobalamin (vitamin B_{12}) and folate deficiency give rise to megaloblastic changes and a macrocytic anemia. Absence of these cofactors of DNA synthesis results in ineffective erythropoiesis by impairing nuclear maturation and division while leaving cytoplasmic protein synthesis intact (nuclear-cytoplasmic asynchrony). Any cell undergoing DNA synthesis is susceptible, especially those in which cellular turnover is particularly rapid (e.g., oral mucosa, gut epithelium, marrow elements). Consequently, systemic findings are not limited to the hematopoietic system and include glossitis, gut epithelial atrophy, and abnormal Papanicolaou smears. Because all elements of the bone marrow are affected (red blood cells, white blood cells, and platelets), the term megaloblastic anemia is somewhat misleading. Pathophysiologically, megaloblastic pancytopenia ensues. The hallmarks of this process are peripheral blood findings of hypersegmented polymorphonuclear leukocytes (any six-lobed poly, >5% five-lobed polys, or a majority of four-lobed polys[6]) and large oval-shaped red blood cells (macroovalocytes) (see Fig. 47–3). The bone marrow reveals a striking arrest of nuclear division in precursor cells, particularly evident in early red blood cells, in which noncondensed chromatin gives a speckled pattern often likened to a slice of salami.

The laboratory and morphologic findings of vitamin B_{12} and folate deficiency are indistinguishable. Vitamin B_{12} is ubiquitous in the food supply (found in red meats and dairy products); consequently, deficiency on a dietary basis alone is extremely uncommon, arising in only fastidious ovolacto-vegetarians (vegans). Instead, impaired absorption is the most important mechanism of depletion. Once ingested, vitamin B_{12} binds to the parietal cell product intrinsic factor in the proximal duodenum, whereby it becomes protected from enzymatic degradation until it reaches its site of absorption in the terminal ileum. Disturbances in any of these steps results in megaloblastic anemia. Immune destruction of parietal cells or intrinsic factor gives rise to a disease named for its former lethal potential, pernicious anemia. Resection of the stomach or terminal ileum, bacterial overgrowth, or severe ileitis also results in depletion of vitamin B_{12} stores, but only after 3 to 5 years (Table 47–2).

In contrast, supplies of folate are short lived, and a diet devoid of green leafy vegetables and legumes will precipitate megaloblastic changes within weeks to months. As folate is absorbed throughout the small intestine, diffuse enteropathy (e.g., celiac sprue) can lead to functional deficiency. Anticonvulsant drugs hinder absorption by interfering with intestinal conjugases that are essential in the transformation of the polyglumate form to the methylated (absorbable) form of folate. Increased demand on a tenuous folate supply, which occurs with pregnancy and chronic he-

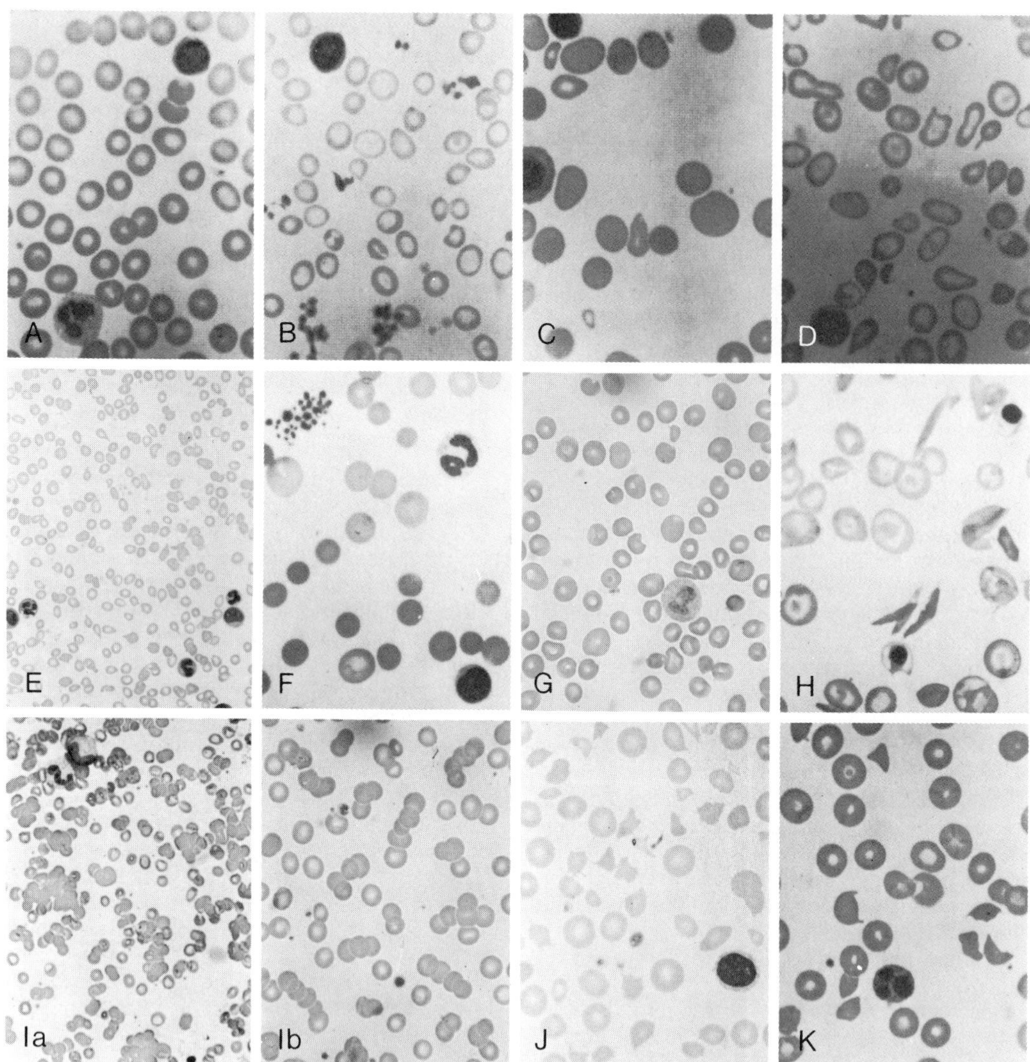

FIGURE 47–3. *A,* Normal peripheral blood. *B,* Iron deficiency: microcytosis and hypochromia. *C,* Megaloblastic changes of folate or vitamin B_{12} deficiency. *D,* Target cells seen in hemoglobinopathies (thalassemia, Hb C, Hb D, Hb E, and liver disease). *E,* Leukoerythroblastic changes consistent with myelophthisic (infiltrative) marrow process. Note the teardrops and nucleated red blood cells. *F,* Spherocytes: hereditary spherocytosis or autoimmune hemolytic anemia. *G,* Bite cells: Heinz body hemolytic anemia. *H,* Sickle cell anemia. *I,* Agglutination versus rouleaux formation. *J* and *K,* Fragmented red blood cells: microangiopathic process (e.g., disseminated intravascular coagulation or thrombotic thrombocytopenic purpura).

TABLE 47–2. COMMON CAUSES OF MEGALOBLASTIC ANEMIA

B_{12} Deficiency
- Pernicious anemia—lack of intrinsic factor
- Gastrectomy
- Resected or diseased ileum
- Transcobalamin deficiency (rare)
- Blind loop syndromes
- Fish tapeworm infestation
- Extreme vegetarian diets (vegans sect)

Folate Deficiency
- Nutritional
- Drugs: *Interfere with absorption:* phenobarbital, diphenylhydantoin, and contraceptives
  - *Competitive inhibition:* methotrexate
- Malabsorption and other diseases of the jejunum
- Increased demand:
  - Hemolytic anemias
  - Pregnancy, infancy
  - Malignancies

molysis, is an important cause of megaloblastic anemia that can be easily preempted (Table 47–2). Liver disease commonly gives rise to mild macrocytosis. Alcohol use, even in the absence of abnormal liver function, can also cause elevation of the MCV.

Another potential cause of macrocytic anemia is stem cell injury, such as aplastic anemia and myelodysplasia. Both diseases are associated with a spectrum of clinical manifestations that range from mild isolated anemia to life-threatening, transfusion-dependent pancytopenia. By unclear mechanisms, hypothyroidism also gives rise to hypoproliferative anemia and minimal elevation in the MCV (100 to 105 fl).

Normocytic (Renal Failure, Infiltrative Bone Marrow Diseases)

Most anemias fall into the normocytic, normochromic category. Erythropoietin (EPO), the glycoprotein hormone synthesized by the kidney and liver in response to hypoxia, is crucial to the regulation of erythropoiesis. In chronic renal insufficiency, levels of EPO fall resulting in depressed red blood cell production. The degree of anemia correlates with the severity of kidney impairment (increasing blood urea nitrogen [BUN] levels[7]) and may be corrected by administration of exogenous recombinant human erythropoietin. Infiltration of the bone marrow by metastatic cancer, fibrosis, granuloma, leukemia, myeloma, or other processes will disrupt or replace normal red blood cell manufacture and give rise to normocytic anemia. There is little that characterizes these anemias, although an examination of the peripheral blood may provide clues to the underlying myelophthisic process, revealing early white blood cells, nucleated red blood cells (leukoerythroblastic picture), and tear drop–shaped red blood cells (see Fig. 47–3).

Increased Destruction (Hemolytic Anemia)

Accelerated destruction of red blood cells arises because of either intrinsic erythrocyte abnormalities or extrinsic, "environmental" stresses. Hemolysis occurs most frequently in the extravascular sinusoids of the reticuloendothelial system (spleen, liver) and less often within the vascular tree (intravascular hemolysis). Intrinsic red blood cell defects are generally inherited and can be classified as membrane, enzyme, or hemoglobin anomalies. In contrast, typically acquired extrinsic causes of premature red blood cell lysis include antibody deposition, parasitic infection, or "hostile" environmental changes.

To compensate for the increased destruction, the normal bone marrow responds with increased production of erythrocytes as manifest by a vigorous reticulocytosis. These early red blood cells are larger than normal and account for the increased MCV that is characteristic of most hemolytic processes. Elevation of indirect bilirubin and serum lactate dehydrogenase with depression of haptoglobin mark the hemolytic process. Free hemoglobin in the serum (hemoglobinemia) or urine (hemoglobinuria) are generally associated with brisk destruction of red blood cells within the intravascular, not extravascular, space (Table 47–3).

The most common familial abnormality of red blood cell membranes is hereditary spherocytosis. This autosomal dominant (rarely autosomal recessive) disease results from deficiency in the skeletal protein spectrin. As a consequence, erythrocytes have decreased surface:volume ratio creating rigid, dense spherical cells with an elevated MCHC (see Fig. 47–3). Hemolysis is mild to moderate and associated with splenomegaly and reactive erythrocytosis. Other anomalies of red blood cell membranes that cause hemolysis include hereditary elliptocytosis, acanthocytosis and spur cell anemia (see Fig. 47–3). Imbalance in cholesterol:phospholipid ratio of erythrocyte membranes as occurs in severe hepatocellular disease gives rise to these misshapen cells whose rigid spicules enhance premature destruction in the conditioning environment of the spleen. Target cells are erythrocytes in which hemoglobin is centralized in the drying process, creating a bull's eye effect. Considered a stigmata of obstructive liver disease, they are also found in certain hemoglobinopathies (e.g., thalassemia, Hb C, Hb D, Hb E) (see Fig. 47–3). In uremia, erythrocytes acquire knobby irregularities (burr cells) that are not well correlated with the degree of anemia or azotemia.

Hemoglobin must be maintained in a reduced (nonoxidized) state. The hexose monophosphate and Embden-Meyerhof pathways protect against oxidation and ensuing accumulation of toxic oxygen radicals and irreversible precipitation of hemoglobin as Heinz bodies. These rigid inclusions, which are apparent only upon supravital staining (Heinz body preparation), adhere to the inner aspect of the red blood cell membrane and yield bite-like deformities as they are extruded from the cell in its tight passage through the splenic sinusoids (see Fig. 47–3). Most frequently, drugs instigate Heinz body hemolytic anemia. Among the many potential culprits, antimalarials, sulfonamides, analgesics, and antipyretics are most notable. Glucose-6-phosphate dehydrogenase (G6PD) deficiency, prevalent in those of African and Mediterranean descent, is sex linked and recessive and is the most common inherited metabolic derangement of erythrocytes. Approximately 10% of black males manifest a mild variant of G6PD that is clinically silent until exposed to oxidant drugs. Heterozygote females are generally unaffected but can develop significant hemolysis due to unequal inactivation of the X chromosomes (lyonization). It is important to remember that during the acute hemolytic episode, studies of enzyme concentration may be falsely normal due to elevated numbers of reticulocytes that are relatively rich in G6PD. Thus, G6PD assays are best performed as screens prior to instituting known oxidant drugs (e.g., dapsone) or after reticulocytosis has resolved. The autosomal recessive disorder pyruvate kinase deficiency and a host of much rarer enzymopathies result in hemolysis of varying severity and chronicity.

Hundreds of hemoglobin variants have been identified, the most notorious of which is sickle hemoglobin (Hb S). Substitution of a single amino acid (valine for glutamic acid) in the sixth position of the β chain predisposes to polymerization of hydrophobic regions of the molecule. This process is hastened in the deoxyhemoglobin state and creates irreversibly misshapened red blood cells (see Fig. 47–3). These rigid, sickled erythrocytes obstruct the microvasculature, precipitating painful hypoxic crises in various tissue beds. Lifelong hemolysis is clinically apparent from early infancy. Other inherited hemoglobin variants (e.g., Hb C, Hb D, and Hb E) are also associated with chronic hemolysis and produce striking peripheral smear changes dominated by target forms (see Fig. 47–3).

Normal red blood cells can be prematurely destroyed when exposed to abnormal environmental processes (e.g., antibodies, parasites, aberrant vascular passageways). Antierythrocyte antibodies develop upon exposure to drugs or infection or in the setting of autoimmune or lymphoprolif-

TABLE 47–3. LABORATORY FINDINGS IN HEMOLYSIS

Characteristics of Intravascular Hemolysis	Characteristics of Extravascular Hemolysis	Characteristics of Both Types
Hemoglobinemia	Splenomegaly	Increased reticulocytes
Hemoglobinuria	Predisposition to bilirubin pigment gallstones	Increased serum LDH
Iron deficiency		Increased indirect bilirubin
		Decreased haptoglobin
Urine hemosiderin		Marrow erythroid hyperplasia

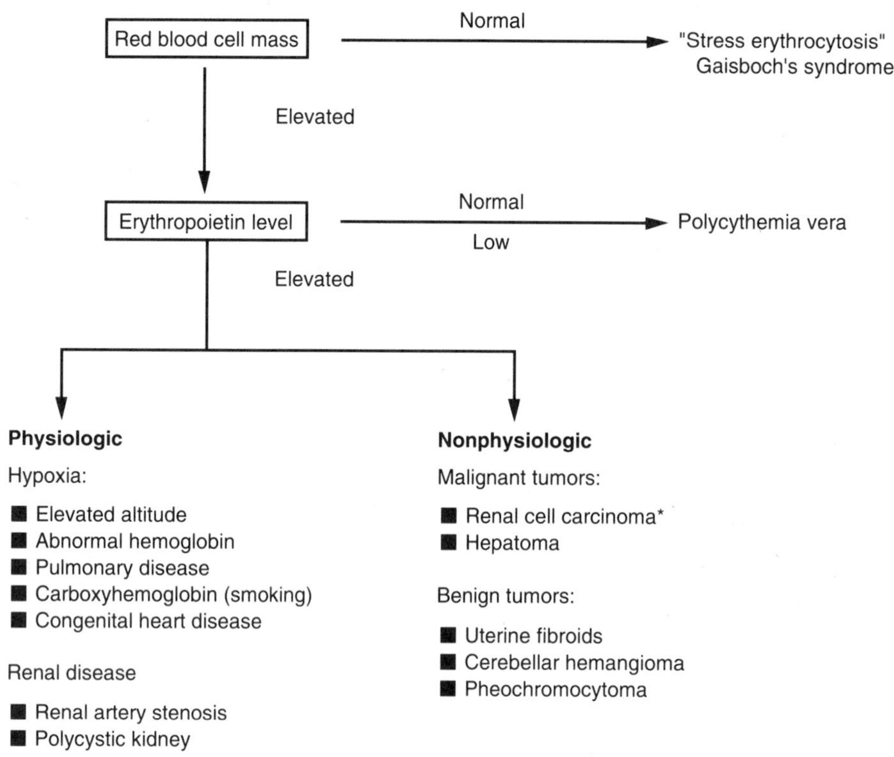

FIGURE 47–4. Physiologic approach to erythrocytosis.

erative diseases. They may be directed against specific red blood cell antigens or may precipitate with antigen on the erythrocyte that serves as an "innocent bystander." IgG antibodies are generally active at body temperatures and induce damage in the extravascular space where macrophages bind to their Fc portion. Progressive trimming of the red blood cell membrane causes a spherocytic deformity that is indistinguishable from the congenital defect. In contrast, IgM antibodies are often "cold reactive." By fixing complement, IgM induces microperforations of cellular structure within the vascular tree (intravascular hemolysis). The larger pentameric IgM antibodies can bridge many red blood cells causing agglutination, whereas rouleaux formation (stacking of red blood cells) is more typical of IgG-coated red blood cells (see Fig. 47–3). The direct antiglobulin test (Coombs' test) detects IgG on the surface of red blood cells in warm hemolytic anemias but often only reveals the presence of complement in cold hemolysis since the inciting IgM antibody disassociates as the temperature rises.

Malaria and babesiosis are common intraerythrocytic parasites that can induce severe and life-threatening hemolytic crises. The peripheral smear (thick or normal preparation) can demonstrate these organisms and confirm the clinical diagnosis.

Perturbations of vascular pathways can injure otherwise normal erythrocytes. Microthrombi deposited during disseminated intravascular coagulation (DIC) and platelet fibrin aggregates characteristic of thrombotic thrombocytopenic purpura (TTP) cause shearing and fragmentation of red blood cells (see Fig. 47–3). Activation of the coagulation cascade in DIC differentiates it from TTP, in which the clinical spectrum of fever, renal failure, and neurologic impairment is present. Schistocytes and helmet cells comprise a microangiopathic picture that is also characteristic of preeclampsia, defective cardiac valves, and severe vasculitis. Hypersplenism, regardless of cause (e.g., portal hypertension, infiltrative diseases), expands the reticuloendothelial sinusoids and results in anemia and mild pancytopenia.

ERYTHROCYTOSIS

Erythrocytosis or polycythemia is defined by a hemoglobin count of more than 16 g/dl in men and more than 14 g/dl in women. It is critical to determine whether the observed values are real or spurious, produced by a relative decrease in plasma volume. This latter condition, relative or stress erythrocytosis (Gaisboch's syndrome), is defined by a normal red blood cell mass. The approach to true polycythemia depends on whether red blood cell production is autonomous (primary polycythemia) or reactive to excess erythropoietin (secondary polycythemia) (Fig. 47–4). A normal physiologic stimulus of erythropoiesis is hypoxia, resulting from chronic obstructive pulmonary disease, elevated altitude, high affinity hemoglobin variant, or congenital cardiac anomalies. In contrast, inappropriate production of erythropoietin generally stems from tumors (benign or malignant). Red blood cell manufacture that escapes hormonal control and proceeds unregulated defines the myeloproliferative disease, polycythemia vera. An elevated red blood cell mass, splenomegaly, and normal oxygen saturation are the diagnostic criteria of this disorder characterized clinically by hyperviscosity and recurrent bouts of hemorrhage or thrombosis.[8]

TABLE 47–4. DIFFERENTIAL DIAGNOSIS IN ABNORMAL WHITE BLOOD CELLS

Leukocytosis (>10.0 × 10^9/l)

Neonate	Anesthesia
Stress	Seizures
Fever	Exercise
Menses	Labor

Neutrophilia (>7.0 × 10^9/l)
Infections: localized or generalized bacterial
Metabolic or chemical intoxication (e.g., uremia and epinephrine stimulation)
Tissue necrosis: gangrene and myocardial infarction
Acute bleeding disorders
Acute hemolytic anemias
Myeloproliferative disorders: polycythemia vera, acute and chronic granulocytic leukemia

Eosinophilia (>0.2 × 10^9/l)
Allergic disorders
Chronic skin diseases
Parasitic diseases
Myeloproliferative disorders
Tumors (e.g., Hodgkin's disease)

Basophilia (>0.04 × 10^9/l)
Myeloproliferative disorders: polycythemia vera, chronic myelogenous leukemia, myeloid metaplasia

Lymphocytosis (>2.5 × 10^9/l)
Infections: such as infectious mononucleosis, toxoplasmosis, cytomegalovirus disease, mumps, measles, infectious hepatitis, brucellosis, pertussis, and syphilis
Leukemia: acute and chronic lymphocytic

Monocytosis (>0.4 × 10^9/l)
Infections: chronic bacterial, subacute bacterial endocarditis (SBE), ulcerative colitis, tuberculosis, and rickettsial infections
Leukemia and myelodysplasia

LEUKOPENIA

A normal total white blood cell count ranges from 4 to 10 × 10^9/l, the majority of which are neutrophils. Leukopenia or neutropenia is not always pathologic. Black individuals typically manifest mean neutrophil counts up to 32% lower than caucasians.[9] As there is no increased risk of infection or other problems, a different scale of normal hematologic values has been proposed for this population.[10]

Neutropenia, like anemia, can be a problem of decreased production or increased destruction. When the reticulocyte count serves as a marker of erythropoietic activity, only an examination of the bone marrow will help to define the pathophysiologic process involved in a lowered white blood cell count.

Isolated hypoproliferative neutropenia is rare and is seen mainly in the setting of congenital hematologic diseases. Infection is probably the most common cause of neutropenia in general practice, presumably arising from direct marrow suppression by viruses (e.g., hepatitis B), bacteria (e.g., *Salmonella*), rickettsia (e.g., Rocky Mountain spotted fever), and other agents. In the setting of severe infection, neutrophils demonstrate distinctive toxic granulations and Dohle bodies (oblong blue cytoplasmic patches representing remnants of rough endoplasmic reticulum). Finally, neutropenia may be the harbinger of an underlying bone marrow disorder. In the elderly, myelodysplasia is foremost on the list of possibilities, although any diffuse marrow process can be implicated.

Increased destruction of neutrophils is most often due to an autoimmune process; however, mechanistic details have been hampered by unreliable and imperfect tests confirming antineutrophil antibodies. Collagen vascular illnesses are prototypic. Examination of the bone marrow in Felty's syndrome (rheumatoid arthritis with splenomegaly and neutropenia) reveals characteristic maturation arrest at the myelocyte stage, supporting the role of antibody mediated destruction of mature as well as immature white blood cell precursors. Medications are the greatest offenders in autoimmune neutropenia. Innumerable agents have been implicated, but frequent culprits include antibiotics (e.g., penicillins, trimethoprim sulfamethoxazole), rheumatologic drugs (e.g., phenylbutazone, gold, indomethacin), antipsychotics (e.g., phenothiazines), and antiepileptics (e.g., phenytoin, tegretol).

LEUKOCYTOSIS

An elevated white blood cell count must be evaluated in the context of the differential. Most frequently one encounters granulocytosis with or without early forms (Table 47–4). Common, yet often overlooked causes of neutrophilia include pregnancy, cigarette smoking, and medication. More than 50% of pregnant women demonstrate some abnormality in their white blood cell count or differential (white blood cell count greater than 10,000 and/or the presence of myelocytes and metamyelocytes).[11] These changes are particularly prominent during the last trimester and resolve postpartum. Smokers develop granulocytosis proportional to the number of cigarettes inhaled and the duration of the habit.[12, 13] Mild leukocytosis can also be induced by oral contraceptives and lithium.

Raised numbers of granulocytes may be secondary to infection. The presence of immature forms suggests the possibility of an underlying bone marrow disorder. Marked elevation of the white blood cell count (> 50,000) or the presence of promyelocytes and myeloblasts is extremely unusual as a secondary reaction and most likely represents a myeloproliferative disease. Accompanying splenomegaly, aberration in other blood counts, basophilia or eosinophilia, serve as corroborative data. The leukocyte alkaline phosphatase (LAP) score is especially helpful in the distinction between a primary marrow derangement and a secondary (leukemoid) process. The LAP score is normal or raised in the setting of inflammation but is distinctively low in chronic myelogenous leukemia. Causes of monocytosis, eosinophilia, basophilia, and lymphocytosis are listed in Table 47–4.

THROMBOCYTOPENIA

Platelets are the mediators of primary hemostasis: platelet plug formation. Thrombocytopenia (platelet count <150,000/µl) can cause bleeding at mucocutaneous surfaces (e.g., oral mucosa, gastrointestinal and genitourinary tracts, skin), which tends to occur promptly after injury. Prolongation of the bleeding time results when platelets fall below 80,000/µl and spontaneous hemorrhage occurs in the 20,000/µl range. A complete discussion of bleeding disorders is found in Chapter 48.

Pseudothrombocytopenia may result from abnormal in vitro clumping of platelets and can be easily recognized by inspection of the peripheral smear. In this case, a true platelet count can be obtained by drawing blood in heparin or sodium citrate (as opposed to ethylenediaminetetraacetic acid [EDTA]). Isolated thrombocytopenia arising from decreased production is uncommon and is relegated

TABLE 47–5. CAUSES OF THROMBOCYTOPENIA

Production	Destruction
I. Congenital Thrombocytopenia with absent radii (TAR syndrome) Fanconi's anemia May-Hegglin anomaly Bernard-Soulier disease X-linked amegakaryocytic thrombocytopenia II. Viral infection HIV, measles, CMV, EBV, etc. III. Drug induced	I. Immune Chronic (including HIV-related) Acute II. Consumptive DIC TTP Kasabach-Merritt syndrome Pre-eclampsia

CMV = cytomegalovirus; DIC = disseminated intravascular coagulation; EBV = Epstein-Barr virus; HIV = human immunodeficiency virus; TTP = thrombotic thrombocytopenic purpura.

mainly to congenital disorders (Table 47–5). Unlike most medications that induce thrombocytopenia via immune mechanisms, thiazide diuretics are unusual, directly affecting megakaryocytes.[14]

The myriad manifestations of human immunodeficiency virus (HIV) infection on thrombopoiesis deserve special mention.[15] The virus has been shown to be capable of infecting bone marrow progenitor cells, thus, presumably directly suppressing megakaryopoiesis.[16] Bone marrows are active, with marked increase in dysplastic, nonfunctioning megakaryocytes. Autoimmune destruction of platelets is also incited by HIV infection. There is debate as to the nature of the process (true autoantibody versus antigen-antibody complex), but response to standard therapy as well as antiviral agents is noted.

Chronic immune thrombocytopenic purpura is now most frequently diagnosed in the HIV-infected population. It is also a disease afflicting otherwise healthy young women and patients with collagen vascular and lymphoproliferative illnesses. Many drugs, most notably quinidine, also mediate immune thrombocytopenia. Consumptive thrombocytopenia accompanies the microangiopathy of DIC and TTP and the rare syndrome, Kasabach-Merritt, in which abnormal endothelial surfaces of giant hemangiomas serve as isolated niches for platelet destruction.

TABLE 47–6. REACTIVE (SECONDARY) CAUSES OF THROMBOCYTOSIS

Bleeding
Acute and chronic (iron deficiency)
Chronic inflammatory diseases
Wegener's granulomatosis
Inflammatory bowel disease
Rheumatoid arthritis
Polyarteritis nodosum
Indolent infections
Drugs
Epinephrine
Vinca alkaloids
Splenectomy and asplenic states
Malignancy
Rebound thrombocytosis:
Following treatment of ITP, pernicious anemia
Exercise
Myelodysplastic states
Chronic hemolytic anemia

ITP = idiopathic thrombocytopenic purpura.

TABLE 47–7. REACTIVE VERSUS ESSENTIAL THROMBOCYTOSIS

	Reactive	Essential
Plt count	$<10^6$	$>600,000$
Plt appearance	Normal	Abnormal
Marrow	Normal	Abnormal
Plt function	Normal	Abnormal
LDH	Variable	Elevated
ESR	Variable	Low

LDH = lactate dehydrogenase; ESR = erythrocyte sedimentation rate; Plt = platelet.

THROMBOCYTOSIS

Platelet counts increase in response to a variety of systemic conditions and as a manifestation of a primary marrow disorder. Iron deficiency results in secondary thrombocytosis, resolving within 1 to 2 weeks after replacement therapy. Acute bleeding, infection, chronic inflammation, malignancy, and hyposplenism are also etiologic (Table 47–6). When the platelet count exceeds $1 \times 10^6/\mu l$ or when the patient develops bleeding or thrombosis, an underlying abnormality in platelet manufacture is suggested. No single laboratory datum will help to distinguish reactive thrombocythemia from primary thrombocythemia, although some studies are helpful (Table 47–7).

REFERENCES

1. Dallman PR, Yip R, and Johnson C: Prevalence and causes of anemia in the United States, 1976 to 1980. Am J Clin Nutr 39:437, 1984.
2. Timiras ML and Brownstein H: Prevalence of anemia and correlation of hemoglobin with age in a geriatric screening population. J Am Geriatr Soc 35:639, 1987.
3. Jandl JH and Kapff CT: Blood, Atlas and Sourcebook of Hematology. Boston, MA, Little Brown, 1981, p 14.
4. Schilling RF: Anemia of chronic disease: A misnomer (Editorial). Ann Intern Med 115:572, 1991.
5. Haurani FI: Anemia of chronic disease: A misnomer (Letter). Ann Intern Med 116:520, 1992.
6. Jandl JH: Megaloblastic Anemias in Blood: Textbook of Hematology. Boston, MA, Little Brown, 1987, p 153.
7. Kaye M: The anemia associated with renal disease. J Lab Clin Med 52:83, 1958.
8. Berlin N: Diagnosis and classification of the polycythemias. Semin Hematol 12:339, 1976.
9. Broun GO, Herbig FK, and Hamilton JR: Leukopenia in Negroes. N Engl J Med 275:1410, 1968.
10. Reed WW and Diehl LF: Leukopenia, neutropenia, and reduced hemoglobin levels in healthy American blacks. Arch Intern Med 151:501, 1991.
11. Kuvin SF and Brecher G: Differential neutrophil counts in pregnancy. N Engl J Med 266:877, 1962.
12. Fisch IR and Freedman SH: Smoking, oral contraceptives and obesity: Effects on white blood cell count. JAMA 234:500, 1975.
13. Corre F, Lellouch J, and Schwartz D: Smoking and leukocyte counts: Results of an epidemiologic survey. Lancet 2:632, 1971.
14. Kutti J and Weinfeld A: The frequency of thrombocytopenia in patients treated with heart disease treated with oral diuretics. Acta Med Scand 183:245, 1968.
15. Scadden DT, Zon LI, and Groopman JE: Pathophysiology and management of HIV-associated hematologic disorders. Blood 74:1455, 1989.
16. Folks TM, Kessler SW, Orenstein JM, et al: Infection and replication of HIV-1 in purified progenitor cells of normal human bone marrow. Science 242:919, 1988.

48

Bleeding and Thrombotic Disorders

ROBERT I. HANDIN, MD
BRUCE M. EWENSTEIN, MD, PhD

Although life-threatening hemorrhage requires emergency hospitalization and treatment, most bleeding disorders are less serious and can be evaluated and treated effectively by the office-based medical practitioner. Furthermore, the physician who delivers primary care has a unique opportunity to discover and define some of the more subtle abnormalities that may have been overlooked or discounted by the patient or by previous physicians. The practitioner can also identify patients with recurrent thrombosis and embolism arising from a disorder in the hemostatic system. The evaluation of most bleeding and thrombotic disorders is straightforward but does require some understanding of the pathophysiology of hemostasis, attention to certain aspects of the history and physical examination, and the ability to select and interpret appropriate laboratory tests. This chapter endeavors to help the primary care physician evaluate bleeding and thrombotic disorders.

The term *hemostasis*—literally, "stopping the blood"—refers to the physiologic system that maintains the integrity of the vascular tree and minimizes the loss of body fluids following injury. Effective hemostasis requires the orderly interaction of components in the vessel wall with blood platelets and circulating plasma proteins. Hemostatic defects lead to hemorrhage by interrupting these interdependent reactions. Conversely, unregulated or excessive hemostasis can predispose patients to thrombosis by creating a "hypercoagulable" state.

Physiology of Hemostasis

Although platelets and plasma coagulation proteins interact continuously during hemostasis, it is easier to discuss each component separately. The initiating event is usually an injury that damages or removes the vascular endothelial lining and exposes subendothelial connective tissue. In the first step of hemostasis, platelets *adhere* to exposed collagen fibrils. Optimal adhesion also requires a specific plasma protein, von Willebrand factor, which binds to the platelet and to subendothelium to facilitate adhesion. The adherent platelets then degranulate, releasing adenosine diphosphate (ADP), which in turn recruits additional platelets to *aggregate* upon the adherent platelet monolayer. Aggregation is due to the binding of fibrinogen to receptor sites on the platelet glycoprotein IIb-IIIa complex. This process can rapidly fill the vessel lumen with a multicellular aggregate or platelet plug (Fig. 48–1). Following activation, the platelets *release* a potent vasoconstrictor, thromboxane A_2, which may minimize blood loss by decreasing vessel diameter. The generation of thromboxane A_2 from arachidonic acid released from platelet membrane phospholipids also induces platelet aggregation.[1,2]

The platelet has additional hemostatic functions that are less well characterized. For example, platelets provide a favorable surface for certain coagulation reactions by binding coagulation proteins to the platelet membrane and facilitating their interactions.[4] One of the least understood, but most vital, platelet functions is the maintenance of vascular endothelial integrity, which is adversely affected when the circulating blood platelet level is decreased.[5] It is this deficiency that leads to hemorrhage into skin, mucous membranes, and other sites seen in patients with severe thrombocytopenia.

The second step in hemostasis is plasma coagulation, which is also activated by vascular injury and amplified by a process of limited proteolysis. The majority of the coagulation proteins are proteolytic or "protein-cutting" enzymes similar to digestive enzymes like trypsin or chymotrypsin. The proteins circulate in a precursor or inactive form and

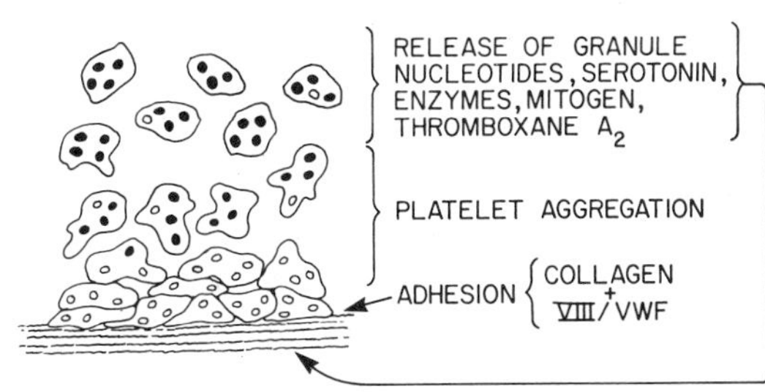

FIGURE 48–1. Injury to the vascular endothelial lining causes platelet *adherence* and degranulation. This is followed by *aggregation* of additional platelets with further *release* of thromboxane A_2 and other substances.

are sequentially activated by the scission of one or two specific peptide bonds.

In addition to the proteolytic clotting proteins, there are specific protein cofactors that regulate reaction rates and a series of inhibitors that neutralize the activated proteins. There is a vast excess of potential coagulation material present in plasma. For example, there is enough potential thrombin in each milliliter of blood to clot the entire blood volume in 15 seconds. This means that a delicate series of checks and balances is necessary to provide the appropriate degree of activation at sites of injury without promoting gross systemic coagulation.

Two mechanisms have been proposed for initiating plasma coagulation. The first pathway, termed the contact or intrinsic pathway, is activated (Fig. 48–2) when Hageman factor (factor XII) binds to collagen fibrils in the vessel wall following damage to its endothelial cell lining. Proteolytic activation steps follow, which involve at least five more proteins and eventually lead to the activation of factor X to Xa. A second pathway, termed the tissue factor or extrinsic pathway, can be activated when factor VII binds to tissue factor, a lipoprotein exposed following more extensive vascular injury. This tissue factor-factor VII complex can directly activate factor X to Xa. These events represent the initiation steps or *first stage* of coagulation.

The *second stage* of coagulation involves the conversion of prothrombin to thrombin by Xa with the aid of calcium, a source of phospholipid, and factor V. Some evidence indicates that the platelet may also produce a highly active form of factor V that is bound to its surface and accelerates prothrombin conversion.[4,6] In the *third stage* of coagulation, thrombin converts fibrinogen to fibrin monomer, which then polymerizes, producing the familiar visible clot. The second and third stages of coagulation are collectively termed the "common pathway." This initial clot is fragile and cannot withstand the shear forces present within the circulation. The individual chains in the fibrin polymer then are cross-linked by another clotting enzyme, factor XIII, to provide a definitive, mechanically stable clot.

Although useful for understanding the screening tests of hemostasis, the division of the coagulation scheme as outlined earlier is clearly an oversimplification. For example,

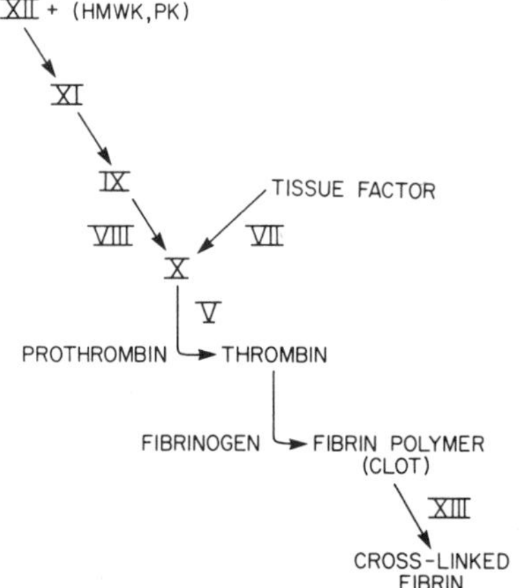

FIGURE 48–2. The two mechanisms for initiating plasma coagulation. The first, intrinsic pathway is activated when factor XII binds to collagen fibrils in the vessel wall. The second, extrinsic pathway is activated when factor VII binds to a tissue factor released after extensive vascular injury. Both pathways lead to activation of factor X, which causes conversion of prothrombin to thrombin (second stage of coagulation) and subsequently conversion by thrombin of fibrinogen to fibrin monomer (third stage of coagulation).

the tissue factor-factor VIIa complex also activates factor IX. This activity is now thought to be the major pathway of factor IX activation in most circumstances, a finding that may explain the variable, and often mild, clinical manifestations that accompany factor XI deficiency. In addition, thrombin activates factors V and VIII and thus provides positive feedback to the intrinsic pathway.

During the past few years, the role of the natural inhibitors that regulate coagulation has become well defined. Furthermore, patients with deficiencies in these natural inhibitors have been identified who have thromboembolism or hemorrhage. Clinically relevant proteins are antithrombin, protein C, protein S, and α_2-antiplasmin. Antithrombin complexes with all of the coagulation proteases except factor VII, in a reaction that is greatly accelerated by heparin. This reaction limits thrombin generation and thereby controls fibrin formation. Proteins C and S are two vitamin K–dependent proteins that work together to inactivate factors V and VIII. Protein C is converted to its active form by thrombin after it is bound to an endothelial cell protein called thrombomodulin. Activated protein C then proteolyzes and inhibits the active forms of factors V and VIII. Protein S enhances protein C activity. Patients with modest deficiencies or dysfunctional forms of antithrombin or proteins C or S have a thrombotic tendency—often referred to as a hypercoagulable state. Conversely, α_2-antiplasmin regulates clot dissolution by binding to and inactivating plasmin. It effectively prevents systemic fibrinolysis and limits plasmin activity to the fibrin clot. As expected, patients with a deficiency in this inhibitor have excessive fibrinolysis and a severe bleeding disorder.

Clinical Types of Bleeding

It is useful to note that the relative importance of platelets and coagulation proteins varies in different vascular beds and at different times after injury. For example, platelet plug formation is critically important in the microcirculation of mucous membranes and skin. Effective hemostasis in larger venules and arterioles requires that the platelet plug be buttressed by fibrin strands. The platelet system, which is a first line of defense, provides initial hemostasis. The coagulation proteins provide a back-up system that is most important several hours after injury. These differences allow the physician to predict tentatively the nature of a hemostatic defect by analyzing the site and pattern of hemorrhage (Table 48–1).

Patients with platelet disorders, who have difficulty generating the initial hemostatic plug, will bleed immediately after any trauma and will bleed primarily into skin and mucous membranes. This superficial bleeding often responds to local pressure or packing. Patients with severe thrombocytopenia also have spontaneous hemorrhage owing to a loss of endothelial integrity often called "capillary fragility."

In contrast, patients with a coagulation protein disorder have no difficulty forming platelet plugs but cannot stabilize them with fibrin strands and will then bleed hours or days after injury. These patients tend to bleed from larger vessels like arterioles and venules and bleed into subcutaneous tissue, muscles, and joints. They also require more intensive treatment and do not readily respond to simple maneuvers like pressure. Unfortunately, clinical symptoms may overlap, and there are patients who present with mixed disorders. However, these basic patterns are still of great utility and can direct the initial laboratory approach.

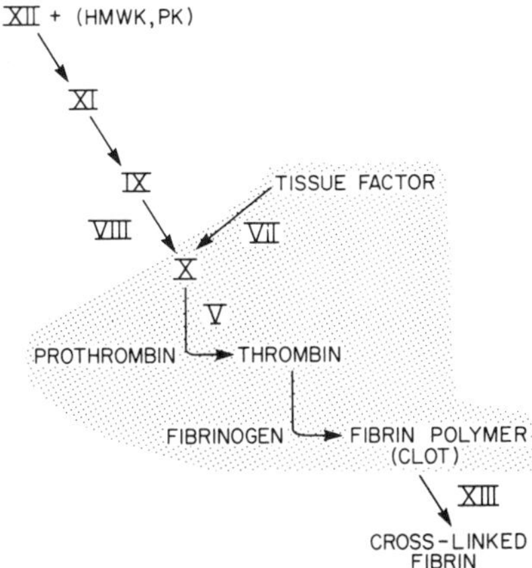

FIGURE 48–3. The prothrombin time (PT) is performed by adding a source of tissue factor to the patient's plasma in the presence of calcium and phospholipid. Normal plasma clots in 10 to 15 seconds. As shown in the figure, the reaction requires factors VII, X, and V and prothrombin and fibrinogen.

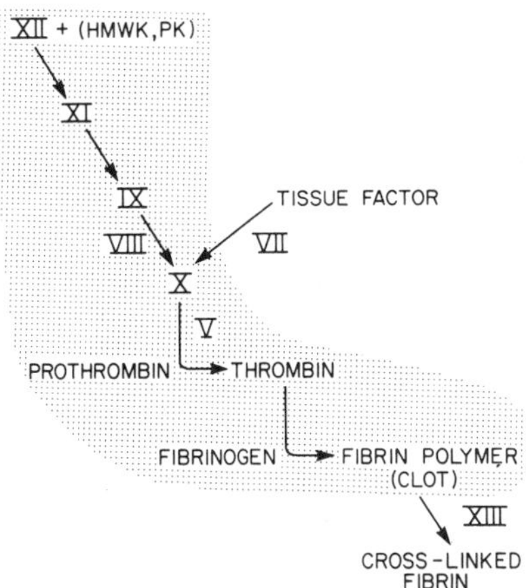

FIGURE 48–4. The partial thromboplastin time (PTT) is performed by adding a foreign material such as celite to plasma along with phospholipid and calcium. The reaction requires activated factor XII, high-molecular-weight kininogen, prekallikrein, and factors XI, IX, and VIII, leading to activation of factor X. Normal plasma clots in 25 to 35 seconds.

Screening Tests of Hemostatic Function

Definitive analysis of coagulation disorders usually requires laboratory testing. Although the detailed biochemistry and physiology, as outlined in this chapter, are quite complex, most of the components of the hemostatic system can be evaluated with four basic tests: the *platelet count, bleeding time, prothrombin time* (PT), and *partial thromboplastin time* (PTT). The platelet count is automatically computed as part of the routine complete blood count in most laboratories. If not available, a good estimate of platelet number can be obtained by examining the dried, stained blood film. The template bleeding time attempts to recreate platelet plug formation in small capillaries by making a standardized skin cut on the forearm. A normal individual will stop bleeding from this incision within 8 minutes. A prolonged bleeding time in a patient with a normal platelet count is a sensitive indicator of a qualitative platelet abnormality.

The screening coagulation tests are designed to survey components of the two pathways depicted in Figure 48–2. Determining the PT (Fig. 48–3) involves adding a source of tissue factor, usually a rabbit brain extract, to plasma in the presence of calcium and phospholipid. Normal plasma will clot in 10 to 15 seconds. As shown in the figure, this reaction requires the presence of factors VII, X, and V and prothrombin and fibrinogen. The PTT is designed to activate the contact or factor XII-dependent pathway. A foreign material like celite or ellagic acid is added to plasma along with phospholipid and calcium. Activated factor XII, in concert with high molecular weight kininogen, prekallikrein, and factors XI, IX, and VIII will lead to activation of factor X (Fig. 48–4). Normal plasma clots in 25 to 35 seconds under these conditions.

The pattern of screening test abnormalities will often pinpoint the defect (Table 48–2). For example, a prolonged PTT and normal PT reflect a defect in initiation or propagation of the contact (or intrinsic) pathway. Similarly, a prolonged PT and normal PTT must be due to a deficiency in the tissue factor–dependent (or extrinsic) pathway. When both tests are prolonged, the abnormality may involve factors in the common pathway, including fibrinogen, or multiple defects such as those seen in severe liver disease or vitamin K deficiency. Further confirmation involves more specialized laboratory tests that quantify the amount and function of each of the individual coagulation proteins.[7]

QUANTITATIVE PLATELET DISORDERS

Abnormalities in the number of circulating platelets can arise from (1) defective platelet production, (2) increased splenic sequestration, or (3) accelerated peripheral destruction. There are many more platelets in the circulation at any time than are needed for hemostasis, thus the platelet count can decrease substantially without impairing hemostasis. For example, patients with more than 50,000 platelets/mm^3 are usually asymptomatic. When the platelet count is between 20,000 and 50,000/mm^3, patients may bruise easily and have mucosal bleeding. Severe bleeding and spontaneous hemorrhage become major problems only when the count is less than 20,000/mm^3.

A clinical approach to the thrombocytopenic patient is outlined in Table 48–3. Certain features should be emphasized. First, patients with *production* defects almost always have associated marrow abnormalities, such as invasion by leukemic cells or fibrosis, which are apparent on bone mar-

TABLE 48–1. THE NATURE OF BLEEDING IN PLATELET AND PLASMA COAGULATION DISORDERS

Clinical Feature	Platelet Disorder	Plasma Coagulation Disorder
Bleeding source	Usually capillary	Usually small artery
Lesion	Cutaneous and mucosal petechiae and/or ecchymoses	Intramuscular and deep subcutaneous hematomas, hemarthroses
Preceding trauma	Unusual	Frequent, with delayed onset of bleeding
Complication of venipuncture	Superficial ecchymoses around site of venipuncture	No ecchymoses, but deep hemorrhage if firm external pressure is not maintained

TABLE 48–2. USE OF LABORATORY TESTS TO IDENTIFY COAGULATION DEFECTS

Test Pattern	Defect
Prolonged PTT; other tests normal	Intrinsic pathway defect History of bleeding: Factors VIII, IX, XI No bleeding: Factors XII, HMWK, PK
Prolonged PTT, PT; other tests normal	Common pathway defect Factors II, V, X Liver disease Vitamin K deficiency/sodium warfarin therapy
Prolonged PT; PTT and other tests normal	Extrinsic pathway defect VII deficiency Mild vitamin K deficiency Mild liver disease Early sodium warfarin therapy
Prolonged TT; PT and PTT often also abnormal	Fibrinogen defect DIC, hypofibrinogenemia Abnormal fibrinogen
Prolonged PTT and PT, which fail to correct with addition of normal plasma	Inhibitor syndromes Specific: Anti-VIII factor, anti-IX factor, anti-V factor Nonspecific: "lupus-like," "antiphospholipid"

row biopsy. This is the only group in which the number of megakaryocytes is diminished. The patient with *splenic sequestration* as a cause of thrombocytopenia has a palpable spleen and an underlying disorder causing splenomegaly, such as lymphoma or liver disease, which should be recognized by its clinical features. Patients with *nonimmune platelet* destruction may have a systemic disorder causing platelet consumption, such as vasculitis or sepsis. Disseminated intravascular coagulation (DIC), thrombotic thrombocytopenic purpura (TTP), and the hemolytic-uremic syndrome are included in this category. The most difficult diagnostic group is that of patients with suspected *immune thrombocytopenia*. Their marrow is usually unremarkable except for an increase in the number of megakaryocytes. The spleen is usually of normal size, and the patient may not have any obvious underlying disease. Three major disorders to consider in this last group are (1) drug-induced thrombocytopenia, (2) postinfectious or acute thrombocytopenia, and (3) chronic or autoimmune thrombocytopenia (ITP).

Drug-Induced Thrombocytopenia

Many of the drugs used in cancer chemotherapy are myelosuppressive and can cause severe bone marrow depression, including thrombocytopenia. In addition, drugs like the chlorothiazides, ethanol, or certain estrogens may selectively inhibit megakaryocyte development and induce thrombocytopenia. These patients will have a decreased number of marrow megakaryocytes; platelet survival is normal, and platelet *production* is diminished. Most drugs cause thrombocytopenia by accelerating peripheral destruction. The usual mechanism involves the formation of drug-antibody complexes that bind to the platelet, fix complement, and rapidly induce platelet lysis. This type of destruction has been well documented in the laboratory for drugs like quinidine and quinine. Many other drugs probably cause thrombocytopenia by this mechanism. A list of drugs that commonly cause thrombocytopenia is given in Table 48–4.

In most cases of drug-induced thrombocytopenia, the platelet count returns to normal within 7 to 10 days of cessation of the offending agent as the drug-antibody complexes are cleared from the circulation.[8] The best approach is to stop all medications, examine the marrow to assess megakaryocyte number, and try to obtain laboratory confirmation of the immune nature of the disorder by ordering specialized tests to demonstrate the presence of a drug-dependent antiplatelet antibody. These tests, although quite useful, detect only a minority of patients with suspected drug-induced thrombocytopenia, thus a typical history, marrow examination, and prompt recovery following drug withdrawal are essential to make this diagnosis. If the bleeding is severe, corticosteroids can be administered, because they can help maintain capillary integrity and decrease bleeding. Platelet transfusions have limited value, until the drug-antibody complexes are cleared from the circulation, because they will be rapidly destroyed by the immune process.

TABLE 48–3. CLINICAL APPROACH TO THE THROMBOCYTOPENIC PATIENT

Clinical Feature	Etiology	Common Diseases
Low Platelet Count and Splenomegaly		
Normal marrow	Splenic sequestration	Congestive splenomegaly, liver disease, storage disease, tumor
Abnormal marrow	Splenic sequestration and decreased production	Hematologic disorders, chronic leukemia, lymphoma, myeloid metaplasia
Low Platelet Count and Normal Spleen		
Normal marrow	Excess destruction	Immune Drug-induced, acute (postinfectious) thrombocytopenia, chronic (autoimmune) thrombocytopenia Nonimmune Sepsis/DIC, TTP, vasculitis, prosthesis
Abnormal marrow	Decreased production	Aplasia, acute leukemia, metastatic carcinoma

TABLE 48–4. COMMON CAUSES OF DRUG-INDUCED THROMBOCYTOPENIA

Mechanism	Drugs
Decreased megakaryocyte production	Thiazide diuretics Ethanol ? Estrogens Chemotherapeutic agents
Immune destruction	Quinidine Quinine Phenytoin (Dilantin) Sulfonamides
? Immune destruction	Gold salts Cephalosporins Heparin

Acute or Postinfectious Thrombocytopenia

The platelet membrane contains a variety of surface antigens, as well as receptors for immunoglobulins and viruses, which may all participate in immunologic reactions. Patients are frequently encountered who have suddenly developed thrombocytopenia and bleeding 2 or 3 weeks after a febrile viral illness. In some cases, the disease can be diagnosed precisely and may be infectious mononucleosis or an exanthem like measles or chickenpox. More often, the nature of the illness is obscure. Most of the cases of acute or postinfectious thrombocytopenia are due to the interaction of viral antigen-antibody complexes with the platelet or to antiviral antibodies that cross-react with platelet antigens. A majority of the antibodies detected in patients with immune thrombocytopenia react with target antigens on the major platelet glycoproteins IIb, IIIa, and Ib. The patients have normal marrow cellularity, except for a slight increase in the number of megakaryocytes, and will recover spontaneously within 14 to 21 days. In fact, any patient whose thrombocytopenia persists for longer than 3 months probably has another underlying disorder.

Most patients with this disorder are children under the age of 10 years. They have a low incidence of complications and are often evaluated in the office and sent home without specific therapy. Although acute postviral thrombocytopenia is much less common in adults, they have a higher incidence of serious bleeding and occasionally have fatal intracranial hemorrhage. Patients should have a marrow aspirate to eliminate other diagnostic possibilities by showing a normal or increased number of megakaryocytes. In addition, serologic tests for mononucleosis, cytomegalovirus, or toxoplasmosis infections may help to clarify some of the cases. If the platelet count is very low and the patient has mucous membrane, retinal, or genitourinary bleeding, corticosteroids should be administered, although there is no evidence that they will shorten the total duration of thrombocytopenia. When given in doses of 1 to 2 mg/kg (prednisone or equivalent), they decrease bleeding by improving endothelial integrity[9] and raise the platelet count in approximately 50% of patients.[10] Some clinicians favor the use of intravenous gamma globulin over high-dose corticosteroids in this setting. It is important to keep in mind, however, that childhood ITP is almost always a self-limiting condition and that most children will regain a normal platelet count within 6 to 12 months. Thus, the goal of therapy is largely one of temporization.

Chronic (Autoimmune or Idiopathic) Thrombocytopenia (AITP or ITP)

Adults usually present a history of easy bruising or mucosal bleeding of several months' duration, although it may be impossible to distinguish this chronic syndrome from the acute variety discussed previously. The patients are usually female and may have a familial history of systemic lupus erythematosus (SLE) or other rheumatic disorders. Bleeding symptoms may become worse following a viral infection, which depresses platelet production, or the ingestion of a medication like aspirin, which interferes with platelet function. Marrow examination is essential to exclude a more serious marrow disorder like aplastic anemia, leukemia, or marrow invasion by tumor. The marrow will show an increased number of megakaryocytes, whereas the number is decreased in infiltrative marrow disorders. A high percentage of these patients may have antibody on their platelets or in their serum, although specific tests to identify them are difficult to perform and are available only in specialized centers. ITP can be readily distinguished from TTP or DIC because of the absence of microangiopathic red blood cell changes or coagulation abnormalities.

Immune thrombocytopenia may also be seen in conjunction with other autoimmune diseases, including SLE and rheumatoid arthritis. The initial evaluation of all patients presenting with unexplained thrombocytopenia should thus include a careful history and laboratory evaluation of these disorders, including antinuclear antibodies, rheumatoid factor, and complement levels. More recently, thrombocytopenia has been seen as a presenting finding in otherwise asymptomatic human immunodeficiency virus (HIV) infection. Thus, the development of immune thrombocytopenia in any individual at risk for HIV warrants evaluation.

Adult patients with ITP are usually treated with corticosteroids, which stimulate a rise in platelet count. Corticosteroids also improve capillary vascular integrity, and thus bleeding symptoms may improve before the platelet count rises. Prednisone is usually begun at an initial dose of 1 to 2 mg/kg/day and tapered slowly once the platelet count has reached 50,000 to 100,000. Unfortunately, as few as 15 to 20% of these patients achieve a durable remission once steroids are discontinued, and the remaining patients are usually referred for splenectomy. Fortunately, a majority respond to this surgical maneuver, although about 10% of patients require additional therapy with immunosuppressive medications.

Patients who fail to achieve adequate platelet counts following splenectomy may be treated with one of several pharmacologic agents, including danazol,[12] vincristine,[13] azathioprine,[14] or cyclophosphamide.[15] The administration of intravenous gamma globulin (1 g/day for 2 days or 400 mg/kg/day for 5 days) results in improved platelet counts in most patients with ITP. However, the salutary effect is usually short lived, and thus this treatment modality is best reserved for the management of acute bleeding episodes or to improve the platelet count in anticipation of splenectomy (see earlier). It is also important to remember that although autoimmune thrombocytopenia may become a chronic disorder, there is a very low incidence of serious hemorrhage after the initial phase, and most patients can live nearly normal lives, even though they continue to have platelet counts in the range of 5000 to 25,000/mm^3.[16]

Case 1. A 24-year-old woman had a vague history of easy bruising for several months and also complained of menorrhagia. There was a history of "morning stiffness," which she attributed to a lack of physical exercise. The only medications she took were occasional aspirin and an oral contraceptive. During the previous week, she also had an upper respiratory infection and noted a marked increase in her bruising, together with a rash on her lower extremities. She stated that she was concerned about the possibility of "leukemia."

Physical examination disclosed bruises of the legs and arms with

TABLE 48–5. LABORATORY TESTS IN QUALITATIVE PLATELET DISORDERS

	Factor or Drug Causing Aggregation				
Disorder	*ADP**	*Epinephrine*	*Collagen*	*Ristocetin*	*vWF Antigen*
Adhesion Defect					
von Willebrand's	Normal	Normal	Normal	↓	↓
First Degree Aggregation Defect					
Thrombasthenia (Glanzmann's disease)	↓	↓	↓	Normal	Normal
Second Degree Aggregation (Release) Defect					
Aspirin-like defect	Normal	↓	↓	Normal	Normal
Storage pool disease	Normal	↓	↓	Normal	Normal

*Assumes use of a high-dose (~10μm) ADP. With lower doses (1–5 μm), pattern is similar to that seen with epinephrine.

multiple petechiae over her legs and the soft palate. Laboratory studies demonstrated a platelet count of 12,000/mm^3 (normal value is 150,000 to 450,000/mm^3), a white blood cell count of 6800 per mm^3 with a normal differential, and a hematocrit of 37 ml/dl. She had a bone marrow aspirate, which showed normal cellularity, normal red and white blood cell maturation, and a slight increase in megakaryocytes. Additional laboratory studies were performed, including an antinuclear antibody titer, latex fixation tests, and a Monospot test, but all results were negative.

This young woman, who had a history of chronic bruising and a low platelet count with a normal marrow aspirate and normal spleen size, most likely had immune platelet destruction. The relation between her increase in symptoms and her recent viral illness raises the possibility of acute thrombocytopenia. However, her symptoms had been present for several months, and it is more likely that her platelet count had fallen owing to viral suppression of hematopoiesis superimposed on a more chronic destructive process. Drug-induced thrombocytopenia might also be considered, since estrogen-containing compounds like the oral contraceptive may lower the platelet count, but megakaryocytes should have been diminished if that were the cause. Aspirin rarely, if ever, causes thrombocytopenia.

The diagnosis of autoimmune thrombocytopenia or ITP is, unfortunately, one of exclusion. The history of morning stiffness is interesting, but the patient had no other objective or laboratory evidence of a rheumatic disorder. The most likely possibility is chronic immune thrombocytopenia with an acute fall in platelet count during the recent viral illness. Treatment was initiated with corticosteroids, but eventually splenectomy proved necessary.

QUALITATIVE PLATELET ABNORMALITIES

Often patients are encountered with normal platelet counts but who exhibit clinical manifestations suggestive of a defect in primary hemostasis or who have a prolonged bleeding time. In such patients, the hemostatic abnormality can arise from a *defect* in platelet *adhesion, aggregation,* or failure to carry out the *release reaction.* It is convenient to discuss the disorders within this physiologic classification. A laboratory approach to the patients with qualitative platelet defects is outlined in Table 48–5. In addition to the bleeding time, the laboratory must be equipped to assess platelet aggregation. This is an in vitro test in which platelet plug formation is stimulated by incubating stirred platelet suspensions with chemicals that are known to cause platelet aggregation and release; these include ADP, collagen, and epinephrine.

Defective Adhesion—Von Willebrand's Disease

The most common platelet adhesion disorder is von Willebrand's disease (vWD), an inherited disorder in which either the quantity or biologic activity of the von Willebrand factor (vWF) is reduced.[17] vWF is essential for optimal platelet adhesion to vascular subendothelium and serves as a carrier for factor VIII (the antihemophilic factor, or AHF), a critical coagulation protein defective in classic hemophilia. These two proteins form a circulating complex in plasma. vWF activity is readily tested by the addition of ristocetin to plasma and reconstituted fixed platelets. The rate and extent of platelet agglutination (ristocetin cofactor activity) parallels the quantity of vWF. The quantity of vWF is measured with various immunoassays, and the amount of associated factor VIII by coagulation assays.

In classic or type I vWD, there is a parallel reduction in the quantity of vWF measured by immunoassay, in vWF activity assessed by the ristocetin test, and in associated factor VIII, sometimes but not always suggested by prolongation of the PTT. This is by far the most common form of vWD and is inherited as an autosomal dominant trait in as many as 1 in 1000 individuals. Clinical manifestations generally correspond to the degree of protein deficiency and are like those of a platelet disorder. Bleeding time is usually prolonged, and mucous membrane bleeding, nose bleeds, menorrhagia, and postoperative bleeding are common symptoms. Hemarthroses and soft-tissue bleeding, which are commonly seen in patients with severe deficiencies of factor VIII, are rarely encountered in vWD.

It has become apparent that vWD is quite heterogeneous and that there are variant forms of the disorder caused by the production of dysfunctional protein. In the variant syndromes (type II disease), the quantity of vWF measured by immunoassay and the amount of associated factor VIII remain normal. The biologic activity with the ristocetin test and the bleeding time are almost always abnormal. The patients have a selective loss in the high molecular forms of vWF, which can be assessed with specialized tests such as agarose gel or crossed immunoelectrophoresis. Of particular note are rare patients with variant vWD (type IIB) arising from a qualitative defect in vWF with increased affinity for platelets and hypersensitivity to ristocetin in laboratory assays. Such patients may present with more severe bleeding manifestations and cannot be treated with 1-deamino-(8-D-arginine)-vasopressin (DDAVP) (see later). An occasional patient will develop an acquired syndrome that mimics inherited vWD caused by antibody directed against vWF or the adsorption of vWF onto tumor or abnormal vascular surfaces.

Most patients with vWD can be treated effectively with DDAVP, a pharmacologic agent that induces the release of vWF from vascular stores.[18] Treatment of patients with type I vWD with DDAVP (0.3 μg/kg in 50 ml of normal saline by slow intravenous infusion) usually results in correction of the bleeding time, factor VIII, and vWF. DDAVP is ineffective in most patients with qualitative defects in vWF (type II) and is contraindicated for use in patients with type IIB. The chief limitation to the use of DDAVP is the rapid tachyphylaxis that develops in most patients. Thus in certain clinical situations, such as major surgery, which require prolonged correction of hemostasis, exogenous sources of vWF are required. Cryoprecipitate (10 units every 12 hours for 2 to 5 days) has for many years been the treatment of choice in such situations.[19] More recently, at least one factor VIII concentrate, Humate-P, has been shown to be effective in patients with vWD.[20] Compared with cryoprecipitate, this product has the advantage of being virally attenuated and of having a long shelf-life. Patients should be treated twice daily with cryoprecipitate or Humate-P for 3 to 5 days after major surgery. Minor hemorrhagic episodes will stop after 24 to 48 hours of therapy.

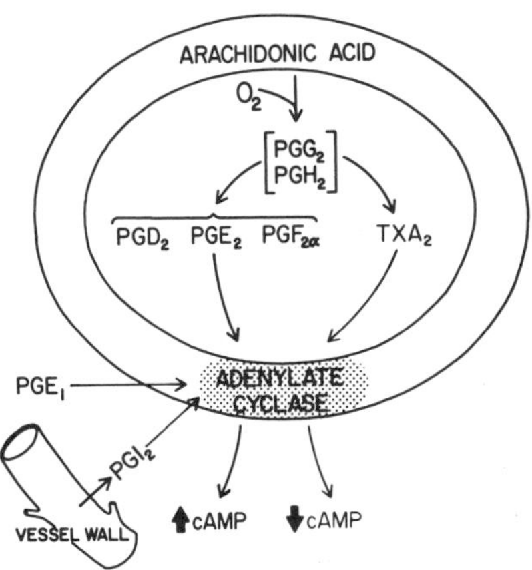

FIGURE 48–5. The biochemical events that control platelet aggregation and release: Aggregating agents first react with specific membrane receptors. The initial step induces changes in membrane adenylate cyclase activity, fluxes in intracellular calcium, and production of prostaglandin derivatives like thromboxane A_2. All induce aggregation and promote release of adenosine diphosphate (ADP). ADP causes further platelet aggregation.

Case 2. A 24-year-old man was seen in the hospital the day after a tonsillectomy. He had bled continuously since surgery, requiring cauterization, sutures, and packed red blood cells. A review of office notes obtained prior to referral for surgery disclosed no history of bleeding, although his sister had had hemorrhage and a few severe nose bleeds. The patient had been receiving narcotics intramuscularly as postoperative analgesia but no other medications.

Laboratory studies showed a bleeding time of 14 minutes (normal is <8 minutes), a platelet count of 457,000/mm^3, a PT of 11 seconds (normal is 10 to 12 seconds), and a PTT of 41 seconds (normal is <38 seconds). The patient's factor VIII level was 25% (normal is 50 to 150%). The tentative diagnosis of vWD was made, and the patient was treated with 10 units of cryoprecipitate twice daily for 4 days, which stopped the bleeding. While treatment was progressing, additional laboratory tests were obtained. The patient's platelets aggregated normally with ADP, epinephrine, or collagen but demonstrated a diminished response to ristocetin. In addition, the patient's factor vWF by immunoassay was 25%.

The clinical presentation and the laboratory tests are all compatible with vWD. The sister should also be tested, because the disease is usually inherited as an autosomal dominant trait. Congenital or acquired disorders of platelet function would usually affect aggregation with ADP, epinephrine, or collagen and not decrease ristocetin-induced aggregation or the vWF antigen level.

Intrinsic Platelet Defects—Aggregation and Release Defects

The biochemical events that control platelet aggregation and secretion are quite complex[21] and only an abbreviated outline is shown in Figure 48–5. Aggregating agents first react with specific membrane receptors. This initial step induces fluxes in intracellular calcium due to breakdown of membrane phospholipids, and production of arachidonic acid derivatives like thromboxane A_2, which all can facilitate aggregation and promote the release of granules containing ADP. ADP, in turn, causes platelet aggregation, by activating platelet membrane receptors that bind fibrinogen. The fibrinogen acts as a bridge between adjacent activated platelets in the evolving aggregate or hemostatic plug. These reactions require normal membrane structure, appropriate regulatory enzymes, and a normal platelet content of secretable ADP.

Occasionally there are patients with a defect in *primary platelet aggregation,* which is called Glanzmann's disease, or thrombasthenia. This total inability of platelets to aggregate to any stimulus is extremely rare and is due to a selective loss in platelet fibrinogen receptors, which are located on the platelet glycoprotein IIb/IIIa complex. Failure to complete the aggregation sequence by undergoing *release* and *secondary aggregation* is a much more common defect. It arises from a deficiency in arachidonate metabolism or from a deficiency in stored ADP within the platelet. Patients with either defect have prolonged bleeding times and platelets that do not aggregate normally when challenged with agents like epinephrine or collagen but that still will respond to high doses of ADP. Patients with these functional platelet abnormalities do not usually have serious bleeding episodes. In fact, they may bleed only when severely challenged by trauma or surgery. Most of these patients do not require specific therapy but usually respond to DDAVP with normalization of the bleeding time and improved clinical hemostasis.[22] Rarely, such patients may require platelet transfusion.

Drug-Induced Platelet Dysfunction

A wide variety of drugs can interfere with the aggregation and release process.[23] Certain drugs that perturb the platelet membrane, such as the phenothiazines or antihistamines, may cause minor bleeding. The most common group of drugs causing clinical bleeding are the nonsteroidal antiinflammatory drugs like aspirin or indomethacin, which block platelet thromboxane biosynthesis. Aspirin, in particular, is a common cause of platelet dysfunction, since it is an irreversible inactivator of the cyclooxygenase enzyme in platelet membranes. A single dose can have a prolonged effect (5 to 7 days), since the platelet cannot regenerate new enzyme. The other nonsteroidal agents have more transient effects, because they are competitive inhibitors, and their effect wanes as the plasma level of the drug declines. The degree of prolongation of the bleeding time varies after ingestion of these drugs. However, those patients with the most marked bleeding time prolongation have the most clinical difficulty. Drug-induced platelet dysfunction can be a serious problem following surgery or trauma, and occasionally patients will need platelet transfusion. More often, drugs cause minor "cosmetic" problems (easy bruising and ecchymosis) that can be corrected by avoiding nonsteroidal analgesic medications.

Case 3. A 30-year-old woman is worried about the frequent occurrence of bruises on her arms and legs. She states that they appear without any known trauma and seem to be more frequent prior to the onset of her menses. She is concerned that she may have a serious blood disorder like leukemia. Her husband has expressed some concern and fears that neighbors and friends will think he has beaten her.

She has no prior history of any serious illness and has had dental extractions, tonsillectomy, and two pregnancies without any unusual bleeding. She is not aware of any family history of bleeding. She occasionally takes acetylsalicylic acid (ASA) for headaches but no other medications.

On physical examination, there are scattered ecchymoses on the flexor and extensor surfaces of the thighs, calves, arms, and forearms. She is otherwise normal. Results of laboratory studies are the following: bleeding time is 7 minutes (normal is <8 minutes); PT is 12 seconds (normal, 10 to 12 sec); and PTT is 28 seconds (normal <38 sec). The platelet count is 450,000/mm^3.

The presence of "easy bruising" in apparently healthy young women is commonly seen in an ambulatory practice. The differential diagnosis includes potentially serious bleeding disorders like vWD; inherited or drug-induced platelet dysfunction, which is usually less troublesome; or the poorly characterized entity of "vascular purpura" or "capillary fragility." The problem facing the practitioner is how to decide which patients need extensive laboratory evaluation and which need minimal laboratory testing and some reassurance.

The case presented here is quite typical. The patient has no prior or family history of bleeding and has a normal physical examination except for her bruises. All laboratory test results of hemostasis are normal. These findings make platelet dysfunction of vWD unlikely, since the bleeding time is a sensitive screening test and correlates well with the risk of clinical bleeding. If it were prolonged, additional tests of vWF activity and platelet function should be ordered. These include factor VIII activity (AHF), vWF antigen level, and vWF activity measured with the ristocetin assay, as well as platelet aggregation.

The syndrome of "vascular purpura" is ill-defined but may be hormonally mediated and involves changes in capillaries and small vessels. Some partially defined examples are (1) "senile purpura," in which skin aging decreases the support of vessels; (2) purpura from prolonged steroid therapy or Cushing's disease, in which there is connective tissue breakdown; and (3) the purpura seen in certain inherited disorders of connective tissue like Marfan's or the Ehlers-Danlos syndrome. It has been postulated that estrogens may have a similar effect on capillaries and small venules, leading to increased bruising.

Finally, the effect of drugs like aspirin on hemostasis must be considered. The biologic effect of aspirin lasts for up to 7 days, thus ingestion of small quantities of aspirin may cause mild bleeding in sensitive individuals. Some physicians screen patients with an "aspirin tolerance test" by doing a bleeding time, administering two aspirin, and repeating the bleeding time 1 or 2 hours later. Sensitive individuals with abnormal baseline bleeding time may have marked prolongation after aspirin ingestion. This test is useful when a history of frequent aspirin ingestion is uncovered or the patient has a markedly prolonged bleeding time following recent aspirin ingestion.

The patient described here most probably has a benign form of vascular fragility, perhaps estrogen-related. She and her husband need only reassurance that she has a cosmetic problem and will not develop serious bleeding or any subsequent blood disorder.

INHERITED COAGULATION DISORDERS

Theoretically, a large number of coagulation disorders could arise from defects in individual plasma proteins. They do not occur with equal frequency, and all the congenital coagulation disorders are rather rare. In fact, it is possible to practice medicine for several decades and not encounter a patient with a congenital coagulation disorder. Of a given patient population, 90% will have hemophilia A, or factor VIII deficiency, and an additional 9% will have factor IX deficiency, which is hemophilia B or Christmas disease. The remaining disorders represent only 1% of the patient population. On the other hand, physicians in subspecialty practice frequently see patients with acquired coagulation deficiencies.

Factors VIII and IX deficiencies are transmitted by sex-linked recessive inheritance, thus they are usually encountered in male patients. Patients with severe factor VIII or IX deficiency usually have episodes of bleeding in early childhood and have the diagnosis established in pediatric centers. These patients have frustrating episodes of recurrent hemarthrosis, which may cause severe orthopedic deformity and lead to serious psychosocial problems. They may have marital, family, and financial difficulties.

Factor concentrates used in the treatment of hemophilia are derived from thousands of individual blood donors. Prior to the introduction of viral attenuation methods, these concentrates were routinely contaminated with hepatitis C and HIV, and the majority of severe hemophiliacs treated in the late 1970s and early 1980s show serologic and clinical manifestations of these infections. Currently, the most widely used products are derived from screened plasma and additionally undergo various heat and biochemical treatments to reduce the infectious risk. The purest concentrates are those which are purified by affinity chromatography. These products appear to be virtually free of risk of transmission of hepatitis and HIV and are the treatment of choice in previously untreated patients.[24] Two new recombinant factor VIII products have been released in the United States. Each appears to be hemostatically effective, although questions surrounding cost and antigenicity have yet to be totally resolved.

Occasionally, patients may present to the practitioner for the first time with a bleeding episode. Although the diagnosis may have been previously established, the physician must carefully review this information. The patient's plasma should be reassayed to confirm the precise protein deficiency, because the plasma products used for infusing patients with factor VIII or IX deficiencies are different, and diagnostic error could seriously impair therapy. In addition, about 10% of patients with VIII or IX deficiency develop an inhibitor, which is an antibody directed against antigens present in transfused factor VIII or IX concentrates or plasma. Thus, any new patient also needs a screening test for the presence of inhibitors. Other complications of therapy include the transmission of hepatitis and AIDS from frequent infusion of plasma fractions if prepared from large numbers of donors and not virally attenuated.

It is more common to see adult patients in whom there

may be a vague family history of hemophilia or a related bleeding disorder. The patient himself may not have any personal history of bleeding following minor trauma and may have had previous minor surgery without bleeding. If the level of VIII or IX is greater than 15 or 20% the screening PTT may also be normal. These patients with so-called mild or minimal hemophilia sometimes bleed following major surgery, with disastrous consequences. The most useful clues to the diagnosis are in the detailed history, especially the family history or the patient's history of bleeding if this occurred after previous surgical or dental procedures. If hemophilia is suspected clinically, extensive laboratory evaluation is in order prior to surgery.

Case 4. A 43-year-old man had recurrent low back pain radiating into the right leg with objective evidence of nerve root compression. He had a myelogram, which showed a disk herniation at the L3–L4 interspace, and was admitted to the hospital for a laminectomy. He had no prior history of any bleeding following trauma and had had a successful herniorrhaphy in the past. He had normal preoperative screening tests, including a PTT of 38 seconds (normal is up to 40 seconds), a PT of 11 seconds (normal is <12 seconds), a platelet count of 458,000, and a bleeding time of 6 minutes (normal is <8 minutes). On the second day after surgery, he suddenly became paraplegic, and repeat myelogram showed extensive hematoma compressing the spinal cord. When the patient's history was reviewed, it was discovered that he had a male cousin with mild hemophilia (a factor VIII of 15%). Repeat laboratory studies were normal (PTT of 35 seconds and a PT of 10 seconds) except for a quantitative factor VIII level of 20%.

This patient had mild hemophilia, which led to postoperative paresis. The only clue to the diagnosis was in the family history. The case also illustrates the limitation of preoperative laboratory screening, since a factor VIII level of 20% may be sufficient to normalize the PTT but not enough to protect the patient from hemorrhage following extensive surgery. Fortunately, this situation is rare.

Factor XI Deficiency

Although it is less common, factor XI deficiency deserves brief comment.[25] It occurs with high frequency in certain populations, notably Eastern European Jews, and is therefore more frequent in cities with large Jewish populations. Unlike factor VIII and IX deficiency, it is inherited as an autosomal recessive trait, and the relationship between laboratory tests and bleeding is not as precise. The patients will often bleed only with surgical stress and usually do not have a history of hemarthroses or muscular bleeding.

Long PTT Syndromes—Laboratory Abnormalities Without Bleeding

Three plasma protein abnormalities are recognized to cause a dramatic prolongation of the PTT without any increase in the incidence of bleeding.[26] This syndrome is caused by defects in three proteins involved in the activation of the intrinsic coagulation pathway: Hageman factor (factor XII), HMW kininogen, and prekallikrein. It is important to emphasize that patients with any of these defects have no known hemorrhagic problems and can tolerate any type of hemostatic stress. The reason for this discrepancy is enigmatic. It has been proposed that there are alternate ways to activate factor XI in vivo or that the trace quantities of proteins present in these deficient individuals are sufficient to support hemostasis. The diagnosis is easy to establish, and these patients should not be confused with the patients discussed previously who have inherited coagulation abnormalities with the potential for serious bleeding.

Case 5. A 22-year-old woman of Swedish descent was referred by an oral surgeon for preoperative evaluation. The patient stated that she did not have any unusual bleeding, had normal menses, had delivered two children successfully, and had had a tonsillectomy without incident. She has two impacted molars that need to be extracted. The oral surgeon obtained preoperative screening tests as a "precaution" and noted a PT of 11 seconds, a PTT of 120 seconds, and a platelet count of 458,000/mm^3.

The presence of a markedly prolonged PTT in the absence of any bleeding is most consistent with one or two diagnostic possibilities. As discussed earlier, deficiencies in the contact factors (factor XII, high molecular weight kininogen, and prekallikrein) lead to prolongation of the PTT but are not associated with clinical bleeding. Alternatively, the presence of an antiphospholipid antibody ("lupus anticoagulant") may prolong the PTT in vitro but is paradoxically associated with an increased incidence of thromboembolic events in vivo (see later). In the case of a simple factor deficiency, the long PTT should correct promptly by addition of normal plasma. This maneuver will eliminate the possibility of an inhibitor. Finally, a specialty laboratory can define the defect further by using congenitally deficient plasma. This patient had a factor XII level of 1% and no other abnormality. She had two uneventful molar extractions under close surveillance by her oral surgeon with no difficulties.

Inhibitors

Occasionally, patients have laboratory abnormalities suggestive of a congenital coagulation disorder but with the history of severe bleeding that is of *recent* onset. These patients often have a circulating anticoagulant or inhibitor that inactivates one of the coagulation proteins.[27] Such inhibitors have been described in patients with autoimmune disorders like systemic lupus erythematosus (SLE), as well as in postpartum females and in patients taking drugs like penicillin or streptomycin. They have also been described in elderly patients with no apparent disease.

Inhibitors, which are antibody molecules, are most commonly directed against factor VIII, although other specificities have been described. The diagnosis is established in the laboratory by demonstrating that the patient's plasma progressively destroys a specific coagulation factor activity in normal plasma. Treatment of this disorder is difficult. If the titer of antifactor VIII is not excessively high (<5 units), restoration of normal hemostasis in the acute setting is best achieved by the use of sufficient quantities of factor VIII concentrate. Often the antibody cross-reacts poorly with porcine factor VIII, allowing for the use of smaller quantities of factor VIII derived from this source. If the titer of inhibiting antibody is greater than 5 units, then products rich in factor VII (e.g., prothrombin complex concentrates) may "bypass" the inhibition. Chronic management is aimed at suppression of the inhibitor with prednisone, cyclophosphamide, or azathioprine.

Patients with these specific inhibitors must be distinguished from those with a nonspecific class of so-called "lupus-like" inhibitors, which interfere with in vitro coagulation tests. It is thought that the antibody produced by these patients binds to the phospholipid component of PT and PTT reagents and prolongs these laboratory tests. Nonspecific inhibitors have been described in patients with systemic lupus erythematosus, or malignancy and in patients who have ingested certain drugs like chlorpromazine.[28] Occasionally, individuals with no apparent abnormalities also have nonspecific inhibitors. It is important to document the nature of the inhibitor, since these patients only exhibit clinical bleeding in the presence of concomitant thrombocytopenia or hypoprothrombinemia. Paradoxically, patients with high titers of antiphospholipid antibody, primarily anticardiolipin antibody, appear to be at a significantly increased risk of thrombosis, stroke, and recurrent fetal loss.[29, 30] The pathogenesis of this syndrome is unknown, but it is thought to arise from interference with one or more of the normal antithrombotic processes associated with vascular endothelial cells. Table 48–6 outlines the diagnostic approach to patients with inhibitors.

Prethrombotic or Hypercoagulable Disorders

In most patients with thromboembolism, it is not possible to identify a specific etiology or an underlying coagulation disorder. Certain systemic illnesses like advanced atherosclerosis, chronic congestive heart failure, or metastatic malignancy increase the risk of thrombosis. Surgical procedures and immobility have a similar effect. In the past few years, however, a small fraction of patients with recurrent thromboembolism have been identified who have inherited specific coagulation defects that predispose them to thrombosis. These patients (1) have a family history of venous and, occasionally, arterial thrombosis; (2) have a personal history of recurrent thrombosis; and (3) usually become symptomatic by their early to middle twenties. The group of identified disorders now includes antithrombin deficiency or dysfunction, deficiency in protein C or S, abnormal fibrinogen or plasminogen molecules, and impaired production or release of tissue plasminogen activator.[31]

Patients suspected of having any of these disorders should be referred for specialized laboratory testing. If a disorder is identified, the patients should be placed on long-term oral anticoagulation and family members should be evaluated, as the disorders are all autosomal dominant traits. At present, these defects account for 10 to 20% of patients with recurrent thromboembolism and about 1 to 2% of all cases of thrombosis.

TABLE 48–6. DIAGNOSTIC APPROACH TO PATIENTS WITH INHIBITORS

Screening Tests

PTT: prolonged
Prothrombin time: slightly prolonged
Thrombin time: usually normal

Test for Anticoagulant Activity

A. Mixture of patient's plasma with normal plasma:
   1. Immediate prolongation of PTT
   2. No progressive loss of clotting factor activity in specific assays
   3. Higher apparent values with dilution of test plasma—multiple factors inhibited
   Conclusion: "Lupus-like" or nonspecific anticoagulant
B. Mixture of patient's plasma with normal plasma:
   1. No immediate prolongation of PTT
   2. Progressive lengthening of PTT and loss of clotting factor activity in specific assays
   3. No change in value with dilution—only *one* factor inhibited
   Conclusion: Specific anticoagulant

REFERENCES

1. Hamburg M, Svensson J, and Samuellson B: Thromboxanes: A new group of biologically active compounds derived from prostaglandin endoperoxides. Proc Natl Acad Sci USA 72:2994, 1975.
2. Smith JB, Ingerman CM, and Silver MJ: Effects of arachidonic acid and some of its metabolites on platelets. *In* Silver MJ, Smith JB, and Kocsis JJ (eds): Prostaglandins in Hematology. New York, Spectrum Publications, 1977, pp 277–292.
3. Ross R and Glomset J: The pathogenesis of atherosclerosis. N Engl J Med 295:369, 1976.
4. Miletich JP, Jackson CN, and Majerus PW: Interaction of coagulation factor Xa with human platelets. Proc Natl Acad Sci USA 74:4035, 1977.
5. Kitchens CS and Weiss L: Ultrastructural changes of endothelium associated with thrombocytopenia. Blood 46:567, 1975.
6. Miletich JP, Majerus DW, and Majerus PW: Patients with congenital factor V deficiency have decreased factor Xa binding site on their platelets. J Clin Invest 62:824, 1978.
7. Williams WJ: Principles of coagulation tests. *In* Williams WJ (ed): Hematology. New York, McGraw-Hill, 1972, pp 1098–1104.
8. Aster RH: Thrombocytopenia due to enhanced platelet destruction. *In* Williams WJ (ed): Hematology. New York, McGraw-Hill, 1972, pp 1131–1158.
9. Kitchens CS: Amelioration of endothelial abnormalities by prednisone in experimental thrombocytopenia in the rabbit. J Clin Invest 60:1129, 1977.
10. Komrower GM and Watson GH: Prognosis in idiopathic thrombocytopenic purpura of childhood. Arch Dis Child 29:502, 1954.
11. Marmont AM and Damasio EE: Clinical experiences with cytotoxic immunosuppressive treatment of idiopathic thrombocytopenic purpura. Acta Haematol (Basel) 46:74, 1971.
12. Ahn YS, Harrington WJ, Simon SR, et al: Danazol for the treatment of idiopathic thrombocytopenia purpura. N Engl J Med 308:1396, 1983.
13. Ahn YS, Harrington WJ, Seelman RC, et al: Vincristine therapy of idiopathic and secondary thrombocytopenias. N Engl J Med 291:376, 1974.
14. Sussman LN: Azathioprine in refractory idiopathic thrombocytopenic purpura. JAMA 202:259, 1967.
15. Verlin M, Laros RK Jr, and Penner JA: Refractory thrombocytopenic purpura treated successfully with cyclophosphamide. Blood 40:971, 1972.
16. Doan CA, Bouroncle BA, and Wiseman RK: Idiopathic and secondary thrombocytopenic purpura: Clinical study and evaluation of 381 cases over a period of 28 years. Ann Intern Med 53:861, 1960.
17. Weiss HJ: Abnormalities of factor VIII and platelet aggregation—use of ristocetin in diagnosing the von Willebrand syndrome. Blood 45:403, 1975.
18. Mannucci PM, Ruggeri ZM, Pareti FI, et al: DDAVP: A new pharmacological approach to the management of haemophilia and von Willebrand's disease. Lancet 1:689, 1977.
19. Perkins HA: Correction of the hemostatic defects in von Willebrand's disease. Blood 30:375, 1967.
20. Fukui H, Nishino M, Terada S, et al: Hemostatic effect of a heat-treated factor VIII concentrate (Haemate P) in von Willebrand's disease. Blut 56:171, 1988.
21. George JN and Shattil SJ: The clinical importance of acquired abnormalities of platelet function. N Engl J Med 324:27, 1991.
22. Kobrinsky NL, Israel ED, Gerrard JM, et al: Shortening of bleeding time by 1-deamino-8-D-arginine vasopressin in various bleeding disorders. Lancet 1:1145, 1984.
23. Roth GJ and Majerus PW: The mechanism of the effect of aspirin on human platelets. I: Acetylation of a platelet particulate fraction protein. J Clin Invest 56:624, 1975.
24. Brettler DB and Levine PH: Factor concentrates for treatment of hemophilia: Which one to choose? Blood 73:2067, 1989.

25. Rimon A, Schiffman S, Feinstein DI, et al: Factor XI activity and factor XI antigen in homozygous and heterozygous factor XI deficiency. Blood 48:165, 1976.
26. Kaplan AP: Initiation of intrinsic coagulation and fibrinolytic pathways of man. Prog Hemost Thromb 4:127, 1979.
27. Feinstein DI and Rapaport SI: Acquired inhibition of blood coagulation. Prog Hemost Thromb 1:75, 1972.
28. Zarrabi MH, Zucker S, Miller F, et al: Immunologic and coagulation disorders in chlorpromazine-treated patients. Ann Intern Med 91:194, 1979.
29. Hughes GRV: Thrombosis, abortion, cerebral disease, and the lupus anticoagulant. BMJ 287:1088, 1983.
30. Lubbe WF, Butler WS, Palmer SJ, and Liggins GC: Lupus anticoagulant in pregnancy. Br J Obstet Gynecol 91:357, 1984.
31. Schafer AI: The hypercoagulable states. Ann Intern Med 102:814, 1985.

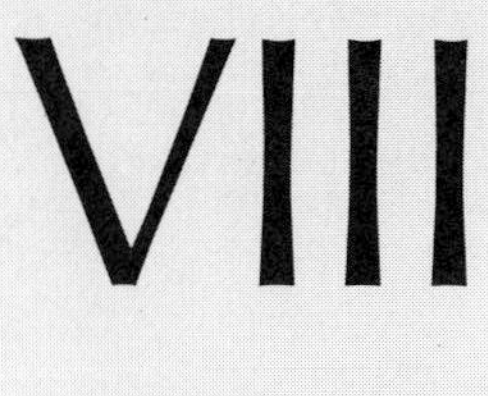

Musculoskeletal Disorders

49

Monoarticular Arthritis and Acute Polyarticular Synovitis

WILLIAM T. BRANCH Jr., MD

This chapter addresses two clinical presentations of joint pain: pain in or near a single joint and acute polyarticular synovitis. The third type of presentation, subacute or chronic arthritis, is the subject of Chapter 50.

PAIN IN OR NEAR A SINGLE JOINT

Conditions that cause *acute* onset of pain localized to or near a single joint are summarized in Table 49–1. Table 49–1 lists additional diagnostic considerations for pain in a single joint that has been persistent or gradual in onset.

Differential Diagnosis

Bursitis

Bursae are synovial membranes that provide nearly frictionless motion between contiguous tendons, muscles, and ligaments. They normally do not communicate with the synovial cavities of joints; thus, inflammation of a bursa does not induce arthritis. Several key findings should allow the clinician to distinguish the periarticular pain of bursitis or tendinitis from synovitis. In synovitis, there is a *generalized* inflammation of the synovium so that the entire joint is involved, with stiffness and diffuse tenderness of the joint capsule. In bursitis and tendinitis, there is point tenderness localized to the site of the tendon or bursa that does not involve the synovial membrane.

Other features characteristic of tendinitis are pain on moving the tendon, including isometric contraction of muscle groups, without moving the joint, and nocturnal pain, resulting from motion or rolling on the inflamed tendon. In acute synovitis, the pain tends to subside at night when the joints are at rest, although nocturnal pain may be a late finding in far-advanced degenerative joint disease.

TABLE 49–1. DIFFERENTIAL DIAGNOSIS OF PAIN NEAR A SINGLE JOINT

Acute Pain
1. Periarticular pain induced by tendinitis or bursitis
2. Joint pain due to trauma
3. Acute monoarticular arthritis
   Crystal-induced synovitis
      Gout
      Pseudogout
   Septic arthritis
   Other inflammatory synovitis

Subacute or Chronic Pain
1. Avascular necrosis
2. Monoarticular osteoarthritis and other monoarticular conditions
3. Reflex sympathetic dystrophy syndrome
4. Tuberculous, neoplastic, or fungal arthritis

Inflammation in tendinitis is generally caused by degeneration or repeated minor trauma but is often induced by a discrete stressful episode. The relatively abrupt onset of pain on motion is most characteristic, but there may be recurrences or chronic intermittent symptoms, usually sharp pains that awaken the patient at night after he or she has rolled on the affected area. The bursal sac can be involved. Olecranon and prepatellar bursitis present the finding of a localized, fluctuant swelling over the patella or olecranon process that is tender but does not limit the motion of the joint, except when the bursa itself is stretched or compressed. Gout, rheumatoid arthritis, or sepsis may involve these bursae, although most cases are caused by repeated trauma, as in "housemaid's knee" and "student's elbow." Ileopsoas bursitis may present as an ultrasonically identifiable inguinal mass, clinically mimicking an inguinal hernia, with variable discomfort.[1] In the case of many other bursae that are contiguous to tendons, there is no important distinction between bursitis and tendinitis, since either and usually both may cause the same clinical findings. In either case, soft tissue calcifications may or may not be present on radiography.

Bursitis or tendinitis often occurs in patients who also have degenerative joint disease. It is important to identify the source of the patient's symptoms correctly, because tendinitis and bursitis may be alleviated completely by anti-inflammatory agents or by a local injection of steroids. The anatomic location of the bursae and tendons that most frequently account for symptoms is illustrated in Figure 49–1.

Joint Pain Due to Trauma

To distinguish trauma from arthritis, one depends on the history of a traumatic event, together with the finding of tenderness localized to that area of the joint that was traumatized or torn. For example, in the knee, sprains of the medial collateral ligament present with swelling and tenderness at the medial aspect of the joint; meniscal injuries produce tenderness localized to the adjacent joint line. Hemarthrosis may result in a generalized synovial effusion following major trauma to the joint capsule and in about 75% of cases is associated with fracture of the joint surface or with ligamentous rupture. Clinical findings of trauma include laxity due to ligamentous tears or locking of the joint if a cartilaginous tear has occurred. Hemarthrosis related to trauma generally develops within several hours of the event; if the effusion develops 12 to 24 hours after the injury, traumatic synovitis remains possible, but one should consider other disorders, such as gout or sepsis. Whenever passive range of motion is relatively free in a joint, compared with what the patient can perform actively, a tendinous tear should be suspected. Figure 49–2 illustrates the principles by which periarticular pain and trauma are distinguished clinically from a true synovitis of the joint.

Other Causes

Neurovascular compromise or referred pain is usually constant and may persist at night. Motor or sensory deficits may be present. Pain may be provoked by motion of the axial skeleton, but the range of motion of the joint is not limited.

Both the medial and the anterior tibial compartments of the leg may be sites of acute ischemia after trauma or of chronic or recurrent pain during and after exertion. The latter (referred to as "shin splints" in the anterior compartment) has been related to increased intracompartmental pressure and, in refractory cases, can be relieved by fasciotomy.[2]

Bone pain caused by fractures is preceded by trauma; tumors and infections of bone usually produce progressively worsening pain. Tenderness is localized to the bone, and x-rays generally show positive findings.

Acute Monoarticular Arthritis

In acute monoarticular arthritis, there is pain and stiffness of the entire joint capsule, often accompanied by heat, swelling, and redness. The onset tends to be abrupt, with stiffness and swelling often developing within a few hours but sometimes over several days. Four major diagnostic categories are gout, chondrocalcinosis, septic arthritis, and "other" causes of inflammatory synovitis.

Gout. In gout, the findings may be characteristic enough to permit a clinical diagnosis. There is an abrupt onset of agonizing, pulsating pain accompanied by exquisitely tender swelling and surrounding hyperemia, commonly referred to as "pseudocellulitis." This most frequently occurs in a middle-aged man, often upon his arising from bed, with severe pain in the first metatarsophalangeal (MTP) joint ("big toe") or another foot joint. Trauma, surgery, ethanol intake,[3] or severe medical illness may provoke an attack. Although the great toe is the most commonly involved joint in gout (in ~ 75% of patients at some time), followed by the ankle and foot (~ 50%), virtually any joint, including the knee (33%), and wrist (10%), with the exceptions of the spine and temporomandibular joints, may be involved at some time during the course of the disease.[4] Bursal sacs may be involved by gout, which may even develop within a Heberden or Bouchard node.

The prevalence of gout increases with increasing blood urate levels—from 0.6% of men with maximum levels below 6 mg/dl, to 2% between 6 and 7 mg/dl, 15% between 7 and 8 mg/dl, and 25% between 8 and 9 mg/dl.[5] But no plasma urate can be diagnostic of gout, and only a fairly low level, perhaps below 4 mg/dl, excludes gout in the patient with acute monoarticular arthritis. In a study of acute polyarticular gout, 38% of patients had urate levels of less than 7 mg/dl at the time of the attack, although in most patients, the levels rose above normal during the intercritical period.[6] Hence, in gouty arthritis, a definitive diagnosis can be established only by finding synovial fluid urate crys-

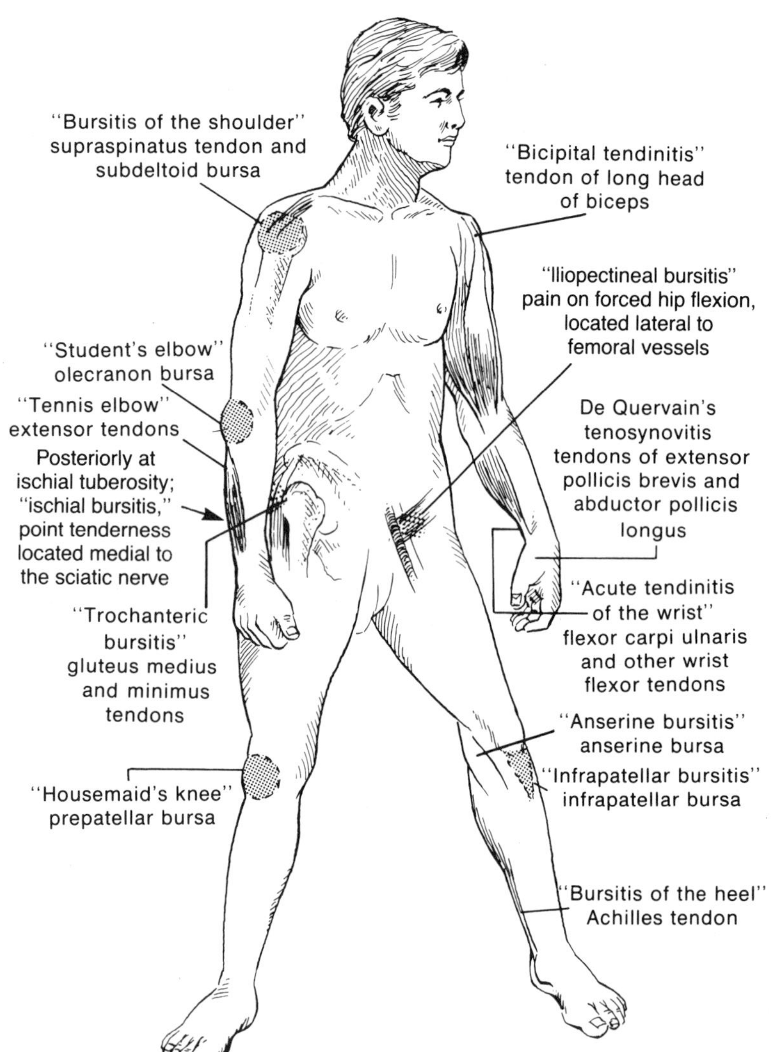

FIGURE 49–1. Common sites for tendinitis or bursitis.

tals that are strongly negatively birefringent in polarized light.

Chondrocalcinosis. The arthritis associated with chondrocalcinosis is called "pseudogout," since it may present an acute synovitis clinically similar to gouty arthritis. Calcific deposits in joints, not necessarily associated with clinical manifestations, were present in 2.2% of adults in one survey.[7] Hyperparathyroidism, acromegaly, Wilson's disease, and hemochromatosis have been associated with chondrocalcinosis; however, most cases are idiopathic. The disease tends to occur in women more than 60 years old and has a predilection for the knee joint. It could well be described as somewhat resembling the clinical picture of degenerative joint disease but with an inflammatory component. When the disease is manifested by an acute monoarticular arthritis, the attack may develop more slowly than in gout, reaching a peak after a few days and lasting for up to a month. These attacks often follow trauma or surgery and may respond dramatically to colchicine. It should be noted, however, that in some cases symptoms are more chronic. Such patients can appear to have a progressive arthritis of the knees, punctuated by bouts of inflammation or by smoldering inflammation. Other joints can be involved, such as the wrists (radiocarpal joints in particular), metacarpophalangeal (MCP) joints, elbows, and shoulders, reported to be accompanied by malaise, morning stiffness, and an increased sedimentation rate.[7] Unlike that in rheumatoid arthritis, the clinical picture in these polyarticular cases of chondrocalcinosis is more that of an inflammatory synovitis that moves from one to another joint "out of phase," as opposed to a smoldering, progressive arthritis involving all of the joints symmetrically. The diagnosis is established by the demonstration of rhomboid-shaped, weakly positively birefringent calcium pyrophosphate dihydrate (CPPD) crystals in joint fluid.

Other Crystal-Induced Arthritis. Acute crystal-induced arthritis may follow intra-articular injection of prednisolone tebutate or triamcinolone hexacetonide crystals.[8–10] A few cases have been described in which needle-shaped crystals resembling hydroxyapatite were noted in synovial fluid examined by electron microscopy.[11] There were four cases of otherwise unexplained acute arthritis in relatively young patients, and four older patients with an inflammatory exacerbation in an osteoarthritic joint. Knee involvement with warm, tender effusions was most common, although other joints may be involved, including the first MTP joint, and one should suspect this etiology in a young woman who develops the clinical features of a crystal-induced arthritis.[12] Joint fluid is generally inflammatory. This arthritis associated with apatite crystals is clinically

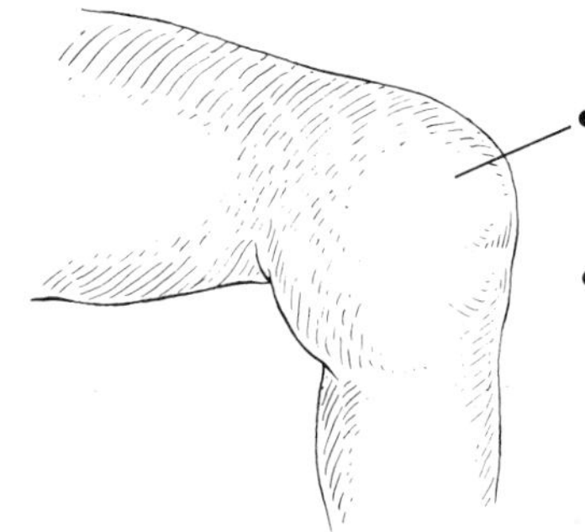

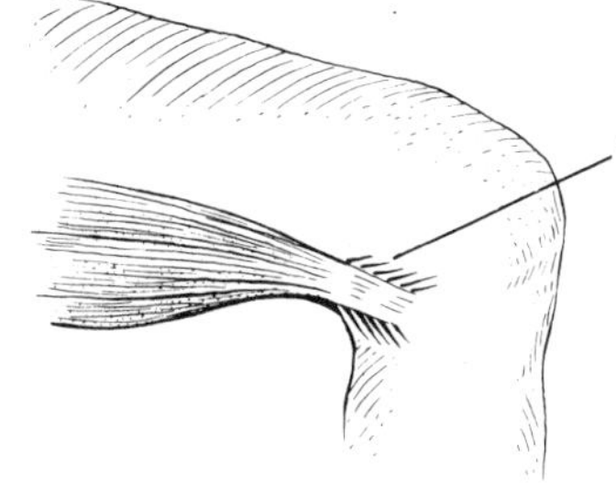

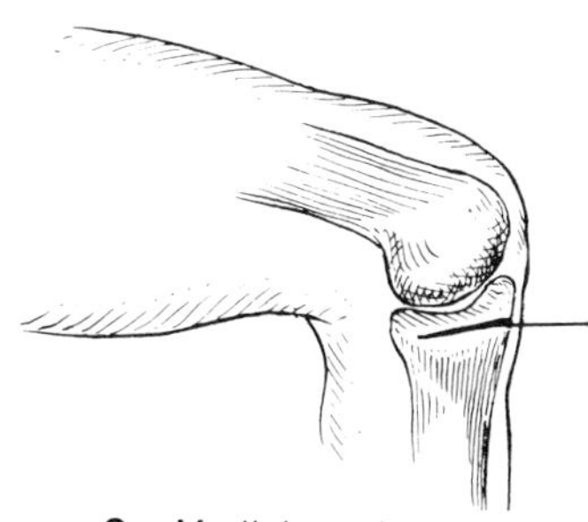

FIGURE 49–2. Differentiating bursitis or tendinitis and trauma to joints from arthritis.

indistinguishable from that associated with chondrocalcinosis, but, of course, crystals are not apparent on routine examination of the synovial fluid by light microscopy.[9]

Septic Arthritis. Community-acquired septic arthritis is rare in the normal host (24 cases of all types encountered from 1947 to 1957 at the Massachusetts General Hospital).[13] When seen initially, it is often confused by the clinician with more common conditions such as traumatic or rheumatoid arthritis. Although usually monoarticular, about 20% of cases involve from two to five joints.[13] Knee, hip, shoulder, elbow, and sternoclavicular joints (in descending order) are the most frequently involved. Peripheral joints in septic arthritis are always limited by painful motion, are swollen, and have effusions, but not all are described as exquisitely tender or "red."[13] The patients with more subtle findings include those with prosthetic joint infections, in whom pain may develop insidiously for several months prior to their presentation,[14] as well as those with rheumatoid arthritis who have received intra-articular steroids prior to developing sepsis. In infections of the hip or sacroiliac joint, the symptoms are limited to stiffness and pain on motion. Pyoarthrosis of the sternoclavicular joint presents with gradually progressive anterior chest discomfort and restricted motion of the shoulder. CT scanning may detect an associated retrosternal abscess.

Conditions that predispose to septic arthritis include steroid therapy (given orally or intraarticularly), underlying chronic arthropathy, such as rheumatoid arthritis, and history of trauma, surgery, or prosthesis of the involved joint, as well as immune deficiency, drug abuse, sickle cell anemia, sepsis, and severe chronic illness. Most adult patients are older than 60 years of age. The most common pathogenic mechanism is probably hematogenous localization of organisms to an already diseased joint. Excluding gonococcal arthritis, *Staphylococcus aureus* is still the most commonly encountered organism, but streptococcal species (group G or group B) and gram-negative bacilli together account for nearly 50% of cases, and *S. epidermidis* is found most commonly in prosthetic joint infections.[14] A furuncle or other obvious source of septicemia may be apparent. If septic chills and fever are present, several joints may be involved and blood culture results are often positive, whereas patients with single joint involvement often present nonspecific prodromal symptoms, a mild anemia, and an elevated sedimentation rate. Gram-negative bacilli as a cause of septic arthritis are usually associated with immunosuppression, debilitating diseases, drug abuse, or urinary tract infection with sepsis.[15] *Pseudomonas* is the most common organism associated with pyoarthrosis of the sternoclavicular joint, encountered in heroin addicts.[16]

The diagnosis in any patient with septic arthritis is established by aspiration of joint fluid. A presumptive diagnosis is made when the fluid is purulent as opposed to an inflammatory exudate, a hemarthrosis, or a noninflammatory fluid. Confirmation of the diagnosis depends on the Gram stain and on cultures of joint fluid.

Infections of periarticular structures should be distinguished from septic arthritis. The olecranon or prepatellar bursa can become infected, usually by direct extension from an overlying skin or subcutaneous infection. In the hand, a puncture wound, crack, or abrasion can lead to suppurative tenosynovitis. The patient generally is febrile, has a leukocytosis, and holds the acutely swollen finger in partial flexion. Midpalmar infections have more subtle findings. Slight swelling and point tenderness are the only signs in early cases; eventually, the dorsal aspect of the hand, the fingers, and even the forearm may swell, since the swelling tends to extend dorsally into soft tissues above the thick palmar fascia. Parenteral antibiotics, usually with surgical drainage, are necessary for these infections. Felons are local infections confined to the pulp of a fingertip, whereas paronychial infections involve the soft tissue along the sides or beneath the cuticle of a fingernail. These can usually be treated by a local incision plus antibiotics.

"Other" Inflammatory Synovitis. Any of the causes of acute synovitis can present with inflammation of a single joint, though more often several or more joints are involved. The differential diagnosis of acute synovitis is discussed in the next section. Some conditions such as familial Mediterranean fever or intermittent hydrarthrosis usually have a self-limited monoarticular synovitis of the knee joint. More commonly encountered conditions, including Lyme arthritis, rheumatic fever, Reiter's syndrome, and systemic lupus erythematosus may begin as monoarticular arthritis but usually develop a characteristic polyarticular involvement of other joints.

Subacute or Persistent Pain Localized to a Joint

Avascular Necrosis (Osteonecrosis). This refers to disruption of blood supply to the bony epiphysis underlying the cartilage of the joint. In general, there is collapse of the joint without loss of joint space (i.e., cartilage). Stasis of blood and bony necrosis are associated with measurable increases in bone marrow pressure. Early medullary decompression may improve the prognosis. This condition should be suspected when unexplained pain and stiffness develop insidiously in a weight-bearing joint. By the time radiographic changes are apparent, collapse of the involved joint with limitation of motion may have occurred, and major disability comes on within 6 to 12 months.

At the hip, avascular necrosis with collapse of the femoral head is associated with diabetes, sickle cell anemia, systemic lupus erythematosus, or corticosteroid therapy; less frequently, the proximal head of the humerus at the shoulder is involved by a similar process. Avascular necrosis of the proximal femoral epiphysis at the hip (Legg-Calvé disease) in a child can result eventually in severe secondary degenerative disease in young adulthood. Elderly persons sometimes develop osteonecrosis of the knee, detectable on bone scanning, with pain at the medial aspect, which may progress to produce secondary degenerative arthritis unless medullary decompression is performed. Avascular necrosis also occurs in the lunate bone of the hand (Kienböck's disease) and at the tarsal navicular (Köhler's disease) or the calcaneal apophysis (Sever's disease) of the foot. Children with these diseases have vague achiness, stiffness, and local tenderness or pain on weight-bearing. Osgood-Schlatter disease, local irritation of the tibial tubercle of the knee in an adolescent, presents with local swelling and tenderness on examination.

Osteochondritis refers to the separation of an avascular segment of subchondral bone, which typically occurs in a child or adolescent, and may form a loose body within the joint. This can involve the knee (medial femoral condyle), the elbow (capitellum of the distal humerus), or the foot (second, third, or fourth metatarsal head [Freiberg's disease]).

Adults may develop symptoms of secondary degenerative joint disease resulting from the avascular necrosis or osteochondritis, or a relatively asymptomatic adult may be noted to have the pronounced x-ray abnormalities of avascular necrosis that occurred in childhood.

Monoarticular Osteoarthritis (Degenerative Joint Disease). Degenerative joint disease resulting from trauma, overuse, or avascular necrosis may develop in any joint. The most characteristic locations are the temporomandibular joint, the acromioclavicular joint, the first carpometacarpal joint, and the first MTP joint (hallux rigidus), as well as the knee and hip joints. These have typical bony enlargement with crepitus and pain on motion. In temporomandibular joint dysfunction, the joint space may be narrowed and the mandibular condyle shaped irregularly; however, the temporomandibular joint is structurally normal in many patients with symptoms of this syndrome, which can be associated with bruxism or dental malocclusion. In the knee, and occasionally in other large joints, degenerative joint disease may be mimicked by two rarely encountered conditions, *pigmented villonodular synovitis* and *synovial osteochondromatosis,* which may present as bouts of painless, recurrent swelling with heat. A Baker cyst, representing communication between the knee joint and the posterior gastrocnemius-semimembranosus bursa, presents as painless swelling located posteriorly to the knee joint and may be associated with rheumatoid arthritis, degenerative arthritis, meniscal tears, or any other condition that produces a knee effusion.[17] In *chondromalacia of the patella,* characteristically there is aching after activity in an adolescent or young person and perhaps some crepitation on moving the patella against the femur.

Table 49–2 provides a list of some of the specific benign conditions that present as chronic or recurrent monoarticular pain and should be recognized from their clinical features. Anatomic locations are indicated in Figure 49–3.

Reflex Sympathetic Dystrophy Syndrome (RSDS). Pain, swelling, and warmth of a distal extremity may result from this syndrome. RSDS is usually associated with another condition such as trauma, fracture, hemiplegia, or peripheral nerve injury. Advanced cases are associated with characteristic patchy demineralization on bone films or increased radionuclide uptake on scanning.[18] In one series of 64 patients suspected of having RSDS, however, 14 had other conditions, including infectious, rheumatoid, and other types of acute arthritis.[18] Arthritis associated with diffuse swelling of the involved hand or foot usually can be distinguished from RSDS by noting that tenderness is localized to one or more joints on careful examination.

Tuberculous Arthritis. This is a monoarticular arthritis characterized by doughy swelling of the joint, often accompanied by marked atrophy of the surrounding muscles from disuse. Mild pain and stiffness are followed by a progressively developing effusion and, eventually, by more severely restricted motion. Fever and other constitutional symptoms are usually absent, and the chest film often shows no evidence of previous tuberculosis. The disease is often confused with degenerative joint disease because of its indolent course. As many as 50% of cases are of greater

TABLE 49–2. SPECIFIC BENIGN CAUSES OF CHRONIC MONOARTICULAR JOINT PAIN

Joint	Major Clinical Features	X-Ray Findings
Temporomandibular		
Temporomandibular joint dysfunction	Intermittent, unilateral pain in the face and temple; snapping of joint; tender pterygoid muscles	Normal or irregular mandibular condyle with narrowing of joint space
Shoulder		
Acromioclavicular osteoarthritis	Pain on abduction of the shoulder > 90°; tender, crepitant joint	Narrowing of joint space with osteophytes
Elbow		
Osteochondritis dissecans	Pain and swelling after activity in a young person	Irregularity of lateral humeral capitellum with loose body fragments in joint
Wrist and Hand		
Avascular necrosis of lunate (Kienböck's disease)	Tenderness and stiffness of wrist in a young person	Dense, irregular, fragmented lunate bone
Osteoarthritis of first carpometacarpal joint	Limited motion of thumb with crepitus	Sclerosis and narrowing of joint
Knee		
Chondromalacia of the patella	Knee aches after activity in an adolescent; crepitus on moving patella	Usually normal
Osteochondritis dissecans	Aching and swelling after activity in an adolescent or child	Clear radiolucent outline around a dense subchondral fragment
Osgood-Schlatter disease	Tenderness, pain, and swelling at the tibial tubercle in an adolescent or child	Fragmented tibial tubercle
Pigmented villonodular synovitis	Recurrent, often painless knee effusions in a young person; dark, bloody joint fluid	Vague soft tissue nodularity of the synovium
Synovial osteochondromatosis	Recurrent, initially painless knee effusion	Calcifications within the joint
Hip		
Avascular necrosis of femoral head or epiphysis (Legg-Calvé disease)	Limping, achiness, and stiffness in adults (avascular necrosis) or children (Legg-Calvé disease)	Flattening of head or widening of epiphyseal line without loss of joint space
Foot		
Avascular necrosis of tarsal navicular (Köhler's disease)	Vague ache and limp in a child	Sclerosis of the navicular without loss of joint space
Avascular necrosis of calcaneal apophysis (Sever's disease)	Pain and tenderness of posterior heel in a child	Fragmented calcaneal apophysis
Osteochondritis of 2nd, 3rd, or 4th metatarsal head (Freiberg's disease)	Pain on weight-bearing in an adolescent	Flat, broadened, sclerotic metatarsal head
Osteoarthritis of 1st metatarsophalangeal joint (hallux rigidus)	Pain on dorsiflexion of great toe	Sclerosis and narrowing of joint space with hypertrophic spurs

than 1 year's duration when diagnosed.[19] Most commonly, the spine and hip joint are involved, but any peripheral joint can be the site of tuberculosis; or it may present as an indolent process involving tendon sheaths. Joint fluid is usually inflammatory rather than septic, so that an adequate biopsy of synovial tissue with culture and microscopic examination is necessary to make the diagnosis.

In addition to tuberculosis, bacterial infections of prosthetic joints may develop subacutely, and occasionally subacute monoarticular arthritis is caused by a primary or metastatic *neoplasm* or by *fungal arthritis.* In the latter, the clinical features are the same as in tuberculous arthritis. Most primary malignancies at or near a joint occur in adolescents or young adults 20 to 40 years of age. Synovial sarcoma presents as a soft tissue mass, usually involving the knee, with progressive swelling and eventually pain. Other neoplasms, including giant cell tumors, osteogenic sarcomas, and chondrosarcomas, tend to involve the distal femur or proximal tibia or fibula near the knee joint, the proximal humerus at the shoulder, or the distal radius at the wrist. These present as warm, tender masses. Fibrosarcomas arise most often from periosteum of the femur or tibia, causing pain from invasion of the bone before a mass is palpable. In addition, joint pain or swelling may be due to benign chondroblastoma. Benign osteoid osteomas can present with nocturnal pain, stiffness, and limited motion of the hip or knee, and no objective findings save for a typical radiolucency within the femur on radiography, surrounded by a rim of sclerotic reactive bone.

Diagnostic Procedures

Radiographic and Radionuclide Studies. The radiographic features are nonspecific in most cases of *acute* monoarticular arthritis. The finding of soft tissue swelling does not distinguish between crystal-induced and septic arthritis or any other form of acute synovitis. Likewise, soft tissue calcification has little diagnostic value in patients suspected of having tendinitis or bursitis, since frequently calcification is absent in symptomatic cases or noted as an incidental finding in asymptomatic individuals. In septic arthritis (Fig. 49–4), there is early destruction of cartilage, as indicated by narrowing of the joint space, and destruction of subchondral bone, sometimes with extensive periosteal new bone formation. These changes do not develop for at least 8 or 9 days, however, so that the radiograph is usually of little diagnostic value other than as a baseline for comparison, since it is important to make the diagnosis before cartilaginous destruction can be noted on the film. Deep-seated sepsis of hip, shoulder, or sacroiliac joints, which are difficult to examine clinically, can be detected by radioisotopic scanning, using technetium polyphosphonate. This method provides a sensitive but nonspecific index of

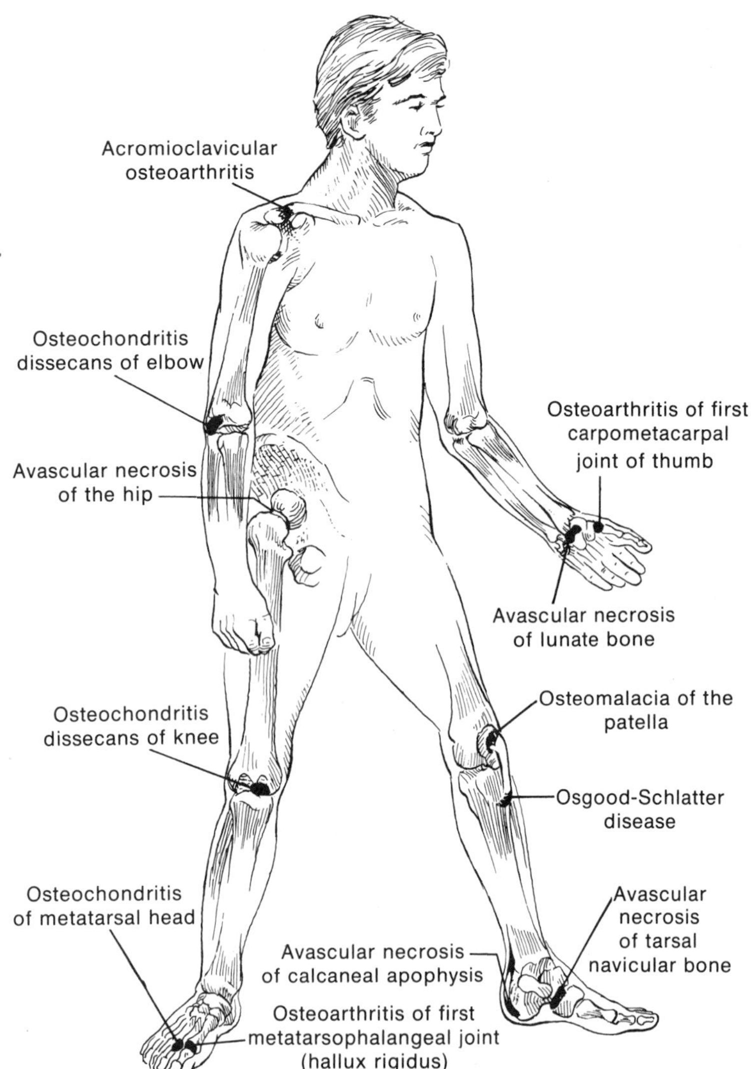

FIGURE 49–3. Anatomic locations of specific benign causes of monoarticular joint pain.

joint involvement.[20] It may be used in conjunction with gallium scanning, as both are positive in septic joint disease as well as in osteomyelitis, whereas only gallium scanning is expected to be positive in cellulitis and only technetium scanning may be positive in degenerative and other nonseptic joint diseases.

Radiographs are valuable for assessing patients with *chronic* monoarticular arthritis. Radiographic findings of rapid bone or cartilage loss suggestive of tuberculous, other infectious or neoplastic joint involvement may lead the clinician to perform biopsies, whereas, often the findings in chronic gout, pseudogout, degenerative joint disease, and osteonecrosis are sufficiently characteristic, together with the clinical picture, to establish a tentative diagnosis (Table 49–3).

In *gout,* bone erosions due to tophi occur. Like erosions in rheumatoid arthritis, these may occur at the margins of joints, where synovium directly abuts bone, but the gouty tophi do not involve each joint symmetrically. Sometimes a spicule of bone grows around the tophus, suggesting a small "overhanging margin." Other key x-ray features that differentiate gouty arthritis from rheumatoid arthritis are the relative lack of osteoporosis and the lack of diffuse joint space narrowing in gout, in which only a few joints have joint space narrowing or erosions (Fig. 49–5).

A fine linear calcification within articular cartilages or fibrocartilages (knee meniscus, triangular cartilage of the wrist, and symphysis pubis) is seen radiologically in *chondrocalcinosis* (Fig. 49–6). Not all patients with chondrocalcinosis have clinical arthritis. When they do, the x-ray picture is similar to that of *degenerative arthritis*; however, the distribution of joint involvement is different. Thus, although both processes involve the knees, osteoarthritis in the hand usually involves only the first carpometacarpal joint of the thumb, together with distal interphalangeal (DIP) and sometimes proximal interphalangeal (PIP) joints. Involvement of midcarpal, all MCP, and particularly the radiocarpal joints is characteristic of pseudogout. In either process, radiographs reveal asymmetric joint space narrowing, bone sclerosis, and cyst formation. The cysts are located within the bone beneath the articular cartilage rather than eroding at the margins.

Avascular necrosis is caused by vascular insufficiency of bone. Most commonly this occurs at the femoral head of the hip. The cartilage itself continues to receive nourishment from synovial fluid. Thus, even in advanced cases with collapse of a portion of the femoral head, the joint space remains intact (Fig. 49–7). Radiologic changes, such as loss of sharpness of the subchondral cortex, may not develop for several weeks. Films of the hip should be taken in forced abduction; and a radiolucent line that parallels the subchondral surface of the joint, with preservation of the joint

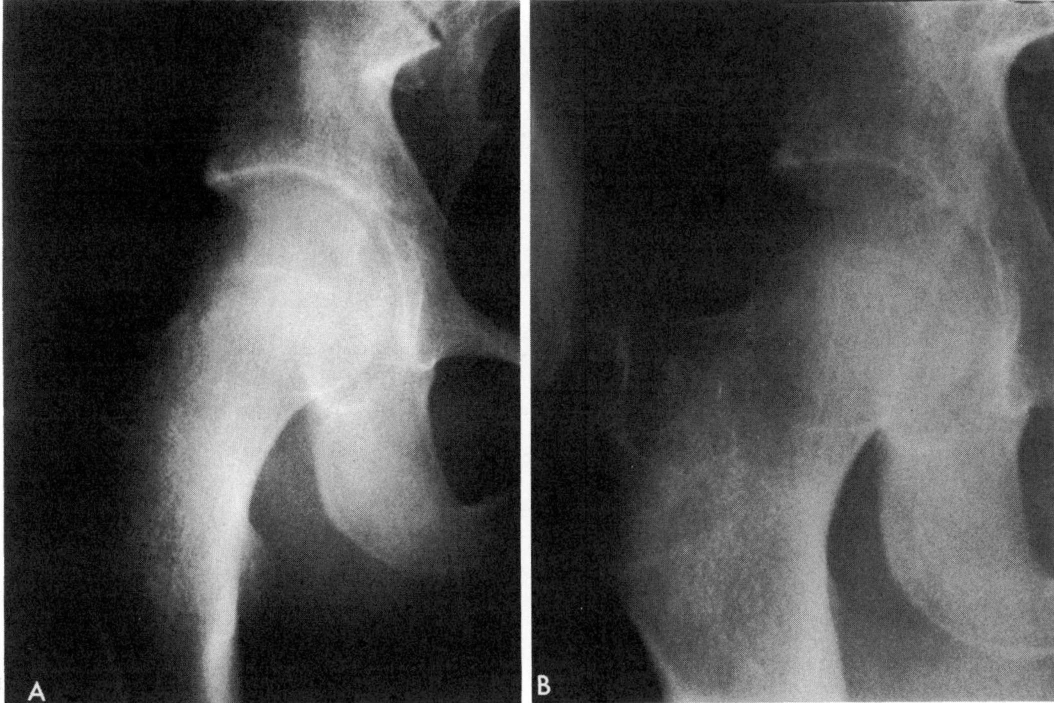

FIGURE 49–4. Radiographic features of septic arthritis. A 24-year-old man complained of stiffness of the hip for 21 days. Only soft tissue swelling appeared on the initial film (*A*). The joint space was normal, although in retrospect there is a slight rarefaction of the femoral head; thus the findings are nonspecific. *B*. A repeat film after 1 week demonstrated narrowing of the joint space and areas of lucency within the femoral head with disruption of the cortex laterally. These later findings are typical of septic arthritis. (X-ray films courtesy of Department of Radiology, Brigham and Women's Hospital, Harvard Medical School, Boston.)

space, is virtually pathognomonic for this condition. Often a secondary synovitis with joint effusion is present; later, with the development of bone fragmentation and collapse, there are secondary degenerative changes.

Radionuclide scanning with ^{99}Tc methylene diphosphonate detects avascular necrosis earlier than plain films. Scanning, usually showing increased uptake but sometimes early on showing an area of decreased uptake, was abnormal in all 14 symptomatic patients with systemic lupus erythematosus with ischemic necrosis, whereas radiographs were abnormal in only 7 of the 14.[21] Magnetic resonance imaging (MRI) is probably the most sensitive method currently available to detect avascular necrosis.[22] Patterns of diminished bone marrow signals may be seen in the subchondral regions of the femoral head prior to bone scanning abnormalities in ischemic necrosis of the hip. Increased uptake on scintigraphy is equally as sensitive (68%) but more specific (86%) than radiographs for recognition of the reflex sympathetic dystrophy syndrome.[18]

Soft tissue swelling, marked demineralization, and loss of bony cortex are the most prominent radiographic findings of *tuberculous arthritis*. Of note, there is little bone sclerosis, and joint spaces are well preserved in the face of a chronic arthritis with extensive demineralization (Fig. 49–8). Later in the disease, joint spaces may be narrowed, with rarefaction of subchondral bone and areas of bone destruction, still with the absence of much sclerosis or osteophyte formation.

TABLE 49–3. RADIOGRAPHIC FEATURES IN MONOARTICULAR JOINT DISEASE

Acute synovitis due to gout, pseudogout, sepsis, or synovitis of other causes	Nonspecific soft tissue swelling
Late manifestations of septic arthritis	Subchondral destruction of bone; periosteal new bone formation; loss of joint space
Late manifestations of gouty arthritis	Asymmetric bony erosions caused by tophi, with an "overhanging margin," relatively little osteoporosis; lack of diffuse joint space narrowing
Late manifestations of chondrocalcinosis	Fine linear calcification within cartilages; asymmetric joint space narrowing; reactive sclerosis and osteophyte formation; subchondral cyst formation; particularly involves knees, hips and radiocarpal, midcarpal, and all MCP joints
Monoarticular degenerative arthritis	Asymmetric joint space narrowing; reactive sclerosis and osteophyte formation; subchondral cyst formation; particularly involves acromioclavicular, 1st carpometacarpal, 1st metatarsophalangeal, and DIP joints
Avascular necrosis	Collapse of bone with preservation of the joint space; radiolucent "crescent" line; eventually, dense sclerosis and secondary degenerative changes
Tuberculous arthritis	Soft tissue swelling; marked demineralization; bony rarefaction; little reactive sclerosis; eventually, bony destruction
Synovial sarcoma	Joint swelling with a soft tissue mass; sometimes small foci of calcification
Primary bone malignancies occurring near a joint	Radiolucency, irregular mottling or rarefaction; sometimes a mass with new bone formation

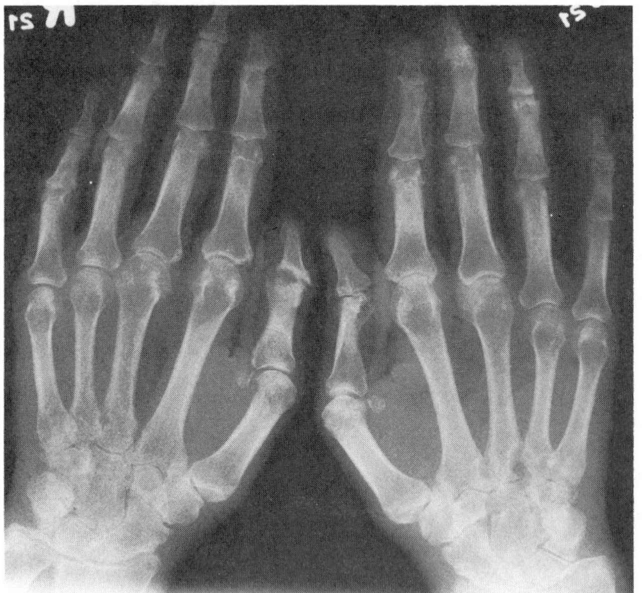

FIGURE 49–5. Chronic gouty arthritis of the hand with x-ray findings. The patient had known gout for 15 years. Several punched-out, sharply marginated erosions are visible, particularly at the interphalangeal joint of the thumb on the right. A tophus is seen at the third left metacarpal head. Despite the finding of erosions, there is little or no osteoporosis of bones in the hand. Most of the joint spaces are well preserved, including those of the metacarpophalangeal (MCP) and proximal interphalangeal (PIP) joints that typically would be narrowed with longstanding destructive rheumatoid arthritis. (X-ray film courtesy of Department of Radiology, Brigham and Women's Hospital, Harvard Medical School, Boston.)

In primary *malignancies* of bone or metastatic malignancies that occur near a joint, radiographic features include radiolucency, irregular mottling, or rarefaction of bone. A mass of new bone formation occurs in osteogenic sarcomas. In synovial sarcomas, a soft tissue mass involves the joint, sometimes containing multiple minute foci of calcification.

Synovial Fluid Analysis. Synovial fluid aspiration in acute monoarticular arthritis may identify patients with septic joint disease or crystal-induced synovitis. One must distinguish a purulent from an inflammatory effusion, such as that found in gout or rheumatoid arthritis. Inflammatory joint effusions average 10,000 to 25,000 white blood cells (WBC)/mm^3 and 25 to 70% polymorphonuclear leukocytes. Purulent or septic fluids characteristically have 50,000 to 100,000 WBC/mm^3, with more than 90% polymorphonuclear leukocytes. There may be considerable overlap, however, with synovial WBC counts greater than 50,000/mm^3 in some cases of gout or pseudogout and very low cell counts in early cases of septic arthritis. Regardless of total cell counts, it is most unusual for septic joint fluid to contain less than 85% polymorphonuclear leukocytes,[23] although fluid from joints infected by the gonococcus or by tuberculosis is usually inflammatory rather than septic. Also, the fluid obtained from septic bursitis of the prepatellar or olecranon bursa is reported to average as few as 3000 WBC/mm^3 and only 52% polymorphonuclear leukocytes.[24] Ordinarily, the bursal fluid leukocyte count of traumatic, nonseptic bursitis is less than 1000 WBC/mm^3.

Gram stains are reported to reveal organisms in 75% of cases with staphylococcal infection, but less often with gram-negative bacillary (50%) and gonococcal (25%) infections.[14] The yield of Gram staining is increased by centrifugation of the synovial fluid.[14] Synovial fluid culture almost always has a positive result in nongonococcal septic arthritis.[14]

The inflammatory fluids of gout and pseudogout are distinguished from those of rheumatoid and other inflammatory synovitis by identification of characteristic crystals within the joint fluid. Repeated aspiration is sometimes necessary, since crystals are not invariably identified on the first attempt. When gout involves a bursa, the fluid may be noninflammatory and average only 4000 WBC/mm^3, with 10% polymorphonuclear leukocytes.[25]

Noninflammatory synovial fluids are found in traumatic arthritis, osteoarthritis, and with relatively early joint involvement in many types of acute synovitis (see Acute Polyarticular Synovitis). In noninflammatory fluids, there are generally fewer than 1000 WBC/mm^3 and less than 25% polymorphonuclear leukocytes.

The number of red blood cells in effusions caused by trauma vary from few to grossly bloody fluid (Table 49–4). Mucin clots, total protein, and glucose in synovial fluid reflect the degree of inflammatory response within the joint rather than providing diagnostic information that is unrelated to the total cell count and differential. The difference between serum and synovial fluid glucose levels averages

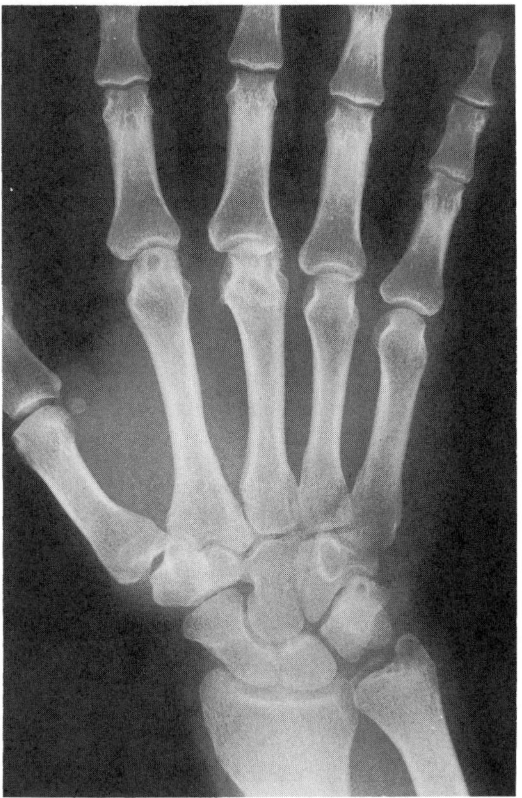

FIGURE 49–6. Chondrocalcinosis of the wrist. The patient had swelling and stiffness of the wrist of relatively abrupt onset during the previous week. Calcium pyrophosphate crystals were found in the joint fluid. The radiographic findings are those of chondrocalcinosis. A fine band of linear calcification is seen within the articular cartilage of the ulnocarpal joint. There is rarefaction of the metacarpal heads (MCP and carpometacarpal involvement), particularly at the proximal head of the fifth metacarpal. A discrete subchondral cyst is noted at the distal second metacarpal head. Asymmetric loss of joint space and reactive sclerosis are most prominent at the third distal metacarpal head. The x-ray features are the same as in degenerative arthritis, but the distribution of joint involvement in this case is typical of chondrocalcinosis involving the hand and wrist. (X-ray film courtesy of Department of Radiology, Brigham and Women's Hospital, Harvard Medical School, Boston.)

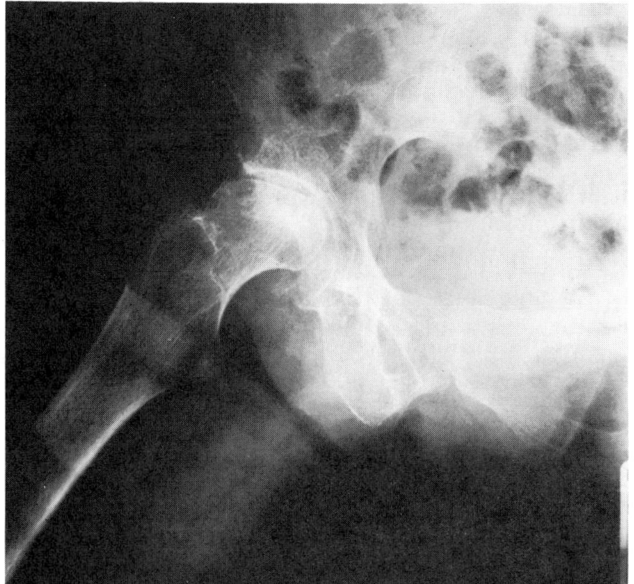

FIGURE 49–7. Aseptic necrosis of the hip. A 76-year-old widow with known mild osteoarthritis but previously normal examinations of the hips complained of the insidious onset, over about 4 weeks, of pain in the right hip. The pain was worse on walking. Severe pain and limited motion were present on internal and external rotation of the hip on examination. The radiograph, which was taken in forced abduction, reveals only flattening and compression of the superior portion of the right femoral head. The joint space remains intact except for slight narrowing. No significant bony spurring is noted. X-ray film of the left hip was normal. The findings are typical of avascular necrosis, although a radiolucent line is not visible in the subchondral bone. After a period of progressive disability and pain of increasing severity, the patient underwent surgical replacement of the right femoral head.

about 90 mg/dl in patients with septic arthritis with more than 50,000 WBC/mm^3 fluid, but averages about 60 mg/dl in those with fewer than 50,000 WBC/mm^3 of fluid.[9]

Approach to Patients With Pain in or Near a Single Joint

Pain of Acute Onset. One depends on the history and clinical findings to distinguish joint pain due to trauma, bursitis, or tendinitis from that caused by synovitis. Septic arthritis is a medical emergency, and diagnostic joint aspiration should be performed in any case with acute monoarticular synovitis and effusion, unless the condition is clearly compatible with or explained by a previously established diagnosis such as gout or pseudogout. It should be recalled that patients with acute gouty arthritis have an exquisitely tender inflammation of the joint and surrounding tissues ("pseudocellulitis"), whereas septic arthritis at times may be more subtle, manifested only by swelling, warmth, and tenderness of the involved joint. If one intends to commit the patient to long-term prophylactic therapy with allopurinol, the diagnosis of gout is best established unequivocally by demonstration of urate crystals within synovial fluid.

Without treatment, in septic arthritis irreversible destruction of cartilage occurs almost invariably after 2 weeks; patients treated within 5 days of the onset of symptoms usually recover fully.[13, 14, 23] This may allow some leeway for a short trial of therapy in some patients with the classic clinical features, as outlined earlier, of a crystal-induced synovitis. Unless the signs of joint involvement resolve within a few days after treatment for gout or pseudogout, however, diagnostic aspiration is advisable, since some improvement may result simply from rest and analgesic therapy even in patients with septic arthritis.

Persistent Monoarticular Arthritis. As mentioned, the clinical picture of pseudogout may be that of an acutely inflamed joint superimposed upon a chronic arthritis. This may also occur with gouty arthritis and with arthritis caused by hydroxyapatite crystals, although chronic tophaceous gouty arthritis is rarely encountered now since the advent of therapy with allopurinol. The picture of acute inflammatory synovitis superimposed upon a chronic arthropathy should be distinguished from the clinical problem of an indolent, persistent, truly monoarticular arthritis. The differential diagnosis of the latter includes tuberculous, fungal, and neoplastic joint involvement, although most cases are caused by degenerative joint disease, osteonecrosis, and other benign entities (see Table 49–2). The diagnosis depends upon the history, the physical findings, and a careful assessment of radiologic features. In order to rule out neoplasms or atypical, smoldering infec-

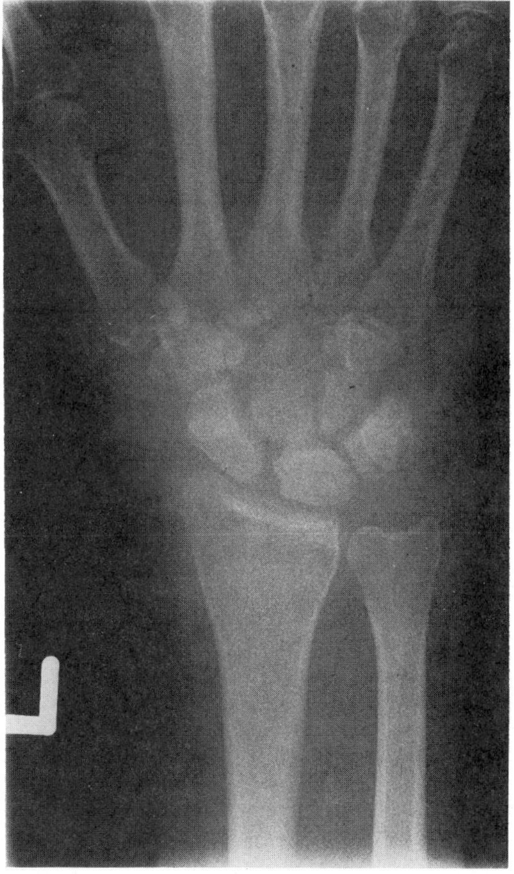

FIGURE 49–8. Tuberculous arthritis of the wrist. A 40-year-old woman first noticed pain, swelling, and warmth of the left wrist after doing push-ups. Three months later, soft tissue swelling is demonstrable. There is marked demineralization of bone with loss of the cortex and trabeculae, particularly at the second and third proximal metacarpal heads and in the distal carpal bones, but with the exception of carpometacarpals, joint spaces are well preserved despite extensive demineralization. There are no marginal erosions and little bony sclerosis. These radiographic features are typical of tuberculous arthritis. Diagnosis was established by biopsy and culture of tissue. (X-ray film courtesy of Department of Radiology, Brigham and Women's Hospital, Harvard Medical School, Boston.)

tious processes, radiographs should be obtained. Unusual or poorly marginated destruction of bone, marked bony decalcification, and evidence of an invasive process are clear indications for biopsy. Biopsy should also be considered in any chronic monoarticular arthritis when the clinical and roentgenographic features are atypical (as in Fig. 49–8) or when local muscle atrophy, soft tissue swelling, and osteoporosis are not accompanied by the expected degree of sclerosis and osteophyte formation that is compatible with the diagnosis of osteoarthritis.

Issues Related to Management

An acute synovitis of the joint or periarticular or traumatic process due to any cause will be helped by an appropriate period of rest, partial removal of weight-bearing (including the use of crutches when indicated), and salicylates or analgesics in moderate doses. In cases with acute bursitis or tendinitis, injection of a corticosteroid (methylprednisolone acetate [Depo-Medrol], 10 to 40 mg, mixed with 1% lidocaine [Xylocaine]) into the affected area generally results in complete subsidence of symptoms. This should be followed by rest for several days until the patient is asymptomatic and then by active range-of-motion exercises.

Traumatic Injuries. The approach to traumatic injuries of joints is governed by the amount of soft tissue swelling and by whether hemarthrosis or ligamentous instability is present. Most injuries result from twisting a weight-bearing joint, such as the knee or ankle. Instability, which can be demonstrated with the patient under anesthesia when pain and swelling prevent an adequate examination, implies complete ligamentous rupture that requires operative repair. Swelling with pain on weight-bearing, in the absence of instability, indicates a ligamentous sprain. For these cases, the principle of management is to immobilize the joint until healing can occur, in order to prevent chronic instability resulting from laxity of the ligament. Joints with moderate-to-severe sprains, as determined by the degree of local soft tissue reaction, should be placed in a cast for a period of up to 3 weeks. Minor sprains, which are manifested only by local tenderness or minimal swelling, can be immobilized for 10 days by using a padded dressing covered by an Ace bandage. If hemarthrosis is present, the examination should include intercondylar, skyline, and stress radiographic views of the joint to exclude fracture of the joint surface, internal derangement, or ligamentous rupture. Negative radiographic examinations, but the presence of a small synovial effusion and joint line tenderness, may indicate a torn meniscus. If the joint is not locked, this injury also can be managed by immobilization using a cast, followed by re-examination in 10 days. After the injured joint is immobilized properly, weight-bearing can be allowed as tolerated. If the knee is involved, it is important for the patient to perform regular isometric quadriceps exercises to avoid muscular atrophy.

TABLE 49–4. DIAGNOSTIC ASSESSMENT OF JOINT FLUID

Septic:	
Staphylococcal	50,000–100,000 WBC/mm³*
Gram-negative bacilli	>85% polymorphonuclear
Other bacterial infections	leukocytes
Some cases of gonococcal arthritis	<40 mg/dl of glucose
Inflammatory:	
Crystal-induced synovitis	10,000–25,000 WBC/mm³*
Rheumatoid arthritis	25%–70% polymorphonuclear
Tuberculous arthritis	leukocytes
Most cases of gonococcal arthritis	>40 mg/dl of glucose
Reiter's syndrome	
Other causes of synovitis, particularly if more than 2 weeks in duration	
Noninflammatory:	
Degenerative joint disease	<100 WBC/mm³*
Trauma (with variable RBC count)†	<25% polymorphonuclear
	leukocytes
Early cases of acute synovitis	Normal glucose

*Typical cell counts are given; there may be overlap between the categories.
†Presence of fat globules within a grossly bloody effusion indicates fracture.

Gout. The management of gout involves both the acute and future attacks. Although colchicine has been used traditionally as therapy for *acute gout,* its associated gastrointestinal side effects and limited effectiveness seem to place it behind the nonsteroidal anti-inflammatory drugs (NSAIDs) as agents of choice for this condition.[26–28] All NSAIDs seem to be effective, especially if given early in the course of the attack. Adrenocorticotropic hormone (ACTH) or a brief course of oral prednisone also aborts an attack, although "rebound" attacks may occur after dissipation of the therapeutic effect. Intravenous administration of colchicine, 1 or 2 mg diluted in 20 ml of normal saline and infused very slowly, was formerly given to circumvent the gastrointestinal side effects of that drug but is usually avoided because it causes severe local necrosis if extravasation occurs, transient granulocytopenia, and, if administered inadvertently in a toxic dose, aplastic anemia or respiratory arrest.

A reasonable program for treating most acute attacks consists of a NSAID, which may be given as a single high dose, followed by 4 daily doses for 1 week or less if inflammation resolves. Colchicine tablets may be given daily for several weeks to prevent recurrent attacks after discontinuing the NSAID.

NSAIDs are often beneficial for patients with *pseudogout.* Complete aspiration of the joint effusion also helps to alleviate symptoms.

In patients with frequently recurrent attacks of gouty arthritis, tophi, or uric acid lithiasis, the decision is usually made to lower the body pool of uric acid. This can be done either by increasing uric acid excretion by means of probenecid or sulfinpyrazone administration or by decreasing uric acid production by the administration of allopurinol. Eighty to 90% of hyperuricemic individuals excrete less than 600 mg/day of uric acid. In these patients, uricosuric agents provide a rational means for reversing underexcretion and restoring the balance of uric acid to normal. On the other hand, uricosuric drugs are limited by the capacity of the kidney to excrete uric acid, and the dosage required to produce an effect varies considerably and must be titrated individually by monitoring 24-hour urinary uric acid excretions. During the initial phase of therapy, prior to restoring balance at a lower serum level of uric acid, there is danger of renal calculus formation; hence, uricosuric agents should be started at low doses while high volumes and perhaps alkalinization of urine are maintained. For these reasons, and because of its relatively low incidence of toxicity, allopurinol seems to be the drug of choice.[29] Many instances of the most common toxic effect of allopurinol, rash, may be avoided by restricting concomitant administration of ampicillin and by giving lower doses of allopurinol to patients with renal insufficiency.[30]

Some clinicians advise therapy for asymptomatic hyperuricemia if the serum urate concentration is greater than 9 mg/dl and the condition is not due to diuretics.[27] However, no appreciable loss of renal function or other adverse effects of asymptomatic hyperuricemia have been noted on prospective studies of nontophaceous subjects,[31, 32] although the data are insufficient to exclude the possibility that long-term adverse effects may develop in persons with unusually high serum urate levels (i.e., >13 or >10 mg/dl in men and women, respectively). Follow-up has revealed a low incidence of renal calculi in persons with asymptomatic hyperuricemia.[32] In patients with gouty attacks, it seems reasonable to weigh the benefits of prophylactic therapy against a policy of treating occasional attacks with indomethacin. When tophi or renal calculi develop or the acute episodes occur frequently, long-term prophylactic therapy should be instituted. Neither allopurinol nor the uricosuric agents are anti-inflammatory, and gouty attacks may occur after the initiation of therapy with these agents, due to increased mobilization of uric acid stores. The prophylactic use of colchicine (1 or 2 tablets per day taken orally) reduces the frequency of such attacks and may be continued until the patient has been attack-free for 3 to 6 months.

The serum uric acid during therapy with hypouricemic agents should fall to below 7 mg/dl, the level at which soluble serum urates precipitate into tophi.[33] If this level is not obtained, the physician can alter the dose of the drug or determine whether the patient is, in fact, taking the drug.

In situations in which massive tophaceous deposits exist, and in the absence of renal insufficiency, both allopurinol and a uricosuric drug may be used concomitantly.

Septic Arthritis. Hospitalization is indicated for patients with purulent or septic joint fluid. Choice of an antibiotic depends on an assessment of the likely source of infection, together with the results of a Gram stain. When these results are not helpful, oxacillin, given intravenously, can be the initial therapy of choice, but in drug abusers and elderly, debilitated, or immunosuppressed patients, parenteral gentamicin should be added until culture results are obtained.[23] Intrasynovial injection of antibiotics is not indicated. In suspected cases of gonococcal arthritis, the initial therapy of choice is ceftriaxone, 1g/day, administered intravenously. Infected joints should be immobilized initially in a position of function, but passive and then active range of motion exercises are started as soon as possible.[14]

Adequate drainage of the joint space must be obtained. Peripheral joints such as the knee or elbow may be drained by repeated aspirations, done at first once or twice daily to relieve large, tense effusions.[14] Surgical drainage is necessary for the hip and other inaccessible joints or in the case of very thick, loculated fluid and is essential in children with septic hips, to prevent ischemia of the femoral neck.[14]

ACUTE POLYARTICULAR SYNOVITIS

The syndrome of acute polyarticular synovitis consists of swelling, warmth, and tenderness involving several or more joints. The number of joints involved varies from a few to widespread inflammation of the hands, wrists, ankles, knees, and other peripheral joints, although some asymmetry often is apparent—for example, a temporomandibular joint on one side only; all the MCPs and PIPs on one hand and only a few on the contralateral side; both knees but only one ankle. The pattern of joint involvement may be "migratory," in which one joint improves or returns to normal while synovitis develops in other joint(s); or the arthritis may follow an "additive" pattern. Multiple small joints of the hands or feet can be involved. Although traditionally distinguishing between "migratory" and "additive" patterns of joint involvement was thought to be helpful, the extent of overlap is such that one cannot rely upon this distinction to make a diagnosis. Repetitive, episodic flare-ups of polyarthritis with intervening subsidence of symptoms occur more commonly in some conditions, including gout, spondylitis, inflammatory bowel diseases, psoriasis, Reiter's syndrome, and Lyme arthritis. Usually the accompanying clinical characteristics and a few laboratory tests lead to establishing the etiology, although at times in acute polyarticular synovitis the objective manifestations are limited to joint involvement or only to diffuse arthralgias at the time of presentation.

Key characteristics that differentiate acute synovitis from rheumatoid arthritis and other chronic articular diseases are the abrupt onset of synovitis (in many cases, within a day or two) and spontaneous remission, often within days to weeks, but occasionally after several months.

The symptoms of rheumatoid arthritis develop insidiously rather than abruptly; the patient usually has morning stiffness for several weeks or months. Joint involvement is bilaterally symmetric, most characteristic being the pattern of involvement of both wrists and all the metacarpophalangeal joints. Figure 49–9 contrasts this typical rheumatoid pattern of joint involvement with that of three patients whose acute synovitis was caused by rubella, sarcoid, and gonococcal arthritis, respectively.

In addition to the subacute onset of joint pain, patients with rheumatoid arthritis have low-grade fevers, malaise, and weight loss, which also generally develop insidiously over a period of weeks to months. Some other features of rheumatoid arthritis may be absent at the time of presentation. Subcutaneous nodules are rare, and the latex fixation test is frequently negative in this initial phase. X-ray films show only nonspecific soft tissue swelling, and the joint fluid exhibits a nonspecific inflammatory pattern. Thus, one often depends on the clinical features outlined earlier to make a diagnosis. In some cases, rheumatoid arthritis has an abrupt onset. If the initial clinical manifestations are nonspecific, it is appropriate to await the development of characteristic findings while providing symptomatic relief with salicylates and physical measures.

There are several accompanying manifestations that help to establish the etiology of polyarteritis in some cases. Raynaud's phenomenon of the hands and feet, involving a two-color change from white to blue, suggests the possibility of an underlying collagen-vascular disease. Photosensitivity, including fever and serositis developing after sunlight exposure, suggests systemic lupus erythematosus. Ocular, oral, nasal and/or vaginal dryness suggests underlying Sjögren's syndrome.

Differential Diagnosis

Acute synovitis may be the presenting manifestation in numerous conditions. My approach to the differential diagnosis is first to discuss four major disease entities: gonococcal arthritis, Lyme disease, Reiter's syndrome, and acute rheumatic fever. Second, I will discuss the joint involvement and manifestations of those cases in which acute synovitis occurs in the course of another specific illness, including viral and other infectious arthritis, the arthritis of inflammatory bowel disease, and hypersensitivity states (Table 49–5). And third, I will address acute synovitis that occurs de novo, in which there are no specific features that identify an associated illness.

Gonococcal Arthritis. Gonococcal arthritis tends to involve multiple small joints with an acute inflammatory

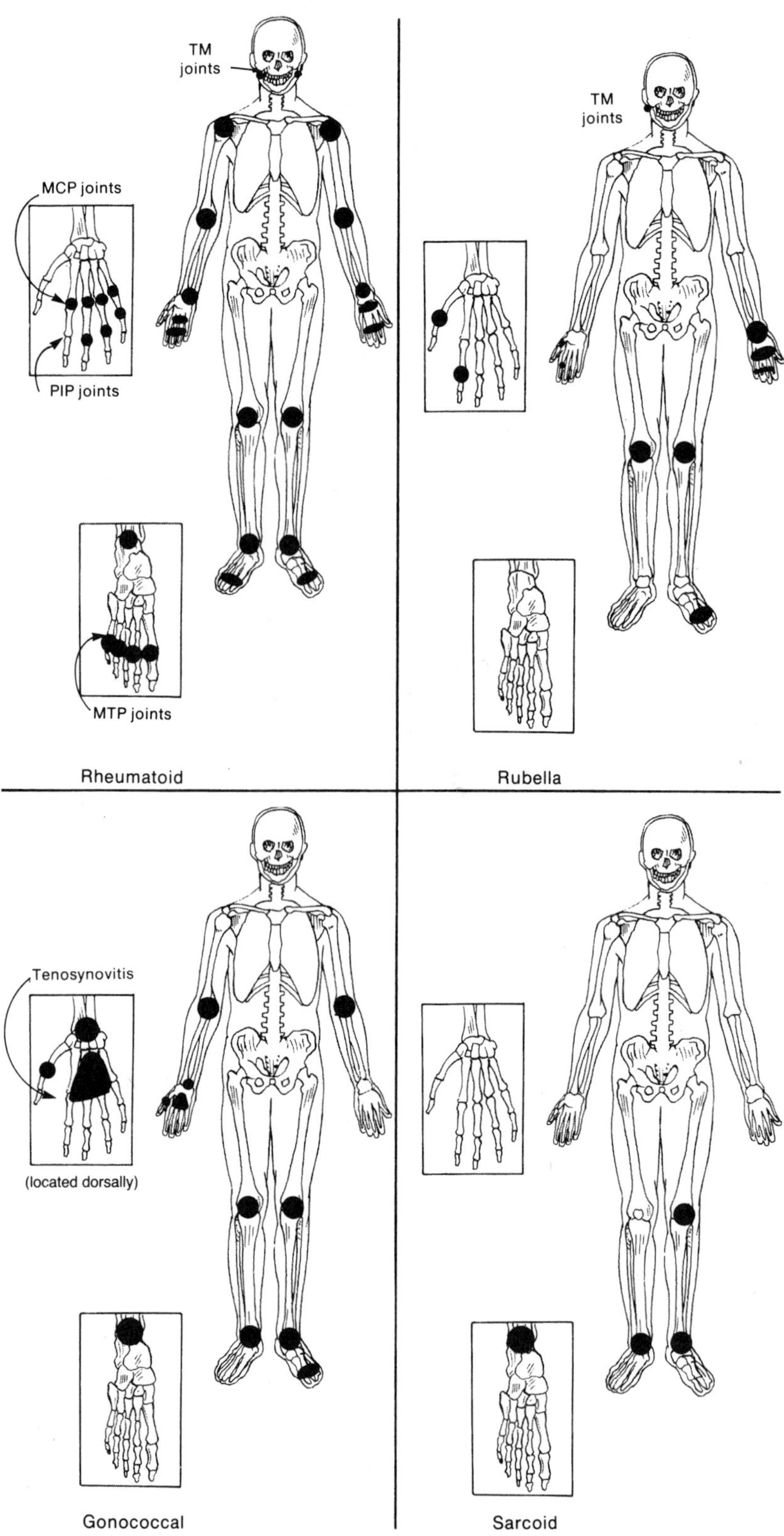

FIGURE 49–9. Patterns of joint involvement in rheumatoid arthritis and in some typical cases with acute polyarticular synovitis. The closed circles are joints with effusions, heat, and tenderness. The patient with rheumatoid arthritis has a symmetric involvement of many small peripheral joints; the diagnosis is also suggested by an insidious onset with gradually developing morning stiffness and synovitis over a period of weeks to months. The onset of acute synovitis is relatively abrupt in rubella, sarcoid, gonococcal, and other forms of acute polyarticular synovitis. Gonococcal arthritis is an acute polyarticular synovitis with asymmetric involvement often accompanied by inflammatory tenosynovitis; rubella arthritis may involve many small peripheral joints but usually with some asymmetry (as shown in the figure); acute synovitis associated with hilar adenopathy and sarcoidosis tends to affect weight-bearing joints such as the knees and ankles in an additive pattern. The patterns shown in the figure are typical for each disease. There is much overlap in the patterns of joint involvement, however, thus one must rely on the associated findings to make a diagnosis.

TABLE 49–5. CLINICAL FEATURES OF DISEASES ASSOCIATED WITH THE SYNDROME OF ACUTE POLYARTICULAR SYNOVITIS

Disease	Major Accompanying Clinical Features
Gonococcal Arthritis	Inflammatory tenosynovitis; shaking chills and fever; small number of papules, pustules, or bullae; onset during menstruation or second or third trimester of pregnancy; positive cervical, rectal, or pharyngeal culture
Reiter's Syndrome	Urethritis; conjunctivitis; mucocutaneous lesions, including circinate balanitis, keratodermia blennorrhagica, and red macules of bucal mucosa; unilateral sacroiliitis; HLA-B27–positive
Rheumatic Fever	Carditis; chorea; subcutaneous nodules; erythema marginatum; increased sedimentation rate; elevated ASO or antideoxyribonuclease B titer
Viral Arthritis	
Rubella	Maculopapular rash
Mumps	Bilateral parotitis
Hepatitis B	Malaise; anorexia; abnormal liver function tests; positive HB_SAg; and eventually jaundice
Others on occasion (see text)	
Presumed Hypersensitivity States and Autoimmune Diseases	
Serum sickness	Eosinophilia; lymphadenopathy; urticaria, and history of receiving foreign protein
Hypersensitivity angiitis	Glomerulonephritis; urticarial, maculopapular, or purpuric rash; colicky abdominal pain
Mixed essential cryoglobulinemia	Raynaud's phenomenon; livedo reticularis; vascular purpura; paresthesias; glomerulonephritis; positive cryoglobulin titer
Erythema multiforme	Red iris-shaped macules, papules, and bullae, mainly of the extremities, face, and lips
Erythema nodosum	Tender subcutaneous nodules of extremities
Systemic lupus erythematosus	Malar rash; alopecia; seizures; polyserositis; glomerulonephritis; hemolytic anemia; positive antinuclear antibody titer
Wegener's granulomatosis, periarteritis, polymyositis, and scleroderma	Polyarthralgias (plus other manifestations)
Inflammatory Bowel Diseases	
Whipple's disease	Lymphadenopathy; hyperpigmentation; gastrointestinal malabsorption
Ulcerative coflitis	Erythema nodosum; bloody diarrhea; proctitis or colitis
Regional enteritis	Erythema nodosum; abdominal colic; diarrhea
Other Infectious Diseases	
Brucellosis, primary coccidioidomycosis, and lymphogranuloma venereum	Erythema nodosum
Rat-bite Fever	Maculopapular rash
Meningococcal sepsis	Chills; fever; petechiae and purpura
Subacute bacterial endocarditis	Fever; murmur; glomerulonephritis; positive blood cultures
Secondary lues	Maculopapular rash involving palms and soles; fever; pharyngitis; lymphadenopathy; positive serologic test for syphilis
Lyme arthritis	Fever; myalgias; headache; erythema chronica migrans
Miscellaneous Conditions	
Type II hyperlipoproteinemia homozygotes	Tendon xanthomata; increased cholesterol levels with hyperlipoproteinemia
Chronic active hepatitis	Abnormal liver function tests
Behçet's syndrome	Aphthous stomatitis (painful); genital ulcers (sometimes painless); erythema nodosum; anterior uveitis; CNS manifestations (meningoencephalitis, intracranial hypertension, focal lesions of the brain stem and spinal cord, cranial nerve palsies, psychosis); thrombophlebitis
Intestinal bypass surgery	Appropriate history
Leukemias and lymphomas	History and findings of leukemia or lymphoma
Sickle cell crises	History and findings of sickle cell anemia
Acute oligoarticular juvenile rheumatoid arthritis	Anterior uveitis; positive antinuclear antibody titer; spondylitis in cases that are HLA-B27–positive
Palindromic rheumatism	Eventually a weakly positive latex titer
Onset of Chronic Arthritis with Acute Synovitis	
Rheumatoid arthritis	Development of chronic synovitis; cartilaginous destruction
Ankylosing spondylitis	Bilateral sacroiliitis and spondylitis; periostitis
Psoriatic arthritis	Psoriatic skin lesions

synovitis and is always a diagnostic consideration in a patient with the abrupt onset of joint pain. Many patients with gonococcal arthritis have a septic phase of fevers, chills, pustulous skin lesions, and migratory polyarthralgias, prior to the development of frank arthritis in one or a few joints. Other patients may present only with arthritis; still others, perhaps the majority, present a mixed picture of simultaneous arthritis and septicemia.[34] Certain features, however, do aid the clinician in recognizing gonococcal arthritis: synovitis accompanied by tender, erythematous swelling of tendon sheaths (inflammatory tenosynovitis); shaking chills or fever in association with synovitis; the characteristic skin lesions of gonococcal sepsis (generally a few scattered lesions that may be papules, pustules, or bullae, sometimes with central necrosis or eschar); and onset in females during menstruation or in the second or third trimester of pregnancy. It is unusual for patients with gonococcal arthritis simultaneously to have active pelvic inflammatory disease or gonococcal urethritis.

Although septic joint fluid has been described in some cases, most have variable cell counts (as low as a few thousand per mm^3) with an inflammatory exudate (usually 70 to 80% polymorphonuclear leukocytes). The results of synovial fluid cultures are positive in about 50% of cases and blood cultures in 20%.[34] The most reliable way to confirm the diagnosis is by a culture of the cervix (also the rectum, urethra, or pharynx when appropriate). The results are positive in 67 to 90% of patients.[34, 35] Hence, culture of the cervix should be considered in any sexually active woman with acute synovitis, since additional clinical features of gonococcal arthritis are not always present.

Lyme Disease. Geographic, familial, and seasonal (summer-fall) clustering of joint manifestations in children in November of 1975 in the community of Lyme, Connecticut, led to the recognition of Lyme disease caused by the spirochete *Borrelia burgdorferi.* The disease is endemic in the northeast (Maryland to northern Massachusetts), upper Midwest (Wisconsin and Minnesota), and far west (northern California and Oregon) and is transmitted by the small ticks, Ixodes dammini and Ixodes pacificus. The ticks are the size of an apple seed, but they swell severalfold when engorged with blood. Infection occurs in about 5% of persons in an endemic area who are bitten by ticks that feed for at least 24 hours.[36]

About two thirds of infected patients have erythema migrans, an expanding red papule at the site of the tick bite, which may be more than 5 cm in diameter, sometimes with central clearing. Patients also have a flu-like illness with fever, headache, chills, arthralgias, or lymphadenopathy.

The diagnosis is made clinically and can be confirmed by the enzyme-linked immunosorbent assay (ELISA), which gives a positive result after several weeks, or the more sensitive antibody capture immunoassay (ELISA capture) for IgM or IgG (currently available in a few centers). False-negative tests occur, especially early after infection or in treated patients, and false-positive test results may occur in patients with syphilis, Rocky Mountain spotted fever, infectious mononucleosis, autoimmune diseases, and some neurologic diseases. A western blot analysis is under development and may be helpful to clarify borderline ELISA results.

Joint involvement includes acute onset of a monoarticular synovitis that is generally followed by the involvement of a few additional joints, with brief exacerbations, remissions, and recurrences. Spontaneous resolution occurs in about 10% of patients annually. Some patients, who are HLA-DR4 or -DR2 positive, may develop chronic erosive joint disease. The synovial fluid in patients with arthritis is inflammatory with a relatively high WBC count of about 25,000 cells, mostly polymorphonuclear leukocytes.

Tick bites may be prevented by taking simple precautions in an endemic area (Table 49–6). Prophylactic treatment following tick bites in patients who have not developed symptoms is of equivocal efficacy,[36] but a cost-effectiveness analysis suggests that such treatment be given when the probability of infection is greater than 4%.[37]

Reiter's Syndrome. Acute Reiter's syndrome is a febrile illness primarily of young men 15 to 35 years old (only about 10% are women) that may be accompanied by rapid and profound weight loss. The most frequent initial symptom is urethritis, and an acute reactive synovitis is the most disabling and persistent feature. The syndrome consists of arthritis plus urethritis, conjunctivitis, and certain mucocutaneous lesions. The arthritis usually involves two to six joints, most characteristically the weight-bearing joints of the lower extremities, although synovitis may occur in the wrists, fingers, toes, and temporomandibular joints. Episodes tend to subside within 2 to 6 weeks, but recurrences, often several times, are very characteristic over a period of 2 to 4 months. Unilateral sacroiliitis is a relatively specific finding present in about one third of acute cases.[38, 39] Periostitis is another feature of Reiter's syndrome that can be an early manifestation, either as heel pain or tenderness (periostitis of the os calcaneus) or as sausage digits (interphalangeal arthritis and periostitis).

Urethritis precedes the onset of arthritis in more than half the cases,[38] but often as a mild symptom manifested only by staining of underwear. However, the picture may include any features of nongonococcal urethritis, including nonspecific prostatitis and seminal vesiculitis; other patients may have a rather severe hemorrhagic cystitis. The conjunctivitis is manifested usually by mild, transient, bilateral conjunctival injection, which should be sought by the examiner after the onset of arthritis and can be expected to subside in a few days.[40] Anterior uveitis may develop during recurrences or after an acute attack.

Mucocutaneous lesions include erythematous macules of the palms and soles, which become waxy plaques and eventually hyperkeratotic lesions (keratodermia blennorrhagica). Painless, circumscribed, red macules appear transiently on the posterior buccal mucosa, or circinate balanitis may occur as a confluent reddened or eroded area of the glans or only as small red spots with central scaling or ulceration. All the skin manifestations of Reiter's syndrome are painless. They can be transient and subtle. Circinate balanitis is the most common,[40] and fully developed keratodermia blennorrhagica is the most characteristic. To be emphasized is the asymptomatic, transient nature of the mucocutaneous manifestations. Typical, for example, would be small pink or brown macules of the soles of the feet, which may disappear in a few days without progressing to a waxy or hyperkeratotic state.[39]

No specific tests establish the diagnosis of Reiter's syndrome. Cell counts from synovial fluid tend to be high

TABLE 49–6. GUIDELINES FOR TICK PREVENTION IN A KNOWN ENDEMIC AREA*

- Wear long sleeve shirts.
- Tuck long pants into socks or boots.
- Wear light colored clothing so that ticks can be easily spotted.
- Stay on hiking paths; avoid brush.
- Once inside, check your skin, particularly skin folds.
- Consider the use of an acaricide, such as DAMMINIX.

*Supplied by Mathew Liang, M.D.

(10,000 to 30,000 WBC/mm^3) with many polymorphonuclear leukocytes (50 to 80%), somewhat decreased glucose levels (60 to 80 mg/dl),[38] and high levels of complement, if measured.[40] Eighty per cent of patients with acute Reiter's syndrome and virtually all those with sacroiliitis, spondylitis, or anterior uveitis are positive for histocompatibility antigen HLA type B27,[41] a finding that sometimes helps to confirm the diagnosis in retrospect. Occasionally patients are encountered with typical articular and other features of Reiter's syndrome who lack either urethritis or conjunctivitis; they can be labeled as cases of incomplete Reiter's syndrome if the diagnosis can be supported by HLA typing.

A reactive, inflammatory polyarthritis with sterile joint fluid similar to that of Reiter's syndrome has been reported in patients following dysentery due to *Salmonella, Shigella flexneri,* or *Yersinia enterocolitica.*[41] In *Salmonella* the stool culture may be positive, whereas in reactive arthritis associated with *Yersinia,* the stool culture is typically negative, and serology is positive.[42] Chlamydial and *Campylobacter* infections are also associated with reactive arthritis.[42] All types of postdysenteric arthritis are associated with the presence of the HLA B27 antigen.[41]

Rheumatic Fever. This still occurs in up to 0.4% of children following untreated, exudative streptococcal pharyngitis.[43] Like Reiter's syndrome, the diagnosis is supported when two or more characteristic clinical features can be recognized. Polyarthralgias and polyarthritis are the most frequent and earliest manifestations of acute rheumatic fever in adults. Pain tends to be more prominent than the objective findings of synovitis. Five or six joints are involved in the average case, most frequently the knees, ankles, or other peripheral joints; but up to 25% of patients have a monoarticular arthritis.[44] Synovitis may follow a migratory or an additive pattern; rarely, however, is a joint affected for more than a few days or more than once during an episode. Organic murmurs, enlargement of the heart, signs of congestive heart failure, or pericarditis occur in less than half of adult cases. Chorea is characterized by abrupt, purposeless involuntary movements. It is a rare manifestation, most often seen in adolescent girls. Subcutaneous nodules are firm, movable nodules on the bony prominences that are smaller and more transient than those of rheumatoid arthritis and occur late in the course of the episode. Erythema marginatum is an evanescent, pink, nonpruritic truncal rash with sharp outer and diffuse inner edges, which occurs early during the episode and is associated with cardiac involvement. Manifestations of systemic illness include fever and elevated sedimentation rate. Only about half the patients with rheumatic fever can recall a preceding sore throat, but although the mean interval between pharyngitis and the onset of joint pain is 18.6 days, the results of cultures of the throat are positive for streptococci in many patients at the time of presentation. Positive cultures, however, may result from asymptomatic carriage of the organism as well as from preceding infection.[45] Serology provides further evidence that rheumatic fever is associated with preceding streptococcal infections in almost all cases, as more than 90% of patients have a fivefold rise or an elevated antistreptolysin O (ASLO), antideoxyribonuclease B, or other titer.[44, 46] An elevated ASLO titer, however, may reflect streptococcal infection at any time up to 12 months of performing the test.[47]

In practice, the clinician may make the diagnosis of rheumatic fever in an adult patient when there are typical joint findings *plus* evidence of a preceding streptococcal infection in the setting of fever, elevated sedimentation rate, and other signs of systemic illness—assuming that no other cause for the synovitis becomes apparent. Suspicion of rheumatic fever is raised if there is a history of a previous episode of rheumatic fever. The major and minor criteria of Jones are sometimes useful but often difficult to apply to adult patients. Whereas arthritis is reported to occur in 90% of adults with acute rheumatic fever, carditis occurs in only about 35%.[46] Conversely, myopericarditis not only is a feature of some cases of rheumatic fever but also may develop in the course of Lyme arthritis, *Yersinia*-associated arthritis, and a variety of viral illnesses (e.g., coxsackie A and B, ECHO type 6 and 8, influenza A, hepatitis B, Epstein-Barr, mumps, polio, varicella) that may frequently or occasionally be associated with arthritis.[48, 49] Erythema marginatum and subcutaneous nodules are infrequently, if ever, present,[46, 50] but erythema nodosum is present in 4 to 7% of adults with rheumatic fever.[46] Suggested revisions of the Jones criteria include both evidence of preceding streptococcal infection[51] and exclusion of other causes of arthritis.[52]

Synovitis in the Course of Other Systemic Illnesses. A large number of diseases are associated with acute synovitis. These are listed in Table 49–5, which also gives key clinical features and laboratory findings. It is conceivable that in many cases the mechanism for the development of synovitis in the course of these illnesses involves deposition of soluble immune complexes within the synovium. There is evidence for this pathogenesis in systemic lupus erythematosus (DNA–anti DNA), serum sickness (foreign protein–antibody), hepatitis B (HB_sAg-antibody), Lyme arthritis (cryoprecipitates), and mixed essential cryoglobulinemia (IgM-IgG), among others.[53]

Rubella, hepatitis B, and *mumps* are the *viral illnesses* most likely to be encountered within the United States that are characteristically associated with acute synovitis; there are also case reports of arthritis following coxsackie, influenza, adenoviral and echoviral infections, rubeola, varicella and, rarely, infectious mononucleosis.[48, 54] Arthritis occurs in 15% of adults at the onset or immediately following development of the rash in rubella. Joint symptoms last 3 to 5 days on the average. Joint symptoms were reported in 25 to 50% of adults at ages 20 to 33 who were vaccinated with attenuated rubella virus because of having an undetectable rubella antibody titer; in a few cases, the joint involvement persisted for months or longer.[48, 55] Typically, the acute symptoms of rubella or postrubella vaccination arthritis include polyarthritis involving multiple small joints, including MCP and PIP, with morning stiffness and effusions. Tenosynovitis can occur, or the only manifestation may be monoarticular synovitis. Early synovial fluid findings are noninflammatory, but an inflammatory effusion identical to that of rheumatoid arthritis is found in cases that persist for weeks to months.[55] The synovitis that occurs with hepatitis B or mumps is similar to that described in rubella. Arthritis in hepatitis B occurs during the prodromal phase of antigen excess (high HB_sAg titers) and tends to resolve as jaundice develops, but it may persist for months in some cases. The occurrence, at the onset, of an urticarial eruption and the finding of reduced total hemolytic complement and C4 levels complete the picture of a disorder involving soluble antigen-antibody complexes.[56] The diagnosis can be established from the transaminase level, which is elevated by the time arthritis develops.

"Other" Polyarticular Synovitis. *Serum sickness* is the prototype of *synovitis associated with hypersensitivity,* but synovitis is associated with a variety of other presumed hypersensitivity states. One depends on associated clinical findings to distinguish among the various conditions. In serum sickness, there are eosinophilia, lymphadenopathy, and urticaria, together with the history of receiving a foreign protein. *Hypersensitivity angiitis,* sometimes caused by a drug allergy, is manifested by glomerulonephritis and an urticarial, macular, or purpuric rash most commonly involving the lower extremities, together with acute synovitis. A similar picture of polyarthritis and rash may develop after intestinal bypass and is thought to reflect immune complexes related to bacterial antigens in a blind intestinal loop.[57,58] The clinical manifestations of *essential mixed cryoglobulinemia* in some cases related to antigenenia from chronic hepatitis, include Raynaud's phenomenon, livedo reticularis, vascular purpura, paresthesias, and glomerulonephritis.[59] Some patients with *erythema multiforme* have associated signs of synovitis. In *erythema nodosum,* fever and synovitis often occur in addition to crops of tender, painful, red, slightly raised nodules on the anterior surfaces of the lower extremities. This syndrome has been associated with primary tuberculosis, streptococcal infections, treatment with sulfonamides, ulcerative colitis, psittacosis, yersinosis, coccidioidomycosis, histoplasmosis, lymphogranuloma venereum, cat-scratch fever, Behçet's syndrome, and the taking of birth control pills.[60] However, synovitis and erythema nodosum are frequently associated with the syndrome of bilateral hilar adenopathy, which is thought to be a self-limited form of sarcoidosis.[60]

Joint symptoms are present during the first episode in two thirds of patients with *systemic lupus erythematosus,* most frequently manifested as polyarthralgias rather than acute synovitis.[44] Polyarthralgias without frank arthritis also are characteristic of *periarteritis, Wegener's granulomatosis, polymyositis, eosinophilic fasciitis* (diffuse fasciitis with eosinophilia),[61] and other connective tissue diseases. In lupus and in *scleroderma,* chronic involvement of joints often develops.

Ulcerative colitis, regional enteritis, and *Whipple's disease* are associated with an acute "migratory" synovitis, which generally occurs during clinically apparent exacerbations, is accompanied by erythema nodosum, and rarely precedes the gastrointestinal symptoms (except in Whipple's disease, in which episodes of transient migratory synovitis may precede bowel symptoms by as long as 5 years). Spondylitis, sacroiliitis, and uveitis develop in the subset of those with inflammatory bowel diseases who are HLA-B27–positive. These latter manifestations progress independently of the activity of the bowel disease, whereas the acute synovitis characteristically begins abruptly, involves a few peripheral joints (often no more than three), persists for weeks to months, and subsides spontaneously, leaving no permanent articular damage.[62]

Lyme disease, an important *infectious* cause of polyarthritis, is discussed in detail earlier. Polyarthralgias may occur at the onset of several other infectious diseases, including *brucellosis, primary coccidioidomycosis,* and *lymphogranuloma venereum.* The mechanism may be the same as that of erythema nodosum. Arthritis is uncommon but has been reported in a few patients with *Mycoplasma pneumoniae* infections.[63] Polyarthralgias and sometimes arthritis occur in *subacute bacterial endocarditis, chronic active hepatitis,* and *secondary lues,* presumably caused by immune complex deposition. In *rat-bite fever,* a maculopapular rash accompanies polyarthralgias that may evolve into an inflammatory polyarthritis. Likewise, *meningococcal sepsis* is characterized by symmetric polyarthralgias, together with petechiae and purpura, followed within a few days by polyarthritis. In both of these infectious diseases, culture of the joint fluid is positive at the time the patient has arthritis. Uncommonly, the patient with meningococcal sepsis may develop a recurrence of polyarthritis 10 to 14 days after treatment of the infection; if the results of diagnostic aspirations and cultures of the joints are negative, the synovitis may be approached as a hypersensitivity reaction, possibly to meningococcal antigen.

Acute synovitis may develop in a large number of other conditions. An acute inflammatory synovitis occurs in patients homozygous for *type II hyperlipoproteinemia.* Acute arthritis and peripheral fat necrosis are reported during acute pancreatitis.[64] Polyarticular acute gout may develop, especially in medically ill patients and usually in those with a prior history of gouty attacks.[65] *Behçet's syndrome* is characterized by aphthous stomatitis and genital ulcers generally accompanied by some combination of polyarthritis, erythema nodosum, anterior uveitis, central nervous system involvement, and thrombophlebitis. The inflammatory polyarthritis in this syndrome is nondestructive but tends to persist for months rather than following a relapsing course.[66] Involvement of the synovium may be implicated in the acute arthritis associated with *leukemias, lymphomas,* and *sickle cell crises.* Both seronegative and seropositive cases with joint involvement resembling rheumatoid arthritis have been reported in association with *solid tumors* and *mesotheliomas,* although the coincidental concurrence of two diseases cannot be excluded in such cases.[67]

Acute Synovitis of Unknown Cause. It should be clear from the preceding discussion that, except for the accompanying clinical manifestations, no characteristics reliably distinguish the acute polyarthritis that may develop in the course of one systemic illness from another. The term palindromic rheumatism is used to describe the occurrence of transient attacks of synovitis without other manifestations. Upper extremity joints are predominantly involved in this entity, which is also characterized by the very brief duration of the synovitis (hours to days). There is no cartilaginous destruction. Initially about 80% of these patients are latex-negative; if followed for 3 years, 90% become at least weakly latex-positive, and about one half have symptoms described as compatible with low-grade rheumatoid arthritis.[68] Either ankylosing spondylitis or psoriatic arthritis, in a minority of cases, also may present as recurrent transient attacks of polyarthritis, with development of characteristic features (see Chapter 50) later in the course of the illness. In a common subtype of juvenile rheumatoid arthritis (JRA), an acute oligoarticular synovitis may be associated with anterior uveitis and a positive antinuclear antibody test. In individuals who are HLA-B27–positive, this form of JRA is also associated with spondylitis.

Since patients with JRA are latex-negative, there is no way in the absence of associated findings to distinguish the acute onset of such a case in a teenager or young adult from any other form of synovitis. Recently, rubella virus was isolated from the blood and synovial fluid mononuclear cells of some children with clinical features of JRA.[69] *Lyme arthritis* provides another example of a specific disease originally mistaken for JRA. A seronegative symmetric polysynovitis associated with pitting edema (RS_3PE) has been described in elderly persons.[70] This condition subsides after several months and responds to treatment with low-dose corticosteroids.

Several other syndromes are in the differential diagnosis of polyarthritis but have little or no joint manifestations. Polymyalgia and giant cell arteritis present with proximal muscle stiffness, often abrupt in onset, without muscle weakness, and with minimal or no accompanying synovitis (see Chapter 50). There are no objective joint findings in fibrositis, although patients may have periarticular pains and tenderness (see Chapter 50). Syndromes resembling polymyositis (e.g., proximal muscle weakness, myalgias, and extreme fatigue) and Sjögren's syndrome (salivary gland enlargement and arthralgias) are associated with HIV-viral infections.

Synovitis of recent onset but with no apparent etiology was described in a group of 24 patients who had joint biopsies, other studies, and clinical follow-up in an effort to establish a diagnosis.[71] Six of the patients eventually developed rheumatoid arthritis. Among the remainder, the following diagnoses were eventually established: juvenile rheumatoid arthritis (three cases), systemic lupus erythematosus (two cases), erythema nodosum (two cases), scleroderma (one case), and hypersensitivity angiitis (one case). In the remaining nine cases (40%), no diagnosis was established. These were termed "transient synovitis." Laboratory values, synovial analyses, and synovial biopsies were nonspecific in all of the cases, so that only by clinical follow-up was an etiology eventually established in the 60% in which there was a specific diagnosis. It was thought that most of the undiagnosed cases were associated with sporadic viral infections.

Diagnostic Procedures

Radiographic Findings. Nonspecific soft tissue swelling around joints appears as a fusiform, symmetric enlargement. Erosion of cartilage with narrowing of joint spaces or destruction of subchondral bone, reactive sclerosis, and osteophyte formation are manifestations of permanent articular damage. When these are present, the differential diagnosis is that of a chronic or subacute arthritis, to be discussed in Chapter 50.

Synovial Fluid Analysis (see Table 49–4). This is noninflammatory (≤ 1000 WBC, ≤ 25% polymorphonuclear leukocytes) in many forms of acute early synovitis, including systemic lupus erythematosus, rubella, inflammatory bowel diseases, erythema nodosum, other hypersensitivity states, and even very early in the course of rheumatoid arthritis in some patients. It may contain 50 to 90% monocytes.[54] Higher cell counts with increased polymorphonuclear leukocytes (inflammatory fluids) are more characteristic of rheumatic fever, gout, Lyme disease, and Reiter's syndrome. Since gout can be polyarticular, the synovial fluid should be examined for crystals. In gonococcal arthritis, the joint fluid is inflammatory or septic (≥50,000 WBC, ≥90% polymorphonuclear leukocytes).

Other Tests. Rheumatoid factor, antinuclear antibodies, hepatitis antigen, cryoglobulin levels, immune complex levels, complement levels, antineutrophil cytoplasmic autoantibody titer (in suspected necrotizing vasculitis),[72] and HLA typing may be helpful in establishing the diagnosis of polyarteritis in persistent cases (see further on and Chapter 50), though in the absence of specific features, may not be indicated in the initial assessment of a patient with this syndrome.

Approach to and Management of Acute Polyarticular Synovitis

The approach to the patient whose chief complaint is acute polyarticular synovitis must take into account the numerous possible etiologies of this syndrome and that the joint involvement itself is usually not diagnostic. The clinician must search carefully for other clinical findings that may help to establish a specific diagnosis (listed in Table 49–5). In general, any condition associated with *circulating soluble immune complexes,* including *infectious diseases,* and any *vasculitis* involving small or medium-sized vessels or *hypersensitivity* state, including the conditions associated with *erythema nodosum,* may present acute polyarticular synovitis. If there are no findings at the time of presentation except polyarthritis, the *initial* approach should exclude conditions requiring *immediate treatment,* including not only those that are medical emergencies but also disorders for which *prophylactic or early therapy* may favorably influence the course of the illness.

Disorders Requiring Immediate Treatment. Gonococcal arthritis is the most commonly encountered bacterial joint disease requiring immediate treatment; others include Lyme disease, subacute bacterial endocarditis, meningococcal sepsis, and septic joint disease with polyarticular involvement caused by staphylococci or other bacteria. To recognize the last group, one must depend on obtaining a history of chills and fever or predisposing factors for endocarditis or septicemia (e.g., previously known valvular heart disease, presence of a local source of infection, debilitation, immunosuppression, including HIV infection, or heroin addiction) or noting a heart murmur, petechiae, purpura, one or two exquisitely painful joints, or other findings that suggest infection on examination. Any of the latter should lead to obtaining blood cultures and/or culture and Gram stain of synovial fluid.

Gonococcal arthritis must be suspected in any sexually active young person, particularly a woman who is within 1 week of menstruation or in the second or third trimester of pregnancy, who develops acute arthritis or inflammatory tenosynovitis. If no features suggest another etiology, cervical, rectal, urethral or pharyngeal gonococcal cultures should be obtained even in the absence of typical gonococcal skin lesions.

Although gonococci isolated from patients with disseminated gonococcal infections are often more susceptible to penicillin than isolates from patients with gonococcal urethritis, resistant organisms (PPNG) are now encountered with sufficient frequency that ceftriaxone 1 g/day administered intravenously is recommended as treatment.[73] Patients who are asymptomatic may be discharged after 24 to 48 hours to complete 7 to 10 days of oral therapy with cefuroxime 500 mg twice daily, 500 mg of amoxicillin plus 125 mg of clavulinic acid (or amoxicillin alone if known sensitive to penicillin) three times daily, or (if nonpregnant) 500 mg of ciprofloxacin twice daily.[73] For pregnant patients allergic to penicillin, erythromycin stearate or estolate (500 mg orally every 6 hours) has been recommended.[73, 74]

Treatment of Lyme disease (Table 49–7) depends on the stage of disease and organ involvement. In early, localized infections with erythema migrans or flu-like illness, doxycycline or amoxicillin can be given for 10 to 21 days.[75] Both are highly effective.[76] Lyme carditis, meningitis, and encephalopathy require parenteral therapy, usually with ceftriaxone, but isolated Bell's palsy can be treated with one of the oral regimens. Intravenous ceftriaxone has been shown to improve most patients with Lyme arthritis, although a response may not be evident for up to 3 months after treatment.[77] Intra-articular corticosteroid injections should be avoided.

Lyme arthritis develops less frequently or is of shorter duration if patients with erythema chronica migrans are treated as soon after its onset as possible with tetracycline, 250 mg four times daily for 10 to 20 days.[78]

A limited course of prednisone has been recommended for patients with cardiomegaly or complete atrioventricular block associated with Lyme arthritis.[49] Hospitalization is advisable for patients with Lyme arthritis who have a PR interval of more than 0.30 second.[49]

TABLE 49–7. RECOMMENDATIONS FOR ANTIBIOTIC TREATMENT*

Early Lyme Disease
- Doxycycline, 100 mg twice daily for 10 to 21 days
- Amoxicillin, 500 mg three times daily for 10 to 21 days
- Erythromycin, 250 mg four times daily for 10 to 21 days (less effective than doxycycline or amoxicillin)

Lyme Carditis
- Ceftriaxone, 2 g daily intravenously for 14 days
- Penicillin G, 20 million units intravenously for 14 days
- Doxycycline, 100 mg orally twice daily for 14 to 21 days may suffice
- Amoxicillin, 500 mg orally three times daily for 14 to 21 days may suffice

Neurologic Manifestations
- Facial nerve paralysis
  - For an isolated finding: oral regimens for early disease, used for at least 21 days may suffice
  - For a finding associated with other neurologic manifestations: intravenous therapy
- Lyme meningitis, radiculoneuropathy, encephalitis, and peripheral neuropathy
  - Ceftriaxone, 2 g daily by single dose for 14 to 21 days
  - Penicillin G, 20 million units daily in divided doses for 10 to 21 days
  - Possible alternatives for Lyme meningitis
    - Doxycycline, 100–200 mg orally or intravenously for 14 to 21 days
    - Chloramphenicol, 1 g intravenously every 6 hours for 10 to 21 days

Lyme Arthritis
- Doxycycline, 100 mg orally twice daily for 30 days
- Amoxicillin and probenecid, 500 mg each orally four times daily for 30 days
- Penicillin G, 20 million units intravenously in divided doses daily for 14 to 21 days
- Ceftriaxone, 2 g intravenously daily for 14 to 21 days

In Pregnant Women
- For localized early Lyme disease: amoxicillin, 500 mg three times daily for 21 days
- For disseminated early Lyme disease or any manifestation of late disease: penicillin G, 20 million units daily for 14 days to 21 days
- For asymptomatic seropositivity: no treatment necessary

*Supplied by Mathew Liang, M.D.

Prophylactic or Early Therapy. Even though manifestations of rheumatic fever are already present, it is reasonable to obtain a throat culture and treat with penicillin if group A β-hemolytic streptococci are recovered. An important objective, in addition, is to make an accurate diagnosis of rheumatic fever so that penicillin prophylaxis can be given to prevent streptococcal infections in the future. Thus, an ASLO and/or other serologic titer to detect preceding streptococcal infection should be performed when the diagnosis is not known in a patient with polyarticular synovitis. Patients with myopericarditis related to either acute rheumatic fever or Lyme arthritis should remain at rest for several weeks.

Secondary syphilis is an uncommon cause of polyarticular synovitis, but because treatment of the patient and his or her contacts is important, a serologic test for syphilis should be obtained in sexually active persons with acute polyarthritis or arthralgias of unknown cause, especially if associated with lymphadenopathy or rash.

Diseases caused by immune complex deposition, vasculitis, or hypersensitivity are associated with a number of complications requiring management. Thus, if the patient has acute polyarthritis of unknown etiology, the initial evaluation should entail searching for manifestations of these complications, which include acute glomerulonephritis, myopericarditis, vasculitic purpura, and neurologic complications. The work-up includes a urinalysis; recording of blood pressure; careful auscultation of the heart, plus an electrocardiogram if there are abnormal findings; search during the physical examination for purpura, rash, or urticaria; and neurologic examination. In addition, hepatitis B has been associated with vasculitis as well as with polyarthritis, and liver function tests should be obtained routinely in all patients with this syndrome.

If the diagnosis remains inapparent after this work-up, treatment may consist of NSAIDs (see Chapter 50), rest, and, when necessary, use of physical measures, such as splinting of exquisitely painful joints. Joint films are of little value other than as a baseline. Diagnostic joint aspiration is not essential unless septic arthritis is suspected, but it is sometimes useful and should be done for easily accessible, persistent effusions.

Persistent or Severe Symptoms. When polyarthritis is recurrent or persists for more than several weeks without a diagnosis, more extensive evaluation is indicated. Diagnostic studies may include latex fixation and antinuclear antibody titers, serum complement, and cryoglobulins. One should also obtain a chest film (to detect hilar adenopathy associated with sarcoidosis), a test for hepatitis B antigen, and, in the most prolonged cases, films of the sacroiliac and other joints to search for manifestations of the spondyloarthropathies associated with sacroiliitis and spondylitis. Careful follow-up is recommended until the clinical course or the diagnosis is established.

At some point, if joint involvement persists or is recurrent but no features of a specific illness develop, the diagnostic hypothesis will become that the patient has seronegative rheumatoid arthritis. The management of chronic but intermittent polyarthritic syndromes (discussed in Chapter 50) can be summarized by saying that most patients respond to salicylates or other NSAIDs, but since polyarthritis associated with many of the conditions listed in Table 49–5 or with seronegative rheumatoid arthritis often is expected to be remitting or of self-limited duration and, therefore, may not require prolonged therapy, corticosteroids sometimes have a role in the management of symptomatic patients.

REFERENCES

1. Underwood PC, McLeod RA, and Ginsburg W: The varied clinical manifestations of ileopsoas bursitis. J Rheumatol 15:1683, 1988.
2. Purgnen J and Alavaikko A: Intracompartment pressure increase on exertion in patients with chronic compartment syndrome in the leg. J Bone Joint Surg 63A:1304, 1981.
3. Faller J and Fox I: Ethanol-induced hyperuricemia: Evidence for increased urate production by activation of adenine nucleotide turnover. N Engl J Med 307:1598, 1982.
4. Grahame R and Scott JT: Clinical survey of 354 patients with gout. Ann Rheum Dis 29:461, 1970.
5. Hall AP, Barry PE, Dawber TA, et al: Epidemiology of gout and hyperuricemia. Am J Med 42:27, 1967.
6. Hadler NM, Frank WA, Bress NM, et al: Acute polyarticular gout. Am J Med 56:715, 1974.
7. McCarty DJ: Calcium pyrophosphate dihydrate crystal deposition disease—1975. Arthritis Rheum 19(Suppl 3):275, 1976.
8. McCarty DJ Jr and Hogan JM: Inflammatory reaction after intrasynovial injection of microcrystalline adrenocorticosteroid esters. Arthritis Rheum 7:359, 1964.
9. Ward PCJ: Interpretation of synovial fluid data. Postgrad Med 68:175, 1980.
10. Gordon GV and Schumacher HR: Electron microscopic study

of depot corticosteroid crystals with clinical studies after intra-articular injection. J Rheumatol 6:7, 1979.
11. Schumacher HR, Smolyo AP, Tse RS, et al: Arthritis associated with apatite crystals. Ann Intern Med 87:411, 1977.
12. Hydroxyapatite pseudopodagra: A syndrome of young women. Arthritis Rheum 32:741, 1989.
13. Ward J, Cohen AS, and Bauer W: The diagnosis and therapy of acute suppurative arthritis. Arthritis Rheum 3:522, 1960.
14. Goldenberg DL and Reed JL: Medical progress: Bacterial arthritis. N Engl J Med 312:764, 1985.
15. Goldenberg DL, Brandt KD, Cathcart ES, et al: Acute arthritis caused by gram-negative bacilli: A clinical characterization. Medicine 53:197, 1974.
16. Bayer AS, Chow AW, Louie JS, et al: Sternoarticular pyoarthrosis due to gram-negative bacilli. Report of 8 cases. Arch Intern Med 137:1036, 1977.
17. Wisley RD: Popliteal cysts: Variations on a theme of Baker. Semin Arthritis Rheum 12:1, 1982.
18. Kozin F. Reflex sympathetic dystrophy syndrome. Bull Rheum Dis 36:1, 1986.
19. Helle PJ and Karlson AG: Musculoskeletal tuberculosis. Mayo Clin Proc 44:73, 1969.
20. Tumeh SS, Aliabadi P, Weissman BN, et al: Chronic osteomyelitis: Bone and gallium scan patterns associated with active disease. Radiology 158:685, 1986.
21. Conklin JJ, Alderson PO, Zizic TM, et al: Comparison of bone scan and radiograph sensitivity in the detection of steroid-induced necrosis of bone. Radiology 147:221, 1983.
22. Kaluniau KC, Hahn BH, and Bassett C: MRI in identified early ischemic necrosis in patients receiving systemic glucocorticoid therapy. J Rheumatol 16:959, 1989.
23. Goldenberg DL and Cohen AS: Acute infectious arthritis: A review of patients with nongonococcal joint infections. Am J Med 60:369, 1976.
24. Ho G, Tia AI, and Kaplan SR: Septic bursitis in the prepatella and olecranon bursi: An analysis of 25 cases. Ann Intern Med 89:21, 1978.
25. Canoso JJ and Yood RA: Acute gouty bursitis: A report of 15 cases. Ann Rheum Dis 38:326, 1979.
26. Gutman AB: Treatment of primary gout: The present status. Arthritis Rheum 8:911, 1965.
27. Boss GR and Seegmiller JE: Hyperuricemia and gout. N Engl J Med 300:1459, 1979.
28. Sturge RA, Scott JT, Hamilton EBP, et al: Multicentre trial of naproxin and phenylbutazone in acute gout. Ann Rheum Dis 36:80, 1977.
29. Wyngaarden JB: Xanthine oxidase inhibitors in the management of gout. Arthritis Rheum 8:883, 1965.
30. Boston Collaborative Drug Surveillance Program: Excess of ampicillin rashes associated with allopurinol or hyperuricemia. N Engl J Med 280:505, 1972.
31. Berger L and Yu T-F: Renal function in gout. IV: An analysis of 524 gouty subjects, including long-term follow-up studies. Am J Med 59:605, 1975.
32. Fessel WJ: Renal outcomes of gout and hyperuricemia. Am J Med 67:74, 1979.
33. Seegmiller JE: The acute attack of gouty arthritis. Arthritis Rheum 8:714, 1965.
34. Brandt KD, Cathcart ES, and Cohen AS: Gonococcal arthritis: Clinical features correlated with blood, synovial fluid, and genitourinary cultures. Arthritis Rheum 17:503, 1974.
35. Holmes K, Counts GW, and Beatty HN: Disseminated gonococcal infections. Ann Intern Med 74:979, 1971.
36. Costello CM, Steere AC, Pinkerton RE, et al: A prospective study of tick bites in an endemic area for Lyme disease. J Infect Dis 159:136, 1989.
37. Magid D, Schwartz B, Craft J, et al: Prevention of Lyme disease after tick bites: A cost-effectiveness analysis. N Engl J Med 327:534, 1992.
38. Weinberger HJ, Ropes MW, Kulka JP, et al: Reiter's syndrome, clinical and pathologic observations. A long-term study of 16 cases. Medicine 41:35, 1962.
39. McCord WC, Nies KM, and Louie JS: Acute venereal arthritis. Comparative study of acute Reiter's syndrome and acute gonococcal arthritis. Arch Intern Med 137:858, 1977.
40. Ford D: Reiter's syndrome. Bull Rheum Dis 20:588, 1970.
41. Brewerton DA, James DCO: The histocompatibility antigen (HL-A B27) and disease. Semin Arthritis Rheum 4:191, 1975.
42. Haunce TJ and Leitisalo-Repa M: Clinical picture of reactive *Salmonella* arthritis. J Rheumatol 15:1668, 1988.
43. Krause RM: Prevention of streptococcal sequelae by penicillin prophylaxis: A reassessment. J Infect Dis 131:592, 1975.
44. McCarty DJ (ed): Arthritis and Allied Conditions, 9th ed. Philadelphia, Lea & Febiger, 1979.
45. Bumfitt W, O'Grady F, and Slater JDH: Benign streptococcal sore throat. Lancet 2:419, 1959.
46. Ben-dov I and Berry E: Acute rheumatic fever in adults over the age of 45 years: An analysis of 23 patients together with a review of the literature. Semin Arthritis Rheum 10:100, 1980.
47. Stollerman GH, Lewis AJ, Schultz I, et al: Relationship of immune response to group A streptococci to the course of acute, chronic and recurrent rheumatic fever. Am J Med 20:163, 1956.
48. Hyer FH and Gottlieb NL: Rheumatic disorders associated with viral infection. Semin Arthritis Rheum 8:17, 1978.
49. Steere AC, Batsford WP, Weinberg M, et al: Lyme carditis: Cardiac abnormalities in Lyme disease. Ann Intern Med 93:8, 1980.
50. Feinstein AR and Spagnuolo M: The clinical patterns of acute rheumatic fever: A reappraisal. Medicine 41:279, 1962.
51. Stollerman GH, Markowitz M, Taranta A, et al: Jones criteria (revised) for guidance in the diagnosis of rheumatic fever. Circulation 32:664, 1965.
52. Ward C: Observation on the diagnosis of isolated rheumatic carditis. Am Heart J 91:545, 1976.
53. Vaughan JH: Rheumatologic disorders due to immune complexes. Postgrad Med 54:129, 1973.
54. Brawer AE and Cathcart ES: Acute monocytic arthritis. Arthritis Rheum 22:294, 1979.
55. Yanez JE, Thompson GR, Mikkelsen WM, et al: Rubella arthritis. Ann Intern Med 64:772, 1966.
56. Alpert E, Isselbacher KJ, and Schur PH: The pathogenesis of arthritis associated with viral hepatitis, complement component studies. N Engl J Med 285:185, 1971.
57. Wands JR, LaMont JT, Mann E, et al: Arthritis associated with intestinal bypass procedure for morbid obesity: Complement activation and characterization of circulation cryoproteins. N Engl J Med 294:122, 1976.
58. Jorizzo JL, Apisarnthanarax P, Subrt P, et al: Bowel bypass syndrome without bowel bypass: Bowel-associated dermatosis-arthritis syndrome. Arch Intern Med 143:457, 1983.
59. Brouet J, Clauvel J, Danon F, et al: Biologic and clinical significance of cryoglobulins: A report of 86 cases. Am J Med 57:775, 1974.
60. Blomgren SE: Erythema nodosum. Semin Arthritis Rheum 4:1, 1974.
61. Solomon G, Barland P, and Rifkin H: Eosinophilic fasciitis responsive to cimetidine. Ann Intern Med 97:547, 1982.
62. McEwan C: Arthritis accompanying ulcerative colitis. Clin Orthop 57:9, 1968.
63. Hernandez LA, Urquhart GED, and Dick WC: *Mycoplasma pneumoniae* infection and arthritis in man. BMJ 2:14, 1977.
64. Wilson WA, Askari AD, Neiderhiser DH, et al: Pancreatitis with arthropathy and subcutaneous fat necrosis: Evidence for pathogenicity of lipolytic enzymes. Arthritis Rheum 26:121, 1983.
65. Raddatz DA, Mahowald ML, and Bilka PJ: Acute polyarticular gout. Ann Rheum Dis 42:117, 1983.
66. Mason RM and Barnes CG: Behçet's syndrome with arthritis. Ann Rheum Dis 28:95, 1969.
67. Hoffman GS: Polyarthritis: The differential diagnosis of rheumatoid arthritis. Semin Arthritis Rheum 8:115, 1978.
68. Williams MH, Sheldon PJH, Torrigiani G, et al: Palindromic rheumatism: Clinical and immunologic studies. Ann Rheum Dis 30:375, 1971.
69. Chantler JK, Tingle AJ, and Petty RE: Persistent rubella virus infection associated with chronic arthritis in children. N Engl J Med 313:1117, 1985.
70. Russell EB, Hunter JB, Pearson L, et al: Remitting seronegative symmetrical synovitis with pitting edema: 13 additional cases. J Rheumatol 17:633, 1990.

71. Schumacher HR and Kitridou RC: Synovitis of recent onset. A clinicopathological study during the first month of disease. Arthritis Rheum 15:465, 1972.
72. Tervaert JWC, Goldschmeding R, Elema JD, et al: Association of assay for antibodies to myeloperoxidase with different forms of vasculitis. Acta Rheumatol 33:1264, 1990.
73. Centers for Disease Control: Supplement 1989 STD Treatment Guidelines. MMWR.
74. Thompson SE, Jakobs NF, Zacarias F, et al: Gonococcal tenosynovitis-dermatitis and septic arthritis. Intravenous penicillin versus oral erythromycin. JAMA 244:1101, 1980.
75. Rahn DW and Malawista SE: Lyme disease: Recommendations for diagnosis and treatment. Ann Intern Med 114:472, 1991.
76. Dattwyler RJ, Volkman DJ, Conaty SM, et al: Amoxicillin plus probenecid versus doxycycline for treatment of erythema migrans borreliosis. Lancet 336:1404, 1990.
77. Dattwyler RJ, Halperin JJ, Volkman DJ, et al: Treatment of late Lyme borreliosis—randomized comparison of ceftriaxone and penicillin. Lancet 1:1191, 1988.
78. Steere AC, Hutchinson GJ, Rahn DW, et al: Treatment of the early manifestations of Lyme disease. Ann Intern Med 99:22, 1983.

50

Chronic Arthritis

RONALD J. ANDERSON, MD

Clinical Assessment

At presentation, it generally will be evident that a patient with chronic polyarthritis or periarticular diseases has one of three major clinical patterns of symptomatology: (1) *chronic inflammation of the joints*, or *synovitis*; (2) *mechanical or cartilaginous lesions*; or (3) *nonarticular rheumatism* (i.e., chronic extra-articular processes that mimic arthritis.) If joint involvement is present, the choice of therapy also depends on whether the symptoms are caused chiefly by inflammation or by mechanical lesions of the cartilaginous surface.

Distinguishing Between Synovial Inflammation and Mechanical Lesions. Rheumatoid arthritis is the most common cause of chronic synovial inflammation; lesions of the cartilaginous surface develop when mechanical stress or chronic inflammation wears out the cartilage, which happens in well-established osteoarthritis or as a result of persistent rheumatoid synovitis leading to cartilaginous erosions. A number of clinical features can be used to distinguish between these two fundamentally different causes of joint pain (outlined in Table 50–1).

The patient with active *synovitis* has symptoms at rest as well as after activity and is helped by anti-inflammatory drugs. The course may fluctuate, so that exacerbations lasting weeks to months are common; morning stiffness persisting for several hours is a prominent feature. Any joint can be involved. The radiographs may be normal or show diffuse loss of cartilage.

Patients with *mechanical lesions* generally experience symptoms only with use of the joint, and anti-inflammatory agents offer less benefit. The course of joint destruction is insidious but always progressively worse, usually without flares or exacerbations. Morning stiffness may be present but lasts for no more than 10 to 20 minutes. In general, the weight-bearing joints are involved; radiographs character-

TABLE 50–1. A COMPARISON OF MECHANICAL AND SYNOVITIC LESIONS

Mechanical Lesions	Synovitic Lesions
1. Symptoms chiefly with use	1. Symptoms at rest also
2. Antiinflammatory Rx of less value	2. Helped by antiinflammatory Rx
3. Persistently worsening course	3. Course may fluctuate
(As cartilage does not have the ability to repair itself, mechanical lesions, once present, become more severe with time. Asymptomatic intervals do not occur.)	
4. No acute exacerbations	4. Flares common
(In mechanical lesions of any etiology, the rate of progression of cartilage loss is usually slow, and changes take months to occur.)	
5. Little morning stiffness	5. Prolonged morning stiffness
(In the chronic inflammatory states [rheumatoid arthritis, spondylitis, and so on] morning stiffness of 2 or more hours is commonly seen, which correlates both with physical findings and with the severity of the disease. As medical therapy is used to combat synovitis, the effect of therapy upon this process is often monitored by changes in the duration of morning stiffness.)	
6. Involvement primarily of weight-bearing joints	6. Any joint involved
(Deformities of nonweight-bearing joints, such as the elbows, wrists, and metacarpophalangeal joints, generally indicate synovitis.)	
7. Cartilage loss and osteophyte formation on radiograph	7. Radiographs are negative or show diffuse cartilage loss and marginal bony erosions but no osteophytes
(Early inflammatory lesions are restricted to the synovium, and no changes are seen radiographically. Osteophyte formation represents new bone formation adjacent to areas of cartilage. These are typically seen in osteoarthritis as opposed to chronic synovitis.)	
8. Noninflammatory fluid WBC <1000	8. Inflammatory fluid WBC >2000

istically show asymmetric loss of cartilage and osteophytic spurring.

Distinguishing Nonarticular Rheumatism from Conditions Involving the Joints. A number of extra-articular conditions have some features that mimic arthritis. Bursitis and other conditions that present acutely are distinguished on physical examination by finding no involvement of the joint itself but only of adjacent or periarticular structures.

Other causes of pain in an extremity have characteristic features. Neuropathic pain is distributed along the course of the nerve and is usually unaltered by use except in a radiculopathy in which motions of the spine may either provoke or relieve symptoms. Pain related to vascular insufficiency is distal in location and related to use. Nocturnal pain suggests tendinitis, lesions of bone, neuropathy, or a nerve root lesion, but it occurs only in far advanced cases of degenerative arthritis. In myositis, weakness of proximal muscles is the major finding, and pain is seldom seen unless severe myonecrosis occurs.

Primary Fibromyalgia (Fibrositis). This refers to a syndrome of pain and stiffness, lasting for at least 3 months, localized chiefly to tendinous insertions, periarticular areas, and bony prominences.[1] Patients are without objective signs of joint involvement, muscle wasting, and abnormal laboratory or radiographic findings but may subjectively report joint swelling. The syndrome occurs more commonly in young women and is a common cause of arthralgias. Muscle stiffness in this syndrome may be worsened by fatigue, immobility, anxiety, insomnia, and chilling but is often relieved by heat, massage, and moderate activity. At least five "tender points" are usually present, most often located at the upper border of the trapezius muscle, the medial aspect of the knees, lateral elbows, iliac crest, or lumbar spinal areas.[1] Other symptoms in many patients include chronic fatigue, sleep disorder, tension headaches, and irritable bowel syndrome.[1]

Whereas rheumatoid arthritis produces gradual exacerbations and remissions of synovial inflammation that typically occur over weeks to months and degenerative arthritis follows a progressively worsening course related to irreversible cartilage loss, symptoms of primary fibromyalgia are seldom progressive.

Fibromyalgia should be distinguished from "psychogenic rheumatism," in which the symptoms are more variable, shift from site to site in an illogical fashion, and typically worsen more in relation to emotional factors than to changes in weather or physical activity.

***Polymyalgia Rheumatica* (PMR).** Patients with PMR (unlike those with fibromyalgia) characteristically have weight loss, fever, anemia, and an elevated sedimentation rate (generally more than 40 mm/h Westergren). This condition occurs almost exclusively in individuals older than 50 years of age. The syndrome involves severe proximal muscle stiffness without weakness or objective evidence of synovitis.[2] Characteristically the symptoms will subside in 2 to 3 days with the institution of 10 mg/day of prednisone. This feature should not be considered diagnostic, however, as a mild synovitis may have a similar initial response to this therapy.

Giant cell arteritis (GCA) was present in 16% of unselected patients with PMR in one series, but almost all had specific features of arteritis, such as visual symptoms, headaches, or tender thickened temporal arteries on physical examination.[3] The risk of permanent blindness is thought to be 1% or less in patients with no features of giant cell arteritis, who are treated with low-dose corticosteroids.[2] Patients suspected of having GCA should have a biopsy done of the superficial temporal artery, which is reported to be positive in approximately 90% of those who at any point require high-dose corticosteroid treatment.[4] Frozen sectioning at the time of biopsy detects all except a few cases with positive results, and, if the results are negative, one may consider proceeding with biopsy of the opposite superficial temporal artery, which has an additional yield of positive results.[4]

Hypertrophic Osteoarthropathy. Patients with hypertrophic osteoarthropathy have deep-seated aching or burning pain and tenderness over the long bones. This condition may be associated with bronchogenic carcinoma, pleural neoplasms, suppurative lung disease, or cyanotic heart disease. Painful swelling and tenderness over the distal long bones is usually seen only in association with carcinoma. A true synovitis even with destruction of cartilage may occur, however, owing to infiltration of synovial membranes adjacent to bone. The clinician may suspect osteoarthropathy when there is clubbing of the nail beds or pronounced bone pain aggravated by dependency. X-ray films usually establish the diagnosis by showing elevation of the periosteum with new bone formation along the margins of metacarpal, metatarsal, and long bones of the legs and forearms.

Reflex Sympathetic Dystrophy Syndrome (RSDS) and Palmar Fasciitis. RSDS produces warmth, swelling, and stiffness of an extremity and may be mistaken for arthritis. Dupuytren's contracture may mimic synovitis. However, the patient maintains the ability to fully flex the hand but is unable to fully extend. The syndrome usually occurs idiopathically with a familial prevalence but is also associated with hepatic disease. A syndrome of bilateral palmar fascial thickening and finger contracture may be seen in association with ovarian neoplasms.

DIFFERENTIAL DIAGNOSIS OF CHRONIC POLYARTHRITIS

Rheumatoid Arthritis. Rheumatoid arthritis begins most frequently as a symmetric peripheral polysynovitis with insidious aching and morning stiffness of the hands and feet. It is particularly characteristic for it to involve bilaterally the wrists, metacarpophalangeal (MCP), and metatarsophalangeal (MTP) joints. In most, but not all, cases a "doughy" synovial thickening can be palpated at those aspects of involved joints where the synovium is not covered by muscle. Constitutional manifestations such as malaise, anorexia, low-grade fever, and an elevated sedimentation rate occur, generally in proportion to the severity of synovitis and multiple joint involvement. In cases involving warmth and swelling of many peripheral joints, including knees, elbows, and shoulders as well as hands and feet, a clinical diagnosis should be made from the history and examination. More indolent cases with subtle clinical features are likely to pose a problem in diagnosis. These cases also tend to be seronegative, with minimal or nonspecific laboratory and x-ray findings.

In early cases, the history may help to convince the examiner that the patient's complaints are related to a true synovitis of the wrist or hand. The patient will have specific dysfunctions such as inability to open a car door or to remove the top from a jar or bottle.

Synovitis at the MCP and proximal interphalangeal (PIP) joints often results in palpable thickening or bulging of the synovium; however, when there is a question about the diagnosis, one should search particularly for very early synovitis at the MCP joints. A subtle finding may be stiffness with limited ability to flex PIP joints when the fingers are held in extension at the MCP joints (Fig. 50–1*A*). This is caused by intrinsic muscle tightness secondary to a minimal MCP joint synovitis.

Another early manifestation may be tenosynovitis of dorsal extensor tendons. This creates an obvious visible bulging on the dorsum of the hands but characteristically is painless (see Fig. 50–1*B*). Extensor tendon subluxation contributes to early ulnar deviation of the digits. Associated tendon sheath involvement, resulting in nodularity of a palmar flexor tendon, may also produce inability to extend a digit that has been flexed (trigger finger) (see Fig. 50–1*E*) Eventually in flexor tenosynovitis, active flexion of the digits is limited, sometimes with preservation of the passive range of motion. A boutonniere deformity at the distal interphalangeal joint may be caused by tenosynovitis with stretching (or rupture) of the extensor mechanism (see Fig. 50–1*D*).

In the wrist, the synovia may not bulge, but the examiner can elicit tenderness by applying pressure dorsally at the radiocarpal joint while twisting and compressing the joint (see Fig. 50–1*C*). There also is not always a visible bulge from flexor tenosynovitis at the wrist. Patients may have a carpal tunnel syndrome caused by median nerve compression.

Spondyloarthropathy and Other Chronic, Sometimes Intermittent Forms of Polyarthritis. The spondyloarthropathies include ankylosing spondylitis, psoriatic arthritis, and chronic or subacute joint involvement in Reiter's syndrome or inflammatory bowel diseases. The most characteristic features of these conditions are spondylitis and sacroiliitis. There is considerable clinical overlap, but all are seronegative forms of polyarthritis in which there is a significant correlation between the occurrence of spondylitis and HLA-type B27. Although present, by definition, in ankylosing spondylitis, spondylitis accompanies the peripheral joint involvement in only 20% of those with psoriatic arthritis,[5] about 15% of those with Reiter's syndrome,[6] and 5 to 20% of those with regional enteritis or chronic ulcerative colitis.[7] As a rule, spondylitis begins in the lower spine, with sacroiliitis—manifested by aching, stiffness, and tenderness over the affected joints—being the most common initial finding. Bouts of anterior uveitis may occur during the course of idiopathic ankylosing spondylitis or of spondylitis associated with inflammatory bowel diseases or Reiter's syndrome. Aortitis with aortic regurgitation can develop in idiopathic, psoriatic, or Reiter's syndrome-associated spondylitis.

Peripheral joint involvement tends to vary. Ulcerative colitis, regional enteritis, and Whipple's disease (the former two may be associated with progressive spondylitis) usually have transient episodes of acute synovitis without permanent destruction of cartilage. Ankylosing spondylitis is generally, and psoriatic arthritis and Reiter's syndrome are sometimes, associated with a chronic inflammatory peripheral arthritis that is destructive of cartilage, thus producing permanent joint deformities.

Peripheral joint synovitis is the first manifestation in 20% of patients with idiopathic ankylosing spondylitis and is indistinguishable from rheumatoid arthritis, except that fewer joints tend to be involved and of those that are involved, hip and knee arthritis is most common. The course may be remitting but is often chronic with erosion of cartilage. There may also be pain and swelling of the temporomandibular, sternomanubrial, and sternoclavicular joints, as well as the heels and the ischial tuberosities. In Reiter's syndrome, a chronic destructive arthritis may persist after several episodes of acute synovitis; and although, in general, the peripheral joint involvement tends to be more intermittent than in ankylosing spondylitis, it may follow a chronic course, and in some cases, may produce severe destructive changes in individual small joints of the hands or feet.

Inflammatory polyarthritis occurs in about 7% of patients with psoriasis.[6] In 16% of these, the joint manifestations antedate the development of psoriasis.[8] Skin involvement may vary from an isolated plaque of the scalp or elbow to widespread exfoliative psoriasis or to pustular psoriasis of the feet indistinguishable from keratodermia blennorrhagica. The joint involvement most often is temporally related to nail involvement, which is present in 80% of patients with psoriatic arthritis. Any number of manifestations can be noted in the nails, ranging from pitting, transverse ridging, or onycholysis, to yellowish discoloration or total destruction. None of these are specific; for example, all may be found with lichen planus or dermatophyte infection. The clinical pattern of joint involvement may be summarized by saying that generally fewer and smaller peripheral joints are affected more severely than in rheumatoid arthritis.[5] Initially, only a few distal interphalangeal joints of the hands and feet most commonly are involved, but this may be followed by involvement of more proximal joints in an asymmetric pattern. The course of patients with this pat-

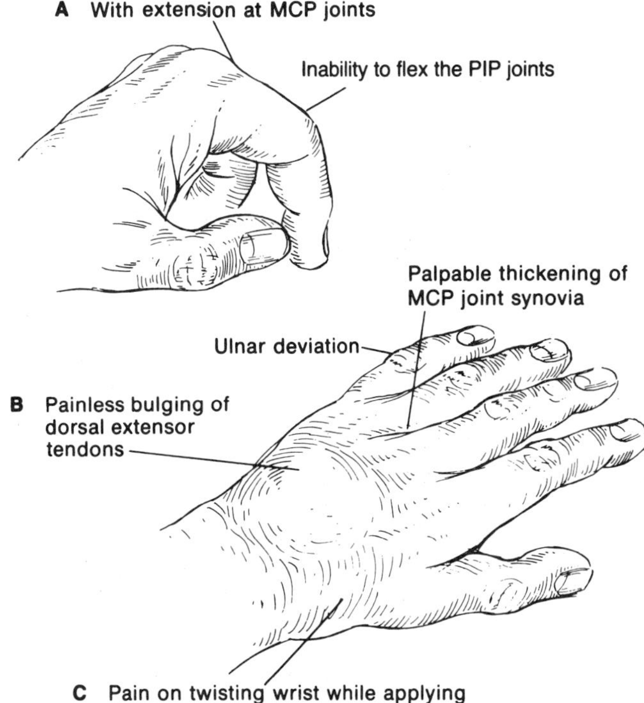

FIGURE 50–1. *A–E,* Findings in rheumatoid arthritis of the hand.

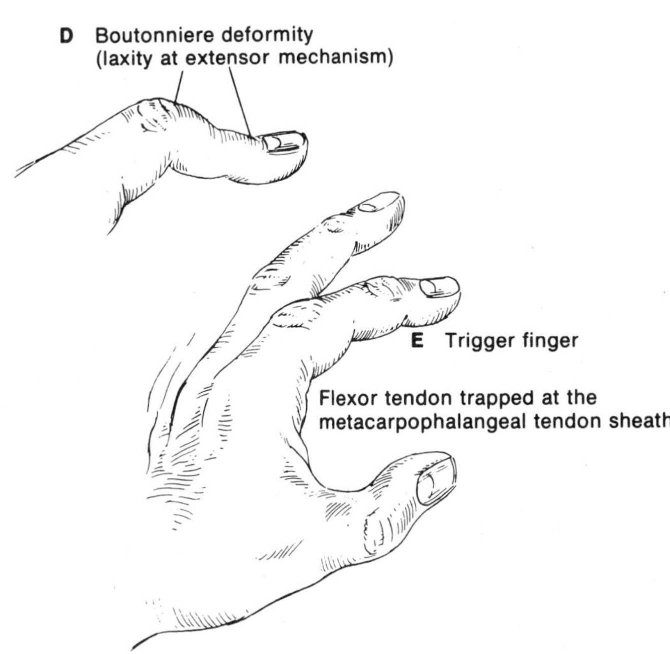

tern of joint involvement is generally characterized by minimal disability and frequent remissions.[8]

A seronegative rheumatoid-like arthritis associated with psoriasis is the second most common clinical pattern of joint involvement; but although such patients may have weight loss, anemia, fever and malaise similar to patients with rheumatoid arthritis, they tend to have more frequent remissions and less severe joint destruction and do not develop the serious extra-articular complications that sometimes occur in rheumatoid arthritis.[8] Other patients with psoriatic arthritis have severe destruction of one or a few distal interphalangeal (DIP) or PIP joints. A few have sausage digits or arthritis mutilans, characterized by severe whittling of phalanges, erosion of terminal phalangeal tufts, and cupping at proximal ends.[5]

In HLA-B27–negative individuals, spondyloarthropathy has been reported in association with hidradenitis suppurativa and acne conglobata.[9] Persistent polyarthritis involving peripheral joints is a feature of many other disorders, including systemic lupus erythematosus (SLE), chronic sarcoidosis, progressive systemic sclerosis (PSS), and mixed connective tissue disease (MCTD). In SLE, periarticular involvement is prominent, manifested by hypermotility of extremities or swan neck deformities, whereas erosive-destructive changes are generally lacking. Similar articular findings, occasionally progressing to permanent deformities, are seen in MCTD, but the extra-articular features include manifestations of two or more disorders, including SLE, PSS, polymyositis, and rheumatoid arthritis. Absorption of terminal phalanges with distal whittling can occur in PSS, similar to that seen in psoriatic arthritis. Otherwise, joint involvement in PSS is rheumatoid-like but rarely accompanied by effusions; rather, there are "leathery" friction rubs, flexion contractures, and synovial fibroses. In sarcoidosis, granulomatous involvement of tendon sheaths and synovia may appear similar to an indolent form of rheumatoid arthritis. Patients are described who developed chronic arthritis of the knees, with pannus formation and cartilaginous erosions that followed bouts of synovitis due to Lyme arthritis.[10] Multicentric reticulohistiocytosis is a rare disorder characterized by an aggressive, erosive synovitis accompanied by reddish-brown or yellow papulonodules of the skin.

Osteoarthritis (Degenerative Joint Disease). Degenerative joint disease may occur secondarily in any joint because of trauma or overuse. Primary osteoarthritis, occurring without such a history, is extremely common in persons older than 55 years of age, develops most frequently in women, and is now the most common cause of chronic disability in the elderly.[11] Repeated trauma and continued use of damaged joints may contribute to its pathogenesis. Obesity is associated with osteoarthritis, but its role in the progression of the disease remains unclear. It is currently postulated that primary osteoarthritis may be related, in part, to hereditary biochemical defects in cartilage structure and that phagocytosis of products of cartilage disintegration by synovial macrophages releases inflammatory mediators that may sometimes hasten further cartilage destruction.[11] Since the disease reflects irreversible damage to cartilage, it tends to produce unrelenting but very gradual progression of pain and disability. Involvement of weight-bearing joints—hips and knees—is most characteristic.

Other joints that may develop characteristic osteoarthritic changes are listed in Table 50–2.

The symptoms are chiefly those of mechanical or cartilaginous lesions. Morning stiffness of several hours' duration is not seen. Discomfort is generally worse after unusual or prolonged activity. Pain at rest and nocturnal pain occur late in the course.

The physical examination reveals enlarged, "bony" joints with crepitus (as opposed to the warm, tender synovitis with effusions found in rheumatoid arthritis.). Osteophyte formation and asymmetric loss of cartilage occur typically; later on, there may be loose bodies ("joint mice") and sometimes instability or "locking" of severely involved joints. No systemic symptoms or laboratory abnormalities appear in patients with degenerative joint disease. The joint fluid is typically noninflammatory.

Occasionally, patients with degenerative joint disease have warmth, swelling, and tenderness of the knees. These findings usually reflect a superimposed inflammatory condition, such as pseudogout or inflammation due to breakdown of loose bodies within the joint. Electron microscopic studies have demonstrated apatite crystals in the joint fluids of a small number of patients with such an "inflammatory osteoarthritis."[12] These crystals are not seen under polarized light.

Osteoarthritis of the hands sometimes is confused with rheumatoid arthritis. The typical DIP joint involvement (Heberden's nodes) is a proliferative process culminating in osteophyte formation restricted to the DIP joints. This familial form of arthropathy chiefly occurs in postmenopausal women and may be present concurrently but is not causally related to degenerative disease of the hips and knees. Sometimes PIP joints (Bouchard's nodes) are involved in this same process, but MCP joints are not involved in typical osteoarthritis (Fig. 50–2). During the proliferative phase, when the joints are involved in sequence, pain and tenderness last an average of 6 to 12 months in each joint. Eventually, the patient is left with painless, enlarged "nodes" but little functional impairment.

Degenerative arthritis commonly occurs in the MC-C joint of the thumb, which serves as a fulcrum in the pinching maneuver. The symptoms are related to instability of the joint and, since stabilizing osteophytes tend to develop over time, in many patients the painful syndrome may run a self-limited course.

"Atypical" osteoarthritis refers to cases with the clinical and radiographic features of osteoarthritis, but with an unusual distribution of joint involvement or severity. Usually this syndrome is associated with a metabolic abnormality of cartilage. The clinical picture sometimes includes thickening or bony enlargement of joints, without the pronounced warmth and morning stiffness that are characteristic of rheumatoid arthritis, whereas the pattern of joint involvement, such as MCPs and wrists, may suggest rheumatoid arthritis (see Table 50–5). Disorders commonly associated with these abnormalities are hemochromatosis, Wilson's disease, onchonosis, and acromegaly. In the majority of these patients, however, no specific etiology can be defined. Radiographic evidence of chondrocalcinosis is not only a universal marker of defective cartilage but is also commonly associated with episodes of acute pseudogout in which an acute inflammatory activity develops superimposed upon or contributing to a degenerative arthritis. In these cases, the radiocarpal, midcarpal, and metacarpophalangeal joints are typically involved. In contrast, osteoarthritis in the wrist usually is limited to the first carpometacarpal joint and possibly the trapezioscaphoid space of the midcarpal joint. Patients with hypothyroidism frequently develop an articular stiffness, which masquerades as arthritis. In addition, the carpal tunnel syndrome frequently is seen in myxedema.

Other conditions may lead secondarily to degenerative joint damage. These include osteonecrosis, hemophilia, Charcot joints (tabes, diabetes, syringomyelia), and Gaucher's disease, in addition to traumatic injuries. Degenerative changes accompanied by pain also have been described in Paget's disease involving bone adjacent to the hips.[13]

Despite the availability of effective hypouricocemic therapy, untreated gouty arthritis occasionally may progress to a chronic polyarthropathy. Patients have a history of previous episodes of acute monoarticular arthritis that resolved completely. Chronic tophaceous arthropathy can develop in a number of peripheral joints, most frequently the first metatarsophalangeal but also other joints of the foot and joints of the hand and wrist, particularly common carpometacarpal joints. Additional features included chroni-

TABLE 50–2. JOINTS CHARACTERISTICALLY INVOLVED BY OSTEOARTHRITIS

Weight-bearing joints: hips and knees
First carpometacarpal joints of thumbs
Distal interphalangeal joints of hands
First metatarsophalangeal joints of feet (hallux rigidus)
Acromioclavicular joints
Facet joints of the spine, in addition to degeneration of intervertebral disks and adjacent vertebral bodies (i.e., spondylosis)

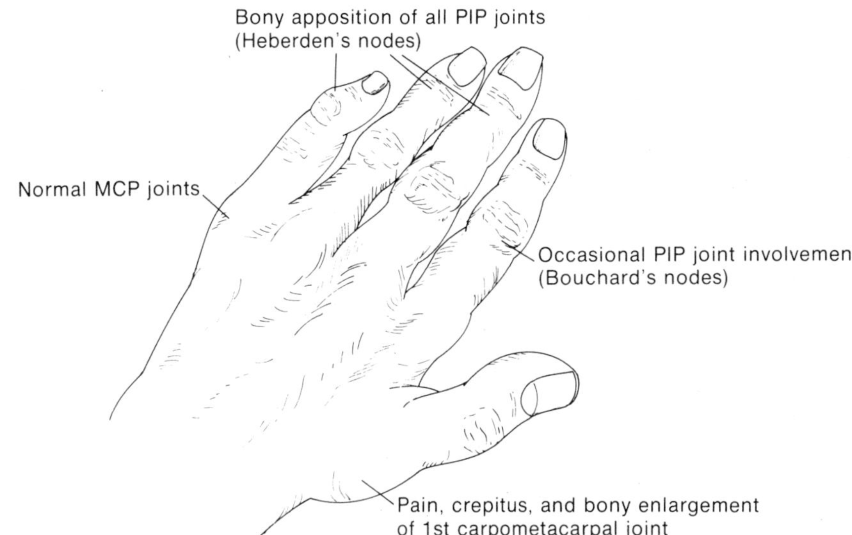

FIGURE 50–2. Typical findings in osteoarthritis of the wrist or hand.

cally enlarged bursal sacs with asymmetric soft tissue swellings representing tophaceous deposits. Today, this picture is uncommon but should not be forgotten in the evaluation of patients with an unexplained atypical arthropathy. Although tophi most commonly are located within the olecranon bursa, and rheumatoid nodules 1 to 2 cm distal to the olecranon, one cannot always rely on their location to distinguish between tophi and nodules; if the deposit is a tophus, microscopic examination of an aspirate will reveal typical needle-shaped monosodium urate crystals.[14]

DIAGNOSTIC STUDIES

Radiographic Studies. The characteristic radiographic features that accompany progressive joint involvement by *rheumatoid arthritis* include (1) soft tissue swelling (synovitis), (2) diffuse early loss of joint spaces (cartilaginous destruction), (3) osteoporosis of the surrounding bone, and (4) marginal erosions. Marginal erosions represent invasion of the joint margins, where bone is unprotected by cartilage, by the rheumatoid pannus. Erosions tend to be bilaterally symmetric and to affect many joints. Except for soft tissue swelling, which is seen better on physical examination, all these findings occur late in the course of the disease.

In *degenerative joint disease*, the major radiographic features are (1) asymmetric loss of cartilage, (2) reactive sclerosis and osteophyte formation, and (3) cysts of subchondral bone rather than marginal erosions. The cysts probably result from microfractures in the subchondral bone plate of the joint. Fingers involved by osteoarthritis may give a radiographic appearance of diffuse loss of joint spaces that can be misleading, but this is accompanied by protruding spicules of bone and a relative lack of osteoporosis. Radiographs of the hand in degenerative joint disease do not reveal the involvement of wrist and MCP joints by arthritis, which usually is characteristic of rheumatoid disease. Patients with rheumatoid arthritis also tend to have foot involvement, with subluxation and fibular deviation at the MTP joints. These radiographic features should allow the clinician to distinguish degenerative from advanced rheumatoid joint involvement. Of course, secondary degenerative changes may develop in longstanding rheumatoid arthritis. However, osteophyte formation is seldom seen.

Table 50–3 contrasts the radiographic features of rheumatoid arthritis with those of degenerative joint disease. Radiographs of the hips in a patient with degenerative joint disease are shown in Figure 50–3.

Almost all patients with symptoms of osteoarthritis will have x-ray abnormalities, but some with advanced changes on radiography have few or no symptoms. For example, in one study, functional impairment in terms of pain, immobility, and the need for support in walking was present in only 22% of those with x-ray abnormalities. In the same study,[15] about 10% of patients with symptoms suggestive of osteoarthritis had joint films that were read as normal.

The earliest radiographic manifestation of *ankylosing spondylitis* and other spondyloarthropathies is usually sacroiliac involvement, with irregularity and "fuzziness" of the joints. Typically, this is bilateral in idiopathic ankylosing spondylitis or spondylitis associated with inflammatory bowel diseases but is often unilateral in Reiter's syndrome

TABLE 50–3. RADIOGRAPHIC FEATURES IN RHEUMATOID ARTHRITIS AND DEGENERATIVE JOINT DISEASE

Rheumatoid Arthritis	Degenerative Joint Disease
Symmetric involvement of many peripheral joints, particularly wrists, MCP, PIP, MTP, and first IP joint of foot	Involvement of weight-bearing (knees and hips), spine, DIP, and isolated first carpometacarpal, first metatarsophalangeal, or acromioclavicular joints
Early fusiform soft tissue swelling (synovitis)	
Osteoporosis of periarticular bone	Lack of osteoporosis
Diffuse loss of joint spaces	Asymmetric loss of joint spaces
Marginal erosions	Subchondral cysts
Little reactive new bone formation	Reactive bony sclerosis and osteophyte formation
Subluxations of MCPs with ulnar deviation and of MTPs with fibular deviation	

DIP = distal interphalangeal; IP = interphalangeal; MCP = metacarpophalangeal; MTP = metatarsophalangeal; PIP = proximal interphalangeal.

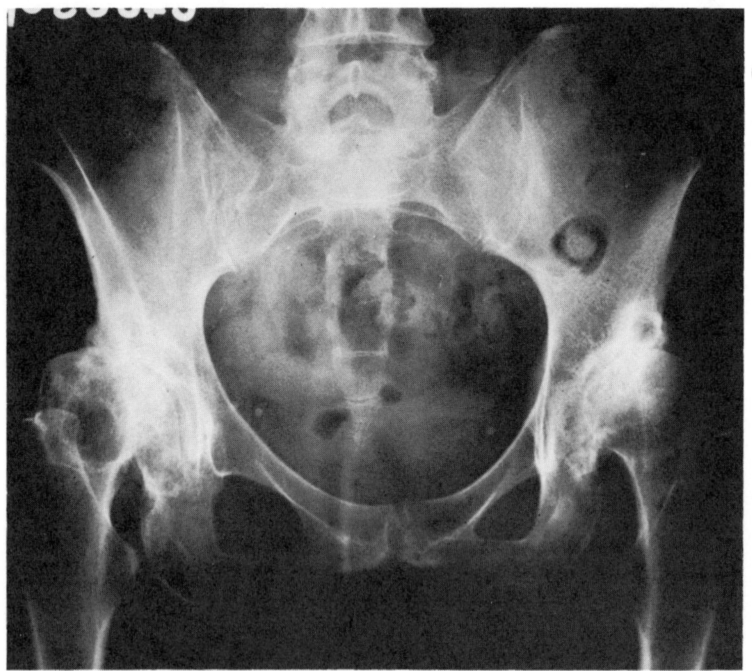

FIGURE 50–3. Degenerative joint disease of the hips. The figure shows an anteroposterior view of the pelvis and hips in a 70-year-old woman with chronic progressive hip pain and disability. The film illustrates asymmetric joint space loss. The most common pattern is asymmetric loss along the superior aspect, with shifting of the femoral head superiorly; this can be seen in both the left and right hip in the film, with relative preservation of the medial aspect of joint space. In rheumatoid arthritis the femoral head migrates axially so that joint space is symmetrically narrowed. This radiograph also shows sclerosis and osteophyte formation typical of degenerative joint disease. On the patient's right, there is an unusually large subchondral cyst of the femoral head.

or psoriatic sacroiliitis. Although specific for the diagnosis of spondyloarthropathy, it may not be demonstrable radiographically until symptoms have been present for several years. In far-advanced disease, the radiographic features of spondylitis related to psoriatic arthritis and Reiter's syndrome may differ from ankylosing spondylitis in that in the former, syndesmophytes are asymmetric and nonmarginal, and there are "skip" areas in which the spine is not involved.

Rheumatoid arthritis of the spine typically is limited to the cervical region, as opposed to the usual onset of lumbosacral involvement in the spondyloarthropathies. In rheumatoid arthritis the cervical disk spaces become narrowed but without the proliferative changes and osteophytic spurring expected with degenerative joint disease. This involvement may progress to atlantoaxial subluxation.

In the peripheral joints, new bone formation with periostitis along the shafts of bones and at the insertions at muscles and tendons characteristic of an enthesiopathy, irregularities at joint margins, and proliferation at the site of bony erosions are the distinguishing features of the spondyloarthropathies. There may be a frayed or "whiskered" appearance at the margins (Fig. 50–4). Calcaneal spurs are especially characteristic of idiopathic ankylosing spondylitis, psoriatic arthritis, and Reiter's syndrome. The radiographic features of the spondyloarthropathies are summarized in Table 50–4.

Chronic gout may be identified by the presence of tophi,

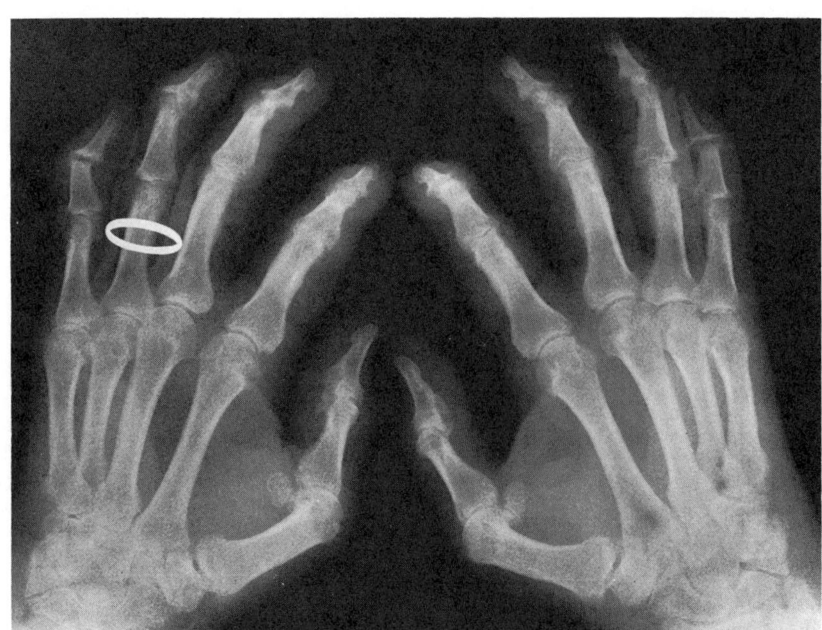

FIGURE 50–4. Psoriatic arthritis. The patient had a 10-year history of psoriasis and joint pains. The radiograph shows typical gross destructive changes with periosteal new bone formation at the involved joints. As is sometimes the case in psoriatic arthritis, involvement is predominantly of distal interphalangeal joints, with sparing of metacarpophalangeal joints and consequently no ulnar deviation. There is minimal periarticular osteoporosis and disuse atrophy of the hand as a whole because of little functional impairment.

TABLE 50–4. RADIOGRAPHIC FEATURES OF THE SPONDYLOARTHROPATHIES

Early irregularity or "fuzziness" of sacroiliac joints
1. Bilateral in ankylosing spondylitis and inflammatory bowel diseases
2. Unilateral in Reiter's syndrome and psoriatic arthritis
Spondylitis beginning in the lumbosacral spine, with late findings of:
1. "squaring" of vertebral bodies
2. ossification of annulus fibrosus ("bamboo spine")
Irregularities and proliferation of joint margins at the site of bony erosions ("whiskered appearance")
Periostitis along the shafts of bones
Calcaneal spurs
In psoriatic arthritis and Reiter's syndrome, gross destruction of joints (particularly DIP and PIP of hand and IP joints of foot) with whittling or cup-and-saucer deformities

DIP = distal interphalangeal; IP = interphalangeal; PIP = proximal interphalangeal.

which appear as asymmetric soft tissue masses, as opposed to the fusiform soft tissue swelling of rheumatoid arthritis (see Fig. 49–5). Additionally, in gout, the erosions are asymmetric (often with overhanging margins related to the intermittency of the condition), and osteoporosis is minimal or absent.

The "atypical" forms of osteoarthritis are not radiographically distinguishable from primary osteoarthritis except that a different pattern of joint involvement occurs. In chondrocalcinosis this usually includes all the MCP joints in addition to the radiocarpal joints (see Fig. 49–6). Table 50–5 summarizes the radiographic features of "atypical" forms of osteoarthritis and compares them with those of gouty arthritis.

In amyloid arthropathy, the chief roentgenographic finding is massive soft tissue swelling due to synovial infiltration; osteolytic lesions from bony replacement by amyloid may also be seen.[16]

Synovial Fluid Analysis. Joint fluid is inflammatory in most conditions characterized by a chronic synovitis, and there are no unique features that allow one to distinguish between the various inflammatory arthritides. However, a relatively low white blood cell (WBC) count in the 2000 to 5000 range is characteristic of but not diagnostic of SLE. In degenerative joint disease and in "atypical" forms of osteoarthritis, joint fluids are noninflammatory with a WBC count at under 1000, unless there is a superimposed crystal-induced synovitis, as in chondrocalcinosis.

Serologic Tests. A variety of serologic tests, including rheumatoid factors, antinuclear antibodies, complement levels, and cryoprecipitates, may be used for diagnostic purposes in patients with persistent polyarthritis. Of these, only rheumatoid factors and antinuclear antibodies are obtained frequently in practice; nevertheless, it is necessary for clinicians to be familiar with the interpretation of all such tests and to know which, if any, are indicated in a particular case.

Rheumatoid Factors. These factors are antibodies to IgG. They are detected by measuring the agglutination of latex particles, bentonite particles, or sheep red blood cells that have been coated with IgG. Using the latex test, 2 to 10% of normal people have positive results. In addition, 25 to 33% of patients with subacute bacterial endocarditis, chronic liver disease, leprosy, or SLE have positive test results. For rheumatoid arthritis, the test result is positive in 90% of those with subcutaneous nodules, in about 80% of otherwise classic cases that lack nodules, and in about 35% of cases thought to be probable or possible rheumatoid arthritis. Extremely high titers tend to be associated with the pulmonary fibrosis, rheumatoid vasculitis, and other extra-articular manifestations of rheumatoid arthritis as well as with a progressive, unrelenting course of joint destruction.[17] Very high rheumatoid titers also may be seen in association with subacute bacterial endocarditis and essential mixed cryoglobulinemia. In summary, the test is neither highly specific nor sensitive for rheumatoid arthritis.

Antinuclear Antibodies. These are detected by exposing a cellular substrate to the patient's serum and by using immunofluorescence to detect binding of antibodies to nuclei. The test has replaced the LE cell procedure in clinical practice. It is chiefly of use in the diagnosis of SLE. Analogous to the latex test in rheumatoid arthritis, antinuclear antibodies are not entirely specific for SLE; however, the test is extremely sensitive, being positive in 99% of patients with SLE.[18] Various patterns of antibody binding within the nucleus may be recognized. Of these, the peripheral pattern is more indicative of SLE, and the speckled pattern of scleroderma, mixed connective tissue disease, or Sjögren's syndrome; the diffuse pattern is more nonspecific. In general, 5 to 10% of normal people have a positive titer in whole serum. Positive titers at 1:10 dilution of serum are found in about 50% of patients with rheumatoid arthritis, juvenile rheumatoid arthritis, scleroderma, and Sjögren's syndrome, or in those taking procainamide hydrochloride (Pronestyl) and other drugs known to produce a lupus-like syndrome. Less than 10% of these patients have a titer of 1:640 or higher, whereas 50% of those with SLE exceed this titer.[18] There is also some correlation between the antinuclear antibody (ANA) titer and disease activity in SLE.

About 75% of patients with active SLE have antibodies to native deoxyribonucleic acid (DNA) and 25% to "Sm" antigens (ribonuclease-resistant antigens).[18] These tests are more specific than the ANA; thus, they may be used to confirm the diagnosis of SLE in patients with symptoms suggestive of SLE and positive ANA titers.[19, 20] MCTD is characterized by the presence of antibodies to soluble ribonucleoprotein but by the absence of anti-"Sm" antibodies or antibodies to native DNA. Most of these patients will evolve clinically into either lupus or scleroderma.

Complement Levels. The CH50 test refers to a bioassay that measures the total amount of complement. This is a screening test to detect patients with reduced levels of com-

TABLE 50–5. RADIOGRAPHIC FEATURES IN CHRONIC GOUTY ARTHRITIS AND "ATYPICAL" FORMS OF OSTEOARTHRITIS

Gouty Arthritis	"Atypical" Osteoarthritis
May involve any joint, especially first MTP, other foot joints, and common carpometacarpal	Involves hips, knees, patellofemoral, MCP, radiocarpals, and midcarpals If etiology is pseudogout, chondrocalcinosis within articular or fibrocartilages
Preservation of joint spaces despite bony erosions	Asymmetric joint space narrowing, bony enlargement, sclerosis, and osteophyte formation
Erosions due to tophi within cartilage and bone, often with a spicule of surrounding bone ("overhanging margin")	Subchondral cyst formation and collapse of bony surface
Lack of osteoporosis	Lack of osteoporosis
Asymmetric soft tissue swelling due to tophaceous deposits	

MCP = metacarpophalangeal; MTP = metatarsophalangeal.

plement, usually as a result of complement utilization in the disease process. The two pathways involving complement consumption are referred to as the classic pathway and the alternate pathway. One may measure specific levels for the various complement molecules. C3, but not C4, is consumed by the alternate pathway. The C4 level is a more sensitive index of consumption via the classic pathway. In general, when complement is involved in the inflammatory joint diseases it is via the classic pathway.

The CH50 test, since it may reflect any immune complex deposition, is probably a better screening test for disease activity in lupus than the native DNA antibody titer.[21] Reduced complement levels sometimes occur in a variety of other disorders that have circulating soluble antigen-antibody complexes. Included among these are serum sickness, hypersensitivity angiitis, mixed cryoglobulinemia, rheumatoid vasculitis, Lyme arthritis, and the prodromal phase of hepatitis B. Detection of reduced complement levels may help to confirm the diagnosis of one of these conditions, but the test is not sensitive. Many such patients have normal or borderline complement levels. More sensitive tests for detecting immune complexes are now available—using either a measurement of the binding of $^{125}IC1_q$ globulin to the immune complexes (labeled $C1_q$ binding) or the binding of immune complexes to Rajii lymphoblastoid cells (Rajii cell radioimmunoassay)[19]—but failure to detect immune complexes by these techniques also does not exclude their presence or possible importance in pathogenesis.

Synovial fluid complement levels are of doubtful diagnostic value in individual patients suspected of having rheumatoid arthritis, because elevated levels do not exclude the diagnosis, whereas clinical findings of severe disease usually are obvious when the synovial fluid complement is low.[22]

Cryoprecipitates. These are circulating immune complexes that become insoluble at low temperatures. These may be monoclonal (either IgA, IgG, or IgM) or mixed (IgM-IgG complexes in which the IgM may be monoclonal or polyclonal). In general, patients with mixed cryoglobulins have vasculitic purpura, together with glomerulonephritis or arthritis, whereas patients with either type of cryoglobulinemia at times may have livedo reticularis, or cold-induced cutaneous ulcers.[23, 24] True vasospastic Raynaud's phenomenon is rare, however, in cryoglobulinemia. Mechanical vascular occlusion occurs only at the very high concentration and associated hyperviscosity sometimes reached by monoclonal cryoglobulins.

Mixed cryoglobulinemia may be idiopathic, or it may be associated with hepatitis C, chronic lymphocytic leukemia, SLE, Sjögren's syndrome, periarteritis nodosa, and autoimmune hemolytic anemia, among others[24]; low titers (usually without clinical manifestations) are found following many viral and other infectious illnesses.

The latex test result is positive in mixed cryoglobulinemia and rarely in hypergammaglobulinemic purpura (due to high titers of monoclonal IgG with anti-IgG activity).[23] Of course, in rheumatoid arthritis there also are circulating rheumatoid factors composed of IgM with anti-IgG activity. These complexes may chiefly be pathogenic within closed joint spaces[25] or in the high titers associated with rheumatoid vasculitis and other extra-articular manifestations.[17]

Cryoglobulins, if present in high titers, can be detected in serum, first by allowing whole blood to clot at 37° C and later by demonstrating a cryoprecipitate of protein at 4° C. The specimen must be handled extremely carefully to prevent cooling, with loss of cryoprecipitate.

SUMMARY OF THE APPROACH TO THE PATIENT

It should be possible to distinguish between chronic synovitis and osteoarthritis, based on the history and a careful physical examination (see Table 50–1). In cases difficult to evaluate, the radiographic features of advanced rheumatoid and degenerative joint disease are sufficiently distinctive to be diagnostically useful.

Patients with osteoarthritic features but an unusual pattern of joint involvement should be scrutinized to be certain that they do not have one of the less common "atypical" osteoarthropathies with a specific etiology.

Patients with chronic synovitis usually have rheumatoid arthritis or one of the seronegative spondyloarthropathies. These latter generally can be recognized because of their accompanying extra-articular manifestations, a different pattern of joint involvement, or the presence of spondylitis and sacroiliitis. In contrast to rheumatoid arthritis, peripheral joint involvement in many spondyloarthropathies tends to be intermittent, to affect fewer joints, and to be more asymmetric. Characteristic radiographic features include periostitis, calcaneal spurs, and bony proliferations at the sites of erosions.

Most patients with chronic synovitis have rheumatoid arthritis. In most cases, this diagnosis will be suggested by the presence of typical clinical features. In such cases, radiographic studies are of less use diagnostically than of use to stage the degree of joint destruction and, thus, help to determine therapy. A latex titer usually should be obtained to complete the evaluation and help in estimating the prognosis, but the finding of a negative latex titer is not a reason to exclude the diagnosis of rheumatoid arthritis.

There is little need to perform diagnostic synovial taps or biopsies in most patients with chronic polyarthritis, since the distinction between rheumatoid-like synovitis and degenerative arthritis should be made on clinical grounds, without an invasive procedure, and since an inflammatory synovial fluid does not distinguish between rheumatoid arthritis and other types of chronic synovitis. Analysis of synovial fluid may help to distinguish chronic synovitis from mechanical lesions of joints or from *acute* synovitis related to SLE, viral infections, or other conditions, when this distinction is difficult to make clinically.

Another type of diagnostic problem is represented by patients whose symptoms consist only of nonspecific arthralgias, general malaise, and, perhaps, vascular instability. When followed over a period of time, some of these patients may develop rheumatoid arthritis, SLE, or other connective tissue diseases. Antinuclear antibody titers should be obtained if there is suspicion of SLE, but a final diagnosis is not usually established until typical clinical features become evident. More elaborate diagnostic studies, including complement and cryoglobulin levels, usually need not be obtained unless there are clinical manifestations of systemic immune complex deposition or cryoglobulinemia. In many of these patients, the symptoms may subside spontaneously; in others, if the clinical course is characterized by morning stiffness and exacerbations lasting for weeks to months but no additional findings develop, the working diagnosis will become seronegative rheumatoid arthritis.

Management

When approaching a patient with chronic polyarthritis, two fundamental questions should be asked:

1. If inflammation is present, what is its natural course and potential response to therapy?
2. Do mechanical lesions exist, and do they merit reconstructive surgery?

The ultimate management (i.e., medical therapy for synovitis or surgical reconstruction of the joint for structural lesions) depends more on an assessment of these factors than on the exact diagnosis. For this reason, the following discussion is divided into two major parts: first, the management of *chronic inflammatory arthritis*; and second, conservative therapy and indications for surgical reconstruction of *mechanical lesions*.

CHRONIC INFLAMMATORY ARTHRITIS

The many conditions leading to chronic synovial inflammation should be separated for the purpose of discussing their management into those that are persistent and those that are intermittent. The former include diseases that, once established, are expected to persist (with continuous activity) for the duration of the patient's life. Examples are rheumatoid arthritis and often ankylosing spondylitis. In the intermittent syndromes, such as Reiter's syndrome, gout, and psoriatic arthritis, symptoms tend to recur but with intermittent activity and at times may be followed by complete remissions.

Persistent Inflammatory Synovitis

The concepts that govern the management of these diseases are:

1. Because persistent synovitis gradually produces erosions and irreversibly damages the structure of joints, the ultimate prognosis for the patient, and specifically for each joint, is predictable within the early years of the disease.
2. The rational selection of agents for management should be determined by the prognosis rather than by the symptoms that a patient is experiencing at the moment.

Rheumatoid Arthritis

Rheumatoid arthritis is the prototype of a persistent chronic polyarthritis. The natural course has been well described.[26–29] Approximately 10% of patients undergo a spontaneous complete remission. This usually occurs in the first 6 months of the disease and always in the first 2 years, if it is to occur at all. The remaining patients will continue with active persistent inflammation. There is a tendency for the specific joints that will eventually become involved by rheumatoid arthritis to "declare" themselves within the first few months of the disease. Therefore, 2 years after the onset in patients with persistently active symptoms, therapy can be based on the likelihood that the disease will not remit spontaneously and that it is highly unlikely for previously uninflamed joints subsequently to become inflamed.[30] Thus, it should be possible, in the course of the disease, to predict the degree of disability if synovitis continues to erode those joints selected and to predict the ultimate options regarding joint replacement.

Nonpharmacologic Therapy. The principles outlined in the following discussion are pertinent to all types of arthritis. Immobilization of a joint by *splinting* not only reduces the pain brought on by joint motion but also reduces the degree of active inflammation from whatever cause. The sacrifice made is a decreased range of motion.[31] Hence, the decision to splint a joint should be predicated on the amount of local relief that can be obtained by decreasing the amount of synovitis, as opposed to the functional importance of maintaining motion in that specific joint. For these reasons, the wrist is usually the optimal joint to splint. Small decrements in wrist inflammation are usually sufficient to relieve the symptoms produced by a carpal tunnel syndrome, a major cause of hand pain in synovitis. With adequate elbow, shoulder, and finger motion, wrist motion is not critical for normal functions. Also, lightweight plastic wrist splints are easy to wear and acceptable to most patients.

Physical *therapeutic exercises* are involved primarily in only two areas of management—that is, increasing or maintaining the range of motion and increasing muscle strength. Range of motion may be benefited by either passive or active exercise; strengthening exercises must be active. It follows that the role of a physical therapist is "active" only in giving passive range of motion. Passive range of motion is required in situations in which the severity of the inflammation prohibits active motion. Once patients are improved, they should be able to continue exercises on their own.

In regard to active range of motion and muscle strengthening, the therapist's role is that of a teacher. In most situations, only the teaching of active range-of-motion and muscle-strengthening exercises is necessary. When the principal deficit is lack of strength, more active participation is required from the patient and not simply more time spent with the therapist.

In ordering exercises, the physician should determine which joints require additional motion and which muscle groups require strengthening. Complete bed rest generally is not indicated. If, in addition to daily activities, the patient learns to perform the full range of motion of involved joints on a daily basis, contractures will be avoided. During periods of severe synovial inflammation, muscular strength can be preserved by teaching the patient to perform daily isometric exercises using at least two-thirds maximal effort maintained for 6 to 10 seconds.

It is important to examine patients in the recumbent posture to detect flexion contractures of the hip or knees. Knee contractures of greater than 10 degrees are major

TABLE 50–6. PHARMACOLOGIC PROPERTIES OF SOME NONSTEROIDAL ANTI-INFLAMMATORY AGENTS

	How Supplied	Usual Daily Dose	Dose Frequency	Cost (Versus Aspirin)
Aspirin	325 mg	4–8 g/day	4 times daily	(about $2/month)
Indomethacin	25,50 mg and 75 mg SR	50–150 mg/day	3 or 4 times daily	about 5 × more
Ibuprofen	300, 400, 600, and 800 mg	900–2400 mg/day	3 or 4 times daily	10–15 × more
Fenoprofen	300 and 600 mg	900–3000 mg/day	3 or 4 times daily	10–15 × more
Naproxen	250, 375, and 500 mg	500–1000 mg/day	Twice daily	10–15 × more
Sulindac	150 and 200 mg	300–400 mg/day	Twice daily	10–15 × more
Piroxicam	10 and 20 mg	10–20 mg/day	Once daily	10–15 × more
Diflunisal	250 and 500 mg	500–1500 mg/day	2 or 3 times daily	10–15 × more
Nabumetone	500 mg	500–1500 mg/day	Once daily	10–15 × more

causes of disability. They result from a tendency of patients to sleep with the hips and knees flexed, often over a pillow, which temporarily reduces tension in the joint capsules and reduces the pain of synovitis. When contractures are detected, the patient should perform range-of-motion exercises and be taught to sleep with the hips and knees extended.

The physician also has an important role in *educating the patient* concerning the course and nature of the illness. In one study, 60% of a population with rheumatoid arthritis who were previously employed and in their prime earning years had become disabled after 10 years of having the disease.[32] In addition to the severity and duration of the illness, the probability of work disability correlated most closely with the degree of autonomy exercised by the patient within the work environment.[32, 33] It was suggested that workers with rheumatoid arthritis may need time off during exacerbations or may need to adjust their work schedule to receive treatment. They may also need assistance in arranging transportation to and from work. The physician can help the patient by informing employers of his or her needs; in some cases, it may be necessary to advise a patient to seek a job with more flexible hours. The physician should also be aware that mortality is significantly increased in patients with rheumatoid arthritis. The mortality correlates not only with extra-articular manifestations of the disease but also with poor functional level.[34]

Pharmacologic Therapy. Drugs available for use in rheumatoid arthritis can be categorized roughly into two groups: suppressive agents and disease-modifying agents that may alter the natural course of the disease.

Suppressive Agents. These are characterized by the inability to produce a remission and, with the exception of the immunosuppressive agents, by their short onsets and durations of action. After a week or two of use, the effectiveness of these agents can be determined. Because rheumatoid arthritis most commonly follows a course of smoldering synovitic activity, and because suppressive agents only decrease the inflammation, which will return full-blown when they are discontinued, one always must consider whether it is reasonable to continue the drug for many years before deciding to initiate therapy. For this reason, it is of paramount importance that the long-term toxicity be minimal.

Salicylates are the standard against which other anti-inflammatory agents are measured.[35] In rheumatoid arthritis, they should be taken regularly in sufficient doses to suppress synovial inflammation (usually 4 to 8 g/day). The limiting factor in their use is gastric intolerance, a feature that usually becomes apparent in the first few weeks. The incidence of gastritis and gastric ulcer is reduced by using enteric-coated aspirin, as well as by using nonacetylated salicylates.[36, 37] The earliest symptoms of salicylate intoxication are usually reversible tinnitus or deafness, most commonly occurring when the optimal therapeutic level of 20 to 25 mg/dl has been exceeded. These reversible side effects may not be evident in the very young, the elderly, or those with pre-existing eighth cranial nerve dysfunction. In these groups, serum salicylate levels may have to be monitored, rather than adhering to the axiom that aspirin may be increased to the point "just before the ears ring."

In recent years, many new nonsteroidal anti-inflammatory agents (NSAIDs) have become available. They include fenoprofen (Nalfon), ibuprofen (Motrin), naproxen (Naprosyn), sulindac (Clinoril), tolmetin (Tolection), meclofenamate (Meclomen), diflunisal (Dolobid), diclofenac (Voltaren), etodolac (Lodine), ketoprofen (Orudis), indomethacin (Indocin), flurbiproten (Ansaid), nambumetone (Relafen), and piroxicam (Feldene) (Table 50–6). Data are not yet adequate on the potential long-term toxicity of these agents, but the following seems apparent in regard to their short-term use: They are not superior to salicylates in anti-inflammatory activity and are five to 20 times as expensive. Although they have less gastric toxicity, the major limitation to their use has been gastric intolerance. The other major advantage of their use is that many of these agents require only once or twice a day administration.

Other side effects of NSAIDs include rash, tinnitus, mental confusion in the elderly, hepatitis, nasal polyposis in sensitive individuals, and renal side effects. The effect of the NSAIDs on prostaglandins may induce reversible renal failure, as well as salt retention leading to edema in elderly patients and those subject to congestive heart failure. Patients being treated with triamterene may be particularly subject to the renal effects of NSAIDs.[38] Sulindac (Clinoril) is possibly less likely to produce renal compromise than the other agents.[39] Uncommon renal toxicities from NSAIDs are papillary necrosis and allergic tubulointerstitial nephritis.

It is believed by some that reproducible individual variation may exist between these agents, so that short (1- to 2-week) clinical trials of different agents have been suggested. I am opposed to this viewpoint and suspect that the combination of a "placebo effect" and the inherent variability of the disease may have created erroneous impressions of comparative efficacy. In addition, to embark upon therapeutic trials with several agents only increases the likelihood of drug-related toxicity. At present, the major indication for changing to a different NSAID should be gastric intolerance and not ineffective anti-inflammatory activity.

Corticosteroids are more potent anti-inflammatory agents whose long-term disadvantages are well known. In general, patients with rheumatoid arthritis benefit from corticosteroids during the initial 1 or 2 years of treatment but "pay for it" later, when the incidences of osteoporosis, muscle wasting, and other adverse effects become substantial, particularly in patients with rheumatoid arthritis.[40] There appear to be two reasonable indications for using prednisone, in doses of over 10 mg qod, for the synovitis of rheumatoid arthritis: first, in the severely inflamed patient who cannot be "mobilized" by other means, and, second, in extremely elderly patients with marginal function in whom one is not concerned about delayed toxicity occurring several years hence.

Intra-articular steroids have been used for more than 30 years. The usual initial result is a dramatic transient benefit producing a happy patient and a heroic physician. On the other hand, there is no evidence that this therapy significantly alters the course of the disease.[41] The major indication for using intra-articular steroids is to suppress inflammation within a specific joint, so that a physical therapeutic goal, such as increasing the range of motion, may be achieved. Complications have been primarily anecdotal but do seem to include an increased risk of infection and local skin atrophy at the injection site.

Immunosuppressive and cytotoxic therapy is also used in the treatment of rheumatoid arthritis. Cyclophosphamide has been studied extensively,[42] and the following principles seem to apply to it and perhaps also to azathioprine: (1) the agents reduce inflammation but usually at doses that are close to toxicity with regard to either leukopenia or hepatic function; (2) inflammation returns upon cessation of the drug; (3) the long-term toxicity is largely unknown and, at present, only anecdotal; however, the consequences of decreased tumor surveillance or hepatic toxicity seem important issues. In summary, these agents are being tried in patients refractory to other forms of therapy[43] but are not indicated for routine anti-inflammatory therapy.

On the other hand, experience during the last decade with low-dose methotrexate given in a single weekly dose of 7.5 to 15 mg has been encouraging. The long-term efficacy in patients who respond has been impressive, and the toxicity does not appear to be cumulative.[44] In addition, evidence suggests that the efficacy may depend on factors other than cytotoxicity and immunosuppression.[45]

Disease-Modifying Agents. Gold salts, hydroxychloroquine, penicillamine, and presumably sulfasalazine all share the common feature of having an onset of action that is delayed until several weeks to months after their initiation. Similarly, their activity persists for a considerable time after they are no longer administered. Therefore, one cannot evaluate the effect of these agents in individual cases simply by observing the clinical effect of abrupt discontinuation or reinitiation of therapy. Difficulty in evaluating the effect of these agents in rheumatoid arthritis is compounded further by features of the disease itself. Synovitic activity tends to follow a pattern in which periods of intense activity are followed by spells of relative quiescence. Because physicians tend to initiate therapy during the periods of exacerbation, subsequent improvement is often ascribed to the effects of the new treatment, rather than to the natural tendency of the disease to subside. In addition, since the manifestations of persistent rheumatoid arthritis are a combination of structural symptoms, which are irreversible, and synovitic symptoms, which are potentially reversible, total remission of synovitic activity may have little measureable effect on deformities or function in some cases.

Gold salts, hydroxychloroquine, sulfasalazine, and penicillamine all have been studied by double-blind controlled trials lasting 6 to 12 months. In each instance, patients receiving the active agent were improved significantly compared with those receiving only salicylates.[46–49] However, for reasons mentioned previously, and because the results were reported as an average for the group as a whole, it is impossible to know from the data whether all the patients were made somewhat better or whether some patients experienced complete remission. This distinction is important, for if the former concept is accepted, these agents will be used continuously under the assumption that many patients might be worse if they do not take the drug. My experience leads me to operate under the concept that these agents either produce a very definite improvement or do little at all. Currently accepted criteria for a remission in rheumatoid arthritis include the following:[50]

1. No morning stiffness (< 15 minutes)
2. No fatigue
3. No joint pain
4. No joint tenderness or pain on motion
5. No soft tissue swelling in joints or tendon sheaths
6. Westergren sedimentation rate less than 30 mm/hr in females or 20mm/hr in males

Five or more of the aforementioned criteria must be met for 2 months with none of these exclusions: vasculitis, pericarditis, pleuritis, myositis, or weight loss or fever attributable to rheumatoid arthritis.[50]

Although there may be a theoretical basis for the action of these drugs, their true mode of action is unknown.

The agents vary greatly in their toxicity. Hydroxychloroquine is virtually nontoxic, its much feared retinal toxicity being rare and not occurring before at least 1 year of use. If the agent is found to be ineffective during the first 6 months, it can be discontinued without risk. If it produces a remission, the small risk of ocular toxicity seems well worth the benefit.

Gold salts and penicillamine seem to have similar toxicities, the most common being dermatitis, stomatitis, and proteinuria, all of which may persist for several months after the discontinuation of the drug. If a remission occurs coexistent with the rash or stomatitis, the benefit usually lasts considerably longer than the toxicity. If the disease exacerbates several months after cessation of the drug, prior rash or stomatitis should not be a contraindication to reinstitution. Thrombocytopenia, due to peripheral destruction of platelets, occurs with both drugs but differs in its severity and temporal pattern. Gold-induced thrombocytopenia is usually abrupt, and severe depression of the platelet count to levels of 5000 to 10,000/mm^3 is the rule. Prompt resolution with corticosteroids is the usual pattern. With penicillamine, thrombocytopenia is usually gradual, and counts under 50,000/mm^3 are rare. Bone marrow hypoplasia has been described with the use of each agent. Myasthenia gravis has been seen with penicillamine use and persists for several weeks to months after the cessation of therapy. Diffuse alveolitis, obliterative bronchiolitis, and pulmonary fibrosis have been described with both agents. However, as these may be systemic features of rheumatoid arthritis, the role of penicillamine or gold is uncertain.

Gold is administered intramuscularly, either in the form of gold thiomaleate (Myochrysine) or gold thioglucose (Solganol), in the following manner: 50 mg is given weekly until a total dose of 1 g is reached. If benefit is seen, the dose is reduced to 50 mg intramuscularly every 4 weeks for an indeterminate period. Most patients who discontinue gold therapy when in remission experience a recrudescence of their disease. Therefore, also because most toxicities to gold occur during the first 6 months, patients in remission on gold therapy are usually continued on it permanently.

Auranofin, an oral form of gold, has been developed within the last decade. Given in doses of 3 mg twice daily, the drug is approximately 25% absorbed from the gastrointestinal tract and reaches a steady-state concentration after 8 to 12 weeks of treatment.[51] It appears to be somewhat less toxic and also somewhat less effective than parenteral gold.[52,53] Rash and proteinuria may occur less often, but diarrhea and other gastrointestinal side effects are common, and thrombocytopenia appears to be equally common when auranofin is used in place of parenteral gold.[51,54] Aplastic anemia has not been reported with oral gold, but insufficient experience exists to be certain of the true incidence of this rare toxicity. If no response occurs after 6 months, the dose of oral gold may be increased to 3 mg tid for an additional month's trial.[51] Auranofin is much more expensive than injectable gold, but the cost of obtaining an injection is avoided. Switching patients who are doing well on parenteral gold therapy to oral gold does not appear indicated.

The precise role of sulfasalazine in the treatment of rheumatoid arthritis is still being determined, but it appears to have a pattern of activity similar to the previously mentioned disease-modifying agents. Toxicities include rash, fever, hemolysis, bone marrow suppression, and hepatic dysfunction. The usual dose is 2 to 3 g/day.

Summary. Basic pharmacotherapy of rheumatoid arthritis should begin with the treatment of all patients by full doses of a suppressive agent (usually aspirin). If the disease appears to be persistent, one then should perform sequential trials of 6 months or more with hydroxychloroquine, gold salts, sulfasalazine, or penicillamine in an attempt to induce a remission. If a remission or major clinical improvement does not occur, these drugs should be discontinued, the suppressive agent should be maintained, weekly methotrexate may be instituted, and surgical therapy considered when appropriate.

Ankylosing Spondylitis

Ankylosing spondylitis does not seem to respond to gold, hydroxychloroquine, or penicillamine. Experience suggests that sulfasalazine may be of value, however, particularly in patients with peripheral synovitis as a major feature.[55] Otherwise, pharmacologic therapy predominantly involves the use of suppressive agents. For unknown reasons, phenylbutazone and indomethacin are significantly more effective than other agents within the same group. Although concern should exist about their potential gastric and hematologic toxicity (with phenylbutazone), greater efficacy seems to warrant long-term use of these agents in persistently active spondylitis.

There is a tendency for the spondylitic patient to stoop forward in flexion, thus opening up the vertebral joints and relieving symptoms. This leads to a fixed flexion deformity when the spine ultimately fuses and to significant dysfunction resulting from the abnormal posture. The physician should routinely measure the patient's height and the distance from the occiput to a vertical axis to determine whether the patient is tilting. If tilting begins to develop, specific exercises should be prescribed and postural habits altered to prevent this deformity. In some situations, the use of a brace may be indicated.

The natural course of spondylitis is progression to complete spinal fusion, usually from the sacroiliac joint cephalad. Fusion is usually associated with loss of pain, and once total ankylosis of the spine occurs, the symptoms become primarily mechanical, although anemia and an elevated erythrocyte sedimentation rate usually persist. Despite loss of spinal mobility in approximately 40% of patients followed for 38 years, more than 90% of patients continued to function well.[56] The identification of the HLA-B27 antigen has broadened the concept of spondylitis, leading to the discovery of mild and intermittent cases of ankylosing spondylitis. Often the process is limited to only a few areas of the spine.[57] However, the ultimate course cannot be predicted, and the basic program of management is the same as for more severe cases.

Chronic but Intermittent Polyarthritic Syndromes

Disorders in this category include psoriatic arthritis, Reiter's syndrome, the arthritis of inflammatory bowel disease, juvenile rheumatoid arthritis, "latex-negative rheumatoid arthritis," and erythema nodosum. Although the pathologic findings are virtually identical to those of rheumatoid arthritis, the clinical course of these conditions differs in view of their common tendency to enter spontaneous and often permanent or prolonged remissions. The management of these disorders follows the same basic principles as discussed previously for rheumatoid arthritis in regard to the use of suppressive agents, physical therapy, and also with regard to indications for surgical reconstruction. The management, however, differs in two distinct areas: the use of disease-modifying agents (hydroxychloroquine, gold salts, and penicillamine) and the use of cytotoxic or immunosuppressive agents and corticosteroids.

The use of disease-modifying agents in these diseases is controversial. Because their action is to provoke a remission after a delay of several months, and because the effects persist after the drug is discontinued, one cannot evaluate their efficacy on the basis of clinical trials of abrupt initiation and cessation of treatment. As the frequency of spontaneous remissions in these disorders within a given period of time appears to be similar to the frequency of drug-induced remissions in rheumatoid arthritis, there are no substantial data with which to assess the value of these agents in the management of these diseases. I believe that the more closely "latex-negative rheumatoid arthritis" resembles classic latex-positive rheumatoid arthritis, the more likely remission-type agents are to be effective. Gold salts, hydroxychloroquine, and penicillamine have been used with success in some patients. On the other hand, in psoriatic arthritis, juvenile rheumatoid arthritis, and the arthritis of inflammatory bowel disease, their effectiveness is questionable. However, because of its low toxicity, hydroxychloroquine is often used when persistent synovitis is the pattern. The results are equivocal.

Corticosteroids and cytotoxic agents sometimes are used for these disorders. The choice of corticosteroids is most rational for conditions that are self-limited in duration and that can be suppressed effectively by relatively low doses. Erythema nodosum, if not associated with tuberculosis, almost invariably meets such criteria; hence, prednisone in doses of 10 to 30 mg/day given for the duration of the disease activity (usually weeks to months) seems to represent optimal therapy.

The cutaneous manifestations of psoriasis can be controlled effectively by cytotoxic agents, namely methotrexate or 6-mercaptopurine,[58, 59] and a similar benefit may be gained in psoriatic arthritis. Arguments for their earlier and more liberal use in psoriatic arthritis as opposed to rheumatoid arthritis are based on the concept that, as the disease is more likely to enter a spontaneous remission, one is not subjecting the patient to a lifetime of potentially toxic therapy. The use of these agents is usually reserved for patients with persistent, severe polyarthritis of greater than 1 year's duration that has not responded to a trial of hydroxychloroquine.

OSTEOARTHRITIS

Medical Management

Physical measures are of relatively greater importance in the management of osteoarthritis, since specific pharmacotherapy to induce remissions is not available, and the NSAIDs are much less beneficial in osteoarthritis than in rheumatoid arthritis. Aspirin and other NSAIDs are usually given in lower doses than in rheumatoid arthritis. Treatment with these agents is most beneficial when more prolonged morning stiffness, warmth, and effusion suggest the presence of superimposed inflammation within the joint(s). There is also evidence that acetaminophen, which has no anti-inflammatory properties, is as effective as ibuprofen in osteoarthritis of the knee.[60] Acetaminophen or propoxyphene may also at times be added to the NSAIDs with benefit.

Since most patients with advanced degenerative joint disease are limited by hip or knee pain, it is important to consider measures that alleviate weight bearing. These may include not only use of a walker, a cane (Fig. 50–5), or crutches, but also use of an elevated toilet seat that avoids the necessity for bending the knees and of handrails around the bathtub to facilitate sitting and standing. Such measures, in addition to chair rest or bed rest, when indicated, will diminish the amount of pain. Patients with involvement of one or both knees should perform daily isometric exercise of the quadriceps muscles (quadriceps setting) to strengthen extra-articular support of the joints.

It is always worthwhile to search for readily treatable sources of pain in patients known to have degenerative joint disease. Bursitis or tendinitis occurs commonly in these patients and may be treated by an injection of corticosteroids into the area of tenderness. Trochanteric bursitis produces tenderness over the prominence of the greater trochanter with pain on forced abduction and adduction but not on rotation of the hip. Anserine bursitis produces a local area of tenderness below and medial to the knee.

Role of Orthopedic Surgery

Synovectomy. Synovectomy is not useful for degenerative joint disease, and although it has been used in the treatment of inflammatory arthritis for more than 75 years, the exact role of synovectomy in the management of this and similar disorders is still uncertain. Knees and wrists are the common sites operated on. In general, the procedure has value only when performed prior to the advent of structural damage to the cartilage. Numerous series have been published describing the value of prophylactic synovectomy.[61] However, the long-term effects of the procedure are essentially unknown, it obviously has no effect on syno-

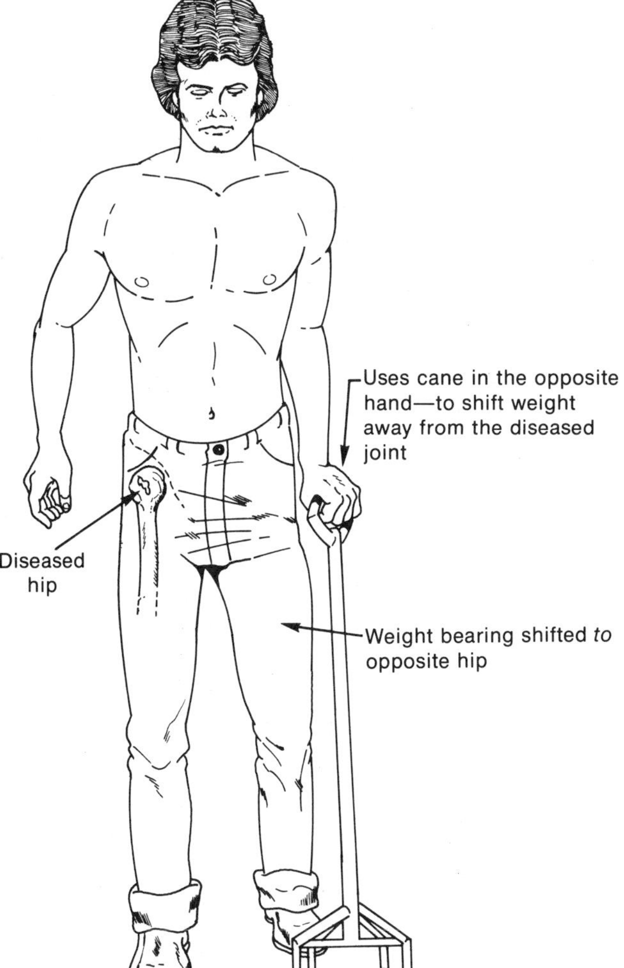

FIGURE 50–5. How to instruct patients to use a cane for disease involving the hip or knee.

vitis in other joints, and, generally speaking, the longer the follow-up, the worse the results. At least 25% of patients eventually will develop recurrent disease in the same joint.[62] When one considers that a knee synovectomy requires 1 to 2 weeks of hospitalization and 2 to 4 months before optimal function is obtained, a reluctance exists to advise this procedure, except in certain situations. Patients who would tend to benefit include (1) those with flagrantly active synovitis predominantly in one or two joints but with no cartilaginous loss radiologically, and (2) individuals with persistent monoarticular or pauciarticular disease in whom the likelihood for involvement of new joints appears to be low.

Reconstructive Surgery. Reconstructive procedures, either arthrodesis or arthroplasty, are indicated for joints in which permanent structural damage has occurred either secondary to degenerative joint disease or from cartilaginous destruction produced by erosive synovitis.

An arthrodesis virtually guarantees total relief from pain in the specific joint but causes inherent loss of joint function. In addition, the adjacent joints, which may also be involved with disease, must bear weight with a longer lever arm. Currently, an arthrodesis is frequently used in four situations:

1. *Wrist*: Wrist motion is not essential, and, with the possible exception of seeing to perineal hygiene, patients with fused wrists have normal function.
2. It may be used as a salvage procedure for joints destroyed by infection.
3. *Interphalangeal joints*: A satisfactory prosthesis has not been developed for interphalangeal joint replacement, and an arthrodesis is often indicated for reconstruction of such a painful and unstable joint.
4. *Talonavicular joint*: When structural destruction has occurred in this joint, little or no motion exists, and satisfactory relief from pain can be obtained by fusion.

Total Joint Replacement. The development of metal to plastic total joint replacement during the last 20 years has completely revolutionized the care of the arthritic patient. This procedure is now available for all joints except the spine. Not only is the degree of pain relief and functional return vastly superior to previous orthopedic procedures but also the duration of hospital stay has been reduced to 1 to 2 weeks for total hip and knee replacements and slightly less for total shoulder, elbow, ankle, and wrist replacements. At this time it should be stated that no arthritic patient, whether afflicted with rheumatoid or degenerative joint disease, should become bedfast. Since there is no specific pharmacotherapy, joint replacement is the only definitive treatment for patients with advanced degenerative joint disease.

In general, 90% of patients who have total hip replacements will be nearly or completely free of pain and have nearly normal or normal ambulation 5 years after the procedure.[63] The knee is a more complex structure, requiring ligamentous support for stability, so that the failure rate of total knee replacement is somewhat higher at present. The surgical mortality rate of joint replacements, using sodium warfarin (Coumadin), dextran, intermittent mechanical pressure, or aspirin to prevent pulmonary embolism, is less than 1%. Current methods have diminished the total incidence of deep sepsis to 1%, although one half of patients who develop it have a late complication, resulting in loss of the joint and a shortened lower extremity. Fractures, particularly in heavy individuals; dislocations; and heterotropic ossification, causing decreased motion, occur in 2 to 4%. The incidence of radiographically demonstrable loosening of the femoral component of total hip replacement or of either component of total knee replacement is about 20%, but to date, this has not produced clinical manifestations in most cases.

The indications for total joint replacement, given radiographic evidence of advanced structural damage, are essentially pain and functional loss. The presence of persistent pain within a given joint, sufficient to interfere consistently with sleep, is virtually an absolute indication for total hip replacement.

The indications for reconstruction of an anatomically destroyed joint, but one that does not cause nocturnal pain, are less clear. In essence, the procedure is indicated when function is limited by an individual joint, either by dysfunction or the pain produced, in a patient whose function would be significantly increased by replacement of that specific joint.

This statement may be clarified by presenting examples of two patients in whom a total knee replacement is *not* indicated. Both patients sleep comfortably throughout the night but have radiographic evidence of total cartilage loss.

1. A patient who develops right knee pain after walking one block, left hip pain after walking one and one half blocks, and left knee pain after walking two blocks. Obviously, to improve the patient's total function, three, rather than one, replacements must be done.
2. A patient who develops right knee pain after one block and occasionally develops dyspnea at the same time, owing to his chronic obstructive lung disease. Dyspnea always occurs after walking two blocks. A total knee replacement is not indicated, because pulmonary disease would replace arthritis as the factor that limits activity.

The decision to perform a joint replacement should be made mutually by the patient and his or her physician. The decision requires a thorough knowledge both of the patient's physical status and of his or her social and economic needs. Although there is no urgency about the procedure and joints replaced early do not necessarily lead to better results, it also is well to remember that structural disease and its symptoms are irreversible and do not improve with time.

ACKNOWLEDGMENT

The author wishes to acknowledge the contributions of William Branch, M.D., to the first two editions of this chapter.

REFERENCES

1. Yunus M, Masi AT, Calabro JJ, et al: Primary fibromyalgia (fibrositis): Clinical study of 50 patients with matched normal controls. Semin Arthritis Rheum 11:151, 1981.
2. Fan PT, David JA, Somer T, et al: A clinical approach to systemic vasculitis. Semin Arthritis Rheum 9:305, 1980.
3. Tsu-Yi C, Hunder GG, and Ilstrup DM: Polmyalgia rheumatica: A ten-year epidemiologic and clinical study. Ann Intern Med 97:672, 1982.
4. Hall S and Hunder GG: Is temporal artery biopsy prudent (Editorial)? Mayo Clin Proc 59:793, 1984.
5. Mol JMH and Wright V: Psoriatic arthritis. Semin Arthritis Rheum 3:55, 1973.
6. Breverton DA and James DCD: The histocompatibility antigen (HLA-B27) and disease. Semin Arthritis Rheum 4:191, 1975.
7. McNab I: Backache. Baltimore, Williams & Wilkins, 1977.

8. Loebl DH, Kirby S, Stephenson CR, et al: Psoriatic arthritis. JAMA 242:447, 1979.
9. Rosner IA, Richter DE, Huettner TL, et al: Spondyloarthropathy associated with hidradenitis suppurativa and acne conglobata. Ann Intern Med 97:520, 1982.
10. Steere AC, Gribofsky A, and Patarroyo ME: Chronic Lyme arthritis: Clinical immunogenetic differentiation of rheumatoid arthritis. Ann Intern Med 90:896, 1979.
11. Hochberg MC: Osteoarthritis: Pathophysiology, clinical features, management. Hosp Pract 19:41, 1984.
12. Schumacker HR, Smolyo AP, Tse RS, et al: Arthritis associated with apatite crystals. Ann Intern Med 87:411, 1977.
13. Franck WA, Bress WM, Singer FR, et al: Rheumatic manifestations of Paget's disease of bone. Am J Med 56:592, 1974.
14. Talbott JH, Altman RD, and Yü TF: Gouty arthritis masquerading as rheumatoid arthritis or vice versa. Semin Arthritis Rheum 8:77, 1978.
15. Gresham GE and Rathey UK: Osteoarthritis in knees of aged persons: Relationship between roentgenographic and clinical manifestations. JAMA 233:168, 1975.
16. Gordon DA, Pruzanski W, Oglyx MA, et al: Amyloid arthritis simulating rheumatoid disease in 5 patients with multiple myeloma. Am J Med 55:142, 1973.
17. Gordon DA, Stein JL, and Broder I: The extra-articular features of rheumatoid arthritis: A systematic analysis of 127 cases. Am J Med 54:445, 1973.
18. Schur PH: Diagnosing SLE. Clin Trends Rheumatol 9:1, 1978.
19. Koffler D: The immunology of rheumatoid diseases. CIBA Clin Symp 31:No. 4, 1979.
20. Moses S: Laboratory criteria for diagnosis of systemic lupus erythematosus. JAMA 242:1039, 1979.
21. Miniter MF, Stolley BD, and Agnello V: Reassessment of the clinical significance of native DNA antibodies in systemic lupus erythematosus. Arthritis Rheum 22:959, 1979.
22. Goldstein IM: Clinical applications of complement measurements in rheumatic disease. Am J Med Sci 269:172, 1975.
23. Vaughan JH: Rheumatologic disorders due to immune complexes. Postgrad Med 54:129, 1973.
24. Brouet J, Clauvel J, Danon F, et al: Biologic and clinical significance of cryoglobulins: A report of 86 cases. Am J Med 57:775, 1974.
25. Zvaifler NJ: Rheumatoid synovitis, an extravascular immune complex disease. Arthritis Rheum 17:297, 1975.
26. Ragan C and Farrington E: The clinical features of rheumatoid arthritis. Prognostic indices. JAMA 2:16, 1959.
27. Short CL and Bauer W: The course of rheumatoid arthritis in patients receiving simple medical and orthopedic measures. N Engl J Med 238:140, 1948.
28. Duthie JJR, Brown PE, Knox JDE, et al: Course and prognosis in rheumatoid arthritis. Ann Rheum Dis 16:411, 1957.
29. Duthie JJR, Brown PE, Truelove LH, et al: Course and prognosis in rheumatoid arthritis. Ann Rheum Dis 23:193, 1964.
30. Roberts WN, Daltroy LH, and Anderson RJ: Stability of normal joint findings in persistent classic rheumatoid arthritis. Arthritis Rheum 31:267, 1988.
31. Partridge REG and Duthie JJR: Controlled trial of the effect of complete immobilization of the joints in rheumatoid arthritis. Ann Rheum Dis 22:91, 1963.
32. Yelin E, Meenan R, Nevitt M, et al: Work disability in rheumatoid arthritis: Effects of disease, social and work factors. Ann Intern Med 93:551, 1980.
33. McDuffie FC: Morbidity impact of rheumatoid arthritis on society. Am J Med 78(Suppl 1A):1, 1985.
34. Pincus T and Callahan LF: Early mortality in RA predicated by poor clinical status. Bull Rheum Dis 41(4):1, 1992.
35. Fremont-Smith K and Bayles TB: Salicylate therapy in rheumatoid arthritis. JAMA 192:1133, 1965.
36. Silvoso GR, Ivey KJ, Butt JH, et al: Incidence of gastric lesions in patients with rheumatic disease on chronic aspirin therapy. Ann Intern Med 91:517, 1979.
37. Lanza FL, Royer GL, and Nelson RS: Endoscopic evaluation of the effects of aspirin, buffered aspirin, and enteric-coated aspirin on gastric and duodenal mucosa. N Engl J Med 303:136, 1980.
38. Clive DM and Stoff JS: Renal syndromes associated with nonsteroidal antiinflammatory drugs. N Engl J Med 310:563, 1984.
39. Ciabattoni G, Cinotti GA, Pierucci A, et al: Effects of sulindac and ibuprofen in patients with chronic glomerular disease: Evidence for dependence of renal function on prostacyclase. N Engl J Med 310:279, 1984.
40. Bernstein CA and Freyberg RH: Rheumatoid patients after five or more years of corticosteroid treatment: A comparative analysis of 183 cases. Ann Intern Med 54:938, 1961.
41. Gristina AG, Pace NA, Kantor TG, et al: Intra-articular Thio-Tepa compared with Depo-Medrol and procaine in the treatment of arthritis. J Bone Joint Surg 52A:1603, 1970.
42. Cooperating Clinics Committee: A controlled trial of cyclophosphamide in rheumatoid arthritis. N Engl J Med 283:883, 1970.
43. McCarty DJ and Carrera GF: Intractable rheumatoid arthritis: Treatment with combined cyclophosphamide, azathioprine, and hydroxychloroquine. JAMA 248:1718, 1982.
44. Weinblatt ME, Weissman BN, Holdsworth DF, et al: Long-term prospective trial of methotrexate in the treatment of rheumatoid arthritis: 84 month update. Arthritis Rheum 35:129, 1992.
45. Sperling RI, Benincaso AL, Anderson RJ, et al: Acute and chronic suppression of leukotriene by synthesis ex vivo in neutrophils of patients with rheumatoid arthritis beginning treatment with methotrexate. Arthritis Rheum 35:376, 1992.
46. Empire Rheumatism Council: Gold therapy in rheumatoid arthritis. Ann Rheum Dis 19:95, 1960.
47. Mainland D and Sutcliffe MI: Hydroxychloroquine sulfate in rheumatoid arthritis: A six month, double-blind trial. Bull Rheum Dis 13:287, 1962.
48. Multicentre Trial Group: Controlled trial of D-penicillamine in severe rheumatoid arthritis. Lancet 1:275, 1973.
49. Pinals RA, Kaplan SB, Lawson JG, and Hepburn B: Sulfasalazine in rheumatoid arthritis: A double-blind, placebo-controlled trial. Arthritis Rheum 29:427, 1986.
50. Pinals RS, Baum J, Bland J, et al: Preliminary criteria for clinical remission in rheumatoid arthritis. Bull Rheum Dis 32:7, 1982.
51. Auranofin (Ridaura). Med Lett 27:89, 1985.
52. Ward JR, Williams HJ, Egger MJ, et al: Comparison of auranofin, gold sodium thiomalate and placebo in the treatment of rheumatoid arthritis: A controlled clinical trial. Arthritis Rheum 26:1303, 1983.
53. Menard HA, Beaudet F, Davis P, et al: Gold therapy in rheumatoid arthritis. Interim report of the Canadian multicenter prospective trial comparing sodium aurothiomalate and auranofin. J Rheumatol 9(Suppl 8):179, 1982.
54. Katz WA, Blodgett RC, and Pietrusko RG: Proteinuria in gold-treated rheumatoid arthritis. Ann Intern Med 101:176, 1984.
55. Ferraz MD, Tugwell P, Goldsmith CH, and Atra E: Meta-analysis of sulfasalazine in ankylosing spondylitis. J Rheumatol 17:1428, 1990.
56. Carette S, Graham D, Little H, et al: Natural course of ankylosing spondylitis. Arthritis Rheum 26:186, 1983.
57. Calia A and Fries JF: Striking prevalence of ankylosing spondylitis in "healthy" B27 positive males and females: A controlled study. N Engl J Med 293:835, 1975.
58. Feldges DH and Barnes CG: Treatment of psoriatic arthropathy with either azathioprine or methotrexate. Rheumatol Rehab 13:120, 1974.
59. Baum J, Hurd E, Lewis D, et al: Treatment of psoriatic arthritis with 6-mercaptopurine. Arthritis Rheum 16:139, 1973.
60. Bradley JD, Brandt KD, Kalasinski LA, and Ryan S: Comparison of anti-inflammatory doses of ibuprofen and analgesic doses of ibuprofen and acetaminophen in the treatment of osteoarthritis of the knee. N Engl J Med 325:87, 1991.
61. Ranawat CS and Desai K: Role of early synovectomy of the knee joint in rheumatoid arthritis. Arthritis Rheum 18:117, 1975.
62. Twenty-third Rheumatism Review. Arthritis Rheum 8(Suppl): 160, 1978.
63. Harris WH: Current concepts: Total joint replacement. N Engl J Med 297:650, 1977.

51

Low Back Pain*

JOYCE E. WIPF, MD
RICHARD A. DEYO, MD, MPH

Back pain is a frustrating problem for patients and clinicians alike. With a lifetime prevalence of approximately 70%, low back pain is a common symptom. Low back pain is an illness, rarely attributable to a specific diagnosis or disease, with an uncertain etiology in most cases.[1, 2] Fortunately, the prognosis is excellent: About 80% of episodes of back pain resolve or greatly improve without specific treatment within 2 to 6 weeks.[3] Only 10% have chronic pain, although recurrences are common. Approximately 2% of patients with back pain have associated lower extremity nerve root symptoms that persist for more than 2 weeks.[4]

Impact on Health Care Delivery. The impact of back pain on health care and disability compensation systems is enormous. Of American adults, 1 to 2% have had back surgery, and most patients followed in referral back pain centers have had at least two back operations.[5] Annual costs of personal medical care for back pain in 1989 were about five times that of acquired immunodeficiency syndrome (AIDS), and back pain is the single greatest cause of lost earnings and productivity for men.[6] Back pain ranks only behind upper respiratory complaints as a reason for symptomatic visits to physicians and is the most common symptom prompting x-rays at office visits.[6] Despite expert opinion that lumbar spine surgery may be performed excessively, surgical rates increased nearly 50% in the United States from 1979 to 1987.[6] Rates in the United States are 30% higher than in Canada and about five times higher than in Britain.

Costs of therapy reflect the poor consensus about diagnosis of certain spine diseases, appropriate therapy, and appropriate use of tests. Expert panels disagree, for example, about criteria for the diagnosis of spinal instability and whether fibrositis or myofascial trigger point syndromes exist.[7] Some elements of the physical examination (e.g., muscle spasm) show very poor interobserver reproducibility.[8] About 20% of normal individuals who have never experienced low back pain show herniated disks on computed tomography (CT), magnetic resonance imaging (MRI), and myelography, and such anatomic variation may often prompt ill-advised testing or invasive therapy.[9–11]

Spinal Anatomy. The normal lumbar spine is shown in Figure 51–1. The anterior elements of the spine (vertebral bodies connected by intervertebral disks) bear weight and absorb shock. The posterior elements include the vertebral arches, transverse and spinous processes, and the articular facets, all of which protect the spinal cord and nerve roots. Ligaments and paravertebral muscles, along with the facets, provide stabilization and balance.

Because of the importance of the intervertebral disk as a cause of back symptoms and radiculopathy, it is important to consider the anatomy and the dynamic forces that affect this structure. The disk consists of the tough lamellar anulus fibrosus and the softer nucleus pulposus. In children the nucleus is gelatinous, but in adults the consistency is that of crab meat. Pressures within the nucleus can be measured and may play a role in the pathogenesis of disk herniation, help to explain some patient symptomatology, and influence the choice of positions and exercises that clinicians prescribe. Figure 51–2 illustrates the marked variations in lumbar intradiskal pressures that occur with various positions and activities.[12]

DIFFERENTIAL DIAGNOSIS

Clinical Syndromes

We use the term "simple back pain" to refer to lumbar pain in patients under age 50, with no evidence of radiculopathy, systemic disease, or cancer history. The vast majority of these patients have nonspecific musculoskeletal etiology and a benign course, requiring little diagnostic testing and primarily symptomatic therapy. Approximately 60% of primary care patients fit this description.[13]

"Complex low back pain" refers to the presence of some clinical feature or risk factor for an underlying infection, neoplastic cause, or inflammatory cause of back pain. About 35% of primary care patients fit this description, although only a small fraction actually prove to have systemic

*Supported in part by grant number HS-06344 (the Back Pain Outcome Assessment Team) from the Agency for Health Care Policy and Research and by the Northwest Health Services Research and Development Field Program, Seattle VA Medical Center, Seattle, WA.

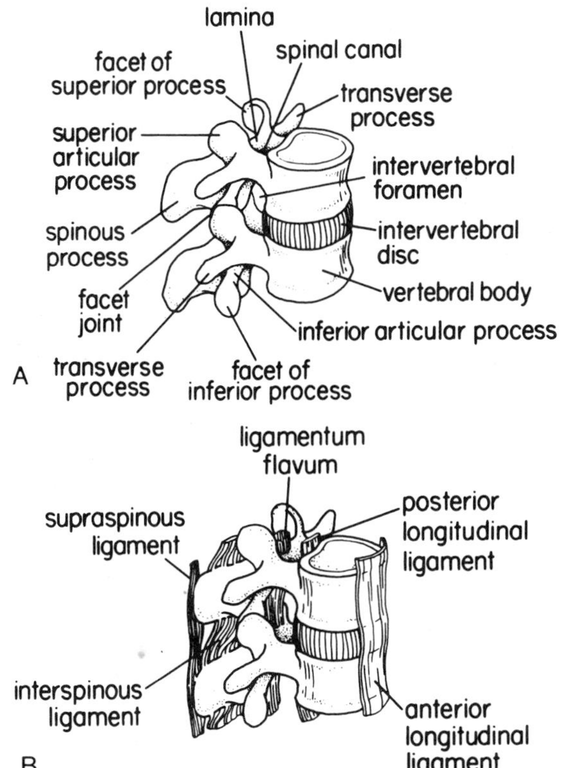

FIGURE 51–1. Anatomy of the spine and associated soft tissues. (From Andersson EBJ and McNeill TW: Lumbar Spine Syndromes: Evaluation and Treatment. New York, Springer-Verlag, 1989, p 7.) *A,* The bony elements and disk of a motion segment. (Adapted from Fine J: Your Guide to Coping with Back Pain. Toronto, McClelland & Stewart, 1985.) *B,* The ligaments of a motion segment. Lateral view. (Adapted from Fine J: Your Guide to Coping with Back Pain. Toronto, McClelland & Stewart, 1985.)

causes. Nonetheless, these patients require some diagnostic testing to rule out serious systemic disease. This category includes individuals older than 50 years of age, those with a history of malignancy or intravenous drug abuse, and those with symptoms such as fever, weight loss, hematuria, or adenopathy.[13]

Radiculopathy (usually sciatica) refers to pain in the distribution of a lumbar nerve root, which is often accompanied by neurosensory and motor deficits. In patients with spinal stenosis, the cardinal symptom may be neurogenic claudication (see later). True sciatica typically radiates to the calf and foot, whereas referred pain from back structures rarely radiates below the knee. Sciatica is usually sharp and is accompanied by paresthesias and numbness. Approximately 3% of primary care patients present with this syndrome.

Simple Back Pain. The differential diagnosis of simple back pain is shown in Table 51–1. Most of these backaches are of uncertain etiology, because of the poor association of symptoms with radiographic or anatomic abnormalities of the spine. Simple back pain is often described by the terms "muscle sprains" and "strains." Degenerative disk disease (spondylosis) may be a cause of simple back pain beginning at approximately 30 years of age. Nonspecific low back pain has also been attributed to fasciitis, fibrositis, myositis, and ligament degeneration or rupture. Radiographic degenerative changes, including osteophytes of vertebral bodies and osteoarthritic changes at the facet joints are common but are equally common in asymptomatic persons. Many congenital radiographic changes, including mild scoliosis, kyphosis, lordosis, sacralization of the fifth lumbar vertebra, lumbarization of the first sacral vertebra, and spina bifida occulta are not clearly associated with back pain.[12, 14–17]

Complex Back Pain. The differential diagnosis of complex back pain includes all of the aforementioned causes, as well as the systemic conditions indicated in Table 51–1. Especially in older adults, the diagnostic spectrum expands to include osteoporosis with vertebral compression fractures, and spinal malignancies. Even among patients with "complex back pain"; however, the prevalence of malignancies and infections is only about 2%.[13]

Visceral referred pain includes back pain secondary to renal causes such as stones or pyelonephritis. Pelvic organ pathology, such as endometriosis, may present with low back pain. Abdominal aortic aneurysm may cause back pain by erosion of vertebral bodies or acute pain with dissection and rupture. Pancreatic disease often presents with back pain.

Radiculopathy. The differential diagnosis includes spinal stenosis (most commonly in older patients) and herniated disks in younger adults. Severe spondylolisthesis and neural tumors are less common causes. It is important to rule out cauda equina syndrome and cord compression early in the evaluation.

SPECIFIC PATHOLOGIC CONDITIONS

Herniated Disk.[18] Structural deterioration of the disk begins early, usually by about 30 years of age. As the annulus fissures and cracks, the nucleus pulposus can become extruded and may irritate or compress adjacent nerve roots. Intradiskal pressure may contribute to this process, and pressure varies substantially with body position and with maneuvers such as straining and coughing. More than 95% of lumbar disk herniations occur at the L4–L5 or L5–S1 levels. L4–L5 disk herniation (L5 root) usually presents with pain and numbness radiating from the back to the posterior thigh, anterolateral leg, medial foot, and great toe (Fig. 51–3). Weakness on dorsiflexion of the foot and toes may be evident, sometimes with atrophy of the anterior compartment. Reflexes are usually unaffected.

L5–S1 disk herniation (S1 root) produces pain and numbness of the posterior thigh and leg, posterolateral foot, and lateral toes. Weakness affects plantar flexion of the foot and toes with subsequent atrophy of the posterior compartment. The Achilles' reflex may be decreased.

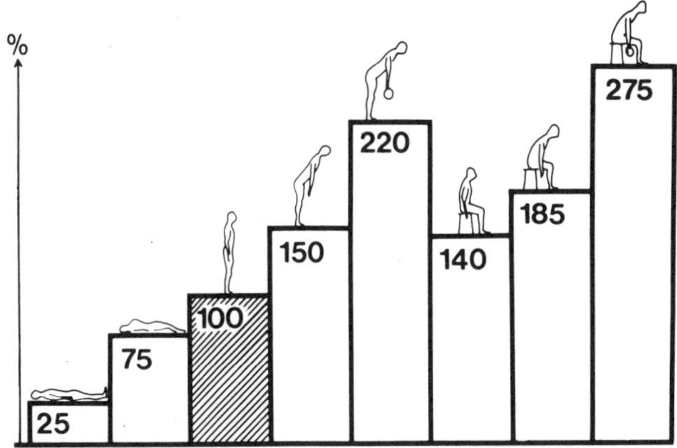

FIGURE 51–2. Relative change in pressure (or load) in the third lumbar disk in various positions in living subjects. (From Nachemson AL: The lumbar spine: An orthopaedic challenge. Spine 1:59–71, 1976.)

TABLE 51–1. DIFFERENTIAL DIAGNOSIS OF CAUSES OF LOW BACK PAIN AS A PRIMARY COMPLAINT AND ESTIMATED PREVALENCE OF EACH CONDITION IN PRIMARY CARE PRACTICES

"Mechanical" Back Pain		Radiculopathy, Pseudoclaudication		Systemic and Visceral Diseases	
Condition	*Prevalence*	*Condition*	*Prevalence*	*Condition*	*Prevalence*
Musculoligamentous strain, degenerative change of disks, vertebrae, or facets	0.85	Herniated disk	0.02	Neoplasia (primary or metastatic, multiple myeloma, metastatic carcinoma, lymphoma and leukemia, spinal cord tumors, retroperitoneal tumors)	0.007
Spondylolisthesis	0.03	Spinal stenosis	0.01	Infection (osteomyelitis, epidural abscess, diskitis)	0.0001
Compression fractures	0.04			Inflammatory spondyloarthritis (e.g., ankylosing or psoriatic spondylitis, Reiter's)	0.003
Severe scoliosis, kyphosis, asymmetric transitional vertebrae	0.04				
				Aortic aneurysm Renal disease (nephrolithiasis, pyelonephritis, perinephric abscess) Pelvic disease (prostatitis, endometriosis) Gastrointestinal disease	0.005
Total	0.96	Total	0.03	Total	0.015

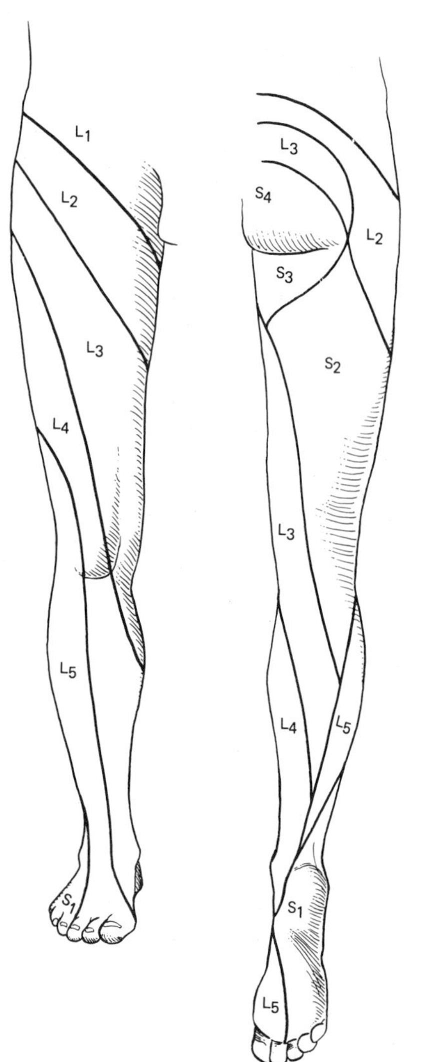

FIGURE 51–3. Lower extremity dermatomes.[50] (From Finneson BE: Low Back Pain, 2nd ed. Philadelphia, JB Lippincott, 1980.)

Higher nerve root compression (L2–L4) is much less common but produces pain and numbness of the posterolateral or anterior thigh extending across the knee and anteromedial leg. Compression of the L4 nerve root may produce weakness of knee extension with atrophy of the quadriceps and decreased knee reflex.

Spinal Stenosis.[19–21] Nerve root entrapment in spinal stenosis is caused by narrowing of the spinal canal (congenital or acquired), nerve root canals, and intervertebral foramina. Most often, this narrowing is produced by bony hypertrophic changes in the facet joints and by thickening of the ligamentum flavum (Fig. 51–4). Symptoms include back pain, transient tingling, and neurogenic claudication (pain that mimics ischemic claudication by occurring with ambulation but that is associated with normal arterial pulses).

Spondylosis. Spondylosis refers to degenerative disk disease, which is radiographically evident as disk space narrowing and associated arthritic changes of the facet joint. Although severe multilevel spondylosis is associated with pain, milder radiographic degenerative changes are equally common in symptomatic and asymptomatic persons. These changes become more common with age and are nearly ubiquitous after 65 years of age.

Spondylolysis. Spondylolysis is a defect in the vertebral pars interarticularis, which joins the superior and inferior facet joints (see Fig. 51–4). Most often the defect is at the level of the fifth lumbar vertebra and is seen on radiographs as a radiolucency. These defects may be congenital or may represent stress fractures. However, in adult populations, the finding is as common in asymptomatic persons as in symptomatic persons, thus it cannot be confidently labeled as the cause of pain in an individual.[15] Bilateral defects may permit forward displacement of the anterior elements, called spondylolisthesis.

Spondylolisthesis. This refers to forward displacement of one or more lumbar vertebrae and may be congenital, traumatic, or degenerative (see Fig. 51–4). Spondylolytic spondylolisthesis occurs in approximately 5% of the population, is usually asymptomatic, and is often found as an incidental finding on x-ray.[15] Degenerative spondylolisthesis occurs in older adults. The slippage in spondylolisthesis

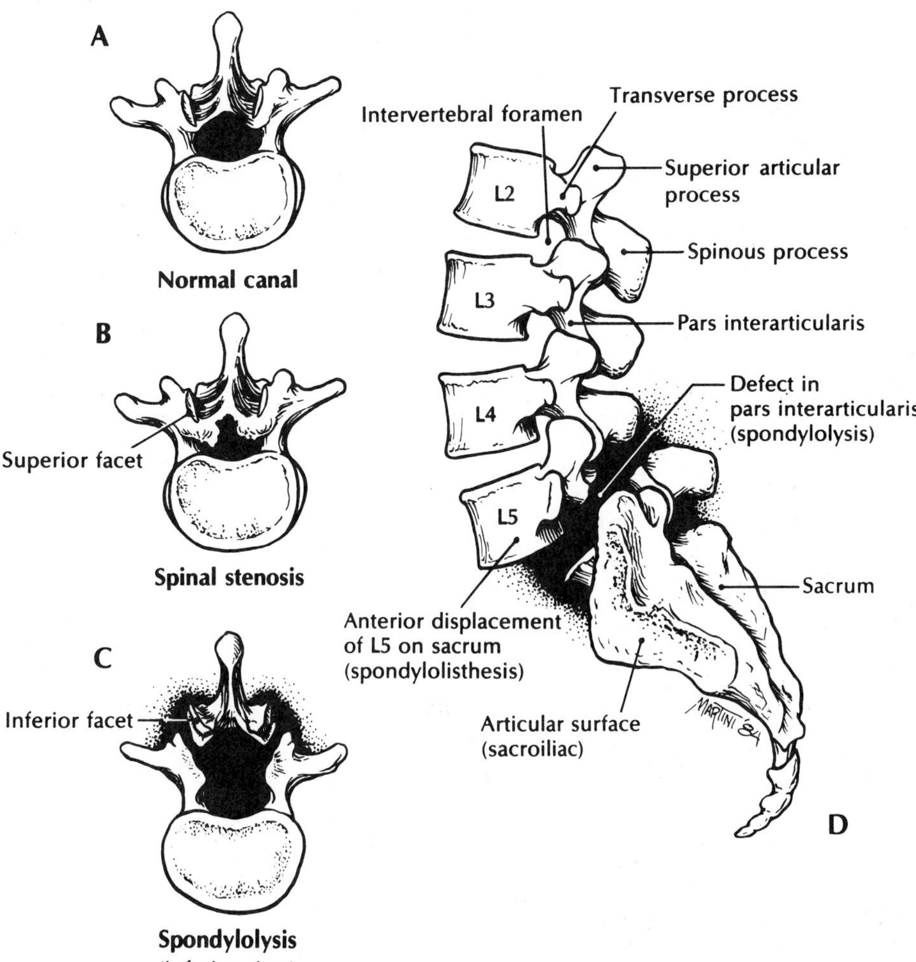

FIGURE 51–4. *A,* Superior view of a lumbar vertebra showing normal anatomy and canal configuration. *B,* Superior view of a lumbar vertebra showing hypertrophic degenerative changes of the facets, resulting in spinal stenosis. *C,* Inferior view of a lumbar vertebra showing bilateral spondylolysis (defects in the pars interarticularis). *D,* Lateral view of the lumbosacral spine illustrating spondylolysis of the L5 vertebra with resulting spondylolisthesis at L5–S1. Spondylolisthesis refers to the anterior displacement of a vertebra on the one beneath it. (From Deyo RA: Early diagnostic evaluation of low back pain. J Gen Intern Med 1:328–338, 1986.)

is characterized as a percentage of vertebral body width, ranging from I (25% of vertebral body width) to IV (100%). Mild spondylolisthesis typically remains stable for many years (often indefinitely). Severe spondylolisthesis is more likely to be associated with radicular symptoms.

Osteoporosis. Osteoporosis is painless unless associated with compression fractures. These typically produce wedge-shaped deformities. Severe osteoporosis may also produce bulging of the disks into the vertebral body in the form of Schmorl's nodes or "codfishing" of lumbar vertebrae. Microfractures may cause acute exacerbations of chronic pain.

Ankylosing Spondylitis. This is the prototypic inflammatory cause of back pain and occurs in less than 1% of most population samples. Typical features include insidious onset of back pain at a young age, usually by 40 years of age.[22] Like other inflammatory arthropathies, pain is worse in the morning and usually improves with exercise. Early radiographic abnormalities include sacroiliac joint sclerosis, with vertebral fusion occurring later in the disease. Psoriatic arthritis, Reiter's syndrome, and the spondyloarthropathy associated with inflammatory bowel disease are less frequent inflammatory causes of low back pain but share many features in common with ankylosing spondylitis.

Cancer. Cancer associated with back pain usually causes gradual and progressive pain and may eventually produce neurologic symptoms. History and examination should focus on patients with systemic symptoms or evidence of a primary neoplasm such as lung, breast, or prostate carcinoma, which commonly metastasize to the spine. Trauma does not rule out a malignancy, because up to 10% of patients with back pain and cancer have a history of trauma. Any compression fracture should be evaluated for possible metastatic malignancy or a primary tumor such as multiple myeloma. Extradural tumors such as lymphoma and spinal neoplasms are associated with intense constant pain and may produce neurologic abnormalities late in the course.

Infection. Infection should be suspected in any patient with fever and backache. Possible causes include subacute bacterial endocarditis, septic diskitis, and vertebral osteomyelitis. *Staphylococcus aureus* is the most common pathogen, although gram-negative osteomyelitis is common in the elderly and in intravenous drug users.[23, 24] Spinal epidural abscess may occur after bacteremia or may be more chronic in association with vertebral osteomyelitis. *Mycobacterium tuberculosis* has a tendency to localize in the anterior disk and vertebral body (Pott's disease). Destruction of vertebrae that extends across a disk space is more likely to be caused by infection than by a tumor.

CLINICAL EVALUATION

Since a specific cause is not identified in up to 85% of patients with low back pain,[2] diagnostic efforts are often disappointing. Rather than seeking a specific mechanical cause, the early evaluation should focus on excluding more serious underlying diseases. Answering three major questions will help to clarify whether further work-up is indicated and help to determine initial therapy: (1) Is there an underlying systemic disease? (2) Is a neurologic deficit present? and (3) Is there evidence of psychosocial distress that may amplify or prolong pain symptoms?[25]

History. Specific details include any history of previous or current malignancy, drug abuse, known arthritic conditions, and underlying medical problems. History of trauma, previous therapy for back pain, and prior back surgery are important diagnostic and prognostic features. Back pain unrelieved by bed rest or unresponsive to conservative therapy may suggest an underlying systemic disease. Fever, weight loss, or neurologic symptoms such as sciatica, weakness, or bowel/bladder incontinence mandate further work-up.

Sciatica or neurogenic "pseudoclaudication" is usually the first clue to possible neurologic impairment. True sciatica (due to radiculopathy) usually radiates below the knee, whereas referred pain from spinal structures may radiate down the buttock and thigh but rarely below the knee and is not associated with numbness of the lower leg or foot. In patients with a herniated disk, back pain usually precedes leg pain, sometimes by months or years. When it begins, the leg pain usually overshadows the back pain. Sciatica is usually unilateral and often associated with numbness and paresthesias. Pseudoclaudication, classically seen with central spinal stenosis, is a syndrome of leg pain and numbness that is precipitated by standing or ambulation. Unlike vascular claudication, peripheral pulses are usually normal and without bruits. Table 51–2 shows the history and physical findings that help to distinguish vascular from neurogenic claudication.[26] Specific neurologic symptoms are determined by the affected nerve root level, and multiple levels are often involved in lumbar stenosis.

Cauda equina syndrome refers to compression of the cauda equina, usually by a massive midline disk herniation. It presents with back pain (in almost 100% of patients), urinary retention (~ 90%), usually bilateral leg paresthesias and neurologic deficits (~80%), and "saddle" anesthesia of the perineal region and posteromedial thighs (75%). Spinal cord compression due to malignancy or infection often presents with similar symptoms. Progressive neurologic deficits or suspicion of cauda equina syndrome require urgent surgical referral.

TABLE 51–2. HISTORY AND PHYSICAL FINDINGS THAT DISTINGUISH NEUROGENIC PSEUDOCLAUDICATION (PRIMARILY DUE TO SPINAL STENOSIS) FROM VASCULAR CLAUDICATION*

	Vascular Claudication (N = 26)	Neurogenic "Pseudoclaudication" (N = 23)
Pain on standing alone (without ambulation)	27%	65%
Pain on cough or sneeze	0%	38%
Distance to claudication constant	88%	38%
Paresthesias on walking	12%	43%
Mean time to relief of walking-induced symptoms	5.0 min	12.7 min
Normal femoral, popliteal, and dorsalis pedis pulses	0%	83%
Femoral or aortic bruit	54%	9%
Sensory deficit	12% (always stocking distribution)	55% (usually dermatomal distribution)
Limited straight leg raising	0%	30%
Muscle weakness	12%	39%

*Data from Hawkes CH and Roberts GM: Neurogenic and vascular claudication. J Neurol Sci 38:337–345, 1978.

Table values are a percentage of patients with each finding (sensitivities).

Various psychosocial features of the patient may affect the duration or perceived severity of pain. Depression, alcoholism, or personal stress (e.g., problems on the job or at home) may exacerbate back pain or result from it. These conditions may suggest important therapeutic opportunities that can moderate symptoms, whether one views back pain as the cause or the result of the psychosocial problem. Back pain is a common complaint of drug-seeking individuals, and physicians should be alert to a pattern of excessive narcotic analgesic use. Litigation and disability compensation claims appear often to affect an individual's recovery time and sense of pain severity.

Frank malingering appears to be extremely rare, but some patients react to back pain with great distress and may exhibit unusual pain behavior. Recognition of this possibility may help to avoid unnecessary testing or ill-advised invasive therapy. Symptoms that suggest an exaggerated behavioral response include whole-leg pain, numbness, or giving way; constant pain for long periods without even transient periods of improvement; emergency hospitalization for low back pain; intolerance of multiple treatments due to worsening or side effects; and excessive bed rest. Screening for depression with standard queries is also important in the face of chronic pain or unusual pain behavior.

Physical Examination. The extent of general and neurologic examination may be determined in part by the history. Those with simple back pain without neurologic complaints or risk factors for systemic illness should have a general examination of the back and only brief screening for lumbar nerve root abnormalities (see later). Spinal examination includes inspection for anatomic abnormalities (e.g., scoliosis, kyphosis, or pelvic tilt), and range of motion. Although limited motion does not distinguish among numerous pathologic causes, it may provide a quantifiable index of therapeutic response. Forward flexion is the most common limitation and is the most reproducibly quantified. Pain on extension is suggestive of spinal stenosis, although the accuracy of this sign has not been tested.

The patient with complex back pain (historical risk factors for systemic disease including persistence of pain beyond several weeks) requires a screening general examination to rule out malignancy, including breast, prostate, and lymph node examinations. It is for this group that laboratory tests and plain x-rays may be most useful (see later).

The patient with back pain and sciatica needs a neurologic examination focused on confirmation of nerve root involvement and on estimation of intervertebral level of abnormality. The maneuver of straight leg raising (SLR) is useful to confirm the impression of radiculopathy. SLR is done with the patient supine and the examiner raising the extended leg, with a positive test result defined as reproducing the sciatica between 30 and 60 degrees of elevation. Use of a goniometer or inclinometer (used in construction work) makes measurement of SLR more accurate and reproducible. Ipsilateral limitation of SLR is a sensitive, but not specific, test for herniated disks (Table 51–3).[27, 28] The crossed SLR test refers to elevation of the unaffected leg causing sciatica in the affected leg. This test is less sensitive for herniated disks but is much more specific.[27, 29, 30]

Neurologic testing should be focused on the L5 and S1 nerve roots, where most disk herniations occur. Testing of the L5 nerve roots can be rapidly accomplished by strength tests of ankle and great toe dorsiflexion. Sensory loss occurs in the medial foot and the web space between first and second toes (see Fig. 51–3). Involvement of the S1 nerve

TABLE 51–3. STRAIGHT LEG RAISING AS A TEST FOR LUMBAR DISK HERNIATION

	No.	Criterion for Positive Test Report	Prevalence of Disk Herniation	Sensitivity*	Specificity*
Ipsilateral SLR					
Hakelius and Hindmarsh[27]	1537	Leg pain at <60 degrees	76%	0.80	0.36
Kosteljanetz et al[28]	100	Leg pain at <60 degrees	58%	0.76	0.45
Crossed SLR					
Spangfort[29]	2157	Contra. leg pain	86%	0.23	0.88
Hakelius and Hindmarsh[27]	1537	Contra. leg pain	76%	0.26	0.88
Hudgins[30]	244	Contra. leg pain	83%	0.24	0.96

*Calculated by ourselves. All results are for surgical series, and in every case the "gold standard" for disk herniation was the surgical finding.
SLR = straight leg raising.

root typically produces diminished ankle reflexes and sensory loss over the posterior calf and lateral foot. Although S1 radiculopathy may produce weakness of foot plantarflexion, this is difficult to detect until relatively advanced.

IMAGING AND LABORATORY TESTS

Plain X-rays. Many textbooks and monographs suggest that every patient with low back pain should receive a multiple-view series of lumbar spine films. Unfortunately, the yield of useful findings on plain radiography is small; many radiologic abnormalities are unrelated to symptoms; high doses of gonadal radiation are involved; the aggregate costs are substantial; and disagreements in interpretation (even among experts) are common. Thus, many experts advocate a selective approach to plain radiography, and the Quebec Task Force suggested that plain radiography is generally inappropriate within the first month of acute low back pain.[31]

Nachemson has summarized several studies that demonstrate that many radiographic abnormalities are equally common in patients with and without low back pain.[12] Table 51–4 illustrates representative findings from these studies.[14–17] In general, single disk space narrowing, apophyseal joint changes, spina bifida occulta, transitional vertebrae, Schmorl's nodes, and even mild spondylolisthesis are probably not associated with back symptoms. Thus, both the physician and the patient may be misled by the presence of such radiographic findings.

Because of such considerations, several authors have suggested selective x-ray criteria. Typical criteria, and their rationale, are shown in Table 51–5.[32] Several studies suggest that in primary care, there would be a very low risk of overlooking serious disease if x-rays were limited to patients with these indications. However, in many settings, primary care physicians appear already to be even more selective than these criteria suggest, with little evidence of harm to patients.[32] One strategy for being even more selective makes use of the erythrocyte sedimentation rate (ESR) as a screening test for patients with "complex" low back pain. A normal ESR and only a single clinical risk factor (e.g., > 50 years of age) for systemic disease make underlying malignancy or infection extremely unlikely. An ESR over 20, or more than two risk factors, suggests a need for plain radiography.[13]

TABLE 51–4. PREVALENCE OF VARIOUS RADIOGRAPHIC ANOMALIES AMONG PERSONS WITH AND WITHOUT LOW BACK PAIN*

Anomaly	No Pain (%)	Pain (%)	Author
Spina bifida occulta	6	4	Splithoff
Spondylolysis	17	7	Magora
Facet joint abnormality	22	19	LaRocca
Degenerative disk	23	32	Biering-Sorenson
	22	26	Splithoff

*See references 14 to 17.

Many patients have come to expect spine x-rays when they have back pain, and physicians may often request them to avoid patient dissatisfaction or anxiety. One study examined the consequences of selective x-ray use in a randomized trial of x-ray strategies.[33] Walk-in patients at low risk for systemic disease by clinical criteria were randomized to receive x-rays or an educational intervention. Those in the latter group received x-rays only if their condition did not improve at a follow-up visit. After 3 weeks, there were no important (or significant) differences in patient satisfaction, worry about serious disease, pain resolution, or functional status. At 3-month follow-up, 31% in the "no x-ray" group had received films, but this was still substantially less than the "x-ray group." No important diagnoses were missed. Thus, a 5-minute educational intervention may allow omission or delay of spine films without adverse consequences, and patient expectations about radiography are reduced.

In many institutions, five views of the lumbar spine are routinely obtained when lumbar radiography is ordered (anteroposterior, lateral, two obliques, and a coned lateral view). A number of studies have demonstrated that omitting the oblique views would result in very few misdiagnoses.[34] Furthermore, diagnoses that were missed (mostly spondylolysis and facet joint changes) have little therapeutic importance (Table 51–6). Similar data suggest that the coned lateral view is rarely of unique benefit. On the basis of such evidence, a World Health Organization report recommended that oblique projections should not be routinely obtained but should be reserved for special problems.[35] Omitting the oblique and coned lateral views would eliminate more than half of the total radiation dose and could save more than $45 million/yr on a national basis.

CT and MRI Scanning. CT and MRI scanning of the lumbar spine have approximately similar sensitivities and specificities for herniated disks or spinal stenosis. Their sensitivity is approximately 90 to 95%, and their specificity is approximately 80%. These are probably superior to traditional myelography, and there is little evidence that CT myelography offers substantial advantages over plain CT scanning.[36] As shown in Table 51–7, the specificity of these tests is limited because herniated disks and spinal stenosis are observed in a substantial number of completely asymptomatic persons.[9, 10] Thus, the mere anatomic finding is not a reason to consider surgery and may not even indicate the true cause of pain. Even these sophisticated imaging re-

TABLE 51–5. CLINICAL FINDINGS THAT SHOULD PROMPT EARLY RADIOGRAPHY*

Finding	Rationale
Age ≥50 yr	More likely to have underlying malignancy, osteoporosis, compression fractures
Significant trauma	Fracture more likely
Neuromotor deficits	Identify underlying spondylolisthesis or malignancy (more common causes such as a herniated disk or spinal stenosis will not be apparent on plain films)
Unexplained weight loss (≥10 lb in 6 mo) or lymphadenopathy	Malignancy or chronic infection more likely
Suspicion of ankylosing spondylitis (see text)	Identify inflammatory spondyloarthropathies
Drug or alcohol abuse	Intravenous drugs increase risk of spinal osteomyelitis; alcohol increases risk of osteoporosis; both increase risk of trauma, often poorly remembered
History of cancer (other than skin cancer)	Metastatic disease more likely
Fever (temperature >100°F or 37.8°C)	Often found with ostemyelitis or epidural abscess
Use of corticosteroids	Increased risk of osteoporosis and infection
Upper lumbar and lower thoracic pain	Possibly increased risk of malignancy
Failure to improve after 2 to 4 wk of conservative therapy	Up to 90% of patients with acute low back pain improve within 1 month; failure to improve may indicate underlying systemic disease
Seeking compensation	Sometimes involves physical injury; x-ray evidence needed for most legal proceedings

*Data from Deyo RA: Lumbar spine films in primary care: Current use and the effects of selective ordering criteria. J Gen Intern Med 1:20–25, 1986.

sults must, therefore, be correlated with clinical findings (e.g., sciatica, neurologic deficits) in order to make accurate pathophysiologic inferences. These false-positive tests are an important reason to avoid early imaging in a patient with back pain, because a finding of disk herniation or spinal stenosis could precipitate a cascade of ill-advised interventions in a patient without clinical indications for surgery. Furthermore, the data in Table 51–7 suggest that most abnormalities of the lumbar spine become more common with age and that bulging and degenerated disks in particular are extremely common in normal persons. Because of these problems, one might reasonably argue that CT and MRI scanning should be kept for patients who appear to be surgical candidates on clinical grounds or who have other evidence to suggest underlying malignancy or infection.

Bone Scanning. Radionuclide bone scanning has a limited role in the evaluation of patients with low back pain. In patients with metastatic cancer or osteomyelitis, the test is more sensitive than is plain radiography and the results become positive earlier in the disease. However, bone scans are relatively nonspecific, with positive findings resulting from a wide variety of conditions, many of which are benign. Furthermore, true positive results on bone scans (for malignancy or infection) almost never occur in the face of both normal plain x-rays and normal laboratory screening (especially the ESR).[37] Thus, bone scans should be used selectively and generally should be reserved for the patient with other evidence of systemic disease.

Electromyography (EMG). Electrodiagnostic tests such as EMG and nerve conduction studies may be useful in patients with equivocal neurologic findings and may help to confirm the presence and level of radiculopathy in patients with definite neurologic abnormalities. This may be particularly useful, for example, in the patient with spinal stenosis, who has variable or uncertain neurologic abnormalities. These tests are not indicated in individuals with simple back pain and usually have little to add for those with obvious radiculopathy in whom surgical referral is planned and anatomic imaging is likely.

Laboratory Tests. Common recommendations include a complete blood count, ESR, creatinine, calcium, phosphate, alkaline phosphatase, acid phosphatase, uric acid, and fasting blood sugar. However, the yields of these tests and their predictive values have not been critically evaluated. Because these tests are nonspecific, and because systemic

TABLE 51–6. STUDIES OF THE YIELDS OF OBLIQUE AND CONED LATERAL VIEWS OF THE LUMBOSACRAL SPINE*

Study	Sample Size	Sampling Frame	Views Considered†	No. of Missed Findings	Missed Diagnoses
Rhea et al, 1980	200 patients	Consecutive studies from emergency room patients	Obliques	4	3 spondylolysis 1 postoperative change
Eisenberg et al, 1980	704 studies	Consecutive veterans examined for disability compensation	Obliques	5	1 spondylolysis 4 mild facet joint changes
Gehweiler et al, 1983	500 studies	Consecutive inpatient and outpatient studies	Obliques	59	33 facet arthritis 22 spondylolysis 2 facet joint anomalies 1 elongated pars interarticularis 1 osteoid osteoma
Scavone et al, 1981	782 patients (993 examinations)	Consecutive inpatient and outpatient studies	Obliques Coned lateral	19	18 spondylolysis 1 congenital anomaly (facet fusion)
Eisenberg et al, 1979	30 patients	Not stated	Coned lateral		Diagnoses not listed; well-centered lateral showed lumbosacral junction as well as coned lateral in 28/30 examinations

*From Deyo RA: Lumbar spine films in primary care: Current use and the effects of selective ordering criteria. J Gen Intern Med 1:20–25, 1986.
†Each examination was read with and without the views listed to determine what diagnoses might be missed.

TABLE 51–7. PREVALENCE OF ABNORMAL IMAGING FINDINGS IN "NORMAL SUBJECTS" WITH NO HISTORY OF LOW BACK PAIN OR SCIATICA*

CT Results (No. = 52)		
	Age	
	<40 Yr of Age	*>40 Yr of Age*
Herniated disk	20%	27%
Spinal stenosis	0%	3%
Facet abnormality	0%	10%
Any abnormality	20%	50%
MRI Results (No. = 67)		
	Age	
	<60 Yr of Age	*>60 Yr of Age*
Herniated disk	22%	36%
Spinal stenosis	1%	21%
Bulging disk	54%	79%
Degenerated disk	46%	93%

*From Boden SD, David DO, Dina TA, et al: Abnormal magnetic resonance scans of the lumbar spine in asymptomatic subjects. J Bone Joint Surg 72A:403–408, 1990 and Wiesel SW, Tsourmas N, Feffer HL, et al: A study of computer-assisted tomography. 1: The incidence of positive CAT scans in an asymptomatic group of patients. Spine 9:549–551, 1984.

CT = computed tomography; MRI = magnetic resonance imaging.

causes of back pain are infrequent, such extensive testing is likely to yield many more false-positive results than true-positive results. False-positive tests may lead to further tests, unnecessary concern, patient dependency, erroneous labeling, or incorrect therapy.

Furthermore, the sensitivity of the hematocrit and the white blood cell count for detecting cancer or infection is limited. Of the commonly recommended tests, the ESR is probably the most sensitive test for detecting these conditions, although the test is relatively nonspecific.[13] Table 51–8 shows the sensitivity and specificity of some common hematologic tests for detecting underlying malignancy in patients with low back pain. Although cancer is the most common systemic cause of low back pain (by severalfold), the ESR is also a sensitive test for osteomyelitis and other spinal infections.

Urinalysis may be useful to rule out suspected urinary tract infection, urolithiasis, or multiple myeloma. Urinary tract disease is usually suggested by a history and physical examination. Dipstick methods are relatively insensitive for the detection of Bence-Jones protein in myeloma, and the ESR is a more sensitive screening test.

The HLA-B27 histocompatibility antigen may be useful in confirming a suspected diagnosis of ankylosing spondylitis. However, it should not be used as a screening test because it is present in about 6% of Caucasians, even though less than 1% have ankylosing spondylitis. Furthermore, unequivocal radiographic findings in the presence of compatible clinical findings establish the diagnosis and obviate the need for the test. It is, therefore, most useful in the face of equivocal x-ray findings and a compatible clinical examination, although a later radiograph would still be necessary to prove the diagnosis.

Early Diagnostic Strategy. Figure 51–5 suggests an early diagnostic strategy, based on the clinical features of the patient. Although diagnostic tests are used selectively, available evidence suggests that the risk of delaying important diagnoses is extremely low.

TABLE 51–8. ACCURACY OF COMMON HEMATOLOGIC TESTS FOR DETECTING MALIGNANCY IN PATIENTS WITH LOW BACK PAIN*†

	Sensitivity	**Specificity**
Erythrocyte Sedimentation Rate		
≥20 mm/hr	0.78	0.67
≥50 mm/hr	0.56	0.97
≥100 mm/hr	0.22	0.996
Anemia (hematocrit <40% for men or 38% for women)	0.54	0.86
Hematocrit <30%	0.09	0.994
WBC ≥12,000/mm^3	0.22	0.94

*Adapted with permission from Deyo RA and Diehl AK: Cancer as a cause of back pain: Frequency, clinical presentation, and diagnostic strategies. J Gen Intern Med 3:230–238, 1988.

†From a study of approximately 1000 walk-in patients with low back pain (the majority of whom were acute cases). There were 13 patients who proved to have an underlying malignancy as the cause of back pain. Data are based on varying patient numbers because not all tests were obtained for every patient.

WBC = white blood cell.

THERAPY

The natural history of acute low back pain without sciatica is for approximately 80% of individuals to improve substantially within 1 month. Even among patients with acute sciatica, about 50% recover in 6 weeks, and most do not require surgical intervention unless massive disk rupture, epidural abscess, or tumor is causing a progressive neurologic deficit. Therefore, reassurance about the good prognosis of most episodes of back pain is a vital part of management and corrects many patients' inaccurate preconceptions. Historically, back pain was treated with long periods of bed rest, inactivity, and prolonged delays in return to work. Evidence suggests a benefit of early activation, very brief bedrest in most cases, and rapid return to work (even if in a temporarily limited capacity). The following treatment suggestions apply to patients with most musculoskeletal causes of back pain.

Bedrest. Bedrest was traditionally regarded as the mainstay of therapy for acute low back pain. This recommendation was based on the clinical observation that many patients obtain temporary relief when supine and on the physiologic observation that supine position minimizes intradiskal pressure. However, many patients with low back pain probably do not have disk herniations as a cause, and the rationale for bedrest in such patients is unclear. Studies have, therefore, challenged the value of the traditional 1- to 2-week recommendation for bedrest.

One study compared a 2-day versus 7-day bedrest recommendation for walk-in clinic patients with acute low back pain but no neurologic deficits. The only significant difference in outcomes between the study groups was that among employed subjects, those given a 2-day recommendation missed 45% fewer days of work than did those given the 7-day recommendation. There were no significant or substantial differences in other functional, physiologic, or perceived outcomes at 3 weeks or at 3 months.[38] Another primary care trial went even further in reducing the bedrest recommendation. Gilbert and colleagues randomly allocated subjects to receive 4 days of bed rest or none at all. There were no detectable differences in the speed or the extent of pain resolution. Although work absenteeism was not directly assessed, the bedrest group required 42% longer to return to "normal activities."[39] These two trials suggest that brief (if any) bedrest is sufficient for most patients without neurologic deficits and that bedrest does not affect the natural history of the illness.

One of these studies examined baseline predictors of sub-

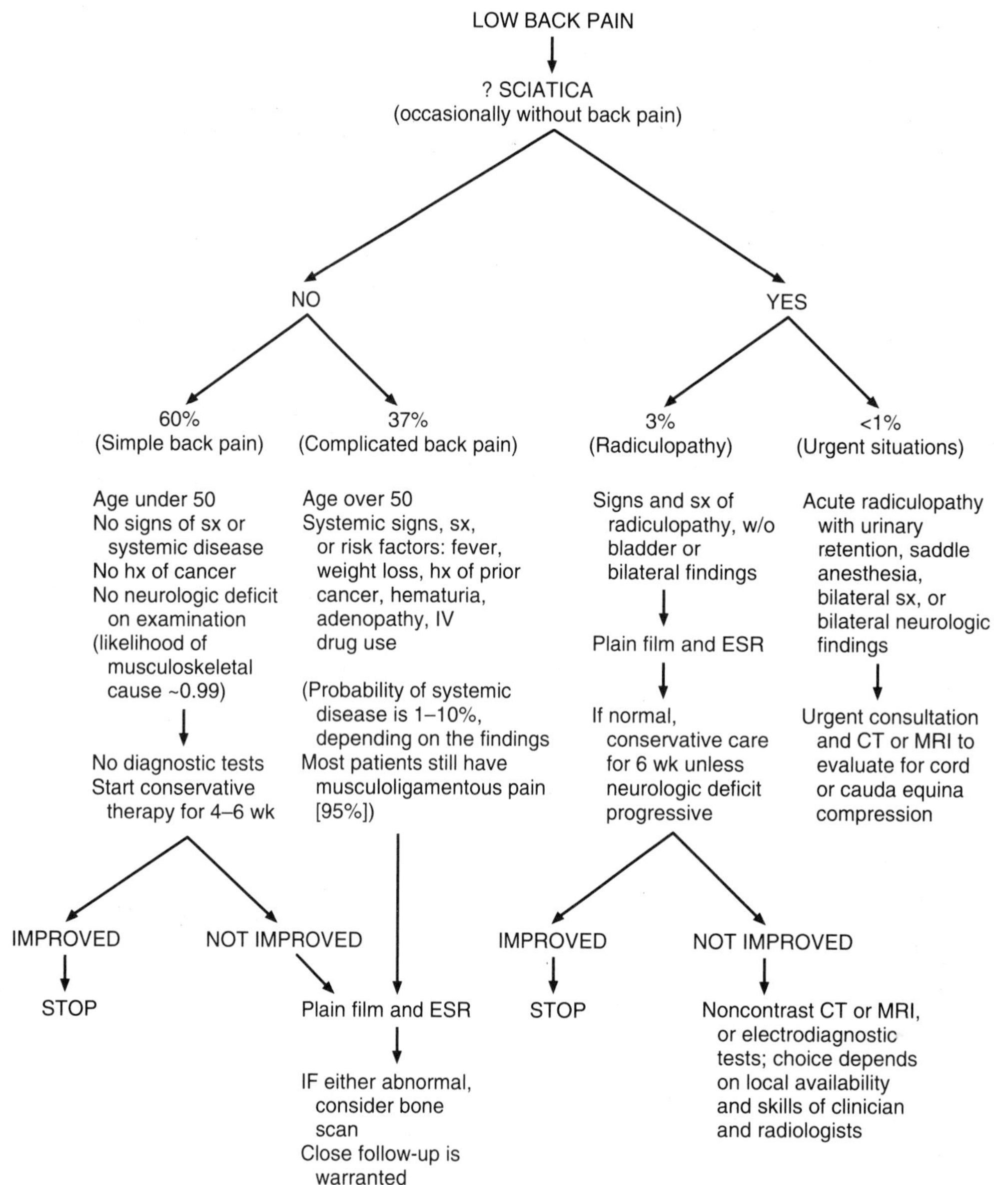

FIGURE 51–5. Diagnostic algorithm of low back pain.

sequent work absenteeism for a 3-month follow-up period. In multivariate analysis, the only significant predictor proved to be the bedrest recommendation given to the patient. Baseline variables such as self-rated pain, duration of pain, prior episodes, spine flexion, and SLR did not significantly predict subsequent work absenteeism. Thus, the physician's recommendation is a powerful determinant of this important outcome.[38]

For patients with a clinical syndrome suggesting a herniated disk with radiculopathy, longer and stricter bedrest may be necessary, although little evidence is available to suggest the optimal duration. Because bedrest results in rapid loss of muscle strength, cardiopulmonary deconditioning, and bone demineralization, we generally advise against bedrest for more than 1 week. Because standing results in disk pressures only slightly higher than the side-lying posture (see Fig. 51–2), it is generally safe to recommend brief periods of standing and walking to prevent deconditioning.

Oral Medication. Several nonsteroidal anti-inflammatory drugs (including naproxen, diflunisal, aspirin, and piroxicam) have been found efficacious in trials of back pain therapy.[31, 32] The evidence for muscle relaxants is inconsistent. There are several trials suggesting a benefit of carisoprodol and some other muscle relaxants, but these studies offer little guidance as to which patients benefit most.[40] Unfortunately, side effects (especially sedation) are common with most drugs in this class, and some are habituating. Thus, prescribing for fixed, time-limited intervals (e.g., 1 week) is desirable in order to avoid creating drug dependency.

Narcotic analgesics are useful for acute severe pain, especially with sciatica. However, most experts advise against prolonged use of narcotics or their use in chronic pain syndromes. Like muscle relaxants, they should be prescribed for brief, fixed, time-limited intervals and should not be used in a pain-contingent manner.

Antidepressant drugs are commonly used for patients with chronic pain, with or without overt evidence of depression. It is unclear whether their benefit derives from primary analgesic effects, treatment of masked depression, or improved sleep. The clinical trials of these drugs for chronic low back pain are flawed, but several trials suggest that they are efficacious.

Exercise. Despite controversy about the optimal exercise regimen, there is a growing consensus that general fitness exercises and back exercises are valuable in treating back pain and preventing recurrences. Even in patients with herniated disks and severe symptoms, it is usually feasible and safe to begin standing and walking by the third day of symptoms or earlier for patients with simple low back pain. We encourage up to 20 minutes of standing and walking for every 3 hours at bedrest.

The ability to sit comfortably usually comes later than does the ability to stand and is a sign of improvement. At this point, controlled endurance training activities are safe. Walking, stationary bicycling, and swimming are particularly appropriate.

More specific back exercises engender greater controversy. Clinical trials are difficult to implement, and most studies have substantial flaws. Nonetheless, there is growing evidence that the traditional Williams' isometric flexion exercises have minimal value for patients with acute back pain. One randomized trial in patients with acute pain suggested that they may even be counterproductive.[39] In contrast, trials have supported rigorous extension exercises and milder stretching exercises.[41, 42] A highly individualized approach advocated by McKenzie has gained popularity among physical therapists.[43] Cohort studies also suggest a benefit to multifaceted exercise programs for patients with chronic pain. Thus, for the patient with persistent pain beyond 4 weeks, or with frequent recurrences, a planned back exercise regimen, in addition to fitness exercises, is probably appropriate. One regimen, based on a program popularized by the YMCA, is illustrated in Figure 51–6.[41] For patients whose pain persists beyond 6 to 8 weeks, referral for physical therapy may be valuable to provide closer supervision of exercises, individualized regimens, and improved patient compliance.

Injection Therapies. Multiple forms of injection are widely practiced, including anesthetic or steroid injections into trigger points, facet joints, and the epidural space. There is growing evidence against the efficacy of facet joint injections, and a single randomized trial suggests that trigger point injections with saline are equivalent to injections of an active drug. There are conflicting results from trials of epidural steroid injections, and their role in the management of herniated disks, spinal stenosis, or other conditions remains uncertain.

Other Physical Treatments. Several randomized trials are remarkably concordant in demonstrating no benefit of conventional lumbar traction for patients with low back pain and sciatica. Controlled trials of inversion devices and other forms of gravity traction have not been reported.

Fewer controlled studies are available for corsets or spinal orthoses. Some observers suggest that prolonged use of these devices could lead to counterproductive abdominal and spinal muscle atrophy. Truly limiting lumbar motion requires a rigid body cast with extension to the legs. The Quebec Task Force on Spinal Disorders concluded that neither traction nor orthoses have scientific support for their efficacy, despite wide use.

Counterstimulation techniques, such as transcutaneous electrical nerve stimulation (TENS) and acupuncture also have unproven benefit. Blinded studies of TENS suggest that most of its benefit may be related to placebo effects.[41] Despite positive results on trials of acupuncture compared with conventional forms of therapy, trials comparing true acupuncture at the proper body meridians with misplaced needling of any sort consistently have negative results.

Spinal manipulation, usually done by chiropractors, is widely sought by patients, who often report dramatic responses. Several randomized trials of manipulation versus conventional treatments have been reported, and some suggest at least a short-term benefit for selected patients.[44] Peculiarities of study design complicate the interpretation of many of these trials, but none suggests that manipulation is inferior to conventional therapy. Even if long-term outcomes were comparable, a faster return to work or other activities might have a substantial benefit. Complications appear to be rare and probably can be avoided with appropriate diagnostic evaluation. Appropriate selection of patients, timing of referral, and duration of therapy remain unclear. Nonetheless, clinicians should keep an open mind about this form of therapy, and a RAND corporation consensus panel of both medical physicians and chiropractors suggested that this treatment may be appropriate for some patients, especially those with simple back pain.[45]

Surgery. Despite a high rate of surgery performed in the United States and a large surgical literature on failed low back surgery, the rate of surgery on the lumbar spine rose substantially from 1979 to 1987.[6] Furthermore, wide geographic variations have been observed with regard to the rates of lumbar spine surgery. In Washington state, even after omitting counties with very small populations, Volinn and coworkers found a sevenfold variation in the rates of

EXERCISE 1.
Loosen up by wobbling your neck, shoulders, arms, thighs, legs and feet. Raise your arms slowly, then let them drop. Repeat these motions with your hands, legs, and feet. Let your head drop to the left, then to the right. Slowly take a deep breath in and breathe out slowly. Now try to feel heavy - let your head, shoulders, arms and legs rest on the your muscles. Breathe deeply again. Close your eyes, let you jaw sag, try to breathe out as slowly as possible, humming or hissing. Tighten your muscles and your neck, then relax. The important part is the relaxing - the letting go - not the tightening. The tightening only helps you to feel the difference between tension and relaxation.

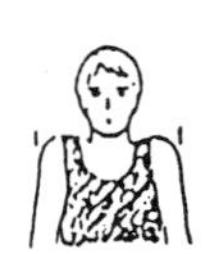

EXERCISE 2.
Sit up on a chair, shrug your shoulders again, and then relax.

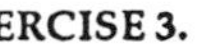

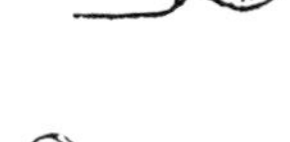

EXERCISE 3.
Lie down once again. Turn you head all the way to the left, then return it to the normal front and center position, and relax. Turn your head all the way to the right, as far as you can, return to normal position, and relax. If you have a stiff neck, also do this exercise in a sitting position.

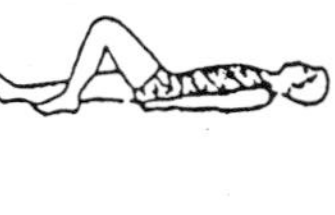

EXERCISE 4.
Lie flat on your back, this time with pillows removed. Bend your knees and slowly draw your right knee up as close to your chest as possible. Slowly straighten your leg, let it fall to the floor limp and relaxed. Pull it up again to the bent starting position. Now do the same thing with the other leg. Repeat the exercise, switching legs.

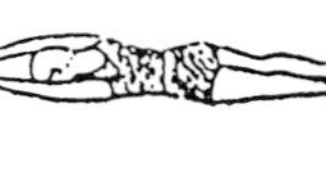

EXERCISE 5. PRONE STRETCH
Lie on your stomach, stretch your left arm and right leg as far as you can along the floor; relax. Repeat the exercise with your right arm and left leg. Then stretch with all four limbs at the same time; relax. (This exercise and the remaining ones are mainly used to stretch muscles, from your back to your heel cords.)

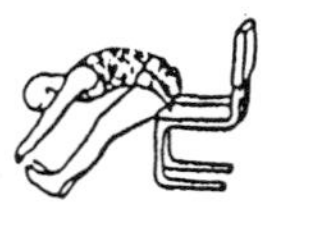

EXERCISE 6. HAMSTRING STRETCH
Sitting on the edge of a chair that is braced against a wall, straighten your legs and try to reach toward the toes. Try not to round the back, but keep the back and legs straight as you reach. Feel as if you are folding in half at the hips.

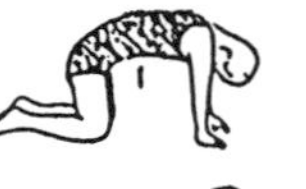

EXERCISE 7. CAT BACK
Kneel down, resting on your hands and knees. Arch your back up like a cat, and drop your head at the same time. Then reverse the arch by bringing your head up and forming a U with your spine.

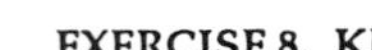

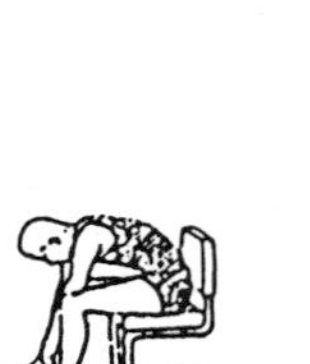

EXERCISE 8. KNEE KISS
Lie on your back with knees bent. Raise both your had and your right knee and try to make them meet. Don't try too hard? At first, you will probably not succeed, but eventually you will. Return to your starting position and do the same exercise with you head and left knee.

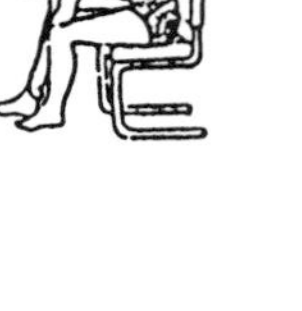

EXERCISE 9. BEND SITTING
Sit on a chair, feet apart on the floor. Let you neck drop, then drop your shoulders and arms, and bend down between your knees, as far as you can. Relax to an upright position, straighten up, and relax.

EXERCISE 10. KNEE-CHEST STRETCH
Lie on the floor with your knees bent. Gradually pull both knees toward your chest, hold for a few seconds, then return to the start position and relax.

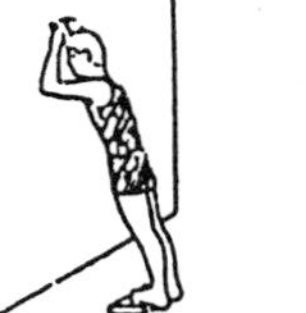

EXERCISE 11. HEEL CORD STRETCH
Near a wall, place books on the floor to make a platform about 2 inches height. Place the balls of the feet on the books. While keeping knees, hips, and back straight, bend the ankles forward so your face touches the wall. The forward bend of the ankles should be slow and gentle, giving a steady stretch on the tendons.

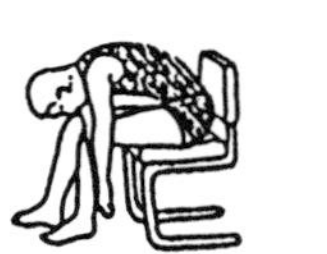

EXERCISE 12. BEND SITTING ROTATION
Sit on a chair and bend down, dropping your head and shoulders. Bend down to the left, then gradually straighten up and rest. Do the exercise again, bending to the right.

FIGURE 51–6. Stretching exercise regimen.

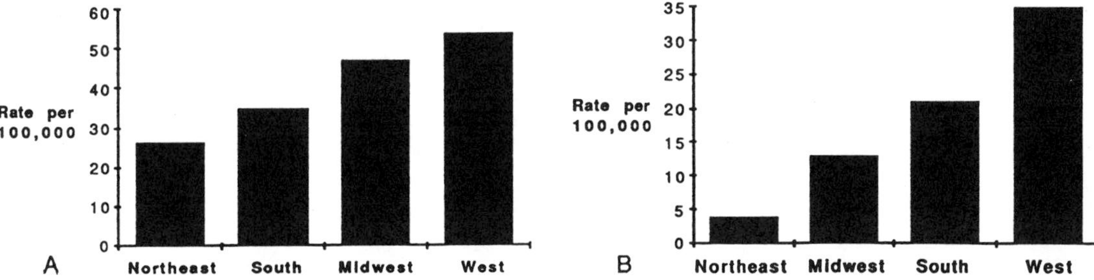

FIGURE 51–7. *A,* Laminectomy rates by geographic region. *B,* Spine fusion rates by geographic region. (From Deyo RA: Nonsurgical care of low back pain. Neurosurg Clin North Am 2(4):851–862, 1991.)

lumbar spine surgery.[46] These rates were essentially unrelated to rates of compensation claims for back pain, the number of spine surgeons in a county, or various indicators of access to medical care. Much of this variability may, therefore, be related to differences in training and practice style among surgeons.

Wide variations in surgical rates have even been observed for large regions of the United States. As shown in Figure 51–7, laminectomy rates varied almost twofold between the northeast and the western United States in 1986.[7] Even more striking were regional variations in the rates of lumbar spine fusion, with ninefold differences between the northeast and the west. These variations suggest a poor consensus on the application of criteria for lumbar spine surgery.

Although there is a reasonable consensus on the general indications for surgery for herniated disks (Table 51–9),[18] there is some inherent ambiguity in these criteria, and they may often be liberalized despite evidence that outcomes are worse under these circumstances. Surgery should not be regarded simply as the last resort for any patient with low back pain. Rather, it should be regarded as a specific therapy for specific lesions. In the absence of these lesions, and history and physical findings related to them, surgery is unlikely to be rewarding. Thus, the existence of chronic pain alone or the observation that "nothing else has worked" are not indications for surgery.

Indications for surgery in the case of spinal stenosis remain more ambiguous than those for herniated disks.[47] The surgical indications for lumbar spine "instability" remain even more uncertain and controversial, and even the diagnostic criteria for instability are hotly debated. Hospital claims data suggest that lumbar spine fusion is associated with increased complications and costs in the short term (compared with laminectomy or diskectomy alone) and that, on average, fusion does not reduce the likelihood of future hospitalization or surgery for low back pain.[48] It seems likely that fusion is essential in some unusual circumstances (e.g., severe spondylolisthesis or surgical removal of multiple facet joints), but its wider use in more routine situations bears critical scrutiny.

In general, the indications for surgical referral shown in Table 51–9 appear most appropriate.[18] Primary care physicians should realize that lumbar spine surgery for herniated disks is almost always elective, since the long-term outcomes, both with regard to symptoms and neurologic function, are roughly equivalent for patients with and without surgery.[49] Tables 51–10 and 51–11 show the results of surgical and nonsurgical treatments from several controlled studies. It appears that the major benefit of surgery is faster relief of sciatica for carefully selected patients, with back pain less consistently relieved.

Patient Education. Patient reassurance and education are major aspects of therapy. Many are unaware of the favorable prognosis or may believe that paralysis is a common sequel to low back problems. Thus, patients should be strongly reassured that rapid recovery is the norm, although recurrences are common. This generalization is true for most musculoskeletal causes of back pain, whether the patient has simple back pain, sciatica, or a demonstrated disk herniation. The major exception may be spinal stenosis, in which symptoms tend to remain stable or gradually worsen after a period of years.

The greatest source of patient dissatisfaction with care for back pain appears to be the lack of adequate explanation about the cause. For some, an explanation of symptoms may be as important as therapy. Although a precise diagnosis is often impossible, the clinician can usually offer a likely explanation based on the clinical evaluation. This explanation may often include a description of soft tissue

TABLE 51–9. INDICATIONS FOR SURGICAL REFERRAL IN THE PATIENT WITH SCIATICA*

- The cauda equina syndrome (a surgical emergency): characterized by bowel and bladder dysfunction (usually urinary retention), saddle anesthesia, bilateral leg weakness and numbness
- Progressive or severe neurologic deficit
- Persistent neuromotor deficit after 4 to 6 weeks of conservative therapy
- Persistent sciatica, sensory deficit, or reflex loss after 4 to 6 weeks in a patient with positive straight leg raising sign, consistent clinical findings, and favorable psychosocial circumstances (e.g., realistic expectations and no evidence of depression, substance abuse, or excessive somatization)

*Reproduced, with permission, from Deyo RA, Loeser JD, and Bigos SJ: Herniated lumbar intervertebral disk. Ann Intern Med 112:598–603, 1990.

Table 51–10. SYMPTOM RESOLUTION IN CONTROLLED STUDIES OF SURGERY OR CHEMONUCLEOLYSIS FOR HERNIATED LUMBAR DISKS (MYELOGRAPHICALLY PROVED)*

Study	Findings	Conservative Care (%)	Surgery or Chemonucleolysis (%)
Hakelius, 1970 (Surgery)	Improved 2 mo after therapy initiated	89	97
	Symptoms entirely gone after 3 mo	76	90
Weber, 1983 (Surgery)	Satisfactory results, 1 yr	79	92
	Satisfactory results, 4 yr	88	82
	Relapses, 4 yr	24	15
Javid et al, 1983 (Chemonucleolysis)	Sciatica improved, 3 wk	38	53
	Sciatica improved, 6 wk	45	73
	Sciatica improved, 6 mo	42	78

*From Deyo RA: Nonsurgical care of low back pain. Neurosurg Clin North Am 2(4):851–862, 1991.

TABLE 51–11. RECOVERY FROM MOTOR WEAKNESS IN RANDOMIZED TRIALS OF DISK DESTRUCTION*

Study	Motor Findings	Conservative Care (%)	Surgery or Chemonucleolysis
Weber, 1983 (Surgery)	Total recovery of dorsiflexion, 4 yr	43	44
	Total recovery of plantar flexion, 4 yr	75	56
	Recovery from all muscle weakness, 10 yr	84	84
Javid et al, 1983 (Chemonucleolysis)	Recovery from muscle weakness, 3 wk	41	64
	Recovery from motor weakness, 6 wk	61	82
	Recovery from motor weakness, 6 mo	66	82

*From Deyo RA: Nonsurgical care of low back pain. Neurosurg Clin North Am 2(4):851–862, 1991.

lesions that cannot be identified by imaging, such as muscular and ligamentous strains or tears.

The language used to describe back pain may often contribute to patient misconceptions, fear, and adverse labeling. The "nominal diagnosis" of a herniated disk was common in the past to explain any episode of severe pain or dysfunction, even without clinical or imaging evidence of nerve root involvement. This diagnosis often carries an implication of severe disease and future disability. The term "ruptured disk" may be even more frightening, implying major trauma and tissue dissolution. Less emotionally laden terms, such as extruded or protruding disk are anatomically descriptive and less alarming. Backache is often referred to as "back injury," implying trauma, possible compensation, and pathophysiologic inferences that are often unfounded. We prefer to use the generic term "backache" or "back pain" to avoid these inferences.

Prevention. Epidemiologic evidence is consistent in suggesting that back pain is more common in the very obese, smokers, and sedentary persons. It is reasonable to assume that these are factors in recurrence as well as first episodes of low back pain, and each seems to carry independent risk. Reasons for the smoking association are unclear but may relate to nicotine effects on diskal metabolism, increases in intradiskal pressure due to coughing, or simply serving as a marker for psychological traits (e.g., anxiety or depression) that amplify or prolong pain. There is at least fragmentary evidence that weight loss, smoking cessation, and improved fitness can reduce the risk of back pain.

Ergonomic factors in the workplace (e.g., requirements for lifting, twisting, or exposure to vibration) are risk factors for back pain. Job modification may help to reduce back pain risk or to facilitate return to work but requires the cooperation of employers. Simple job modifications may sometimes be possible, whereas others may be prohibitively expensive. There is no evidence that training in lifting techniques or x-ray screening can prevent occupational back problems.

REFERENCES

1. Quinet RJ and Hadler NM: Diagnosis and treatment of back pain. Semin Arthritis Rheum 8:261–247, 1979.
2. White AA III and Gordon SL: Synopsis: Workshop on idiopathic low-back pain. Spine 7:141–149, 1982.
3. Frymoyer JW: Back pain and sciatica. N Engl J Med 318:291–300, 1988.
4. Deyo RA and Tsui-Wu YJ: Descriptive epidemiology of low-back pain and its related medical care in the United States. Spine 12:264–268, 1987.
5. Newman RI, Seres JL, Yospe LP, and Garlington B: Multidisciplinary treatment of chronic pain: Long-term follow-up of low-back pain patients. Pain 4:283–292, 1978.
6. Deyo RA, Cherkin D, Conrad D, and Volinn E: Cost, controversy, crisis: Low back pain and the health of the public. Ann Rev Publ Health 12:141–156, 1990.
7. Deyo RA: Nonsurgical care of low back pain. Neurosurg Clin North Am 2(4):851–861, 1991.
8. Waddell G, Main CJ, Morris EW, et al: Normality and reliability in the clinical assessment of backache. BMJ 284:1519–1523, 1982.
9. Boden SD, David DO, Dina TA, et al: Abnormal magnetic resonance scans of the lumbar spine in asymptomatic subjects. J Bone Joint Surg 72A:403–408, 1990.
10. Wiesel SW, Tsourmas N, Feffer HL, et al: A study of computer-assisted tomography. 1: The incidence of positive CAT scans in an asymptomatic group of patients. Spine 9:549–551, 1984.
11. Hitselberger WE and Witten RM: Abnormal myelograms in asymptomatic patients. J Neurosurg 28:204–206, 1968.
12. Nachemson AL: The lumbar spine: An orthopaedic challenge. Spine 1:59–71, 1976.
13. Deyo RA and Diehl AK: Cancer as a cause of back pain: Frequency, clinical presentation, and diagnostic strategies. J Gen Intern Med 3:230–238, 1988.
14. Splithoff CA: Lumbosacral junction: Roentgenographic comparison of patients with and without backache. JAMA 152:1610, 1953.
15. Magora A and Schwartz A: Relation between low back pain and x-ray changes. 4: Lysis and Olisthesis. Scand J Rehab Med 12:47–52, 1980.
16. LaRocca H and MacNab I: Value of pre-employment radiographic assessment of the lumbar spine. Can Med Assoc J 101:49, 1969.
17. Biering-Sorenson F, Hansen FR, Schroll M, and Runeborg O: The relation of spinal x-ray to low back pain and physical activity among 60 year old men and women. Spine 10:445, 1985.
18. Deyo RA, Loeser JD, and Bigos SJ: Herniated lumbar intervertebral disc. Ann Intern Med 112:598–603, 1990.
19. Moreland LW: Spinal stenosis: A comprehensive review of the literature. Semin Arthritis Rheum 19:127–149, 1989.
20. Hall S, Bartleson JD, Onofrio BM, et al: Lumbar spinal stenosis: Clinical features, diagnostic procedure, and results of surgical treatment in 68 patients. Ann Intern Med 103:271–275, 1985.
21. Spengler DM: Current concepts review: Degenerative stenosis of the lumbar spine. J Bone Joint Surg 69-A:305–308, 1987.
22. Gran JT: An epidemiological survey of the signs and symptoms of ankylosing spondylitis. Clin Rheum 4:161–169, 1985.
23. Sapico FL and Montgomerie JZ: Pyogenic vertebral osteomyelitis: Report of nine cases and a review of the literature. Rev Infect Dis 1:754–776, 1979.
24. Waldvogel FA and Vasey H: Osteomyelitis: The past decade. N Engl J Med 303:360–370, 1980.
25. Deyo RA, Rainville J, and Kent DL: What can the history and physical examination tell us about low back pain? JAMA 268:760–765, 1992.
26. Hawkes CH and Roberts GM: Neurogenic and vascular claudication. J Neurol Sci 38:337–345, 1978.
27. Hakelius A and Hindmarsh J: The significance of neurological signs and myelographic findings in the diagnosis of lumbar root compression. Acta Orthop Scand 43:239–246, 1972.
28. Kosteljanetz M, Espersen JO, Halaburt H, and Miletic T: Predictive value of clinical and surgical findings in patients with lumbago-sciatica: A prospective study, Part 1. Acta Neurochir 73:67–76, 1984.

29. Spangfort EV: Lumbar disc herniation: A computer aided analysis of 2504 operations. Acta Orthop Scand 142 (Suppl):1–93, 1972.
30. Hudgins RW: The crossed straight leg raising test: A diagnostic sign of herniated disc. 21:407–408, 1979.
31. Quebec Task Force on Spinal Disorders: Scientific approach to the assessment and management of activity-related spinal disorders: A monograph for clinicians. Report of the Quebec Task Force on Spinal Disorders. Spine 12:S1–S59, 1987.
32. Deyo RA: Lumbar spine films in primary care: Current use and the effects of selective ordering criteria. J Gen Intern Med 1:20–25, 1986.
33. Deyo RA, Diehl AK, and Rosenthal M: Reducing roentgenography use: Can patient expectations be altered? Arch Intern Med 147:141–145, 1987.
34. Deyo RA: Early diagnostic evaluation of low back pain. J Gen Intern Med 1:328–338, 1986.
35. World Health Organization: A rational approach to radiodiagnostic investigations. World Health Organization Technical Report Series 689, World Health Organization, Geneva, 1983, p 31.
36. Kent DL, Haynor DR, Larson EB, and Deyo RA: Diagnosis of lumbar spinal stenosis in adults: A meta-analysis of the accuracy of CT, MR, and myelography. Am J Roentgenol 158:1135–1144, 1992.
37. Schutte HE and Park WM: The diagnostic value of bone scintigraphy in patients with low back pain. Skeletal Radiol 10:1–4, 1983.
38. Deyo RA, Diehl AK, and Rosenthal M: How many days of bed rest for acute low back pain? A randomized clinical trial. N Engl J Med 315:1064–1070, 1986.
39. Gilbert JR, Taylor DW, Hildebrand A, and Evans C: Clinical trial of common treatments for low back pain in family practice. BMJ 66:100–102, 1985.
40. Deyo RA: Conservative therapy for low back pain: Distinguishing useful from useless therapy. JAMA 250:1057–1062, 1983.
41. Deyo RA, Walsh N, Martin D, et al: A controlled trial of transcutaneous electronic nerve stimulation (TENS) and exercise for chronic low back pain. N Engl J Med 322:1627–1634, 1990.
42. Manniche C, Hellelsoe G, Bentzen L, et al: Clinical trial of intensive muscle training for chronic low back pain. Lancet 2:1473–1476, 1988.
43. McKenzie RA: Prophylaxis in recurrent low back pain. N Z Med J 89:22–23, 1979.
44. Hadler NM, Curtis P, Gillings DB, and Stinnett S: A benefit of spinal manipulation as adjunctive therapy for acute low-back pain: A stratified controlled trial. Spine 12:703–706, 1987.
45. Shekelle PG, Adams AH, Chassin MR, et al: The appropriateness of spinal manipulation for low-back pain: Indications and ratings by a multi-disciplinary expert panel. R-4025/2-CCR/FLER. Santa Monica, CA, RAND Corp, 1992.
46. Volinn E, Mayer J, Diehr P, et al: Small area analysis of surgery for low back pain. Spine (In press).
47. Turner JA, Ersek M, Herron L, and Deyo R: Surgery for lumbar spinal stenosis: Attempted meta-analysis of the literature. Spine 17:1–8, 1992.
48. Deyo RA, Cherkin D, Loeser JD, et al: The morbidity and mortality of lumbar spine surgery: Influences of age, diagnosis and procedure. J Bone Joint Surg 74A:536–543, 1992.
49. Weber H: Lumbar disc herniation: A controlled, prospective study with ten years of observation. Spine 8:131–139, 1983.
50. Finneson BE: Low Back Pain, 2nd ed. Philadelphia, JB Lippincott, 1980.

52

Pain in the Shoulder, Neck, and Arm

WILLIAM T. BRANCH, Jr., MD

Pain in the neck or shoulder is a frequently encountered and sometimes difficult to treat complaint. The pain may be quite severe, or it may become chronic or recurrent, resulting in a frustrating problem for the patient. The physician must be able to localize the site of pain accurately, which can be difficult because neck and shoulder pains are often confused with one another. Not only are the structures contiguous, but also cervical spine disease frequently leads to tender muscle spasm and stiffness in the muscles of the shoulder girdle. For this reason, the chief complaint of many patients with cervical spondylosis is "shoulder pain." It is usually possible to localize the source of the pain from the patient's history and from an examination of the patient's neck, shoulder, and arm.

SHOULDER PAIN

The shoulder joint (glenohumeral joint) usually is not the source of shoulder pain. It is involved occasionally by rheumatoid, septic, and other types of arthritis but virtually never is involved, except for cases associated with specific occupations, by degenerative arthritis. Degenerative arthritis often develops in the acromioclavicular joint, which should be examined for tenderness, enlargement, or crepitant motion in any patient with shoulder pain. When this joint is not the source of symptoms, pain in the shoulder generally arises from periarticular structures. These include the musculotendinous insertion of the rotator cuff, the subdeltoid (subacromial) bursa, and the long head of the biceps tendon. If one can exclude traumatic dislocations, sprains, and fractures, nearly all intrinsic shoulder pain is caused by one of four conditions:

1. Supraspinatus tendinitis and subdeltoid bursitis
2. Torn rotator cuff
3. Bicipital tendinitis
4. Adhesive capsulitis

Assessment of the Patient

Figure 52–1 illustrates how the periarticular structures fit into a relatively small space beneath the acromion and the coracoid ligament. The subdeltoid bursa lies within this space. Arising from beneath the bursa, in an anterolateral position, is the tendon of the long head of the biceps. The joint itself is very shallow and has a loose joint capsule, allowing a wide range of motion. Figure 52–2 shows the musculotendinous insertion of the rotator cuff muscles (supraspinatus, infraspinatus, and teres major); these pass beneath the acromion to insert on the humerus. Thus, the important structures involved in shoulder pain are contiguous to one another. The subdeltoid bursa lies beneath the deltoid muscle. The floor of the subdeltoid bursa is contiguous with fibrous tissue of the musculotendinous rotator cuff insertion. This tendinous insertion likewise forms a part of the joint capsule laterally. More anteriorly, the long head of the biceps tendon arises from within fibrous tissue of the joint capsule and passes beneath the subdeltoid bursa into the arm. Although a single tendon or structure may be the source of symptoms, often several contiguous tissues are involved, particularly in adhesive capsulitis, which can be considered the end process of any painful condition that immobilizes these structures.

Figure 52–3 shows the range of motion of the shoulder joint. Painful conditions of the periarticular structures are distinguished from those arising from the cervical spine by showing that symptoms are reproduced by this motion. The conditions listed previously produce pain during passive range of motion—particularly during abduction of the shoulder in supraspinatus tendinitis, torn rotator cuff, and adhesive capsulitis, and during pronation-supination of the forearm in bicipital tendinitis (Fig. 52–4); however, the extent to which passive or active motion is more limited can be helpful in making the diagnosis. Both passive and active ranges of motion are painful in synovitis of the shoulder joint. Adhesive capsulitis also restricts both passive and active motion of the shoulder. In patients with tendinitis, the range of motion can be performed actively and passively, but pain characteristically becomes more severe when the tendon is employed in *actively* moving the joint. To the extent that a patient cannot initiate or maintain abduction of the shoulder but passive motion can be done, one should suspect a torn rotator cuff mechanism (Table 52–1).

When it has been determined that the source of pain is from the shoulder, the most practical approach is to consider whether the pain is acute, intermittent, or chronic.

Acutely Painful Conditions. These are generally accompanied by focal tenderness. The diagnosis is usually either *bicipital tendinitis, supraspinatus tendinitis,* or *subdeltoid bursitis.* One can confirm the diagnosis of bicipital tendinitis by demonstrating tenderness when rolling the biceps tendon beneath the fingers as it passes from within the joint down the biceps groove anteriorly. In supraspinatus tendinitis and subdeltoid bursitis, pain is reproduced by pressing laterally beneath the acromion at the insertion of the supraspinatus tendon and subdeltoid bursa. The diagnosis should be made from these clinical findings and is not aided by obtaining radiographs of the shoulder; the finding of calcification within the subdeltoid bursa by x-ray is of no help to the clinician, because many asymptomatic individuals have calcifications and symptomatic patients at times do not. Because the subdeltoid bursa is adjacent to and its floor forms a part of the fibrous insertion of the supraspinatus tendon, there is no practical distinction between tendinitis and bursitis in this region. As inflammation spreads into the bursa, pain and tenderness will involve a larger area of the arm.[1]

Dislocations of the shoulder generally occur in the anterior direction and give the shoulder a "squared-off" appearance. The patient is usually in intense pain after a fall or injury, holds the injured arm across the chest or abdomen with the opposite arm, and will resist any attempt to move the arm. Often a hollow can be felt just below the acromion, and in thin people, the humeral head can be palpated anterior, medial, and distal to its normal position. Anterior dislocations are relatively easily recognizable on an anteroposterior film. Posterior dislocations occur rarely but are more difficult to diagnose. If the patient is an epileptic or for some reason cannot supply the history of a traumatic dislocation, posterior dislocations are often mistaken for adhesive capsulitis. The correct diagnosis should be suspected, however, because the head of the humerus can no longer be felt at the anterior prominence of the shoulder.[2] Lateral radiographic views are needed to identify the dislocation.[2] Radiographs should be obtained to detect fracture prior to attempted manual reduction of dislocation; neurovascular examination of the hand is mandatory as well. Recurrent dislocations of the shoulder are common.

The remaining consideration in patients with acutely painful shoulders is whether there is a *tear* in the *rotator cuff mechanism.* These rarely occur in individuals younger than 50 years of age.[1] Partial tears result from the combination of minor or repetitive trauma and muscular or tendinous degeneration. These tears may produce the same manifestations as supraspinatus tendinitis: pain, local tenderness, and abduction limited by pain. Complete tears of the rotator cuff often result from more significant trauma and occasionally occur in younger individuals. The patient at times may note a "snap" during some strenuous motion

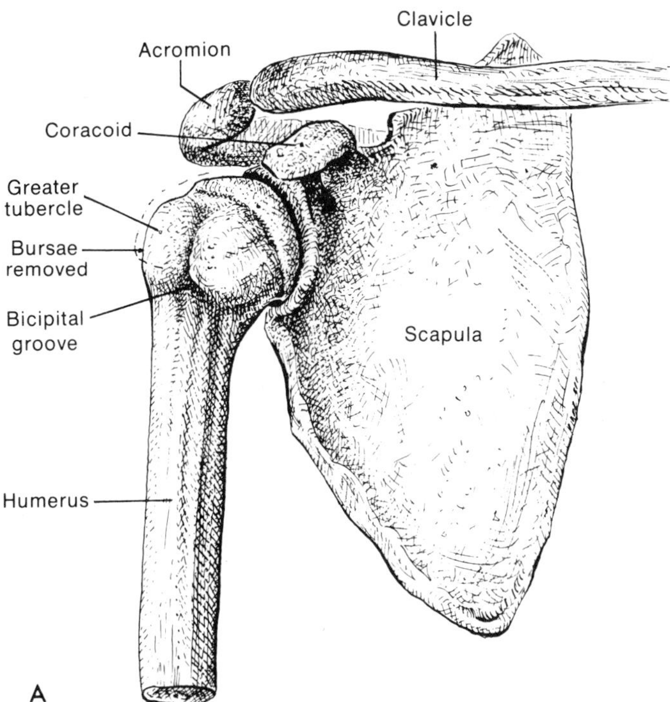

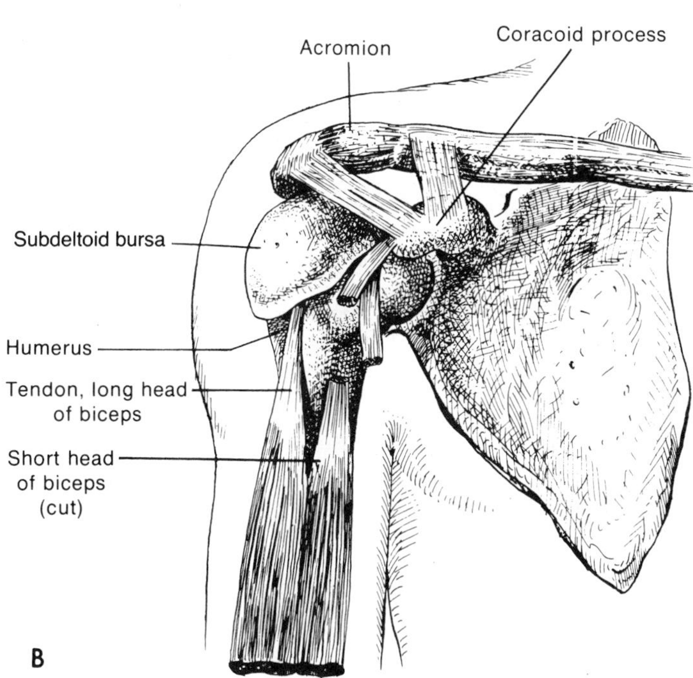

FIGURE 52–1. *A,* The bony structures and *B,* the subdeltoid or subacromial bursa at the shoulder joint. The bursa, lying beneath the deltoid muscle, is located above the musculotendinous insertion of the rotator cuff and also above the origin of the tendon of the long head of the biceps. The bursa and tendons of the rotator cuff are beneath the acromion and corocoid ligament; hence, these structures are subject to compression on motion of the shoulder, because they must fit between the acromion and the head of the humerus.

that is followed by gradually increasing pain and spasm of the shoulder muscles. When the patient appears for examination, often 6 to 12 hours after the event, the arm will be held in adduction, and movement of the shoulder is accomplished by "shrugging." Small or incomplete rotator cuff tears probably occur more frequently than was previously thought but are mistakenly diagnosed as tendinitis or bursitis. If a patient with shoulder pain has not improved substantially after 6 weeks of conservative management, one should consider the possibility of rotator cuff tear.

It is most important to distinguish minor or partial rotator cuff tears, which can be managed with rest, analgesics, and physical therapy, from complete tears, which may benefit from surgical repair. To make this distinction, it may be necessary to anesthetize the area with lidocaine (Xylocaine) or procaine so that one can compare the passive with the active range of motion. Discomfort may also be relieved temporarily by the pendulum position (see Fig. 52–6), which tends to separate the painful structures gently.[1] Once pain is relieved, it will be apparent that the patient with a complete tear cannot initiate abduction. In addition, although the patient may be able to maintain the arm at more than 90 degrees' abduction by using the deltoid, if he or she attempts to move the arm downward slowly, there will ensue a jerky collapse at the point below 90 degrees, where rotator cuff musculature replaces the deltoid in maintaining abduction (see Fig. 52–4). The diagnosis of a complete tear can be confirmed by demonstrating that con-

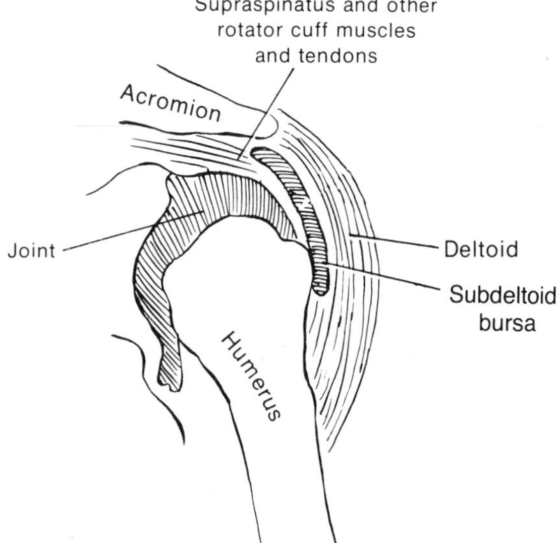

FIGURE 52–2. The musculotendinous insertion of the rotator cuff muscles. The tendons of the teres major, infraspinatus, and supraspinatus insert onto the humerus. This tendinous insertion becomes contiguous with the joint capsule. Superiorly, it also becomes contiguous with the floor of the subdeltoid bursa. The tendons pass beneath the acromion, where they are subject to compression. Usually, it is the supraspinatus tendon that becomes inflamed or torn.

trast material injected into the joint space during arthrography enters the subdeltoid bursa through the tear in the rotator cuff.

Intermittent Pain in the Shoulder. This often results from "chronic" bursitis or tendinitis. The typical case involves an elderly person who complains of being awakened at night by rolling on the shoulder or recurrently experiencing pain during certain motions involving the joint, such as putting on a coat. These intermittent symptoms are usually caused by tendinitis. If the tendon is not tender on palpation, the diagnosis can be made by resisted supination of the wrist, which reproduces pain in bicipital tendinitis, or by fully abducting the shoulder and reproducing pain beneath the acromion at the site of the supraspinatus tendon.

Chronic Symptoms of Stiffness and Pain in the Shoulder. If stiffness develops gradually, persists for weeks or months, and is poorly localized around the joint, the physician must suspect adhesive capsulitis. The full manifestations of adhesive capsulitis include a gradually worsening soreness of the shoulder that increases until the patient is in constant pain and unable to sleep comfortably; this is accompanied by limitation of mobility of the joint. There may follow a gradual lessening of pain itself, but the patient will continue to be moderately uncomfortable with decreased motion on a chronic basis.

The cause of adhesive capsulitis is unknown, but it may be related to reflex sympathetic dystrophy[1] or possibly simply to adhesions that form in the joint capsule when immobility occurs for any reason. The condition is said to remit spontaneously within 2 years in up to 60% of patients.[3] It causes disability, however, by producing atrophy of the shoulder musculature, and some authorities believe that spontaneous complete remissions are actually rare.[1] It is important, therefore, that adhesive capsulitis be diagnosed at an early stage before motion is entirely lost. In this way, many patients with poorly localized pain in the shoulder and fairly subtle limitations of motion may be suspected of having an early stage of adhesive capsulitis, may be treated vigorously, and possibly may be prevented from developing the complete syndrome. If it becomes necessary to establish the diagnosis of adhesive capsulitis, one may obtain arthrography, which reveals contraction of the joint capsule and reduction, by 60 to 90%, in the volume of contrast agent that can be injected.[3]

Management of Tendinitis and Capsulitis of the Shoulder

The principles of management of shoulder pain are as follows: (1) anti-inflammatory agents are used to relieve acute pain; (2) rest is advised for very painful shoulders, but only as briefly as possible; and (3) gradually increasing, regular range-of-motion exercises are given to maintain or improve mobility and prevent adhesive capsulitis. Most authorities agree that the optimal treatment for acute tendinitis is injection of a long-acting corticosteroid preparation (e.g., methylprednisone acetate [Depo-Medrol] or betamethasone sodium phosphate [Celestone, Soluspan], 20 to 40 mg) into the vicinity of the local pain. Many clinicians inject the subdeltoid bursa from the lateral aspect where the maximal tenderness is located, at the point below the acromion. The bursa can also be injected by advancing the needle from a posterior site and having it enter the bursa beneath the acromion (Fig. 52–5). The latter probably is the preferred method because it allows one to judge the depth of the injection more accurately. To inject for bicipital tendinitis, one places the needle at the site of maximal tenderness adjacent to but not within the tendon. Having the patient pronate and supinate the forearm can verify that one is near the tendon by causing movement of the needle and syringe. It is reasonable to be concerned that frequent steroid injections might induce local atrophy with weakening of the tendon. We advise that injections be limited to no more than a total of six to eight to a joint or tendon and no more than three in a single year.

Nonsteroidal anti-inflammatory drugs (NSAIDs) probably are less effective but can be used for treatment of tendinitis in addition to or instead of corticosteroid injection, especially when the area of tenderness is difficult to localize precisely enough to be confident in using the injection.

The patient with an acutely painful shoulder may require a short period of immobilization to relieve discomfort (Fig. 52–6). After a few days, properly injected local corticosteroids or effective doses of a NSAID should diminish symptoms sufficiently so that exercises can be done. Three commonly used exercises—pendulum, broomstick, and wall climbing—are shown in Figure 52–7. It is best to simplify the instructions. I usually initiate exercise with pendulum movements, which are least painful to perform and can be

TABLE 52–1. PASSIVE AND ACTIVE RANGE OF MOTION INVOLVING THE SHOULDER JOINT

Condition	Passive Motion	Active Motion
Synovitis	Painful	Painful
Adhesive capsulitis	Limited	Limited
Tendinitis or bursitis	Painful at the point where the tendon or bursa is compressed or moved	More painful than passive motion
Torn rotator cuff	Unlimited after anesthetization or subsidence of acute pain	Unable to perform

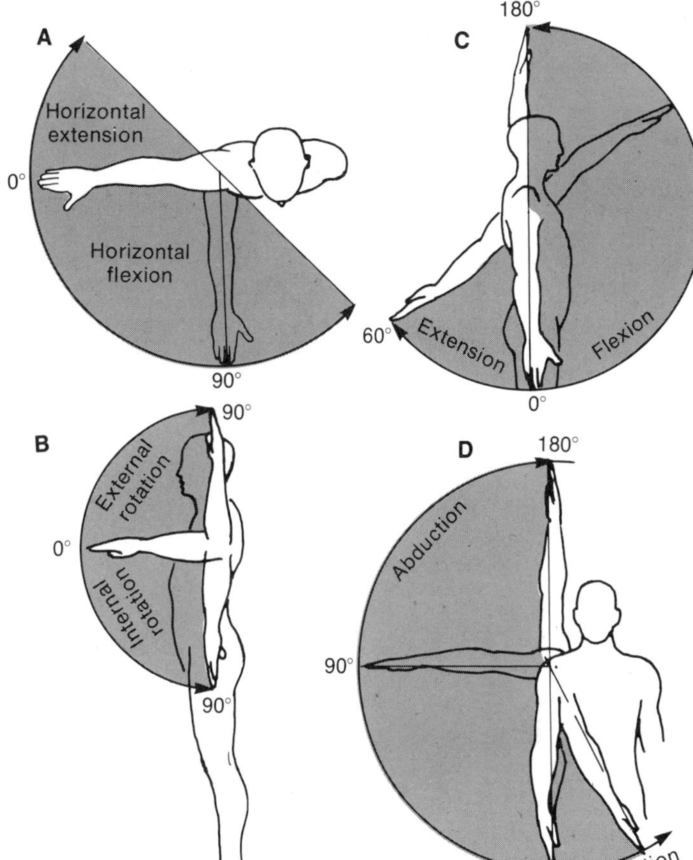

FIGURE 52–3. Range of motion of the shoulder joint.

increased gradually. As soon as possible, I instruct the patient also to begin broomstick exercises to achieve complete abduction. These can be done in a few minutes once or twice a day. It is possible that the regular performance of active range-of-motion exercises promotes the absorption of local calcifications and thus may prevent recurrent attacks of tendinitis and bursitis in the shoulder.

The intermittent symptoms of "chronic" bursitis or tendinitis respond less readily to anti-inflammatory drugs. If one can localize the symptoms to a specific tendon, injection of corticosteroids—either in the vicinity of the subdeltoid bursa or in a fan-shaped distribution along the bicipital tendon—benefits some, but not all, patients. Several corticosteroid injections or several 1- to 2-week courses of NSAIDs may suppress the symptoms, after which the patient can begin regular exercises.

Adhesive capsulitis, including the nonspecifically, chronically diffusely painful or restricted shoulder, requires a more vigorous approach. If the symptoms appear somewhat localized to the area of a single tendon or bursa, one may try injecting this area with corticosteroids and then prescribing physical therapy. Even patients with mild cases might be referred to a physical therapist at least for several sessions in order to be instructed properly in performing exercises. In patients with more diffuse restriction of shoulder motion, a course of oral corticosteroids (e.g., prednisone, 40 mg, tapered over 2 to 6 weeks and discontinued after) is beneficial, in addition to physical therapy.[1] Alternatively, one may utilize an injection containing 40 mg of a long-acting corticosteroid, 3 ml of lidocaine (Xylocaine), and enough sterile saline solution to distend the joint capsule. After instillation of this into the joint space under pressure, physical therapy should be started immediately, and the patient should continue to be seen regularly in physical therapy to have vigorous passive range-of-motion exercises designed to mobilize the joint. This combination of steroid injection and physical therapy is said to produce good results in patients with adhesive capsulitis, although no randomized controlled study has been conducted.[3] The surgical procedure of forcefully restoring motion under general anesthesia is no longer recommended for patients with adhesive capsulitis, because of the frequent recurrence of the condition following this approach.

NECK AND ARM PAIN

The range of motion of the cervical spine—90 degrees rotation in each direction, 60 degrees extension, 30 degrees flexion, and 70 degrees lateral bending (Fig. 52–8)—is limited in most patients with cervical spine disease. Stiffness and tender muscle spasm also are characteristic of these patients. Often this spasm and tenderness may be localized to one side of the cervical spinous processes or may be palpable in the posterior neck or at the angle of the neck and trapezius muscle ridge (Fig. 52–9). The patient whose "shoulder pain" consists of muscle spasm above the scapula or over the scapula can be recognized if one observes shoulder abduction from behind; this patient will abduct the shoulder but may limit motion of the scapula. Conversely, when the origin of pain is from the shoulder rather than the cervical spine, there is a "shrugging" motion in which the scapula moves vigorously, accompanied by relatively little motion of the joint itself (Fig. 52–10). In practice,

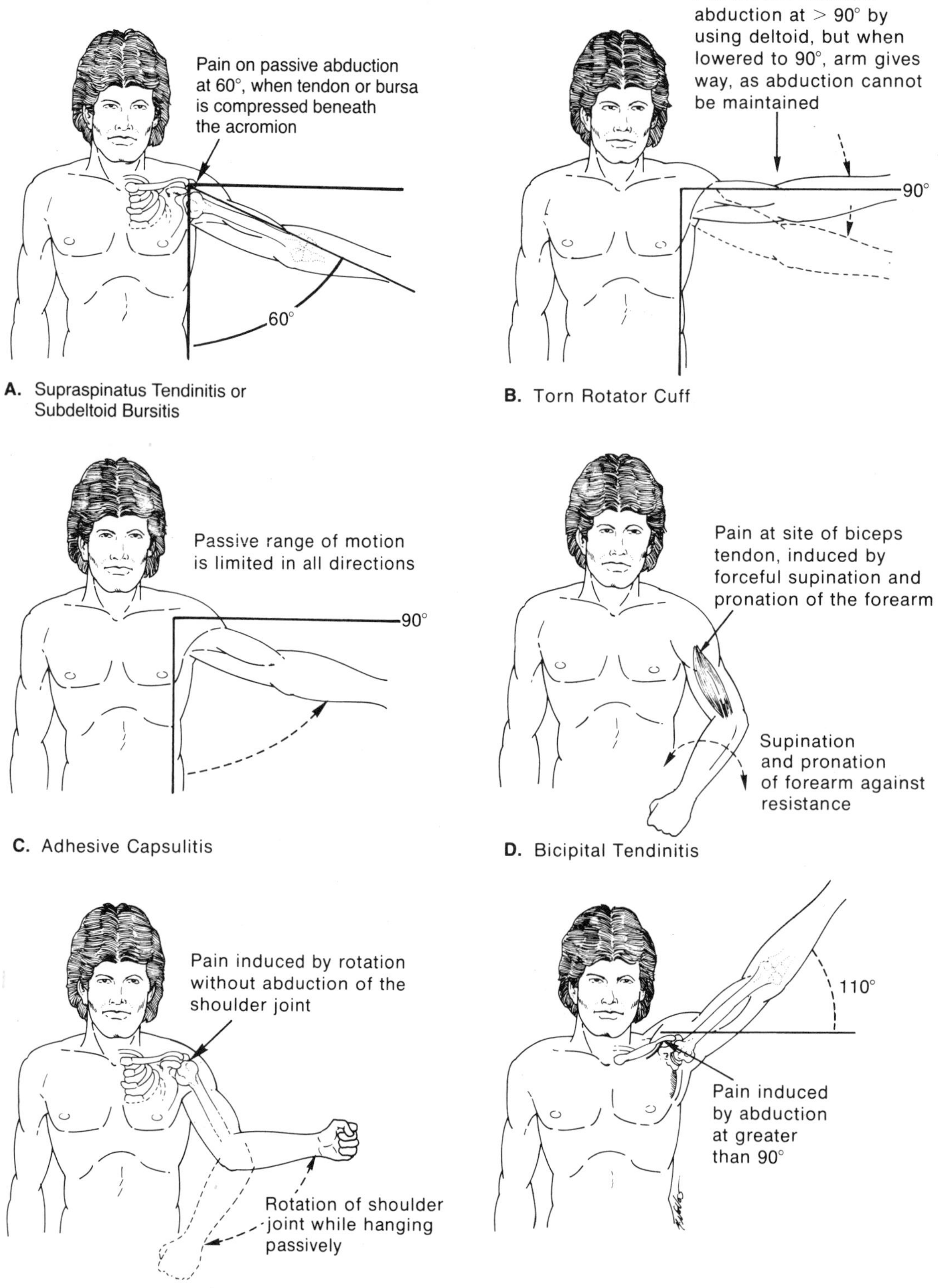

FIGURE 52–4. Reproduction of symptoms in various conditions that cause shoulder pain. *A,* In acute tendinitis and bursitis, more severe inflammation can cause pain to occur at lesser degrees of motion of the shoulder. *B,* The arm "gives way" because the abduction cannot be maintained at this angle without use of the rotator cuff muscles. In incomplete tears, this sign may not be present. In *E,* pain is induced by rotation in patients with synovitis of the shoulder joint (e.g., rheumatoid, tuberculous, or septic arthritis). In *F,* pain with crepitus noted at greater than 90 degrees of abduction suggests the possibility of acromioclavicular arthritis.

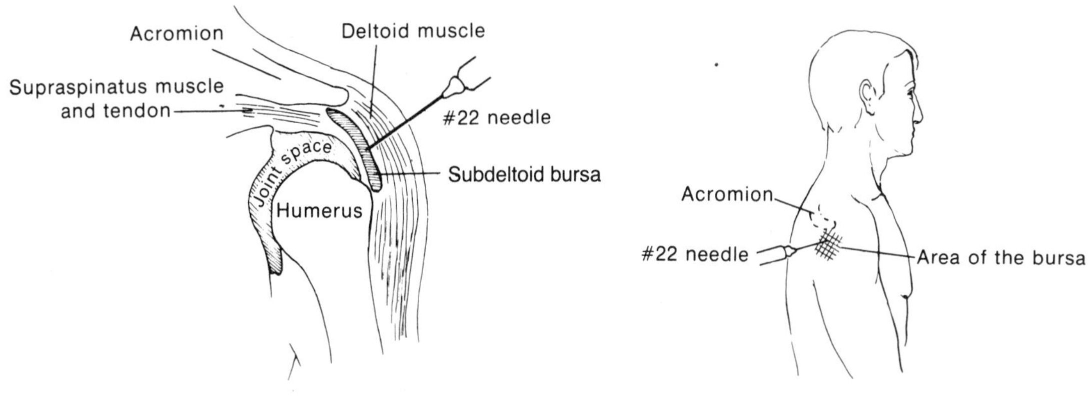

FIGURE 52–5. *A,* Injection of the subdeltoid bursa can be accomplished by passing the needle through the deltoid and into the bursa as it lies beneath the acromion. *B,* From the posterior aspect of the shoulder, one may insert the needle beneath the acromion, and entry into the bursa may be accomplished somewhat more easily than if the injection is made from directly above the bursa.

tender muscle spasm generally is recognizable in patients with cervical spine disease when one palpates the muscles behind the neck, the paraspinal muscles, and the back muscles over the scapula. "Trigger points," locally painful knots of muscle spasm, are characteristically noted in this condition and usually are identified easily by the experienced examiner who is aware of the usefulness of this finding.

Some particular features of the anatomy of the cervical spine are clinically important. Figure 52–11 shows a cervical vertebra, spinal cord, nerve root, and sympathetic ganglion. Unlike the lumbar region, through which pass the multiple cauda equina nerve roots (one or several of which may be involved by a herniated disk), the spinal cord itself passes through the cervical region, so that a syndrome of cord rather than root compression results when any process

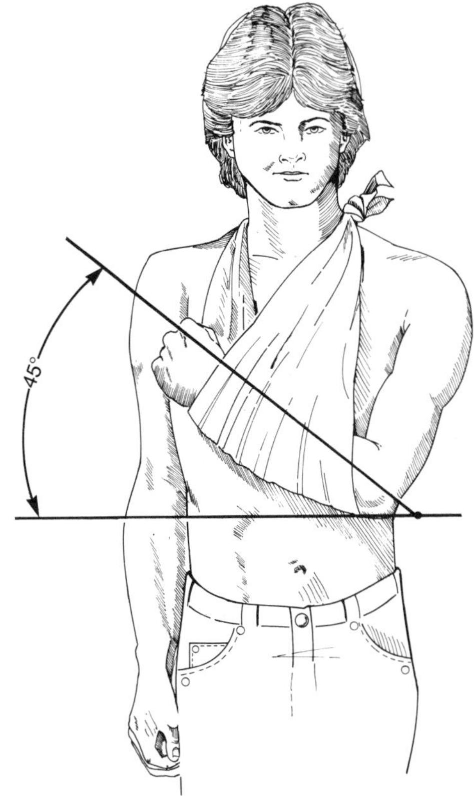

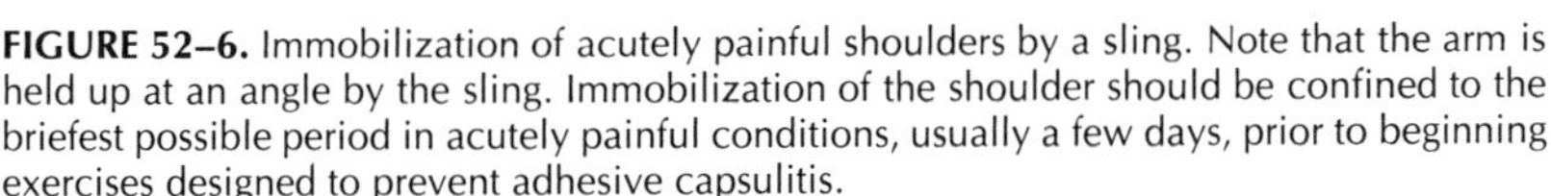

FIGURE 52–6. Immobilization of acutely painful shoulders by a sling. Note that the arm is held up at an angle by the sling. Immobilization of the shoulder should be confined to the briefest possible period in acutely painful conditions, usually a few days, prior to beginning exercises designed to prevent adhesive capsulitis.

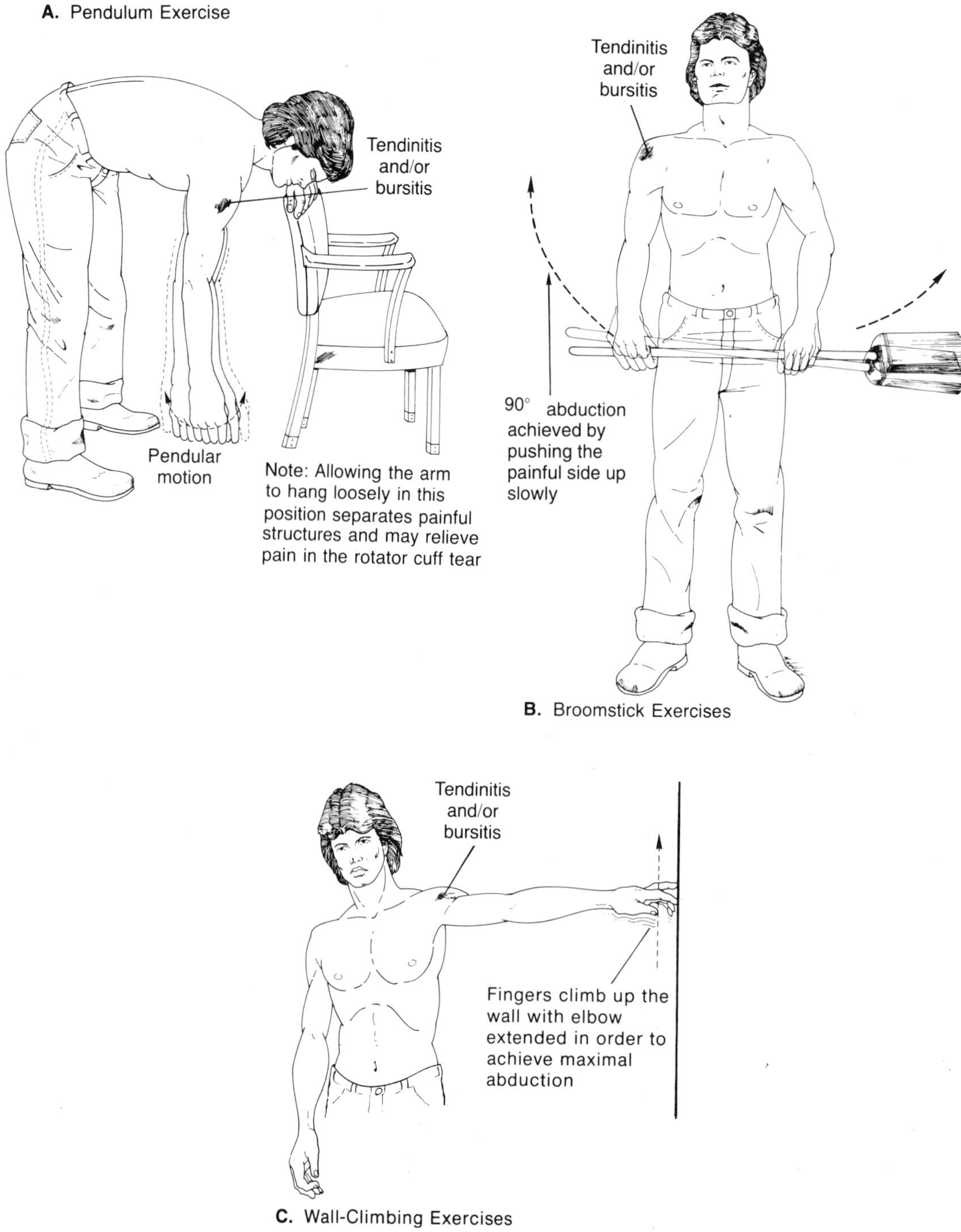

A. Pendulum Exercise

Tendinitis and/or bursitis

Pendular motion

Note: Allowing the arm to hang loosely in this position separates painful structures and may relieve pain in the rotator cuff tear

Tendinitis and/or bursitis

90° abduction achieved by pushing the painful side up slowly

B. Broomstick Exercises

Tendinitis and/or bursitis

Fingers climb up the wall with elbow extended in order to achieve maximal abduction

C. Wall-Climbing Exercises

FIGURE 52–7. Active range-of-motion exercises for patients with tendinitis or bursitis of the shoulder. *A,* Pendulum exercise. The patient relaxes by leaning and supporting his weight on a chair. This allows the affected arm to hang freely. If a tear of the rotator cuff is present, this may relieve discomfort. For performing exercises, with the arm hanging freely, a pendulum motion is initiated by moving the body and can be gradually increased to extend the range of motion, first for flexion-extension and later for abduction-adduction. This is the least painful exercise to perform when acute tendinitis is present. *B,* Broomstick exercise. The patient holds the broomstick in front of the body and initiates motion by pushing upward with the nonpainful arm. This motion can be repeated in a backward and forward manner. By pushing with the unaffected arm, one can achieve more abduction of the affected shoulder. *C,* Wall-climbing exercises. The patient stands next to the wall and "walks up the wall with his fingers." If the elbow is extended and the patient moves at the shoulder joint rather than by shrugging, significant abduction can be achieved.

impinges upon the canal. However, in the cervical region, the posterior longitudinal ligament is extremely well developed and extends laterally to the intervertebral foramina, so that the anterolateral disk herniations that often occur in the lumbar spine are virtually nonexistent in the cervical spine. In addition, in the cervical spine, two joints of Luschka (lateral interbody joints) are located between the vertebral bodies and protect against lateral disk herniation (see Fig. 52–11). Disease that does develop in the cervical spine is often caused by the combination of disk degeneration and osteoarthritis of joints and vertebrae, which is termed spondylosis. Spondylosis produces lipping and spur-

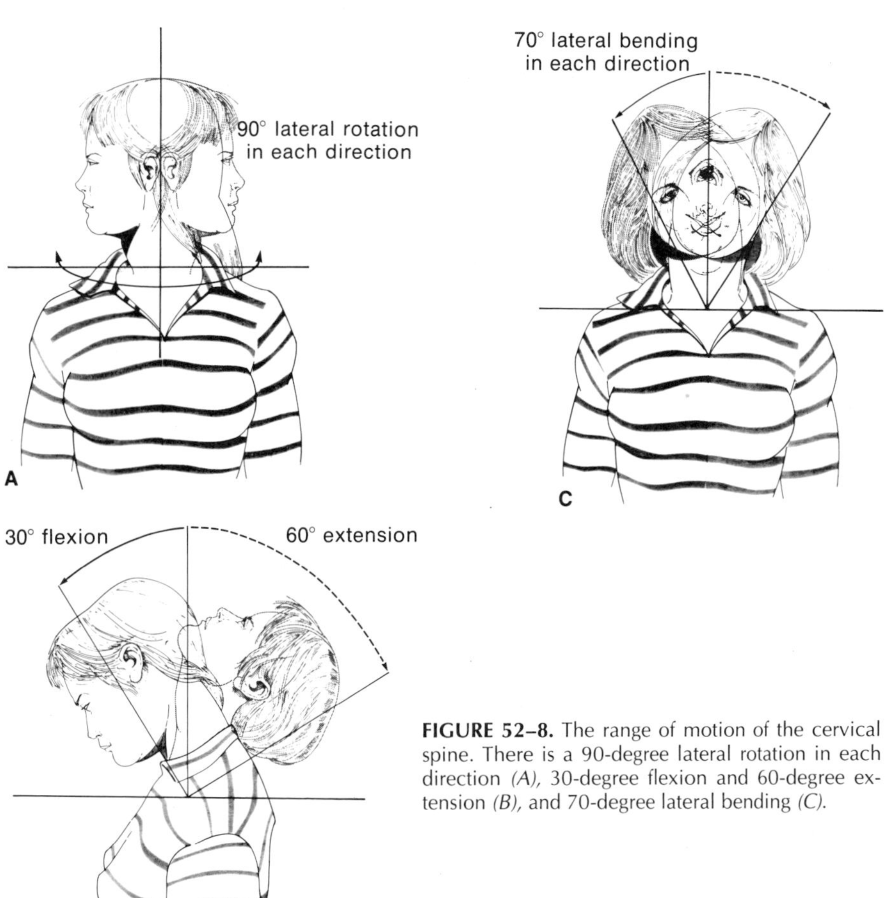

FIGURE 52–8. The range of motion of the cervical spine. There is a 90-degree lateral rotation in each direction *(A)*, 30-degree flexion and 60-degree extension *(B)*, and 70-degree lateral bending *(C)*.

ring of the vertebral bodies anteriorly and degenerative sclerosis of the facet joints and the joints of Luschka. With degeneration of the disk, the annulus fibrosus may become fragmented, causing its nuclear material to become dehydrated and assume a more flattened configuration. Disk material may tend to extrude through the fragmented annulus fibrosus. This flattening also will displace the joints of Luschka to some extent, resulting in wear and tear and osteoarthritis. Soft disk material that extrudes beneath the posterior longitudinal ligament generally will be forced far laterally by the strong posterior longitudinal ligament. The result is impingement upon the intervertebral foramen. In some cases the disk material itself is extruded in such a way as to cause impingement; frequently, it is the gradual build-up of osteoarthritic spurs and calcified hardened disk material, resulting from the combination of disk degeneration and osteoarthritis of the joints of Luschka, that causes impingement at the foramen. Less commonly, extensive disk degeneration, with thinning and buckling of the ligament and posterior bulging of the annulus fibrosus, forms a median bar of degenerative material across the entire width of the disk, in which case there is also the potential for compression of the spinal cord within the spinal canal.

Assessment of the Patient

Symptoms may arise from the cervical spine because of injury, consisting of a "whip-lash" type of trauma or of repetitive minor stresses. This may result in sprain, usually without the subluxation that would result from actual buckling or rupture of the ligaments and dislocation of the facet joints. Disk degeneration or extrusion may result in impingement of a nerve root within the intervertebral foramen by osteophytic spurs, hard disk material, or soft extruded disk. More extensive degeneration forming a median bar across the spinal canal may impinge on the spinal cord. Excluding rheumatoid arthritis of the atlantoaxial joint and rare conditions such as tumor or osteomyelitis, the three mechanisms listed earlier probably account for most symptoms of cervical spine disease. The combination of osteophytic spurs within the foramen plus minor stress or trauma (e.g., leaning backward to paint a ceiling, sleeping with the head twisted, or riding over bumpy roads) often leads to an exacerbation of symptoms. A nerve root previously accommodated to a gradually narrowing foramen becomes acutely traumatized by the unusual position or motion.

Major Clinical Patterns in Cervical Spine Disease

Cervical Sprain or Strain

This syndrome is defined by the presence of neck pain or muscle spasm of the posterior neck, back, and shoulder

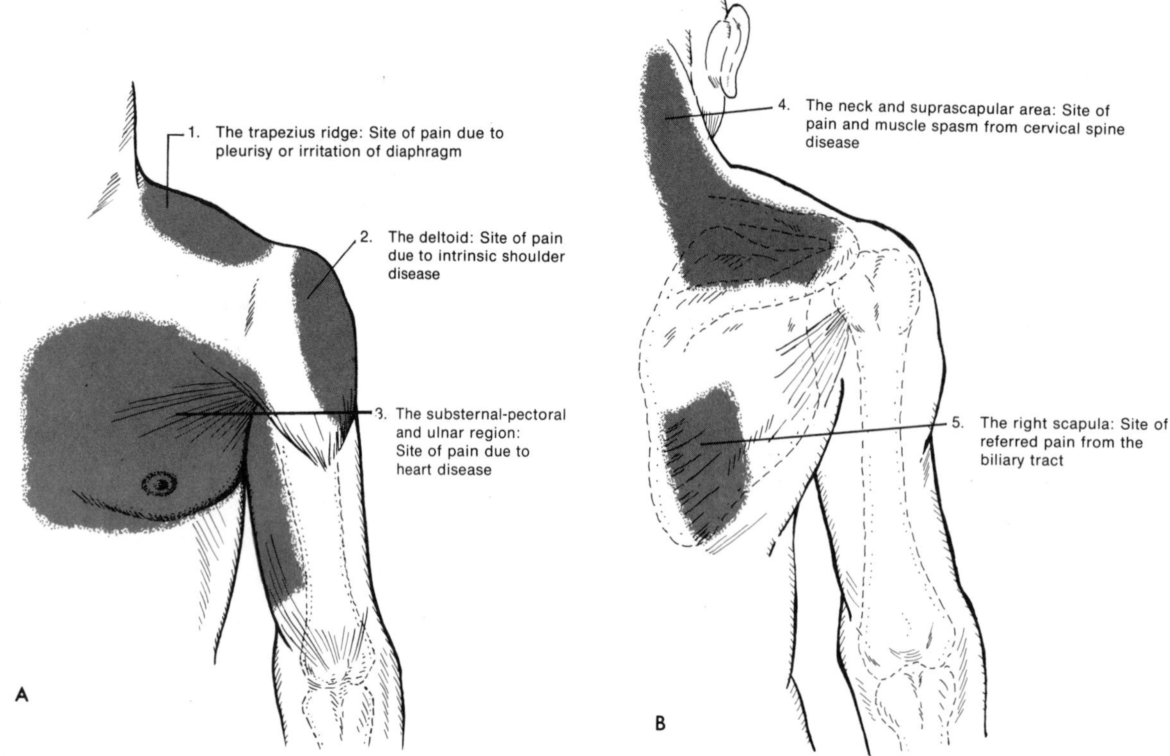

FIGURE 52–9. Typical sites of pain in the neck and shoulder region. (Adapted from Kozin F: Painful shoulder and reflex sympathetic dystrophy syndrome. *In* McCarty DJ [ed]: Arthritis and Allied Conditions. Philadelphia, Lea & Febiger, 1979.)

girdle without radicular symptoms radiating to the arm. Presumably, the cause is a traumatic "sprain" of joints or ligaments unaccompanied by narrowing of the foramen; however, there is often no history of a single traumatic event, and in many such cases the cause may be "strain" of cervical musculotendinous insertions rather than ligamentous or capsular sprain. The identical clinical picture also occurs in cervical spondylosis or disk extrusion but is usually accompanied by nerve root findings. The approach to the treatment can be based on the clinical findings, although it may not be possible to know the exact pathology in individual cases.

Cervical sprain follows a pattern of exacerbations and remissions, with symptoms persisting for several weeks and tending to recur. Sprain resulting from severe "whiplash" injuries may be accompanied by multiple manifesta-

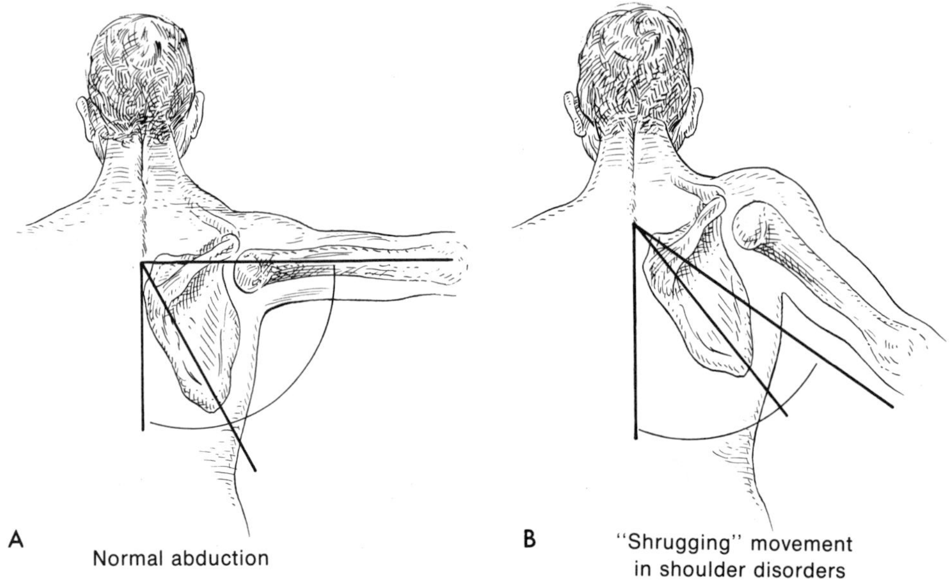

FIGURE 52–10. Movement of the shoulder joint in patients with neck or shoulder pain. *A,* The patient with cervical spine disease will abduct the shoulder normally, but if pain is severe, motion of the scapula may be limited. *B,* The patient with intrinsic disease of the shoulder will abduct the arm chiefly through a "shrugging" motion in which the scapula moves vigorously but the shoulder joint moves less.

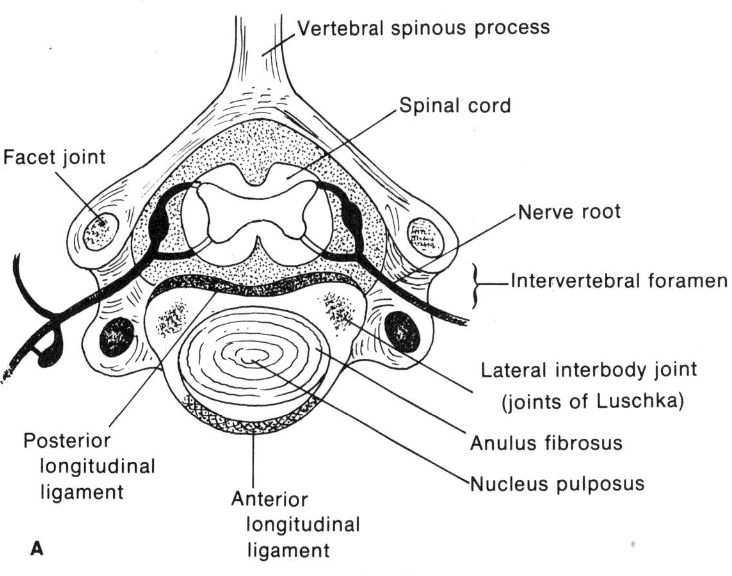

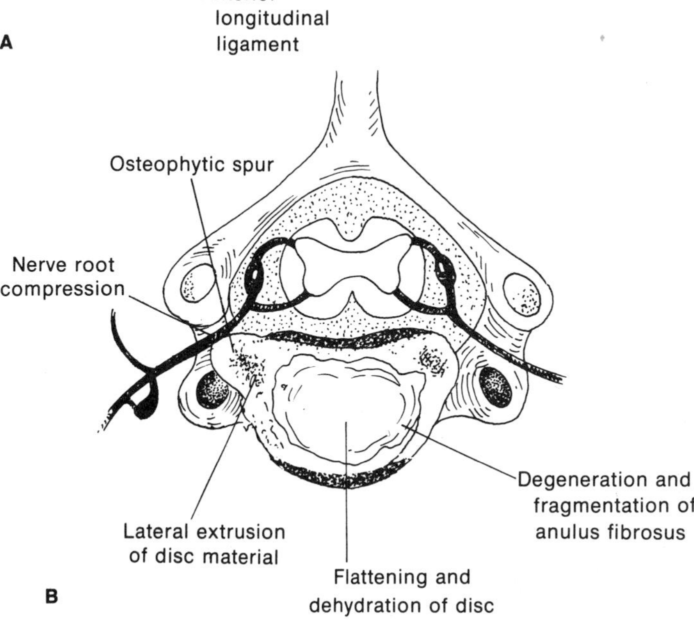

FIGURE 52–11. *A,* A cervical vertebra, the spinal cord, and nerve root, showing the relationship of the lateral interbody joints (joints of Luschka) to the intervertebral disk. *B,* Cervical spondylosis or disk extrusion.

tions similar to those of the postconcussion syndrome, including anxiety and depression, insomnia, vertigo, and tinnitus. In the usual cases, in which there is not a history of notable trauma, pain and stiffness are the only clinical features. Episodes of pain in these patients are commonly precipitated by heavy lifting, poor posture, overly tight clothing, exposure to cold, or sudden, unprotected motion. In some cases, anxiety could be a contributory factor, possibly by causing unconscious tensing of muscles and initiating a cycle of spasm and neck pain, although in general an organic source of pain is also present if symptoms of this type ensue. The natural history of cervical sprain or strain probably concludes when there is a spontaneous resolution after several or more exacerbations precipitated by the factors just mentioned. More persistent or chronic symptoms, even without manifestations of nerve root compression, are attributed usually to underlying spondylosis.

Cervical Nerve Root Compression

Neck, back, and shoulder pain, identical to that noted in patients with cervical sprain, also occurs in patients with cervical spondylosis or disk extrusion. Many of these patients have additional manifestations of nerve root compression, and the course is usually more prolonged. Our discussion focuses on the radicular symptoms. The clinical problem includes developing a differential diagnosis for pain radiating to or in the arm, because at times this will be the presenting complaint in patients with cervical spine disease. In others, there may be some stiffness or limited motion of the neck, but it must be determined that the upper extremity symptoms also are caused by cervical spine disease rather than by another disorder. Lateral bending of the neck toward the side of discomfort is usually more painful when there is nerve root compression, whereas bending the neck away from the side of discomfort, which stretches involved muscles, may be more painful in patients whose symptoms are only due to muscle spasm, without nerve root compression.

In many cases of pain radiating to the arm, it is possible to distinguish between a neuritic type of pain, which is localized and has a “burning” or “tingling” quality, and pain caused by local tendinitis and arthritis, which may have a more aching, diffuse quality. In tendinitis and arthritis, symptoms are reproduced by maneuvers that specifically move the involved tendon or joint. In compression of a peripheral nerve, such as in carpal tunnel syndrome, the area of numbness or “tingling” usually can be localized more precisely than in nerve root compression because dermatomes overlap somewhat in the latter.

When the chief complaint at the time of presentation is burning or tingling of the hand, the differential diagnosis includes (1) spondylosis, disk extrusion, or other disease of the cervical spine, (2) carpal tunnel syndrome and other compression neuropathies of the upper extremity, (3) thoracic outlet syndromes, (4) brachial neuritis, and (5) reflex sympathetic dystrophy.

Differential Diagnosis. ***Cervical Spondylosis or Disk Extrusion.*** Stiffness, pain, or decreased range of motion on extension, flexion, and rotation of the neck implies that disease is present in the cervical spine. In addition, as noted previously, tender muscle spasm elicited by palpation over the exit of nerve roots in the neck or over the rhomboid and trapezius muscles, particularly in the suprascapular region and at the medial angle of the scapula, is a sign implicating cervical spine disease. Some additional observations at times may be helpful. Patients with nerve root pain, if severe, will tend to avoid motion of the involved extremity and prefer to sit with the neck, shoulder, and arm at rest. Reproduction of radicular pain by having the patient cough or perform the Valsalva maneuver also implies that nerve root compression is present. In severe cases, forceful talking and deep breathing may be painful. Whether or not these features are present, a neurologic examination should be done to localize the symptoms. The patient should describe as precisely as possible the zone of hypesthesia or numbness. In many cases, this is the only neurologic manifestation; motor weakness without painful paresthesias is unusual in patients with cervical disk disease.

The nerve roots of C6, C7, and C8 are most commonly involved by cervical spondylosis or disk extrusion and accounted for 96% of cases in one series.[4] The clinical manifestations of patients with impingement localized to each of these roots include: paresthesias of the thumb and index finger, loss of biceps reflex, and weakness of the deltoid and biceps muscles indicate C6 involvement; paresthesias of index and middle fingers, loss of triceps reflex, and weakness of the triceps muscle indicate C7 involvement; and paresthesias of little finger and inner forearm, no reflex loss, and weakness of finger interossei indicate C8 involvement (Fig. 52–12). Symptoms may be difficult to localize when only subjective paresthesias are present.

Carpal Tunnel Syndrome and Other Entrapment Neuropathies. Carpal tunnel syndrome is the most commonly encountered entrapment neuropathy; other entrapment neuropathies of the upper extremity include median nerve entrapment at the elbow, ulnar entrapment at the medial epicondyle of the elbow or in the pisiform-hamate tunnel in the hand, and radial nerve entrapment at the supinator muscle near the lateral epicondyle in the forearm. The neurologic findings of the entrapment neuropathies are illustrated in Chapter 60.

There are some common clinical features of entrapment neuropathies. Those that occur in the hand usually first produce sensory symptoms—tingling or burning—that typically awaken the patient at night, presumably because nerve compression is greatest during sleep, when the wrist is flexed or when some edema occurs. In these cases, patients tend to shake the involved hand, trying to "bring it to life," whereas the typical patient with nerve root compression sits rigidly and avoids even the slightest movement of the extremity or cervical spine.

The provocative test is to reproduce the symptoms, usually tingling paresthesias in the distribution of the nerve, by manual compression at the involved site. The clinical diagnosis of entrapment neuropathies is based on eliciting a typical history plus the provocative maneuver. Manual pressure over the nerve may produce some tenderness in normal individuals but should not produce paresthesias in the distribution of the nerve unless there is an entrapment. Tapping over the carpal tunnel with a reflex hammer is not thought to be as sensitive or as reliable a provocative test for carpal tunnel syndrome as having the patient flex the wrist maximally for several minutes or simply pressing firmly over the median nerve at the transverse carpal ligament. It should be noted that the transverse carpal ligament is quite broad, extending from the wrist crease two thirds of the way over the thenar eminence. Additional details of diagnosis and management of this and other entrapment neuropathies are found in Chapter 60.

Thoracic Outlet Syndromes. Manifestations are essentially the same in all three thoracic outlet syndromes—scalenus anticus, costoclavicular, and pectoralis minor. There are paresthesias in the arm, hand, and fingers, and sometimes an "aching" of the hand, but generally no objective findings of either numbness or motor weakness. The symptoms occur intermittently and are related to posture. Management consists mainly of physical therapy* plus education and reassurance of the patient. Resection of a cervical rib and other surgical procedures designed to alleviate thoracic outlet compression seldom are necessary and should be reserved for only the most unusually severely affected patients. The chief problem for the clinician is to determine that the symptoms are due to thoracic outlet compression of the neurovascular bundle and are not caused by some other lesion of the cervical roots or peripheral nerves. This is done by provocative testing, as illustrated in Figure 52–13. For the scalenus anticus syndrome, the patient extends the neck and rotates the head toward the side on which the symptoms occur while abducting the arm fully and inhaling deeply. Retraction and depression of the shoulder girdles in order to assume an exaggerated military posture is done for the costoclavicular syndrome. The provocative test for the pectoralis minor syndrome involves holding the arms overhead and abducted backward. When the sensory symptoms are reproduced by these provocative maneuvers, in the absence of another explanation, one may reassure patients that the diagnosis is thoracic outlet syndrome. Diminution or absence of the radial pulse during provocative testing is a nonspecific finding and does not establish the diagnosis.

Brachial Neuritis. Brachial neuritis refers to inflammation of the brachial plexus. At one time this was encountered most frequently as a complication of serum sickness; currently, most cases are idiopathic or result from trauma. Any number of branches of the brachial plexus may be involved, although most frequently muscles supplied by C5

---

*Shoulder-girdle exercises for thoracic outlet syndrome: (1) Stand erect with arms at sides holding 2-lb weight in each hand: (a) shrug shoulders forward and upward; (b) relax; (c) shrug shoulders backward and upward; (d) relax; (e) shrug shoulders upward; (f) relax, and repeat each exercise 10 times. (2) Stand erect with arms out straight at shoulder level and 2-lb weight in each hand: (a) raise arms sideways and up until hands meet over head with elbows extended; (b) relax and repeat 10 times. (3) Stand facing a corner with one hand on each wall: (a) slowly let upper body lean forward and press chest into corner while inhaling; (b) push body back to original position while exhaling. (4) Stand erect with arms at sides: (a) attempt to touch the left ear to the left shoulder without shrugging the shoulder; (b) repeat with right ear to right shoulder. Each exercise can be repeated 10 times twice daily. As strength improves, the number of times can be increased, and the weights can be increased to 5 lb and then to 10 lb.

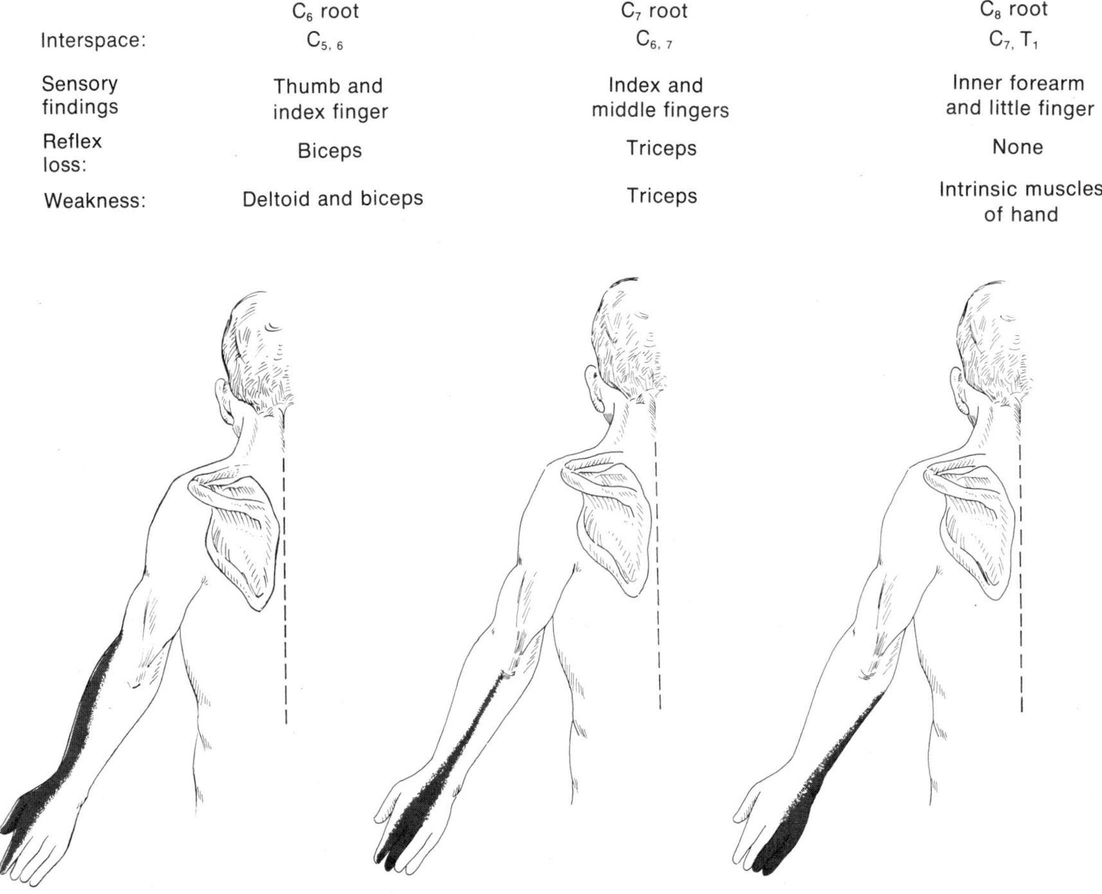

FIGURE 52–12. Neurology findings in compression of the C6, C7, and C8 cervical roots.

and C6 are affected. The diagnosis is generally suggested by several typical features. As opposed to the outlet syndromes and entrapment neuropathies, in which symptoms occur sporadically, the onset of brachial neuritis is abrupt and the findings are persistent, often present for weeks or months before resolving spontaneously. In addition, unlike outlet syndromes and entrapment neuropathies, there is often excruciating pain with tenderness near the brachial plexus. A third characteristic of brachial neuritis, which helps to differentiate it from nerve root or peripheral nerve problems, is early and prominent findings of motor weakness. Although motor weakness also occurs in other lesions, it is more often a late manifestation and is usually preceded by sensory symptoms. Since brachial neuritis may involve several combinations of branches in the brachial plexus, the most important aspect of the neurologic examination is to test for each dermatome. A brachial plexus lesion (as opposed to a nerve root lesion) would be suspected if several or more dermatomes were involved.

Reflex Sympathetic Dystrophy Syndrome (RSDS). RSDS, often referred to as "causalgia" when the cause is specifically traumatic, is a disorder involving sympathetic innervation of the hand and arm. Although the pathologic mechanism by which RSDS is produced remains unclear, the full clinical syndrome should be recognized easily. There is thickening, edema, and atrophy of skin in the hand, with loss of normal skinfold creases. This is eventually accompanied by muscular atrophy, immobility, contractures, and osteoporosis. Patients with this syndrome sometimes improve spontaneously after several years, but most are left with disability from permanent residual contractures. Because treatment is more effective in early stages and is ineffective once contractures have occurred, the clinician should consider the possibility of RSDS in any patient with persistent paresthesias, "burning" pain, or stiffness of the hand (Table 52–2). Advanced changes will not be present in the early stages; instead, one must rely on finding cutaneous sensitivity, swelling, and vasomotor changes of coolness and perspiration, which help to distinguish RSDS from paresthesias caused by nerve root compression, peripheral nerve entrapments, or thoracic outlet syndromes (if unaccompanied by RSDS). Often it is the history of a preceding myocardial infarction, significant trauma, hemiplegia, or another process known to be associated with RSDS that leads one to suspect the diagnosis (although 23% of cases are idiopathic[3]). Most patients should be diagnosed and treated on the basis of their history and findings. Nerve conduction studies are not helpful diagnostically and generally are normal in these patients.[3] In a few instances, one may resort to referring the patient to an anesthesiologist for a trial stellate ganglion block performed using the anterior paratracheal approach. This may confirm the diagnosis of early RSDS if it is effective in abolishing the symptoms. Treatment generally consists of the combination of orally administered corticosteroids (initially 60 to 80 mg of prednisone), tapered over a period of 6 weeks, and maximal movement of the arm and shoulder that should be achieved during physical therapy.[1]

Diagnostic Studies for Cervical Spine Disease

The standard cervical spine series includes a variety of views, but in practice only several of these are necessary to

Symptoms: paresthesias of arm, hand and fingers
deep "aching" pain

Findings: usually none
sometimes vasomotor changes

Provocative tests:

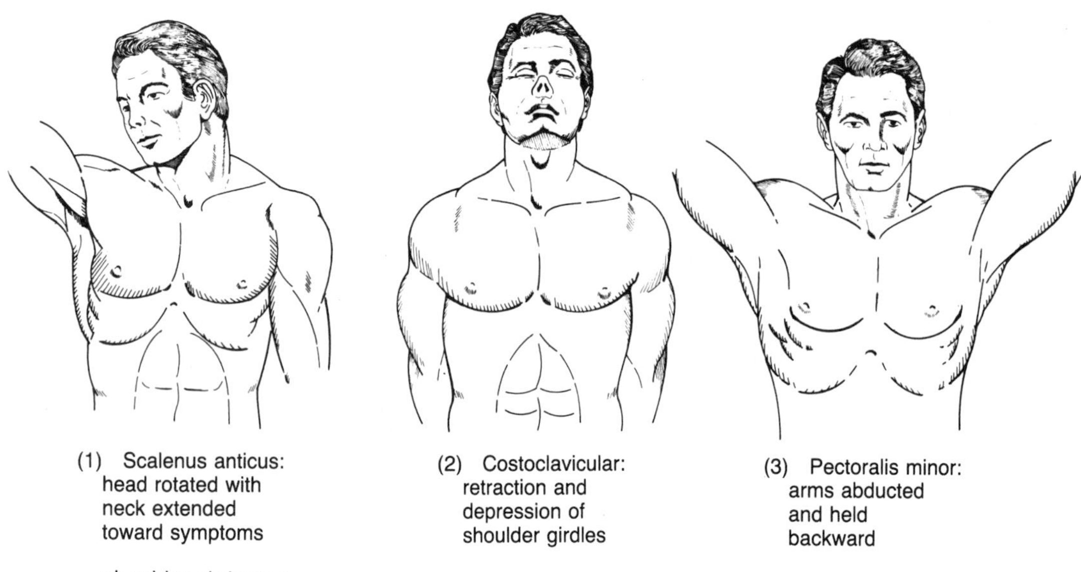

FIGURE 52–13. Symptoms, findings, and provocative tests for thoracic outlet syndromes. (1) Scalenus anticus: head rotated with neck extended toward symptoms; (2) Costoclavicular: retraction and depression of shoulder girdles; (3) Pectoralis minor: arms abducted and held backward.

evaluate patients with chronic symptoms. Anteroposterior and lateral views (Fig. 52–14) show whether there is normal cervical lordosis or straightening of the spine due to muscle spasm. They also show osteophytic spurs, compression fractures, and metastatic or other invasive processes of the vertebral bodies. Narrowing of disk interspaces due to degenerative spondylosis can also be identified on anteroposterior or lateral views, and major subluxations are seen on the lateral.

Oblique views are superior to the lateral for identifying osteophytic spurs encroaching upon the intervertebral foramina. Because these spurs arise near the joints of Luschka, located in the vertebral bodies, one should examine the posterior aspects of the disks and vertebral bodies to identify them. The foramina are seen as oval shapes that may appear as dumbbells when encroached upon. This can be seen at the C5–C6 interspace in Figure 52–15. Soft disk material extruded into the foramen is not visible radiographically.

When patients were carefully studied in one series, 50% with proved nerve root compression had no narrowing of the disk interspace and no encroachment on the foramen that could be identified radiographically. In this group of patients, 20% had disk space narrowing or foraminal osteophytes at interspaces that subsequently were proved not to be the site of nerve root compression.[4] Therefore, although spinal radiographs do detect osteophytic spurring caused by cervical spondylosis, they are of little use clinically, because the degree of spondylosis noted radiographically cannot be correlated with the presence or absence of symptoms. Nor is the radiograph likely to be helpful for the purpose of localizing a specific interspace as the site of nerve root compression. In practice, the usefulness of cervical spine films probably is limited to excluding other

TABLE 52–2. SYMPTOMS IN THE EARLY, MIDDLE, AND LATE STAGES OF REFLEX SYMPATHETIC DYSTROPHY

Stage 1 (First 6 Months)	Stage 2 (Additional Period of Months)	Stage 3 (Chronic)
Burning pain; dry, hot, tender skin	Decreased edema and pain	Cool, cyanotic, atrophied skin
Dusky red edema of hand and fingers	Atrophy of skin, muscles, and subcutaneous tissue in the hand	Brittle nail edges
Early limitation of movement, stiffness of the fingers	Palmar fascial contractures similar to Dupuytren's contractures, and joint contractures	Flexion contractures of the hand
Sometimes early osteoporosis on x-ray film		Advanced osteoporosis
Often accompanied by stiffness and pain in shoulder	Often accompanied by adhesive capsulitis of the shoulder	Often accompanied by adhesive capsulitis of the shoulder

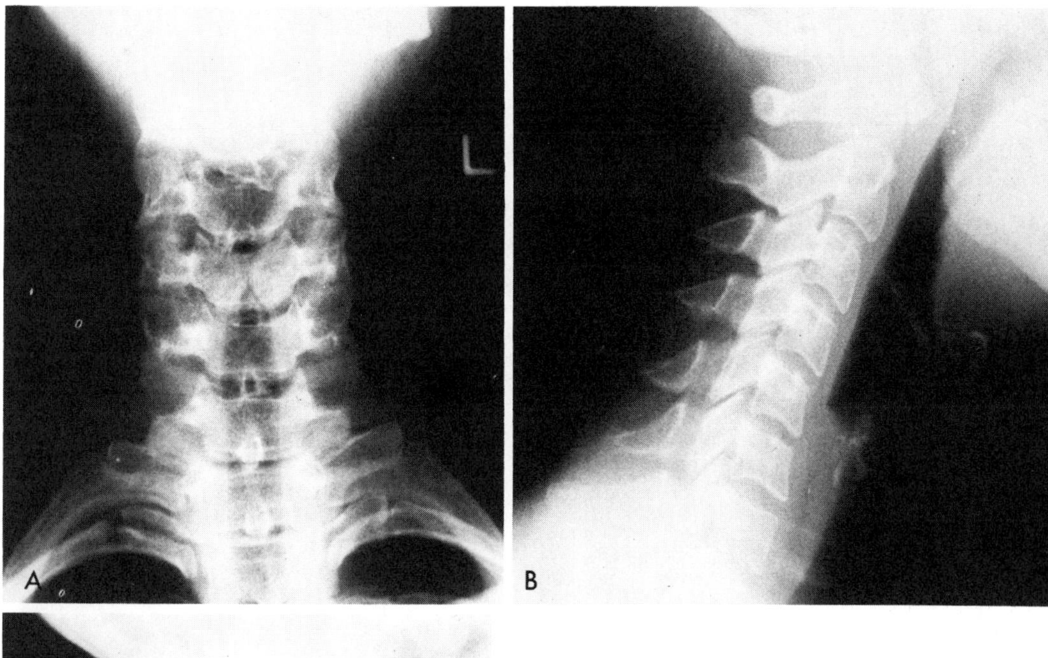

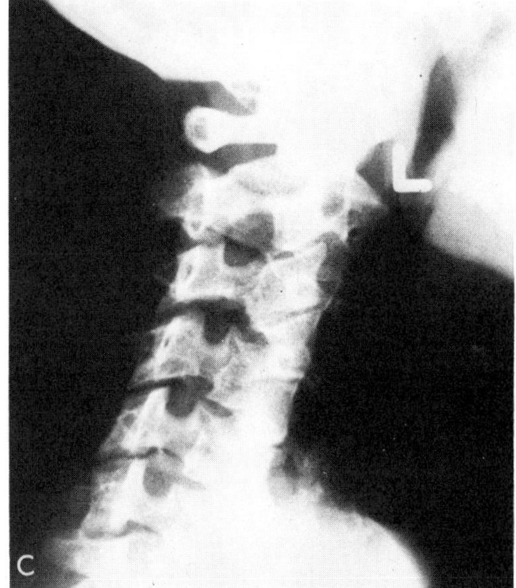

FIGURE 52–14. *A–C,* Cervical spinal radiographs of a young woman following "whiplash" injury. The lateral view reveals straightening of the normal cervical lordosis, a radiologic sign of pain, and muscle spasm in the cervical spine. No major subluxations are present. The oblique and lateral views reveal normal intervertebral foramina.

pathologic conditions, such as metastases, traumatic subluxations, or congenital abnormalities in patients with neck pain (Fig. 52–16). Obtaining x-ray films is unnecessary in young patients with uncomplicated cervical muscle spasm syndromes that are unrelated to significant trauma and neither recurrent nor particularly severe.

Additional views of the cervical spine can be included in the x-ray series when indicated. In general, these views are useful in patients with trauma or rheumatoid arthritis. The open mouth view will show fractures of the odontoid process or lateral subluxation of the atlas on the axis. Flexed or hyperextended lateral views demonstrate incomplete subluxations and angulations that are not seen on the straight lateral view, but these maneuvers should not be performed until a major subluxation has been excluded by examining the lateral view. The caudad-angled view identifies fractures of the posterior articular processes. In the cervical spine, if one knows the nerve root involved, one can be certain of knowing the disk interspace, because a specific nerve root emerges at each interspace. This is unlike the lumbar spine, where several roots of the cauda equina cross near each interspace.

Bone scanning is more sensitive than plain radiographs for detecting a metastasis, vertebral osteomyelitis, or other invasive disease of the spine. A normal bone scan excludes most tumors and virtually all infections of the spine.

Computed tomographic (CT) scanning using thin (1 to 2 mm) slices has been reported to detect cervical disk herniation with accuracy comparable with myelography.[5] Magnetic resonance imaging (MRI) provides excellent detailed anatomy of the spinal cord and detects herniated disk material but is inferior to CT scanning for detection of bony spurs.[6] In special situations, such as syringomyelia, cervical spinal myelopathy (see later), or fractures not identifiable on plain x-ray films, the use of CT scanning during myelography of the cervical spine provides a sensitive and precise diagnostic technique.

Cervical myelograms with CT scanning are often used preoperatively to help identify the involved interspace in patients with nerve root compression and to ensure that the spinal cord is not compressed. The water-soluble contrast agent metrizamide (Amipaque) has replaced Pantopaque for use in myelography in most institutions. Amipaque may offer a better view of nerve root sleeves, but its

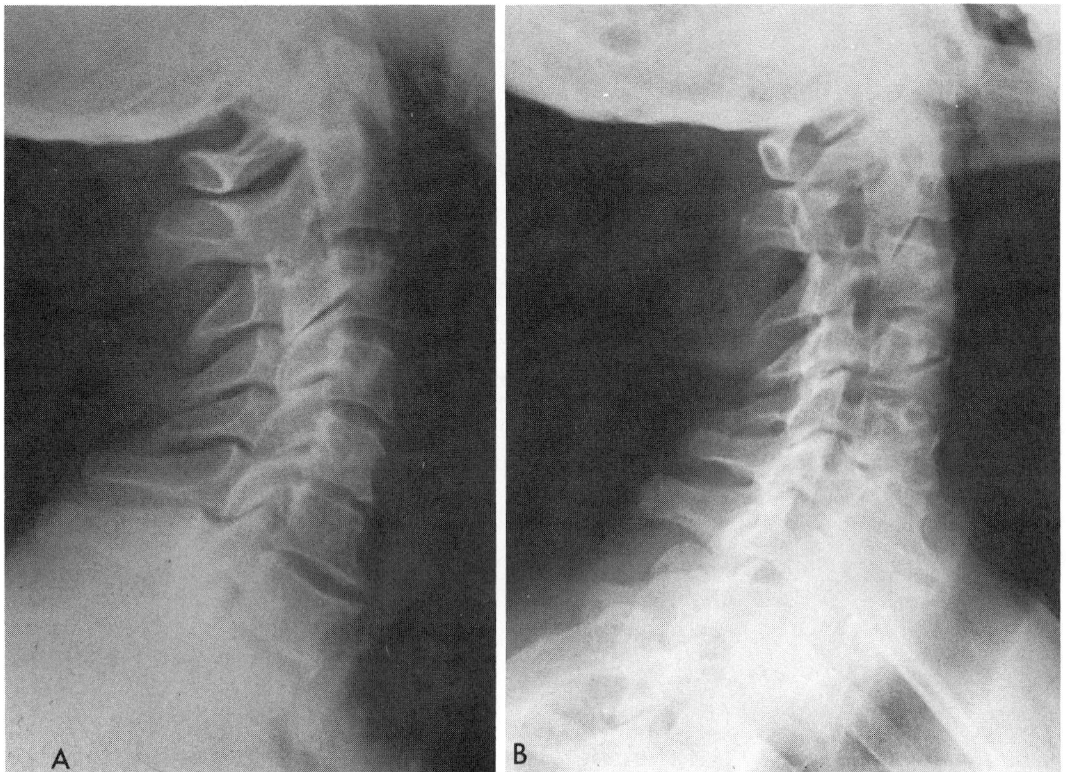

FIGURE 52–15. Oblique view of the cervical spine in a patient with spondylosis at the C5–C6 interspace. The patient had complained of tingling and numbness at the radial aspect of the forearm. His biceps reflex was noted to be diminished, although there was no weakness of the deltoid or biceps muscles. These findings correspond to the C6 nerve root. On the oblique films, an osteophytic spur can be identified at the C5–C6 interspace. The finding is of interest but, in general, in a population of persons who have neck radiographs, cervical spondylosis demonstrated radiographically does not correlate well with the site or the severity of symptoms.

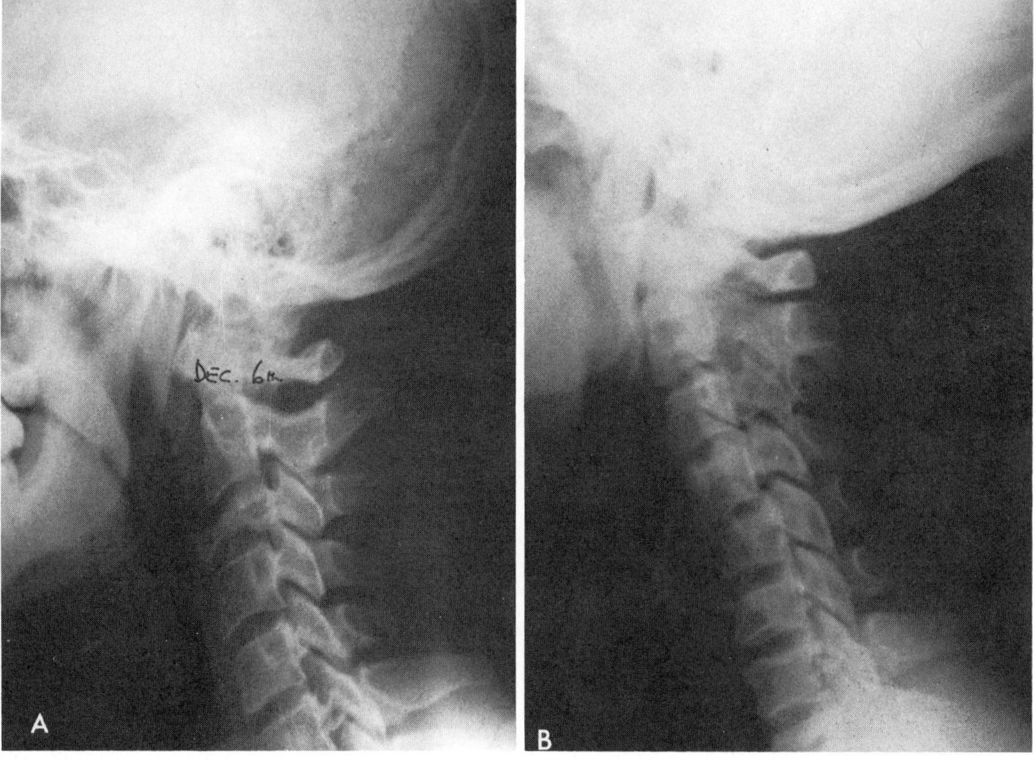

FIGURE 52–16. *A,* Radiograph showing metastasis to the cervical spine by collapse of the vertebral body. *B,* Traumatic subluxation of the cervical spine.

major advantage over Pantopaque appears to be that, despite greater cost and an increased incidence of headache, nausea, and vomiting, long-term sequelae related to arachnoiditis have not been noted in humans following the use of this agent.[7,8]

Cervical Spinal Myelopathy and Other Cervical Conditions That Produce Spinal Cord or Central Nervous System Manifestations

Only about half of patients with cervical spinal myelopathy have a history of neck pain, and only one fourth have a history of root symptoms.[9] The diagnosis of myelopathy depends on finding signs of spinal cord compression involving the corticospinal tract, the spinothalamic tract, or the posterior columns. Most frequently, the patient has signs of corticospinal tract involvement, such as ankle clonus, spasticity, extensor plantar reflexes, or gait disorders of the lower extremities. Some have a level of sensory loss as the only manifestation or, more frequently, associated with spastic motor symptoms. Others have loss of vibratory or position sensation or a disturbance of micturition usually occurring with other signs but rarely as a single manifestation. Usually this is a slowly progressive disorder of the elderly. Acute prolapse of a disk producing spinal cord compression occurs less commonly, sometimes related to trauma or previous cervical fusion, in middle-aged persons.

Only a minority of patients with cervical spinal myelopathy also have manifestations of nerve root compression. There are some patients who have shoulder girdle atrophy, diminished upper extremity reflexes, or atrophy of muscles in the hands (caused by compression of central gray matter in the cervical spinal cord) in addition to the long tract signs. When these findings are present together with neck pain, the diagnosis is suggested, but any patient with unexplained bilateral or unilateral long tract signs should be suspected of having cervical spinal myelopathy.

In patients with cervical spinal myelopathy, the radiographically determined sagittal diameter of the spinal canal generally is less than 11 mm. An MRI or a myelogram with CT scanning is usually necessary to establish the diagnosis because impingement can be caused by soft tissue not identifiable by plain films. It is important to identify every level involved before proceeding with surgery. More than half have cord compression at two or more disk interspaces, and higher interspaces are involved than those that typically produce spondylotic nerve root compression. In one large series, almost half of the patients had cord compression at the C3–C4 or the C4–C5 interspace.[10]

It is necessary to exclude other disorders of the brain or spinal cord before making the diagnosis of cervical spinal myelopathy. Progressive or severe symptoms of cord compression or persistent pain localized to the thoracic spine are suggestive of neoplastic involvement, which can be confirmed by bone scanning or myelography. Vitamin B_{12} deficiency must be excluded in all patients with unexplained bilateral signs of disease involving the posterior columns. Very similar neurologic findings, related to spinal cord compression and varying from minimal proprioceptive losses or the presence of Babinski's signs to frank quadriplegia, also may be seen in patients in whom rheumatoid arthritis causes subluxation at the atlantoaxial or other cervical articulations. Subluxation is related to rheumatoid involvement and subsequent loss of integrity of the spinal ligaments. Occasionally, sudden death may occur as the first known manifestation of this problem, and, therefore, it is warranted to obtain cervical spinal radiographs, including flexed and hyperextended lateral views, in every individual with longstanding or chronically active rheumatoid arthritis.

Another syndrome related to cervical spondylosis is vertebrobasilar arterial insufficiency due to compression of the vertebral arteries in the neck by osteoarthritic spurs. The hallmark of this condition is the occurrence of transient neurologic symptoms—most often sudden falling, with or without loss of consciousness ("drop attacks")—provoked by movement of the head. This syndrome is actually rare, because vertebral arterial compression has to occur bilaterally or one vertebral artery has to be hypoplastic for symptoms to develop. Among 50 suspected cases in one series, the diagnosis could be confirmed ultimately in only six, by reproducing the symptoms during head motion and by documenting the interception of vertebral arterial flow during angiography.[11]

Management of Cervical Spine Disease

The principles of management are the same for most patients, whether they have cervical sprain or strain, disk extrusion, or cervical spondylosis with nerve root compression. First, there are a number of measures for conservative management. Second, surgery is a consideration for those with nerve root compression. The same considerations apply in the management of cervical spinal myelopathy, but since the indications for surgery are somewhat different, this condition is discussed separately.

Conservative Management. The conservative management of neck pain and muscle spasm with or without radiculopathy chiefly depends on the severity of pain. Bedrest is employed when pain is most severe at the onset of an episode. The patient must adopt a comfortable position for the head or neck and remain off the feet as much as possible but may sit propped on pillows, lie on a couch, or adopt any other position that is comfortable, reduces intradisk pressure, and immobilizes the neck. This may be necessary for only a few days. After pain becomes less severe or intermittent, the patient should resume activity gradually while wearing a cervical collar. Soft collars provide support for the neck and partially limit motion but allow the patient to talk, eat, and perform other activities. For patients with nerve root compression, a hard plastic collar properly fitted genuinely restricts motion, which can be especially helpful during travel and at other active times. Usually the patient can gradually cease wearing the collar as symptoms become minimal or occur only occasionally after a period of several weeks.

The cervical collar may be fitted in several ways, but for most cases about 20 degrees of neck flexion is best. To achieve this, the collar occasionally must be worn "backward," fastened in front. This flexed position opens the foramina, relieving nerve root compression, and stretches the posterior neck muscles. A neutral position is preferred for patients with fractures, subluxations, or cervical spinal myelopathy. In patients whose problem is limited to pronounced muscle spasm of the posterior neck, more benefit sometimes results from wearing the collar with slight extension of the neck, which shortens and relaxes the posterior muscles.[12]

A number of ancillary measures seem to be helpful. NSAIDs provide some analgesia and may reduce associated inflammation; however, I believe that pharmaceutical measures rarely provide major relief and must be combined with bedrest, a cervical collar, and the physical therapeutic modalities to be described later if maximal benefit is to be achieved. In the initial few days, however, codeine, meperidine, or another strong analgesic sometimes is indicated. Symptoms may also be diminished temporarily by measures designed to relieve muscle spasm in the neck and back. Diazepam (Valium) can be given in a therapeutic dose regularly while the patient is at rest and then for several weeks as needed to provide more relaxed sleep. The usefulness of this drug probably is more related to achieving sedation and perhaps promoting bedrest than to a specific muscle-relaxing property. A heating pad may also relieve muscle spasms, and, when the patient has resumed activity, can be used for a single 20-minute session each afternoon to provide a period of rest at the time when tension may be increasing. For patients who remain symptomatic after several weeks of using the program of heat and bedrest followed by the wearing of a cervical collar, one may prescribe cervical traction at home. Commercial kits are available with a head halter that can be fitted to a door. These provide 30 minutes of traction using 5 to 7 lb (2.3 to 3.2 kg) up to several times a day. Gentle massage done by a physiotherapist may also provide temporary relief from muscle spasm but should be avoided in patients with severe nerve root inflammation producing tenderness of the posterior neck. We usually avoid massage, traction, or other manipulations and rely on bedrest alone during the earlier period when the patient's painful radicular symptoms are excruciating.

There are various methods for cervical traction, but using 5 to 7 lb for 30 minutes is least troublesome and difficult. Other methods employ 10 to 15 lb (4.5 to 6.8 kg) for 25 minutes, 5 to 7 lb (2.3 to 3.2 kg) for 24 hours, or 25 lb (22.4 kg) for 7 seconds, with 5-second rest periods, given as intermittent traction over 50 minutes.[13] Whatever the method, the neck should be flexed at about 20 degrees to minimize nerve root compression during the traction. In hospital, traction can be maintained with the patient supine, which helps to immobilize the cervical spine if it is severely painful; home traction, using 5 to 7 lb for 30 minutes while the patient is sitting, probably works by relaxing posterior neck muscles. It is doubtful whether any method of traction produces elongation of the spine, which in theory would diminish nerve root compression. At least one neurosurgeon reports that cervical traction was detrimental in many patients with nerve root compression.[14]

The efficacy of cervical traction, collars, and posture and positioning exercises given by physiotherapists has been tested in a randomized trial.[15] This study also defines the natural history of acute episodes. There were 493 patients in the study (57% enrolled after the first attack). Detailed questionnaires and clinical examinations revealed *no differences* in the outcomes of patients treated by traction, collars, or postural exercises compared with the outcome in those treated with placebo (an untuned diathermy instrument). Twenty to 25% were asymptomatic in every group after 4 weeks, at which time 50% continued to have mild symptomatology, 20% had moderate symptoms, and 3 to 5% had severe symptoms. The neck pain, rather than root symptoms, persisted chiefly. The investigators concluded that there was no proven benefit from any ancillary measures in treating neck pain. Whereas some patients felt "better" wearing a collar, others experienced temporary relief from symptoms after traction or after heat and massage. Such treatments, therefore, do not shorten the duration of episodes or alter the long-term course.

Following an episode of neck pain, the patient remains vulnerable, so that even slight trauma or sudden, unanticipated motion may lead to relapse. The most vulnerable time is while the patient is sleeping, when neck muscles relax, leaving the spine susceptible to motions or awkward postures. It may be advisable to wear a soft cervical collar during sleep. Special pillows are available that stabilize the head and hold it in a slightly flexed position while the patient sleeps on his or her back. Sleeping on the stomach can be detrimental. The patient must be particularly careful when first arising in the morning; a hot shower may help to warm up and relax the neck. Anything leading to muscle tension can precipitate a setback. This may include emotional upsets; sitting in an uncomfortable chair or some other awkward position; exposing the neck to drafts or cold; wearing tight or ill-fitting clothing; and, certainly, heavy lifting, push-ups, or other strenuous activity. If care is taken, however, it is usually possible to have sexual intercourse. Driving or riding over bumpy roads can be particularly detrimental. Patients should be instructed to use the cervical collar temporarily while driving or riding, or at any other time muscle spasm begins to worsen in the neck or back.

Several reports discuss the long-term natural history of cervical spine disease. In the multicentric trial of physiotherapy,[15] one third of the patients were asymptomatic and another one third only minimally symptomatic after 6 months. The course over 6 to 10 years was observed in another study of 51 patients with cervical disk disease or spondylosis.[16] In this small group, 43% ultimately became asymptomatic, 30% had mild or intermittent symptoms, and 27% showed moderately severe, persistent symptomatology. None of the patients were disabled in terms of employment, and only one (an 86-year-old man) developed cervical spinal myelopathy during the period of follow-up. The study suggests that generally the course of cervical spondylosis consists of symptomatic episodes lasting for weeks to months with subsidence and few or no symptoms between episodes.

Surgery. The surgical literature contains reports describing anterior and posterior approaches, but no randomized study has compared their efficacy. Given the benign natural history, there is agreement that surgery is generally indicated only if there are persistent findings that can be localized to a nerve root that exits a foramen with demonstrable pathology by MRI or CT scanning and that are unresponsive to medical management. Many surgeons employ an anterior approach to enter the disk space and remove disk material; some visualize and resect spurs or disk material from the vertebral bodies near the foramen. Then, some surgeons perform a spinal fusion at the explored interspaces.[17,18] Posterior approaches enlarge the foramina to better accommodate nerve root exit without necessarily removing anteriorly located spurs. Successful surgery generally relieves pain. Surgery rarely restores sensation to areas of numbness or leads to recovery of lost reflexes, but motor weakness may be improved following surgery, as documented in one series in which two thirds of 24 patients recovered some strength.[17]

Overall surgical results for neck pain and root compression may be summarized as follows. The mortality rate is 0.2 to 0.4%. Complications occur in about 5%. These include vocal cord paresis caused by injury to the recurrent laryngeal nerve, bone infections, extrusion of bone grafts, wound infections, persistent pain due to fractured spine, postoperative hematoma, spinal cord or nerve root injuries, pneumothorax, carotid artery injury, cerebrospinal fluid fistula, and Horner's syndrome. Spinal fusions sometimes fail to fuse or develop pseudoarthroses. The long-term results after 5 or more years seem to be, in general, that about two thirds of patients have no or few symptoms but that the remainder are either no better (20 to 30%) or worse (5 to 8%) after surgery.[14,17–21] One surgeon, using the relatively conservative approach of posterolateral foraminotomy, reported good-to-excellent results in 91.5% of patients, with 1.5% complications, and 13.9% requiring reoperations after a mean follow-up of 11 years.[22] Others, using the more technically difficult anterior approach to remove disk protrusions or osteophytes, reported benefit in 44 of 47 patients after 6 months.[23] Taking all patients, surgical results would seem about equal to the natural history of the disease, so that surgery is usually reserved for patients with progressive motor weakness or severe or disabling pain unresponsive to 3 months or longer of conservative therapy. Those undergoing surgery should be advised that their pain may be only partially alleviated. The average patient returns to work about 4.2 weeks after the operation.

In *cervical spinal myelopathy,* the major question is whether or in what patients there is a progressive course that would justify surgical intervention. Medical therapy using immobilization with a hard cervical collar leads to some resolution of long tract findings in about half of patients.[24] Most patients with rheumatoid involvement of the cervical spine also can be managed by using a cervical collar, especially when riding in an automobile or otherwise at risk for sudden neck motion. Those with neurologic deficits may improve with hospitalization, during which gentle cervical traction is employed to prevent flexion of the neck; for more severe cases, a halo collar is used.[25]

The natural history of cervical spinal myelopathy was defined in 44 patients, half of whom were followed for more than 10 years.[16] Of these patients, few improved, most remained unchanged, but very few worsened. There tended to be long periods of stability punctuated by episodes with temporarily worsened findings. However, more than likely the disease is slowly progressive for the first several years and only tends to stabilize thereafter.[26]

Surgical results for cervical spinal myelopathy may be summarized as follows. The surgical mortality is 3%.[10] An additional 6.5% are worse following the operation.[10] Of those remaining, about two thirds improve at least somewhat following surgery, but the neurologic picture is unchanged in the remaining patients.[9, 10] Thus, since the natural history may be nonprogressive or the findings improved by medical immobilization, leaving many patients with minimal residual symptoms, and since about one third of patients are worse or no better following surgery, operations should be reserved for those who are young, have severe deficits, or have progressive findings. In most patients who improve following surgery, the improvement is only partial. On the other hand, partial recovery is of most importance for the most severely affected patients; thus, in general, the more severe the neurologic deficits, the more likely one will be able to recommend a surgical approach.

REFERENCES

1. Bland JJ, Merrit JA, and Boushey DR: The painful shoulder. Semin Arthritis Rheum 7:21, 1977.
2. Paton DF: Posterior dislocation of the shoulder: A diagnostic pitfall for physicians. Practitioner 223:111, 1979.
3. Kozin F: Painful shoulder and reflex sympathetic dystrophy syndrome. *In* McCarty DJ (ed): Arthritis and Allied Conditions. Philadelphia, Lea & Febiger, 1979, pp 1091–1120.
4. Scoville WB, Dohrmann GJ, and Corkill G: Late results of cervical disc surgery. J Neurosurg 45:203, 1976.
5. Coin CG and Coin JT: Computed tomography of cervical disk disease: Technical considerations with representative case reports. J Comput Assist Tomogr 5:275, 1981.
6. Han JS, Kaufman B, El Yousef SJ, et al: NMR imaging of the spine. Am J Neuroradiol 4:1151, 1983.
7. Nickel AR and Salem JJ: Clinical experience in North America with metrizamide: Evaluation of 1850 subarachnoid examinations. Acta Radiol (Suppl 355):409, 1977.
8. Baker RA, Hillman BJ, McLennan JE, et al: Sequelae of metrizamide myelography in 200 examinations. Am J Roentgenol 130:499, 1978.
9. Crandall PH and Batzdorf U: Cervical spondylotic myelopathy. J Neurosurg 25:57, 1966.
10. Gonzalez-Feria L and Peraita-Peraita P: Cervical spondylotic myelopathy: A cooperative study. Clin Neurol Neurosurg 78:19, 1975.
11. Pasztor E: Decompression of vertebral artery in cases of cervical spondylosis. Surg Neurol 9:371, 1978.
12. Gibson JW: Cervical syndromes: Use of a comfortable cervical collar as an adjunct in their management. South Med J 67:205, 1974.
13. Harris PR: Cervical traction: A review of literature and treatment guidelines. Phys Ther 57:910, 1977.
14. Fager CA: Rationale and techniques of posterior approaches to cervical disc lesions and spondylosis. Surg Clin North Am 56:581, 1976.
15. British Association of Physical Medicine: Pain in the neck and arm: A multicentric trial of the effects of physiotherapy. BMJ 1:253, 1966.
16. Lees F and Aldren Turner JW: Natural history and prognosis of cervical spondylosis. BMJ 2:1607, 1963.
17. Green PWB: Anterior cervical fusion: A review of 33 patients with cervical disc degeneration. J Bone Joint Surg 59B:263, 1977.
18. Rish BL, McFadden JT, and Penix JO: Anterior cervical fusion using homologous bone grafts: A comparative study. Surg Neurol 5:119, 1976.
19. Martins AJ: Anterior cervical discectomy with and without interbody bone graft. J Neurosurg 44:290, 1976.
20. Hakuba A: Trans-unco-discal approach: A combined anterior and lateral approach for cervical discs. J Neurosurg 45:284, 1976.
21. Tew J and Mayfield FH: Complications of surgery of the anterior cervical spine. Clin Neurosurg 23:424, 1976.
22. Henderson CM, Hennessy RG, Shuey HM Jr, et al: Posterior-lateral foraminotomy as an exclusive operative technique for cervical radiculopathy: A review of 846 consecutively operated cases. Neurosurgery 13:504, 1983.
23. Bollati A, Galli G, Gandolfini M, et al: Microsurgical anterior cervical disk removal without interbody fusion. Surg Neurol 19:329, 1983.
24. Peterson DI and Dayes LA: Myelopathy associated with cervical spondylosis: A frequently unrecognized disease. J Fam Pract 4:233, 1977.
25. Thomas WH: Surgical management of the rheumatoid cervical spine. Orthop Clin North Am 6:793, 1975.
26. Wilkinson M: The clinical aspects of myelopathy due to cervical spondylosis. Acta Neurol Belg 76:276, 1976.

53

Elbow, Hand, Knee, Hip, and Foot Pain

PAUL R. FORTIN, MD, MPH
MATTHEW H. LIANG, MD, MPH
WILLIAM T. BRANCH, Jr., MD

This chapter focuses on acute and subacute musculoskeletal pain of specific joints and their structures, including ligaments, tendons, muscles, bursae, and bone itself. The most common causes of pain represent more than 95% of the problems encountered in clinical practice. To treat these conditions properly, an understanding of the anatomy, pathophysiology, and healing process is vital.

ANATOMIC STRUCTURES AND ASSOCIATED INJURIES

Ligaments are collagenous structures that originate on one bone and insert on another. They stabilize the joint and limit motion in certain planes. The fibrous portion of the joint capsule (as distinct from the synovial lining) is the primary "ligament" of any joint. In many joints, this capsule is supplemented by intra-articular or extra-articular fibrous bands. For example, the medial and lateral collateral ligaments prevent side-to-side wobble of the knee, whereas the intra-articular anterior and posterior cruciate ligaments prevent the tibia from sliding forward or backward on the femur. The knee capsule itself limits extension of the knee.

Ligaments are composed of collagen bundles running parallel to the stress that the ligament resists. Their strength depends on the number of fibers in the ligament and the cross-linking between the fibrils. Ligaments are weaker than bone but are much more elastic. They are strongest when pulled, relatively weak under shear (force at right angles to the axis of the fibers), and have no compressive strength. These differences determine the type of injury that is likely to occur in a given situation: a high-velocity injury (auto accident, fall from a height) will probably produce a fracture because bone is brittle; a low-velocity injury (athletic injury or minor fall) will generally produce a ligamentous injury. Torsional injuries are particularly likely to tear ligaments under tension. Purely compressive forces (e.g., fall from a height) usually produce fracture and not ligamentous injury.

Any injury to a ligament is defined as a sprain. For both accuracy and deciding treatment, this type of injury must be distinguished from a "strain," which is defined as an injury to the musculotendinous unit. A sprain occurs when the tensed ligament gives way at its attachments or at some point in its substance. If the force is reduced early, only a few fibers may be torn, but if it continues, all fibers may be torn. In general, three degrees of sprain are recognized (Fig. 53–1): A first-degree sprain consists of tears of only a few fibers of the ligament. In second-degree sprain, less than half of the fibers are torn. In third-degree or severe sprain, all the fibers are torn, with resulting loss of stability.

The *musculotendinous unit*, like the ligament, has an origin on one bone and an insertion on another. Its function is to stabilize the joint and also to move the joint through its range of motion. Though its component parts (origin, muscle belly, tendon, and insertion) are structurally different from one another, functionally it acts as one unit. Injury to the structure is of two types: chronic strain, resulting from overuse, and acute strain, resulting from overstress. *Chronic strain* occurs when the repetitive demands placed on the unit are greater than its capacity to comply. This results in fatigue and ischemia, causing muscle spasm and inflammation. It may also result in irritation of the synovial sheath (tenosynovitis) or irritation at the tendinous attachment (e.g., epicondylitis in "tennis elbow"). *Acute strain*, on the other hand, is the result of a single stress. It results in physical tearing of muscle or tendon fibers and may be classified as mild, or first-degree (involving less than half the fibers); moderate, or second-degree; and severe, or third-degree (involving all the fibers).

Contusion of muscle, tendon, or tendon sheath may also occur, usually as the result of a direct blow. Here, a hematoma within the fiber bundles, rather than discontinuity of

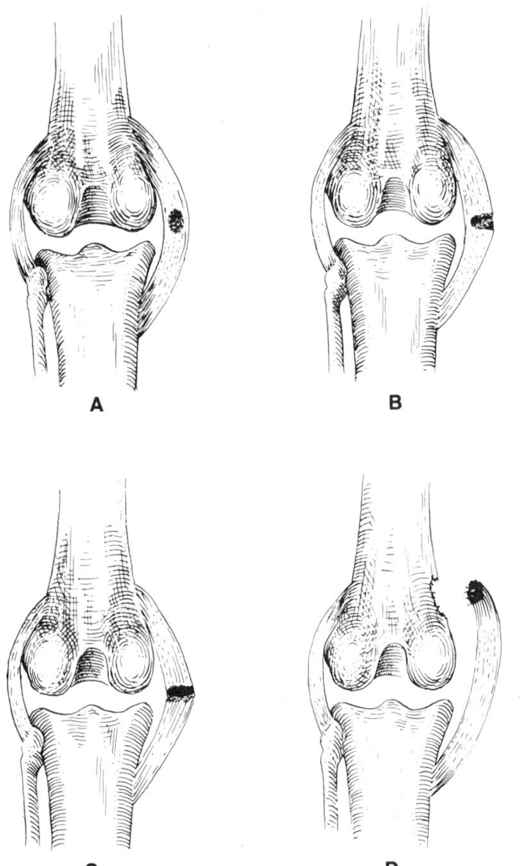

FIGURE 53–1. Types of sprains. *A*, Mild (first-degree) sprain in which there is a localized hematoma in the ligament, with a few fibers torn. *B*, Moderate (second-degree) sprain in which the tear is larger but at least half the fibers are intact. *C*, Severe (third-degree) sprain in which the tear is complete, with the torn ends of the fibers separated. *D*, Sprain fracture (avulsion fracture) in which the ligament is torn at its attachment to the bone, with a fragment of bone still attached to the ligament fibers.

the fibers, is the problem. Trauma to the tendon sheath may cause *tenosynovitis* with inflammation and occasionally adhesions between the tendon and its sheath. If treated initially with rest and slow rehabilitation, tenosynovitis will resolve. Occasionally, however, chronic disability may develop because of repeated trauma, severity of the injury, or lack of proper care. In chronic *adhesive tenosynovitis*, the tendon, its sheath, and surrounding structures become bound in an adherent inflammatory mass. This causes restricted and painful motion and may be extremely difficult to treat. Frozen shoulder (adhesive capsulitis) is probably the most common example. Tenosynovitis may result in progressive thickening of the walls of the sheath. This tends to happen in an area in which more than one tendon passes through the same sheath. For example, in trigger finger, the gliding action of the tendon through the sheath is impeded and may require surgical release.

Bursitis is an inflammatory process within a bursa. Bursae are closed synovial sacs that facilitate motion between adjacent tissues. Inflammation occurs within the sac as the result of external trauma (housemaid's knee) or from inflammatory disease (gout).

Fracture refers to bone, but breaks may also occur in cartilage and result in chondral or osteochondral fractures. Fractures may be gross or microscopic (stress or microfractures).

Stress fractures in weight-bearing bones subjected to unusual stress occur most commonly in the "weekend warrior" who places unaccustomed demands on his or her skeletal system, in people in training who attempt to progress too rapidly to a new level of activity beyond the capability of their bone, or in individuals with osteopenia (e.g., in women with exercise-induced amenorrhea). Stress fractures may not be visualized on a routine roentgenogram.

Bone scans may reveal a "hot spot" at a stress fracture site weeks before the radiograph result is positive. Alternatively, a repeat radiograph 2 to 3 weeks after a fracture may show the callus of a healed fracture.

Chondral fractures may be partial or complete. Meniscal tears are partial chondral fractures. In complete chondral fractures, pieces of cartilage, so-called loose bodies or joint mice, may float freely within the joint. These may interfere with normal joint motion and can produce locking and lead to accelerated degenerative changes.

Bone, ligament, and muscle injuries are capable of repair and healing; however, in cartilage, the chondrocytes are nourished by synovial fluid and have no blood supply; thus, they are incapable of forming new matrix. Unless the injury is sufficiently extensive to allow new vessels and fibroblasts to penetrate the subchondral plate and manufacture fibrocartilage, cartilage may never heal completely.

HEALING PROCESS

An understanding of how injuries heal underlies rational therapy to restore function. Healing occurs in ordered stages in all tissues just discussed except cartilage, in which healing does not occur.

The first stage begins at the time of injury and continues for 7 to 10 days. First, a hematoma forms from ruptured blood vessels. If clotting is normal and the vessels are small, the hematoma reaches maximum size by 6 hours. If clotting is abnormal, if the torn vessels are large, or if there is excessive movement of the injured extremity, bleeding may continue for several days. Bleeding is followed by swelling caused by fluid accumulating within the soft tissue. This is usually maximal within 36 hours but may increase thereafter if the injured limb is moved excessively or is left in a dependent position. The first stage of healing, consisting of migration of phagocytic cells to remove extravasated blood and other necrotic debris, begins 5 to 10 days after injury. The first fibroblasts also appear at this time.

On occasion, the combined effects of bleeding and edema in fascial compartments of the arm or leg can create enough pressure to lead to ischemic changes and even necrosis of muscle.

The second stage of healing begins when fibroblasts form new collagen fibers. In complete tears of the ligament or musculotendinous unit, the process of healing requires about 8 weeks. If the injury is a fracture of bone, calcification of this collagen matrix may take much longer.

The final step in the healing process is that of remodeling. Once the collagenous scar (or bony callus in the case of a fracture) has been formed, the involved structure remodels. Scar tissue, previously laid down as randomly oriented collagen fibers, will be replaced by new collagen fibers oriented along lines of stress, a process that extends over many months and depends on the patient's use of the extremity. Similar remodeling takes place in a "healed" fracture but takes even longer.

The implications of these stages of healing are important. The object of treatment during the first 24 to 36 hours after injury is to minimize bleeding and swelling to prevent further injury. Ice may be used to cause vasoconstriction and minimize bleeding and edema. Immobilization in a splint, dressing, or cast will prevent further injury but must not be so tight as to constrict venous circulation. Finally, simple elevation of the extremity is important because dependency will increase swelling, whereas elevation will decrease it.

In order to heal properly fractures must be immobilized in casts or by other means. In a ligamentous injury, all too often the patient is told that it is "only a sprain," and the joint is not immobilized during the 6 to 8 weeks of healing. The consequence of this is *nonunion* or *malunion* of the ligament or tendon, leaving the patient with an unstable knee, an unstable ankle, or a shoulder that repeatedly dislocates with minor trauma.

The crucial point is that whenever the physician suspects that a ligament, tendon, or muscle is torn significantly, the area must be immobilized until healing can take place (for at least 6 weeks). If less than 50% of the structure is torn, the remaining fibers will sufficiently immobilize the area to allow adequate healing without external immobilization. Even in this situation, the patient must understand that major stresses (as in sports activities) during the initial 6 to 8 weeks of healing may further damage the weakened structure and complete the tear.

Complete tears require surgical repair within a week of injury. Surgery is performed to reapproximate the torn ends so that healing can take place.

The final phase of healing, remodeling, can also be aided by the physician. Simply removing the splint or cast and sending the patient away "healed" may prolong disability. A planned program to regain joint motion and muscle strength will lead to an earlier return to full activity. Exercises to regain both motion and strength should be performed to tolerance daily. If a patient has not regained nearly normal strength, stability, and function 2 weeks after immobilization, physical or occupational therapy should be prescribed.

MUSCULOSKELETAL PAIN WITHOUT ANTECEDENT TRAUMA

The sudden or gradual onset of pain or functional loss with no identifiable preceding event or systemic illness is frequently a diagnostic puzzle. These problems most often result from repeated minor trauma occurring over long periods of time. "Degenerative" meniscal tears in the knee and tendinitis and bursitis are common examples. Stress fractures, shin splints, iliotibial band friction syndrome, hamstring pulls, plantar fascitis, and the like have become more common with the increasing popularity of exercise. Generally, these problems are related to lack of stretching, poor conditioning followed by vigorous exercise, repetitive atypical motion (e.g., shoulder or low back pain from carrying heavy objects), uncoordinated or poorly executed motions (e.g., tennis elbow from a poor backhand), and minor anatomic variations leading to unusual stress (e.g., foot or knee pain in runners with pronated feet).

ELBOW PAIN

Elbow pain is caused by intra-articular and extra-articular conditions (Table 53–1). A screening examination can be done by having the patient flex and extend the elbow while the joint capsule and the radiohumeral articulation are palpated (Fig. 53–2). Normally, one may palpate the sulcus (in thin persons) or the bones (in obese persons) of the olecranon and the humerus. Tenderness, "sponginess," or warmth and painful or incomplete elbow extension suggest synovitis or an intra-articular process. Intra-articular loose bodies, synovitis, radial head fractures, and elbow dislocations are the common intra-articular conditions. Point tenderness without these findings suggests an extra-articular process. No findings of the joint suggests referred pain or an osseous lesion.

TABLE 53–1. CAUSES OF ELBOW PAIN

Extra-articular Conditions
Medial and lateral epicondylitis
Olecranon bursitis
Intra-articular Conditions
Synovitis of any etiology (elbow and radiohumeral joints)
Loose bodies
Elbow subluxations
Dislocations and fractures

Epicondylitis

Among the most common elbow complaints is lateral epicondylitis, or "tennis elbow." Medial epicondylitis or "golfer's elbow" is a similar complaint that occurs with less frequency on the medial side of the elbow. Both result from repeated trauma at the origin of the conjoint tendons of the forearm extensors or flexors. In epicondylitis, the initiating event is probably a tear in the attachment of the tendon to the epicondyle of the humerus brought about by overuse or misuse. Continued use prevents healing and results in chronic inflammation.

The pain is typically associated with, or accentuated by, activity. It can be reproduced by elbow or wrist extension and by direct pressure over the tendon attachment to the epicondyle. The pain may be localized to the epicondylar area or may radiate down the dorsum of the forearm to the hand.

The pain of medial epicondylitis is made worse by wrist or elbow flexion and radiates from the medial side of the elbow down the palmar surface of the forearm. The findings on examination are localized tenderness and, occasionally, mild swelling over the medial epicondyle and atrophy of forearm muscles. On the lateral side, the most tender spot is usually slightly distal and anterior to the most prominent bony area of the distal humerus. On the medial side, the tender area is distal to the bony prominence. Elbow and wrist motion are normal. Radiographs are of little value.

Initial treatment consists of rest and anti-inflammatory agents. Rest means cessation of all painful activities for 4 to 6 weeks. Splinting the wrist in dorsiflexion reduces the tension on the tendon and usually relieves the pain. Anti-inflammatory agents are effective in fewer than 50% of cases. Injection of a steroid preparation into the most tender spot is effective in 80 to 90% of cases, but recurrences are common.

Following injection, the patient should rest the arm even if the pain is gone. After 4 to 6 weeks, a rehabilitative program can be instituted. The involved muscle group should be strengthened by a program of weight-lifting (primarily wrist curls) or by isometric exercise. The patient should continue exercising for 8 to 12 weeks, or until the circumference of the forearm is equal in both arms. An external support may be used during vigorous activity. The tennis elbow support consists of a bandage wrapped firmly

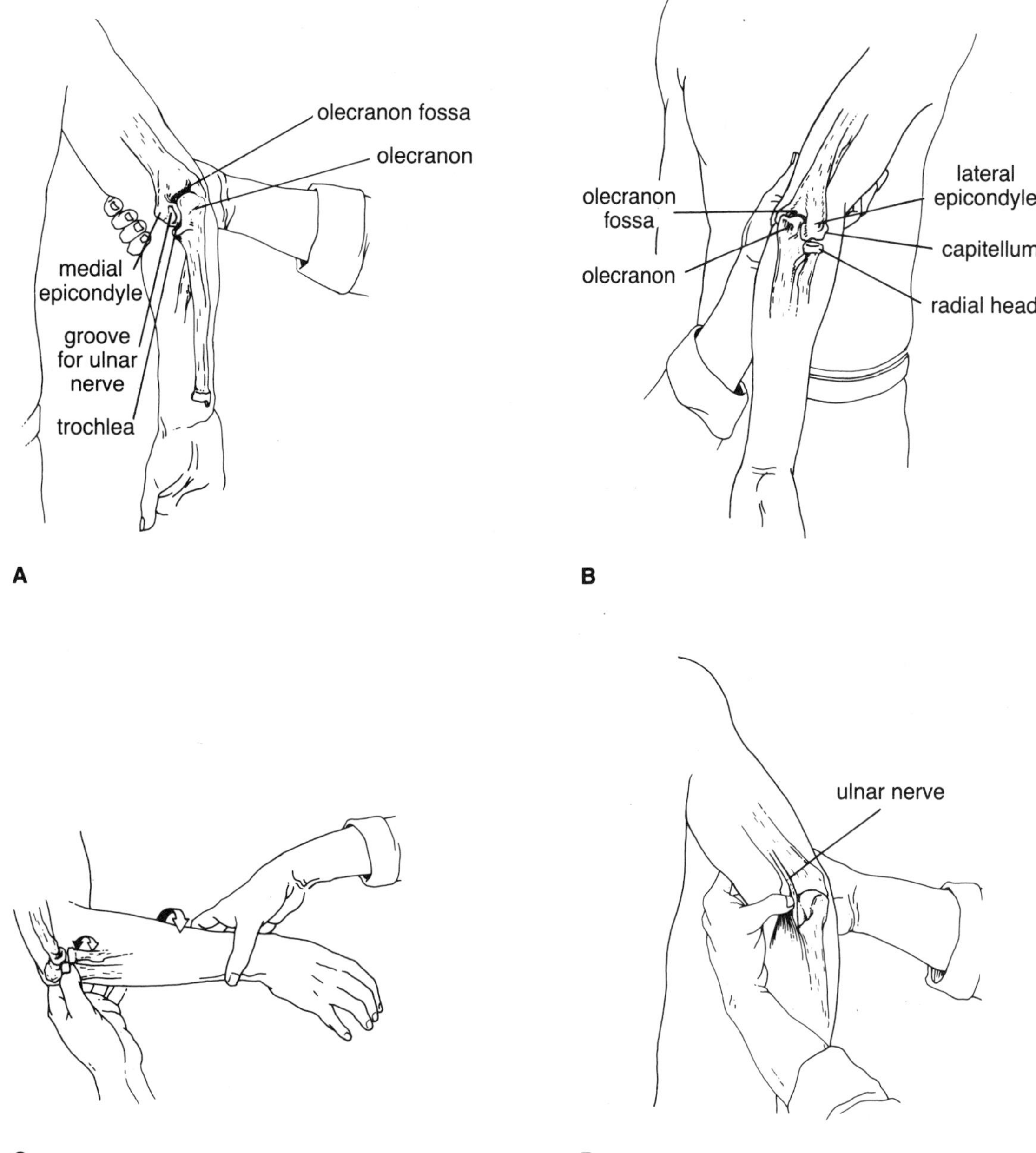

FIGURE 53–2. Examination of the elbow. The joint capsule is palpated in the groove between the olecranon and the epicondyles. The olecranon bursa lies over the hard tip of the elbow. The joint capsule can be felt medially and laterally. The conjoint tendon of the forearm extensors arises from the lateral epicondyle and is locally tender with pain reproduced at this site by forceful extension of the wrist in lateral epicondylitis. Medial epicondylitis (not shown in figure) refers to pain that is located at the origin of tendons from the medial epicondyle and is reproduced by forceful flexion of the wrist. The ulnar nerve passes in a groove beneath the medial epicondyle where it may be entrapped; palpation at this point may reproduce paresthesias radiating down the forearm to the fingers.
A, Posterior aspect of the elbow.
B, Lateral aspect of the elbow.
C, Palpation of radial head during supination and pronation of forearm.
D, Palpation of ulnar nerve.

about the upper forearm. The bandage transfers the force of the muscle "origin" distally and places less stress on the conjoint tendon origin. In the long term, patient activity should be changed to lessen the stress at the tendon origin. For example, the patient may take tennis lessons to improve the backhand or may change to a two-handed backhand stroke. At work, repetitive actions may be avoided or changed to prevent recurrence.

Recurrence of epicondylitis usually indicates that complete healing has not occurred or that the area has been subjected to repeated trauma. Rarely, the cause may be a large tear in the tendon, which may require surgery.

Olecranon Bursitis

The olecranon is the large bony prominence at the tip of the elbow. The triceps attaches here. Overlying the fascia of the triceps and the periosteum of the olecranon is a large bursa that allows the free movement of these structures. The olecranon bursa begins about 2 cm proximal to the elbow and ends 4 to 5 cm distal to the joint. It does not communicate with the elbow joint. Because it is located subcutaneously over a large bony prominence, the bursa is easily traumatized, which leads to a bursal inflammation with pain and swelling. The bursa may also become infected, usually from a local portal of entry (e.g., scratches, laceration, or foreign bodies).

Depending on the degree of inflammation, olecranon bursitis may present as a painless accumulation of fluid within the bursal sac or as an acutely painful, erythematous, warm swelling. Chronic bursitis is usually painless. Elbow flexion and extension are normal.

The first task of the clinician is to make sure that the swelling is not infected. Septic bursitis is suggested by pain at rest, redness or warmth over the bursa, or constitutional symptoms, including fever, regional adenopathy, purulent drainage, or a skin break over the bursa. When in doubt, one should aspirate the bursa. Frank pus, of course, is diagnostic of a septic bursitis, but more often the fluid will simply be cloudy. Cell count, culture, crystal examination and Gram stain should be carried out routinely. The synovial fluid cell count in septic bursitis is always greater than 1000 leukocytes/mm^3 and usually is greater than 10,000/mm^3, with 52 to 98% polymorphonuclear leukocytes.[1] A positive Gram stain or culture is diagnostic. *Staphylococcus aureus* is the causative organism in about 90% of cases.[1]

Once the diagnosis of septic bursitis is made, the patient should begin oral antibiotic therapy (usually one of the penicillinase-resistant semi-synthetic penicillins) until sensitivities are determined. The bursa should be reaspirated in 24 to 48 hours. If a significant amount of purulent material has reaccumulated, strong consideration must be given to open drainage and intravenous antibiotics. Repeat aspiration may be an alternative to open drainage and is often done with lavage of the bursa. Antibiotics, either oral or parenteral, should be continued for 7 to 10 days.

Bland, or noninfected, olecranon bursitis can be left alone or can be aspirated dry, injected with a corticosteroid, then wrapped with an elastic bandage.

Intra-articular Conditions

Synovitis of the elbow joint may be produced by any inflammatory or septic process. Degenerative arthritis of the elbow is very unusual except as the result of previous trauma. Elbow effusions may be palpable anteriorly, medially, or laterally and indicate intra-articular pathology. Range of motion is usually limited, with loss of full extension being most common.

Several other conditions should be considered. *Osteochondritis dissecans*, a disorder of adolescence, is manifested by recurrent swelling of the joint following exercise. Occasionally, a fragment of subchondral bone or cartilage separates and forms a loose body within the joint. Adolescents engaged in sports activities such as baseball pitching are particularly susceptible to this type of injury. The chief complaint of a patient with a loose body is "locking" of the joint; surgical removal relieves the symptoms.

Elbow subluxation occurs most commonly in young children and results from sudden jerking or pulling on the child's arm, usually by someone who is trying to pull the child from danger suddenly. The subluxation of the radial head can be reduced by extending the elbow using manual traction along with gentle supination of the forearm. Recurrent subluxations, osteochondritis dissecans, previous trauma, or joint damage from a previous infection of the elbow may lead to *secondary degenerative arthritis.* This may produce osteophytes that limit the motion of the joint. Isolated *synovitis of the elbow* is very unusual and may be caused by inflammatory arthritis or infection (see Chapter 49). *Pigmented villonodular synovitis*, a rare synovial tumor, can cause elbow pain, swelling, or locking.

Significant trauma to the elbow or forearm requires that radiographs be made to identify *fractures.* The films should include the elbow joint and the forearm when a fracture is suspected because *dislocation* of the radial head is associated with fracture of the ulna. Although isolated subluxation of the radial head cannot be recognized on radiographic films, dislocation associated with a fracture is identifiable radiographically as dorsal displacement of the radial head. Undisplaced fractures do not require reduction but must be immobilized to prevent displacement when healing occurs.

WRIST AND HAND

Wrist Pain (Table 53–2)

Osteoarthritis rarely develops in the wrist unless it is secondary to trauma, fracture, previous synovitis, or avascular necrosis of the lunate bone (Kienböck's disease). The wrist may be inflamed from rheumatoid arthritis, gout, pseudogout, or infection (see Chapter 49). One may elicit pain from synovitis by palpating the joint line. Normally, dorsiflexion of the radiocarpal joint can be achieved to 90 degrees, volar flexion to 50 degrees, ulnar deviation to 40 degrees, and radial deviation to 25 degrees. Because the wrist joint includes articulations of seven different bones, numerous dislocations are possible. Most commonly, the ulna, lunate, and navicular bones are involved. These dislocations are easily missed both clinically and radiographically; therefore, following injury one should obtain stress views of the joint and refer patients with persistent wrist pain to a hand surgeon.

Extra-articular causes of wrist pain include tendinitis, carpal tunnel syndrome (discussed in Chapter 60), de Quervain's tenosynovitis, and ganglions (Fig. 53–3). Acute *tendinitis* involving flexors of the wrist and fingers presents with pain and local tenderness. The local nature of the involvement, the history of trauma, and the reproduction of pain by resisted isometric flexion of the wrist and fingers helps distinguish isolated tendinitis from true synovitis of the wrist. Tendinitis responds to immobilization, using a

TABLE 53–2. CAUSES OF WRIST AND HAND PAIN

Wrist Pain
Degenerative joint disease
Synovitis
Tendinitis
Carpal tunnel syndrome
De Quervain's tenosynovitis
Ganglion
Hand Pain
Osteoarthritis
Paronychias, felons, suppurative tenosynovitis, and midpalmar infection
Soft tissue injuries
Trigger finger
Ruptured tendon
Dupuytren's contracture

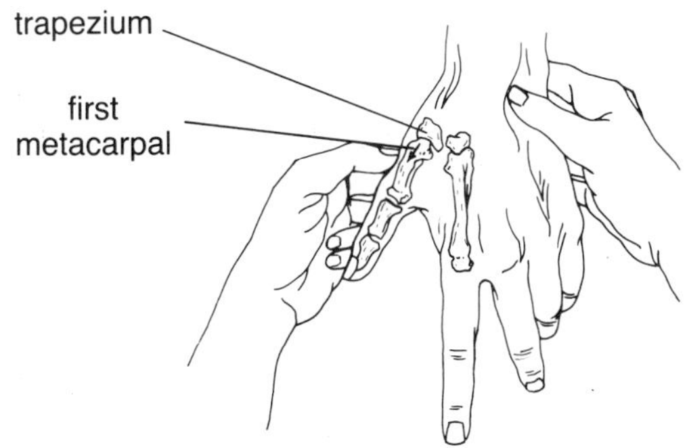

A Palpation of the first metacarpal joint

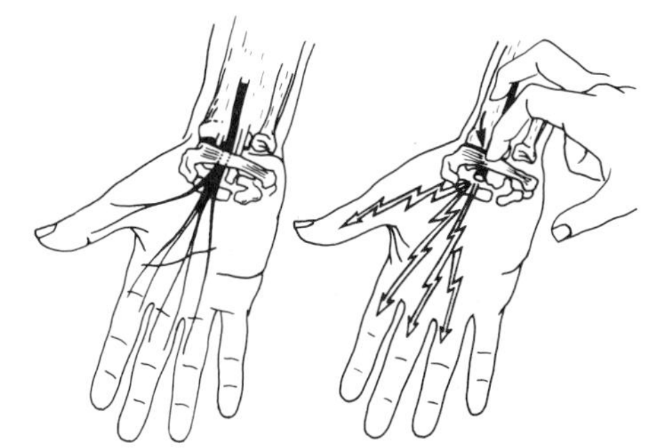

B Elicitation of Tinel's sign in carpal tunnel syndrome

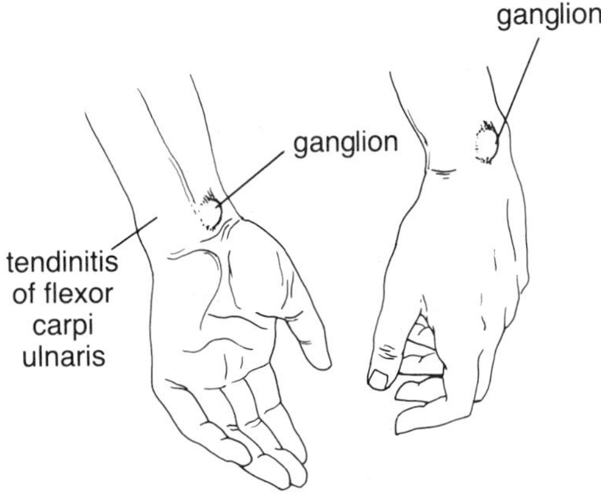

C Sites of ganglia of the dorsal or volar surfaces and tendinitis of the wrist

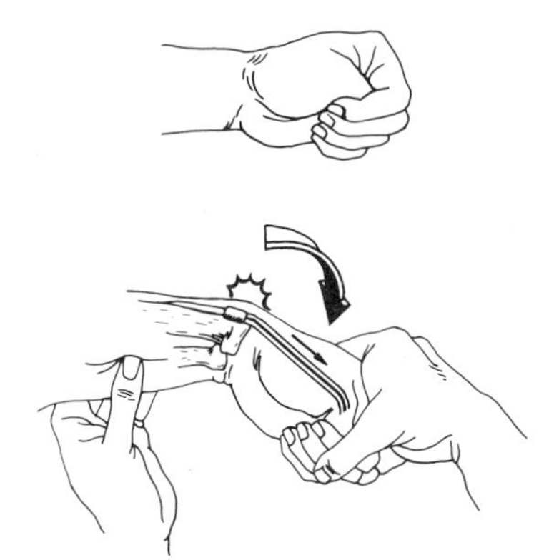

D Finkelstein test

FIGURE 53–3. Examination of the patient with pain in the wrist or hand. *A,* Osteoarthritis of the wrist is most commonly located at the first metacarpal joint, where crepitus and limitation of motion may be elicited on rotation of the thumb. *B,* In carpal tunnel syndrome (discussed in Chapter 60), the median nerve is compressed by the transverse carpal ligament. Symptoms include paresthesias of the first four digits, with thenar atrophy in more advanced cases. *C,* A ganglion may be appreciated as a nontender cystic mass located in connection with a tendon sheath or joint capsule. Acute tendinitis of the wrist most commonly involves the tendon of the flexor carpi ulnaris but may also involve other flexor tendons, which are locally tender with pain elicited by forceful isometric flexion of the wrist. *D,* De Quervain's tenosynovitis refers to inflammation of the extensor pollicis brevis and abductor pollicis longus near the first carpometacarpal joint; in tenosynovitis, pain is reproduced by palpating the tendon or with the Finkelstein test.

splint to hold the wrist in 20 degrees of dorsiflexion, plus either local corticosteroid injection or nonsteroidal anti-inflammatory agents.

De Quervain's tenosynovitis refers to inflammation of the tendons of the extensor pollicis brevis and abductor pollicis longus as they pass between two bony prominences on the distal radius. This area is just proximal to the anatomic "snuff box." Tenderness is present over the snuff box and just proximal to it, and crepitus of the tendons may be palpable during active thumb motion. Pain can be reproduced by active abduction and hyperextension of the thumb or by passive flexion and adduction of the metacarpophalangeal joint (Finklestein's test). Immobilization in a radial gutter splint including thumb and wrist, together with nonsteroidal anti-inflammatory agents or local corticosteroid injection, is effective in most cases. Occasionally, surgical release is needed to relieve persistent symptoms.

A *ganglion* is a discrete, slightly movable firm cystic structure connected to the joint space or tendon, as can be shown by moving the joint or tendon. It represents a synovial herniation of either a tendon sheath or joint capsule. Ganglions are usually asymptomatic but may occasionally be painful when pressure is applied. Usually no treatment is required. Symptomatic ganglions may be treated by aspiration or surgery. Aspiration using a large-bore needle will collapse the ganglion, but recurrence is frequent.

Hand Pain (see Table 53–2)

Degenerative arthritis of the hand commonly involves the first carpometacarpal joint and patients complain of wrist pain on activities that require a forceful grip. The base of the thumb has a squared appearance, and motion of the thumb produces crepitus and pain. The lack of tenderness of the tendon sheaths themselves distinguishes degenerative arthritis of this joint from de Quervain's tenosynovitis. The radiograph shows unequal joint space narrowing, osteophytes, and eburnation. Treatment includes immobilization with a splint and analgesics as needed; for patients with unusually severe persistent pain, arthrodesis or prosthetic replacement of the greater multangular bone can be of benefit.

A related form of osteoarthritis of the hands primarily involves the distal and proximal interphalangeal joints (Heberden's and Bouchard's nodes). Patients may complain of pain and stiffness. Deformity and signs of inflammation may occasionally be seen. Women in the fourth to sixth decades are most commonly affected. Patients can be reassured that the pain, but not the deformity, will resolve, and that this condition does not evolve into a diffuse crippling process, a concern of many patients that is more often felt than stated. Treatment with joint rest, acetaminophen, or nonsteroidal agents may be required. Morning stiffness may be relieved by immersing the hands in warm water.

Infections of the fingers are classified as paronychia, which is an infection of the side of the nail, or felon, which is a deep infection of the pulp of a fingertip. Both conditions may be treated by orally administered antibiotics and warm soaks. Paronychia sometimes requires drainage by incision. Felon may respond to conservative therapy, but if an abscess has formed, a "fishmouth incision" of the fingertip will be necessary. In *suppurative tenosynovitis*, infection involves the tendon sheath. The entire finger is swollen and acutely tender and will be held in semiflexion. Active or passive motion of the finger is exquisitely painful. Early infection may be treated with warm soaks and antibiotics; however, open surgical drainage will be required if the process fails to resolve promptly or spreads proximally. Extension of suppurative tenosynovitis to the midpalm results in swelling of the dorsum of the hand because the volar aspect is protected by the palmar fascia. Midpalmar infection may also result from a deep puncture wound. Slight swelling and tenderness of the palm should prompt inspection of the dorsum of the hand and fingers for swelling. This infection requires adequate drainage of the abscess in addition to antibiotics given systemically. Failure of adequate or timely treatment of either of the latter two infections may result in permanent damage to the hand.

Deformity of a finger may result from rupture or thickening of a tendon. This is more likely to occur in patients with rheumatoid arthritis whose tendons are nodular or weakened by the inflammatory process. *Rupture of the extensor pollicis longus tendon* produces weakness on extension of the distal thumb, and repair consists of suturing or, when this is not possible, grafting the tendon. *Rupture of an extensor tendon* of the fingers at its insertion into the distal phalanx, resulting usually from a blow to the tip of the extended finger, produces a "mallet" or "baseball" finger. The tip of the involved finger classically droops and cannot be actively extended (passive extension is normal). Mallet finger is treated by splinting in extension for 6 to 8 weeks. Occasionally, if a large fragment of bone has been pulled off with the tendon, surgical repair is needed. A trigger finger occurs when the gliding of a flexor tendon is obstructed by thickening of the tendon sheath or a nodule of the tendon itself. A snapping sensation occurs with flexion or extension of the finger, or it becomes "locked" in flexion. The condition may be treated by local corticosteroid injection or surgical division of the tendon sheath under local anesthesia. *Dupuytren's contracture* is usually an idiopathic condition that is commonly encountered in men and manifested by thickening and nodularity of the palmar fascia with contraction of the tendon sheaths, usually of the fourth and fifth fingers. Other fingers are occasionally involved. Although the etiology is unknown, heredity is thought to play a role in some cases; in others, the disorder has been associated with reflex sympathetic dystrophy, liver disease, and epilepsy. The diagnosis is made by physical examination, in which thickening of the palmar tendon sheaths is palpable, and the contraction prevents full extension of the fingers. Severe deformity related to Dupuytren's contracture may be released surgically.

Management of injuries to the hand is often complex. Thorough cleansing of even trivial lacerations is essential to prevent infection. Certain injuries require prompt referral to a surgeon experienced in their management. These include extensive laceration with skin loss, "potential nerve" lacerations, and lacerated flexor or extensor tendons. Flexor tendons lacerated in "no-man's land" (between the proximal interphalangeal joints and the midpalmar crease) must be sutured secondarily because of the high rate of scarring and the resultant poor finger function.

Fractures of the hand and carpal bones are usually treated by closed reduction. Open reduction may be necessary if problems are encountered in the alignment of the bones, but this does not need to be done immediately. Acute splinting and referral in 1 to 3 days are adequate treatment.

HIP PAIN

Pain originating from the hip joint may be referred to the knee, groin, or thigh. The hip is involved if there are no findings at the site to which pain is referred, and the patient has an antalgic gait or an adductor lurch. In an antalgic gait, the affected leg is left on the ground for a shorter time than the opposite side (producing a hop-like gait). In an adductor gait, the patient shifts body weight toward the affected side, reducing stress across the joint by reducing muscle force needed to remain upright.

The origin of the pain can be confirmed by physical examination. The most important maneuver during the examination is to determine whether motion of the hip joint is limited or reproduces pain. This may be tested by rotating the hip internally and externally with the patient lying flat and the hip and knee partially flexed (Fig. 53–4*A*). Loss of normal internal rotation is the most sensitive sign of hip disease. One should also test for abduction and adduction of the hip, with the knee extended, and for flexion and extension of the hip.

When examining a patient suspected of having hip pain, it is important to exclude other conditions, such as pain arising from the lumbosacral spine or knee or from bursitis. Discogenic pain from the lumbosacral spine may be reproduced by straight leg raising but not by internal and external rotation of the hip (see Fig. 53–4*B*). Trochanteric and ischial bursitis can be recognized because the pain is localized (see Fig. 53–4*C*) and reproduced by pressure over these structures. The pain of trochanteric bursitis is also reproduced by contraction of the musculotendinous insertion during forced abduction and adduction of the hip but not by passive movement of the hip joint. The iliopectineal bursa lies anterior to the hip joint and may, in some cases, communicate with it. Inflammation of this bursa causes inguinal pain and tenderness and is sometimes difficult to differentiate from intra-articular disease without aspiration and arthrography. Symphysis pubis inflammation often produces anterior or medial thigh pain that is exacerbated by attempted adduction of the thighs against resistance. The symphysis itself may be tender to direct palpation. Pathologic fracture from metastatic cancer or fracture of the pelvic ramus causes pain on weight bearing reproduced by applying pressure to the pelvic bone with the patient lying on his or her side but not by rotation of the hip joint. The differential diagnosis of hip pain usually depends on whether the symptoms are acute, subacute, or chronic (Table 53–3).

Acute Hip Pain

Commonly, the etiology of pain will be trochanteric, ischial or iliopectineal bursitis. These conditions can be di-

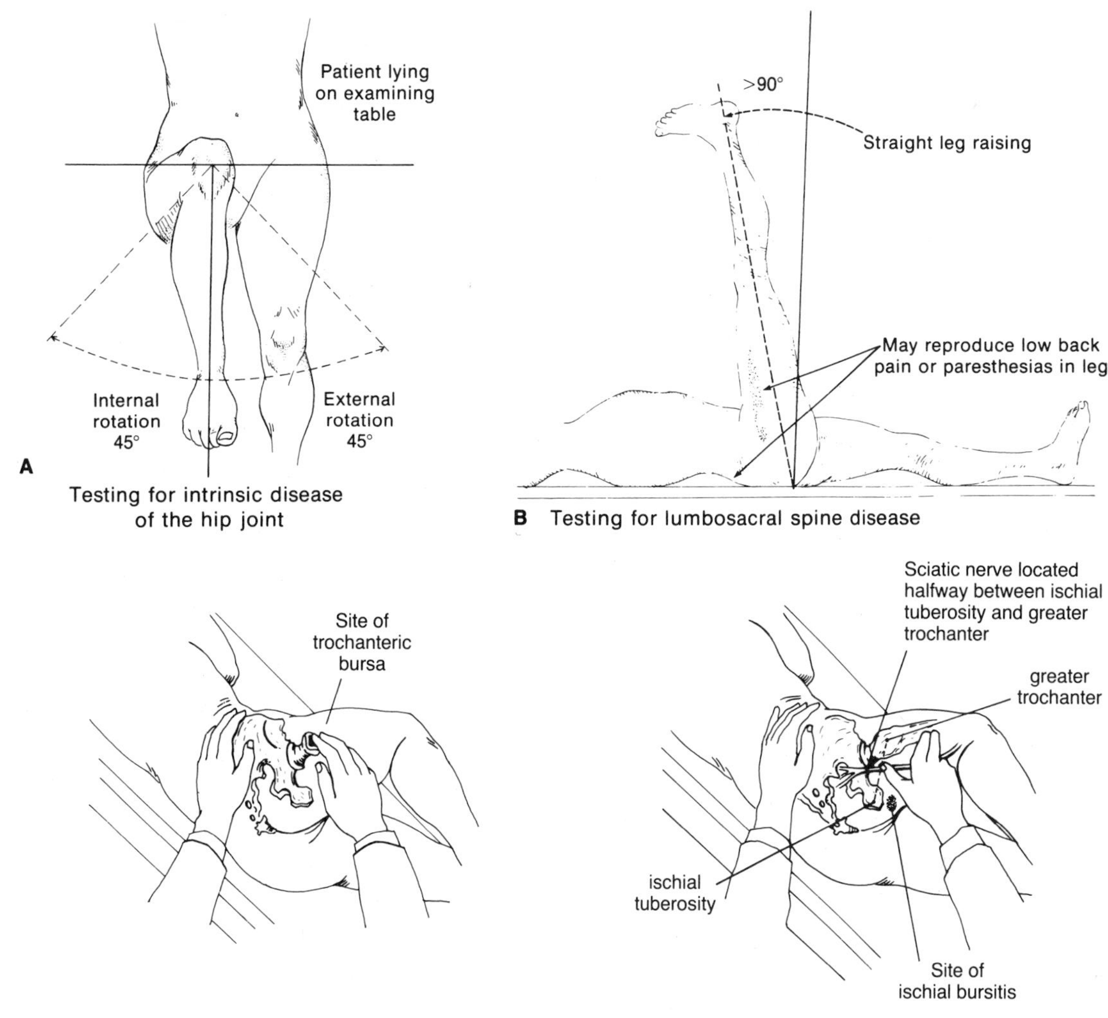

FIGURE 53–4. Examination of the patient with pain in the groin, hip, buttock or trochanter area. *A*, With the patient sitting or lying on the table and the hip partially flexed, the examiner tests for internal and external rotation. This is limited or reproduces pain in intrinsic diseases of the hip joint. *B*, With the patient lying on the table, the hip is fully flexed with the knee extended (straight leg raising); this reproduces low back pain or radiating paresthesias in disease of the lumbosacral spine. *C*, With the patient lying on the table, the examiner palpates for tenderness at the site of the trochanteric bursa. *D*, With the patient lying on the table, the examiner may palpate for local tenderness at the ischial bursa located medial to the sciatic notch, and at the sciatic notch reproducing sciatica manifested by paresthesias radiating to the lower extremity in addition to local tenderness.

TABLE 53–3. CAUSES OF HIP PAIN

Acute Pain in the Hip
- Trauma, including fracture
- Referred pain from the lumbosacral spine
- Bursitis (trochanteric, ischial, iliopectineal)
- Synovitis, caused by infection, rheumatoid arthritis, crystal-induced arthritis, or other conditions

Chronic or Subacute Pain in the Hip
- Chronic trochanteric or ischial bursitis or tendinitis
- Degenerative joint disease
- Congenital and acquired conditions that predispose to early development of degenerative arthritis
    - Legg-Calvé-Perthes disease
    - Slipped femoral epiphysis
    - Coxa vara
    - Congenital hip dislocation or subluxation
- Tuberculous or fungal infection
- Avascular necrosis
- Referred pain from the lumbosacral spine

agnosed on physical examination alone (see Fig. 53–4*D*) and may be treated by rest and oral anti-inflammatory agents (such as indomethacin) or by injection of corticosteroids into the bursa. For ischial bursitis, systemic agents are preferred because of the proximity of the bursa to the sciatic nerve, which might be damaged if inadvertently injected. Iliopectineal bursitis can be confirmed by ultrasound and needs to be injected under radiographic guidance.

When pain arises from the hip itself and is of acute or subacute onset, one must suspect *septic arthritis* or *avascular necrosis*. The organism most often encountered in septic arthritis is *Staphylococcus aureus*. Except in drug addicts, gram-negative bacilli and other organisms such as *Mycobacterium tuberculosis* are rare but must be kept in mind. Other forms of acute synovitis may also affect the hip joint but are usually accompanied by involvement of other joints. Gout is unusual in the hip. The patient with septic arthritis of the hip will usually describe the onset of pain over a few days and will hold the hip in flexion.

Because the joint cannot be palpated directly, radiographic changes may not develop for several weeks (see Fig. 49–5). All patients with acute onset of unexplained hip pain should undergo diagnostic aspiration of the hip joint. Hip arthrocentesis should be done under fluoroscopy to document that the synovial space has been entered; arthrocentesis without fluoroscopy cannot be considered successful unless synovial fluid is obtained. After the diagnosis of septic arthritis has been established by examination of the synovial fluid, the patient should be treated with antibiotics administered parenterally; incision and drainage of the infected joint will often be required in nongonococcal infection.

The diagnosis of avascular necrosis of the hip should be considered in patients with recent worsening or new subacute onset of hip pain.[1a] Initial radiographs may be normal. Flattening of the femoral head or development of a subchondral radiolucent line with preservation of the joint space (see Fig. 49–9) can be seen on radiograph in the advanced phase. Bone scan or magnetic resonance imaging are the best techniques to diagnose avascular necrosis before plain radiographic changes become apparent. Alcoholism, oral corticosteroids (for as short a period as 15 days), fracture or dislocation of the hip, hemodialysis, and diabetes are conditions associated with avascular necrosis.

Chronic Hip Pain

Bursitis and lumbosacral spine conditions may cause chronic or intermittent as well as acute symptoms. If chronic symptoms are localized to the hip joint, the most likely etiology is *degenerative joint disease*. This most often develops in older persons and presents with intermittent pain on weight bearing, which is appreciated in the groin, anterior thigh, the trochanter and/or the knee; later, stiffness following periods of inactivity develops, then limping, and eventually, more severe nocturnal pain or pain with any weight bearing. The radiograph may show asymmetric narrowing of the joint space, eburnation, osteophyte formation, and subchondral cysts. Obtaining the radiograph is important to exclude other causes of intra-articular hip pain, such as tumor, avascular necrosis, or infection.

Numerous congenital and acquired disorders of children and adolescents may predispose patients to early development of degenerative joint disease of the hips, particularly if they are not adequately managed or diagnosed. These conditions include Legg-Calvé-Perthes disease, or coxa plana, slipped femoral capital epiphysis, coxa vara, and congenital dislocation or subluxation of the hip. *Coxa plana* is caused by avascular necrosis of the proximal femoral epiphysis in childhood; this may occur unilaterally or bilaterally and tends to develop most often in boys. *Slipped femoral capital epiphysis* is a condition of teenagers in which the head of the femur slips over the epiphyseal plate. The condition should be suspected when an adolescent complains of groin, thigh, or knee pain without precipitating trauma. The diagnosis is made by radiography, which demonstrates a slippage of the femoral head (commonly described as the "ice cream falling off the cone," an appearance suggested by the position of the femoral head relative to the shaft). It is important to review both anteroposterior and lateral (frog lateral) films. Treatment is surgical, by fixation of the "slipped" femoral head with a screw or multiple pins. *Coxa vara* refers to a congenitally, usually bilaterally increased angle of the femoral neck and shaft, which generally presents as hip pain in childhood; if severe, osteotomy should be considered to prevent future arthritis. *Congenital dislocation and subluxation* of the hip occurs in infants; if not diagnosed and treated at that time, these conditions also may lead to degenerative joint disease in early adulthood.

Management

Once degenerative joint disease of the hip becomes symptomatic, one can predict that the course will be one of progressive worsening, but the rate varies greatly.

Early osteoarthritis is usually associated with mild stiffness that improves with repeated use of the joint and is worse after prolonged weight bearing. Acetaminophen or nonsteroidal anti-inflammatory drugs, joint rest during painful periods, and ways to reduce the forces across the hips, such as weight reduction or a cane in the opposite hand[2] are usually adequate to control the symptoms. In contrast, joint pain that is due to severe structural damage does not respond to medications and occurs with any weight bearing. Physical examination of the end-stage joint reveals coarse "bone-on-bone" crepitus during passive movement, and the radiographic film shows marked destruction of the cartilage.

When joint destruction is advanced and pain or disability is refractory to treatment, joint surgery should be considered. The decision to have surgery and its timing depend on various clinical factors: is the damaged joint the primary limiting condition; will the total joint replacement "outlive" the patient; are there any contraindications or other options?

A patient with angina may not be benefited by improved function and diminished pain in the hip if function is limited by coronary insufficiency. A young, active man may not be an appropriate candidate for total joint replacement because of the increased likelihood that the prosthesis will need surgical revision, with its increased risk of a bad result and infection.

The only absolute contraindications for primary total joint replacement are the presence of active infection or severe neurosensory deficit, such as a Charcot joint. Relative contraindications include youth, high activity level, inadequate bone stock, severe peripheral vascular disease, morbid obesity, dementia, drug abuse, alcoholism, and compromised muscular control (polio, cerebral palsy, stroke). Peripheral vascular disease may compromise wound healing. Loss of muscular control may make the patient unable to protect the operated limb.

Using modern techniques to review published surgical series with more than 50 patients followed for a minimum of 2 years reveals excellent results for total joint replacement for degenerative disease of the hip.[2] Patients can expect significant pain relief in over 90% of the cases and good functional outcome, with very low operative mortality. Deep infections vary between centers but usually average less than 4% over the long term. Loosening, as indicated radiographically by a radiolucent zone around the cement-bone interface of greater than 1 mm, may occur in 20 to 50% of patients at 10 to 15 years, but surgical revision is necessary in only about 2% of patients. Less frequent complications include heterotopic bone formation, hemarthrosis, nerve palsies, stress fractures, and component wear.[3, 4]

Operative mortality in total joint replacement ranges from 0.5 to 1.9%, with centers doing fewer than or equal to 50 patients a year having the higher mortalities.[3] Isolated femoral thrombosis occurs in as many as 50% of total hip reconstructions, but the incidence of pulmonary embolism is about 10% and of fatal embolism, less than 2%.

In younger or obese patients or in those with less severe disease, osteotomy of the femoral neck, to reposition the femoral head and give a better "fit" between the femoral head and the acetabulum, may be preferred. Results, although less predictable than those of total hip replacement, avoid the late problems of loosening of the total hip replacement.

KNEE PAIN

The knee has a hingelike motion, and the tibia rotates on the femur during flexion and extension. Flexion is chiefly accomplished by the hamstring muscles, whereas extension is controlled by the quadriceps, whose tendinous expansion inserts onto the patella. The infrapatellar tendon joins the lower pole of the patella and the tibial tubercle. This tendon transfers the force of contraction of the quadriceps to the tibia. The gliding motion of the patella across the femur allows smooth extension at the knee and increases the mechanical advantage of the quadriceps. The joint capsule itself attaches to the patellar margin and extends proximally to form the suprapatellar pouch and distally to attach to the tibia. Four ligaments provide stability to the joint. In the anterior and posterior directions, stability depends on the anterior and posterior cruciate ligaments. The medial and lateral aspects of the joint are stabilized by the tibial and fibular collateral ligaments, respectively. Hyperextension and rotation of the tibia are limited by the posterior joint capsule. Within the joint space, two fibrocartilaginous menisci, the medial and lateral menisci, are attached to the tibia and articulate with the femur. Numerous bursae also facilitate motion, the most important of which, from a clinical standpoint, are the prepatellar, infrapatellar, and anserine bursae.

Complete examination of the joint includes localization of pain, search for synovial effusion, testing of stability of the ligaments in the anteroposterior and lateral directions, and assessment of meniscal integrity. Tenderness of the knee, if present, should be accurately localized to a specific ligament, meniscus, or bursa, or to the entire joint space (Fig. 53–5). The hip joint should also be examined because hip disorders may present only with pain referred to the knee.

The approach to the patient with knee pain depends upon whether (1) spontaneously occurring pain or swelling is of acute onset or is an acute recurrence of previous pain or swelling, (2) the symptoms are related to trauma, (3) the pain or swelling is chronic, or (4) mechanical symptoms, such as locking or giving way, are present (Table 53–4).

TABLE 53–4. CAUSES OF KNEE PAIN

Acute Knee Pain
Synovitis (e.g., rheumatoid arthritis, gout, pseudogout, Reiter's syndrome, rheumatic fever, viral arthritis, systemic lupus erythematosus, septic arthritis)
Intermittent hydrarthrosis
Baker's cyst
Acute anserine, prepatellar, or infrapatellar bursitis
Subluxation of patella
Osgood-Schlatter disease (osteochondritis of tibial tubercle)
Discoid meniscus
Osteochondritis dissecans
Spontaneous osteonecrosis of the knee
Tumor (synovial chondromatosis, pigmented villonodular synovitis)
Traumatic Injuries
Hemarthrosis
Ligamentous sprains or tears
Meniscal tears
Fracture of tibial plateau or patella
Chronic Knee Pain
Degenerative arthritis
Genu valgum, varum (ligament sprain)
Chronic infection (e.g., tuberculosis)
Chondromalacia of patella
Tumor of bone or synovium
Synovitis
Torn meniscus

Spontaneous Recurrent or Acute Knee Pain

Distinguishing between intra-articular and extra-articular problems is the most important goal of the evaluation. The most reliable sign of an *intra-articular problem* is a joint effusion. It is important to remember that the most distensible portion of the knee joint is the suprapatellar pouch, which is an extension of the knee joint itself. Thus, moderate-to-large effusions are most easily found by examination of the area proximal to the patella. To detect small knee effusions, one milks the fluid from the knee joint into the suprapatellar pouch by stroking the medial and lateral aspects of the joint cephalad. Then, one strokes downward from the suprapatellar pouch to the lateral aspect of the joint while observing for a bulge sign on the medial aspect.

As discussed in Chapter 49, any type of synovitis may affect the knee joint. If an effusion is present, a diagnostic synovial tap and analysis of synovial fluid are helpful in distinguishing synovitis associated with low cell counts, such as osteoarthritis and early rheumatic fever, viral arthritis, or systemic lupus erythematosus; from that characteristically associated with higher cell counts (i.e., inflammatory fluid), such as rheumatoid arthritis, gout, pseudogout, and Reiter's syndrome; and from septic arthritis.

A patient with a single "hot" knee and effusion should undergo arthrocentesis to rule out infection. Infection must be kept in mind even in patients with chronic joint disorders because chronically abnormal joints are more likely to become infected. Monoarticular gonococcal arthritis commonly involves the knee; cultures may be negative, and the synovial white cell count is often less than 50,000/mm^3.

Baker's cysts usually represent a communication between the joint space and a synovial hernia or bursa located posteromedially at the knee. They present as transient or intermittent swelling in the popliteal fossa and may be accentuated by extension of the knee. About half the cases of Baker's cysts are associated with degenerative, rheumatoid, and other joint disorders.

Several patellar conditions may cause knee pain in adolescents. That the patella is the origin of the difficulty may be suggested by the distinctive pattern of what activities induce the pain. Patellar pain is worse going down stairs or inclines than up. *Chondromalacia* of the patella is manifested by retropatellar aching pain, which recurs particularly after exercise. The undersurface of the patella is roughened and may produce crepitus when the knee is flexed and extended. A small, bland effusion may be present. *Traumatic subluxation of the patella* may predispose to recurrent subluxations, in which case sudden discomfort or alarm may be reproduced by having the patient relax and then pushing the patella laterally (the so-called appre-

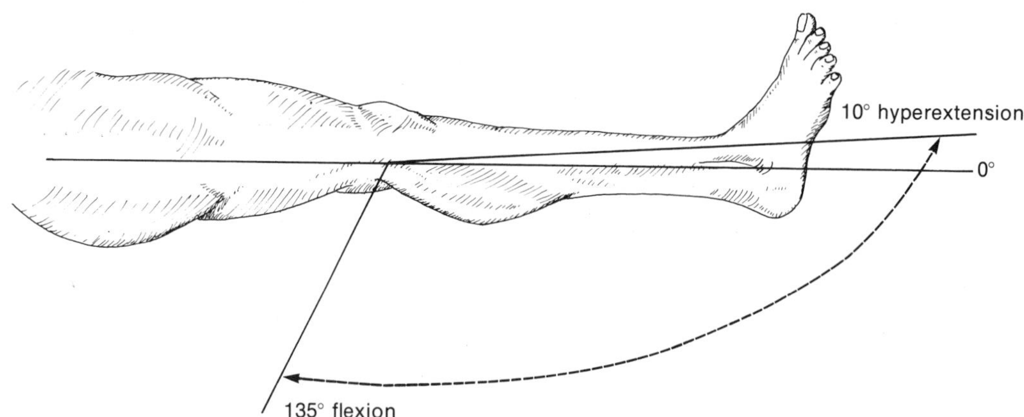

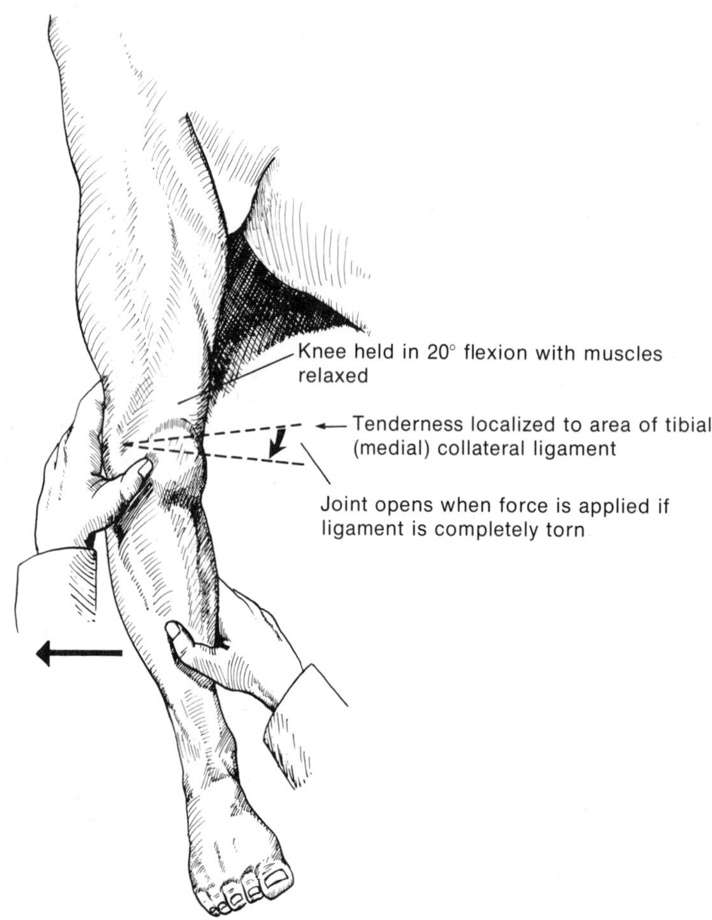

FIGURE 53–5. Examination of the knee joint. *A,* Following inspection, palpation of the suprapatellar pouch, and ballottement of the patella to detect joint effusion, the range of motion of the joint should be tested while feeling for crepitus during flexion. *B,* The stability of the tibial (medial) collateral and fibular (lateral) collateral ligaments should be tested with the knee held in 20 degrees of flexion. Force is applied, and if the ligaments are intact, even though sprained, pain but not instability results. Complete ligamentous tear results in instability of the joint as illustrated in the figure.

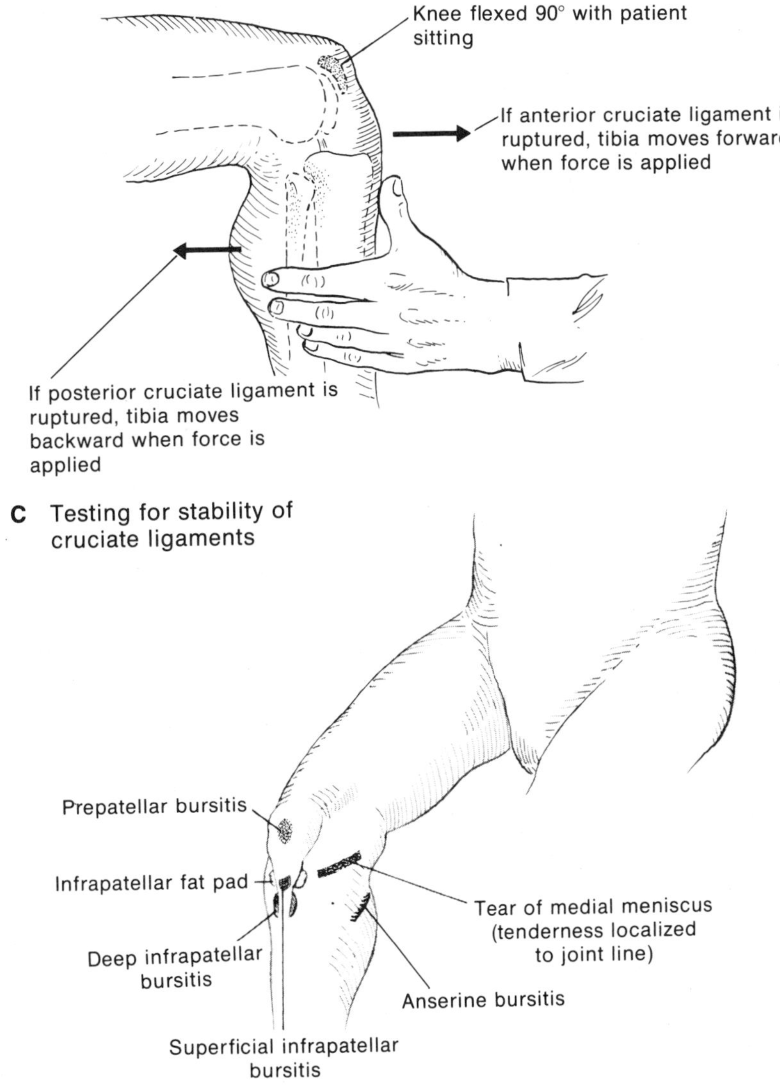

FIGURE 53–5 *Continued C,* Testing for integrity of the anterior and posterior cruciate ligaments is accomplished with the patient sitting and the knee flexed at 90 degrees. The examiner applies pressure in the posterior direction to detect abnormal movement of the joint, which is present in complete tear of the posterior cruciate ligament, and applies force in the anterior direction to detect abnormal movement of the joint and complete tear of the anterior cruciate ligament. *D,* Sites of local tenderness in bursitis and meniscal injuries of the knee. In bursitis, tenderness is localized (as shown) to the area of the prepatellar, superficial or deep infrapatellar, or anserine bursa. Tear of the medial meniscus results in tenderness localized to the tibial joint line. Likewise, tenderness is localized laterally in sprain or tear of the lateral meniscus, but this injury is less common than injury of the medial meniscus.

hension sign). The patient's chief complaint may be that "the knee gives way when I step down," not to be confused with the sudden locking or "giving way" that occurs in meniscal injuries. Both chondromalacia patella and recurrent subluxation of the patella can be treated with rest, anti-inflammatory agents, and unresisted exercises to maintain the strength of the quadriceps. Particularly important is the avoidance of activities requiring deep knee bends. A surgical approach is rarely necessary. In most cases, the condition will resolve after several years.

In middle-aged to elderly patients, a *degenerative meniscal tear* may occur without a history of trauma and usually presents as recurrent pain with weight bearing. Most young patients, will have a history of previous trauma and will complain of symptoms of instability—either locking or "giving way." Physical findings include an effusion, tenderness localized to the joint line (usually medially but sometimes laterally), and a positive McMurray test (see page 691).

Aching and localized pain at the midlateral joint line that fluctuates and is aggravated by weight bearing may be due to a *cyst of the lateral meniscus.* These are usually degenerative, and often a cystic swelling can be palpated at the lateral joint line. On radiography, a soft tissue bulge may be seen laterally, corresponding to the swelling noted clinically.

Discoid lateral meniscus is a congenital disorder in which the lateral meniscus is abnormally large and often not perforated in its central portion. These menisci cause lateral pain and are unusually prone to tear. The diagnosis should be entertained in any younger patient with recurrent lateral knee pain or subluxation and no history of trauma.

When a symptomatic torn meniscus, meniscal cyst, or discoid meniscus is suspected, a magnetic resonance image of the knee can define the anatomic derangement. The patient should be referred to an orthopedic surgeon for consultation concerning management if symptoms persist with conservative treatment (i.e., partial or full non–weight bearing for several months). Not all patients with meniscal tears related to degeneration or trauma should have surgical meniscectomy. An autopsy study showed that 34% of persons older than 55 years of age dying of unrelated causes, had meniscal lesions, which apparently had been asymptomatic and were compatible with normal functioning.[5] In a study of patients over the age of 40 years who underwent meniscectomy because of recurrent symptoms, more than half had developed degenerative arthritis on the side of the surgery within 10 years.[6] Limited surgical removal (sometimes by arthroscopy) of meniscal tears has theoretical advantages and may have a better long-term outcome.

Recurrent swelling, mild discomfort, and aching of the knee aggravated by weight-bearing activities, usually occurring in a young person or adolescent, sometimes with locking or giving way, may be due to osteochondritis dissecans. In this disorder, a devitalized fragment of bone and articular cartilage detach from the medial femoral condyle. The classic radiographic finding in this condition is a bony sequestrum located within a cavity in the medial condyle. Symptoms result from a loose body within the joint.

In adults over the age of 60 years, knee pain can result from *spontaneous osteonecrosis of the medial femoral condyle*, which presents with abrupt onset of pain at the medial aspect of the knee, followed by stiffness, persistence of pain, local tenderness, and effusion. Non–weight bearing is the preferred treatment if the condition can be diagnosed early. About a quarter of patients will progress to advanced osteoarthrosis.[7] *Synovial osteochondromatosis* is a metaplasia of the cartilage that creates detached loose bodies within the joint. The radiograph reveals multiple rounded opacities within an otherwise normal joint. This condition generally requires synovectomy. *Pigmented villonodular synovitis* most commonly involves the knee. Focal masses may be palpable, and the radiograph, though not infrequently normal, may reveal lobulation of the synovial tissues. Joint fluid in this condition is characteristically dark brown and bloody. Synovectomy, sometimes followed by radiotherapy, or radiation synovectomy alone is indicated.

Arthrocentesis is important in the diagnosis and treatment of patients with acute intra-articular knee pain. Arthrocentesis must be done under sterile conditions with careful skin preparation with povidone-iodine and alcohol. Aspiration is done from the medial aspect by inserting a needle beneath the patella (Fig. 53–6). The needle should be at least 20 gauge to ensure that some viscous joint effusions can be aspirated easily.

Corticosteroid injection is useful in the patient with an acutely painful inflammatory condition (e.g., pseudogout) that is not expected to cause persistent joint inflammation. Local steroid injection is also useful in chronic synovitis, such as rheumatoid arthritis for flares, but the symptoms may recur. Injections should not be repeated more than three to six times in the lifetime of a single joint. One should not inject corticosteroids into a possibly septic joint.

Extra-articular conditions about the knee that produce pain are encountered commonly. Prepatellar bursitis (housemaid's knee) is diagnosed by inspection and palpation of the bursa, which is subcutaneous and overlies the patella. The condition is common in people whose work involves bearing weight on the bended knee (such as carpet layers or roofers). Aspiration and corticosteroid injection of the bursa are the most efficient methods of treatment, but anti-inflammatory agents are also useful. Septic bursitis may occasionally occur in this bursa and can be managed like septic olecranon bursitis (see page 682).

The other clinically important bursae at the knee are the infrapatellar or patellar tendon bursae (superficial and deep) and the pes anserinus bursa (under the tendons of the sartorius gracilis and semitendinosus on the medial side of the knee joint). The diagnosis is made by finding point tenderness in the area of the bursa. Infrapatellar and patellar bursitis, seen most often in young people who do jumping sports, such as basketball or volleyball, can be treated with rest, ice, and nonsteroidal anti-inflammatory agents. Pes anserine bursitis responds dramatically and often for prolonged periods with an injection of corticosteroids into the painful area. Anserine bursitis is commonly associated with obesity, degenerative disease, and valgus deformity of the knee.

Osgood-Schlatter disease or osteochondritis at the apophysis of the tibial tubercle occurs in adolescents 10 to 15 years old. It is occasionally confused with chondromalacia, in which symptoms may be similar; however, in Osgood-Schlatter disease, distinct, well-localized tenderness will be palpable over the tibial tubercle (not the patella), and on inspection the tubercle is often larger than normal. Fragmentation of the apophysis is sometimes evident on radiographic film.

Overuse syndromes about the knee occur commonly as a result of the increased popularity of jogging and other physical activities. Painful areas, often poorly localized about the knee, occur after vigorous physical activity. Most often, they are localized to muscle insertions. Shin splints or pain of the shins is probably a mild form of anterior compartment syndrome. Usually all that is needed is rest followed by *gradual* resumption of activity. Recurrence of a particular area of pain or shin splints over time is less common. When it does occur, both the leg and the foot should be evaluated for anatomic abnormalities leading to chronic strain (bow legs, short leg, pronated feet, and the like).

Traumatic Injury to the Knee

A direct blow or injury to the knee may produce a *hemarthrosis*. The knee becomes stiff and swollen, with a bloody effusion. Aspiration of the blood through a large-bore needle may relieve pain considerably, after which an ice pack may be applied during the first 12 hours following injury. With isometric exercises and use of a crutch or cane, the symptoms should subside without sequelae. Any knee that has a hemarthrosis must be carefully examined to rule out ligamentous damage, particularly injuries of the cruciate ligaments, and subtle fractures. The presence of fat droplets in the aspirate is strongly suggestive of an intra-articular fracture, often of the tibial spines or tibial plateau, which may result in formation of a loose body within the joint.

Less severe injury also requires careful evaluation of the supporting tendons, ligaments, and menisci. Traumatic dislocation of the patella can generally be treated by closed reduction and immobilization.[8] Minor sprain or partial tear of a ligament may result from an injury in which the knee has been twisted. Maneuvers do not reveal instability of the joint but produce pain at the site of the ligamentous sprain. Complete or nearly complete tear of a cruciate ligament is associated with frank hemarthrosis and instability of the knee joint, and can be elicited by anterior and poste-

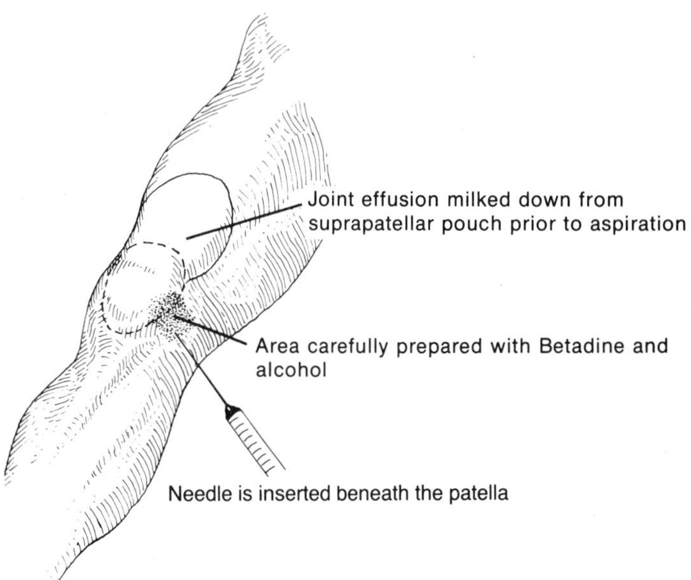

FIGURE 53–6. Arthrocentesis of the knee joint. The area is carefully prepared with Betadine and alcohol. The operator passes the needle beneath the patella to enter the joint space from its medial aspect. Synovial fluid may be obtained for diagnostic purposes, or corticosteroids may be injected.

rior drawer tests. Complete tear of one of the collateral ligaments also must be tested for by determining the stability of the joint (see Fig. 53–5*B* and *C*). Meniscal tears generally occur medially. A torn medial meniscus may act as a loose body within the joint and cause locking, a small joint effusion, and tenderness localized to the medial joint line. Posterior meniscal tear is difficult to diagnose clinically. It may be suspected if one can palpate or hear a click when the flexed knee is externally rotated and brought to full extension (McMurray test). Blows to the anterior knee can tear the patella or quadriceps tendon or can fracture the patella. Diagnosis of a fractured patella can usually be made on the lateral radiographic view, but longitudinal fractures may be seen only on the "sunrise" view, taken with the x-ray beam directed tangentially to the patella and the knee flexed at 90 degrees.

The principles of management for ligamentous injuries of the knee are the same as those for ligamentous injuries in other areas. Because the knee is a weight-bearing joint, it is essential that the ligaments be allowed to heal prior to resuming activity, with a period of immobilization. Sprains with no instability can be treated initially with cold application, followed by rest and isometric exercise for strengthening the quadriceps. If there is also significant tenderness and pain on weight bearing in such cases, a dressing or cast is applied to stabilize the joint in extension, and the patient must use crutches for 10 days to 3 weeks (Fig. 53–7). Following complete tear of a ligament leading to frank instability of the joint, surgical repair may be needed, and this should be carried out promptly. Surgery is usually necessary for major acute meniscal tears, although the surgery need not be carried out immediately, and the patient may

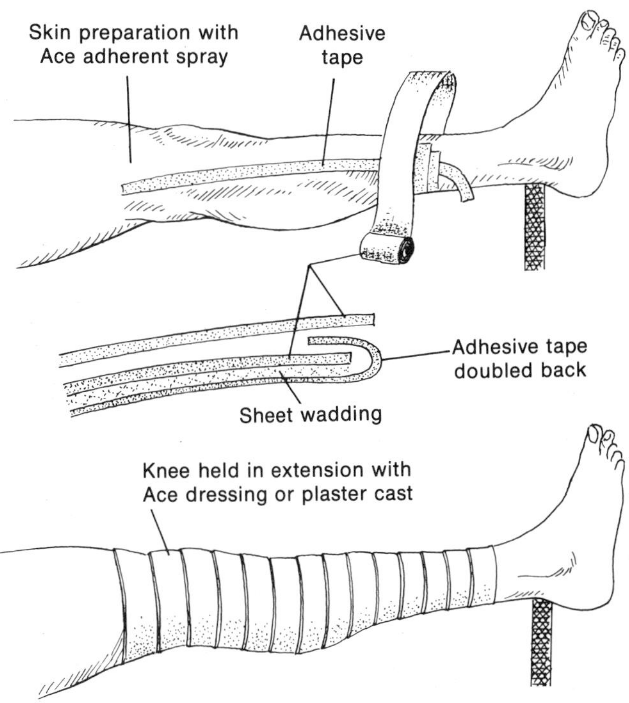

FIGURE 53–7. Application of an Ace (Jones) dressing for ligamentous injury of the knee in which there is no demonstrable instability of any of the knee ligaments but there is considerable pain. The dressing should be worn for 2 to 3 weeks until pain abates. If instability is present on clinical examination, a cylinder cast is necessary and should be worn for 6 to 8 weeks until ligamentous healing is complete. To apply the Jones dressing, the skin is first prepared with Ace adherent spray and a strip of 1-inch adhesive is applied from the upper thigh to the ankle. Sheet wadding is applied next, wrapped in a circular fashion from the upper thigh to above the malleolus in at least four thicknesses. An Ace bandage is then wrapped over this. The adhesive tape is placed between layers of Ace bandage to prevent the dressing from slipping downward. The patient can then walk on crutches while the ligamentous sprain is given time to heal. (Adapted from Hill GJ: Outpatient Surgery, 2nd ed. Philadelphia, WB Saunders, 1980, p 543.)

be followed. Minor meniscal tears, particularly in elderly persons, may not require surgery, although chronic pain occasionally necessitates it.

If any doubt exists concerning the presence of meniscal or ligament tear or fracture in the setting of acute injury, the patient should be referred promptly to a physician experienced in the diagnosis and treatment of such injuries. Results of late reconstruction of torn knee ligaments are much less satisfactory than those that have repair within the first 3 days after injury.

Chronic Knee Pain

The patient with chronic knee pain and no localizing findings around the knee or effusion should be examined carefully for anatomic abnormalities, such as genu valgum, varum, tibial torsion, or the possibility of a hip or osseous problem (Fig. 53–8). If a malalignment is recognized in childhood or adolescence, the patient should be sent to an orthopedic surgeon with expertise in developmental problems because the question is always whether a conservative or surgical approach should be undertaken to prevent the development of degenerative arthritis. In a chronic monoarthritis of the knee, joint aspiration with synovial biopsy and culture should be done to exclude indolent infections, such as tuberculosis and tumor. In children, the presenting complaint of lymphoma or leukemia may occasionally be persistent knee pain. Radiographs taken of these children may reveal only demineralization of the tibia or femur, and bone biopsy may be needed to make the diagnosis.

Degenerative arthritis commonly involves the knee. Typical findings are bony enlargement of the joint and crepitation with little or no warmth, erythema, or morning stiffness. Management consists of exercises designed to strengthen the quadriceps mechanism, and thereby stabilize the joint, together with periods of rest or relief from weight bearing during painful exacerbations. Reducing loads exerted on the knee by weight reduction and use of a cane in the opposite hand is useful. Acetaminophen is as efficient as a nonsteroidal anti-inflammatory drug to control pain,[9] but if signs of inflammation are obvious, the latter may be a better choice. It is important to prevent flexion contractures in all patients with chronic knee involvement. This is best done by teaching the patient to take his or her knee through a full range of motion often and to avoid prolonged periods with the knees in a flexed position. Weight reduction should be encouraged in the obese.

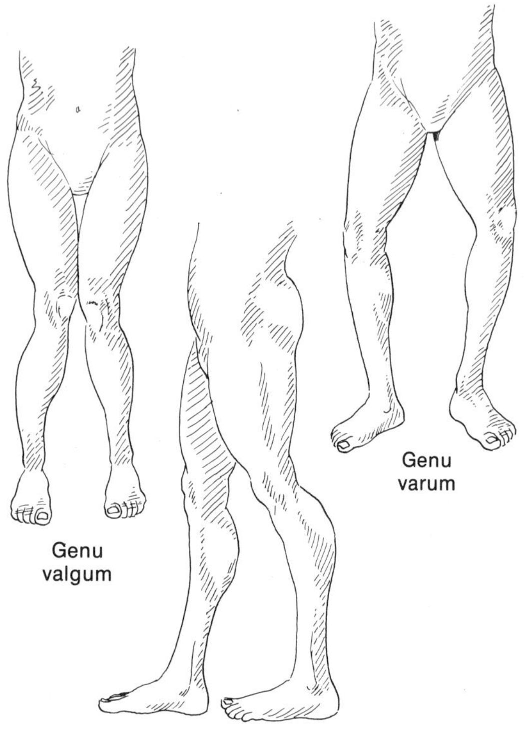

FIGURE 53–8. Genu valgum and genu varum. Chronic pain associated with minor deformities can be treated by use of a heel-and-sole wedge in the shoe or, in the case of genu recurvatum, a long leg brace. (Adapted with permission from MacAusland WR Jr and Mayo RA: Orthopedics: A Concise Guide to Clinical Practices. Boston, Little, Brown and Company, 1965, pp 245–247.)

Episodes of synovitis sometimes occur in osteoarthritis and may be related to inflammation due to cartilage debris or hydroxyapatite crystals. They respond to nonsteroidal agents and to judicious use of intra-articular steroids.

The same indications and contraindications discussed for total replacement of the hip apply to the knee as well. Knee replacements, more so than hip replacements, require considerable skill in both the surgery itself and in the rehabilitation process. Published series of cases using modern techniques and prostheses and with adequate follow-up indicate that approximately 90% of the patients having surgery experienced significant pain relief. Functionally, good ambulation is achieved in roughly 80% of patients. Morbidity, short and long term, is similar to that of hip replacements. After knee replacement surgery, about half the patients have evidence of calf vein thrombosis by venography, but extension of the clot proximally is rare and usually occurs 1 to 3 weeks after surgery. Because of the difficulty of salvaging the joint when a complication or infection supervenes, total knee replacement is sometimes withheld in young persons (less than 55 years of age) or obese individuals. Arthroscopic débridement or osteotomy may be used.[11]

Patients with persistent knee symptoms may also have a surgically correctable torn meniscus or cruciate ligament or a loose body within the joint. This should be suspected when there is a history of "locking" (sudden but temporary inability to extend the knee) or "giving way" (sudden falling). Magnetic resonance imaging is an excellent technique to visualize internal derangements or loose bodies and is now widely available. Arthrography or arthroscopy is useful to complement the information obtained by magnetic resonance.[10, 11] Arthrography is rarely associated with an allergic reaction (hives). The major complication, septic arthritis, occurs only about once per 10,000 procedures using either arthrography or arthroscopy.[12] Arthroscopy has been reported to be slightly more accurate than arthrography.[13] Arthroscopy is limited in the assessment of the posterior third of the medial meniscus.[10] If a tear in this area is suspected, arthrography or magnetic resonance imaging may be needed. About 50% of loose bodies and meniscal tears can be treated arthroscopically and morbidity from the procedure is substantially lower than that following an arthrotomy.

ANKLE PAIN

In practice, the most commonly encountered problems of the ankle and foot are sprains and traumatic injuries (Table 53–5). When there is no obvious history of trauma, ankle pain may be related to chronic ligamentous instabil-

TABLE 53–5. CAUSES OF ANKLE PAIN

Traumatic Injuries
- Sprains of lateral, medial, or cruciate ligaments
- Avulsion fracture of medial malleolus
- Fracture of fibula and/or tibia accompanied by sprain of ligaments

Ankle Pain Not Associated with Trauma
- Chronic ligamentous instability
- Degenerative joint disease, usually of subtalar and tarsal joints
- Synovitis (gout, pseudogout, rheumatoid, sarcoid, Reiter's syndrome, sepsis)
- Osteomyelitis of distal tibia
- Unusual causes: chronic infectious arthritis (tuberculosis, brucellosis), tumor of bone or joint (villonodular synovitis)

ity or to arthritis such as rheumatoid arthritis, crystalline synovitis, Reiter's syndrome, or infection. Primary degenerative joint disease of the ankle is uncommon. Sorting out the cause of ankle pain is done by getting the history of its onset and course and by identifying which joint is involved. Goals of the examination are to determine whether there is instability, point tenderness, or pain or limitation of motion of the three principal groups of joints: the ankle, the midfoot (subtalar), and the metatarsophalangeal joints. Figure 53–9 illustrates the key maneuvers. An effusion and signs of inflammation over the joint line define synovitis and require further diagnostic studies. Occasionally, edema needs to be distinguished from synovitis of the ankle. In edema, the swelling may pit and involve the entire foot and is not confined to the joint lines. In cellulitis, heat, erythema, and tenderness are also not confined to the periarticular tissues; although stretching or applying pressure to the skin will cause pain in cellulitis, pain is not specifically related to the motion of the ankle joint.

Sprains and Other Traumatic Injuries

The majority of ankle sprains involve the ligaments stabilizing the lateral aspect of the ankle (see Fig. 53–9*A*). The medial aspect of the ankle is stabilized by the medial collateral or deltoid ligament (see Fig. 53–9*B*). Sprains of the medial collateral ligament are uncommon (6% of cases). They are accompanied by an avulsion fracture of the tip of the medial malleolus in almost 60% of cases. A third set of ligaments (tibiofibular or interosseous ligaments) connects the tibia and fibula but is affected only by severe trauma to the ankle associated with fracture of the fibula.

To assess the extent of an ankle injury, a physical examination should be performed as soon as possible, so that the findings will not be obscured by swelling or hematoma. Palpating for tenderness and swelling localizes the site of a ligamentous tear (Fig. 53–10*A*). The most important part of the examination is testing for stability of the joint. The anterior talofibular ligament, stabilizing the lateral aspect of the joint, is most commonly ruptured. Rupture of the talofibular ligament is suggested when the talus can move forward more than 4 mm as the foot is pulled forward and into slight internal rotation (see Fig. 53–10*B*). Rupture of both the anterior talofibular and the calcaneofibular ligaments laterally can be demonstrated by forced inversion of the foot. The ability to tilt or invert the foot by more than 25 to 30 degrees implies rupture of these ligaments.[14] One may test for fracture of the tibia by compressing the tibia and fibula with the thumb and fingers of one hand. Pain, crepitation, and soft tissue swelling directly over the bone suggest presence of a fracture, which should be confirmed with a radiograph.[15] These should include anteroposterior and lateral projections and a mortise view. The anteroposterior and lateral views demonstrate fractures of the tibia or the fibula. The mortise view, a true anteroposterior view of the ankle joint and talus, evaluates whether lateral subluxation of the talus from a complete tear of the deltoid ligament has occurred. The position of the talus is judged by the appearance of the cartilage space. The normal space is the same medially, superiorly, and laterally. If the medial space is greater than the superior, the talus has been displaced laterally. Stress radiographs of the ankle using weights in an attempt to provoke anterior displacement or inversion of the foot are also useful for demonstrating instability caused by tears of the lateral ligaments. Such radiographs are reported to detect 90% of complete liga-

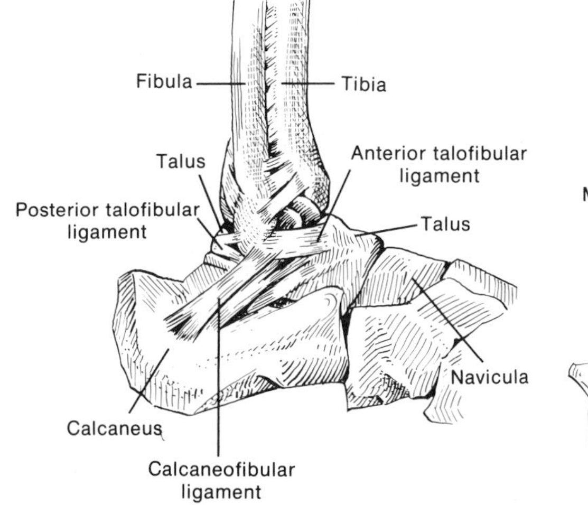

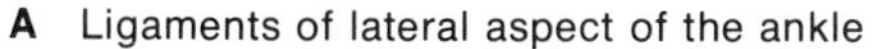

A Ligaments of lateral aspect of the ankle

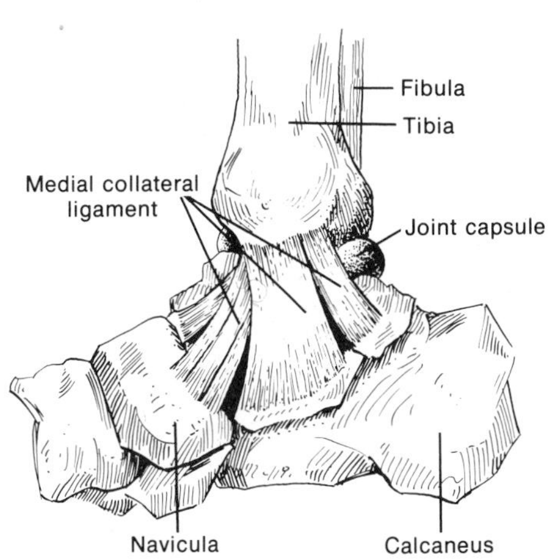

B Ligaments of medial aspect of the ankle

FIGURE 53–9. Ligaments stabilizing the ankle. *A*, The lateral aspect of the ankle is stabilized by the anterior talofibular ligament, calcaneofibular ligament, and posterior talofibular ligament. Most ankle sprains involve the anterior talofibular ligament, sprain or rupture of which is often accompanied by a partial tear of the calcaneofibular ligament. *B*, The medial aspect of the ankle is stabilized by the medial collateral ligament, which because of its integrity is usually only minimally sprained except in major trauma involving fracture.

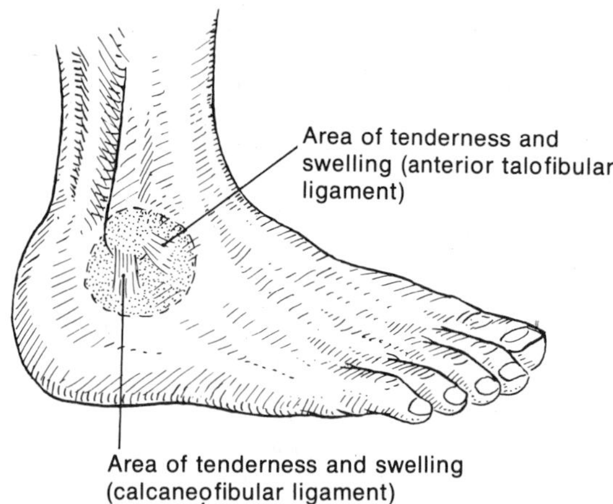

A Palpation to detect swelling and tenderness in ankle injuries

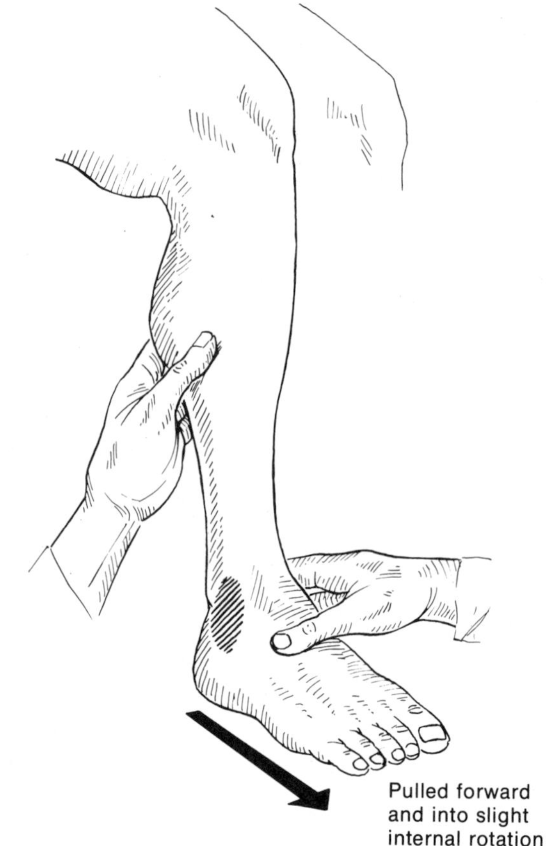

B Testing for stability of anterior talofibular ligament

FIGURE 53–10. Physical examination of the sprained ankle. Most sprains involve the lateral aspect of the ankle. *A,* Swelling and tenderness can be palpated in the area of the anterior talofibular ligament and, sometimes, of the calcaneofibular ligament. *B,* To test for stability of the anterior talofibular ligament, one grasps the foot and, with the patient relaxed, pulls it forward and into slight internal rotation. More than 4 mm of forward motion suggests rupture of the ligament.

mentous tears but are occasionally falsely negative due to insufficient muscle relaxation.[16]

Therapy depends on the degree of sprain. Partial ligamentous tears are manifested by tenderness, swelling, and pain localized to a discrete area of a single ligament, and by good stability. Treatment consists of elevating the foot and applying ice to the ankle for 1 day, followed by taping the ankle or wrapping an Ace bandage from the base of the toes to the midcalf. The patient should use crutches while the ankle is painful. The patient may resume activity as symptoms allow but should be restricted from vigorous activities or sports for 6 to 8 weeks because stress on a partially torn incompletely healed ligament may complete the tear.

Complete tears are manifested by marked tenderness, swelling, and ecchymosis over the entire lateral aspect of the ankle, and by instability. Treatment of complete sprains is somewhat controversial. Most orthopedists believe that treatment should be nonsurgical, using elevation, ice, and posterior splinting until swelling subsides. Patients are placed in a short leg cast for a minimum of 6 weeks and on crutches for 2 to 3 weeks until weight bearing is pain-free. Some orthopedists recommend surgical repair of the ligament within 10 days, reporting that 20 to 40% of patients treated conservatively have some recurrent instability of the ankle.[14] Surgical repair is reported to produce long-term stability in all but 15% of cases.[17] Others believe that with *good* conservative management, chronic instability is quite rare.

Mild sprains of the medial collateral or deltoid ligament, although rare, are treated in the same way as lateral sprains. Most medial injuries are accompanied by a fracture, usually of the proximal fibula. These and any ankle injury with displacement of the talus, the medial malleolus, the lateral malleolus, the entire fibula (interosseous ligamentous tears), or dislocation of the ankle, are severe injuries and need an assessment of whether there is impending skin necrosis and vascular compromise. Prompt referral to restore normal anatomic relationships must be done to avoid late post-traumatic arthritis.

Ankle Pain Not Associated with Trauma

Ankle synovitis alone is unusual and, if present, is generally a manifestation of rheumatoid arthritis, gout, sarcoid, one of the B-27–related spondyloarthropathies, or gonococcal arthritis. The signs of synovitis are warmth, swelling, and an effusion. Marked limitation of the range of motion of the ankle joint is unusual. When a patient has signs of synovitis in just one ankle and has no history of trauma, gout, or other explanation, joint infection should be suspected and diagnostic joint aspiration performed. Localized pain at the medial malleolus, particularly in children, may indicate osteomyelitis of the distal tibia. If this cannot be diagnosed by aspiration of the ankle joint, a technetium or gallium scan can be confirmatory. Gradual onset of a painful ankle, even with little or no warmth and erythema around the synovium, may suggest a chronic infection, such as tuberculosis or brucellosis, whereas focal tenderness or pain suggests the possibility of a tumor of the bone or synovium. Erythema nodosum and hypertrophic osteoarthropathy are associated with periarthritis of the ankles.

Chronic ankle pain most frequently results from chronic instability from recurrent injury or inadequately treated partial or complete ligamentous tear or inflammatory arthritis. In the former, pain is usually localized to the ligaments of the lateral aspect of the joint. Use of a lateral heel wedge may be considered in such patients in order to reduce the frequency of recurrent injury.[14] Surgical repair is not likely to produce an excellent result because of the difficulty in identifying the ends of the ligaments, whereas nonoperative treatment results only in re-establishing the level of stability that was present prior to the most recent injury. Degenerative arthritis may result from recurrent injury or ligamentous laxity. Surgical fusion of the ankle is the alternative to medical management in patients with severe degenerative arthritis of the ankle and disabling pain.

FOOT PAIN

The etiology of foot pain may be traumatic, inflammatory, neuropathic, or circulatory (Table 53–6). Thus, the evaluation of foot pain begins with careful inspection of the foot, assessment of the circulation, and testing for sensation (Fig. 53–11). In practice, foot pain can be divided into three general categories: heel pain, midfoot pain, and anterior foot and toe pain.

Heel Pain

The most common causes of heel pain are plantar fasciitis, bursitis of the heel, and Achilles tendinitis. *Plantar fasciitis* seen alone or as a manifestation of Reiter's syndrome and other spondyloarthropathies (Chapter 50) can be diagnosed by eliciting point tenderness at the insertion of the plantar fascia into the calcaneal tuberosity (Fig. 53–12). An exostosis of the calcaneus may be present radiographically but does not change management. Treatment includes use of a "doughnut" heel insert, nonsteroidal anti-inflammatory agents, and local corticosteroid injection in refractory cases.

The bursae that lie in front and in back of the Achilles tendon at its insertion into the calcaneus may become traumatized. The most common situation is produced by friction against the shoe top; in such cases, bursitis can be treated by use of a lift on the inner side of the heel. Calcaneal bursitis is characterized by point tenderness at the insertion of the Achilles tendon into the calcaneal tuberosity (see Fig. 53–12).

Achilles tendinitis causes posterior heel pain. It may occur after vigorous exercise or during less strenuous exercise if there are underlying degenerative changes of the tendon. The diagnosis is made by finding tenderness and swelling along the tendon, occasionally accompanied by audible crepitus, and by reproducing tenderness with passive stretching of the tendon. Achilles tendinitis is also seen in the spondyloarthropathies. Apophysitis of the calcaneus, a condition seen in adolescents, is a form of osteochondritis analogous to Osgood Schlatter disease of the knee.

Rupture of the Achilles tendon may occur after vigorous exercise. The patient tells a story of an acutely painful "snap," and of inability to flex the sole of the foot. Examination discloses that squeezing the calf muscle fails to flex the sole of the foot, and a defect in the continuity of the tendon may be appreciated about 1 inch above its insertion at the heel. Fresh rupture requires prompt surgical referral.

Rupture of the plantaris tendon produces rapid onset of localized swelling of the midcalf without loss of power but with pain on plantar flexion. The integrity of the Achilles tendon should be checked as earlier. Days after the injury, there may be pitting edema and a crescent-shaped ecchymosis along the malleolus. In the first day, ice should be applied and the leg elevated. Aspirin and nonsteroidal agents should be avoided, as they may increase deep hemorrhage and prolong recovery. After the acute phase, treatment includes crutches, analgesics, and a 1- to 1.5-inch heel lift, for 6 weeks.

TABLE 53–6. CAUSES OF FOOT PAIN

Heel Pain
Plantar fasciitis
Bursitis
Apophysitis
Ruptured Achilles or plantaris tendon
Midfoot Pain
Subtalar arthritis
Tarsal coalition
Chronic ligamentous strain
Anterior Foot Pain and Toe Pain
Metatarsalgia
Plantar neuroma
Plantar warts
Synovitis (e.g., rheumatoid, gout, septic)
Infection, cellulitis, septic arthritis, or osteomyelitis
Peripheral neuropathies
Vascular problems (e.g., arterial insufficiency, including phlebitis and chronic venous insufficiency)
Painful Toes
Hallux valgus and rigidus
Ingrown toenail
Subluxation, particularly of metatarsophalangeal joints
Osteochondritis of metatarsal head

Midfoot Pain

Midfoot pain is most commonly the result of chronic foot strain related to intrinsic ligamentous laxity or, infrequently, to problems of the subtalar joint and the tarsal bones (see Fig. 53–11). Flat feet without symptoms should be ignored, as they usually do not cause symptoms in the future. For instance, black people often have flat feet but rarely have arch pain.

The midfoot can be examined by observing the arch with the patient sitting. The subtalar and midfoot joints may be assessed by immobilizing the ankle and inverting and everting the forefoot. Limitation of full range of motion or pain suggests problems of the subtalar or midfoot joints; radiographs should be obtained for signs of arthritis, tarsal coalition, and other osseous lesions.

Subtalar arthritis is secondary to inflammatory arthritis, degenerative joint disease, sepsis, or congenital tarsal coalition (incomplete separation of the tarsal bones). These conditions are treated with analgesics or nonsteroidal anti-inflammatory agents, and if inflammation exists, a heel cup to limit foot inversion and eversion. A podiatry consultation should be sought when initial treatment fails.

If radiographs reveal congenital tarsal coalition or other congenital fusion of the tarsal bones, initial treatment is the same as for subtalar arthritis, but consultation is advised if symptoms persist.

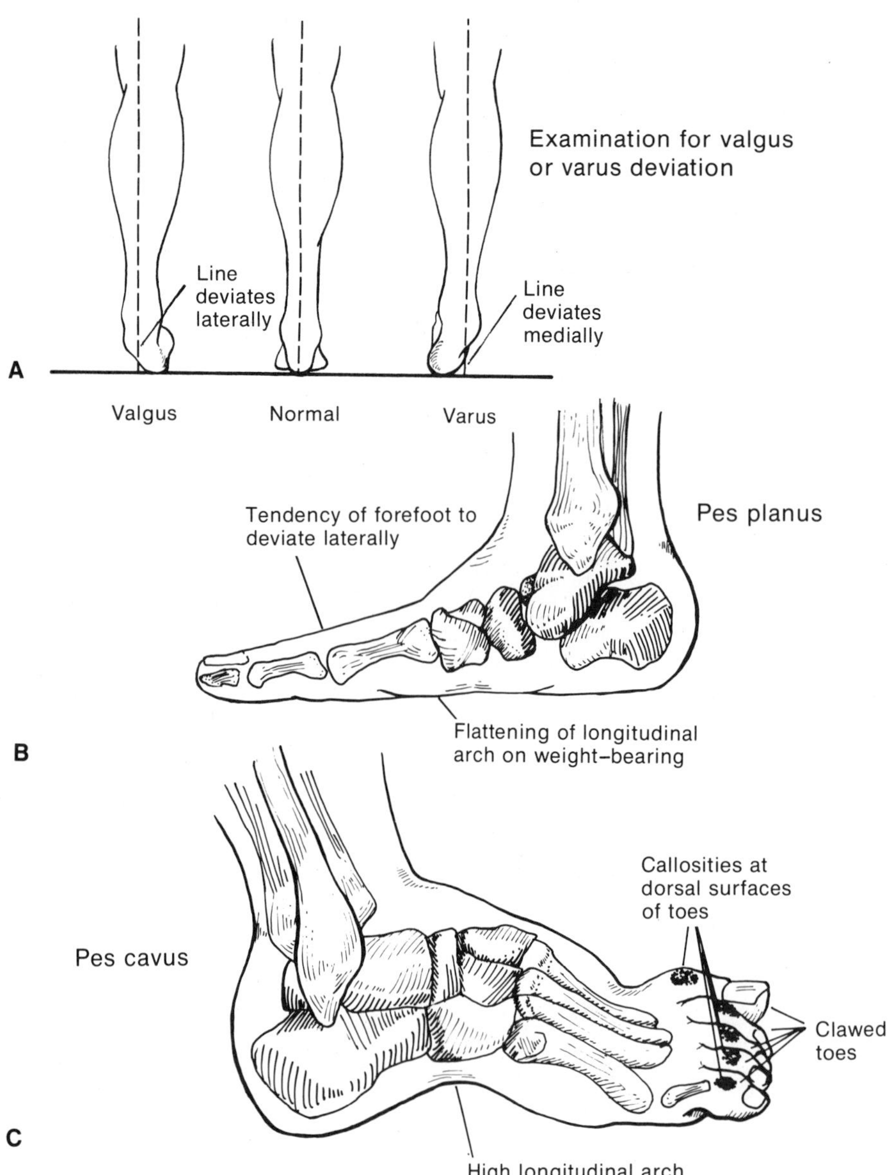

FIGURE 53–11. Inspection of the foot. The skin is examined for abrasions, swelling, callus, and adequacy of the pedal pulses and peripheral sensation. *A*, Valgus or varus deformity can be determined by standing behind the patient and observing any deviation. *B*, Pes planus, a flat or weak foot, refers to flattening of the longitudinal arch often with a slight valgus deviation. *C*, Pes cavus refers to increased angle of the longitudinal arch with clawing of the toes, hyperextension of the metatarsophalangeal joints, and flexion of the proximal interphalangeal joints. This deformity may be related to poliomyelitis, spina bifida, and other neurologic diseases or may be idiopathic. It is usually encountered in adolescents and predisposes to secondary degenerative arthritis of the tarsal joints and the formation of callosities on the dorsal surface of the proximal interphalangeal joints. (Adapted with permission from MacAusland WR Jr and Mayo RA: Orthopedics: A Concise Guide to Clinical Practices. Boston, Little, Brown and Company, 1965, pp 265–300.)

Anterior Foot or Toe Pain

The evaluation of anterior foot or toe pain begins with checking the peripheral pulses and performing a neurologic examination of the foot. The patient should stand to assess the presence of deformities. The metatarsal heads can be squeezed as a group to elicit pain from neuroma, metatarsalgia, and osteochondritis of the metatarsal heads. The big toe should be assessed for its range of motion and whether movement elicits pain. Finally, the bottom of the foot should be examined for warts and calluses. Normally, calluses and thickened skin are located at the points of a triangle formed by the big toe, the small toe, and the heel. Any deviation from this pattern suggests altered biomechanics or structural abnormalities.

Any of the inflammatory forms of arthritis discussed previously can affect the metatarsophalangeal joints and cause metatarsal pain. These are suggested by the existence of other inflamed joints and will not be discussed further here. *Metatarsalgia* is a static foot disorder producing symptoms in the absence of synovitis (Fig. 53–13*A*). It is a common disorder of middle-aged individuals, frequently those who have cocked-up deformities of their toes from inappropriate shoes or from soft tissue contractures. When associated with deformity, metatarsalgia should be treated with a program of active and passive stretching to stretch and strengthen the musculature and other soft tissues. A proper shoe should be prescribed, particularly if there is evidence of unusual wear of the shoe or if calluses are located in unusual places. For symptomatic treatment, patients with metatarsal pain can be provided with a metatarsal bar to shift the weight posteriorly away from the metatarsal heads. Resection of the metatarsal heads is an effective procedure in patients with refractory arthritic pain of the metatarsophalangeal joints.

A plantar or *Morton's neuroma* involves the interdigital nerve supplying the third and fourth digits (see Fig. 53–13*B*). The diagnosis is made by reproducing the lancinating pain in the third and fourth toes by metatarsal compression. Similar symptoms occur in the absence of an actual neuroma, and they may be related to nerve compression from soft tissue structures. A Morton's neuroma is treated initially by the use of a lift or bar to remove pressure from the metatarsal heads and occasionally by local injection of

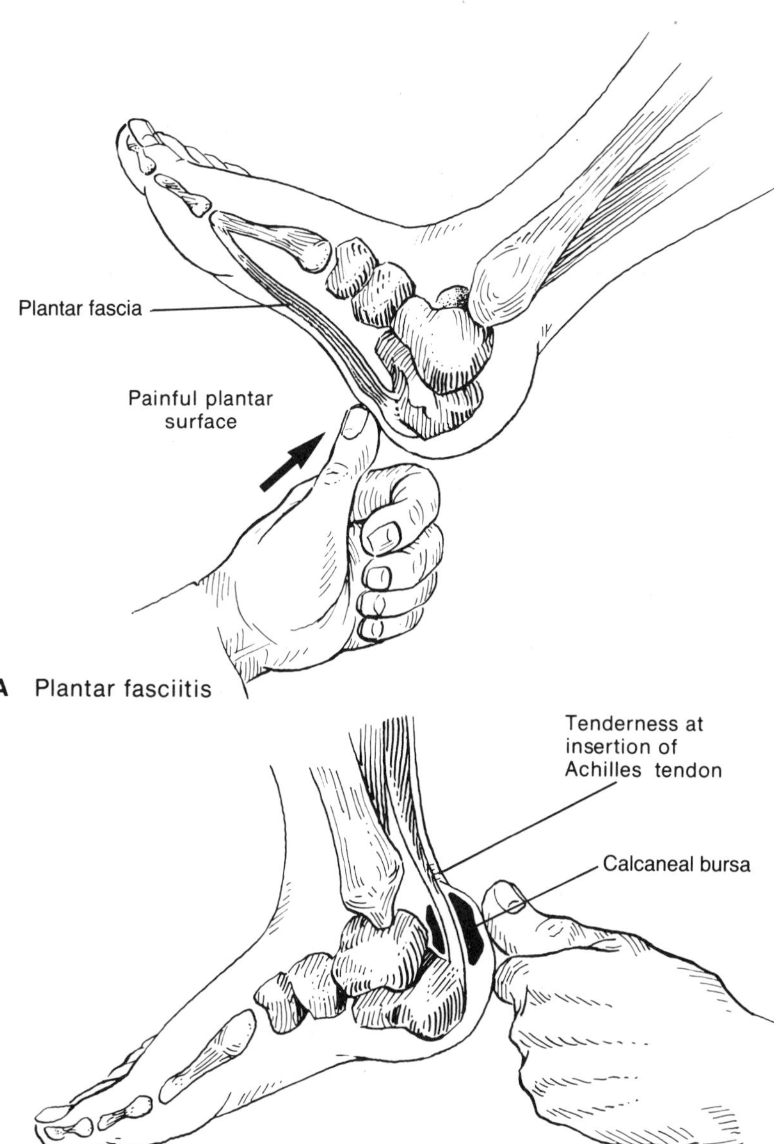

FIGURE 53–12. Examination of the patient with heel pain. *A*, Pressure exerted by the thumb beneath the plantar fascia elicits tenderness in patients with plantar fasciitis. *B*, Pressure over the insertion of the Achilles tendon into the calcaneus reproduces tenderness in bursitis of the heel.

the neuroma with corticosteroids. A surgical approach produces unsatisfactory results in 10 to 15% of instances and should be reserved for refractory cases.[18] *Plantar warts* are diagnosed by inspection. In contrast to a callus one sees abnormal skin with fine blood vessels viewed on end and a cleavage between the wart and the surrounding skin (see Fig. 53–13*C*). If painful, warts are best treated by chemical removal or curettage.

Osteochondritis of the metatarsal heads (Freiberg's disease) usually occurs during adolescence but also may become symptomatic in an adult. Left alone, the symptoms usually resolve, but they can be treated locally with a metatarsal bar, anti-inflammatory agents, and occasionally, a local steroid injection. Metatarsal head resection is necessary in refractory cases.

The big toe is the battleground for many insults. Because it takes the brunt of pressure during walking, the first metatarsophalangeal joint commonly develops degenerative arthritis. The metatarsophalangeal joint is enlarged without signs of synovitis and frequently demonstrates (limited) motion with pain. If restriction is extreme, the condition is called hallux rigidus (Fig. 53–14*A*). Acute inflammation of the first metatarsophalangeal joint suggests gout (podagra).

Ingrown toenails may occur anywhere but frequently involve the big toe and result from improper cutting of the nail (see Fig. 53–14*B*). When infected, they should be treated with antibiotics and drained surgically.

Hammer toes or cocked-up toes result from intrinsic muscle shortening or capsular contraction (see Fig. 53–14*C*). They are most commonly painless abnormalities in women who wear high heels. Symptomatic patients should be fitted with a better shoe that accommodates the deformity. If pain is present, one needs to identify whether its source is the metatarsal or the interphalangeal joint. For metatarsal discomfort, a good shoe and a metatarsal bar are indicated.

The common bunion or callus usually suggests underlying structural abnormalities. Almost always, calluses come from altered biomechanics in combination with ill-fitting shoes. It is important to refer diabetics and patients with peripheral neuropathies for preventive podiatric treatment. Normally, calluses and bunions are not painful; painful

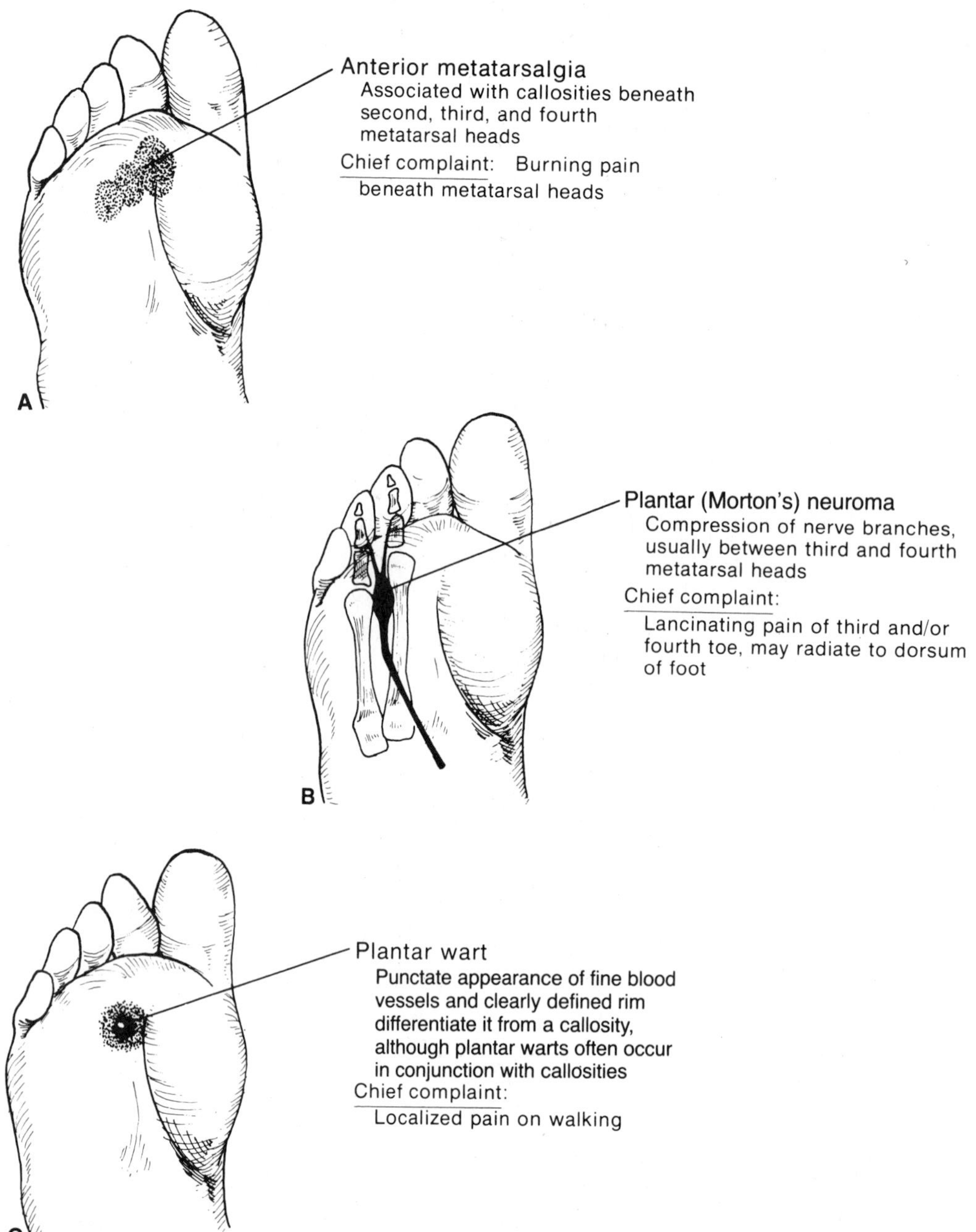

FIGURE 53–13. Examination of the patient with pain in the anterior foot. *A,* Anterior metatarsalgia produces burning pain and is associated with callosities beneath the metatarsal heads. *B,* Plantar neuroma produces lancinating pain radiating to the third or fourth toe or dorsum of the foot. *C,* Plantar warts are punctate in appearance with clearly defined margins but may be associated with a callosity; they produce localized pain on walking.

ones suggest underlying infection or inflammation. One of the most common bunions occurs at the bony prominence of the first metatarsal head. These prominences, present in everyone, become accentuated in patients who have a congenital first metatarsal varus with a greater than normal angle between the first and second metatarsal shafts. With tight shoes, the great toe is pushed laterally, creating the *hallux valgus* deformity. The metatarsal head becomes more prominent and, through shoe irritation, a bony exostosis develops with an overlying painful bursa (see Fig. 53–14*D*). Treatment consists of shoes with adequate toe width to accommodate the forefoot. If modification of shoes is not effective in relieving symptoms, corrective surgery can be done to realign the first metatarsal bone and great toe.

It is important to emphasize the principles of foot care for patients with vascular insufficiency and/or peripheral neuropathy.[19] Because sensation is impaired so that the patient may not be aware of trauma, avoidance of ill-fitting shoes and breaking-in of shoes is essential. The skin of the foot should be carefully inspected daily by the patient to identify abrasions, blisters, or paronychias. Daily applications of a water-soluble cream may be applied to the autonomically denervated foot, and lamb's wool may be used between toes to prevent maceration of tissues. Warm soaks, if used, should be tested first with the patient's finger to avoid burning the heat-insensitive foot. Nails should be cut and corns shaved only by a podiatrist. Infections may be less painful than one would expect, due to the decreased

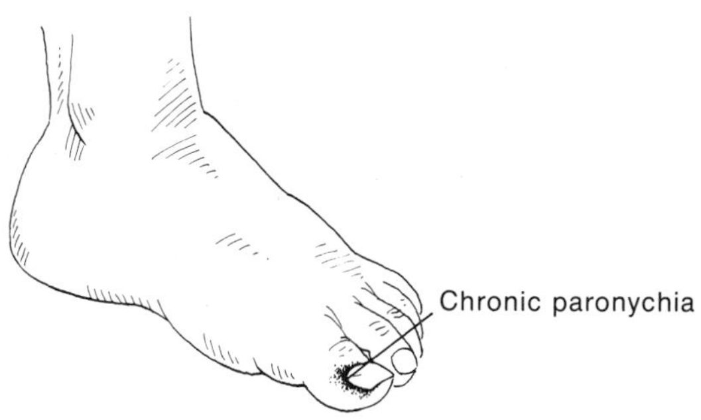

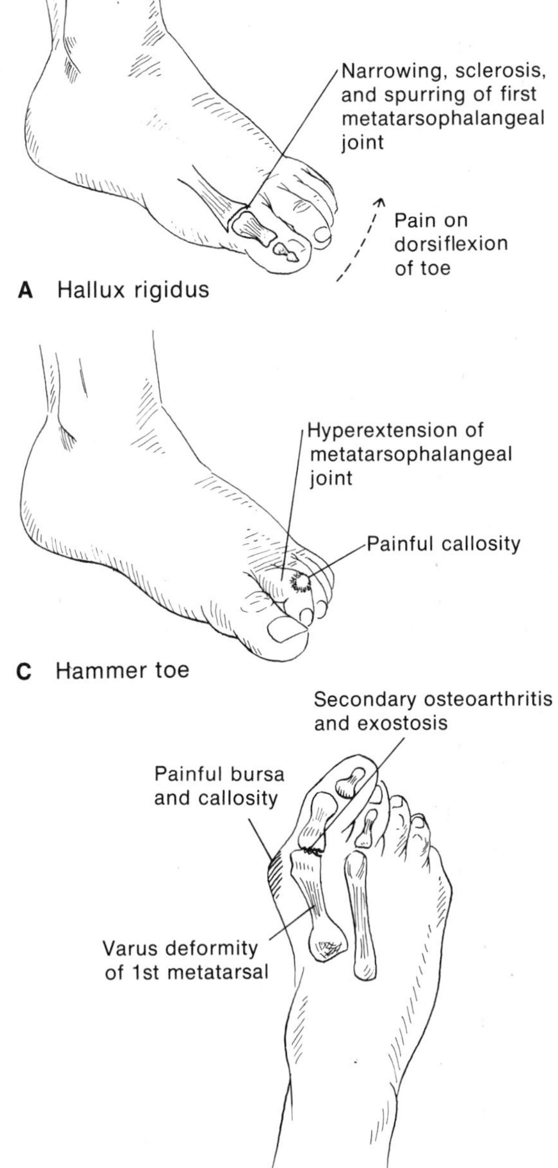

FIGURE 53–14. Examination of the patient with painful toes. *A,* Hallux rigidus refers to degenerative joint disease of the first metatarsophalangeal joint. Pain is produced on dorsiflexion of the toe. *B,* Paronychia refers to soft tissue infection at the side of a toenail, often associated with an ingrown nail. *C,* Hammer toe is produced by hyperextension of the metatarsophalangeal joint, usually of unknown etiology, and may result in formation of a callus at the hyperextended joint. *D,* Hallux valgus is produced by varus deformity of the first metatarsal bone with associated valgus deformity of the phalanges of the first toe. A painful bursa and callous form on the side of the toe, accompanied by secondary degenerative arthritis of the first metatarsophalangeal joint.

sensation. If infection develops, intravenous antibiotics should be considered. Cellulitis in diabetics is usually caused by streptococci or staphylococci, whereas deep-seated infections of the foot are often caused by mixed aerobic and anaerobic organisms.

REFERENCES

1. Ho G, Tice AD, and Kaplan SR: Septic bursitis in the prepatellar and olecranon bursae. An analysis of 25 cases. Ann Intern Med 89:21, 1978.
1a. Mankin HJ: Nontraumatic necrosis of bone (osteonecrosis). N Engl J Med 326:1473, 1992.
2. Liang MH and Fortin PR: Management of osteoarthritis of the hip and knee. N Engl J Med 325:125, 1991.
3. Liang MH, Cullen KE, and Poff R: Primary total hip or knee replacement: Evaluation of patients. Ann Intern Med 97:735, 1982.
4. Harris WH and Sledge CB: Total hip and total knee replacement. N Engl J Med 323:725, 1990.
5. Noble J: Lesions of the menisci: Autopsy incidence in adults from 55 years old. J Bone Joint Surg Am 59(A):480, 1977.
6. Jones RE, Smith EC, and Reisch JS: Effects of medial meniscectomy in patients older than 40 years. J Bone Joint Surg Am 60(A):783, 1978.
7. Haupt JB, Pritzker KPH, Alpert B, et al: Natural history of spontaneous osteonecrosis of the knee (SONK): A review. Semin Arthritis Rheum 13:212, 1983.
8. Cofield RH and Bryan RS: Acute dislocation of the patella. Results of conservative treatment. J Trauma 17:526, 1977.
9. Bradley JD, Brandt KD, Katz BP, et al: Comparison of an antiiflammatory dose of ibuprofen, an analgesic dose of ibuprofen and acetaminophen in the treatment of patients with osteoarthritis of the knee. N Engl J Med 325:87, 1991.
10. Ireland J, Trickey EL, and Stoker DJ: Arthroscopy of the knee: A critical review. J Bone Joint Surg Br 62B:3, 1980.
11. Schonholtz GJ: Arthroscopic debridement of the knee joint. Orthop Clin North Am 20:257, 1989.
12. Poehling GG, Bassett FH, and Goldner JL: Arthroscopy: Its role in treating nontraumatic and traumatic lesions of the knee. South Med J 70:465, 1977.
13. Korn MW, Spitzer RM, and Robinson KE: Correlations of ar-

thrography and arthroscopy. Orthop Clin North Am 10:535, 1979.
14. Saunders EA: Ligamentous injuries of the ankle. Am Fam Pract 22:132, 1980.
15. Brand DA, Frazier WH, Kohlhepp WC, et al: A protocol for selecting patients with injured extremities who need x-rays. N Engl J Med 306:333, 1982.
16. Lindstrand A and Mortensson W: Anterior instability in ankle joint acute lateral sprain. Acta Radiol 18:529, 1977.
17. Redlir I, Brown GG Jr, and Williams JT: Operative treatment of the acutely ruptured lateral ligament of the ankle. South Med J 70:1168, 1977.
18. Bradley N, Miller WA, and Evans PA: Plantar neuroma: Analysis of results following surgical excision in 145 patients. South Med J 69:853, 1976.
19. Lippmann HI, Perotto A, and Farrar R: The neuropathic foot of the diabetic. Bull NY Acad Med 52:1159, 1976.

54

Osteoporosis and Paget's Disease of Bone

MERYL S. LEBOFF, MD
GHADA EL-HAJJ FULEIHAN, MD
EDWARD M. BROWN, MD

Under normal circumstances, the skeleton serves both structural and homeostatic functions. It provides support and protection for soft tissue and serves as a rigid framework for muscular activity and locomotion. The skeleton also acts as a large and readily available reservoir for calcium and phosphate, both of which are essential for normal cellular function.

Bone is constantly being remodelled, with areas of resorption resulting from osteoclastic action being replaced by bone laid down by osteoblasts over a period of 3 to 4 months. Bone formation has been regarded as being determined primarily by the concentrations of calcium and phosphate in extracellular fluids, by mechanical forces on the skeleton, and perhaps by vitamin D metabolites. Bone resorption is also known to be regulated by systemic factors, being stimulated by parathyroid hormone (PTH) as well as 1,25-dihydroxyvitamin D and inhibited by calcitonin. Recently, however, it has been recognized that local factors may be even more important than systemic hormones for the regulation of bone formation and resorption as well as the coupling of these two parameters. Factors that may be involved in these processes include prostaglandins, interleukins (e.g., IL-1 and IL-6), lymphotoxins, tumor necrosis factors (TNF), and transforming growth factor-β.

The skeleton contains 80% cortical bone, concentrated in the long bones, and 20% trabecular bone representing a greater fraction of the spine, epiphyses, and pelvis. Bone accretion occurs during childhood and early adulthood, with the greatest increment taking place during puberty. After peak bone mass is achieved during the second and third decades of life, bone loss ensues with decreases of about 10% of trabecular bone and 2 to 4% of cortical bone per decade in both sexes (Fig. 54–1).[1, 2] However, at the time of the menopause, an acceleration of bone loss occurs

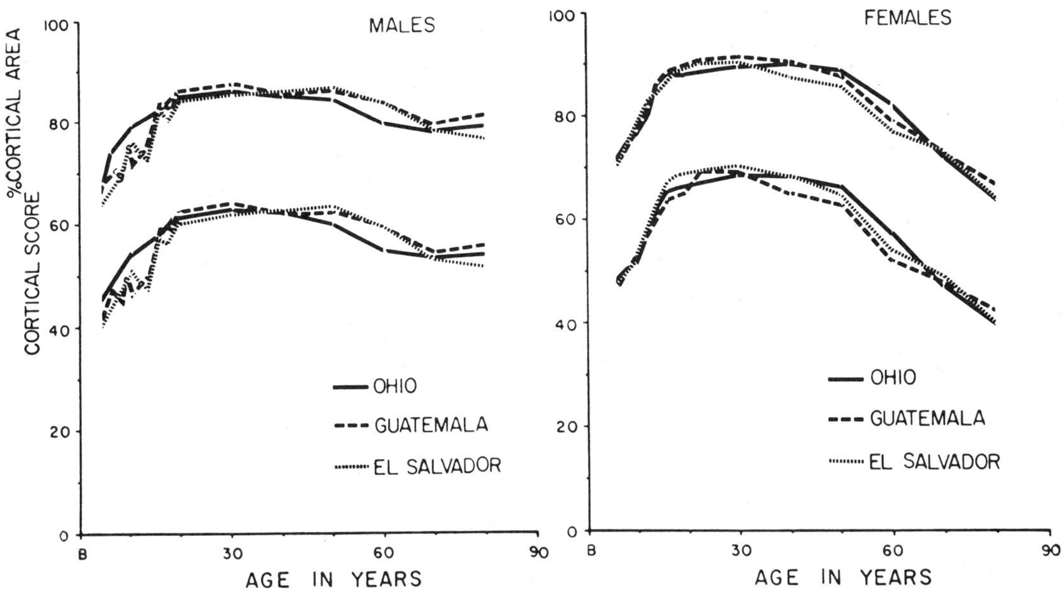

FIGURE 54–1. Changes in bone mass with age in men and women from various geographic locations. (From Garn SM, Rohman CG, and Wagner B: Bone loss as a general phenomenon in man. Fed Proc 26:1749, 1967.)

over approximately 5 to 8 years with a loss of 2 to 5% of trabecular bone and 1 to 2% of cortical bone per year.[3, 4] Over a lifetime, women lose approximately 50% of their trabecular bone and 30% of their cortical bone, whereas men lose two thirds as much.[2, 5, 6]

Although many metabolic bone diseases are uncommon and seldom encountered disorders in clinical practice, two commonly encountered ones, which are discussed here, are osteoporosis and Paget's disease of bone. Both reflect the clinical consequences of defects in the normal orderly sequence of events involved in bone turnover; that is, the regulation of bone formation, resorption, and the coupling of these processes. Discussions of the less common metabolic bone disorders may be found in excellent texts.[7, 8]

OSTEOPOROSIS

Osteoporosis is a disorder in which bone is normally mineralized but is reduced in quantity to the point where fractures occur with minimal or no trauma. This may occur as a result of a low peak bone mass or accelerated bone loss. It must be distinguished from osteomalacia (e.g., defectively mineralized bone), in which the radiographic appearance may be similar. It has been estimated that approximately one third of white women will suffer a vertebral fracture by 65 years of age or a hip fracture by 90 years of age. Of the 1.5 million fractures occurring annually in the United States (~ 500,000 are vertebral and 300,000 are hip fractures), the majority seem to be related to pre-existing osteoporosis.[6] One fifth of elderly patients suffering a hip fracture will die within 4 months of their injury. Although it remains unclear to what extent hip fractures are the cause of mortality, as opposed to resulting from the underlying morbid conditions that predispose to falling, osteoporosis clearly produces significant morbidity and imposes a large financial burden related to the care of fractures and their sequelae. The annual cost to the United States health care system of osteoporosis and its complications is estimated at $10 billion annually. Moreover, owing to the aging population, such costs are projected to more than double in the next 30 years.[9]

In addition to aging and gonadal status, there appear to be a number of other risk factors for osteoporosis, including racial and genetic factors. Blacks have a 5 to 10% higher skeletal mass than do whites; they exhibit a lower rate of bone loss and have one third to one half of the incidence of fractures.[10, 11] Daughters of women with osteoporosis have low bone densities compared with those of a control population.[12] Moreover, studies in twins suggest a higher concordance in bone mass in monozygotic twins than in dizygotic twins.[13] Thin women may be at increased risk of osteoporosis. In addition, other risk factors such as cigarette smoking and excessive intake of alcohol may be deleterious to skeletal health.

Osteoporosis traditionally has been subdivided into primary (juvenile, postmenopausal, and involutional) or secondary osteoporosis. In all types of osteoporosis, the loss of bone mass results from an aberration in the normal balance between bone breakdown and formation with deep osteoclastic resorption cavities or diminished osteoblast-mediated bone formation.[14] This net bone loss may be quite subtle, since a 30 mg/day negative balance of calcium may result in a 10% decrease in skeletal calcium per decade.

Juvenile osteoporosis is defined as otherwise unexplained, excessive loss of bone occurring during the first 2 decades of life. It occurs characteristically in individuals between the ages of 8 and 12 years, frequently with a self-limited course followed by spontaneous improvement at the time of puberty. The commonest forms of osteoporosis are those that occur in women after menopause and in elderly women and men. After the age of 50 in women, there is an exponential rise in osteoporotic fractures as bone density decreases with menopause and advancing age. With menopause, estrogen deficiency and other factors lead to excessive bone resorption and fractures (called postmenopausal or type I osteoporosis). Data show that peripheral monocytes from postmenopausal and osteoporotic women release an elevated rate of IL-1 activity when incubated in vitro. These cytokines are known to stimulate bone resorption in vitro and estrogen therapy suppresses them, suggesting that cytokines may be involved in postmenopausal bone loss and fractures, although further studies to elucidate the role of these factors in skeletal metabolism are necessary.[15]

Patients with postmenopausal osteoporosis generally present within 10 to 15 years after menopause with fractures of areas rich in trabecular bone, such as distal radial (Colles' fracture) or spinal fractures, following minimal or no trauma. Women with the "crush fracture" syndrome note a progressive loss of height, which is often accompanied by kyphosis or a "dowager's hump." In severely affected individuals, the lower ribs may abut the iliac crests. Episodes of spinal collapse may be totally asymptomatic, may produce acute back pain that resolves within several weeks, or may be the source of chronic back pain. Osteoporosis that occurs in older women and in elderly men (otherwise called involutional or type 2 osteoporosis) has been associated with decreased osteoblast function, a deficiency of 1,25-dihydroxyvitamin D, and decreased intestinal calcium absorption accompanied by increasing PTH levels. This type of osteoporosis produces loss of both cortical and trabecular bone.[6] The incidence of hip fractures rises in older patients in whom bone loss is compounded by the tendency to fall because of poor eyesight, failing coordination, or other factors. A sharp increase in these fractures takes place around 65 years of age.

A wide variety of secondary causes of osteoporosis may impinge on the normal changes in bone mass occurring with age and may produce symptomatic disease by themselves or by exacerbating underlying primary osteoporosis (Table 54–1). The bone loss that takes place with menopause occurs with any estrogen-deficient or hypogonadal state (e.g., use of gonadotropin-releasing hormone agonists, anorexia nervosa, athletic amenorrhea, or hyperprolactinemia). With hyperthyroidism or exogenous overreplacement with thyroid hormone, the ensuing high bone turnover may result in bone loss. Such skeletal loss may occur when the thyroid-stimulating hormone is suppressed even without a frankly elevated T4 level.[16] In several of the secondary forms of osteoporosis, osteolytic agents include osteoclast-activating factors such as lymphotoxin, TNF, or IL-1 in multiple myeloma and other hematologic malignancies, or $1,25(OH)_2$ vitamin D in some lymphomas, and heparin in mastocytosis (see Table 54–1). The mechanisms for glucocorticoid-induced bone loss are multiple and include decreased intestinal calcium absorption, increased urinary calcium excretion, depressed osteoblast function, and enhanced bone resorption.[17] Cyclosporine A produces a dose-dependent bone loss in rats, and therapy with both cyclosporine and prednisone is associated with the development of osteoporosis in humans.[18, 19] Patients with rheumatoid arthritis may have periarticular and generalized bone loss caused by immobilization or by the action of inflammatory bone-resorbing cytokines.[20, 21] Smokers have low bone mass in conjunction with a thin body habitus and lower estrogen levels. The low bone mass in alcoholics may reflect malnutrition and malabsorption in addition to the direct suppressive effect of ethanol on osteoblast function. The abnormal collagen formation in the various connective tissue disorders listed in Table 54–1 may be the basis for a reduced peak bone mass or suboptimal skeletal integrity. In many other secondary forms of osteoporosis, however, the cause of the changes in bone dynamics has not been fully established.

TABLE 54–1. CAUSES OF OSTEOPOROSIS/OSTEOPENIA

1. Cause unknown (primary osteoporosis)
   - Juvenile osteoporosis
   - Idiopathic osteoporosis
   - Postmenopausal osteoporosis
   - Involutional osteoporosis
2. Endocrine abnormalities
   - Glucocorticoid excess
   - Thyrotoxicosis
   - Hypogonadism
   - Primary hyperparathyroidism
   - Prolactinomas
   - Hypercalciuria
3. Process affecting the marrow
   - Multiple myeloma
   - Leukemia, lymphoma
   - Anemias—sickle cell disease, thalassemia minor
4. Immobilization
5. Gastrointestinal diseases
   - Postgastrectomy
   - Primary biliary or alcoholic cirrhosis
6. Drugs
   - Anticonvulsants
   - Heparin
   - Methotrexate
   - Glucocorticoids
   - Thyroid hormone (supraphysiologic)
   - Gonadotropin-releasing hormone (GnRH) agonist
   - Lithium
   - Cyclosporine-A
7. Connective tissue disorders
   - Osteogenesis imperfecta
   - Scurvy
   - Homocystinuria
   - Ehlers-Danlos syndrome
8. Rheumatologic disorders
   - Ankylosing spondylitis
   - Rheumatoid arthritis

Approach to the Patient

The goals of the evaluation of the osteoporotic patient are to rule out other forms of bone disease and to determine the principal causes of bone loss so that appropriate treatment can be instituted to mitigate or even reverse any further decrease in skeletal mass. In addition, the basis for acute or chronic musculoskeletal pain must be established so that appropriate medical or orthopedic interventions can be made.

The differential diagnosis of osteoporosis varies with the age and sex of the patient. In children, the most likely possibilities are Cushing's syndrome and exogenous glucocorticoids, immobilization, hypogonadism (e.g., Turner's syndrome or Klinefelter's syndrome), hematologic malignancies (leukemias and lymphomas), as well as occasional cases of idiopathic juvenile osteoporosis. In young and middle-aged adults, particularly among blacks, men, and young women, the most common causes of osteoporosis, other than idiopathic causes, are glucocorticoid excess, premature menopause, or male hypogonadism.[22] Other contributing diagnoses in this age group as well as in older individuals are hyperthyroidism, primary hyperparathyroidism, liver diseases (primary biliary and alcoholic cirrhosis), multiple myeloma, and hematologic malignancies.[22] In older individuals, the osteoporoses associated with menopause and aging are by far the commonest and only identifiable causes of this disorder.

Diagnostic Studies

The discovery of osteoporosis is frequently made from routine radiographs. The spine often shows demineralization with collapse or anterior wedging of one or more vertebral bodies (Fig. 54–2). In more advanced cases, the re-

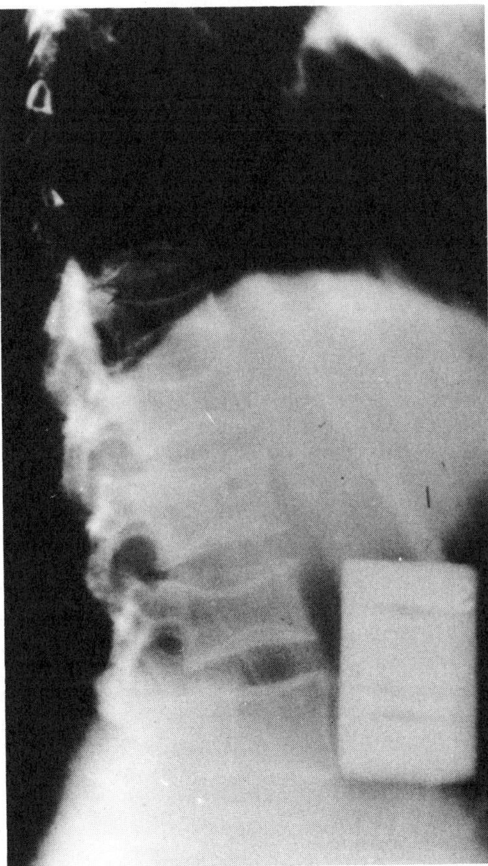

FIGURE 54–2. Spinal osteoporosis. Note the demineralization of the spine with "codfish" vertebrae. In contrast, in malignant disease, focal lytic lesions are frequently seen.

mainder of the skeleton also shows loss of bone mass with cortical thinning of the long bones and thinning and loss of trabeculae in areas of cancellous bone. Conventional radiography, however, is insensitive (an estimated 20 to 50% of bone mass must be lost to be detectable) and is not helpful in defining early stages of the disease. It may, nevertheless, provide clues to possible causes, such as the presence of subperiosteal resorption in primary hyperparathyroidism, localized bone destruction in malignancy, or pseudofractures (Looser's zones) in osteomalacia. If, after the interpretation of the plain radiographs and a review of the clinical features, there is still doubt concerning the diagnosis and, for example, one is unable to differentiate between osteoporosis and osteomalacia, a bone biopsy should be obtained to establish the diagnosis histologically. Iliac crest biopsies are generally performed, and an evaluation should be made of properly stained undecalcified sections. The differentiation of osteoporosis from osteomalacia and other metabolic bone diseases is therapeutically important and generally requires prebiopsy tetracycline labeling of sites of new bone formation. Common causes of osteomalacia in the United States are chronic renal insufficiency, nutritional vitamin D deficiency, and abnormalities of vitamin D metabolism.

Serial measurements of height provide a crude but simple index of changes in vertebral body integrity. More accurate and precise techniques for evaluating skeletal mass include single photon absorptiometry (SPA) and dual photon absorptiometry (DPA), dual x-ray absorptiometry (DXA), and quantitative computed tomographic (QCT) scanning of the spine.[1–3, 23–26] These are summarized in Table 54–2. SPA of the forearm is simple and inexpensive; however, as with DPA, SPA requires the use of an isotope. With both techniques the precision is not generally as good as with DXA. QCT scanning has made it possible to quantify directly the age-related loss of trabecular bone per se in the spine, but the procedure entails a relatively high radiation exposure and time.[3] DXA is currently the technique of choice, allowing measurement of spine, hip, and forearm bone densities as well as total body bone mass to be performed in a short time with very good precision and minimal exposure to radiation (see Table 54–2). The bone density data in a given patient are compared with age-matched controls and young normal controls. This information permits the assessment of bone density compared with age-matched normal subjects and determines whether there is a reduction in bone density compared with these normal subjects of the same age; it also establishes whether there is a reduction in bone density compared with the peak bone mass of young normal controls. There is an inverse relationship between bone density and the risk of fracture at multiple sites.[27] With QCT and DPA there appear to be theoretical fracture "thresholds"—that is, an estimated 90% of all patients who have had a vertebral fracture fall below a value of bone mineral density of about 100 mg/cm^3 by QCT, 1 g/cm^2 by DPA, and about 0.85 g/cm^2 for DXA using extrapolated data from DPA. (Different standards are used to calibrate bone density with these three techniques, accounting for the differences in the absolute values.) Using DXA, however, this fracture threshold is now reported as 2 standard deviations below peak bone density for all bone density sites (Fig. 54–3). The fracture threshold must be interpreted as the level of bone density at which there is an increased gradient of risk for fracture. There are likely to be factors in addition to bone density, such as trabecular integrity, that contribute to bone strength but cannot be quantified using bone densitometry. Whereas some studies show no significant difference in the predictive value for a fracture of a site-specific bone density determination (e.g., spine, forearm, or proximal femur), additional long-term data including spine fractures and large numbers of hip fractures are necessary.[28, 29] We currently, however, recommend a spinal bone density determination in patients younger than 65 years of age in whom vertebral fractures are preponderant and a proximal femur bone density measurement in patients older than 65 years of age in whom there is an exponential rise in hip fractures.

At present, it is not feasible to screen all patients for osteoporosis. The Scientific Advisory Board of the National Osteoporosis Foundation has identified the following four indications for bone mass measurements that are considered to be justified by available data[25]: (1) in estrogen-deficient women, to identify those at risk for a low bone mass and to help in the clinical decision-making regarding hormone replacement therapy (see later); (2) in patients with vertebral abnormalities or x-ray evidence of osteopenia in order to obtain information that will be useful for making decisions regarding evaluation and therapy; (3) in patients receiving long-term therapy with glucocorticoids in order to identify those with a low bone mass; (4) in patients with asymptomatic primary hyperparathyroidism in order to identify subjects who have a low bone mass and who may be candidates for surgery. In these latter patients a forearm bone density measurement is useful because cortical bone loss is greatest. Bone densitometry is also useful for monitoring the clinical response to a therapeutic intervention. Screening asymptomatic premenopausal women (without established risk factors) for low bone density is not considered to be cost-effective at the present time.

TABLE 54–2. COMPARISON OF DENSITOMETRY TECHNIQUES*

Technique	Bone Site	Bone Type	Precision† (%)	Duration of Examination (min)	Absorbed Dose (mrem/scan)	Cost ($)
SPA	Proximal radius	Mostly cortical	1–3	15	5–10	50–75
DPA	Spine (L2–L4)	Mostly trabecular	2	20–40	5–10	150–200
	Hip (femur neck, trochanter)	Mixed	2–4	20–40	5–10	150–200
	Total body	Mostly cortical	1–2	60	5–10	200–250
DXA	Spine	Mostly trabecular	0.7–1.5	6	2–4	150–200
	Hip (femur neck, trochanter)	Mixed	1.0–2	6	2–4	150–200
	Total body	Mostly cortical	0.5–1	20	2–4	200–250
QCT	Spine	Trabecular	4–6	10	200–1000	300–400

*Modified from Wahner HW: Measurement of bone mass and bone density. Endocr Clin North Am 18:996, 1989.
†Shown as the coefficient of variation (CV).
SPA = single-photon absorptiometry; DPA = dual-photon absorptiometry; DXA = dual x-ray absorptiometry; QCT = quantitative computed tomography.

Patients with clinically significant osteoporosis (symptoms or fractures) should be screened to exclude treatable causes (Table 54–3). The work-up includes a determination of a serum calcium level, PTH level, liver function tests, a complete blood count to detect hematologic disorders, a serum protein electrophoresis, a 1, 25-dihydroxyvitamin D level, a urinary calcium and creatinine level, and an overnight dexamethasone suppression test if there are any features of Cushing's syndrome. In addition, we routinely measure a sensitive TSH level to screen for hyperthyroidism and, if suppressed, we obtain T4 and T3 levels. In the case of a postmenopausal woman, further work-up is probably not necessary if these tests are unrevealing. If any tests are abnormal, however, or if the patient is a young man or premenopausal woman, an additional definitive evaluation should be considered. If the serum calcium level is elevated, but the PTH is suppressed, such testing would include, for example, appropriate work-up for non–PTH-mediated hypercalcemia. If an infiltrative process of bone is suspected (e.g., multiple myeloma, other hematologic disorders), a urinary protein electrophoresis and bone marrow aspiration and biopsy should be carried out. If a patient has an abnormal result on an overnight dexamethasone suppression test, the possibility of Cushing's disease should be definitely confirmed or excluded by performing low- and high-dose dexamethasone suppression tests. Such ancillary testing for secondary osteoporosis is particularly important in children, premenopausal women, men younger than 60 years of age, and blacks in whom the occurrence of primary osteoporosis is unusual. Moreover, the correction of the underlying basis for secondary osteoporosis may yield substantial improvements in bone mass.

Management

The management of osteoporosis is directed at treating the acute complications while attempting to halt the progression of the disease (see Table 54–3). Fractures, particularly the collapse of vertebral bodies, should be treated with brief immobilization designed only to achieve symptomatic relief. Chronic pain and instability may be alleviated with braces or by other orthopedic measures. Long-term bedrest is inadvisable because of the rapid increase in bone resorption attendant upon immobilization. A physical therapy program designed to increase flexibility and overall fitness and to strengthen back and abdominal muscles may improve the patient's overall sense of well-being and posture and relieve chronic back discomfort caused by paravertebral muscle spasm.

Double-blind randomized trials have been carried out to establish the efficacy of several forms of drug therapy for osteoporosis.[6] In the absence of any contraindications, estrogen is the therapy of choice for the prevention and treatment of established osteoporosis. As determined by various bone densitometry measurements, low-dose estrogen replacement (at least 0.625 mg of conjugated estrogens or 25 to 50 μg/day of ethinyl estradiol) retards bone loss in postmenopausal women primarily by inhibiting bone loss rather than by increasing new bone formation (Fig. 54–4*A*).[30, 31] Even when therapy is initiated many years after menopause, when considerable bone loss has taken place, increases in bone mass can still be observed.[32] Cessation of therapy is associated with resumption of rapid bone loss, approximating that of untreated controls (see Fig. 54–4*B*). Estrogen therapy is also associated with an approximately 50% reduction in osteoporotic fractures.[33] Of great importance to postmenopausal women in whom heart disease is the leading cause of death are the data from several observational studies indicating that estrogen therapy decreases the risk of cardiovascular disease by approximately 50%, although further randomized studies on the effects of estrogen and progesterone on cardiovascular disease are needed.[34, 35] This cardioprotective effect of estrogens is mediated, in part, by changes in lipoprotein profiles (a reduction in total cholesterol and low-density lipoprotein [LDL] levels and an increase in high-density lipoprotein [HDL] concentrations) and by other mechanisms such as direct vascular effects.[36] Transdermal estrogens are as efficacious as oral preparations in the prevention of bone loss but produce less beneficial effects on lipoprotein profiles.[37] Additional effects of estrogens include a decrease in hot flushes and atrophic vaginitis.

In women with an intact uterus, however, estrogen replacement with sequential or continuous administration of a progestin will minimize the risk of endometrial hyperplasia or carcinoma, although the addition of a progestin may abrogate some of the estrogen-induced rise in HDL levels.[38] Use of sequential estrogen and progesterone regimen often mimics the normal menstrual cycle and induces cyclical bleeding. Because many women do not wish to resume menses, daily continuous estrogen or progesterone regimens are now used. With this approach, endometrial atrophy is generally produced. Commonly used oral estorgen or progesterone regimens include: (1) 0.625 mg/day of Premarin with 10 mg of Provera being added on days 1 to 13 each month; and (2) 0.625 mg/day of Premarin plus 2.5 or 5 mg of Provera. Some but not all studies show that sequential 10 mg of Provera with estrogen raises HDL levels. Because the use of continuous estrogen plus 2.5 mg (but not 5 mg) of Provera produces a significant rise in HDL levels, we often initiate treatment with the first of these treatment regimens.[39] In the daily continuous estrogen plus

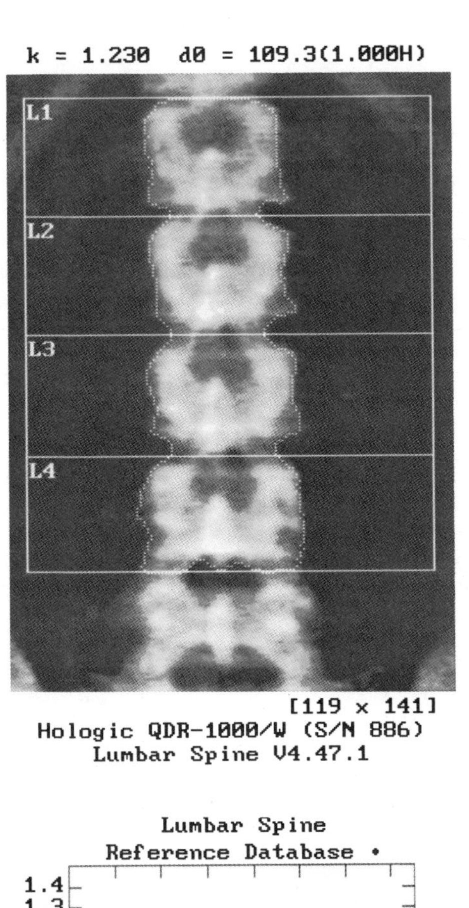

K05069204 Wed 08:05
Name:
Comment:
I.D.: Sex: F
S.S.#: Ethnic:
ZIP Code: Height:5' 4"
Scan Code: Weight: 108
BirthDate: Age:
Physician:

TOTAL BMD CV FOR L1 - L4 1.0%

C.F. 1.000 1.059 1.000

Region	Area (cm^2)	BMC (grams)	BMD (gms/cm^2)
L1	12.25	8.81	0.719
L2	12.40	11.05	0.891
L3	13.47	11.05	0.821
L4	14.47	12.81	0.885
TOTAL	52.59	43.71	0.831

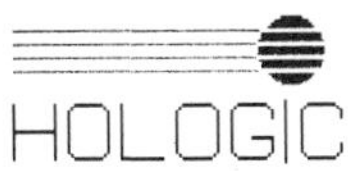

Lumbar Spine
Reference Database ♦

BMD 1.4 1.3 1.2 1.1 1.0 0.9 0.8 0.7 0.6 0.5 0.4 0.3

10 20 30 40 50 60 70 80
Age

BMD(L1-L4) = 0.831 g/cm^2

Region	BMD	T(30.0)		Z	
L1	0.719	-1.88	78%	-1.67	80%
L2	0.891	-1.25	87%	-1.01	89%
L3	0.821	-2.39	76%	-2.15	78%
L4	0.885	-2.10	79%	-1.85	81%
L1-L4	0.831	-1.96	79%	-1.72	81%

♦ Age and sex matched
T = peak bone mass
Z = age matched TK 11/04/91

K05069204 Wed 08:05
Name:
Comment:
I.D.: Sex: F
S.S.#: Ethnic:
ZIP Code: Height:5' 4"
Scan Code: Weight: 108
BirthDate: Age:
Physician:

Physician Comment:

Technique	Good Fair Marginal
	Uninterpretable
Z Score	Expected Bone Loss
	Borderline
	More than Expected
T Score	No Osteopenia Borderline
	Osteopenia
Other	Scoliosis Compression FX
Factors:	Osteo-Arthritis Calcif.
	Laminectomy Other

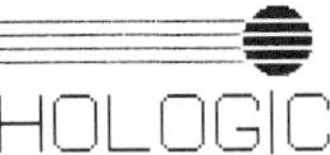

FIGURE 54–3. Use of dual x-ray absorptiometry (DXA) to quantify bone density in the spine. Bone density is compared with peak bone mass and age-matched controls. The T score and Z score indicate the number of standard deviations below young-normal and age-matched controls, respectively.

TABLE 54–3. DIAGNOSIS AND MANAGEMENT OF OSTEOPOROSIS

Establish Diagnosis
1. Routine x-ray studies for symptoms or suspected fracture
2. Bone mineral density
3. Bone biopsy (iliac crest) with tetracycline labelling necessary in some cases

Rule Out Secondary Causes
1. CBC,* SMA, thyroid tests, 1, 25-dihydroxyvitamin D, serum/urine protein electrophoresis, parathyroid hormone, urinary calcium levels; overnight dexamethasone suppression or urinary free cortisol if Cushing's syndrome suspected
2. More definitive tests if screening is abnormal

Treat Acute Complications
1. Limited bedrest and conservative measures for fractures
2. Avoid prolonged immobilization and use conservative treatment for chronic pain (e.g., physical therapy, braces)

Attempt to Halt Disease Progression
1. Encourage exercises against gravity
2. Calcium supplementation (1–1.5 g of elemental calcium/day) and a multivitamin with adequate vitamin D (400 IU)
3. Estrogens (± progesterone) in selected postmenopausal women
4. Calcitonin
5. Bisphosphonates (intermittent)
6. Vitamin D supplementation in select cases (? for those on long-term glucocorticoid therapy, those with malabsorption of vitamin D)
7. Others (see text)

*CBC = complete blood count.

progesterone regimens, approximately 26 to 40% of women develop irregular bleeding in the first 4 to 6 months of treatment, but most are amenorrheic by 1 year.[40] Endometrial biopsies are now generally not considered necessary prior to starting estrogen or progesterone therapy according to the guidelines of the American College of Obstetrics and Gynecology.[41] If a woman is overweight, which may result in high estrone levels, or has irregular bleeding before initiating hormone replacement therapy, an endometrial biopsy should be performed to exclude endometrial pathology. An endometrial biopsy is also indicated if a woman develops unexpected or severe vaginal bleeding concurrent with estrogen or progesterone therapy. Estrogen therapy can be given without progesterone to women who have had a hysterectomy. Because of the possibility of a slight increase in the incidence of breast cancer with estrogen use, annual mammograms and monthly self-breast examinations are mandatory.[42] Contraindications to estrogen therapy are previous or concurrent carcinoma of the breast; active liver disease; vascular thrombosis or embolus; or endometrial carcinoma. Data suggest that use of the estrogen antagonist tamoxifen, which exerts estrogen agonist-like properties on bone, lipids, and the endometrium, may be an alternative to estrogen therapy for preserving bone mass in a woman with a history of breast cancer, although further studies are necessary to evaluate the effects of this therapy on each of these parameters.[43]

The data on the effects of calcium on bone mass have been controversial. Several studies suggest that calcium may prevent bone loss, although there may be a threshold dose for the effects of calcium on different skeletal compartments and at different ages. In prepubertal children calcium supplementation can increase bone density, which may subsequently improve peak bone mass and reduce the risk of fracture later in life.[44] In early postmenopausal women, calcium tends to produce a small reduction in cortical bone loss but does not prevent trabecular bone loss.[45] In later postmenopausal women, calcium supplementation appears to stabilize bone density at multiple sites.[45, 46] If the amount of calcium absorbed is not sufficient to balance the obligatory losses in the urine and feces, bone loss ensues. To maintain zero calcium balance, Heaney and associates showed that premenopausal women between the ages of 35 and 50 require approximately 1000 mg/day of elemental calcium and that postmenopausal women need 1500 mg/day to offset these losses.[47] Thus, calcium supplementation in these doses appears to be beneficial and is usually without appreciable risk. Renal lithiasis and hypercalcemia are not generally of concern in nonazotemic women who have no disorders of calcium balance. Immobilization, excessive doses of calcium (> 2 g/day), or concurrent vitamin D excess does enhance the risk of hypercalcemia.

Several calcium preparations may be used to provide 1 to 1.5 mg/day of elemental calcium. From dietary sources, milk contains about 1200 mg/qt of calcium; foods that are relatively high in calcium include other milk products, sardines (with bones), turnip greens, molasses, tofu, and broccoli. Calcium carbonate is the most widely used supplement, containing 40% of elemental calcium by weight. Evidence indicates that not all formulations of calcium are readily dissolved and therefore absorbable. The dissolution of a given preparation can be tested by examining whether more than 75% of the tablet dissolves in vinegar within 30 minutes. Tums and Os-Cal are two preparations that do meet the USP standards. The calcium content per tablet is 200 mg with Tums, 300 mg with extra-strength Tums, and 500 mg with Os-Cal, although concern has been expressed by some people that "natural" forms of calcium (e.g., oyster shell or dolomite) may be contaminated with heavy metals, such as lead. Calcium carbonate preparations should optimally be taken at mealtime, because some older patients are achlorhydric, a condition that diminishes the absorption of calcium on an empty stomach.[48] The major side effects are flatulence and constipation. Calcium citrate, which contains only 24% of elemental calcium, is more expensive than calcium carbonate, but is preferable because of its enhanced bioavailability, fewer gastrointestinal side effects, and good absorption on an empty stomach.[48, 49] Calcium citrate is distributed in 200-mg tablets and as an effervescent preparation containing 500 mg of elemental calcium. Calcium gluconate may also reduce the possibility of flatulence and constipation. Neo-Calglucon has 115 mg/5 ml of calcium as calcium gluconate.

Salmon calcitonin, a potent inhibitor of osteoclastic-mediated bone resorption, is the only other available therapy approved by the Food and Drug Administration (FDA) for the treatment of osteoporosis other than estrogen. Parenteral calcitonin (100 IU every other day or daily) generally prevents bone loss or produces a small increment in the bone density in the forearm, vertebrae, femoral diaphysis, or total body.[50, 51] In addition, the other beneficial response to calcitonin includes a possible analgesic effect. Side effects of calcitonin include nausea in approximately 10 to 15% of subjects, flushing, and inflammation at the injection site. Resistance to salmon calcitonin may develop in some patients after approximately 18 months of therapy as a consequence of filling in of the remodeling spaces or down-regulation of the receptors. Compared with parenteral calcitonin, nasal spray calcitonin provides a better-tolerated mode of drug delivery and is associated with fewer side effects. The efficacy of calcitonin in reducing fractures is currently being investigated in large multicenter trials.

Bisphosphonates are also inhibitors of bone resorption that are adsorbed onto the hydroxyapatite of bone, where they remain for a long time. The first-generation bisphos-

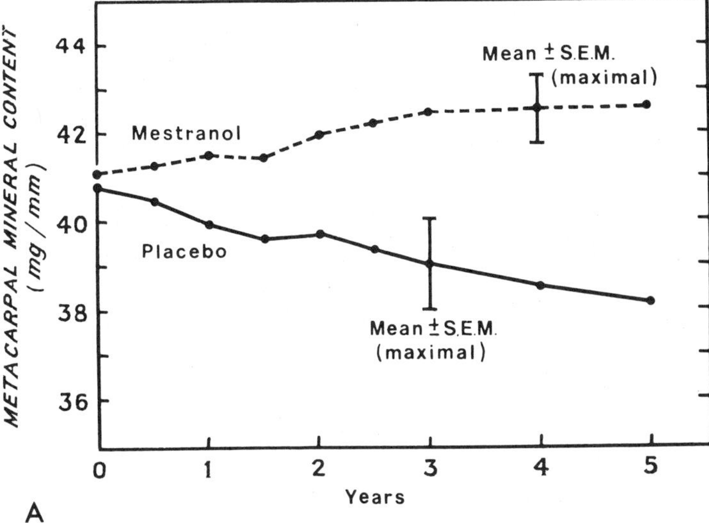

Mean metacarpal mineral content during 5-year follow-up of group observed from 3 years after bilateral oophorectomy (zero time).

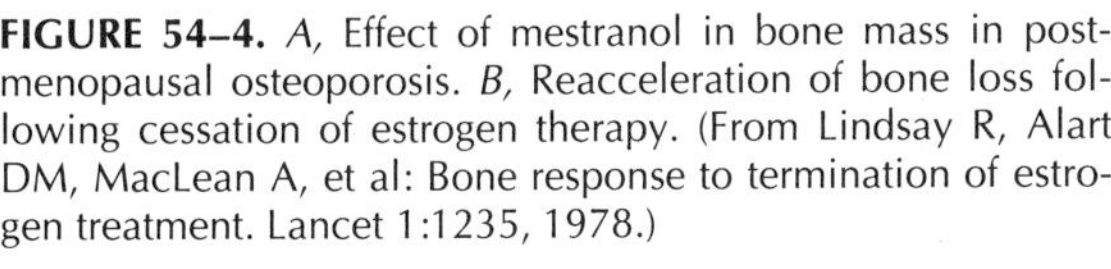

FIGURE 54–4. *A,* Effect of mestranol in bone mass in postmenopausal osteoporosis. *B,* Reacceleration of bone loss following cessation of estrogen therapy. (From Lindsay R, Alart DM, MacLean A, et al: Bone response to termination of estrogen treatment. Lancet 1:1235, 1978.)

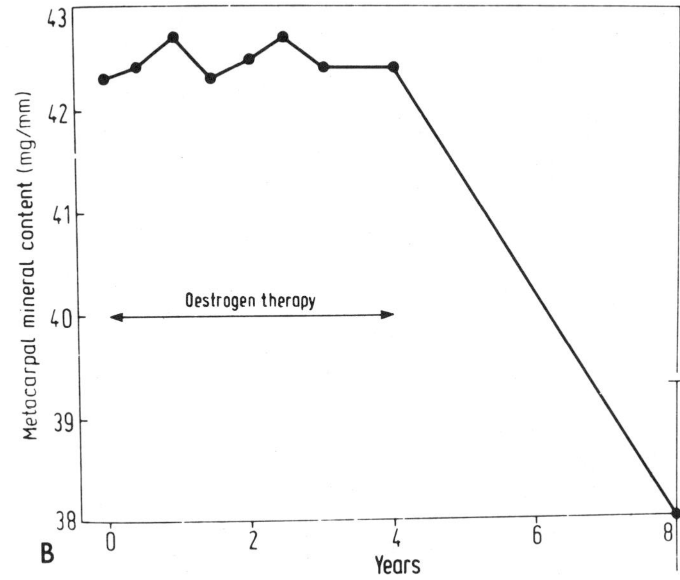

phonate compounds including etidronate disodium (Didronel) also inhibit bone mineralization at the high doses used clinically. In two clinical trials, etidronate disodium, administered intermittently at a dose of 400 mg on an empty stomach for 2 weeks alternating with 11 or 13 weeks of no therapy, led to small increases in spinal bone mass and decreased vertebral fractures at 2 years.[52, 53] Preliminary data on the efficacy of etidronate disodium in reducing the incidence of fractures after 4 years of follow-up showed no significant reduction in fractures compared with the baseline; however, there were a few fractures in these patients. In both studies, patients were given calcium supplements, although in one study the calcium supplement was not administered during the therapy with etidronate disodium. Because calcium inhibits the absorption of etidronate disodium, the calcium supplementation should not be taken within 2 hours of drug ingestion. Second- and third-generation bisphosphonates (e.g., Pamidronate, Tiludronate, Residronate, Alendronate) are being tested because these drugs are potent inhibitors of bone resorption at much lower doses than are those that impair bone mineralization. There is some concern that these agents may interfere with the ability of the skeleton to heal fractures, because they have a long half-life and they can completely suppress bone resorption at high doses. If their safety and efficacy are established, however, they could also act as an alternative to estrogen therapy.

In a subset of elderly subjects, a decreased calcium intake and low vitamin D levels may account for the negative calcium balance and the bone loss that these individuals experience. One study demonstrated that the administration of 1.2 g of supplemental calcium and 800 IU of vitamin D_3 decreased the incidence of hip fractures by 43% in elderly ambulatory nursing home subjects.[54]

There is some evidence that administration of calcitriol, the active metabolite of vitamin D, in higher doses preserves or increases bone mass and reduces fractures even at low doses.[55, 56] Other studies, however, show that it is no more effective than is calcium. In addition, there is a narrow therapeutic window with potential serious risks of hypercalciuria, hypercalcemia, and renal damage. We generally recommend only physiologic doses of vitamin D (400 units/day), which may be provided by a multivitamin, except in patients with malabsorption or on chronic glucocorticoid therapy (see later).

In contrast to the predominantly antiresorptive effects of estrogen, calcitonin, and bisphosphonates, sodium fluoride increases bone formation. Compared with controls, sodium fluoride (75 mg/day) increased vertebral bone density by 35% and proximal femur bone mass by 12% over 4 years, but cortical bone density in the forearm decreased by 4% during this time interval.[57] Moreover, despite this large increment in bone mass, vertebral fractures did not decrease and nonvertebral fractures increased, indicating greater bone fragility. Side effects, including gastrointestinal intolerance and lower extremity pain syndrome, occur commonly in approximately 40% of patients treated with sodium fluoride. Slow-release fluoride and monofluorophosphate produce fewer side effects than do sodium fluoride. Ongoing protocols are geared toward determining whether lower doses and better absorbed and tolerated fluoride preparations are effective in the treatment of osteoporosis. Until its safety and efficacy are determined, the use of fluoride should be limited to clinical investigation. Various other agents have been tried for postmenopausal osteoporosis, including growth hormone, which is generally not beneficial, and the synthetic 1-34 fragment of human PTH, which may increase bone mass in the spine but can compromise cortical bone mass.[58] The effects of daily parenteral PTH on the incidence of fractures has not been ascertained.

Osteoporosis develops in an estimated 30 to 50% of glucocorticoid-treated subjects.[17] Glucocorticoids may produce an early loss of trabecular bone with less effect on cortical bone. For prevention of glucocorticoid-induced bone loss, we generally recommend using the lowest glucocorticoid dose possible, providing adequate calcium intake, and reducing other risk factors for osteoporosis (see later). As hypercalciuria and nephrolithiasis occur commonly in glucocorticoid-treated subjects, if the urine calcium levels are elevated (> 4 mg/kg) the addition of hydrochlorothiazide (25 to 50 mg twice daily) may be necessary. Because data from Hahn and associates indicate that vitamin D may produce an increase in bone density of the forearm, in a patient at high risk for bone loss (with a normal urinary calcium level and no history of nephrolithiasis), we generally administer vitamin D (50,000 units once or twice weekly) to raise the 1, 25-dihydroxyvitamin D level to the upper range of normal. It is important with vitamin D therapy to ensure that the serum and urinary calcium concentrations remain within the normal range.[59] Several small studies and preliminary data from a large multicentered prospective placebo-controlled trial indicate that calcitonin therapy produces a small increment in bone mass or retards bone loss in patients treated with moderate doses of glucocorticoids.[60, 61] The bisphosphonate pamidronate administered orally in an investigative protocol increased vertebral bone density in a prospective randomized study in glucocorticoid-treated subjects, and preliminary data suggest that etidronate disodium may also prevent bone loss.[62, 63] In a retrospective study, estrogen replacement therapy prevented bone loss in women treated with glucocorticoids. At present there is no FDA-approved treatment for this common secondary cause of osteoporosis, although calcitonin, hormone replacement therapy in postmenopausal women, and possibly a bisphosphonate (preferably the newer compounds) may be beneficial in these patients.

Weight-bearing exercise (e.g., aerobics, running, walking, and mixed programs) may modestly increase bone density in older subjects. The optimal form and duration of exercise remain to be determined, but exercises three or more times weekly for 30 to 60 minutes should be beneficial. In a patient with a reduced bone mass, flexion exercises of the back may increase the risk of fracture. Patients who have already had fractures should gradually increase the intensity of their exercise. Prevention is the therapy of choice for optimizing skeletal health and preventing osteoporosis. Attempts directed at increasing peak bone mass (e.g., good calcium intake), reducing risk factors for bone loss such as menstrual abnormalities, thin body habitus, decreased physical activity or excessive alcohol intake, and slowing down bone loss and reversing any causes of secondary bone loss should be pursued vigorously. In practice, all patients should be encouraged to get regular exercise as well as adequate vitamin D (at least 400 IU/day) and calcium intake. Estrogen today is the mainstay for the prevention and treatment of osteoporosis in women without contraindications who wish to commence this therapy. Other antiresorptive agents are available as alternative therapies to estrogen. Therapies that increase bone formation (other than fluoride), including the possible use of skeletal growth factors, are not currently available. Such interventions, however, used in conjunction with an antiresorptive therapy, offer the potential to enhance bone mass and may hold a promise for the treatment of osteoporosis in the future.

PAGET'S DISEASE OF BONE

This relatively common disorder appears to result from a primary overactivity of osteoclasts.[7, 8, 64] At the onset of the disease, excessive resorption of bone is manifested by localized rarefaction on radiographs and by increased urinary hydroxyproline excretion, reflecting the breakdown of bone collagen. A mixed osteoblastic-osteoclastic phase follows, with elevated alkaline phosphatase levels originating from osteoblasts and the formation of disorganized, structurally defective bone. Late in the course, a sclerotic phase of the disorder may be seen, in which abnormal but now metabolically inactive bone persists. Although the cause of Paget's disease remains obscure, intranuclear inclusions, raising the possibility of a slow viral disease, have been demonstrated in abnormal osteoclasts but not in normal osteoclasts or in bone cells within unaffected areas of the skeleton.

Clinical Features

Paget's disease is virtually unheard of in individuals younger than 20 years of age, rare before the age of 40 years, and increasingly common thereafter (3 to 4% of the population). It is likely that the majority of affected persons are asymptomatic, but the frequency of asymptomatic involvement is unknown. The clinical presentation in symptomatic Paget's disease is related to the signs and symptoms of skeletal involvement per se as well as to skeletal, metabolic, cardiovascular, and neurologic complications (Fig. 54–5). The natural history of symptomatic Paget's disease appears to be progression at a pace varying widely among different individuals.

Commonly affected areas of the skeleton include the skull, spine, sacrum, pelvis, femur, and tibia. It is uncommon for the disorder to affect additional bones beyond those involved at the time of the patient's presentation, although the extent of involvement in a given bone may progress with time. The usual presenting symptoms are deformity

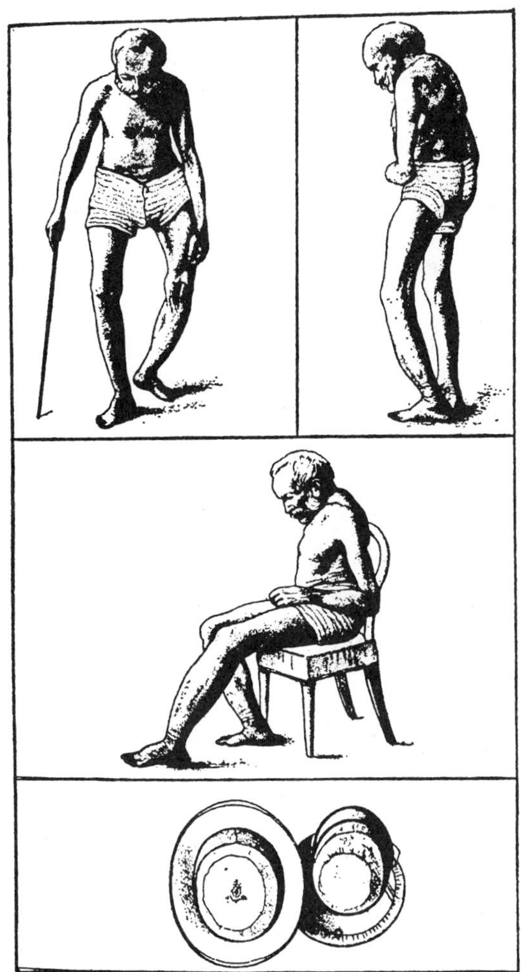

Plate from Paget's original article. Patient, aged 68, is shown 6 months before his death from a "cancerous growth round the radius." Lower part of the figure depicts patient's cap worn in 1844, and hat worn in 1876, measuring inside respectively 22½ inches and 27¼ inches: "nearly every year, for many years, his hat needed to be enlarged."

FIGURE 54–5. Paget's original patient, showing bowing and deformity of long bones and gross increase in size of skull (note the increase in hat size). (From Nagant de Deuxchaisnes CN and Krane SM: Paget's disease of bone: Clinical and metabolic observations. Medicine 43:233, 1964.)

and pain, the latter probably arising from periosteal stretching, microfractures, degenerative joint disease, or direct neural compression. Involvement of the skull may be asymptomatic but is not uncommonly accompanied by an increase in the circumference and weight of the skull. Patients may note progressively enlarging hat size and may even have difficulty in keeping their heads erect. Softening of pagetic bone at the base of the skull can result in basilar impression, which has a variety of neurologic sequelae (see later). Rare patients with massive involvement of the facial bones develop leontiasis ossea ("lion-like facies"). Ten to 15% of patients have angioid streaks on funduscopic examination.

Paget's disease of the spine is most often asymptomatic but may result in pain, vertebral collapse with loss of height, or, in a few patients, compression of spinal cord and nerves. Rare patients with involvement of multiple adjacent vertebrae may develop a clinical picture, with back pain and stiffness, mimicking ankylosing spondylitis.[65] The lumbar spine is involved most commonly, followed by the dorsal and cervical spine, in that order. On x-ray examination, the vertebral bodies may appear enlarged, with thickened, irregular cortices and coarse vertical striations.

Paget's disease of the pelvis is most commonly complicated by the development of hip disease. Softening of the bone around the hip joint may result in protrusio acetabuli (protrusion of the hip joint farther than normal into the pelvic cavity). The gross disorganization of pagetic bone in the pelvis may mimic metastatic disease radiographically; a helpful sign in Paget's disease is thickening of the ileopectineal line, the "brim sign."

Involvement of the lower extremities occurs frequently and may be accompanied by pain on weight bearing as well as by knee pain related to abnormal stress on the joint from bone deformity. Enlargement and bowing of the femur and tibia are frequently seen; increased warmth and sweating of the skin overlying affected bones may be observed. The upper extremities are infrequently involved and almost always are asymptomatic, while the hands and feet are hardly ever involved.

Skeletal complications include fractures (10 to 30%), and development of osteogenic sarcoma (0.1 to 1%) as well as degenerative joint disease.[64, 66] Fractures are characteristically transverse and perpendicular to the cortex and may be preceded by asymptomatic or painful fissure fractures, which only extend part of the way through the involved bone. The most common sites are the femur, just below the lesser trochanter, and the tibia. Fractures tend to heal with exuberant callus formation, but recurrence may be a problem. The prognosis of osteogenic sarcoma in Paget's disease remains dismal, with a 1-year survival rate of 50% or less.[67] The onset of this complication may be marked by a new onset of pain, a sudden rise in alkaline phosphatase levels, or a soft tissue mass.

Metabolic complications include hypercalcemia (rare, but it may occur during immobilization), hypercalciuria, and hyperuricosuria and hyperuricemia, perhaps related to increased turnover of abnormal osteoclasts. Hypercalcemia in ambulatory patients with Paget's disease is most commonly caused by primary hyperparathyroidism, which occurs relatively frequently in the age group at risk for Paget's disease. Since elevated levels of PTH can further enhance the increased rate of bone turnover in pagetic patients, parathyroidectomy is generally indicated in this setting. The incidence of renal stones in Paget's disease is probably only slightly, if at all, increased, since bone formation is generally closely coupled to breakdown.

The chief cardiovascular complication is the development of high output cardiac failure in a few patients. The increased blood flow is not due to shunting but to increased vascularity in the affected bones and overlying skin. The incidence of cardiac dysfunction per se is probably not increased in Paget's disease.

Neurologic complications result primarily from compression of nerves running through pagetic bone. A variety of cranial nerves may be involved, most commonly resulting in extraocular muscle palsies or lower cranial nerve dysfunction. Hearing loss is common and related to cochlear dysfunction, involvement of the stapes, or compression of the eighth cranial nerve. Basilar impression may result in cerebellar compression and dysfunction or obstructive hydrocephalus with gait disturbance, incontinence, and progressive dementia. Occasionally, excessive blood flow to involved bones of the skull through the external carotid system has led to a "pagetic steal" with resultant cerebral hypoxia. A similar syndrome has produced symptoms of spinal cord dysfunction in the dorsal spine. Dorsal spinal involvement more commonly results in cord compression (the cord has the least clearance in this area), whereas Paget's disease of the lumbar spine more commonly affects the cauda equina. Both of these complications, however, are relatively rare.

Laboratory Findings and Diagnosis

The diagnosis of Paget's disease can usually be made from the characteristic clinical picture (see Fig. 54–5) and x-ray findings (Fig. 54–6), associated with an elevated alkaline phosphatase level of bone origin. Alkaline phosphatase activity, reflecting osteoblastic bone formation combined with excessive bone breakdown, is almost always elevated with clinically significant Paget's disease and may be ten or more times the upper limit of normal with polyostotic disease. It tends to correlate with the extent of pagetic involvement but may be disproportionately elevated with isolated Paget's disease of the skull; it may be normal in some cases of monostotic disease. Urinary hydroxyproline is a direct indicator of the resorptive activity of osteoclasts, but the test is expensive and usually changes in parallel with the alkaline phosphatase level. In the future, the measurement of pyridinium cross-links, which are also breakdown products of collagen, may be a more specific marker of osteoclastic activity than hydroxyproline.[68] Serum and urine calcium values should be measured, particularly during periods of immobilization. Serum uric acid level should also be determined to assess the risk of gouty arthritis and uric acid nephrolithiasis.

In some cases of Paget's disease, the disorganized bone structure, which is apparent radiographically, may be confused with other metabolic bone diseases or with malignant involvement of bone, particularly osteoblastic metastatic carcinoma of the prostate or lymphoma. In a few cases, bone biopsy may be necessary for histologic confirmation of the diagnosis. In most instances, the differentiation can be made radiographically. Osteoblastic metastases show new bone formation in the medulla as well as in the cortex, and the increase in the size of the bone, typical of Paget's dis-

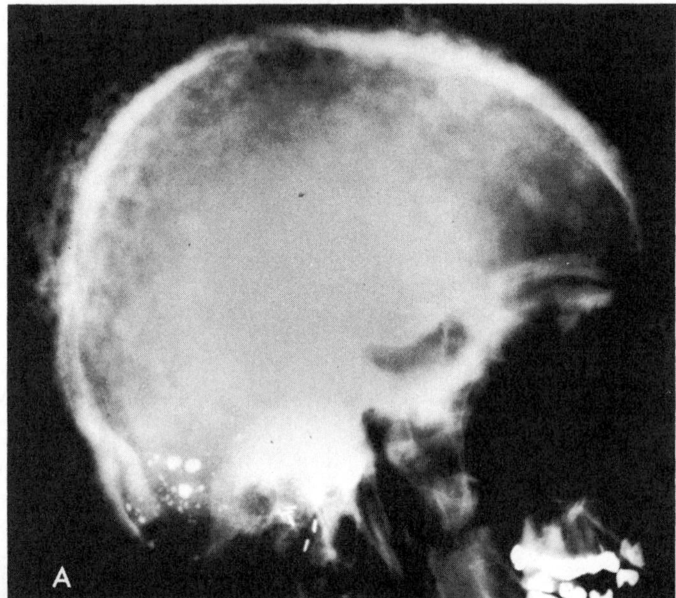

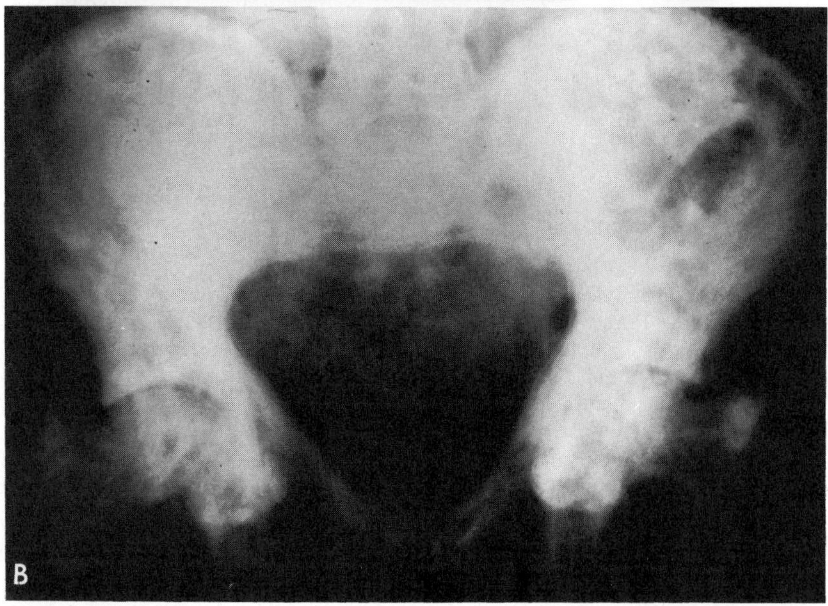

FIGURE 54–6. *A,* Paget's disease of the skull. Note the honeycomb appearance of the skull and increased thickness of the cortex. Radiodense material and clips at the base of the skull are from previous diagnostic studies and a posterior fossa decompression for basilar impression. *B,* Paget's disease of the pelvis with gross disorganization of the bone architecture. With involvement of the pelvis, a helpful sign distinguishing Paget's disease from malignancy is thickening of the iliopectineal line (the "brim sign" is not seen well here).

ease, is not seen in malignancies involving bone. Osteogenic sarcoma, if associated with Paget's disease, is usually associated with lytic lesions and a soft tissue mass that can be seen on x-ray examination.

Although routine x-rays generally are sufficient to establish the diagnosis of Paget's disease, they do not provide information on the cellular activity of the diseased bone. Bone scans with technetium-labeled diphosphonates usually demonstrate areas of metabolically active bone (Fig. 54–7), which correlate well with symptoms, and this study is a useful baseline to obtain in a symptomatic patient or prior to initiating therapy.[7, 8, 69] Audiograms may disclose subclinical hearing loss. A lateral film showing the base of the skull should be obtained in any patient whose bone scan indicates that the disease is active in that area. Computed tomography scanning may be helpful to rule out hydrocephalus in patients with changes in mental status.

TABLE 54–4. DIAGNOSIS AND MANAGEMENT OF PAGET'S DISEASE

Diagnosis
1. Skeletal radiographs
2. Alkaline phosphatase, serum and urine calcium, uric acid determinations
3. Bone biopsy if diagnosis uncertain
4. Bone scan to assess disease activity
5. Audiogram, myelogram, CT* scan, etc., if specific neurologic complications arise (see text)

Treatment
1. No therapy for asymptomatic disease
2. Specific therapy (bisphosphonates or calcitonin) for pain, deformity, or complications
3. Consider orthopedic surgery for fixed skeletal or articular deformities
4. Consider neurosurgical intervention for posterior fossa compression or cord compression

*CT = computed tomography.

Management

Because of the uncertain natural history of mild Paget's disease, asymptomatic patients generally have not been treated, except in cases of involvement in areas of the skeleton where future serious complications might ensue (i.e., long bone fractures, arthritis, or neurologic complications). Several definite or possible indications have been suggested for starting therapy in symptomatic patients: (1) severe bone pain in areas of skeletal involvement, (2) high output cardiac failure, (3) hypercalcemia due to Paget's disease, (4) hypercalciuria with renal calculi, (5) multiple pathologic fractures, (6) nerve compression, and (7) prior to an orthopedic procedure involving pagetic bone.[7, 8, 63] Effective forms of therapy are now available (Tables 54–4 and 54–5).[70–74] These include calcitonin and the bisphosphonates (formerly called diphosphonates). All have as their principal mechanism of action the inhibition of bone resorption through effects on the action of osteoclasts.

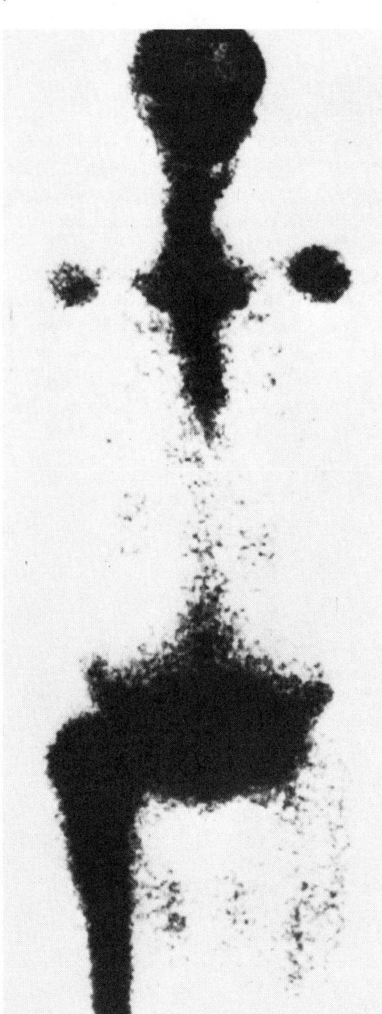

FIGURE 54–7. A bone scan in a patient with active Paget's disease. Note the increased uptake in the skull, upper spine, pelvis, and proximal femur. Areas of uptake frequently correlate with symptoms and respond well to medical therapy.

Salmon (Calcimar, Miacalcin) and human calcitonin (Cibacalcin) have as their physiologic actions a diminution in the number and action of osteoclasts. Treatment is usually initiated with salmon calcitonin in doses of 50 to 100 MRC units/day given subcutaneously or intramuscularly. It may be possible to decrease the dose to three times per week in patients showing a good response. About 80% of patients show symptomatic improvement, and the serum alkaline phosphatase level decreases by 50% or more in about two thirds of patients after 2 to 6 months of therapy. During this initial period of treatment, the biochemical response is conveniently monitored by measuring serum alkaline phosphatase every 1 to 2 months. The maintenance of the response can be documented with a measurement of alkaline phosphatase every 3 to 4 months. Some patients will have a complete biochemical and clinical remission, whereas a larger second group shows an initial response followed by a plateau despite continued therapy. A third group responds transiently but subsequently relapses to pretreatment symptoms and blood chemistry values. Such resistance to the action of calcitonin is poorly understood. More than half of patients develop antibodies to heterologous calcitonin, and a minority of these (5 to 20%) develop clinically significant titers of antibodies. Changing from salmon to human calcitonin may overcome the resistance to the drug in this group of patients. Toxicity has been mild and limited to local reactions at the injection site, flushing, nausea, and transient erythema and swelling of the hands. The need for parenteral administration and the expense of calcitonin (see Table 53–4) are the principal drawbacks of this form of therapy, although a formulation of calcitonin, which is administered by nasal spray, has been developed. The latter may require higher doses than parenteral forms of calcitonin, however, to achieve an equivalent therapeutic re-

TABLE 54–5. AGENTS USEFUL IN THE THERAPY OF PAGET'S DISEASE

	Bisphosphonates	Calcitonin
Action	Inhibit osteoclastic bone resorption	Inhibits osteoclastic bone resorption
Dose	5–7.5 mg/kg/day 6 months on, at least 6 months off	50–100 MRC units/day or 3 times/wk
Route of administration	Oral	Subcutaneous or intramuscular
Time to clinical response	2 wk–3 mo	2 wk–3 mo
Patients responding	60–80%	60–80%
Maximum decrease in alkaline phosphatase	40–60%	40–60%
Resistance	Rare	Downregulation of receptors, filling in remodeling spaces. Occasionally caused by neutralizing antibodies
Toxicity	Abdominal pain, diarrhea, pathologic fractures (with doses of > 10 mg/kg/day)	Nausea, flushing, inflammation at the injection site
Cost	$55/wk	$87/wk

sponse. Patients are usually administered a 1- to 2-year course of treatment, followed by withdrawal of therapy until a relapse occurs. The latter is accompanied by a recrudescence of symptoms and by an increase in alkaline phosphatase, which should be measured every 3 to 6 months after therapy is stopped. Unfortunately, the cost of therapy with calcitonin remains high.

A less expensive and orally administered form of therapy is etidronate disodium (EHDP) (Didronel). It is often the first agent employed in the treatment of Paget's disease for these two reasons. This agent is one of a series of bisphosphonates, which are nonhydrolyzable analogs of pyrophosphate, a natural inhibitor of bone mineralization. These compounds interact directly with bone mineral matrix to retard bone breakdown, although direct effects on osteoclasts may also exist. In doses of 5 to 20 mg/kg/day, EHDP produces biochemical and clinical improvement in patients with Paget's disease comparable in time course and magnitude to improvement observed in patients treated with calcitonin (Fig. 54–8). Unlike with the latter agent, resistance does not develop. At higher does (10 to 20 mg/kg/day), however, defective mineralization of bone may lead to osteomalacia, increased bone pain, and pathologic fractures. Lower doses, therefore, should be used (5 to 7.5 mg/kg/day).[73] The use of etidronate is contraindicated in patients recovering from fractures, in the presence of fissure fractures in long bones, or with overt lytic lesions that might predispose to fractures. Cessation of therapy after 6 months or more may lead to prolonged remission of disease activity, but relapse is common. Reinstitution of therapy will once again reduce symptoms. Many clinicians now alternate 6 months of treatment with EHDP with 6 months off the drug. Newer, second- and third-generation bisphosphonates, such as aminohydroxypropylidine bisphosphonate, are 100 times more potent or greater in inhibiting bone resorption than is etidronate and do not impair mineralization. While not yet approved by the FDA for use in the treatment of Paget's disease, clinical trials in Europe have shown them to be highly effective agents that can induce prolonged remissions of disease activity after one or only a few intravenous infusions of 15 to 60 mg.[74]

Specific therapy with calcitonin or etidronate generally leads to about 50% decrease in alkaline phosphatase in about two thirds of patients and improvements in symptoms in a comparable fraction of patients, although only a few double-blind, controlled studies have been performed.[73] In the case of calcitonin, the drug appears to exert direct analgesic effects in addition to its action at the level of

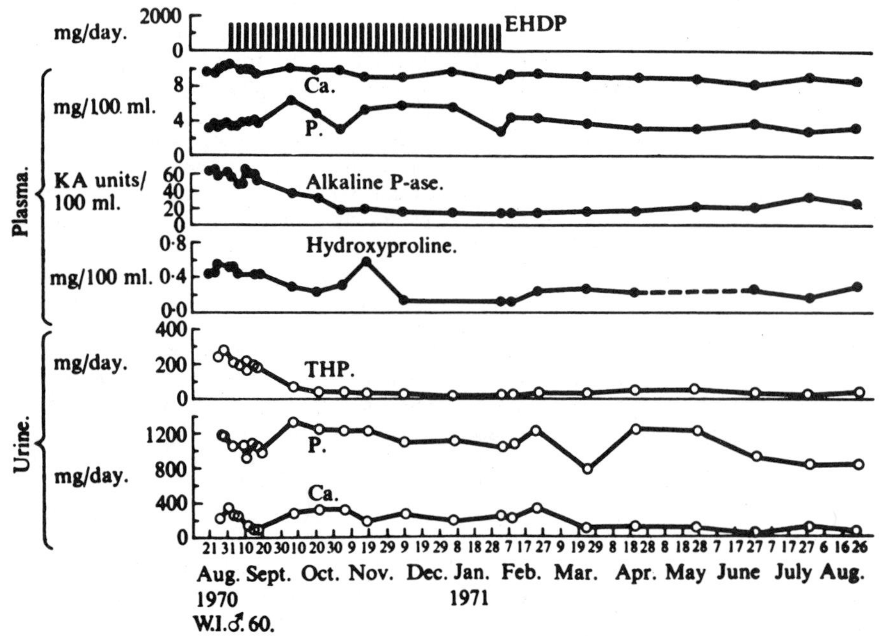

FIGURE 54–8. Biochemical response to sodium etidronate (EHDP) in a 60-year-old man with Paget's disease. Note that alkaline phosphatase and urinary hydroxyproline (THP) values remain low after cessation of therapy. (From Smith R, Russell RG, Bishop MC, et al: Paget's disease of bone: Experience with a diphosphonate [etidronate disodium] in treatment. Q J Med 42:235, 1973.)

bone. Prolonged therapy has led to histologic improvement in patients treated with either EHDP or calcitonin as well as radiologic improvement in patients treated with calcitonin.[72] Fixed bone deformity and osteoarthritis respond poorly to medical therapy, because this type of damage is usually irreversible. Pain caused by arthritis and pain that is not relieved by EHDP or by calcitonin may respond to therapy with nonsteroidal anti-inflammatory agents.

Several types of pagetic complications have been found to respond to medical therapy. Hypercalcemia and hypercalciuria frequently improve with administration of calcitonin. High output cardiac failure has responded dramatically to calcitonin. Therapy with calcitonin combined with immobilization may forestall an impending long bone fracture. A number of reports have documented rapid improvement in neurologic complications, such as cord compression, with medical therapy.[75] Patients with hearing loss may not show improvements although treatment may arrest its progression. Neurosurgical intervention following appropriate diagnostic testing (myelogram or computed tomography scan), however, remains the standard therapy for rapidly developing cord compression or posterior fossa compression secondary to basilar impression. An important unanswered question is whether long-term therapy with calcitonin or bisphosphonates will change the incidence of bone tumors in Paget's disease.

When the long-term safety of the agents has been established, it will be possible to make more definitive recommendations. Improved forms of therapy, either combinations of several agents (calcitonin and bisphosphonates have been successfully used) or newer bisphosphonates that cause less inhibition of mineralization, will probably become available for clinical use within the next several years.

Progress has also been made in the orthopedic management of skeletal complications.[76] Orthopedic intervention is most often warranted for the management of painful, transverse fissure fractures in long bones or true fractures, of skeletal deformity, particularly of the lower extremities, and of secondary degenerative arthritis. Procedures such as osteotomy of the tibia and fibula for knee pain or total hip replacement appear to have a lower risk of bleeding and other complications if performed after medical treatment of the Paget's disease (generally with calcitonin for 4 to 6 weeks). Unfortunately, the prognosis for patients who develop osteogenic sarcoma remains poor despite early amputation. Radiotherapy has only a palliative role in the treatment of this complication; chemotherapeutic regimens similar to those used successfully in childhood osteogenic sarcoma continue to be investigated.

REFERENCES

1. Mazess RB, Barden HS, Ettinger M, et al: Spine and femur density using dual photon absorptiometry in US women. Bone Miner 2:211, 1987.
2. Mazess RB: Bone densitometry of the axial skeleton. Orthop Clin North Am 21:51, 1990.
3. Genant HK, Cann CE, Ettinger B, and Gordon GS: Quantitative tomography of vertebral spongiosa: A sensitive method for detecting early bone loss after oophorectomy. Ann Intern Med 97:699, 1982.
4. Lindsay R, Hart DM, and Aiken JM: Long-term prevention of postmenopausal osteoporosis. Lancet 1:1038–1042, 1976.
5. Riggs BL, Wahner HW, Dunn WL, et al: Differential changes in bone mineral density of the appendicular and axial skeleton with aging: Relationship to spinal osteoporosis. J Clin Invest 67:328, 1981.
6. Riggs BL and Melton LJ III: The prevention and treatment of osteoporosis. N Engl J Med 327:620, 1992.
7. Favus MJ (ed): Primer of the Metabolic Diseases and Disorders of Mineral Metabolism. Richmond, VA, Byrd Press, 1990.
8. Avioli LN and Krane SM (eds): Metabolic Bone Disease and Clinically Related Disorders. Philadelphia, WB Saunders, 1990.
9. Cummings SR, Rubin SM, and Blank D: The future of hip fractures in the United States: Numbers, cost, and potential effects of postmenopausal estrogen. Clin Orthop 252:163, 1990.
10. Luckey MM, Meier DE, Mandeli JP, et al: Radial and vertebral bone density in white and black women: Evidence for racial differences in premenopausal bone homeostasis. J Clin Endocrinol Metab 69:762, 1989.
11. Cummings SR, Kelsey JL, Nevitt MC, and O'David KJ: Epidemiology of osteoporosis and osteoporotic fractures. Epidemiol Rev 7:178, 1985.
12. Seeman E, Hopper JL, Bach L, et al: Reduced bone mass in daughters of women with osteoporosis. N Engl J Med 320:554, 1989.
13. Slemenda CW, Christian JC, Williams CJ, et al: Genetic determination of bone mass in adult women: A re-evaluation of the twin model and the potential importance of the gene interaction on heritability estimates. J Bone Miner Res 7(6):561, 1991.
14. Parfitt AM: Bone remodeling: Relationship to the amount and structure of bone, and the pathogenesis and prevention of fractures. *In* Riggs BL and Melton LJ III (eds): Osteoporosis: Etiology, Diagnosis, and Management. New York, Raven Press, 1988, pp 45–93.
15. Pacifici R, Rifas L, Teitelbaum S, et al: Spontaneous release of interleukin-1 from human blood monocytes reflects bone resorption in idiopathic osteoporosis. Proc Natl Acad Sci 84:4616, 1987.
16. Ross DS, Neer RM, and Ridgway EC: Subclinical hyperthyroidism and reduced bone density as a possible result of prolonged suppression of the pituitary-thyroid axis with L-thyroxine. Am J Med 82:1167, 1987.
17. Lukert BP and Raisz LG: Glucocorticoid-induced osteoporosis: Pathogenesis and management. Ann Intern Med 112:352, 1990.
18. Movsowitz C, Epstein S, Fallon M, et al: Cyclosporin-A in vivo produces severe osteopenia in the rat: Effect of dose and duration of administration. Endocrinology 123:2571, 1988.
19. Rich GM, Mudge GH, Laffel GL, and LeBoff MS: Cyclosporine A and prednisone-associated osteoporosis in heart transplant recipients. J Heart Lung Transplant 11(5):950, 1992.
20. Als OS, Godfredsen A, Christiansen C: The effect of glucocorticoids on bone mass in rheumatoid arthritis patients: Influence of menopausal state. Arthritis Rheum 28:369, 1985.
21. Sambrook PN, Eisman JA, Champion GD, et al: Determinants of axial bone loss in rheumatoid arthritis. Arthritis Rheum 30:721, 1987.
22. Johnson BE, Lucasey B, Robinson RG, and Lukert B: Contributing diagnoses in osteoporosis. Arch Intern Med 149:1069, 1989.
23. Sartoris DJ and Resnick D: Dual-energy radiographic absorptiometry for bone densitometry: Current status and perspective. Am J Roentgenol 152:241, 1989.
24. Hui SL, Slemenda CW, and Johnston CC: Baseline measurement of bone mass predicts fracture in white women. Ann Intern Med 111(5):355, 1989.
25. Johnston CC, Slemenda CW, and Melton LJ: Clinical use of bone densitometry. N Engl J Med 324:1105, 1991.
26. LeBoff MS, El-Hajj Fuleihan G, Angell J, et al: Dual energy x-ray absorptiometry of the forearm: Reproducibility and correlation with single photon absorptiometry. J Bone Miner Res 7:841, 1992.
27. Melton LJ III, Wahner HW, Richelson LS, et al: Osteoporosis and the risk of hip fracture. Am J Epidemiol 124:254, 1986.
28. Black DM, Cummings SR, Genant HK, et al: Axial and appendicular bone density predict fractures in older women. J Bone Miner Res 7:633, 1992.
29. Black DM, Cummings SR, and Melton JL: Appendicular bone mineral and a woman's lifetime risk fo hip fracture. J Bone Miner Res 7:639, 1992.

30. Horsman A, Gallagher J, Simpson M, et al: Prospective trial of estrogen and calcium in postmenopausal women. BMJ 2:789, 1977.
31. Lindsay R, Aitken JM, Anderson JB, et al: Long-term prevention of postmenopausal osteoporosis by estrogen: Evidence for an increased bone mass after delayed onset of estrogen treatment. Lancet 1:1038, 1976.
32. Lindsay R and Tohme JF: Estrogen treatment of patients with established postmenopausal osteoporosis. Obstet Gynecol 76:290, 1990.
33. Kiel DP, Felson DT, Anderson JJ, et al: Hip fractures and the use of estrogen in postmenopausal women. N Engl J Med 317:1169, 1987.
34. Stampfer JM, Colidtz GP, and Willet WC: Postmenopausal estrogen therapy and cardiovascular disease: Ten year follow-up from the Nurse's Health Study. N Engl J Med 325:756, 1991.
35. Weinstein MC: Estrogen use in postmenopausal women, costs risks, and benefits. N Engl J Med 303:308, 1980.
36. Barnes RB, Roy S, and Lobo RA: Comparison of lipid and androgen levels after conjugated estrogen or depo-medroxyprogesterone acetate treatment in postmenopausal women. Obstet Gynecol 66:216, 1985.
37. Stevenson JC, Cust MP, Gangar KF, et al: Effect of transdermal versus oral hormone replacement therapy on bone density in spine and proximal femur in postmenopausal women. Lancet 336:265, 1990.
38. Hiroven E, Malkonen M, and Manninen V: Effects of different progestogens on lipoproteins during postmenopausal replacement therapy. N Engl J Med 304:560, 1981.
39. Gibbons WE, Judd HL, Luciano AA, et al: Comparison of sequential versus continuous estrogen/progestin replacement therapy on serum lipid patterns: Multiuniversity National Upjohn Study Collaborative. Washington, DC, Society for Gynecologic Investigation, 1991.
40. Weinstein L: Efficacy of continuous estrogen-progestin regimen in the menopausal patient. Obstet Gynecol 69:929, 1987.
41. Hormone replacement therapy. ACOG Technical Bull 166:1, 1992.
42. Steinberg KK, Thacker SB, Smith SJ, et al: A meta-analysis of the effect of estrogen replacement therapy on the risk of breast cancer. JAMA 265:1985, 1991.
43. Love RR, Mazess RB, Borden HS, et al: Effects of tamoxifen on bone mineral density in postmenopausal women with breast cancer. N Engl J Med 326:852, 1992.
44. Johnston CC, Meller JZ, Slemenda CW, et al: Calcium supplementation and increases in bone mineral density in children. N Engl J Med 327:82, 1992.
45. Dawson-Hughes B, Dallal GE, Krall EA, et al: A controlled trial of the effect of calcium supplementation on bone density in postmenopausal women. N Engl J Med 323:878, 1990.
46. Reid IA, Ames RW, Evans MC, et al: Effect of calcium supplementation on bone loss in postmenopausal women. N Engl J Med 328:400, 1993.
47. Heaney RP, Recker RR, and Saville PD: Menopausal changes in calcium balance performance. J Lab Clin Med 92:953, 1978.
48. Recker RR: Calcium absorption and achlorhydria. N Engl J Med 313:70, 1985.
49. Nicar MJ and Pak CYC: Calcium bioavailability from calcium carbonate and calcium citrate. J Clin Endocrinol Metab 61:391, 1985.
50. Gruber HE, Ivey JL, Baylink DJ, et al: Long-term calcitonin therapy in post menopausal osteoporosis. Metabolism 33:295, 1984.
51. Gennari C, Chierichetti SM, Bigazzi S, et al: Comparative effects on bone mineral content of calcium and calcium plus salmon calcitonin given in two different regimens in postmenopausal osteoporosis. Curr Ther Res 38:455, 1985.
52. Storm T, Thamsborg G, Steiniche T, et al: Effect of intermittent cyclical etidronate therapy on bone mass, and fracture rate in women with postmenopausal osteoporosis. N Engl J Med 322:1265, 1990.
53. Watts WB, Harris ST, Genant HK, et al: Intermittent cyclical etidronate treatment of postmenopausal osteoporosis. N Engl J Med 328:73, 1990.
54. Chapuy MC, Arlot ME, DuBreuf F, et al: Vitamin D_3 and calcium to prevent hip fractures in elderly women. N Engl J Med 327:1837, 1992.
55. Gallagher JC and Goldgar O: Treatment of postmenopausal osteoporosis with high doses of synthetic calcitriol. Ann Intern Med 113:649, 1990.
56. Tylard MW, Spears GF, Com BA, et al: Treatment of postmenopausal osteoporosis with calcitriol and calcium. N Engl J Med 326:357, 1992.
57. Riggs BL, Hodgson SF, and O'Fallon WM: Effect of fluoride treatment on the fracture rate in postmenopausal women with osteoporosis. N Engl J Med 322:802, 1990.
58. Slovik DM, Rosenthal DI, Doppelt SH, et al: Restoration of spinal bone in osteoporotic men by treatment with human parathyroid hormone (1-34) and 1,25-dihydroxyvitamin D. J Bone Miner Res 4:377, 1986.
59. Hahn TJ: Steroid and drug induced osteopenia. *In* Favus MJ (ed): Primer of the Metabolic Diseases and Disorders of Mineral Metabolism. Richmond, VA, Byrd Press, 1990, p 158.
60. Ringe JD and Welzel D: Salmon calcitonin in the therapy of corticoid-induced osteoporosis. Eur J Clin Pharmacol 33:35, 1987.
61. Silverman SL, Gallaher JC, Healy L, et al: A multicenter study of the treatment of corticosteroid induced osteoporosis with injectable calcitonin: An interim analysis (Abstract). Am Coll Rheumatol 1992.
62. Reid IR, King AR, Ibbertson HK: Prevention of steroid-induced osteoporosis with (3-amino-1-hydroxypropylidene)-1,1-bisphosphonate (APD). Lancet 1:143, 1988.
63. Mudler H and Snelder HAA: Effects of cyclical etidronate regimen on prophylaxis of bone loss of glucocorticoid (prednisone) therapy in postmenopausal women (Abstract). Am Soc Bone Miner Res 1992.
64. Singer FR: Paget's Disease of Bone. New York, Plenum, 1976.
65. Franck WA, Bress NM, Singer FR, et al: Rheumatic manifestations of Paget's disease of bone. Am J Med 56:592, 1974.
66. Nagant de Deuxchaisnes C and Krane SM: Paget's disease of bone: Clinical and metabolic observations. Medicine 43:233, 1964.
67. Porretta CA, Dahlin DC, and Janes JM: Sarcoma in Paget's disease of bone. J Bone Joint Surg 39A:1314, 1957.
68. Black D, Farquharson C, and Robins SP: Excretion of pyridinium crosslinks of collagen in ovariectomized rats as urinary markers for increased bone resorption. Calcif Tiss Int 74:343, 1989.
69. Khairi MRA, Wellman HN, Robb JA, et al: Paget's disease of bone (osteitis deformans): Symptomatic lesions and bone scan. Ann Intern Med 79:348, 1973.
70. Ryan WG, Schwartz TB, and Northrup G: Experiences in the treatment of Paget's disease of bone with mithramycin. JAMA 213:1153, 1970.
71. DeRose J, Singer FR, Avramides A, et al: Response of Paget's disease to porcine and salmon calcitonin. Am J Med 56:858, 1974.
72. Doyle FH, Pennock J, Greenberg PB, et al: Radiological evidence of a dose-related response to long-term treatment of Paget's disease with human calcitonin. Br J Radiol 47:1, 1974.
73. Khairi MRA, Altman RD, DeRosa GP, et al: Sodium etidronate in the treatment of Paget's disease of bone: A study of long-term results. Ann Intern Med 87:656, 1977.
74. Hosking DJ: Advances in the management of Paget's disease of bone. Drugs 40:829, 1990.
75. Chen JR, Rhee RSC, Wallach S, et al: Neurologic disturbances in Paget's disease of bone: Response to calcitonin. Neurology 29:448, 1979.
76. Stauffer RN and Sim FH: Total hip arthroplasty in Paget's disease of the hip. J Bone Joint Surg 58A:476, 1976.

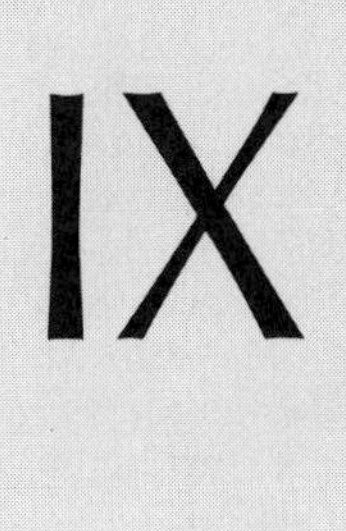

Neurologic Disorders

55

Vertigo

WILLIAM T. BRANCH, Jr., MD

Vertigo can be defined as an illusory sensation of motion. Some patients have a "spinning" or "whirling" sensation; others perceive a sense of tilting or moving. Patients having vertigo are alert but generally prefer to remain motionless; they do not experience syncope or impending loss of consciousness. Autonomic manifestations, such as pallor, faintness, and diaphoresis, may appear during severe episodes of vertigo but will not precede the attack, as they may in syncope. The duration of vertigo varies from a few seconds to hours or days, and this information may be useful in determining the etiology. Whatever the duration, episodes of vertigo are often paroxysmal; that is, they begin and end abruptly, as opposed to developing gradually.

Of all patients with dizziness severe or persistent enough to require referral to a neurology clinic, almost half (45%) were found to have vertigo (Table 55–1).[1] It is important to emphasize that in the majority of patients (85%) in this series, the vertigo was of peripheral or vestibular origin (Fig. 55–1), as opposed to that caused by diseases of the central nervous system or eighth cranial nerve. The majority of these will follow a self-limited course. In most cases, a practitioner can establish a workable hypothesis for the diagnosis from the history and physical examination, without resorting to additional studies. What remains of paramount importance is to identify, among the many patients with vertigo, the small number with lesions of the central nervous system or eighth cranial nerve, as well as the very small number with cholesteatoma or other treatable or potentially serious causes of peripherally induced vertigo.

From the patient's description of the vertigo and associated symptoms, the physician can usually recognize a clinical pattern and formulate an initial diagnostic hypothesis. This hypothesis then will be tested by asking additional questions concerning the history, aspects of the physical examination, or diagnostic maneuvers, either to confirm or to reject it. In every case with vertigo, the additional information sought should include examination of the tympanic membranes, gross testing for hearing, and a neurologic examination. In some cases, depending on how much information is needed to confirm the diagnosis and exclude other

TABLE 55–1. CAUSES OF VERTIGO IN 45 SELECTED CASES*†

		%
Vestibular disorders		
Benign positional vertigo		25
Acute vestibular neuronitis		8
Recurrent vestibular neuronitis		13
Meniere's disease		8
Chronic labyrinthine imbalance		6
Others		25
	TOTAL	85
Brain stem cerebrovascular accidents		10
Other lesions of the central nervous system including multiple sclerosis		4

*Adapted from Drachman DA and Hart CW: An approach to the dizzy patient. Neurology 22:323, 1972.

†All patients were selected by referral to a neurology clinic.

conditions, positional maneuvers, a fistula test, and radiographic or other studies may also be employed (Fig. 55–2). The remainder of this chapter will consist of a description of the major clinical patterns of vertigo, followed by a discussion of less commonly encountered etiologies and of the special diagnostic studies needed in their evaluation.

THE MAJOR CLINICAL PATTERNS OF VERTIGO

In the series of Drachman and Hart (see Table 55–1), more than half the patients had one of three clinical patterns of vestibular-induced vertigo.[1] These included (1) brief episodes that were attributed to benign positional vertigo (25%); (2) more prolonged vertigo without cochlear manifestations, attributed to vestibular neuronitis or labyrinthitis (21%); and (3) severe, episodic vertigo with cochlear manifestations, attributed to Meniere's disease (8%). These common syndromes can be recognized from the patient's description of vertigo and other symptoms; usually, the diagnosis can be made without the need for diagnostic studies other than the physical examination, testing for hearing, and positional maneuvers done in the physician's office.

Brief Episodes of Positional Vertigo

The syndrome of benign positional vertigo is defined as episodes of vertigo that occur only on changes of position and are without other manifestations or findings except for accompanying horizontal or horizontorotatory direction-fixed nystagmus. The nystagmus develops on positional maneuvers after a latency of 5 to 15 seconds, diminishes in intensity within 2 to 30 seconds, and fatigues on repetitive positional testing (Fig. 55–3).[2] The syndrome, if conforming to this precise definition, is thought to be a benign, self-limited disorder most likely related to an abnormality—debris, cupilolithiasis—of the posterior semicircular canal.[3] Vertigo that is sometimes induced or made worse by positional changes occurs in many disorders. It is emphasized that a syndrome of brief positional vertigo identical to benign positional vertigo can also be associated with head injury, ear diseases, and various other disorders. In two large series, 60 to 66% of cases were idiopathic (benign positional vertigo), 17 to 23% were post-traumatic, 4 to 11% were secondary to ear disease, and 5 to 13% were secondary to miscellaneous conditions, including sinus infection, cervical spondylosis, and central nervous system (CNS) lesions.[4, 5]

Once it was realized that the syndrome of brief positional vertigo was common, it was thought that one might avoid extensive diagnostic testing by reproducing the symptoms on positional testing according to the criteria listed above. Thus, the Bárány maneuver, as illustrated in Figure 55–3*A*, could be employed to establish the diagnosis of benign positional vertigo, in the absence of a history of trauma or findings of ear disease. In one large series, only 3.6% of patients with vertigo of this type whose nystagmus was fixed in its direction had CNS lesions, whereas 30% of those whose nystagmus changed its direction with different positions had CNS lesions.[5] Direction-changing nystagmus is far less common than nystagmus of fixed direction in these patients.[2] Other findings that raise the suspicion of a CNS lesions in these patients are spontaneous nystagmus without change in position and nystagmus persisting for much longer than 30 seconds.

In practice, it may be advisable to rely primarily on a careful neurologic examination to detect or exclude CNS disease in patients with this syndrome. Because CNS lesions are rare to begin with in such patients, the Bárány maneuver would need to be highly reliable to avoid yielding many more false than true results suggesting CNS disease. However, it is difficult to obtain patient cooperation for repeated positional testing to demonstrate the direction and "fatigability" of nystagmus. Direction and duration of nystagmus are also hard to observe reliably in the office setting—they can be much better documented during electronystagmography. Reproduction of a brief, vertiginous spell with transient nystagmus during a simple positional change, as illustrated in Figure 55–3*B*, does help clarify the nature of the symptoms being experienced by the patient. In addition to meeting this criterion and having a normal neurologic examination, patients with benign positional vertigo experience no tinnitus, hearing loss, or other cochlear symptoms and have no abnormality of the tympanic membrane on examination that would explain their symptom of vertigo.

More Prolonged Vertigo Without Cochlear Manifestations

Quite frequently, young patients have attacks of vertigo that are accompanied either by mild tinnitus or by no cochlear symptoms (e.g., transient sensations of "fullness" in the ear, fluctuating or permanent hearing loss, or hyperacusis). In addition, these patients usually have normal caloric responses and attacks of relatively brief duration, usually lasting for hours but sometimes for days. Often, the vertigo is initially nonpositional but as it resolves may begin to resemble benign positional vertigo. These cases, if they resolve without developing other manifestations, are usually termed *vestibular neuronitis* or *labyrinthitis*.[6] The etiology is unknown, though seasonal clustering of cases and frequent association with preceding upper respiratory symptoms suggest an infectious pathogenesis.[7] Positional or nonpositional vertigo of this type occurs in many vestibular disorders, however. It is not limited to the benign type, and sometimes is induced by diseases of the central nervous system. In such cases, clinicians must consider diagnoses of transient ischemic attack, multiple sclerosis, or neoplasm of the central nervous system, especially if the patient is elderly or if the episodes are recurrent or prolonged. The diagnosis of vestibular neuronitis or labyrinthi-

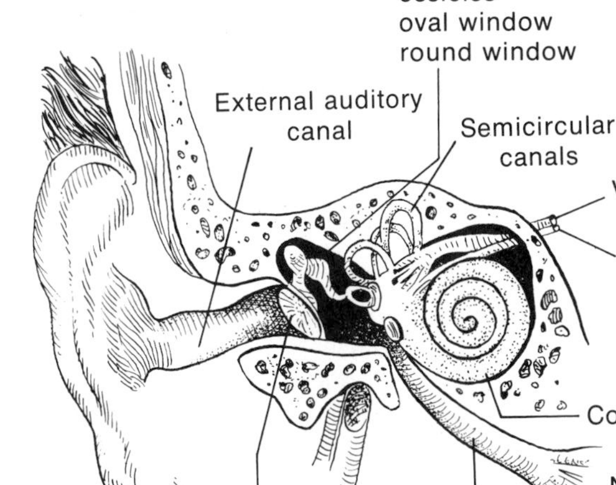

FIGURE 55–1. Clinical anatomy of the vestibular apparatus and its relationships. The close proximity of the cochlea to the vestibular apparatus can be seen. Thus, any process that actually invades or destroys the labyrinth or its vestibular nerve is likely, in addition, to produce hearing loss. Only disorders of the central nervous system and those confined to the vestibular portion of the nerve or labyrinth (e.g., benign positional vertigo or vestibular neuronitis) are expected to cause vertigo without affecting hearing. The middle ear cavity is also closely related to the labyrinth.

tis should be made only after occurrence of other neurologic or otolaryngologic symptoms and signs is excluded by a carefully conducted history and examination.

Attacks of Severe Vertigo with Cochlear Symptoms

Meniere's disease is a degenerative disorder (endolymphatic hydrops) of the inner ear.[8] Both the cochlear and vestibular apparatuses are involved. Vertigo tends to be severe, accompanied by roaring tinnitus and associated with hearing loss. The symptoms at times are violent, including diaphoresis and vomiting. Recurrent episodes of vertigo, each several hours or more in duration, may be the most prominent manifestation in some individuals; other patients present chiefly with hearing loss, sometimes sudden in onset. The sensation of fullness in the ear experienced by many patients during attacks may be a manifestation of the fluctuating hearing loss that occurs early in the course of the disease. Within 1 to 2 years, a pattern of hearing loss becomes established in most cases. Low tones are affected in 70 to 85% of patients, but high tones also may be affected, sometimes because of superimposed presbycusis.[9] Involvement of the contralateral ear develops within several years of onset in about 10% of cases.[9]

Whereas the diagnosis of benign positional vertigo or vestibular neuronitis is usually made in the office, Meniere's disease may require additional testing. If unilateral hearing loss is suggested by gross testing (Fig. 55–4), it should be documented by pure tone audiogram and one may characterize it further with an audiometric battery and brain stem–evoked audiometry. Computed tomographic (CT) scanning or magnetic resonance imaging (MRI) may be performed if these tests suggest a retrocochlear eighth-nerve lesion (see further on).

MANAGEMENT OF VERTIGO

Patients may be treated with antivertigo drugs, such as meclizine (Antivert, Bonine), dimenhydrinate (Dramamine), cyclizine (Marezine), scopolamine, or promethazine (Phenergan) (see Table 55–2). These drugs form the cornerstone of therapy for patients with Meniere's disease and other disorders causing vertigo, although their benefit is sometimes difficult to assess because of the unpredictable natural history of the disease. In a study of motion sickness, scopolamine (0.6 mg) and promethazine (25 mg) were most effective, but the others were helpful under moderate-to-mild conditions.[10] Individuals who remain severely afflicted with vertigo may receive a brief trial of dextroamphetamine (5 mg) in addition to promethazine (25 mg) if there are no contraindications. Various other treatments, such as dietary salt restriction, nicotinic acid, diuretics, oxygen, corticosteroids, vasodilators, and infusions of histamine have been tried but are without proved efficacy.[11] Individuals with severe disability related to vertigo may be treated by surgery, intratympanally applied streptomycin, or ultrasonic irradiation of the round window.[8, 12, 13] These treatments have the potential complication of producing additional hearing loss. Vestibular neuronectomy may be considered for some patients with persistent imbalance when the disease already has progressed to complete, nonfluctuating hearing loss.[14]

Tinnitus is persistent enough in some patients with Meniere's disease and other cochlear disorders to become incapacitating. At times, such patients are aided in falling asleep by use of radio music, taped cassettes, or even the static of an FM radio. The most severely affected individuals may require a hearing aid–masker matched to the frequency of the tinnitus. Approximately half these patients are helped by use of the masker, but the remaining half prefer tinnitus to the noise of the masker or have tinnitus at frequencies that are not matched sufficiently for the masker to be effective.[15]

OTHER CAUSES OF VERTIGO

Various other vestibular disorders may produce vertigo. Unless additional manifestations are present, many must be placed within the poorly defined diagnostic categories of recurrent vestibular neuronitis or chronic labyrinthine imbalance.[1] In some cases, the etiology of the labyrinthine disorder is toxic or drug induced. Episodic vertigo of varia-

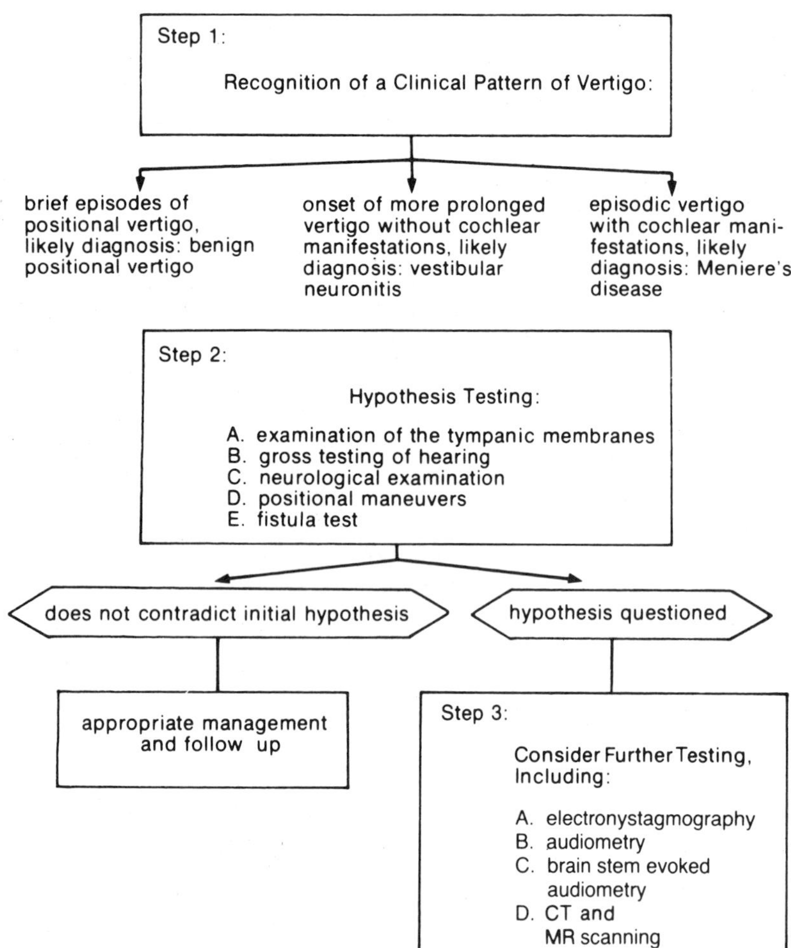

FIGURE 55–2. Summary of the clinical approach to a patient with vertigo.

ble duration also may follow head or neck injury. In one series of 129 patients, all of whom had suffered major concussions followed by post-traumatic amnesia, 34% had vertigo, and 59% of these continued to have some positional attacks 5 years after the injury.[16] In all patients with vertigo, no matter what the clinical pattern of presentation, it is most important to exclude invasive or destructive processes that affect vestibular function.

In general, these processes may be divided into three categories: (1) otitis and other local conditions that affect labyrinthine function, (2) lesions of the central nervous system, and (3) lesions of the eighth cranial nerve. As discussed previously, these conditions are encountered less frequently than are the vestibular causes of vertigo but are often treatable or have potentially serious outcomes.

When the etiology of vertigo is not apparent, its differential diagnosis depends on whether hearing loss is present. Diseases of the brain stem and cerebellum that cause vertigo do not also produce hearing loss, unless associated with extensive damage sufficient to suggest the presence of a lesion within the CNS. Conversely, most diseases that invade and anatomically disrupt the labyrinth affect the cochlear apparatus as well and produce hearing loss in addition to vertigo. Lesions of the eighth cranial nerve, generally early in their course, are also associated with hearing loss. When hearing loss is present in the absence of positive neurologic signs indicative of a lesion of the central nervous system, its etiology will be further suggested by determining whether it (1) has the characteristics of a conductive or mixed conductive-sensorineural hearing loss, suggesting diseases localized to the middle ear or causing cochlear destruction, or (2) has characteristics of pure sensorineural hearing loss, suggesting either cochlear dysfunction without anatomic disruption of the middle-inner ear (Meniere's disease), or involvement of the eighth cranial nerve.

When there has been severe destruction by any disease or surgical ablation of the labyrinth, a sense of disequilibrium may be persistent, particularly in patients with visual deficits, even to the point of producing disability[17] because vision is necessary for compensation by patients with labyrinthine disorders. Such patients generally describe their symptoms as tilting sensations, a sense of imbalance, or drop attacks rather than classic vertigo.

Otitis and Other Causes of Vertigo Associated with Conductive or Mixed Conductive-Sensorineural Hearing Loss

The most commonly encountered diseases of the middle ear only occasionally if at all produce vertigo that is mild, brief, and not a major component of the clinical picture. This applies to patients with cerumen or other material completely obstructing the external auditory canal, who present chiefly with conductive hearing loss, as well as to those with acute otitis media, who generally complain of a painful ear. However, in some instances, acute otitis media causes more pronounced vertigo by producing serous and, rarely, suppurative labyrinthitis.

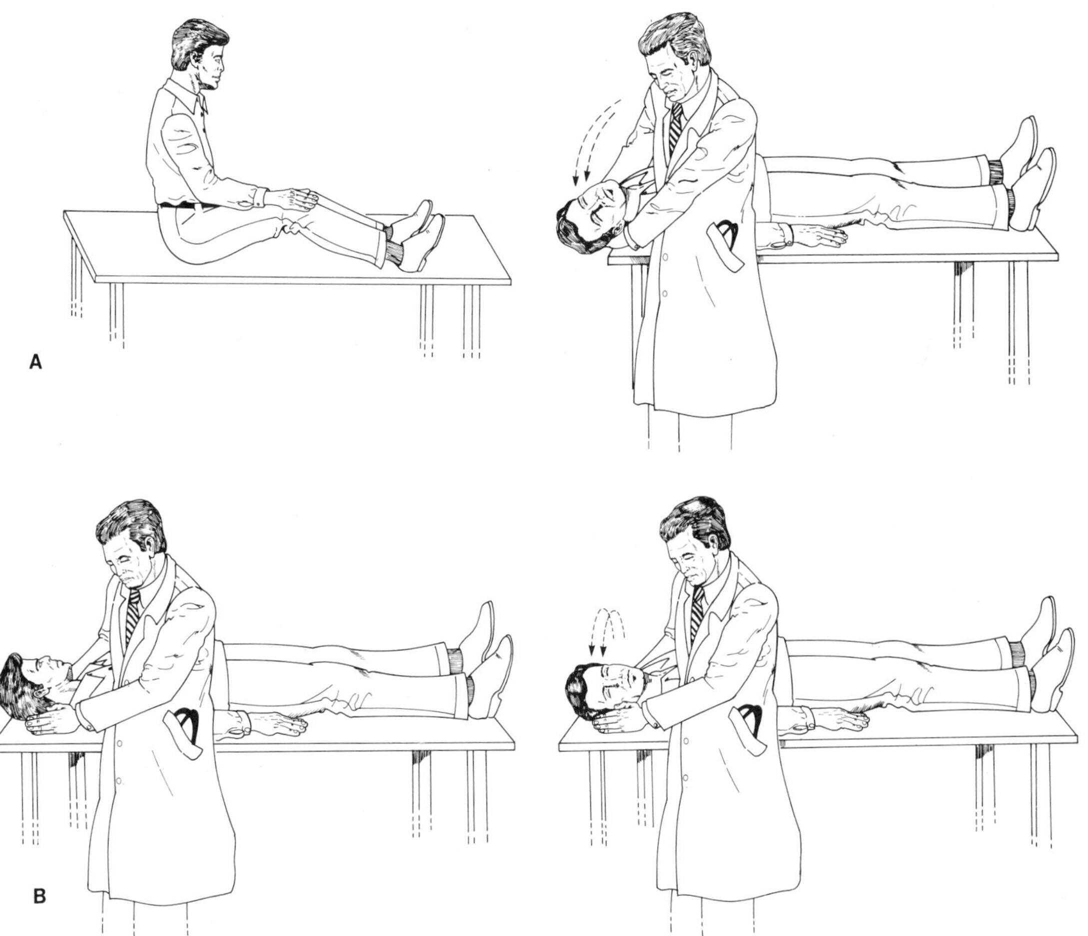

FIGURE 55–3. Benign positional vertigo. *A,* The Bárány response. With the eyes open, the subject is moved rapidly from the sitting position to the lying position. Nystagmus develops that is maximal with one ear down, has a quick component in one direction only, and is brief in duration with fatigue of the response. *B,* The head is moved from side to side while the patient is lying down. Positional vertigo and nystagmus may be produced. No specific diagnosis is implied, although positional vertigo with transient nystagmus is usually peripheral, indicating vestibular pathology.

Vertigo occurring in the setting of chronic otitis media requires careful evaluation because it rarely, if ever, is a prominent feature of such cases in the absence of complications. If present, vertigo may be associated with a serous or sclerotic labyrinthitis produced by chronic irritation but always should prompt consideration of the diagnosis of two potentially serious complications: suppurative labyrinthitis, which generally is associated with otogenic meningitis, and cholesteatoma with labyrinthine fistula. These conditions fall into the category of "can't miss" diagnoses that must be recognized when present. They will not be overlooked if a careful otoscopic examination of the tympanic membranes, gross testing for conductive hearing loss using a tuning fork, and the fistula test are done at the time of presentation.

Examination of the Tympanic Membranes. Acute otitis media will be recognized by most physicians from the bulging and erythematous appearance of the tympanic membrane with distortion of the normal anatomic landmarks. This appearance, and its differentiation from serous or secretory otitis media, is described in Chapter 18. The four types of chronic otitis media (Fig. 55–5) are all recognizable from clinical assessment and examination of the tympanic membrane. The latter will reveal evidence of perforation in almost every case. However, as mentioned earlier, vertigo is not a common manifestation of uncomplicated chronic otitis media, and all patients with this symptom, no matter which type of perforation is present, should be referred for otolaryngologic evaluation.

The Fistula Test. The fistula test, using the pneumatic otoscope, is designed to detect conditions in which trauma or an invasive process has disrupted the anatomic integrity of the inner ear. During a positive test, vertigo and nystagmus are reproduced by applying pressure with the pneumatic otoscope. The maneuver is particularly important not only in patients with a perforated tympanic membrane, but also in those with vertigo or disequilibrium that is nondescript in character. Trauma to the head or neck may cause vertigo, which at times presents with a clinical pattern of brief positional vertigo but more often with nondescript features.[5, 17] Recently, some of these cases have been discovered to have a leakage of perilymph from the round or oval window, which may follow diving or other exposure to high pressure, stapedectomy, or strenuous exertion, in addition to trauma.[18] Cases were detected by finding a positive result on a fistula test in patients with vertigo but normal-appearing tympanic membranes. When persistent, symptomatic relief can be obtained by plugging the leak surgically using a piece of adipose tissue.

Testing for Conductive Hearing Loss. Conditions of the external or middle ear that cause vertigo are often associated with conductive hearing losses. In some cases, conductive hearing loss is the most prominent finding. An example is acute serous otitis media, if retraction or dull-

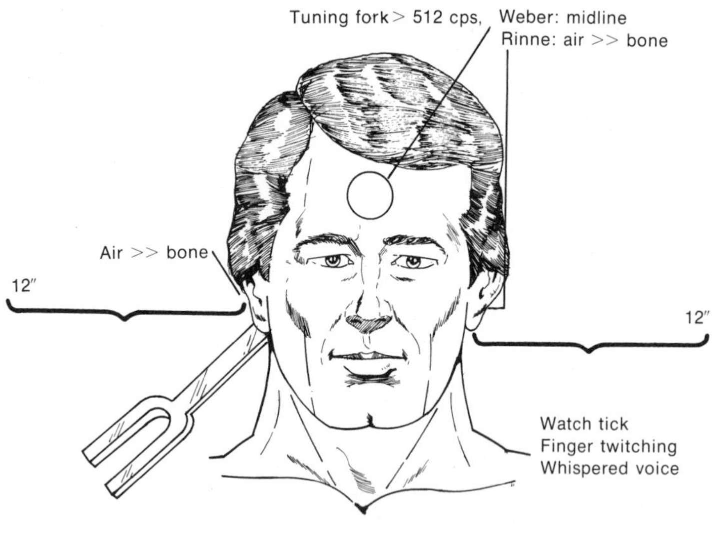

NORMAL

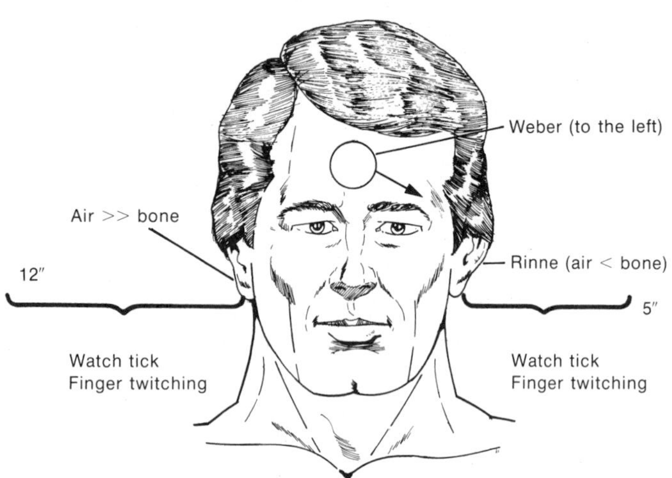

CONDUCTIVE LOSS

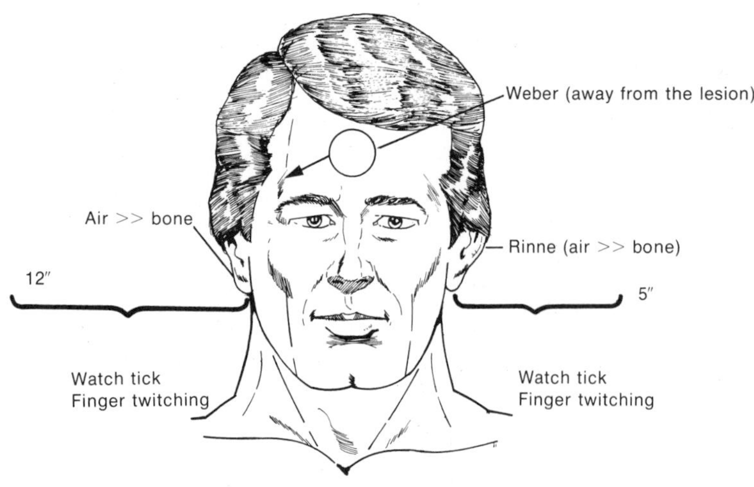

SENSORINEURAL LOSS

FIGURE 55–4. Approximate results from gross hearing tests. The side with the deficit is identified by gross testing with watch tick, finger twitching, or whispered voice. The tuning fork in midforehead (Weber) is perceived best on the diseased side in conductive losses and on the nondiseased side in sensorineural losses. The Rinne test confirms that bone conduction exceeds air conduction with conductive losses and vice versa with sensorineural losses.

TABLE 55-2. ANTIVERTIGO DRUGS

Meclizine (Bonine, Antivert)	12.5–50 mg PO, given twice daily
Dimenhydrinate (Dramamine)	50 mg PO, given each 4–6 hr
Cyclizine (Marezine)	25–50 mg PO, given each 4–6 hr
Scopolamine (Transderm-Scop)	Disk placed behind ear, may replace each 3 days, avoid eye contact
Promethazine (Phenergan)	25–50 mg PO, given each 4–6 hr, or 25 mg rectal suppository
Dextroamphetamine (Dexedrine)	5–10 mg PO, given each 6–8 hr

ness of the tympanic membrane is subtle, while a conductive hearing loss is detectable. In a series of 255 cases of brief positional vertigo,[5] 1% were associated with otosclerosis, the diagnosis of which is suggested by finding conductive hearing loss but a normal-appearing tympanic membrane.

Vertigo Caused by Lesions of the Central Nervous System or Eighth Cranial Nerve

It is necessary to exclude diseases of the central nervous system or eighth cranial nerve in patients with vertigo. Lesions within the central nervous system include infarctions, hemorrhages, or transient ischemic attacks involving the brain stem or cerebellum; neoplasms or other mass lesions of the posterior fossa; and multiple sclerosis. Lesions involving the eighth cranial nerve include tumors located at the cerebellopontine angle or in the internal auditory canal, and a recently described syndrome of vascular loops compressing the nerve near the brain stem.[19] Although these "central" causes are encountered infrequently, compared with the previously discussed vestibular or "peripheral" causes of vertigo, they may be life threatening and should be diagnosed accurately, if possible, at the time of presentation.

The usual approach is to depend on the clinical assessment and neurologic examination to detect lesions of the central nervous system. It is more difficult to exclude tumors of the cerebellopontine angle or internal auditory canal compressing the eighth nerve based on an office evaluation alone. When such a lesion is suspected because of unilateral sensorineural hearing loss, tinnitus, or other findings, one may perform screening tests, such as pure tone audiometry, brain stem–evoked audiometry, an audiometric battery, and electronystagmography, or proceed to MRI or CT scanning if the screening test results are positive or if clinical suspicion is high.

Lesions of the Central Nervous System

Some clinical features suggest the presence of a lesion within the CNS in patients with vertigo. The vertigo may be of any duration, including brief positional episodes but generally will be less severe and more prolonged than when induced by vestibular causes. Patients often experience the waxing and waning sensations of disequilibrium or loss of balance rather than whirling or spinning. Tinnitus is less likely to accompany the vertigo, and hearing loss is less likely to occur. Vertigo of CNS origin also is somewhat less likely to be strongly influenced by positional changes. If induced by the Bárány or other positional maneuvers, vertigo or nystagmus may be prolonged atypically, may be vertical or bidirectional, or fail to fatigue as expected. In general, nystagmus is more prominent, and vertigo is less prominent in CNS disease than in vestibular disease.

There are a few absolute and many relative distinctions between nystagmus of vestibular and that of CNS origin (Table 55-3). The quick component of vestibular nystagmus does not alter with changes in the direction of gaze, that is, the nystagmus is direction fixed. This type of nystagmus usually is accompanied by vertigo, often is induced by positional changes, and may be either horizontal, rotatory, or horizontorotatory in character. CNS-related nystagmus often is of long duration or present without vertigo; it is somewhat less commonly induced by positional changes and may change its direction with changes in the direction of gaze. An example of the latter is nystagmus related to drug toxicity, which is an exaggeration of the normal physiologic nystagmus with rapid jerks that alter toward the direction of lateral gaze. Certain types of nystagmus are virtually always of CNS origin, including vertical or oblique nystagmus and nystagmus in one eye only (internuclear ophthalmoplegia), in which, on looking to one side, the opposite eye fails to adduct, and nystagmus develops only in the abducting eye. One may suspect a CNS lesion on the basis of the findings listed previously, but confirmation generally depends on the demonstration of localizing signs on neurologic examination or by history.

It is unusual for a patient to have vertigo as the *sole* manifestation of a transient cerebral ischemic attack involving the brain stem or cerebellum. In addition to vertigo, most such patients also have dysarthria, loss of vision, diplopia, ataxia, or long tract signs in some combination dur-

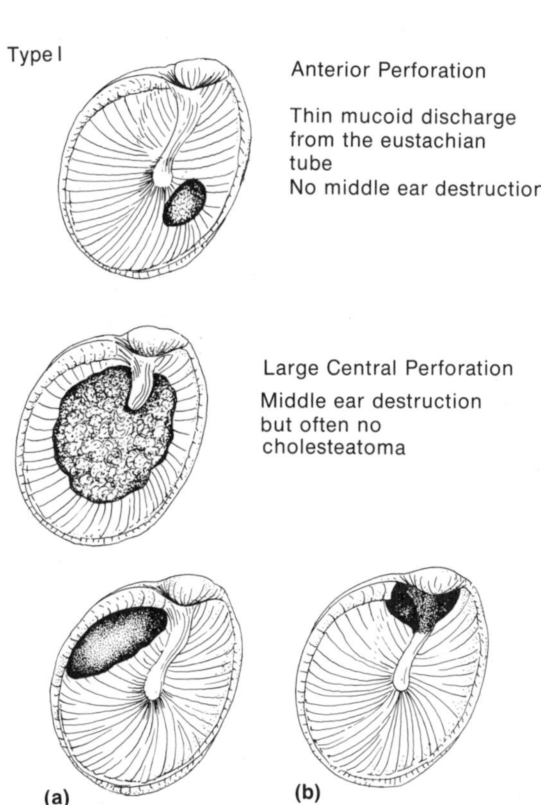

FIGURE 55-5. Types of perforations of the tympanic membrane.

TABLE 55–3. CHARACTERISTIC FEATURES OF VERTIGO AND NYSTAGMUS

Feature	Vestibular Lesions	Central Lesions
Vertigo	Abrupt onset of whirling or spinning	Less clear onset of disequilibrium
	Severe	Less severe
	Paroxysmal	May be continuous
	Seconds to weeks in duration	Often prolonged
	Usually positional	Somewhat less likely to be positional
Tinnitus	Common	Less common
Nystagmus	Horizontal, rotatory, or horizontorotatory	Vertical, oblique (also rotatory, horizontal, or horizontorotatory)
	Accompanied by vertigo	Of long duration or present without vertigo
	Turning eyes toward quick component increases its amplitude but does not alter its direction	Direction of nystagmus may change with changes in gaze. May resemble exaggerated physiologic nystagmus (especially in drug toxicity)
	Always in both eyes	May be in one eye only (internuclear ophthalmoplegia)
	May cease with fixation of vision, more pronounced with eyes closed	Not suppressed by fixating, equally pronounced with eyes open
	Gradually diminishes	May wax and wane or begin spontaneously after ceasing

ing the attack. However, because the labyrinthine circulation is derived from the vertebrobasilar system, in a few cases with underlying vertebrobasilar atherosclerosis, the only clinical manifestation may be vertigo or sudden loss of hearing resulting from ischemia or infarction involving only the labyrinthine artery. In rare instances, interruption of the labyrinthine circulation leads to a clinical presentation similar to that of benign positional vertigo, but the caloric response and hearing generally also are diminished on the affected side.

Small, completed infarctions or multiple sclerosis involving the brain stem should be accompanied by neurologic signs at the time of presentation. However, these signs may be subtle. Pontine lesions may produce Horner's syndrome, loss of sensation on one side of the face and the opposite side of the body, or motor ataxia on one side and loss of sensation on the other. Midline lesions of the cerebellum tend to produce truncal ataxia and abnormalities of tandem walking. Hemispheric cerebellar lesions more often cause clumsy rapid alternating movements and dysmetria of the ipsilateral extremities.

Individuals with cerebellar hemorrhages generally present with a sudden onset of headache and nausea and vomiting, followed shortly by inability to stand or walk, and ultimately, by loss of consciousness. Headache, nausea, vomiting, and inability to walk usually are less severe and may be absent in patients with cerebellar infarction. Ataxia of a limb and bidirectional horizontal, as opposed to vertical, nystagmus, if present without neurologic signs localized to the brain stem, usually are indicative of a cerebellar lesion. Patients with vascular accidents of the brain stem generally do not present with headache, vertigo, and nystagmus alone but will have additional focal neurologic findings. When cerebellar hemorrhage is suspected on clinical grounds, emergency MRI or CT scanning is indicated to identify the lesion and distinguish it from infarction.

Vertigo caused by a pontine or cerebellar lesion tends to resolve slowly because adaptation due to visual compensation is slow to develop. Consequently, ataxia induced by a brain stem–related or cerebellar lesion is equally pronounced in light or dark, whereas vestibular ataxia may be more severe in the dark than when the patient can see adequately. Tandem walking is abnormal initially with both CNS-related and vestibular lesions, but when the lesions are chronically present, tandem walking in patients with vestibular lesions may be more nearly normal when the eyes are open than when they are closed.[20]

Once a lesion has been detected, further evaluation, usually by MRI or CT scanning, will be necessary. In some cases, however, the clinican is concerned about the possibility of a central CNS-related lesion, but there are no unequivocally positive neurologic signs on examination. Electronystagmography may be useful in such instances.

Electronystagmography. Using the electronystagmogram, the amplitude, velocity, or duration of nystagmus may be recorded with a precision that is never possible using clinical testing. In this way, spontaneous or positionally induced nystagmus can be detected and its direction recorded precisely, the velocity of the slow component can be compared with eyes open and closed, very exact caloric testing can be performed, and one may record the patient's ability to track a moving object.

Since the advent of electronystagmography, many exceptions to the rules previously cited for interpreting nystagmus and caloric testing have been documented. Transient positional nystagmus could be detected in 60% of patients with brain stem–related lesions.[21] Spontaneous nystagmus occurs almost as frequently in peripheral as in central disorders. Rarely, patients with unilateral vestibular diseases have been noted to have vertical nystagmus.[21] Caloric testing also does not distinguish between peripheral and central disorders, and canal paresis was noted in one study in 60% of patients with brain stem–related pathology.[21] Nevertheless, an entire battery of electronystagmographic studies usually helps to confirm the suspicion of a lesion of the CNS or may strongly suggest that the patient has a peripheral disorder (Table 55–4).

If the nystagmus is vertical, changes its quick component according to the direction of gaze, or ceases and then starts again after the primary nystagmic response, it is very likely that the patient has a lesion related to the CNS. Persistence of spontaneous nystagmus with the eyes opened also correlates with diseases of the CNS. If the ratio of velocity of the slow component with the eyes opened to that with eyes closed exceeds 0.7, a lesion of the CNS or the effect of a drug or other toxin on the brain is suggested.[20] Lesions of the eighth nerve are often associated with electronystagmographic findings similar to those of vestibular (peripheral) disorders, but if the eighth nerve lesion also compresses the brain stem, the electronystagmographic features of a central lesion may coexist.

A most helpful test involves recording movements of the eyes while the patient attempts to follow a target moving at constant angular velocity. Irregular tracking patterns or brief, rapid movements in the direction of the target suggest disease related to the CNS. However, many normal older individuals have abnormal but nonspecific tracking patterns. The most specific finding is the presence of pro-

TABLE 55–4. RESULTS OF ELECTRONYSTAGMOGRAPHIC TESTING*

Finding	Patients with Unilateral Vestibular Lesions (%)	Patients with Brain Stem Lesions (%)
Spontaneous nystagmus with eyes open†	3	58
Spontaneous nystagmus with eyes closed	58	64
Greater velocity with eyes open than eyes closed†	0	13
Vertical nystagmus†	3	9
Positional nystagmus present with eyes open	24	69
Vertical nystagmus after positional maneuvers†	9	52
Reduced caloric response in one ear	94	60
Directional preponderance of caloric nystagmus	60	60
Irregular tracking† patterns	3	30
One or more abnormalities characteristic of brain stem lesion present by electronystagmography	30	100

*Adapted from Parker SW and Weiss AD: Some electronystagmographic manifestations of central nervous system disease. Ann Otol Rhinol Laryngol 85:127, 1976.
†ENG responses that were associated with lesions of the brain stem ($P < .05$).

nounced saccades. These are high-velocity movements that occur during tracking that may be associated with even moderate use of barbiturates and other sedatives but, when pronounced, virtually always are related to the CNS.[22] Figures 55–6 and 55–7 provide examples of the electronystagmographic findings in patients with peripherally and centrally induced nystagmus.

Acoustic Neuromas and Other Lesions Involving the Eighth Nerve

Acoustic neuromas constitute 8% of all brain tumors. Most are unilateral and occur in the fourth and fifth decades of life. Other tumors of the cerebellopontine angle, including meningiomas and the neurofibromas associated with von Recklinghausen's disease, may cause similar manifestations. The neurofibromas are often bilateral and present at a younger age.[23] All but 1 to 2% of affected individuals have hearing loss at presentation,[24, 25] and progressive unilateral hearing loss is the initial complaint in 70% of patients with acoustic neuromas.[23] Tinnitus, experienced in 80% of cases, is the presenting complaint for 20%, whereas only 10% complain at onset of an unsteadiness or episodic "veering" of gait; very few have whirling or spinning sensations as the initial manifestation.[23]

Patients with an acoustic neuroma can develop edema or ischemia of the vestibular nerve, causing classic episodes of vertigo. Hence, the diagnosis of acoustic neuroma should be considered in a patient complaining of vertigo, especially if there is unilateral sensorineural hearing loss or tinnitus.

Patients with small tumors (< 2 cm in diameter) rarely have neurologic or other physical findings except for hearing loss; in one series, all nine patients with small tumors had normal corneal reflexes.[23] When the tumor reaches an intermediate size (up to 3.5 cm), the corneal reflex is usually diminished, and other signs may develop, such as numbness in the region of the anterior mandible (fifth nerve), slowly progressive facial muscle weakness (seventh nerve), numbness and metallic taste of the tongue (chorda tympani), dull ache in the ear (sensory seventh), instability of tandem walking, and nystagmus.

The pure tone audiogram is an excellent initial screening test for detection of acoustic neuroma or other cerebellopontine angle tumor. Eighty-eight per cent of 117 patients with acoustic neuromas reported from the Mayo Clinic had audiometrically demonstrable hearing loss.[26] In another series, all patients had unilateral sensorineural hearing loss that averaged 60 decibels at 8000 Hz and 50 decibels at 1000 Hz.[27] If the audiogram confirms the possibility of an acoustic neuroma, MRI or CT scanning may be performed. If suspicion remains despite a normal audiogram, further testing may include screening by more extensive audiometric battery, brain stem–evoked audiometry, electronystagmographic caloric testing, or going directly to MRI or CT scanning. Nowadays, when suspicion is reasonably high, one may proceed to an MRI study. The other studies are discussed here for completeness and historical interest.

Audiometric Battery. Audiometric testing includes the pure tone audiogram and a battery of other tests designed to elucidate the characteristics of sensorineural hearing loss. The pure tone audiogram compares the patient's threshold for tones at a given frequency with that of a normal standard. The patient should be within 20 decibels of the normal standard. Bone conduction (using a different standard baseline) can be compared and should be equal to, but no better than, air conduction; if bone conduction is better, there is a conductive rather than a sensorineural hearing loss, and the pathologic process will be located peripherally to the cochlea (e.g., external canal obstruction, otitis media, and otosclerosis). Once the patient is found to have sensorineural hearing loss, a battery of tests may help distinguish cochlear disease (Meniere's disorder or presbycusis) from retrocochlear disease (e.g., acoustic neuroma or other central lesions).

Intensity of loudness may be varied until a patient can correctly identify 50% of polysyllabic words from a recorded tape. This is the speech reception threshold. A marked discrepancy, in which the patient's threshold for speech is diminished out of proportion to that for pure tones, is suggestive of retrocochlear disease. One can test this grossly by having the patient identify words whispered on each side.

A second way to distinguish between a cochlear and a retrocochlear disorder involves the presence or absence of recruitment. One may use the alternate binaural loudness balance test, in which the loudness of a pure tone above the threshold is adjusted until it is equal in both ears at the same frequency. A known increment on the good side is compared with the increase in loudness required to equal this on the bad side. The patient can adjust the loudness subjectively until the sounds are equal. If recruitment is present, a small increment on the diseased side will be equal to a larger increment in the nondiseased ear. Recruitment is indicative of cochlear disease, as opposed to retrocochlear disease.

There are several other components of the audiometric battery, but these will not be discussed in detail because reliability using the audiometric battery for distinguishing between Meniere's disease and acoustic neuroma is not

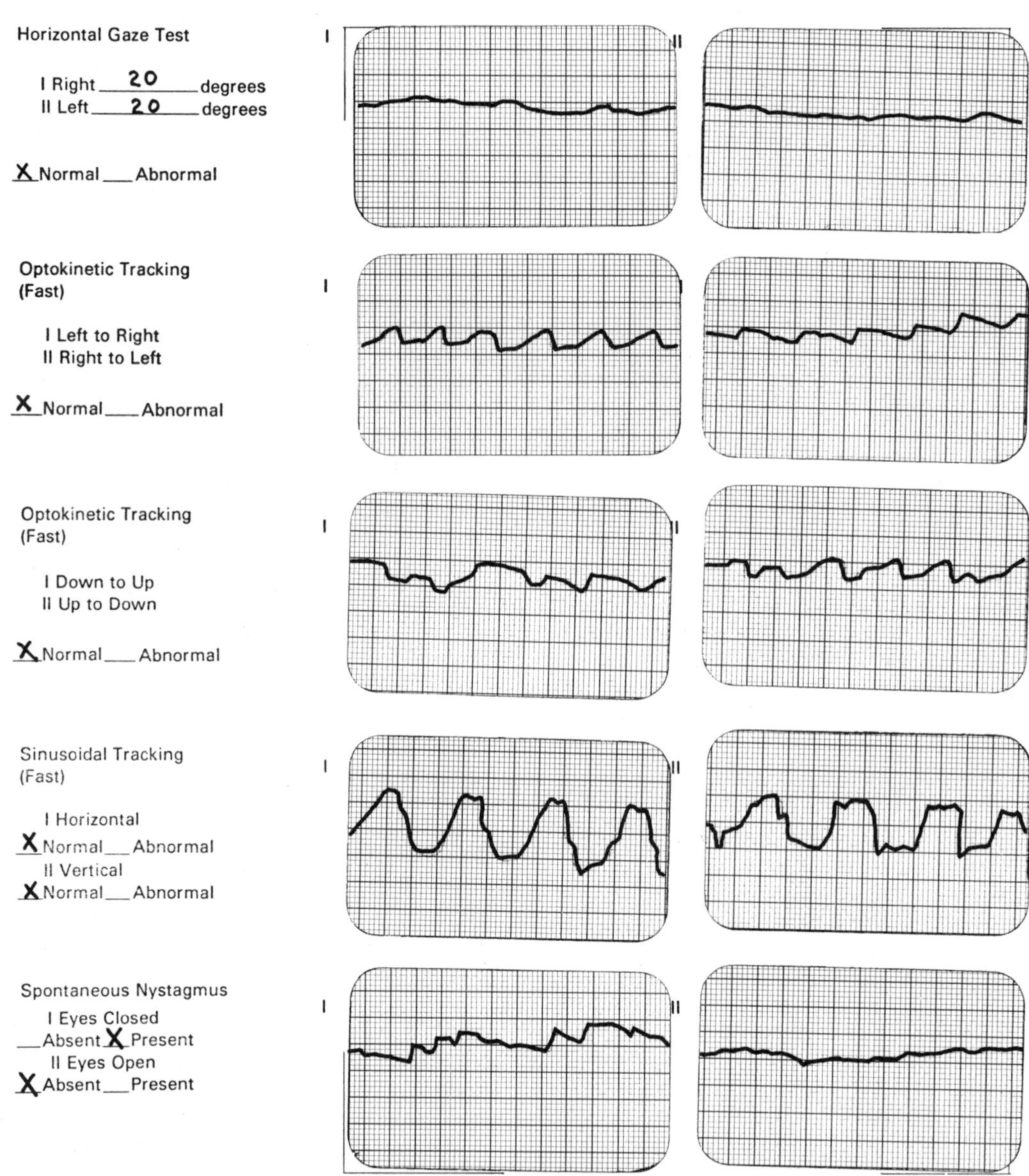

FIGURE 55–6. Electronystagmographic findings in peripherally induced nystagmus.

high.[28, 29] Among 155 patients with surgically confirmed acoustic neuromas, only 45% showed a complete retrocochlear audiometric pattern, and in 13%, the pattern was totally of the cochlear type.[28] Small tumors are more likely to give mixed or misleading results. Hence, although the audiometric battery may sometimes aid in making the assessment, it cannot be relied on to exclude an acoustic neuroma.

Brain Stem–Evoked Audiometry. This test, which measures the electrical response to a sound passing from the cochlea to the brain stem, is highly sensitive for detection of acoustic neuromas. Of patients with neuromas, 90 to 95% have an abnormal response in which the usual pattern is absent or prolonged.[26, 27] The pattern of response of the brain stem may be distorted, however, by any type of sensorineural hearing loss and does not distinguish between cochlear and retrocochlear disease. Twenty-five per cent of 229 patients with Meniere's disease, unknown-type sensorineural hearing loss, otosclerosis, and various other conditions had abnormal brain stem–evoked responses that could not be distinguished from those of acoustic neuro-

ELECTRONYSTAGMOGRAPHY LABORATORY

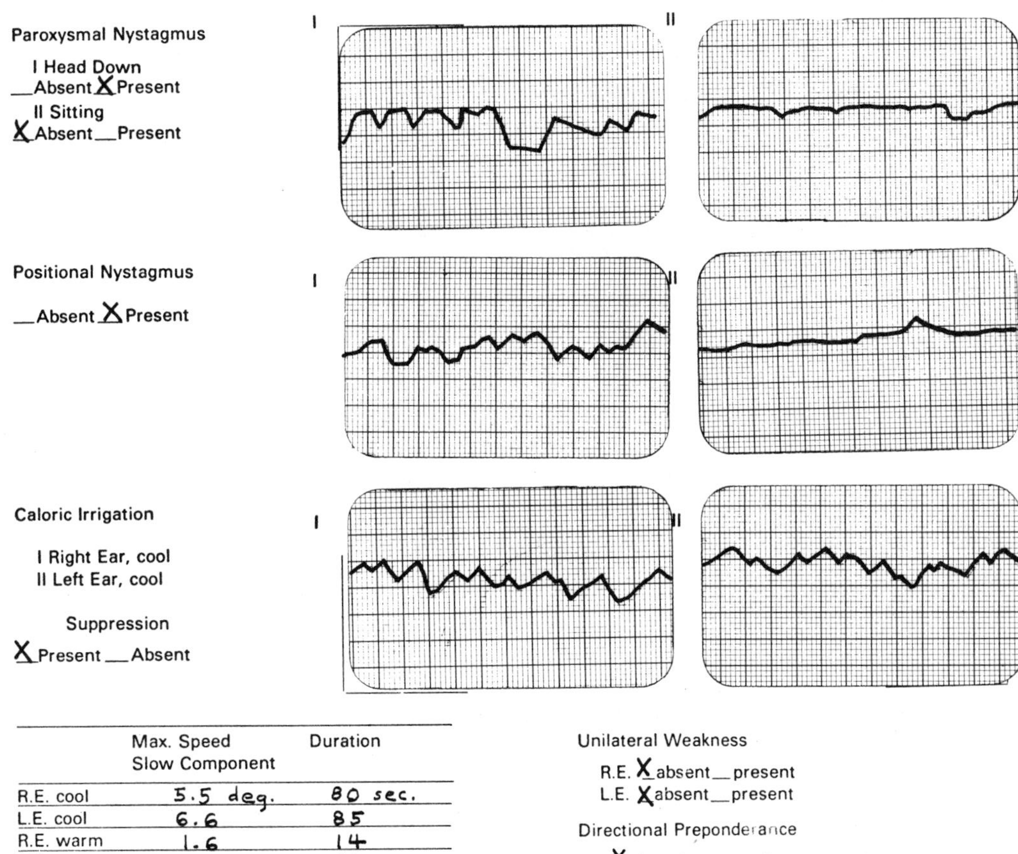

Paroxysmal Nystagmus

I Head Down
__Absent X Present
II Sitting
X Absent __Present

Positional Nystagmus

__Absent X Present

Caloric Irrigation

I Right Ear, cool
II Left Ear, cool

Suppression
X Present __Absent

	Max. Speed Slow Component	Duration
R.E. cool	5.5 deg.	80 sec.
L.E. cool	6.6	85
R.E. warm	1.6	14
L.E. warm	2.6	32

Unilateral Weakness

R.E. X absent __present
L.E. X absent __present

Directional Preponderance

X absent __present

Technical Summary Right-beating spontaneous nystagmus augmented by downward movement of head to right and by static right head position. Nystagmus fatigues after first trial and is suppressed by visual fixation. Bithermal irrigations are equal and approach borderline bilateral weakness.

Interpretation

Abnormal electronystagmogram indicative of right peripheral disorder, end-organ or nerve.

________________ Ph.D. ________________ M.D.

MEDI-TRACE GRAPHIC CONTROLS CORPORATION BUFFALO NEW YORK PRINTED IN CANADA MED 213-421 (ECF 30015)

FIGURE 55–6 *Continued*

mas.[30] Thus, a normal brain stem–evoked audiometric pattern provides strong evidence against acoustic neuroma, but an abnormal result is nonspecific.

Caloric Testing and Electronystagmography. Office caloric testing in the evaluation of vertigo is of historical interest. To be useful, the test must be done with precision, using warm (44° C) and cool (30° C) water in both ears with at least 6 minutes, preferably more, between each of the perfusions and exercising care that the external canals are not obstructed and that the time of perfusion (1 to 2 minutes) is equal for each test. The quick component of nystagmus is toward the ear being perfused when warm water is used and away from the ear when cool water is used. Unilateral weakness (canal paresis) refers to a lesser duration of nystagmus evoked with both cool and warm water in one side compared with the other side. Directional preponderance refers to greater duration of nystagmus in one direction—for example, as occurs with cool water in the left ear

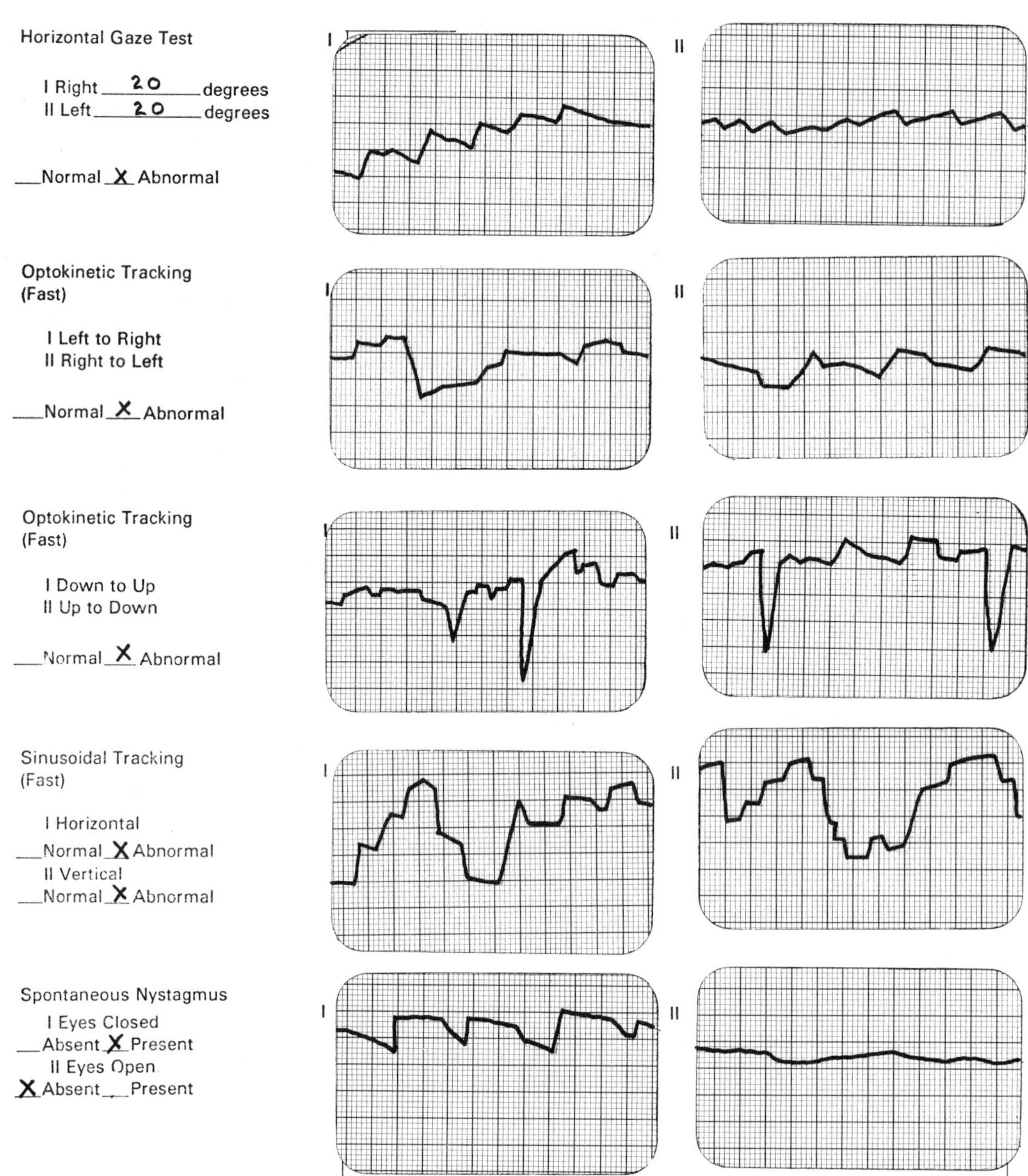
Peter Bent Brigham Hospital
A Division of the Affiliated Hospital Center, Inc.

NAME:
HOSP #:
REF. PHYS:

ELECTRONYSTAGMOGRAPHY LABORATORY

Horizontal Gaze Test

I Right 20 degrees
II Left 20 degrees

___Normal X Abnormal

Optokinetic Tracking (Fast)

I Left to Right
II Right to Left

___Normal X Abnormal

Optokinetic Tracking (Fast)

I Down to Up
II Up to Down

___Normal X Abnormal

Sinusoidal Tracking (Fast)

I Horizontal
___Normal X Abnormal
II Vertical
___Normal X Abnormal

Spontaneous Nystagmus

I Eyes Closed
___Absent X Present
II Eyes Open
X Absent ___Present

FIGURE 55–7. Electronystagmographic findings in central nervous system–induced nystagmus.

(when the quick component is away from the ear being perfused) and with warm water in the right ear (when the quick component is toward the ear being perfused). Duration of nystagmus should be timed using a stopwatch and a second observer. Even so, there is probably a 15% error in the method. When the reactions are equal in both ears, even if very weak or very prolonged, no conclusion should be drawn. Patients also may have vertigo and demonstrate pass pointing after caloric testing. These symptoms may be taken as evidence for vestibular response; however, they are not quantifiable.

The interpretation of caloric testing is as follows (Fig. 55–8): The caloric response is always normal in idiopathic benign positional vertigo but also can be normal in many other vestibular disorders, including early Meniere's disease, acute vestibular neuronitis, and in lesions of the central nervous system. If there is decreased caloric responsiveness on one side, with or without directional preponderance, then the presence of a lesion on that side is suggested, but it may be located in the vestibular apparatus, the eighth nerve, or the CNS. If there is directional preponderance without canal paresis, no specific conclusion can be drawn.

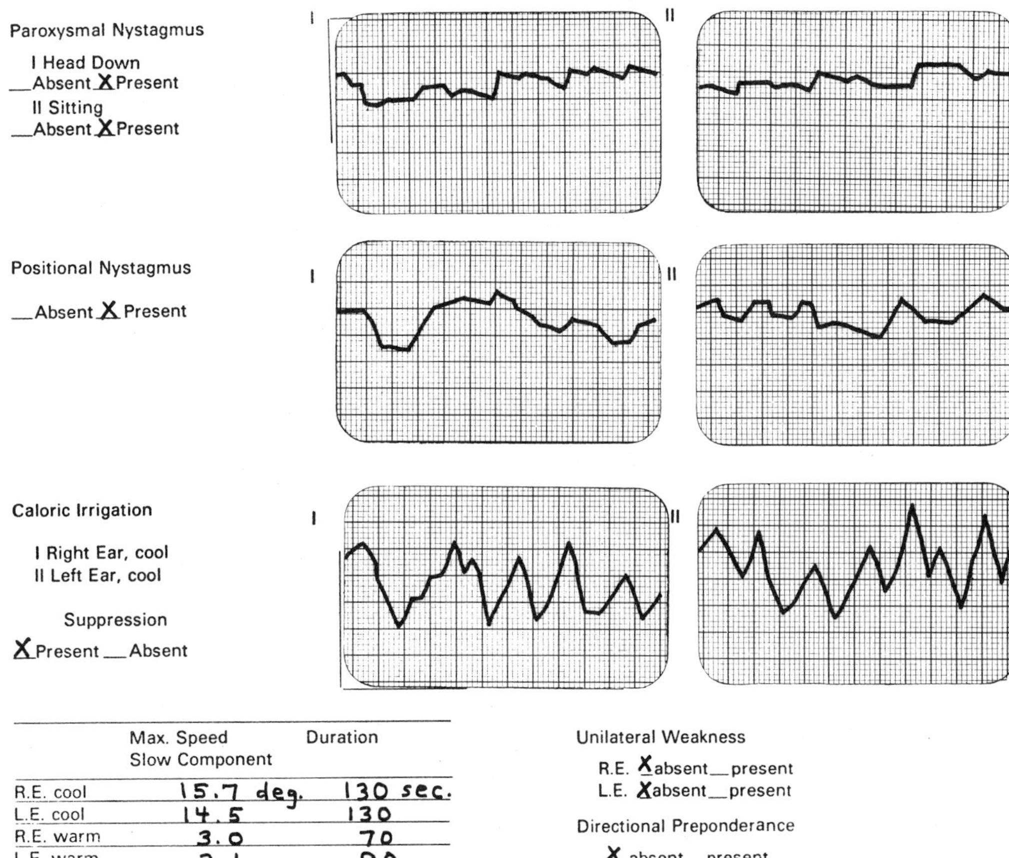

ELECTRONYSTAGMOGRAPHY LABORATORY

Paroxysmal Nystagmus

I Head Down
__Absent X Present

II Sitting
__Absent X Present

Positional Nystagmus

__Absent X Present

Caloric Irrigation

I Right Ear, cool
II Left Ear, cool

Suppression

X Present __Absent

	Max. Speed Slow Component	Duration
R.E. cool	15.7 deg.	130 sec.
L.E. cool	14.5	130
R.E. warm	3.0	70
L.E. warm	3.1	90

Unilateral Weakness

R.E. X absent __present
L.E. X absent __present

Directional Preponderance

X absent __present

Technical Summary Bilateral direction-changing gaze nystagmus, right greater than left. Asymmetric OKN. Breakup of sinusoidal tracking. Direction-changing spontaneous nystagmus, predominantly right-beating, eradicated by visual fixation. Paroxysmal and positional nystagmus, which do not fatigue and do not elicit subjective vertigo. Bithermal calorics are equal.

Interpretation Abnormal electronystagmogram indicative of central pathology, brain stem or cerebellar.

__________ Ph.D. __________ M.D.

MEDI-TRACE GRAPHIC CONTROLS CORPORATION BUFFALO NEW YORK PRINTED IN CANADA MED 213-421 (ECF 30015)

FIGURE 55–7 *Continued*

The combination of directional preponderance and canal paresis may lead to complex patterns, and irrigating one canal more forcefully or for a longer period, may create a falsely exaggerated response. Thus, the clinical usefulness of the test is limited. In practice, it has been supplanted by electronystagmography.

In the evaluation of patients suspected of having an acoustic neuroma, caloric testing by electronystagmography, in which the speed of the slow component and the total number of beats can be quantified more precisely, has advantages. The major question is whether finding a reduced caloric response as determined by electronystagmography is a sensitive enough index, so that one may exclude acoustic neuroma if the caloric response is normal. The results of two series reveal that 16 to 21% of patients with acoustic neuromas had normal vestibular responses on the side of the tumor.[26, 27] Only 40% of patients with the small acoustic neuromas had abnormal caloric responses.[26] Thirty

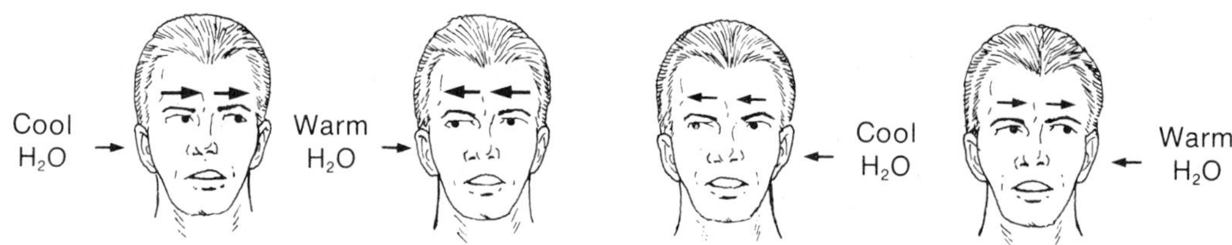

Decreased caloric response (or canal paresis): Duration of nystagmus is absent or less for cool and warm perfusions of one ear. Suggests vestibular pathology, lesion of the eighth cranial nerve, or CNS pathology on the affected side (where duration is diminished or nystagmus is absent).

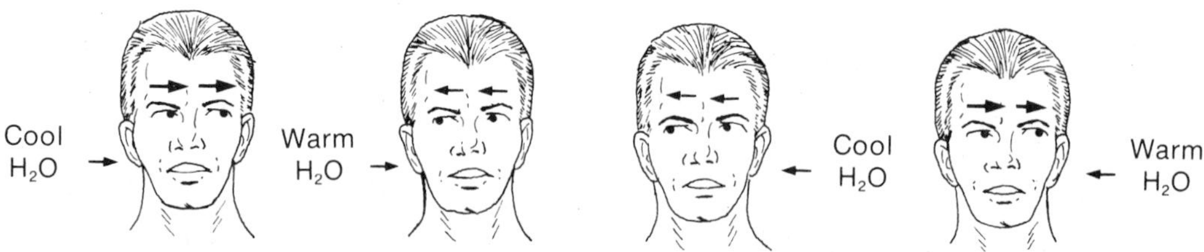

Directional preponderance: Duration of nystagmus is greater for cool on one side and warm on the other, so that duration is accentuated in one direction. No definite conclusion can be drawn, as this can be normal or can occur in central nervous system disorders.

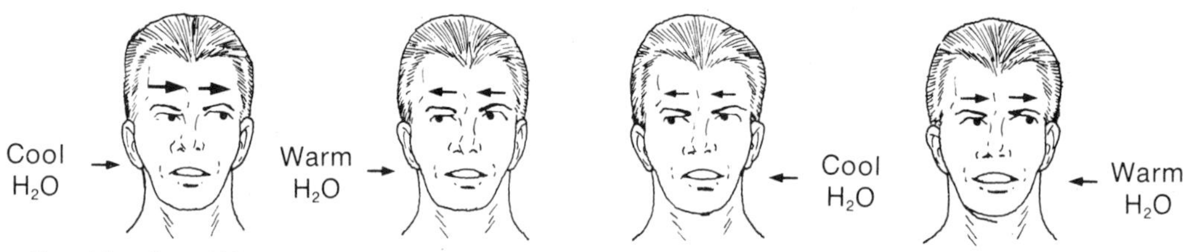

Combination: With canal paresis on the left and directional preponderance to the left, cool water in the right ear provokes the greatest response. Responses may reflect any of the possible combinations of paresis and preponderance. Suggests vestibular, eighth cranial nerve, or central pathology.

FIGURE 55–8. Interpretation of office caloric testing.

per cent of patients with other disorders causing unilateral hearing loss had diminished caloric responses[27]; hence, the test made no distinction between cochlear and retrocochlear disorders. As a screening test for acoustic neuroma, caloric testing is less sensitive than brain stem–evoked audiometry.

Magnetic Resonance Imaging and Computed Tomographic Scanning. MRI is now the procedure of choice in suspected acoustic neuroma and is the gold standard for making the diagnosis. Sensitivity and specificity were 100% in two recent series.[31] On a high-resolution MRI scan of the skull base using gadolinium diethylenetriamine pentaacetic acid enhancement, the eighth nerve can be traced through the internal auditory canal, and small tumors can even be identified. When MRI cannot be performed because of metallic implants or claustrophobia, CT scanning using bone windows is the alternative procedure of choice and can identify widening of the canal or contrast-enhancing tumors at the cerebellopontine angle. In two series, CT detected 58 and 65% of the tumors detected by MRI scanning.[31]

Summary and Example of the Presentation of an Acoustic Neuroma

A 68-year-old woman complained of "imbalance" for 3 to 4 weeks. She had spontaneous horizontal nystagmus on left lateral gaze and instability on tandem walking, but no other neurologic signs. Further history revealed chronic tinnitus of the right ear. A right sensorineural hearing loss had been documented 3 years previously, and an audiometric battery had revealed the presence of recruitment, suggesting Meniere's disease as the diagnosis.

In the past, this was not an unusual presentation for the patient with an acoustic neuroma. All too frequently, as in this case, the symptoms were neglected until the tumor was quite large. Here, acoustic neuroma was suspected when it was noted that the patient, who had a disorder of gait, also had unilateral hearing loss. The finding of recruitment on the previous audiogram did not exclude this possibility. CT scanning (Fig. 55–9) confirmed that a large neuroma was located at the cerebellopontine angle.

Improved technology now allows the diagnosis of acoustic

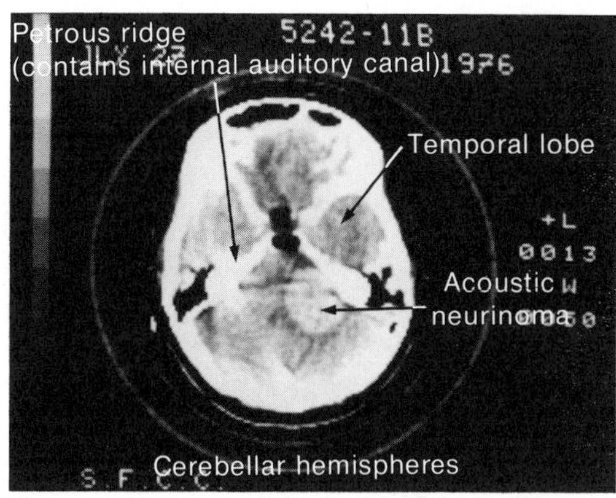

FIGURE 55–9. A large cerebellopontine angle lesion enhanced with contrast and most likely representing acoustic neuroma.

neuroma to be made when the tumor is very small in the majority of cases.[31] The tumor was removed successfully in 98% of 129 patients seen at the Mayo Clinic.[26] The diagnosis can generally be made by MRI or CT scanning after initial screening, if necessary, by pure tone audiometry, and/or brain stem–evoked audiometry.

REFERENCES

1. Drachman EA and Hart CW: An approach to the dizzy patient. Neurology 22:323, 1972.
2. Dix MR and Hallpike CS: The pathology, symptomatology and diagnosis of certain common disorders of the vestibular system. Proc R Soc Med 45:341, 1952.
3. Hall SF, Ruby RKF, and McClure JA: The mechanics of benign positional vertigo. J Otolaryngol 8:151, 1979.
4. Harrison MS and Ozsahinoglu C: Positional vertigo. Arch Otolaryngol 101:675, 1975.
5. Katsarkas A and Kirkham PH: Paroxysmal positional vertigo—a study of 255 cases. J Otolaryngol 7:320, 1978.
6. Slater R: Benign recurrent vertigo. J Neurol Neurosurg Psychiatr 42:363, 1979.
7. Anttinen A, Lang AH, Aantag E, et al: Vestibular neuronitis: A neurologic and neurophysiologic evaluation. Acta Neurol Scand 67:90, 1983.
8. Pulec JL: Meniere's disease: Etiology, natural history and results of treatment. Otolaryngol Clin North Am 6:25, 1973.
9. Eliachar I, Keels E, and Wolfson RJ: Basic audiometric findings in Meniere's disease. Otolaryngol Clin North AM 6:41, 1973.
10. Wood CD, Cramer DB, and Graybiel A: Antimotion sickness drug efficacy. Otolaryngol Head Neck Surg 89:1041, 1981.
11. Marlowe FI: Drug treatment of Meniere's disease. Otolaryngol Clin North Am 6:119, 1973.
12. Beck C and Schmidt CL: Ten years of experience with intratympanally applied streptomycin (gentamicin) in therapy of morbus Meniere. Arch Otorhinolaryngol 221:149, 1978.
13. Tabb HG, Nurris CH, and Hagan WE: Round window ultrasonic irradiation of Meniere's disease with ENG monitoring. Laryngoscope 88:460, 1978.
14. Palva T: Vestibular neuronectomy. Acta Otolaryngol 360 (Suppl):51, 1979.
15. Longridge NS: A tinnitus clinic. J Otolaryngol 8:390, 1979.
16. Berman JM and Frederickson JM: Vertigo after head injury: 5 year follow-up. J Otolaryngol 7:237, 1978.
17. Foley J: Vestibulogenic imbalance. BMJ 1:1244, 1978.
18. Editorial: Nonspecific disturbance of balance. Lancet ii:237, 1979.
19. Jannetta PJ, Moller MB, Moller AR: Disabling positional vertigo. N Engl J Med 310:1700, 1984.
20. Barber HO: Current ideas on vestibular diagnosis. Otolaryngol Clin North Am 11:283, 1978.
21. Parker SW and Weiss AD: Some electronystagmographic manifestations of central nervous system disease. Ann Otol Rhinol Laryngol 85:127, 1976.
22. Afzelius LE, Henriksson NG, and Wahlgren L: Vertigo as reflected by the nystagmogram: A clinical analysis. Acta Otolaryngol 86:123, 1978.
23. Shiffman F, Dancer J, Rothballer AB, et al: The diagnosis and evaluation of acoustic neuromas. Otolaryngol Clin North Am 6:189, 1973.
24. Lundborg T: Diagnostic problems concerning acoustic tumors. Acta Otolaryngol 99(Suppl):1, 1952.
25. Edwards CH and Paterson JH: A review of the symptoms and signs of acoustic neurofibromata. Brain 74:144, 1951.
26. Harner SG: Clinical findings in patients with acoustic neuroma. Mayo Clin Proc 58:721, 1983.
27. Selters WA and Brackmann DE: Acoustic tumor detection with brain-stem electric response audiometry. Arch Otolaryngol 103:181, 1977.
28. Johnson EW: Auditory findings in 200 cases of acoustic neuromas. Arch Otolaryngol 88:598, 1968.
29. Clemis JD and Mactricola PG: Special audiometric test battery in 121 proved acoustic tumors. Arch Otolaryngol 102:654, 1976.
30. Bausch CD, Rose DE, and Harner SJ: Auditory brain-stem response results from 255 patients with suspected retrocochlear involvement. Ear Hear 3:83, 1982.
31. Shaffer, K: The temporal bone. *In* Latchaw RE (ed): MR and CT Imaging of the Head, Neck and Spine, 2nd ed. St. Louis, Mosby–Year Book, 1991, p 929.

56

Seizure Disorders

SHAHRAM KHOSHBIN, MD

Seizures and epilepsy are either the presenting issue or complicating problem in a large and diverse group of disorders that come to medical attention in an office practice.

Approximately 2% of the population give a history of having had a seizure at some time in their lives; in the Mayo Clinic study of Rochester, Minnesota, six of 1000 subjects either were taking antiseizure medications or had experienced a seizure within the preceding 5 years.[1] Extrapolated to the total population, these data reveal that 1 million Americans are being treated for a seizure disorder at any one time. It is estimated that one third of individuals with a history of a seizure do not reach medical attention. Among patients visiting an outpatient neurology facility, seizure disorder or epilepsy constitutes one of the five most common conditions. In terms of physical and emotional disability, as well as the expense involved in evaluation and drug treatment, seizures constitute a major public health problem.

Despite their prevalence and importance, seizure disorders are poorly understood by the general public and inadequately managed by some general physicians. This situation arises in part from the variety of neurologic manifestations that may result from seizures, ranging from the sudden loss of consciousness to complex patterns of seemingly meaningful behavior. In addition, epilepsy is not one entity, but it represents diverse conditions with varied etiologies and mechanisms. A further source of difficulty is the large and fairly recent body of data regarding the pharmacology and optimal use of anticovulsant drugs and imminent appearance of newer anticonvulsants. This chapter emphasizes these two problem areas.

A seizure is a transient alteration in neurologic function consequent on a sudden, abnormal, excessive discharge in the cerebral cortex or underlying hemispheric structure.[2] Implicit in this definition is the notion that diseases causing seizures affect the cerebral hemispheres and are not confined to the brain stem, cerebellum, or spinal cord. The term *seizure disorder* refers to all forms of seizures, regardless of their cause or clinical manifestations; *epilepsy* is generally reserved for patients with a lifelong or prolonged tendency to seizures, often genetically based, in distinction to patients with seizures related to such events as stroke, head injury, or metabolic abnormality. Patients frequently prefer the term *seizure disorder* to *epilepsy* because it does not suggest the image of mental deterioration and the prospect of social ostracism that still unfortunately cling to the latter term.

CLASSIFICATION

Since 1970, seizures have been classified by most neurologists according to the International Classification described by Gastaut.[3] Its most recent modification, in 1981, separates partial from generalized seizures.[4]

- I. Partial seizures (focal)
  - A. Simple partial seizures
    1. With motor signs
    2. With somatosensory or special sensory symptoms
    3. With autonomic symptoms or signs
    4. With psychic symptoms
  - B. Complex partial seizures
    1. Simple partial onset followed by impairment of consciousness
    2. With impairment of consciousness at onset
  - C. Partial seizures evolving to generalized tonic-clonic (GTC)
    1. Simple partial seizures (A) evolving to GTC
    2. Complex partial seizures (B) evolving to GTC
    3. Simple partial seizures evolving to complex partial seizures evolving to GTC
- II. Generalized seizures
  - A. Absence seizures ("petit mal")
  - B. Atypical absence seizures
  - C. Myoclonic seizures
  - D. Tonic seizures
  - E. Tonic-clonic seizures ("grand mal")
  - F. Atonic seizures

According to this scheme, febrile convulsions are tonic-clonic seizures (grand mal) occurring in children aged 0 to 6 years in the context of a rapidly rising body temperature; *temporal lobe epilepsy* (a common term for seizures with atypical cognitive or physical symptoms) is either simple partial seizures or, if associated with impairment of consciousness, complex partial seizures.

CLINICAL DIAGNOSIS

Accurate characterization of the seizure type is crucial to effective management, both for diagnostic evaluation and for choice of drug therapy. In seizures characterized by alterations of consciousness—particularly generalized seizures and psychomotor seizures—reports from both the patient and bystanders may contribute to accurate classification. As a general rule, the electroencephalogram (EEG) does not establish the type of seizure except in the case of petit mal absence attacks, in which bilateral, synchronous 3-per-second spike-and-wave activity during the absence is required for the diagnosis. It is crucial to recognize that there is frequently a progression from one seizure type to another. This progression may be quite rapid. The clinical clue is the patient reporting an "aura" of almost any kind; this indicates a simple partial or complex partial onset.

The distinction between the different seizure types primarily has an etiologic significance. Generalized seizures primarily denote metabolic or genetic etiologies, partial seizures, primarily structural anomalies or damage to the cortex. Generalized seizures have childhood onset, whereas partial seizures are more prevalent in adults and usually are of adult onset. Pharmacologic therapy is directed toward this group of seizures.

DIFFERENTIAL DIAGNOSIS

Absence seizures, so-called petit mal, are a disorder of children, beginning after the age of 4 years and before puberty, often with tens or hundreds of episodes per day. Each episode consists of a sudden, very brief (1 to several seconds) interruption of consciousness, during which the patient stops attending, stares, and may undergo several clonic movements of eyelids, facial muscles, or arms, or automatisms in the form of lip smacking, chewing, or fumbling movements of the fingers. Simultaneous with the absence is bilateral, synchronous 3-per-second spike-and-wave activity in the EEG. Both the absence and the EEG changes may frequently be induced by 2 or 3 minutes of hyperventilation. Such patients rarely fall during an episode and may continue their activity immediately after the spell because they do not experience postictal confusion.

True petit mal is not a common disease. In one pediatric clinic, such patients accounted for only 5% of all seizure patients.[5] Petit mal is most often confused with partial seizures of the psychomotor type, in which the only manifestation of the seizure, at least from the patient's point of view, is a gap in his or her experience. If prolonged, partial complex seizures may present as nothing more dramatic to the patient than a period of several minutes (rarely hours) for which the patient has no recollection. To observers, the behavior during that period may have been characterized by continuation of well-practiced skills, such as driving or riding a bicycle, accompanied by a vacant stare and lack of contact with the surroundings. Unlike petit mal, such episodes are not invariably related to 3-per-second spike-and-wave activity, and they occur much less frequently.

Petit mal seizures invariably begin before the age of 15 years and cease by the age of 20 years in 80 to 90% of individuals afflicted. Absence attacks persisting beyond the age of 25 or 30 years should suggest a diagnosis of partial complex seizures. Approximately 50% of children with petit mal seizures develop grand mal seizures that may persist into adult life.

Petit mal seizures may be complicated by the occurrence of other types of seizure, including episodes of myoclonic jerking and drop attacks. If the petit mal episodes in such patients display typical 3-per-second synchronous spike-and-wave activity, the prognosis is quite good. On the other hand, association of petit mal episodes with atypical spike-and-wave activity (2 to 2.5 Hz) constitutes the petit mal variant or petit mal triad of Lennox syndrome and is frequently associated with cerebral pathology and a high incidence of mental deterioration.

Petit mal status—that is, attacks occurring for hours with no intervening normal mentation—is an uncommon disorder, described as frequently in adults as in children.[6] An EEG showing the 3-per-second spike-and-wave activity is diagnostic in this condition.

Grand mal seizures are easily diagnosable to the bystander, although the patient may be unaware of anything other than a "black out" and the sore muscles, headache, confusion, and fatigue that often follow. The prodrome may extend over a period of hours, marked by a feeling of apathy, irritability, or a sense of foreboding. Myoclonic jerks of the arms or trunk muscles may precede the actual seizure. The aura, which immediately precedes the loss of consciousness, may involve a turning of the head or eyes, a strange feeling of fullness in the epigastrium, palpitation, or generalized malaise. No aura is experienced in about half of grand mal seizures, presumably because of the rapid spread of seizure activity. The actual seizure is usually heralded by forceful tonic contractions of the limbs and jaw, a strangled cry, arrest of respiration, pupillary dilation, and a sudden fall to the ground, during which there is mild generalized trembling or shivering, succeeded by forceful rhythmic contractions of the arms and legs and facial grimacing, accompanied by cyanosis, grunting, and salivation. Incontinence may occur, as may subconjunctival hemorrhages.

After 2 or 3 minutes, the clonic phase ends with a deep inspiration, the musculature relaxes, and color returns to the face and extremities. After another few minutes, consciousness returns, although the person is often confused and may be agitated. Complete recovery follows a period of several hours of sleep, although some patients may exhibit focal neurologic deficits, such as hemiparesis, hemisensory loss, or aphasia that gradually resolve over 48 to 72 hours. This postictal paralysis of nervous function, a so-called Todd's paralysis, has important localizing value, although the lesion that is localized may be old or new. Some patients with a "new" stroke may in fact have a postical paralysis following a seizure from the scar left by a previous stroke.

Grand mal seizures frequently occur in small flurries of several seizures over a few hours; this is a common pattern in alcohol withdrawal seizures during the first 6 to 36 hours after the sudden cessation or reduction in the consumption of alcohol. A small percentage of epileptic patients, about 5%, will at some time have a series of seizures between which consciousness is not recovered—*status epilepticus.* This life-threatening condition most frequently results from sudden reduction in anticovulsant medication.[7] However, withdrawal from other drugs (sedatives, hypnotics) or alcohol, exposure to drugs known to precipitate epilepsy (like penicillin) and metabolic disorders (hypocalcemia, hypernatremia, hyponatremia—especially if rapidly developed—hypoglycemia, and hyperglycemia with hyperosmolality), and uremia may also precipitate status.[8]

The diagnosis of grand mal seizure is readily apparent in fully developed cases that have been witnessed; otherwise, a diagnosis of *transient ischemic attacks* or *syncope* due to any cause may be considered when the patient can report only a loss of consciousness or is found in the postictal phase. However, transient ischemic attacks rarely lead to loss of consciousness, whereas prolonged confusion or postictal sleepiness does not follow syncope. Moreover, the patient with vasodepressor syncope has a more prolonged premonitory phase consisting of non-neurologic symptoms that include weakness, nausea, dizziness, and diaphoresis, as opposed to the sudden loss of consciousness that can occur in seizures. Although a brief tonic phase sometimes followed by a few clonic jerks can occur in syncope of any cause, when it is accompanied by cerebral hypoxia, fecal incontinence, cyanosis, stertorous breathing, and a prolonged course (over a minute), it usually implies a true seizure occurrence.

Generalized myoclonic seizures consist of sudden flexion of head and neck with upward jerking of the arms, sometimes of sufficient force to throw a child to the ground; occasionally, the movements are asymmetric or even unilateral. Seizures of this type may complicate the course of petit mal or of the petit mal variant previously described.

Tonic and atonic seizures, as well as infantile spasms, are seen primarily in certain pediatric conditions and will not be discussed further.

Partial (i.e., focal) seizures are classified according to the predominant symptomatology. Such seizures reflect a specific cortical lesion, either macroscopic or microscopic, that serves as an autonomous focus for excessive electrical discharge, which becomes symptomatic when it spreads beyond the local epileptic focus, either to a sufficient number of adjacent neurons or via white matter pathways to distant portions of the cerebrum.

Partial motor seizures generally arise from the frontal or rolandic cortex, although similar movements may be induced experimentally by cortical stimulation at quite distant sites from the frontal lobes. Simple motor seizures often consist of adversive movements of head, eyes, and trunk in a tonic fashion away from the hemisphere involved, after which clonic movements or progression to a generalized seizure may occur. This should be distinguished from the *jacksonian* form of motor seizure, in which a tonic contraction of one side of the face, the fingers, or one foot is followed immediately by clonic movements of the extremity, which then spread or march in a regular fashion up the extremity to involve eventually the adjacent extremity and finally, if the seizure persists, all the muscles on one side. This condition may persist for some minutes and then subside, or it may progress to a generalized seizure.

Such a march is held by most neurologists to indicate a macroscopic lesion in a very high percentage of cases, usually involving the opposite rolandic cortex or adjacent portions of the cerebrum. Such patients should undergo extensive investigation for a lesion and be followed closely for many years if a lesion is not initially demonstrated. Simple focal seizures, without jacksonian march, are frequently associated with a pathologic condition in adults, although they may emanate from old microscopic or macroscopic lesions and are occasionally seen in states of metabolic derangement, especially hyperglycemia. In children, simple focal seizures and even Todd's postictal paralysis may be associated with no demonstrable pathologic condition in many cases.

In some cases, especially following cerebral infarction, focal motor seizures may persist for hours or days without impairing consciousness. This condition, *epilepsia partialis continua,* should not be confused with status epilepticus, as it rarely poses the threat to survival that the latter does. The treatment is quite different.

Other partial seizures depend on the location of the inciting lesion. Disturbances in the rolandic area may give rise to episodes of numbness, tingling, or prickling sensations, which may also march in a fashion characteristic of jacksonian seizures. Occipital lesions may rarely produce visual phenomena, usually of an elemental nature and positive in character. Colored or white lights, moving or stationary, in the opposite visual field or straight ahead, have been described. On the other hand, complex visual hallucinations, such as distortions of size (micropsia or macropsia), shape, or arrangement, arise from the posterior temporal lobe. Uncinate seizures consist of brief sensations of unusual or disagreeable smells or tastes; they reflect discharge in the most medial portion of the temporal lobe, usually secondary to a discrete lesion in that area. Auditory phenomena and vertiginous sensations have been described but occur infrequently and are usually accompanied by other seizure manifestations.

Because of their focal nature and the variety of their manifestations, partial seizures may be mistaken for *transient ischemic attacks* or for neurologic symptoms associated with *migraine.* In general, transient ischemic attacks are distinguished from partial seizures because they do not involve convulsive movements, occur in an older age group, and exhibit a full range of prominent neurologic deficits at the start. Migraine is usually distinguished by the initial visual manifestations of fortification scintillations and visual field defects, both of which are extremely rare in seizure disorders; by the more gradual march of the neurologic symptoms over a 15- to 20-minute period; by the absence of convulsive movements in an extremity; and by the prolonged, pulsating headache that usually follows the neurologic symptoms in migraine.

Compared to the relative simplicity of the symptomatology in simple seizure disorders, psychomotor seizures present such a bewildering variety of clinical phenomena that the precise boundaries of the diagnosis are still unclear.[9]

Typically, a psychomotor seizure has three elements: (1) an *aura,* which is usually a complex hallucination, perception, or emotional feeling and actually constitutes a part of the seizure itself; (2) a *dreamy state,* in which consciousness is altered, and contact with the surroundings deficient, although not completely suspended; and (3) *behavioral automatisms.* The aura, the content of which can frequently be recalled by the patient, may consist of a complex hallucination—visual, auditory, olfactory, or vertiginous; a perceptual distortion; a feeling of unreality *(jamais vu)* or familiarity *(déjá vu)*; or an affective state such as fear, anxiety, or rage. Automatisms frequently involve either repetitive inappropriate acts (washing hands, repeating incoherent words, or pacing) or movements around the mouth, such as sucking, chewing, or swallowing. Highly practiced motor acts, such as driving or dressing, may actually continue during a seizure. In such cases, only the failure to respond to a question or a suggestion indicates the altered consciousness. Rarely, such individuals will become hostile if restrained, but persistent, directed aggressive behavior is most unusual.

Fully two thirds of patients with psychomotor seizures will experience generalized seizures at some time in their lives, and the conjunction of these two phenomena frequently permits one to make the correct diagnosis regarding complex partial seizures. Whereas a population of patients with psychomotor seizures exhibits a seemingly endless variety of seizure patterns, the pattern in any given patient is frequently quite stereotyped.

Recently, attention has been focused on a disturbance of personality in patients with temporal lobe seizures, referred to as "Geschwinds syndrome."[9–13] These patients sometimes display a socially "viscous" quality, hyper-religiosity, tendency to abstraction in their concerns, hyposexuality, and proclivity to engage in excessive literary composition in their spare time.[10] These changes certainly occur in only a minority of patients with complex partial seizures, and their relationship to the seizures is problematic. There is general agreement, however, that the changes are interictal and are not direct manifestations of a discharging focus in the temporal lobe. However, the hyposexuality, a loss of interest as well as performance, appears to reflect the degree on ongoing seizure activity; control of the seizures may increase sexual drive. The other behavioral characteristics are not closely linked to the seizure frequency, and in some cases may be exacerbated by tighter seizure control.

Psychiatric disorders may be difficult to distinguish at times from partial seizures with complex symptomatology; this is particularly true of extreme anxiety states, disorders of impulse control, hysteria, and schizophrenia. In these psychiatric conditions, the frequently normal EEG result and the absence of a clear history of convulsive disorder may help in the diagnosis, but distinction is sometimes difficult.

There is no question that temporal lobe epileptics are more prone to develop eventual psychosis, which may be difficult to distinguish from more classic schizophrenia.[12] Prolonged episodes lasting days without intervening periods of lucidity suggest schizophrenia and are unusual in psychomotor seizures, as is the performance of psychologically meaningful behavior of a complex nature. Amnesia for at least part of the episode is common in seizure disorders but relatively uncommon in psychiatric disease. During interictal periods, patients with psychomotor epilepsy can be distinguished from those with schizophrenia if they display a normal and appropriate affect, maintain close interpersonal relationships, and are capable of clear, logical thinking.

The diagnosis of psychogenic or behavioral seizures poses special problems. Many patients presently seen with these seizures have a genuine seizure disorder as well, making the differentiation of their spells both important and doubly difficult. Behavioral seizures should be suspected when frequent seizure episodes are accompanied by a normal EEG result; when seizures occur frequently, although friends and relatives are unaware of the seizure disorder; when consciousness is preserved, despite bilateral movements or movements during the seizure consisting of alternately flailing each arm or leg or side-to-side movement of the head, and typically, pelvic thrusting (Fig. 56–1); when generalized seizures are not followed by confusion, dilated pupils, extensor plantars, and increased tendon reflexes; and when medication produces no improvement and results in bizarre reactions. From the foregoing, it follows that the differentiation between true grand mal and hysterical grand mal seizures is often much easier than that between psychomotor seizures and unusual subjective experiences. One requirement for the diagnosis of hysterical seizures, pointed out by Charcot in the last century, is familiarity with the pattern of an actual seizure, gained either from a friend or relative or from work in a medical facility. Despite this familiarity, however, the imitation is rarely so good that it cannot be differentiated from a true grand mal seizure if the examiner has a chance to witness the episode.

DIAGNOSTIC STUDIES AND EVALUATION

The etiology of seizure disorders may be genetic, congenital, or acquired; it may reflect either concurrent systemic disease or disorders confined to the central nervous system.

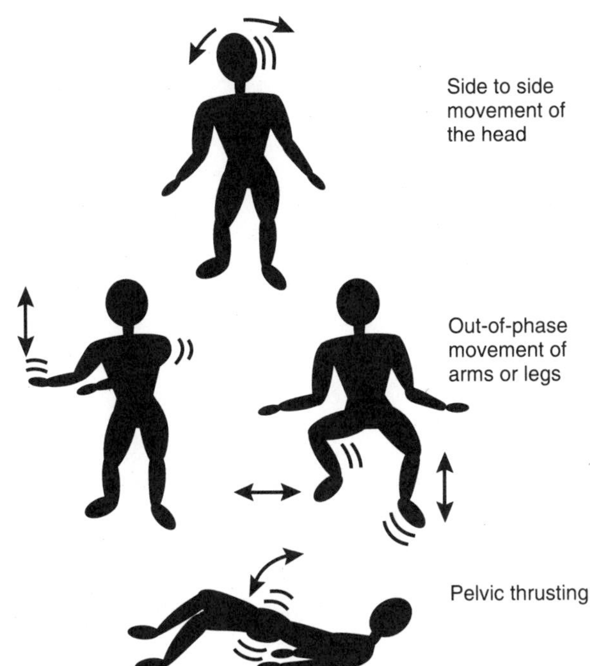

FIGURE 56–1. Movements suggestive of psychogenic seizures.

In a given patient, the likelihood of the various causes depends on both the age of onset and the type of seizure. By age group, the most common causes are the following:

Infancy: congenital lesions, perinatal encephalopathy, pyridoxine deficiency, and metabolic abnormalities (hypocalcemia, hypoglycemia)
Childhood: perinatal trauma or anoxia, febrile condition, and idiopathic disorder
Adulthood: idiopathic disorder, alcohol or drug withdrawal, tumor, and trauma
Old age: vascular infarct, tumor, trauma, and degenerative disorder

The older the patient, the more likely it is that a cause will be found in unselected adult populations with grand mal seizures. The largest group of causes is related to vascular disease in those over 50 years old, but tumor remains an important concern. If evaluation with noninvasive tests and a thorough neurologic examination are undertaken at the onset and close follow-up is ensured for the first 5 years, it is quite unlikely that serious correctable lesions will be missed.

Certain aspects of the clinical situation should alert one to the possibility of a tumor manifesting itself as a seizure. Abnormalities on the neurologic examination, especially if focal and if suggestive of a hemispheric lesion, should prompt the ordering of magnetic resonance imaging (MRI) or computed tomography (CT). Age of the patient plays a role. Tumors of the cerebral cortex are rare in children; unless the examination or EEG points to a focal disorder, studies beyond EEG and MRI are not likely to be helpful. In adults, the percentage of patients with tumors increases with age but varies considerably from series to series. Estimates range from 30%[14] down to 4%[15] for groups over 35 to 40 years old. For those with partial (i.e., focal) seizures in the same age group, the percentages are from 70%[16] down to 35%.[17] Two studies indicated, however, that with generalized seizures commencing after the age of 35 years, when there is no preceding aura or partial seizure evolving

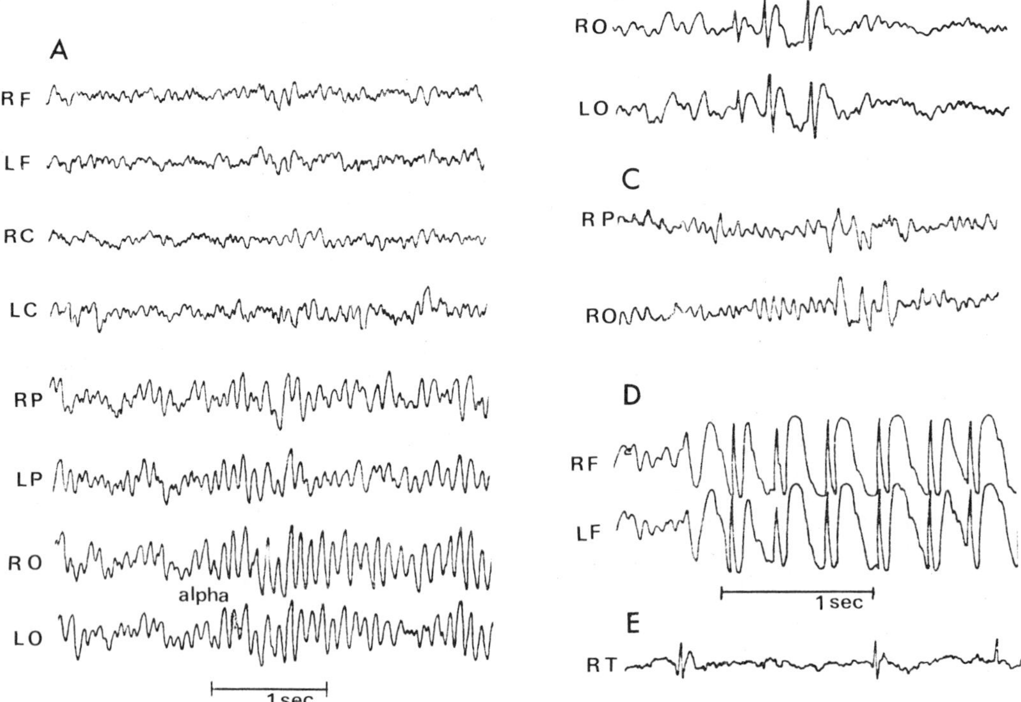

FIGURE 56–2. *A,* Normal waking adult tracing. *B,* Multiple occipital spike foci. *C,* Sharp waves and spikes. *D,* Three per second spike and wave. *E,* Small, sharp spikes.
RF-right frontal; LF-left frontal; RC-right central; LC-left central; RP-right parietal; LP-left parietal; RO-right occipital; LO-left occipital; RT-right temporal.

to a generalized seizure, and when both the neurologic examination and the EEG indicate a nonfocal disorder, an ultimate diagnosis of tumor is extremely uncommon.[18–19]

With partial seizures other than the temporal lobe type, the yield in terms of new central nervous system lesions is much higher; this is especially true if either focal EEG abnormalities or focal neurologic abnormalities are present (see percentages in the preceding paragraph). In summary, focal seizure disorders deserve more careful and extended scrutiny than do generalized seizure disorders.

The first step in evaluation is a careful history, both of the seizures themselves and of past infections, trauma, perinatal injury, strokes, and drug usage. In hospitalized patients, hyponatremia, hypoglycemia, hyperglycemia, hypocalcemia, and respiratory alkalosis are frequent causes of new-onset seizures, as is the adminstration of certain drugs, such as lidocaine and theophylline.

A number of blood tests, including complete blood count, serology, electrolytes, blood urea nitrogen, blood sugar, and calcium, are required at the time of initial evaluation as screening for occult medical disease. A complete neurologic evaluation, including some assessment of cortical function (language, visual fields, construction, calculation, praxis), is mandatory.

Using a Wood lamp to examine the back for ash-leaf spots will find about one new case of tuberous sclerosis per year in a large neurologic clinic. Lumbar puncture should be performed in any patient in whom acute or chronic infection is possible, as judged by the medical history or the neurologic examination; in others, its yield is extremely low.

An EEG should be performed initially in every patient suspected of having seizures for several reasons: first, to add further evidence for a diagnosis of seizure disorder in patients in whom this diagnosis is uncertain; second, to search for focal abnormalities of cortical function in the form of local slow waves or a spike or sharp-wave focus; third, to serve as a baseline assessment for comparison if seizures become more frequent or harder to control; and fourth, to distinguish partial complex seizures from classic petit mal. An EEG taken in the sleep-deprived patient is useful in documenting the seizure disorder but is less useful in searching for focal abnormalities. The prior administration of anti-convulsants may marginally reduce the yield of paroxysmal EEG abnormalities but will not significantly alter the chances of finding a focal abnormality. For this reason, anticonvulsants should not be withheld pending completing of an EEG when the presence of a seizure disorder is certain. The types of abnormalities seen on EEG in patients with seizure disorders are shown in Figure 56–2.

The reliability of EEG in diagnosing seizure disorders varies according to the type of seizure exhibited by the patient. In grand mal seizures, the EEG reading is invariably abnormal during the seizure, usually showing a high-frequency train of spikes initially, followed by spike-and-wave or sharp-and-slow activity, which is succeeded after some seconds or minutes by high-amplitude, irregular, diffuse slowing (postictal phase). The interictal record, on the other hand, may or may not be abnormal. Ajmone-Marsan and Zivin found that only 56% of epileptic patients had epileptiform patterns on a single EEG, although a higher percentage had some abnormality.[20] The percentage of EEG results positive for epileptic activity decreases with age and increases with the frequency of the seizures. Curiously, these same investigators found that the administration of anticonvulsant medication did not significantly lower the incidence of epileptiform abnormalities in the EEG. Repeat EEGs, especially if performed during a period of maximum seizure susceptibility, may increase the yield of positive results, but provocative techniques are more useful. Not only does sleep deprivation provide a record of cerebral activity in sleep, which may reveal abnormalities, but also the waking tracing with sleep deprivation is more likely to show epileptiform activity. Mattson and associates found that 34% of a group of epileptic patients with previously normal tracings showed epileptiform patterns after a single night of sleep deprivation.[21] Hyperventilation will disclose paroxysmal activity in a small percentage of the rest and will almost invariably evoke spike-and-wave activity in children with petit mal seizure disorder. Photic stimulation at varying frequencies with eyes open and closed may disclose recruitment of slow-wave activity or spiking, the so-called photoconvulsive response.

The diagnosis of partial complex seizures is more difficult because partial (or focal) seizures may present a normal record even during the occurrence of a seizure. Both sleep deprivation and the use of nasopharyngeal leads produce a higher yield of epileptiform tracings. The efficacy of nasopharyngeal leads is based on their proximity to the mesial temporal lobe, a common site for the origin of seizure discharges that is not easily accessible to the conventional EEG leads. In DeJesus and Masland's series, 17.5% of patients had significant EEG abnormalities seen only in the nasopharyngeal leads.[22] Recently, zygomatic leads, anterior to the usual temporal leads, have been found to be as sensitive as nasopharyngeal electrodes in detecting temporal lobe discharges; their placement is not as traumatic to the patient as that of nasopharyngeal leads. Light sleep, either following sleep deprivation or after a small dose of chloral hydrate, may further enhance the procedure. Recent evidence indicates that an adequate sleep tracing is just as effective in eliciting paroxysmal activity as is the intravenous administration of methohexital.

In withdrawal states, the EEG is frequently normal or marked by abundant low-voltage fast activity. In metabolic encephalopathies, the EEG is usually diffusely slow, and seizure discharges may not be apparent or apparent only as sharp waves or periodic discharges superimposed on the background.

The major purpose of the diagnostic evaluation in patients known to have seizures is the exclusion of brain neoplasms or other focal pathologic conditions that might be correctable. MRI or CT, especially in those with focal abnormalities on EEG or neurologic examination are now routinely done. More than 95% of brain neoplasms are detected by MRI; however, when there is a very strong suspicion of a focal lesion, such as in a young person with repeated partial motor seizures, especially jacksonian, without other explanation, cerebral angiography can be considered even if the results of MRI or CT scanning are negative.

MRI has dramatically improved the evaluation of epilepsy. MRI is clearly advantageous over CT in the evaluation of partial seizures because it allows additional planes of evaluation to the transverse cuts of CT. Coronal sections have made it possible to study the hippocampal gyri, a frequent site of pathology in these seizures. Also, lack of bone artifact allows for better resolution of the contents of middle cranial fossa, especially the cranial edges of the temporal lobe. It also provides a better anatomic resolution to distinguish small areas of sclerosis or vascular malformations (Table 56–1).

The MRI has been particularly revolutionary in diagnosis of hippocampal sclerosis, especially prior to surgery.[23, 24] In patients with partial seizures or focal findings, repeating the MRI or CT scan after an appropriate interval of a year or so, especially if seizures are difficult to control, is appropriate.

TABLE 56–1. MAGNETIC RESONANCE IMAGING FINDINGS IN PATIENTS WITH SIMPLE OR COMPLEX PARTIAL SEIZURES

Nonspecific
Asymmetry of lateral and temporal horns (coronal cuts)
Focal areas of cerebral atrophy
Compensatory enlargement of adjacent ventricle
Compensatory enlargement of adjacent sulci
Subarachnoid cysts (compensatory)
Specific
Heterotopic gray matter
Foreign tissue
Tumors (high grade, low grade)
Hamartomas
Tuberous sclerosis
Vascular malformation
Arteriovenous malformations
Cavernous hemangiomas
Hippocampal sclerosis

MANAGEMENT

As a general rule, the diagnosis of a seizure disorder is sufficient indication for treatment. There are rare exceptions. Some authorities consider a single seizure in an otherwise healthy patient with a normal or nearly normal EEG to require nothing more than close follow-up; needless to say, a substantial number of such patients will develop further seizures.[25] When seizures have occurred in the context of an intercurrent medical illness with hypoglycemia, severe electrolyte or blood gas abnormality, or other precipitating factors, a work-up should be undertaken to exclude an underlying seizure focus within the cortex. In the absence of such a focus, treatment of the medical problem may be more reasonable than commitment to long-term anticonvulsants. Withdrawal seizures from barbiturates, tranquilizers, or alcohol have usually run their course after a series of one or a few grand mal seizures by the time the patient is seen by the physician. Animal experiments in the past had suggested that drug withdrawal seizures are relatively impervious to anticonvulsant medication, but a study of alcoholics in a drug detoxification center indicates that early prophylactic use of phenytoin may markedly reduce the tendency to have withdrawal seizures, although the withdrawal state is not aborted.[26] Some alcoholics, often because of suffering previous head trauma, have an underlying seizure disorder. This poses a difficult problem in management because the seizures may be exacerbated by varying alcohol intake and erratic compliance with antiseizure medications. Except for these patients, once withdrawal seizures have run their course, long-term anticonvulsant therapy is useful only to help prevent seizures if another period of drug or alcohol abuse is followed by a period of abstinence. Unfortunately, patient compliance with anticonvulsant therapy is generally poor in alcohol or drug abuse populations.

Several principles guide the selection and administration of chronic anticonvulsant therapy. First, therapy should be initiated with a single drug, which is gradually increased at intervals of several days or weeks until either toxicity supervenes or control occurs. When seizures persist despite therapeutic levels of one drug, a second drug may be added and the first drug can often be carefully discontinued if seizure control is attained. Simple grand mal seizures, especially if occurring infrequently before the initiation of therapy, may require only a single drug in therapeutic dosage for complete control. However, partial seizures and psychomotor epilepsy more often require more than one drug for satisfactory control. In some cases, when complete control can be obtained only by using multiple drugs with resulting significant side effects, a compromise may be desirable in which occasional innocuous spells are preferred to a permanent state of reduced alertness from excessive drug intake. In many cases, addition of a third or fourth drug does not result in substantially better control.

The choice of drugs is guided by the type of seizures, the patient's previous response to the medication, and the relative desirability or undesirability of particular side effects. For example, a patient with liver dysfunction due to a medical condition should avoid drugs such as carbamazepine (Tegretol) or valproic acid (Depakene), which have the potential for further serious hepatic toxicity. The basic decision regarding treatment concerns two major seizure types: petit mal and grand mal. Partial seizures are treated with essentially the same drugs as grand mal seizures, although some authorities would contend that partial seizures with complex symptomatology (psychomotor seizures) are better treated with phenytoin (Dilantin), carbamazepine, or primidone (Mysoline) than with phenobarbital. Myoclonic and akinetic seizures, chiefly of concern in a pediatric practice, are best treated with the benzodiazepines; they will not be discussed further.

Treatment for grand mal seizures is usually initiated with either phenytoin or phenobarbital. The latter has the advantage of extremely low long-term toxicity, but a considerable overlap between the toxic range for its sedative properties and the therapeutic range make it less desirable for some vigorous patients. In the very old and the very young, phenobarbital may cause paradoxical excitement. Phenytoin, on the other hand, rarely produces significant drowsiness or incoordination in the therapeutic range. Gum hypertrophy and hirsutism may present unacceptable problems for some patients concerned about their appearance, especially young females. The former can usually be managed by adjusting the dose, daily attention to dental hygiene, and regular visits to the dentist. The latter complication is fortunately not common. Carbamazepine or primidone constitute third-choice or accessory drugs for the control of grand mal or partial seizures. The use of combinations of phenobarbital and primidone or mephobarbital (Mebaral) and primidone is illogical in view of the rapid metabolism of primidone to phenobarbital in most subjects.

With true petit mal seizures, ethosuximide (Zarontin) or sodium valproate are the drugs of choice. Sodium valproate has been used successfully for over 10 years for the control of petit mal seizures and as an accessory drug in the control of virtually all other forms of seizure disorder.[27] This wide spectrum of usefulness, coupled with its low incidence of side effects, makes sodium valproate an important addition to the anticonvulsant formulary. At present the indications for the use of oxazolidinediones (trimethadione [Tridione] and paramethadione [Paradione]) are unclear; only rare patients intolerant of the aforementioned first-line drugs should be exposed to the greater risk of side effects, including nephrotic syndrome, posed by the oxazolidinediones. In some cases, supplementation of the regimen with acetazolamide (Diamox) may improve control in petit mal epilepsy.

Anticonvulsant drugs should be administered in the simplest possible schedule. Except for sodium valproate, most of the drugs have long biologic half-lives and therefore require only once or at most twice daily administration. This has the advantage of ensuring compliance by relieving the patient of the necessity of carrying pills to work or school to be taken in the middle of the day. In some patients, especially those on phenobarbital and primidone, an acute dose-related sedation may complicate the administration of large single doses and lead to the use of small doses during the day with a larger dose at bedtime.

Patients taking anticonvulsants should be monitored closely to ensure adequate blood levels of the drug. There is a wide range of individual variability, both in the rapidity with which drugs are metabolized and in the degree to which concurrent administration of other drugs alters the rate of metabolism of the drug in question. Blood levels should be checked at intervals of several months and especially 7 to 10 half-lives after an alteration in dosage. A number of studies have demonstrated that serum levels from most anticonvulsants correlate well in a group of patients with therapeutic efficacy and with the presence of side effects.[28] For this reason, measurement of the blood level can monitor the adequacy of intake and can serve to distinguish toxicity of one drug from another. It should be emphasized, however, that for any given patient the proper blood level depends on individual factors: a patient without nystagmus who achieves control of seizures with a slightly high phenytoin level should not be subjected to the risk of further seizures in order to lower the level to the therapeutic range. Similarly, a patient whose seizures have been completely controlled for years need not have the dosage of medication increased because a blood level is slightly below the usual therapeutic range, nor should complaints of excessive sedation be ignored because a blood level lies in the therapeutic range. Absence of seizures and freedom from side effects are the goals of treatment; blood levels are only a guide, albeit an important one, toward achieving those goals.

Although individual laboratories differ in the precise range accepted as therapeutic for a given anticonvulsant, the levels given in Table 56–2 are close to those found in most institutions.[29–31]

The relationship between the blood level of an agent and the dose administered is not always linear. This is particularly true of phenytoin. Once binding sites, renal excretory capacity, or metabolic enzymes become saturated, the blood level tends to rise more markedly with smaller increments in dosage (saturation kinetics). Thus, if the level of phenytoin is 6 μg/ml and one desires a level of 12 to 15, doubling the intake—for example, from 300 to 600 mg/day—may result in a substantial rise in the level to the toxic range. As a general rule, changes in phenytoin dosage in the therapeutic range should be made gradually, in 50- or 30-mg increments.

In summary, blood levels may be useful in any of the following situations: (1) checking the adequacy of dose (individual daily doses of phenytoin to achieve the same blood level may vary from 200 to 600 mg); (2) checking on patient compliance with the medication regimen; (3) assessing the effect of newly added drugs on the levels of previously administered ones; (4) spotting rare individuals who fail to absorb sufficient amounts of the drug; and (5) confirming the diagnosis of toxic side effects, such as drowsiness, ataxia, dizziness, diplopia, and dysarthria, which usually represent excessive blood levels.

Finally, patients treated with anticonvulsants should undergo periodic physical examinations to spot early idiosyncratic side effects and to ensure that no lesion missed in the initial evaluation has now become evident. EEGs should be performed every few years to assess the nature of the abnormal activity and to monitor the appearance of new focal abnormalities. However, frequent use of EEGs in

TABLE 56–2. ANTICONVULSANT DRUGS*

Drug	Half-life in Adults (hr)	Time to Steady State (days)	Therapeutic Range of Serum Concentration (μg/ml)	Protein Binding (%)	Daily Dosage (mg/kg)	Indications	Common Adverse Effects	Idiosyncratic Effects
Phenobarbital	45–136	14–21	15–40	40–60	1.5–3	Still used in treatment of status and as secondary drug of choice for major motor seizures. No longer a primary drug for any seizure in adults.	Sedation (in adults); hyperactivity (in children); behavior changes (depression); cognitive dysfunction; lethargy; osteopenia.	Morbidiform rash, exfoliative dermatitis (Stevens-Johnson), hepatic failure, granulocyte suppression.
Primidone†	6–18	4–7	5–12	0	5–12	Used same as phenobarbital but also secondary drug in complex partial seizures. (Metabolites include phenobarbital.)	Sedation, dizziness, nausea, and GI‡ irritability, ataxia, loss of libido, cognitive changes.	Same as phenobarbital
Phenytoin	10–34	7–8	10–20	69–96	3–8	Still widely used for generalized tonic-clonic seizures. Also for simple partial and complex partial seizures.	Drowsiness, cognitive changes, ataxia, dyskinesias, hirsutism, coarse facial features, gingival hyperplasia, osteopenia, lymphadenopathy, anemia (megaloblastic), neuropathy. Teratogenic.	Allergic/exfoliative dermatitis, hepatic failure, agranulocytosis, aplastic anemia, lupus-like reactions, hyperglycemia.
Carbamazepine	14–27	3–4	4–12	66–89	10–15	First-line drug for complex partial seizures and simple seizures. Also used in major motor (generalized tonic-clonic) seizures.	Blurred/double vision, dizziness, lethargy, loss of energy, behavior changes, cognitive changes, dyskinesias, conduction blocks. Teratogenic.	Agranulocytosis and granulocyte suppression, aplastic anemia, morbidiform rash, exfoliative dermatitis, hepatic failure, kidney failure.
Valproate	6–15	1–2	50–100	80–95	20–30	Drug of choice in absence seizure, myoclonic, atonic, and generalized tonic-clonic. Also used in simple and complex partial seizures.	GI upset (with Depakene), hepatic toxicity, hyperammonemia, behavior changes, tremor, nausea, weight gain, hair loss. Teratogenic.	Pancreatitis, hepatic failure, coma.
Clonazepam	20–40	—	>.03	47	.05–0.1	As a second drug of choice in minor motor and absence seizures. Also in complex partial seizures.	Drowsiness, ataxia, behavior disorders.	

*From Khoshbin S., Seizure disorders. Intensive Rev Intern Med, 29, 30, 31, 1993.
†Metabolized to phenobarbital and phenylethylmalonamide. Both of these derivatives have antiepileptic activity.
‡GI = gastrointestinal.

the management of patients with seizures not yet controlled by medication is not likely to prove helpful in deciding the next therapeutic step and may cause unnecessary alarm owing to drug-induced slowing.

Anticonvulsant Drugs[29–31]

Phenytoin (formerly called diphenylhydantoin) is a major anticonvulsant, most useful because of its relative freedom from sedation and its long half-life (average, about 22 hours). It is usually administered in divided or single doses, the latter particularly advisable because of the greater ease of patient compliance. (Some generic preparations of phenytoin require multiple daily dosing; confusion between the long-acting form and these generic forms may result in a loss of seizure control.) Total daily dose in an adult ranges from 200 to 800 mg/day, usually 300 to 400 mg/day. The elderly may require only 200 mg/day. At therapeutic concentrations (10 to 20 μg/ml), the enzyme system responsible for its hydroxylation is nearly saturated, so that small increments in daily dosage may produce large changes in plasma concentration. At low plasma levels, similar changes in daily intake may have modest effects on plasma concentration. A plasma concentration in the therapeutic range is well correlated with both a reduction in seizure frequency and relative freedom from toxic side effects. The presence of nystagmus and mild difficulty with tandem gait are convenient clinical means of assessing therapeutic concentrations.

Early toxicity is usually manifested as gastrointestinal irritation, which passes, or a skin rash, most commonly morbilliform, which usually necessitates discontinuation of the drug. Excessive blood levels are associated with dizziness, ataxia, slurred speech, and lethargy. A number of idiosyncratic reations occur infrequently with phenytoin usage. Megaloblastic anemia, probably reflecting interference with folic acid utilization, may be overcome by large doses of folate (50 to 100 mg/day). Osteomalacia in children results from either increased hepatic metabolism of vitamin D, reduced absorption of calcium, or both; it is accompanied by reduced serum calcium and elevated alkaline phosphatase levels. Treatment consists of vitamin D supplementation, usually 50,000 units/month.

In some individuals, hirsutism or gingival hypertrophy may limit the usefulness of phenytoin; serious consideration should be given to alternative drugs in young, growing women. Scrupulous attention to dental hygiene and modification of dose may minimize the development of gingival hyperplasia.

Rarely, during the first few months of administration, a generalized painless lymphadenopathy may develop, accompanied by systemic symptoms. Similarity to lymphoma often causes unnecessary concern, but no Reed-Sternberg cells are seen on biopsy, and the condition resolves spontaneously after discontinuing phenytoin.

Of the present major anticonvulsants, phenobarbital has been used the longest. Its half-life is comparable to that of phenytoin, and once or twice daily administration is usually sufficient to obtain therapeutic levels (15 to 40 μg/ml) in most patients. Divided dosage, with the largest dose at bedtime, may help some individuals cope with the sedative side effects of large single doses. As a single drug, dosages of 90 to 180 mg/day are recommended; as an adjunct to other drugs, slightly lower doses may be used.

The major advantage of phenobarbital is its relative freedom from long-term side effects. On the other hand, it is more likely to produce sedation at therapeutic levels than either phenytoin or carbamazepine. In children and elderly adults, this sedation may produce a paradoxic excitement or behavior disorders. Interference with vitamin K metabolism may require supplemental vitamin K administration in pregnant women just before term.

With both phenytoin and phenobarbital, changes in daily dosage may require 4 to 7 days before a new steady state is achieved. Using phenytoin, with which dose-related sedation is usually not a problem, more rapid attainment of higher levels may be accomplished by temporary administration of higher doses for 3 to 4 days. In the case of patients not previously taking phenytoin, or in those with very low levels, intravenous loading, with up to 1000 mg at 25 to 50 mg/min, or rapid oral loading, 400 mg every 6 hours for 24 hours, may be helpful when rapid attainment of therapeutic levels is desirable.

Carbamazepine has been used for 20 years in the treatment of generalized and focal seizures, especially partial complex seizures. It is given in divided doses, usually 600 to 1200 mg/day, to attain a therapeutic level of 4 to 12 μg/ml. Plasma levels, unlike those with phenytoin, are linearly related to the level of oral intake. Establishment of a stable dosage should be approached gradually over several days to avoid gastrointestinal side effects. Sedation is uncommon in the therapeutic range, but diplopia is frequent with toxic levels. There are two major adverse effects of carbamazepine: cutaneous reactions, which may become severe and desquamative in character if the medication is not discontinued; and bone marrow depression, although true aplastic anemia persisting after withdrawal of the drug is extremely rare (estimated at 1 in 40,000 to 100,000 individuals exposed to the drug). Routine blood counts should be performed at 3 weeks, 6 weeks, 3 months, and 6 months after the initiation of therapy, and at greater intervals thereafter. Serious blood reactions have not been recorded after 1 year's continuous administration.[32]

Carbamazepine is the drug of choice in partial complex seizures (psychomotor seizures). Not only does it control seizures more effectively than other major anticonvulsants, but it also appears to have certain desirable psychotropic effects on behavior, perhaps as a result of its similarity to tricyclic antidepressants. Its relative freedom from sedation is another advantage, especially in patients subject to seizures in the drowsy state. Carbamazepine is often useful in focal seizure disorders that are refractory to phenytoin or phenobarbital.

Primidone is closely related to phenobarbital, into which it is converted in vivo. It is quite likely that primidone itself possesses anticonvulsant properties, as does its other metabolite, phenylethylmalonamide. In different individuals, the relative amounts of primidone and phenobarbital differ; close monitoring of blood levels therefore requires simultaneous determination of both compounds. The therapeutic level of primidone lies between 5 and 12 μg/ml.

Primidone is useful in the treatment, especially adjunctive treatment, of both tonic-clonic seizures and partial seizures. There is no convincing evidence that it is superior to other drugs for partial complex seizures, and many authorities would recommend phenytoin or carbamazepine rather than phenobarbital or primidone.

The drug is given three or four times a day, commencing therapy with a low dose (125 mg two or three times a day) and gradually increasing by 125-mg increments to therapeutic doses (250 mg three or four times a day in adults). The major disadvantages of primidone relate to the necessity of multiple doses per day, transient but frequently annoying sedation, and gastrointestinal upset, as well as the necessity for two drug determinations to monitor levels, which are not always well correlated with toxic manifestations.

Side effects of primidone include nausea, vomiting, central nervous system depression (ataxia, nystagmus, dysarthria), megaloblastic anemia secondary to folic acid deficiency, and skin rashes. Any side effect of phenobarbital is potentially applicable to primidone.

The treatment of petit mal disorder is largely confined to the administration of ethosuximide or sodium valproate; trimethadione and paramethadione are only infrequently employed at present. Ethosuximide, in addition to its effectiveness against petit mal seizures, may be useful in the treatment, alone or in combination with other drugs, of minor absences associated with atypical petit mal seizures and of myoclonic seizures. Ethosuximide is well absorbed orally and has a long half-life in both adults and children. Despite this, it is usually given two to three times a day, commencing therapy with one capsule (250 mg) each day and continuing with an additional capsule every week to 10 days until a therapeutic response is achieved or therapeutic levels are attained. These levels range from 40 to 100 μg/ml. Different individuals may require quite different dosages to achieve these levels.

Side effects are infrequent, consisting most frequently of nausea, vomiting, and sedation. Transient leukopenia may occur, as well as other blood dyscrasias, skin reactions, and, rarely, lupus erythematosus.

Valproic acid was introduced to the United States in 1978 after 10 years of use in Europe. It differs from other anticonvulsants in its relatively simple structure (eight-carbon branched-chain carboxylic acid), its relatively short half-life (8 to 15 hours), requiring multiple doses per day, and its efficacy against a wide range of seizure types, including petit mal, generalized tonic-clonic seizures, and partial seizures, both simple and complex. Except for typical petit mal, valproate is usually given with other anticonvulsants as adjunctive therapy. Only myoclonic seizures (best treated with clonazepam or other benzodiazepines) seem resistant to its effects. Treatment is usually begun with 250 mg two or three times a day, with increases by 250 mg every 3 to 4 days until a therapeutic effect is obtained or the therapeutic range is reached. Therapeutic levels range from 50 to 100 μg/ml, levels that are usually attained in adults by dosages of 1500 to 2000 mg/day in three or four doses. Profound alterations in the levels of other anticonvulsants given concurrently have been observed—either to the point of toxicity (phenobarbital) or ineffectiveness (phenytoin); follow-up blood levels are required when adding valproate to an anticonvulsant regimen, especially if seizures are not controlled or toxicity appears.

Early side effects are usually gastrointestinal; they may be alleviated in many cases by taking the medicine with meals or a snack. An enteric-coated preparation (Depakote) is frequently better tolerated. Transient alopecia and thrombocytopenia have been reported. The most common serious side effect has been liver toxicity, with a hepatocellular profile that often reverts to normal with downward adjustment of the dose. Rarely, progressive parenchymal liver damage results in liver failure.

Recently two benzodiazepine derivatives have become available in this country: clonazepam (Klonopin) and nitrazepam (Mogadon). Clonazepam is effective against minor motor seizures (myoclonic, akinetic) in children and myoclonic seizures in adults (for example, in uremia). In addition, it may be used as an adjunctive drug in the management of partial complex seizures, especially in patients whose EEG is characterized by spike-wave abnormalities. Dosage should be initiated at 0.5 mg three times a day, with gradual increases up to 2 mg three times a day; dosages above 6 mg/day are rarely justified. Therapeutic blood levels lie above 0.03 μg/ml, but these levels should be treated only as guidelines in the patient who is taking other anticonvulsants. Side effects are primarily sedation and ataxia. Hypersecretion from the upper respiratory tract and excessive salivation may result in serious problems for individuals with chronic respiratory disease, asthma, or difficulty in handling secretions. Most individuals placed on clonazepam develop tolerance to its effects within 6 to 12 months; restarting the drug after a brief "holiday" may restore its efficacy.[33]

Nitrazepam has recently become available in this country for the management of myoclonic and akinetic attacks; it appears to be the most effective drug against myoclonic seizures. The dose is 5 to 10 mg/day; peak blood levels are obtained within about 2 hours; 85% of the circulating drug is bound to plasma protein. Side effects are confined to drowsiness and confusion, the latter especially in the elderly.[34]

New Anticonvulsants

As we gain a clearer understanding of cellular mechanisms of epilepsy, new drugs are being added to the antiepileptic armamentarium after a long hiatus. These are mostly based on inhibitor effects of γ-aminobutyric acid (GABA), calcium channel activity, and effect on *N*-methyl-D-aspartate (NMDA) receptors. Although not quite on the market yet, most of these are in the last stages of clinical trials.

GABAergic Drugs. GABA constitutes the main inhibitory neurotransmitter. A number of drugs are being tried that effect GABA concentration.

Vigabatrin. Vigabatrin inhibits GABA transaminase and therefore increases GABA concentration.

GABApentin. Gabapentin, an amino acid structurally similar to GABA, has shown promise as an adjunct in treatment of generalized tonic-clonic and partial complex seizures.

Clobazam. This new benzodiazepine, like others of its class, has a broad spectrum with fewer of the common benzodiazepine side effects and a longer half-life specifically effective against reading epilepsy.

Other promising new anticonvulsants are felbamate (structurally related to meprobamate), effective in partial seizures, and lamotrigine (an antifolate drug), again, effective in partial seizures.

Also, new variations on established anticonvulsants to give fewer side effects and longer half-lives are eterobarb (a barbiturate) with less of a hypnotic effect; carbamazepine-OROS, a slow releasing carbamazepine; stiripentol (an alcohol), shows a synergistic effect with carbamazepine in the treatment of complex partial seizures. And finally a new calcium channel blocker, flunarizine, has shown antiepileptic properties, but adverse effects are still being evaluated.[35]

Refractory and Recurrent Seizures

In patients with refractory seizures, a systemic trial of a wide spectrum of suitable drugs should be made, each drug being pushed to tolerance or high therapeutic levels before another is tried. Drugs that do not reduce the seizure frequency appreciably should be discontinued; it is rarely necessary to have the patient taking more than three drugs at a time. In discontinuing medication, even of an auxiliary drug, dosage should be gradually tapered over several weeks. The most common cause of status epilepticus is sudden withdrawal of medication.

Failure to control seizures despite therapeutic levels of two or more drugs may result from numerous factors: (1) wrong choice of medication—for example, use of a major anticonvulsant to control petit mal seizures; (2) paradoxic increase in seizures with increased medication, sometimes seen with phenytoin but recently reported for carbamazepine; (3) excessive sedation, which may lead to seizures in some patients, especially those with partial complex seizures; (4) hysterical seizures replacing true seizures; (5) progression of an underlying neurologic disorder that may require discovery or further definition; and (6) drug-resistant epilepsy. Porter has used simultaneous video recording of seizures and EEG, EEG telemetry, and frequent assessment of plasma anticonvulsant concentrations to improve seizure control in 70%, reduce drug toxicity in 83%, and improve social adjustment in 50% of 23 patients with intractable epilepsy.[36]

As a general rule, failure to control seizures despite additional drugs in higher doses should lead to a reassessment of the whole regimen and gradual simplification of the regimen. Shifts from one drug to another or discontinuation of a major drug should be undertaken gradually; in those with a serious potential for frequent grand mal seizures, this may have to be accomplished in the hospital.

The recurrence of seizures after a period of good control should prompt a diligent search for complicating factors. Most commonly, these include inadequate dosage to maintain therapeutic levels, lapses in patient compliance, or intercurrent illness, such as electrolyte abnormalities, infection, or liver or kidney disease. Worsening of the condition that led to the seizure disorder may be evaluated by repeating the EEG and MRI or CT scan. A patient whose results on initial neurologic evaluation for central nervous system pathology were negative may experience a reappearance of seizures as the sole manifestation of a slowly growing tumor, especially a glioma or oligodendroglioma.

Over time, on the same dose, plasma levels may decline, and the initial inclination will often be to attribute any recurrence of seizures to inadequate anticonvulsant levels. One must be careful in such patients, however, to exclude intercurrent illness, for example, pneumonia, which may be responsible for precipitating attacks in a person whose seizures had previously been controlled by barely therapeutic drug levels.

Surgical Management

Most major medical centers have now established epilepsy surgery and long-term inpatient monitoring units because of a resurgence of interest in the surgical therapy for epilepsy. These evaluations are obviously costly, and in the current economic circumstances, there is controversy regarding the cost-benefit aspects of monitoring and surgery in epilepsy.[37]

In patients with intractable, disabling epilepsy from focal cortical lesions or from a discrete temporal lobe focus, surgery may be considered when drug therapy fails. Two major types of resection surgery are performed: local excision of seizure foci associated with cortical scars and temporal lobectomy for seizures occurring in the temporal lobe. Rasmussen reviewed the results of local excision in focal epilepsy and concluded that 32 to 46% became seizure-free, depending on the site of the excision, and 63 to 69% improved.[38] Falconer has been the major advocate of temporal lobectomy for intractable temporal lobe epilepsy, when the discharge could be localized reliably to one side and when conventional therapy had failed. In his first 100 cases, 39 were free of seizures (follow-up of 2 to 10 years), 14 were markedly improved, and 17 did not respond; in the second 100 cases, 62 were improved or free of seizures, and 10 did not respond.[39] Curiously, patients with mesial temporal sclerosis had a better outcome than those with no identifiable lesion. Selective amygdalahippocampectomy, which allows for nonrestrictive ablation, has recently been tried.[40]

Interest in surgical therapy is high in patients with frontal lobe foci because this is a surgically approachable area. Other surgical procedures previously abandoned because of complications are returning as more sophisticated evaluation prior to surgery makes patient selection more reasonable. These are hemispherectomy and corpus collosotomy, especially for seizures with secondary generalization.[41]

Pregnancy

Pregnancy in a woman under treatment for seizures raises important questions regarding the efficacy and safety of anticonvulsants in this situation, as well as the effects of the seizure disorder on the fetus. In patients with established seizures before pregnancy, seizure frequency will increase in 45%, decrease in 5%, and remain unchanged in 50%. Not surprisingly, a greater degree of seizure control prior to pregnancy is associated with a better prognosis during pregnancy, but exceptions occur.[42]

One of the major factors contributing to impaired seizure control during pregnancy is the alteration of anti-convulsant distribution and metabolism. Plasma levels of phenytoin and phenobarbital fall progressively during pregnancy secondary to fluid retention, increased hepatic metabolism, and poor intake due to nausea.[43]

There seems little question that epileptics suffer more problems during pregnancy than comparable nonepileptic mothers, but the precise role of seizures as opposed to that of anticonvulsant medication is unclear. These problems include vaginal bleeding, toxemia, and excessive vomiting. Moreover, delivery is marked by an increased incidence of prematurity, small-for-dates babies, and perinatal mortality and morbidity. However, most of the increased seizure rate is due to noncompliance or sleep deprivation.

Greatest attention, both by lay persons and physicians, has focused on the occurrence of congenital malformations, which occur in 1 to 6% of babies born to non–drug-treated mothers. Cardiac defects, especially atrial and ventricular septal defects, cleft lips, and cleft palates are the most common abnormalities. The fetal hydantoin syndrome includes cranial abnormalities (epicanthal folds; hypertelorism; short, upturned nose; ptosis; malformed, low-set ears; and altered cranial configuration), strabismus, limb defects (hypoplastic fingers and malformed thumbs), intrauterine growth retardation, and frequent mental retardation. A different syndrome has been seen in infants of mothers taking trimethadione, as well as occasionally phenobarbital or primidone. No syndrome related to carbamazepine has been reported, though there may be increased risk of spina bifida and other malformations in these mothers.

Management of the pregnant epileptic involves the establishment of therapeutic levels of the minimum number of drugs required to establish good seizure control. Preferably, only one drug is used. Trimethadione is highly teratogenic and should be avoided; valproic acid is relatively contraindicated because of its high teratogenic potential. Switching between phenytoin, phenobarbital, and carbamazepine in anticipation of pregnancy or after attainment of pregnancy probably makes little sense because their potential for teratogenesis is comparable, and the threat of seizures from the transition may pose problems. Plasma levels should be checked frequently, about every 4 to 6 weeks, especially toward the end of pregnancy, and intake adjusted appropriately to maintain therapeutic levels. Changes in regimen should occur only when seizure control is poor despite therapeutic levels. Tonic-clonic seizures during pregnancy increase the risk of miscarriage, premature labor, and future learning disabilities in the child.

Infants exposed to phenytoin, barbiturates, or trimethadione sometimes manifest bleeding disorders in the first 24 hours of life, probably related to drug-induced depression of vitamin K–dependent clotting factors. This can be treated with one or more injections of vitamin K and routine evaluation of clotting parameters. Fresh frozen plasma is required if hemorrhage occurs.

SOCIAL AND LEGAL ISSUES

No discussion of the management of seizure disorders would be complete without some reference to the considerable social and legal implications of the diagnosis. Each state differs in its precise requirements, but most states impose obligations on both the physician and the patient in regard to driving. Every physician who treats seizure disorders should become familiar with the laws of his or her state. Most states require a period of abstention from driving following the diagnosis of a seizure disorder and a minimum period of seizure-free status before the resumption of driving. These requirements are generally binding on patients with an element of impaired consciousness during their seizures; the strictures may be less severe in the case of focal seizures without loss of consciousness.

Engaging in sports or occupations in which a sudden impairment of consciousness would lead to almost certain injury should be discouraged. Skiing, bobsledding, mountain climbing, and swimming without a companion pose hazards that are frequently unacceptable; operating milling machines, lathes, saws, or other dangerous equipment is in the same class. Further restrictions usually depend on the nature of the seizures (rate of onset and degree of impairment) and their frequency. Finally, it is essential that patients receive a thorough explanation of the nature of epilepsy or seizures and that efforts be made to dispel the mistaken but nonetheless prevalent popular notions regarding this illness. Family members are entitled to the same complete explanation and will often require instruction in the proper steps to take if a seizure should occur.

STOPPING MEDIATIONS

In many patients, complete control of seizures for a period of years leads to the inevitable question: *When can I stop the medicine?* Unfortunately, although guidelines exist,[44] their application to a particular patient's situation is often difficult. The end result is frequently a semienlightened form of gambling with the odds. Certain factors in the history raise the risk of discontinuing therapy. More severe seizure disorder, as measured by frequency of seizures before medication is instituted or by frequent seizures while on medication, is associated with increased risk of recurrence. A long history of seizures, even if infrequent, should suggest an ongoing seizure diathesis as opposed to the patient with a similar number of seizures over a short period. Onset of seizures after the age of 30 years has a higher incidence of recurrence when no medication is being taken. EEG abnormalities, such as focal slowing or bilateral paroxysmal spike or sharp-wave activity, either before the institution of therapy, during therapy, or following withdrawal of medication, are usually associated with an increased risk of recurrence. In one series in which 200 patients were withdrawn from medication after 2 or more years of control, 40% had recurrences, 75% of those within the first year.[45] Most investigators agree that the risk of further seizures is greater in those with partial seizures than in those with generalized seizures of the grand mal type.

Practice varies in different clinics, but a seizure-free period of at least 2 years and possibly longer (in the patient with a longer history of seizures) should be achieved before drug withdrawal is considered. In suitable candidates, an EEG before tapering the medication over several months and a satisfactory EEG result (absence of focal slowing or bilateral paroxysmal changes) after the cessation of all drugs are necessary conditions for the further withholding of anticonvulsants. However, a normal or mildly abnormal EEG result is no guarantee of a sustained remission. Patients should avoid driving during the period of tapering and for several months thereafter. In many cases, a frank discussion of the risks and potential difficulties involved will lead to a mutual decision to continue the medication indefinitely.

PROGNOSIS

With the increasing availability of reasonably safe medications for the control of seizures, the ancient prospect of social disruption and intellectual deterioration—possibly resulting from anoxia or other complications of uncontrolled seizures—no longer fits this disorder. Provided physicians realize that the goal of treatment is the prevention of all seizures, suitable adjustments of medication will render a large percentage of patients with epilepsy free of all seizures or only minimally inconvenienced by minor episodes. Even psychomotor seizures, sometimes dismayingly refractory to anticonvulsant therapy, can be satisfactorily controlled in many patients. A study from England showed that 88% of patients with the diagnosis of psychomotor epilepsy followed up in a clinic were working and productive.[46] Many individuals will become seizure-free over a period of many years, whether given medications or not. Further understanding of the pathogenesis of seizure disorders as well as newer anticonvulsant drugs should improve even this optimistic prognosis.

ACKNOWLEDGMENT

The author acknowledges with gratitude the contributions of Harris Funkenstein, MD.

REFERENCES

1. Kurland L: The incidence and prevalence of convulsive disorders in a small urban community. Epilepsia 1:143, 1959.
2. Jackson H: On convulsive seizure: Lecture I. BMJ 1:703, 1890.
3. Gastaut H: Clinical and electroencephalographic classification of epileptic seizures. Epilepsia 11:102, 1970.
4. Commission on Classification and Terminology of the International League Against Epilepsy: Proposal for revised clinical

and electroencephalographic classification of epileptic seizures. Epilepsia 22:489, 1981.
5. Livingston S: Comprehensive Management of Epilepsy in Infancy, Childhood and Adolescence. Springfield, IL, Charles C. Thomas, 1972.
6. Thompson SW and Greenhouse HA: Petit mal status in adults. Ann Intern Med 68:1271, 1968.
7. Orbery JM and Whitty CWM: Causes and consequences of status epilepticus in adults: A study of 86 cases. Brain 94:733, 1971.
8. Delgado-Escutea AV, Wasterlain CG, Treiman DM, and Porter RJ (eds): Status epilepticus, mechanisms of brain damage and treatment. Adv Neurol 34 (entire volume), 1983.
9. Williams D: Temporal lobe epilepsy. BMJ 1:1439, 1966.
10. Blumer D: Temporal lobe epilepsy and its psychiatric significance. In Benson DF and Blumer D (eds): Psychiatric Aspects of Neurological Disease. New York, Grune & Stratton, 1975, pp 171–198.
11. Waxman SG and Geschwind N: Hypergraphia in temporal lobe epilepsy. Neurology 24:629, 1974.
12. McKenna P, Kane J, and Parrish K: Psychotic syndromes in epilepsy. Am J Psychiatry 142:895, 1985.
13. Khoshbin S: VanGogh's malady and other cases of Geschwind's syndrome. Neurology 36:213, 1986.
14. Martin H and McDowell F: Evaluation of seizures in the adult. Arch Neurol Psychiatr 71:101, 1954.
15. Ang R and Utterback R: Seizures with onset after forty years of age-role of cerebrovascular disease. South Med J 59:1404, 1966.
16. Raynor RB, Paine RS, and Carmichael EA: Epilepsy of late onset. Neurology 9:111, 1959.
17. Sumi S and Teasdall R: Focal seizures—a review of 150 cases. Neurology 13:582, 1963.
18. Berlin L: Significance of grand mal seizures developing in patients over thirty-five years of age. JAMA 152:794, 1953.
19. Woodcock S and Cosgrove JBR: Epilepsy after the age of 50: A five-year follow-up study. Neurology 14:34, 1964.
20. Ajmore-Marsan C and Zivin L: Factors related to the occurrence of typical paroxysmal abnormalities in the EEG records of epileptic patients. Epilepsia 11:361, 1970.
21. Mattson R, Pratt K, and Calverley J: Electroencephalograms of epileptics following sleep deprivation. Arch Neurol 13:310, 1965.
22. DeJesus P and Masland W: The role of nasopharyngeal electrodes in clinical electroencephalography. Neurology 20:869, 1970.
23. Kuzniecky R, de la Sayette V, Ethier R, et al: Magnetic imaging in temporal lobe epilepsy: Pathologic correlations. Ann Neurol 22:341, 1987.
24. Lencz T, McCarthy G, et al: Quantitative magnetic resonance imaging in temporal lobe epilepsy: Relationship to neuropathology and neuropsychological function. Ann Neurol 31:629, 1992.
25. Livingston S: Convulsive disorders in infants and children. *In* Levine SZ (ed): Advances in Pediatrics, Vol 10. Chicago, Year Book Medical Publishers, 1958.
26. Sampliner R and Iber FL: Diphenylhydantoin control of alcohol withdrawal seizures: Results of a controlled study. JAMA 230:1430, 1974.
27. Pinder RM, Brogden RM, Speight TM, et al: Sodium valproate: A review of its pharmacological properties and therapeutic efficacy in epilepsy. Drugs 13:81, 1977.
28. Kutt H and Penry JK: Usefulness of blood levels of antiepileptic drugs. Arch Neurol 31:283, 1974.
29. Browne TR: Clinical pharmacology of antiepileptic drugs. Drug Ther Rev 2:474, 1979.
30. Funkenstein HH: Anticonvulsant drugs. *In* Miller RR, Greenblatt DJ (eds): Handbook of Drug Therapy. New York, Elsevier, 1979, pp 585–603.
31. Eadie MJ and Tyrer JH: Anticonvulsant Therapy: Pharmacologic Basis and Practice, 2nd ed. Edinburgh, Churchill-Livingstone, 1980.
32. Hart RG and Easton JD: Carbamazepine and hematological monitoring. Ann Neurol 11:309, 1982.
33. Browne TR: Clonazepam. N Engl J Med 299:812, 1978.
34. Baruzzi A, Michelucci R, and Tassinari CA: Benzodiazopines: Nitrazepam. *In* Woodbury DM, Penry JK, and Pippenger CE (eds): Anti-Epileptic Drug. New York, Raven Press, 1982, pp 753–769.
35. Porter RJ: Mechanisms of action of new antiepileptic drugs. Epilepsia 30:S29, 1989.
36. Porter RJ, Penry JK, and Lacy JR: Diagnostic and therapeutic re-evaluation of patients with intractable epilepsy. Neurology 27:1006, 1977.
37. Silfrenius H: Economic costs of epilepsy: Treatment benefits. Acta Neurol Scand 78(Supp 117):136, 1988.
38. Rasmussen T: The role of surgery in the treatment of focal epilepsy. Clin Neurosurg 16:288, 1969.
39. Falconer MA: The surgical treatment of temporal lobe epilepsy. *In* Herrington RN (ed): Current Problems in Neuropsychiatry. London, Headley Bros, 1969, p 95.
40. Wieser HG: Selective amygdalo-hippocampectomy for temporal lobe epilepsy. Epilepsia 29(Supp 2):S100, 1988.
41. Spencer SS: Corpus callosum section and other disconnection procedures for medically intractable epilepsy. Epilepsia 29(Supp 2):S85, 1988.
42. Montouris GD, Fenichel GM, and McLain LW Jr: The pregnant epileptic. Arch Neurol 36:601, 1979.
43. Dalessio DJ: Seizure disorders and pregnancy. N Engl J Med 312:559, 1985.
44. Juul-Jansen P: Frequency of recurrence after discontinuance of anticonvulsant therapy in patients with epileptic seizures. Epilepsia 5:352, 1964.
45. Juul-Jansen P: Frequency of recurrence after discontinuance of anticonvulsant therapy in patients with epileptic seizures—A new follow-up study after 5 years. Epilepsia 9:11, 1968.
46. Currie S, Heathfield KWG, Henson RA, et al: Clinical course and prognosis of temporal lobe epilepsy: A survey of 666 patients. Brain 94:173, 1971.

57

Dementia

JAMES D. BOWEN, MD
ERIC B. LARSON, MD, MPH
WAYNE C. McCORMICK, MD, MPH

Cognitively impaired elderly patients are an increasingly common problem as the number of aged in our population rises. It is estimated that by the year 2000, 13% of the population will exceed 65 years of age, compared with 9% in 1960.[1] The age group over 85 years of age is the fastest growing age stratum in the population, expected to increase by 80% by the year 2000. The incidence of dementia increases with age; greater numbers of aging individuals and their later retirement will therefore magnify the personal and social consequences of dementing illnesses. In the United States, prevalence rates for dementia in those aged 65 or older range from 2.2 to 10.3%.[2, 3] It is estimated that between 17 and 47% of those aged 85 or older have dementia.[3, 4] National expenditures for care of the 2.4 million demented Americans in 1985 are estimated to be $35.8 billion. By 2040, this expenditure is expected to increase to $92 to $149 billion (in 1985 dollars) for 6.1 to 9.8 million demented Americans.[5] Faced with a problem of such obvious magnitude, clinicians require a logical and consistent approach.

DEFINITION

The most widely used definition of dementia is that of the *Diagnostic and Statistical Manual*, third edition, revised (DSM-III-R) of the American Psychiatric Association.[6] Dementia

1. Is acquired (excludes congenital disorders)
2. Includes impairment in short- and long-term memory
3. Is associated with impairment of one of the following: abstract thinking, impaired judgment, other disturbances of higher cortical function (aphasia, apraxia, agnosia, or contructional difficulties), or personality change (excludes isolated memory loss syndromes, such as amnestic syndrome)
4. Interferes significantly with work or usual social activities or relationships with others (excludes benign forgetfulness)
5. Does not occur exclusively during the course of delirium
6. Either an organic factor is identified that is judged to be etiologically related to the disturbance or the disturbance cannot be accounted for by any nonorganic mental disorder (e.g., major depression)

In addition to poor performance on mental status testing, the history and demeanor of the individual may fit a characteristic pattern seen in dementing illnesses. The symptoms have frequently been slowly progressive for a considerable time. The patient may seem relatively unconcerned about the problem or may try to conceal the disabilities by a defensiveness, resistance to testing, or a casual attempt to dodge the significance of the failure ("Oh, everyone knows that!"). If pressed, the patient's answers may initially be wide of the mark, then be corrected to more reasonable, though not always accurate, responses. In milder cases, memory for remote events may be better than for recent events. Inability to recall information tends to be persistent, unlike the normal elderly person who is temporarily unable to recall some familiar name or object but can remember it a few moments later. The demented patient may retain social skills until late in the course of the illness. Symptoms may temporarily worsen at night or in unfamiliar surroundings. Dementia-producing illnesses sometimes impair other functions in addition to those of cognition. Personality changes may include a reduced motivation, reduced interest in work and hobbies, irritability, inappropriate euphoria, and occasional paranoia. Mood may vary from elation to depression, even in the same individual within a few minutes (lability of affect).

SCREENING TESTS FOR DEMENTIA

Many tests have been developed to screen for dementia, each designed for specific clinical situations. The most widely used tool for screening patients suspected of having dementia is the mini–mental state examination (Fig. 57–1).[7] The performance on this screening varies with age and education.[8] We studied 150 patients complaining of memory loss, using full clinical and neuropsychological exami-

ORIENTATION

Maximum Score

5 What is the (year)(season)(date)(day)(month)?

5 Where are we: (state)(country)(town)(hospital)(floor)?

REGISTRATION

3 Name 3 objects. Give 1 second to say each. Then ask the patient all 3 after you have said them. Give 1 point for each correct answer. Then repeat them until the patient learns all 3 count trials and record.

ATTENTION AND CALCULATION

5 Serial 7s. 1 point for each correct. Stop after 5 answers. Alternatively spell "world" backwards.

RECALL

3 Ask for the 3 objects repeated above. Give 1 point for each correct answer.

LANGUAGE

9 Names a pencil, and watch (2 points)
Repeat the following "No ifs, ands, or buts." (1 point)
Follow a 3-stage command:
"Take a paper in your right hand, fold it in half, and put it on the floor." (3 points)

Read and obey the following:

CLOSE YOUR EYES. (1 point)

Write a sentence. (1 point)

Copy design. (1 point)

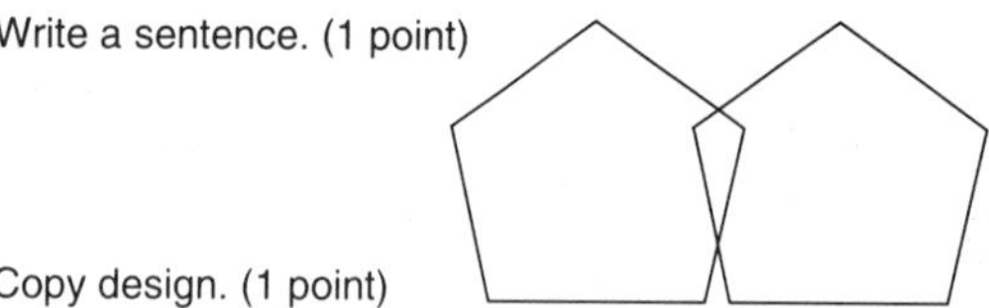

FIGURE 57–1. Mini–mental state examination.

nations as a gold standard. Considering a score of 24 or lower to be abnormal, we found a sensitivity of 61% and a specificity of 95% in those with a high school education. In those without a high school education, sensitivity rose to 75% and specificity fell to 75%. Thus, clinical judgment must be used in interpreting test results. In most persons with suspected dementia, systematic mental status examination or a screening test like the mini–mental state examination will be sufficient to diagnose the presence of dementia. Occasionally, additional formal neuropsychological testing will be helpful in patients who are not clearly demented and not clearly normal on bedside evaluation or after screening.

TABLE 57–1. PROBLEMS PRESENTING AS MEMORY LOSS

Dementia
Worried well
Normal aging
Depression
Delirium
Stroke syndromes
Bradykinesia
Abulia
Seizure
Excessive daytime somnolence
Amnestic syndrome

DIFFERENTIAL DIAGNOSIS OF MEMORY LOSS

Numerous conditions lead to complaints of memory loss (Table 57–1). In our series, 27% of those complaining of memory loss were not demented. These cases must be differentiated from those with true dementia.

Depression presenting as memory loss has been recognized since at least 1961.[9] Clinical items suggesting depression rather than dementia are listed in Table 57–2. In

TABLE 57–2. CLINICAL ITEMS FAVORING DEPRESSION RATHER THAN DEMENTIA

Depression precedes memory complaints
Past history of depression
Complaints are exaggerated
"Don't know" answers to questions
"Near miss" answers are uncommon
Orientation, memory, and physical examination are normal
Results of electroencephalogram are normal
Abrupt onset of symptoms
Short duration of symptoms
Fluctuating cognitive performance
Recent and remote memory losses are equally affected

several large series, the number of nondemented patients complaining of memory loss ranges from 7 to 15%. Of those not demented, about half are depressed.[10–12] There is no consensus on diagnostic criteria for depression in patients complaining of memory loss. Most studies have relied on clinical impression; some use DSM-III-R criteria for depression. Clinical screening tools for depression are available. Use of the dexamethasone suppression test to diagnose depression in demented patients may be misleading and is not recommended because half of elderly demented patients without depression have abnormal test results.[13] Abnormal dexamethasone suppression tests were noted in seven of 13 elderly depressed, 11 of 25 demented and seven of 12 combined depression-dementia patients.[14]

It is noteworthy that of patients with dementia, 10 to 15% have a concomitant depression.[15–17] Accompanying depression is more common in early dementia than in late disease, thus complicating the early diagnosis.[18] In one study, Reding and colleagues found that 24 of 85 patients referred to a dementia service were not demented. Of these 24, 15 were depressed. However, after 1 year, eight of these 15 depressed "nondemented" patients had intellectual impairment. None of the seven nondepressed nondemented patients deteriorated.[19]

Delirium is recognized by clouding of consciousness and reduced ability to sustain attention or shift focus. Illusions and hallucinations may be seen, speech may be incoherent at times, sleep-wake cycles are often disturbed, and psychomotor activity is increased or decreased. Metabolic alterations or infections, drug intoxications or withdrawal, or diffuse brain abnormalities are often responsible. *Stroke syndromes* refer to single infarctions rather than multi-infarct states. Isolated cognitive deficits are seen with stroke syndromes, allowing differentiation from dementia with its global deficits. Strokes with language dysfunction (aphasia) or spatial-constructional dysfunction (apraxia) may be mislabeled as dementia. Stroke syndromes with predominant cognitive changes include the "top of the basilar" stroke with bilateral hippocampal infarction (usually with cortical visual loss) and paramedian or tuberothalamic strokes of the thalamus. *Bradykinesia* may be mislabeled as dementia because of slowness in responses. Responses are typically correct however. Many parkinsonian syndromes also have a true dementia. *Abulia* refers to reduced spontaneous motor and verbal activity with responses occurring after a prolonged latency. The content of thought may be surprisingly intact. Abulia is usually seen in frontal lobe disease and hydrocephalus. *Seizures* are rarely mislabeled as dementia. These clearly episodic events are more likely to be confused with delirium. *Excessive daytime somnolence* is a symptom of many conditions, such as sleep apnea, narcolepsy, and stimulant withdrawal. These patients may appear demented due to their extreme sleepiness. The *amnestic syndrome* consists of an isolated loss of both short- and long-term memory. It is most commonly seen with alcohol abuse (Korsakoff's syndrome).

ETIOLOGIES

Dementia is a syndrome, not an etiologic diagnosis. Many different diseases are potentially capable of producing the clinical syndrome of dementia (Table 57–3). Many of these diseases may be recognized by historical clues, associated neurologic abnormalities, inheritance, or associated systemic illness. Of the multitude of dementing illnesses, only a few are common (Table 57–4).

IDIOPATHIC DEMENTIA

Alzheimer's disease is the most common dementia-producing illness. The distinction between presenile and senile forms of the disease is not presently tenable because both forms display similar pathologic changes in the brain. Its clinical features fit the typical picture of a dementing illness. The onset is usually gradual and hence obscure. Only later do relatives comment on the increased apathy, impaired judgment, forgetfulness, the aimless, repetitive quality of daily activity, and the easy confusion in the face of new problems or situations. In the early stages (which can last for months or years), mental and behavioral changes dominate the clinical picture. Late in the disease, corticospinal tract signs, motor slowing, and gait difficulty emerge, with eventual death from respiratory or other infections brought on by immobility and rigidity. A few cases may present with deficits of only a portion of cognition, only to develop more typical global cognitive deficits over time. For example, 10% of cases initially have a relatively pure amnesic disorder. Others subtypes of disease include a rigid and bradykinetic form resembling Parkinson's disease, and familial forms. Helpful criteria for diagnosis of Alzheimer's disease have been published.[20]

Pathologically, the disease is characterized by widespread cortical changes, including atrophy, sulcal enlargement, and ventricular dilatation. Histologically, neurofibrillary tangles, senile plaques, and granulovacuolar degeneration are seen, the last especially prominent in the hippocampus. Plaques contain a protein core made of β-amyloid protein, which is capable of causing cell injury in animal models.[21, 22] Several mutations involving β-amyloid or related proteins and that appear to account for several forms of familial Alzheimer's disease[23] have been discovered. Amyloid deposition may also occur in blood vessels. Numerous laboratories have confirmed a disproportionate reduction in the level of enzymes associated with cholinergic transmission, suggesting that some of the clinical deficits of Alzheimer's disease reflect a cholinergic deficiency state.[24] Computed tomography (CT) frequently demonstrates atrophy. Although the presence of atrophy is nonspecific, and the degree of atrophy is not related to cognitive performance, the progression of atrophy is more rapid in patients with Alzheimer's disease,[25] reflecting progressive cellular and brain volume loss. Magnetic resonance imaging (MRI) also demonstrates atrophy. In addition, MRI may demonstrate periventricular and subcortical white matter lesions of uncertain significance. These lesions are no different in quality or quantity in demented patients than in normal subjects and are not related to degree of dementia.[26] Electroencephalography typically shows diffuse slowing. Spinal fluid examination is unremarkable. Although positron-emission tomography and single-photon emission computed tomography often demonstrate decreases in parietal-temporal blood flow, these techniques have uncertain diagnostic benefit in everyday practice and are best reserved for research protocols.[27–31]

Pick's disease is rare compared with Alzheimer's disease and is difficult to clinically distinguish from Alzheimer's disease. Patients with Pick's disease tend to have more prominent frontal lobe signs, behavioral changes, and language disturbances. Pathologically, atrophy is strikingly confined to the frontal and inferolateral temporal lobes. Pick's bodies (cytoplasmic inclusions) and giant cortical neurons are added to the frequent presence of neurofibrillary tangles and plaques. The diagnosis may be suspected when frontal and temporal atrophy is seen on imaging but is certain only after biopsy or autopsy.

TABLE 57–3. DISORDERS THAT MAY PRODUCE DEMENTIA

Idiopathic
- Alzheimer's disease
- Pick's disease

Focal Brain Pathology
- Multi-infarct dementia
- Binswanger's disease
- Multiple sclerosis
- Mass lesions (tumors, abscess, hematoma, AVM*)
- Hydrocephalus

Infection
- AIDS†
- Syphilis
- Lyme disease
- Prion disease (kuru, Creutzfeldt-Jakob)
- Chronic meningitis
- Encephalitis
- Progressive multifocal leukoencephalopathy
- Subacute sclerosing panencephalitis
- Progressive rubella panencephalitis

Toxins
- Drugs
- Alcohol
- Heavy metals
- Industrial toxins
- Domoic acid

Inherited Disease
- Huntington's disease
- Gerstmann-Straussler syndrome
- Porphyria
- Propionic aciduria
- Adult-onset lysosomal storage diseases
  - Hexosaminidase
  - Arylsulfatase (metachromatic leukodystrophy)
  - Kufs's disease
  - Adrenoleukodystrophy
  - Others
- Myotonic muscular dystrophy
- Down syndrome
- Hereditary ataxias
- Hereditary spastic paraplegias
- Cerebrotendinous xanthomatosis

Systemic Disease
- Cardiac
- Pulmonary
- Renal
  - Renal failure
  - Dialysis dementia
- Hepatic
  - Hepatic failure
  - Hepatocerebral degeneration
  - Wilson's disease
- Endocrine
  - Hyper/hypothyroid
  - Hyper/hypoparathyroid
  - Hyper/hypoadrenalism
  - SIADH‡
- Rheumatologic
  - Vasculitis (including SLE§)
  - Giant cell arteritis
  - Hypereosinophilia syndromes
  - Sarcoidosis
  - Amyloidosis
- Neoplastic
  - Metastasis—see tumors above
  - Carcinomatous meningitis
  - Paraneoplastic (limbic encephalitis)

Associated Movement Disorder
- Huntington's disease
- Parkinsonian syndromes
  - Parkinson's disease
  - Progressive supranuclear palsy
  - Postencephalitic dementia
  - Post-traumatic (dementia pugilistica)
  - Diffuse Lewy body disease
- Myoclonus
  - Creutzfeldt-Jakob disease
  - Alzheimer's disease
  - Metabolic derangement
- Other movement disorder
  - Hereditary ataxias
  - Hereditary spastic paraplegia
  - Kuru
  - Wilson's disease
  - Seizures
  - Kufs's disease

Deficiency
- Vitamin B_{12} deficiency
- Thiamine
- Niacin (pellagra)

*AVM = arteriovenous malformations.
†AIDS = acquired immunodeficiency syndrome.
‡SIADH = syndrome of inappropriate antidiuretic hormone.
§SLE = systemic lupus erythematosus.

TABLE 57–4. CAUSES OF DEMENTIA IN REPRESENTATIVE SERIES (%)

Disease	Series (%)						
	Marsden	*Marletta*	*Smith*	*Larson**	*Katzman*	*Freemon*	*Wells†*
Alzheimer's disease	57	60	83	80	70	43	52
Multi-infarct dementia	10	14	0	2	7	8	10
Alcohol	7	10	0	4	5	7	11
Drug toxicity	0	0	0	10	0	8	3
Normal pressure hydrocephalus	6	1	5	0	4	12	7
Huntington's disease	4	3	3	0	5	7	3
Other	16	12	9	10	9	15	14

*n = 300.
†n = 382.

DEMENTIA DUE TO FOCAL BRAIN PATHOLOGY

Until recently, the role of vascular disease in producing dementia was overemphasized. The notion that senile cortical atrophy or "senility" can result from diffuse atherosclerosis in the absence in infarction has been conclusively refuted. The degree of dementia due to Alzheimer's disease correlates highly with the density of senile plaques and neurofibrillary tangles, not with the degree of atherosclerosis.[32] The reduction in cerebral blood flow seen in cortical atrophy is a secondary, not primary, change. The term "atherosclerotic dementia" should be dropped from the nosologic lexicon.

Multiple strokes, on the other hand, may produce such extensive cerebral damage that dementia ensues.[33] These strokes may result from multiple embolic infarction or from small thrombotic infarcts (lacunes). Approximately 20% may have an insidious onset without histories of acute strokes.[34] To the dementia is conjoined a constellation of neurologic signs, including pseudobulbar palsy; dysarthria; bilateral corticospinal tract signs, including weakness, spasticity, and hyper-reflexia; and a gait abnormality called *marche à petits pas*, consisting of small, shuffling steps. The picture resembles Parkinson's disease save for the prominent corticospinal tract findings, and the fact that the tremor of Parkinson's disease is absent. Multi-infarct dementia should be suspected whenever dementia is marked by a fluctuating course, stepwise worsening, one or more clear strokes, focal neurologic signs, or imaging evidence of multiple areas of cerebral infarction. Treatment is aimed at preventing further cerebral damage by control of blood pressure or by prevention of further emboli with antiplatelet or anticoagulant therapy.

Hydrocephalus leads to dementia, gait difficulty, and incontinence.[35] This clinical picture does not specify a unique disease; in fact, most patients with the triad do not have hydrocephalus. The diagnosis is suspected in those with the clinical triad in whom imaging demonstrates hydrocephalus. Radionuclide cysternography lends support for the diagnosis and, together with CT or MRI, allows classification into noncommunicating or communicating (normal pressure) hydrocephalus. Other diagnostic tests including extended cerebrospinal fluid pressure monitoring, cerebrospinal fluid infusion tests, and therapeutic lumbar punctures have not been uniformly adopted. Treatment consists of surgical cerebrospinal fluid shunting. Results are dependent on careful case selection.

INFECTION

Most infectious causes of cognitive dysfunction are acute or associated with systemic illness. However, indolent infections may occasionally lead to dementia. Although syphilis has historically been the most prominent of these diseases, human immunodeficiency–virus infection is now the most prevalent cause of infectious dementia.

Creutzfeldt-Jakob disease (spongiform encephalopathy) is a subacute disorder characterized by rapidly progressing dementia, visual difficulties, myoclonus (especially startle myoclonus in which a loud noise elicits a generalized jerk of the body musculature), and cerebellar ataxia. The diagnosis should be considered in cases with a rapid decline over a few weeks. Characteristic generalized periodic epileptiform discharges are seen on electroencephalography. Detection of prion protein has been reported in the cerebrospinal fluid.[36] The disease is transmissible by infectious proteinaceous agents.

TOXINS

Drugs prescribed by physicians are the most common toxic agents responsible for dementia. In addition, patients with other causes of dementia may have worsened cognitive performance due to the use of medications. Medications commonly leading to cognitive impairment include benzodiazepines, followed by meprobamate, antipsychotic drugs, cimetidine, methyldopa, aspirin, insulin, meperidine, amoxapine, amantadine, propranolol, hydrochlorothiazide, and reserpine.[37]

INHERITED DISEASE

Huntington's chorea is only rarely encountered by the internal medicine or family practitioner. Behavior and personality abnormalities, choreiform movements, and dementia may each occur as the initial symptom leading to misdiagnosis. Correct diagnosis depends on a careful family history for this dominantly inherited condition. Neuroimaging shows atrophy of the caudate nuclei in many patients. Decreased blood flow to the caudate nuclei is an early sign detectable on positron-emission tomographic scanning.[38] Patients with suitable families may have the diagnosis confirmed through DNA linkage analysis with 96% accuracy.[39] The responsible gene has now been cloned and a clinical test is expected soon.

DEMENTIAS ASSOCIATED WITH MOVEMENT DISORDERS

Parkinsonian disorders are frequently associated with dementia in advanced stages. The coexistence of dementia and parkinsonism in early disease suggests a multi-infarct state, Alzheimer's disease with Parkinsonian features, or diffuse Lewy body disease.

DEFICIENCY STATES

Although most patients with dementia due to vitamin B_{12} deficiency have obvious neurologic and hematologic abnormalities, vitamin B_{12} deficiency may lead to dementia in the absence of other neurologic or hematologic findings. Thiamine deficiency may be primarily responsible for the dementia associated with alcohol abuse.

LABORATORY STUDIES

In light of these diagnostic considerations, the minimum evaluation of a person newly diagnosed as suffering from dementia should include a complete blood count; urinalysis; treponemal syphilis test; determination of blood urea nitrogen, glucose, calcium, electrolytes, and B_{12}; and thyroid function tests. CT scanning and electroencephalography are considered ancillary tests that should be used selectively.[11, 40] For example, CT may be of benefit in unusual cases, such as in patients with early-onset dementia, a stuttering course, prominent gait abnormality, incontinence, or in those with focal neurologic signs, whereas in patients with slowly progressive dementia over several years and normal neurologic examinations in whom the diagnosis of Alzheimer's disease is highly likely, the clinician can forgo brain imaging studies with confidence. Electroencephalography is chiefly of value in patients in whom concurrent or concomitant seizures are suspected or in patients with rapid progression and prominent myoclonus. Selective use of tests, especially brain imaging tests, can yield substantial cost savings with minimal risk. Imaging with MRI, positron-emission tomography, and single-photon emission tomography may be useful in selected cases but should not be performed indiscriminately.

Using standard diagnostic criteria and the techniques described, the overall accuracy of clinical diagnosis can be 80 to 85% and will improve based on long-term follow-up.[41, 42] Most errors are due to misclassification of multi-infarct dementia.[43] If cases without confusing aspects are excluded, it is possible to obtain a series of essentially pure Alzheimer's cases.[44] Ultimately, autopsy confirmation is the best diagnostic method and may be quite helpful to interested families and clinicians.

MANAGEMENT

The use of pharmacologic agents for the treatment of cognitive failure has proved disappointing. At best, modest improvements in cognitive function have been demonstrated, often at the expense of significant side effects. Studies have been limited by small numbers of subjects, brief periods of follow-up, and limited controls. The Food and Drug Administration has attempted to streamline the approval of drugs used to treat dementia. This has led to an increased interest in developing these drugs by the pharmaceutical industry. A relatively large number of drugs are in various stages of evaluation worldwide.

Cognitive-enhancing drugs may be divided into four groups: blood flow enhancers, those that augment acetylcholine, nootropics, and miscellaneous.[45] Many of the agents used were originally recommended as a means of *enhancing cerebral blood flow*; the most commonly used such agent is a combination of ergot alkaloids, Hydergine. The discovery that reduced blood flow plays no role in causing most cases of dementia has seriously undermined the rationale for using these agents. The most recent studies of Hydergine have found no benefit. Other vascular enhancers under study include nicergoline and nimodipine. *Drugs that augment acetylcholine* have received recent attention. The benefits of acetylcholine precursors (choline and lecithin) have been offset by gastrointestinal discomfort. *N*-Acetylcarnitine increases acetylcholine and has shown a modest degree of cognitive improvement in preliminary reports. *Inhibitors of acetylcholinesterase* have also been used.[46] Physostigmine was associated with nausea, vomiting, diaphoresis, and tachycardia. Tetrahydroaminoacridine (THA, Tacrine) has recently received FDA approval for use in patients with Alzheimer's disease, but it has significant side effects (e.g., gastrointestinal distress and elevation of transaminase levels). Combining precursors and acetylcholinesterase inhibitors has not resulted in enhanced benefits. *Cholinergic muscarinic agonists* under study include RS-86 and bethanechol. *Nootropics* are drugs that increase neuronal metabolic activity. Piracetam is being evaluated. Oxiracetam proved to be of no benefit. *Miscellaneous drugs* that require further study include selegiline, nerve growth factor, phosphatidylserine, thiamine, naloxone, somatostatin, and aluminum chelators. Clinicians should expect to receive reports on the efficacy of these and other drugs in the next 5 years.

The successful management of the demented patient requires as much compassion and patience as scientific sophistication. The physician's responsibilities to both patient and family lie in five major areas: specific therapy, removal of factors exaggerating disability, management of specific behavior problems, pharmacotherapy of complications, and advice regarding residential and legal arrangements.

Specific Therapy, as Indicated by the Results of the Evaluation. Strokes may be treated with risk factor modification, antiplatelet agents (aspirin, ticlopidine), anticoagulants, or surgery. Mass lesions must be diagnosed and treated. Hydrocephalus may be treated with cerebrospinal fluid shunting. Many infections respond to antimicrobial drugs. Systemic diseases, such as hypothyroidism and vitamin deficiency states, should be corrected.

Removal of Factors Exaggerating Disability. In particular, including medical illness as well as nutrition and fitness, drugs that worsen cognitive performance should be minimized or avoided. Overall health should be optimized. In a study of 200 demented patients, 10% had previously unrecognized hypertension, urinary tract infection, chronic lung disease, strokes, congestive heart failure, or peptic ulcer disease.[47] Thus, periodic health assesments and access to care from a general physician should be provided. The high prevalence of hypothyroidism and folate deficiency among these patients most often reflects the neglect of their health and nutritional status because treatment of these disorders may not reverse the dementia.[48] Correcting conditions so that cognitive ability is partially restored may provide a measure of independence to the patient's daily activities. Specific therapy for anemia, infection, vitamin deficiency, constipation, congestive heart failure, dehydration, electrolyte abnormality, and respiratory insufficiency is often remarkably effective in reversing the acute confusional episodes that frequently complicate the course of dementia. Vision and hearing deficits may further hinder a tenuous cognitive status.

Management of Specific Behavior Problems. Nonpharmacologic therapies may suffice for many behavior problems. Detailed explanation of the biologic nature of the disease and its expected course often measurably assists the family in coping with the inevitable problems they encounter. Suggesting that the patient is not in full control of his or her behavior will often defuse the anger that family members exhibit in the face of paranoia, agitation, incontinence, and slowness. This anger, if allowed to grow, may result in reduced caring, frank neglect, or abuse. Referral of the family to the local chapter of the Alzheimer's Association or to a local support group for families of demented individuals may provide them with further information and coping skills, as well as permit them to share their frustration and loss. The home should be made safe, with locks on certain doors, gas cutoffs for appliances (or the removal of knobs), use of nonskid floors and rugs, stairwell maintenance, and proper footwear. Home safety evaluations by occupational therapists are often helpful. Wandering within the home may be tolerated to some degree as long as safety is addressed. An identification bracelet may be useful if wandering away from home is a concern. A clear-cut daily routine, including time for bowel and bladder functioning, rest periods, and meals, is usually best for demented persons. Driving safety is a personal as well as public safety concern.[49] It may be necessary to remove car keys or to disable the car. Incontinence may improve with scheduled voidings but may require disposable shields. Both family members and patients may benefit from counselling regarding frustration, loss, and depression. Adult day care and community support services may provide the family with relief from the continual burdens of caregiving as well as provide patients with an escape from isolation and sensory deprivation.

Pharmacotherapy of Complications. Pharmacologic control of behavior may be necessary for extreme agitation or aggressiveness. Neuroleptic medications are preferred; haloperidol for patients not needing sedation or thioridazine for those requiring sedation. Though best treated with nonpharmacologic methods, insomnia may be treated with sedatives. Unfortunately, all sedatives may, and often do, worsen confusion. In particular, potent benzodiazepines with short half-lives have been associated with confusion. Cyclic antidepressants may be helpful for depression or sleep. Antidepressants that are strongly anticholinergic may exacerbate cognitive deficits. Likewise, anticholinergic agents used to treat incontinence may lead to cognitive worsening. In general, demented patients are more likely to respond to and tolerate lower doses of psychotropic drugs, especially those with anticholinergic effects. We typically use half of the lowest dose available as initial therapy.

Advice Regarding Residential and Legal Arrangements. It is important that a legal proxy be established in the event that the patient becomes incompetent to manage his or her own affairs. This may range from a revocable power of attorney to custodianship. A durable power of attorney for health care is recommended. Financial planning is also important early in the course because dementia can be an immense financial drain. The physician also can help the family deal with the inevitable question of custodial care as the patient's helplessness increases. The advantages and disadvantages of continued home care versus nursing home or chronic hospital placement need to be explored, often with the assistance of a social worker. As a rule, continued existence in familiar surroundings results in less confusion and a higher level of personal self-care. Although the patient's own wishes must not be neglected, they must not constitute the sole factor in decisions about placement. End-of-life issues and financial matters are ideally addressed in the presence of the proxy early in the course of the disease while the patient is still able to express preferences and even participate in discussions. As a general rule, the physician and family function best when future problems are anticipated and their possible solutions agreed to in advance. The physician should seek out the questions and concerns of demented patients and their families. Clarifying their concerns helps relieve the anxiety, guilt, and uncertainty that such families bear and will make future care more effective.

REFERENCES

1. Guralnik J and FitzSimmons S: Aging in America: A demographic perspective. Cardiol Clin 4:175–183, 1986.
2. Schoenberg B, Anderson D, and Haerer A: Severe dementia. Prevalence and clinical features in a biracial US population. Arch Neurol 42:740–743, 1985.
3. Evans D, Funkenstein H, and Albert M: Prevalence of Alzheimer's disease in a community population of older persons. JAMA 262:2551–2556, 1989.
4. Mortimer J and Hutton J: Epidemiology and etiology of Alzheimer's disease. *In* Hutton J and Kenny A (eds): Senile Dementia of the Alzheimer Type. New York, Alan R. Liss, 1985, pp 177–196.
5. Schneider E and Geralnik J: The aging of America: Impact on health care costs. JAMA 263:2335–2340, 1990.
6. American Psychiatric Association: Diagnostic and Statistical Manual of Mental Disorders, 3rd ed., revised. Washington, DC, American Psychiatric Association, 1987.
7. Folstein M, Folstein S, and McHugh P: Mini-mental state: A practical method for grading the cognitive state of patients for the clinician. J Psychiatr Res 12:189–198, 1975.
8. Anthony J, LeResche L, Niaz U, et al: Limits of the "mini-mental state" as a screening test for dementia and delirium among hospital patients. Psychol Med 12:397–408, 1982.
9. Kiloh L: Pseudo-dementia. Acta Psychiatr Scand 37:336–351, 1961.
10. Smith J and Kiloh L: The investigation of dementia: Results in 200 consecutive admissions. Lancet 1:824–827, 1981.
11. Larson E, Reifler B, Sumi S, et al: Diagnostic tests in the evaluation of dementia: A prospective study of 200 elderly outpatients. Arch Intern Med 146:1917–1922, 1986.
12. Reding M, Haycox J, and Blass J: Depression in patients referred to a dementia clinic. Arch Neurol 42:894–896, 1985.
13. Spar J and Gerner R: Does the dexamethasone suppression test distinguish dementia from depression? Am J Psychiatry 139:238–240, 1982.
14. Shrimankar J, Soni S, and McMurray J: Dexamethasone suppression test in dementia and depression. Clinical and biological correlates. Br J Psychiatry 154:372–377, 1989.
15. Greenwald B, Kramer-Ginsberg E, Marin D, et al: Dementia with coexistent major depression. Am J Psychiatry 146:1472–1478, 1989.
16. Krol V: The relationship between senile dementia (Alzheimer type) and depression. Can J Psychiatry 28:304–306, 1983.
17. Rovner B, Broadhead J, Spencer M, et al: Depression and Alzheimer's disease. Am J Psychiatry 146:350–353, 1989.
18. Reifler B, Larson E, and Hanley R: Coexistence of cognitive impairment and depression in geriatric outpatients. Am J Psychiatry 139:623–626, 1982.
19. Reding M, Haycox J, Wigforss K, et al: Follow up of patients referred to a dementia service. J Am Geriatr Soc 32:265–268, 1984.
20. McKhann G, Drachman D, Folstein M, et al: Clinical diagnosis of Alzheimer's disease: Report of the NINCDS-ADRDA work group under the auspices of department of health and human services task force on Alzheimer's disease. Neurology 34:939–944, 1984.
21. Frautschy S, Baird A, and Cole G: Effects of injected Alzheimer beta-amyloid cores in rat brain. Proc Natl Acad Sci USA 88:8362–8366, 1991.
22. Kowall N, Beal M, Busciglio J, et al: An in vivo model for the neurodegenerative effects of beta amyloid and protection by substance P. Proc Natl Acad Sci USA 88:7247–7251, 1991.
23. Harrington M, Merril C, Asher D, and Gadjusek D: Abnormal proteins in the cerebrospinal fluid of patients with Creutzfeldt-Jakob disease. N Engl J Med 315:279–283, 1986.
24. Whitehouse P, Gambetti P, Harik S, et al: Neurochemistry of dementia: Establishing the links. Prog Clin Biol Res 317:131–142, 1989.
25. DeCarli C, Kaye J, Horwitz B, and Rapoport S: Critical analysis of the use of computer-assisted transverse axial tomography to study human brain in aging and dementia of the Alzheimer type. Neurology 40:872–883, 1990.
26. Leys D, Soetaert G, Petit H, et al: Periventricular and white matter magnetic resonance imaging hyperintensities do not differ between Alzheimer's disease and normal aging. Arch Neurol 47:524–527, 1990.
27. Duara R, Barker W, Loewenstein D, et al: Sensitivity and specificity of positron emission tomography and magnetic resonance imaging studies in Alzheimer's disease and multi-infarct dementia. Eur Neurol 29(Suppl 3):9–15, 1989.
28. Fazekas F, Alavi A, Chawluk J, et al: Comparison of CT, MR, and PET in Alzheimer's dementia and normal aging. J Nucl Med 30:1607–1615, 1983.
29. Haxby J, Grady C, Duara R, et al: Neocortical metabolic abnormalities precede nonmemory cognitive defects in early Alzheimer's-type dementia. Arch Neurol 43:882–885, 1986.
30. Johnson K, Holman B, Mueller S, et al: Single photon emission computed tomography in Alzheimer's disease. Arch Neurol 45:392–396, 1988.
31. Sharp P, Gemmell H, Cherryman G, et al: Application of io-

dine-123-labeled isopropylamphetamine imaging to the study of dementia. J Nucl Med 27:761–768, 1986.
32. Roth M, Tomlinson B, and Blessed G: Correlation between scores for dementia and counts of "senile plaques" in cerebral gray matter of elderly subjects. Nature 209:109–110, 1966.
33. Hachinski V, Lassen N, and Marshall J: Multi-infarct dementia. Lancet 2:207–210, 1974.
34. Erkinjuntii T and Sulkava R: Diagnosis of multi-infarct dementia. Alzheimer Dis Assoc Disord 5:112–121, 1991.
35. St Laurent M: Normal pressure hydrocephalus in geriatric medicine: A challenge. J Geriatr Psychiatry Neurol 1:163–168, 1988.
36. Goate A, Chartier-Harlin M, Mullan M, et al: Segregation of a missense mutation in the amyloid precursor protein gene with familial Alzheimer's disease. Nature 349:704–706, 1991.
37. Larson E, Kukull W, Buchner D, and Reifler B: Adverse drug reactions associated with global cognitive impairment in elderly persons. Ann Intern Med 107:169–173, 1987.
38. Mazziotta J, Phelps M, Pahl J, et al: Reduced cerebral glucose metabolism in asymptomatic subjects at risk for Huntington's disease. N Engl J Med 316:357–362, 1987.
39. Meissen G, Myers R, Mastromauro C, et al: Predictive testing for Huntington's disease with use of a linked DNA marker. N Engl J Med 318:535–542, 1988.
40. Differential diagnosis of dementing diseases. Nat Inst Health Consensus Dev Conf Consensus Statement 6:1–9, 1987.
41. Rocca W, Amaducci L, and Shoenberg B: Epidemiology of clinically diagnosed Alzheimer's disease. Ann Neurol 19:415–424, 1986.
42. Ettlin T, Staihelin H, Kischka U, et al: Computed tomography, electroencephalography and clinical features in the differential diagnosis of senile dementia. Arch Neurol 46:1217–1220, 1989.
43. Wade J, Mirsen T, Hachincki V, et al: The clinical diagnosis of Alzheimer's disease. Arch Neurol 44:24–29, 1987.
44. Morris J, McKeel D, Fulling K, et al: Validation of clinical diagnostic criteria for Alzheimer's disease. Ann Neurol 24:17–22, 1988.
45. Cooper J: Drug treatment of Alzheimer's disease. Arch Intern Med 151:245–249, 1991.
46. Kumar V and Calache M: Treatment of Alzheimer's disease with cholinergic drugs. Int J Clin Pharmacol Ther Toxicol 29:23–37, 1991.
47. Larson E, Lo B, and Williams M: Evaluation and care of elderly patients with dementia: A comprehensive review. J Gen Intern Med 1:116–126, 1986.
48. Larson E, Reifler B, Featherstone H, et al: Dementia in elderly outpatients: A prospective study. Ann Intern Med 100:417–423, 1984.
49. Friedland R, Koss E, Kumar A, et al: Motor vehicle crashes in dementia of the Alzheimer type. Ann Neurol 24:782–786, 1988.

58

Headache

EGILIUS L. H. SPIERINGS, MD, PhD

In the absence of harm done to it, the head hurts more often than any other part of the body. Seventy to 80% of the population, men and women alike, experience headaches. Fifty per cent of the population experience headaches at least once/mo, 15%, at least once/wk, and 5%, daily.

Headaches can be of different intensities and are, for the sake of simplicity, generally divided into three categories: mild, moderate, and severe. Moderate and severe headaches occur twice as frequently in women than in men and are related to the menstrual cycle in women. Moderate headaches occur in 13% of men and 23% of women, and severe headaches, in 6 and 12%, respectively.[1] The prevalence of migraine lies between those of moderate and severe headaches and is 9% for men and 16% for women.

Headache, independent of its frequency of occurrence, is familial in nature. The strongest positive family history is found for the parents, of whom one or both are affected in 61%.[2] The mother is affected almost twice as frequently as the father (46% versus 26%). The positive family history of migraine is the same as that for headache in general, suggesting that the familial occurrence of headache is also independent of headache intensity.

The high frequency of occurrence makes headache a common complaint in medical practice. There, it presents itself as an acute, subacute, or chronic condition. The acute headache is generally severe in intensity and is presented in the emergency department. The subacute and chronic headaches, on the other hand, are presented in the office.

The diagnostic considerations depend to a great extent on the presentation of the headache. Therefore, the differential diagnosis of headache will be discussed for the three presentations separately. It is important to remember, however, that whatever the presentation, headache is *always* a valid complaint. It should always be investigated seriously and never considered merely a product of the imagination.

ACUTE HEADACHE

Headache not caused by trauma is responsible for 1 to 2% of visits to the emergency department.[3] Men and women are equally represented, and 80% of the patients are between 15 and 54 years of age. Muscle-contraction headache is the most common cause (32%), followed by migraine (22%) and upper respiratory infection (12%). The following diagnoses each account for 5% or fewer of nontraumatic headaches in the emergency department: sinusitis, hypertension, gastroenteritis, cerebral tumor, and cervical degeneration. Apart from cerebral tumor, the neurologic causes of headache, that is, subarachnoid hemorrhage, meningitis, temporal arteritis, and subdural hematoma, each account for fewer than 1%.

Headache, as it is presented in the emergency department, may be encountered at home when house visits are performed. Temperature, blood pressure, and pulse rate should be obtained first, and the neck should be examined for meningeal irritation. The examination of the neck should be done gently, with the back of the head resting in the palm of the hands. The neck is first gently rotated to each side, after which it is carefully bent forward so that the chin touches the chest. While the neck is being bent forward, the face of the patient is watched for indications of pain and the legs, for signs of flexion. Limitation of forward flexion of the neck is of significance only when rotation of the neck is intact. Otherwise, it is merely an indication of tightness of the neck muscles, from which many patients with headache suffer.

The presence of fever aids in making the diagnosis, which could be upper respiratory infection, sinusitis, or gastroenteritis. Each of these conditions comes with specific symptoms, such as throat ache, cough, purulent nasal discharge, nausea, vomiting, or diarrhea. The combination of fever with meningeal irritation raises suspicion of meningitis, either viral or bacterial. Lumbar puncture should be performed once cerebral involvement (encephalitis, cerebral abscess) has been excluded by neurologic examination or neurodiagnostic imaging (computed tomography or magnetic resonance imaging). Meningeal irritation without fever may be indicative of subarachnoid hemorrhage, for which computed tomography without contrast should be performed, and if the results are negative, a lumbar puncture.

Cerebral tumor is a cause of subacute headache but may present with acute headache when complicated by hemorrhage. This is seen particularly with chromophobe adenomas of the pituitary gland and cerebral metastases of malignant melanoma. With hemorrhage into a pituitary adenoma, there may be no other symptoms than severe headache. Therefore, neurodiagnostic imaging may be necessary to make this diagnosis. With cerebral tumors, there are generally neurologic symptoms or abnormalities on neurologic examination.

Temporal arteritis and subdural hematoma should be looked for in patients with subacute headache over the age of 60. Temporal arteritis is generally associated with a significantly elevated sedimentation rate of 50 mm or higher. Therefore, it is important to perform this simple test in *all* patients older than 60 years of age who present with headache. Muscle-contraction headache and migraine are chronic headache conditions. Hence, if they are diagnosed in acute headache, there must be a previous history of similar headaches.

Cerebral tumor, temporal arteritis, and subdural hematoma as causes of headache are further discussed under subacute headache. Meningitis and subarachnoid hemorrhage are discussed here as causes of acute headache.

Meningitis

The incidence of meningitis in the United States is estimated to be 10 to 20 cases per 100,000 population per year. Children below the age of 5 account for 70% of all cases. About half of the cases are caused by a bacterial infection, usually *Haemophilus influenzae, Neisseria meningitidis,* or *Streptococcus pneumoniae.* The infection is generally hematogenic, and the site of entry of the organisms into the blood is usually the upper respiratory tract. When not caused by a bacterial infection, the meningitis is usually viral. The infections are mostly caused by the enteroviruses, followed by the mumps virus, arboviruses, and herpes simplex virus.

Meningitis develops acutely over hours or days. It may, or may not, be preceded by a respiratory or gastrointestinal illness, and may be either bacterial or viral in nature. Severe, bilateral headache associated with photophobia, nausea, and vomiting is its main presentation. When the cause is bacterial, altered sensorium with drowsiness, disorientation, and confusion is also common. Fever is present in 80% of patients with meningitis, and in 80%, signs of meningeal irritation are found on physical examination. Diagnosis is made by lumbar puncture and analysis of spinal fluid, which should be performed in *every* suspected case.

Patients with bacterial meningitis are usually sicker than those with viral meningitis. However, a distinction between the two can often only be made by spinal fluid analysis. In bacterial meningitis, the cell count is generally more than 1000/mm^3 with 90% polymorphonuclear leukocytes. The protein level is usually significantly elevated and the glucose level decreased. In viral meningitis, the cell count is generally less than 1000/mm^3 with mostly lymphocytes, and the protein and glucose levels are normal. If no distinction can be made and the patient is not seriously ill, the spinal fluid should be re-examined after 6 hours. Bacterial meningitis is treated with antibiotics; treatment of viral meningitis is symptomatic only.

Subarachnoid Hemorrhage

The incidence of subarachnoid hemorrhage in the United States is estimated at 10 to 15 cases per 100,000 population per year. In 75%, the hemorrhage occurs from a ruptured aneurysm, and in the remainder, it is caused by an arteriovenous malformation or bleeding disorder. Two thirds of the patients affected are between the ages of 40 and 60. Women are affected slightly more frequently than men, possibly because of the higher prevalence of hypertension in women. Sometimes, the hemorrhage is precipitated by activities, such as lifting, straining, intercourse, or emotional excitement. However, it can also occur during sleep, probably related to the increase in blood pressure as it occurs during rapid eye movement sleep.

Headache of hyperacute onset is the characteristic presentation of subarachnoid hemorrhage. The rapidity in onset of the headache is also the key feature in diagnosing the condition. The patient should be asked explicitly how fast the headache came about in terms of seconds, minutes, or hours. The headache of subarachnoid hemorrhage comes about in a matter of seconds, like a blow on the head or neck. If this history is obtained, the diagnostic process should be pursued to the point of lumbar puncture. The lumbar puncture should, however, always be preceded by computed tomography without contrast and only be performed when the results are negative.

On physical examination, the key finding in subarachnoid hemorrhage is limited forward flexion of the neck with intact rotation. The limitation in forward flexion is due to chemical inflammation of the meninges and takes several hours to develop. Preretinal hemorrhages on examination of the fundi are seen in large hemorrhages only. The ultimate diagnostic test in subarachnoid hemorrhage is lumbar puncture and spinal fluid analysis. If the patient is not seriously ill, it is important to wait 6 hours after the onset of the headache before performing the lumbar puncture. This will make it easier to distinguish a positive result from a traumatic puncture when the cerebrospinal fluid is hemorrhagic. Centrifugation of the spinal fluid will reveal yellow fluid in the first case and colorless fluid in the latter.

Treatment of Acute Headache

For the treatment of headache in the emergency department, generally parenterally administered medications are used. The medications are presented in order of their efficacy, usually in decreasing headache intensity within 1 hour of administration (Table 58–1). Most patients studied had severe migraine headaches. Prochlorperazine edisylate (Compazine), given slowly intravenously in a dose of 10 mg, seems most effective, with an efficacy of 88% in providing complete or partial pain relief.[4] Second is chlorpromazine hydrochloride (Thorazine), also given intravenously, which has an efficacy of 80%.[5] The chlorpromazine was given in intravenous boluses of 12.5 mg, if necessary, repeated twice at intervals of 20 minutes with a maximum dose of 37.5 mg. Prior to the administration of the medication, the patients were given 500 ml of normal saline intravenously. This may have decreased the frequency of hypotension often seen with intravenous administration of chlorpromazine, and less commonly with prochlorperazine. Other adverse effects occurring with the use of either prochlorperazine or chlorpromazine, both phenothiazines, are drowsiness and dystonia.

Next in line with regard to efficacy is metoclopramide hydrochloride (Reglan), either alone or in combination with dihydroergotamine mesylate (DHE 45). Metoclopramide, when given in a dose of 10 mg intravenously, has an efficacy of 67% in providing effective pain relief.[6] Adding dihydroergotamine in a dose of 1 mg intravenously increases the efficacy in relieving headache to 70%.[7] Dihydroergotamine alone, in a dose of 1 or 2 mg intravenously, has an efficacy of only 37%.[5] The medication should *never* be given without prior administration of an antinausea medication because it is very potent in causing nausea and vomiting. When given alone, the occurrence of these adverse affects may, to a great extent, reduce the beneficial effect obtained with the medication.

Of the narcotic medications studied, only butorphanol tartrate (Stadol) had a relatively good efficacy of 64%.[7] The combination of meperidine hydrochloride (Demerol) plus hydroxyzine pamoate (Vistaril) has an efficacy of only 45%.[7] Nevertheless, this is the treatment of acute headache most commonly used in the emergency department. The new nonsteroidal anti-inflammatory analgesic ketorolac tromethamine (Toradol), which is available for parenteral administration, has a somewhat better efficacy of 55%.[8] However, my own experience with the use of this medication for acute headache has been disappointing. More promising is the new antimigraine medication sumatriptan succinate (Imitrex). The efficacy of this medication, in a dose of 6 mg subcutaneously, in decreasing the intensity of moderate and severe headaches to no or mild headache is 70%.[9]

My approach is to start by giving the patient 10 mg of metoclopramide (Reglan) intravenously. Metoclopramide is an effective antinausea medication without contraindications and with few adverse effects. It does not have cardiovascular effects and therefore can be safely given as an intravenous bolus. Sometimes it causes restlessness as an adverse effect and rarely, dystonia. The dystonia usually occurs in adolescent and young adult women and usually

TABLE 58–1. TREATMENT OF ACUTE HEADACHE IN THE EMERGENCY DEPARTMENT

Generic and Brand Name	Dose	Efficacy	Study
Prochlorperazine edisylate (Compazine)	10 mg IV	88%	Jones et al[4]
Chlorpromazine hydrochloride (Thorazine)	12.5–37.5 mg IV*	80%	Bell et al[5]
Dihydroergotamine mesylate (DHE 45) plus metoclopramide hydrochloride (Reglan)	1 mg IV and 10 mg IV	70%	Belgrade et al[7]
Metoclopramide hydrochloride (Reglan)	10 mg IV	67%	Tek et al[6]
Butorphanol tartrate (Stadol)	2 mg IM†	64%	Belgrade et al[7]
Ketorolac tromethamine (Toradol)	60 mg IM	55%	Harden et al[8]
Lidocaine hydrochloride (Xylocaine)	50–150 mg IV	50%	Bell et al[5]
Meperidine hydrochloride (Demerol) plus hydroxyzine pamoate (Vistaril)	75 mg IM and 50 mg IM	45%	Belgrade et al[7]
Dihydroergotamine mesylate (DHE 45)	1–2 mg IV	37%	Bell et al[5]

*IV = intravenously.
†IM = intramuscularly.

involves the tongue, which becomes stiff. It can be easily reversed with diphenhydramine hydrochloride (Benadryl), administered in a dose of 50 to 100 mg intravenously.

Metoclopramide does not cause drowsiness and therefore can be given to the patient with acute headache before the diagnostic process is initiated. Acute headache is generally severe in intensity, and, as a result, is often associated with nausea and vomiting. Metoclopramide will effectively relieve the gastrointestinal symptoms and make it easier for the patient *and* the physician to go through the diagnostic process. Once the diagnostic process is completed and treatment can be continued, I give 5 to 10 mg of diazepam (Valium) intravenously when muscular symptoms, such as tightness of the neck muscles, are prominent. Otherwise or with any remaining headache, I give dihydroergotamine, 0.5 mg intramuscularly, which I repeat, if necessary, after 30 minutes. In my experience, giving the dihydroergotamine intravenously does not provide better relief. On the other hand, gastrointestinal, and possibly cardiac,[10] adverse effects occur more often with intravenous than with intramuscular administration of the medication.

SUBACUTE HEADACHE

Subacute headache develops over a course of days or weeks, as opposed to acute headache, which develops over hours or days. Cerebral tumor, temporal arteritis, and subdural hematoma are possible etiologies of subacute headache. Cerebral tumor is especially a concern in children with subacute headache. In adults, cerebral tumors are usually located in a hemisphere and give rise to neurologic symptoms early in the course of the illness. In children, they are often located in the posterior fossa. There, they easily obstruct the flow of cerebrospinal fluid, giving rise to headache without neurologic symptoms.

The most common cerebral tumors in childhood are medulloblastoma, a malignant tumor of the cerebellar vermis; ependymoma, a tumor of the fourth ventricle; cerebellar astrocytoma, a malignant tumor of the cerebellar hemisphere; and pontine glioma, a malignant tumor of the pons. Particulars in the history that in children should raise suspicion of cerebral tumor as the cause of headache are: (1) having a headache on awakening in the morning, (2) being awakened by headache at night, (3) persistence of headache in high intensity, and (4) a changing nature or frequency of the headache.[11] From the general history, a change in behavior or school performance, or both, can be added to this list.

In the evaluation of headache in childhood, the neurologic examination is very important and should include evaluation of visual acuity and fundi.[11] In children with headache due to cerebral tumor, 55% show abnormalities on the examination within 2 weeks of headache onset. Within 2 months of onset of the headache, 85% of children have neurologic abnormalities. After half a year, *all* children with headache due to cerebral tumor have abnormalities on the neurologic examination.

Cerebral Tumor

Cerebral tumors are divided into primary and secondary, or metastatic. Metastatic tumors reach the brain through hematogenic seeding, most notoriously from lung or breast cancer. Much less common sources of metastatic cerebral tumors are hypernephroma and melanoma. By the time the cerebral metastasis occurs, the primary tumor is generally known. However, particularly with lung cancer, a cerebral metastasis may be the first manifestation of the illness.

The incidence of primary cerebral tumors in the United States is estimated at 5 to 10 cases per 100,000 population per year. Those affected are mostly between the ages of 50 and 70. In half the cases, the tumor originates from the glial cells of the brain and is a glioma. In 60%, this glioma is a so-called malignant glioma, or glioma multiforme, which is a glioma characterized by a high degree of pleomorphism of the cells, invasiveness of growth, mitotic figures, vessel proliferation, hemorrhages, and necrosis. It is a very malignant tumor that causes a short duration of illness, often leading to death within half a year.

The initial manifestation of malignant glioma is generally not headache but neurologic symptoms or seizure. A seizure without obvious cause in adulthood should *always* be considered a symptom of cerebral pathology until proven otherwise. The other gliomas, that is, astrocytoma and oligodendroglioma, have a much less disastrous course than malignant glioma but are still malignant. They grow slowly but invasively, generally leading to death within 3 to 5 years. They generally also present with neurologic symptoms or seizure, but the symptoms progress slowly and can be very subtle. Abnormalities on the neurologic examination may be found early in the course of illness if the examination is performed meticulously and, if necessary, repeated.

The cerebral tumor occurring almost as frequently as glioma is meningioma, a benign tumor that originates from the dura mater. It occurs three times more frequently in women than in men. It is often localized over the cerebral hemisphere and manifests itself through headache or seizure. Nonfocal neurologic symptoms, such as lack of perseverance, irritability, emotional lability, and memory impairment, generally occur before focal symptoms develop. The nonfocal neurologic symptoms are due to edema, which occurs in the cerebral tissue adjacent to the tumor.

Headache caused by meningioma is localized to the side of the tumor but is not necessarily limited to its exact location. It may be intermittent or continuous, but it usually progresses in intensity over weeks or months. Gastrointestinal symptoms associated with this headache are generally not very prominent. The headache may be very easily mistaken for a muscle-contraction or migraine headache. The localization of the headache always to the same side as well as its gradually progressive nature should raise suspicion of meningioma. The preferential diagnostic test for meningioma is neurodiagnostic imaging. Computed tomography shows the tumor as a hyperdense lesion that further increases in density after administration of iodine contrast.

When a cerebral tumor leads to increased intracranial pressure due to its size, induction of edema, or obstruction of spinal fluid flow, generalized headache develops independent of the location of the tumor. Vomiting, typically explosive and with minimal or no associated nausea, may also occur, as well as a decrease in the level of consciousness. On neurologic examination, the increased intracranial pressure will be evident from the congested optic disks (papilledema).

Temporal Arteritis

Temporal arteritis is a condition affecting the elastic arteries, with a preference for those of the head ("cranial arteritis"). Anatomically, it is characterized by necrosis of the media, which, in elastic arteries, is predominantly made up of elastine. The necrosis is associated with the formation of granulomatous tissue and giant cells (giant-cell arteritis). The cause of the condition is unknown but probably involves the generation of (auto)antibodies against elastine.

Temporal arteritis almost exclusively occurs over the age of 60 and equally affects men and women. It is a relatively rare condition, of which the incidence increases with age. The symptoms can be divided into those specific for the arteries involved and those reflecting the systemic, inflammatory nature of the condition. The systemic symptoms include general malaise, generalized weakness, easy fatigability, lack of appetite, weight loss, and low-grade fever. The low-grade fever can often be detected only by having the patient measure his or her temperature several times daily.

Headache is probably the most common of the specific symptoms of temporal arteritis, primarily because of the preference of the condition for the arteries of the head, in particular, the temporal arteries. The headache is often severe in intensity and described as a deep, burning pain, sometimes with a throbbing quality. It is caused by dilatation of the larger extracranial arteries, of which the lumens are narrowed by swelling of the vessel wall. In addition, the vessel wall is very sensitive to stretch because of the inflammatory process affecting the arteries. Ischemia of the scalp is another contributing factor to the headache of temporal arteritis. It also explains why heat applied to the head often diminishes the intensity of the pain.

Another specific symptom of temporal arteritis is "claudication" of the muscles of mastication. The patient complains of pain in the jaw muscles on prolonged chewing due to ischemia of the muscles. This symptom is considered to be pathognomonic for temporal arteritis. Sometimes, the condition affects the cerebral arteries, resulting in encephalopathy, with symptoms of apathy, confusion, and disorientation. Also, when the cerebral arteries are involved, ischemic stroke may occur with focal neurologic symptoms, such as aphasia, hemiparesis, or hemianopia.

On physical examination, very little is generally found in terms of specific abnormalities. A low-grade fever may be present but is easily missed because of its fluctuating course. The temporal arteries may be more clearly visible or more pronounced on palpation but characteristically have absent or diminished pulsations. Routine laboratory testing generally reveals a strongly elevated sedimentation rate, slight anemia, and a slightly elevated alkaline phosphatase. The sedimentation rate is generally increased to between 50 and 100 mm but may also be normal. This means that in cases of high clinical suspicion for temporal arteritis, even with a normal sedimentation rate, a biopsy of the temporal artery should be performed. For the biopsy, a reasonably long segment of the temporal artery should be excised, as the lesions may not be present along the entire course of the blood vessel.

In 30% of cases, temporal arteritis also affects the ophthalmic arteries, leading to partial or total blindness due to retinal ischemia. Because of this potential complication, the condition, once diagnosed, should be treated as soon as possible. Treatment consists of corticosteroids, which generally have a positive effect on the course of the illness. Otherwise, the condition is self-limiting, and the symptoms gradually disappear over the course of several months. Nonsteroidal anti-inflammatory analgesics are often effective in relieving the symptoms of temporal arteritis, such as the headache. However, they do not reduce the potential risk of blindness!

Subdural Hematoma

Subdural hematoma is *always* the result of head injury. However, in the elderly, the injury may be minimal and easily forgotten by the patient. Also, confusion and impairment of memory are common symptoms of the condition, making it difficult to obtain an accurate history. Subdural hematoma is a hematoma of venous origin located between the dura mater and arachnoidea. It is generally located over the cerebral hemisphere and can be unilateral or bilateral. The cause of the hematoma is rupture of a so-called bridging vein resulting from trauma of the head. However, it is almost never associated with fracture of the skull, indicating the generally mild nature of the head injury.

Apart from infants, subdural hematoma predominantly occurs over the age of 50, and its incidence, like that of temporal arteritis, increases with age. The particular relationship of the condition with age is related to the progressive shrinkage of the brain that occurs with age. As a result, the bridging veins of the brain become more and more stretched, rendering them progressively susceptible to injury. The use of anticoagulants as well as alcohol abuse is a further contributing factor to the occurrence of subdural hematoma.

Subdural hematoma is more common in men than in women. Headache is most frequently its presenting symptom but may also be absent. It is generally mild in intensity, present continuously, and localized to the side of the hematoma. There are usually no other symptoms associated with it. Mental symptoms, in particular confusion and disorientation, as well as drowsiness, are also common presenting symptoms of the condition. Focal neurologic symptoms or signs, such as hemiparesis or asymmetric or pathologic reflexes, are much less common. Also, papilledema is hardly ever seen with subdural hematoma because of the fact that it predominantly affects the elderly. In the elderly, papilledema generally does not occur with space-occupying intracranial lesions because of the large volume of cerebrospinal fluid.

Subdural hematoma is diagnosed with neurodiagnostic imaging. Computed tomography, depending on the age of the hematoma, shows it as hyperdense, isodense, or hypodense. When isodense, the only manifestation of the hematoma may be a shift of midline structures without further abnormalities. Magnetic resonance imaging or angiography may then be necessary to establish the presence of the hematoma.

Subdural hematoma can be treated either medically or surgically. Medical treatment consists of corticosteroids that in the very old patient may be preferred over surgical treatment. Surgical treatment consists of evacuation of the hematoma and is associated with the general risks of surgery. Also, in the very old patient, the brain may not expand after evacuation of the hematoma, resulting in a subdural space filled with air. Generally, patients improve with either treatment, but the improvement may be slow and only partial.

CHRONIC HEADACHE

In patients with chronic headache, the headache has been present, either intermittently or continuously, for months, years, or sometimes decades. The patient is generally between 20 and 50 years of age, as these are the years of highest headache prevalence. The prevalence of headache sharply increases during the second decade of life to remain stable until the age of 50. After the age of 50, the prevalence of headache gradually decreases with the advancement of age. The patient is also more likely to be a woman than a man because of the fact that headaches in women are more intense than in men. Men and women suffer from headache equally frequently, but headaches of moderate and severe intensity are twice as common in women than in men.

Chronic headache is related to abnormal functioning of extracranial tissues, in particular, the muscles and arteries. Patients who suffer from chronic headache have increased tightness of the neck and jaw muscles, as was shown in a study that looked at 164 headache patients and compared them with 108 age- and sex-matched controls.[12] The patients had suffered from headache for an average of 14 years. Tightness of the neck muscles was reported by 49% of the headache patients, as compared with 30% of the control subjects. The tightness of the neck muscles increased to 69% in the headache patients when headache was present. Tightness of the jaw muscles was equally present in the headache patients and the control subjects (17%) but was increased in the headache patients when headache was present (30%). Similar observations were made in an electromyographic study that involved 19 patients with headache and 12 controls.[13] No differences were found between patients with muscle-contraction headache and those with migraine.

Arterial vasodilatation causes pain by stretching of the nerve fibers that coil around the blood vessels. This is the mechanism that has been implicated in the headache of migraine and cluster headache. It particularly involves the frontal branch of the superficial temporal artery, giving rise to the characteristic throbbing migraine pain in the temple. Another prominent location of the headache that involves a vascular mechanism is in or behind the eye. This is typically the location of the headache in cluster headache, which is generally considered a migraine-related condition. Cluster headache is a chronic headache condition with a well-defined presentation and treatment.

The two most common chronic headache conditions, muscle-contraction headache and migraine, are not as well defined. The distinction between the two is relatively arbitrary and generally of little or no relevance to treatment. This is in spite of the fact that the International Headache Society has recently come out with strict criteria for the diagnoses of these conditions.[14] The criteria for the two conditions are summarized in Table 58–2 and are presented here for the sake of completeness. They are arbitrary and overlapping, lack biologic validity, and have not been tested clinically.[15]

Clinically, muscle-contraction headache and migraine fall on a continuum that is schematically shown in Figure 58–1. The episodic form of muscle-contraction headache stands on one side of the continuum and migraine on the other. Between them are chronic muscle-contraction headache and muscle-contraction vascular headache. The latter condition is also referred to as chronic muscle-contraction headache with coexisting migraine, mixed, or combined headache. Patients with chronic headache can present anywhere on the continuum and can, in the course of time, move along it, as indicated by the arrows.

The basis of the continuum is the interaction between the muscular and vascular mechanisms of headache. In this interaction, the vascular mechanism, through the intense pain it generates, activates the muscular mechanism. The activation of the muscular mechanism consists of voluntary and involuntary contraction of the muscles of the head, face, and neck. The muscular mechanism in turn activates the vascular mechanism through the interference with muscle blood flow. The body responds to the decrease in blood flow of the muscles by dilating the feeding arteries, such as the frontal branch of the superficial temporal artery, which overlies the powerful temporalis muscle.

TABLE 58–2. DIAGNOSTIC CRITERIA FOR MIGRAINE AND TENSION-TYPE (MUSCLE-CONTRACTION) HEADACHE AS PROPOSED BY THE INTERNATIONAL HEADACHE SOCIETY*

Migraine (code 1.1)

A. At least five attacks fulfill criteria B–D
B. Attacks last from 4 to 72 hours
C. Headache has at least two of the following characteristics:
   1. Unilateral location
   2. Pulsating quality
   3. Moderate or severe intensity
   4. Aggravation by routine physical activity
D. At least one of the following occurs during headache:
   1. Nausea or vomiting
   2. Photophobia and phonophobia

Tension-type headache (code 2.1)

A. At least 10 episodes fulfill criteria B–D
B. Episodes last from 30 minutes to 7 days
C. Headache has at least two of the following characteristics:
   1. Pressing or tightening quality
   2. Mild to moderate intensity
   3. Bilateral location
   4. No aggravation by routine physical activity
D. Both of the following occur during headache:
   1. No nausea or vomiting
   2. No photophobia or phonophobia

*From Headache Classification Committee of the International Headache Society: Classification and diagnostic criteria for headache disorders, cranial neuralgias and facial pain. Cephalalgia 8(Suppl 7):1–96, 1988; with permission.

The muscular mechanism is generally responsible for mild-to-moderate headaches of diffuse location and pressing quality. The headaches usually occur during the day, often in the afternoon, and gradually build in intensity as the day progresses. They usually lack associated symptoms, such as photophobia or nausea, because of the relatively low intensity of the pain. The vascular mechanism, on the other hand, is generally responsible for moderate-to-severe headaches. These headaches are often localized, usually to the temple or behind the eye, and are throbbing in nature. They are usually associated with other symptoms, such as photophobia and phonophobia as well as nausea and vomiting. The headaches are often present on awakening in the morning or wake the patient out of sleep in the early morning.

Muscle-Contraction Headache

Muscle-contraction headache is divided into episodic and chronic, depending on the frequency of occurrence of the headaches. In chronic muscle-contraction headache, the headaches occur daily or almost daily. Chronic muscle-contraction headache is more often secondary than primary, that is, it generally develops out of episodic muscle-contraction headache. When the chronic muscle-contraction headache is primary, there is often a precipitating physical event, such as a whiplash injury of the neck or a flu-like illness. Sometimes, the event is meningitis, subarachnoid hemorrhage, or myelography, with the meningeal irritation initiating the contraction of the craniocervical muscles. The most common cause of progression of episodic into chronic muscle-contraction headache is treatment that relies on analgesics. Analgesics, whether over-the-counter or pre-

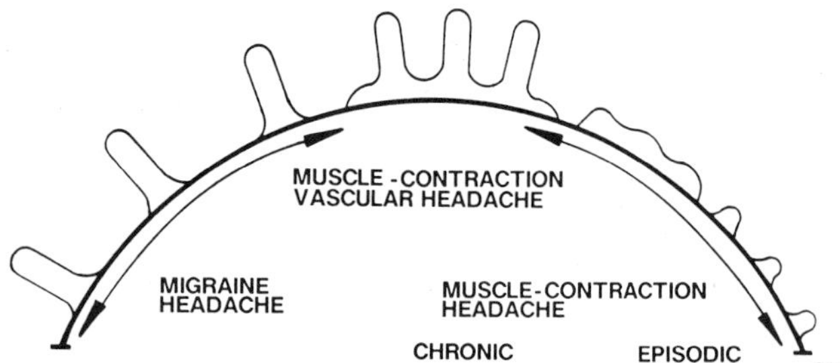

FIGURE 58–1. The continuum of muscle-contraction headache and migraine, covering episodic and chronic muscle-contraction headache (right), muscle-contraction vascular headache (middle), and migraine (left).

scription, address the pain of the headache but neglect the underlying mechanism. As a result of this neglect of the underlying mechanism, the headaches gradually increase in frequency over time.

Frequent use of analgesics for headache also has an impact on the efficacy of preventive treatments, that is, treatments aimed at decreasing the frequency, intensity, or duration of the headaches. This was demonstrated for the first time in an elegant study by Kudrow[16] on the effect of amitriptyline on chronic muscle-contraction headache. He showed that the efficacy of the medication was less than half (30% versus 72%) in the patients who were allowed to take analgesics for their headaches, as compared with those who were not. This negative effect of analgesics when used frequently for headache is, however, not limited to amitriptyline and extends to all pharmacologic and nonpharmacologic preventive treatments for headache. Therefore, it is important that with frequently occurring headaches, even when these headaches are mild in intensity, accurate information is obtained on the intake of both over-the-counter *and* prescription analgesics. The information needs to include the number of tablets taken per day and the number of days per week or per month that the medications are taken. When analgesics are taken more often than 1 or 2 days/wk, these analgesics need to be discontinued as the first step of treatment.

Discontinuation of analgesic use is often followed by an improvement of the headaches, even without the prescription of preventive treatment. The analgesics are generally best discontinued abruptly rather than in a tapered fashion. Abrupt discontinuation of the analgesics is, however, often followed by an initial worsening of the headaches for 2 or 3 days. Patients have to be informed about this so that they know what to expect. They can be prescribed muscle-relaxant medications, such as carisoprodol (Soma), for their headaches.

The two medications that have been shown to be effective in the preventive treatment of chronic muscle-contraction headache are amitriptyline hydrochloride (Elavil)[17, 18] and doxepin hydrochloride (Sinequan).[19] These medications are best prescribed once daily at bed time because they cause sedation. The doses used for the treatment of headache are lower than those for depression and range from 25 to 75 mg/day. Apart from sedation, the medications cause dry mouth, constipation, and weight gain. They are particularly helpful in patients who also have problems falling asleep or sleeping through the night. I usually initiate treatment with a dose of 25 mg at bedtime and gradually increase the dose until some dryness of the mouth occurs. At the same time, I watch for the effect on the headaches and the occurrence of other adverse effects, in particular, weight gain. Once the headaches are under control, I gradually decrease the dose to see whether the patient can do without the medication or to find the minimal effective dose. Both amitriptyline and doxepin increase serotonin in the central nervous system and by doing so inhibit central pain transmission. The medications may also have a muscle-relaxant effect, possibly mediated by their anticholinergic activity.

Treatments other than medication that relax the craniocervical muscles and prevent muscle-contraction headache are physical and relaxation therapy. The simplest form of physical therapy is to have the patient use a heating pad daily for the neck and shoulder muscles. This is an effective way of decreasing the tightness of the neck and shoulder muscles, provided it is applied regularly, preferably daily. Exercises can be added to the daily use of the heating pad to stretch and strengthen the neck and shoulder muscles. More formal physical therapy modalities for these muscles include massage, ultrasound, and traction. Injection of the muscles, for example, the trapezius muscles, with a local anesthetic can further help relax the muscles. Relaxation therapies that can be used are autogenic and biofeedback training. In autogenic training, suggestions of warmth and heaviness are used to relax successive parts of the body. Biofeedback training makes use of information on the state of contraction of the muscles, thereby enabling the patient to relax the muscles more effectively. The relaxation therapies, however, are effective only when practiced regularly, preferably daily, as with the preventive medications, which have to be taken daily.

Migraine

Migraine is a condition of recurring moderate-to-severe headaches. The headaches last from several hours to a few days and occur at greatly varying frequency. When occurring frequently, i.e., more than once or twice per month, they are often interspersed with muscle-contraction headaches. The headache condition may subsequently gradually develop into a muscle-contraction vascular headache (see earlier). In women, the migraine headaches often occur in relation to the menstrual cycle, that is, with menstruation and ovulation. The estrogens seem to be at fault here because their withdrawal has been related to the occurrence of migraine.[20] Stress is also a common precipitating factor of migraine, and typically the headaches come afterward.

Other important precipitating factors of migraine are the vasoactive agents, which can be either vasodilator or vasoconstrictor in nature. Examples of vasodilator agents causing migraine are alcohol and sodium nitrite. Sodium nitrite is a food additive used to preserve meat and is present in cured meat products. Vasoconstrictor agents causing migraine are caffeine and the sympathomimetic amines, tyramine and phenylethylamine. Caffeine causes headache on withdrawal (weekend migraine) when consumed in a quantity of more that 200 to 300 mg/day, which is the equivalent of two cups of coffee.[21] Tyramine and phenylethylamine are chemicals present in dietary products, such as aged cheese, red wine, and dark chocolate. They act on the sympathetic nerve fibers and release from them the neurotransmitter substances, noradrenaline and adrenaline. These neurotransmitter substances cause vasoconstriction, and the headache occurs as a result of the rebound vasodilatation following the vasoconstriction.

In classic migraine, or migraine with aura, the headaches are preceded by transient focal neurologic symptoms, generally known as aura symptoms. These aura symptoms are sensory in nature, either visual or somatosensory, although occasionally a speech disturbance occurs. The visual disturbance typical of migraine is the scintillating scotoma, also called teichopsia or fortification spectra. The scintillating scotoma generally starts near the center of vision as a small spot surrounded by bright, often flickering and sometimes colorful zigzag lines. After slight enlargement, the circle of zigzag lines breaks open on the inside to take the form of a horseshoe, which gradually further expands into the periphery of the visual field. Vision is usually obscured not only by the zigzag lines but also by a band of dimness that lies against it on the inside of the horseshoe (Fig. 58–2).

From its onset near the center of vision to its disappearance in the periphery of the visual field, the scintillating scotoma lasts from 10 to 30 minutes, with an average of 20 minutes. This is also the approximate duration of the somatosensory disturbance that typically presents itself in the form of digitolingual paresthesias. These paresthesias consist of a feeling of numbness or pins-and-needles that starts in the fingers of one hand. They gradually extend upward into the arm, ultimately to involve the face, especially the nose-mouth area, on the same side. The somatosensory disturbance follows the visual disturbance but can also occur alone, although this is less common. The headache follows the visual or somatosensory disturbance right away or occurs after a certain interval, for example, after 1 hour. The headache is often unilateral in location and can be on the same side as the visual or somatosensory disturbance or on the opposite side.

The aura symptoms of migraine have long been thought to result from localized spasm of cerebral arteries, leading to transient brain hypoxia. This notion is based on experiments in which it was shown that inhalation of a cerebral vasodilator, such as carbon dioxide or amyl nitrite, is followed by a temporary regression of the symptoms. However, cerebral blood flow studies have shown an initial *increase* in blood flow in the occipitoparietal area, followed by a decrease and a gradual spreading of the decrease toward the frontal pole.[22] The decrease was 25%, which is not enough to cause neuronal dysfunction by ischemia.[23] The decrease was therefore referred to as oligemia, and the rate of forward spreading of the oligemia was determined to be approximately 2.2 mm/min.

The particular nature of the cerebral blood flow changes of the migraine aura has shed new light on a hypothesis that ascribes the migraine aura to the neurophysiologic phenomenon of spreading depression.[24] Spreading depression is a wave of inhibition of neuronal activity that travels over the cerebral cortex at a rate of 2 to 5 mm/min and is preceded by a short-lasting phase of intense neuronal activity. The vascular changes accompanying spreading depression are similar to those of the migraine aura and consist of a short-lasting increase in cerebral blood flow, followed by a longer-lasting decrease in the order of 20 to 25%.[25] Spasm of cerebral arteries is the mechanism probably related to complicated migraine, in which a stroke occurs during a migraine attack.[26] The stroke generally leaves a permanent neurologic deficit, such as a homonymous hemianopia or hemiparesis.

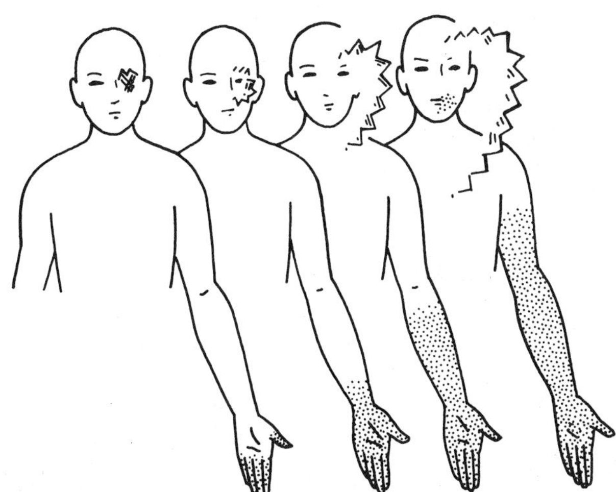

FIGURE 58–2. The two most typical aura symptoms of migraine, the scintillating scotoma and digitolingual paresthesias, shown from left to right in their successive stages of development.

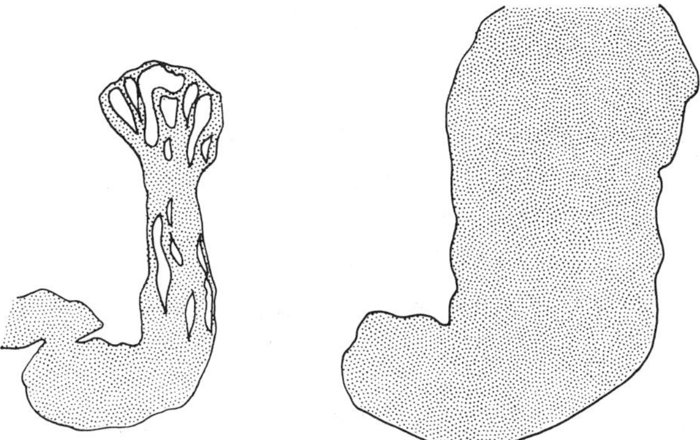

FIGURE 58–3. The stomach between (left) and during migraine (right) showing dilatation and atony with closure of the pyloric sphincter during the attack.

The treatment of migraine, as of headaches in general, can be divided into abortive and preventive. Abortive treatment is always indicated when headaches are moderate or severe in intensity, as is generally the case in migraine. For the abortive treatment of migraine, analgesic and vasoconstrictor medications are the most effective. When these medications are taken by mouth, as is often the case, absorption has to be considered. It has been shown for several medications that absorption during migraine is impaired because of dysfunction of the gastrointestinal tract.[27] This dysfunction consists of atony and dilatation of the stomach with closure of the pyloric sphincter, as shown in Figure 58–3. The dysfunction probably results from increased activity of the sympathetic nervous system secondary to the pain.[28]

The gastrointestinal dysfunction of migraine can be addressed with metoclopramide hydrochloride (Reglan), which is an antinausea medication with gastrokinetic properties. It stimulates the gastrointestinal tract and by doing so corrects the impaired absorption of oral medications during migraine.[29] It can be taken in a dose of 10 mg by mouth but needs to be taken early in the onset of migraine to get absorbed. It generally does not cause drowsiness or any other adverse effects and, therefore, can be taken early. Medications for headache will be more effective if taken 15 minutes after the metoclopramide.[30]

A useful oral medication for the treatment of migraine is Midrin, which is a combination of isometheptene mucate, dichloralphenazone, and acetaminophen.[31] Isometheptene is an indirectly acting sympathomimetic with vasoconstrictor properties, and dichloralphenazone is a mild sedative. Midrin is generally well tolerated with few if any adverse effects. It is taken in a dose of two capsules at the onset of headache, followed by one capsule every half hour, with a maximum of six. A step up in potency as an oral medication for migraine is acetaminophen with codeine, or Tylenol #3.

Codeine often causes nausea as an adverse effect, which is an additional reason for prior treatment with metoclopramide. A step up again from acetaminophen with codeine is Fiorinal, which is a combination of aspirin, caffeine, and butalbital. It is generally well tolerated and without adverse effects but, more so than acetaminophen with codeine, is potentially addicting.

When oral medications fail to relieve migraine, usually the impaired absorption is at fault. Rather than increasing the strength of the medication, it is generally more effective to alter the route of administration. Administration of a medication other than by mouth is also more effective once the migraine has already established itself, for example, when it is present on awakening in the morning or when it wakes the patient out of sleep at night. An effective way of administering a medication under these circumstances is by rectal suppository. The suppositories that can be used for this purpose are indomethacin (Indocin) and ergotamine tartrate with caffeine (Cafergot). Indomethacin is a potent anti-inflammatory analgesic with mild constrictor effect on the cerebral and extracranial arteries.[32] It is available as a 50-mg suppository, of which one can be taken every half hour, with a maximum of four in 1 day.[33]

The Cafergot suppository contains 2 mg of ergotamine tartrate in combination with 100 mg of caffeine to improve its absorption. Ergotamine is a very potent vasoconstrictor and is, therefore, contraindicated in hypertension and coronary artery disease. In a dose of 1 mg, that is, one half of a Cafergot suppository, it has been shown to relieve migraine within 3 hours in 73% of patients.[34] Nausea and vomiting are common adverse effects of ergotamine, therefore, it is important to administer the medication with care. I usually advise patients to take one quarter or one third of a suppository at a time and to repeat the dose every half to 1 hour, with a maximum of two suppositories. Taken in that way, the Cafergot suppository often provides effective relief of migraine without causing significant gastrointestinal adverse effects.

Ergotamine is a long-acting medication, and its vasoconstrictor effect has been shown to last at least 3 days.[35] This means that the medication should not be used more frequently than once/wk. If used more frequently, the wearing off of the effect of the medication is followed by rebound vasodilatation and headache that is indistinguishable from migraine. A cycle is thus created in which occurrence of headache and intake of ergotamine gradually increase over time, ultimately leading to what is often referred to as migraine status. This is an intractable condition in which headaches occur frequently, requiring daily or almost daily intake of ergotamine. The only way this condition can be treated is by total discontinuation of the use of ergotamine, for which hospitalization may be necessary. A dramatic reduction in the frequency of occurrence of the migraine headaches usually follows, once the withdrawal has been accomplished.[36]

Another route of administering a medication for the abortive treatment of migraine other than by mouth is by injection. An abortive antimigraine medication that is available for administration by subcutaneous injection is sumatriptan succinate (Imitrex). It is available in a prefilled syringe that contains 6 mg of the medication. It is supplied with an autoinjector device for easy administration by the patient. The efficacy of the medication has been shown to be 70% in decreasing the intensity of moderate and severe headaches to no or mild headache.[9] The administration of the medication can be repeated after 1 hour; it has been shown that this does *not* increase the efficacy. As the duration of action of the medication is relatively short, the headache can recur. If the headache does recur, this usually happens between 8 and 12 hours after the injection. The injection can be repeated at this point, or a longer-acting medication, such as the ergotamine (Cafergot) suppository, can be administered. Adverse effects of the medication are a hot, tight, or tingling sensation, generally in the upper chest, anterior neck, and face; and lightheadedness. Sumatriptan, like ergotamine, is a potent vasoconstrictor and, therefore, is contraindicated in hypertension and coronary artery disease.

When migraine headaches occur frequently, that is, more than twice/mo, preventive treatment may be indicated. Preventive treatment may also be indicated when the attacks are intense or prolonged and abortive treatment is ineffective. The medications that have been shown to be effective in migraine prevention are methysergide maleate (Sansert),[37–39] the β-blockers that lack partial agonist activity,[40] amitriptyline hydrochloride (Elavil),[41, 42] and verapamil hydrochloride (Isoptin).[43, 44]

Methysergide is available in 2-mg tablets. Treatment is usually initiated with a dose of one tablet twice daily, after which the dose is increased to one tablet four times per day. The medication is given in divided doses because of its relatively short duration of action. It is taken with the meals and at bedtime with some food because it can cause nausea and indigestion. With long-term use, the medication can give rise to retroperitoneal, pleuropulmonary, or endocardial fibrosis.[45, 46] Methysergide should therefore not be taken for longer than 4 to 6 months, after which it should be discontinued for 2 to 4 weeks. The medication is contraindicated in hypertension, vascular disease, valvular heart disease, chronic pulmonary disease, collagen disease, and fibrotic conditions.

The β-blockers that lack partial agonist activity are atenolol (Tenormin), metoprolol tartrate (Lopressor), nadolol (Corgard), propranolol hydrochloride (Inderal), and timolol maleate (Blocadren). Of these medications, propranolol is most commonly used, generally in doses ranging from 80 to 160 mg/day. When use is made of the long-acting capsule, the medication can be given once daily. Adverse effects of propranolol are fatigue, depression, insomnia, and impotence. The medication is contraindicated in sinus bradycardia, atrioventricular block, congestive heart failure, obstructive pulmonary disease, and diabetes mellitus. Atenolol and metoprolol are cardioselective and therefore can be used, with care, in obstructive pulmonary disease, such as asthma. I prefer the use of nadolol because it is generally better tolerated than propranolol, and it seems as effective. Nadolol is long-acting and therefore can be given once daily. I usually initiate treatment with a dose of 40 mg/day, after which I gradually increase the dosage. While increasing the dose, I monitor the effect of the medication on the pulse rate, which I bring down, if necessary, to 50 or 60.

Amitriptyline is best prescribed once daily at bedtime as it causes sedation. I usually initiate treatment with 25 mg and gradually increase the dose until some dryness of the mouth occurs. The medication is particularly helpful in patients who also have problems falling asleep or sleeping through the night. Apart from sedation and dry mouth, amitriptyline can cause constipation and weight gain. The medication is contraindicated in patients with glaucoma, prostate hypertrophy, epilepsy, or cardiac arrhythmias.

With regard to verapamil, I usually prescribe the 240-mg slow-release tablet, which can be given twice daily. I initiate treatment with a dose of 240 mg/day, after which I increase the dosage to 480 mg/day. Verapamil is generally well tolerated, and constipation is its most common adverse effect. The medication is contraindicated in patients with atrioventricular block and sick sinus syndrome because it slows down atrioventricular conduction.

Of the preventive antimigraine medications, the β-blockers are probably the most effective and best tolerated. Verapamil is probably the least effective, and amitriptyline falls somewhere in between. It should always be tried first to manage the migraine condition preventively with a single medication. However, the medications can also be combined, and a good combination is that of a β-blocker with amitriptyline. Special care should be taken when a β-blocker is combined with methysergide (which can cause peripheral vasoconstriction) or with verapamil (which can cause bradycardia).

Cluster Headache

Cluster headache is a chronic headache condition related to migraine but is much less common. Its prevalence in the general population is estimated at 70/100,000, with a male-to-female ratio of 14 to 1.[47] The clinical presentation of cluster headache is very constant; therefore, it is a condition generally easy to diagnose. The headaches of cluster headache last from a half to 2 hours and occur once or twice/24 hr. They have a tendency to occur during the early night, waking the patient out of sleep 1 or 2 hours after retiring. In 85% of the patients, the headaches occur in episodes lasting from a half to 2 months, separated by remissions of a half to 1 year. In the remaining 15%, the headaches occur for longer than 1 year without remission. In these cases, the condition is referred to as chronic, as opposed to episodic cluster headache. The onset of cluster headache occurs, for the majority of patients, in the second to fourth decade of life.

The pain of cluster headache is *always* unilateral and in 90% of the patients, always affects the same side of the head, with a slight preference for the right. The pain is usually located in and around the eye, in the forehead, temple, or in the face. In these areas, autonomic symptoms, such as reddening and tearing of the eye, edematous swelling and drooping of the upper eye lid, narrowing of the pupil, increased sweating over the forehead, and stuffiness and running of the nose, often occur. In general, these symptoms occur only on the side of the headache and only during the presence of pain. However, the symptoms are *not* pathognomonic for cluster headache, and their presence is not required for the diagnosis. Systemic symptoms, such as nausea and vomiting, which are common in migraine, are rare in cluster headache. Another prominent distinction between cluster headache and migraine is the behavior of the patient during the headache: whereas the patient with migraine usually lies down, the patient with cluster headache typically paces the floor.

The most consistent precipitating factors of the headache in cluster headache are alcohol and daytime napping. When a headache is triggered by alcohol, it generally occurs 30 to 45 minutes after ingestion of the alcohol. The occurrence of episodes has been related to the seasons of spring and fall. The psychophysical make-up of patients with cluster headache has been described as the leonine-mouse syndrome.[48] This refers to the husky appearance of many of the patients, with leonine facial features, such as ruddy complexion, deep furrows, and prominent eyebrows. In contrast to this supermasculine appearance stands the timid personality with increased dependency needs. Cluster headache patients often also smoke and drink alcohol excessively, possibly accounting for the increased incidence of coronary heart disease, peptic ulcer disease, and cancer in these patients.

Apart from instructing the patients to avoid alcohol and daytime napping during the episodes, treatment of cluster headache is pharmacologic in nature. The pharmacologic treatment can be divided into abortive and preventive, and although generally both are applied, the emphasis is on preventive treatment. Four medications, methysergide maleate (Sansert),[49] verapamil hydrochloride (Isoptin),[50] prednisone (Deltasone), and lithium carbonate (Lithobid),[49] are effective in preventing cluster headache. The three medications that are effective in aborting the headaches of cluster headache are ergotamine tartrate, oxygen,[51] and sumatriptan succinate.[52]

Ergotamine is most effective in cluster headache when taken as a sublingual tablet that contains 2 mg of the medication (Ergomar). It aborts at least seven of 10 headaches in 70% of patients, mostly within 10 to 12 minutes of treatment. The most common adverse effects of the medication are nausea, leg cramps, and a bad aftertaste. The medication is contraindicated in patients with hypertension and coronary artery disease. Inhalation of 100% oxygen is somewhat more effective than ergotamine. It is inhaled through a face mask at a rate of eight to 10 l/min for 15 minutes at the onset of headache. It aborts at least seven of 10 headaches in 82% of patients, within 6 minutes of treatment in more than 50%. There are no adverse effects or contraindications to the use of oxygen. Sumatriptan, in a dose of 6 mg subcutaneously, aborts 74% of cluster headaches within 15 minutes of treatment.[52]

Methysergide is least effective as a preventive medication for cluster headache. In a dose of 8 mg/day, it has an efficacy of 53% in episodic and 7% in chronic cluster headache. Efficacy is determined as a reduction in headache frequency of at least 75%. Verapamil has an efficacy of 73% in episodic and 60% in chronic cluster headache. The daily dose of verapamil to obtain this effect ranges from 240 to 600 mg in episodic and from 240 to 1200 mg (sustained-release tablets) in chronic cluster headache. With the use of doses higher than 480 mg/day, an echocardiogram should be performed to exclude heart muscle disease. It is also recommended that an electrocardiogram be performed several days after every dose increase to determine any impact on atrioventricular conduction.

When prednisone is used for the preventive treatment of cluster headache, it is usually given in a course of 3 or 4 weeks. The initial dose is 40 to 60 mg/day, which is maintained for 3 to 5 days. Subsequently, the dose is gradually decreased in steps of 5 mg/2 days. The efficacy of prednisone is 77% in episodic and 40% in chronic cluster headache. Adverse effects are insomnia, fluid retention, mood changes, and abdominal pain. The medication is contraindicated in patients with hypertension, diabetes mellitus, infections, peptic ulcer disease, and diverticulosis.

Lithium is particularly effective in treating chronic cluster headache; it has an efficacy of 87%. The therapeutic dose is generally between 600 and 1200 mg/day. Lithium is contraindicated in cases of electrolyte imbalance or when sodium restriction or diuretic therapy are required. In the latter cases, lithium intoxication easily develops as a result of increased tubular reabsorption of the medication, leading to symptoms ranging from tremor to convulsion. Common adverse effects of lithium are gastrointestinal symptoms, such as nausea, abdominal discomfort, and diarrhea. These symptoms, however, often respond rapidly to a slight lowering of the dose of the medication. The maintenance dose of lithium in the treatment of cluster headache does not depend on the serum level of the medication. It is, however, advisable to keep the serum level below 1.5 mEq/l and to determine it regularly, together with the serum electrolyte levels and kidney and thyroid functions.

Paroxysmal Hemicrania

Paroxysmal hemicrania is a variant of cluster headache that is rare but easy to diagnose and treat.[53] It consists of severe unilateral headaches similar to cluster headache, but the headaches are shorter in duration and occur more frequently. The headaches last from 10 to 30 minutes and occur five to 15 times/24 hr. They often occur like clockwork every 2 hours during the day and at night. The headaches occur in episodes with remissions or daily for years, that is, chronically. The headaches are totally relieved by preventive treatment with indomethacin. The dose generally required is 25 mg, four times per day, or 75 mg, sustained-release, twice daily. The beneficial effect is usually apparent within 2 to 5 days of treatment. Indomethacin is contraindicated in patients with peptic ulcer disease and bleeding disorders.

REFERENCES

1. Goldstein M and Chen TC: The epidemiology of disabling headache. Adv Neurol 33:377–390, 1982.
2. Messinger HB, Spierings ELH, Vincent AJP, and Lebbink J: Headache and family history. Cephalalgia 11:13–18, 1991.
3. Leicht MJ: Non-traumatic headache in the emergency department. Ann Emerg 9:404–409, 1980.
4. Jones J, Sklar D, Dougherty J, and White W: Randomized double-blind trial of intravenous prochlorperazine for the treatment of acute headache. JAMA 261:1174–1176, 1989.
5. Bell R, Montoya D, Shuaib A, and Lee MA: A comparative trial of three agents in the treatment of acute migraine headache. Ann Emerg Med 19:1079–1082, 1990.
6. Tek DS, McClellan DS, Olshaker JS, et al: A prospective, double-blind study of metoclopramide hydrochloride for the control of migraine in the emergency department. Ann Emerg Med 19:1083–1087, 1990.
7. Belgrade MJ, Ling LJ, Schleevogt MB, et al: Comparison of single-dose meperidine, butorphanol, and dihydroergotamine in the treatment of vascular headache. Neurology 39:590–592, 1989.
8. Harden RN, Carter TD, Gilman CS, et al: Ketorolac in acute headache management. Headache 31:463–464, 1991.
9. Cady RK, Wendt JK, Kirchner JR, et al: Treatment of acute migraine with subcutaneous sumatriptan. JAMA 265:2831–2835, 1991.
10. Galer BS, Lipton RB, Solomon S, et al: Myocardial ischemia related to ergot alkaloids: A case report and literature review. Headache 31:446–450, 1991.
11. Honig PJ and Charney EB: Children with brain tumor headache. Am J Dis Child 136:121–124, 1982.
12. Lebbink J, Spierings ELH, and Messinger HB: A questionnaire survey of muscular symptoms in chronic headache. Clin J Pain 7:95–101, 1991.
13. Pritchard DW: EMG cranial muscle levels in headache sufferers before and during headache. Headache 29:103–108, 1989.
14. Headache Classification Committee of the International Headache Society: Classification and diagnostic criteria for headache disorders, cranial neuralgias and facial pain. Cephalalgia 8(Suppl 7):1–96, 1988.
15. Messinger HB, Spierings ELH, and Vincent AJP: Overlap of migraine and tension-type headache in the International Headache Society classification. Cephalalgia 11:233–237, 1991.
16. Kudrow L: Paradoxical effects of frequent analgesic use. Adv Neurol 33:335–341, 1982.
17. Lance JW and Curran DA: Treatment of chronic tension headache. Lancet i:1236–1239, 1964.
18. Diamond S and Baltes BJ: Chronic tension headache—treated with amitriptyline—a double-blind study. Headache 11:110–116, 1971.
19. Morland TJ, Storli OV, and Mogstad TE: Doxepin in the prophylactic treatment of mixed "vascular" and tension headache. Headache 19:382–383, 1979.
20. Sommerville BW: The role of estradiol withdrawal in the etiology of menstrual migraine. Neurology 22:355–365, 1972.
21. Shirlow MJ and Mathers CD: A study of caffeine consumption and symptoms: Indigestion, palpitations, tremor, headache and insomnia. Int J Epidemiol 14:239–248, 1985.
22. Olesen J, Larsen B, and Lauritzen M: Focal hyperemia followed by spreading oligemia and impaired activation of rCBF in classic migraine. Ann Neurol 9:344–352, 1981.
23. Lauritzen M, Olsen TS, Lassen NA, and Paulson OB: Changes in regional cerebral blood flow during the course of classic migraine attacks. Ann Neurol 13:633–641, 1983.
24. Milner PM: Note on a possible correspondence between the scotomas of migraine and spreading depression of Leao. Electroencephalogr Clin Neurophysiol 10:705, 1958.
25. Lauritzen M, Jorgensen MB, Diemer NH, et al: Persistent oligemia of rat cerebral cortex in the wake of spreading depression. Ann Neurol 12:469–474, 1982.
26. Spierings ELH: Angiographic changes suggestive of vasospasm in migraine complicated by stroke. Headache 30:727–728, 1990.
27. Volans GN: Absorption of effervescent aspirin during migraine. BMJ 4:265–269, 1974.
28. Anthony M: Biochemical indices of sympathetic activity in migraine. Cephalalgia 1:83–89, 1981.
29. Volans GN: The effect of metoclopramide on the absorption of effervescent aspirin in migraine. Br J Clin Pharmacol 2:57–63, 1975.
30. Tfelt-Hansen P and Olesen J: Effervescent metoclopramide and aspirin (Migravess) versus effervescent aspirin or placebo for migraine attacks: A double-blind study. Cephalalgia 4:107–111, 1984.
31. Diamond S: Treatment of migraine with isometheptene, acetaminophen, and dichloralphenazone combination: A double-blind, crossover trial. Headache 15:282–287, 1976.
32. Sicuteri F, Michelacci S, and Anselmi B: Termination of migraine headache by a new anti-inflammatory vasoconstrictor agent. Clin Pharmacol Ther 6:336–344, 1965.
33. Nelemans F: Een technisch gelukt onderzoek met indomethacine bij patienten lijdende aan migraine. Een dubbelblind onderzoek versus placebo. Huisarts Wetenschap 14:337–340, 1971.
34. Graham JR: Rectal use of ergotamine tartrate and caffeine alkaloid for the relief of migraine. N Engl J Med 250:936–938, 1954.
35. Tfelt-Hansen P and Paalzow L: Intramuscular ergotamine: Plasma levels and dynamic activity. Clin Pharmacol Ther 37:29–35, 1985.
36. Tfelt-Hansen P and Aebelholt Krabbe A: Ergotamine abuse. Do patients benefit from withdrawal? Cephalalgia 1:29–32, 1981.
37. Shekelle RB and Ostfeld AM: Methysergide in the migraine syndrome. Clin Pharmacol Ther 5:201–204, 1964.
38. Southwell N, Williams JD, and Mackenzie I: Methysergide in the prophylaxis of migraine. Lancet i:523–524, 1964.
39. Pedersen E and Moller CE: Methysergide in migraine prophylaxis. Clin Pharmacol Ther 7:520–526, 1966.
40. Weerasuriya K, Patel L, and Turner P: Beta-adrenoceptor blockade and migraine. Cephalalgia 2:33–45, 1982.
41. Gomersall JD and Stuart A: Amitriptyline in migraine prophylaxis. Changes in pattern of attacks during a controlled clinical trial. J Neurol Neurosurg Psychiatry 36:684–690, 1973.
42. Couch JR and Hassanein RS: Amitriptyline in migraine prophylaxis. Arch Neurol 36:695–699, 1979.
43. Solomon GD, Steel JG, and Spaccavento LJ: Verapamil prophylaxis of migraine. A double-blind, placebo-controlled study. JAMA 250:2500–2502, 1983.
44. Markley HG, Cheroms JCD, and Piepho RW: Verapamil in prophylactic therapy of migraine. Neurology 34:973–976, 1984.
45. Graham JR: Methysergide for prevention of migraine. Experience in five hundred patients over three years. N Engl J Med 270:67–72, 1964.

46. Graham JR: Cardiac and pulmonary fibrosis during methysergide therapy for headache. Am J Med Sci 254:23–34, 1967.
47. D'Alessandro R, Gamberini G, Benassi G, et al: Cluster headache in the Republic of San Marino. Cephalalgia 6:159–162, 1986.
48. Graham JR: Cluster headache. Headache 11:175–185, 1972.
49. Kudrow L: Comparative results of prednisone, methysergide and lithium therapy in cluster headache. *In* Greene R (ed): Current Concepts in Migraine Research. New York, Raven Press, 1978, pp 159–163.
50. Gabai IJ and Spierings ELH: Prophylactic treatment of cluster headache with verapamil. Headache 29:167–168, 1989.
51. Kudrow L: Response of cluster headache attacks to oxygen inhalation. Headache 12:1–4, 1981.
52. Sumatriptan Cluster Headache Study Group: Treatment of acute cluster headache with sumatriptan. N Engl J Med 325:322–326, 1991.
53. Spierings ELH: Episodic and chronic paroxysmal hemicrania. Clin J Pain 8:44–48, 1992.

59

Parkinsonism, Tremors, and Gait Disorders

LEWIS SUDARSKY, MD

Parkinson's disease is common, affecting 1.5% of the population older than 65 years of age. Exciting advances in the study of Parkinson's disease will change the way patients are managed and teach us something about how the motor system changes with age. Other movement disorders,. at one time the province of the neurologic specialist, are increasingly a part of office practice. Patients with essential tremor, focal dystonias, dyskinesias, and odd gait disorders routinely seek medical attention.

This chapter focuses on facets of parkinsonism. Parkinson's disease is recognized by its four cardinal clinical features: bradykinesia, rigidity, tremor, and gait disorder. Each of these symptoms can be the presenting manifestation of Parkinson's disease or some related disorder (Fig. 59–1). This chapter considers first patients presenting with bradykinesia-rigidity, the differential diagnosis, and the management of idiopathic Parkinson's disease. A discussion of tremor, its diagnosis, and treatment follows. Finally, we will consider the approach to the patient with a gait disorder, with special reference to gait and balance problems of the elderly.

PARKINSON'S DISEASE

The diagnosis of Parkinson's disease is often one of impressions. Patients display masked facial expression, hypophonic speech, and a characteristic simian posture. Activities of daily life (buttoning, dressing, washing) take extra time. Handwriting degenerates into micrographia, a poorly legible scrawl. As noted, the four cardinal features are: bradykinesia, rigidity, tremor, and a characteristic disorder of posture and gait. Bradykinesia (slowness and difficulty initiating movement) is the most disabling feature of the illness. Slowness and inertia are pervasive in everyday activities. Rigidity with cogwheeling is uniform through the range of movement. Extrapyramidal rigidity is most easily appreciated in the wrist and neck. Tremor, the most distictive feature, and gait are considered separately.

Parkinson's disease remains a clinical diagnosis. No laboratory tests are done routinely. Because 10 to 20% of patients who present with a bradykinetic-rigid disorder will ultimately turn out to have another illness,[1] magnetic resonance imaging is sometimes used to screen patients with atypical parkinsonism.

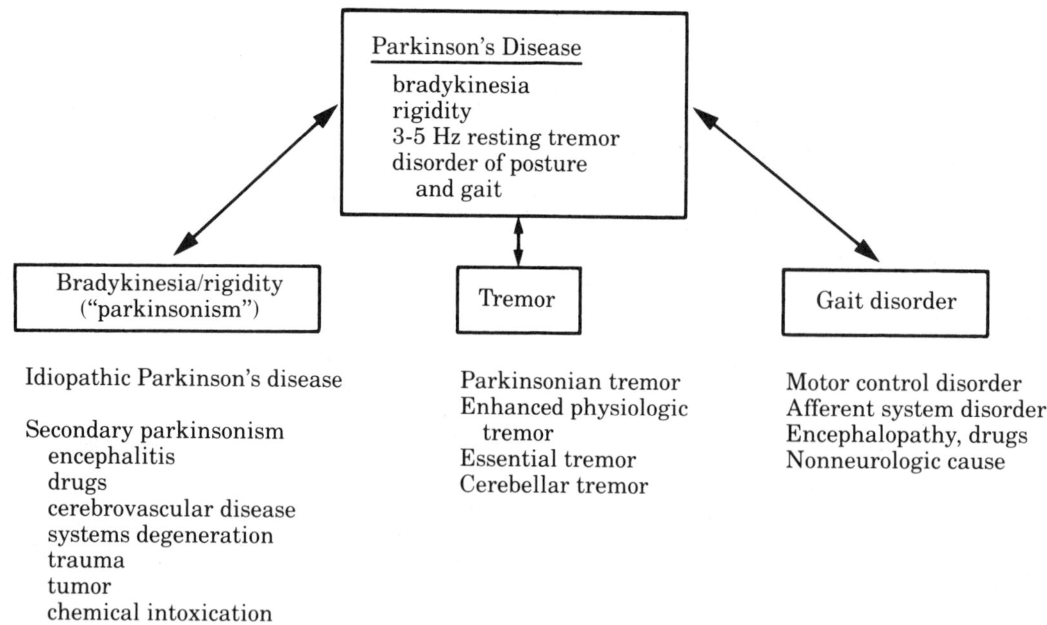

FIGURE 59–1. Differential diagnosis of the various presenting features in Parkinson's disease.

The differential diagnosis of bradykinesia-rigidity (parkinsonism) is summarized in Table 59–1. Secondary causes of parkinsonism include encephalitis, trauma, and vascular disease. Neuroleptic antipsychotic drugs and dopamine-depleting agents like reserpine can cause a parkinsonian syndrome with long-term use. Drug-induced parkinsonism is important to recognize because it is reversible over weeks.[2] Anticholinergic medications, such as benztropine and trihexyphenidyl, are used to reduce rigidity and tremor. Five to 10% of patients with parkinsonism will have a related systems degeneration, sometimes referred to as a Parkinson's plus syndrome. Progressive supranuclear palsy may present with axial rigidity, poor balance, and a tendency to fall (a late feature in idiopathic Parkinson's disease). Difficulty with downward gaze usually develops within a year or two. Striatonigral degeneration, olivopontocerebellar atrophy, and Shy-Drager syndrome can all be mistaken for Parkinson's disease early on in the disease course. Response to dopamine replacement (levodopa and carbidopa [Sinemet]) is usually disappointing.

Etiology and Pathogenesis

The clinical syndrome of bradykinesia and rigidity results from a deficiency of neurotransmitter dopamine in the basal ganglia. The ultimate cause is the loss of pigmented cells in the pars compacta of the substantia nigra. This limited cell population is the source of dopamine projections for the motor system (Fig. 59–2). Some of these cells are lost through attrition with normal aging, but not enough to cause difficulty. When 75% of nigral neurons are lost, there is a critical deficiency of striatal dopamine, and patients exhibit clinical signs. The disorder is progressive, and the cells do not regenerate. Preclinical dopamine depletion can be imaged with the use of positron-emission tomography.

The etiology of Parkinson's disease is still not understood. The incidence increases sharply with age, approaching 2.5% at age 80. Results of twin studies argue against inheritance and suggest that Parkinson's disease is somehow acquired in postnatal life.[3] The experience in the 1970s with *N*-methyl-4-phenyl-tetrahydropyridine (MPTP)–induced parkinsonism has emphasized the biologic vulnerabilities of the nigral cell population. There is considerable interest in the possibility that idiopathic Parkinson's disease may result from exposure to an environmental toxin or free radical by-products of dopamine oxidation. In some patients with Parkinson's disease, abnormalities of the mitochondrial respiratory chain have been documented.[4]

TABLE 59–1. DIFFERENTIAL DIAGNOSIS OF BRADYKINESIA-RIGIDITY

Idiopathic Parkinson's disease

Secondary parkinsonism
- Toxic
  - MPTP (*N*-methyl-4-phenyl-tetrahydropyridine)
  - Manganese
  - Carbon monoxide
- Drug-induced
  - Neuroleptic drugs
  - Metaclopramide, prochlorperazine
  - Reserpine
- Vascular disease ("arteriosclerotic parkinsonism")
  - Basal ganglia lacunes
  - Binswanger's disease
- Hydrocephalus
- Trauma
- Tumor
- Chronic hepatocerebral degeneration
- Wilson's disease
- Infectious
  - Post-encephalitic parkinsonism
  - Creutzfeldt-Jakob disease
  - Acquired immunodeficiency syndrome

Systems degeneration (Parkinson's plus syndrome)
- Progressive supranuclear palsy
- Multisystem atrophy
  - Shy-Drager syndrome
  - Striatonigral degeneration
  - Olivopontocerebellar atrophy
- Parkinson's-ALS*-dementia of Guam
- Generalized Lewy body disease
- Cortical-basal ganglionic degeneration
- Alzheimer's/Parkinson's overlap syndrome
- Huntington's disease: rigid variant
- Hallervorden-Spatz disease
- Gerstmann-Strausler syndrome

*ALS = amyotrophic lateral sclerosis.

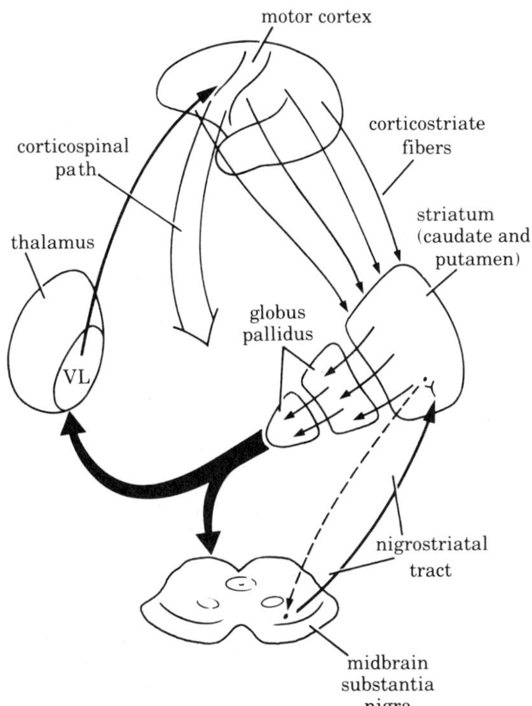

FIGURE 59–2. The striatal loop is involved in the elaboration of voluntary movement. Cortical impulses are fed to the neostriatum (caudate and putamen). Output through the globus pallidus to the thalamus influences the execution of movement by the corticospinal tract.

Midbrain substantia nigra neurons, via the nigrostriatal pathway, control the flow of process through the striatal loop. Dopamine is the principal neurotransmitter of nigral afferents to the striatum.

If oxidative damage is important in the pathogenesis of Parkinson's disease, then it might be possible to retard the progression of the illness with antioxidants or inhibitors of the monoamine oxidase (MAO) enzyme. Early diagnosis and institution of treatment might then become important. This strategy of *neuroprotective therapy* was examined in a large multicenter clinical trial (DATATOP study), the results of which were published in 1989.[5] Daily use of selegiline, a MAO B-isoenzyme inhibitor, significantly slowed the evolution of disability in treated patients. The study does not establish a neuroprotective mechanism for the drug effect, however, and its interpretation has been controversial.[6]

Management

For consideration of management, we divide patients into three groups: those with early, moderate, and advanced disease. The patient with early disease, often newly diagnosed, is easily able to work and perform daily activities. Such patients primarily experience symptoms at a nuisance level, some social embarrassment, and a great deal of anxiety about the outlook. Moderate parkinsonism begins to impinge on function as the patient shows a change in mobility. Daily activities require more time. Advanced disease is marked by limitations in daily activities *despite drug treatment.* Such patients may develop fluctuations, treatment-limiting side effects, and a loss of independence in activities of daily living.

Although controversy persists about the interpretation of the DATATOP study, most movement disorder specialists would recommend the use of selegiline in all newly diagnosed patients. The drug is usually well tolerated; the standard dose is 5 mg twice/day (morning and midday). At this dose, the MAO B-isoenzyme is selectively inhibited, and no dietary restrictions are necessary. Five to 10% of patients experience insomnia or nausea. Selegiline can cause confusion in older, demented patients. It also aggravates postural hypotension when used with other antiparkinsonian medications. Although it is not intended as symptomatic therapy, selegiline will improve motor function (and mood) in some patients. Most new patients will do well without requiring other medication for about a year. Patients need to understand the rationale for an expensive medication that is not dramatic in its effect on motor performance.

Moderate Disease

Symptomatic therapy (some form of dopamine replacement) is added as soon as slowness or disability has begun to interfere with the patient's occupation or daily activities. Large studies have not demonstrated any advantage to withholding levodopa at this stage, although the best results are generally achieved in the first 5 or 6 years of its use. It is curious to think that one can influence the function of the brain by the oral loading (by feeding) of neurotransmitter precursors, yet this is precisely the mechanism of action of levodopa. Levodopa enters the nervous system by facilitated transport and is converted directly into neurotransmitter dopamine. The regulatory step in catecholamine synthesis is bypassed, so that large quantities of neurotransmitter dopamine can be made and stored presynaptically. Peripheral inhibitors of dopa decarboxylase enhance the central accumulation of transmitter and diminish side effects caused by receptors in the periphery. For this reason, levodopa is usually given in combination with 75 to 150 mg/24 hr of carbidopa (Table 59–2). It is best to begin with a small dose (half of a 25/100 Sinemet tablet, twice a day; or half of a Sinemet CR). If nausea is a problem, options include reducing selegiline to 5 mg, adding extra carbidopa (available from the manufacturer), or adding an antiemetic. There is less nausea with Sinemet CR, which does not cause a rapid surge in plasma levodopa level.

Authorities on the treatment of Parkinson's disease increasingly recommend early introduction of a dopamine receptor agonist drug, such as bromocriptine (10 to 15 mg) or pergolide (1.0 to 1.5 mg) together with levodopa. The principal advantage of this approach is that it allows the levodopa dose to remain in the low range (300 to 500 mg/day) for most patients. (For theoretical reasons, smaller doses of levodopa may be preferable.) In one frequently cited study, Rinne demonstrated that patients treated with bromocriptine from the onset had less difficulty in subsequent years with response fluctuations and dyskinesias.[7]

One point against this strategy is the greater toxicity and expense of the dopamine agonists, which are generally less potent therapeutic agents than the levodopa-carbidopa combination. Synthetic dopamine agonists can cause cutaneous manifestations, nausea, dizziness, leg edema, orthostatic hypotension, confusion, and dyskinesias. In large doses, they can produce symptoms of ergotism, including digital vasospasm and chest pain. Best results are obtained by starting with a small dose (1.25 mg of bromocriptine, 0.05 mg of pergolide) and gradually increasing the dosage over 2 to 3 weeks into the desired dose range. The agonist drugs have the advantage of a longer half-life, and used together with levodopa, they provide a smoother response. Few patients succeed with these drugs as primary therapy.

TABLE 59–2. DRUGS USEFUL IN THE TREATMENT OF PARKINSON'S DISEASE

Preparation	Available Form	Average Daily Dose
Levodopa	100, 250, 500 mg	1.5–8.0 g
Levodopa and carbidopa (Sinemet)	100/10, 100/25, 250/25 mg	200–1200 mg
Sinemet CR	200/50 mg	200–1500 mg
Amantadine (Symmetrel)	100 mg	100–300 mg
Trihexyphenidyl (Artane)	2, 5 mg	2–15 mg
Benztropine (Cogentin)	0.5, 1, 2 mg	1.0–6.0 mg
Ethopropazine (Parsidol)	50 mg	100–400 mg
Bromocriptine (Parlodel)	1.25, 2.5, 5 mg	10–25 mg
Pergolide (Permax)	0.05, 0.25, 1 mg	2–4 mg
Selegiline (Eldepryl)	5 mg	5–10 mg

Advanced Disease

The transition to advanced Parkinson's disease is often marked by the development of response fluctuations. Patients have trouble maintaining an even response to levodopa after 5 or 6 years of therapy. The half-life of levodopa is short (90 to 120 minutes), and many late-stage patients experience "wearing off" of its effect 2 to 3 hours after a dose. At the same time, they may be more sensitive to central nervous system toxicity at the peak dose. Because of the narrow therapeutic window, replacement of neurotransmitter dopamine by interval administration of precursor is unphysiologic and unsatisfactory for these patients. The solution to the problem of end of dose wearing off is a greater reliance on long-acting medications. Dopamine agonists are a useful adjunct in this situation. Sinemet CR, a sustained-release preparation, provides delayed enteric absorption over 4 to 6 hours. Sinemet CR can be expected to last twice as long as regular Sinemet, though individuals differ with respect to their response to this medication. Selegiline has not been as successful, and we rarely use it for this purpose in late-stage patients.

Other patterns of response fluctuation are more difficult to manage. Some patients describe transient freezing or episodes of "sudden off," which resolve over minutes without additional medication. Other patients develop a pattern of diphasic dyskinesia, in which involuntary movements accompany medication onset and wearing off. Greater reliance on dopamine agonist medications is often helpful, especially if the levodopa-carbidopa dose can be reduced.

Patients with late-stage Parkinson's disease are quite often disabled by postural instability and falls. Postural reflexes are poorly responsive to medication, and such patients must be more cautious. They should be encouraged to use a cane or walker when ambulation is unstable. Autonomic symptoms, such as postural hypotension and constipation, require attention in some patients.

Mental Status Changes

Although James Parkinson described a motor disorder, it is increasingly apparent that some patients with Parkinson's disease suffer mental change (delirium, depression, dementia). Delirium is generally transient and reversible and related to medications. All the commonly used antiparkinsonian medications have the potential to cause delirium, even transient psychosis. Anticholinergic drugs are the worst offenders; it may be best to avoid them altogether in patients over 75 years of age. In the patient prone to confusion, the preferred strategy is to avoid polytherapy and focus on the single drug with the greatest therapeutic index (i.e., the levodopa-carbidopa combination).

Depression occurs in a substantial number of patients. It is generally mild to moderate in degree but can be a difficult management problem. Depression is not correlated with the magnitude of disability and is often a feature in early-stage Parkinson's disease. Selegiline elevates mood for some patients, but a tricyclic antidepressant may be required if depression is significant.

The natural history of Parkinson's disease has changed in the levodopa era. More late-stage patients are alive and functioning, and it is apparent that 10 to 20% have a dementia syndrome as part of their illness. Episodic confusion (even off medication), slowness, and frontal behavioral features are most often observed. Neuropathologic examination reveals cortical plaques and tangles in about half such cases.[8] Some will have only lesions of Parkinson's disease, with widespread involvement of subcortical structures (locus ceruleus, ventral tegmental area, basal nucleus). It is best to avoid antipsychotic drugs, if possible; their prolonged use will inevitably worsen motor symptoms.

TREMOR

The term *tremor* has different meaning to engineers, geologists, and health professionals. For medical purposes, tremor can be defined as an oscillating involuntary movement about a joint. This definition encompasses the very slight movements seen with anxiety or stimulant drugs and the large-amplitude movements of cerebellar ataxia. The motor system is complex, and a slight disturbance of targeting or timing of muscle activation can easily result in instability. In practice, most tremors are not associated with gross central nervous system pathology.

Tremor phenomena can be classified at the bedside into four principal types: parkinsonian tremor, physiologic tremor, essential tremor, and cerebellar tremor (Table 59–3).[9] To draw this distinction, note first the frequency and distribution of the movements. Observe the patient sitting quietly with his or her arms relaxed, hands in his or her lap. Only Parkinson's tremor is present in an attitude of quiet repose (at rest). Next, ask the patient to extend his or her arms and spread his or her fingers and observe the postural component. Enhanced physiologic tremor and essential tremor are postural, brought out by tonic innervation of limb muscles. Essential tremor is somewhat slower and more intrusive by virtue of its higher amplitude. Finally, observe tremor movements during the finger-to-nose test as the finger approaches its target. Intention tremor, the most characteristic of the cerebellar tremors, is a side-to-side movement that increases in amplitude as the endpoint is approached, in a manner most suggestive of a defective servomechanism. On first inspection, the patient with essential tremor may appear to have a terminal exac-

TABLE 59–3. CLASSIFICATION OF TREMOR TYPE

	Parkinsonian Tremor	Physiologic Tremor	Essential Tremor	Cerebellar Tremor
Tremor appears	At rest	Tonic innervation, anxiety, stress	Tonic innervation (postural or action tremor)	Target-seeking
Frequency	3–7 Hz	8–12 Hz	4–8 Hz	3–8 Hz
EMG pattern*	Alternating	Synchronous	Synchronous	Alternating
Relieving factors	Levodopa, anticholinergics	Diazepam, propranolol	Alcohol, diazepam, propranolol	Limb weighting

*Surface electromyography (EMG) records the pattern of activation in antagonist muscle groups, such as biceps and triceps, pronator and supinator. An alternating pattern of activation is seen with parkinsonian tremor (see text).

erbation. Repeat trials should demonstrate that tremor amplitude (and direction) is inconsistent and varies with the attitude or position of the limb in space.

This descriptive sorting of tremor type will resolve 80 to 90% of the tremor problems seen clinically. There is some overlap, and an occasional patient will have more than one tremor. Tremors that defy classification can be further evaluated with physiologic tests or by response to medication.[10] Accelerometric recording is the simplest way to study tremor, although elegant studies have been done using surface electromyography in agonist and antagonist muscles.

Family history and history of medication exposure should be reviewed. Essential tremor is quite commonly a familial disorder. Patients often report improvement after ingesting alcohol. A minimum of laboratory tests are used in the evaluation. Thyroid function tests are obtained routinely. Patients with acute-onset Parkinson's disease should have toxicologic analysis of serum dose for drugs or alcohol. Serum copper studies for Wilson's disease are expensive and reserved for coarse proximal tremor of unknown etiology and for patients with liver disease. Patients with cerebellar signs require a more detailed etiologic evaluation, including computed tomographic scanning or magnetic resonance imaging of the posterior fossa to exclude a structural lesion (Table 59–4).

Parkinsonian Tremor

The characteristic tremor of Parkinson's disease occurs at rest, at 3 to 5 Hz (tremor cycles/sec). Some degree of tone is required to produce the tremor, so it will abate when the limb is truly relaxed or the patient asleep. The distal extremities are usually first. The tremor commonly begins as a pill-rolling tremor of one hand, sometimes intermittent, recruiting a pronation-supination motion of the forearm. The jaw and perioral area may be involved, especially in drug-induced parkinsonism. Whole-head tremor is not seen in Parkinson's disease. Physiologic studies demonstrate alternating contractions of agonist and antagonist muscles, brief bursts of muscle activity with a frequency of 3 to 5 Hz.

In studies on the natural history of Parkinson's disease, patients presenting with tremor may have a slower rate of progression.[11] The tremor often responds best to anticholinergic medications. When levodopa is necessary for the treatment of other symptoms, tremor characteristically improves as well. For the majority of patients with Parkinson's disease, tremor is not the most limiting feature of the illness.

A significant degree of action tremor, resembling essential tremor, can often be observed in Parkinson's disease. A few patients present with essential tremor and subsequently evolve features more characteristic of Parkinson's disease. Consequently, it is difficult to reassure the patient with essential tremor that he or she does not, or will not ever have, Parkinson's disease. In such patients, the tremor usually responds to β-blockers, and initial management is the same as for other patients with essential tremor. Lance and McLeod suggest that the cogwheeling phenomenon experienced when ranging the limbs of the patient with Parkinson's disease corresponds with the essential tremor.[12]

Enhanced Physiologic Tremor

A small-amplitude, high-frequency tremor (8 to 12 Hz) is present among asymptomatic normal persons. It can be observed by placing a 3 × 5″ card over the fingers of the fully extended limb. This tremor is enhanced by catecholamines (coffee, stress, thyroid hormone), drug or alcohol withdrawal, nicotine, numerous other medications, and muscular fatigue. The electrophysiology is difficult to study, because the tremor is generally buried in the normal interference pattern of the muscle.

This tremor can be improved by small doses of propranolol, a common practice among performing artists. Young and colleagues suggest a peripheral mechanism involving β-receptors in skeletal muscle because intra-arterial injection can often quiet this tremor in a single limb.[13] The preferred management of the symptomatic patient with en-

TABLE 59–4. TREMOR TYPE AND ETIOLOGY

Parkinsonian tremor
- Idiopathic Parkinson's disease
- Secondary parkinsonism, especially drug induced

Enhanced physiologic tremor
- Stress induced
- Endocrine: thyrotoxicosis, pheochromocytoma, hypoglycemia
- Drug induced:
  - xanthines; epinephrine, adrenergic agonists; nicotine; tricyclic antidepressants; lithium; phenothiazines; alcohol withdrawal

Essential tremor
- Inherited
- Sporadic
- Senile head tremor
- Associated with neurologic disease (Roussey-Lévy syndrome, spasmodic torticollis)

Cerebellar tremor
- Intention tremor: cerebellar degeneration, brain stem–cerebellar infarct, multiple sclerosis, neoplasm
- Cerebellar postural tremor: midbrain infarct, multiple sclerosis, Wilson's disease

Other
- Neuropathic tremor
- Primary writing tremor

Other movement disorders commonly mistaken for tremor
- Asterixis
- Myoclonus

hanced physiologic tremor is treatment of the underlying disorder. Anxiety and hyperthyroidism are common; such a tremor is often drug related.

Essential Tremor

Essential tremor is a 4- to 8-Hz action tremor similar to the physiologic tremor but often slightly slower and of greater amplitude. It may appear in the head, neck, voice, or upper limbs, and rarely, in postural or lower extremity muscles. Physiology shows cocontraction of the agonist and antagonist muscles. Most patients have a positive family history. Essential tremor may be sporadic or may be associated with other neurologic disease. In particular, focal dystonias, such as torticollis and spastic dysphonia, are sometimes associated with essential tremor. There are no neuropathologic findings at the light microscope level.[14]

Patients discover on their own the beneficial effect of alcohol. Alcohol attenuates the tremor for most patients. Propranolol is the preferred treatment. A central mechanism has been proposed, and sustained trials of high doses are often required. A dosage of 240 to 300 mg/day should be attempted before the patient is considered to be a nonresponder. An alternate medication is primidone, which is effective in low doses (50 to 125 mg/day). The subcategory of senile head tremors is notoriously difficult to treat. Both the yes-yes and no-no variety are observed. The tremor frequency is lower in patients with head tremors and among older patients in general.

Cerebellar Tremor

Patients with cerebellar system disease manifest a complex disorder of motor control that includes tremor. The ataxic patient has dysmetria, a tendency to overshoot or undershoot when executing a voluntary movement. Erratic movement is often more disabling to the patient than is his or her tremor. With intention tremor, the amplitude of oscillation increases as the goal, or desired final position of the limb, is approached. A coarse, high-amplitude, 3- to 5-Hz postural tremor may be seen with lesions of cerebellar outflow, particularly at the level of the red nucleus. This cerebellar postural tremor (sometimes called rubral tremor or midbrain tremor) is especially disabling.

The slow, high-amplitude oscillations of cerebellar tremor are difficult to treat. Limb weighting may be more helpful than pharmacologic treatment. Mechanical damping is used to design devices to assist patients in daily activities.

Other Characteristics

This nosology of tremor is by no means exhaustive. Patients with neuropathy may have a tremor, the mechanism of which is ill understood. Patients with motor neuron disease often display fasciculation tremor, the irregular action of a small pool of giant motor units on an extended limb. Particularly perplexing are patients with tremors restricted to one movement, such as primary writing tremor. Myoclonus and asterixis are sometimes associated with tremor in patients with metabolic encephalopathy. Asterixis is a 35- to 200-msec lapse in tonic activation of a muscle, which produces an arrhythmic movement, often somewhat tremorous in appearance.

GAIT DISORDERS

The office evaluation of the patient with impaired gait is one of the more troublesome problems in medical practice. Disorders of stance and gait are a source of considerable morbidity, particularly among the elderly. Gait disorders place patients at increased risk for disabling injury due to falls.[15] Progressive failure of ambulation may compromise the patient's independence and require long-term nursing care. Nonambulatory patients have excess morbidity and mortality.

Normal walking is a complex performance that calls on a range of neural systems. The production of a stable gait involves coordinated control of locomotion and balance. Spinal pattern generators contribute to locomotion in quadrupedal animals, but independent spinal walking is not observed in primates.[16] The mesencephalic locomotor region depends on afferent information from the motor cortex, basal ganglia, and cerebellum.[17] Dynamic balance calls on numerous postural control systems, known in the older literature as *righting reflexes*.[18] Postural control systems, in turn, depend on afferent sensory information from the visual system, vestibular system, and proprioceptive information from the lower limbs. A stable body architecture and normal vasomotor reflexes are also necessary for upright stance and gait.

Because so many neural systems participate in the performance, there is a great potential for mischief. An enormous diversity of gait disorders is observed clinically. This heterogeneity creates a challenge in diagnosis. Table 59–5 provides a partial listing of conditions presenting with chronic disturbance of gait. Some gait problems are multifactorial, particularly among the elderly. In one study of patients over 70 years of age, 28% met criteria for more than one etiologic diagnosis.[19] Fourteen per cent of gait disorders in this study were labeled as idiopathic (Table 59–6).[19] For purposes of discussion, locomotor disorders,

TABLE 59–5. COMMON ETIOLOGIES FOR CHRONIC GAIT DISORDER

Disorders affecting motor control
Parkinson's disease
Huntington's disease
Progressive supranuclear palsy
Wilson's disease
Cerebellar degeneration
Other system degenerations
Normal pressure hydrocephalus
Stroke
Subdural hematoma
Cervical spondylitic myelopathy
Multiple sclerosis
Subacute combined-systems disease
Neuromuscular disorders
Afferent system disorders
Peripheral neuropathy
Multiple sensory deficits
Tabetic neurosyphilis
Encephalopathy
Metabolic encephalopathy
Drugs, especially phenothiazine tranquilizers
Non-neurologic causes
Arthritis
Intermittent claudication
Spinal stenosis
Depression

TABLE 59–6. PRINCIPAL ETIOLOGIES OF GAIT DISORDER IN ELDERLY PATIENTS*

Disorder	%
Myelopathy	16
Parkinson's disease†	10
Hydrocephalus†	4
Multiple cerebral infarcts	16
Cerebellar atrophy	8
Sensory disorders	18
Encephalopathy†	4
Drug toxicity†	2
Depression†	2
Other	6
Essential (idiopathic)	14

*Adapted from Sudarsky L and Ronthal M: Gait disorders among elderly patients. Arch Neurol 40:740, 1983.
†Denotes treatable disorder.

balance disorders, encephalopathies, and non-neurologic causes are considered separately.

Etiologic Considerations

Primary degenerative disease (systems degeneration) can present with motor deficits that compromise gait. The causes of an extrapyramidal syndrome (atypical parkinsonism) are reviewed in Table 59–1. Such diseases can be familial (Huntington's disease) or sporadic (Parkinson's disease, progressive supranuclear palsy). Cerebellar deficits have a dramatic effect on gait, whether caused by a cerebellar degeneration, alcohol, or toxin exposure.

Cerebrovascular disease is easy to appreciate when it presents with an acute hemiparesis or an obvious stroke. Some patients presenting with gait disorders have suffered a series of small, nonparalyzing strokes, which have a cumulative effect on motor performance. Hypertensive patients with subcortical strokes may present in this fashion; only in retrospect is the step-wise incremental nature of their deficits appreciated. Adams and colleagues introduced the syndrome of normal-pressure hydrocephalus in 1965.[20] Fisher has contributed further to our understanding of hydrocephalus as an etiology of isolated gait disorder; some elderly patients with normal-pressure hydrocephalus lack dementia and incontinence.[21] An occasional patient with a frontal gait disorder will have a mass lesion.

Locomotor control is impaired when disease affects the descending pathways in the spinal cord. Cervical spondylosis is the commonest cause of myelopathy in older people; autopsy studies suggest that compression of the cervical cord by spondylitic bars is common.[22] Vitamin B_{12} deficiency also needs to be considered because it is a treatable disorder. In younger patients, demyelinating disease and trauma are the most common spinal disorders. Paty and colleagues reviewed a group of patients, mean age, 42, in whom chronic progressive myelopathy was often found to be due to otherwise unapparent multiple sclerosis.[23] Neuromuscular disease can compromise locomotor performance. Rarely, a late-onset limb girdle muscular dystrophy will be detected by virtue of excessive sway of the pelvis during gait.

A large number of patients who present with gait disorder suffer primarily from a disturbance of balance. Falls are particularly common in this group. Failure of afferent systems may compromise stability. Peripheral neuropathy of severe degree will result in a positive Romberg test and abnormal gait. Drachman and Hart noted a group of patients, generally elderly, in whom multiple sensory deficits involving vestibular, visual, and proprioceptive afferent systems resulted in chronic imbalance.[24] Tabetic neurosyphilis, formerly a common source of sensory ataxia, is now an infrequent occurrence in outpatient practice. Nevertheless, a high-stepping, wide, foot-slapping gait should suggest a sensory neuropathic disorder.

An important diagnosis to consider because of its frequent reversibility is metabolic encephalopathy. In patients with chronic liver disease or patients on hemodialysis, motor symptoms may be manifestations of an underlying encephalopathy. The phenothiazine tranquilizers and other neuroleptic medications can produce parkinsonism and cause a range of stereotypic gait disorders related to tardive dyskinesia. These medications are the principal cause of the odd gait disorders seen at extended care psychiatric hospitals and nursing homes. Depressed patients can present with psychomotor retardation and a slow-paced, head-hanging gait.[25] There is no simple screening test for the psychogenic gait disorder, but knowledge of a psychiatric history is helpful.

Finally, it is important to remember that patients may have abnormal gait because of skeletal and joint disorders. Arthritis produces pain and limitation of motion, evident as an "antalgic gait." Minor degrees of orthopedic deformity are unquestionably the commonest cause of slight gait disorder in office practice. The spinal stenosis syndrome causes pain that effectively limits ambulation.

Approach to the Diagnostic Evaluation

It is important to separate the chronic progressive disorder of gait from the acute failure of ambulation. Rapidly evolving gait difficulty, with a history measured in hours, days, or at most, a few weeks, represents a higher order of urgency and a medical problem of substantially different character. Stroke, subdural hematoma, and tumors of the brain and spinal cord are etiologies to be considered, as are acute encephalopathy and intoxication.

For the patient with a chronic and slowly progressive disorder, falls are an important landmark in the history. Abrupt, step-wise, incremental onset of deficits suggests vascular disease. Weakness in the legs is typically evident as difficulty getting up from a chair or climbing stairs. Incontinence and dementia often accompany frontal disorders of gait, as seen in a multi-infarct state or with normal pressure hydrocephalus. The patient's medications and drinking history should be reviewed; gait problems are commonly seen with phenytoin, barbiturates, sedatives, and the phenothiazine tranquilizers. It is helpful to check for postural hypotension, which may be related to medications.

The neurologic examination is the single most informative procedure. Corticospinal signs are sought by examining for hyperreflexia or palpable spasticity in the legs; an extensor plantar sign is useful corroborating evidence. Extrapyramidal disease is evident in the posture, an attitude of flexion in the trunk and upper limbs. Cerebellar signs may be absent in the upper limbs of patients with alcoholic cerebellar degeneration; it is essential to examine truncal stability in walking tandem, heel to toe. Romberg's test is a good bedside measure of adequacy of proprioceptive afferent from the legs. Peripheral neuropathy can be appreciated if the patient has absent ankle jerks and a stocking loss to sensation.

Watching the failing gait may be quite useful, although many features are merely those of biomechanical compensation for loss of competence. Most patients with poor gait will display widened stance, short steps, and a tendency to be easily displaced back. Huntington's disease and Parkinson's disease cause unique and characteristic gait abnormalities. Festination, start hesitation, and en bloc turning are features peculiar to parkinsonism. The choreic gait of Huntington's disease is also unique. The adequacy of postural righting reflexes can be tested in the office, by stressing stance with a gentle push on the sternum.[26] It is useful to stand behind the patient, to provide back-up support and prevent falls.

Laboratory tests of particular utility in the diagnosis of gait disorder include the cranial computed tomographic scan, magnetic resonance imaging, and radiologic studies of the spine. Brain imaging studies are used to search for occult hydrocephalus, lacunes, or white-matter abnormalities seen in patients with demyelination or small-vessel disease. An occasional patient presenting with a gait disorder will have a mass lesion or subdural hematoma. Cervical spine films and magnetic resonance are of particular importance in patients with bilateral long tract signs in the absence of dysarthria or mental change. Plain films of the cervical spine are often informative in cervical spondylitic myelopathy. Spondylitic bars and spondylolisthesis can be seen well, as can C1–C2 subluxation in the rheumatoid patient. Ligamentous hypertrophy and impression on the cord from a cervical disk are evident only with myelography or magnetic resonance imaging.

Treatment

In studies of the elderly, roughly one patient in four will have a treatable disorder. This ratio compares favorably with the yield in dementia evaluation. Psychogenic gait disorders and those due to toxic or metabolic encephalopathy are generally reversible. Parkinson's and related disorders often respond to some form of dopaminergic therapy. The management of cervical myelopathy and the various surgical procedures is considered in another chapter. Likewise, the treatment of multiple sclerosis, which threatens ambulation, is controversial. Studies suggest a role for immunotherapy in the management of progressing disease.[27] Brief treatment with adrenocorticotropic hormone or corticosteroids is commonly prescribed for acute exacerbations. Lioresal or diazepam are prescribed for patients whose function is limited by spasticity, although these medications do not always benefit ambulatory patients.

Hydrocephalus can be treated surgically, with best results achieved in patients with a history of head trauma, meningitis, or subarachnoid hemorrhage. Such symptomatic hydrocephalus may be more responsive than the idiopathic case. The prediction of outcome from shunting will otherwise require dynamic tests. A noninvasive assessment is often obtained by clinical response to lumbar puncture and removal of cerebrospinal fluid.[28] Many institutions shunt idiopathic late-life hydrocephalus infrequently, fearing the complications of shunt infection and subdural hematoma in elderly patients.

Even in the absence of specific treatment, numerous general measures are employed in rehabilitation. Patients should have appropriate footwear, with support and an intermediate degree of friction. (High-friction soles increase the risk of tripping falls.) Mechanical aids to walking are available, such as the four-prong cane and hinged and rolling walkers. Their use should be encouraged to reluctant patients who repeatedly experience falls.

Gait evaluation and training with a physical therapist are often helpful. At minimum, these sessions provide instruction in the best use of cane and walker. Those patients with sensory or balance disorders and those with high motivation often obtain substantial benefit. Programs that strengthen skeletal muscle through resistance and weight training may be helpful in patients who are sedentary and deconditioned.[29] Otherwise, the management of the patient with progressive failure of ambulation consists in the successful mobilization of family, community, and social services.

REFERENCES

1. Marsden CD: Parkinson's disease. Lancet i:948–952, 1990.
2. Stephen PJ and Williamson J: Drug-induced parkinsonism in the elderly. Lancet ii:1082–1083, 1984.
3. Ward CD, Duvoisin RC, Ince SE, et al: Parkinson's disease in 65 pairs of twins and in a set of quadruplets. Neurology 33:815–824, 1983.
4. Boyson SJ: Parkinson's disease and the electron transport chain. Ann Neurol 30:330–331, 1991.
5. Parkinson Study Group: Effect of deprenyl on the progression of disability in early Parkinson's disease. N Engl J Med 321:1364–1371, 1989.
6. Landau WM: Clinical neuromythology IX: Pyramid sale in the bucket shop. Neurology 40:1337–1339, 1990. DATATOP authors' response: Neurology 41:771–777, 1991.
7. Rinne UK: Combined bromocriptine-levodopa therapy early in Parkinson's disease. Neurology 35:1196–1198, 1985.
8. Boller F, Mizutani T, Roessmann U, et al: Parkinson's disease, dementia, and Alzheimer's disease: Clinicopathologic correlations. Ann Neurol 7:329–335, 1980.
9. Jankovic J and Fahn S: Physiologic and pathologic tremors. Ann Intern Med 93:460–465, 1980.
10. Shahani BT and Young RR: Physiologic and pharmacologic aids in the differential diagnosis of tremor. J Neurol Neurosurg Psychiatry 39:460–465, 1976.
11. Hoehn M and Yahr M: Parkinsonism: Onset, progression, and mortality. Neurology 17:427–442, 1967.
12. Lance J and McLeod J: A Physiologic Approach to Clinical Neurology, 3rd ed. London, Butterworths, 1981.
13. Young RR, Growdon JH, and Shahani BT: Beta-adrenergic mechanisms in action tremor. N Engl J Med 293:950–953, 1975.
14. Rajput AH, Rozdilsky B, Ang L, and Rajput A: Clinicopathologic observation in essential tremor: Report of six cases. Neurology 41:1422–1424, 1991.
15. Rubenstein LZ, Robbins AS, Josephson KR, et al: The value of assessing falls in an elderly population. Ann Intern Med 113:308–316, 1990.
16. Eidelberg E, Walden JG, and Nguyen LH: Locomotor control in Macaque monkeys. Brain 104:647–663, 1981.
17. Armstrong DM: The supraspinal control of mammalian locomotion. J Physiol 405:1–37, 1988.
18. Nashner LM: Balance adjustments of humans perturbed while walking. J Neurophysiol 8:915–917, 1980.
19. Sudarsky L and Ronthal M: Gait disorders among elderly patients: A survey study of 50 patients. Arch Neurol 40:740–743, 1983.
20. Adams RD, Fisher CM, Hakim S, et al: Symptomatic occult hydrocephalus with "normal" cerebrospinal fluid pressure: A treatable syndrome. N Engl J Med 273:117–126, 1965.
21. Fisher CM: Hydrocephalus as a cause of disturbances of gait in the elderly. Neurology 32:1358–1363, 1982.
22. Brownell B and Hughes JT: Necropsy observations on the damage to the nervous system in degenerative disease of the C-spine. Presented at the Fifth International Congress of Neuropathology, Zurich, 1965.

23. Paty DW, Blume WT, Brown WF, et al: Chronic progressive myelopathy: Investigation with CSF electrophoresis, evoked potentials, and CT scan. Ann Neurol 6:419–424, 1979.
24. Drachman DA and Hart CW: An approach to the dizzy patient. Neurology 22:323–334, 1972.
25. Sloman L, Berridge M, Homatidis MA, et al: Gait patterns of depressed patients and normal subjects. Am J Psychiatry 139:94–97, 1982.
26. Weiner WJ, Nora LM, and Glantz RH: Elderly inpatients: Postural reflex impairment. Neurology 34:945–947, 1984.
27. Noseworthy JH, Seland TP, and Ebers GC: Therapeutic trials in multiple sclerosis. Can J Neurol Sci 11:355–362, 1984.
28. Wikkelso C, Andersson J, Blomstrand C, and Lindqvist G: The clinical effect of lumbar puncture in normal pressure hydrocephalus. J Neurol Neurosurg Psychiatry 45:64–69, 1982.
29. Fiatarone M, Marks E, Ryan N, et al: High-intensity strength training in nonagenerians. JAMA 22:3029–3034, 1990.

60

Peripheral Nerve Disorders

SHAHRAM KHOSHBIN, MD
DAVID C. PRESTON, MD

Clinical problems resulting from peripheral nerve disorders are presently among the most common neurologic conditions seen by physicians in general practice.[1] The individual with bilateral numbness or tingling in the feet, or with isolated numbness of an extremity, frequently suffers from a peripheral nerve disorder. Although some patients with these symptoms suffer from central nervous system disorders (e.g., multiple sclerosis, tumors, migraine, or focal seizures), the majority are caused by afflictions of the peripheral nerves, either diffuse or localized. Because the differential diagnosis is considerable in these disorders, the combination of a directed neurologic history and exam and relatively simple ancillary testing is required to quickly narrow the diagnostic possibilities. Because many of these disorders are potentially treatable or curable, prompt recognition, especially early in the clinical course, is important.

This chapter presents an approach to the diagnosis of peripheral nerve problems, looking first at the anatomy of the peripheral nervous system, then at the types of pathologic processes affecting peripheral nerves. The major patterns of nerve disorders and the role of electrical diagnostic studies are considered next. Finally, several specific peripheral nerve disorders are described.

ANATOMY AND PATHOLOGY

The peripheral nervous system (PNS) includes neuronal elements existing outside the spinal cord and brain stem (excluding the olfactory and optic nerves, which are part of the central nervous system). The central processes of these peripheral structures, including the anterior horn cells, are also considered part of the PNS. The PNS consists of both myelinated and unmyelinated fibers. The myelin sheath, which invests the fastest conducting fibers, is derived exclusively from Schwann cells for all such fibers in the PNS, in contrast to oligodendroglia cells, which serve a similar function in the central nervous system.

All peripheral nerves are ultimately derived from the spinal nerve roots. The dorsal (sensory) and ventral (motor) nerve roots exit from the spinal cord and travel within the subarachnoid space, where they lie in contact with the cerebrospinal fluid (CSF). At the level of the neural foramen are the dorsal root ganglion cells. These are bipolar structures whose central axons form the sensory root and ultimately synapse in the spinal cord or the gracile and cuneate nuclei in the medulla. Their peripheral axons form the sensory component of peripheral nerves. This sensory component joins with the motor nerve root distal to the dorsal root ganglion to form the spinal nerve. Figure 60–1 is a simplified diagram of a spinal nerve and its components. The spinal nerves quickly divide into the dorsal and ventral rami, which each contain both motor and sensory fibers. Autonomic fibers, originating from either the sympathetic neurons in the thoracic-lumbar cord or from parasympathetic nuclei originating in the brain stem and sacral cord, also run with most peripheral nerves. The *dorsal rami* supply cutaneous sensation over the back as well as innervate the underlying midline musculature, whereas the *ventral rami* supply (1) the brachial plexus, which subsequently forms the upper extremity peripheral nerves, (2) the intercostal nerves, which supply the anterolateral thorax, and (3) the lumbosacral plexus, which subsequently forms the lower extremity peripheral nerves.

A *dermatome* is the cutaneous distribution of a single spinal segment (i.e., spinal nerve or dorsal root), whereas a *myotome* contains all the muscles derived from a single spinal segment (i.e., a single spinal nerve or ventral root). There is a high degree of overlap between adjacent dermatomes. Thus, anesthesia is never caused from a single root lesion. Likewise, most muscles are derived from multiple myotomes (i.e., the quadriceps muscle is derived from L2, L3, and L4 myotomes). Thus, a single root lesion rarely results in paralysis, only in paresis. Commonly there is a poor geographic correlation between myotomes and the dermatomes (i.e., the dermatome over a muscle commonly does not correspond to the same myotome that innervates that muscle).

From a pathologic perspective, several processes may affect the peripheral nervous system, as outlined in Figure 60–2. Physical injury to a nerve trunk resulting in transection causes degeneration of both axon and myelin distal to the site of injury, a process called *wallerian degeneration.* This is accompanied by chromatolysis within the parent cell body of the nerve fibers affected (i.e., the Nissl substance is dispersed, and the nucleus becomes eccentric). Although clinical symptoms occur immediately after nerve injury or transection, the process of distal axonal degeneration is slow, requiring five to nine days after complete transection. Nerve conduction studies will demonstrate abnormalities following this period. However, the subsequent electrical changes in the muscles innervated by the injured nerve, as seen during electromyography, may be delayed for several more weeks.

Many disease processes may preferentially attack either the axon or the myelin sheath. As a rule, peripheral neuropathies affecting the axon affect the longest axons first. These are the so-called dying-back neuropathies. Transport of proteins and nutrients from the cell body is affected early, with subsequent breakdown and loss of the most distal peripheral nerve fibers. Patients develop numbness or weakness of the toes and feet initially, which then slowly progresses up the leg. When the process reaches the upper calf, the finger tips become involved as well (i.e., the length from the spinal cord to upper calf is the same as that from spinal cord to finger tips). Unless very severe, this process produces no or only very slight slowing of nerve conduction velocity. In contrast, disease processes affecting the myelin sheath are usually associated with marked slowing of conduction velocity and may affect the proximal and distal segments of the peripheral nerve at the same time.

Symptoms and Signs

When nerve is diseased, it can react in a limited number of ways. Thus, many peripheral nerve disorders present with similar symptoms. Peripheral nerve may be viewed as supplying motor, sensory, as well as autonomic function. In addition, it is helpful to consider nerve on the basis of large and small fibers. All motor fibers are large fibers. All autonomic fibers are small fibers. However, sensory fibers are both of the large- and small-fiber types. Large sensory fibers mediate vibration, proprioception, and touch, whereas small sensory fibers convey pain and temperature sensations. Pathology of these fiber types may create symptoms and signs by lack of function (negative symptoms and signs) or by extra or abnormal function (positive symptoms and signs). All people can relate to falling asleep on their arm, which initially causes numbness or lack of feeling (negative symptom) followed by intense pins-and-needles paresthesias (positive symptom). Likewise, symptoms and signs in the different nerve fiber types can be divided into positive and negative (Table 60–1).

The assessment of muscle weakness is always begun during the clinical history. Although the physical examination remains important, in most instances, the history gives key information. Patients often relate difficulties doing daily activities, which will clue the physician into which muscle groups are weak, long before formal testing reveals any abnormality. Depending on the muscle groups involved, dif-

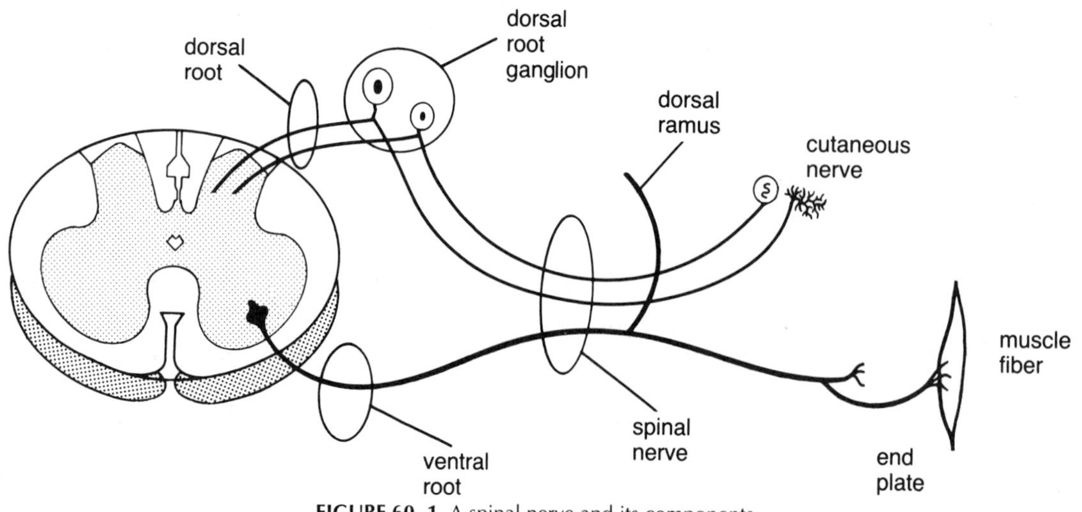

FIGURE 60–1. A spinal nerve and its components.

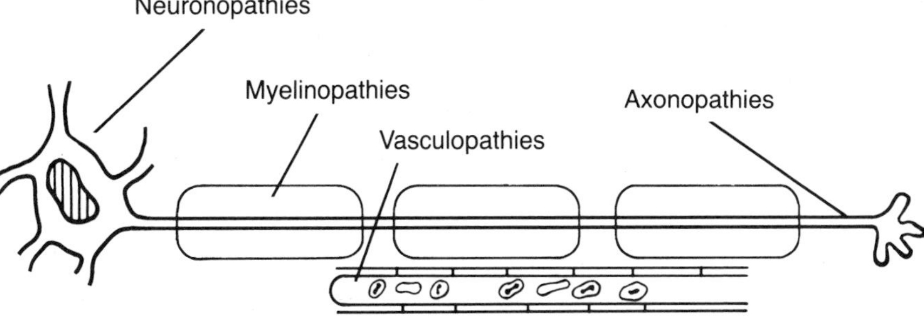

FIGURE 60–2. Processes affecting the peripheral nervous system.

ferent patients will characteristically report the same symptoms (Table 60–2).

The examination of reflexes and muscle tone are important in evaluating the PNS. Distal reflexes, especially the ankle reflex, tend to be diminished in most neuropathies. Demyelinating neuropathies are commonly associated with generalized areflexia. Although reduced or absent reflexes together with muscle hypotonia are generally associated with disorders of the PNS, it is important to remember that these may exist in a central nervous system lesion where there has been a massive or acute insult. For instance, in an acute massive spinal cord injury, it is not unusual for the paralyzed limbs to be hypotonic and areflexic for the first several days to weeks, before spasticity and hyperreflexia develop.

The presence or absence of sensory findings are important in recognizing a peripheral nerve disorder. Almost all neuropathies will have some sensory involvement. The absence of sensory symptoms or signs in a patient with weakness suggests a pure motor syndrome: either motor neuron disease, myopathy, or disease of neuromuscular junction. All patients with a suspected PNS disorder need to be examined for the presence of muscle wasting. When looking for wasting, the best muscles to inspect are the distal intrinsic hand and foot muscles. The extensor digitorum brevis is a small muscle on the dorsum of the foot, which tends to waste early in polyneuropathy. An equally important finding is the presence of foot deformities. *Pes cavus* (high arched sole and foreshortened foot) and hammer toes result from intrinsic foot muscle weakness present during development as a child. This finding in a patient with a neuropathy usually signifies a long-standing, most likely inherited, neuropathy.

TABLE 60–1. PERIPHERAL NERVE SYMPTOMS AND SIGNS

Symptoms and Signs	Negative	Positive
Motor	Weakness	Fasciculation
	Fatigue	Cramp
	Areflexia	Myokymia
	Hypotonia	Restless legs
	Deformities	Tightness
Sensory		
Large fiber	↓ Vibration, joint position sense	Tingling
		Pins and needles
	Areflexia	
	Ataxia	
	Hypotonia	
Small fiber	↓ Pain, temperature	Burning, jabbing
Autonomic	Hypotension	Hyperhidrosis
	Decreased sweat	
	Impotence	
	Urinary retention	Urinary frequency
	Constipation	Diarrhea

CLASSIFICATION OF PERIPHERAL NERVE PROBLEMS

Peripheral nerve disorders divide into three basic groups: mononeuropathy, mononeuropathy multiplex, and peripheral neuropathy. In a *mononeuropathy,* a single peripheral nerve is affected. Depending on whether this nerve is a sensory nerve, a motor nerve, or a mixed sensorimotor nerve, the manifestations will be sensory, motor, or a combination of the two. In some cases, autonomic symptoms in the distribution of the nerve may occur. A mononeuropathy may result from compression of the nerve (tumors, bony prominences, ligaments, solid external objects) or division of the nerve (penetrating injury). The pathologic response to injury depends on the severity and the type of injury. If the injury involves axonal loss and wallerian generation, recovery is invariably slow, beginning from the intact segment of nerve and proceeding at a rate of less than 1 mm/day. Recovery of large nerves in the lower extremity after an axonal injury may require as long as 2 years or more. On the other hand, demyelination may repair much faster, usually over days to weeks.

In a *mononeuropathy multiplex,* isolated peripheral nerves are affected individually, but multiple nerves are affected during the course of a single illness. Manifestations depend on the particular nerves involved and the degree to which the nerve is affected. Mononeuropathy multiplex is rare compared with the other two types of peripheral nerve problem; only a few disease processes are capable of producing this picture. They include diabetes mellitus, serum sickness, systemic vasculitis, sarcoidosis,

TABLE 60–2. MOTOR SYMPTOMS AND SIGNS BY MUSCLE GROUP

Bulbar muscles	Slurred or nasal speech
	Drooling
	Nasal regurgitation of liquids
	Difficulty whistling or smiling
	Difficulty swallowing or weight loss
Extraocular muscles	Diplopia
	Ptosis
Proximal upper extremity muscles	Trouble reaching
	Trouble holding a razor, comb, or hair dryer
	Trouble putting away dishes in high cabinets
Distal upper extremity muscles	Difficulty with jars, keys, silverware, or doors
	Trouble buttoning clothes
Proximal lower extremity muscles	Trouble getting out of chairs or the car
	Trouble getting out of bath or off toilet
	Trouble with stairs
Distal lower extremity muscles	Tripping
	Sprained ankles

TABLE 60–3. ACUTE PERIPHERAL NEUROPATHIES

Acute inflammatory demyelinating polyradiculoneuropathy
Porphyria
Diphtheria
Drugs (dapsone, nitrofurantoin, vincristine)
Toxins (arsenic, thallium, triorthocresylphosphate)
Tick paralysis

multiple entrapment neuropathies (e.g., rheumatoid arthritis), and acquired demyelinating neuropathies. The diagnosis of mononeuropathy multiplex depends primarily on the clinical recognition of the syndrome and the subsequent ancillary tests used to narrow the differential diagnosis.

Peripheral neuropathies, on the other hand, reflect more diffuse injury to the peripheral nervous system. Clinically peripheral neuropathies can be characterized along a number of different dimensions:

Temporal course (acute, subacute, chronic; progressive, relapsing, or remitting)
Fiber types involved (motor, sensory large fiber, sensory small fiber, autonomic)
Localization (neuron, root, plexus, nerve; symmetric or asymmetric; proximal or distal)
Pathology (axonal, demyelinating, or mixed)

This information can be obtained primarily from the history and physical examination. Knowledge of the temporal course of a neuropathy will narrow the differential diagnosis considerably. Most neuropathies are chronic, and the onset cannot be easily determined. Acute polyneuropathies are notably less common (Table 60–3), with acute inflammatory demyelinating polyradiculoneuropathy (AIDP) being the most distinctive, with onset over a few days or a few weeks at most. Likewise, most neuropathies are progressive. The history of a relapsing or remitting course is unusual and suggests either an exposure or intoxication or an autoimmune inflammatory neuropathy.

Polyneuropathies usually involve both sensory and motor fibers. However, most distal axonal neuropathies have sensory symptoms and findings long before the disease process becomes sufficiently severe to cause actual weakness. Certain hereditary neuropathies (e.g., Charcot-Marie-Tooth) and conditions such as lead poisoning, porphyria, and AIDP may exhibit predominantly motor symptoms and signs. Entrapment neuropathies, depending on the nerve involved, may also present with motor findings. Involvement of small fibers almost invariably reflects a pathologic process directed against axons. Its manifestations include a distal sensory deficit, particularly for pin prick and touch, often with dysesthesia, as well as autonomic changes distally in the extremities. Several neuropathies are associated with predominantly small sensory fiber dysfunction (Table 60–4). Involvement of large fibers produces loss of reflexes, a distal sensory deficit, particularly to vibration and touch, little or no autonomic involvement, and distal weakness if severe enough.

TABLE 60–4. SMALL-FIBER PERIPHERAL NEUROPATHIES

Diabetes
Amyloidosis (inherited and acquired)
Alcohol
Hereditary sensory neuropathies
Tangier disease
Fabry's disease

TABLE 60–5. DEMYELINATING NEUROPATHIES

Hereditary
Hereditary motor sensory neuropathy, type I (Charcot-Marie-Tooth disease)
Hereditary motor sensory neuropathy, type III (Déjerine-Sottas disease)
Hereditary motor sensory neuropathy, type IV (Refsum's disease)
Metachromatic leukodystrophy
Krabbe's disease
Adrenoleukodystrophy
Cockayne's syndrome
Niemann-Pick disease
Cerebrotendinous xanthomatosis
Acquired
Acute inflammatory demyelinating polyradiculoneuropathy (Guillain-Barré syndrome)
Chronic inflammatory demyelinating polyradiculoneuropathy
Idiopathic
Associated with HIV* infection
Associated with MGUS† (especially IgM)‡
Associated with anti-MAG§ antibodies
Associated with osteosclerotic myeloma
Associated with GM_1 antibodies
Diphtheria

*HIV = human immunodeficiency virus.
†MGUS = monoclonal gammopathy of undetermined significance.
‡IgM = gamma M immunoglobulin.
§MAG = myelin-associated glycoprotein.

Localization is based largely on the clinical examination and can be supplemented by electromyographic and nerve conduction studies. In the case of a single limb that is weak and numb, knowledge of the sensory and motor innervations of each peripheral nerve and nerve root is necessary to recognize certain patterns of weakness and numbness. In analyzing polyneuropathies, one needs to concentrate on the overall pattern. Is there a distal or proximal gradient? Distal symptoms and findings occur in most neuropathies, in part reflecting the frequency with which dying-back or axonal degeneration is the underlying pathologic process. However, some neuropathies, such as porphyria, may show proximal involvement, as may some mononeuropathies (e.g., femoral neuropathy). Most neuropathies are symmetric. The presence of any asymmetry is a key finding because this commonly excludes a large number of toxic, metabolic, and genetic abnormalities that cause only a symmetric pattern. Asymmetry implies the possibility of a mononeuritis multiplex pattern, a superimposed radiculopathy or mononeuropathy, or an acquired demyelinating neuropathy. Nerve conduction studies are frequently useful in this regard.

Pathologically, injury to nerves may consist of two major processes: axonal degeneration or demyelination. In axonal neuropathies, the metabolic function of the nerve fiber is impaired, with relative preservation of conduction velocity. Most neuropathies are primarily axonal. In demyelinating neuropathies, the initial injury to the nerves reflects damage to, or dysfunction of, the Schwann cells and the myelin sheaths. As a consequence of demyelination, saltatory conduction is impaired, and conduction is markedly slowed. In the differential diagnosis of a peripheral nerve disorder, the presence of demyelination is a key finding (Table 60–5). Demyelination may be demonstrated either by pathologic examination of nerve or more easily by electrophysiologic testing. Demyelination may be diffuse, as in inherited disorders, or patchy, as in acquired disorders, which are usually inflammatory or immune mediated.

In addition, it is also important to inquire about *family*

history and *occupational or exposure history*. A large number of difficult-to-diagnose neuropathies will ultimately be shown to be secondary to one of these.

The differential diagnosis of peripheral nerve disease is outlined in Table 60–6. Using the four dimensions discussed earlier, it is often possible to narrow this list to a small number of plausible candidates. Final determination of the etiology will then depend on a detailed history, a careful neurologic examination, appropriate laboratory tests, including nerve conductions and electromyography, and possibly, spinal fluid examination or nerve biopsy.

Laboratory tests in the evaluation of peripheral neuropathy should be chosen according to the type of neuropathy present. Complete blood count, liver function tests, glucose tolerance test, vitamin B_{12} levels, thyroid function tests, levels of heavy metals in blood and urine, and serum and immunoprotein electrophoresis are all helpful in selected cases. A search for an occult neoplasm should be considered in a middle-aged or elderly individual with a subacute or chronic neuropathy of unclear etiology. Pathologic processes affecting nerve roots may alter spinal fluid composition. Examination of the spinal fluid is particularly helpful in demyelinating neuropathies such as AIDP, in which the protein is elevated despite few or no cells.

In selected cases, nerve biopsy may be indicated. Biopsy is useful in documenting the presence of a demyelinating neuropathy and in identifying certain neuropathies due to vasculitis, amyloid, sarcoid, leprosy, or metachromatic leukodystrophy. Usually the sural nerve is selected for biopsy, which leaves the patient with an area of numbness along the lateral foot. Nerve biopsies should be reviewed by an experienced pathologist. Routine biopsy of nerve in cases of axonal neuropathy is usually not helpful.

TABLE 60–6. DIFFERENTIAL DIAGNOSIS OF PERIPHERAL NERVE DISEASE

- Trauma
  - Direct
  - Indirect
- Metabolic disorders
  - Diabetes mellitus
  - Acute intermittent porphyria
  - Uremia
  - Hepatic failure
  - Thyroid disease
  - Hypoglycemia
- Infection
  - Leprosy
  - Diphtheria
  - Lyme disease
  - Human immunodeficiency virus
- Vitamin deficiencies
  - Thiamine in alcoholics
  - B_{12} deficiency in subacute combined degeneration
  - Malabsorption
- Toxins
  - Chemicals, including solvents, pesticides, and drugs
  - Heavy metals
- Hereditary conditions
  - Charcot-Marie-Tooth disease (peroneal muscular atrophy)
  - Refsum's disease
  - Hereditary sensory neuropathy
  - Amyloidosis
- Acquired inflammatory demyelinating neuropathies
  - Acute and chronic inflammatory demyelinating neuropathy
  - GM_1 antibodies
- Paraneoplastic disorders
- Collagen vascular disease and vasculitis
- Dysproteinemias
- Tumors involving nerve, primarily or secondarily

Nerve Conduction Studies and Electromyography. Nerve conduction studies and electromyography are routinely employed in the evaluation of peripheral nerve disorders. These studies are useful to confirm the presence of a neuropathy and will often suggest the underlying type of pathology (axonal, demyelinating, or mixed), in addition to aiding in the assessment of severity and chronicity. In some cases of demyelinating neuropathy, nerve conduction studies can further distinguish between an acquired and an inherited condition. In cases of mononeuropathy, nerve conduction studies are extremely useful to clarify the exact location of the nerve injury or entrapment.

Sensory Nerve Conduction Studies. An action potential produced by stimulation of a sensory nerve can be recorded at a site along the nerve both distal and proximal to the site of stimulation. The amplitude of the recorded action potential reflects the number of functioning axons. It is possible to calculate a conduction velocity by measuring the distance between the site of stimulation and the site of recording and dividing by the time involved in traversing the segment measured. The conduction velocity reflects the integrity of the myelin in that segment. A reduction in the amplitude of sensory action potential is frequently seen in both axonal and demyelinating neuropathies, where individual nerve fibers may be degenerated and blocked, respectively. Furthermore, in demyelinating neuropathies, a slowing of conduction velocity occurs. One of the most important findings in sensory conduction studies is the preservation of the sensory action potential in all lesions proximal to the dorsal root ganglion (i.e., nerve root or spinal cord). In these cases, because the integrity of the dorsal root ganglion cell and its peripheral axon remains intact, sensory conduction study results remain normal.

Motor Nerve Conduction Studies. Electrical stimulation of a mixed nerve results in contraction of the muscles innervated by that nerve. A compound motor action potential can be recorded by placing recording electrodes over such a muscle. The potential obtained represents the number of activated muscle fibers. It is possible to obtain conduction velocities along a nerve by stimulating at different sites and dividing the distance between these sites by the difference in latency of the onset of the muscle action potential. This process may help in localizing lesions along the length of a peripheral nerve (e.g., in entrapment neuropathies), as well as provide information about the integrity of the axons and myelin.

Late Responses. Late responses are used to study the proximal segments of nerve. The H-reflex is a monosynaptic reflex similar to the tendon jerk. In normal adults, an H-reflex can be obtained in the leg only by stimulating the tibial nerve and recording over the soleus muscle, and is therefore most useful in assessing S1 radiculopathies. The F-wave is produced by antidromic stimulation of a motor nerve. The nerve action potential travels antidromically to the anterior horn cell and then back down again orthodromically to produce a delayed muscle response. Hence, to produce an F-response the potential must travel twice through the proximal segment of a motor nerve. The F-response can be obtained in most motor nerves and is most useful in documenting proximal involvement of the nerve, such as in early AIDP.

Electromyography. With the use of concentric needle electrodes, one can look for abnormal spontaneous activity (e.g., fibrillations or fasciculations) in muscle as well as evaluate the number and quality of the muscle action potentials. It is frequently possible to distinguish between neuropathic (due to disease of peripheral nerve, root, or motor neuron) and myopathic disorders (see Fig. 61–1). The type and distribution of muscle abnormalities are used in arriving at the correct anatomic diagnosis (i.e., are the changes restricted to the innervation of one nerve, one nerve root, many individual nerves, or all nerves?). Electromyography may also be used to document recovery from peripheral nerve lesions.

Therapy

The treatment of peripheral nerve disorders may be divided into therapy of the underlying disorder versus symptomatic therapy. When the correct etiology can be found, treatment of the underlying disorder is always preferable, such as hemodialysis in uremic neuropathies, thyroid replacement for hypothyroid neuropathy, or immunosuppression for autoimmune or acquired demyelinating neuropathy. In patients with entrapment neuropathy, surgical decompression may be useful in selected cases. In cases in which treatment for the underlying condition does not exist (e.g., inherited neuropathies) or the diagnosis is uncertain, symptomatic therapy must be employed. Motor function may be improved by splinting, bracing, and other physical appliances. In most instances, physical therapy is useful in making the most of the remaining muscle function. Treatment of painful or other paresthesias is frequently difficult. Simple analgesics, low-dose tricyclic antidepressants, anticonvulsants, and baclofen may be tried with varying success. Narcotics are useful in selected cases but are best avoided. Transcutaneous nerve stimulation and acupuncture are also useful in some patients.

POLYNEUROPATHIES

Diabetic Neuropathy

Neuropathies associated with diabetes are probably the most common types of neuropathy the clinician encounters. Three different neuropathies are commonly seen in diabetes: (1) diabetic polyneuropathy: a symmetric, sensory-motor, autonomic neuropathy; (2) mononeuropathies, mononeuritis multiplex, and radiculopathies; and (3) diabetic amyotrophy (proximal motor neuropathy).

Diabetic Polyneuropathy

Diabetic polyneuropathy is predominantly sensory. Clinically, patients show a stocking-glove loss of sensory function. Both large and small sensory fibers may be affected, although many patients show primarily pain and temperature involvement. Symptoms of severe pain and dysesthesias are common. Patients describe the pain as a disturbing and burning sensation. Hypersensitivity to all stimuli is common. The ankle jerks are usually absent. Motor signs and weakness are not usually very prominent, if present at all. Muscle cramps may also be present. Cranial nerves are very rarely affected. Rarely, patients with diabetic polyneuropathy present with a disturbance of gait due to position-sense disturbance (sensory ataxia). Secondary arthropathy involving the distal joints (Charcot's joints) can be seen. Autonomic signs and symptoms including impotence may also be present, and examination may show evidence of orthostatic hypotension. Electrodiagnostic tests, as well as pathologic studies, show that diabetic polyneuropathy is primarily an axonal neuropathy with some evidence of secondary segmental demyelination.

A primarily autonomic neuropathy without sensorimotor symptoms can be seen rarely and is present only in insulin-dependent diabetics. Here, signs and symptoms of autonomic disturbance are prevalent: impotence, abnormalities of sweating (hypohidrosis or hyperhidrosis), detrusor dysfunction (increased residual urine), postprandial diarrhea, postural hypotension, and tachycardia.[2] The possibility of sudden death from cardiac arrest exists in these patients.

Diabetic Mononeuropathies, Mononeuropathy Multiplex, and Radiculopathies

Diabetics show a much higher frequency of compression and entrapment neuropathies than do nondiabetics. The sites of involvement are the same as in nondiabetics, and the common presentations are those of carpal tunnel syndrome (median nerve), cubital tunnel syndrome (ulnar nerve), and peroneal palsy below the fibular head. Femoral neuropathy is also seen in diabetes, especially in patients whose blood glucose level is poorly controlled.[3]

Cranial Nerves. Diabetic palsy of the sixth or third cranial nerve is common. The disorder is usually of sudden onset and is painful. In diabetic third-nerve palsy, the pupil is relatively spared. The seventh nerve and also the fourth nerve have been involved. The course is usually that of resolution of symptoms in a few months.

Radiculopathies and Intercostal Neuropathies. These have a sudden onset and present difficulties in differential diagnosis.[4] Intercostal neuropathies may present as abdominal pain or as chest pain and have been known to mimic both cardiac and gall bladder pain. Radicular patterns may be difficult to distinguish from common discogenic disease.

Diabetic Amyotrophy

A rare, asymmetric, predominantly motor neuropathy is seen in diabetes that affects the upper lumbar nerve roots and lumbar plexus.[5] The disorder may have either a gradual or subacute onset and is often associated with severe pain and weight loss. Proximal weakness is noted in the lower extremities, mainly in the quadriceps, adductors, and iliopsoas muscles. Often, knee jerks are absent. Clinically, the distribution of weakness may mimic a myopathy, but electromyography reveals signs of neuropathic disease. Diabetic amyotrophy often improves with time, although insulin therapy and closer diabetic control may help as well.[6]

Various pathogenic mechanisms have been suggested for the different neuropathies of diabetes. Ischemia and nerve infarction are the likely etiologies in mononeuropathies, cranial neuropathies, radiculopathies, and also in amyotrophy.[7] However, the sensorimotor-autonomic polyneuropathy likely has a metabolic pathogenesis. Abnormalities in the sorbitol pathway and inhibition of *myo*-inositol uptake have both been suggested.[8, 9]

Therapy

Adequate control of diabetes is the first step in management. Patients with new-onset diabetes and peripheral nerve symptoms respond better than do patients with chronic diabetes. Monitoring of blood sugar at home and checking hemoglobin A_{1C} levels have made follow-up easier. A number of studies that use nerve conductions to follow the course of the patients' neuropathies seem to indicate that good diabetic control halts the progression of the disease, although it does not result in improvement in the neuropathy.[10] Trials using *myo*-inositol have not shown a definite improvement in the course of the illness.[11] Symptomatic therapy, in particular, treatment of neuropathic pain, is the next most important step. Most patients respond to treatment with carbamazepine (Tegretol) or phenytoin (Dilantin). Addition of nightly doses of amitriptyline improves the response. These medicines should be prescribed in the minimal dosage range and adjusted upward until symptomatic relief is obtained or side effects are unacceptable. Narcotic analgesics do not seem to be effective and are best avoided. Some individuals may benefit from the use of local capsaicin cream applied to the affected painful areas three to four times a day. Simple maneuvers, such as elevation of the feet and use of elastic stockings are also helpful. In patients with sensory ataxia, early intervention with gait training and the simple use of a cane may avoid some future complications.

Uremic Neuropathy

An axonal polyneuropathy is seen in patients with chronic renal failure. Clinically, this is a symmetric, sensorimotor polyneuropathy. The patients are usually on hemodialysis.[12] Multiple factors have been implicated in the pathogenesis of uremic neuropathy. Transketolase and *myo*-inositol inhibition have been suggested, as in diabetic polyneuropathy.[13] Increased parathyroid hormone has also been implicated, although no theory has been proved. Uremic neuropathy has a subacute or gradual onset. It is seen mainly in male patients who complain of dysesthetic symptoms (burning feet and restless leg syndrome). Motor symptoms are more prominent than in diabetic neuropathy, and in some cases, moderate weakness may be seen. The neuropathy is not related to the degree of uremia, although high levels of blood urea nitrogen and a creatinine clearance level below 5 ml/min are present before patients show symptoms. Nerve conduction studies are uniformly abnormal, even in patients who are not symptomatic with regard to neuropathy. Mononeuropathies, including carpal tunnel syndrome and other entrapment neuropathies, are noted with higher frequency in uremic patients.

Therapy. Although hemodialysis stabilizes the symptoms of neuropathy, it does not result in marked improvement and commonly does not improve nerve conductions. In contrast, successful renal transplantation improves nerve conduction studies as well as symptomatology.[14, 15] Symptomatic treatment of pain with phenytoin, carbamazepine, or amitriptyline may be needed. Surgical therapy for carpal tunnel syndrome has resulted in relief in most patients on dialysis.

Vitamin Deficiency and Alcoholic Neuropathies

B_{12} Deficiency

An axonal neuropathy is seen in pernicious anemia and in B_{12} deficiency of other etiology. Symptoms are predominantly sensory. Patients complain of distal numbness and tingling.[16] Signs and symptoms of peripheral neuropathy accompanied by long-track signs (i.e., Babinski's signs, increased reflexes) indicate the presence of combined-systems disease in a patient with B_{12} deficiency.

Therapy. Treatment is begun with 5 days of intramuscular injections of B_{12} at 1000 μg/day. A rather rapid recovery of the peripheral nervous system symptoms ensues except in combined-systems disease, in which case the myelopathy may not improve as rapidly. Unless a reversible etiology is discovered, patients will require lifelong monthly B_{12} injections.

Thiamine Deficiency (Nutritional Beri-Beri)

Thiamine deficiency is seen in starvation, in malabsorption syndromes, and even in cases of persistent vomiting. Patients whose diets are high in carbohydrate and deficient in vitamins manifest symptoms of thiamine deficiency. Electrodiagnostic studies indicate that this is an axonal neuropathy. Alcoholic neuropathy is similar to thiamine deficiency neuropathy. Both the vitamin-deficient and high-calorie carbohydrate diet of the alcoholic patient, and the direct toxic effect of alcohol result in a symmetric sensory neuropathy that is at times resistant to replacement by thiamine.

Therapy. Thiamine replacement is given at 100 mg/day, and a balanced diet is indicated. Hyperpathic leg pain may respond to acetylsalicylic acid. Anticonvulsants and amitriptyline are also helpful. Sympathetic block in the lumbar area has been used in some cases of severe pain. Recovery is slow, and in the alcoholic patient there is the danger of returning to alcohol abuse.

Other Vitamin Deficiencies

Other vitamin deficiencies are most commonly associated with malabsorption syndromes or highly restricted diets. Neuropathies associated with vitamin deficiencies are typically distal, symmetric, predominantly sensory polyneuropathies. In addition, vitamin deficiencies may be seen as a side effect of certain medications. Isoniazid-induced polyneuropathy is presumed secondary to pyridoxine deficiency, which results in a sensory polyneuropathy.

It may be prudent to treat with multivitamin supplementation in either single- or multiple-vitamin deficiencies. A suggested daily schedule is oral thiamine, 25 mg; niacin, 100 mg; riboflavin, 10 mg; pantothenic acid, 10 mg; pyridoxine, 5 mg; folic acid, 5 mg; and intramuscular B_{12}, 1000 μg/month.[17] Treatment is continued at high doses until the patient is asymptomatic.

Porphyric Neuropathy

The porphyrias are rare disorders of heme metabolism. Variegate porphyria, acute intermittent porphyria, and hereditary coproporphyria are associated with a severe, acute polyneuropathy. These disorders are separated on the basis of different enzymatic defects and the pattern of porphyrin metabolites in the serum and urine.

Each of these disorders is rare. Acute intermittent porphyria is the most common. Inheritance is usually autosomal dominant. Attacks are commonly precipitated by drugs (especially barbiturates, estrogens, and sulfonamides), fever, or fasting. Abdominal crises (abdominal pain, fever, or constipation) and psychiatric illness (psychosis or delirium) are common. Most patients who present with acute neuropathy will have had previous attacks or will have coexistent attacks of abdominal crisis.

The clinical features of the neuropathy can be quite varied. It is usually an acute, predominantly motor neuropathy involving the proximal muscles first, and commonly the upper extremities before the lower extremities. The weakness can be symmetric or asymmetric. Most progress to quadriplegia and respiratory compromise. Facial and bulbar weakness can be present. Rarely, other cranial nerves can be involved. Reflexes may be absent or present.[18] Sensory loss often accompanies the motor weakness in a similar distribution. Autonomic dysfunction is extremely common, with tachycardia, blood pressure instability, sphincter dysfunction, and fever.

Laboratory studies show an elevated CSF protein. δ-Aminolevulinic acid (δ-ALA) and porphobilinogen are usually present in the urine during an acute attack. Electromyography shows evidence of an acute axonopathy, usually most prominent in the proximal muscles.

Differential diagnosis includes intoxication (especially lead) and AIDP. The history of prior abdominal or psychiatric illness should always suggest the diagnosis.

Therapy. Avoidance of drugs that precipitate attacks is the most important first step. These include alcohol, barbiturates, carbamazepine, chloramphenicol, chlorpropamide, ergotamine, imipramine, meprobamate, methyldopa, oral contraceptives, phenytoin, and sulfonamides. Chlorpromazine has been used to treat both the severe pain and the behavioral disturbance seen during attacks. Trials with intravenous glucose and hematin have resulted in improvements during attacks of neuropathy.[19]

Hepatic Neuropathy

In both viral hepatitis and chronic liver disease, peripheral neuropathies are seen. Neuropathy is common in chronic alcoholic liver disease and other cirrhotic conditions. Most are axonal sensory greater than motor distal polyneuropathies.[20] Pathologic study shows lipid infiltration of the peripheral nerves. In both type A and type B viral hepatitis, a mild sensory polyneuropathy can be seen. In addition, AIDP, which has been associated with many viral infections, can be seen in both hepatitis A and B.

Hypothyroid Neuropathy

The most common neuropathy of thyroid disease is bilateral carpal tunnel syndrome, seen in myxedema, but also at times seen in milder hypothyroid disease. The neuropathy responds to treatment with hormone replacement. A diffuse polyneuropathy can also be seen in hypothyroid states.[21] This is primarily a distal neuropathy, with sensory symptoms and loss of reflexes. Cerebrospinal fluid protein may be slightly elevated. The myopathy seen with hypothyroid states can be concomitant. Therapy is primarily replacement of hormone. The peripheral neuropathy responds within a few months. It is of note that in thyrotoxicosis, a predominantly myopathic picture is seen, although electrodiagnostic studies have also shown the presence of a mild peripheral neuropathy.

Sarcoid Neuropathy

Sarcoid neuropathy has an atypical peripheral neuropathy with cranial neuropathies. Although the most common finding is that of a facial palsy, a polyneuropathy more in the nature of mononeuritis multiplex can be seen. Patients develop large areas of sensory loss and dysesthesias, usually in an atypical distribution on the body.[22] Onset of the disorder may be acute, and at times a clinical picture similar to that of AIDP can be seen. In evaluation of sarcoid neuropathy, one should look for associated findings of parotitis, hilar lymphadenopathy, and uveitis. Nerve biopsy may be needed for the diagnosis. As in central nervous system sarcoid, treatment is generally with steroids.

Carcinomatous Neuropathy

Patients with cancer are susceptible to a wide variety of neuromuscular complications either by direct effect of the tumor, its therapy, or by secondary systemic effects. Tumor can infiltrate nerve roots or nerve or cause extrinsic compression from a mass lesion. Chemotherapy has well-known side effects on nerve and muscle. Secondary metabolic, infectious, and vascular complications can also affect peripheral nerves. In addition, patients with cancer have an increased incidence of peripheral nervous system dysfunction as a result of distant toxic or autoimmune effects of carcinoma (i.e., paraneoplastic).[23, 24] These may take the form of a neuropathy, neuronopathy, myelopathy, or neuromuscular junction disorder.

Paraneoplastic neuropathies may precede or follow the diagnosis of cancer. The most common neuropathy is a sensorimotor polyneuropathy. Although associated most often with lung cancer, it can be found with carcinoma from any site. It is a mild distal axonal neuropathy that is very difficult to differentiate from other toxic or metabolic etiologies. Disability is usually quite mild. The most distinctive paraneoplastic neuropathy is that of sensory neuropathy or neuronopathy. Patients present acutely or subacutely with prominent sensory loss involving all modalities. Presentation may be symmetric or patchy. Reflexes are lost early. Sensory ataxia and gait disturbance are common. Although patients may appear weak, most of their disability is actually secondary to loss of joint position sense. Pain and paresthesias may occur. Electrodiagnostically, this condition is a sensory neuronopathy with preservation of the motor system. This syndrome is most commonly associated with small-cell carcinoma, and in some cases, anti-Hu antibodies can be demonstrated. Rarely, this condition may exist as a primary autoimmune disorder in the absence of carcinoma. However, any patient who presents with this syndrome needs to be evaluated aggressively for small-cell carcinoma. Denny-Brown showed degeneration of dorsal root ganglion cells, dorsal roots, and the dorsal column to be present pathologically.[25] Unfortunately, recovery is usually poor, as destruction of dorsal root ganglion cells precludes any peripheral regeneration.

Acute and chronic inflammatory demyelinating neuropathies are also seen in greater frequency in patients with carcinoma and lymphoma. Diagnosis and treatment is similar to patients without carcinoma (see later). Rarely, vasculitic neuropathy has also been seen as a paraneoplastic syndrome.

Inflammatory Demyelinating Neuropathies

Acute Inflammatory Demyelinating Polyradiculoneuropathy (Guillain-Barré Syndrome)

AIDP is considered a neurologic emergency.[26] There is an acute onset and a rapid progression, with a clinical picture of a polyradiculoneuropathy. However, the course of the illness may be quite varied. Most patients give a history of viral infection (typically an upper respiratory infection or gastroenteritis) 3 to 4 weeks prior to the onset of weakness. Cytomegalovirus, Epstein-Barr virus, human immunodeficiency virus (HIV), vaccination, surgery, trauma, and malignancy (especially lymphoma) have also been associated with AIDP. Motor involvement is profound. Usually an ascending weakness is seen, progressing from the lower extremities to the upper extremities, with gradual involvement of the respiratory muscles and cranial neuropathies (bifacial paralysis and ophthalmoplegia). The rapidly progressive course eventually requires artificial ventilation in 30% of patients. Diffuse weakness at onset may be present.

The sensory findings are usually not as prominent. Pain in the lower extremities or the lower back is common. Patients complain of paresthesias that start in the feet and hands at the same time and progressively ascend. There is always a marked hyporeflexia and then areflexia. Any weak limb with preserved reflexes should lead the clinician to seriously question the diagnosis. Autonomic signs and symptoms may also occur, including tachycardia and cardiogenic shock, bladder dysfunction (retention), and hypotension; papilledema may also be seen in the early phases. The disease usually lasts 1 to 4 weeks, and then improvement begins gradually. Some patients may relapse from 2 to 4 weeks after recovery.

In their original description, Guillain, Barré, and Strohl pointed out the CSF findings:[27] there is elevated protein with absence of pleocytosis. However, in 20% of patients, a small number of cells can be seen. Greater than 50 cells/mm^3 would be an unusual finding for this illness, and would call into question HIV-associated AIDP, where a CSF pleocytosis is common. The CSF protein is usually most elevated 10 days after the onset of the symptoms. The Fisher variant of Guillain-Barré syndrome shows areflexia, ophthalmoplegia, and ataxia.[28] The clinician should consider the differential diagnosis of porphyria, lead neuropathy, and diphtheritic neuropathy and, in cases with ophthalmoplegia, myasthenia gravis.

Electrodiagnostic studies are most helpful in the diagnosis of this syndrome. Nerve conduction studies eventually show electrophysiologic evidence of segmental demyelination (markedly prolonged distal latencies, markedly slowed conduction velocities, and conduction block or temporal dispersion) in 85% of patients by 3 weeks. However there is a large range, with some patients having unexcitable nerves early on. This may be from either wallerian degeneration or presumed very distal demyelination. The most useful findings early in the course are abnormally prolonged or absent late responses (F-response and H-reflex) in the presence of normal distal conductions. This pattern strongly suggests the presence of proximal demyelination.

The pathogenesis of the Guillain-Barré syndrome is not known. However, an autoimmune process is most likely. Pathologic study reveals an inflammatory infiltrate in the nerve roots and the peripheral nerve, with evidence of marked segmental demyelination and rarely axonal involvement.

Therapy. Management involves plasma exchange, respiratory support, and prevention of medical complications. Most seriously ill or progressing patients are treated with 5 to 6 large volume plasma exchanges over 2 weeks.[29, 30] This treatment is most effective early in the course and in patients requiring intubation. Length of intubation, clinical course, and outcome are improved with plasma exchange. Respiratory management involves careful serial testing of vital capacity by a trained respiratory technician, and the use of early intubation. All agree that early intubation when a falling vital capacity reaches 15 ml/kg is beneficial and reduces the risk of further pulmonary complications (aspiration, atelectasis, and pneumonia). Arterial blood gases are too insensitive, becoming abnormal only late after considerable pulmonary atelectasis has taken place. Of course, prominent bulbar weakness with the corresponding risk of aspiration should lower the threshold to intubate. Otherwise routine, meticulous intensive care unit care is the mainstay of treatment (chest physiotherapy, bladder management, adequate caloric intake, and frequent positional changes to avoid bed sores or pressure palsies). In addition, all patients should receive low-dose subcutaneous heparin for deep venous thrombosis and pulmonary embolus prophylaxis. Severely affected patients who require a prolonged hospitalization are most easily treated with warfarin (Coumadin) until they regain mobility.

Recently, intravenous immune globulin, which has been used successfully in other autoimmune disorders, has been studied in patients with AIDP.[31] In one large trial, intravenous immune globulin was shown to be as effective as treatment with plasma exchange. This therapy, which has little in the way of side effects or potential complications, may replace plasma exchange in patients with AIDP because of its ease of administration.

Chronic Inflammatory Demyelinating Polyradiculoneuropathy

Chronic inflammatory demyelinating polyradiculoneuropathy (CIDP) is a demyelinating motor and sensory neuropathy that is presumed to be immune mediated.[32] All ages can be affected, but most patients present in their fifth to sixth decades. Proximal and distal muscles are both affected. The time course in CIDP is longer than that of AIDP (>6 weeks) and may follow either a monophasic progression, a step-wise progression, or a relapsing and remitting course. Early in the illness, it may not be possible to differentiate AIDP from the initial presentation of CIDP. Patients with CIDP generally progress slowly (weeks to months). The major disability is usually gait disturbance. Areflexia or hyporeflexia is the rule. Large-fiber sensory loss (touch, vibration, position sense) is more common than small-fiber loss (pain, temperature). A Romberg sign is commonly present. It is unusual to have significant bulbar or respiratory weakness.

CIDP may be idiopathic or occur in association with HIV infection, osteosclerotic myeloma, monoclonal gammopathy of undetermined significance or antibodies to myelin-associated glycoprotein. Therefore, all patients should undergo skeletal survey for osteosclerotic myeloma and have blood studies, including serum protein, and immunoelectrophoresis, and antibodies to myelin-associated glycoprotein and HIV.

As in AIDP, nerve conduction studies in patients with CIDP show electrophysiologic evidence of segmental demyelination, and CSF studies reveal protein elevation with the absence of a pleocytosis (with the exception of HIV-associated CIDP). Pathologic examination may demonstrate perivascular or diffuse mononuclear infiltration of nerve, without vasculitis, and segmental demyelination, although many biopsy results are nonspecific.

Therapy. CIDP patients are commonly treated with immunosuppressive therapy. Idiopathic CIDP may respond to prednisone, azathioprine (Imuran), intravenous immune globulin, or plasma exchange. Patients with myelin-associated glycoprotein antibody are often not responsive to these measures and may require cyclophosphamide (see later).[33] In patients with osteosclerotic myeloma–associated CIDP, surgery or radiation therapy directed toward the plasmacytoma frequently results in improvement of the neuropathy.

GM_1 Antibody Associated CIDP/Atypical Motor Neuron Disease

In recent years, new attention has been focused on the role of antiganglioside antibodies (especially GM_1) in patients with either neuropathy or motor neuron disease. It is now clear that there are a group of patients with elevated titers of antiganglioside antibodies who resemble patients with motor neuron disease clinically, but whose electrophysiologic studies show evidence of an acquired segmental demyelinating neuropathy, similar to CIDP. It is unclear if these patients simply are a variant of CIDP or represent a unique new syndrome.

Initially, a number of investigators suggested an association between atypical motor neuron disease and monoclonal gammopathies. Early anecdotal case reports drew attention to the unusual coincidence of monoclonal gammopathies, usually gamma M immunoglobulin (IgM), and progressive lower motor neuron syndromes, resembling variants of amyotrophic lateral sclerosis.[34–36] This association was further strengthened when individual patients were described with progressive lower motor neuron syndromes and IgM proteins directed against gangliosides. Further studies suggested that these antiganglioside antibodies, usually polyclonal IgM anti-GM_1 antibodies, may cause motor dysfunction either by paranodal demyelination or interference with the sodium channels at the nodes of Ranvier. Increasing attention to anti-GM_1 antibodies grew when other patients were reported with lower motor neuron syndromes, anti-GM_1 antibodies, and evidence of multifocal conduction block (i.e., segmental acquired demyelination) on nerve conduction studies that responded to immunosuppressive therapy.[37] These patients presented with asymmetric upper extremity weakness in the distribution, more or less, of named nerves. Reflexes were either reduced or inappropriately brisk for the level of weakness and wasting. No other definite upper motor neuron signs were present. Sensory symptoms were minimal or absent. Nerve conduction studies showed evidence of segmental demyelination on motor studies. No clinical or serologic response followed either prednisone or plasma exchange. However, treatment with cyclophosphamide lowered anti-GM_1 titers and accompanied clinical improvement. Although these patients were initially thought to have motor neuron disease clinically, they electrophysiologically demonstrated a demyelinating disorder of motor nerve, rather than motor neuron, with changes consistent with an acquired demyelinating neuropathy. However, the asymmetry, upper extremity predominance, relative absence of sensory findings, and lack of response to prednisone all suggested a disorder unique from the usual presentation of CIDP.

Subsequent reports have continued to emphasize the triad of antiganglioside antibodies, lower motor neuron dysfunction, and multifocal motor conduction block on nerve conduction studies as a treatable syndrome that can mimic motor neuron disease. Clinically, these cases present with progressive, asymmetric weakness and wasting. Distal upper extremity muscles are often affected first. Many of the patients are younger (<50 years old) than typical motor neuron disease patients. At times, it may be possible to detect weakness in the distribution of named motor nerves with sparing of others in the same myotome (clinical multifocal motor neuropathy). Definite upper motor neuron signs are absent, although some have retained or relatively brisk reflexes in a weak and wasted limb. Bulbar function and sensation are usually spared, although some mild or transient sensory symptoms may be present.

These patients are an important group to identify because treatment with immunosuppression may be associated with improvement. Antiganglioside titers have been shown to be unaffected by prednisone but responsive to treatment with intravenous or oral cyclophosphamide. Lowering the antiganglioside titers by 75% or more is usually required to effect a response and often requires many months of treatment.[38] In addition, some patients have been shown to respond to therapy with intravenous immune globulin, which is far less toxic than cyclophosphamide.

These studies suggest that a patient with a lower motor neuron syndrome, with or without sensory loss, should be screened for anti-GM_1 antibodies. The presence of anti-GM_1 antibodies in high titers clearly over control levels as well as over those of patients with other neurologic diseases and non-neurologic autoimmune diseases raises a possible autoimmune etiology for the syndrome. Conversely, the presence of multifocal conduction block or other evidence of demyelination on nerve conduction studies in a patient suspected of having motor neuron disease should prompt a search for antiganglioside antibodies.

Dysproteinemic Neuropathies

One of the major advances in recent years has been the recognition that monoclonal proteins may be responsible for a large number of undiagnosed polyneuropathies.[39] In the adult population, between 0.1 and 3% of individuals will have a monoclonal protein; however, 10% of idiopathic polyneuropathy patients will have a monoclonal protein. Of all patients with an IgM monoclonal protein, 50% will have an associated polyneuropathy, and of that group, 50% will have a type of monoclonal protein that can be demonstrated to have direct antinerve activity. It is now estimated that as many as 5% of all polyneuropathies may be due to the presence of a monoclonal protein. These studies suggest that all patients with an undiagnosed polyneuropathy should undergo screening using serum protein electrophoresis. Even if these results are normal, all patients should then have both serum and urine immunoelectrophoresis, as many small monoclonal proteins may be missed if these studies are not performed. If a monoclonal protein is discovered, then appropriate hematologic evaluation (e.g., bone marrow biopsy, skeletal survey) should be performed to type the monoclonal protein as part of a specific plasma cell dyscrasia, including multiple myeloma, Waldenström's macroglobulinemia, primary systemic amyloidosis, or a nonmalignant plasma cell dyscrasia.

Myeloma

Polyneuropathy is uncommon in multiple myeloma and occurs in only 3 to 5% of patients.[40, 41] More commonly, the peripheral nervous system is involved by direct infiltration of nerve root or spinal cord. Radiculopathies may also be seen from involvement of the vertebral bones with subsequent compression or pathologic fracture. The neuropathy associated with myeloma can be quite heterogeneous. Some cases are due to associated amyloid deposition and present similarly to the neuropathy of primary systemic amyloidosis (see later). In cases without amyloid, the neuropathy is usually a mild distal, axonal sensory motor polyneuropathy, similar to other paraneoplastic polyneuropathies. In addition, rare patients will have a primary sensory neuronopathy or an associated demyelinating polyneuropathy similar to CIDP. *Osteosclerotic myeloma* is a rare variant of myeloma and represents only between 0.3 and 3% of all myeloma cases. However, 50% of these patients will have an associated demyelinating neuropathy similar to CIDP. Clinically, this neuropathy presents as a chronic, slowly progressive, motor > sensory polyneuropathy. Generally, patients are not systemically ill, as in multiple myeloma.

Nerve conduction studies demonstrate acquired segmental demyelination. In most cases, there is a small monoclonal protein. Osteosclerotic myeloma usually involves a single or, less commonly, multiple lesions of the axial skeleton with sclerotic or mixed features. Some patients develop organomegaly, adenopathy, dermatologic, and endocrine abnormalities (POEMS syndrome). Treatment of a solitary lesion with surgery or chemotherapy often results in improvement of the neuropathy. Multiple lesions often require aggressive chemotherapy.

Primary Systemic Amyloidosis

Acquired systemic amyloidosis frequently presents with a polyneuropathy. The neuropathy is predominantly a small-fiber neuropathy, affecting small sensory and autonomic fibers. Clinically, patients present with a symmetric distal painful polyneuropathy, frequently with autonomic features (e.g., hypotension, impotence) and bilateral carpal tunnel syndrome. It is more common among older men. More than 90% will have a low level of serum monoclonal protein, but without bone marrow evidence of malignancy. Other organs, including liver, spleen, kidney, bone marrow, and heart, are commonly involved and may overshadow the neuropathy. Diagnosis is made by demonstrating amyloid deposition in nerve, rectal, or fat pad biopsy. The illness continues, with progressive organ infiltration with amyloid. Response to chemotherapy is generally poor, and over 50% of patients die within 36 months.

Monoclonal Gammopathy of Undetermined Significance

The most frequent association of neuropathy with a monoclonal protein is seen in patients with monoclonal gammopathy of undetermined significance, a syndrome characterized by a benign plasma cell dyscrasia and the production of low levels of monoclonal protein. Most of these patients with an associated neuropathy have an IgM monoclonal protein. Patients can be separated into two groups: those with and those without antimyelin associated glycoprotein activity. The non–myelin-associated glycoprotein group is heterogeneous, with some patients similar to those with idiopathic CIDP. The myelin-associated glycoprotein group of patients are more homogeneous. This neuropathy is usually very chronic, affecting predominantly large sensory fibers. Patients are usually older men who present with ataxia of gait, tremor, and distal loss of vibration and proprioception. CSF protein is elevated, and nerve conductions demonstrate a demyelinating neuropathy with very prolonged distal latencies. Treatment involves immunosuppression, often with cytotoxic drugs. Following the level of the monoclonal protein is useful and many times will parallel the activity of the neuropathy.

Waldenström's Macroglobulinemia

Patients with Waldenström's macroglobulinemia also may develop an associated polyneuropathy.[42] The neuropathy is usually similar to the IgM neuropathy in monoclonal gammopathy of undetermined significance and may present as a demyelinating neuropathy. Rarely, secondary amyloid infiltration or axonal degeneration may also be seen.

Infectious Neuropathies

Diphtheria

For the clinician in developed countries, diphtheria is a disease of the past. *Corynebacterium diphtheriae* causes an atypical pharyngitis. However, it also produces a very potent neurotoxin, which in turn produces a profound neuropathy. The pathology is that of severe segmental demyelination, causing conduction block and paralysis.

The polyneuropathy in diphtheria can present with two distinct syndromes. The first is a local effect on the palate, leading to palatal weakness and nasal speech. This can occur within the first 2 weeks of the illness. Other cranial nerves (extraocular, facial, vagus) and the phrenic nerve can then rarely become involved. Loss of accommodation with preservation of pupillary light responses can occur.

Later in the course (3 to 12 weeks), a diffuse sensorimotor demyelinating polyradiculoneuropathy may develop, with hyporeflexia or areflexia. CSF protein is markedly elevated, with an occasional lymphocytosis. Nerve conduction studies eventually show electrophysiologic evidence of a demyelinating polyneuropathy. Treatment is primarily supportive. If antitoxin is given early in the course of the respiratory infection, the incidence of polyneuropathy can be substantially reduced.

Leprosy

In the United States and other Western countries, leprosy is seen only in immigrants from endemic areas.[43] However, it is the most common treatable neuropathy in the world. *Mycobacterium leprae* is found in the lesions of the skin and also in peripheral nerves. There are three clinical forms of leprosy: the lepromatous, the tuberculoid, and the intermediate. The lepromatous variety is the diffuse and severe form. Leprosy is predominantly a small-fiber neuropathy affecting very small cutaneous nerve twigs. Pain and temperature sensations are lost early, with relative preservation of vibration and joint position sense. Cooler areas of the body (e.g., ears and extensor surfaces) tend to be affected first.[44] Later, nerve trunks become involved and weakness appears. Nerves may become enlarged and palpable. Neuropathic changes are noted in the same areas as the skin changes. Biopsy of either skin or nerve is required for the diagnosis.

Therapy. Leprosy is a reportable disorder; however, only in the lepromatous and intermediate varieties is there need for treatment of contacts. The current therapy is dapsone, started at 25 mg, twice a week for 21 weeks, gradually increasing to 100 mg twice a week for 2 years. Higher dosages (100 mg, six times per week) are used for the lepromatous variety and continued for many years or life. Rifampin in dosages of 600 mg/day has been used in combination with dapsone.[45]

Herpetic Neuropathy

Seen usually in the elderly and the immunosuppressed patient, herpes zoster invades dorsal root ganglia, primarily in the thoracic area. Cranial neuropathy may occur, mainly in the first division of the trigeminal nerve. The neuropathic picture of postinfectious neuralgia can continue for a long period of time.

Therapy. Steroids and acyclovir have been used during the acute infection, with the goal of decreasing the likelihood of delayed postherpetic neuralgia. Postherpetic neuralgia is frequently very difficult to treat. Anticonvulsants,

TABLE 60–7. PERIPHERAL NERVE COMPLICATIONS OF HIV*

Distal symmetrical polyneuropathy
Acute inflammatory demyelinating polyradiculoneuropathy†‡
Chronic inflammatory demyelinating polyradiculoneuropathy‡
Mononeuritis multiplex
Vasculitis
CIDP§ variant
Lymphomatous infiltration of nerve
Progressive CMV‖-associated polyradiculopathy‡
Autonomic neuropathy
ddI¶ and ddC** neuropathy
Herpes zoster
Facial palsy†

*HIV = human immunodeficiency virus.
†May be associated with HIV seroconversion.
‡May be associated with asymptomatic HIV infection.
§CIDP = chronic inflammatory demyelinating polyradiculoneuropathy.
‖CMV = cytomegalovirus.
¶ddI = dideoxyinosine.
**ddC = 2′,3′-dideoxycytidine.

antidepressants, capsaicin cream, and thoracic nerve blocks have been used with mixed results.

Lyme Neuropathy

Lyme disease is a systemic illness caused by the tick-borne spirochete *Borrelia burgdorferi.* Lyme disease may affect many organs but preferentially involves skin, joints, heart, and nervous system. Peripheral neuropathy is common in Lyme disease and can occur in the acute or chronic setting.[46] Acutely, Lyme neuropathy is an axonal polyradiculoneuropathy often involving the cranial nerves as well. Although all cranial nerves can be involved, the facial nerve, especially bilaterally, is the most frequently affected. The neuropathy is frequently asymmetric from superimposed radiculopathies. Patients present with pain, numbness, and weakness in the distribution of multiple nerve roots. Thoracic radiculopathies are common. These patients usually present along with a lymphocytic meningitis, often following erythema migrans, the classic dermatologic manifestation of Lyme.

The chronic neuropathy is much more mild and far less dramatic. Patients have either a mild distal axonal neuropathy with predominantly nonpainful sensory paresthesias, or a mild polyradiculopathy often associated with radicular and muscular pain. Typically, the physical examination is fairly unremarkable. Cranial nerve palsies and CSF pleocytosis are unusual. In general, these patients have very mild changes on nerve conduction studies and electromyography.

Although the acute neuropathy will subside without intervention, antibiotics may hasten the recovery and prevent later complications. In patients with late Lyme neuropathy, clinical symptoms and electrophysiologic abnormalities show improvement after prolonged treatment with intravenous antibiotics.

HIV-Associated Neuropathy

There are a wide variety of neurologic disorders associated with HIV infection and acquired immunodeficiency syndrome (AIDS).[47] Although initial reports focused on the central nervous system, PNS complications of HIV infection are common and, indeed, may be the initial presentation of HIV infection (Table 60–7).

Peripheral neuropathy has been reported as 5 to 20% of the neurologic complications seen in patients with AIDS, with this figure probably being an underestimate.[48] Many peripheral nerve disorders have been overlooked in seriously ill patients. It is important to differentiate between the various HIV-associated neuropathies when considering prognosis and therapy. Several distinct clinical, laboratory, and electrophysiologic syndromes have been elucidated (Tables 60–8, 60–9). Some can be treated only symptomatically, whereas others have definitive and possibly life-saving treatment. Peripheral neurologic disease may manifest at any stage of the infection from initial seroconversion through fully established AIDS. Like the disorders affecting the central nervous system in patients with AIDS, many of the peripheral disorders are not mutually exclusive; some patients have more than one complication at the same time.

Distal Sensory Polyneuropathy

Distal sensory polyneuropathy is probably the most common neuropathy associated with HIV infection. It is typi-

TABLE 60–8. CLINICAL FEATURES OF HIV*-RELATED PERIPHERAL NERVE DISORDERS

			Mononeuritis Multiplex		
	DSP†	**AIDP/CIDP‡**	*Vasculitis*	*Early CIDP*	**CMV§**
Setting	AIDS‖	SC¶, ASYMP**, AIDS	AIDS	AIDS	AIDS
Fiber type	S†† >> M‡‡	M > S	M/S	S > M	M/S
Hypesthesia	Distal	Distal	Multifocal	Multifocal	Saddle
Sensory level	−§§	−	−	−	+‖‖
Urinary retention	−	− (Rare)	−	−	++¶¶
Tendon areflexia	Ankle	Generalized	Multifocal	Multifocal	Caudal
Cranial nerves	−	+	+	−	+ (late)
Weakness	Distal	Generalized	Multifocal	Multifocal	Caudal

*HIV = human immunodeficiency virus.
†DSP = distal sensory polyneuropathy.
‡AIDP/CIDP = acute and chronic inflammatory demyelinating polyneuropathy.
§CMV = cytomegalovirus-associated polyradiculopathy.
‖AIDS = acquired immunodeficiency syndrome.
¶SC = seroconversion.
**ASYMP = asymptomatic HIV infection.
††S = sensory.
‡‡M = motor.
§§(−) = not involved.
‖‖(+) = occasionally involved.
¶¶(++) = frequently involved.

TABLE 60–9. LABORATORY FEATURES OF HIV-RELATED PERIPHERAL NERVE DISORDERS

			Mononeuritis Multiplex		
	DSP	**AIDP/CIDP**	*Vasculitis*	*Early CIDP*	**CMV**
CSF					
WBC	NL	↑	NL/↑	↑	↑↑
PMN	NL	NL	NL/↑	NL	↑↑
Glucose	NL	NL	NL/↓	NL	↓/↓↓
Protein	NL/↑	↑/↑↑	NL/↑	NL/↑	↑/↑↑
NCS	Distal axonal	Demyelinating	Multifocal axonal	Multifocal axonal or demyelinating	Axonal
EMG	Distal denervation	Generalized denervation (late)	Multifocal denervation	Multifocal denervation	Caudal denervation
Sural nerve biopsy					
Inflammation	+	++	++	+/++	+/−
Vasculitis	−	−	++	−	−

DSP = distal sensory polyneuropathy.
AIDP/CIDP = acute and chronic inflammatory demyelinating polyneuropathy.
CMV = cytomegalovirus-associated polyradiculopathy.
NL = normal.
WBC = white blood cells.
PMN = polymorphonuclear cells.
NCS = nerve conduction studies.
EMG = electromyography.
(↑/↑↑) = increased moderately/markedly.
(↓/↓↓) = decreased moderately/markedly.
(−) = not involved.
(+) = occasionally involved.
(++) = frequently involved.

cally seen in well-established AIDS, and in many cases will coincide with AIDS dementia.[48] In one study, 35% of 40 unselected patients with AIDS had distal sensory polyneuropathy.[47]

Clinically, distal sensory polyneuropathy presents with distal symmetrical lower extremity numbness and painful paresthesias, which are often described as burning. Pain is most prominent in the soles and rarely ascends above the level of the ankles.[49] Contact hypersensitivity to walking, and to simply wearing socks and shoes, is common. A sensory loss to all modalities in a stocking, or stocking-glove, distribution is present. The most common neurologic sign is reduced or absent ankle jerks. There may be distal muscle atrophy, but rarely is weakness or atrophy prominent.

Electromyography and nerve conduction studies are consistent with a distal sensory and motor axonal polyneuropathy.[47, 49–51] CSF protein is normal or slightly elevated (46 to 105 mg/dl in one study[49]). No pleocytosis is present.

Pathology demonstrates axonal degeneration of large and small myelinated fibers, and less prominent demyelination and perivascular mononuclear inflammation.[47, 51–53] Although the pathologies in distal sensory polyneuropathy and CIDP are similar, the intensity of inflammation is less prominent in distal sensory polyneuropathy.[53] Pathology of the spinal cord shows gracile tract degeneration, likely reflecting distal dying back of the central axon.[54] HIV can rarely be cultured from nerve, and in these cases, it is unknown if HIV is from the inflammatory infiltrate, nerve, or Schwann cell.[47, 53]

The pathogenesis of distal sensory polyneuropathy is unknown. Possibilities include a direct viral infection, an opportunistic infection (e.g., cytomegalovirus), or secondary immune attack.[47] Most investigators feel that the most likely explanation is direct HIV infection of nerve and secondary T-cell– and macrophage-mediated tissue destruction.[53]

In nearly all patients with established AIDS and a distal painful neuropathy, distal sensory polyneuropathy will be the correct diagnosis. Other conditions that cause a distal painful axonal neuropathy should be considered, including diabetes, amyloid, nutritional deficiency (especially thiamine), and rare intoxications (e.g., thallium).[49] These alternative diagnoses are usually suggested by associated symptoms, past medical history, and physical examination.

Distal sensory polyneuropathy does not respond to steroids or immunosuppression.[53] Rare cases improve with zidovudine, although the majority of patients show no clinical and electrophysiologic improvement with zidovudine.[49, 50, 55] Treatment remains primarily symptomatic. Simple analgesics, tricyclics, and antiepileptics (carbamazepine, phenytoin) are the mainstay of therapy.[49] A trial of topical capsaicin cream may be worthwhile, because other neuropathies with prominent small-fiber paresthesias (pain and burning), such as diabetes and zoster, may respond to this treatment.

Inflammatory Demyelinating Polyradiculoneuropathy

Inflammatory demyelinating neuropathies occur in HIV-infected patients in both the acute (AIDP, or Guillain-Barré syndrome) and chronic forms (CIDP). The clinical presentation, treatment, and prognosis are similar to that of seronegative patients (see earlier). In many cases, only the CSF pleocytosis suggests the diagnosis of HIV-associated demyelinating polyradiculoneuropathy. Although both of these disorders can occur in well-established AIDS, they differ from distal sensory polyneuropathy in that they most commonly occur at the time of initial HIV seroconversion (typically, 30 to 150 days after infection) or during asymptomatic HIV infection.[47, 48, 56]

The most important laboratory tests in HIV-associated AIDP and CIDP are the CSF exam and electromyography. CSF protein is increased in most patients (range of 24 to 516 mg/dl), although it may be normal in the first few days.[57] The critical discriminating point is the presence of a CSF pleocytosis (mean of 25 cells; range of 1 to 50).[47, 48, 51, 56–58] A CSF pleocytosis in a patient with otherwise typical

AIDP or CIDP should strongly suggest the possibility of HIV infection. Nerve conduction studies show electrophysiologic evidence of segmental demyelination. Sural nerve biopsy demonstrates segmental demyelination and perivascular cellular infiltrates.[47, 51] Some reports have demonstrated direct IgM immunofluorescence of the perineurium.[51] Although the pathogenesis is not entirely known, it is likely autoimmune. Direct viral invasion appears unlikely, considering that improvement can occur spontaneously or following immunosuppressive therapy (see later).[57]

Management is similar to that for seronegative patients. Although steroids have been successfully used in some HIV-associated CIDP patients, one is always hesitant to further immunosuppress these patients. Patients with asymptomatic HIV infection probably can be safely managed with steroids. However, patients with established AIDS who do not respond to plasma exchange may be given a trial of intravenous γ-globulin prior to consideration of treatment with steroids.[59] Thus, recognition of the inflammatory demyelinating neuropathies is important because effective treatment is available. The prognosis in most patients is generally good, although the recovery may be longer than in seronegative patients.[50]

Mononeuritis Multiplex

Mononeuritis multiplex is a rare peripheral nervous system complication of HIV infection and is usually associated with well-established AIDS. The clinical presentation is distinctive: there is an asymmetric step-wise progression of individual cranial or peripheral neuropathies.[47, 48] Over time, a confluent pattern will develop that is difficult to distinguish from a generalized polyneuropathy. In most cases, the individual neuropathies are of named nerves (e.g., median, ulnar, and peroneal) as opposed to small nerve twigs. Of note, the pattern of mononeuritis multiplex in non-HIV patients is classically associated with either a necrotizing vasculitis, an early variant of CIDP, or less commonly, direct infiltration of nerve by tumor (e.g., lymphoma) or infection (e.g., leprosy). The differential diagnosis in HIV patients is the same.

The mononeuritis multiplex pattern in HIV may be associated with a necrotizing vasculitis.[47, 48, 53, 60] Fever, weight loss, and cachexia are frequently present. The CSF shows a pleocytosis. The electromyographic result is consistent with that of an acute or subacute axonal degeneration of multiple peripheral nerves. Sural nerve biopsy demonstrates a necrotizing arteritis similar to polyarteritis nodosa.[47, 50, 60] The pathogenesis of this syndrome is obscure. Inflammatory cells surrounding the blood vessels have been identified as HIV positive.[53] There are similar cases demonstrating cytomegalovirus inclusions in peripheral nerves, with one case report of a patient responding to ganciclovir.[47] At this time, the proper therapy is not known. Antiviral or immunosuppressive therapy may be worth trying, although prognosis in most of these cases is frequently poor.

CIDP may present with a mononeuritis multiplex pattern, but it has a far better prognosis than vasculitis.[50, 51, 60] These patients most frequently present with multifocal sensory loss without systemic symptoms. CSF shows a pleocytosis and elevated protein. Electromyography may demonstrate electrophysiologic evidence of demyelination. Sural nerve biopsy shows axonal loss, demyelination, and perivascular infiltration. Some cases will progress to typical CIDP, whereas others spontaneously improve. Improvement may occur with plasma exchange.

Although most HIV-associated mononeuritis multiplex patients will have either underlying vasculitis or early CIDP, it is important to consider the possibility of unusual infiltration of nerve by tumor (lymphoma) or by infection (herpes zoster, leprosy). Dermatologic manifestations may accompany zoster or leprosy. Leprosy may be further suggested by patches of small-fiber sensory loss (pain, temperature) in the distribution of small unnamed nerve twigs, especially in relatively cooler body parts (e.g., ear lobes, extensor surfaces). Nerve biopsy is usually required to diagnose direct infiltration by tumor or leprosy.

Progressive CMV-Associated Polyradiculopathy

Progressive CMV-associated polyradiculopathy is a dramatic syndrome usually seen in well-established AIDS (average time since AIDS diagnosis, 18 months), although rare cases may be seen in asymptomatic HIV infection.[61] Early clinical recognition is imperative because this formerly universally fatal condition can be successfully treated with antiviral therapy.

These patients present with a cauda equina syndrome (rapidly progressive motor and sensory dysfunction affecting the lower extremities and sacral myotomes).[47, 48, 51, 61, 62] Pelvic pain and saddle paresthesias (perineum, buttock, inner thighs) may be prominent early. A flaccid paraparesis follows with early bladder and bowel dysfunction. The initial presentation may be asymmetric. The course progresses in days and may last several weeks (mean of 5.8 weeks; range of 3 to 15 weeks).[61, 62] There may be an early loss of lower extremity, cremasteric, and anal reflexes. Untreated, the illness relentlessly spreads rostral to involve the thoracic and cervical myotomes and may be associated with a sensory level. During the course of the illness, the legs may be paralyzed and the arms spared, a pattern not seen in the inflammatory demyelinating polyneuropathies.[61]

The CSF examination is the most helpful laboratory test. In nearly all cases, a CSF pleocytosis with predominantly polymorphonuclear neutrophils is present (typically 100 to 1500 cells).[47, 51, 61, 62] CSF protein is elevated (65 to 630 mg/dl), and CSF glucose is frequently depressed. Occasionally, CSF culture results may be positive for cytomegalovirus (four of seven patients in one study).[61] Myelography is normal or shows only thickened nerve roots. Electromyography typically shows an axonal pattern affecting the lower extremities, although some cases may be confused with AIDP.[63]

Pathology at autopsy shows extensive acute and chronic multifocal necrotic inflammation of nerve root parenchyma and endothelial cells, with congestion and edema.[47, 51, 52, 61] Inclusion bodies immunocytochemically positive for cytomegalovirus are found in endothelial, Schwann, and inflammatory cells.[61] Frank vasculitis with segmental thrombosis may be present. In some cases, a coexistent focal myelitis is present. Spinal nerves distal to the dorsal root ganglion show inflammation and inclusion bodies, implying that this syndrome is actually a polyradiculoneuropathy. Similar but less marked pathologic changes are present in the thoracic and cervical roots. Pathologic cytomegalovirus encephalitis may be present. Sural nerve biopsy has failed to demonstrate cytomegalovirus, occasionally showing only perivascular inflammation.[25]

Patients may respond to early treatment with ganciclovir. Empiric therapy is indicated prior to culture results because most patients need to be treated within 48 hours of onset to effect improvement.[47, 61] When ganciclovir is started late, patients have no response. Similarly, steroids and plasma exchange have no effect.[47] Ganciclovir is given intravenously in a dose of 2.5 mg/kg every 8 hours for a 10-day course.[61] Some may require maintenance therapy.

Cytomegalovirus is responsible for an unknown number of peripheral nerve disorders in HIV patients.[64] In addition to polyradiculopathy, cytomegalovirus has been associated with some cases of mononeuritis multiplex (see earlier). Many times, it is difficult based on culture results to implicate cytomegalovirus as the causative factor because cytomegalovirus may be found in various body fluids without other pathology.[64] Most agree with empiric therapy with ganciclovir in any HIV-positive patient with a subacute severe multifocal sensory motor neuropathy, especially when it is associated with fever, polymorphonuclear neutrophils in the CSF, hypoglycorrhacia, or other evidence of cytomegalovirus infection (e.g., retinitis, esophagitis, pneumonitis).[64]

The differential diagnosis of cytomegalovirus polyradiculopathy includes spinal cord syndromes and other causes of polyradiculopathy. In AIDS, the spinal cord may be involved by direct HIV infection (vacuolar myelopathy) or by secondary infection (herpes simplex virus 1, human T-cell lymphotrophic virus, herpes zoster).[61] Polyradiculopathy may be caused by neurosyphilis (positive results on Venereal Disease Research Laboratories) or direct infiltration by lymphoma (positive CSF cytology, no polymorphonuclear neutrophils in CSF).[47, 61] Finally, cytomegalovirus polyradiculopathy must be differentiated from the more common inflammatory demyelinating neuropathies (AIDP or CIDP). Clinical, laboratory, and electrophysiologic studies usually allow easy separation (Tables 60–10 and 60–11).

Autonomic Neuropathy

It is not unusual for HIV-infected patients to have autonomic complaints (presyncope, bladder, bowel, or sexual dysfunction).[47, 65] The etiology is likely multifactorial, including medicines, systemic illness, and central nervous system disease. In addition, a small-fiber autonomic neuropathy may be present. This neuropathy usually coexists with distal sensory polyneuropathy in AIDS patients.[47, 56, 65]

ddI and ddC Neuropathy

Both the HIV drugs dideoxyinosine (ddI) and 2′,3′-dideoxycytidine (ddC) have polyneuropathy as a major dose-limiting factor.[47, 66] Both are associated with an acute onset of distal painful neuropathy with intense burning. Examination shows a distal stocking sensory loss and loss of ankle jerks. Improvement usually occurs several weeks to months after withdrawal of the offending drug. Patients may be rechallenged successfully at lower dosages.[47] Both of these compounds are likely axonal toxins. In one study, all patients receiving a dose of ddC of greater than 0.03 mg/kg every 4 hours developed a neuropathy.[47] In another study of ddI, neuropathy was frequently associated with a daily dose of more than 12 mg/kg and/or a total dose of more than 2 g/kg.[47]

TABLE 60–10. CMV RADICULOPATHY: CLINICAL FEATURES*

Feature	No.
AIDS†	7/7
Progressive severe weakness	7/7
Early sacral paresthesias	7/7
Early urinary retention	7/7
CMV‡ retinitis	3/7
Sensory level	2/7
Pyramidal signs	0/7
Treated with AZT§	3/7
Duration of illness (days)	40 (29–56)

*From Miller RG, Storey JR, and Greco CM: Ganciclovir in the treatment of progressive AIDS-related polyradiculopathy. Neurology 40:569–574, 1990.
†AIDS = acquired immunodeficiency syndrome.
‡CMV = cytomegalovirus.
§AZT = zidovudine.

TABLE 60–11. CMV RADICULOPATHY: LABORATORY FEATURES*

Feature	No.
CSF† cell count (cells/mm³)	449 (29–1,500)
% Polymorphonuclear cells	71 (58–94)
CSF protein (mg/dl)	274 (113–630)
CSF glucose (mg/dl)	29 (15–47)
CMV‡ culture, positive	4/7
VDRL§	0/7
Acute denervation on EMG‖	7/7
Small motor amplitudes on lower extremity nerve conduction studies	7/7
CMV at autopsy	5/5

*From Miller RG, Storey JR, and Greco CM: Ganciclovir in the treatment of progressive AIDS-related polyradiculopathy. Neurology 40:569–574, 1990.
†CSF = cerebrospinal fluid.
‡CMV = cytomegalovirus.
§VDRL = Venereal Disease Research Laboratory.
‖EMG = electromyography.

Neuropathy of Connective Tissue Disorders

In most of the connective tissue disorders and related conditions, peripheral neuropathy is a major component of the disease, and in a significant proportion, it is the presenting sign.[67] Moreover, it may be, along with arthritis, the most disturbing chronic symptom to the patient.

Systemic Vasculitis

This group of disorders, exemplified by polyarteritis nodosa, also includes Churg-Strauss syndrome, Wegener's granulomatosis, hypersensitivity vasculitis, and vasculitis associated with malignancy or infection (specifically HIV). The peripheral nervous system is involved in a high percentage of these cases. Although a number of different clinical patterns are noted, multiple mononeuropathies superimposed on a distal symmetric polyneuropathy is the most common.

The pathology in vasculitic neuropathy is presumed to be an immune complex–triggered leukocytoclastic reaction in a vessel wall, resulting in a segmental infarction from occlusion of the vasa nervosum. This process results in predominantly axonal damage. Electrodiagnostic studies are often helpful in diagnosis. Electromyographic findings are more extensive than expected, and nerve conduction study results are consistent with axonal damage, showing relatively normal conduction velocity but reduced compound muscle action potential amplitudes.

Therapy. Immunosuppressive therapy frequently results in dramatic improvement of the neuropathy. A combination of cyclophosphamide and prednisone is usually required, with 80% of patients showing improvement.

Rheumatoid Arthritis

Different patterns of peripheral neuropathy are seen in rheumatoid arthritis: (1) mononeuropathies, including compression and entrapment neuropathies, and digital neuropathies; (2) distal sensory polyneuropathy; and (3) progressive sensorimotor polyneuropathy. The most common peripheral nervous system involvement is that of entrapment neuropathies.[68] Carpal tunnel syndrome, cubital tunnel syndrome, digital neuropathies of the ulnar and median nerves, anterior and posterior interosseous nerve syndrome, and tarsal tunnel syndrome are seen. One entrapment peculiar to rheumatoid arthritis is when a Baker cyst in the popliteal fossa gives rise to a posterior tibial or a peroneal nerve palsy.

There are two polyneuropathies associated with rheumatoid arthritis: a mild, slowly progressive distal sensory neuropathy, and a rapidly progressive sensorimotor neuropathy associated with vasculitis and mononeuritis multiplex. An elevated rheumatoid factor and decreased serum complement are usually present.

Therapy. Local steroid injection and splinting are the first steps for the treatment of compression neuropathies. Anti-inflammatory agents used concomitantly reduce the discomfort. In the severe sensorimotor neuropathy, steroids in high doses and other immunosuppressives have been effective.

Lupus Neuropathy

The involvement of the nervous system in lupus neuropathy is mainly central. However, as in rheumatoid arthritis, different patterns of neuropathy can be seen: (1) mononeuropathies and mononeuritis multiplex, including cranial neuropathies and (2) distal sensory polyneuropathy.[69] A Guillain-Barré–like syndrome has also been noted with lupus. The pathogenesis of the polyneuropathy is not understood. However, deposition of immune complexes is thought to be the underlying problem in the mononeuropathies. In most patients, there is evidence for a lupus flare-up when symptoms of peripheral neuropathy worsen. However, there is often little connection between serologic titers and the clinical picture.

Therapy. As in rheumatoid neuropathy, corticosteroids have been used with varying results. When the polyneuropathy is severe and progressive, high doses of corticosteroids have been useful.

Other Collagen Vascular Disorders

In most other collagen vascular disorders, the pathogenesis of neuropathy is considered to be due to vasculitis. In scleroderma, peripheral neuropathy is rare, and, when present, it is mild. A mild sensory motor neuropathy may be seen in Sjögren's syndrome. Recently, the association of a sensory neuronopathy has been appreciated in patients with Sjögren's syndrome. A mononeuritis multiplex picture may be seen in polyarteritis nodosa, which also may present with a sensorimotor neuropathy of acute onset, akin to that of Guillain-Barré syndrome. Trigeminal sensory neuropathy is also reported in up to 25% of these patients.

Therapy. Corticosteroids have been used in high dosages. However, frequently other immunosuppressive therapies, especially oral cyclophosphamide, are required to control the neuropathies associated with vasculitis.[70]

Toxic Neuropathies

A number of agents produce toxic damage to the peripheral nervous system, resulting at times in severe peripheral neuropathy. Recent increasing awareness of environmental and workplace pollutants has resulted in a growing list of agents that may cause peripheral neuropathies. In all cases, the patient should first be removed from the source of intoxication.

Lead Neuropathy

This is primarily a motor neuropathy; it predominantly affects the upper extremities and presents as a radial nerve palsy or sometimes as a foot drop. Patients are usually adults (children develop lead encephalopathy), and the condition is seen usually in workers exposed to environmental lead. In addition, patients frequently have a mild encephalopathy (i.e., mild impairment in memory, mood, or behavior), gastrointestinal disturbance, and abnormalities on routine chemistries and blood counts.

Therapy. Chelation with ethylenediaminetetraacetic acid (EDTA) or British antilewisite (BAL) is used only when blood levels exceed 100 μg/100 g.[71] In chronic cases, treatment with penicillamine has been effective.

Arsenic Neuropathy

Arsenic causes a primarily sensory neuropathy, with pain and paresthesias dominating the picture. Intoxication in large doses results in severe abdominal pain and acute renal failure. Chronic poisoning may be seen in industrial workers and in those exposed to insecticides.[72]

Therapy. Urine and hair samples are used to monitor arsenic levels (toxicity occurs when urine excretion exceeds 25 μg/24 hr). As in lead neuropathy, British antilewisite is used at dosages of 2.5 mg/kg intramuscularly. Oral penicillamine has been used as an adjunct therapy.

Other Heavy Metals

Mercury, thallium, gold, and platinum may cause various different neuropathies.[73] Manifestations often vary, depending on the dose and length of exposure. Commonly, other organ systems may be involved as well, including the central nervous system. Treatment usually involves avoidance of further exposure, and in some cases, chelating agents.

Drug-Induced Neuropathies

Drug-induced neuropathies are usually symmetric, distal sensory, or sensorimotor neuropathies. Motor symptoms and autonomic dysfunction are rare. Electrodiagnostic studies show an axonal process. Some of the commonly used drugs that cause toxic neuropathies are isoniazid, phenytoin, nitrofurantoin, ethambutol, vincristine, vinblastine, imipramine, disulfiram, dapsone, hydralazine, platinum, gold, metronidazole, and thalidomide.[74] In isoniazid and disulfiram neuropathies, pyridoxine at dosages of 50 mg/day has been effective in stabilizing the neuropathy.

Industrial Toxins

Solvents and other hydrocarbons, such as carbon tetrachloride, trichlorethylene, and toluene, cause different degrees of peripheral neuropathy. The list of industrial compounds causing neurotoxicity is growing by the day. The clinician should inquire into the possibility of symptoms occurring in more than one worker in a work place and then use state agencies to investigate the possibility of neurotoxin pollution.[75]

Insecticides and Organophosphorus Compounds

Insecticides and organophosphorus compounds have both central nervous system and PNS effects. The epidemic of triorthocresyl phosphate in the 1930s was a good example of an epidemic peripheral neuropathy. Organophosphates, which are used in insecticides, petroleum additives, plastics, and nerve gases, are cholinesterase inhibitors. Overdose of these compounds can cause acute cholinergic crisis. A delayed polyneuropathy will follow in some patients. The peripheral neuropathy may be moderately severe or rapidly progressive, with predominantly motor weakness and some paresthesias. It may be difficult to distinguish clinically from AIDP unless a history of ingestion or exposure is obtained.

Inherited Neuropathies

A large number of disorders come under this heading, including porphyric neuropathy, which has already been discussed.[76–80] Most have no specific therapy at this time, and only symptomatic therapy is available. However, correct diagnosis is important in genetic counseling and advising on prognosis. Neuropathies associated with disorders of metabolism, such as metachromatic leukodystrophy, Krabbe's, Refsum's, Bassen-Kornzweig, Tangier, and Fabry's diseases are now well described. In most of these disorders, the central nervous system abnormality predominates; however the PNS evaluation and nerve biopsy result may greatly assist in the diagnosis and avoid further, more complicated or invasive tests.[81]

Although most are extremely rare, several inherited neuropathies account for a large percent of the difficult-to-diagnose neuropathies. It is now apparent that inherited neuropathies may affect certain individuals so minimally, or progress so slowly over an individual's lifetime, that they may never seek medical attention. In a patient with a difficult-to-diagnose neuropathy, particular attention must be paid to family history. In addition, it is frequently beneficial to examine family members or study them with nerve conduction studies and electromyography.

Hereditary Motor Sensory Neuropathy (Charcot-Marie-Tooth Disease)

Hereditary motor sensory neuropathy is the most common type of inherited neuropathy. The nomenclature of this neuropathy, like those of many other inherited neuropathies, is complex. Hereditary motor sensory neuropathy is synonymous with Charcot-Marie-Tooth and peroneal muscular atrophy.

The most common subtypes of hereditary motor sensory neuropathy are types I and II, which are demyelinating and axonal neuropathies, respectively. This neuropathy is a slowly progressive, distal, predominantly motor neuropathy, associated with pes cavus and hammer toes. Sensory symptoms are uncommon, although mild sensory signs are usually discovered on careful examination. There are no cranial nerve signs. Hereditary motor sensory neuropathy predominantly affects the intrinsic foot and lower leg anterior compartment musculature. Ankle reflexes are absent. In well-established cases, all reflexes are absent. The onset is commonly in early childhood for type I and in adolescence or adulthood for type II, and typically presents as a foot deformity, delay in motor milestones, or bilateral foot drop.

The genetics in hereditary motor sensory neuropathy are heterogeneous. The inheritance in most families is autosomal dominant, although rare cases of autosomal recessive and x-linked recessive inheritance have been documented. Nerve conduction studies in type I show marked slowing of conduction velocity. Slowing is uniform in all nerves, without evidence of temporal dispersion or conduction block. There is often little correlation between the degree of slowing and clinical symptoms. Sensory studies are abnormal and generally show low or absent amplitudes. Electromyography typically shows little spontaneous activity, with evidence consistent with distal reinnervation. Type II looks like a typical chronic distal axonal sensory and motor neuropathy on nerve conductions and electromyography.

The prognosis is most cases is relatively benign. Although occasional patients are confined to a wheelchair, most remain ambulatory with the use of simple bracing and have little impairment in functional strength.

Déjerine-Sottas Disease

Déjerine-Sottas disease, also known as hereditary motor sensory neuropathy type III or hypertrophic neuropathy of infancy, is a severe demyelinating neuropathy, with onset usually in infancy. Patients present with prominent sensory loss, ataxia, distal weakness, pes cavus, hyporeflexia or areflexia, and hypertrophic nerves.

The typical presentation during infancy is usually a delay in motor milestones and a disturbed gait. Children do not walk until the age of 3 or 4.[76] Patients are often of short stature. Occasionally, nystagmus, deafness, bifacial weakness, and pupillary abnormalities may be present.[78, 79] Scoliosis and foot deformities are common. Inheritance is usually autosomal recessive. Nerve conduction studies show profoundly slow conduction velocities, as low as 2 to 6 m/sec. CSF protein is commonly mildly elevated. These patients are much more severely affected than the other more common hereditary motor sensory neuropathies and are usually totally disabled in early youth.

Familial Amyloid Polyneuropathy

The neuropathy associated with acquired systemic amyloidosis has previously been discussed. More rarely, amyloidosis may occur as an inherited neuropathy. The diagnosis of familial amyloid polyneuropathy has been based traditionally on attempts to classify patients based on clinical features and ancestry or geographic origin of cases. Four types of familial amyloid polyneuropathy (Andrade, Rukavina, Van Allen, and Meretoja) have been described in various ethnic groups. Each is autosomal dominant. The most frequently reported type, Andrade, resembles the neuropathy of primary systemic amyloidosis, with early loss of small fiber function, autonomic symptoms, and pain. Ulceration and injury to the feet is common. The disorder is slowly progressive, ultimately resulting in infiltration of other organs.

Most cases of familial amyloid polyneuropathy are associated with extracellular deposition of abnormal prealbumin (also known as transthyretin). Recent molecular studies have demonstrated point mutations in the prealbumin gene on the long arm of chromosome 18. Diagnostic testing using recombinant DNA methods is now commercially available.[82]

MONONEUROPATHIES

Traumatic Neuropathies

The peripheral nerves are generally well protected by surrounding tissues. However, in certain locations, the nerves may be exposed to trauma or to injuries secondary to bone fractures. Therapy is dictated by the type and extent of injury. Two common classifications have been used to characterize the type of injury. In one, Seddon classified injury into (1) neurapraxia, (2) axonotmesis, and (3) neurotmesis.[83] A more detailed classification by Sunderland divides injury into five categories.[84]

Category 1 *(neurapraxia):* implies that there is only demyelination and conduction block with intact axonal continuity. Recovery is usually complete over days to weeks.
Category 2 *(axonotmesis):* axons are damaged, but with the endoneurium intact. Regeneration occurs but is slowed to a rate of 1 to 2 mm/day.
Category 3: axons and endoneurium are damaged, but the perineurium is preserved. Regeneration is still possible, but it is commonly not complete.
Category 4: axons, endoneurium, and perineurium are damaged, but the epineurium is preserved. Regeneration, if it occurs, is rather poor.
Category 5: axons, endoneurium, perineurium, and epineurium are damaged. Recovery is often minimal or absent.

Compression and Entrapment Neuropathies

Mononeuropathies that occur secondary to direct trauma or fractures are easily localized clinically because of the obvious anatomic correlation between site of lesion and disturbed function. However, lesions due to compression and thereby intermittent, indirect trauma are not as easily recognizable clinically. The clinical course is variable, and the presentation relates to the degree of compression or entrapment and to the chronicity. Distinguishing these from common radiculopathies may be difficult. Occupational etiologies are frequently involved, and careful review of work habits is necessary. Table 60–12 and Figure 60–3 list some of the more common entrapment neuropathies. Some of these are discussed later. For a more comprehensive review, see major texts.[85, 86]

Common Compression and Entrapment Neuropathies of the Upper Extremity

Carpal Tunnel Syndrome

Carpal tunnel syndrome is the most common entrapment neuropathy and often is misdiagnosed. The median nerve becomes entrapped by the transverse carpal ligament, which is a tough fibrous tissue with sharp edges and forms the roof of the carpal tunnel.

Patients present with arm and wrist pain, with paresthesias in the thumb and first two or three fingers. The paresthesias usually awaken the patient at night because of sustained flexion of the wrist during sleep. Symptoms often worsen after the use of the hand (especially with driving or holding the phone or a book). The involvement is usually bilateral but worse in the dominant hand. Percussing the nerve at the wrist (Tinel's sign) and flexing the patient's hand at the wrist (Phalen's maneuver) should reproduce the symptoms. In severe cases, there is atrophy and weakness of thenar muscles and numbness involving the thumb and the first two and one-half digits, but sparing the thenar eminence (Fig. 60–4).

Electrodiagnostic studies show a slowed median sensory conduction velocity and prolonged median distal motor latency.

The etiology is usually an anatomically small carpal tunnel or nonspecific flexor tenosynovitis. However, some conditions predispose the patient to carpal tunnel syndrome. In pregnancy and in patients with hypothyroidism, rheumatoid arthritis, diabetes, and amyloidosis, carpal tunnel syndrome is a common finding. Recently, carpal tunnel syndrome has become increasingly recognized as an occupational disorder. In industries where workers make repeated wrist motions or use computer keyboards excessively, carpal tunnel syndrome cases have reached epidemic proportions.

Treatment. In mild cases, splinting the wrist in neutral position at night and use of nonsteroidal anti-inflammatory agents are sufficient to relieve symptoms. If symptoms persist, local injection of corticosteroids may be of use. Surgery for carpal tunnel syndrome is recommended if these maneuvers fail or if there is significant sensory loss or signifi-

TABLE 60–12. COMMON COMPRESSION AND ENTRAPMENT NEUROPATHIES*

Nerve	Syndrome	Primary Clinical Feature
Upper Extremity		
Median	Carpal tunnel	Weakness in thenar muscles, sensory loss in thumb and index and middle fingers
	Pronator	Pain over the pronator muscle, weakness of wrist flexion and pronation, sensory loss over palm, thumb, and index and middle fingers
	Anterior interosseous	Weakness in thumb and index finger flexion
Ulnar	Guyon's canal	Weakness in interossei, sensory loss in ring and little fingers
	Cubital tunnel	Same as above plus weakness in ulnar wrist flexion and flexion of ring and little fingers
Radial	Saturday night palsy	Wrist and finger drop, numbness over dorsum of the hand
	Posterior interosseous	Wrist and finger drop, sparing radial wrist extension
Brachial plexus	Thoracic outlet	Ulnar sensory loss, weakness of ulnar and distal median muscles
	Long thoracic	Winging of the scapula
Lower Extremity		
Sciatic	Piriformis muscle	Sciatica, foot drop, decreased ankle jerk
Peroneal	Fibular head or Baker's cyst	Foot drop, sensory loss in lateral calf and dorsum of the foot
Posterior tibial	Tarsal tunnel	Burning heel, weakness of intrinsic foot muscles
Lateral femoral cutaneous	Meralgia paresthetica	Numbness and burning in lateral thigh
Femoral	Femoral neuropathy	Weakness of knee extension, decreased knee jerk, numbness over anterior thigh

*Adapted from Nakano K: The entrapment neuropathies. Muscle Nerve 1:264, 1978.

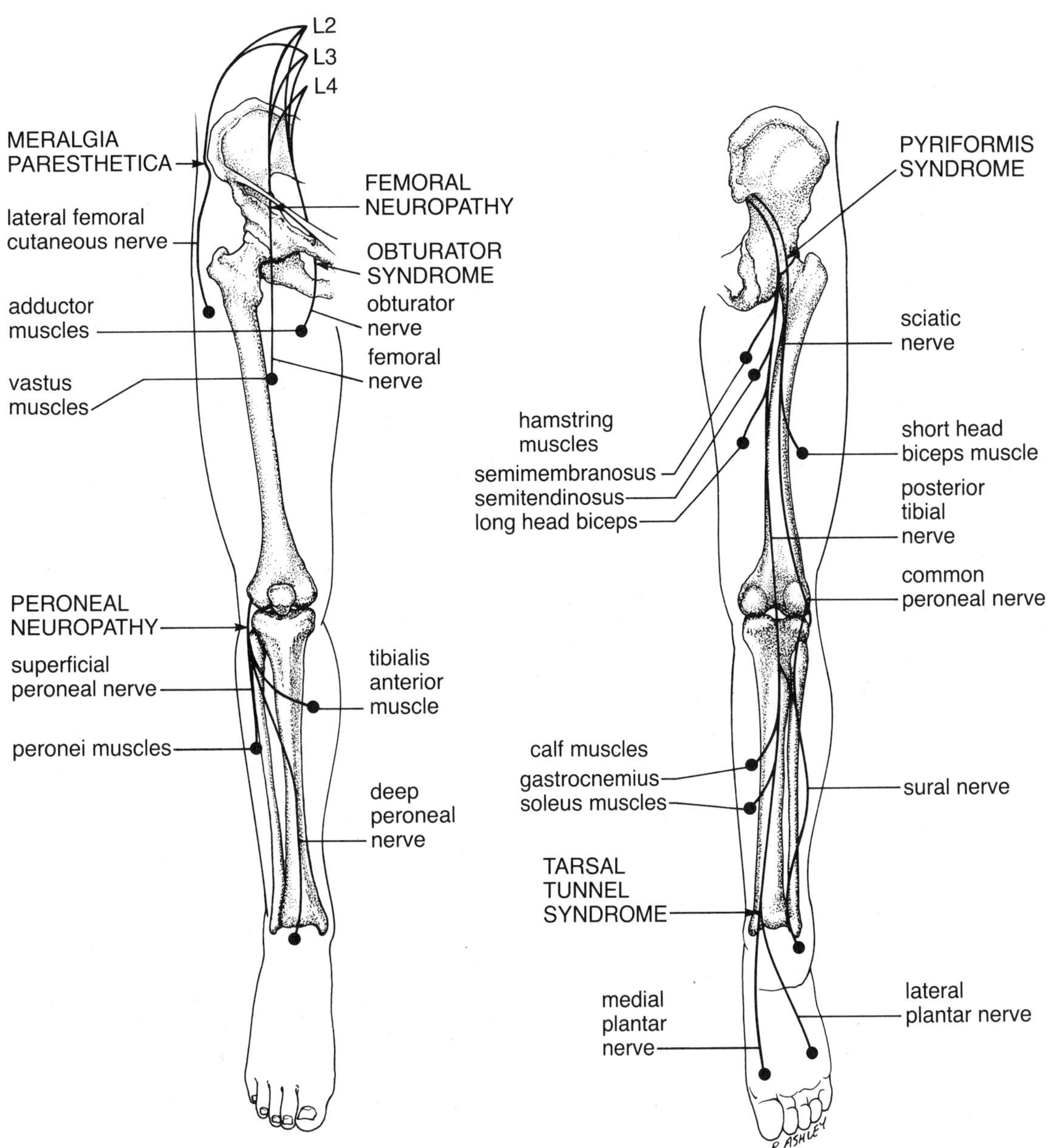

FIGURE 60–3. Major nerves and muscles of the lower extremities. Arrows mark sites of common compression syndromes.

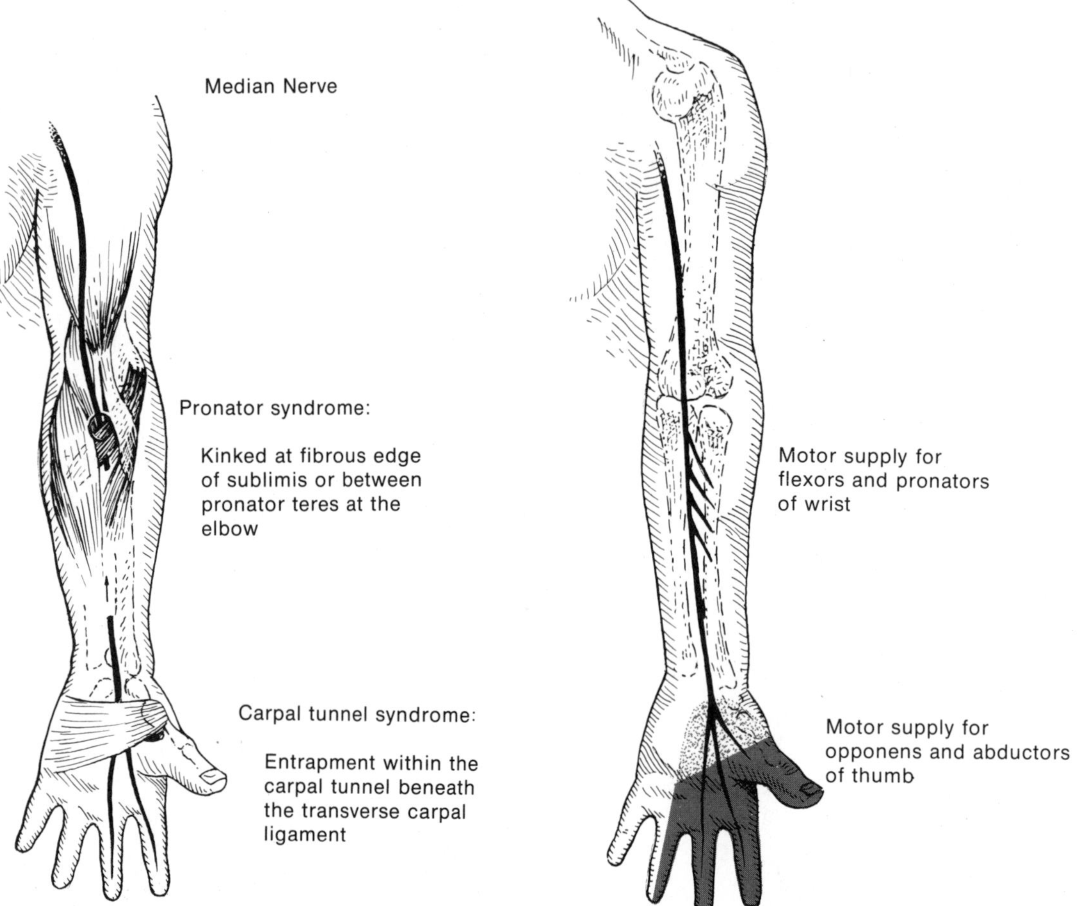

FIGURE 60–4. Entrapment neuropathies involving the median nerve. *A,* The median nerve may be trapped at the fibrous edge of the sublimis muscle at the elbow (pronator syndrome) or beneath the transverse carpal ligament (carpal tunnel syndrome). *B,* Sensory findings include "tingling" of the palm of the hand and numbness of the distal palmar aspects of the first four digits (thumb, index, middle, and fourth fingers). Compression at the carpal tunnel produces weakness of the opponens and abductors of the thumb and wasting of the thenar eminence. Compression near the elbow also causes weakness of the flexors and pronators of the wrist and forearm.

cant weakness of thenar muscles. A great majority of patients show excellent results.

Pronator Teres Syndrome

Entrapment of the median nerve may rarely occur at the elbow as it passes between the two heads of the pronator teres and beneath the sublimis muscle ("pronator syndrome," see Fig. 60–4). The pronator syndrome has been associated with trauma, fracture, rheumatoid arthritis, and other lesions, but also may result from "honeymoon" paralysis when the spouse rests his or her head on the other's forearm while sleeping. Pronator syndrome has also been seen in manual laborers who perform repetitive pronation and supination. In this syndrome, numbness involves the upper palm as well as the fingers. Palpation of the median nerve over the pronator teres muscle elicits tenderness and radiating paresthesias along the course of the nerve. There may be weakness on flexing the wrist or pronating the forearm.

Ulnar Nerve Entrapment

Ulnar neuropathy at the elbow is the second most common entrapment neuropathy of the upper extremity. At the elbow, the ulnar nerve runs in a groove between the medial epicondyle and the olecranon before entering between the two heads of the flexor carpi ulnaris muscle ("cubital tunnel"). Entrapment at the elbow is usually related either to minor trauma, such as leaning on the elbow, or to repetitive elbow flexion, such as when playing tennis, hammering, or using other tools (Fig. 60–5). Symptoms include numbness of the fourth and fifth digits and the ulnar aspect of the palm. Paresthesias may be reproduced by applying pressure to the groove behind the medial epicondyle. Ulnar entrapment may rarely also occur distally in the wrist at the pisiform-hamate tunnel (Guyon's canal). Paresthesias involve the fourth and fifth digits but spare the palm. Motor signs in either case include interosseus and hypothenar atrophy, weakness on "pinching" with the thumb, and loss of fine hand movements. Insidious motor loss may occur in some cases, without sensory symptoms, particularly in those with slowly worsening mechanical compression or in patients with a ganglion. Ulnar neuropathy is also common in patients who have been immobilized because of surgery and shift themselves in bed on their elbows, or in patients who sustain compression during anesthesia or coma.

Therapy. In mild cases, conservative therapy is recommended, with avoidance of repetitive elbow flexion and use of an elbow pad. Splinting the elbow in an extended position may be tried but is seldom well tolerated. In patients unresponsive to these measures and in patients with atrophy, weakness, or persistent sensory loss, surgery is required. In cases with entrapment at the cubital tunnel, a simple release procedure may be used. In others, anterior submuscular transposition of the ulnar nerve is performed. Patients with underlying neuropathy of any cause with coexistent ulnar neuropathy may not respond as well to surgical intervention.

Radial Nerve Entrapment

Radial nerve compression may occur in the axilla as a result of improper use of crutches. The famous "Saturday Night Palsy" occurs in intoxicated patients who fall asleep in chairs, compressing the radial nerve in the axilla, or against the lateral aspect of the humerus where the nerve passes along the spiral groove (Fig. 60–6). The extensors of the wrist and fingers may be weak, with numbness involving the dorsal aspect of the hand and first four digits. Radial neuropathies secondary to transient compression usually improve spontaneously over weeks.

Posterior Interosseous Entrapment

This condition results from a lesion of the deep motor branch of the radial nerve, which can become entrapped at the level of the supinator muscle. It may also be seen in patients with rheumatoid arthritis, trauma, and soft tissue masses or fibrous bands. The patient is unable to extend the digits at the metacarpophalangeal joints, and there is radial deviation of the wrist on extension. Surgical exploration and decompression of the posterior interosseous nerve may become necessary.

Common Entrapment and Compression Neuropathies of the Lower Extremity

Sciatic Neuropathy

Compression of the sciatic nerve can occur in the setting of obstetric complications, hip surgery, immobility, neoplasms, intramuscular injections, and prolonged squatting or stretching.[68] There is a possibility of entrapment as the nerve courses over the sciatic notch and at the edge of the piriformis muscle, although the existence of a piriformis syndrome is still debated by many. Clinically, the picture is similar to a root lesion from disk herniation at the L5–S1 interspace (Fig. 60–7*A*). Electromyographic studies are helpful in distinguishing a sciatic nerve lesion from a radiculopathy. On rare occasions in patients with clinical and electrophysiologic evidence of a progressive sciatic neuropathy of unclear etiology, exploratory surgery may be required.

Peroneal Neuropathy

The most common mononeuropathy in the lower extremity is peroneal neuropathy. Clinically, patients present with a painless foot drop and paresthesias over the dorsum of the foot.[87] On examination, one notes weakness of dorsiflexion and eversion of the foot, and sensory loss over the dorsum of the foot (see Fig. 60–7*B*). Distinction from an L5 radiculopathy may be very difficult. Compression is usually below the fibular head, often secondary to crossing of the leg in the sitting position. Popliteal (Baker's) cyst may be a cause, especially in patients with rheumatoid arthritis.[88] Other etiologies include fractures, direct trauma, nerve sheath tumors, ganglia, and compression by casts or braces below the knee. If the superficial branch is involved, the sensory loss is more extensive and covers most of the lateral calf. Electrodiagnostic studies are essential for diagnosis and are useful in excluding a sciatic neuropathy, lumbosacral plexopathy, or radiculopathy. Motor nerve conductions may demonstrate a conduction block of the peroneal nerve below the fibular head. Therapy is mainly directed toward removing the compressing agent and splinting or bracing. Early surgical exploration and decompression in patients with cysts or ganglia may be needed.

Posterior Tibial Neuropathy

The entrapment of the posterior tibial nerve at the ankle as it passes under the flexor retinaculum is referred to as *tarsal tunnel syndrome.* This is a rare condition. Patients

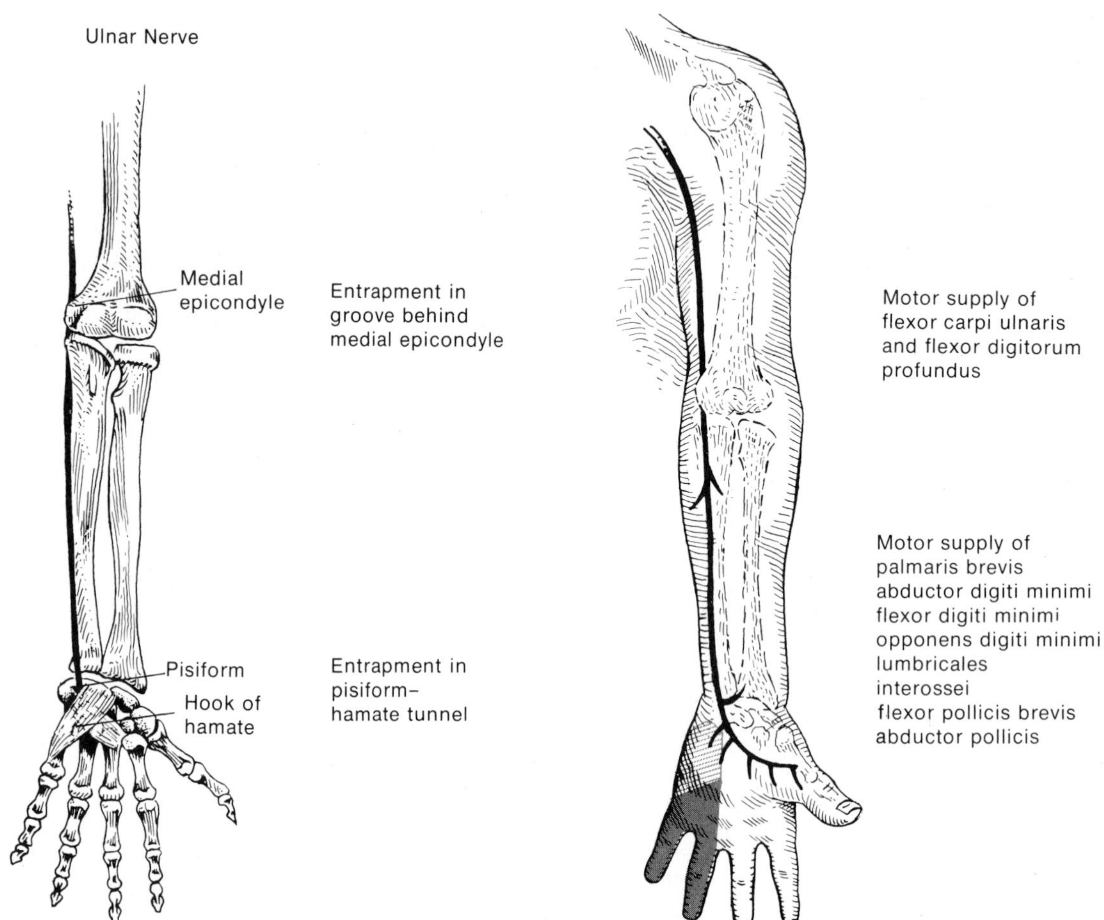

FIGURE 60–5. Entrapment neuropathies of the ulnar nerve. *A,* Sites of entrapment neuropathy. *B,* Motor and sensory findings. Entrapment at the elbow induces numbness of the palmar fourth and fifth digits and ulnar aspect of the palm. The palm itself is spared in entrapment at the pisiform-hamate tunnel. In either case, motor signs include interosseous and hypothenar atrophy, weakness on "pinching" with thumb, and loss of fine hand movements.

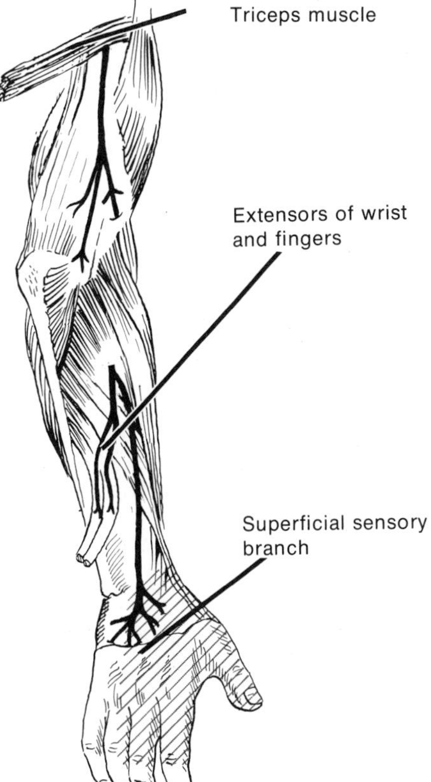

FIGURE 60–6. Entrapment of the radial nerve. Entrapment may occur if the nerve is damaged by hanging the arm over a chair ("Saturday night palsy") or by compression at the fibrous slit of the supinator near the lateral epicondyle at the elbow. Numbness is produced on the dorsal aspect of the hand and the first four digits. Motor findings include weakness of extension of the wrist (wrist drop).

usually complain of a burning sensation in the heel that is worse at night (see Fig. 60–7*C*). Weakness and atrophy of the intrinsic muscles of the foot may be noted on examination.[89] The condition can be seen in patients with direct trauma and in rheumatoid arthritis. It may also be seen during pregnancy. Therapy is often conservative. Improvement is mainly noted with rest, arch support, and orthotics. Steroid injection occasionally may help. Surgical exploration has shown mixed results.[90]

Meralgia Paresthetica

Meralgia paresthetica is a common syndrome caused by compression of the lateral femoral cutaneous nerve, which supplies the sensation to the lateral thigh. Constriction by tight belts, corsets, or garments, as well as sudden weight gain or pregnancy may cause compression of this nerve at the lateral end of the inguinal ligament. Patients complain of numbness, paresthesias, and an unpleasant burning sen-

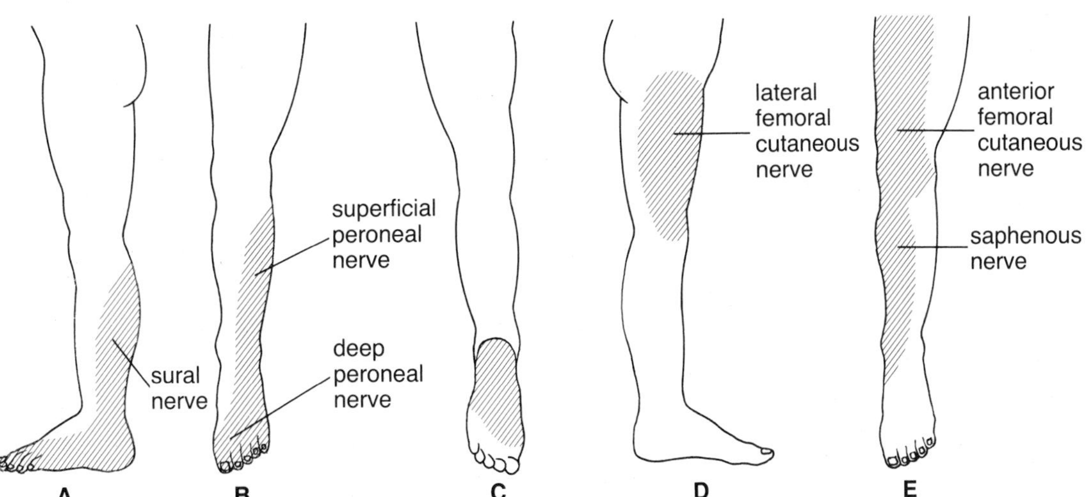

FIGURE 60–7. Approximate distribution of sensory changes in compression syndromes of lower extremities. *A,* Sciatic neuropathy; *B,* Peroneal neuropathy; *C,* Posterior tibial neuropathy; *D,* Meralgia paresthetica; *E,* Femoral neuropathy.

sation on contact with clothing in the lateral thigh (see Fig. 60–7*D*). On examination, sensory loss is noted over the lateral aspect of the thigh. The condition is usually considered in the differential diagnosis of L3–L4 radiculopathy or femoral neuropathy. It has also been seen in retroperitoneal tumors.[68] Electrodiagnostic studies of sensory action potentials of the lateral femoral cutaneous nerve may be of help with the diagnosis. Therapy is usually conservative and consists of weight loss and mild analgesics. In more severe cases, local injection of anesthetics is often helpful. Surgical exploration is seldom required.

Femoral Neuropathy

Femoral neuropathy is a relatively uncommon neuropathy (see Fig. 60–7*E*). Patients may complain of pain in the groin or thigh, weakness of knee extension, knee buckling and falls. Examination discloses quadriceps muscle weakness and atrophy and loss of the knee jerk on the symptomatic side. Etiologies include compression secondary to a mass, hemorrhage (in hemophilia or anticoagulation), diabetes, nerve infarction, or trauma at the level of the inguinal ligament. Distinction from an L4 root lesion or lumbar plexopathy is often difficult and may often be sorted out with electrodiagnostic studies.

Miscellaneous Neuropathies

A number of other compression neuropathy syndromes have been described in the lower extremities. These are quite uncommon and mostly result from direct trauma. Clinically, pain and paresthesias in the distribution of the nerve are the most common clinical features. The obturator nerve, which supplies sensation to the medial thigh, may become entrapped in the obturator canal. Patients complain of pain radiating into the inner thigh. Electromyography shows involvement of adductor and gracilis muscles. Etiologies include trauma, genitourinary surgery, hernia, or osteitis pubis. Therapy is conservative, and improvement is seen with rest and analgesia. In severe cases, surgical exploration with resection of the nerve may be considered. The ilioinguinal nerve may be damaged by trauma or genitourinary surgical procedures. Patients usually complain of groin pain aggravated by hip motion. Sensory changes along the iliac crest and in the scrotum or the labia can be seen on examination. Therapy is usually conservative and consists of rest and analgesia.

REFERENCES

1. Miller JQ: Neurologic content of family practice. Arch Neurol 43:286, 1986.
2. Bradley W: Aspects of diabetic autonomic neuropathy. Ann Intern Med 992:289, 1980.
3. Raff MD and Asbury AK: Ischemic mononeuropathy and mononeuropathy multiplex in diabetes mellitus. N Engl J Med 279:17, 1968.
4. Waxman SG: Diabetic radiculoneuropathy: Clinical patterns of sensory loss and distal paresthesias. Acta Diabetol 19:199, 1982.
5. Locke S and Lawrence DG: Diabetic amyotrophy. Am J Med 34:774, 1963.
6. Hamilton CR, Dobson HL, and Marsha J: Diabetic amyotrophy: Clinical and electron microscopic studies of six patients. Am J Med Sci 256:81, 1968.
7. Thomas PK and Ehasson SG: Diabetic neuropathy. *In* Dyck PJ, Thomas PK, and Lambert EH (eds): Peripheral Neuropathy. Philadelphia, WB Saunders, 1975, pp 956–981.
8. Gabbey KH: Role of sorbitol pathway in neuropathy. *In* Camerrin-Duralos RA and Cole HS (eds): Vascular and Neurological Changes in Early Diabetes. New York, Academic Press, 1973, pp 417–432.
9. Brown MJ and Greene DA: Diabetic neuropathy: Pathophysiology and management. *In* Asbury AK and Gilliatt RW (eds): Peripheral Nerve Disorders. London, Butterworths, 1984, pp 126–153.
10. Ward JD, Barnes CG, Fisher DJ, et al: Improvement in neuroconduction following treatment in newly diagnosed diabetics. Lancet i:428, 1971.
11. Clements RS, Vourganti B, Kuba T, et al: Dietary myo-inositol intake and peripheral nerve function in diabetic nerve. Metabolism 28:477, 1979.
12. Tyler HR: Neurologic disorders in renal failure. Am J Med 44:734, 1968.
13. Egan JD and Wells IC: Transketolase inhibition and uremic peripheral sensory neuropathy. J Neurol Sci 41:379, 1979.
14. Oh SJ, Clements RS, Lee YW, et al: Rapid improvement in neuroconduction velocity following renal transplantation. Ann Neurol 4:369, 1978.
15. Asbury AK, Victor M, and Adams RD: Uremic polyneuropathy. Trans Am Neurol Assoc 87:100, 1962.
16. Mayer RF: Peripheral nerve function in vitamin B_{12} deficiency. Arch Neurol 13:355, 1965.
17. Victor M: Polyneuropathy due to nutritional deficiency and alcoholism. *In* Dyck P, Thomas PK, and Lambert EH (eds): Peripheral Neuropathy. Philadelphia, WB Saunders, 1975, pp 1030–1066.
18. Ridely A: The neuropathy of acute intermittent porphyria. Q J Med 38:307, 1969.
19. Brodie MJ, Moore MR, Thompson GC, et al: The treatment of acute porphyria with laevulose. Clin Sci 53:365, 1977.
20. Knill-Jones RP, Goodwill CJ, Dayan AD, et al: Peripheral neuropathy in chronic liver disease: Clinical electrodiagnostic and nerve biopsy findings. J Neurol Neurosurg Psychiatry 35:22, 1972.
21. Dyck PJ and Lambert EH: Polyneuropathy associated with hypothyroidism. J Neuropathol Exp Neurol 29:631, 1970.
22. Mathews WB: Sarcoid neuropathy. *In* Dyck PJ, Thomas PK, and Lambert EH (eds): Peripheral Neuropathy. Philadelphia, WB Saunders, 1975, pp 21–28.
23. Kelly JJ: Paraneoplastic and paraproteinemic neuropathies. 1987 American Association of Electrodiagnostic Medicine Course C.
24. Croft PB, Urich H, and Wilkinson M: Peripheral neuropathy of sensorimotor type associated with malignant disease. Brain 90:307, 1971.
25. Denny-Brown D: Primary sensory neuropathy with muscular changes associated with carcinoma. JNNP 11:73, 1948.
26. Ropper AH: Current concepts: The Guillain-Barré syndrome. N Engl J Med 326:1130, 1992.
27. Guillain G, Barré J, and Strohl H: Sur un syndrome des radiculonévrite avec hyperalbuminose du liquid cephalorachidien sans réaction cellulaire. Bulletin et mémoires de la Société medicale des hôpitaux de Paris, 1462, 1916.
28. Fisher CM: An unusual variant of acute idiopathic polyneuritis. N Engl J Med 255:57, 1956.
29. Ropper AJ, Shahani B, and Huggins CE: Improvement in four patients with acute Guillain-Barré syndrome after plasma exchange. Neurology 20:361, 1980.
30. The Guillain-Barré Study Group: Plasmapheresis and acute Guillain-Barré syndrome. Neurology 35:1096, 1985.
31. Van der Meche FGA and Schmitz PIM: A randomized trial comparing intravenous immune globulin and plasma exchange in Guillain-Barré syndrome. N Engl J Med 326:1123, 1992.
32. Dyck PJ, Lais AC, Ohta M, et al: Chronic inflammatory polyradiculoneuropathy. Mayo Clin Proc 50:621, 1975.
33. Server AC, Stein SA, Braine H, et al: Experience with plasma exchange and cyclophosphamide in the treatment of chronic relapsing inflammatory polyradiculoneuropathy. Neurology 30:362, 1980.
34. Rowland LP, Defendini R, Sherman W, et al: Macroglobulinemia with peripheral neuropathy simulating motor neuron disease. Ann Neurol 11:532, 1982.
35. Parry GJ, Holtz SJ, Ben-Zeev D, et al: Gammopathy with proximal motor axonopathy simulating motor neuron disease. Neurology 36:273, 1986.

36. Rudnicki S, Chad DA, Drachman DA, et al: Motor neuron disease and paraproteinemia. Neurology 37:335, 1987.
37. Pestronk A, Cornblath DR, Ilyas AA, et al: A treatable multifocal motor neuropathy with antibodies to GM_1 gangliosides. Ann Neurol 24:73, 1988.
38. Pestronk A, Adams RN, Kuncl RW, et al: Differential effects of prednisone and cyclophosphamide on autoantibodies in human neuromuscular disorders. Neurology 39:628, 1989.
39. Kelly JJ: Peripheral neuropathies associated with monoclonal proteins: A clinical review. Muscle Nerve 8:138, 1985.
40. Kelly JJ, Kyle RA, Miles JM, et al: The spectrum of peripheral neuropathy in myeloma. Neurology 31:24, 1981.
41. Kelly JJ, Kyle RA, O'Brien PC, et al: The prevalence of monoclonal protein in peripheral neuropathy. Neurology 21:1480, 1981.
42. Logothetis J, Silverstein P, and Coe J: Neurologic aspects of Waldenström's macroglobulinemia. Arch Neurol 5:564, 1960.
43. Dawson DM: Weekly clinicopathological exercise case 10-1979. N Engl J Med 300:546, 1979.
44. Sabin TD: Temperature linked sensory loss: A unique pattern in leprosy. Arch Neurol 20:251, 1969.
45. Sabin TD and Swift TR: Leprosy in peripheral neuropathy. *In* Dyck PJ, Thomas PK, and Lambert EH (eds): Peripheral Neuropathy. Philadelphia, WB Saunders, 1975, pp 1166–1198.
46. Logigian EL and Steere AC: Clinical and electrophysiologic findings in chronic neuropathy of Lyme disease. Neurology 42:303, 1992.
47. Simpson DM and Wolfe DE: Neuromuscular complications of HIV infection and its treatment. AIDS 5:917, 1991.
48. Dalakas MD: Neuromuscular aspects of acquired immunodeficiency syndrome (AIDS). National Institute of Neurologic and Communicative disorders and Stroke, National Institutes of Health, Bethesda, 1986.
49. Cornblath DR and McArthur JC: Predominantly sensory neuropathy in patients with AIDS and AIDS-related complex. Neurology 38:794, 1988.
50. Cornblath DR: Treatment of neuromuscular complications of human immunodeficiency virus infection. Ann Neurol 23(Suppl):S88, 1988.
51. Miller RG, Parry GJ, Pfaeffl W, et al: The spectrum of peripheral neuropathy associated with ARC and AIDS. Muscle Nerve 1:857, 1988.
52. de la Monte SM, Gabuzda DH, and Ho DD: Peripheral neuropathy in the acquired immunodeficiency syndrome. Ann Neurol 23:485, 1988.
53. Gherardi R, Lebargy F, Gaulard P, et al: Necrotizing vasculitis and HIV replication. N Engl J Med 321:685–686, 1987.
54. Rance NE, McArthur JC, Cornblath DR, et al: Gracile tract degeneration in patients with sensory neuropathy and AIDS. Neurology 38:265, 1988.
55. Smith T, Jakobsen J, Gaub J, and Trojaborg W: Symptomatic polyneuropathy in human immunodeficiency virus antibody seropositive men with and without immune deficiency: A comparative electrophysiologic study. J Neurol Neurosurg Psychiatry 53:1056, 1990.
56. Parry G: Peripheral neuropathies associated with human immunodeficiency virus infection. Ann Neurol 23(Suppl):S49, 1988.
57. Cornblath DR, McArthur JC, Kennedy PG, et al: Inflammatory demyelinating peripheral neuropathy associated with human T-cell lymphotropic virus type III infection. Ann Neurol 21:32, 1987.
58. Piette AM, Tusseau F, Vignon D, et al: Acute neuropathy coincident with seroconversion for anti-LAV/HTLV-III. Lancet i:852, 1986.
59. Panicker R, Bloom AL, and Compston DA: Inflammatory demyelinating polyneuropathy in a hemophiliac associated with human immunodeficiency virus infection, responding to high dose intravenous immunoglobulin. Postgrad Med J 64:699, 1988.
60. Lipkin WI, Parry G, Kiprov D, and Abrams D: Inflammatory neuropathy in homosexual men with lymphadenopathy. Neurology 35:1479, 1985.
61. Miller RG, Storey JR, and Greco CM: Ganciclovir in the treatment of progressive AIDS-related polyradiculopathy. Neurology 40:569, 1990.
62. Eidelberg D, Sotrel A, Vogel AT, et al: Progressive polyradiculopathy in acquired immune deficiency syndrome. Neurology 36:912, 1986.
63. Beydoun SR: Misdiagnosis of cytomegalovirus polyradiculopathy, coexisting with HIV neuropathy. Muscle Nerve 14:575, 1991.
64. Said G, Lacroix C, Chemouilli P, et al: Cytomegalovirus neuropathy in acquired immunodeficiency syndrome: A clinical and pathologic study. Ann Neurol 29:139, 1991.
65. Freeman R, Roberts MS, and Friedman LS: Autonomic function and human immunodeficiency virus infection. Neurology 40:575, 1990.
66. Dubinsky RM, Yarchoan R, Dalakas M, and Broder S: Reversible axonal neuropathy from the treatment of AIDS and related disorders with 2′,3′-dideoxycytidine (ddC). Muscle Nerve 12:856, 1989.
67. Olney RK: Neuropathies in connective tissue disease. Muscle Nerve 15:531, 1992.
68. Nakano KK: The entrapment neuropathies. Muscle Nerve 1:264, 1978.
69. Johnson RT and Richardson EP: The neurologic manifestations of systemic lupus erythematosus. Medicine 47:337, 1968.
70. Fauci AS, Haynes BF, and Katz P: The spectrum of vasculitis: Clinical, pathologic, immunologic, and therapeutic considerations. Ann Intern Med 84:271, 1976.
71. Feldman RG, Hayes MK, Younes R, et al: Lead neuropathy in adults and children. Arch Neurol 34:481, 1977.
72. Feldman RG, Niles CA, Kelly-Haynes M, et al: Peripheral neuropathy in arsenic smelter workers. Neurology 29:939, 1979.
73. Goldstein NP, McCall JI, and Dyck PJ: Metal neuropathy. *In* Dyck PJ, Thomas PK, and Lambert EH (eds): Peripheral Neuropathy. Philadelphia, WB Saunders, 1975, pp 1237–1262.
74. Argov Z and Mastraglia FL: Drug-induced peripheral neuropathies. BMJ 1:663, 1979.
75. Hopkins A: Toxic neuropathy due to industrial agents. *In* Dyck PJ, Thomas PK, and Lambert EH (eds): Peripheral Neuropathy. Philadelphia, WB Saunders, 1975, p 825.
76. Miller RG, Gutmann L, Lewis RA, and Sumner AJ: Acquired versus familial demyelinative neuropathies in children. Muscle Nerve 8:205, 1985.
77. Miller RG: Hereditary and acquired polyneuropathies. Neurol Clin 3:543, 1985.
78. Schaumburg HH, Spencer PS, and Thomas PK: Disorders of Peripheral Nerves. Philadelphia, FA Davis, 1986.
79. Menkes JH: Textbook of Child Neurology. Philadelphia, Lea & Febiger, 1985.
80. Ouvrier RA, McLeod JG, and Pollard JD: Peripheral Neuropathy in Childhood. New York, Raven Press, 1990.
81. Dyck PJ: Inherited neuronal degeneration and atrophy affecting peripheral motor, sensory, and autonomic neurons. *In* Dyck PJ, Thomas PK, and Lambert EH (eds): Peripheral Neuropathy. Philadelphia, WB Saunders, 1975, pp 1207–1226.
82. Mendell JR, Jiang XS, Warmolts JR, et al: Diagnosis of Maryland/German familial amyloidotic polyneuropathy using allele-specific, enzymatically amplified, genomic DNA. Ann Neurol 27:553, 1990.
83. Seddon HJ: Three types of nerve injury. Brain 66:237, 1943.
84. Sunderland S: Nerves and Nerve Injury. London, Churchill-Livingstone, 1978.
85. Dawson D, Hallet M, and Millender L: Entrapment Neuropathies. Boston, Little Brown, 1983.
86. Kopell H, and Thompson W: Peripheral Entrapment Neuropathies. Baltimore, Williams & Wilkins, 1963.
87. Berry H, and Richardson P: Common peroneal palsy: A clinical and electrophysiologic review. J Neurol Neurosurg Psychiatry 3:1162, 1976.
88. Nakano K: Entrapment neuropathy from Baker's cyst. JAMA 239:135, 1978.
89. Keck C: The tarsal tunnel syndrome. J Bone Joint Surg Am 44A:180, 1962.
90. Kaplan K and Kernahan W: Tarsal tunnel syndrome: An electrodiagnostic and surgical correlation. J Bone Joint Surg Am 63A:96, 1981.

61

Muscular Weakness

DAVID M. DAWSON, MD

The primary care physician may encounter several different types of symptoms and signs in patients with neuromuscular diseases. The commonest symptom is weakness, which is to be sharply distinguished from fatigue or tiredness. Fatigue is a manifestation of abnormality of the central nervous system, not the muscles. Cramps, myalgia, muscle twitching, and diffuse or focal atrophy are other symptoms that may be observed.

MUSCLE DISEASES

Symptoms

Weakness

Weakness in muscle diseases is often insidious; the capacity of the central nervous system to compensate for weakness of the peripheral nervous system allows for many adaptations that may prevent its early detection. Patients with weakness of the shoulder girdle experience difficulty lifting objects above their heads, for example, placing a heavy set of dishes onto a shelf. Women may have trouble managing their hair because the arms cannot be held elevated for long periods of time. A weakness of the hip girdle is frequently expressed as trouble climbing onto steps that are widely separated, or as difficulty on climbing into an automobile or truck with a high step. The patient may notice instability around the hips, and this may seem to the patient like poor balance. Patients with distal weakness will complain of more familiar symptoms, such as difficulty gripping a hammer or a door handle, or foot drop if the feet are weak.

Patients with disease of the neuromuscular junctions, particularly myasthenia gravis, have fluctuating weakness. The weakness will be worse in the afternoon and after long usage of the affected extremity and will improve with rest. Some patients with myasthenia gravis or with myasthenic syndrome will have surprisingly focal symptoms: weakness of one hand or even of several fingers of one hand, so that the generalized character of the weakness, often demonstrable on testing, may not be known to the patient.

Cramps

A cramp consists of a painful, tight contraction of a group of muscle fibers, commonly lasting several minutes to half an hour and usually relieved by massage, stretching of the muscle, and use of the extremity. Patients with cramp will try to "walk it off" or "rub it out." Following a cramp, residual soreness and tenderness in the affected muscles are frequent and may last for many hours or even days. Muscle cramps do not reflect disease of the muscle fiber but result from a defect in innervation of muscle and may occur with amyotrophic lateral sclerosis, polyneuritis, or various electrolyte disorders, such as hypocalcemia. In most instances, cramp is a benign syndrome that does not imply serious etiology.

Myalgia

Muscle pain may occur in some patients with inflammatory myopathy. However, it is not a common symptom in that syndrome, and most patients with myalgia do not have polymyositis. Myalgia occurs in many viral diseases. Usually, it does not reflect any disease of muscle itself, although occasionally, in patients with intercurrent viral illness, an elevation of serum enzymes indicates that the virus has affected muscle. The differential diagnosis of muscle pain includes disease of the nerve innervating muscle, the fascia overlying it, and the blood vessels. The pain of polymyalgia rheumatica is frequently felt in the muscles of the neck, upper thorax, and shoulder girdle. The muscles may be tender, and local tenderness may be an important diagnostic feature. It is believed that the pain is due to the granulomatous arteritis that is sometimes found on biopsy. Patients with nerve root pain produced by cervical spondylosis or by lumbar disc disease frequently have pain in muscles. In patients with sciatica, pain may be referred to the posterior thigh muscles, the buttocks, or occasionally, the calf muscles. Patients with the common nerve root compressions affecting cervical 6 or cervical 7 nerve roots will experience pain in the triceps, the wrist extensors, and other large muscles of the arm and forearm. Local tenderness may mislead both patient and doctor. The characteristic symptoms of paresthesias and sensory loss help clarify the nature of this complaint, as does the radiating quality of the pain.

Fatigue

Generalized fatigue is not a common complaint of patients with muscular disease; usually the symptom is on a central nervous system basis. It may reflect depression or anxiety and is also observed in patients with Parkinson's disease or dementia; it is particularly common in patients with multiple sclerosis. Fatigue should be distinguished from the fatigability seen in patients with myasthenia gravis; myasthenic patients do not complain of fatigue but say that their muscles are weak.

Muscle Necrosis

Acute rhabdomyolysis (acute necrosis of muscle fibers) may occur in drug intoxication, severe injury to an extremity, heat stress, acute alcoholic myopathy, McArdle's disease, carnitine deficiency of muscle fibers, and a host of other circumstances. In all these situations, diffuse muscular pain, tenderness, and weakness occur, and visible myoglobinuria accompanied by very marked elevation of serum muscle enzymes is found. Myoglobin discolors the urine to a coffee color. The compound rapidly clears from the circulation, and even in severe instances of muscle necrosis, myoglobinuria is observed for a matter of only 6 to 12 hours.

Signs

Weakness

A characteristic pattern of muscular weakness is seen in many diseases of muscle, including dystrophy, polymyositis, sarcoidosis, and other common and rare diseases of muscle. The muscle groups often affected are neck flexors, the deltoid, triceps, and quadriceps muscles, hip flexors, knee flexors, and foot dorsiflexors. Often the weakness will be symmetric and will affect these muscle groups, whereas others are normal.

Reflexes

In most instances of primary muscle disease, including polymyositis, and in diseases of neuromuscular junction, the reflexes are reduced but still present. An exception to this rule is the patient with Eaton-Lambert syndrome (a form of the myasthenic syndrome). In these patients, total areflexia occurs, with signs of autonomic disorder.

Fasciculations

Fasciculations (muscle twitches) are not a symptom of muscular disease. They should be carefully looked for because, if observed, they indicate that the disorder is likely to be in the anterior horn cells, the nerve roots, or the peripheral nerve. The fasciculations seen with amyotrophic lateral sclerosis and other widespread diseases causing muscle denervation are scattered and erratic in their location. The physician will notice a flicker in one spot, only to have attention drawn quickly to a flicker in another place. The fasciculations are best seen in muscles near the surface, such as the pectorals and muscles of the shoulder girdle, the forearm, or the calf. Muscle fasciculations affecting intrinsic muscles of the hand will cause rapid quivering of fingers or of the thumb, which may be observed when the hands are held outstretched. Muscle fasciculations in the tongue are very important in confirming that motor nuclei are affected because the tongue is not affected in cervical spondylosis, neuropathy, or other diseases that may cause local fasciculations. Irritation of a nerve root (e.g., by cervical spondylosis) causes fasciculations that fire repeatedly in the same area for several seconds.

Tests

Serum Enzymes

The primary test for the presence of muscle necrosis is serum creatine kinase (CK). CK is primarily found in muscle and in brain; small amounts of the enzyme are also present in the thyroid and in tissues containing smooth muscle. In clinical practice, an elevation of CK nearly always indicates disease of heart or skeletal muscle. The brain form of the enzyme escapes into the circulation only with widespread severe brain injury.

Two isoenzymes of CK are observed in the serum. The MM or muscle form of the enzyme is present in skeletal muscle, whereas both MM and MB isoenzymes are present in cardiac muscle, often in approximately equal amounts. Therefore, in diseases of skeletal muscle, the MM isoenzyme predominates.

Other enzymes sometimes have been measured. Aldolase occurs in every tissue, and its usefulness in muscle disease is slight. Other serum enzymes, such as transaminase and lactate dehydrogenase are present in muscle in smaller quantities than CK; the elevation of CK should always be higher in proportion than that of other enzymes.

Electromyography

Electromyography (EMG) is a widely used technique for detecting muscle disease. It consists of the insertion of a needle electrode into muscle; from the tip of the needle, a sphere of neighboring muscle fibers will be recorded. With graded amounts of muscle contraction, individual motor units can be tested. The size and shape of muscle action potentials are the data used by electromyographers to make an assessment of the intactness of the muscle fibers (Fig. 61–1). In primary disease of muscle, EMG typically will show small, brief action potentials because damaged muscle fibers cannot summate to produce a large-sized motor unit. The small, brief action potentials of myopathy are no different from those of a distant motor unit, so the complete absence of large normal units defines the electromyogram as that of primary muscle disease. Spontaneous fibrillations of individual fibers occur because of local loss of their nerve supply within the muscle, either due to inflammation (polymyositis) or denervation (lower motor neuron lesion).

Electromyography results depend a good deal on the skill and experience of the electromyographer. To make a judgment about the presence of myopathy, as well as to obtain the distribution of the changes in many muscles, considerable recording time is required.

A separate type of testing is required to test for myasthenia gravis. A routine EMG, done with the presumed diagnosis of myopathy, will miss myasthenia gravis completely. Myasthenia gravis is tested for with a "single-fiber" EMG, or by means of recording the overall action potential from a group of muscle fibers while stimulating a nerve repetitively. The same type of testing is also required to detect the presence of Eaton-Lambert syndrome (myasthenic syndrome).

Nerve conduction testing also may be necessary to dem-

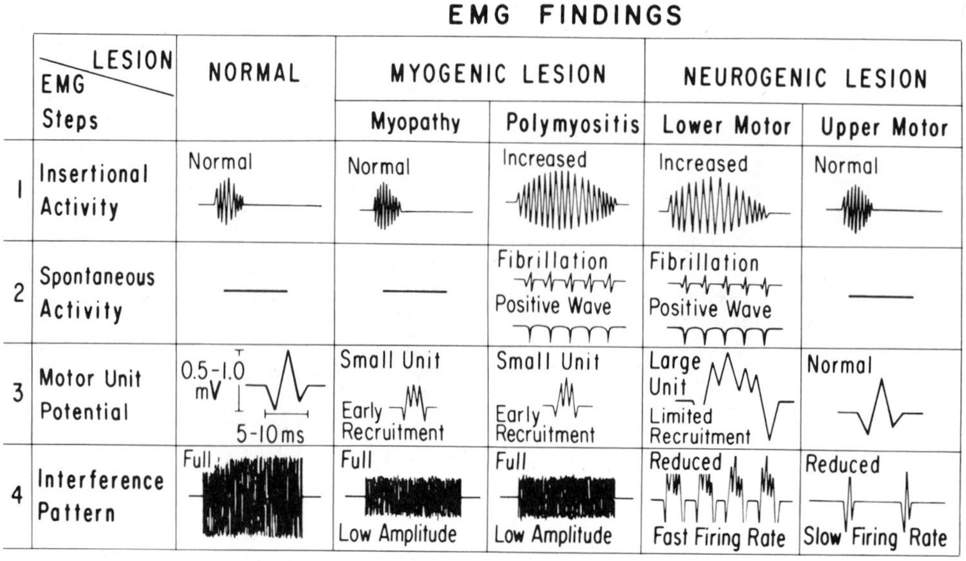

EMG FINDINGS

EMG Steps \ LESION	NORMAL	MYOGENIC LESION		NEUROGENIC LESION	
		Myopathy	Polymyositis	Lower Motor	Upper Motor
1 Insertional Activity	Normal	Normal	Increased	Increased	Normal
2 Spontaneous Activity	—	—	Fibrillation; Positive Wave	Fibrillation; Positive Wave	—
3 Motor Unit Potential	0.5–1.0 mV; 5–10 ms	Small Unit; Early Recruitment	Small Unit; Early Recruitment	Large Unit; Limited Recruitment	Normal
4 Interference Pattern	Full	Full; Low Amplitude	Full; Low Amplitude	Reduced; Fast Firing Rate	Reduced; Slow Firing Rate

FIGURE 61–1. EMG findings of typical myogenic and neurogenic lesions. (Adapted from Kimura J: Electrodiagnosis in Diseases of Nerve and Muscle: Principles and Practice. Philadelphia, FA Davis, 1983.)

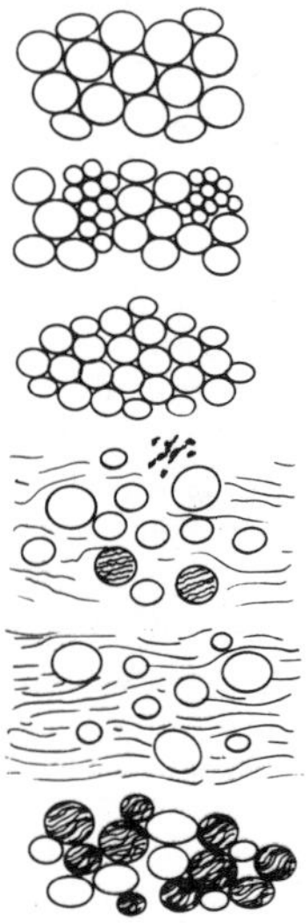

APPEARANCE	DESCRIPTION	CLINICAL DIAGNOSIS
	Normal fibers	None
	Grouped atrophy, indicating denervation plus reinnervation	Chronic denervation, often ALS
	Normal, except small size of all fibers	Normal, or metabolic myopathy (steroid, thyrotoxic, etc.)
	Variation in fiber size, necrosis of some fibers, foci of histiocytes	Myopathy, probably polymyositis
	Variation in fiber size, increase in fibrous tissue	Myopathy, could be dystrophy or inactive polymyositis
	Widespread necrosis of many fibers	Acute rhabdomyolysis

FIGURE 61–2. Cross-sectional appearance of muscle biopsies.

onstrate the reduction of sensory action potential and the slowing of motor nerve conduction in neuropathy. In muscle disease itself, all values in nerve conduction testing are normal, and the only abnormalities are in the EMG reading.

Muscle Biopsy

Muscle biopsy may be required to establish a final diagnosis when a diagnosis of myopathy is seriously considered and the histologic features need to be established. It should be done with care. A muscle that is clinically affected and that is undergoing active recent change should be chosen for biopsy, if possible. The muscle needs to be treated carefully by the surgeon, placed in fixative in a position of stretch, and handled by the pathologist so that longitudinal and cross-sectional cuts are available.

Figure 61–2 shows some of the main features that should be looked for in a muscle biopsy. Muscle biopsies are frequently used at the simplest level to answer two questions: (1) myopathy versus denervation—that is, the difference between a primary muscle disease and a disease of peripheral nerve or anterior horn cells, and (2) inflammatory versus noninflammatory muscle disease—that is, distinguishing between polymyositis and other muscle diseases (dystrophy, metabolic myopathy, or some of the congenital myopathies).

The reliability of muscle biopsy is high; unfortunately, muscle biopsy results may be negative in the presence of myopathy that is clearly present by other criteria; presumably, this result reflects the presence of focal disease that is missed. In some centers, two muscle biopsies are taken at the same time from different muscles; however, this method increases the yield of positive information only slightly and is not a widespread practice.

Guidelines for Evaluation

In evaluating patients with complaints possibly referable to muscle disease, the following general guidelines may be helpful. Patients with muscle cramps usually do not require a full-scale evaluation. Cramps sometimes reflect a metabolic disorder and, rarely, are an early manifestation of denervation of muscles, such as occurs with amyotrophic lateral sclerosis. The best initial approach to a patient with cramps is to check calcium, electrolyte, and CK levels and then follow the patient. It is rare for EMG or muscle biopsy results to be helpful in this setting.

Patients with complaints of muscular fatigue should be examined to see if they have proximal weakness. If they do not, the complaint most likely reflects depression, anxiety, or some other psychological state. Rarely is an evaluation for myopathy necessary unless weakness is detectable. Occasionally, patients with myasthenia gravis will have complaints of fatigue and will have normal results on examination; complaints referred to eye movements or bulbar muscles require further examinations or neurologic referral.

Patients with periodic muscular weakness present special problems. Some of them have familial periodic paralysis. Some patients have periodic mild or moderate rhabdomyolysis; this may occur in patients taking diuretics or in patients who undergo heat stress or have recurrent alcoholic myopathy. In such patients, measurement of CK is the best screening test because elevation of CK is always far more sensitive than is the presence of myoglobin in the urine or EMG abnormalities.

In patients who have diffuse muscular weakness and visible muscular atrophy, the starting point of the investigation should probably be an EMG. In that setting, one would be seeking evidence of denervation caused by peripheral neuropathy, congenital disorders of muscle, or primary myopathy, such as polymyositis.

Inflammatory Myopathy

A set of criteria for the diagnosis of polymyositis includes the following:

1. Increasing weakness, usually proximal, usually progressive over the course of weeks or months; swallowing dysfunction; and myalgia, muscle tenderness, and rarely, arthralgias and evidence of systemic disease are occasionally present.
2. Electromyography shows a pattern compatible with myopathy (brief short-duration action potentials).
3. Serum muscle enzymes are elevated (in practice, CK is the only relevant enzyme).
4. Increased erythrocyte sedimentation rates and elevated γ-globulin levels are present in some patients; positive antinuclear antibodies or lupus erythematosus cell test results are present in a minority of patients.
5. The family history is negative for muscular disease, and no other metabolic myopathy or endocrine disease is present.
6. A reddish macular rash on the cheeks, eyelids, dorsum of the fingers, or extensor surfaces is present in dermatomyositis.

Because polymyositis is a syndrome, usually of unknown cause, it is not possible to give universally agreed on diagnostic criteria. Bohan and Peter, taking an approach that resembles the criteria for diagnosis of rheumatic fever, use five major criteria for the diagnosis of polymyositis: (1) symmetric proximal weakness, (2) muscle biopsy evidence of necrosis of fibers and inflammatory exudate, (3) elevation of serum enzymes, particularly CK, (4) EMG evidence of "myopathic" motor units, and (5) a dermatitis of a characteristic type.[1–5]

When three or four of these criteria are present, the diagnosis of polymyositis is very probable. The most clinically significant criterion is symmetric weakness because this is liable to be the only symptom the patient will experience, and the degree of weakness usually defines the aggressiveness of treatment. Approximately 10 to 20% of patients have a skin rash.

Patients with inclusion-body myopathy constitute an important subgroup of polymyositis patients often unresponsive to treatment.[6, 8] Toxins (alcohol, clofibrate, colchicine) should always be considered as an etiology. AIDS is associated with myopathy.[7]

About 50% of patients with a polymyositis syndrome have no associated disease. Observed diseases present in patients with polymyositis include systemic lupus erythematosus, sarcoidosis, rheumatoid arthritis, and progressive systemic sclerosis.

A review of 153 patients at the University of California, Los Angeles, demonstrated that only 8.5% had a malignancy (most commonly, cancer of the lung).[2] In contrast to earlier reports, this association was as common in polymyositis as in dermatomyositis, and as common in women as in men. In another study of 118 patients in England, 8% had malignancy.[3]

Treatment. The response to prednisone in patients with polymyositis is basically unknown. An important review[1] pointed out that prior studies have been marked by insufficient adherence to diagnostic criteria, and the lack of controlled trials of corticosteroids makes it clear that the natural history of the untreated disease is unknown. A study from Columbia Neurological Institute indicated improvement on steroid therapy in about one third of patients, which is much lower than is commonly accepted in clinical medicine. In the UCLA series, 124 of the 153 patients received prednisone.[2] In 40 (32%) of these patients, prednisone treatment seemed to maintain or increase the strength of muscles in a significant manner.

The use of cytotoxic immunosuppressive drugs, either methotrexate or azathioprine, has become fairly common. Improvement was observed in 48 of 56 patients with either dermatomyositis or polymyositis who were treated with immunosuppression.[2] However, such studies, like those with steroids, lack prospective controls.

Because of the uncertain usefulness of steroids or cytotoxic agents and the uncertain natural history of the disease, it is difficult to be precise in recommending treatment.[4, 5] The decision may involve balancing the severity of the disability against the risk of the therapy. In most instances, patients are given a trial of steroids that lasts a minimum of 3 months; probably a dose of 60 mg/day of prednisone or its equivalent is necessary to demonstrate steroid unresponsiveness. Following that treatment, the use of cytotoxic agents may be considered. If the patient has mild disease, appears to be stable, and shows no sign of serious disability, watchful waiting or no treatment is certainly possible.[9, 10]

Myasthenia Gravis

Myasthenia gravis is a disease that affects individuals of any age. It tends to have two main incidence peaks—in young adults and then in older people aged 50 years and above. In both instances, the clinical picture is often dominated by weakness of ocular and bulbar muscles. Well over 95% of myasthenic patients have double vision, ptosis, or weakness of ocular movements; frequently, weakness of the face and of swallowing is obvious. A few patients will present with generalized weakness, and occasionally, patients will have marked generalized weakness requiring hospitalization; in these, the diagnosis is difficult and may be established only by EMG. Patients with myasthenia gravis nearly always have normal-appearing muscle bulk, normal reflexes, normal CK levels, and, by routine testing, a normal EMG result. Repetitive stimulation or single-fiber EMGs will demonstrate the physiologic defect. Ninety per cent of patients with myasthenia will have antibodies to acetylcholine receptor protein.

Metabolic Myopathies

Thyrotoxic myopathy is a well-known, although infrequently observed, condition. Like the closely allied condition of steroid myopathy, thyrotoxic myopathy presents as mild-to-moderate proximal weakness, usually more marked in the legs, accompanied by normal serum enzymes, normal EMG results, and lack of reflex change. In some instances, the degree of visible atrophy seems greater than does the loss of strength. Thyroid myopathy, like steroid myopathy, seems to reflect the abnormal turnover and replacement of muscle proteins. It is reversible.

Steroid myopathy causes a painless, symmetric weakness of proximal muscles. With time, the muscles are atrophic as well as weak. It is probably more common with long-term use of dexamethasone than with prednisone; doses of prednisone greater than 60 mg/day are usually necessary before myopathy appears. The changes of Cushing's syndrome are, of course, visible. If the steroid is withdrawn, muscular strength will slowly return to normal over the next 2 to 6 weeks.

It is rare for steroid myopathy to complicate the treatment of primary myopathy. Occasionally, this occurs with myasthenia gravis or with severe lupus erythematosus, in which doses of prednisone above 120 mg/day may be required. No specific test for steroid myopathy exists other than the withdrawal of the steroid.

In some patients with hyperparathyroidism, a proximal muscle weakness (Vicale's syndrome) has been observed in those who are normocalcemic, as well as in those who are hypercalcemic; the normocalcemic patients tend to be those with chronic renal failure and secondary hyperparathyroidism undergoing dialysis. In either instance, the illness presents as proximal muscle weakness, without abnormalities of serum enzymes, and with unimpressive or minor changes on EMG. Hypercalcemic patients may also com-

TABLE 61–1. TYPES OF MUSCULAR DYSTROPHY OBSERVED IN ADULTS

Type	Age of Onset (Yr)	Course	CK* Level	Unusual Features	Inheritance
Duchenne	2–6	Wheelchair by age 12 years	20–100 times normal	Female carrier can be detected Low intelligence in many affected boys	Sex-linked
Becker	4–20	Benign	2–10 times normal	Mild version of Duchenne's	Sex-linked
Emery-Dreifuss	2–10	Benign	Slight elevation	Muscle contractures at neck, elbow, spine	Sex-linked
Facioscapulohumeral	7–20	Benign, variable	Slight elevation	Either sex, findings may be slight in degree, facial weakness commonest	Dominant
Myotonic	birth–50	Variable, age-dependent	May be normal	Myotonia on examination or EMG,† cataracts, hypogonadism, etc.	Dominant
Ocular	50 and up	Benign	Normal	Ptosis, ocular palsy, may include pharynx	Dominant
Limb-girdle	10–40	Variable	Slight elevation	May resemble many other diseases: spinal muscular atrophy, enzyme defects, etc.	Dominant in most families

*CK = creatine kinase.
†EMG = electromyography.

plain of fatigue or weakness of central nervous system origin.

Another group of metabolic myopathies include the muscular weaknesses that occur with diseases of the mitochondria. In some instances, this presents as progressive ocular muscular weakness in adult life, possibly accompanied by retinal pigmentary degeneration, spastic weakness of the legs, heart block, sometimes cerebellar ataxia, and a spongiform encephalopathy. All these unusual conditions appear to be related to an abnormality of mitochondrial function, which is present in brain, spinal cord, peripheral nerve, liver, and muscle. Of the clinically significant features, cardiac arrhythmia, progressive ophthalmoplegia, and mental retardation are the most important.

The periodic paralyses may be classified as metabolic disorders, although their cause remains unknown. Patients with either hyperkalemic or hypokalemic varieties of periodic paralysis in time may have attacks of weakness sometimes lasting days to weeks, and later in life, some of these patients develop slowly progressive muscular weakness. The changes in the serum electrolytes are mild in degree and often require careful study on a metabolic ward to demonstrate the change. In either instance, the use of acetazolamide may be useful for prevention of the attacks. The patients with hyperkalemic paralysis may have an associated myotonia of the eyelids or the face. The etiologies of these syndromes remain elusive.

Muscular Dystrophy

Muscular dystrophy in the adult is a slowly progressive condition, often present for many decades, and often appearing to be static when observed for shorter periods of time. The common types of adult dystrophy include myotonic dystrophy, facioscapulohumeral dystrophy, and limb girdle dystrophy (Table 61–1). Myotonic dystrophy is a systemic disorder accompanied by abnormalities of the limbs, of pulmonary function, of gastrointestinal function, and of reproductive function. Often, patients with myotonic dystrophy appear to have mild mental retardation, compared with their more normal siblings. If the disease comes on in infancy, as many do, it may be fatal in the early days or weeks of life. In adulthood, the presenting features are weakness and stiffness of muscles, especially in the hands and forearms, the face, the tongue, and the trunk muscles. Facioscapulohumeral dystrophy and limb-girdle dystrophy present as mild-to-moderate proximal weakness, usually with a family history. The diagnosis may be extremely difficult to establish, even by biopsy, which is usually required for confirmation. No therapy of any value is available for dystrophy. The myotonia of myotonic dystrophy may be slightly improved by the use of quinine or phenytoin.

REFERENCES

1. Bohan A and Peter JB: Polymyositis and dermatomyositis. N Engl J Med 292:344, 1975.
2. Bohan A, Peter J, Bowman R, et al: A computer-assisted analysis of 153 patients with polymyositis and dermatomyositis. Medicine 56:255, 1977.
3. DeVere R and Bradley WG: Polymyositis—its presentation, morbidity and mortality. Brain 98:637, 1975.
4. Brooke MA: A Clinician's View of Neuromuscular Diseases. Baltimore, Williams & Wilkins, 1986.
5. Mastaglio FL and Ojeda VJ: Inflammatory myopathies. Ann Neurol 17:215, 306, 1985.
6. Carpenter S, Karpati G, Heller I, and Eisen A: Inclusion body myositis: A distinct variety of idiopathic inflammatory myopathy. Neurology 28:8, 1978.
7. Dalakas MC and Pezeshkpour GH: Neuromuscular diseases associated with human immunodeficiency virus infection. Ann Neurol 23:538, 1988.
8. Ringel SP, Kenny CE, Neville HE, et al: Spectrum of inclusion body myositis. Arch Neurol 44:1154, 1987.
9. Ramirez G, Asherson RA, Khamashta MA, et al: Adult onset polymyositis/dermatomyositis: Description of 25 patients with emphasis on treatment. Semin Arthritis Rheum 20:114, 1990.
10. Urbano-Marquez A, Casademont J, and Grau JM: Polymyositis/dermatomyositis: The current position. Ann Rheum Dis 50:191, 1991.

62

Transient Ischemic Attacks

THOMAS M. WALSHE, MD

There is no single cause for transient neurologic deficits. Each case needs a specific evaluation to separate the ischemic from the nonischemic deficit and to identify the cause of the ischemic event when present. The evaluation derives from an understanding of the pathophysiology of cerebral ischemia and an awareness of the other possibilities.

Transient neurologic deficits may be important warnings of serious underlying atherosclerotic vascular disease. A transient ischemic attack (TIA) is by definition harmless in itself because it is short lived; the threat of stroke and myocardial infarction causes the concern. The current treatment for cerebral infarction lies in its prevention. TIA gives the physician a warning that sometimes enables actions that avert impending stroke.

The distribution, timing, and natural history of TIA are not homogeneous but depend on the vessel affected and the underlying cause of the ischemia. TIA can warn of several types of cerebrovascular disease; therefore, one cannot approach transient ischemia as a target of therapy but as a clinical phenomenon that leads to a specific pathology.

The duration of the neurologic deficit in transient ischemia has been defined ranging from minutes to a maximum of 24 hours. The deficit usually lasts for less than 10 minutes in cases of tight stenosis of a large vessel. When embolism from an arterial source is the cause, the deficit may last longer, and in cases in which the deficit lasts for hours, there is often an associated infarction. The longest TIAs are in fact infarcts with short-lived deficits, many of which are embolic. Most data about TIA lump the short stroke with the TIA, although they may arise from different pathologies. Both warn of a potentially serious stroke.

EPIDEMIOLOGY

Transient ischemia occurs in 50 to 75% of patients with extracranial carotid artery disease. The occurrence of TIA among all strokes is only 10 to 20%. The incidence reported for all first TIAs in Rochester, Minnesota during a 12-year period was 237/100,000 population.[1] The incidence and prevalence ranges widely among studies because of the definitions used, the inclusion of transient retinal ischemia with transient hemispheric ischemia, and the population studied. The prevalence of all types of TIAs (total number/population) ranges from 1.1 to 77/1000 persons, depending on the criteria and the population studied. In the elderly "poor" of Chicago, the prevalence rate was 63/1000.[2] No definite sex predominance has been found. There is almost certainly an increasing frequency with age.[3,4] The incidence of stroke per se is related to cholesterol level, blood pressure, and smoking.[5] Recent decline in the incidence of stroke is attributed chiefly to treatment of hypertension.[6]

CLINICAL SYNDROMES

TIAs are grouped into those that follow ischemia in the carotid circulation and those from ischemia in the vertebrobasilar circulation. In the carotid type, attacks are further divided into hemispheric attacks and transient monocular blindness (amaurosis fugax).

Carotid Artery Ischemia

Hemispheric Attacks

A transient unilateral disturbance of sensory or motor function is typical of ischemia in the carotid circulation. The distribution and degree of the neurologic deficit depends on the location of the arterial obstruction and the availability of collateral circulation. For example, occlusion of the internal carotid artery in the neck may cause no clinical deficit if there is adequate collateral blood flow through the circle of Willis. Obstruction more distally in the middle cerebral artery will usually cause a sensorimotor deficit because there is less collateral at that level. Very distal obstruction by small emboli may cause cortical deficits (aphasia, apraxia) without motor findings. Such small infarcts may cause short-lived signs despite the presence of an infarction. In general, however, transient deficits are related to temporary ischemia rather than to infarction. In TIAs, a partial syndrome is the rule; face and hand weakness or numbness with an aphasia is one of the common transient deficits associated with anterior ischemia. Table 62–1 lists symptoms of the carotid artery TIA. If symptoms are repetitive, there are often small differences between attacks. One may affect the whole side and others, just the face or the hand. Some patients describe "bigger" or

TABLE 62–1. CAROTID ARTERY TRANSIENT ISCHEMIC ATTACKS: PRESENTING SYMPTOMS IN 133 PATIENTS*

	%
Paresis (mono, hemi)	61
Paresthesia (mono, hemi)	57
Monocular visual symptoms	32
Paresthesia (facial)	30
Paresis (facial)	22
Dysphasia	17
Dysarthria	16
Headache	12
Lightheadedness	3 each
Dizziness	
Convulsion (focal)	
Convulsion (grand mal)	
Binocular visual (hemianopia) symptoms	
Visual hallucinations	
Dysphagia	
Mental changes	

*From Genton E, Barnett HJM, Field WS, et al: XIV. Cerebral ischemia: The role of thrombosis and antithrombotic therapy. Stroke 8:150, 1977.

"smaller" episodes and seem to get a warning before the full deficit appears. When examined during the attack, the patients display clearly identifiable neurologic signs, although most attacks go unexamined. Recurrent attacks of aphasia are pathognomonic of anterior ischemia in the carotid or middle cerebral artery, whereas dysarthria can occur with changes in either carotid or vertebrobasilar circulation. Aphasia causes an abnormality in writing comparable to the deficit in spoken language; dysarthria does not.

Transient Monocular Blindness (Amaurosis Fugax)

A transient episode of uniocular blindness, partial or complete, means ischemia of the retina either from failure of the blood flow through the ophthalmic artery or its distal branches. Transient monocular blindness (TMB) usually comes on suddenly and without warning. It may affect only half of a field (usually the superior, rarely the inferior field) of vision. In many cases, it is first noted peripherally, and then vision fades toward the horizontal meridian of the eye. It can last from 30 seconds to 10 minutes but usually lasts for 3 or 4 minutes. Platelet emboli have been observed traversing the retinal arteries during an attack. Ophthalmoscopic examination may also reveal white or yellow glistening particles in the retinal artery usually at a bifurcation, which probably represent embolic cholesterol fragments.

Because the ophthalmic artery is the first major branch of the internal carotid, TMB raises the suspicion of ipsilateral, proximal carotid artery atherosclerosis. About 50% of patients with TMB will have a systolic bruit in the neck, and 50% will have angiographically demonstrable lesions of the carotid artery. If there are separate episodes of transient hemiparesis and of monocular blindness, there is a high probability of tight stenosis of the carotid artery.[7] Local stenosis of the ophthalmic artery without carotid artery disease is also a cause of transient retinal ischemia. In one series in which 80 patients with amaurosis fugax were followed for 3 to 120 months, five of the 80 had a cerebrovascular accident, and nine subsequently developed blindness.[8] "Silent" cerebral emboli occur in patients whose only symptoms are ocular. Asymptomatic cerebral emboli appear on angiograms, indirectly by electroencephalogram, or as blood flow abnormalities.[9]

Vertebrobasilar Syndromes

If bilateral hemispheric signs, crossed signs (i.e., ipsilateral face, contralateral limb), or bilateral visual symptoms are present, the vascular territory is usually vertebrobasilar. Stenosis or occlusion may occur in a single vertebral artery, both vertebral arteries, or the basilar trunk. The deficit depends on the available collateral flow. Small-branch occlusions cause discrete syndromes that localize to a small region of the brain stem. The larger branches of the vertebral and basilar arteries (posterior inferior cerebellar, anterior inferior cerebellar, and superior cerebellar arteries) may cause cerebellar ataxia as well as specific segmental signs.

Acute vertigo raises the suspicion of vertebrobasilar ischemia. The labyrinth receives blood supply through the internal auditory artery via the anterior inferior cerebellar artery, a branch of the basilar artery. However, in patients with isolated vertigo, only about 3% will have a basilar thrombosis in the next year. Presumably, the majority of patients with isolated vertigo have a peripheral or labyrinthine cause for their symptoms, and in the others, vascular insufficiency is limited to the internal auditory artery. However, up to 35% of all patients with basilar thrombosis do experience vertigo in the year preceding the stroke. Symptoms of the vertebrobasilar TIA are listed in Table 62–2.

When vertigo occurs with other signs and symptoms, vertebrobasilar ischemia becomes a major concern. Dysarthria together with vertigo always implies a lesion of a large vessel, and patients with these symptoms should be hospitalized for evaluation and treatment. For example, dysarthria and bilateral leg weakness or right facial and left arm and leg weakness would imply a brain stem localization and vertebrobasilar ischemia.

Diplopia is also a commanding feature of basilar ischemia either of the main trunk or a penetrating branch. Visual field deficits from ischemia in the distribution of both posterior cerebral arteries clearly imply a disorder in the

TABLE 62–2. VERTEBROBASILAR TRANSIENT ISCHEMIC ATTACKS: PRESENTING SYMPTOMS IN 54 PATIENTS*

	%
Binocular visual symptoms	57
Vertigo	50
Paresthesia	40
Diplopia	38
Ataxia	33
Paresis	33
Dizziness	20
Headache	18
Nausea/vomiting	14
Dysarthria	14
Loss of consciousness	14
Visual hallucinations	7
Tinnitus	5
Mental changes	5
Dysphonia	3
Drop attack	3
Drowsiness	<3 each
Lightheadedness	
Hearing loss	
Hyperacusis	
Dysphagia	
Weakness (generalized)	

*From Genton E, Barnett HJM, Field WS, et al: XIV. Cerebral ischemia: The role of thrombosis and antithrombotic therapy. Stroke 8:150, 1977.

vertebrobasilar circulation: sudden total blindness can only be from compromised vertebrobasilar circulation. On the other hand, a homonymous field defect can be either carotid or basilar in origin.

Recurrent transient deficits of increasing severity and duration almost always suggest that a major vessel occlusion is imminent and therefore demand prompt evaluation and treatment. A single TIA warrants prompt evaluation but may not portend immediate disaster.

PATHOGENESIS

Transient ischemia indicates underlying cerebrovascular disease and cardiovascular disease. The loss of neurologic function implies an arterial obstruction with inadequate collateral flow to a specific arterial territory. The duration of the obstruction and the availability of collateral flow determines if ischemia or infarction occurs. No single mechanism causes transient arterial obstruction.

Emboli (platelet aggregates, cholesterol, or fibrin) from various sources account for some TIAs. The major evidence for embolization as the cause of TIA is the occasional visualization of emboli in the fundi,[10] their responsiveness to antiplatelet agents and anticoagulants, the frequent finding of an ulcerated or grumous plaque on angiography, and cessation of symptoms following surgery of the lesion in the proximal vessel. When the carotid artery is the source of the embolus, the lesion is often at the bifurcation, especially in the internal carotid artery; less frequently, the source is in the aortic arch or in the heart itself. In addition, when TIA occurs after complete occlusion of a partially occluded artery, the emboli may arise from the external carotid[11] or from the residual internal carotid.[12] TIA from emboli usually last longer than 5 to 10 minutes, which is the anticipated timing for TIA associated with tight stenosis of the carotid artery. Emboli from sources other than the large vessels cause deficits that last even longer.[13] Embolic events not related to disease of the carotid arteries may be associated with myocardial infarction, mitral stenosis, chronic sinoatrial disorder, atrial fibrillation even in the absence of valvular heart disease, myocardial muscle dysfunction, and mitral valve prolapse.[14]

Perfusion failure through a stenotic or compromised artery is another explanation for transient ischemia. Only severe stenosis can cause symptoms, but a decrease in blood pressure or a cardiac arrhythmia might decrease the blood pressure enough to decrease distal circulation behind a severely narrowed carotid artery.[15]

Other hemodynamic variations include orthostatic hypotension, cardiac arrhythmias, increased blood viscosity, low perfusion states, and vascular steal syndromes. Most patients with hemodynamic problems suffer a generalized cerebral ischemia, with loss of consciousness (faintness) rather than focal symptoms. In one series of 290 patients with dysrhythmias, only 1.4% had a TIA as a presenting symptom, as opposed to 81% who had syncope, fainting, or other generalized symptoms.[15] The basilar arterial circulation appears more vulnerable to general hypoperfusion, so that patients who faint report visual blurring, vertigo, distortion of hearing, and eventually, loss of consciousness. There is usually a history of pallor of the face during syncope, which implies a deficit in blood supply via the external carotid arteries. This observation may help differentiate a faint from a TIA. It is more difficult to separate seizure disorder from syncope than from TIA.

Cerebral arterial spasm causes ischemia in patients with subarachnoid hemorrhage. The internal carotid and basilar arteries and the proximal one third of all major primary branches from these vessels may be affected. The more distal branches do not appear to go into spasm, except in patients with exceedingly high blood pressures. Vasospasm is an unlikely mechanism of TIA, unless the diastolic blood pressure is greater than 130 mm Hg or unless it is the result of the irritating effect of free blood in the subarachnoid space. Localized vasospasm may be a cause of TIA if it is induced by vasoconstrictors (serotonin, thromboxane) released by platelet aggregates in the distal arteries. However, this explanation is speculative. Vasospasm has been described in cases of TMB.[16]

Modern imaging techniques have illustrated that some patients with typical TIA have infarctions in the appropriate distribution despite clearing of the clinical deficit. The etiology of such transient strokes is unclear but may be from embolism.

A series of TIAs is difficult to distinguish from a progressing stroke, but both imply thrombosis of a large vessel. In the progressing stroke, there are usually stepwise incremental increases in neurologic deficit over several hours, and at least in some cases, the pathogenesis involves disruption of collateral circulation by a thrombus extending from its site of origin.[15]

Carotid occlusion can occur without any initial symptoms when there is enough collateral circulation through the circle of Willis or the leptomeningeal anastomotic circulation. Signs of cerebral ischemia may occur later when a change in blood pressure, blood volume, or increased viscosity of the blood reduces collateral flow.

Lacunar infarctions are caused by abnormalities in the small penetrating arteries that go to the basal ganglia and brain stem. The arterial pathology is induced by hypertension. About 20% of patients with a lacunar stroke have transient signs and symptoms (usually sensory) resembling a TIA from large-vessel disease.[17]

Differential Diagnosis

Transient neurologic dysfunction occurs with several nonischemic processes. These conditions can be identified by their clinical features and results of laboratory tests.

Migrainous Accompaniments

Migraine may occur with or without a headache. Typically beginning in young adulthood, the headaches tend to disappear at menopause in women and after age 50 to 60 years in men. The migrainous aura usually precedes the headache and may last for up to 20 minutes. The aura is usually unilateral and may cause visual, sensory, motor, aphasic, or other signs. The onset is abrupt, worsening over minutes and disappearing within 20 to 30 minutes. On rare occasions, the aura may last longer than 2 hours, but this duration increases the clinical suspicion of some other pathology. The visual aura usually appear as scotomata but may cause unilateral or homonymous field defects. Most often there are "zigzags," scintillating lights, or movements distally in the field of vision affected. These "fortification" spectra are very characteristic of migraine and, if present, make any other etiology unlikely. Visual phenomena of the scotomata develop at a rate that would be unusually slow for a seizure or cerebrovascular insufficiency. The patient often gives a deliberate and detailed account of how the phenomenon slowly changes, enlarges, and shifts. The visual phenomenon associated with the aura of a seizure or with an episode of vascular insufficiency usually develops rapidly (in less than 1 to 3 minutes) and ends within this period.

Progressing somatic sensory phenomena in migraine are usually one sided and slowly spread up or down an extremity. If the sensory symptoms are on the right side, aphasia or confusional states may develop. Migrainous spells can be difficult to distinguish from transient ischemic attacks, although anterior circulation TIAs seldom cause a headache. The history of other migraine phenomena or the development of a unilateral headache in young patients helps to make the distinction. It is unusual to see a pure motor weakness as the only sign of a migrainous aura without the subsequent development of a headache. Visual and sensory auras, however, can occur repeatedly as isolated phenomena without headache. In some patients, headaches may be a minor feature, and the visual and sensory auras are the symptoms that bring them to the physician. Hemiparesis may occur as a finding in complicated migraine and at times may not resolve.[18]

Focal Seizures

Focal seizures can also cause transient neurologic dysfunction that may be very difficult to distinguish from vascular insufficiency. Focal seizures will often have positive phenomena associated with them (i.e., active twitching of an arm or hand), and the episode may be followed by transient confusion or headache. Cerebral embolism may cause focal seizures but usually after the deficit has appeared.

Other Causes

The brain requires effective blood flow, oxygen, and glucose to supply its metabolic needs. Any marked change in cardiac output resulting from *cardiac arrhythmias, myocardial infarction, hypoglycemia,* or *hypoxia* from any cause can result in generalized transient neurologic dysfunction. Because such factors tend to affect the whole brain, symptoms are not focal.

Unusual causes of TIA can be elusive in patients who seem to have none of the usual risk factors. Tendency for platelet aggregation or hypercoagulable states accounts for some cases in young patients.[19, 20] Oral contraceptives,[21] spontaneous dissection of the craniocerebral vessels,[22] acquired immunodeficiency syndrome,[23] drug abuse,[24] and sickle cell disease[25] are other subtle causes of stroke and transient ischemia.

NATURAL HISTORY

Over 25 studies of the natural history of TIAs have been made, but the data are unclear because all pathologies are considered together. The natural history of the TIA depends on the underlying arterial pathology. TIAs in the carotid distribution are twice as frequent as those in the basilar. Because of variable criteria and pathogenesis, the reported incidence of stroke following a TIA ranges from 4 to 75% and a fatal stroke, from 0 to 18.6%.[26, 27] In the Framingham Study,[5] in which 5184 men and women were followed for 18 years, 6% had a TIA. Of 800 patients recorded in the Harvard Stroke Registry, only 55 had a preceding recognized TIA.[28]

In the National Cooperative Study, 50% of patients with repetitive TIAs stopped having attacks in the first month, 70% of patients in the second month, and 80 to 85% in the third month. Marshall also noted that 50% of patients with carotid symptoms and 28% of patients with vertebrobasilar symptoms cleared after only one or two episodes.[29] Current consensus seems to put the overall risk of stroke following TIA of all types at about 5 to 6%/y,[30] but the risk for an individual depends on the vessel involved and pathology causing the TIA.

It appears that the risk of stroke in the first month is the highest. Of 72 patients with a stroke following a TIA, 51% had the stroke in the first year and 21% in the first month.[31] Of patients with transient ischemic attacks who die, one third die of stroke, and two thirds die of cardiac disease.

When patients with normal results on angiograms after TIAs were followed up for 5 years, approximately 20% had further attacks, 13% had a stroke, and 22% died over a 5-year period, more often a cardiac rather than a cerebral death.[32, 33] A stroke is more likely to occur shortly after a transient attack if the symptoms were carotid rather than basilar. Marshall showed that 76% of patients with a carotid territory attack and 52% of patients with vertebrobasilar attack who subsequently had a cerebrovascular accident did so after no more than one or two transient attacks.[34]

PHYSICAL EXAMINATION

All patients must have a complete medical and neurologic examination. Special attention should be paid to the carotid arteries. Although the physical examination of the arterial system is notoriously unreliable, when signs are present, they can guide the clinician to pursue more definitive tests and speed the diagnosis.

Palpation

Direct palpation of the carotid artery is a normal part of a routine physical examination. In most instances, the common carotid can be felt, and pulsation is noted below, at, and above the bifurcation. Thrills can be detected. The internal carotid is normally not palpable because it swings medially and posteriorly from the bifurcation. Palpation of the carotid artery in the neck is not a reliable means of detecting carotid disease and is inaccurate even in patients in whom carotid occlusion is later demonstrated. The total absence or marked decrease of pulsation above the middle of the neck and strong pulsation below suggest occlusion.

Palpation of Branches of the External Carotid

Many tests for internal carotid stenosis depend on the hypothesis that as pressure in the internal carotid falls, there will be collateral flow from anastomotic channels derived from the external carotid. Palpable pulses of branches of the external carotid may indicate that this flow has developed (Fig. 62–1).

Preauricular and Superficial Temporal Pulses. A segment of the superficial temporal artery is palpable just in front of the tragus of the ear. In a few patients with unilateral internal carotid stenosis, this pulse, or the superficial temporal pulse located over the temporalis muscle, will increase in volume on the affected side. In patients with occlusion of the common carotid, they will often be reduced. The latter patients, in most instances, are not surgical candidates.

Orbital Pulses. The supratrochlear pulse is felt at the inner rim of the orbit, whereas the supraorbital pulse is more lateral, usually at the supraorbital notch, one third of

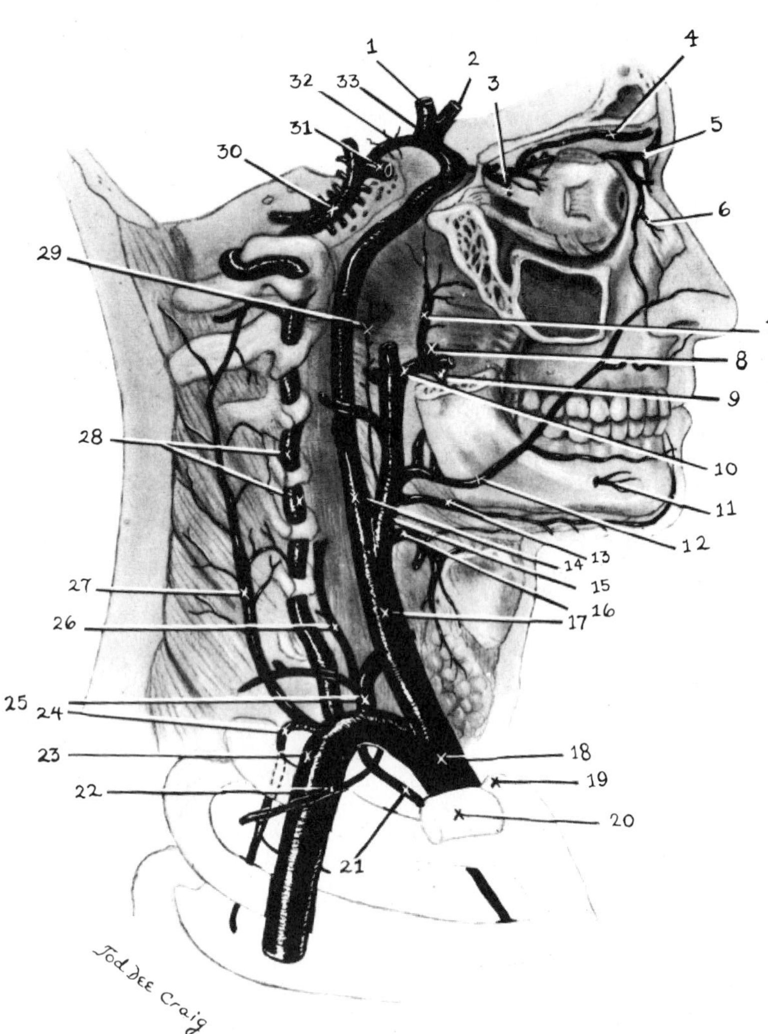

FIGURE 62–1. Diagram of branches of the carotid and vertebral arteries. The palpable pulses referred to in the text are as follows: (4) supraorbital artery, (5) supratrochlear artery, (12) facial artery. For orientation, (17) common carotid, (14) internal carotid, (28) vertebral artery, (30) basilar artery.

the way along the upper rim of the orbit. These two arteries are terminal branches of the ophthalmic artery. Normally, the flow is outward from within the orbit. The arteries may hypertrophy if there is reversal of flow caused by occlusion of the internal carotid or ophthalmic artery.

Carotid Auscultation

Carotid bruits begin over the bifurcation and are transmitted upward. They occur in early systole or are pansystolic. A harsh, high-pitched "cooing" bruit with a diastolic component nearly always implies a very stenotic but not totally occluded carotid artery.

In many instances, it is not possible to determine the origin of a carotid bruit. Some are transmitted from the heart, large proximal vessels, or the common carotid artery. Bilateral carotid bruits with a systolic cardiac murmur at the base are particularly difficult to interpret. Approximately 35% of patients at risk by age for TIAs will have a bruit over one of the major vessels in the neck. Although the bruits indicate atherosclerotic disease, the risk of stroke or the presence of significant stenosis is not known. Moreover, absence of a bruit does not imply absence of a carotid lesion because low-grade stenosis, ulcerated plaques, or lesions that occlude the carotid totally or by more than 85% may be silent. A localized bruit at the midportion or upper area of the neck is suggestive of a carotid lesion; other noises are less helpful.

Asymptomatic Bruit

About 4% of persons older than 65 years of age have a localized, easily audible *carotid bruit.* One half of these have carotid stenosis with at least a 50% narrowing of the artery, but fewer than 10% have stenosis with a residual lumen of 1.5 mm or less. In the patient with an asymptomatic carotid bruit, further noninvasive testing may be indicated. It is debatable whether endarterectomy is advisable.[35, 36] Follow-up studies reveal a high incidence of stroke (5.5% in 1 year) in persons with bruits associated with tight carotid stenosis as shown by noninvasive tests, but strokes were usually preceded by TIA symptoms.[37] Very close follow-up and angiography to determine the feasibility of endarterectomy if TIA symptoms occur is certainly recommended for patients in this subgroup.[38] Recent data suggest a benefit of endarterectomy in selected asymptomatic patients for the reduction of the incidence of ipsilateral TIAs and transient monocular blindness.[39] Endarterectomy also may reduce the risk of significant hemispheric stroke.[39]

Ocular Findings

A cholesterol embolus seen in a retinal artery is highly suggestive of carotid artery atherosclerosis. Carotid occlusion or severe stenosis can prevent hypertensive fundic changes on the blocked side in a severely hypertensive patient. When present, this occlusion or stenosis helps support the suspicion of carotid artery disease.

DIAGNOSTIC TESTS

The history and neurologic findings during an attack are crucial in identifying patients with transient ischemia, but to determine the pathogenesis, special diagnostic tests are essential. The tests are aimed at identifying the possible causes of TIA: carotid or basilar disease, cerebral embolism, or lacunar disease. Because disease of the carotid artery is dangerous and treatable, it becomes the first target of inquiry.

Many procedures, short of conventional angiography, attempt to identify a focal lesion in the carotid artery. Bruits and TIAs occur without carotid disease. One would like to select the most likely patients for angiography rather than study all cases. In general, there is no consensus yet of the best tests with which to image the carotid. Each clinic develops its special competence in certain procedures.

Noninvasive

Periorbital Doppler (Doppler Sonometry, Doppler Ophthalmosonometry). The direction of blood flow in the arteries around the orbit can be checked using bidirectional Doppler probe. Normally, blood flows from the ophthalmic artery out into the supraorbital and supratrochlear arteries. If the pressure falls within the ophthalmic territory because of a proximal stenosis in the internal carotid in the neck, the blood flow will be reversed in these small branches. This reversal of flow can be easily assessed by the Doppler technique.[39]

The test will frequently detect total occlusion or very high-grade stenosis in the internal carotid artery. False-positive test results sometimes occur through improper technique; false-positives also occur with stenosis or occlusion of the ophthalmic artery. False-negative test results occur in up to 30% of patients and make it mandatory that this test be combined with one or more additional tests.

Carotid Imaging by Doppler Technique. Doppler ultrasound devices image the direction and rate of flow of the blood in the carotid. The characteristics of flow in the common, internal, and external carotid arteries imply the status of the artery. In a high-grade stenosis, the flow will accelerate and may be as much as four to five times the normal velocity.

The reliability of the readings increases with the experience of the technician. When done by an experienced observer, the Doppler probe can recognize the common, internal, and external carotids in over 95% of cases and can identify significant arterial pathology.[40, 41]

Because the flow rate does not begin to increase markedly until stenosis of at least 70% has occurred, the continuous-wave Doppler systems are not accurate in detecting minor degrees of stenosis and will not detect ulcerated plaques in the absence of stenosis.

With complete occlusion, there is no flow, and the carotid artery is silent by the Doppler technique. Likewise, a very high-grade stenosis of the internal carotid—in the range of 98%—will be missed by Doppler continuous-wave techniques because the flow is small enough in amount (although very rapid) such that it cannot be detected by the operator. Sometimes, dense calcification of the carotid artery can also make the sounds inaudible.

The vertebral artery and subclavian and other large vessels cannot be usefully assessed by this technique because they are not near enough to the probe to give reliable signals.

Carotid Imaging by B-Mode Sonography. The ultrasonic approach to investigating carotid artery disease also will produce an image by the B-mode technique. This gives a visual image of the wall of the carotid artery.[42] The B-mode scanner, unlike the continuous-wave Doppler ultrasound technique, will identify plaques and show craters or breaks in the surface of the arterial wall. Some correlation exists between the ultrasonic appearance (reflective or shadowed) of the plaque and whether it is hemorrhagic, fibrotic, calcified, or collagenized.

Normal arteries are easy to image, and small plaques are also easy to see, but large plaques, sometimes heavily calcified, have a more mixed composition and may scatter the sound wave and deteriorate the image.

Transcranial Doppler Ultrasonography. Transcranial Doppler ultrasonography offers a means of detecting abnormal blood flow in the ophthalmic artery, carotid siphon, and the circle of Willis as well as the intracranial parts of the vertebral and basilar arteries. In experienced hands, transcranial Doppler can detect abnormal intracranial collateral flow with 85% sensitivity. Increases in blood velocity arise from conditions that reduce the arterial lumen (vasospasm) or that increase flow through the artery (arteriovenous malformation). Reduced velocity occurs when blood flow is reduced either globally (increased intracranial pressure) or regionally (proximal occlusion). Tight stenosis or occlusion of the distal internal carotid artery can be detected with a sensitivity of 86% and specificity of 97%.[43] Vertebral and basilar arterial stenoses are less reliably detected. Transcranial Doppler is an inexpensive and portable method of analyzing vascular disease in the distal large vessels.

Magnetic Resonance Angiography. Magnetic resonance (MR) angiography is rapidly becoming available with resolution adequate to effectively depict the extracranial and the intracranial arteries. MR angiography promises to be the safest means to identify a stenosis or occlusion in the extracranial arteries. It is expensive and requires patient cooperation.

Combined Noninvasive Tests. The noninvasive tests are often performed as a battery, including carotid imaging by Doppler, B-mode sonography, and sometimes, periorbital Doppler. The tests at times are complementary because periorbital Doppler is highly sensitive only for tight stenosis or occlusion, whereas Doppler and sonographic imaging may miss the latter but are more sensitive for detecting mild-to-moderate stenosis or ulcerative plaque.

Invasive

Digital Subtraction Venous Angiography. Digital subtraction angiography visualizes the carotid arteries using intravenous injection of contrast material. By the use of a computer and an image intensifier, a visualization of the carotid arteries can be achieved in about 85% of patients.

The large amount of contrast agent used is a hazard in patients with renal or cardiac disease. The resolution of the venous studies is variable and often marred by motion artifact caused by reflex swallowing induced by the circulating dye. Elderly, confused, or uncooperative patients cannot be studied by this technique. Venous subtraction angiography has not supplanted the noninvasive tests that offer similar sensitivity and specificity.

Arterial Angiography. Conventional arteriography visualizes the carotid artery and its intracranial branches. It clearly identifies carotid artery stenosis and ulceration without stenosis. Angiography also images lesions of the vertebral and basilar arteries and their distal intracranial branches. Aneurysms, vascular dissections, moya moya disease, fibromuscular dysplasia, and occlusions in distal branches can be identified on angiography. Angiography is usually done to ascertain the degree of carotid stenosis in patients whose noninvasive tests show tight stenosis. Arterial puncture, catheterization, and dye load are risks to patients, especially those who have atherosclerotic disease. Stroke and other serious morbidity were reported in 0.65% of patients undergoing traditional arteriography.[44] Transient neurologic deficits occurred in about 4%.[45] In most departments, dye load is diminished to one third by using digital subtraction technique for arterial study. The risk of arterial catheterization remains dependent on the experience of the radiologist. Arteriography is usually reserved for patients who are considered for carotid endarterectomy. Carotid stenosis with residual lumen of 2-mm diameter or less, usually with evidence of plaque, is considered a surgical target. (Fig. 62–2). Interpretation of atherosclerotic plaque without stenosis is more difficult, and interpretation of the characteristics of the ulcerated plaque is not fully reliable. Patients with a typical history of TIA (often lasting hours) may have normal noninvasive test and angiographic results. These patients have a rate of subsequent stroke, probably from cardiac or large-vessel emboli, nearly the same as those of patients with clear-cut angiographic lesions in the carotid artery.

Summary

Using the history and an understanding of its characteristics, one separates transient ischemia from other causes of transient neurologic signs. Then, assessment of the underlying cause of the ischemia is the focus of the evaluation. Patients who are having active ischemia should be evaluated immediately in the hospital. Patients with a single episode days or weeks before and who are asymptomatic can have the evaluation as an outpatient. The neurologic findings during the ischemic attack separate carotid from basilar lesions in most cases. The physician is eager to identify a carotid artery lesion to account for the findings because there is therapy available. In the patient with *clear-cut history of carotid territory TIA,* a full examination—including palpation of pulses and auscultation for carotid bruit, electrocardiogram, and noninvasive images of the carotid are done, and if they suggest a lesion, angiography is done to delineate the lesion fully. If the carotid

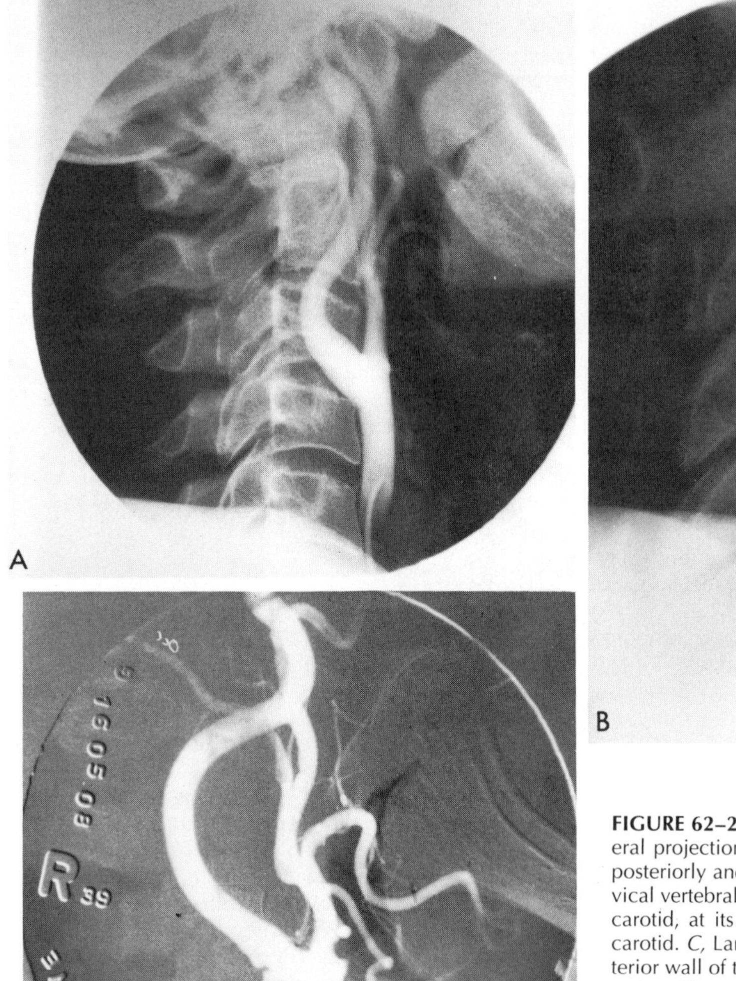

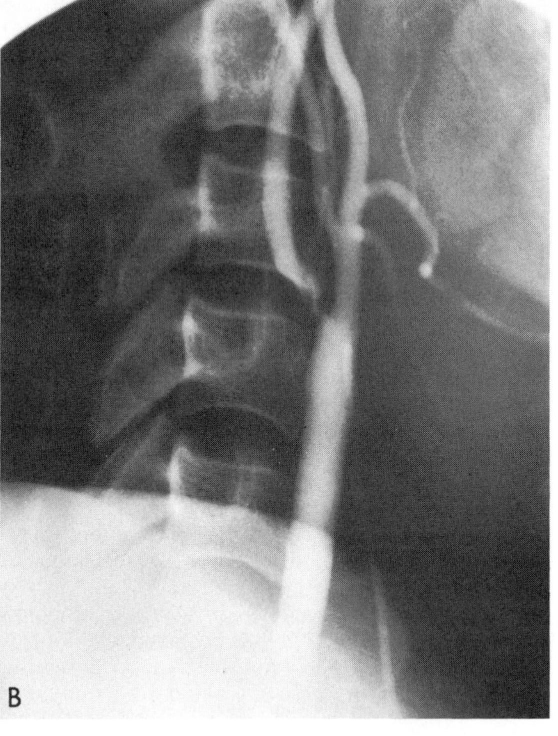

FIGURE 62–2. *A,* Normal selective carotid angiogram, lateral projection. The internal carotid is visualized swinging posteriorly and is projected over the second and third cervical vertebral bodies. *B,* High-grade stenosis of the internal carotid, at its origin from the bifurcation of the common carotid. *C,* Large, ulcerated plaque of the interior and posterior wall of the internal carotid artery soon after the bifurcation. There is additional plaque on the anterior wall of the external carotid subtraction view.

artery is found to be normal, a search for an embolic source is the next step. Twenty-four–hour monitoring for occult arrhythmia sometimes identifies a source of embolism. A transesophageal echocardiogram is recommended to detect occult sources of embolism in patients with unexplained TIAs.[46] Evidence of recent myocardial infarction or cardiomyopathy suggests a cardiac source of emboli.

In patients with hypertension, the consideration of a lacunar lesion must be made, but there are no tests to identify the lacune that has not caused an infarct. An MR image or computed tomographic scan may show the small infarct that caused the transient signs but became asymptomatic.

Treatment is usually coupled with the evaluation, especially in patients with multiple transient attacks in the carotid territory. In such patients, rapid assessment of the carotid artery by noninvasive imaging techniques or angiography is needed; if a tight stenosis is identified, the patient goes for endarterectomy. In patients without multiple, continuing TIAs the evaluation can proceed with less haste.

Patients suspected of having basilar or vertebral ischemia should be hospitalized and observed for progression. MR angiography is a useful method to image the posterior circulation, but the software needed for the studies is available in only a few centers. The noninvasive methods used for imaging the carotid arteries are not reliable in the basilar artery and are limited in the vertebral. When the neurologic syndrome suggests ischemia of the distal branches of the basilar artery (posterior cerebral or cerebellar arteries), search for an embolic source is indicated. Computed tomographic scanning and MR imaging can identify basilar artery aneurysms and small infarcts in the brain stem caused by branch occlusions.

MEDICAL TREATMENT

General Medical Care

When the TIA is single and remote (occurring days before), an outpatient evaluation is acceptable once the physician has determined from the history and examination that there is no other obvious evidence of immediate risk for stroke. The outpatient evaluation must be done expeditiously and the patient warned to return at once if deficits recur. A single or recurrent acute TIA should also provoke admission because there is no way to anticipate the onset of an associated stroke.

Treatment of underlying medical problems, such as hypertension, is essential. In patients with lacunar infarction, treatment of hypertension is the primary mode of therapy. The necessity for correction of dehydration, hyperglycemia, cardiac problems, and hyperlipidemia underlies sound management. Atrial fibrillation is an important cause of cerebral embolization and if present, requires treatment with anticoagulation.[47] Treatment of high-grade cardiac arrhythmias of other types, when present, should be considered in patients with recurrent TIAs.[48] An interesting study suggested that lowering the hematocrit level from the range of 47 to 53 ml/dl to the range of 36 to 46 ml/dl increased cerebral blood flow in some patients.[49] Phlebotomies are certainly indicated for patients with TIAs associated with polycythemia. Other medical conditions that cause stroke include increased blood viscosity, thrombocytosis, giant cell arteritis, and bacterial endocarditis. When determined to be the cause of TIA, these conditions require specific treatments.

Management of Transient Monocular Blindness[50]

In patients older than 40 years, TMB requires a rapid evaluation that begins with an ophthalmologic consultation to insure that there is no intrinsic ocular disorder. Sedimentation rate, complete blood count, and serum glucose and lipid levels are used to search for systemic illness that can cause transient blindness. In young patients and those with malignancies or other chronic illness, tests for a hypercoagulable state may give a clue to the underlying problem. Patients without systemic cause, such as temporal arteritis or specific ocular disease, (e.g., narrow-angle glaucoma) need imaging of the carotid arteries by noninvasive testing. If there is evidence of carotid artery disease, MR angiography or convential angiography is done to define a surgical lesion. In cases of complete occlusion of the ipsilateral carotid artery, aspirin is often adequate treatment. In patients over 40 years without obvious cause for the TMB, aspirin is also indicated. In patients younger than 40 years without obvious cause for TMB, the prognosis is usually good, and no treatment is needed. Young patients with TMB should be asked about illicit drug use.

Anticoagulant Therapy

Anticoagulants have been used to prevent emboli and to prevent propagation of a thrombus in large vessels.[51, 52] The efficacy of anticoagulation in TIA is not clear because the results of different studies are not in agreement. Almost all studies on anticoagulants in patients who have had a TIA have used sodium warfarin (Coumadin). Contraindications generally agreed on include hypertension, blood in the cerebrospinal fluid, advanced age, cognitive deficits, and peptic ulceration.

Patients who have inoperable, symptomatic carotid stenosis may benefit from anticoagulation; however, there is no consensus in the data so far collected.[53, 54] Likewise, patients with acute symptomatic basilar artery stenosis may benefit from heparin, but concrete data are lacking. Patients with lacunar disease either in the anterior or posterior circulation (including basilar branch occlusions) are not treated with anticoagulants.

Patients with cardiogenic embolism receive anticoagulation immediately with heparin and then for at least 6 months with warfarin. Patients with chronic atrial fibrillation are treated with warfarin over long periods.[55] Patients with TIA and no identifiable cause do not receive anticoagulation.

Antiplatelet Agents

Acetylsalicylic acid, clofibrate, dipyridamole, and sulfinpyrazone have been studied in regard to TIAs. These agents inhibit platelet aggregation in vitro and intra-arterial clot formation in vivo. Dipyridamole in doses of up to 800 mg/day was studied in one series,[56] and no clear-cut beneficial results were obtained. A similar failure was noted for clofibrate.[57] The evidence to date suggests that aspirin, combined with control of hypertension and other risk factors, can reduce the recurrence rate of TIAs, and there is now evidence it may prevent strokes or death; the Canadian study demonstrated a protective effect of aspirin in carotid and basilar ischemia against a combined measurement of stroke and death.[58] Sulfinpyrazone gave no added benefit. For unknown reasons, in the Canadian study women did not benefit. The United States multicenter study noted the effect of aspirin and placebo in both surgically and nonsurgically treated patients with carotid TIAs.[59] All patients in the study had carotid distribution symptoms, and four-vessel arteriography had been performed. After 6 months of therapy, there was a striking decrease in the incidence of recurrent TIAs but no effect on stroke or death. One trial using aspirin, 330 mg/day, in patients with small completed strokes or TIAs revealed approximately 40% fewer strokes compared with use of placebo.[60] It has been shown that 30 mg of aspirin, compared with 283 mg, is equally effective in preventing vascular events following an initial TIA or minor stroke.[61]

Unless there are reasons to the contrary, it seems desirable to place most patients with TIAs not caused by tight carotid stenosis or by cardiogenic embolism on a low dose of aspirin once per day.

Ticlopidine has been released as a platelet antiaggregate for use in stroke and TIA. In the 1529 cases treated with ticlopidine in one study, 11% had fatal or nonfatal strokes in the 2- to 6-year follow-up period; in 1540 patients treated with 1300 mg of aspirin, 14% had stroke. Efficacy analysis emphasizes the difference between aspirin and ticlopidine, so that the risk reduction appears as 27% overall in favor of ticlopidine.[62] Ticlopidine is as effective as aspirin, if not more, but has greater risk and side effects than 1300 mg of aspirin; the cost is also much greater. Besides skin rashes and gastrointestinal side effects, ticlopidine causes severe neutropenia in some patients. Ticlopidine may be of value in patients who are allergic to aspirin.

SURGICAL TREATMENT

Patients who have symptomatic stenosis of the carotid artery that is greater than 70% benefit from endarterectomy. The North American Symptomatic Carotid Endarterectomy (NASCE) Trial[63] showed the efficacy of endarterectomy and identified the risk factors that influenced stroke rate for patients who had a tight stenosis of the carotid artery and a TIA or minor stroke. The factors that increase the risk of future stroke are age greater than 70 years, male sex, systolic blood pressure greater than 160 mm Hg, diastolic blood pressure greater than 90 mm Hg, interval of less than 31 days since primary event, previous stroke rather than TIA, greater than 80% carotid stenosis, ulceration of plaque on angiogram, intermittent claudication, and high blood lipid level. The NASCE data help establish the risk of stroke in medically treated patients with symptomatic carotid artery disease. The data show that in aspirin-treated patients with zero to five risk factors, the stroke rate over 2 years was 17%; in patients with six risk factors, the stroke rate in medical patients was 23%; in patients with more than seven risk factors, the stroke rate was 39% during the 2 years. Risk of stroke was diminished by endarterectomy. Among the endarterectomy group, the risk reduction for stroke was greatest in the highest degrees of stenosis: in patients with 90 to 99% stenosis, the risk reduction was 26% over 2 years; in those with 80 to 89% stenosis, it was 18%; in those with 70 to 79%, it was 12%. There are little data to support carotid endarterectomy in cases other than tight carotid stenosis, but some believe that complex ulcerated plaques presumed to be the source of embolism are also acceptable targets for surgery.[64]

Summary

The controversy and disagreement in the management of patients with TIAs rises out of the diversity of pathogenesis. Identification of specific arterial pathology when possible helps direct the management. Patients with TIA and minor stroke in the setting of high-grade carotid artery stenosis receive endarterectomy when possible. When recurrent embolism is from chronic atrial fibrillation or another cardiac source, chronic anticoagulation is appropriate. Management of acute basilar thrombosis usually includes heparin, but there are no controlled data. Thrombolytic therapy is now under investigation in these patients but will require instillation at the site of the thrombus. There is no consensus on treatment for other types of lesions, but aspirin in low doses may be adequate to prevent recurrence in many patients. Patients who have no clear cause for TIA need special attention in future studies to determine the risk of stroke.

The immediate concern in patients with TIA is the prevention of a fixed neurologic deficit. The management depends on the type of lesion, the patient's health, the availability of diagnostic tests, and surgical skill.

REFERENCES

1. Whisnant JP, Melton LJ, Davis PH, et al: Comparison of case ascertainment by medical record linkage and cohort follow up to determine the incidence rates for transient ischemic attacks and stroke. J Clin Epidemiol 43:791, 1990.
2. Ostfield AM, Shekelle RB, and Klawans HL: Transient ischemic attacks and risk of stroke in an elderly poor population. Stroke 4:980, 1973.
3. Whisnant JP, Matsumoto N, and Elveback LR: Transient ischemic attacks in a community. Mayo Clin Proc 48:194, 1973.
4. Friedman GD, Wilson WS, Mosier JM, et al: Transient ischemic attacks in a community. JAMA 210:1428, 1969.
5. Wolf PA: Hypertension as a risk factor. *In* Whisnant JP and Sandok BA (eds): Cerebrovascular Disease 9th Conference. New York, Grune & Stratton, 1974, pp 105–112.
6. Whisnant JP: The decline of stroke. Stroke 15:160, 1984.
7. Pessin MS, Duncan GW, Mohr JP, and Poskanzer DC: Clinical and angiographic features of carotid transient ischemic attacks. N Engl J Med 296:358, 1977.
8. Mungas JE and Baker WH: Amaurosis fugax. Stroke 8:232, 1977.
9. Harrison MJG and Marshall J: Evidence of silent cerebral embolism in patients with amaurosis fugax. J Neurol Neurosurg Psychiatry 40:651, 1977.
10. Milliken CH, Bauer RB, Gaodschmidt R, et al: A classification of cerebrovascular diseases. Stroke 6:564, 1975.
11. Fisher CM: Observations of the fundus oculi in transient monocular blindness. Neurology 9:333, 1959.
12. Burnbaum M, Selhorst JB, Harbison JW, et al: Amaurosis fugax from disease of the external carotid artery. Arch Neurol 34:532, 1977.
13. Barnett HJM: Transient cerebral ischemia: Pathogenesis, prognosis and management. Ann R Coll Phys Surg Can 7:153, 1974.
14. Byer JA and Easton JD: Therapy of ischemic cerebrovascular disease. Ann Intern Med 93:742, 1980.
15. Reed RL, Siekert RG, and Meredith J: Rarity of transient focal cerebral ischemia in cardiac dysrhythmia. JAMA 223:893, 1973.
16. Burger SK, Saul RF, Selhorst JB, et al: Transient monocular blindness caused by vasospasm. N Engl J Med 325:870, 1991.
17. Fisher CM: Lacunar strokes and infarcts: A review. Neurology 32:871, 1982.
18. Larsen BH, Sorensen PS, and Marquardsen J: Transient ischemic attacks in young patients: A thromboembolic or migrainous manifestation? A 10 year follow up study of 46 patients. J Neurol Neurosurg Psychiatry 53:1029, 1990.
19. Hess DC, Krauss J, Adams RJ, et al: Anticardiolipin antibodies: A study of frequency in TIA and stroke. Neurology 41:525, 1991.
20. Levine SR, Deegan MJ, Futrell N, and Welch KM: Cerebrovas-

cular and neurologic disease associated with antiphospholipid antibodies: 48 cases. Neurology 40:1181, 1990.
21. Muzal S: Transient ischemic attack and increased platelet aggregability associated with oral contraceptives: Treatment with dipyridamide and aspirin. J Neurol Neurosurg Psychiatry 40:9, 1977.
22. Ojemann RG, Roberson GH, and Fisher CM: "Spontaneous" dissection of cervicocerebral arteries. Stroke 8:15, 1977.
23. Berger JR, Harris JO, Gregorios J, and Norenberg M: Cerebrovascular disease in AIDS: A case control study. AIDS 4:239, 1990.
24. Kaku DA and Lowenstein DH: Emergence of recreational drug abuse as a major risk factor for stroke in young adults. Ann Intern Med 113:821, 1990.
25. Finelli PF: Sickle cell trait and transient monocular blindness. Am J Ophthalmol 81:850, 1976.
26. Cartlidge NEF, Whisnant JP, and Elveback LR: Carotid and vertebro-basilar transient ischemic attacks. A community study, Rochester, Minnesota. Mayo Clin Proc 52:117, 1977.
27. Brust JCM: Transient ischemic attacks. Natural history and anticoagulation. Neurology 27:701, 1977.
28. Mohr JP, Caplan LF, Mielski J, et al: Cases of carotid artery stroke in the Harvard Stroke Registry. Stroke 8:142, 1977.
29. Marshall J: The natural history of transient ischemic cerebrovascular attacks. Q J Med 35:309, 1964.
30. Whisnant JP, Matsumoto N, and Elveback LR: The effect of anticoagulant therapy on the prognosis of patients with transient cerebral ischemic attacks in a community: Rochester, Minnesota, 1955–1969. Mayo Clin Proc 48:844, 1973.
31. Meyer JS, Guirand B, and Bauer R: Clinical and pathophysiological considerations of atherosclerotic thrombotic disease of the carotid arteries. *In* Vinken PJ and Bruyn GW (eds): Vascular Disease of the Nervous System. Handbook of Neurology, Vol 11. New York, Elsevier, 1972, pp 327–365.
32. Marshall J and Wilkinson MS: The prognosis of carotid transient ischemic attacks in patients with normal angiograms. Brain 94:395, 1971.
33. Toole JF and Yuson CP: Transient ischemic attacks with normal arteriogram: Serious or benign prognosis. Ann Neurol 1:100, 1977.
34. Marshall J: The natural history of transient ischemic cerebrovascular attacks. Q J Med 35:309, 1964.
35. Ropper AH, Wechsler LR, and Wilson LS: Carotid bruit and the risk of stroke. N Engl J Med 307:1388, 1982.
36. Mohr JP: Asymptomatic carotid artery disease. Stroke 13:431, 1982.
37. Chambers BR and Norris JW: Outcome in patients with asymptomatic neck bruits. N Engl J Med 315:860, 1986.
38. Wise B, Parker J, and Burkholder J: Supraorbital Doppler studies, carotid bruits, and arteriography in unilateral ocular or cerebral ischemic disorders. Neurology 29:34, 1979.
39. Hobson RW, Weiss DO, Fields WS, et al: Efficacy of carotid endarterectomy for asymptomatic carotid stenosis. N Engl J Med 328:221, 1993.
40. Garth KE, Carrol BA, Sommer FG, et al: Duplex ultrasound scanning of the carotid arteries with velocity spectrum analysis. Radiology 147:823, 1983.
41. Wiebel WJ, Austin CW, Sackett JF, et al: Correlation of high-resolution, B-mode and continuous-wave Doppler sonography with arteriography in the diagnosis of carotid stenosis. Radiology 149:523, 1983.
42. Comerata AJ, Cranley JJ, Katz ML, et al: Real-time B-mode carotid imaging. J Vasc Surg 1:84, 1984.
43. Ley-Pozo J and Ringelstein EB: Noninvasive detection of occlusive disease of the carotid siphon and middle cerebral artery. Ann Neurol 28:640, 1990.
44. Swansen PD, Calanchini PR, Dyken ML, et al: A cooperative study of hospital frequency and character of transient ischemic attacks. II. Performance of angiography among six centers. JAMA 237:2202, 1977.
45. Hankey GJ, Warlow CP, and Sellar RJ: Cerebral angiographic risk in mild cerebrovascular disease. Stroke 21:209, 1990.
46. Pearson AC, Labovitz AJ, Tatineni S, and Gomez CR: Superiority of transesophageal echocardiography in detecting cardiac source of embolism in patients with cerebral ischemia of uncertain etiology. J Am Coll Cardiol 17:66, 1991.
47. Kitchens JM and Flegel KM: Atrial fibrillation, stroke and anticoagulation. J Gen Intern Med 1:126, 1986.
48. Francis DA, Heron JR, and Clarke M: Ambulatory electrocardiographic monitoring in patients with transient focal cerebral ischemia. J Neurol Neurosurg Psychiatry 47:256, 1984.
49. Thomas DJ, Marshall J, Ross-Russeel RW, et al: Effect of haematocrit on cerebral blood flow in man. Lancet ii:941, 1972.
50. The Amaurosis Fugax Study Group: Current management of amaurosis fugax. Stroke 21:201, 1990.
51. Baker RN: An evaluation of anticoagulant therapy in the treatment of cerebrovascular disease: Report of the Veterans Administration Cooperative Study on Atherosclerosis. Neurology 17:132, 1961.
52. Baker RN, Browand J, Fang HC, et al: Anticoagulant therapy in cerebral infarction. Report on cooperative study. Neurology 12:823, 1962.
53. Pearce JMS, Gulby SS, and Walton JN: Long-term anticoagulant therapy in transient ischaemic attacks. Lancet i:6, 1965.
54. Keller L: The transient ischemic attack: A critical review of anticoagulant and surgical therapy. Current concepts of cerebrovascular disease. Stroke 5:23, 1974.
55. The Boston Area Anticoagulation Trial for Atrial Fibrillation Investigators: The effect of low dose warfarin on the risk of stroke in patients with nonrheumatic atrial fibrillation. N Engl J Med 323:1505, 1990.
56. Acheson J, Danta G, and Hutchinson EC: Controlled trial of dipyridamole in cerebral vascular disease. BMJ 1:614, 1969.
57. Acheson J and Hutchinson EC: Controlled trials of clofibrate in cerebral vascular disease. Atherosclerosis 15:177, 1972.
58. Barnett HJM, McDonald JWD, and Sackett DL: Aspirin effective in males threatened with stroke. Stroke 9:295, 1978.
59. Fields WS, Lenuch NA, Frankonski RF, et al: Controlled trial of aspirin in cerebral ischemia. Stroke 8:301, 1977.
60. Bousser MG, Eschwege E, Haguenau M, et al: "AICLA" controlled trial of aspirin and dipyridamole in the secondary prevention of atherothrombotic cerebral ischemia. Stroke 14:5, 1983.
61. The Dutch TIA Trial Study Group: A comparison of two doses of aspirin (30 mg vs 283 mg a day) in patients after a transient ischemic attack or a minor ischemic stroke. N Engl J Med 325:1261, 1991.
62. Hass WK, Easton JD, Adams HP, et al: A randomized trial comparing ticlopidine hydrochloride with aspirin for the prevention of stroke in high risk patients. N Engl J Med 321:501, 1989.
63. North American Symptomatic Carotid Endarterectomy Trial Collaborators: Beneficial effect of carotid endarterectomy in symptomatic patients with high grade stenosis. N Engl J Med 325:445, 1991.
64. Dixon S, Pais SO, Raviola C, et al: Natural history of nonstenotic symptomatic ulcerative lesions of the carotid artery: A further analysis. Arch Surg 117:1493, 1982.

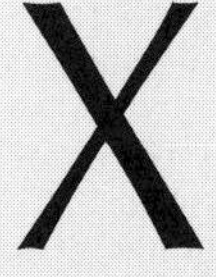

X

Clinical Primary Care Problems

63

Fatigue and Chronic Fatigue Syndrome

ANTHONY L. KOMAROFF, MD

FRUSTRATIONS OF FATIGUE

Chronic fatigue is a common problem in general medical practice,[1–6] accounting for 10 to 15 million office visits annually in the United States. It is one of the most frustrating problems for a physician to deal with, for several reasons. For one, the complaint of "fatigue" does not mean the same thing to all people. Some people mean that they feel like they want to sleep. Others mean that they have trouble finding the energy to start new tasks. Others mean that they have difficulty concentrating and that they are experiencing a kind of mental fatigue. Still others mean that their muscles are weak or that they get tired easily.

Another reason that the complaint of fatigue is a frustrating one for the physician is that patients who seek medical care for fatigue are often the "worried well." A physician may naturally respond by thinking: "You're tired? Well, so am I." Indeed, everyone gets tired. Fatigue is a universal human experience. Moreover, many people often feel tired: In one British survey, 20% of adults said that they had "always felt tired" during the preceding month.[7] The pace of life in the late 20th century is fast, and most people (including physicians) have multiple competing demands on their time. A careful study of Americans concludes that, far from evolving toward a "leisure society," we are working increasingly longer hours, with less time for relaxation.[8] Moreover, some sleep physiologists believe that many citizens of the developed nations suffer from a chronic state of sleep deprivation.[9]

Fatigue is a frustrating complaint, too, because the diagnosis is often obscure. Although there may be hints of an underlying psychological or physical disorder, the evidence is often inconclusive. Finally, fatigue is frustrating because attempts at treatment are often unsuccessful.[10] This is especially discouraging because patients with chronic fatigue often have remarkable degrees of functional impairment and often are as restricted in their levels of activity as are patients with well-characterized major medical disorders.[1]

Causes of fatigue sufficient to induce a patient to go to a doctor's office are summarized in Table 63–1. The available literature and common experience makes it clear that "lifestyle" (e.g., the pace of life, substance abuse) along with depression and other psychiatric disorders are the most common causes of fatigue. After that, a variety of well-characterized organic illnesses as well as a few poorly understood illnesses account for the rest of the cases.

DEPRESSION AND FATIGUE

Physicians also find the complaint of fatigue frustrating because they know that the patient is often suffering from depression. Indeed, in the patient whose presenting complaint is chronic fatigue, the first three diagnoses on the differential diagnosis list are depression, depression, and depression (often with associated anxiety or somatization disorder).[11–16]

If the physician diagnoses depression in a patient, it can be frustrating because the patient may find the diagnosis stigmatizing and, therefore, have trouble accepting it. Thus, making the diagnosis and talking with the patient about the diagnosis will require a lot of work and may also involve conflict with the patient. Particularly if the patient will not accept a diagnosis of depression, the complaint of fatigue will also be frustrating because it will be difficult to treat.

The diagnosis and treatment of depression, anxiety disorders, and somatization disorder in a primary care practice is not the subject of this chapter; rather, these topics are covered in Chapters 77 to 81. But it is important to emphasize that, as primary care physicians, we do not do a good job of identifying and treating depression as it presents in a primary care practice.[17, 18] The principal reason for this is that many patients with depression do not overtly state that they are "depressed," "sad," "down," and so forth. Rather, they present with headache, myalgias, abdominal pain, fatigue, and other symptoms. They express their suffering by somatizing their suffering.

ORGANIC ILLNESS AND FATIGUE

Fatigue can reflect disorder of almost any organ system (see Table 63–1). Although the list is long, most of the conditions mentioned cause the presenting complaint of fatigue only rarely. Indeed, most systematic studies of the

TABLE 63–1. CAUSES OF FATIGUE*

Physiologic	**Endocrine Disorders**
Increased physical exertion	Hyperparathyroidism
Inadequate rest	Hypothyroidism
Sedentary lifestyle	Apathetic "hyperthyroidism"
Environmental stress (e.g., noise, vibration, heat)	Adrenal insufficiency
New physical disability, recent illness, surgery, trauma	Cushing syndrome
	Hypopituitarism
Habit Patterns	Diabetes mellitus
Caffeinism	**Syndromes of Uncertain Etiology**
Alcoholism	Chronic fatigue syndrome
Other substance abuse	Fibromyalgia (fibrositis)
	Sarcoidosis
Psychosocial	Wegener granulomatosis
Depression	**Occult Malignancy**
Dysthymia and grief	**Hematologic Problems**
Anxiety-related disorders	Anemia
Stress reaction	Myeloproliferative syndromes
Pregnancy	**Hepatic Disease**
	Alcoholic hepatitis or cirrhosis
Autoimmune Disorders	**Cardiovascular Disease**
Systemic lupus erythematosus	Low output states
Multiple sclerosis	"Silent" myocardial infarction
Thyroiditis (with or without thyroid dysfunction)	Bradycardias
Rheumatoid arthritis	Mitral valve dysfunction
Myasthenia gravis	**Metabolic Disorders**
Sleep Disorders	Hyponatremia
Sleep apnea	Hypokalemia
Narcolepsy	Hypercalcemia
Infectious Diseases	**Renal Disease**
Mononucleosis	Chronic renal failure
Human immunodeficiency virus infection	**Respiratory Disorders**
Chronic hepatitis B or C virus infection	Chronic obstructive pulmonary disease
Lyme disease	**Miscellaneous**
Fungal disease	Medications
Chronic parasitic infection	Autonomic overactivity
Tuberculosis	Reactive hypoglycemia
Subacute bacterial endocarditis	

*Adapted from a chapter on this subject in the second edition by W. T. Branch, Jr and B. Lown. This list is not meant to be an exhaustive catalog of every illness that can cause chronic fatigue. Rather, it is intended to highlight some of the illnesses that most commonly do so.

complaint of fatigue in a primary care practice indicate that well-characterized organic diseases of any type explain the complaint of fatigue in fewer than 10% of patients.[1–5] This poses a dilemma for the physician. Many diseases, each of which may require a number of different diagnostic tests to help establish the diagnosis, may be present; however, the odds are that none are present. Thus to what extent should the physician go in pursuing organic illness? We address this question later.

Most of the organic diseases that can present with the chief complaint of fatigue are discussed in detail elsewhere in this book and are not discussed in detail here. Only a few points relative to these well-recognized organic diseases are emphasized here.

In our experience, fatigue that has lasted 2 to 6 months after some type of apparently infectious illness is one of the more frequent "organic" conditions found. In patients with a fatigue that is more chronic (lasting 6 months or more), various autoimmune diseases and hypothyroidism (whether of clearly autoimmune etiology, or not) are the most common organic disorders (see Table 63–1). The other organic illnesses listed in Table 63–1 appear to be more infrequent causes of chronic fatigue. Most organic diseases that produce fatigue are usually far enough advanced to be recognizable on history, physical examination, or laboratory testing. For example, fatigue caused by cardiac or respiratory insufficiency is generally accompanied by physical signs (except for occult mitral stenosis), is predictably reproduced by exercise and relieved by rest, and becomes progressively more severe over time. Infectious, neoplastic, and hematologic diseases that produce fatigue also do so in the setting of progressive deterioration and are usually severe or widespread enough to be associated with weight loss, fever, and other symptoms or findings like pallor and lymphadenopathy. Since mild, stable anemia (hematocrit of 32 or greater) produces no more tiredness than is present in age- and sex-matched nonanemic persons,[19] chronic anemia is severe before producing fatigue. Fortunately, many of these conditions can be diagnosed by inexpensive, routine blood tests.

NEITHER CLEARLY ORGANIC NOR PSYCHIATRIC: THE GRAY ZONE OF FATIGUE

Another cause of frustration for the physician, when caring for the patient with fatigue, is that a substantial fraction of patients do not have evidence of either organic nor psychiatric causes of fatigue. In a landmark study of fatigue, Kroenke and colleagues performed a systematic evaluation, including an assessment of organic and psychiatric illness, in several hundred patients.[1] Despite an extensive evaluation, they could not establish a diagnosis in a substantial fraction of the patients: The patients fell into a gray zone in which some features of their illness suggested organic or psychiatric diseases, but they did not meet established diagnostic criteria for any organic or psychiatric disease.

One reason for this is that most organic and psychiatric illnesses become recognizable and definitively diagnosable only when they are at their most severe point. For example, although multiple sclerosis (MS) and lupus are well-recognized organic illnesses, it can be very difficult to make the diagnosis of either disease when the disease is less than full-blown. Indeed, in many patients with mild MS or lupus, the predominant symptom for which they seek medical care is not a focal neurologic deficit, a malar rash, or other characteristic manifestation of the illness; instead, the predominant symptom is fatigue. Sometimes such mild cases of MS and lupus progress over time to the point when the diagnosis becomes clear; in other cases, the illness remains in a gray zone in which clinicians cannot make a definitive diagnosis or in which different clinicians make different diagnoses.

There are also a group of illnesses that remain in a gray zone and that at this time have few objective criteria by which they are defined. These illnesses are of unknown etiology. Although the illnesses have been described by different names in the medical literature for more than 100 years, they are sufficiently similar that some observers suspect that they are all part of the same syndrome. The pathogenesis of this illness (or these illnesses) has not been elucidated. Indeed, no reasonably specific and sensitive diagnostic tests have been developed. Finally, many (but not all) of the symptoms of these illnesses are shared in common with a variety of organic diseases and are also seen frequently in patients with psychiatric illness, particularly depression, anxiety, and somatization disorder. For that reason, some clinicians question whether there really is an underlying organic disorder. The name currently used for this illness is *chronic fatigue syndrome* (CFS).

CHRONIC FATIGUE SYNDROME

Similar Illnesses Throughout History

Neurasthenia (or neurocirculatory asthenia), first described in the mid-19th century, was typically an affliction of young adults, usually women.[20] Patients with neurasthenia complained of chronic malaise that often had started with an acute infectious illness. In the early 20th century, the illness was ascribed to "weakness" of the nervous system and cardiovascular system. When no characteristic objective deficits of the neurologic or cardiovascular system were identified, however, physicians stopped using neurasthenia as a diagnostic label.

Myalgic encephalomyelitis is a very similar chronic fatiguing illness that typically has been described as occurring in epidemic form, affecting hundreds of individuals living in small towns in most parts of the world, or large numbers of coworkers in a large institution.[21–27] Many of these outbreaks have been studied by national public health organizations such as the United States Centers for Disease Control (CDC) and have been described in the medical literature. Myalgic encephalomyelitis has also gone by a variety of other names, including epidemic neuromyasthenia, Akureyri disease, and Icelandic disease.

Typically the illness is heralded by acute respiratory infection symptoms, followed by months or years of profound fatigue, muscular weakness and twitching, muscular pain (especially in the neck, shoulder girdle, low back, and thighs), pharyngitis, nausea, vomiting, abdominal cramps, swelling in the fingers and feet, cognitive problems, emotional instability, depression, insomnia, paresthesias, and a tendency to transpose words. Not infrequently, these patients note that their symptoms worsen in damp weather or in the premenstrual period. A physical examination is often entirely unremarkable, but a substantial number of patients have been reported to have low-grade fevers, adenopathy (especially in the posterior cervical chain), splenomegaly, and nystagmus. Earlier outbreaks have led to disability and work loss lasting for many months or years. The few long-term follow-up studies that have been done suggest gradual improvement in the following years, although many patients continue to experience mild but similar episodes of illness. No particular viral agent has been definitively associated with these syndromes.

Fibromyalgia, originally called fibrositis, is a very common cause of chronic musculoskeletal pain and fatigue. Up to 5% of patients at a general medical clinic and 12% of new patients seen by rheumatologists may have fibromyalgia.[28–32] Indeed, some rheumatologists believe that primary fibromyalgia is the most common rheumatologic condition seen in their practice, particularly in women younger than 50 years of age.[28–32] It has been estimated that 3 to 6 million people in the United States have fibromyalgia.[28, 33, 34]

The chronic pain is accompanied by morning stiffness and increased tenderness at specific sites known as "tender points." A large, systematic study of fibromyalgia conducted by American College of Rheumatology has demonstrated that the tender points occur at characteristic locations and that tenderness is not elicited at other "control" points.[35] Along with the musculoskeletal pain, fibromyalgia is also characterized by poor sleep, headaches, irritable bowel syndrome, and fatigue. Partial or total work disability is common.[36, 37]

Patients with fibromyalgia often have the symptoms characteristic of chronic fatigue syndrome (described later), particularly the sudden onset of their syndrome with an "infectious-like" illness, chronic fevers, sore throat, cough, and adenopathy.[38] Moreover, patients with chronic fatigue syndrome have detectable tender points with a frequency approaching that seen in fibromyalgia and much more often than in healthy control subjects.[39]

In fibromyalgia there is a disturbance in stage 4 deep sleep, in which α waves (typical of the awake, alert state) intrude on the δ wave electroencephalogram (EEG) pattern characteristic of deep sleep; moreover, repeatedly interrupting sleep as healthy volunteers slip into stage 4 sleep produces symptoms and the tender point findings on examination that are consistent with fibromyalgia.[17] This α wave intrusion on δ waves has been seen in most patients studied with chronic fatigue syndrome (described later) and is not characteristically seen in depression. The shortened latency until rapid-eye movement (REM) sleep, which is often seen in depression, is not characteristically seen in fibromyalgia.

Chronic Epstein-Barr Virus Infection Syndrome. Infection with Epstein-Barr virus (EBV) is ubiquitous and permanent: More than 90% of adults in the developed nations are infected. This chronic infection is not associated with illness in most individuals. The virus is generally dormant: The viral DNA takes up residence in B lymphocytes and other cells, but the virus does not reproduce itself. In the mid-1980s, several reports associated increased levels of antibodies to EBV, an antibody pattern suggesting that the virus had been reactivated from its normally dormant state, with a syndrome characterized by chronic fatigue and other symptoms.[40–47] This led some to conclude that the syndrome might be caused by reactivation of EBV. Subsequent research has indicated, however, that reactivation of EBV (associated with modest elevations of EBV-VCA-IgG and anti-early antigens, such as had been noted in the patients with chronic fatigue) is not uncommon in healthy individuals.[48] The syndrome originally misnamed "chronic EBV infection" syndrome is better called CFS because there is no convincing evidence that the illness is caused by EBV, except perhaps in a few cases.

Chronic mononucleosis may be an example of a chronic, fatiguing illness associated with EBV.[49, 50] First described 40 years ago, chronic mononucleosis starts with classical acute infectious mononucleosis, as characterized by clinical, hematologic, and serologic features.[51] However, instead of recovering, these patients remain ill for years. Some of them have serologic evidence of persistently active EBV infection (persistent heterophil antibody or clearly elevated antibodies to EBV), although in our experience there are some patients who remain chronically ill but whose EBV serologic studies become unremarkable. For this reason, although this chronic illness clearly begins with a well-characterized acute viral infection—mononucleosis caused by EBV—the role of EBV, or other organic factors, in producing the chronic fatiguing illness remains uncertain.

Severe chronic active EBV infection is a rare illness that can produce chronic fatigue.[42, 52] This illness often, but not always, follows acute infectious mononucleosis, like chronic mononucleosis. Indeed, it may represent the most severe form of chronic mononucleosis. These patients all have strikingly abnormal levels of antibodies against EBV, particularly IgG antibodies to the viral capsid antigen and viral early antigens. Many of these patients also have evidence of major organ involvement, such as recurrent interstitial pneumonia, persistent non-A, non-B hepatitis, splenomegaly and adenopathy, or pancytopenia or selective cytopenia. Again, the parsimonious explanation is that these patients have an illness related to EBV infection in which immunologic containment of EBV is impaired.

Clinical Presentation of Chronic Fatigue Syndrome

Case Definitions. As stated earlier, the illness now called CFS was defined in a case definition developed by the CDC, and summarized in Table 63–2.[53] Somewhat less restrictive case definitions also have been developed by British and Australian investigators.[54, 55] The CDC case definition relies entirely on a combination of symptoms and signs (not laboratory data) and on the exclusion of chronic active organic or psychiatric illnesses that can produce chronic fatigue.

Symptoms. As summarized in Table 63–3, CFS is characterized by varying degrees of chronic fatigue, and chronic or recurrent fever, pharyngitis, myalgias, headache, arthralgias, paresthesias, depression, and cognitive deficits. These symptoms are regularly experienced by most patients in the months and years *after* the acute onset of the illness but were not experienced regularly by these patients in the years *before* the onset of the illness.[56] Typically, the chronic illness begins abruptly with an acute "infectious-like" syndrome that includes respiratory or gastrointestinal symptoms, with associated fever, myalgias, and arthralgias. The onset of the syndrome typically seems to be in young adulthood,[40–42, 44–47] although it may also begin in childhood or later in life.[46] By definition (see Table 63–2), there is no evidence of rheumatologic, endocrinologic, infectious, malignant, or other chronic diseases and no pre-existing and chronic psychiatric disease. The diagnosis has been made about twice as often in women as in men. Almost all patients perceive themselves to be impaired in some way. Some patients are completely disabled by the fatigue, muscular weakness, and pain.

Of the principal symptoms of CFS (see Table 63–2) three are particularly remarkable: (1) the sudden onset with a "flu-like" illness; (2) the chronic postexertional malaise; and (3) chronic night sweats. In more than 85% of the patients who we have seen with this illness, the chronic debility began suddenly with a "flu-like" illness; the patient had been functioning very well, then one day became acutely ill

TABLE 63–2. WORKING CASE DEFINITION OF CHRONIC FATIGUE SYNDROME*

A case of chronic fatigue syndrome must fulfill major criteria 1 and 2 and the following minor criteria: 6 or more of the 11-symptom criteria and 2 or more of the 3 physical criteria; or 8 or more of the 11-symptom criteria.

Major Criteria

1. New onset of persistent or relapsing, debilitating fatigue or easy fatigability in a person who has no previous history of similar symptoms that do not resolve with bedrest and that are severe enough to produce or impair average daily activity below 50% of the patient's premorbid activity level, for a period of at least 6 months.
2. Other clinical conditions that may produce similar symptoms must be excluded by thorough evaluation, based on history, physical examination, and appropriate laboratory findings. These conditions include malignancy; autoimmune disease; localized infection (e.g., occult abscess); chronic or subacute bacterial disease (e.g., endocarditis, Lyme disease, or tuberculosis), fungal disease (e.g., histoplasmosis, blastomycosis, or coccidioidomycosis), and parasitic disease (e.g., toxoplasmosis, amebiasis, giardiasis, or helminthic infestation); disease related to human immunodeficiency virus (HIV) infection; chronic psychiatric disease, either newly diagnosed by history (e.g., endogenous depression; hysterical personality disorder; anxiety neurosis; schizophrenia) or inferred from chronic use of major tranquilizers, lithium, or antidepressive medications; chronic inflammatory disease (e.g., sarcoidosis, Wegener's granulomatosis, or chronic hepatitis); neuromuscular disease (e.g., multiple sclerosis or myasthenia gravis); endocrine disease (e.g., hypothyroidism, Addison's disease, Cushing's syndrome, or diabetes mellitus); drug dependency or abuse (e.g., alcohol, controlled prescription drugs, or illicit drugs); side effects of a chronic medication or other toxic agent (e.g., a chemical solvent, pesticide, or heavy metal); or other known or defined chronic pulmonary, cardiac, gastrointestinal, hepatic, renal, or hematologic disease.

Minor Criteria

Symptom Criteria

To fulfill a symptom criterion, a symptom must have begun at or after the time of onset of increased fatigability and must have persisted or recurred for at least 6 months (individual symptoms may or may not have occurred simultaneously).

Symptoms include:

1. Mild fever—oral temperature between 37.5° C and 38.6° C, if measured by the patient—or chills (Note: oral temperatures of greater than 38.6° C are less compatible with chronic fatigue syndrome and should prompt studies for other causes of illness.)
2. Sore throat
3. Painful lymph nodes in the anterior or posterior cervical or axillary distribution
4. Unexplained generalized muscle weakness
5. Muscle discomfort or myalgia
6. Prolonged (24 hours or greater) generalized fatigue after levels of exercise that would have been easily tolerated in the patient's premorbid state
7. Generalized headaches (of a type, severity, or pattern that is different from headaches that the patient may have had in the premorbid state)
8. Migratory arthralgia without joint swelling or redness
9. Neuropsychological complaints (one or more of the following: photophobia, transient visual scotomata, forgetfulness, excessive irritability, confusion, difficulty thinking, inability to concentrate, depression)
10. Sleep disturbance (hypersomnia or insomnia)
11. Description of the main symptom complex as initially developing over a few hours to a few days (this is not a true symptom but may be considered as equivalent to the aforementioned symptoms in meeting the requirements of the case definition)

Physical Examination Criteria

Physical criteria must be documented by a physician on at least two occasions, at least 1 month apart.

1. Low-grade fever—oral temperature between 37.6° C and 38.6° C or rectal temperature between 37.8° C and 38.8° C (see note under Symptom Criterion 1)
2. Nonexudative pharyngitis
3. Palpable or tender anterior or posterior cervical or axillary lymph nodes. (Note: lymph nodes greater than 2 cm in diameter suggest other causes. Further evaluation is warranted.)

*Reproduced with permission, from Holmes GP, Kaplan JE, Gant NM, et al: Chronic fatigue syndrome: A working case definition. Ann Intern Med 108:387–389, 1988.

TABLE 63–3. FREQUENCY OF SYMPTOMS AND SIGNS IN CHRONIC FATIGUE SYNDROME*

Symptom/sign	Frequency (%)
Fatigue	75–100
Low-grade fever (by self-report)	60–95
Low-grade fever (at the time of examination)	5–30
Myalgias	30–95
Depression (following the onset of CFS)	70–85
Headaches	35–85
Pharyngitis	50–70
Impaired cognition	50–70
Sleep disorder	15–70
Anxiety (following the onset of CFS)	50–70
Adenopathy	40–60
Nausea	50–60
Arthralgias	40–60
Diarrhea	30–40
Cough	30–40
Odd skin sensations	30–40
Rash	30–40
Weight loss	20–30
Weight gain	50–70
Low basal body temperature (95.0–97.6° F)	10–20

*Adapted from our experience plus that of others.[45–47]
CFS = chronic fatigue syndrome.

(patients can often remember the exact day and date) and have been seriously impaired for at least 6 months thereafter. Patients typically say that their CFS "all began with that virus."

The postexertional malaise is characterized not only by symptoms that could simply represent deconditioning—pain and weakness of the involved muscles—but also by exacerbation of "systemic" symptoms (e.g., fatigue, fevers, pharyngitis, adenopathy, and impaired cognition). The night sweats are drenching and require changes of bedclothes and sheets.

While some of the symptoms of CFS are also characteristic of depression, generalized anxiety disorder, and somatization disorder (e.g., headaches, myalgias, sleep disturbance, difficulty with concentration), other symptoms are not (e.g., the sudden onset, recurrent fevers, adenopathy, arthralgias, photophobia). Moreover, several investigators have argued that the fact that these symptoms typically started abruptly in the context of an acute "infectious"-type illness also suggests that the symptoms are not likely to be caused exclusively by a psychiatric disorder.

In our experience, a few patients with this disorder have had transient acute neurologic events, typically in the first 6 months of the illness: primary seizures; acute, profound ataxia; focal weakness; transient blindness; and unilateral paresthesias (not in a dermatomal distribution). Similar acute and transient neurologic events have also been reported occasionally in outbreaks of myalgic encephalomyelitis.

Past Medical History. Although most elements of the past medical history are unremarkable in patients with CFS, there is a strikingly high frequency of atopic or allergic illness: 60 to 80% of patients with CFS have longstanding atopic disorders versus approximately 10% of the general population.[57–59]

Physical Examination. A few physical examination findings may be seen more often in patients with CFS than in healthy subjects, although this remains to be determined from controlled studies with blinded observers: fevers; unusually low basal body temperature ($< 97°F$); posterior cervical adenopathy; and abnormal tests of balance (Romberg and tandem gait).

Standard Laboratory Testing. Standard laboratory testing is generally unremarkable in CFS. Controlled studies have demonstrated that a few abnormalities may occur more frequently in patients with CFS than in healthy control subjects of similar age and sex: circulating immune complexes, elevated levels of IgG, atypical lymphocytosis; elevated alkaline phosphatase; depressed lactic dehydrogenase; and elevated total cholesterol.[60] However, none of these abnormalities is seen in more than 50% of patients with CFS; thus, none constitutes a sufficiently sensitive diagnostic test. Moreover, each can be seen in other disorders; thus, none is a sufficiently specific test.

Immunologic Testing. A large and growing literature reports immunologic abnormalities in patients with CFS.[61] In general, the picture that is emerging indicates that in many patients with CFS all arms of the immune system seem to be chronically activated, with cytotoxic T lymphocytes and natural killer lymphocytes demonstrating impaired function that could be interpreted as exhaustion secondary to a state of chronic activation. Thus, it appears that the immune system is chronically waging a battle against antigens that it perceives as foreign.

Although not all reports of immune function in CFS come to consistent conclusions, a few immunologic abnormalities have been found by multiple investigators studying different groups of patients with CFS. The first is impaired function of natural killer cells.[62–66] Since these lymphocytes play a central role in the immunologic containment of viral infections, the observation that they have impaired function in CFS is of particular interest. The second is circulating immune complexes,[47] in low levels and without evidence of immune-complex–mediated disease; these immune complexes are considered to represent some chronic immunologic response to antigens that are perceived by the immune system as foreign. Several investigators also have reported T lymphocyte dysfunction, as reflected by anergy and reduced T cell lymphoproliferative responses after stimulation with various mitogens and antigens.[65, 67, 68]

A widely held hypothesis is that the state of chronic immune activation leads to the chronic "overproduction" of various immune system mediators, cytokines such as interferon-α, interleukin-6, tumor necrosis factor, interleukin-1, and interleukin-2. It is well established that many of these cytokines can produce most of the symptoms that are characteristic of CFS: fatigue, fevers, adenopathy, myalgias, arthralgias, sleep disorders, cognitive impairment, and mood disorders. Technical problems have limited careful study of this hypothesis, and to date the results have been inconclusive.

Whereas these studies have all demonstrated objective differences in immunologic parameters among patients with CFS and healthy control subjects, more work needs to be done to determine whether these abnormalities also distinguish CFS from various organic and psychiatric diseases that can also produce chronic fatigue.

Neurologic Studies. One large study of patients from one geographic area has found areas of abnormal signal in the white matter of the central nervous system by magnetic resonance images (MRI); such areas of abnormal signal were seen much more often in patients with CFS than in healthy control subjects of similar age and sex.[61] Studies are underway of other neurologic tests of the brain—particularly evoked potentials, cognitive evoked potentials, BEAM-scanning, and single photon-emission positron tomography (SPECT)—because of preliminary data suggesting abnormalities of these tests in patients with CFS.

Neuroendocrine Studies. An abnormality of the hypothalamic-pituitary-adrenal (HPA) axis has been demonstrated in CFS: diminished secretion by the hypothalamus of corticotropin-releasing hormone (CRH), leading to diminished secretion of adrenocorticotropic hormone (ACTH) by the pituitary, leading to diminished production of cortisol by the adrenal glands.[69] The basal hypocortisolism is not in the Addisonian range but is clearly different from what is seen in healthy control subjects. Either the low cortisol levels or the low CRH levels could produce fatigue. This abnormality of the HPA axis is the opposite of what is seen in patients suffering from major depression.

Infectious Disease Studies. Although CFS can apparently begin following a variety of stressful noninfectious events (e.g., major surgery, accidents, and severe allergic reactions), it typically begins suddenly with an "infectious-like" illness. However, in most cases of CFS, the "infectious-like" illness that has allegedly initiated the chronic illness has not been carefully studied. For this reason, some observers are skeptical that CFS is associated with infection.

Yet, as stated earlier, an illness like CFS can be associated with very well-characterized EBV infection. CFS has also been seen following documented influenza virus infection and acute parvovirus infection.[70, 71] CFS has also been found in patients with proven Lyme disease who have received adequate antibacterial treatment and in whom the cardinal manifestations of Lyme disease (e.g., arthritis, carditis) have resolved.[72] CFS also has been described following in the wake of a variety of acute infections.[43, 73–77]

At this time, these associations between specific infectious agents and CFS are anecdotal case reports. It is not clear how frequently these infectious agents may trigger CFS; however, these cases document that an acute infection can trigger a chronic illness, even though the nature of the chronic illness, including the ongoing role of the triggering agent, remains obscure.

In addition to these studies that document an acute infection as the initiating event in CFS, there are a variety of studies of infectious agents in patients long after the CFS has begun. Several studies have incriminated the *enteroviruses* in some cases of CFS. Enteroviral nucleic acid has been found much more often in the muscle of patients with CFS than in healthy control subjects,[78–80] and enteroviral antigen has been found more frequently in the stool and serum of patients with CFS.[81] Enteroviruses can produce chronic, persistent infection and are both lymphotropic and neurotropic.

A recently discovered member of the herpesvirus family—*human herpesvirus-6* (HHV-6)—has been found to be actively replicating more often in patients with CFS than in matched healthy control subjects.[61] Most humans become permanently infected with HHV-6 in childhood. To date, the evidence indicates that reactivation of a long dor-

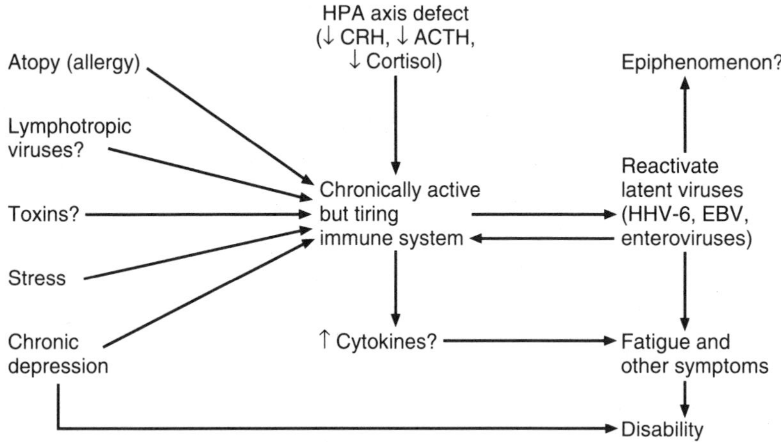

FIGURE 63–1. Current favorite model.

mant infection with HHV-6, rather than new infection with HHV-6, is present in CFS. Thus, the active HHV-6 infection most likely represents a secondary phenomenon in CFS. As such, it could be an epiphenomenon that has nothing to do with the illness. Alternatively, even if the reactivation of HHV-6 is a secondary phenomenon, the reactivated virus could contribute to the symptoms of the illness: HHV-6, too, is a lymphotropic and neurotropic virus.

Several research teams are evaluating the possibility that novel *retroviruses* are involved in some cases of CFS. A few cases of chronic human T cell lymphotropic virus type 1 (HTLV-I) and HTLV-II infection have been documented in patients who have CFS and no other HTLV-associated illness. Surely, an occasional individual must develop a CFS-like syndrome following human immunodeficiency virus (HIV) infection, and before acquired immunodeficiency syndrome (AIDS)–related complications develop, although no such case has yet been reported. One team has found indirect evidence that a novel retrovirus, related to but different from HTLV-II, may be related to some cases of CFS[82]; as of this writing, no direct evidence of a novel retrovirus has been found, however, and recent research has contradicted even the previously reported indirect evidence.[82a]

Psychological Studies. Much confusion has resulted from a failure to distinguish chronic fatigue, a common problem for which patients seek medical attention, from CFS. As stated at the outset, most patients seeking medical care for chronic fatigue are probably suffering from depression or anxiety disorders or somatization disorder. Moreover, most patients seeking medical care for chronic fatigue probably do not have CFS.[1, 83]

But, however rare they are among all patients with fatigue, do patients with CFS have psychiatric disorders? If so, how often? Have they suffered from psychiatric disorders in the years *before* the onset of their CFS, or only *after*? Most studies of the question find that most patients with CFS *become* depressed and anxious following the (usually sudden) onset of their disorder.[84–88] For many patients, the depression and anxiety become the most debilitating parts of their illness. At the same time, these studies also indicate that a substantial fraction of patients with CFS (25 to 50%) have no evidence of any active psychiatric disorder since the onset of CFS.

By and large the studies find a higher past history of psychiatric disorders in patients with CFS than in the population at large: The average across all studies is around 30% (range of 20 to 50%) of patients with CFS.[84–89] On one hand, this past history of psychiatric disorders is greater than is found in the population at large (range of 5 to 10%); on the other hand, despite extensive psychiatric evaluation, no evidence of a pre-existing psychiatric disorder can be found in most patients with CFS.

Model for the Pathogenesis of Chronic Fatigue Syndrome

Most students of CFS believe that the illness can have both physical and psychological factors. And, as with any illness, the degree of disability seen in CFS must be due, in part, to physical and psychological factors. As summarized in Figure 63–1, many believe that CFS is mainly an immunologic disturbance—one that allows reactivation of latent and ineradicable infectious agents, particularly viruses. The reactivation of these viruses may only be an epiphenomenon. Alternatively, once secondarily reactivated, these viruses may contribute to the morbidity of CFS—directly, by damaging certain tissues (e.g., the pharyngeal mucosa), and indirectly, by eliciting an ongoing immunologic response in which a variety of cytokines are chronically elaborated, as discussed earlier.

What triggers the immune dysfunction in the first place? As summarized in Figure 63–1, many factors could do so: atopic disorders, exogenous lymphotropic infectious agents, environmental toxins, stress, and even the biology of an underlying affective disorder. The recently described neuraxis abnormality that results in a basal hypocortisolism could also render the immune system "hyper-responsive" to antigenic stimulation, contributing to the state of chronic activation and partial exhaustion described earlier. Clearly, CFS seems likely to have a multifactorial etiology, like most illnesses.

Although psychological illness is not found in a substantial fraction of patients with CFS, it could well be playing a role in other patients with CFS. The somewhat higher history of psychiatric illness in patients with CFS than in the population at large could indicate that in some patients CFS is depression expressed with predominantly somatic symptoms; or it could indicate that CFS is triggered by an organic illness (e.g., an infection) that is followed and perhaps supplanted by the re-emergence of an underlying depression; or it could indicate that the biologic underpinnings of depression somehow render one vulnerable to the "organic" abnormalities (e.g., the immunologic and virologic findings) seen in CFS; or, in the individual patient, more than one of these factors may be operative.

Instead of asking whether CFS is a disease of the mind or the body, it may be more useful to consider CFS and other illnesses as conditions in which mind and body are inevitably linked. In the case of CFS, biologic forces that increase the likelihood of affective disorder may also increase vulnerability to disorders of immunity. In patients with CFS, who have a current or past affective disorder and who also have evidence of immune dysfunction and active viral infection, it may never be possible to determine whether the affective disorder, the immune dysfunction, or the viral infection came first. Rather, the practical question is what form of management will be most effective: psychotherapy, pharmacotherapy of the affective disorder, "immune modulating" pharmacotherapy, antimicrobial therapy, or some combination of these. There are no good studies of these important issues at this time.

TABLE 63–4. SYMPTOMS AND SIGNS SUGGESTING UNDERLYING ORGANIC DISORDER

Symptoms
Weight loss >10%
Persistent or recurrent fevers
Adenopathy
Rashes
Arthralgias
Arthritis
Morning stiffness
Gelling (stiffness after remaining in one position, such as lying or sitting, for several hours)
Persistent vomiting
Persistent diarrhea
Night sweats
Postexertional malaise
Photophobia
Paresthesias
Transient focal neurologic deficits

MANAGEMENT OF FATIGUE

Initial Interview

Assessment of Underlying Psychiatric Disorders. For the very commonly encountered patient with fatigue or other somatic symptoms related to depression or anxiety, the interview serves as both a diagnostic and therapeutic tool. The process of making the psychiatric diagnosis also serves to make the patient aware of how his or her feelings relate to the symptoms, which is an essential first step in management. Thus, the patient's emotional status is explored while the medical history is being obtained. A simple interviewing technique can be based on the biopsychosocial approach developed by Engel and by the medical interviewing techniques developed by Bird and Cohen-Cole.[90–92] These techniques are discussed in detail in Chapters 76 and 81. In attempting to elicit submerged information, it is important to remember that occult alcohol abuse (and other forms of substance abuse) often produces chronic fatigue, either directly as a result of chronic intoxication, or indirectly through its disruptive effects on sleep or its production of inflammatory disease of the liver. The subject of substance abuse is covered in Chapter 83.

Assessment of Underlying Organic Disorders. Although underlying psychiatric disorders are very common in patients with fatigue, and even though the interview may suggest that the patient has a current or lifetime psychiatric diagnosis, it is nevertheless important to assess the possible presence of concomitant organic illness. The depression itself can result from the patient's awareness of an impending or actual change in health status (see Chapter 77). Any symptom that is not consistent with the psychological diagnosis or any finding on physical examination must be rigorously assessed. A list of such symptoms is contained in Table 63–4. All symptoms greatly raise the likelihood of an underlying organic disorder.

In the patient with fatigue of modest severity and relatively short duration (e.g., 1 to 3 months) who probably is most typical of patients seeking medical care for fatigue, no laboratory testing may be warranted. This is particularly true when the patient clearly has enough "lifestyle" features to explain fatigue, when a psychological disorder is deemed likely, and when no other symptoms suggest an organic abnormality.

In patients with fatigue of greater duration (6 months or more) or severity (significantly interfering with their ability to work or maintain their responsibilities at home), a modest screening evaluation is warranted to look for evidence of an underlying organic disorder. A panel of tests recommended by a National Institute of Health conference is shown in Table 63–5. Although not all of these tests are highly sensitive for organic disease (e.g., erythrocyte sedimentation rate) nor highly specific for any particular disease, they serve as a useful screen for organic illness. The various immunologic, neurologic, and virologic tests mentioned in the discussion of CFS should be considered experimental and not appropriate for general use at this time.

Treatment of Suspected Chronic Fatigue Syndrome

Low-Dose Tricyclic Drugs. Few treatments have been carefully studied in CFS. Randomized, controlled trials have shown that low-dose tricyclic drugs reduce the level of fatigue, musculoskeletal pain, and objectively demonstrable tender points in patients with fibromyalgia.[93] Given the similarities between CFS and fibromyalgia, many physicians have tried the same therapy in CFS. While no controlled trial of low-dose tricyclics has been mounted in CFS, it is the general experience of most physicians that such treatment clearly improves the quality of sleep; as a consequence, perhaps, many patients state that their fatigue, myalgias, arthralgias, and cognitive problems also improve. The α-δ sleep disorder that has been found in both fibromyalgia and CFS improves with low-dose tricyclic therapy; thus, there is objective confirmation of the experience reported by patients.

The tricyclics most often used for CFS are either amitriptyline or doxepin, 10 to 20 mg po before bedtime. Interest-

TABLE 63–5. CASE-FINDING LABORATORY TESTS*

Complete blood count
Manual differential white blood cell count (unless automated counts accurately determine atypical lymphocytes)
Erythrocyte sedimentation rate (Westergren technique)
Chemistry panel including assessment of renal and hepatic function, glucose, electrolytes, calcium, phosphate, total cholesterol, albumin, and globulin
Thyroid function tests (highly sensitive thyroid-stimulating hormone is sufficient)
Antinuclear antibodies and rheumatoid factor, if there are prominent arthralgias and myalgias
Urinalysis

*Adapted from National Institutes of Health conference, March 1991.

ingly, most patients with CFS cannot tolerate doses of tricyclic drugs usually used for depression (e.g., amitriptyline, 100 to 300 mg/day). Indeed, few can tolerate more than 50 mg of amitriptyline. Even with low doses, such as 10 mg of amitriptyline at bedtime, most patients with CFS report increased somnolence and fatigue in the morning for about the first week of therapy. Patients should be warned of this transient adverse effect and urged to continue for at least 1 to 2 months before drawing any conclusions about the efficacy of the therapy.

In patients with concomitant depression and a sleep disorder, we have often used sertraline 25 to 50 mg each morning combined with low-dose tricyclics at bedtime. As with tricyclics and all other central nervous system–active substances, patients with CFS often cannot tolerate usual doses of sertraline. Also, the sleep-disruptive potential of sertraline may be greater in CFS, leading to the recommendation that this medication be taken in the morning.

In our experience, treatment of a concomitant depression by psychotherapy or pharmacotherapy, in patients with CFS, often reduces the mood disorder; however, it rarely eliminates the fatigue, cognitive problems, myalgias, arthralgias, postexertional malaise, respiratory tract symptoms, fevers, and adenopathy.

Other Treatments. One controlled study has shown no benefit from one antiviral agent, acyclovir[94]; that medication, however, has little in vitro effect on the viruses that have been associated with CFS. Controlled trials of gamma globulin have come to conflicting conclusions.[95, 96] One randomized study reported a magnesium deficiency in CFS and a benefit from magnesium therapy[97]; that study was subsequently subjected to much criticism. A large number of treatments, some of which have a reasonable conceptual basis, have been proposed but not studied. As with any illness for which no definitive therapy exists, a variety of unconventional therapies have been used.

Nonpharmaceutical Treatments. Patients should be encouraged to be as active as possible but to avoid activities that involve intensive physical or emotional stress. The role of exercise in CFS is controversial. Limbering exercises are recommended by almost all physicians who are experienced in treating this disorder. Some physicians recommend a program of very gradually increasing aerobic exercises. In some patients, this seems to be well tolerated, but in others it leads to relapses, including recurrence of fevers and adenopathy. Cognitive behavior therapy is beneficial in some patients.[98]

REFERENCES

1. Kroenke K, Wood DR, Mangelsdorff AD, et al: Chronic fatigue in primary care: Prevalence, patient characteristics, and outcome. JAMA 260:929–934, 1988.
2. Allan FN: The differential diagnosis of weakness and fatigue. N Engl J Med 231:414–418, 1944.
3. Morrison JD: Fatigue as a presenting complaint in family practice. J Fam Pract 10:795–801, 1980.
4. Katerndahl DA: Fatigue of uncertain etiology. Fam Med Rev 1:26–38, 1983.
5. Nelson E, Kirk J, McHugo G, et al: Chief complaint fatigue: A longitudinal study from the patient's perspective. Fam Pract Res J 6:175–188, 1987.
6. Solberg LI: Lassitude: A primary care evaluation. JAMA 251:3272–3276, 1984.
7. Cox B, Blaxter M, Buckle A, et al: The Health and Lifestyle Survey. London, Health Promotion Research Trust, 1987, pp 61–62.
8. Schor JB: The Overworked American: The Unexpected Decline of Leisure. New York, Basic Books, 1992.
9. Dement W: The Sleepwatchers. Stanford CA, Stanford University Press, 1992.
10. Kroenke K, Arrington ME, and Mangelsdorff AD: The prevalence of symptoms in medical outpatients and the adequacy of therapy. Arch Intern Med 150:1685–1689, 1990.
11. Stoeckle JD, Zola IK, and Davidson GE: The quantity and significance of psychological distress in medical patients. J Chronic Dis 17:959–970, 1964.
12. Reifler BV, Okimoto JT, Heidrich FE, and Inui TS: Recognition of depression in a university-based family medicine residency program. J Fam Pract 9:623–628, 1979.
13. Hoeper EW, Nycz GR, Cleary PD, et al: Estimated prevalence of RDC mental disorder in primary medical care. Int J Ment Health 8:6–15, 1979.
14. Nielsen ACI and Williams TA: Depression in ambulatory medical patients. Arch Gen Psychiatry 37:999–1004, 1980.
15. Kessler LG, Cleary PD, and Burke JD: Psychiatric disorders in primary care. Arch Gen Psychiatry 42:583–587, 1985.
16. Barsky AJI: Hidden reasons some patients visit doctors. Ann Intern Med 94:492–498, 1981.
17. Moldofsky H and Scarisbrick P: Induction of neurasthenic musculoskeletal pain syndrome by selective sleep stage deprivation. Psychosom Med 38:35–44, 1976.
18. Littlejohn GO, Weinstein C, and Helme RD: Increased neurogenic inflammation in fibrositis syndrome. J Rheumatol 14:1022–1025, 1987.
19. Elwood PC, Waters WE, Greene WJW, and Sweetnam P: Symptoms and circulating haemoglobin level. J Chronic Dis 21:615–628, 1969.
20. Paul O: DaCosta's syndrome or neurocirculatory asthenia. Br Heart J 58:306–315, 1987.
21. Sigurdsson B, Sigurjonsson J, Sigurdsson JHJ, et al: A disease epidemic in Iceland simulating poliomyelitis. Am J Hyg 52:222–238, 1950.
22. Sigurdsson B and Gudmundsson KR: Clinical findings six years after outbreak of Akureyri disease. Lancet i:766–767, 1956.
23. Shelokov A, Habel K, Verder E, and Welsh W: Epidemic neuromyasthenia: An outbreak of poliomyelitis-like illness in student nurses. N Engl J Med 257:345–355, 1957.
24. Poskanzer DC, Henderson DA, Kunkle EC, et al: Epidemic neuromyasthenia: An outbreak in Punta Gorda, Florida. N Engl J Med 257:356–364, 1957.
25. Medical staff of the Royal Free Hospital: An outbreak of encephalomyelitis in the Royal Free Hospital Group, London, in 1955. BMJ 2:895–904, 1957.
26. Acheson ED: The clinical syndrome variously called benign myalgic encephalomyelitis, Iceland disease and epidemic neuromyasthenia. Am J Med 4:569–595, 1959.
27. Henderson DA, and Shelokov A: Epidemic neuromyasthenia—clinical syndrome. N Engl J Med 260:757–764, 1959.
28. Yunus M, Masi AT, Calabro JJ, et al: Primary fibromyalgia (fibrositis): Clinical study of 50 patients with matched normal controls. Semin Arthritis Rheum 11:151–171, 1981.
29. Goldenberg DL: Fibromyalgia syndrome: An emerging but controversial condition. JAMA 257:2782–2803, 1987.
30. Wolfe F, Cathey MA, and Kleinheksel SM: Fibrositis (fibromyalgia) in rheumatoid arthritis. J Rheumatol 11:814–818, 1984.
31. Dinerman H, Goldenberg DL, and Felson DT: A prospective evaluation of 118 patients with the fibromyalgia syndrome: Prevalence of Raynaud's phenomenon, sicca symptoms, ANA, low complement, and Ig deposition at the dermal-epidermal junction. J Rheumatol 13:368–373, 1986.
32. Felson DT and Goldenberg DL: The natural history of fibromyalgia. Arthritis Rheum 29:1522–1526, 1986.
33. Wolfe F and Cathey MA: Prevalence of primary and secondary fibrositis. J Rheumatol 10:965–968, 1983.
34. Campbell SM, Clark S, Tindall ES, et al: Clinical characteristics of fibrositis. I: A "blinded" controlled study of symptoms and tender points. Arthritis Rheum 26:132–137, 1983.
35. Wolfe F, Smythe HA, Yunus MB, et al: The American College of Rheumatology 1990 criteria for the classification of fibromyalgia. Report of the Multicenter Criteria Committee. Arthritis Rheum 33:160–172, 1990.
36. Cathey MA, Wolfe F, Kleinheksel SM, and Hawley DJ: Socioeconomic impact of fibrositis. Am J Med 81:578–584, 1986.

37. Wolfe F and Cathey MA: Assessment of functional ability in patients with fibromyalgia. Arch Intern Med 150:460, 1990.
38. Buchwald D, Goldenberg DL, Sullivan JL, and Komaroff AL: The "chronic, active Epstein-Barr virus infection" syndrome and primary fibromyalgia. Arthritis Rheum 30:1132–1136, 1987.
39. Goldenberg DL, Simms RW, Geiger A, and Komaroff AL: High frequency of fibromyalgia in patients with chronic fatigue seen in a primary care practice. Arthritis Rheum 33:381–387, 1990.
40. Tobi M, Morag A, Ravid Z, et al: Prolonged atypical illness associated with serologic evidence of persistent Epstein-Barr virus infection. Lancet i:61–64, 1982.
41. Ballow M, Seeley J, Purtilo DT, et al: Familial chronic mononucleosis. Ann Intern Med 97:821–825, 1982.
42. Edson CM, Cohen LK, Henle W, and Strominger JL: An unusually high-titer human anti-Epstein Barr virus (EBV) serum and its use in the study of EBV-specific proteins synthesized in vitro and in vivo. J Immunol 130:919–924, 1983.
43. Salit IE: Sporadic postinfectious neuromyasthenia. Can Med Assoc J 133:659–663, 1985.
44. Hamblin TJ, Hussain J, Akbar AN, et al: Immunological reason for chronic ill health after infectious mononucleosis. BMJ 287:85–88, 1983.
45. DuBois RE, Seeley JK, Brus I, et al: Chronic mononucleosis syndrome. South Med J 77:1376–1382, 1984.
46. Jones JF, Ray CG, Minnich LL, et al: Evidence for active Epstein-Barr virus infection in patients with persistent unexplained illnesses: Elevated anti-early antigen antibodies. Ann Intern Med 102:1–7, 1985.
47. Straus SE, Tosato G, Armstrong G, et al: Persisting illness and fatigue in adults with evidence of Epstein-Barr virus infection. Ann Intern Med 102:7–16, 1985.
48. Horwitz CA, Henle W, Henle G, et al: Long-term serological follow-up of patients for Epstein-Barr virus after recovery from infectious mononucleosis. J Infect Dis 151:1150–1153, 1985.
49. Komaroff AL: The "chronic mononucleosis" syndromes. Hosp Pract 22:71–75, 1987.
50. Straus SE: The chronic mononucleosis syndrome. J Infect Dis 157:405–412, 1988.
51. Isaacs R: Chronic infectious mononucleosis. Blood 3:858–861, 1948.
52. Schooley RT, Carey RW, Miller G, et al: Chronic Epstein-Barr virus infection associated with fever and interstitial pneumonitis: Clinical and serologic features and response to antiviral chemotherapy. Ann Intern Med 104:636–643, 1986.
53. Holmes GP, Kaplan JE, Gantz NM, et al: Chronic fatigue syndrome: A working case definition. Ann Intern Med 108:387–389, 1988.
54. Sharpe MC, Archard LC, Banatvala JE, et al: A report—chronic fatigue syndrome: Guidelines in research. J R Soc Med 84:118–121, 1991.
55. Lloyd AR, Hickie I, Boughton CR, et al: Prevalence of chronic fatigue syndrome in an Australian population. Med J Aust 153:522–528, 1990.
56. Komaroff AL and Buchwald D: Symptoms and signs of chronic fatigue syndrome. Rev Infect Dis 13:S8–S11, 1991.
57. Olson GB, Kanaan MN, Gersuk GM, et al: Correlation between allergy and persistent Epstein-Barr virus infections in chronic active Epstein-Barr virus-infected patients. J Allergy Clin Immunol 78:308–314, 1986.
58. Olson GB, Kanaan MN, Kelley LM, and Jones JF: Specific allergen-induced Epstein-Barr nuclear antigen-positive B cells from patients with chronic-active Epstein-Barr virus infections. J Allergy Clin Immunol 78:315–320, 1986.
59. Straus SE, Dale JK, Wright R, and Metcalfe DD: Allergy and the chronic fatigue syndrome. J Allergy Clin Immunol 81:791–795, 1988.
60. Bates DW, Buchwald D, Lee J, et al: Laboratory abnormalities in patients with the chronic fatigue syndrome. Clin Res 40:552A, 1992.
61. Buchwald D, Cheney PR, Peterson DL, et al: A chronic illness characterized by fatigue, neurologic and immunologic disorders, and active human herpesvirus type 6 infection. Ann Intern Med 116:103–113, 1992.
62. Caligiuri M, Murray C, Buchwald D, et al: Phenotypic and functional deficiency of natural killer cells in patients with chronic fatigue syndrome. J Immunol 139:3306–3313, 1987.
63. Aoki T, Usuda Y, Miyakoshi H, et al: Low natural killer syndrome: Clinical and immunologic features. Nat Immun Cell Growth Regul 6:116–128, 1987.
64. Kibler R, Lucas DO, Hicks MJ, et al: Immune function in chronic active Epstein-Barr virus infection. J Clin Immunol 5:46–54, 1985.
65. Klimas NG, Salvato FR, Morgan R, and Fletcher M: Immunologic abnormalities in chronic fatigue syndrome. J Clin Microbiol 28:1403–1410, 1990.
66. Whiteside TL and Herberman RB: The role of natural killer cells in human disease. Clin Immunol Immunopathol 53:1–23, 1989.
67. Murdoch JC: Cell-mediated immunity in patients with myalgic encephalomyelitis syndrome. N Z Med J 101:511–512, 1988.
68. Lloyd AR, Wakefield D, Boughton CR, and Dwyer JM: Immunological abnormalities in the chronic fatigue syndrome. Med J Aust 151:122–124, 1989.
69. Demitrack MA, Dale JK, Straus SE, et al: Evidence for impaired activation of the hypothalamic-pituitary-adrenal axis in patients with chronic fatigue syndrome. J Clin Endocrinol Metab 73:1224–1234, 1991.
70. Imboden JB, Canter A, and Cluff LE: Convalescence from influenza. Arch Intern Med 108:393–399, 1961.
71. Leventhal LJ, Naides SJ, and Freundlich B: Fibromyalgia and parvovirus infection. Arthritis Rheum 34:1319–1324, 1991.
72. Coyle PK and Krupp LB: *Borrelia burgdorferi* infection in the chronic fatigue syndrome. Ann Neurol 28:243–244, 1990.
73. Benjamin JE and Hoyt RC: Disability following postvaccinal (yellow fever) hepatitis. JAMA 128:319–324, 1945.
74. Lawton AH, Rich TA, McLendon S, et al: Follow-up studies of St. Louis encephalitis in Florida: Reevaluation of the emotional and health status of the survivors five years after acute illness. South Med J 63:66–71, 1970.
75. Rosene KA, Copass MK, Kastner LS, et al: Persistent neuropsychological sequelae of toxic shock syndrome. Ann Intern Med 96:865–870, 1982.
76. Cluff LE, Trever RW, Imboden JB, and Canter A: Brucellosis. II: Medical aspects of delayed convalescence. Arch Intern Med 103:393–405, 1959.
77. Imboden JB, Canter A, Cluff LE, and Trever RW: Brucellosis. III: Psychologic aspects of delayed convalescence. Arch Intern Med 103:406–414, 1959.
78. Archard LC, Bowles NE, Behan PO, et al: Postviral fatigue syndrome: Persistence of enterovirus RNA in muscle and elevated creatine kinase. J R Soc Med 81:326–329, 1988.
79. Cunningham L, Bowles NE, Lane RJM, et al: Persistence of enteroviral RNA in chronic fatigue syndrome is associated with the abnormal production of equal amounts of positive and negative strands of enteroviral RNA. J Gen Virol 71:1399–1402, 1990.
80. Gow JW, Behan WMH, Clements GB, et al: Enteroviral RNA sequences detected by polymerase chain reaction in muscle of patients with postviral fatigue syndrome. BMJ 302:692–696, 1991.
81. Yousef GE, Bell EJ, Mann GF, et al: Chronic enterovirus infection in patients with postviral fatigue syndrome. Lancet i:146–150, 1988.
82. DeFreitas E, Hilliard B, Cheney PR, et al: Retroviral sequences related to human T-lymphotropic virus type II in patients with chronic fatigue immune dysfunction syndrome. Proc Natl Acad Sci U S A 88:2922–2926, 1991.
82a. Khan AS, Heneine WM, Chapman LE, et al: Assessment of a retrovirus sequence and other possible risk factors for the chronic fatigue syndrome. Ann Intern Med 118:241–245, 1993.
83. Manu P, Lane TJ, and Matthews DA: The frequency of the chronic fatigue syndrome in patients with symptoms of persistent fatigue. Ann Intern Med 109:554–556, 1988.
84. Taerk GS, Toner BB, Salit IE, et al: Depression in patients with neuromyasthenia (benign myalgic encephalomyelitis). Int J Psychiatry Med 17:49–56, 1987.
85. Kruesi MJP, Dale J, and Straus SE: Psychiatric diagnoses in patients who have chronic fatigue syndrome. J Clin Psychiatry 50:53–56, 1989.
86. Wessely S and Powell R: Fatigue syndromes: A comparison of chronic "postviral" fatigue with neuromuscular and affective disorders. J Neurol Neurosurg Psychiatry 52:940–948, 1989.

87. Hickie I, Lloyd A, Wakefield D, and Parker G: The psychiatric status of patients with the chronic fatigue syndrome. Br J Psychiatry 156:534–540, 1990.
88. Gold D, Bowden R, Sixbey J, et al: Chronic fatigue: A prospective clinical and virologic study. JAMA 264:48–53, 1990.
89. Robins LN, Helzer JE, Weissman MM, et al: Lifetime prevalence of specific psychiatric disorders in three sites. Arch Gen Psychiatry 41:949–958, 1984.
90. Engel GL: The need for a new medical model: A challenge for biomedicine. Science 196:129–136, 1977.
91. Bird J, Cohen-Cole SA, Boker J, and Freeman A: Teaching psychiatry to non-psychiatrists. I: The application of educational methodology. Gen Hosp Psychiatry 5:247–253, 1983.
92. Cohen-Cole SA and Bird J: Teaching psychiatry to nonpsychiatrists. II: A model curriculum. Gen Hosp Psychiatry 6:1–11, 1984.
93. Goldenberg DL, Felson DT, and Dinerman H: A randomized, controlled trial of amitriptyline and naproxen in the treatment of patients with fibromyalgia. Arthritis Rheum 29:1371–1377, 1986.
94. Straus SE, Dale JK, Tobi M, et al: Acyclovir treatment of the chronic fatigue syndrome: Lack of efficacy in a placebo-controlled trial. N Engl J Med 319:1692–1698, 1988.
95. Lloyd AR, Hickie I, Wakefield D, et al: A double-blind, placebo-controlled trial of intravenous immunoglobulin therapy in patients with chronic fatigue syndrome. Am J Med 89:561–568, 1990.
96. Peterson PK, Shepard J, Macres M, et al: A controlled trial of intravenous immunoglobulin G in chronic fatigue syndrome. Am J Med 89:554–560, 1990.
97. Cox IM, Campbell MJ, and Dowson D: Red blood cell magnesium and chronic fatigue syndrome. Lancet 337:757–760, 1991.
98. Butler S, Chalder T, Ron M, and Wessely S: Cognitive behaviour therapy in chronic fatigue syndrome. J Neurol Neurosurg Psychiatry 54:153–158, 1991.

64

Addressing HIV Infection in Office Practice

HARVEY J. MAKADON, MD
THOMAS G. COONEY, MD

There are currently over 1 million individuals infected with the human immunodeficiency virus (HIV) in the United States; estimates are that there are anywhere from 40,000 to 80,000 new infections occurring in this country each year.[1] Globally, there are an estimated 10 million people already infected with HIV, a number projected to grow to at least 40 million and possibly as high as 110 million by the end of the century.[2, 3] From the perspective of the primary care provider, it is challenging to consider how to be most effective at working with patients to identify those who may be at risk of HIV infection, how to prevent new infections from occurring, and how to care for those who already have HIV disease.

This chapter focuses specifically on the needs of practitioners who are working in industrialized nations because both the epidemiology of HIV disease and the resources available for evaluation and management of HIV-related conditions vary considerably from developing nations. We address the following questions: What are approaches to risk assessment, counseling, and testing in the office? What is the natural history of HIV disease? What constitutes the clinical evaluation of a patient with early HIV infection? What are basic therapeutic interventions for all individuals with HIV disease? How do you evaluate common symptoms in later-stage disease?

ASSESSING RISK OF HIV INFECTION

HIV infection has been shown to be transmitted in three ways.[4]

1. Sexually, either homosexually or heterosexually, when individuals engage in unsafe sexual practices
2. By exposure to contaminated blood when intravenous drugs are used and needles are shared, or by an occupational needle stick (individuals who received transfusion of blood or blood products prior to 1985, when routine screening of the blood supply was initialized, are also at risk for HIV infection)
3. Perinatally during pregnancy or breast-feeding

Given advances in treatment of HIV disease with both antiretroviral therapy and prophylaxis against opportunistic infections, it has become advantageous for individuals to know about infection as soon as possible, and to seek access to care and treatment. For this reason, it is essential that primary care providers assess all their patients for behaviors that may have put them at risk for HIV disease and recommend that those who are at high risk be tested for HIV infection.[5]

Determining whether patients are at high risk can be complex, particularly in situations where patients are those of long standing, and assumptions about their lifelong behavior may or may not have been clarified over years of care. Nevertheless, it is always important to address behaviors that may put individuals at high risk for HIV infection. These include whether patients or their partners have had multiple sexual partners or a history of sexually transmitted diseases, whether they have practiced anal or vaginal intercourse without condoms, whether they have used injectable drugs and shared needles or other drug equipment, and whether they received blood transfusions between 1978 and 1985. HIV is transmitted homosexually most frequently through receptive anal intercourse. Transmission during insertive anal intercourse appears to occur less commonly. There are reports of transmission during oral sex when ejaculation has occurred. Heterosexual transmission appears to occur during vaginal intercourse more efficiently from man to woman rather than vice versa. Partners of injecting drug users and bisexual men are at highest risk because of the prevalence of HIV infections in those populations. At all times, the history of such behaviors can be most effectively elicited in a nonjudgmental way, combined with reassuring individuals about the confidentiality of the interview. It is helpful to reassure individuals that this history taking is now routine because of the risk of HIV disease. There are excellent reviews on how to take such a history.[4] All women of child-bearing age should receive information about perinatal transmission of HIV and the implications of neonatal HIV infection,[6] particularly in higher-prevalence areas. They should be offered the opportunity to be tested for HIV.

Because HIV infection carries with it a great deal of stigma and potential for discrimination, and because of the medical and psychological consequences of testing positive, it is recommended that before diagnostic testing is performed, individuals have an opportunity for counseling. Many states provide counseling programs as part of anonymous or confidential test sites, which can be accessed by individuals on their own or at the recommendation of their primary care provider. Some states have published guidelines on HIV counseling for use by primary care providers. Table 64–1 summarizes the objectives of pretest and post-test counseling as suggested by the Massachusetts Department of Public Health.[7] Following counseling, patients can be tested voluntarily.[8] HIV antibody testing consists of two tests done in sequence. These are an enzyme-linked immunoassay (ELISA) test, which is repeated when the results are positive and subsequently confirmed by a Western Blot test. The sensitivity and specificity of the combined tests are 99% and 100%, respectively.[7] When used in individuals at high risk, the predictive value of a positive test result exceeds 99%. When screening a population with a lower risk of HIV, the predictive value of a positive test result can be substantially lower.[8]

Tests should be done at confidential or anonymous test sites where patients can get their own results and take them to their primary care provider for further follow-up. Particularly in situations in which follow-up is initiated by patients or access to care is problematic, tying the counseling and testing process more closely to rapid access to primary care may lead to more effective care.

When test results are negative, many providers do not enter this information into the medical record because even information that an individual was felt to be at risk for HIV infection and subsequently tested has led to discrimination in applications for insurance or employment. Nevertheless, a negative test result in an individual at high risk for HIV infection does need to be followed up with ongoing counseling to help eliminate the behavior that initially put the person at risk for infection. Specifically, it is important to emphasize the need to engage in safer sex, using latex condoms when there is exchange of body fluids during anal, vaginal, or oral sex. Condoms should be used in conjunction with a spermicidal jelly during anal or vaginal intercourse. As stated earlier, although there are clearly documented cases of HIV transmission related to oral sex, the extent to which this occurs is uncertain. Safer sex guidelines from the American College Health Association are included in Table 64–2. Drug and alcohol counseling is a necessary component of post-test HIV counseling because the related disinhibition that occurs in the setting of alcohol or drug use is associated with a higher rate of unsafe behavior. It is also important to be able to refer individuals using injectable drugs to appropriate treatment programs. In many communities, availability of treatment programs has been limited.

For individuals who test positive for HIV, the primary care provider must initiate care that encompasses both a comprehensive medical and psychological assessment. A multidisciplinary approach to care may often be appropriate; its precise configuration will depend on resources available in a given practice or community. Providers who are beginning to see people with HIV disease should contact local acquired immunodeficiency syndrome (AIDS) service organizations to understand more about services that may supplement or complement their own, including counseling services, case management services, and drug treatment programs. Information about local resources can also be obtained by calling the National AIDS Information Clearinghouse at 1-800-458-5231.

THE NATURAL HISTORY OF HIV DISEASE

As the HIV epidemic developed in the early 1980s, its diverse manifestations were grouped and described as specific syndromes. Patients with significant opportunistic infections or malignancies were described as having AIDS. Others who had less significant symptoms were described as having AIDS-related complex. Once testing was available, those who tested positive but had few or no medical symptoms were often deemed asymptomatic HIV positive. The Centers for Disease Control (CDC) defined specific criteria for the first two categories in 1982. These criteria have been revised several times, most recently in January 1993.[9]

TABLE 64–1. COUNSELING INDIVIDUALS BEFORE AND AFTER HIV TESTING—RECOMMENDATIONS OF THE MASSACHUSETTS DEPARTMENT OF PUBLIC HEALTH*

Physicians traditionally counsel patients on a variety of topics: HIV/AIDS†‡ counseling should be incorporated into the physician's established patterns.

Pretest Counseling

Before testing, the physician should assess the patient's understanding of the test and its implications, and his or her ability to deal with the results and the benefits of obtaining the information. If there are emotional contraindications to testing a patient, counseling should nevertheless be provided on how to reduce the risk of HIV transmission.

It is important to note that prevention efforts are strengthened when an individual has exercised choice and personal responsibility in seeking counseling and testing.

Because patients who receive positive HIV test results often cannot fully comprehend new information at the time of receiving them, and because some patients may not return to get their test results, good counseling practice suggests covering the following information in the pretest session:

1. Explain the nature of AIDS and its related illness.
2. Explain the advantages of knowing one's antibody status in terms of medical management of HIV infection and other conditions.
3. Explain which behaviors put one at risk for HIV infection.
4. Ascertain the patient's understanding of how he or she can reduce the risk of infection, including the use of condoms.
5. Try to understand what, if anything, prevents the adoption of these risk-reduction practices.
6. Explain what an HIV-antibody test result means.
7. Learn what the patient expects his or her test results to be.
8. Ask how the patient plans to change his or her behavior.
9. How will the patient cope with the psychosocial ramifications of a positive test result? Does the patient have health insurance? Should he or she obtain health insurance before being tested?
10. If the test result is positive, how will the patient tell his or her partners?
11. Discuss the importance of partner notification and the availability of the Department of Public Health to help with this task.
12. Discuss the possibilities of discrimination that may result from disclosure of a patient's antibody status.
13. Finally, your patient should be encouraged to identify
    a. One person who knows the patient is being tested.
    b. One person with whom he or she can discuss the test.
    c. What he or she plans to do in the 24 hours immediately following receipt of the test result.

Post-test Counseling

Post-test counseling should always be provided, regardless of the test result. It is an opportunity for the physician to emphasize the important of risk-reduction practices (e.g., the use of condoms) to both seropositive and seronegative patients.

For persons who test positive, post-test counseling offers the patient the opportunity to express his or her feelings and concerns and permits the provider to clarify the implications for the patient's health and to plan medical follow-up and management.

Post-test counseling for HIV-positive individuals should cover

1. Information on available medical treatment and counseling services.
2. Development of a comprehensive care plan for the patient.
3. Coping with emotional consequences of learning the test results, including development of a social support plan.
4. Behavioral change to prevent transmission, including how to use condoms and, where appropriate, how to enter drug and alcohol abuse treatment programs.
5. Discrimination problems that could be caused by disclosure of the patient's antibody status. (In general, patients should be encouraged to share positive test results only with their closest intimates and to wait before telling others. Discussing disclosure with professional or peer support group or systems is helpful in making such decisions.)
6. The need to notify sex partners.

*From Massachusetts Department of Health: Guidelines for Physicians and Health Care Providers on HIV Counseling, Testing, and Early Treatment. Boston, Massachusetts Department of Health, 1990. Publication 16202-52-20,000-2-90 CR.

†HIV = human immunodeficiency virus.

‡AIDS = acquired immunodeficiency syndrome.

Now, more than 10 years after the first AIDS cases were described, it is clear that the diverse infections and malignancies that appear with increasing frequency correlate with a progressive but variable decline in immune function that occurs in infected individuals. This decline in immune function can be measured by following one of a number of surrogate markers of immunologic function. The most commonly used marker is the number of absolute CD4 helper cells, or the percentage of CD4 cells as a fraction of total lymphocytes.[10] Despite the usefulness of this test, it is important to keep in mind that the results of CD4 tests are variable and not well standardized, and there is a great deal of clinical variation in the development of manifestations of HIV disease as immune function declines.

Although various staging systems for HIV disease have been developed, it is most useful to think of HIV disease as a continuum (Table 64–3). HIV is often first manifested clinically during the time of acute seroconversion. Shortly after initial exposure to HIV, an acute clinical syndrome has been detected in 20 to 30% of newly infected individuals.[11, 12] During this self-limited illness, individuals experience what has been described as a flu-like or mononucleosis-like syndrome or aseptic meningitis. This state generally lasts several weeks. In most cases, a specific diagnosis of seroconversion is not made unless individuals are seen in clinics where there is a high prevalence of new infections being seen, or individuals relate a specific incident of behavior that leads them to believe they may be at high risk for recent HIV infection. At the time of seroconversion, p24 antigen, a protein related to the viral core of HIV, is measurable in individuals' blood, whereas HIV antibodies are not present.

Following seroconversion, individuals with HIV infection enter a chronic phase of HIV disease. HIV antibodies measured by a combination of ELISA and Western Blot testing will appear in over 99% of cases by 6 months.[13] Individuals can live for a long time with few or no clinical symptoms. Cohort studies have revealed that individuals who are HIV infected can remain in this stage for well over a decade. Studies of the San Francisco cohort of gay men show that after 10 years of infection, approximately 50% of infected individuals developed AIDS (using the 1987 case defini-

TABLE 64–2. SEXUAL CONTACT*

Anal and Vaginal Intercourse: HIV† is more likely to be transmitted by unprotected anal or vaginal intercourse than by other sexual activities. Anal intercourse (penis in anus) is more likely to allow HIV transmission because HIV can attach itself to cells in the lower rectum. HIV may be easier to transmit to the receptive partner than to the insertive partner. However, an intact latex condom, properly used, substantially reduces the risk of transmitting HIV during anal or vaginal intercourse.

Oral Sex (oral-genital contact): The risk of acquiring HIV infection by performing oral sex on a man (fellatio) is uncertain. There seems to be some risk, but it is clearly much lower than the risk of vaginal or anal intercourse. Since pre-ejaculate ("pre-cum") may contain HIV, it is not necessarily any safer to stop before the man ejaculates. The chance of acquiring HIV by performing oral sex on a woman (cunnilingus) is not precisely known but also seems small. Whether you are a man or a woman, the risk of contracting HIV by having oral sex performed on you seems extremely low.

Kissing: Although HIV is very rarely present in the saliva of people with HIV infection, there is absolutely no evidence that kissing can transmit the virus. *No case of HIV infection has been traced to exposure to saliva in any circumstances.*

There is no chance of transmitting HIV through sexual activities that do not involve direct contact of semen, vaginal secretions, or blood with mucous membranes. *Touching, stroking, massage, and masturbation, alone or with a partner, do not transmit HIV.*

*Reprinted with permission from American College Health Association: HIV Infection and AIDS—What Everyone Should Know. Rockville, MD, 1990.
†HIV = human immunodeficiency virus.

tion), whereas approximately half of those remaining will have non–AIDS-defining clinical symptoms associated with HIV infection. Many remain asymptomatic from a medical perspective.[14]

The second phase of chronic HIV disease, in which individuals have few or no symptoms, could be divided at the point that it has been shown individuals begin to benefit from antiretroviral therapy.[15] This will be discussed in the section on therapeutics later. Currently, it is generally recommended that antiretroviral therapy be considered when an individual's CD4 count is below 500 per mm^3. Although studies show that viral replication occurs in individuals prior to this point,[16] there are no proven therapies for early chronic disease. Therapeutic vaccines with viral antigens and other techniques to modulate immune function are being evaluated in this population.

A third stage of chronic HIV disease begins when individuals are at higher risk for development of significant opportunistic infections. This generally occurs when CD4 counts are less than 200 to 250. In some cases, individuals will have already experienced significant symptoms or developed opportunistic infections or malignancies prior to this point. When either situation occurs, there is indication for prophylaxis against *Pneumocystis carinii* pneumonia (PCP). There are growing indications for prophylaxis against other opportunistic infections, particularly for individuals with CD4 counts of less than 75 to 100.

The CDC's most recent definition of AIDS includes all individuals with fewer than 200 CD4 cells, as well as those with tuberculosis, certain bacterial infections, and invasive cervical cancer in the setting of HIV infection.[17] The major impact of this change on clinicians will be concomitant changes in reporting requirements based on individuals who now meet the AIDS definition. Although access to some government benefits programs were heretofore tied automatically to an AIDS diagnosis, based on changes by the Social Security Administration in 1991, this is no longer the case.[18] Clinically, the redefinition may have the greatest impact on individuals with HIV who experience a significant emotional response to an earlier "AIDS" diagnosis, even when they feel well. Nevertheless, the medical challenge will be to continue to follow individuals and initiate antiretroviral therapies and prophylaxis and treatment for opportunistic infections at appropriate times. Median survival following a first episode of PCP was 10.2 months before 1985; it now appears to be closer to 2 years.[19] This is likely due to a combination of earlier testing, access to care, and treatment with both antiretroviral therapy and prophylaxis. Current emphasis on primary prophylaxis not only for PCP but also for other opportunistic infections, as well as a slow increase in options for antiretroviral therapy, holds out the promise of a continued increase in overall survival for those with HIV disease.

During the last, terminal phase of HIV disease, individuals will usually continue to be treated for chronic problems but also begin to prepare for death. Optimally, issues concerning durable powers of attorney and advanced directives will already have been discussed, but it is always important to ensure that you reassess these with patients as they experience changes in their stage of illness. It also may be important to consider ways to help patients with both physical and emotional pain and possibly consider options for care, such as hospice, which will allow maximum comfort. Even though hospice traditionally has provided narrowly defined palliative care and comfort measures, in the case of people with HIV disease, there has been a greater willingness to consider use of medication to prevent blindness from cytomegalovirus, as well as prophylactic and antiretroviral therapies. Once again, it is important to consider multidisciplinary resources in the community that are available to support individuals in this stage of their illness. Helping patients find ways to address their emotional and spiritual needs is a necessary complement to

TABLE 64–3. CLINICAL CONTINUUM OF HIV* INFECTION

Stage	Clinical Presentation	Treatment
I. Acute seroconversion syndrome	Acute illness, p24 antigenemia.	?
II. Chronic HIV disease		
A. CD4 > 500	Few clinical symptoms, viral replication occurring	?
B. CD4 < 500	Symptoms may be present; higher risk for HIV-associated malignancies, infections	Antiretroviral therapy should be considered; PCP† prophylaxis with constitutional symptoms or AIDS‡-defining illness
C. CD4 < 200	Symptoms common	Antiretroviral therapy and PCP prophylaxis
D. CD4 < 75–100	Symptoms, OIs§ common	Surveillance, prophylaxis against OIs.
III. Advanced HIV disease	Chronic opportunistic infections	Continue therapies; advance directives

*HIV = human immunodeficiency virus.
†PCP = *Pneumocystis carinii* pneumonia.
‡AIDS = acquired immunodeficiency syndrome.
§OI = opportunistic infection.

medical care and may facilitate discussions around transitions in care.

THE CLINICAL EVALUATION

When patients present with new knowledge of HIV disease, it is important to work with them about the diagnosis in many ways. First, it is important that individuals understand the natural history of HIV infection; the variability in clinical manifestations from individual to individual must be emphasized. Acknowledging both the reality that most individuals, once diagnosed with AIDS, have died within several years of diagnosis, as well as the hope that with earlier access to care and the availability of new treatments people may go on to live for many years, can be important. As part of this discussion, it is useful to describe methods of monitoring the progression of HIV disease, as are described later.

An integral part of this initial evaluation should be an assessment of an individual's psychological state to determine how he or she is adapting and to ensure that he or she is not depressed or suicidal. Often, this is a greater problem shortly after finding out about a diagnosis than in later stages of disease. In addition, patients may need advice with respect to available resources, and they should be aware of their own status with respect to health, disability, and life insurance. Many patients do not realize that if they change jobs, they may lose health coverage due to preexisting exclusion clauses in some health insurance plans.

Patients must have an ongoing opportunity for counseling about high-risk behavior, the importance of practicing safer sex, and using drugs in ways that do not put others at risk for infection. Whether there is an ethical or legal obligation of the primary care provider to inform sexual partners of a patient's seropositive status, or to ask a public health department to do so, is a complex question. The answer may depend on state law.[20] In some states, public health departments take on responsibility for contact tracing following required reports from health care providers. Aside from state regulations, primary care providers can be very helpful by working with their patients to help them become more comfortable about imparting this information both to intimate relations as well as friends and acquaintances. In addition to contributing to reducing the spread of HIV, this counseling can be an important part of the process of adjustment to a diagnosis of HIV disease.

Unfortunately, many patients present for their first visit with symptoms already suggestive of later-stage disease. The evaluation of such symptoms is described in the last section of this chapter. Others will have few or no symptoms, in which case more attention can be focused on doing a careful baseline history and physical examination and ensuring that routine diagnostic testing and immunizations are complete (Table 64–4).

TABLE 64–4. INITIAL EVALUATION OF AN INDIVIDUAL WITH HIV* INFECTION

Comprehensive history and physical examination
Diagnostic tests
CD4 count (see Table 64–5)
CBC†, electrolyte levels, liver function
Hepatitis B serology
Purified protein derivative and controls
Syphilis serology (RPR‡ or VDRL§)
Antitoxoplasmosis IgG‖ antibodies
Cytomegalovirus antibodies
Immunizations

*HIV = human immunodeficiency virus.
†CBC = complete blood count.
‡RPR = rapid plasma reagin.
§VDRL = Venereal Disease Research Laboratories.
‖IgG = gamma G immunoglobulin.

History and Physical Examination

An individual with early HIV disease who presents with few or no clinical symptoms should have a complete history and physical examination to establish a clinical baseline and to review any seemingly minor issues that may be harbingers of advancing disease. There are several areas to highlight in this initial evaluation.

Constitutional Symptoms. Low-grade fevers, fatigue, sweats, mild weight loss and diarrhea are legion in people with early HIV disease. In many cases, they are self-limited and disappear without a clear etiology. They may often be related to concurrent infection with other viruses or bacteria but receive heightened attention from both providers and patients in the context of HIV disease. It is important to evaluate each of these symptoms. If no clear explanation is found, it is helpful to reassure patients that these kind of symptoms may come and go and do not have a clear prognostic meaning. Certainly, if fevers are sustained and increase in severity, or if sweats continue, they will need to be re-evaluated. Concomitant HIV-related illnesses, such as tuberculosis, must be considered. If weight loss exceeds 10% of body weight and there is no other explanation, it may be AIDS-defining wasting syndrome. Such findings are rare, however, in an individual with early-stage disease and a high CD4 count.

Lymphadenopathy. Generalized lymphadenopathy is present in the majority of individuals at some stage of their HIV disease. When such lymphadenopathy is diffuse, and all nodes are less than 2 cm without any accompanying significant constitutional symptoms, the diagnosis of generalized lymphadenopathy syndrome can be made without further evaluation.[21, 22] Nevertheless, if nodes continue to grow, cause pain or other symptoms, or are accompanied by other persistent constitutional symptoms, a lymph node biopsy is indicated to evaluate the possibility of lymphoma or other HIV-related infections that may cause adenopathy, such as tuberculosis, toxoplasmosis, or syphilis.

Mucocutaneous Lesions. Skin and mucosal lesions are extremely common in people with HIV disease and are often the first harbingers of a decline in immune function. In many cases, they are still the first symptom that brings individuals to seek medical attention. Any such lesion can cause a great deal of anxiety, even if it is not obvious to others.

Common skin manifestations include many problems that are also common in non–HIV-infected individuals. Therefore, without knowledge of an individual's HIV status, their presence should not lead to a conclusion that someone is HIV infected. Nevertheless, it should lead clinicians to review a patient's history for behavior that might put him or her at risk for HIV disease.[23, 24]

Psoriasis, folliculitis, eczema, seborrheic dermatitis, herpes simplex virus, and herpes zoster virus are all more common in individuals with HIV infection. Treatment for patients with HIV disease may vary somewhat from standard therapy. For example, there is evidence that seborrheic dermatitis may be caused by a fungal skin irritation, and that treatment with local antifungal medication is of benefit. Immediate treatment of lesions secondary to herpes simplex virus with acyclovir is generally extremely helpful. An acute case of herpes simplex can be treated with 1 to 2 g of oral acylcovir daily. Herpes simplex virus resistance to acylcovir has been described.[25] Research on ways to avoid this resistance is needed. In such cases, individuals may need therapy with foscarnet. The recommended dose of acyclovir to prevent dissemination of herpes zoster is 4 grams per day. Another viral lesion, molluscum contagiosum, is a common problem in people with HIV disease. Although this lesion is generally benign and characterized by umbilicated papules in the non–HIV-infected population, in individuals with HIV disease these do not resolve and often increase in size and severity. Early treatment with cryotherapy is helpful in limiting spread.

Prior to 1982, Kaposi's sarcoma was previously considered to be a relatively unaggressive lesion found on the skin of the lower extremities of elderly men of Mediterranean origin. It has now been diagnosed commonly, generally in homosexual men with HIV disease, although its incidence has been declining in this population. Although Kaposi's sarcoma has been an AIDS-defining condition, it clearly develops earlier in the course of HIV disease than other AIDS-defining conditions. Its course can still be relatively benign, and prominent lesions can be treated with local injections of chemotherapy or cryotherapy, with good results. Radiation therapy has also been used for specific lesions. When Kaposi's sarcoma becomes more aggressive or causes significant pain or lymphedema, systemic chemotherapy can be helpful. There are studies indicating that use of interferon alfa can be helpful in people with Kaposi's sarcoma with CD4 counts higher than 200.[26]

Mucosal lesions related to immunologic deterioration accompanying HIV disease are common. Persistent oral or vaginal yeast infections without a history of antibiotic use often are one of the first signs of immune dysfunctions in HIV disease. The most common presentation is the fluffy white exudate diagnostic of oral thrush or vaginal candidiasis.[27, 28] These lesions are usually easily distinguished from other oral lesions by the fact that they can be easily removed with a cotton swab. Oral thrush can be treated initially with clotrimazole troches five times daily or oral nystatin. Vaginal candidiasis is best treated with vaginal miconazole cream. It is important to keep in mind that oral candidiasis may present in other, less typical ways. Atrophic candidiasis can present as an erythematous atrophic area in the oral cavity that can be painful or produce a metallic taste. Even without the presence of typical lesions of thrush, antiyeast treatment can be helpful. Finally, thrush can cause angular cheilitis, an inflammation of the corners of the mouth. Such a presentation in an individual with HIV disease should be treated with local anticandidal cream in addition to a hydrocortisone cream.

When first-line therapies for mucosal candidal infection are no longer effective, oral therapy with ketoconazole or fluconazole is generally effective. Use of various antibiotics for other opportunistic infections has led to oral and esophageal candidiasis which is more difficult to treat. Higher doses of oral therapy (up to 400 mg/day of fluconazole) can be used. Some antibiotics do alter the metabolism of antifungal azoles. At times, particularly in later-stage disease in the context of concomitant antibiotic use, oral systemic therapy is no longer effective, and it may be necessary to treat patients with very low doses of intravenous amphotericin (10 to 15 mg/day) for short periods.

Another oral lesion almost pathognomonic of HIV disease is hairy leukoplakia, a white plaque-like lesion that appears in vertical bands along the lateral aspect of the tongue.[28] This is known to be caused by the Epstein-Barr virus. This lesion is generally benign and does not require treatment. Nevertheless, it does lead to a great deal of concern because of its prominent location and its clinical significance as a harbinger of immunologic deterioration. In severe cases, acyclovir may be helpful.

Human papilloma virus has traditionally caused venereal warts. It is also a risk factor for cervical intraepithelial neoplasm. There is growing evidence of the risk of cervical neoplasia in HIV-infected women and, on this basis, more aggressive screening with Papanicolaou's smear and potentially, colposcopy are recommended.[27]

Gingivitis is also commonly seen in people with HIV disease. Routine use of antiseptic oral solutions such as Peridex and periodontal care is recommended.

Ophthalmologic Findings. In early HIV disease, retinal findings consisting of benign cotton wool spots are common. These are often small fluffy exudates that are transient and do not progress or cause any visual disturbance. They are of note in part because of a need to distinguish them from lesions secondary to cytomegalovirus infection, which may start off with a similar appearance, but which progress, often become hemorrhagic, and leads to visual change. Early symptoms of cytomegalovirus retinitis commonly consist of floaters but may be more severe, depending on the extent of retinal involvement. Although lesions of cytomegalovirus retinitis typically do not occur until individuals' CD4 counts are less than 100, any retinal findings should prompt primary care providers to seek an ophthalmologic evaluation. This is particularly true if lesions persist, enlarge, or impair vision. When individuals have CD4 counts of less than 100, it is important to pay particular attention to all visual symptoms. Some authorities recommend regular ophthalmologic examinations regardless of symptoms. Other opportunistic infections that can present with retinal findings include toxoplasmosis and syphilis.[29, 30]

Neuropsychological Evaluation. Although there has been a great deal of attention paid to the presence of cognitive deficits in people with early HIV disease, their occurrence is rare. In an individual who demonstrates some change in cognitive function, neuropsychological evaluation may be indicated. Of greater concern for people with early HIV disease is an evaluation for depression and suicidal ideation. In such cases, medication and psychotherapy can be extremely helpful at treating depression and helping individuals adjust to their diagnosis. In fact, most individuals with HIV disease can benefit from ongoing counseling to help them with the numerous situational adjustments that they need to make not only initially but also as they progress through various stages of HIV disease.[31, 32]

Diagnostic Evaluation

The laboratory and diagnostic evaluation of someone with early HIV disease is straightforward.

Immunologic Monitoring. There is much in the literature about various tests to assess the level of immune function and prognosis in people with HIV disease. The test most often used is the CD4 count. The pathophysiology of HIV infection is closely related to the virus' infection of cells that possess CD4 membrane receptors. The clinical stage of illness appears to relate almost directly to the decline in the number of CD4 lymphocytes. There is debate about the best way to monitor CD4 cells. There is some indication that looking at CD4 cells as a percentage of total lymphocytes is less variable than monitoring absolute numbers of CD4 cells. Nevertheless, studies of clinical effectiveness of various therapies have been correlated with the absolute numbers of CD4 cells, and this test is currently the most widely used. As the absolute numbers of cells have been shown to vary in an individual from day to day as well as from laboratory to laboratory, it is recommended to try to maintain as much consistency in terms of time of testing and the laboratory used. The use of this test will be much improved when it is better standardized.[10, 33]

CD4 testing is recommended every 4 to 6 months, unless an individual is close (i.e., within 100 CD4 cells) to a point where therapeutic decisions should be considered.[34] At this time, testing may need to be more frequent (Table 64–5). It is also important to check CD4 counts more frequently in individuals who have had great variability in their results to establish a reasonably stable baseline.

Although numerous other tests in the literature have been used to establish prognosis or level of immune function, including testing for p24 antigen and β_2-microglobulin and monitoring CD8 and neopterin levels, none of these is currently recommended for initial testing.[35–37] Some clinicians use them to determine when individuals are no longer responding to their current treatment regimens and therefore may benefit from some change.[38]

Complete Blood Counts. Hematologic abnormalities are common in people with HIV disease. A complete blood count can help clinicians both establish a baseline and look for evidence of cytopenias, even in individuals who are relatively asymptomatic. A complete blood count is also important in monitoring patients who are taking various treatments, such as zidovudine and ganciclovir, which can affect the bone marrow. Therefore, the periodicity of complete blood count monitoring once a baseline is established must depend on a patient's clinical course and therapeutic regimen.

Baseline Electrolytes and Liver Function Tests. Various renal and liver abnormalities are associated with HIV disease. It is important to establish a baseline for all individuals with HIV infection. This is particularly true given the toxicity of many medications. Again, periodicity of testing is dependent on clinical status and current therapeutics.

***Mycobacterium tuberculosis* Exposure.** Reports have shown a steady increase in the number of cases of *Mycobacterium tuberculosis* being diagnosed, particularly in people with HIV infection.[39] This organism is most common in populations already at risk for tuberculosis. In light of this, it is extremely important that individuals with HIV infection or at high risk for HIV infection be screened for previous exposure to tuberculosis. In taking a history, particular attention should be paid to whether an individual has been treated for tuberculosis, has had household contact with infectious tuberculosis, or lives in a setting, such as congregate living facilities, homeless shelters, or health care settings, where outbreaks have been reported.

CDC recommendations are that everyone have an intermediate purified protein derivative with two controls, including individuals with a history of bacille Calmette Guérin vaccination. Testing is best done as early in the course of HIV disease as possible because the prevalence of anergy increases with advanced disease. The standard for interpreting the purified protein derivative has been changed for individuals who are HIV infected, for whom 5 mm of induration should be considered a positive reaction.[40] Any induration in response to the controls is considered significant. Individuals with a positive test should have a chest x-ray. The CDC also recommends a routine chest x-ray in anergic patients to look for signs of latent tuberculosis. This is particularly important in individuals who may be receiving aerosolized pentamidine as a form of PCP prophylaxis. This is further discussed later.

Although most cases of tuberculosis represent reactivation of latent infection, new cases of tuberculosis in people with HIV infection are becoming increasingly common.[41] Therefore, individuals with HIV should continue to be screened for recent exposure by history and repeated skin testing.

Hepatitis B Virus. Individuals at risk for HIV are also commonly at risk for hepatitis B virus. Therefore, screening people for prior evidence of hepatitis B infection or a history of a vaccination should be done as part of an initial evaluation. Individuals without evidence of prior infection or immunity should be immunized.[42]

Syphilis. Concomitance of syphilis in HIV-infected populations and its subtle manifestations make early screening important. All patients should be asked specifically about a history of syphilis or a history of treatments suggestive of this diagnosis. If possible, records documenting treatment given may be helpful.[38] With respect to screening, the standard recommendation is that all HIV-infected individuals have at least a nontreponemal screening test (Venereal Disease Research Laboratory [VDRL] or rapid plasma reagin). There is some evidence that nonspecific tests may be falsely negative in late-stage HIV disease (CD4 counts less than 200) and that in such individuals it may be reasonable to use both a nonspecific and a specific trepenomal test as a screen.[43]

Toxoplasmosis. Individuals with past exposure to toxoplasmosis, documented by gamma G immunoglobulin antibodies to toxoplasmosis in the blood, have a greater risk of developing cerebral toxoplasmosis and may benefit from prophylaxis. Therefore, a baseline titer is indicated. Although there are no clear recommendations with respect to toxoplasmosis prevention for those who have a positive titer, numerous ongoing studies are looking at drugs such as pyrimethamine and trimethaprim-sulfamethoxazole as forms of prophylaxis. In addition, it is recommended that individuals without prior exposure to toxoplasmosis should avoid contact with cat feces and undercooked food. Titers should be rechecked at approximately yearly intervals.[44]

Cytomegalovirus. Individuals who do not have cytomegalovirus antibodies in their blood should not receive blood products that contain cytomegalovirus antibodies.[45]

TABLE 64–5. USE OF CD4 TESTING TO INITIATE ANTIRETROVIRAL THERAPY AND O.I. PROPHYLAXIS*

Result†	Management
CD4 > 600/mm³	No proven therapies; consider investigational studies
CD4 500–600/mm³	Antiretroviral therapy may be indicated soon; closer surveillance needed
CD4 300–500/mm³	Antiretroviral therapy to be considered; new constitutional symptoms or oral candidiasis are indications for PCP‡ prophylaxis
CD4 200–300/mm³	Antiretroviral therapy indicated; PCP prophylaxis may be needed soon; closer surveillance needed
CD4 < 200/mm³	PCP prophylaxis and antiretroviral therapy indicated; monitor for risk of other OIs§
CD4 < 100/mm³	Begin MAC prophylaxis

*Adapted from Hecht FM and Soloway B: HIV Infection: A Primary Care Approach. Waltham, MA, Massachusetts Medical Society, 1992.

†If the initial CD4 count is <600/mm³, or results at any time do not fit previous trends, the test should be repeated and results confirmed before management is changed.

‡PCP = *Pneumocystis carinii* pneumonia.

§OI = opportunistic infection.

Although there is no current recommendation with respect to prophylaxis against cytomegalovirus, there are ongoing efforts to look at ways to prevent cytomegalovirus retinitis.

IMMUNIZATIONS

Individuals with HIV infection are often at increased risk of hepatitis B exposure, and of developing infections due to encapsulated organisms. They have also been shown to have severe cases of measles when they have been previously unvaccinated. In addition, HIV-infected individuals may be more vulnerable to developing severe influenza. Finally, individuals with HIV need to have routine vaccinations that would be recommended even if they were not infected. In light of this, immunizations described in Table 64–6 are recommended for people with HIV infection. Although there has been some concern that antigenic stimulation from vaccinations might accelerate HIV infection, this has not been found to be the case. Given that measles is a live virus vaccine, it is recommended in individuals with a high risk of exposure (i.e., children, health care workers). It is also important to note that response rates to vaccinations in people with HIV infection seem to be lower as immunologic dysfunction progresses. Therefore, vaccines should be given as early in the course of HIV as possible.[46–48]

Therapeutics in Early HIV Infection

Studies have shown that the use of antiretroviral therapy in early HIV infection combined with prophylaxis against opportunistic infections has slowed the progression of HIV disease and the development of AIDS. The Food and Drug Administration (FDA) has licensed three antiretroviral agents. All of these are nucleoside analogs that act as reverse-transcriptase inhibitors. The first of these to be licensed, zidovudine (3′-ZDV, formerly AZT) was found to be effective in both preventing opportunistic infections and prolonging survival in patients with advanced AIDS-related complex in 1987[49]; it was licensed for use in these populations at that time. The first evidence that it may be an effective agent in earlier HIV infection came in 1990 when a study showed that individuals who are asymptomatic with CD4 counts less than 500 progressed to AIDS and advanced AIDS-related complex about half as quickly as individuals treated with placebo. In addition, the study showed that there was no difference in terms of effectiveness between a 500-mg dose and a 1500-mg dose of zidovudine, and the lower dose had less toxicity.[50]

Recent studies differ with respect to the point at which individuals benefit from therapy with zidovudine (ZDV) while they are asymptomatic and to how long they sustain a benefit from such therapy.[51, 51a, 51b] The National Institute of Allergy and Infectious Disease recommends that therapy be considered by doctor and patient when an individual's CD4 count is below 500.[52]

Most clinicians will initiate zidovudine at either 100 mg every 4 hours while awake or will use 200 mg three times a day for better compliance. Even at this dose, many individuals experience side effects, including anemia and neutropenia, nausea, headaches, fatigue, and insomnia. Anemia can often be managed by dose modification, transfusion, or use of erythropoietin. Neutropenia may also respond to dose reduction or growth colony stimulating factor. Often the latter symptomatic effects of zidovudine disappear within 4 to 6 weeks. Rarely, they require discontinuation of the drug.

At this time, in addition to zidovudine, two other nucleoside analogs have been licensed for use. These are didanosine and zalcitabine. Didanosine has been licensed to be used as a single agent. Initially licensed for individuals who could not tolerate or were no longer responsive to zidovudine, one study suggests its effectiveness in slowing progression of disease in HIV-infected patients who had tolerated zidovudine for a median of 13 to 14 months.[53] Studies are now taking place comparing therapy with zidovudine and didanosine as single agents. Zalcitabine has been licensed to be used only in combination with zidovudine.[54] Side effects of both didanosine and zalcitabine include peripheral neuropathy and pancreatitis. In addition, many patients experience diarrhea when taking didanosine, largely due to the buffer with which it is compounded, because it is inactive in an acid environment.

It appears that individuals do develop resistance to these drugs after prolonged use.[55] This raises the question of how long anyone should be treated with one particular regimen. Numerous ongoing studies compare these drugs used sequentially or in combination. Hopefully, the results of these trials will yield more information on whether combination therapy enhances the duration of effectiveness of early antiretroviral therapy.

Practically speaking, there are few data from clinical trials to suggest when to change from one antiretroviral agent to another. Most clinicians will begin with zidovudine as a single agent. Some will start with didanosine based on a patient's clinical profile or preference. Clinicians will either change to didanosine or add zalcitabine to zidovudine when a patient's CD4 count shows a clear decline or when there is clinical evidence of progressive immune dysfunction. Some clinicians do begin treatment with combination therapy with the hope that this will lead to prolonged clinical effectiveness.

Given limitations in the effectiveness of currently available nucleoside analogs, evaluation of other classes of antiretroviral agents, immunomodulators, and therapeutic vaccines may suggest new ways to minimize the development of viral resistance and extend the effectiveness of therapy against HIV.

TABLE 64–6. IMMUNIZATIONS FOR HIV-INFECTED ADULTS*

Vaccine	Frequency	Comments
Pneumococcal vaccine	Once	HIV† infection predisposes to pneumococcal infections
Hepatitis B vaccine	Series of 3	Indicated if there is no prior hepatitis B exposure
Influenza vaccine	Yearly	Early fall is the optimal time for maximizing protection
Diptheria and tetanus vaccine	Every 10 years	Administer if a booster is indicated
Haemophilus influenzae vaccine	Once	Should be considered; efficacy is uncertain
Measles vaccine	Once	Consider if patient was born after 1956, particularly if at high risk. However, safety and efficacy are unknown in HIV infection

*Adapted from Hecht FM and Soloway B: HIV Infection: A Primary Care Approach. Waltham, MA, Massachusetts Medical Society, 1992.

†HIV = human immunodeficiency virus.

Prophylaxis Against HIV-Related Infections

It has become clearer that infections associated with HIV occur in rough correlation with progressive decline in immune function. This decline is usually correlated with measurement of CD4 counts as shown in Figure 64–1. Based on this predictable occurrence, ongoing efforts are looking at effective ways to prevent the development of these infections, which cause significant morbidity and mortality in people with HIV disease. It is clearly important to consider prevention of both opportunistic and nonopportunistic infections.

Pneumocystis carinii *Pneumonia*

During the first decade of the AIDS epidemic, *Pneumocystis* pneumonia was the greatest cause of morbidity and mortality among people with HIV disease. Although this infection is still an extremely common occurrence, its rates have decreased dramatically in response to efforts to provide prophylaxis. Currently, the U.S. Public Health Service recommends that all individuals with HIV disease and CD4 counts of less than 200 should receive prophylaxis. In addition, those with new constitutional symptoms, such as oral candidiasis or concomitant malignancies, as well as all individuals with a prior episode of PCP, should receive prophylaxis.

With regard to prophylactic regimes, oral trimethaprim-sulfamethoxazole (TMP-SMX) has been proved to be effective for both primary and secondary prophylaxis against PCP. Several recent studies have shown that TMP-SMX was significantly more effective than aerosolized pentamidine in preventing PCP. Although recommended doses vary from one study to another, most prefer using one double-strength TMP-SMX tablet each day as prophylaxis against PCP.[56, 57] TMP-SMX has the advantage of being readily available, inexpensive, and systemic. Some believe that it may also offer protection against cerebral toxoplasmosis, but the data for this are preliminary and not conclusive. Disadvantages of TMP-SMX are that many individuals do not tolerate it due to development of severe rash, hematologic toxicity, and elevated liver enzymes. If TMP-SMX is not tolerated, some recommend desensitization.[58]

Alternative regimens for PCP include use of aerosolized pentamidine and dapsone. Generally speaking, aerosolized pentamidine is used at a dose of 300 mg once monthly using the Respigard II jet nebulizer. This appears to be generally well tolerated with few systemic side effects. Nevertheless, this medication and its delivery are expensive, and there appears to be a higher recurrence rate for second episodes of PCP than with patients taking TMP-SMX. The administration of aerosolized pentamidine, with its induced coughing, may increase the risk of spread of tuberculosis. Anyone receiving aerosolized pentamidine should be evaluated for tuberculosis before administration. Health care workers administering aerosolized pentamidine should take appropriate precautions.

Particularly in light of concerns about the spread of tuberculosis during the administration of aerosolized pentamidine, as well as costs, oral dapsone has been used as an alternative to TMP-SMX. There are no prospective controlled studies of its use, and it is not currently approved by the FDA for this purpose. Clinicians use a dose of 50 to 100 mg/day. Individuals who are G6PD deficient should not receive dapsone. There is also a risk of methemoglobinemia.

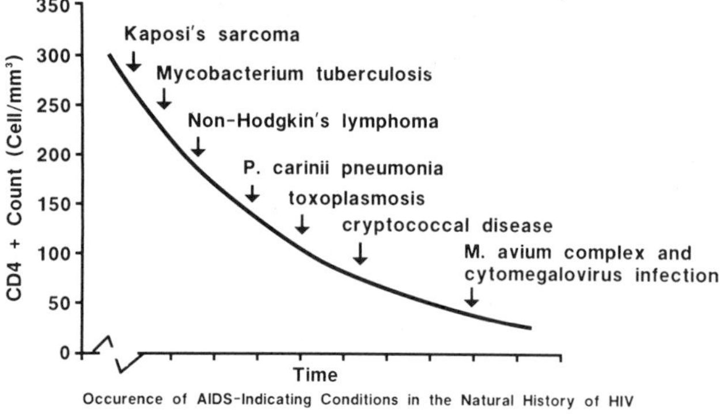

FIGURE 64–1. Correlation of opportunistic infection with CD4. Occurrence of AIDS-indicating conditions in the natural history of HIV infection, according to CD4+ cell count. (From Horsburgh CR, Jr: *Mycobacterium avium* complex infection in the acquired immunodeficiency syndrome. Reprinted, by permission, from the New England Journal of Medicine 324:1332, 1991.)

Other Opportunistic Infections

Studies are currently underway evaluating ways to prevent other opportunistic infections, including *Mycobacterium avium* complex (MAC), cryptococcal disease, and cytomegalovirus infection.[59] Rifabutin, a rifampin-like drug, has been shown to be effective in individuals with CD4 counts less than 100 as prophylaxis against MAC in a dose of 300 mg per day.[59a, 59b] Trials looking at the use of pyrimethamine and TMP-SMX to prevent toxoplasmosis in individuals who are toxoplasmosis antibody positive are underway. Although acyclovir has not been shown to be effective at preventing clinical evidence of cytomegalovirus disease, individuals who do not have cytomegalovirus antibodies should not receive blood transfusions unless blood is screened to ensure that it does not have the antibodies.[45]

Tuberculosis

Current CDC recommendations are that all individuals who have a history of a positive purified protein derivative or recent exposure to tuberculosis receive a year of prophylaxis with isoniazid.[60] Some also advocate that all anergic individuals at high risk for tuberculosis who are HIV positive receive isoniazid prophylaxis.[61] There are also recommendations being developed for prophylaxis among people who have been exposed to multiple drug-resistant tuberculosis. It is anticipated that these recommendations will soon be released by the CDC.

Syphilis

Treatment of syphilis in individuals with HIV is complex. Most recommend traditional therapy with penicillin for early-stage disease.[38, 62] Nevertheless, because the central nervous system can be a reservoir for syphilis, aggressive evaluation of cerebrospinal fluid is recommended in any patient with HIV who has had syphilis for an uncertain period of time or who was treated for syphilis in the past with a regimen inadequate to treat neurosyphilis. Some investigators recommend a regimen to treat neurosyphilis in all patients with HIV.[63] Treated patients should be followed clinically and with quantitative, nontreponemal serologic tests. Individuals treated for early disease whose titers do not respond should be retreated and undergo cerebrospinal fluid evaluation.

TABLE 64–7. PULMONARY COMPLICATIONS ASSOCIATED WITH HIV* DISEASE

Opportunistic Infections
Pneumocystis carinii pneumonia
Cytomegalovirus pneumonia
Mycobacterium avium complex (MAC), disseminated
Pulmonary cryptococcosis
Disseminated histoplasmosis
Pulmonary coccidioidomycosis
HIV-related pulmonary infections
Tuberculosis
Nocardiosis
Streptoccal pneumonia
Haemophilus pneumonia
Neoplasia
Kaposi's sarcoma
Lymphoma
HIV-related pulmonary disorders
Nonspecific interstitial pneumonitis

*HIV = human immunodeficiency virus.

EVALUATING SYMPTOMS IN INDIVIDUALS WITH HIV DISEASE

The diverse complications of HIV disease result in common symptoms that require a systematic diagnostic approach. The following sections detail approaches to many common HIV-related symptoms.

Pulmonary Symptoms

Pulmonary complications are among the most common problems encountered in the care of HIV-infected patients. Their diverse etiologies, detailed in Table 64–7, emphasize the importance of a systematic approach to patients presenting with respiratory symptoms, such as cough or dyspnea.[64]

The relative frequencies of various pulmonary complications are changing.[65] Early in the epidemic, PCP was the most commonly recognized pulmonary complication; increasingly, non–AIDS-defining infections, including *M. tuberculosis* and pyogenic bacterial pneumonias (e.g., streptococcal pneumonia) account for the respiratory complications of HIV infection, particularly in individuals with CD4 counts higher than 200. Nonetheless, despite widespread use of antiretroviral therapy and PCP prophylaxis, PCP remains a major cause of morbidity and mortality.

Dyspnea and Cough

The individual with, or at risk for, HIV infection who presents with dyspnea or cough should undergo a careful clinical evaluation. This evaluation should be guided by several factors. First, if known, the patients' CD4 count may help stratify their risk of various complications. A CD4 count of less than 250 indicates that a patient is at risk for the full spectrum of pulmonary complications.[66] CD4 counts of more than 250 to 300 suggest that other complications, such as bacterial pneumonia or tuberculosis, are more likely. Second, the administration of inhaled pentamidine will alter the clinical and radiographic presentation of PCP; upper lobe involvement and pneumothorax may be presenting symptoms. A clinical strategy for evaluating respiratory symptoms in a patient with CD4 counts of less than 250 is shown in Figure 64–2.

The initial step is the chest x-ray. Generally, one of three basic patterns will be found: normal; segmental or lobar infiltrates; or diffuse infiltrates. If the chest x-ray reveals lobar or segmental infiltrates, a sputum examination for Gram stain and acid-fast bacilli should be performed and therapy initiated for presumed bacterial pneumonia, pending results of cultures.[67] In individuals at high risk for tuberculosis, multiple samples for acid-fast bacilli should be obtained. Sputum should also be evaluated for PCP.

If the initial chest x-ray shows a diffuse or patchy interstitial infiltrate, efforts should be directed toward obtaining sputum to evaluate the possibility of PCP as well as routine Gram's stain, acid-fast bacilli, and special stains for *Legionella* and fungi. Treatment should be initiated based on the results of these tests, though empiric therapy should not be delayed in seriously ill patients pending performance of tests to obtain respiratory secretions. For severe cases of PCP, intravenous therapy with TMP-SMX or pentamidine is recommended initial therapy. Generally, treatment is for 21 days. In less severe cases, oral therapy can be initiated with either a combination of trimethaprim and dapsone or TMP-SMX. There are alternatives for individuals who do not tolerate these regimens. In addition to antibiotic therapy, treatment should include corticosteroids when there is a reduction in oxygen saturation (PaO_2) (<70 mm Hg in room air) or an increased alveolar-arterial oxygen (A-a) gradient (>35 mm Hg).[68]

If the x-ray is normal, additional evaluation should include noninvasive testing because 10 to 15% of patients with proven PCP may present with normal chest x-rays. Numerous noninvasive tests have been reported for the evaluation of suspected PCP.[64, 69] No one test appears to have sufficient sensitivity to exclude PCP or other opportu-

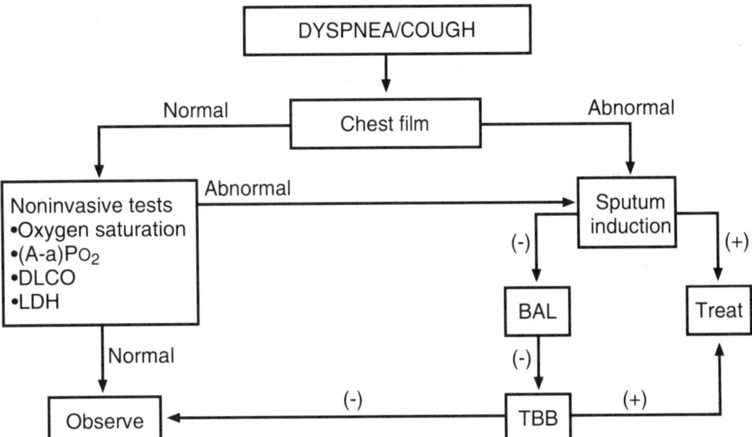

FIGURE 64–2. Evaluation of dyspnea and cough. BAL = bronchoalveolar lavage; TBB = transbronchial biopsy.

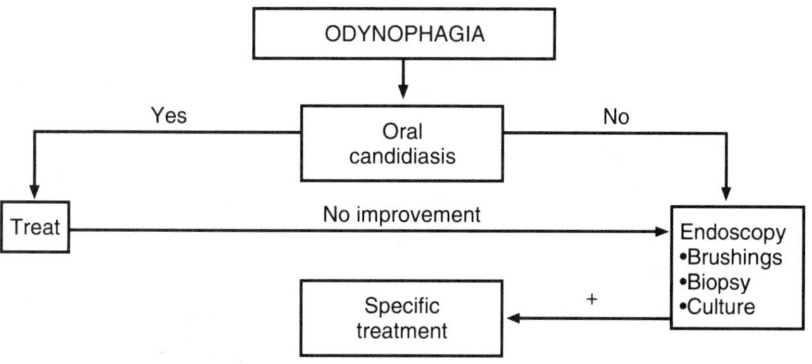

FIGURE 64–3. Evaluation of odynophagia.

nistic infections. A low PaO_2 or increase in the A-a gradient (>10 mm Hg) has only moderate sensitivity and low specificity; sensitivity is improved when the test is performed following 3 minutes of exercise. The diffusing capacity for carbon monoxide (DL_{CO}) is more sensitive but again lacks specificity. It is also expensive and not available in many care sites. Finally, serum lactate dehydrogenase has high sensitivity and moderate specificity for PCP but not for other opportunistic infections.[70] Significantly, no screening strategies have been evaluated prospectively. Based on existing data, noninvasive tests can be used, when the results are normal, to help rule out serious opportunistic infections, such as PCP. When any are abnormal, or when the clinical picture is suggestive, the evaluation should proceed to obtaining pulmonary secretions, as noted in Figure 64–2. Evaluation of induced sputum by using monoclonal antibodies is highly sensitive. If the results are negative, bronchoscopy with bronchoalveolar lavage will increase sensitivity.

Gastrointestinal Symptoms

During the course of their illness, most patients with HIV infection will develop clinically significant gastrointestinal symptoms. These symptoms include dysphagia, odynophagia, diarrhea, abdominal pain, and jaundice.[71] Among those symptoms, diarrhea and odynophagia occur most frequently, and both produce substantial morbidity.

Odynophagia

Odynophagia (pain on swallowing) indicates that there is an inflammatory process involving the esophagus; in HIV-infected patients, this is most often infectious in origin. Infectious agents that cause odynophagia include *Candida albicans,* herpes simplex virus, and cytomegalovirus.[72, 73] Although less common, dysphagia also may be caused by these infectious agents, but its occurrence suggests neoplastic involvement (Kaposi's sarcoma, lymphoma).

A strategy for evaluating and managing odynophagia is shown in Figure 64–3. This strategy assumes that a patient who has odynophagia and oral candidiasis is most likely to have esophageal candidiasis.[71, 72] In this circumstance, empiric therapy (ketaconazole, 200 to 600 mg/day; fluconazole, 100 mg/day) is indicated.[74] If there is no improvement, or only partial improvement, gastroduodenoscopy is indicated because the patient may have cytomegalovirus or herpes simplex virus esophagitis, either alone or accompanying candidal esophagitis. Finally, if esophageal ulcerations are detected but no infectious agent is identified, the patient may have primary HIV infection of the esophagus, which has been reported to respond to prednisone or antiretroviral therapy.[75, 76]

Diarrhea

At some time in the course of their disease, many patients with HIV disease develop diarrhea.[71, 77, 78] Numerous microorganisms have been linked to diarrheal illnesses in HIV-infected patients (Table 64–8).[77, 78] Risk for infection with these organisms is dependent on the magnitude of immune dysfunction. For example, cytomegalovirus colitis or MAC-associated diarrhea is seen largely in patients with advanced disease (CD4 counts <100), whereas enteric bacterial infections may have been seen at all stages of disease.

Figure 64–4 demonstrates a stepwise strategy for the evaluation of an HIV-infected patient with diarrhea. Although this strategy produces an excellent diagnostic yield, it may not represent the most cost-effective approach when one considers the likelihood of response to specific therapy, the diagnostic yield, and the costs and associated discomfort of diagnosis and treatment. For some patients, an empiric trial of antidiarrheal therapy with loperamide or diphenoxylate after obtaining initial stool specimens for culture may be optimal.[79] Additional diagnostic evaluation may be reserved for patients whose symptoms are progressive or are not controlled. The more intensive diagnostic evaluation is most likely to yield the discovery of cytomegalovirus, *Microsporida,* MAC, and *Giardia.* Effective therapy for *Microsporida* infection is still being sought, although some preliminary data suggest that an abendazole may be effective. Cytomegalovirus requires lifelong intravenous therapy with either ganciclovir or foscarnet. Therapy for MAC is showing increasing promise with multidrug combinations that include the new macrolide antibiotics azithromycin and clarithromycin.

Neurologic Symptoms

Neuropsychiatric symptoms are assuming an increasingly important role in HIV-infected individuals.[80–82] Nearly

TABLE 64–8. CAUSES OF DIARRHEA ASSOCIATED WITH HIV* DISEASE

Small intestine	*Cryptosporidium, Microsporidium, Isospora belli, Mycobacterium avium-intracellulare, Salmonella, Campylobacter*
Colon	Cytomegalovirus, *Cryptosporidium, Mycobacterium avium* complex (MAC), *Shigella, Clostridium difficile, Campylobacter,* adenovirus

*HIV = human immunodeficiency virus.

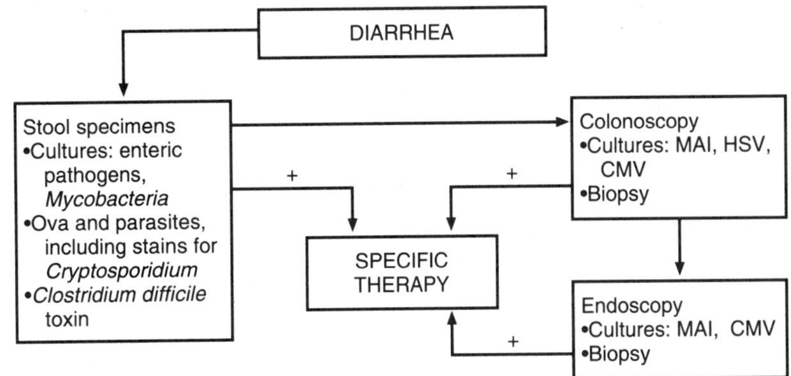

FIGURE 64–4. Evaluation of diarrhea.

10% of patients with AIDS present with neurologic symptoms, and up to 40% will develop neurologic complications during the course of their illness. Central nervous system dysfunction in HIV infection can be divided into two broad categories based on the associated symptom complex. One is an encephalopathy syndrome, with mental status changes, with or without associated fever and headache. The second is the development of focal deficits, with or without associated fevers, headaches, and seizures.[80]

Encephalopathy syndromes may be caused by various agents, including toxoplasmosis, cryptococcal meningitis, tuberculosis meningitis, herpes simplex virus, syphilis, and HIV itself. The HIV-AIDS dementia complex is a slowly progressive subcortical dementia typically seen in individuals with advanced HIV disease. Though it initially presents with cognitive defects, in advanced cases there may also be associated weakness, tremor, and seizures, in addition to a severe dementia.[81]

Focal neurologic deficits and seizures are caused most commonly by cerebral toxoplasmosis; less common causes include central nervous system lymphoma, progressive multifocal leukoencephalopathy, and various infectious etiologies, including cryptococcoma, tuberculoma, and pyogenic brain abscess.[80, 82, 83]

Patients who present with clinical findings suggestive of central nervous system dysfunction should undergo a careful, systemic evaluation and appropriate blood tests, imaging procedures, and studies of cerebrospinal fluid. Figure 64–5 outlines a strategy for evaluation of an HIV-infected individual with advanced HIV disease (CD4 <250 to 200).

The initial step, after a careful clinical evaluation and appropriate blood tests, including serum cryptococcal antigen, is to perform a computed tomographic (CT) scan with contrast or magnetic resonance imaging (MRI). Which is the most cost-effective test is unknown; the CT scan is less expensive but also less sensitive than MRI. However, when the CT scan is negative in the face of demonstrable neurologic deficits, an MRI scan is usually indicated because it may detect lesions not seen on a CT scan (e.g., lymphoma, smaller lesions of toxoplasmosis). If the CT scan or MRI is normal or shows only atrophy, the cerebrospinal fluid should be examined for cell count and differential, protein and glucose, cryptococcal antigen, VDRL, and appropriate bacterial, mycobacterial, and viral cultures.

If the CT or MRI demonstrates a mass lesion, further evaluation is based on the presence or absence of ring enhancement or multiple lesions. If either are present, empiric therapy for *Toxoplasma gondii* should be initiated and continued if there is clinical response. If there is only a solitary lesion, or if the lesions do not respond to empiric therapy, stereotactic brain biopsy should be considered, taking into account the patient's overall condition, prognosis, and clinical and epidemiologic likelihood of harboring treatable causes, such as a tuberculoma.

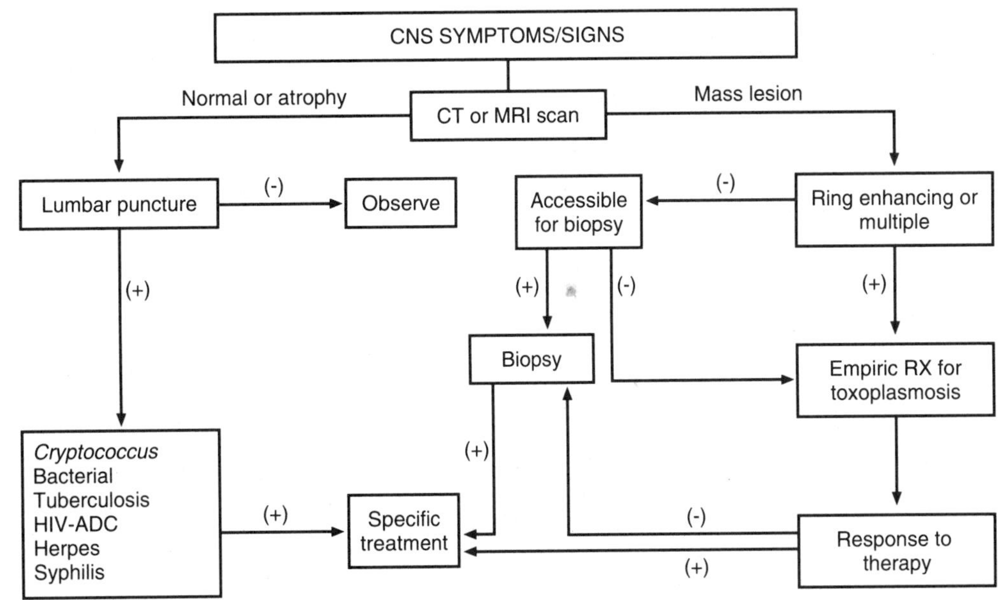

FIGURE 64–5. Evaluation of central nervous symptoms. HIV-ADC = HIV-AIDS dementia complex.

REFERENCES

1. Centers for Disease Control: HIV prevalence estimates and AIDS case projections for the United States: Report based upon a workshop. MMWR 39:1–30, 1990.
2. World Health Organization: Global Program on AIDS.
3. Mann J, Tarantola D, and Netter TW (eds): AIDS in the World. Global AIDS Policy Coalition, Boston, Harvard University Press, 1992.
4. Kassler WJ and Wu AW: Addressing HIV in office practice: Assessing risk, counseling, and testing. *In* Makadon HJ (ed): Primary Care: AIDS and HIV Infection in Office Practice. Philadelphia, WB Saunders, 1992, pp. 19–33.
5. Makadon HJ: Assessing HIV infection in primary care practice. J Gen Intern Med 6(Suppl):S2–S7, 1991.
6. American College of Gynecology: Human Immunodeficiency Virus Infections. Washington, D.C., American College of Gynecology, 1992.
7. Massachusetts Department of Health: Guidelines for Physicians and Health Care Providers on HIV Counseling, Testing, and Early Treatment. Boston, Massachusetts Department of Health, 1990. Publication 16202-52-20, 000-2-90ER.
8. Lo B, Steinbrook RL, Cooke M, et al: Voluntary screening for human immunodeficiency virus (HIV) infection. Ann Intern Med 105:969, 1986.
9. Centers for Disease Control: 1992 Revised Classification System for HIV Infection and Expanded AIDS Surveillance Case Definition for Adolescents and Adults (Draft). Washington, D.C., Public Health Service, U.S. Department of Health and Human Services, November 15, 1991.
10. Stein DS: CD4 lymphocyte cell enumeration for prediction of clinical course of human immunodeficiency virus disease: A review. J Infect Dis 165:352–363, 1992.
11. Cooper DA, Gold J, Maclean P, et al: Acute AIDS retrovirus infection: Definition of a clinical illness associated with seroconversion. Lancet i:537–540, 1985.
12. Ho DD, Sarngadharan MG, Resnick L, et al: Primary human T-lymphotropic virus type III. Ann Intern Med 103:880, 1985.
13. Cooper DA, Imrie AA, and Penny R: Antibody response to human immunodeficiency virus after primary infection. J Infect Dis 115:1113–1118, 1987.
14. Moss AR, Bacchetti P, Osmond D, et al: Seropositivity for HIV and the development of AIDS or AIDS related condition: Three year follow up of the San Francisco General Hospital Cohort. BMJ 297:745–750, 1988.
15. Volberding PA, Lagakos SW, Koch MA, et al: Zidovudine in asymptomatic human immunodeficiency virus infection: A controlled trial in persons with fewer than 500 CD4-positive cells per cubic millimeter. N Engl J Med 322:941–949, 1990.
16. Fox CH, Tenner-Racz K, Racz P, et al: Lymphoid germinal centers are reservoirs of human immunodeficiency virus type 1 RNA. J Infect Dis 164:1051–1057, 1991.
17. Centers for Disease Control: 1992 Revised Classification System for HIV Infection and Expanded AIDS Surveillance Case Definition for Adolescents and Adults (Draft). Washington, D.C., Public Health Service, U.S. Department of Health and Human Services, November 15, 1991.
18. U.S. Department of Health and Human Services, Social Security Administration: A Guide to Social Security with SSI Disability Benefits for People with HIV Infection. February, 1992. Document 05-10020.
19. Lemp GF, Hirosawa AM, Araneta MR, et al: Improved survival for persons with AIDS in San Francisco. Department of Public Health, San Francisco, California. VI International Conference on AIDS, Florence, Italy 1991 1:66, 1991.
20. Brennan TA: Legal and insurance issues. *In* Makadon HJ (ed): Primary Care: Aids and HIV Infection in Office Practice. Philadelphia, WB Saunders, 1992, pp 217–229.
21. Lang W, Anderson RE, Perkins H, et al: Clinical immunology and serologic findings in men at risk for acquired immune deficiency syndrome. JAMA 257:326–330, 1987.
22. Cooney T: Clinical management of the complication of HIV infection: Incorporating HIV infection into primary care practice. J Gen Intern Med 6(Suppl):S12–18, 1992.
23. Berger RS, Stoner MF, Hobbs ER, et al: Cutaneous manifestations of early human immunodeficiency virus exposure. J Am Acad Dermatol 19:298–303, 1988.
24. Kaplan MH, Sadick N, McNutt NS, et al: Dermatologic findings and manifestations of acquired immunodeficiency syndrome (AIDS). J Am Acad Dermatol 16:485–506, 1987.
25. Schnipper LE, Crumpacker CS, Marlowe SI, et al: Drug resistant herpes simplex virus in vitro and after acyclovir treatment in an immunocompromised patient. Am J Med 73:387–392, 1982.
26. Heyer DM, Kahn JO, and Volberding PA: HIV-related Kaposi's sarcoma. *In* Cohen PT, Sande MA, and Volberding PA (eds): The AIDS Knowledge Base. Waltham, MA, Medical Publishing Group, 1990, pp 1–19.
27. Minkoff HL and Dehovitz JA: Care of women infected with HIV. JAMA 266:2253–2300, 1991.
28. Pandborg JJ: Oral candidiasis in HIV infection. *In* Robertson PB and Greenspan JS (eds): Perspectives on Oral Manifestations of AIDS. Littleton, MA, PSG Publishing Company, 1988, pp 28–37.
29. Bloom JN and Palestine AG: The diagnosis of cytomegalovirus retinitis. Ann Intern Med 109:963–969, 1988.
30. Northfelt DW: Evaluation and treatment of later manifestations of HIV infection. *In* Makadon HJ (ed): Primary Care: AIDS and HIV Infection in Office Practice. Philadelphia, WB Saunders, 1992, pp 57–85.
31. Forstein M: The Neuropsychiatric aspects of HIV infection. *In* Makadon HJ (ed): Primary Care: AIDS and HIV Infection in Office Practice. Philadelphia, WB Saunders, 1992, pp 97–117.
32. Marzuk PM, Tierney H, Tardiff K, et al: Increased risk of suicide in persons with AIDS. JAMA 259:1333–1337, 1988.
33. Centers for Disease Control: Guidelines for the performance of CD4+ T-cell determinations in persons with human immunodeficiency virus infection. MMWR 41(RR-8):1–17, 1992.
34. National Institutes of Health: State of the art conference on azidothymidine therapy of early HIV infection. Am J Med 89:335–344, 1990.
35. Polk BF: Predictors of the acquired human immunodeficiency syndrome developing in a cohort of sero-positive homosexual men. N Engl J Med 158:615–622, 1987.
36. MacDonell KB: Predicting progression to AIDS: Combined usefulness of CD4 lymphocyte counts and p24 antigenemia. Am J Med 89:706–712, 1990.
37. Fahey JL: The prognostic value of cellular and serologic markers in infection with human immunodeficiency virus type I. N Engl J Med 332:166–172, 1990.
38. HIV Guideline Panel Agency for Health Care Policy and Research: Guidelines for Evaluation and Management of Early HIV Infection (In press).
39. Selwyn PA, Hartel D, Lewis VA, et al: A prospective study of the risk of tuberculosis among intravenous drug users with human immunodeficiency virus infection. N Engl J Med 320:545–550, 1989.
40. Centers for Disease Control: Tuberculosis and human immunodeficiency virus infection: Recommendations of the Advisory Committee for the Elimination of Tuberculosis (ACET). MMWR 38:236–250, 1989.
41. Small PM, Schecter GF, and Goodman PC: Treatment of tuberculosis in patients with advanced human immunodeficiency virus infection. N Engl J Med 324:289–294, 1991.
42. Centers for Disease Control: Update on hepatitis B prevention. MMWR 36:353–366, 1987.
43. Haas JS, Bolan G, and Larsen SA, et al: Sensitivity of treponemal tests for detecting prior treated syphilis during human immunodeficiency virus infection. J Infect Dis 162:862–826, 1990.
44. Hecht FM and Soloway B: Laboratory tests for monitoring HIV infection. *In* Cotton DJ and Friedland GH (eds): HIV Infection: A Primary Care Approach. Waltham, MA, Massachusetts Medical Society, 1992, p 17.
45. DiNubile MJ: Screening HIV-infected recipients of blood transfusions for CMV infection. N Engl J Med 323:1282–1283, 1990.
46. Centers for Disease Control: General recommendations for immunizations. Ann Intern Med 111:133–142, 1989.
47. Poland GA, Love KR, and Hughes CE: Routine immunization of the HIV-positive asymptomatic patient. J Gen Intern Med 5:147–152, 1990.

48. Steinhoff MC, Aurerbach BS, and Nelson KE: Antibody responses to *Haemophilus influenza* type B vaccines in men with human immunodeficiency virus infection. N Engl J Med 325:1837–1842, 1991.
49. Fischl MA: The efficacy of azidothymidine in the treatment of patients with AIDS and AIDS-related complex. N Engl J Med 317:185–192, 1987.
50. Volberding PA, Lagakos SW, Koch MA, et al: Zidovudine in asymptomatic human immunodeficiency virus infection: A controlled trial in persons with fewer than 500 CD4-positive cells per cubic millimeter. N Engl J Med 322:941–949, 1990.
51. Hamilton JD: A controlled trial of early versus late treatment with zidovudine in symptomatic human immunodeficiency virus infection. N Engl J Med 326:437–443, 1992.
51a. Aboulker J-P, Swart AM: Preliminary analysis of the Concorde trial. Lancet 341:889–890, 1993.
51b. Cooper DA, Gatell JM, Kroon S, et al: Zidovudine in persons with asymptomatic HIV infection and CD4+ cell counts greater than 400 per cubic millimeter. N Engl J Med 329:297–303, 1993.
52. Sande MA, Carpenter CCJ, Cobbs CG, et al: State-of-the-Art Conference on Antiretroviral Therapy for Adult HIV-Infected Patients: Final Report. JAMA (In press).
53. Kahn JO, Lagakos SW, Richman DD, et al: A controlled trial comparing continued zidovudine with didanosine in human immunodeficiency virus infection. N Engl J Med 327:581–587, 1992.
54. Meng T-C, Fischl MA, Boota AM, et al: Combination therapy with zidovudine and dideoxycytidine in patients with advanced human immunodeficiency virus infection. A phase I/II study. Ann Intern Med 116:13–20, 1992.
55. Richman DD: Effect of stage of disease and drug dose on zidovudine susceptibilities of isolates of human immunodeficiency virus. J Acquir Immune Defic Syndr 3:743–746, 1990.
56. Hardy WD: Trimethoprim-sulfamethoxazole versus aerosolized pentamidine for secondary prophylaxis of *Pneumocystis carinii* pneumonia in AIDS patients (In preparation).
57. Carr A: Trimethoprim-sulfamethoxazole appears more effective than aerosolized pentamidine as secondary prophylaxis against *Pneumocystis carinii* pneumonia in patients with AIDS. AIDS 6:165–171, 1992.
58. Conant MA and Allen B: Oral desensitization to trimethaprim-sulfamethoxazole. (Personal communication, 1992)
59. Pierce P: O.I. prophylaxis overview: Treatment issues—The gay men's health crisis. Newsletter of Experimental AIDS Therapies 6(4):1–6, 1992.
59a. Nightingale SD, Byrd LT, Southern PM, et al: Incidence of *Mycobacterium avium intracellulare* complex bacteremia in human immunodeficiency virus-positive patients. J Infect Dis 165:1082–1085, 1992.
59b. Gordin F, Nightingale S, Wynne B, et al: Rifabutin monotherapy prevents or delays *Mycobacterium avium* complex (MAC) bacteremia in patients with AIDS. Eighth International Conference on AIDS, Amsterdam 1992; 3081: abstract.
60. Advisory Committee for Elimination of Tuberculosis: The use of preventive therapy for tuberculosis infection in the United States: Recommendations of the Advisory Committee for Elimination of Tuberculosis. MMWR 39(RR-8):9–12, 1990.
61. Selwyn P, et al: High risk of active tuberculosis in HIV infected drug users with cutaneous anergy. JAMA 268:504–509, 1992.
62. Centers for Disease Control: Guidelines for prophylaxis against *Pneumocystis carinii* pneumonia for persons infected with human immonodeficiency virus. MMWR 38(Suppl 5):1–9, 1989.
63. Musher DM, Hamill RJ, and Baughn RE: Effect of human immunodeficiency virus (HIV) on the course of syphilis and on the response to treatment. Ann Intern Med 113:276–282, 1990.
64. Freedberg KA, Tosteson AN, Cotton DJ, and Goldman L: Optimal management strategies for HIV-infected patients who present with cough or dyspnea: A cost-effectiveness analysis. J Gen Intern Med 7:261–272, 1992.
65. Farizo KM, Buehler JW, Chamberland ME, et al: Spectrum of disease in persons with human immunodeficiency virus infection in the United States. JAMA 267:1798–1805, 1992.
66. Masur H, Ognibene FA, Yarchoan R, et al: CD4 counts as predictors of opportunistic pneumonias in human immunodefeciency virus (HIV) infection. Ann Intern Med 111:223–231, 1989.
67. Polsky B, Gold JWM, Whimbey E, et al: Bacterial pneumonia in patients with acquired immunodeficiency syndrome. Ann Intern Med 104:38–41, 1986.
68. National Institutes of Health, University of California Expert Panel for Corticosteroids as Adjunctive Therapy for *Pneumocystis* Pneumonia: Consensus statement on the use of corticosteroids as adjunctive therapy for *Pneumocystis* pneumonia in the acquired immunodeficiency syndrome. N Engl J Med 323:1500–1504, 1990.
69. Katz MH, Baron RB, and Grady D: Risk stratification of ambulatory patients suspected of *Pneumocystis* pneumonia. Arch Intern Med 151:105–110, 1991.
70. Zaman MK and White DA: Serum lactate dehydrogenase levels and *Pneumocystis carinii* pneumonia. Am Rev Respir Dis 137:796–800, 1988.
71. Kotler DP: Intestinal and hepatic manifestations of AIDS. Adv Intern Med 34:43–72, 1989.
72. Raufman JP: Odynophagia/dysphagia in AIDS. Gastroenterol Clin North Am 17:599–614, 1988.
73. Wilcox CM, Diehl DL, Cello JP, et al: Cytomegalovirus esophagitis in patients with AIDS: A clinical, endoscopic and pathologic correlation. Ann Intern Med 113:589–593, 1990.
74. De Wit S, Weerts D, Goosens H, and Clumeck N: Comparison of fluconazole and ketoconazole for oro-pharyngeal candidiasis in AIDS. Lancet i:746–748, 1989.
75. Rabeneck L, Popovic M, Gartner S, et al: Acute HIV infection presenting with painful swallowing and esophageal ulcers. JAMA 263:2318–2322, 1990.
76. Bach MC, Howell PD, and Valenti AJ: Apthous ulceration of the gastro-intestinal tract in patients with the acquired immunodeficiency syndrome (AIDS). Ann Intern Med 112:465–467, 1990.
77. Smith PD: Gastrointestinal infections in AIDS. Ann Intern Med 116:63–77, 1992.
78. Smith PD and Janoff EN: Infectious diarrhea in human immunodeficiency virus infection. Gasteroenterol Clin North Am 17:587–598, 1988.
79. Johanson JF and Sonnenberg A: Efficient management of diarrhea in the acquired deficiency syndrome (AIDS). A medical decision analysis. Ann Intern Med 112:942–948, 1990.
80. Hollander H: Neurologic and psychiatric manifestations of HIV disease. J Gen Intern Med 6:S24–S31, 1991.
81. Navia BA and Price RW: The AIDS dementia complex. I. Clinical features. Ann Neurol 19:517–524, 1986.
82. McArthur JC: Neurologic manifestations of AIDS. Medicine 66:407–437, 1987.
83. Snider WD, Simpson DM, Nielson SL, et al: Neurologic complications of acquired immune deficiency syndrome: Analysis of 50 patients. Ann Neurol 14:403–418, 1988.

65

Clinical Problems in Geriatrics

DAVID F. POLAKOFF, MD, MSPH
KENNETH MINAKER, MD

Medical care of the elderly, both inpatient and outpatient, will dominate the internal medicine of the 21st century because of demographic trends and the increased rates of utilization of health care resources by elderly patients.[1] Between 1960 and 1980 a 55% increase was seen in the number of individuals older than 65 years of age. By the year 2000, the elderly will number 36.3 million, and by 2040, 67.3 million.[2] Within the elderly as a group, those older than 85 years of age, often referred to as the oldest-old, are the most medically dependent and are increasing more rapidly than are those in any other population group. By 2000, those older than 85 years of age will have tripled from present numbers to 13.3 million, and by 2040 will comprise 4% of the population in the United States.

Americans older than 65 years of age account for 40% of acute hospital days, buy 20% of all prescription drugs, and spend 30% of our entire health care budget, which presently represents 13% of the Gross National Product. Annual physician visits per capita increase from 4.4 at ages 17 to 44 to 5.5 at ages 45 to 64 and peak at 6.6 over 64 years of age. Hospitalizations per year for various age groups increase from 13.4% at ages 17 to 44 years to 21.9% at ages 45 to 64 years and peak at 30.4% over age 64 years.[3] Long-term care and rehabilitation settings are essentially geriatric programs. Increased knowledge of physiologic and pathologic changes that contribute to disability and complicate therapy in the elderly has led to the development of general principles of geriatric assessment and management. A practical approach to several common geriatric syndromes encountered in the office setting is presented.

IMPACT OF AGING ON HEALTH

True aging changes occur with advancing age in all members of a species. Physiologic aging exerts a broad, yet contínous, spectrum of influences that range from insignificant to changes that actually represent disease inasmuch as they have direct, predictable, adverse clinical sequelae.[4] Several specific, clinically relevant points along the continuum can be identified. Physiologic aging may cause no changes in clinical parameters, may increase the vulnerability to disease, or may alter the expression of clinical illness.

Perhaps the most important change that occurs with age, from a clinical standpoint, is no change at all. Routine hematologic parameters of hematocrit, total neutrophil, lymphocyte count, and platelet count are unaltered with age. There is no "anemia of old age," and reductions in hematocrit signify the presence of illness that deserves proper investigation and treatment. Iron deficiency anemia due to blood loss, anemia of chronic diseases such as renal failure, nutritional anemias such as pernicious anemia, and myeloproliferative disorders are frequent in the elderly. Cardiac output at rest or during vigorous exercise is not limited by the aging process. Measures of hepatic function and electrolytes and most basal hormonal values are unaltered with aging. Aging does not affect basal levels of testosterone, the glucoregulatory hormones, insulin, glucagon, growth hormone, or cortisol. Thyroxine levels are generally considered to be unaltered with age.[5] A major progressive, and uniformly silent, impact of aging is the normative decline in organ function required for homeostasis during acute medical illness. Maximum ventilatory capacity, glomerular filtration rate, many measures of immune competence, ability to maintain a stable upright posture, and carbohydrate tolerance all demonstrate progressive normative decrements of nearly 10% per decade starting at the peak of homeostatic capacity near 30 years of age (Fig. 65–1). These changes in organ function become clinically relevant not during everyday living, but when reserve organ function must be acutely drawn upon or when the magnitude of a chronic demand is large. Simultaneous linear reductions in reserve function of many organs result in a geometric reduction in total homeostatic capacity. The markedly enhanced vulnerability of the elderly to the morbid effects of acute illness such as head injury, major surgery, trauma, burns, and administration of medications is explained in part by these normal changes with age.[6] Additionally, advances in therapy may not extend equally to all ages of patients, accounting, in part, for the age-related slowing of the improvement in survival from burns in the past decade.[7]

Altered presentation of disease in the elderly has long been recognized as a consequence of changes produced by

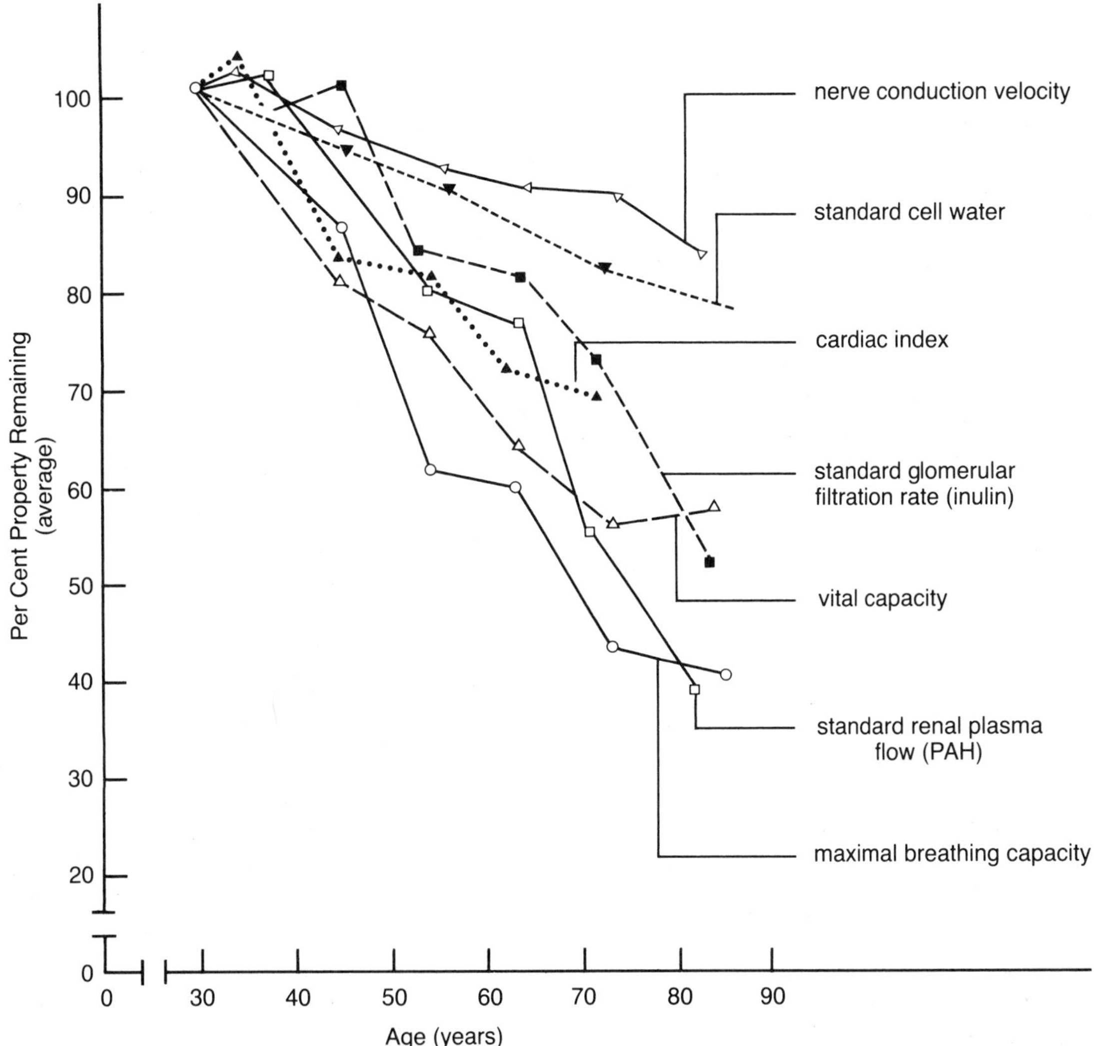

FIGURE 65–1. Decline with age in selected physiologic functions in humans. (Adapted from Shock NW: Discussion on mortality and measurement. *In* Strehler BL, Ebert JD, Glass HB, et al: The Biology of Aging: A Symposium. Washington, DC, American Institute of Biological Sciences, 1960, pp 22–23.)

the aging process. One example is hyperthyroidism. Whereas in this condition younger individuals present a generalized symptom complex of agitation, hyperkinesis, goiter, hyperdynamic circulation, and hyperphagia, older individuals seldom appear activated, frequently show no thyromegaly, often appear "apathetic," and commonly show a deterioration in cardiac function.[8] The major clinical importance relates to increasing the recognition of hyperthyroidism in the elderly because treatment of this condition brings the same excellent results as in younger patients. Another example in which physiologic changes lead to differing presentations of illness in late life is hyperosmolar, nonketotic, hyperglycemic coma. This diabetic state, which has been shown to be a largely geriatric illness, may present without the polydipsia and polyuric complaints that accompany the common hyperglycemic stresses in the young. Indeed, perhaps one third of elderly individuals with this condition have not previously been characterized as diabetic.

An overriding principle of gerontologic physiology is the marked inter- and intraindividual variability in rates of true aging changes in different persons.[9] Thus, organs such as kidney, heart, and lung age at different rates in different individuals, and within the same individuals the rates of aging may vary greatly from one organ to another. In contrast, certain physiologic functions remain largely intact into extreme old age without detectable differences among individuals, that is, young and old or within old. Finally, some changes that occur during aging are the result of accumulated exposure over time and are not aging changes per se. The development of skin cancer on ultraviolet light–damaged skin, pulmonary cancer secondary to smoking for many years, and the appearance of polycystic renal disease represent changes secondary to toxin exposure or delayed expression of genetic disease.

ASSESSMENT OF THE ELDERLY PATIENT

Comprehensive assessment of the geriatric patient identifies a patient's difficulties and the resultant impact on functional capacity. Geriatric assessment requires systematic consideration of function in three dimensions: physical/medical, mental/psychiatric, and social/financial. Even though the physical/medical evaluation is most familiar to practitioners, special care and knowledge are necessary even in this area when assessing frail elderly individuals.

Physical/Medical Assessment

History. History-taking in the elderly must be flexible and tap resources that are not frequently used in the rest of adult medicine. History-taking for patients in the geriatric age range has the same purpose as it does at younger ages: to gather information leading to appropriate diagnostic and therapeutic strategies. Certainly, we all see in clinical practice previously healthy elderly patients who give a lucid history of new-onset exertional chest pain, radiating to the neck, associated with shortness of breath, and all relieved by 5 minutes' rest. These patients require no change in history-taking technique. Much more common, and leading to substantial frustration for the physician, is the patient with nonfocal symptoms who is unable to provide necessary information leading to an efficient evaluation. The interview process must be able to accommodate this challenge.

As in most complex procedures, preparation is essential before the patient interview begins. The problem geriatric patient is not a single independent individual with a localized symptom but rather a fragile, slowly deteriorating patient highly dependent on family and other community supports. Before the patient enters the examining room, the similarity and quality of the agendas that patient, family, and community resource persons have for the medical evaluation should be ascertained. For example, a patient may indicate that shortness of breath is the complaint to be addressed; his daughter indicates that associated with shortness of breath is confusion leading to panicked phone calls, alteration in the sleep/wake cycle, and three falls in the past 2 weeks; and finally, the visiting nurse may be having great difficulty monitoring the multiple medications the patient is taking. Failure to appreciate the agendas beyond the elderly patient's chief complaint will lead to an overnarrow interview and doom therapy to ineffectiveness.

The gathering of historical material should have begun before the interview and is based on the four Rs: *records* (your own and relevant hospital records); *relatives; respect* for the individually appropriate objective for health and social care; and finally, during the interview, patient *recall.* The major barriers to incorporating the four Rs into history taking in elderly subjects are the time required to assemble these data and the lack of reimbursement for this effort. Necessity, common sense, and physician competition are leading to a fuller incorporation of the four Rs in the geriatric interview process.

Patients with complex histories should be accompanied by a relative, and the professional should have access to their previous records. Four or five chronic illnesses commonly coexist in older patients. The time span over which these illnesses commonly exist, the modernization and sophistication of therapies (e.g., varied pharmacologic agents for hypertension during the past 20 years), the complications and intolerances, and the interrelatedness of illnesses all tax even a very lucid elder person's memory, making the patient's past records an important data base from which to continue care.

Relatives should be encouraged to provide their historical perspective for a number of reasons. In the majority of complex geriatric patients, relatives obtain, maintain, and retain prosthetic or pharmacologic interventions, and they assume progressively greater responsibility in determining the health care utilization patterns of the elderly patient. Supportive relatives are, in most cases, your case managers, assurers of compliance, and monitors of therapy. They should be given access to the physician before investigation and therapy begin.

Improvement in functional status has supplanted prolongation of life as the primary objective of medical care in the geriatric population. Respect for an individual's lifestyle (and, therefore, deathstyle) must be present, and an appropriate consensus should be established.

The interview technique can be expanded beyond the doctor-patient interview in several ways. First, secretarial staff should be trained to emphasize during a preappointment telephone call the necessity to obtain all past medical records and for all of the patient's medications to be identified and brought to the interview. A family resource person should be identified and be encouraged to accompany the patient. Increasing use of self- or family-completed questionnaires, which include demographic, functional, and medical components specifically designed for the elderly, are becoming available and can serve as a checklist for the physician and assist the family and patient to crystallize the elements of a deteriorating situation.

For a more detailed evaluation, physician-extending professionally administered interview tools are available to evaluate mental status and functional capacity, essential facts that can be in place prior to physician evaluation but are crucial to an efficient physician-patient interview. It is crucial to enlist the assistance of responsible relatives by having them participate in the interview at some point, to emphasize their responsibilities, and to reward their caregiving at the end of your examination. They become your extensions and monitors and will ensure compliance with any recommended therapy. In practical terms, if no medical emergency exists it is best to conduct the interview over a comfortable series of visits, which permits familiarity to develop, some short-term longitudinal impressions to be gained, and completion of a sound data base.

The physician-patient interaction assumes a distinctly different ambiance with the background thus obtained. Rapport is gracefully and tactfully established in this setting, and one can rapidly focus on the patient's subjective chief complaint, with little likelihood of frustration if history-taking cannot extend beyond the chief complaint or the history of present illness. The major skills in interview technique that require special attention in the elderly relate primarily to communication and patient comfort. The deaf, blind, confused, or immobile patient must be comfortably positioned, and sensitivity to and compensation for sensory deficits must be made. We keep a hearing tube available, avoid backlighting ourselves, simplify the history, and carefully position patients for each clinical problem.

Although it has been demonstrated that in the United States the elderly patient spends less time per visit with his or her physician than does a younger individual, complex patients clearly require more time. With family presence, good background data, and a reasonably cooperative patient, we believe that direct physician-patient time will generally be in the 30-minute range for an initial interview, which, done properly, leads to dramatically shorter and progressively more successful subsequent follow-up appointments.

Examination. The physical examination requires a number of modifications to successfully evaluate elderly patients. As the examination is commonly more lengthy than in younger individuals, it is best to establish priorities in the initial examination for urgent medical problems and aim to complete the evaluation in subsequent visits.[10] The components of special relevance to the physical examination in the older patient are the mental status examination, the functional assessment, and quantification of the impact of sensory impairment.

The mental status examination is an important adjunct to physical examination in the elderly because 10% of Americans older than 65 years of age will suffer from some form of progressive memory failure. Impaired cognition has a broad range of impacts on medical care, including reliability of the history, compliance with therapies, and reporting of complications.[11] The principal areas of cognitive function that should be evaluated include attention, language, memory, visuospatial ability, conceptualization, and executive function. For clinicians in the office setting, the most practical approach is to employ a standardized, valid testing instrument that has been shown to be useful for mild-to-moderate degrees of cognitive impairment. From the patient care perspective, mild-to-moderate impairment is the most clinically relevant because it leads to the greatest degree of medical management problems. Severe degrees of memory failure are obvious. Subtle changes in memory often require formal neuropsychological testing for full characterization.

Although a variety of tests are available, perhaps the most widely applied test is Folstein's "Mini–Mental State" examination (see also Chapter 57).[12] It provides a general overview of the major areas of cognitive assessment, is reliable and reproducible, and can be completed in less than 10 minutes. The score generated is a quick way to document changes over time. As any test of this kind can be perceived as threatening, it is best to introduce such testing as standard practice for older patients.

An essential component of the clinical assessment of the ill elderly is measurement of the functional impact of an unweighted list of diagnoses. This is necessary because diagnosis or physical findings provide an inadequate index of health because the range of functional impact of a given diagnosis is very great in the elderly.

Functional assessment for older patients helps the clinician to understand health capacities of frail older patients. The goal in modern health care is not the complete elimination of illness but facilitation of the highest level of personal function that is possible. Familiarity with this component of geriatric assessment orients the clinicians to management goals for older patients. Several types of function are assessed.[13] The first set of functions or activities of daily living include the patient's ability to feed, toilet, dress, and perform personal hygiene together with an assessment of mobility. The second set of functional abilities, termed instrumental activities, include shopping, cooking, managing money, housekeeping, and traveling. The history is important in identifying the need to evaluate function, but its formal observation and quantitation are crucial.[14] For example, the elderly patient with arthritic hands should be observed opening pill bottles and performing self-hygiene if the history suggests clinically important impairment. The local visiting nurse is skilled in completion of this type of evaluation in the home, where success in these activities is most relevant.[15] Detailed knowledge of a patient's function often leads to the procurement of focused support services that actually promote or increase function, improve hygiene, and permit the patient to remain at home.

Unfortunately, no clear choices are presently available in standardized measures of function, but this area has become a high priority in technology assessment for the elderly.[13]

The third area of physical assessment of special importance to the elderly is the documentation of sensory impairment. Visual impairment affects 15% of the elderly and is a major contributor to falls and functional impairment in late life. There is a slight decline in visual acuity up to the age of 60 years, which accelerates between the ages of 60 and 80 years.[16] Constriction of visual fields also shows dramatic acceleration after 60 years of age.[17] Other visual parameters documented to show progressive impairments with advancing age include color sensitivity (particularly to blue light), accommodation, and oculomotor function with progressive failure of upward gaze.[18] Physicians capable of performing ocular examinations of their older patients and aware of the age-related physiologic changes will be able to facilitate appropriate referrals. Visual acuity testing, retinoscopy, and tonometry are the major skills required.

The elderly are particularly susceptible to several syndromes requiring prompt care, which the aforementioned data base and skills will prepare the clinician to handle. Giant cell arteritis can produce an ophthalmic catastrophe and occurs exclusively in the elderly. It most commonly produces ischemic optic neuritis (75% of ocular events) due to arteritis of the posterior ciliary artery. Therapy with high-dose steroids, followed by temporal artery biopsy, should be initiated immediately. Acute monocular blindness may be caused by other illnesses common in the elderly, such as retinal detachment, hemorrhage, and vascular occlusion. Like ischemic optic neuritis, these are geriatric ophthalmic emergencies.

Amaurosis fugax, a syndrome characterized by transient monocular visual loss, is three times more common in the elderly than in younger individuals, and half the cases in the elderly may have underlying operable disease, a much higher percentage than in younger individuals.[19] Cataract and glaucoma are frequent causes of visual impairment in the elderly, and it is the careful internist who can guide the elderly, who often have limited contact with subspecialty care, to important preventive visual care.

One half of those with significant hearing loss are older than 65 years of age. With advancing age, a progressive sensorineural hearing loss occurs beginning at 20 years of age but becoming clinically relevant only at 60 to 70 years of age when deficits in the spoken voice frequencies (500 to 4000 cps) appear.[20] In the 45- to 64-year age group, the incidence of hearing loss is 114 per 1000; in the 64- to 74-year age groups, 231 per 1000; and this nearly doubles in the over 75-year group to 399 per 1000. The practicing physician is responsible for the initial evaluation of hearing loss and appropriate referral for further care. The otologic examination should include examination for ceruminous impaction, thickened or perforated ear drums, and otitis media or externa. If hearing loss remains after appropriate therapy for the foregoing conditions, a baseline audiogram should be obtained. This will include air and bone conduction evaluation for pure tones initially. An air/bone gap will confirm a conductive loss, and sensorineural loss is characterized by overlapping air and bone conduction thresholds.

Subsequent components of a formal audiologic examination are determination of a speech reception threshold and a speech discrimination test. The successful prescription of a hearing aid for the elderly presbycusic patient requires a thoughtful trial of an aid under careful supervision by an audiologist. Ability to master the controls, adjustment to the altered character of the transmitted sound, and the stigma of the aid may all make hearing rehabilitation difficult, but an attempt is always justified.

The components of the hearing aid include the microphone, receiver, amplifier, and volume and on/off switches. Differing aids can be matched to individual patient needs.

The tiny canal-type unit will compensate for mild hearing loss of up to 45 decibels; the "conch" variety accommodates moderate hearing loss of up to 60 decibels; and the postauricular prosthesis is the most powerful type and is able to help with severe loss of up to 90 decibels (see Chapter 70). For those failing amplification of sound by an aid, amplifier controls on telephones and other transmitters may help to prevent major degrees of sensory deprivation.

Psychosocial Assessment. Physicians who have had little training in psychiatry may lead management teams for the elderly with psychiatric problems. The incidence of psychopathology increases with advancing age.[21] Between 5 and 15% of the elderly are depressed. Suicide rates are highest in elderly white men.[22] According to the Biometry Branch of the National Institute of Mental Health, about 80% of elderly people who need psychiatric assistance are not currently being served. Perhaps 2% of psychiatrists' time in private practice is spent with older patients. The interplay of physical, mental, and social function justifies psychiatric assessment for its influence on other realms of function as well as for its own sake.

An individual's quality of life has four elements: life satisfaction, self-esteem, general health and functional status, and socioeconomic characteristics. Social function (relationships with family and friends, and community interactions) is viewed as an important creator of self-esteem. Although social assessment tools exist, there is a general lack of support for specific measurements.[13] It is important to recognize that 80% of the long-term care needs of elderly individuals are provided by family and friends. The practical elements of social assessment are focused clearly, then, on the quality of support that family members are able to provide and on their ability to satisfy the usually increasing needs of the elderly homebound patient. Growing out of this interaction, and crucial to the treatment plan, is consideration of the morale of the relatives and of any services that might be designed to provide them with respite and education.

The impact of social forces on the physical well-being of an individual has been best described for the loss of a spouse—the clearest social support of all. The link between bereavement and mortality due to suicide was first emphasized in British studies.[23] In early studies of overall mortality during widowhood, widowers suffered increased mortality during the 6 months following the death of a spouse.[24] Widows experience a less dramatic early mortality, and their peak mortality is in the second year of bereavement. Even when the effects of homogamy (the sick marrying the sick), common infections (i.e., tuberculosis), and joint unfavorable environment were considered as causes for this excess mortality, other factors seem more causally attractive. As the causes of death seem to parallel the usual causes of death for the respective age groups, it is conceptually consistent that grief acts as a stress that can unmask established disease. The pathophysiologic mechanism may be found in neuroendocrine or immune changes.

The management of the grief reaction is based on awareness of bereavement's capacity to induce morbid events, and the recognition that 25 to 50% of recently widowed individuals will visit their physicians early with nonspecific symptoms.[25] This presents to the physician an opportunity to practice a preventive approach. Such an approach would treat bereavement as a normal and self-limited reaction to the recent loss. The bereaved individual should be followed closely for signs of deepening depression or development of a comorbid illness. If the symptoms of bereavement fail to clear after 6 months, or are so severe as to cause impairments in physical, cognitive, or social function, pharmacotherapy for major depression should be considered. It must be emphasized that at present few data exist on the efficacy of this or any other approach; fruitful research in this area can be anticipated.

In summary, geriatric assessment involves a multidisciplinary approach, often extending over several patient visits, to make a complex clinical situation understandable and thus therapeutically approachable.

USE OF MEDICATIONS BY THE ELDERLY

Geriatric patients consume 25% of all prescribed and over-the-counter medications in the United States, an amount disproportionate to their numbers (currently 11% of the population). This drug consumption is not evenly distributed among all older individuals. In the previous 2 years, 12.4% of older Americans have not seen a physician because of good health and would not be expected to be significant consumers of pharmacologic agents. A further 55% consider themselves unlimited in daily activities, and although they are probably moderate consumers of medications, particularly antihypertensives and diuretics, they would not account for a major amount of the disproportionate use of medications by the elderly. This leaves a remaining 20 to 25% of the elderly who have major functional disabilities (~3% of the United States population) to be the predominant consumers of 25% of all medications. These patients, usually older than 75 years of age, have a 20% chance of having an adverse drug reaction with the initiation of therapy and, if taking more than three medications initially, a moderate likelihood of noncompliance. Failure to take medication is the commonest noncompliant response, but suicidal overdosage is another potential response. Because medication is the second highest out-of-pocket health care expense for the elderly (after physician fees), compliance will also be influenced by prescribing practices of physicians.

The effects of medication are determined by pharmacokinetic and pharmacodynamic factors. The elderly show significant alterations in both, leading to specific changes in prescribing practices for certain drug groups. Drugs eliminated by the kidney must be decreased in dosage to prevent their accumulation in elderly individuals who are likely to have a 50% reduction in glomerular filtration rate from 30 to 80 years of age. Examples of such medications include aminoglycoside antibiotics, acetohexamide, chlorpropamide, vancomycin, nitrofurantoin, tetracycline, digoxin, procainamide, cephaloridine, lithium, and cimetidine. Several drugs are metabolized more slowly by the liver with age, particularly those requiring phase I reactions such as hydroxylation, *N*-dealkylation, sulfoxidation, nitroreduction, and hydrolysis. Antipyrine, phenytoin, quinidine, phenobarbital, imipramine, amitryptiline, desipramine, nortryptiline, diazepam, and chlordiazepoxide are proven examples of drugs less well metabolized by the aging liver.[26]

A larger and difficult-to-study group are those drugs that show pharmacodynamic changes with age. Drugs in this group are more potent in the elderly, because of either greater therapeutic or greater adverse effects. These alterations in pharmacodynamic effects are secondary to heightened sensitivity at drug receptor sites or decreased homeostatic capacity. Analgesics, particularly pentazocine and morphine, are more potent in the elderly, and reductions in dosages by one third are recommended in the very old. Oral anticoagulants are more potent in the elderly, and maintenance dosages are usually 60% less in the old. The large group of medications in the neuroleptic group find an important role in managing a variety of behavioral disturbances in the elderly, including delirium, dementia, late paraphrenia, schizophrenia, and major affective disorders. As access of elderly patients to psychiatric assistance is limited, the introduction and management of these medications falls to the physician. Pharmacokinetic changes largely due to modest reduction in hepatic metabolism of these agents produce higher levels in older patients, but a major secondary effect is due to diminished dopaminergic and cholinergic neurotransmission that occurs with aging. These reductions result in the equivalent of enhanced sensitivity to side effects of these agents (see Chapter 82). Other medications show greater effects with advancing age, including most antihypertensive agents, which should be initiated in general at one half of the usual dosages. Growing directly from these clinically important changes in drug effects with age are a series of general principles of drug therapy in the elderly (Table 65–1). Adherence to these principles will improve the effectiveness of pharmacotherapy in the elderly.[27]

CLINICAL PROBLEMS

Urinary Incontinence

Urinary incontinence is a prevalent and particularly distressing symptom in the elderly, with major psychosocial, economic, and health consequences. Largely because of the social stigma attached, as well as a misunderstanding of potential causes and treatment outcomes, the symptoms of incontinence are often disguised and underreported.[28] Estimates of its prevalence in the elderly range from 5 to 20% among persons living in the community[28] and from 40 to 75% among those in long-term care facilities.[29] Incontinence is associated with an increased incidence of pressure sores, use of indwelling catheters, and subsequent urinary infection. Psychosocially, incontinence can cause embarrassment, isolation, and regression, and it contributes to the decision to institutionalize an elderly person.

Incontinence may be characterized as either reversible or fixed (Table 65–2). The elderly are particularly susceptible to reversible causes of incontinence, because the capacity of the bladder and competency of the urethral mechanism are diminished in elderly persons; hence, the first step in the assessment of urinary incontinence of the aged is to identify and remove all reversible causes, even if irreversible causes are also present. Fixed or irreversible incontinence may result from diminished central nervous system (CNS) inhibition of the bladder, spinal cord lesions, peripheral neuropathy, or local lesions such as bladder tumor, outlet obstruction, and pelvic floor laxity. Up-going toes, hyperreflexia, and spasticity of the lower extremities are signs of CNS or spinal cord lesions. Both the afferent and efferent limbs of sacral innervation are tested by the anal wink reflex. Voluntary anal sphincter contraction and sacral pin sensation should also be tested. A careful history, pelvic and urologic examination, and urinalysis should detect most local causes of incontinence. The cystometrogram can help to establish the cause of incontinence and should be performed before surgical intervention in most cases, but it is poorly standardized in the aged, so that clinical evaluation, removal of reversible causes, and a trial of therapy are generally indicated prior to cystometrography.

After decades of neglect of the topic, studies of incontinence suggest that the fixed or chronic type, which is unrelated to the causes of reversible incontinence listed in Table 65–2, can be treated successfully in many patients. The most common subtype, accounting for approximately 50% of cases, is *urge incontinence*.[30] In these cases, the patient senses an urge to void but is unable to prevent voiding; cystometric evaluation shows uninhibited contractions of the bladder. Decreased CNS or spinal cord inhibition of bladder contraction or local bladder disorders are the usual causes (see Table 65–2). Urge incontinence can often be substantially improved by smooth muscle relaxants, such as calcium channel blockers,[31] or by administration of anticholinergic medications, such as oxybutynin,[32] which are effective in decreasing bladder contractions but often have troublesome anticholinergic side effects. In one preliminary study in the elderly, low-dose imipramine, a tricyclic antidepressant, was beneficial, probably because of the combined anticholinergic and direct smooth muscle relaxant effects on the detrusor, along with the drug's α-adrenergic

TABLE 65–1. PRINCIPLES OF PHARMACOTHERAPY IN THE ELDERLY

- Before prescribing new drugs, thoroughly review all medication the patient is presently taking.
- Before prescribing a drug for a specific symptom, consider the possibility that the symptom is an adverse reaction to a medication. In general, stopping a drug is more beneficial than starting one.
- Before prescribing a drug, consider the patient's age and the presence of any specific disease states, particularly cardiac disease and impaired renal function.
- Keep drug regimens as simple as possible.
- Use the lowest effective dose and increase the dose slowly.
- Do not withhold drugs because of age.
- Assess therapeutic response frequently and discontinue unneeded drugs.
- Perform thorough, frequent reviews of the medication regimen.
- Consider the cost of medications and use generic preparations when appropriate.

TABLE 65–2. CAUSES OF INCONTINENCE IN THE ELDERLY

Reversible Causes
- Acute confusional state
- Marked immobility
- Fecal impaction
- Symptomatic bladder infection
- Metabolic abnormalities (hypercalcemia, hyperglycemia)
- Medications (sedatives, anticholinergic drugs, α-adrenergic agonists and antagonists, calcium channel blocking agents)

Urge Incontinence due to Detrusor Instability or Hyperreflexia
- Lack of central nervous system inhibition (Alzheimer's disease, Parkinson's disease, other central nervous system disorders)
- Interference with spinal inhibitory pathways (cervical spinal myelopathy due to spondylosis, other spinal cord lesions)
- Local bladder disorders (interstitial cystitis, postradiation effects, bladder tumor or obstruction)

Stress Incontinence
- Pelvic laxity from overstretching of pelvic musculature in childbirth, age-related weakness, or previous surgical damage
- Atrophic urethritis, urethral caruncle, and vaginitis
- Stress-induced detrusor instability (suggested by delay between stress and leakage, treated as urge incontinence)

Overflow Incontinence
- Bladder outlet obstruction (prostatic hypertrophy, urethral stricture)
- Neurogenic bladder (peripheral neuropathy due to diabetes, tabes, vitamin B_{12} deficiency, or herniated disk or other sacral nerve root lesions)

Reflex Incontinence
- Spinal cord lesions (spondylosis, tumor)
- Disorders of the cerebral cortex

agonist properties, which would be expected to increase bladder outlet tone. However, this agent is associated with orthostatic hypotension and must be used with caution in the elderly. In an innovative, nonpharmacologic approach, McGuire and associates employed transcutaneous electrical stimulation of the peroneal or posterior tibial nerve, by means of a portable unit similar to that used for pain control, in 22 patients with documented detrusor instability.[33] Urinary incontinence was completely controlled in 12 patients and was improved in seven, with no adverse effects. It appears that bladder emptying is inhibited as the nerve stimulation traverses the sacral cord and inhibits the center that controls detrusor contraction. This effective, simple, and relatively inexpensive treatment holds promise for incontinent patients whose cognitive function permits initiation of nerve stimulation with the onset of the urge to void.

A second major form of chronic incontinence in the elderly is *stress incontinence,* the involuntary loss of urine only when intra-abdominal pressure is transiently increased. The underlying abnormality is usually incompetence of the bladder outlet secondary to overstretching of pelvic musculature during childbirth, age-related weakening of the pelvic musculature, or damage from previous surgery (see Table 65–2).

Though stress incontinence is often unreported by embarrassed patients and ignored by physicians, effective treatments are now available for this common disorder. Since the urethral mucosa contributes to outlet resistance and is maintained in women by estrogens, postmenopausal estrogen deficiency with atrophic urethritis can be an important contributing cause of stress incontinence. Local (vaginal cream) or systemic estrogens improve stress incontinence in many patients, although widespread use of estrogens for this disorder has been tempered by concerns about their long-term adverse effects.

More recently, pelvic floor exercises have been shown to be a very effective adjunct to estrogen in stress incontinence.[34] Patients are trained to discontinue the flow of urine several times during each voiding. Once the patient can easily contract the necessary muscles, the contractions are repeated frequently throughout the day. In 44 of 46 postmenopausal women with stress incontinence, a combined regimen of regular pelvic floor exercises and estrogen eliminated or markedly reduced incontinence in 3 months. Stress incontinence recurred in all 11 patients who discontinued the exercises and was again controlled with resumption of the exercise regimen.[34] In patients who are not responsive to this regimen, improved surgical techniques, requiring less than 30 minutes, are very effective, even in frail, institutionalized patients.

Leakage of small amounts of urine throughout the night and day suggests *overflow incontinence.* The diagnosis is confirmed by finding a palpable, distended bladder and large, postvoiding urinary residual volume. As a rule, overflow incontinence is caused by bladder outlet obstruction or neurogenic bladder. Complete evaluation including cystometrography is usually indicated. Treatment includes intermittent or indwelling catheterization to decompress the bladder for several weeks, maneuvers such as the Credé maneuver for voiding, use of an α-blocker such as prazosin, or cholinergic agents such as bethanechol, and surgical correction of obstruction if feasible.[30] *Reflex incontinence* refers to frequent involuntary voidings throughout the day and night without warning. Because sacral reflexes are preserved, a moderate volume of urine is expressed, unlike the small, more continuous urinary leakage associated with overflow incontinence. Reflex incontinence is usually caused by spinal cord lesions but may be due to cerebral cortical damage.[30] Bladder decompression with prazosin, terazosin, muscle relaxants (diazepam or baclofen), or intermittent catheterization is indicated.[30] Since residual urine is present in overflow incontinence and reflex incontinence, treatment or prophylaxis of urinary tract infection may be indicated.

Clinical Disorders of Water Balance in the Elderly

Clinical disorders of water balance are more frequent in elderly patients than in young adults, suggesting that age-related alterations in the homeostatic mechanisms regulate the volume and composition of extracellular fluid. A variety of physiologic and pathophysiologic conditions predispose to the common clinical disorders associated with impaired water homeostasis.

With the possible exception of the lung, changes in kidney function during normal aging are the most dramatic of any human organ or organ system. Although it is substantially diminished in old age, renal function still provides for adequate regulation of the volume and composition of extracellular fluid under ordinary circumstances but may fail under illness or stress. The major clinically relevant functional defect arising from these histologic and physiologic changes is a progressive decline in the glomerular filtration rate, estimated by the clearance of either inulin or creatinine. Creatinine clearance is stable until the middle of the fourth decade, then a linear decrease of about 8 ml/min per 1.73 m^2 per decade begins.[35] Because of the age-related loss of muscle mass and perhaps decreased protein turnover with age, this rather drastic age-related loss of renal function is not reflected in an elevation of serum creatinine. Depressions of glomerular filtration rate so severe as to result in elevation of serum creatinine above 1.5 mg/dl are rarely due to normal aging and thus indicate a coexisting disease.

Urine-concentrating ability during water deprivation has been shown to decline with advancing age, and a modest age-related impairment in maximal excretion of free water after water loading has been demonstrated.[36] The extrarenal modulators of water balance show alterations with advancing age. Under physiologic circumstances, vasopressin modulates water balance, and thirst functions primarily to repair actual deficits. During two specific sets of circumstances, the thirst mechanism has been described as impaired with advancing age. In one study, during simple dehydration elderly subjects failed to express the degree of severity of thirst that younger individuals expressed. During hypertonic stress, there is a striking age-related increase in the threshold for thirst production, with a high prevalence of elderly individuals not expressing thirst at all during dramatic increases in osmolality. During aging, there is no decline in hypothalamic vasopressin content, and, indeed, vasopressin concentrations after hypertonic stimulation show heightened responsiveness in the elderly. The pharmacokinetics of vasopressin in young and old subjects are identical.

These physiologic alterations in water homeostasis are insufficient alone to account for the disproportionate occurrence of clinical disorders of water balance among older individuals but serve to increase the vulnerability of the elderly. When combined with illnesses limiting renal perfusion, such as hypertension and congestive heart failure, these physiologic changes increase the risk of the elderly.

The symptoms associated with hypo- or hypernatremia are often misinterpreted by the physician because of their nonspecific features. Lethargy, apathy, disorientation, anorexia, agitation, depressed sensorium, altered patterns of respiration, hypothermia, pathologic reflexes, and seizures are all part of the clinical symptomatology of disorders of water metabolism.[37] It is difficult to evaluate volume status by physical examination in elderly individuals because of their lax subcutaneous tissues.

The incidence of severe *hypernatremia* among the elderly exceeds one case per hospital per month. Clinical experience suggests that patients likely to present in this manner are institutionalized, cognitively impaired persons who may have impaired thirst mechanisms and may be receiving sedatives and major tranquilizers likely to contribute to hypodipsia.[38] Many renal diseases impair urine-concentrating ability and accelerate the age-related decline in glomerular filtration rate. When the glomerular filtration rate decreases below 60 ml/min, urinary-concentrating ability is significantly limited. Obstructive uropathy secondary to prostatic hypertrophy, chronic pyelonephritis, renal amyloidosis, and the tubulointerstitial diseases associated with excretion of Bence Jones protein in multiple myeloma are conditions frequently seen in advanced age and further reduce renal concentrating ability. Chronically ill elderly patients are at risk for protein-calorie malnutrition and sodium depletion, both of which further reduce medullary tonicity. The result of hypertonicity is brain shrinkage, capillary hemorrhages, and permanent neurologic injury if deficits are severe and prolonged. Data on the rate at which hypernatremia can be corrected for elderly patients are lacking. Rapid correction of hypertonicity to serum osmolality of approximately 300 Osm/kg is suggested, which can then be followed by a more gradual repletion of remaining free water deficits over 36 to 48 hours.

Although age-related alterations of the maximal diluting capacity of the senescent kidney are less than the decreases of concentrating ability, the most commonly encountered electrolyte disturbance among elderly individuals is *hyponatremia*.[39] Eleven per cent of elderly individuals in a 683-bed geriatric service were found to have serum sodium concentrations of less than 130 mEq/l. Sixty-one per cent of those individuals were symptomatic, albeit with nonspecific complaints. It has been suggested that symptoms are determined by both the magnitude and rate of development of hyponatremia. Subclinical brain edema occurs after a 7% increase in brain water (at sodium concentrations below 125 mEq/l).[40] The result can be seizures or permanent neurologic injury. Age has been implicated as a factor in the syndrome of idiopathic excess vasopressin secretion in which volume status is generally euvolemic to slightly volume-expanded.[41] In this syndrome, the mechanism causing the hyponatremia is known as "vasopressin leak," in which vasopressin continues to be released at a time when it should be completely suppressed. It is seen in the absence of conditions or medications commonly associated with the syndrome of inappropriate vasopressin secretion. Both anesthesia and surgery predispose older individuals to hyponatremic states. The usual cause is sustained vasopressin secretion plus the administration of hypotonic fluids. Chloropropamide-induced hyponatremia secondary to prolonged stimulation of vasopressin release occurs in 4% of the general clinic population, yet advanced age is the dominant feature of the cases of severe hyponatremia associated with this drug. Other conditions with protean manifestations in the elderly, such as tuberculosis and hypothyroidism, are commonly associated with hyponatremia and excess vasopressin release. Diuretics, especially thiazides, impair free water excretion. In one series, diuretics were identified as the causative agent in 64% of elderly patients admitted with hyponatremia.

The first step in treating elderly patients with hyponatremia is the discontinuation of medications or intravenous fluids that are frequent causes of this condition. Standard therapeutic measures such as fluid restriction or demeclocycline can then be used. The present morbidity and mortality that accompany severe hyponatremia (serum sodium less than 120 mEq/l) indicate an aggressive approach using hypertonic saline (3%) to raise serum sodium to 125 mEq/l, with slower correction subsequently.[42]

Systolic Hypertension

Systolic hypertension can be defined as a systolic pressure of more than 160 mm Hg in the presence of a diastolic pressure of less than 95 mm Hg. In most western countries, advancing age is associated with progressive increases in systolic pressure throughout the adult years, unaccompanied by increases in diastolic pressure. Average systolic pressures of populations older than 65 years of age are in the 155 to 165 mm Hg range, while average diastolic pressures are maintained in the range of 80 to 90 mm Hg from 50 years of age onward. Estimates from the Framingham study and other relevant literature indicate that isolated systolic hypertension occurs with increasing prevalence with advancing age, reaching a peak prevalence of approximately 25% in both men and women at 75 years of age. When combined with the similarly high prevalence of diastolic hypertension, the total prevalence of hypertension in the elderly is nearly 60%.

It is important to recognize that the pathophysiology of isolated systolic hypertension is age dependent. Young adults with this disorder generally have a hyperdynamic circulation with increases in pulse rate and cardiac output. The elderly, on the other hand, generally display increases in peripheral resistance with no changes in cardiac output or heart rate. There is general agreement that isolated systolic hypertension in the elderly most likely results from age-related decreases in compliance of major vessels like the aorta and its branches. Secondary causes of hypertension are generally not of major importance in elderly individuals with systolic hypertension, but renal vascular disease deserves special attention and should be excluded when the clinical situation suggests that it is an underlying possibility. One of the major "myths" regarding systolic hypertension in the elderly is that it is "harmless." A number of large, well-designed studies of community-dwelling populations have shown that the progressive increases in systolic blood pressure in the middle-aged and elderly are associated with an increased risk of adverse cardiovascular and cerebrovascular events, especially stroke. Studies indicate that there is no specific cut-off point at which risk of systolic hypertension increases abruptly but that there is a continuous increase of risk with increasing pressures. The Framingham study attempted to differentiate the risk of stiffening of vessels versus the risk of increases of systolic pressure by analysis of the incidence of stroke according to age, systolic pressure, and alterations in the carotid arterial pulse tracing that was used as an indirect index of vessel thickening. The study showed that the systolic pressure is a much greater determinant of a stroke risk than age or vessel thickening.[43] Another major myth regarding systolic hypertension in the elderly is that elderly individuals tolerate antihypertensive treatment poorly. A large number of trials have shown a low incidence of adverse effects in elderly patients treated with antihypertensives.[44]

A 12-year double-blind randomized placebo-controlled trial of antihypertensive treatment for 840 patients older than 60 years of age was conducted by a consortium of European investigators.[45] Eight hundred and forty patients (70% women) were randomized to 25 mg of hydrochlorothiazide, 50 mg of triamterene, or matching placebo if sitting blood pressures on entry were in the range of 180 ± 17 mm Hg systolic and 101 ± 7 mm Hg diastolic. If the blood pressure remained elevated, a second pill was added. At 1 month, if blood pressure remained elevated, methyldopa, 250 mg, was started and increased slowly to a maximum of 2000 mg/day. In the treatment group at the end of the trial, one half of the patients were taking one diuretic pill, and 45% were taking two. Sixty-five per cent did not require methyldopa, and less than 10% were taking 1000 mg of methyldopa or more. Mean blood pressure reductions of 20 mm Hg systolic and 10 mm Hg diastolic were achieved in this group, with modest increases in blood sugars, uric acid, and creatinine documented. Based on the intention-to-treat analysis, all causes of mortality and stroke mortality decreased insignificantly. Fatal cardiac events decreased significantly. In the patients randomized to active treatment, there were 29 fewer cardiovascular events and 14 fewer cardiovascular deaths per 1000 patient years during the double-blind part of the trial. Further information is expected on subgroups of this large study of individuals with a range of initial blood pressures and differing funtional status. The data favored active treatment, although benefit was not demonstrated in persons older than 80 years of age.

The Systolic Hypertension in the Elderly Program has examined the efficacy of antihypertensive therapy in patients older than 60 years of age who have isolated systolic hypertension.[46] Study participants (551 of 2130 patients initially screened) were randomized to 12.5 mg/day of chlorthalidone or placebo, which was increased to two capsules per day after 1 month if the patients were free of side effects and if blood pressure goals were not achieved. Eighty-eight per cent of the actively treated patients reached goal blood pressures on this routine, and most required only 25 mg/day of chlorthalidone. An overall mean difference of 17 mm Hg systolic and 16 mm Hg diastolic pressures was achieved between randomized groups. As noted by prior studies, asymptomatic reductions in serum potassium (0.5 mEq/kg) and increases in uric acid (0.9 mg/dl) and creatinine (0.08 mg/l) were noted. After an average 4.5 years of follow-up, the incidence of stroke was 36% lower in the active treatment group than in the placebo group. The incidence of nonfatal myocardial infarction was decreased by 28%, and the risk of death from all causes was reduced by 13%. This provides the first credible evidence not only that the elevated systolic blood pressure levels that frequently occur in aged individuals can be safely lowered but also that such reduction results in substantial and measurable reductions in morbidity and mortality.[47] In these two large trials, relatively small doses of diuretic agents seem to be effective in reducing blood pressure safely in the great majority of older individuals; they thus represent first-line treatment agents. No clear consensus exists regarding second-line agents (Table 65–3). However, a common observation is that lower dosages are required for blood pressure reduction in the elderly.

At least two studies suggest that clonidine can be an effective drug when used alone in elderly patients with isolated systolic hypertension. We do not generally recommend β-blockers for isolated systolic hypertension in the elderly since these agents can worsen peripheral vascular disease, cardiac failure, and obstructive respiratory disease, which are common in the elderly. Agents that are not highly water soluble may cause confusion and depression in older individuals because of penetration into the CNS. Hydralazine is an effective second-line agent for isolated systolic hypertension. Since baroreflex sensitivity is impaired with advancing age, older individuals do not usually develop the reflex tachycardia in response to hydralazine that younger individuals do. Low doses—10 mg two or three times a day—are often most effective in reducing blood pressure in older patients. Although calcium channel blockers are thought to be excellent choices for elderly individuals with isolated systolic hypertension for several pharmacologic reasons, no studies of their usefulness in this condition have been reported.

TABLE 65–3. ANTIHYPERTENSIVE THERAPY IN ELDERLY PATIENTS

	Dosage Ranges	
Diuretics	Chlorthalidone	12.5–50 mg/day
	Hydrochlorothiazide, 25 mg, plus triamterene, 50 mg	Daily
Vasodilators	Hydralazine	25–50 mg bid
	Nifedipine	10–20 mg tid, qid
Central Sympatholytics	Clonidine	0.1–0.2 mg/day
	Methyldopa	250–500 mg/day to qid
β-Blockers	Labetolol	Titrate dose
	Atenolol	50–100 mg/day to bid
Converting-Enzyme Inhibitor	Captopril	12.5–50 mg bid to tid

If one chooses to treat systolic hypertension in the elderly, the following issues should be addressed. First, there is no general consensus of the blood pressure at which to initiate treatment. Pressures of over 170 mm Hg seem to be a reasonable place to start. Second, the goal of therapy is not clear, but it is important not to try to lower systolic blood pressure to levels normally seen in younger individuals, that is, 120 to 130 mm Hg. A reasonable goal in the elderly is 160 mm Hg. Third, because of the marked variability in blood pressure in individual elderly patients, the prescreening of patients is important. Several basal blood pressure determinations should be taken before initiation of treatment. It is also important to obtain a standing blood pressure, most conveniently taken 3 minutes after assuming the upright posture, to evaluate for orthostatic hypotension before beginning antihypertensive therapy.

Falls

Falls are a highly prevalent geriatric syndrome. The annual incidence of falls in women rises from 30% at 65 to 69 years of age to 50% in those older than 85 years of age. In men, the annual incidence rises from 13% at age 65 to 69 years to 31% in those aged 80 to 84 years.[48] The consequences of serious falls are dramatic. The annual incidence of femur fracture increases from 100 per 100,000 population at 40 years of age to greater than 500 per 100,000 after 60 years of age. Seventy-two per cent of deaths due to falls in the United States occur in the population older than 75 years of age (< 10% of the entire population). Falls not only result in physical injury but may also erode confidence, encouraging withdrawal and depression, and lead to the complications associated with immobility. The statistics clearly indicate the special vulnerability of elderly women, which is related in large part to osteoporosis.

A variety of age-related changes contribute to declines in postural stability with age, including impairment in cervical mechanoreceptors and peripheral vision.

Sheldon was the first to conduct systematic quantitative studies of postural stability in the elderly.[49] He demonstrated a progressive age-related increase in the degree of sway. Frail elderly people are placed at increased risk of falling by medications that produce confusion, orthostatic hypotension, vertigo, lethargy, or sluggishness. Alcohol use is often unreported and thus must be specifically sought in the history. The literature provides a clear consensus on the specific causes of falls in the elderly. Four of ten falls are accidental. A trip over a throw rug, poor lighting, recently waxed floors, and icy streets may result in falls. Drop attacks, which cause up to 25% of falls in outpatient populations, are characterized by the sudden loss of body tone with the patient finding herself or himself on the ground, somewhat surprised but alert, often transiently paralyzed or at least very clumsy in the legs and unable to get up. Incoordination and weakness may last several minutes; normal strength returns with application of pressure on the feet and assistance. The mechanism of the fall appears to be a sudden loss of postural tone. As some episodes have been associated with turning of the head or trunk or looking upward, particularly in individuals with cervical arthritis, it has been hypothesized that neural or vascular spinal cord pressure is causative. A careful clinical examination of the neck and cervical spine films are useful. A trial of soft collar bracing is sometimes very effective in preventing further episodes.

A large portion of falls result from multiple sensory deficits. As described earlier, the constriction of visual fields, worsening of visual acuity, and impairment of visual tracking place the elderly at risk for tripping over unseen obstructions. Peripheral neuropathy and impaired hearing may contribute to older patients' unawareness of the dangers of falling. A host of lesser causes of falls include the causes of syncope, severe postural hypotension, alcoholism, painful arthritis, parkinsonism, and drug overdosage. An interesting observation is that postural hypotension in the elderly, if occurring after meals, is partially ameliorated by caffeine.

The practical evaluation of falls requires a careful history, for many episodes are unwitnessed, and many of the diagnostic clues are in the history. A decision tree based initially on a history of giddiness, postural symptoms, palpitations, or the presence of drug intoxication can then lead to a focused clinical examination that will confirm the diagnosis of sufficient cause for falling. Laboratory evaluation appropriate for the most likely possibilities is always indicated. Since the etiology may be multifactorial, one should seek to identify and remedy all contributing factors. Corrective therapy, which may include discontinuation of drugs, use of a cervical collar, correction of visual deficits, or a home visit to remove obstacles and loose rugs, should be initiated. A very helpful modality in the management of falls is having a physical therapist teach the patient how to handle the consequences because, for the most part, complete correction of all underlying causes is not achievable. If patients can develop confidence that they can right themselves or signal for help, the morbidity of the event is lessened.

Acute Confusional States

Since the first clear description of postoperative disturbances of mental status in the 1800s, the syndrome of acute confusion has been recognized as a morbid one even though it often fails to appear in health statistics. Many synonyms, including delirium, toxic psychosis, and acute brain syndrome, may tend to obscure the basic features of this syndrome, which consists of the potentially reversible inability to maintain a coherent stream of thought and behavior. The clinical picture is dominated by an inability to maintain attention appropriately to the tasks at hand. The vulnerability of the elderly to the development of this syndrome is documented in several studies,[50] and clinical experience in geriatric consultation has identified the acute confusional state as a major management problem in hospitalized patients.

The elderly are vulnerable to the development of this syndrome for several reasons. The heightened autonomic arousal in the elderly may provoke a failure to adjust to the stress of acute illness. There is a definite decline during aging in the ability to handle new information (fluid intelligence), particularly when speed or attention to multiple elements of the task are required. Added to those normal facets of aging is the high prevalence of cognitive and mental disorders in the elderly. Pre-existing dementia almost certainly predisposes to the development of acute confusion during the stress of an illness.

The differential diagnosis of acute confusion is broad, with the majority of precipitating causes originating outside the central nervous system (Table 65–4). Pneumonia, cardiac failure, urinary infections, neoplasia, and depression appear to be the commonest causes. Hyponatremia, a syndrome common to the first four causes just listed, is often found in hospitalized elderly and clearly contributes to acute confusion. Postoperatively confused patients have generally received more medications than nonconfused patients, and the elderly are particularly sensitive to developing drug toxicity.

The therapeutic approach is multidisciplinary. The first responsibility is to diagnose and treat any underlying medical problem after taking a careful history and performing

TABLE 65–4. ETIOLOGIC FACTORS IN ACUTE CONFUSIONAL STATES OF THE ELDERLY*

Drugs: Sedatives-hypnotics; anticholinergics, including phenothiazines, tricyclic antidepressants, and antihistamines; narcotics; diuretics; digitalis; antiparkinsonism drugs; antihypertensives; chlorpropramide; cimetidine
Alcohol and Drug Withdrawal
Cardiac Disease: Cardiac failure, myocardial infarction, cardiac arrhythmia, endocarditis
Infection: Especially pulmonary and urinary infection; bacteremia, septicemia, meningitis, encephalitis
Metabolic Disorders: Electrolyte, fluid, and acid-base imbalance; hepatic, renal, and respiratory failure; hypoglycemia, hyperglycemia; hypothyroidism, thyrotoxicosis; hypothermia, hyperthermia; vitamin B complex deficiency
Cerebrovascular Disorders: Stroke, transient ischemic attacks; subdural hematoma; temporal arteritis; cerebral vasculitis
Neoplasm: Intracranial, extracranial (especially bronchogenic carcinoma)
Trauma: Head injury, burns, hip fracture, surgery
Epilepsy

*From Lipowski ZJ: Acute confusional states (delirium) in the elderly. *In* Albert MC (ed): Clinical Neurology of Aging. New York, Oxford University Press, 1984, pp 277–297.

physical and laboratory testing. Historical review of the premorbid mental status is imperative, and there is good reason to suggest a formal mental status test on every aged individual preoperatively.

Concurrent with the investigative initiative is attention to the patients' physical and social comfort with nonpharmacologic and supportive measures, most recently termed *milieu therapy* and in general implemented by nursing staff. Careful control of extraneous stimuli, provision of familiar objects, facilitation of interaction with family members, adequate control of pain, and provision of a supportive relationship with primary caregivers form the basis of this approach. Drug treatment when necessary usually involves major tranquilizers, chosen for their capacity to control agitation without altering the level of consciousness. Choices within the group are dictated by the type of side effects desirable to avoid (see Chapter 82). Restraints, properly applied and supervised, occasionally are necessary, but are to be avoided whenever possible. They have been shown to be largely ineffective in preventing injuries from falls, cause patients and families emotional distress, and result in significant injuries when patients become entangled.

The prognosis in the elderly depends on the underlying cause but in general is less optimistic than that in younger populations. In one study,[50] 25% of patients died, 35% recovered to be discharged; the remainder remained in hospital at the study's termination. A study of postoperative patients of all ages revealed a 7.8% incidence of acute confusion; of those, 32% had not fully recovered by the time of discharge.

The genuine reversibility of a significant proportion of acute confusional states justifies a thorough investigation for this common geriatric syndrome.

REFERENCES

1. Hazzard WR: Geriatric medicine—Leading the health care team of the elderly. *In* Braunwald E (ed): Harrison's Textbook of Internal Medicine. New York, McGraw-Hill, 1983.
2. Soldo BJ and Manton KG: Dynamics of health changes in the extreme elderly: New perspectives and evidence. Milbank Memorial Fund Quarterly 63:286, 1985.
3. Office of Health Research, Statistics and Technology: Health. Washington, DC, US Department of Health and Human Services, Public Health Service, 1981.
4. Rowe JW and Minaker KL: Geriatric medicine. *In* Finch C and Schneider E (eds): Handbook of the Biology of Aging, Vol II. New York, Van Nostrand, Reinhold, 1985, pp 932–959.
5. Minaker KL, Meneilly GS, and Rowe JW: Endocrine systems. *In* Finch C and Schneider E (eds): Handbook of the Biology of Aging, Vol II. New York, Van Nostrand, Reinhold, 1985, pp 433–456.
6. Feller I, Flora JD, and Baurol R: Baseline results of therapy for burned patients. JAMA 130:1943, 1976.
7. Feller I, Thalen D, and Cornell RG: Improvements in burn care, 1965 to 1979. JAMA 244:2074, 1980.
8. Davis PJ and Davis PG: Hyperthyroidism in patients over the age of 60 years: Clinical features in 85 patients. Medicine 53:161, 1974.
9. Maddox GL and Douglass EB: Aging and individual differences: A longitudinal analysis of social, psychological, and physiological indicators. J Gerontol 29:555, 1974.
10. Minaker KL: Geriatric assessment—Consider the interaction of aging and disease. Consultant 24:328, 1984.
11. Grimley Evans J: Prevention of age-associated loss of autonomy: Epidemiologic approaches. J Chron Dis 37:353, 1984.
12. Folstein MF, Folstein SE, and McHugh PR: "Mini-Mental State." A practical method for grading the cognitive state of patients for the clinician. J Psychiatr Res 12:189, 1975.
13. Kane RA and Kane RL: Assessing the Elderly: A Practical Guide to Measurement. Lexington, MA, Lexington Books, 1981.
14. Linn BS and Linn MW: Objective and self-assessed health in the young and very old. Soc Sci Med 14:311, 1980.
15. Brocklehurst JC, Carthy MH, Leeming JT, et al: Medical screening of old people accepted for residential care. Lancet 1:141, 1978.
16. Anderson B and Palmore E: Longitudinal evaluation of ocular function. *In* Palmore E (ed): Normal Aging II: Reports from the Duke Longitudinal Studies, 1970–1973. Durham, NC, Duke University Press, 1974, pp 24–32.
17. Harrington DO: The Visual Fields: A Textbook and Atlas of Clinical Perimetry. St Louis, CV Mosby, p 102.
18. Chamberlain W: Restriction in upward gaze with advancing age. Trans Am Ophthalmol Soc 68:235, 1970.
19. Wilson LA and Russell RW: Amaurosis fugax and carotid artery disease: Indications for angiography. BMJ 2:435, 1977.
20. Osterhammel D: High frequency audiometry: Clinical aspects. Scand Audiol 9:249, 1980.
21. Butler RN and Lewis MI: Aging and Mental Health. St Louis, CV Mosby, 1973.
22. Miller M: Geriatric suicide: The Arizona study. Gerontologist 18:488, 1978.
23. Durkheim E: Suicide: A Study in Sociology (translated by JA Spaulding and G Simpson). Glencoe, IL, Free Press, 1951.
24. Young M, Benjamin B, and Wallis C: The mortality of widowers. Lancet 2:454, 1963.
25. Lipowski ZJ: Psychiatry of somatic diseases: Epidemiology, pathogenesis, classification. Comp Psychiatry 16:105, 1975.
26. Greenblatt DJ and Shader RI: Pharmacokinetics in old age: Principles and problems of assessment. *In* Jarvik LF, Greenblatt DJ, and Harmon D (eds): Clinical Pharmacology and the Aged Patient. New York, Raven Press, 1981, pp 27–46.
27. Rowe JW and Besdine RW (eds): Health and Disease in Old Age. Boston, Little, Brown, 1982, pp 39–53.
28. Thomas TM, Plymat KR, Blannin J, et al: Prevalence of urinary incontinence. BMJ 281:1243, 1980.
29. Ouslander JG, Kane RL and Abrass IB: Urinary incontinence in elderly nursing home patients. JAMA 248:1194, 1982.
30. Resnick NM and Yalla SV: Managemet of urinary incontinence in the elderly (Current Concepts). N Engl J Med 313:800, 1985.
31. Palmer JH, Worth PHL, and Exton-Smith AN: Flunarizine: A once-daily therapy for urinary incontinence. Lancet 2:279, 1981.
32. Moisey CU, Stephenson TP, and Brendler CB: The urodynamic and subjective results of treatment of detrusor instability with oxybutynin chloride. Br J Urol 125:318, 1981.
33. McGuire EJ, Shi-Chun Z, Horwinski ER, et al: Treatment of motor and sensory detrusor instability by electrical stimulation. J Urol 129:78, 1983.
34. Mohr JA, Rogers J Jr, Brown TN, et al: Stress urinary incontinence: A simple and practical approach to diagnosis and treatment. J Am Geriatr Soc 31:476, 1983.
35. Rowe JW, Andres R, Tobin J, et al: The effect of age on creatinine clearance in man: A cross-sectional and longitudinal study. J Gerontol 31:155, 1976.
36. Rowe JW, Shock NW, and DeFronzo RA: The influence of age on the renal response to water deprivation in man. Nephron 17:270, 1976.
37. Weiner MW and Epstein FH: Signs and symptoms of electrolyte disorders. *In* Maxwell MH and Kleeman CR (eds): Clinical Disorders of Fluid and Electrolyte Metabolism. New York, McGraw-Hill, 1972, pp 629–661.
38. Miller PD, Krebs RA, Neal BS, et al: Hypodipsia in geriatric patients. Am J Med 73:354, 1982.
39. Sunderam SG and Mankikar GD: Hyponatremia in the elderly. Age Ageing 12:77, 1983.
40. Arieff A, Llach F, and Massry S: Neurologic manifestations and morbidity of hyponatremia: Correlation with brain water and electrolytes. Medicine 55:121, 1976.
41. Goldstein CS, Braunstein S, and Goldfarb S: Idiopathic syndrome of inappropriate antidiuretic hormone secretion possibly related to advanced age. Ann Intern Med 99:185, 1983.
42. Ayus JC, Olivero S, and Frommer JP: Rapid correction of severe hyponatremia with intravenous hypertonic saline solutions. Am J Med 72:43, 1982.

43. Kannel WB, Wolf PA, McGee DL, et al: Systolic blood pressure, arterial rigidity, and risk of stroke: The Framingham Study. JAMA 245:1225, 1981.
44. Amery A, Berhaux P, Birkenhager W, et al: Antihypertensive therapy in patients above 60 years. Fourth Interim Report of the European Working Party on High Blood Pressure in the Elderly (EWPHE). Clin Sci 55(Suppl):263s, 1978.
45. Mortality and morbidity results from European Working Party on High Blood Pressure in the Elderly trial. Lancet 2:1349, 1985.
46. Hulley SB, Furberg CD, et al: Systolic Hypertension in the Elderly Program (SHEP): Antihypertensive efficacy of chlorthalidone. Am J Cardiol 56:913, 1985.
47. SHEP Cooperative Research Group: Prevention of stroke by antihypertensive drug treatment in older persons with isolated systolic hypertension. JAMA 265:24, 1991.
48. Gryfe CI, Amies A, and Ashley MJ: A longitudinal study of falls in an elderly population. I: Incidence and morbidity. Age Ageing 6:201, 1977.
49. Sheldon JH: The effect of age on the control of sway. Gerontol Clin 5:129, 1963.
50. Hodkinson HM: Mental impairment in the elderly. J R Coll Physicians Lond 7:305, 1973.

66

Fever of Unknown Origin

JAMES L. BREELING, MD
LOUIS WEINSTEIN, MD, PhD

One of the most difficult problems in clinical medicine is the patient with cryptic fever of prolonged duration. Various investigators have defined such fever of unknown origin (FUO) as body temperature higher than 100.5 to 101° F (38.05 to 38.3° C) lasting for at least 3 weeks without clear cause despite investigation. The criteria employed by Petersdorf and Beeson required a 1-week in-hospital study but may no longer be applicable in many current ambulatory settings.[1]

The pathogenesis of fever is understood to depend on the elaboration of humoral substances formerly called endogenous pyrogen; including interleukin-1, tumor necrosis factor, gamma-interferon, and other cytokines.[2] These pyrogenic cytokines may be released in response to infection, inflammation, tissue necrosis, or other stimuli. Their site of action is the preoptic nucleus of the anterior hypothalamus, where they bind to specific membrane receptors to promote phospholipase-dependent production of arachidonic acid and prostaglandin synthesis. The hypothalamic "set point" rises, leading to heat conservation (decreased sweating and increased cutaneous vasoconstriction) and increased heat production (increased muscle tone and shivering).

NORMAL TEMPERATURE VARIATION

Many physicians and patients are under the impression that "normal" daily maximal oral and rectal temperatures are 37° C (98.6° F) and 37.5° C (99.6° F), respectively. In actuality, daily fluctuations of body temperature are greater than these "normal" numbers suggest. A study of a number of schoolchildren indicated an oral temperature of 37° C or below in only 24.5%.[3] Normal temperature has been found to be closer to 36.3° C in girls who are 12 to 17 years of age.[4] Temperatures determined between 8:00 and 9:00 AM in medical students have been noted to range between 35.8 and 37.4° C with a mean of 36.7° C.[5] Of patients visiting physicians' offices, 17% had a maximal oral temperature of 37° C; in 42%, the temperature reached 37.7° C. Maximal daily temperature in elderly persons may be as low as 35.8° C in the morning and may not exceed 36.4° C late in the day. Unless these variations are appreciated, physicians may misinterpret 37.5° C as a fever in a young adult and fail to recognize the possibility of disease in an older individual with a maximal temperature of 37.2° C. It should be noted that tachypnea (>20 breaths/min) lowers an oral temperature by approximately 1.5 degrees.

In the elderly, there may be a delay in the onset of fever in the presence of significant infection. The main clinical features of fever in the elderly include headaches, restlessness, dizziness, confusion, hallucinations, and delusions.

CLINICALLY BENIGN FEVER OF UNKNOWN ORIGIN

A benign FUO is usually characterized by minimal elevations of temperature and rarely indicates the presence of organic or life-threatening disease.[6] Patients who seek medical attention because of "low-grade fevers" may not have determined their temperature but have a subjective sensation of "feverishness." If they have determined their temperature, they may not recognize that oral temperatures are elevated by as much as 0.55° C if taken after a substantial meal, a hot beverage, a cigarette, pipe, or cigar. Many women may note an elevation of temperature to 37.8° C for 2 weeks every month before menstruation and may not be aware that this represents normal ovulatory cycles.[7]

The fact that exercise increases body temperature is also well documented.[8] Temperatures of 38.3° C after strenuous exercise such as rowing, long-distance running, or football can be found. The normal circadian variation usually takes afternoon body temperatures over 37.5° C. Whether mental stress can also elevate body temperature is questionable. An older syndrome called "psychogenic fever," with persistent temperatures of over 37.7° C, was described in patients with anxiety and was thought to respond to sedation with phenobarbital.[9] In some patients with low-grade oral temperatures occurring soon after the patient's admission to hospital, the entity of "admission fever" was thought to relate to anxiety as well. Another entity known as "essential oral hyperthermia," in which oral temperatures are reported to be elevated by 0.2 to 0.4° C over rectal temperatures, was also thought to represent a benign variant that disappeared over time.[10] Modern observation has not recorded many of these phenomena.

All physicians must be aware of the possibility that an FUO may be produced factitiously.[11, 12] Typically, the temperatures are quite high and are associated with headache, generalized aching of the muscles, and fatigue. If the factitious disorder has been present for a long time, some patients will have weight loss and anemia, but most patients appear surprisingly well.

A mercury thermometer can be manipulated in various ways to produce a factitious fever by artificially heating it (e.g., in hot water, near a light bulb, or by vigorous rubbing). Modern use of electronic thermometers that give readings in a few seconds while the provider watches has largely eliminated this ruse, but ingestion of a hot beverage prior to recording the temperature still occurs. Taking rectal temperatures can overcome this strategy. Although most cases of factitious fever are benign, they are occasionally featured by self-induced disorders (very often infections) that are potentially life-threatening.

Drug fever, or fever related to sensitization or to idiosyncratic reactions to drugs, is common. The temperature may be low- or high-grade, sustained, remittent, or intermittent. Chills preceding an elevation of temperature do not rule out the possibility of drug fever. Cessation of exposure is followed by a return to normal temperature—related to the time required for a drug to be completely excreted or metabolized; this may require 3 to 4 weeks in some cases. Rash and eosinophilia may be totally absent.

Almost all therapeutic agents may produce fever.[13] Table 66–1 lists drugs that frequently cause drug fever. Antibiotics appear prominently on the list. The fever induced by iodine may persist for 3 to 4 weeks after its ingestion has been discontinued, because of the very slow rate at which it is excreted. Even salicylate may be responsible for fever—usually in the setting of overdosage. Digitalis appears to be the only commonly used agent that is not associated with fever.

Exposure to industrial agents (e.g., metals, plastics, fumes, solvents) may lead to "occupational fever" presenting as an FUO. Polymer fume fever has been described in individuals working in plastics factories, and similar syndromes have been reported for workers in brass foundries, welders, and individuals exposed to zinc, nickel, or other metal dusts. A careful review of the patient's occupational exposure might reveal the cause.[14] A temporal relationship with work also would be an indication of occupational fever ("Monday morning fever").

CLINICALLY SIGNIFICANT FEVER OF UNKNOWN ORIGIN

The modern classification of an FUO defines five major categories: infection, neoplasm, collagen-vascular disease, granulomatous disease, and a miscellaneous group (Table 66–2). With improved diagnostic testing available in many areas (e.g., blood culture technology, computed tomography, nuclear medicine), the diseases commonly represented in lists of patients with FUO has changed since the 1950s, with fewer cases of syphilis, typhoid fever, endocarditis, and increased incidence of neoplasms.[15] Because of the number of different diagnostic possibilities, it is impossible to initiate a broad and simultaneous search for all causes. The approach to diagnosis must, therefore, be systematic and focused first on the most common causes of FUO.

Infectious Fever of Unknown Origin

Approximately one third of FUOs can ultimately be traced to an infectious illness. Most papers about FUO describe tuberculosis, subacute endocarditis, intra-abdomi-

TABLE 66–1. DRUGS ASSOCIATED WITH FEVER

Antihistamines
Aspirin and other salicylate compounds
Barbiturates
H_2 blockers
Hydralazine
Ibuprofen
Methyldopa
Nitrofurantoin
β-Lactam antibiotics
Phenolphthalein-containing laxatives
Phenytoin
Procainamide
Quinidine
Sulfonamide
Vancomycin
Streptomycin
Isoniazid
Amphotericin B
Tetracyclines
Clindamycin
Bleomycin
Interferon

TABLE 66–2. CAUSES OF CLINICALLY SIGNIFICANT FEVER OF UNKNOWN ORIGIN

Infectious Causes
Tuberculosis
Infective endocarditis
Hepatobiliary infection
Genitourinary infection
Typhoid fever
Typhoidal form of mononucleosis or cytomegalovirus
Rheumatic fever
Intra-abdominal abscess
Neoplastic Disease
Hodgkin's disease
Chronic myelogenous leukemia
Primary or metastatic tumors of the liver
Hypernephroma
Metastatic carcinoma of the thyroid
Connective Tissue Disease
Polyarteritis nodosa
Systemic lupus erythematosus
Juvenile rheumatoid arthritis
Temporal arteritis/giant cell arteritis
Granulomatous Disease
Sarcoidosis
Granulomatous hepatitis
Crohn's disease
Miscellaneous Diseases
Congenital ectodermal dysplasia of the anhidrotic type
Hypothalamic dysfunction
Dorsolumbar sympathectomy
Hyperthyroidism
Subacute thyroiditis
Factitious fever
Multiple pulmonary emboli
Large hematoma
Familial Mediterranean fever

nal infection, viral illness, and systemic mycoses as the most frequent causes.

Tuberculosis, especially miliary tuberculosis in the elderly, should be suspected even with a negative result on a first-strength tuberculin test.[16] By retesting in 1 to 2 weeks, some patients mount a positive PPD via the "booster" phenomenon.[17] The presentation of fever, weight loss, cough, confusion or delirium, and/or hepatomegaly may be accompanied by a normal chest x-ray. Bone marrow or liver biopsy for culture and histology is usually diagnostic; the presence of miliary tubercles in the retina may be an important clue. Extrapulmonary tuberculosis may also be associated with FUO, such as genitourinary tuberculosis, pericardial tuberculosis, or mesenteric tuberculosis. The presence of sterile pyuria, unexplained pericardial effusion or constriction, or abdominal pain would be important indicators for further evaluation.

Subacute endocarditis must always be considered when an FUO is present. Murmurs may be absent, trivial, or unchanged from baseline examination. Fever is commonly not striking in the elderly (37.5 to 37.8° C) and may be present for weeks or months before the diagnosis is established. The frequent use of oral antibiotics for an FUO makes the possibility of culture-negative endocarditis from antibiotic pretreatment a likelihood. When suspected, at least three blood cultures in a 24-hour period should be obtained, and if antibiotics have been inadvertently administered prior to the suspicion of endocarditis, another culture should be taken from the patient in several days. In the setting of prolonged or unexplained fever in a patient with a prosthetic heart valve in which culture-negative endocarditis is clinically likely, an empiric course of intravenous antibiotics for endocarditis may have a limited role after other causes have been exhausted.

With the advent of computed tomography, intra-abdominal infection as a cause of FUO has become less common. Four chief causes should be considered: biliary tract disease, diverticulitis, appendicitis, and abscess in the liver or spleen. Atypical presentations such as retrocecal appendicitis, posterior perforation of gastric ulcer, and Crohn's disease in the elderly should be considered. Perinephric collections of pus from nephrolithiasis or pyelonephritis may present with fever alone and a normal urinary sediment. Several weeks may elapse before the characteristic bulge in the flank of a renal carbuncle or xanthogranulomatous pyelonephritis develops. Other sites of infection include the pelvis (in women especially after cesarean section or hysterectomy), prostatic abscess (which may not be associated with enlargement or tenderness of the gland, especially in the elderly), and splenic abscess (from endocarditis, typhoid fever, brucellosis, or bacteremia of other causes).

Fever persisting for several weeks may be the only manifestation of typhoid fever. In some cases, the elevation of temperature is relatively small. Symptoms may be so mild that patients go about their normal activities complaining only of fatigue and persistent low-grade fever; this is the syndrome of "walking typhoid fever." Other *Salmonella* species may produce a typhoidal picture, especially *Salmonella typhimurium* and *S. choleraesuis*, and blood culture results are usually positive, indicating an endovascular source of infection such as mycotic aneurysm.

The typhoidal form of infectious mononucleosis almost always presents as an FUO. In patients older than 45 years of age, primary mononucleosis without exudative pharyngitis or marked lymphadenopathy can occur. The monospot test and specific viral IgM antibody test remain important diagnostic tests. Cytomegalovirus, toxoplasmosis, or primary human immunodeficiency virus (HIV) infection should be suspected if atypical mononuclear cells are seen on a peripheral smear but the result of the monospot test is negative.

Neoplastic Disease

Certain neoplasms have been associated with fever,[18] most commonly with Hodgkin's disease, other lymphomas, acute and chronic myelogenous and lymphocytic leukemia, primary and metastatic tumors of the liver, carcinoma of the lung, hypernephroma, and metastatic carcinoma of the thyroid. Neoplastic fevers represent approximately one third of FUO cases. The febrile reaction may be sustained or intermittent, abrupt in onset or insidious, and associated with rigors or not. A Pel-Ebstein fever (a single high temperature every day) has been classically associated with Hodgkin's disease.

The possibility of complicating cryptic bacterial, viral, mycotic, and parasitic infections must receive serious consideration in patients with "tumor fever." The immunosuppression produced by malignant lesions, often exaggerated by chemotherapy, increases the susceptibility to microbial invasion. All patients should have a "tumor fever" initially evaluated by blood cultures, urine cultures, sputum examination and chest radiographs, and additional testing as required by the clinical setting. Fever from neoplastic disease appears to respond dramatically to naproxen, which is a nonsteroidal anti-inflammatory drug. This almost complete "fever lysis" has been proposed as a diagnostic test for neoplastic fever.[19]

Connective Tissue Disease

Patients with inflammatory diseases of the blood vessels, joints, muscles, skin, lungs, heart, and kidneys may have fever as a manifestation of their illness. Sometimes, fever is the only manifestation of a connective-tissue disease before other manifestations become clinically obvious. Patients with allergic vasculitis, various forms of polyarteritis, and systemic lupus erythematosus (SLE) may present in this manner. High-positive titers of antinuclear antibodies may increase the suspicion of SLE, but often the diagnosis becomes confirmed only when other manifestations develop. Patients with severe juvenile rheumatoid arthritis (JRA) may exhibit striking elevations of temperature over prolonged periods, well before arthritis develops. The presence of a variety of skin eruptions, including petechiae or purpura, in some cases may lead to a mistaken diagnosis of infection. Still's disease is JRA presenting in a young adult. Usually after observation, arthritis finally develops in a matter of months and the diagnosis can be made. In the elderly, temporal arteritis and polymyalgia rheumatica may initially present as an FUO. Weight loss, malaise, depression, anemia, elevated sedimentation rate, and fever may be the only clues. Characteristic headache or jaw claudication may be absent. The diagnosis depends on clinical suspicion and temporal artery biopsy.[20]

Granulomatous Causes

Diffuse sarcoidosis, on rare occasions, may occur with FUO when arthritis, lesions of the skin, hila, and other lymphadenopathy; or pulmonary infiltration is absent. Ulcerative colitis and regional enteritis or Crohn's disease may also present in the absence of diarrhea or abdominal pain, with fever being the initial sign.[21] Whipple's disease has been associated with FUO. Granulomatous lesions on liver biopsy are a frequent finding in patients with FUO. Granulomatous hepatitis has multiple causes including Hodgkin's disease, tuberculosis, brucellosis, Crohn's disease, parasitic infections, fungal infections, reactions to drugs (sulfonamide and others), Q fever, vasculitis/arteritis, primary biliary cirrhosis, and syphilis. When a specific cause cannot be identified, one should consider treatment for tuberculosis. If defervescence does not occur after 6 weeks, one could consider administration of prednisone.

Miscellaneous Causes

Processes that alter water balance or disturb the mechanisms that control body temperature may be responsible for the development of a significant and persistent fever. Tumors of the brain near the hypothalamus, viral encephalitis, dorsolumbar sympathectomy, and malignant neuroleptic syndrome are examples of this. In addition, some diffuse skin diseases prevent normal radiational cooling and may be associated with prolonged cryptic fever, such as diffuse ichthyosis, scleroderma, and congenital ectodermal dysplasia of the anhidrotic type. Temperature elevations in these disorders are higher during the warm summer months.

Some metabolic disorders may lead to fever. The most frequent is hyperthyroidism, with the usual presentation of subacute thyroiditis, generalized malaise, overwhelming fatigue, and recurrent throat pain that can be localized to the thyroid without thyroid enlargement. Progesterone itself is also associated with a higher body temperature "set-point."

Multiple pulmonary emboli should be considered in any case of cryptic fever, especially if the patient has been pregnant or has undergone pelvic surgery. The classical findings of abdominal pain, pelvic mass, and pulmonary infarction or cavitation may not be present. Large hematomas also have been associated with fever, even when the hematoma is bland or noninfected. Examples include subarachnoid hemorrhage, multiple trauma of the long bones, and large retroperitoneal hemorrhages.

Familial Mediterranean fever (FMF) is characterized by intermittent episodes of moderate-to-high fever, alone or together with diffuse abdominal pain or arthritis or both. It involves primarily ethnic groups whose origin is in countries bordering the Mediterranean Sea.[22] Colchicine has been shown to treat the fever and prevent recurrences.

Factitious fever from self-induced infection can be serious and even life-threatening. Examples of methods used by patients with this disorder include injection of urine, soil, yeast, and saliva leading to bacteremia, cystitis, pyelonephritis, multiple dermal abscesses, and septic pulmonary emboli. In a study of factitious fever in a teaching hospital,[11] most patients were found to have some medical knowledge or training.

WORK-UP OF FEVER OF UNKNOWN ORIGIN

An evaluation of FUO should begin only when the strict case definition is met, because most cryptic fevers are caused by atypical manifestations of common diseases that manifest themselves over time. Most patients with clinically significant causes of FUO can be evaluated as outpatients, especially when the fever is relatively low grade and the patients are able to carry on their usual activities. A wide variety of radiologic and surgical/biopsy procedures can be done out of hospital or in a day surgery suite. Studies and biopsies should be directed by clinical suspicion and laboratory evidence of an abnormality. Culture of the blood is one of the most important approaches to elucidation of the cause of FUO, although cultures may have negative results in cases of endocarditis pretreated with antibiotics and in cases of *Brucella* in which cultures should be held for 4 to 6 weeks before being discarded. Serologic testing should not be indiscriminate but focused by elements of the history, clinical findings, epidemiology, and exposures of the particular patient.

The decision to admit a patient for evaluation has changed since the initial studies of Petersdorf and Beeson. Admission to hospital for debilitated or elderly patients may be necessary or for surgical indications such as exploratory laparotomy. The yield of laparotomy has declined in the era of computed tomography and magnetic resonance imaging (with or without guided biopsy) and should be reserved as a "last resort" in patients who have undiagnosed fevers and who are in clinical decline. "Fever alone is no cause for haste in diagnosis."[23]

SUMMARY

FUO, the cause of which is not established over a prolonged period, is a trying experience not only for patients but also for physicians engaged in attempts to unravel its etiology. Because the problem may remain unsolved for long periods, it tends to induce a progressive loss of interest and even unconscious medical neglect because the patients are now "chronic cases" and because they may come to represent a varying degree of diagnostic defeat for the physician. Despite the fact that its solution is often complex, there is a role for cautious waiting and careful periodic reexamination in solving the riddle.

REFERENCES

1. Petersdorf RG and Beeson PB: Fever of unexplained origin: Report on 100 cases. Medicine 40:1, 1961.
2. Dinarello CA, Cannon JG, and Wolf SM: New concepts on the pathogenesis of fever. Rev Inf Dis 10:168, 1988.
3. Williams MH: A note on the temperature of 1,000 children. Lancet i:1192, 1912.
4. Paton JHP: The mean temperature of healthy girls. BMJ 2:142, 1932.
5. Ivy AC: What is the normal body temperature? Gastroenterology 5:326, 1945.
6. Weinstein L: Clinically benign fever of unknown origin: A personal retrospective. Rev Inf Dis 7:692, 1985.
7. Tompkins P: The use of basal temperature graphs in determining the date of ovulation. JAMA 124:698, 1944.
8. Bardswell NE and Chapman JE: Some observations upon the deep temperature of the human body at rest and after exercise. BMJ 1:1106, 1911.
9. Falcon-Lesses M and Proger SH: Psychogenic fever. N Engl J Med 203:1034, 1930.
10. Molave A and Weinstein L: Persistent perplexing pyrexia: Some comments on etiology and diagnosis. Med Clin North Am 54:379, 1970.
11. Petersdorf RG and Bennett IL: Factitious fever. Ann Intern Med 46:1039, 1957.
12. Reich P and Gottfried LA: Factitious disorders in a teaching hospital. Ann Intern Med 99:240, 1983.
13. Cluff LE and Johnson JE: Drug fever. Prog Allergy 8:149, 1964.
14. Lewis C and Kerby G: An epidemic of polymer fever. JAMA 191:375, 1965.
15. Larson EB, Featherstone HJ, and Petersdorf RG: Fever of undetermined origin: Diagnosis and follow-up of 105 cases. 1970–1980. Medicine 61:269, 1982.
16. Holden M, Dubin MR, and Diamond PH: Frequency of negative intermediate-strength tuberculin sensitivity in patients with active tuberculosis. N Engl J Med 285:1506, 1971.
17. Thompson NJ, Glassroth JL, Snider DE, et al: The booster phenomenon in serial tuberculin testing. Am Rev Respir Dis 119:587, 1979.
18. Browder AA, Huff JW, and Petersdorf RG: The significance of fever in neoplastic disease. Ann Intern Med 55:932, 1961.
19. Chang JC: Neoplastic fever: A proposal for diagnosis. Arch Intern Med 149:1728, 1989.
20. Allen NB and Studenski SA: Polymyalgia rheumatica and temporal arteritis. Med Clin North Am 70:369, 1982.
21. Lee FI and Davids DM: Crohn's disease presenting as pyrexia of unknown origin. Lancet i:1205, 1961.
22. Heller H, Sohar E, and Sherf L: Familial Mediterranean fever. Arch Intern Med 102:50, 1958.
23. Baker RR, Tumulty PA, and Shelley WM: The value of exploratory laparotomy in fever of undetermined etiology. Johns Hopkins Med J 125:159, 1969.

67

Lymph Nodes and Subcutaneous Masses

ROBERT OSTEEN, MD
MONICA BERTAGNOLLI, MD

The diagnostic possibilities presented by subcutaneous masses range from trivial lipomas to lymphomas and sarcomas. For most of these lesions, the patient's history, physical examination, and biopsy are the only important diagnostic tests. Thus, without obtaining helpful additional information from radiographs or laboratory tests in most cases, the physician must decide whether a lesion is sufficiently indicative of malignancy to justify a biopsy. Although there are many possible diagnoses, the therapeutic options are limited to observation, antibiotic administration, or excision. We will try to provide a basis on which one can decide which lesions to observe, which lesions to treat with antibiotics, and for which to recommend a biopsy.

HISTORY

Because lymph nodes and other subcutaneous masses are superficial, the patient usually finds the mass. The patient may complain of pain, irritation by clothing, or concern about cancer or cosmesis, or may display idle curiosity. It is important to identify which is of most concern to the patient. A lipoma that is clearly benign to the physician can require excision to allay anxiety of a patient concerned about cancer. A change in the size of a lesion or in symptoms will alert both the patient and the physician to the possibility of malignancy. A history of fluctuation in size should be sought as an indication of inflammation.

If a lesion is felt to be a lymph node, it is important to inquire about possible antecedent infections, including systemic viral illnesses as well as bacterial infections in the regional drainage bed. If lymphadenopathy has been observed by the patient for a period longer than several months, the possibility of chronic infections, such as acquired immunodeficiency syndrome (AIDS), tuberculosis, or fungus, should be considered. Systemic symptoms such as fever, weight loss, night sweats, and pruritus may be symptoms of a lymphoma. It may be difficult by history alone to distinguish mononucleosis from lymphoma.

Metastatic malignant melanoma to lymph nodes can occur from a long-forgotten mole treated in a physician's office without biopsy. Therefore, a history of surgical manipulation of skin lesions should be sought if not volunteered spontaneously.

PHYSICAL EXAMINATION

The physical findings of subcutaneous cysts have been summarized in Table 67–1. A major initial step in the identification of subcutaneous masses is precise anatomic location. Is the mass limited to the subcutaneous tissue, or is it attached to the skin above or muscle below? Masses confined to the subcutaneous space without fixation can be rolled between the fingers and palpated on all aspects. Attachment to muscle can be detected by having the patient contract the muscle in question and demonstrate fixation of the mass, which may be mobile otherwise.

Fixation to overlying skin usually indicates inflammation, malignant invasion, or origin of the mass from a dermal appendage, e.g., sebaceous cyst. Attachment to the skin is indicated by the inability to pinch skin free of the mass and by skin dimpling when the mass is displaced to either side. Attachment to the skin at a number of points will produce a peau d'orange appearance when the mass is displaced. Invasion of the skin by a malignant tumor results in a plaque, which may be elevated or depressed.

Skin changes may occur even though the mass is not attached to the skin. When the skin is stretched tightly over a subcutaneous mass, it may become atrophic, thin, or shiny. Initially, infection produces edema in the skin. As an abscess matures and enlarges, the skin becomes stretched, atrophic, and hot. Venous congestion gives the skin a violaceous hue, and, finally, the skin becomes necrotic. In the nonimmunosuppressed patient, an abscess in the subcutaneous space can be assumed to result from a foreign body, an area of decreased blood supply (e.g., the center of an infected lymph node), or a cyst. Pain and tenderness are generally signs of inflammation, but as lymph nodes swell with lymphoma, there is a period when these lesions are tender. Some sarcomas with necrotic centers also mimic an abscess or a cyst.

Firmness of a mass is one of the findings that increases the examiner's suspicion of malignancy. Lymph nodes infiltrated with lymphoma are often described as "rubbery," whereas metastatic carcinoma is "rocky hard." Although there is a slight difference in feel between these two pathologic processes, the difference is so subtle as to have little practical value. Histopathologic examination is much more useful. Lipomas are distinguished from liposarcomas primarily by the firmer consistency of the latter. It is a mistake to think of all subcutaneous malignancies as "rocky hard." Many sarcomas have enough myxoid elements to give the tumor a soft consistency, but they are never as soft as a benign lipoma. Fibrosis within a lipoma can give a degree of firmness that is lacking in the more liquid fat of the usual lipoma.

Fluctuance describes the sensation of fluid within a capsule. The thumb and forefinger are placed on either side of a superficial lump. The index finger of the other hand presses on the lump. Transmission of a force by liquid causes the thumb and forefinger to separate. The term is most commonly used to describe the liquefied center of an abscess, but it is a common finding with dermoid cysts, lipomas, and normal muscle. Fluctuance is a late finding in an abscess. Preceding the development of fluctuance is a long period when an abscess is merely hard. It is not necessary to delay drainage of an abscess until fluctuance develops.

A distinct border is characteristic of most uninflamed, benign lesions in the subcutaneous tissue. Indistinct borders occur when inflammation causes a border of edema around the mass or when malignant lesions invade the surrounding tissue. A mass arising beneath the fascia or a mass that is attached to muscle cannot be pinched up and have its borders clearly identified. Distinctness of the border should be distinguished from mobility. Fascial fixation will inhibit mobility and blur the distinctness of the borders, but a freely movable mass with indistinct borders should also raise concern over the possibility of malignancy.

TABLE 67–1. SUMMARY OF PHYSICAL FINDINGS INDICATING THAT A MASS IS BENIGN, INFECTED, OR MALIGNANT

Feature	Benign	Infected	Malignant
Skin fixation	+	+ + +	+
Muscle fixation	+	+	+ + +
Skin edema	−	+ + +	−
Skin erythema	−	+ + +	±
Skin warmth	−	+ + +	−
Tenderness	−	+ + +	±
Firmness	+	+ +	+ + +
Fluctuance	+	+ +	
Distinct border	+ + +	−	+

BIOPSY TECHNIQUES

Selection of the appropriate technique for sampling tissue is important if evaluation of a mass is to proceed as expeditiously and inexpensively as possible. Most biopsy procedures can be performed in the office or as outpatient surgical operations. The cost of hospitalization and the risks of general anesthesia are rarely justified for biopsy of subcutaneous masses or superficial lymph nodes. When a lesion is felt to arise from deeper structures and an extensive dissection is anticipated, general anesthesia may be necessary. Selection of the type of anesthesia and the biopsy technique is based on the surgeon's opinion regarding the likely diagnosis, the amount of tissue necessary to establish the diagnosis, and the desirability of totally removing the lesion.

Needle Aspiration

For this technique, a 20-gauge needle attached to a syringe is inserted into the mass. Suction is applied, and the needle is withdrawn. Anesthesia is usually not necessary. The scanty amount of material obtained is ejected onto an albuminized slide and fixed in 95% alcohol. The albuminized slide is necessary to prevent the cells from floating off in the fixative. By this technique, one obtains individual cells and small clusters of cells for cytologic examination.

Needle aspiration is a highly accurate method for the diagnosis of epithelial malignancies. Kline and colleagues[1] have reported that 95% of 88 malignant neoplasms were diagnosed as positive and that there were no false-positive results among 42 benign specimens. Needle aspiration is particularly useful in evaluation of cervical masses, where excisional or incisional biopsies are best avoided to preserve tissue planes for definitive surgery of malignancies. Shaha and associates[2] report 96% diagnostic accuracy in 140 needle aspiration biopsies of cervical adenopathy. In the management of young patients with peripheral adenopathy, Kardos and associates report that needle aspiration provides 95% specificity and 93% sensitivity in the diagnosis of both malignant and benign lymphadenopathy.[3]

The limitation of aspiration biopsy is that it yields cytologic, not histologic, information. It is possible to distinguish benign from malignant disease, but inferences about the specific type of cancer are not as certain as diagnoses made by examination of sections from a whole piece of tissue. The aspiration biopsy technique is particularly useful for the patient who has an established diagnosis of cancer. Lymph nodes or subcutaneous nodules can be proved to contain tumor but are left intact as an indicator of response to chemotherapy. The technique is relatively free of complications. Engzell and associates[4] found no evidence of recurrent tumor in biopsy needle tracks in 641 patients. This is opposed to the findings of Ackerman and Wheat,[5] who found tumor implants in tracks of needle biopsies of the parotid. Although it is possible for tumor cells to spread along the needle biopsy tracks, the clinical implications are minimal because most malignant tumors, including the area of the needle tract, are subjected to subsequent surgical excision or radiotherapy.

Needle Biopsy

A small core of tissue can be obtained with any of several available biopsy needles. These instruments are primarily used to obtain biopsies from such organs as liver, kidney, or prostate but can be used to obtain biopsies from superficial masses and superficial organs, such as the thyroid. The Silverman needle, which has been used for this purpose for many years, is a 14-gauge needle that has an inner, split, flexible stylet that holds the tissue as it is sheared from its surroundings by an outer needle. This technique offers the possibility of obtaining tissue for histologic examination without making an incision. Local anesthesia is required, but the patient may experience some discomfort because of the force required to insert the large needle and because it is difficult to anesthetize the center of a mass. Bleeding is not a problem if the patient's clotting mechanisms are normal. The specimen obtained is small, about 25 mg, and has the diameter of the bore of a 14-gauge needle. The distinction between benign and malignant can be made, but the specimen is often inadequate to establish the specific type of malignant neoplasm. In a series reported from the Brigham and Women's Hospital, it was found that when a malignant neoplasm was suspected but the histopathology was unknown, a needle biopsy yielded a specimen that was adequate for definitive diagnosis in only three of 19 instances.[6] Therefore, like aspiration biopsy, this technique seems most applicable to situations in which the diagnosis is established, but verification of a metastasis without an incision is desirable. It has also been used for the diagnosis of cold thyroid nodules,[7] although it has been supplanted in many centers by less complicated "skinny-needle biopsies."

Incisional and Excisional Biopsies

Open biopsy techniques trade the disadvantages of an incision for the advantages of a more generous specimen. The choice between an incisional biopsy and an excisional biopsy depends on the size and location of the lesion, the adequacy of anesthesia, the vascularity of the lesion, and the type of information desired. Benign lesions should be completely excised to avoid the necessity for second operation. It is desirable to excise malignant lesions completely to avoid spreading tumor cells. However, a deforming, major operation is rarely justified to remove a suspected, unproven malignancy. An adequate margin around a malignant lesion can rarely be obtained with an excisional biopsy. It is generally preferable to make a diagnosis by means of a small incision that can be encompassed by a more radical resection if that is indicated by the pathology.

The initial biopsy incision should be planned in a manner that avoids excessive skin loss and deformity and minimizes problems of wound healing if a wider excision becomes necessary. Complete excision of lymph nodes is advisable to avoid lymph leaks (lymphoceles) and to provide adequate nodal architecture for the diagnosis of lymphomas. Major decisions for the treatment of lymphomas are made on the basis of the histologic pattern. It is helpful to have a whole, intact lymph node to distinguish the subcategories of lymphomas. Complete excision of a large cluster of lymph nodes is not justified for diagnostic purposes.

Most biopsies of superficial masses and lymph nodes can be performed as outpatient procedures with the patient under local anesthesia. For deeper lesions, particularly when muscle retraction is necessary and for repeat biopsies, general anesthesia is required.

Tissue Processing

Consultation with the pathologist and possibly a frozen section are helpful to ensure that an adequate representative tissue sample has been taken. In addition to hematoxylin-eosin staining, numerous techniques are available to the pathologist that aid in a complicated diagnosis. These techniques require both planning and fresh, unfixed tissue.

Communication with the pathologist is essential if these techniques are to be effective.

"Touch preps" that are made by touching the cut surface of the specimen to a glass slide are an excellent way to assess the morphology of individual cells, particularly in cases of suspected lymphoma.

Cell-surface markers for subsets of lymphocytes (T and B cells) have diagnostic significance.[8] Immunofluorescence studies with commercially available monoclonal antibodies can identify proliferating clones of lymphocytes. Myeloid cells can be distinguished from lymphoid cells by their characteristic enzymes.

Electron microscopy may be useful if there is reason to include melanoma or sarcoma in the differential diagnosis. The melanosomes of a melanoma are visible with electron microscopy even though the lesion is grossly amelanotic.[9] Similarly, identification of myofibrils may clarify the diagnosis of rhabdomyosarcoma. Tissue for electron microscopy should be fixed in glutaraldehyde instead of the usual fixation in formalin or Zenker's solution.

The diagnosis of breast cancer metastatic to lymph nodes can be supported by assay of the specimen for estrogen receptor protein.[10] The identification of estrogen receptor protein may also have important diagnostic and therapeutic implications.[11, 12] Tissue for that assay must be fresh or rapidly frozen in liquid nitrogen. The identification of organ-specific cell-surface antigens by monoclonal antibodies such as S-100 and HMB-45 for melanomas,[13] prostate-specific antigen for carcinomas of prostatic origin,[14] and gross cystic disease fluid protein for breast carcinoma,[15] is a promising new technique for finding the tissue of origin for metastases from an unknown primary.

Unless the diagnosis of lymphoma or metastatic malignancy is evident on frozen section of a lymph node, nodal tissue should be cultured for tuberculosis, fungi, and aerobic and anaerobic bacteria. Approximately 0.5 to 1.0 g of tissue, sterilely divided into equal portions, should be adequate for bacteriologic examination.

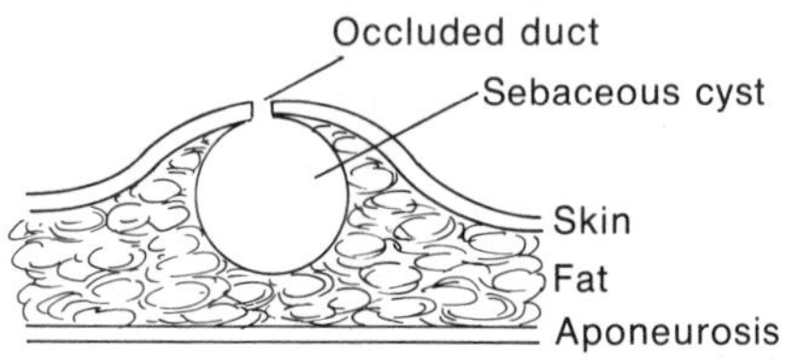

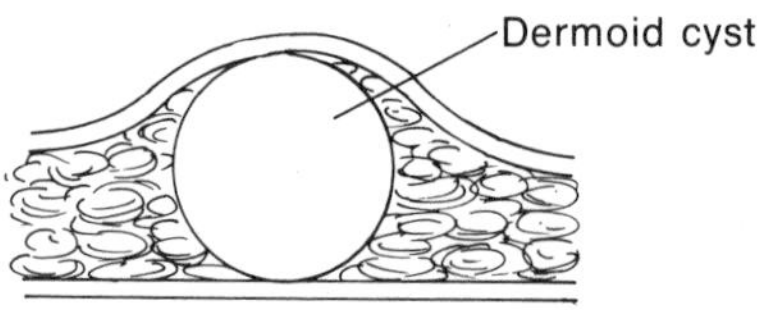

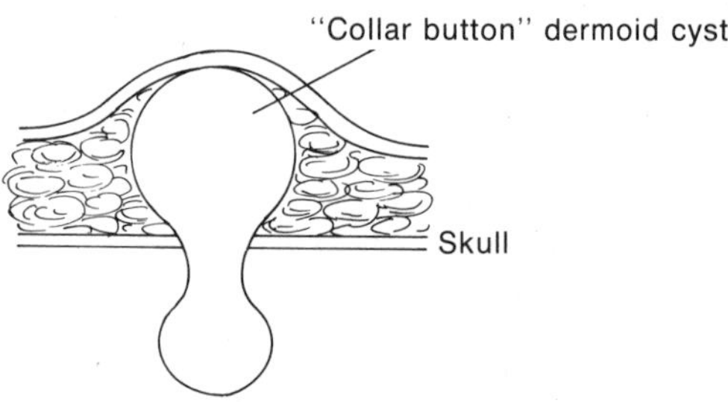

FIGURE 67–1. Subcutaneous cysts.

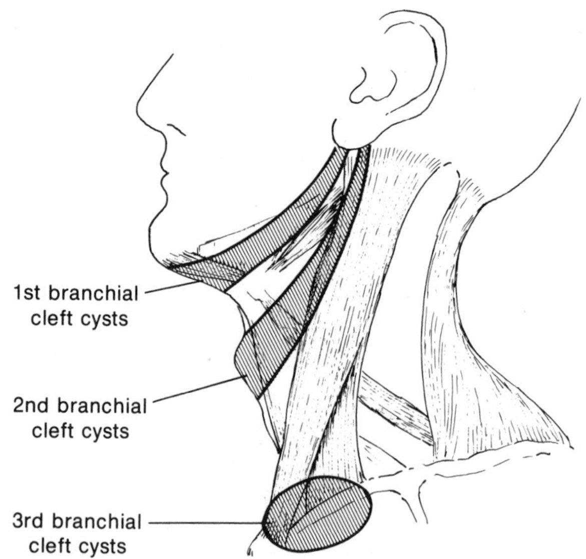

FIGURE 67–2. Sites of cysts and sinuses that arise from incomplete obliteration of embryonic branchial clefts.

Recently, the cellular DNA content of soft tissue tumors has been shown by flow cytometry to aid in histopathologic staging.[16] Evidence suggests that benign and low-grade tumors are diploid, whereas high-grade tumors tend to be aneuploid. The prognostic significance of flow cytometry in soft tissue tumors has not yet been established.

NONLYMPHOID SUBCUTANEOUS MASSES

Cysts and Other Benign Neoplasms

Sebaceous cysts result from plugging of a sebaceous duct (Fig. 67–1). The resulting mass is attached to the skin at one small point. The unattached skin will slide over the smooth wall of the cyst, and there is no attachment to the deep fascia. These characteristics are usually preserved except when the cyst becomes infected. Epidermoid (inclusion) cysts have similar physical findings. Robbins and colleagues[17] believe that epidermoid cysts merely result from a change of a sebaceous cyst to a squamous epithelium, which can produce keratin. Cysts occurring on the fingers or palms are usually the result of trauma.

Dermoid cysts tend to occur in the midline of the body. They have no obvious skin attachments, are lined by squamous epithelium, and are often fluid filled (see Fig. 67–1). Cysts in the midline of the skull should be viewed with some caution because they may have an intracranial extension of a collar button configuration. The fluid-filled center of a dermoid cyst gives it a fluctuant feel. Both dermoid and sebaceous cysts become infected. Although antibiotics against the staphylococcus may help reduce the surrounding cellulitis, an infected cyst can rarely be cured by antibiotics without drainage. Occasionally it is possible to extrude the cyst wall when an infected cyst is drained, but, more commonly, pain and hemorrhage prevent manipulation of the cyst wall. After the inflammation has subsided, the cyst should be excised to prevent reinfection.

Patients with congenital branchiogenic cysts (Fig. 67–2) usually present with an infection in the neck or an annoying secretion from a sinus. Cysts arising from the first branchial cleft produce a sinus near the ear that follows

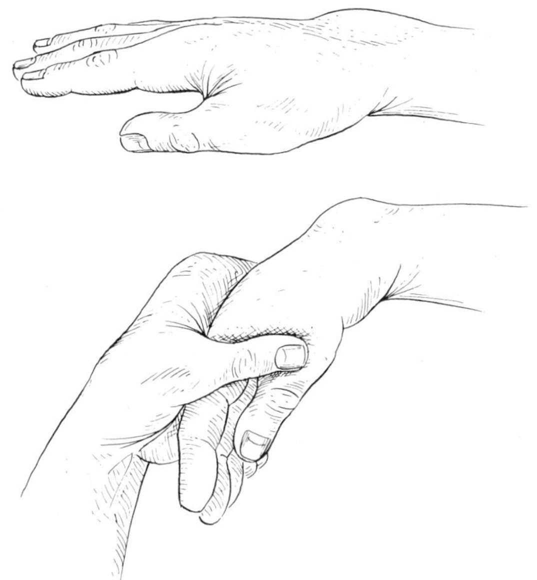

FIGURE 67–3. Ganglion of the wrist made more prominent by flexion.

the external auditory canal medially. Cysts arising from the second branchial cleft occur in the midportion of the neck and track between the internal and external carotids into the tonsilla fossa. Cysts arising from the third brachial cleft occur either above or below the clavicle and near the head of the sternocleidomastoid muscle. Although branchiogenic cysts may develop into a primary carcinoma, most cases thought to be a branchiogenic carcinoma are in fact metastases from oropharyngeal or lung cancer to cervical lymph nodes.

Thyroglossal duct cysts are congenital anomalies resulting from retention of an epithelial track between the thyroid gland and its origin at the foramen cecum in the floor of the pharynx. These lesions, therefore, occur in the midline, in the midportion of the neck, and track upward through the hyoid bone into the base of the tongue. These lesions will move with tongue protrusion or deglutition. Thyroglossal duct cysts are most commonly diagnosed in the pediatric-aged group but can present at any age. Fine-needle aspiration may be useful in distinguishing thyroglossal duct cysts from midline dermoid cysts. General anesthesia is required for excision. The malignant potential of a thyroglossal duct cyst is low.

Ganglia or cysts resulting from degeneration of synovium are found in association with the joints and tendons of the hands and feet (Fig. 67–3). These cysts do not communicate with joint cavities or synovial spaces around tendons, and the contents are not the same as synovial fluid. The cavities contain a highly viscous, clear fluid. Aspiration of a ganglion will produce temporary disappearance of the lesion, but cure requires complete excision of the cyst and the surrounding area of dense connective tissue from which it arose. This is not a procedure that can be done in the office. Tourniquet hemostasis and careful dissection are required for good long-term results.

Lipomas are among the most common benign subcutaneous masses. These tumors consist of normal fat enclosed in a capsule. Lipomas have a soft, fluctuant feel and are not attached to underlying fascia. Lateral compression of a lipoma may produce a characteristic peau d'orange appearance (Fig. 67–4).

Benign solid tumors can arise from any of the dermal or subcuticular elements. These tumors are almost invariably hard enough to raise the suspicion of malignancy. Only with biopsy can one be sure that such lesions are benign.

Malignant Subcutaneous Masses

Malignant tumors can arise from any of the elements of the skin or subcutaneous tissue. The most common primary tumors of the subcutaneous space are liposarcomas, malignant fibrous histiocytomas, leiomyosarcomas, and fibrosarcomas. The various tumor types are grouped together under the term *soft tissue sarcomas.* These tumors share a tendency to spread along fascial planes and metastasize by hematogenous dissemination. Many of these tumors are surrounded by a pseudocapsule of tumor and compressed normal tissue. The tendency to local recurrence can be prevented only by adequate, usually radical, excision. Adequate excision frequently involves removal of entire muscle groups or amputation of the limb.

In the past, pretreatment evaluation and staging of soft tissue sarcomas has been primarily determined by computed tomography. Recently, however, magnetic resonance imaging (MRI) has largely replaced computed tomography, especially for the evaluation of the extremities.[18] Biopsy is important to establish histologic grade. Open biopsy is preferred, with incisional biopsy for large lesions and wide excisional biopsy for small (<2 cm) superficial lesions.[19]

Although each individual cell type has its own presenting features and prognosis, the investigations of Russell and colleagues[20] have tended to group all soft tissue sarcomas together and emphasize the importance of histologic grade as well as size and nodal status in the staging. High-grade lesions with an aggressive histologic appearance require a multimodality approach combining the efforts of the surgeon, radiation therapist, medical oncologist, and pathologist. A discussion of the various ways that surgery, chemotherapy, and radiation therapy can be integrated in the treatment of high-grade, soft tissue sarcomas is beyond the scope of this chapter. However, for such an approach to be successful, it is essential that all the interested parties become involved as early as possible in the evaluation of the patient.

Although most sarcomas present as painless, hard

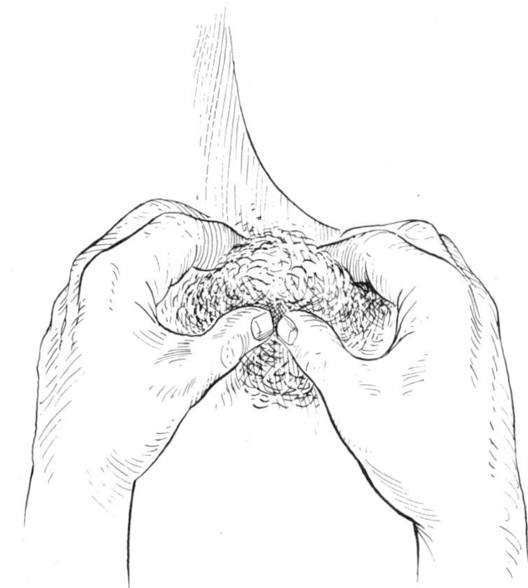

FIGURE 67–4. Peau d'orange sign of a lipoma. Lateral compression lifts the skin upward, putting tension on the vertical trabeculae.

masses, some resemble an abscess, with pain, heat, and skin changes. If an infection fails to clear with antibiotics or if the contents of an abscess look like cheesy, necrotic tissue, the diagnosis of sarcoma should be considered. Several common soft tissue sarcomas are discussed next.

Liposarcoma. Liposarcomas arise from adipose tissue and are softer than some other malignant tumors, but they are never as soft as a lipoma. They lose the liquid feel so characteristic of a lipoma. Liposarcomas frequently occur in the gluteal and popliteal regions.

Fibrous Histiocytoma. Fibrous histiocytomas have been identified with increasing frequency. Many arise in the skin and subcutaneous tissues. The malignancy of these tumors varies from well-differentiated types with virtually no tendency to metastasize to highly malignant, rapidly metastasizing types. Histologic grade is the key to identifying the aggressiveness of the individual tumor.

Fibrosarcoma. Fibrosarcomas arise from connective tissue anywhere in the body but are common in the superficial layers of the extremities and trunk. They are composed of fibroblasts and collagen. They occur at any age and may grow slowly for many years. The tumors are pseudoencapsulated and are often of low histologic grade. These less aggressive tumors can be treated by wide local excision. Higher-grade tumors require a multimodality approach.

Synovial Sarcoma. Many synovial sarcomas occur in younger adults. They originate from synovium and are commonly found about tendon sheaths and joints. They are frequently mistaken for ganglion cysts but lack the smooth, round character and myxoid contents of a benign ganglion. Although synovial sarcomas are not strictly a tumor of the subcutaneous tissue, they are superficial and must be included in the differential diagnosis. Many synovial sarcomas are aggressive tumors with a poor prognosis. Lymph node metastases are somewhat more common from synovial sarcomas than from other soft tissue sarcomas.

Rhabdomyosarcoma. Rhabdomyosarcomas arise from striated muscle. They frequently present as a superficial mass that is diffusely attached to the muscle below. The popliteal, gluteal, inguinal, and interscapular areas are common sites of presentation. They are frequently confused with other soft tissue sarcomas by gross appearance. The tumors are soft and may be slightly fluctuant from hemorrhage within the center. Electron microscopy is useful for making the diagnosis.

Kaposi's Sarcoma. This once rare neoplasm is associated with human immunodeficiency virus (HIV) infection and presents as a painful, bluish-black lesion of the skin or oral mucosa. Diagnosis is confirmed by fine-needle aspiration, revealing overlapping spindle cells with nuclear distortion and ill-defined cytologic borders.[21] Kaposi's sarcoma associated with AIDS differs considerably from the classic tumor. In patients with AIDS, the disease may be anywhere on the skin or mucous membranes, as well as in lymph nodes and viscera. Radiotherapy or chemotherapy offers palliative therapy in patients with this virulent disease.[22]

Metastatic Cancer. Metastases from breast, colon, and ovary as well as carcinoids and malignant melanomas may occur in the subcutaneous space. These tumor deposits initially present as a plaque in the subcutaneous tissues with attachment to the skin. As they enlarge, the mass assumes a rounder configuration and protrudes superficially.

Summary. Sebaceous and dermoid cysts should be drained when they are infected and excised after inflammation has subsided. Lipomas should be excised with the patient under local or general anesthesia, depending on the size, when the patient complains of an annoying mass or a cosmetic problem. Firm, irregular, fixed masses should be biopsied (incisional or excisional) to rule out a malignant tumor. Needle biopsies are useful and appropriate for the confirmation of subcutaneous metastasis from a known primary site.

LYMPH NODES

One of the most important decisions made during a physical examination is whether a subcutaneous mass is a lymph node. From that decision numerous actions, tests, and assumptions follow. The freely movable "lima bean" palpated in the normal groin or axilla is not easily mistaken. However, as lymph nodes become larger and rounder or if they occur beneath fascia, or if mobility is lost, they can be difficult to distinguish from other masses. Lymph nodes tend to retain their round, smooth surface characteristics until quite late in the disease process. Only when tumor or infection has broken through the capsule of a lymph node will that round, smooth character be lost. Even when a group of nodes is fused by lymphoma or carcinoma, the "knobbiness" of a mass is imparted by the basic round shape of the individual nodes. This roundness can be helpful for identifying masses deep in the supraclavicular fossa or presenting deep to the pectoralis muscles in the infraclavicular area.

Lymph nodes enlarge in response to either a regional or a systemic antigen challenge or because of infiltration by lymphoma or metastatic cancer. The need to obtain a biopsy of an enlarged lymph node varies with the clinical setting and the physician's suspicion that a lymph node may harbor a primary or metastatic malignancy.

Enlargement of the lymph nodes that drain a regional infection is identified by a history of infection, lymphangitis, spontaneous resolution, or improvement with antibiotics. Lymphadenopathy in response to chronic irritation may be more difficult to identify. For instance, isolated enlargement of posterior cervical lymph nodes in a patient without systemic symptoms is commonly due to seborrheic dermatitis of the scalp and will respond to a more effective shampoo. Such inflammatory nodes are rarely over 1 cm in diameter. Larger nodes and nodes that fail to respond to antibiotics raise the possibility of an abscess in the center of an inflammatory node or of infiltration by a neoplastic process. Although normal lymph nodes may be palpable in a thin individual, enlarged lymph nodes usually indicate some type of pathologic condition. That pathologic condition may be minor in the case of reactive lymph nodes stimulated by an unnoticed infection. In general, lymph nodes greater than 2 cm in their largest diameter deserve further investigation.

Generalized Lymphadenopathy

Generalized lymphadenopathy may develop as part of a syndrome of systemic illness, or it may be noted in the absence or presence of only nonspecific symptoms. A clinical diagnosis is possible in many cases of generalized lymphadenopathy caused by infectious mononucleosis and mononucleosis-like illness (toxoplasmosis, cytomegaloviral infection), hepatitis B, or secondary syphilis. Other conditions that cause this syndrome and are accompanied by specific features include disseminated tuberculosis or histoplasmosis, drug reaction such as that from phenytoin (Dilantin), heroin addiction, sarcoidosis, systemic lupus erythematosus, rheumatoid arthritis, hyperthyroidism, serum sickness, chronic lymphocytic leukemia, lymphoma, and rare diseases like brucellosis and leptospirosis. Thus, one should search specifically for the history or findings of pharyngitis, hepatosplenomegaly, chorioretinitis, rash, condyloma latum, fever, cough, weight loss, anorexia, synovitis, goiter, exophthalmos or the history of drug intake.

In addition to lymphoma, diseases related to HIV infection are certainly considerations in patients with known risk factors for this infection (homosexual or bisexual patients, intravenous drug users, or regular recipients of blood products) who have generalized lymphadenopathy. The patient may present with weight loss, fever, fatigue, and diarrhea in addition to generalized lymphadenopathy, prior to the appearance of an AIDS-defining illness. Additional clinical features include unexplained oral thrush and herpes zoster, lymphopenia, mild anemia, hypergammaglobulinemia, hypoalbuminemia, and decreased T helper (T4) to T suppressor (T8) ratio.[23] Such patients, and any patient with persistent, unexplained generalized lymphadenopathy who is possibly at risk for HIV, should be tested for HIV.

The lymph nodes in patients with HIV infection are usually soft, and the average size of biopsy specimens is relatively small (~1.5 cm).[24] Patients with AIDS-related complex frequently exhibit the pattern of follicular and paracortical hyperplasia in lymph nodes.[25] Nodes from patients with AIDS typically reveal effacement of nodal architecture, small-vessel proliferation, and atypical lymphoid proliferation. However, histologic examination of lymph nodes has not yielded prognostic information in addition to that already obtained by noninvasive studies, except for the identification of secondary infections and neoplasms in approximately 10% of patients.[26] For this reason, lymph node biopsy in patients with AIDS or AIDS-related complex is reserved for HIV-infected patients with unexplained generalized symptoms or atypical lymph node enlargement. AIDS is associated with a high rate of neoplastic complications, including aggressive lymphomas, plasmacytomas, Hodgkin's disease, and monoclonal B cell proliferation,[27] in addition to infection with *Mycobacterium avium-intracellulare* (also known as *Mycobacterium avium* complex, or MAC).

Regarding the issue of when to perform a biopsy of lymph nodes in patients with generalized lymphadenopathy, Greenfield and Jordan suggested biopsy if there are supraclavicular nodes.[28] Otherwise, the initial evaluation includes culture for streptococcus if pharyngitis is present, culture for gonorrhea if oral-genital contact was established, and testing for heterophil antibodies, repeated in 1 week if results are negative. The initial evaluation may also include the complete blood count with white blood cell count differential, liver function tests, hepatitis B surface antigen, serology for syphilis, chest film, urinalysis, and tuberculin tests. Thyroid function tests are indicated if there is any suspicion of hyperthyroidism, and blood should be cultured if the patient is febrile. Greenfield and Jordan also suggested searching for scratches or other evidence of cat-scratch fever if nodes are localized to the axillary area, and a complement-fixation test for lymphogranuloma venereum plus searching for other sexually transmitted diseases if localized inguinal nodes are present. Patients with fever, chills, weight loss, and nodes present for 1 week should have serologic studies for *Toxoplasma* (complement fixation >16, indirect hemagglutination >256, or indirect fluorescent antibody >256) and cytomegalovirus complement fixation (complement fixation >64 to 128), a chest film, and intermediate purified protein derivative. Drugs such as phenytoin, hydralazine, or allopurinol should be discontinued. Greenfield and Jordan suggest that persistence of unexplained nodes should then lead to biopsy.[28] Slap and associates also addressed this issue in 123 patients, aged 9 to 25 years, who had biopsies for enlarged peripheral lymph nodes.[29] In these young patients, they suggested that an abnormal chest film, lymph node size of more than 2.0 cm, history of night sweats, history of weight loss, or hemoglobin of 10.0 or less g/dl identified patients with granulomatous or neoplastic disease, whereas a history of ear, nose, and throat infection identified those likely to have negative biopsy specimens.[29]

Hodgkin's disease and non-Hodgkin's lymphoma are major considerations in any patient with persistent lymphadenopathy, regardless of whether HIV is suspected. Such patients may be symptomatic or asymptomatic. Epitrochlear nodes may be involved, as may Waldeyer's ring in the pharynx. Libman summarizes the question of when to do a biopsy by suggesting that patients with generalized lymphadenopathy of unclear etiology after thorough evaluation be observed for 4 weeks and then undergo lymph node biopsy if lymphadenopathy fails to regress.[30]

Some lymph nodes biopsies are nondiagnostic. Sinclair and colleagues reported that a specific diagnosis could be made in 63% of their patients who had biopsies of enlarged, superficial lymph nodes.[31] Of the patients with nondiagnostic specimens, 25% eventually developed a disease related to the indication for biopsy, usually lymphoma. Saltzstein found that 17% of patients who had nondiagnostic biopsies for adenopathy eventually developed lymphomas.[32]

If an adequate sample of a suspicious lymph node is nondiagnostic, the patient should be followed up carefully, and biopsies should be done of new lesions. Most patients who develop lymphoproliferative disorders after an initial nondiagnostic biopsy do so within 6 to 8 months.[31, 32]

Regional Lymph Node Enlargement

It is evident that biopsy of persistently enlarged, superficial lymph nodes is advisable, but how much evaluation should be done prior to a biopsy? If it is likely that the nodal hypertrophy is a response to regional or systemic antigen stimulation, then the biopsy should be deferred until the effects of treatment or potential spontaneous resolution can be observed. Under these circumstances, one would expect significant diminution in size within a few weeks. Kaplan has pointed out that lymph nodes infiltrated with lymphoma may also fluctuate in size.[33] The type and extent of evaluation must be governed by the probability of finding a given diagnosis. There are differences in the order of the differential diagnosis, depending on the anatomic location of the enlarged lymph nodes. Therefore, inguinal, axillary, and cervical lymph nodes will be considered separately.

Inguinal Adenopathy

Inguinal lymph nodes are found below the inguinal ligament and usually medial to the femoral pulse. This is also the site of femoral hernias, and at times it is difficult to distinguish a hernia from a single enlarged lymph node. Hernias can usually be reduced, and bowel sounds may be heard by auscultation over the mass.

Biopsy of inguinal adenopathy is generally regarded as less productive than biopsy of other nodal groups, probably because low-grade infections in the feet stimulate chronic reactive changes in draining lymph nodes. Enlarged inguinal nodes seen on lymphangiogram do not carry the diagnostic significance of nodes of the same size elsewhere.[34] However, Sinclair and colleagues[31] found significant disease in 16 of 22 inguinal lymph node specimens that were presented for biopsy only because they were enlarged. Zaren and Copeland[35] reviewed the records of 2232 patients with inguinal node metastases. The primary sites of malignancy were, in order of frequency, the skin of the lower extremities, the cervix, vulva, skin of the trunk, rectum and anus, ovary, and penis. Malignant melanoma was the most common histologic diagnosis, followed by squamous cell carcinoma. Of particular interest in that series were 22 patients whose metastases arose from an unknown primary. The 3-year survival in the group was 50% after lymph node dissection. These studies suggest that the proper approach to inguinal adenopathy should be biopsy of unilaterally enlarged nodes greater than 2 cm in diameter after a careful search of the skin of the trunk and extremities and examination of the perineum and pelvis for a primary cancer or site of infection. The biopsies should be done in such a way that the incision does not interfere with a subsequent, wider, inguinal node dissection.

Axillary Adenopathy

Examination for lymph nodes in the axilla should be performed with the patient's arm held comfortably at the side. If the arm is held in abduction at greater than 45°, the axillary fascia is too tense for adequate examination of lymph nodes high in the axilla. The fingers of the examiner's hand should be slightly cupped and an effort made to gently sweep the axillary contents inferiorly. The lymph nodes can be felt to roll under the examiner's hand as the tethering vessels pull the nodes back up into the apex of the axilla. There are nodes lower in the axilla palpable against the chest wall and others located behind the anterior axillary fold formed by the lateral border of the pectoralis major muscle. A diffuse bulge or an indistinct mass may be produced in the infraclavicular area by nodes that are deep to the pectoralis major muscle.

An inflammatory response in axillary lymph nodes is often predicted by an enlarged epitrochlear node. The axillary nodes are a common site for presentation of Hodgkin's disease and non-Hodgkin's lymphomas. In women with undifferentiated carcinoma or adenocarcinoma metastatic to axillary lymph nodes, the most likely source is the breast.[36] Axillary metastases from an occult breast cancer should have a favorable prognosis because one is treating a regional disease that has the possibility of long-term cure. Accurate and adequate histologic study is the key to management. Early axillary lymph node biopsy will indicate what routes to follow in the evaluation, how to evaluate for other sites of disease, and what definitive therapy to employ. For example, patients with melanoma localized to axillary lymph nodes will require an axillary dissection, as will men with unclassified malignancies. Copeland and McBride reported long-term survival of nine of 42 patients whose axillary nodes were treated with surgical excision or radiation therapy for metastases with no known primary site.[37] Women with adenocarcinoma or unclassified malignancies should have treatment directed at the breast as well as the axilla. Campana and colleagues treated 31 women presenting with isolated axillary lymphadenopathy of probable metastatic origin from the breast, but without clinical or radiologic evidence of breast tumor or other primary tumor. Treatment with axillary surgery and radiotherapy to the breast or a combination of radiotherapy and systemic adjuvant chemotherapy resulted in 5- and 10-year survival rates of 73 and 71%, respectively.[38]

When large, rubbery axillary lymph nodes are associated with supraclavicular or cervical adenopathy, it is preferable to do a biopsy of the axillary nodes so that the incision is less conspicuous. Biopsies should be performed on unilateral, nontender, hard axillary lymph nodes larger than 1.5 cm in diameter and matted nodes.

Cervical Adenopathy

Lymph nodes in the posterior triangle of the neck are superficial, but in the anterior parts of the neck, nodes may be quite deep. To examine for these deeper nodes, it may be helpful to stand behind the patient. As nodes in the supraclavicular fossa enlarge, they may initially appear only as a diffuse puffiness, but later distinct, fixed masses become palpable. Lymph nodes originating along the internal jugular chain are poorly defined because only a small portion of the circumference of the node is palpable. Submental and digastric nodes may be very difficult to distinguish from other structures in the area, such as the submaxillary glands. Lymph nodes are usually rounder, more mobile, and less distinctly palpated with an intraoral finger than are salivary glands. In the midcervical area, enlarged lymph nodes may transmit a brisk pulsation from the carotid artery.

Systemic inflammatory processes, especially viral infections, may produce cervical adenopathy. Rubella and toxoplasmosis, as well as infectious mononucleosis, commonly cause enlargement of posterior cervical, posterior auricular, and suboccipital lymph nodes. Tuberculosis can be found in cervical and supraclavicular nodes. Sarcoidosis is often identified in mediastinal nodes on radiography, and involved lymph nodes can be palpated in the supraclavicular fossa.

Lymph nodes in different parts of the neck drain specific areas and can be expected to enlarge with inflammation or cancer arising in the drained area (Figs. 67–5, 67–6). Lymphomas may arise in any lymph node. When lymph nodes high in the neck contain lymphoma, one should also anticipate involvement of the circumoral collection of lymphatic tissue known as Waldeyer's ring. In the absence of inflammation, a firm lymph node in the middle or upper third of the neck may contain either lymphoma or regional metastasis from a carcinoma. It was thought that squamous cell carcinoma in an upper or middle cervical node was "branchiogenic carcinoma" arising in a branchial cleft cyst. Although malignant degeneration of branchial cysts can occur, we now believe that such a change is very rare. Largely through the efforts of Martin and Morfit,[39] it is now recognized that most of these branchiogenic carcinomas are regional metastases from carcinomas of the nasopharynx or upper digestive tract.

Primary oropharyngeal cancers may be difficult to find even with repeated examinations of the nose, oropharynx, and larynx with the patient under topical anesthesia and sedation. If a lymph node is strongly suspected to contain metastatic carcinoma, aspiration biopsy is usually recommended for confirmation of the diagnosis. Excisional biopsy is to be avoided in this circumstance because the ensuing inflammation may make examination under anesthesia confusing, and the incision may interfere with a subsequent radical neck dissection. Recently, development of a new needle designed specifically for use with MRI has improved the accuracy of MRI-guided fine-needle aspiration of cervical masses.[40] If after confirmation of a carcinoma in a cer-

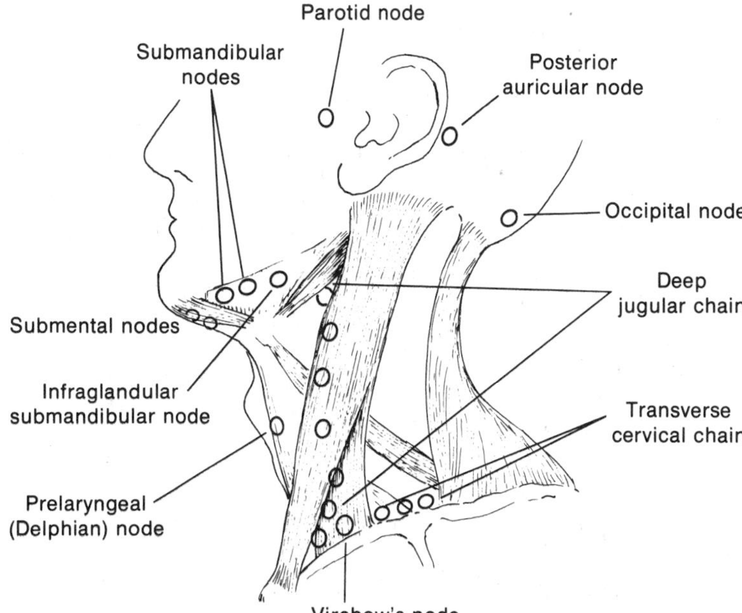

FIGURE 67–5. Anatomy of the cervical lymph nodes.

vical node the primary site is still unknown, then examination of the patient while under anesthesia and blind biopsy of the nasopharynx are indicated.

Even after an extensive evaluation, a small number (approximately 5%) of patients will still have cervical metastases from an undetected primary site.[41] Patients who have early lesions can be treated with radical neck dissections with or without irradiation of potential primary sites, with surprisingly good results. Coker and colleagues[42] reported that survival is related to the degree of nodal involvement. The 5-year survival for patients with squamous cell carcinoma or anaplastic carcinoma was 48% in their series. Adenocarcinoma in a supraclavicular lymph node is likely to be a systemic metastasis and has a more ominous prognosis. Until more effective systemic therapy becomes available, there appears to be little reason to conduct an expensive evaluation of asymptomatic patients in search of the unknown primary site that has given off metastatic adenocarcinoma to supraclavicular lymph nodes.[6]

SUPERFICIAL ENDOCRINE AND EXOCRINE GLANDS

Salivary Glands

Parotid Glands

The salivary glands are included in a discussion of subcutaneous masses because they are often confused with lymph nodes by the inexperienced or unwary examiner. The parotid gland sits on the ramus of the mandible ante-

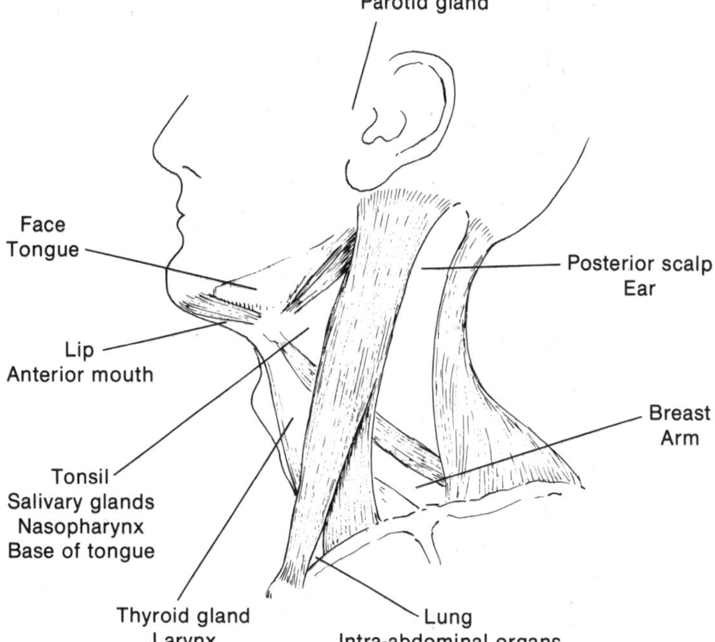

FIGURE 67–6. Common sites for metastases to lymph nodes.

rior to the ear and extends down to or just below the angle of the mandible. The normal parotid is not palpable as a discrete entity. Inflammatory changes in the parotid are usually obvious. They are tender, hot, swollen masses anterior and slightly inferior to the ear. If the gland is massaged, pus can be expressed from Stensen's duct. Mass lesions arising in the parotid are more subtle. Such masses bulge from the anterior surface of the gland, which is normally concave. A parotid tumor may appear either as a swelling anterior to the ear or as a mass in the upper neck. Some parotid tumors are freely movable, with only a small connection to the main parotid gland. Approximately 70% of parotid neoplasms are benign. Paralysis of the facial nerve is uncommon even when the tumor is malignant.[43] Sialography is of little help in distinguishing benign from malignant lesions.[43] Even with a history of acute parotitis, it may be impossible to distinguish a mass of chronic parotitis from a neoplasm by physical examination. In that circumstance, a biopsy is indicated. Biopsy of a parotid mass is done with the patient under general anesthesia to excise the lesion completely with a margin of normal tissue. Even benign parotid tumors tend to recur locally if the margin is inadequate. The need for superficial parotidectomy, in which all of the gland superficial to the nerve is removed, is determined at the time of operation by frozen-section diagnosis. Total parotidectomy with sacrifice of the facial nerve is indicated only for invasion of the nerve by tumor. Radical neck dissection is indicated if there are palpable cervical nodes.

Submaxillary (Submandibular) Gland

The submaxillary glands lie deep in the floor of the mouth but relatively superficial in the neck (Fig. 67–7). Each gland is located in a triangle bounded by the digastric muscle and the mandible. Like the parotid, the normal submaxillary gland is not palpable. Inflammation commonly results from an impacted stone in the duct. The diagnosis can be made by expressing pus from the intraoral opening of the duct or by radiologic visualization of stones. The acute situation can be treated with heat and antibiotics. Stones can often be removed by incising the duct directly over the stone through the floor of the mouth. Sialography should be avoided in the acute situation. Chronic inflammation may result in a hard, palpable gland. As with the parotid gland, chronic inflammation of the submaxillary gland may be indistinguishable from a neoplasm by physical examination. Most neoplasms of the submaxillary gland are malignant, which is not true in the parotid. There were 116 malignant tumors in the collection of 230 submandibular neoplasms studied by Rafla.[44]

Sublingual Glands

Sublingual glands lie immediately beneath the buccal mucosa along the body of the mandible. They have the same disposition to infection as the parotid and submandibular glands. Neoplasms are likely to be malignant.

Thyroid and Parathyroid

The evaluation of thyroid disease is discussed in Chapter 44. Parathyroid glands are rarely palpable even when significantly enlarged.

Chemodectoma

Tumors arising from the paraganglionic cells are rare. Most of these tumors are concentrated in the area of the carotid bifurcation and lie within the adventitial coat of the artery. Carotid body tumors occur as palpable lesions that transmit pulsations from the adjacent artery. They have lateral mobility but limited vertical movement. Although most of these tumors are benign, slowly growing lesions, excision is recommended for symptomatic lesions, when malignancy is suspected, or when the diagnosis is unclear.[45] Westbrook and colleagues[46] have advocated arteriography rather than percutaneous biopsy. Fine-needle aspiration biopsy, made safer by localization with ultrasonic or MRI guidance, may also be used for preoperative diagnosis.[47] Because these lesions are easier to resect when small, resection of small-to-moderate–sized tumors in low-risk patients has been recommended.

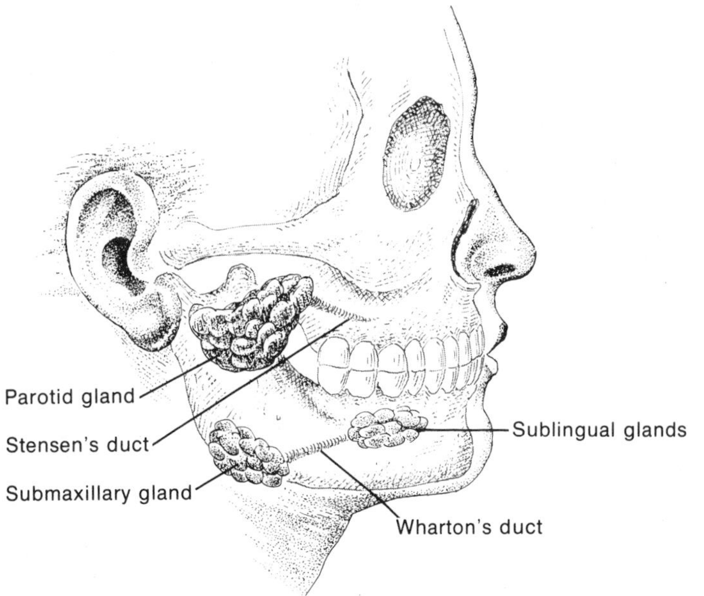

FIGURE 67–7. Anatomic location of the salivary glands.

MISCELLANEOUS SUBCUTANEOUS MASSES

Gout. Irregular masses overlying the joints may be produced by the chronic deposition of urate crystals in cartilage, tendons, synovium, or soft tissue. These deposits build up slowly over a period of years. There should rarely be any confusion regarding the diagnosis. Needle aspiration will produce urate crystals. Allopurinol and uricosuric agents will mobilize urate deposits. Occasionally, surgical removal of large tophi may be indicated.[48]

Weber-Christian Disease. Weber-Christian panniculitis forms inflammatory subcutaneous nodules, which become attached to the skin by inflammatory reactions.

Erythema Nodosum. Lesions of erythema nodosum are characterized as acute, tender, erythematous nodules commonly appearing on the legs. Erythema nodosum is associated with various primary diseases, including tuberculosis, fungal infections, sarcoidosis, inflammatory bowel disorders, and drug reactions.

Arteritis. The necrotizing inflammation of arteries may result in the formation of small aneurysms. This results in nodularity along the course of the artery.

Rheumatoid Nodules. Rheumatoid nodules appear in the subcutaneous tissue overlying pressure points. Vasculitis involving small vessels is probably the initiating phenomenon.

Traumatic Fat Necrosis. The combination of hemorrhage, fat necrosis, and calcification resulting from trauma may be indistinguishable from cancer by physical examination. A biopsy is indicated to establish the diagnosis.

Vascular Tumors. Aneurysms of small, superficial arteries, such as the radial artery, are uncommon but can be recognized by expansile pulsations. Prominent vessels often result from kinking of the vessel by atherosclerotic lengthening. A kinked subclavian artery projecting into the supraclavicular space may be confused with the rounded surface of a deep lymph node.

Arteriovenous fistulas usually result from trauma. They can be identified by a palpable thrill and audible murmur. Proximal and distal compression of the artery should diminish the size of the mass.

Thrombosis of superficial veins can produce small, subcutaneous nodules that may or may not be tender. The vein is often visible but not distended because collaterals relieve any pressure that results from the block. Venous thrombosis causes subcutaneous nodules that have lateral mobility but cannot be moved easily in the long access of the vessel.

REFERENCES

1. Kline TA, Neal HS, and Holroyde CP: Needle aspiration biopsy. Diagnosis of subcutaneous nodules and lymph nodes. JAMA 235:2848, 1976.
2. Shaha A, Webber C, and Marti J: Fine-needle aspiration in the diagnosis of cervical lymphadenopathy. Am J Surg 152:420, 1986.
3. Kardos TF, Maygarden SJ, Blumberg AK, et al: Fine-needle aspiration biopsy in the management of children and young adults with peripheral lymphadenopathy. Cancer 63:703, 1989.
4. Engzell U, Jakobsson PA, Sigurdson A, et al: Aspiration biopsy of metastatic carcinoma in lymph nodes of the neck. Arch Otolaryngol 72:138, 1971.
5. Ackerman LV and Wheat MW: The implantation of cancer—An avoidable surgical risk? Surgery 37:341, 1955.
6. Osteen RT, Kopf G, and Wilson RE: In pursuit of the unknown primary. Am J Surg 135:494, 1978.
7. Hamburger JI: Consistency of sequential needle biopsy findings for thyroid nodules: Management implications. Arch Intern Med 147:97, 1987.
8. Whiteside T and Rowlands DT: T-cell and B-cell identification in the diagnosis of lymphoproliferative disease. Am J Pathol 88:754, 1977.
9. Ghadially SN: Ultrastructural pathology of the cell. London, Butterworth, 1975.
10. Golomb HM and Thomsen S: Estrogen receptor. Therapeutic guide in undifferentiated metastatic carcinoma in women. Arch Intern Med 135:942, 1975.
11. Millis RR: The relationship between the pathology of breast cancer and hormone sensitivity. Rev Endocrinol Rel Cancer 20(Suppl):13, 1987.
12. National Institutes of Health Consensus Development Panel on Adjuvant Chemotherapy and Endocrine Therapy for Breast Cancer: Introductions and conclusions. NCI Monogr 1:1, 1986.
13. Gown AM, Vogel AM, Hoak D, et al: Monoclonal antibodies specific for melanotic tumors distinguish subpopulations of melanocytes. Am J Path 123:195, 1986.
14. Gentile PS, Carloss HW, Huang TY, et al: Disseminated prostatic carcinoma simulating primary lung cancer. Cancer 62:711, 1988.
15. Wick MR, Lillemoe TJ, Copland GT, et al: Gross cystic disease fluid protein-15 as a marker for breast cancer. Hum Pathol 20:281, 1989.
16. Kriecbergs A, Tribukait B, Willems J, and Bauer HCF: DNA flow analysis of soft tissue tumors. Cancer 59:128, 1987.
17. Robbins SL, Cotran RS, and Kumar V: Pathologic Basis of Disease, 4th ed. Philadelphia, WB Saunders, 1989.
18. Berquist TH: Magnetic resonance imaging of musculoskeletal neoplasms. Clin Orthop 244:101, 1989.
19. Brennan MF: Management of extremity soft-tissue sarcoma. Am J Surg 158:71, 1989.
20. Russell WO, Cohen J, Enzinger F, et al: Clinical and pathological staging system for soft tissue sarcomas. Cancer 49:1562, 1977.
21. Hales M, Bottles K, Miller T, et al: Diagnosis of Kaposi's sarcoma by fine-needle aspiration biopsy. Am J Clin Pathol 88:20, 1987.
22. Hommel DJ, Brown ML, and Kinzie JJ: Response to radiotherapy of head and neck tumors in AIDS patients. Am J Surg 154:443, 1987.
23. Spira TJ, Kaplan JE, Holman RC, et al: Deterioration in immunologic status of human immunodeficiency virus (HIV)-infected homosexual men with lymphadenopathy: Prognostic implications. J Clin Immunol 9:132, 1989.
24. Davis JM, Mouradian J, Fernandez RD, et al: Acquired immune deficiency syndrome: A surgical perspective. Arch Surg 119:90, 1984.
25. Byrnes RK, Chan WC, Spira TJ, et al: Value of lymph node biopsy in unexplained lymphadenopathy in homosexual men. JAMA 250:1313, 1983.
26. Gerstoft J, Pallesen G, Mathiesen LR, et al: The value of lymph node histology in human immunodeficiency virus related persistent generalized lymphadenopathy. APMIS Suppl 8:24, 1989.
27. Kaplan MH, Susin M, Pahwa SG, et al: Neoplastic complications of HTLV-III infection. Am J Med 82:389, 1987.
28. Greenfield S and Jordan MC: The clinical investigation of lymphadenopathy in primary care practice. JAMA 240:1388, 1978.
29. Slap JB, Brooks JSJ, and Schwartz JS: When to perform biopsies of enlarged peripheral lymph nodes in young patients. JAMA 252:1321, 1984.
30. Libman H: Generalized lymphadenopathy. J Gen Intern Med 2:48, 1987.
31. Sinclair S, Beckman E, and Ellman E: Biopsy of enlarged, superficial lymph nodes. JAMA 228:602, 1974.
32. Saltzstein SL: The fate of patients with nondiagnostic lymph node biopsies. Surgery 58:659, 1965.
33. Kaplan H: Hodgkin's Disease. Cambridge, Harvard University Press, 1972.
34. Fuchs WA: Neoplasms of epithelial origin. *In* Abrams HL (ed): Angiography, Vol 2. Boston, Little, Brown, 1977.
35. Zaren HA and Copeland EM: Inguinal node metastases. Cancer 41:919, 1978.

36. Feuerman L, Attie JN, and Rosenberg B: Carcinoma in axillary lymph nodes. Surg Gynecol Obstet 114:5, 1962.
37. Copeland EM and McBride CM: Axillary metastases from unknown primary sites. Ann Surg 177:25, 1973.
38. Campana F, Fourquet A, Ashby MA, et al: Presentation of axillary lymphadenopathy without detectable breast primary (T_oN_{Ib} breast cancer): Experience at Institut Curie. Radiother Oncol 15:321, 1989.
39. Martin H and Morfit HM: Cervical lymph node metastases as the first symptom of cancer. Surg Gynecol Obstet 78:133, 1944.
40. Duckwiler G, Lufkin RB, Teresi L, et al: Head and neck lesions: MR-guided aspiration biopsy. Radiology 170:519, 1989.
41. Winegar LK and Griffen W: The occult primary tumor. Arch Otolaryngol 98:159, 1973.
42. Coker DD, Casterline PF, Chambers RG, et al: Metastases to lymph nodes of the head and neck from an unknown primary site. Am J Surg 134:517, 1977.
43. Bardwill JM: Tumors of the parotid gland. Am J Surg 114: 498, 1967.
44. Rafla S: Submaxillary gland tumors. Cancer 26:821, 1970.
45. Conley JJ: The carotid body tumors. Arch Otolaryngol 81:187, 1965.
46. Westbrook KC, Guillamondegui OM, Medellin H, et al: Chemodectomas of the neck. Selective management. Am J Surg 124:760, 1972.
47. Chen LT and Hwang WS: Fine needle aspiration of carotid body paraganglioma. Acta Cytol 33:681, 1989.
48. Rothschild BM and Round MJ: Subcutaneous crystal deposition in pseudogout. JAMA 244:2079, 1980.

68

Ophthalmologic Problems

DON C. BIENFANG, MD

EYE EXAMINATION

Some general comments about eye disease are useful before one deals with the anatomic subdivisions of the eye (Fig. 68–1). First, serious eye *disease usually decreases vision.* Second, significant eye *pain is almost always generated in the cornea or iris,* unless the pain is referred from the central nervous system. The final point worth remembering is that the eyes retain a remarkable *luster* and *clarity* throughout life. One of the rules of examining eyes is to expect the best of them and to question it when this clarity is disturbed.

Measurement of Visual Acuity

The importance of *measuring central vision in all cases of eye disease* cannot be overemphasized. Doing this has important medical, legal, and diagnostic implications. The standard method of measuring a patient's visual acuity is the use of a Snellen chart. One is easily obtainable through medical retailing houses. They need not be used in a 20-ft room, but if they are not, the fractions that are given with each line of type must be adjusted so that the numerator reflects the true distance from the patient to the chart. If a Snellen chart if not available, a record of the patient's visual acuity can be obtained by the use of newspaper print. One must measure the size of the print and then record what size print the patient can see and at what distance.

Of somewhat less importance is the *recording of peripheral vision.* The central few degrees of field can be tested by asking the patient to stare with one eye at the examiner's face and remark on the ability to see all details well as he or she stares at the nose. The physician may test peripheral fields by confronting the patient, staring in the patient's eyes, and having the patient stare in his or her eye with one eye as small test objects are brought in from the periphery; thus, the physician simultaneously compares his or her visual field with the patient's.

External Examination

The lids should be carefully inspected for evidence of localized swelling and for exudates along the lash margins. It is of particular value in cases of conjunctivitis to evert

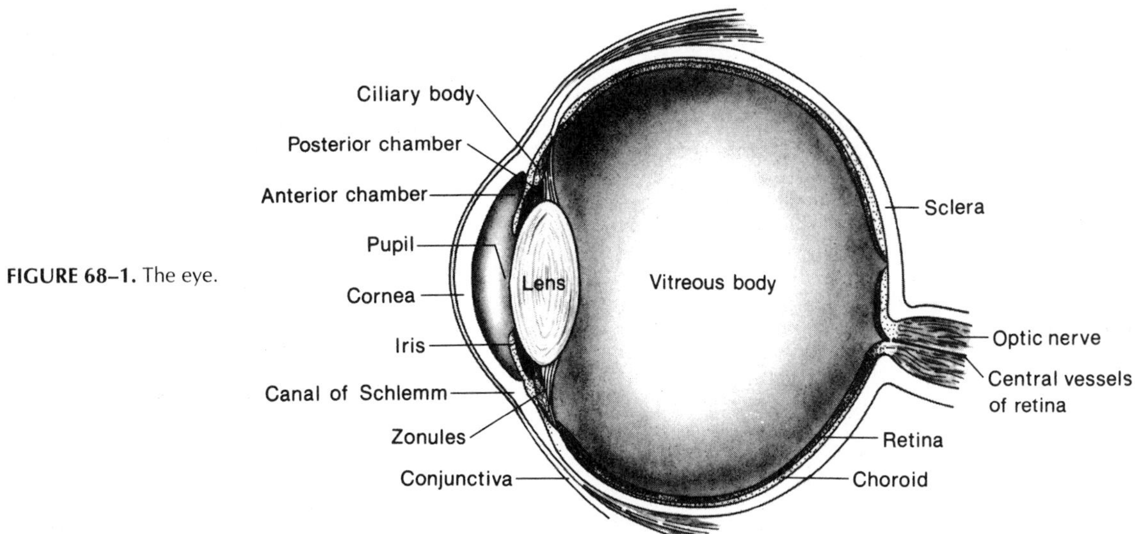

FIGURE 68–1. The eye.

the lower lid and examine the lid for the presence of follicles, which are a clue to the presence of a viral or allergic conjunctivitis. One should palpate the area in front of the ear to determine the presence of a preauricular node, which is another clue to viral disease. The presence of purulence in the tear film should be noted.

The conjunctiva of the globe should be inspected for the presence of foreign bodies, accumulation of edematous fluid in the conjunctiva (known as chemosis), and the pattern of injection of the conjunctiva. Infections of the surface of the eye result in a broad, superficial tangle of blood vessels. With deep inflammatory conditions of the eye, such as iridocyclitis, one sees rather a dusky pattern of blood vessels that are radial and not random. The blood in these vessels has a purplish hue rather than bright red.

Cornea

The cornea should be inspected with a flashlight, but one can also make use of a pair of special tests that are most useful. If the patient is complaining of significant ocular pain, and if this pain is largely relieved by a drop of topical anesthetic, one can safely assume that the pain is probably generated in the cornea. The use of fluorescein-impregnated strips to stain areas of epithelial loss of the cornea is likewise useful.

Anterior Segment

One should use the flashlight to try to gain information about the depth of the anterior chamber and the clarity of the aqueous humor. These are difficult assessments to make with a flashlight alone but suffice to detect abnormalities when these two parameters are profoundly disturbed.

It is very useful to examine the front of the eye with a direct ophthalmoscope. One uses the high magnification afforded by putting in the plus or black No. 15 diopter lens.

Pupil

The pupil should be examined for size and symmetry. It is important to write down the *size of each pupil and the lighting conditions* under which that measurement has been made. One should determine the pupillary response to light, both direct and consensual. An afferent pupillary defect is a useful clue to the presence of optic nerve disease. This is elicited by swinging a flashlight from one pupil to the other and noting whether both pupils constrict when the light is shined upon the pupil. If both pupils dilate when the light shines into one eye, this is a sign that the optic nerve on the side that is being illuminated is somehow deficient in its transmission compared with the optic nerve on the opposite side. In other words, the consensual response was greater than the direct response.

Fundus

Two maneuvers make the direct ophthalmoscope easier to use. The first is the physician's closeness to the patient. If one thinks of the pupil as a window, one can see that a larger view of the fundus is obtained as the examiner moves closer and closer to the patient. It is difficult to obtain a good view of the fundus without actually making physical contact with the patient's face. Second, the patient's body position is important. It is most useful to have the patient sitting on the edge of the bed or in an examining chair. In this manner, the examiner can merely bend over and examine the patient's eye without obstructing the patient's line of sight and without having great difficulty in maintaining balance. If it is important to examine the fundus, and if the fundus cannot be viewed through the undilated pupil, pupillary dilatation should be carried out. The best eyedrop to use for this is 2.5% phenylephrine, which affords excellent pupillary dilatation, has a rapid onset, and wears off rapidly. The fact that the effect wears off rapidly is a distinct advantage in cases of potential angle-closure glaucoma.

Extraocular Muscles

Extraocular muscle testing should be carried out in all cases. However, in most cases a deficiency in individual extraocular muscle function will be obvious merely by asking whether the patient has double vision. Much can be gained from extraocular muscle testing if one remembers the prime movers of the eye in each field of gaze. The muscle that moves the eye outward is the lateral rectus (cranial nerve VI); the muscle that moves the eye inward is the medical rectus (cranial nerve III). The prime mover of the eye upward is the superior rectus (cranial nerve III); the prime mover of the eye downward is the inferior rectus (cranial nerve III). The superior oblique muscle (cranial nerve IV) has some effect in moving the eye downward when the eye is turned in toward the nose. Likewise, the inferior oblique muscle (cranial nerve III) moves the eye somewhat upward when the eye is turned in toward the nose.

Intraocular Pressure

The physician will find it useful to become acquainted with the Schiotz tonometer, most comfortably used with the patient lying down. A local anesthetic is placed in each eye, and without much fuss the pressure is measured with the examiner spreading the lids. It is useful to have the patient fixate on some object on the ceiling or on his or her own thumb to keep the eye steady. I have found that prolonged descriptions of what one is going to do actually make the patient more tense and the testing more difficult.

Conditions that result in abnormally high intraocular pressure are synonymous with acute attacks of glaucoma. It is worth pointing out, however, that it takes a considerable amount of pressure to cause pain in glaucoma. In most patients a pressure of 50 mm Hg or more must be obtained before the eye hurts.

Conditions that result in low intraocular pressure are iritis, retinal detachment, and a perforated eye.

INFLAMED EYE—A LOGICAL APPROACH TO THE DIAGNOSIS

Collection of Data. When the physician is faced with a patient with an inflamed eye, six special areas of information will greatly help in making the correct diagnosis (Table 68–1). Two are historical and relate to the presence or absence of *pain* and the *tempo* of the illness. Is the patient consulting the physician at the onset of the illness or several days after it has started? Two questions relate to the physical examination and concern the presence of a *preauricular node* and the *pupillary size.* Finally, two special tests are useful: the response of the patient's pain to use of a *topical anesthetic* and the presence or absence of *fluorescein staining.*

Inflamed, Painful Eye

Short Interval Between Onset and Office Visit. An inflamed painful eye for which the patient seeks immediate medical attention almost always means a mechanical or toxic insult to the corneal epithelium. The most common problems are foreign bodies of the cornea or upper lid and corneal abrasions. In the same category, however, are radiant energy burns, typified by sunlamp injuries, ultraviolet light and welder's flash injuries, and accidental chemical injuries. The patient seeks medical attention so promptly because the pain comes on immediately and is particularly intense. If the patient cannot seek attention immediately, the pain will gradually diminish with time in most cases, and as time passes the patient is less likely to come into the office. If no foreign body is present, corneal abrasions and ultraviolet energy burns—including those from sunlamps, welder's flashes, and known ultraviolet exposures—can be treated with the expectation of prompt recovery. The physician's task is to make the patient as comfortable as possible during the recovery period and to instruct the patient to return if there is not a steady improvement in his or her symptoms. Missed diagnoses and infection are common reasons for lack of improvement. Depending on the severity of the injury, the physician may wish merely to patch the eye and give a mild pain medication, which the patient will probably need for only approximately 24 hours. If the epithelial loss is large, the addition of cycloplegia to reduce the ciliary body spasm will help as well. For this purpose, a short-acting cycloplegic agent should be used. Cyclopentolate and homatropine are both good choices. Eye patching is indicated mainly because it keeps light and air from reaching the sensitive abrasion. The patient in most cases may remove the patch in 24 hours and at that point should experience a sandy or scratchy sensation, which should disappear in the following 24 hours. A single application of a topical antibiotic is probably more reassuring to the physician than beneficial to the patient.

The treatment for *retained foreign bodies* under the upper lid or on the cornea is their removal. Some of these can be easily wiped away with a cotton-tipped applicator. Those that are more firmly embedded will undoubtedly require the attention of an ophthalmologist, who has available higher magnification and more experience.

The first line of defense against *chemical injuries* is copious irrigation, which should be instituted at the time of injury without delay, because it is the most effective ther-

TABLE 68–1. RED EYE—DIFFERENTIAL DIAGNOSIS

	Discharge	Vision	Pupil	Pain	Lymph Node	Duration of Symptoms Prior to Visit	Response to Topical Anesthetic
Bacterial conjunctivitis	Purulent	Mildly reduced	Normal	Little	None	2–3 days	Little
Viral conjunctivitis	Less purulent, watery	Slight reduction unless cornea is also infected	Normal	Little	Preauricular or submental	Variable, usually patient comes late in course of disease	Little, unless cornea involved, then gets relief
Corneal abrasion or foreign body	Tears only	Reduced if lesion is central	Bilaterally small	Severe, acute, superficial	None	Hours	Marked relief
Acute iridocyclitis	Tears only	Moderate reduction	Bilaterally small	Deep ache	None	Several days	No change
Acute angle-closure glaucoma	Tears only	Severe reduction	Dilated and fixed on side affected	Deep ache	None	Hours to days	No change

apy available. The irrigating fluid need be nothing more than plain water; most emergency wards have normal saline or dextrose in water, both of which are excellent choices. Irrigation should be carried out for at least half an hour. The instillation of a topical anesthetic allows the patient to tolerate the procedure more easily, and a thorough irrigation can be carried out. Depending on the nature of the chemical, an ophthalmologist may need to see the patient. Severe chemical injuries are largely restricted to the stronger acids and stronger alkalis. The other most commonly encountered chemicals, though irritating, are not in general particularly toxic.

Interval of Several Days Between Onset and Office Visit. ***Cornea Stains with Fluorescein and Significant Relief from Topical Anesthetic.*** Occasionally one will encounter a patient with a *corneal abrasion* or retained corneal foreign body who has waited several days before seeking attention. For the reasons indicated previously, this is unusual and should always raise the possibility of an infected ulcer of the cornea. The most common corneal ulcer occurring this way will be the *viral ulcer of herpes simplex keratitis.* The patient with an herpetic ulcer may delay seeking treatment for two reasons. Often a relative anesthesia of the cornea is associated with the herpetic infection, and the onset of the illness is insidious in contrast to the acute abrasion. Herpes simplex infections of the cornea stain vividly with fluorescein and usually have a branched, arborized distribution.

Because repeated episodes of herpetic keratitis may cause corneal scarring, treatment with topical antiviral agents, such as 5-iodo-2-deoxyuridine, trifluorothymidine, or adenine arabinoside, ointment or drops, given fives times daily, should be started as soon as possible. Acyclovir should not be used. Bacterial ulcers of the cornea—characterized by a relatively large ulcer with a white center and frequently by a collection of white blood cells in the anterior chamber—are so dramatic that their very appearance alerts the physician to the seriousness of this disease. Patients with bacterial corneal ulcers or herpetic corneal ulcers should be referred to an ophthalmologist.

No Staining of the Cornea with Fluorescein and No Significant Relief from a Topical Anesthetic. Ocular pain that is not significantly relieved by application of a topical anesthetic is probably generated in most cases in the ciliary body. Two main entities can cause this: the pain of the increased pressure of *acute glaucoma* and the pain of *acute iridocyclitis.* Patients with these disorders will have reduced vision. In angle-closure glaucoma, the pupil will be semidilated, and in iridocyclitis the pupil will be small. A clue to the internal origin of the ocular pain is the radiating pattern of darkly colored blood vessels coming from the limbus, the "ciliary flush."

Inflamed, Nonpainful Eye

Subconjunctival Hemorrhage. One should remember that hemorrhage under the conjunctiva of the eye has a dramatic appearance to the patient. The clue to the existence of this problem is the sharp demarcation between the edge of the blood and the white sclera. It looks like red paint. The so-called inflammation extends up to the limbus as well and stops abruptly. No therapy is necessary for this condition. Although it is occasionally associated with hypertension and bleeding dyscrasias, more frequently it is not and one need only reassure the patient.

Itchy, Inflamed Eye. If the eye is red and itchiness is the most prominent symptom, it may be assumed that one is dealing with an allergic reaction. Many of these patients have experienced this before at the same time of the year or know what contact they have made to precipitate it, thus it is not common for them to seek medical attention. When they do, however, use of an ocular decongestant (e.g., Naphazoline) without steroids is indicated. It is probably best to reserve topical steroid therapy for the ophthalmologist to consider, because the ocular side effects of the use of topical steroids will require his or her management.

Inflamed Eye with a Purulent Discharge and No Preauricular Nodes. It can be safely assumed, given this set of conditions, that one is dealing with a bacterial infection of the conjunctiva. Such infections are uncomfortable, but pain is not a leading symptom. These infections frequently start out unilaterally, but they go on to become bilateral in most cases and are usually unassociated with any other systemic illness. The copiousness of the discharge is manifested by the patient's inability to open the eyes in the morning without the use of warm compresses. The therapy for acute bacterial conjunctivitis is hot compresses.

Following use of hot, moist compresses, the patient should instill a topical antibiotic in the inflamed eye, and the whole process can be repeated three or more times a day. A good choice for a topical antibiotic in this situation is erythromycin ointment, because most bacteria *(Pneumococcus, Haemophilus, Staphylococcus)* encountered is this type of ocular infection are sensitive to the drug in the high concentrations used. The drug is not sensitizing to the patient and not irritating to the eye. The physician should avoid combinations of antibiotics and steroids and should also avoid all ophthalmic preparations containing neomycin, because neomycin is routinely irritating to the corneal epithelium.

Gonococcal conjunctivitis should be suspected in a sexually active person with conjunctivitis that is accompanied by copious amounts of a purulent discharge. A Gram stain and culture are necessary to confirm the diagnosis. Then, because corneal perforation may result from inadequately treated gonococcal conjunctivitis, the patient should be hospitalized and treated with systemic as well as topical antibiotics.

Inflamed Eye with a Watery Discharge and a Preauricular Node. This symptom complex is characteristic of viral infections of the eye. One sees relatively fewer of these than bacterial infections, mainly because the patient correctly recognizes that the ocular symptoms are part of a generalized virus infection. Thus, the lay interpretation that the eye has a "cold" in it is in many ways correct. One can do little for this condition, and fortunately in most cases the symptoms are relatively mild. Occasionally the cornea is afflicted by the virus, and in this case the symptoms are quite prominent and similar to those of corneal abrasion. This patient will require ophthalmic care.

Swollen Lids

Diffusely Swollen Lids. This is the appearance of an acute blepharitis, although in certain hemodynamic states that increase the venous pressure or cause facial edema one may see a similar picture. It is often more prominent in the eye under these circumstances because of the relative softness of the tissues of the lid. When one is dealing with an acute infectious process of the lid (being careful to distinguish it from acute infection of the lacrimal sacs located on the side of the nose), topical application of a moist, hot washcloth is indicated. If the infection appears to be spreading to the face or is present in a patient who is at risk because of a generalized depressed physical state, the use of systemic antibiotics may be considered. In these cases, topical antibiotics have little value. It is not uncommon, however, for this diffuse process to progress to the next stage, which is covered in the following paragraph.

Limited Swelling with Pain. This situation may be the sequela of a diffuse swelling of the lid and is the result of a localization of the infectious process to an abscess formation (hordeolum). Occasionally, the acute processes may appear spontaneously, but in most cases, if there is noticeable inflammation and pain, one may expect that the lesion will resolve spontaneously and disappear or will drain with resolution. Once again, topical application of moist heat is beneficial.

Limited Swelling Without Pain. If a patient spontaneously develops a nonpainful lump in the lid, the prognosis for rapid recovery is less favorable. Most of these lumps will turn out to be chalazia, which are lipogranulomata of unknown etiology, and although there is a general tendency for them to resolve spontaneously, the process usually takes several months or a year. Some of these lumps are large enough to present a cosmetic problem or even a visual problem, because they may induce astigmatism. In such cases an ophthalmologist will be able to drain and curette the walls of the cyst cavity and hasten its resolution. A small number of these lumps, of course, will turn out to be localized tumors of the lid, thus it may be wise to refer patients who have painless lid swellings to an ophthalmologist.

SUDDEN, PAINLESS, PERSISTENT LOSS OF VISION

The diagnostic features of painless and sudden loss of vision are outlined in Figure 68–2.

Assessment of Vision

Since loss of vision can mean many things to different people, one must first determine what part of the vision has been lost. For some, loss of vision will mean a *refractive error,* and the existence of this refractive error can be suggested by a marked improvement in visual acuity when the test letters are viewed through a small hole, the so-called "pinhole test." A pinhole used in this manner acts as a universal lens, and although it sacrifices brightness, it puts all objects in relative focus. It is also useful to determine the visual field in such a patient, because a few patients will say they have loss of vision when in reality they have a *loss of visual field.* In any case, careful visual field testing can aid greatly in the anatomic localization of visual loss, since certain types of disease cause characteristic types of field loss. For example, compressive lesions or inflammatory lesions of the optic nerve typically cause loss of macular vision, with a resultant central scotoma, which may or may not break out into the periphery. Disorders that cause an opacity within the media of the eye—in particular, the cornea, lens, and vitreous—tend to cause a generalized constriction of the visual field, with no localized scotoma. Although retinal diseases can give cleanly defined scotomas, they frequently result in unusually shaped visual fields that seem to bear no relationship to any anatomic organization. Compressive lesions in the region of the chiasm result in temporal hemianopic field defects. Lesions from the lateral geniculate body to the occipital lobes cause more or less congruous loss of visual field on the same side in both eyes.

Ophthalmoscopic Examination

Once the vision has been assessed, the ophthalmoscope may be used to assess the clarity of the media and the appearance of the fundus. If the fundus cannot be seen and the pupil does not seem to be abnormally small, one can assume that there is an opacity in the media, probably a cataract or an opacification of the vitreous, most commonly blood.

If the fundus can be seen, attention should be directed to the macula and to the optic nerve head. These are the two areas that cause loss of central vision. One should look in the macula for the presence of swelling, inflammation, and hemorrhage and in the optic nerve for the presence of atrophy or swelling.

Some Major Causes of Persistent Loss of Vision

Central Retinal Artery Occlusion. Acute occlusion of the central retinal artery has a characteristic appearance. The arteries are thin and almost devoid of blood. The veins are slightly larger, but though a blood column can be detected, frequently there is segmentation of the blood within the vein, giving evidence for the stagnant flow. Within a few hours after the occlusion, if it is complete, the entire retina will become edematous and translucent. The only area where the normal red retinal pigment epithelium can be seen is at the fovea, which is devoid of the ganglion cells that are swelling to cause the retinal opacity in the rest of the retina. This gives rise to the so-called *cherry-red spot.* Within a few days after the occlusion, the previously described appearance is replaced by atrophy of the retinal nerve fiber layer, which is difficult to detect, and optic atrophy, which will give the optic nerve head a dead, white appearance. In most cases, after several days some retinal circulation will return, although function probably will not. In exceptional cases, usually in younger persons, vision may be restored if flow can be returned even several hours or days after the occlusion has occurred. However, these cases are unusual, and most patients do not respond as well.

Occlusions of the central retinal artery are usually due to either embolic disease or local atherosclerosis of the vessel immediately behind the lamina cribrosa of the optic nerve. Therapy is directed toward dislodging a possible embolus. The maneuvers are aimed at rapid lowering of the intraocular pressure to increase the pressure head behind the embolus. Also an attempt may be made to dilate the retinal arteries by increasing the percentage of carbon dioxide in the inspired air. Rapid lowering of the intraocular pressure and manipulation of the embolus within the blood vessel are accomplished by ocular massage, which is best carried out by the patient. The patient should press firmly upon the eye for a count of five and then release for a count of three. While the patient is doing this, intravenous acetazolamide (Diamox), 500 mg, should be given, and the patient may be instructed to rebreathe the expired air through a rebreathing bag, or he or she may breathe a mixture of 90% oxygen with 10% carbon dioxide, if available, given by face mask. An ophthalmologist should be called, and he or she may wish to lower the intraocular pressure rapidly by removing some of the aqueous humor

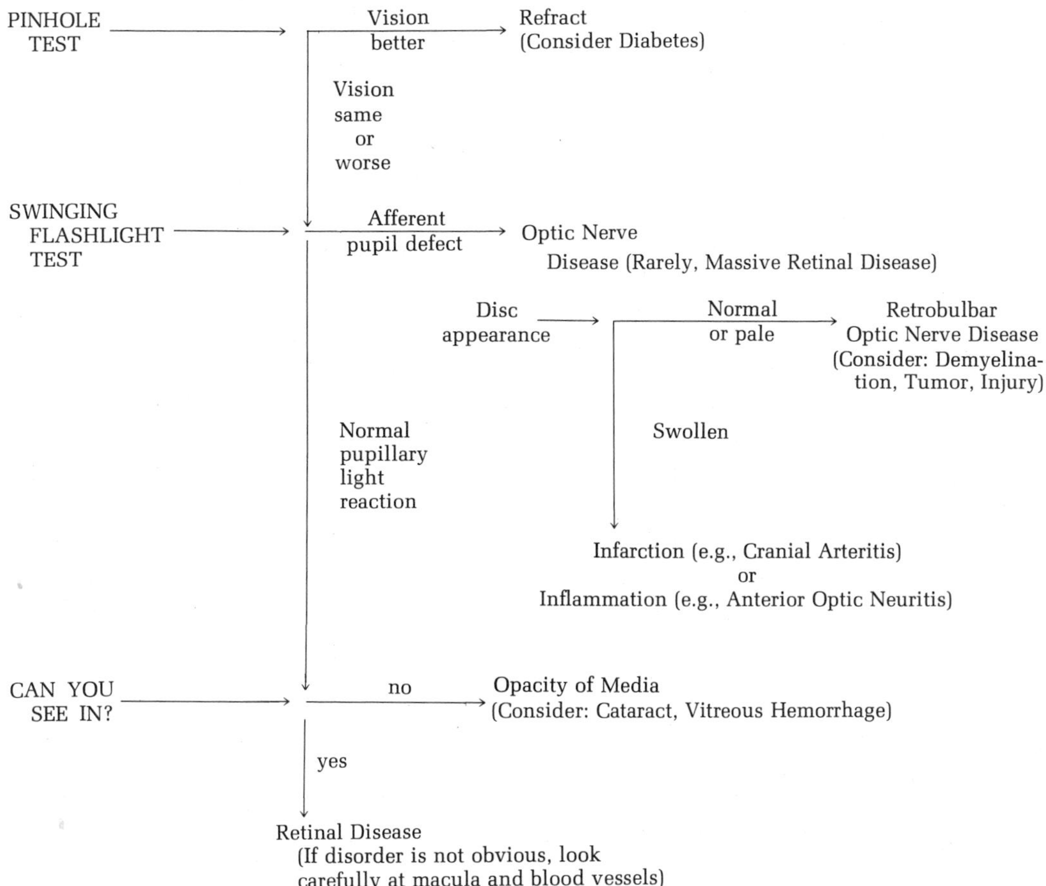

FIGURE 68–2. A diagnostic flow sheet for painless loss of sight in one eye.

from the anterior chamber. The aforementioned maneuvers are more successful in cases of embolus than in cases of local atherosclerotic disease of the artery. In all cases the sedimentation rate should be measured, because a small percentage of these cases of local narrowing of the central retinal artery are caused by cranial arteritis.

Retinal Detachment. Retinal detachment is characterized by a slowly moving shade passing across the vision, usually coming upward from below as the retina detaches from above. The etiology is almost always due to a retinal hole, which may appear spontaneously or may follow trauma or ocular surgery. The treatment of retinal detachments has improved, so that a high success rate can be expected. However, *an emergency situation exists when central vision is still retained,* since the prognosis for good vision in the affected eye is improved if the surgery is done before the macula has detached. Certain warning symptoms that occur when the retinal hole appears should be promptly attended to, because the prognosis is best of all when the holes are sealed before detachment. Such warning signals are the sudden appearance of a flashing spot of light or a prominent floater in the vision.

Nontraumatic (Spontaneous) Intraocular Hemorrhages. The appearance of the eye in these cases is relatively normal to inspection. The patient will have decreased vision and will frequently describe a red cloud before his or her sight. On attempting to examine the fundus, the physician will note that the fundus view is obscured by something in the media. Most of these patients have diabetes and are bleeding from abnormal blood vessels as part of proliferative diabetic retinopathy. However, a few patients with sickle cell retinopathy will be encountered, as well as patients with leukemia. Patients with persistent intraocular hemorrhage may benefit from vitrectomy, although many hemorrhages clear spontaneously as well. Once a clear view of the fundus can be obtained, the ophthalmologist may wish to treat the offending vessels with laser photocoagulation.

It is important that all diabetic patients be referred for regular ophthalmologic examination, because evidence has shown that diabetic retinopathy can be treated successfully by local or panretinal photocoagulation.

Central Retinal Vein Occlusion. The appearance of a central retinal vein occlusion is that of profound dilatation of the veins, with extensive hemorrhages on the surface of the retina extending far out into the periphery. It bears a certain coarse similarity to papilledema, except that the hemorrhages extend much farther out and the vision is more commonly reduced. In addition, there tends to be much more hemorrhage in central retinal vein occlusion. Although the name implies an occlusion limited to the central retinal vein, in the more severe cases there is usually an element of arterial occlusion as well. Most of the severe cases are due to an atherosclerotic plaque that has partially occluded the artery and totally occluded the vein at a point where the artery and vein lie close to one another in the optic nerve. A branch vein occlusion has a similar clinical picture, except that the hemorrhages are associated with only a portion of the venous tree. It is always distal to an arteriovenous crossing and reflects the influence of the artery on the vein. In all central retinal vein cases, however, a search should be carried out for possible causes other than atherosclerosis. Central retinal vein occlusions are strongly associated with glaucoma and are also seen in systemic conditions that cause increased sludging of the blood, such as hyperviscosity states.

Therapy is directed toward reversal of any systemic condition, such as polycythemia, that is leading to increased viscosity of the blood, toward relief of elevated intraocular pressure if present, and toward improvement of the circulatory status if localized atherosclerosis is suspected. In the last case, certain maneuvers similar to those previously described in the Central Retinal Artery Occlusion section may prove useful. The less severe forms of central retinal vein occlusion that really are in fact due to poor circulation on the venous side can be detected by the relative preservation of the visual acuity, or in those cases in which the fundal hemorrhages are profound, by preservation of the electroretinogram.

Ischemic Optic Neuropathy. Ischemic optic neuropathy is characterized by a swollen, pale yellow, or even white optic nerve head, which is anatomic evidence for *ischemia of the anterior portion of the optic nerve.* There are two main etiologies. First is cranial arteritis, which usually produces profound loss of vision occurring suddenly or over a few days. It is associated with a markedly elevated sedimentation rate and usually a prodrome of malaise, fever, headache, and anemia. There is an urgency in the detection of this disease, because although vision usually cannot be restored to the affected eye, the unaffected eye is at risk if treatment with large doses of systemic corticosteroids is not initiated. A similar picture can be generated by atherosclerotic changes in the feeder vessels to the anterior portion of the optic nerve and is usually seen in middle-aged hypertensive patients. Little can be done in the way of therapy for this latter group, but the prognosis is much better for these patients, since the visual loss tends to be less profound in the affected eye.

"Optic Neuritis." Optic neuritis is a term used by many physicians to apply to a loss of central vision associated with a relatively normal-appearing optic nerve head. It is emphasized, however, that although the term optic neuritis implies an inflammatory etiology, in many cases it may be difficult to distinguish a compressive lesion from an inflammatory one.

A typical case of true inflammatory optic nerve disease will have an abrupt onset and be associated with a modest amount of pain, especially on movement of the eye, and with recovery within several days to several weeks. In all cases, however, the possibility of compression of the optic nerve by a tumor, which may give an identical appearance in terms of visual loss and loss of central field, should be suspected. It may be necessary to have magnetic resonance imaging with contrast of the optic nerves and chiasm.

Therapy depends on the findings. Corticosteroids should in general be avoided in treating this condition. Oral prednisone has been shown to increase recurrences of this condition. If the patient has profound visual loss in the only seeing eye, recovery can be hastened by a few days of intravenous glucocorticosteroid administration followed by oral prednisone administration for a limited period of time. This therapy does not improve the amount of long-term visual recovery.

CATARACT

Diagnostic Features

Symptoms. The symptoms of cataract are almost always *loss of central acuity.* The patient may choose a descriptive phrase to characterize this loss of vision, and the one I have heard most often is that the vision is distorted as though one were looking through a screen. Frequently patients describe the blurred vision as seeming as though it could be wiped away, as if there were some mucus in the eye or their glasses were dirty. In the early stages of a special type of cataract, the nuclear cataract, the patient may experience a dramatic change in visual acuity as he or she becomes more myopic. This will blur distance vision, but the patient may experience the ability to read at close range without glasses for the first time. A common symptom with posterior subcapsular cataracts is vision that becomes especially blurred under those circumstances in which the pupil becomes constricted, such as reading and in bright illumination. These patients typically describe better vision indoors than outdoors.

Signs. One will probably be able to detect a decrease in central visual acuity that is unimproved by a change in glasses. In advanced cases of cataract, the opacity may be easily visible within the pupil or against the red reflex using the direct ophthalmoscope with a +10 lens. There may be extreme difficulty in visualizing the fundus of the eye. The ability to visualize the fundus of the eye through the undilated pupil is probably the single best test for the effect that the cataract is having upon vision, next to testing of the visual acuity itself. It should be emphasized also, however, that in all cases of cataract the pupillary response to light is preserved. One does not see an afferent pupillary defect due to a cataract alone. Cataracts may be translucent, but they are never opaque. They largely distort the light rather than preventing it from reaching the retina. The presence of an afferent pupillary defect coexistent with a cataract should suggest that there is also disease in the retina or the optic nerve.

Types. Three main types of cataract are found. The *nuclear cataract* has a hard, usually brown or even mahogany-colored center and is frequently associated with the second type of cataract, which is *cortical* in nature. At the slit lamp the cortical cataract appears to have radiating spokes. Both these types are so-called senile cataracts; they have a relatively slow progression and are commonly observed in most elderly patients. The third type of cataract, the *posterior subcapsular cataract,* is more typically seen in younger persons and in those taking corticosteroids. It has a much more rapid progression and is much more debilitating. This is because it is located on the back surface of the lens in the center and has an irregular, rough quality that diffuses and diffracts the light to a much greater extent.

Causes

Age. Almost all cataracts are associated with age. One may typically expect to see some type of cataractous changes in most patients older than 50 years of age. Of course, the presence of a cataract is not a mandate for its removal; it is only when the cataract interferes with the patient's lifestyle that surgery is warranted.

Association with Local and Systemic Diseases and Medicines. ***Local.*** Although most cataracts are associated with simple aging of the patient, a variety of local conditions of the eye may accelerate the development of a cataract or may be sufficient in themselves to cause cataract. Certainly, surgery of the interior of the eye, such as glaucoma filtering surgery, may hasten the development of a cataract. Prior inflammation of the anterior portions of the eye, such as iridocyclitis, may be a cause of cataract. Injury to the front of the eye may precipitate a cataract, and chronic use of topical steroids may cause cataractous changes.

Systemic. Systemic causes of cataract include the chronic use of systemic corticosteroids. Insulin-dependent diabetes mellitus may be associated with cataract formation, expecially during periods of hyperglycemia. This cataract may be partially reversed when the glucose level returns to normal. Hepatolenticular degeneration and myotonic dystrophy are also associated with cataracts.

Treatment

Medical Treatment. Those types of cataract that are associated with significant refractive changes, especially the nuclear cataract, may be managed temporarily by a change in the prescription of the glasses. All types of cataract, but especially posterior subcapsular cataracts, may be benefited for a short time by dilating the pupil so that some undiffracted light may pass around the opacity. When the posterior subcapsular cataract is not changing, as in patients who have been on high doses of systemic corticosteroids for only a brief time and who develop the cataract during the period of the high-dose steroids, such therapy may be enough to return useful vision. In most cases, however, these maneuvers are only temporarily effective.

Indications for Surgery. Cataract surgery used to be limited by the problem of aphakic vision—that is, vision after the natural lens has been removed. The most commonly performed operation today, extracapsular cataract surgery with posterior chamber implant, avoids this problem.

Surgery without lens implant will still produce aphakia. A particularly severe problem is that of monocular aphakia, when one eye has no cataract and the other eye has had cataract surgery. An aphakic spectacle magnifies the image observed through it by 25%. Most people cannot fuse this large image with the smaller image perceived through the normal eye. Thus, when considering cataract extraction without lens implant in one eye alone, if the other is normal the physician must also take care to ensure postoperative fusion of images. One way to get around the magnification problem is through the use of a contact lens, which may be difficult for an elderly person to manage but is a practical solution in young individuals. An intraocular lens, preferably the posterior chamber implant, is usually placed in older persons. Prior to the development of this operation, it was common for the ophthalmologist to delay surgery until there were signs of a significant cataract in the fellow eye.

The decision to perform surgery depends on an assessment of disability and should be individualized. It is generally wise to wait until the patient asks to be helped because the annoying loss of side vision, a disturbing glare from the cataract itself, or the inability to ignore the blurred, distorted image obtained from that eye has made life so difficult that he or she cannot function normally. Surgery should *only* be done when the patient feels the cataract is interfering with his or her lifestyle. Although one might expect that in cases of bilateral cataracts the restoration of good vision in one eye by successful surgery would be enough to satisfy most people, when they find out how benign the procedure is most patients wish the other cataract to be operated upon to restore binocular vision and a full, useful field.

Some mandatory reasons exist to operate upon a cataract even though the fellow eye does not have a significant cataract. It is generally agreed that a completely opaque and white mature lens is an indication for surgery. Such lenses are likely to swell and narrow the anterior chamber and may thus cause angle-closure glaucoma. They frequently leak proteins into the anterior chamber and precipitate an iritis with synechia formation. A lens need not be mature to swell and close the anterior chamber, and this by itself is an indication for surgery. Similarly, a lens that is leaking protein and causing iridocyclitis, whether it is mature or not, is an indication for cataract surgery.

Types of Surgery. ***Intracapsular Cataract Extraction.*** An older type of surgery is intracapsular cataract extraction. In this technique the entire lens is removed from the eye, including the capsule of the lens. This surgery requires a large opening into the eye but has the advantage that secondary opacification of a retained membrane does not occur.

Extracapsular Cataract Extraction. A revived operation made better by vastly improved technology is the extracapsular cataract extraction. In this technique a small incision is made into the eye, the anterior capsule of the lens is opened, and the contents of the lens are removed from the anterior chamber. The posterior capsule is left intact, or a small opening may be made in it. A high percentage of patients develop a secondary opacification of the posterior capsule, which may require a second operation to make a small opening in the posterior capsule. This type of operation can be done with a knife or with the laser. The laser, however, currently does not have a role in the initial extracapsular operation. The idea that it does has been impossible to eliminate from the public's mind.

Intraocular Lenses. If an intraocular lens is to be placed, it is usually done at the time of cataract extraction. It is an additional step at the end of surgery before the eye is closed, and the lens to be placed in the eye must be carefully measured to match the refractive needs of the aphakic eye. With the use of this technique, patients avoid many of the problems of aphakic vision and usually need to wear only a low-power final correction in their spectacle lenses. The intraocular lens may be placed in the anterior chamber, pupil, or posterior chamber, depending in part on whether an intracapsular or extracapsular extraction has been done. Because the problems of chronic iritis and glaucoma related to mechanical problems with the lens are avoided, the most common placement today is a posterior chamber implant after extracapsular extraction.

Rehabilitation. The key to successful rehabilitation of the cataract patient after surgery is the timing of the surgery. Patients who have surgery when they need it and who can recognize its benefits are usually happier with the surgery.

Contact lenses, which must be removed daily, are seldom successful in patients older than 60 years of age. Prolonged-wear aphakic contact lenses are available, but the failure rate is alarmingly high (30 to 40%). Problems with infection, dislocation and even loss, accumulation of deposits on the lens surface, and corneal decompensation make them unpredictable. With spectacle lenses as a correction for aphakia, the patient will be aware of difficulty with side vision. The patient will be aware of distortion and difficulty in walking until he or she grows accustomed to the lenses. Unfortunately, a small percentage of patients never adjust to aphakic vision and could properly be called aphakic cripples. This group has served as a stimulus for the development of aphakic contact lenses and intraocular lenses.

Unless there is an ocular condition that precludes their use (e.g., chronic iritis or corneal disease), the intraocular lens is probably the most satisfactory method of visual rehabilitation available today.

GLAUCOMA

Angle-Closure Glaucoma

Pathophysiology. Angle-closure glaucoma is usually heralded by an acute event in which there is a sudden obstruction to most or all of the aqueous outflow from the anterior chamber. In angle-closure glaucoma, this obstruction is due to the apposition of the iris to the filtering meshwork. Aqueous continues to be produced by the ciliary body, and the pressure rises to great heights in a matter of a few hours.

History. There tends to be a rather strong family history for angle-closure glaucoma. This is undoubtedly because an anatomic predisposition to angle-closure glaucoma establishes the proper conditions for the acute attack. In some cases, careful questioning reveals that more modest attacks with spontaneous resolutions were experienced previously. In addition, one may obtain from the patient a recent history of prolonged face-down position, especially in the dark, or exposure to drugs that may cause the pupil to dilate, such as systemic atropine given preoperatively. Symptoms at the time of the attack are dramatic. The patient experiences extreme *ocular pain* and *blurred vision.* There is often *nausea* and *vomiting* associated with acute attacks of angle-closure glaucoma, so much so in some cases that the patient may be directed to an immediate surgical service with the mistaken diagnosis of acute cholecystitis.

Physical Examination. The patient undergoing an attack of angle-closure glaucoma will have an extremely high intraocular pressure. This can be perceived by palpation with the fingers or with a Schiotz tonometer. It is not infrequent to measure pressures of 70 mm Hg or higher. This high pressure will cause the cornea to become edematous, and it will be difficult to observe fine details of the iris through the cloudy cornea. The eye will be injected, and there will be a radiate-type pattern of blood vessels extending out from the limbus, similar to that which is seen in acute iritis. These blood vessels will be dusky in color. The pupil will be semidilated and unreactive. The patient will almost always be middle-aged or older. Vision will always be decreased, and fundus examination may be difficult; the high pressure may cause the development of a visible pulse within the arterial system of the retina.

Management

It is emphasized that the correct management of angle-closure glaucoma is always *surgical.* The fallacy of continuing to attempt to lower the intraocular pressure by medical means has been well demonstrated. Attempted medical management frequently results in chronic angle-closure glaucoma with formation of synechiae, which prevent a successful surgical outcome at a later date. It is true that the initial approach to an attack of angle-closure glaucoma is to attempt to lower the intraocular pressure rapidly by medical means. These medical maneuvers include constriction of the pupil with pilocarpine, reduction of aqueous humor formation with the use of acetazolamide, and shrinking of the vitreous volume to allow the anterior chamber to deepen with the use of an osmotic agent such as glycerol. These maneuvers are carried out because it is much safer to operate on a noncongested eye electively than on a congested eye as an emergency.

The patient must be informed that he or she will need surgery not only on the eye that is having the acute attack, but in almost all cases also on the fellow eye, since the anatomic predisposition is present in both eyes. The surgery is remarkably simple. It involves creation of a second pupil at the periphery of the iris. This new opening in the iris can be created in the operating room through an incision in the eye, but now the laser is more frequently used. Laser iridotomy, when possible, can be done in the office with topical anesthesia. Some irides are too thick to be penetrated with a laser and require a surgical incision.

If the attack has been of brief duration and no synechiae have formed, one can expect that creation of a peripheral iridectomy will prevent further attacks of angle-closure glaucoma, and the patient will need no further therapy. With prolonged attacks of angle-closure glaucoma and scar formation, one may have to supplement the peripheral iridectomy with medical therapy for the residual glaucoma.

Open-Angle Glaucoma

Pathophysiology. In open-angle glaucoma, there is no visible obstruction to the filtering meshwork. Presumably the obstruction to aqueous outflow occurs at the microscopic level within the fine tubules of the filtering meshwork or even Schlemm's canal, which drains the aqueous back into the blood vessels. This type of glaucoma is of gradual onset. In most cases, the pressure elevation tends to be less than that associated with angle-closure glaucoma, but in certain instances it may attain remarkably high levels. The pressure, however, is attained usually at a much slower rate than with angle-closure glaucoma.

History. A family history, especially in siblings or parents, may be obtained in many cases. One should also ask about drug exposure, especially to topical or systemic corticosteroids. Ocular injuries or prior ocular surgery may contribute to chronic open-angle glaucoma. Overt symptoms of chronic open-angle glaucoma are usually found only in far-advanced cases. The modest elevation of pressure itself does not cause any perceivable problems until visual field is lost. Unfortunately, even loss of peripheral vision, which is characteristic of glaucoma, may not be perceived by the patient, and the patient unfortunately frequently presents when he or she has lost the last bit of visual field, the central vision.

Physical Examination. In open-angle glaucoma the pressure may merely be abnormal. It is difficult to establish firm standards for normal intraocular pressure. *Glaucoma is usually defined as elevated intraocular pressure combined with pathologic cupping of the optic nerve head.* This somewhat strict definition has developed because it is clear that some people have elevated intraocular pressure who never develop pathologic cupping. For these people, the term *ocular hypertension* is reserved. These patients have a pressure above the normal range, which is usually taken to be approximately 22 mm Hg, but it is also usually less than 30 mm Hg. Most physicians will want to treat any intraocular pressure greater than 30 mm Hg whether the patient has pathologic cupping or not. In any case, the elevated intraocular pressure above 30, combined with the passage of time, in most cases will lead to pathologic cupping. In pathologic cupping from glaucoma, there is true loss of substance of the optic nerve head; even with the direct ophthalmoscope one can visualize that the normal physiologic cup is extended, usually in the superior and inferior temporal quadrants, so that it may reach the rim of the optic nerve (Fig. 68–3). Associated with this displacement toward the rim of the optic nerve is a deepening of the cup, so that the lamina cribosa, the scleral fibers passing through the optic nerve, may be visible. Associated with the pathologic cupping when the rim of the optic nerve has

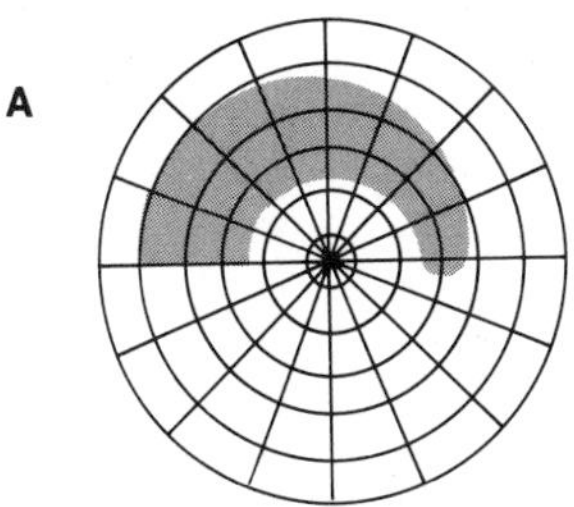

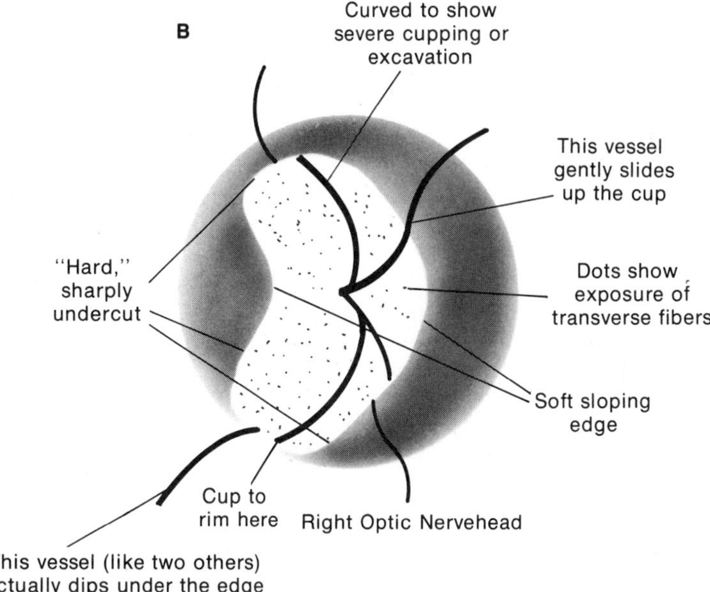

FIGURE 68–3. Optic nerve damage from glaucoma. *A,* The visual field loss that might be expected from the damage done to the disk shown in *B.* Note that the pathologic cupping extends to the rim inferotemporally and that the deep cupping causes some of the blood vessels to disappear under the edge of the cup. Superotemporally, the pathologic cup does not reach the rim of the disk, and one would expect no field loss corresponding to this part of the disk. The deep cupping has exposed the transverse scleral fibers at the depth of the cup.

been reached is the development of arcuate scotomata extending from the blind spot on the tangent screen under or over the macula to reach the median raphe on the opposite side. In more advanced cases, these arcuate scotomata completely dominate the entire upper or lower visual fields, giving rise to an altitudinal field defect. When altitudinal field defects in the upper and lower fields meet, the patient has lost central visual acuity. Prior to meeting, the patient may have only a small island of central field, with relatively good preservation of central acuity.

Management

Drugs. A drug still commonly used in older patients with open-angle glaucoma is *pilocarpine.* This drug has a long history of successful use in treatment of open-angle glaucoma, and our experience with the complications of pilocarpine use is well known. In younger patients pilocarpine has certain disadvantages: induced myopia and refractive changes are probably the most troublesome. In the elderly patient with cataracts, induced miosis of the pupil further reduces vision. The drug acts by increasing the ability of the eye to filter aqueous humor. *Phospholine iodide* acts in a manner similar to but more intense than that of pilocarpine and produces numerous complications. It is used less today than it once was. The miosis is intense, it is believed that the drug itself creates cataracts, and finally, chronic use of topical phospholine iodide results in a drop in serum pseudocholinesterase levels and may result in a dramatically prolonged effect of succinyl choline if this drug is given as a muscle blocker when anesthesia is administered.

Another popular drug is *epinephrine* or the epinephrine precursor dipivefrin hydrochloride, which when applied topically results in a decrease in aqueous humor formation and a lowering of the intraocular pressure. It does have the annoying side effect of usually being irritating and also causing chronic redness of the eyes. Because of the nature of the drug, an occasional patient will develop a hypersensitive cardiovascular response to the drug. Epinephrine is also the most likely drug of the antiglaucoma drugs to cause ocular local allergy. The *β-adrenergic blockers* are the first line of defense in the treatment of elevated intraocular pressure. There are almost no ocular side effects, and they may be used as little as once a day, thus enhancing compliance. β-Adrenergic blockers, however, should be used with caution, if at all, in patients with known asthma or borderline congestive heart failure. *Acetazolamide* is a carbonic anhydrase inhibitor that acts directly on ciliary bodies to decrease aqueous humor formation. It is given orally and is usually reserved for cases of glaucoma that are unresponsive to topical medications. Potassium loss is a major long-term problem with this drug. Most patients experience temporarily some numbness and tingling of the extremities and fatigue. The drugs just discussed can be used singly or in combination.

Laser Trabeculoplasty. A newer treatment for chronic open-angle glaucoma is the application of tiny laser burns to the trabecular meshwork of the eye. This form of therapy is usually successful for about 2 years and has provided a much-needed intermediate level of therapy before resorting to filtering surgery.

Surgery. If the patient continues to lose visual fields, despite what is considered to be maximal medical and laser therapy, glaucoma filtering surgery should be considered. The principle of surgery involves creation of a small hole between the anterior chamber and the subconjunctival space. The aqueous humor then leaves the anterior chamber via this new route and is absorbed by the blood vessels of the conjunctiva. Filtering surgery is associated with a number of perioperative complications, and for this reason it is usually reserved for patients who cannot be managed comfortably by the aforementioned methods.

OCULAR MANIFESTATIONS OF SYSTEMIC DISEASE

Iridocyclitis

Diagnostic Features

History and Symptoms. Iridocyclitis has a gradual onset over several hours or several days and is associated with a deep injection of the globe. The patient will notice, in addition to blurred vision and a deep, aching pain in the eye, the symptom of photophobia, which is prominent in this disease and characteristic of it.

Physical Examination. One will routinely be able to record a decrease in the visual acuity in the affected eye. There will be a radiate pattern of deep purple blood vessels extending from the limbus outward. The pupil will be small, and one may be able to detect precipitates of the anterior chamber reaction on the corneal endothelium. With the slit lamp, one will be able to see the presence of cells and protein, which is manifested by a flare in the anterior chamber.

Clinical Tests. Ophthalmologists frequently refer patients with iridocyclitis to an internist for evaluation, especially those with repeated attacks. There is a reluctance to refer all cases for evaluation, because with the exception of a few diseases to be discussed further on, iridocyclitis is often unrelated to other systemic disease. In addition to a careful medical history, a few tests are usually indicated: a chest radiograph, a toxoplasmosis titer, and a serologic test for syphilis.

Varieties

Nongranulomatous Iridocyclitis. As previously stated, most iridocyclitis is idiopathic, and this applies to both the monocular and the binocular varieties of the disease. Nongranulomatous iridocyclitis is characterized by small cells in the anterior chamber, which precipitate out in fine, small, white keratic precipitates. This is in contrast to granulomatous iridocyclitis, in which the keratic precipitates tend to be large and waxy yellow in appearance. In juvenile rheumatoid arthritis (JRA), the iridocyclitis is often asymptomatic, and this is a feature of this type of iridocyclitis in contrast to all others. However, just as frequently it has the typical injection, pain, and blurred vision that is characteristic of ordinary iridocyclitis. In JRA, the iridocyclitis tends to be seen more frequently in patients with monoarticular rather than polyarticular forms. The adult form of arthritis associated with iridocyclitis is ankylosing spondylitis. Behçet's syndrome is characterized by a posterior uveitis with hypopion in the anterior chamber, aphthous lesions in the mouth, and genital ulcerations. Posterior uveitis implies that the major area of attack for the uveitis is in the retina and choroid, and the basic lesion is a vasculitis that obliterates the blood vessels, resulting in infarction, hemorrhage, and retinal detachment. The hypopion is a layering of white blood cells in the anterior chamber.

Granulomatous Iritis. The two entities to consider under this heading are *sarcoidosis* and *tuberculosis.* Granulomatous iritis refers to a form of iritis in which the cells in the anterior chamber are somewhat larger, and in particular they precipitate out as large, greasy keratic precipitates, in contrast to the fine keratic precipitates seen on slit-lamp examination of patients with nongranulomatous iritis. Because of the two diagnostic entities, it is usual that a more detailed and exhaustive work-up be carried out with this form of iridocyclitis than with the nongranulomatous iritis, because in many cases when large, greasy keratic precipitates are seen, one should be able to determine that the patient has either sarcoidosis or tuberculosis.

Complications

In all cases of persistent iridocyclitis, a number of serious changes can occur in the anterior segement of the eye. The most common early changes to be observed are synechiae to the anterior capsule of the lens. These synechiae are attachments between the iris and the lens capsule, which can completely occlude the communication between the anterior and posterior chambers and result in a form of angle-closure glaucoma. It is for better management of synechiae that dilatation is a routine part of the treatment of iridocyclitis. When the iridocyclitis is active, the pressure of the eye is usually low because in most cases the ciliary body can be considered to be sick, and as a result of this, less aqueous humor is created and the pressure drops. However, the inflammation of the iridocyclitis may block the outflow channels of the eye and drive the pressure upward. Patients with iridocyclitis may thus have an intraocular pressure that reflects a balance between these two forces. With chronic low pressure, a frank papilledema may develop. In addition, chronic low pressure or some combination of chronic low pressure and chronic iridocyclitis may result in the formation of keratopathy and cataract.

Treatment

Treatment is aimed at suppressing the inflammation and preventing complications during the usually self-limited course of the iridocyclitis. If a systemically treatable diagnosis is reached, treatment should be aimed primarily at this. In most cases, however, as indicated previously, the treatment is nonspecific and largely aimed at suppression of the inflammation. Dilating the pupil with a long-acting parasympatholytic drug such as atropine is useful in putting the ciliary body musculature at rest and also in enlarging the pupil so that synechia formation will be at the periphery of the lens and out of the visual axis. If synechiae do form with a pupil widely dilated, there will be less opportunity for them to occlude the pupil completely. Topical steroids are useful in suppressing the inflammation. Occasionally, however, with more severe cases systemic corticosteroids may be necessary. Cataract surgery should be deferred until the eye is completely quiet, since surgery on an eye with active iritis is fraught with complications.

Complications. Unfortunately, the treatment of dilatation and cycloplegia may cause problems. This is a particular problem for children with JRA, since with chronic use of a cycloplegic agent the eye may become disused and amblyopic. Some of this can be avoided with the proper use of glasses; a bifocal may be necessary. Topical use of corticosteroids may induce glaucoma by itself in certain sensitive individuals and may lead to cataract formation. In addition, chronic use of topical corticosteroids is an inducement for reactivation of herpes simplex keratitis.

Systemic Vascular Disease

Diabetes Mellitus

The ocular complications and implications of diabetes mellitus are in Chapter 46 on diabetes.

Lupus Retinopathy

The characteristic finding with lupus retinovasculitis is the cotton wool patch. This is in fact an infarction of the nerve fiber layer of the retina and indicates a localized vascular insufficiency of the retina. Fortunately, this relatively mild problem is the most common manifestation of lupus retinopathy. A few patients have much more severe complications, consisting of broad areas of vascular insufficiency in the retina leading to loss of central visual acuity. Lupus vasculitis of the retina generally does not respond to steroid therapy, although other modes of suppression of the inflammatory response may be indicated in certain individuals.

Cranial Giant Cell Arteritis

Symptoms. This systemic disease of the elderly is in typical cases characterized by a prodrome of malaise, anemia, weight loss, and a number of diverse, ill-defined systemic symptoms that generally indicate that the patient is not feeling well. Some patients present manifestations of polymyalgia rheumatica. In any case, the sometimes ill-defined prodromes, which may include headache, usually precede the more acute and dramatic vascular occlusions, which form the serious aspect of this disease.

Signs. The physical signs in giant cell arteritis largely relate to the inflammatory response within the blood vessels. Fortunately, the superficial temporal artery is often involved in the disease process and provides a useful clue to the nature of the patient's problem. The palpatory changes in the superficial temporal artery consist of, at one extreme, a conversion of the artery into a hard, tender cord with no pulse and, at the other, less severe extreme, a thickening of the walls of the artery. In all suspected cases, a temporal artery biopsy should be done to confirm the diagnosis. The relatively poor circulation in the distribution of these branches of the external carotid gives rise, in more severe cases, to a headache in the temple or even a claudication of the masseter muscles, which appears when the patient talks or chews. The latter finding is quite characteristic, when present, of giant cell arteritis. Finally, the patient may suffer an occlusion of the terminal branches of the ophthalmic artery, resulting in an infarction of the optic nerve head or, less commonly, the central retinal artery, both of which give rise to the most common disastrous complication of giant cell arteritis, which is blindness in one or both eyes.

Laboratory Findings. One should expect that in almost all cases of giant cell arteritis there would be a striking elevation of the sedimentation rate, usually in excess of 70 mm/hr and frequently well above 100. Unfortunately, there are well-documented cases without an elevation of the erythrocyte sedimentation rate. Other laboratory findings in giant cell arteritis are largely a reflection of the inflammatory response that is occurring, but in addition one regularly sees a depression of the hematocrit.

Complications. The most common complication of untreated giant cell arteritis is infarction of the optic nerve head in both eyes. Usually the disaster occurs in the second eye a few days following its attack on the first eye. There may be prodromal warnings of vascular insufficiency consisting of transient obscuring of vision. Any medium-sized artery may be affected, and infarctions of the coronary artery distribution have also been recorded. Cerebral infarction, particularly in the distribution of the basilar artery, is a well-known complication as well.

Management. Once the diagnosis of giant cell arteritis is confirmed, systemic corticosteroids in high doses should be started immediately. It has been shown that systemic corticosteroids have a significant influence in preventing the ischemic complications of this disease, and, in particular, use of these drugs dramatically reduces the incidence of involvement of the second eye following ischemic optic neuropathy in the first eye. The disease, however, has a long course, and although the responsiveness of the disease to the steroids may be monitored by following the sedimentation rate, it should be expected that therapy will have to be carried out for many months, and in some cases for more than 1 year. The risk for development of ischemic optic neuropathy in the second eye probably is highest during the first 2 months after the onset of the attack in the first eye. It is important to note that alternate-day steroids are ineffective in the treatment of giant cell arteritis, and therefore they cannot be substituted for every-day therapy. Alternate-day use of steroids are, therefore, useful only in re-establishment of adrenal function as the patient is being brought off steroid therapy. In all cases an effort should be made to confirm the diagnosis through superficial temporal artery biopsy. However, since this artery is not universally involved, the diagnosis can be established without confirmatory biopsy if the clinical impression is strong enough. Usually, however, the physician will at some point in the course of the disease wish to have histologic confirmation of the clinical suspicion. The biopsy must be done within a few days of or prior to starting steroid therapy, since the corticosteroid therapy itself will cause changes in the artery that may cause it to regress to a nondiagnostic appearance.

Sarcoidosis

Sarcoidosis causes major ophthalmic complications by induction of an iridocyclitis or a retinal periphlebitis. Sarcoid nodules can occasionally be seen in the conjunctiva and thus may be useful in establishing the diagnosis, but blind biopsy of the conjunctiva has not proved to be as useful in the absence of obvious clinical changes. In suspected cases, biopsy of an enlarged lacrimal gland is more useful. The iridocyclitis of sarcoidosis, as mentioned previously, is classically a granulomatous iridocyclitis. It is treated in much the same way as idiopathic iridocyclitis. Many patients with sarcoidosis will be treated with systemic corticosteroids for the systemic aspects of the disease, which may also be adequate treatment for the iridocyclitis. Retinal periphlebitis has a characteristic appearance, consisting of waxy exudates that line the edges of the veins or arteries far out into the periphery of the eye. These exudates are interrupted along their course, giving rise to the description of their appearance as candle wax drippings. Retinal periphlebitis likewise responds to treatment with systemic corticosteroids.

Sickle Cell Retinopathy

Although *SS hemoglobinopathy* has severe systemic complications, the ocular complications of this form of sickling disease are for some reason less severe than those seen with SC disease. Sickle cell retinopathy is usually restricted to the posterior pole. There is less chance of visual loss. One sees a spotty arteriolar occlusion, venous dilatations, some arteriovenous anastomoses, and occasional choroidal infarctions.

By contrast, *SC disease* is associated with proliferative retinopathy, and the characteristic appearance is that of a peripheral "sea fan" arcade of new vessels that extends into the vitreous and may result in ultimate retinal detachment or vitreous hemorrhage. Because of this, the diagnosis of SC retinopathy requires dilatation of the pupil, and this should be done routinely in all patients with this type of hemoglobinopathy, since the new vessel proliferations are treatable with laser photocoagulation if they are observed early.

Graves' Disease

Definition. Graves' disease accompanies prior or current thyroid dysfunction. The pathophysiology is infiltration of the periocular tissues with lymphocytes, mucopolysaccharides, and edema fluid, with resultant exophthalmos, limitation of extraocular muscle function, and even compression of the optic nerve. The disease most typically is seen in patients who have had prior thyroid disease, usually hyperthyroidism, and who have undergone therapy for their hyperthyroidism, either surgery or radiation to the thyroid gland. Some patients who are hyperthyroid at the time of developing Graves' disease respond to management of the hyperthyroidism itself. However, many patients with Graves' disease are euthyroid or even hypothyroid, so that therapy for the ocular manifestations may be directed at the inflammatory response itself.

Symptoms. The most common symptom of Graves' disease is a sandy or scratchy sensation on the surface of the eye, worse on arising in the morning. If the patient is having extraocular muscle dysfunction, he or she may experience diplopia, which is typically vertical, since the inferior rectus muscle is commonly involved. The visual loss experienced in Graves' disease is largely caused by corneal changes due to exposure of the cornea or optic nerve dysfunction, presumably resulting from compression of the nerve by the inflammatory response within the orbit. In all cases, however, it is typical for the symptoms and signs of Graves' disease to wax and wane under influences that are as yet obscure.

Signs. The signs of Graves' disease may be bilateral, asymmetric, or apparently unilateral. One may see a retraction of the upper lid and a lagging of the upper lid in downward gaze. In all forms of Graves' disease, a diffuse sausage-like swelling of the upper lids is characteristic. The orbit, because of the infiltration with lymphocytes, is more tightly packed than usual, and this is manifested by a difficulty in repositioning the globe within the orbit or by frank exophthalmos. If the lids do not adequately protect the surface of the cornea, one may see exposure keratitis, which is usually manifested by ulceration of the corneal epithelium, usually inferiorly. In some cases these ulcerations may be severe enough to result in corneal perforation. The stiffness of the ocular musculature can be demonstrated by the subjective complaint of diplopia, but also by attempting to move the eye with forceps; the physician will encounter resistance when trying to stretch the stiff muscle. The tightness of the muscles may be so severe in Graves' disease that frank glaucoma can develop. Another reason why patients with Graves' disease may lose vision is the optic neuropathy of Graves' disease, presumed to result from a compressive effect from the packed orbit upon the optic nerve.

Complications. The most serious complications of Graves' disease are those that threaten sight; these are primarily corneal perforations and the optic neuropathy. The patient will be disturbed by the appearance of the eyes, by the sandy sensation, and by the double vision, but these can be managed more easily.

Management. Most patients will have a scratchy or a dry sensation on the surface of the eye. They will need ocular lubrication, usually with a viscous eyedrop. Some patients with the sight-threatening forms of Graves' disease will need orbital decompression, which can be dramatic in its effect on the exposure keratitis and the optic neuropathy. It is also true, however, that because of the nature of the pathophysiologic process in the orbit, the sight-threatening manifestations of Graves' disease are sensitive to the use of drugs that suppress the lymphocytic response. The most commonly used drugs of this type are systemic corticosteroids. In like manner, however, the ocular complications may be sensitive to orbital radiation, and in some cases steroids, radiation, and decompression may be necessary. Extraocular muscle problems can be managed expectantly, but if they establish themselves as a consistent pattern over 6 or more months, extraocular muscle surgery can be considered. It is highly successful.

Acquired Immunodeficiency Syndrome in the Eye

The effect of acquired immunodeficiency syndrome (AIDS) on the eye and on the visual and oculomotor system is mediated by so many unusual infections and tumors that the description of what can be seen in patients with this disease would cover pages. Two entities are seen commonly. About half of patients with known AIDS have small retinal infarcts (cotton wool patches) and small hemorrhages. The most devastating problem, however, is infection of the retina with cytomegalovirus. The retina has areas of necrosis with hemorrhage. Foscarnet and ganciclovir (given intravenously) can be used for treatment. Unfortunately, ganciclovir, like zidovudine, which the patient may be receiving concurrently, is toxic to the bone marrow.

References

1. Duane TD (ed): Clinical Ophthalmology. Hagerstown, MD, Harper & Row, 1978.
2. Grant WM: Toxicology of the Eye. Springfield, IL, Charles C Thomas, 1974.
3. Scheie HG and Albert DM: Textbook of Ophthalmology. Philadelphia, WB Saunders, 1977.
4. Walsh FB and Hoyt WF: Clinical Neuro-Ophthalmology. Baltimore, Williams & Wilkins, 1969.

69

Dermatology in Primary Care

HARLEY A. HAYNES, MD
WILLIAM T. BRANCH, Jr., MD

As few as nine diagnostic categories account for 85% of dermatologic problems seen by primary care physicians (Table 69–1).[1] Dermatologists encounter similar types of problems.[2] Dermatologists and primary care physicians employ chiefly the same diagnostic and treatment modalities for patients with skin problems.[1, 2] Of primary care patients with skin problems, about 80% are treated by the primary care physician and 20% are referred to dermatologists.[1]

PRINCIPLES OF DIAGNOSIS AND MANAGEMENT

Dermatologic diagnoses are made largely according to the distribution and morphologic classification of lesions.[3–7]

TABLE 69–1. DIAGNOSTIC CATEGORIES OF SKIN DISORDERS ENCOUNTERED IN PRIMARY CARE AND DERMATOLOGIC PRACTICES*

Category	Primary Care (%)	Dermatology (%)
Tumors of skin	19.1	21.8
Eczematous dermatitis	18.5	19.6
Fungal diseases of skin	17.1	3.8
Viral diseases of skin	6.8	10.2
Bacterial infections of skin	4.8	5
Acneiform lesions	5.5	9.8
Disorders of epidermal proliferation	4.8	8.8
Alopecia	4.1	3
Xerosis	5.5	2
Urticaria	†	1.4
Parasitic diseases of skin	†	1.4
Cutaneous manifestations of systemic disease	†	1.2

*From Branch WT Jr, Collins M, and Wintroub BU: Dermatologic practice: Implications for a primary care residency curriculum. J Med Educ 58:136, 1983.

†Primary care categories were obtained by a survey of 495 patients, 111 of whom (22.4%) had one or more dermatologic problems in the course of a single year. Categories in dermatology were determined by chart review of 370 patients seen in dermatology clinic. No primary care patients had urticaria, parasitic diseases, or cutaneous manifestations of systemic diseases in this survey.

A *papule* is a solid, elevated, circumscribed lesion less than 1 cm in diameter, with most of the lesion above the plane of the surrounding skin rather than deep within it. The surface of the papule may be dome-shaped, flat-topped (as in lichen planus), or umbilicated (as in molluscum contagiosum). When papules become confluent and produce an elevation that occupies a relatively large surface area, the lesion is termed a *plaque*.

A *macule* is a flat, circumscribed lesion 1 cm or less in diameter. Larger, flat discolorations or lesions are termed *patches*.

Comedomes are papules with whitish or blackish material plugging a hair follicle.

Edema is swelling resulting from abnormal amounts of tissue fluid in the dermis. Edema may or may not be associated with other discrete lesions, including erythema.

Edema with erythema is the term for edema combined with excessive redness of the skin and/or mucous membranes. Erythema is due to vasodilatation and, therefore, blanches with pressure from the examiner's finger or a transparent instrument. The presence of extravascular blood under the skin surface that does not blanch on pressure is termed *purpura*.

Wheals and *hives* are edematous, transitory papules, or plaques.

Atrophy indicates a reduction in normal tissue elements. In the skin, there may be epidermal atrophy with normal dermis, and normal skin markings are usually absent. In dermal atrophy, there is a decrease in dermal connective tissue, and the lesion is manifested as a depression in the skin. *Scarring* indicates a fibrotic reaction that may be atrophic or hypertrophic. Epidermis covering a scar is generally without normal skin markings and without appendages.

A *pigmented plaque or nodule* refers to a raised lesion with increased pigmentation from melanin. At times an old ecchymosis with dark-colored purpura may simulate melanin pigmentation.

A *nodule* is a palpable, solid lesion located deeper than a papule, either in the dermis or in the subcutaneous tissue.

Tumors are solid lesions extending into the dermis or subcutaneous tissue and are greater than 1 cm in size.

An *erosion (with or without crusts)* is a lesion in which

TABLE 69–2. TREATMENTS USED BY PRIMARY CARE PHYSICIANS AND DERMATOLOGISTS FOR SKIN DISORDERS*

	Primary Care (% of Patients)	Dermatology (% of Patients)
Topical corticosteroids	22.5	37.6
Topical absorbent and water-repellent ointments (e.g., lanolin-stearin, petrolatum)	7.2	18.9
Orally administered antihistamines	7.2	12.7
Cryotherapy with liquid nitrogen	1.8	11.4
Topical antibiotics (e.g., bacitracin, erythromycin, clindamycin)	2.7	8.4
Systemic antibiotics	4.5	9.2
Topical preparations for acne (e.g., retinoic acid, benzoyl peroxide)	4.5	8.1
Baths and soaps (e.g., Alpha-Keri, Nivea, Aveeno)	4.5	6.5
Wet dressings (e.g., Burrow's solution)	5.4	6.2
Keratolytic agents (e.g., salicylic acid, propylene glycol, lactic acid, or urea-containing lotions)	†	5.7
Shampoos (e.g., selenium sulfide, zinc pyrithione)	1.8	5.4
Topical antifungal agents (e.g., Tinactin, Halotex, Lotrimin)	14.4	2.2
Antipruritic agents (e.g., menthol, camphor- and phenol-containing lotions)	0.9	1.9

*From Branch WT Jr, Collins M, and Wintroub BU: Dermatologic practice: Implications for a primary care residency curriculum. J Med Educ 58:136, 1983.
†Survey includes 63 treatments prescribed for 111 patients with dermatologic problems encountered by primary care physicians. None employed keratolytic agents in this survey.

part of the epidermis is removed but at least one cell layer of epidermis remains at the base. Erosions allow tissue fluid to rise to the surface since the stratum corneum is absent, but bleeding does not occur because the dermis is not exposed. When the tissue fluid dries, it forms a crust. When tissue fluid is mixed with numerous white blood cells, a seropurulent crust will form.

Ulcers are lesions in which the entire epidermis is missing, exposing the dermis. Very superficial ulcerations are difficult to distinguish from erosions and often have a similar diagnostic value.

In *erythema and scaling with or without edema*, erythema of varying degrees of intensity is always seen as well as the presence on the surface of the lesion of flaking of stratum corneum, called scaling. It is necessary to differentiate scaling from crusting.

A *vesicle* is simply a blister filled with reasonably clear fluid approximating serum. In a vesicle, either (1) part of the epidermis forms the roof and part the base, termed an intraepidermal vesicle, or (2) the entire epidermis forms the roof and the dermis forms the base. In herpes simplex and zoster, impetigo, and contact dermatitis, vesicles are intraepidermal. In the case of suction, fixed drug eruption, and many of the primary dermatologic blistering diseases, blisters are subepidermal.

A *pustule* is a circumscribed elevation of skin, usually less than 0.5 cm in diameter. It contains a purulent exudate that may be white, yellow, or greenish-yellow. Any condition capable of producing a vesicle can result in a pustule provided the vesicle is not promptly ruptured, and the fluid becomes turbid and relatively opaque owing to the presence of significant numbers of cells.

Diagnostic Procedures

Skin scraping for identification of fungal infection and skin biopsy are performed in more than one quarter of dermatologic patients.[1]

Scraping for the Diagnosis of Fungal Infections. The specimen is obtained from the margin of the lesion. Hold a No. 15 scalpel blade perpendicular to the surface and stroke in a lateral fashion across the lesion. Scales are collected on a clear microscopic slide. A drop of potassium hydroxide (KOH) or Swartz-Lamkins stain (much superior) is applied to the slide, then a coverslip. The preparation is heated gently over a flame until tiny bubbles begin to form, at which point the slide is immediately placed on the counter to cool and prevent boiling. Once cooled, the slide is turned upside down onto a paper towel placed flat on the counter and pressed firmly to squeeze out excess fluid and to thin and flatten the specimen. The slide is then turned right side up and examined under the microscope using reduced illumination and a low-power lens, with high-power employed as needed to evaluate suspicious areas. All superficial fungal infections and inflammatory candidal infections show separate branching hyphae. If in a relatively quiescent phase, *Candida* will show budding yeast forms, and the lesions of tinea versicolor will appear similarly. If any of these features are found, the diagnosis is straightforward. Currently, it is no longer essential to differentiate between tinea and candidal infections, because now therapeutic agents are effective for both.

Skin Biopsy. Punch biopsy is the most commonly performed dermatologic office procedure. For entirely removing a lesion, surgical excisional biopsy with suturing is utilized; if cosmetic effects are not primary, elevated lesions may be excised using sharp-pointed scissors, with bleeding stopped by pressure, Gelfoam, Monsel's solution, or electrocautery. A shave biopsy of an elevated lesion can be done with a No. 15 blade held even with the surface of the normal skin. Punch biopsies are easily performed. A special instrument is used after injection of a small amount of local anesthetic. To create a linear scar, giving best cosmetic results, one should stretch the skin perpendicularly to the desired line of the scar. The biopsy generally should be taken from an actively involved margin of the lesion. One penetrates the skin by rotating the punch-biopsy instrument while stretching the skin as described and excising a circle of tissue. Bleeding is controlled by application of pressure for a few minutes. Specimens are placed in 10% formalin solution for delivery to the laboratory. Suturing is not essential but results in speedier wound closure and a smaller scar. Application of bacitracin or erythromycin ointment twice daily until the wound heals may prevent infection and thus enhance the cosmetic result.

Treatment Modalities

Thirteen therapeutic categories account for the majority of treatments prescribed for skin lesions by primary care and dermatologic physicians (Table 69–2).[1] Some of the agents—topical antibiotics, preparations for acne, shampoos, and antifungal agents—are discussed later in sections on specific disease categories. Here, we address principles involved in using some of the most important categories of dermatologic therapy.

Topical Corticosteroids. Topical corticosteroids are divided into several groups by potency (Table 69–3). Adrenal insufficiency resulting from topical corticosteroid usage is extremely rare, but local atrophy and telangiectasia may occur at the application sites, especially if applied to fine skin of the face, axilla, or genitalia. Hydrocortisone at 1% or less concentration is generally free of this side effect. The other generally fluorinated preparations are more potent therapeutically and produce more local side effects—apparently these potencies are linked. The most potent agents should never be used on thin skin or under occlusive dressings. Almost all preparations are supplied as ointments, creams, or lotions.

Ointment vehicles produce higher bioavailability of the steroid and are hydrating. Thus, dry lesions respond best to an ointment. Patients often dislike greasy-feeling medications and prefer the vanishing cream vehicles, at least for daytime use, unless therapeutic results require an ointment. Intertriginous areas are usually naturally moist and respond well to cream or lotion. Hairy areas are most easily treated with lotion in most patients, but black patients often prefer an ointment for use on the scalp. Treatment consists of thoroughly rubbing a small amount of preparation into the surface of the lesion. Very scaly lesions generally require the more potent compounds to achieve a therapeutic effect. The advantage of the weaker hydrocortisone preparations is that they may be used on the face, intertriginous areas, mucous membranes, or other areas of fine skin without producing atrophy. Stronger preparations decrease collagen synthesis, leading to loss of normal elements and thinning and depression of skin if applied for as few as several weeks to facial or intertriginous skin. The potency of topical corticosteroids is further increased when used with occlusive plastic dressings. This is useful in treating localized, difficult-to-clear lesions of psoriasis or eczema.

Topical Absorbent and Water-Repellent Ointments. Lanolin-stearin and petrolatum-containing *ointments* are examples of preparations that hydrate and thus soften skin surfaces; they are used on dry, scaly lesions. Petrolatum ointment is occlusive and waterproof. This barrier effect increases the water retention in treated lesional or nonle-

TABLE 69–3. CURRENTLY AVAILABLE TOPICAL CORTICOSTEROIDS LISTED BY POTENCY

Most potent	Betamethasone dipropionate cream, ointment 0.05% (optimized vehicle) (Diprolene) Clobetasol propionate cream, ointment 0.05% (Temovate) Diflorasone diacetate ointment 0.05% (optimized vehicle) (Psorcon) Halobetasol propionate cream, ointment 0.05% (Ultravate)
	Amcinonide ointment 0.1% (Cyclocort) Betamethasone dipropionate ointment 0.05% (Diprosone) Desoximetasone cream, ointment 0.25% (Topicort) Desoximetasone gel 0.05% (Topicort) Diflorasone diacetate ointment 0.05% (Florone, Maxiflor) Fluocinonide cream, ointment, gel 0.05% (Lidex) Halcinonide cream 0.1% (Halog)
	Betamethasone benzoate gel 0.025% (Benisone, Uticort) Betamethasone dipropionate cream 0.05% (Diprosone) Betamethasone valerate ointment 0.1% (Valisone) Diflorasone diacetate cream 0.05% (Florone, Maxiflor) Triamcinolone acetate ointment 0.1% (Aristocort A), cream 0.5% (Aristocort HP)
	Amcinonide cream 0.1% (Cyclocort) Betamethasone benzoate ointment 0.025% (Benisone, Uticort) Betamethasone valerate lotion 0.1% (Valisone) Desoximetasone cream 0.05% (Topicort-LP) Fluocinolone acetonide cream 0.2% (Synalar-HP) Fluocinolone acetonide ointment 0.025% (Synalar) Flurandrenolide ointment 0.05% (Cordran) Hydrocortisone valerate ointment 0.2% (Westcort) Triamcinolone acetonide ointment 0.1% (Aristocort, Kenalog)
	Betamethasone benzoate cream 0.025% (Benisone, Uticort) Betamethasone dipropionate lotion 0.02% (Diprosone) Betamethasone valerate cream, lotion 0.1% (Valisone) Clocortolone cream 0.1% (Cloderm) Fluocinolone acetonide cream 0.025% (Fluonid, Synalar) Flurandrenolide cream 0.05% (Cordran) Hydrocortisone butyrate cream 0.1% (Locoid) Hydrocortisone valerate cream 0.2% (Westcort) Triamcinolone acetonide cream, lotion 0.1% (Kenalog) Triamcinolone acetonide cream 0.025% (Aristocort)
Least potent	Alclometason dipropionate cream 0.05% (Aclovate) Betamethasone valerate lotion 0.05% (Valisone) Desonide cream 0.05% (Tridesilon) Flumethasone cream 0.03% (Locorten) Fluocinolone acetonide solution 0.01% (Synalar) Dexamethasone 0.1% (Decadron Phosphate) Hydrocortisone 0.5%, 1.0%, 2.5% (generic, Hytone, others) Methylprednisolone 1% (Medrol)

sional epidermis. This softens stratum corneum and scales, reduces the adherence of scales, and increases the penetration of topical medications through the stratum corneum.

Creams are less occlusive or waterproof and have less wetting effect but are more pleasant for the patient to use. *Shake lotions,* such as calamine lotion, are more drying than creams and may be used for a cooling effect on large areas or widespread, oozing, mildly inflamed dermatoses such as those associated with herpes zoster or poison ivy.

Keratolytic Agents. Salicylic acid, propylene glycol, lactic acid, or ammonium lactate preparations are useful to remove or soften heaped-up keratin or scales and thus allow penetration of therapeutic agents applied afterward. Psoriasis, seborrheic dermatitis, and localized chronic eczematous dermatitis are examples of problems that may not respond to medication without the prior application of a keratolytic agent. Such agents, however, should be avoided on the face and in intertriginous areas.

Wet Dressings. Crusting, oozing vesicular lesions are commonly treated with wet dressings, which promote drying and healing by débriding the lesion when removed. The solutions are applied to gauze covering the lesion, which should be removed while still damp. Use of gauze prevents maceration that would occur using "closed" dressings covered by plastic sheeting. Gauze is first applied, after which it may be moistened by pouring aluminum acetate (Burow's solution) (1 tablet or packet of Domeboro to 2 pints of tap water or a 1:40 dilution) onto the dressing.

Baths and Soaps. Baths have a soothing effect on generalized pruritus or dry skin of any etiology but tend to have a drying effect afterward. A lubricating bath appropriate for dry skin or eczema may be achieved by adding 1 or 2 tablespoons of Alpha-Keri or Nivea to the tub of water. This helps to avoid the drying effect of an ordinary bath in patients with ichthyosis or atopic eczema. For generalized pruritus, one may achieve an antipruritic effect with 1 cup of colloidal oatmeal (Aveeno) or one half a box of starch added to a tub of cool or at most lukewarm water. The patient must be cautious on entering and leaving the tub, because the tub becomes slippery when these agents are used. Dove soap is considered by many to be the least irritating and drying for most people.

Cryotherapy with Liquid Nitrogen. Superficial small lesions, such as warts and actinic or seborrheic keratoses, may be treated in the office by application of liquid nitrogen, either via cotton swab or by fine spray from a cryosurgical device. Nitrogen is applied to the surface of the lesion for a few (about 30) seconds, long enough to freeze the lesion. There is some pain. With or without blister formation, the lesion generally peels away and is replaced by normal skin over approximately a 2-week period. Topical antibiotics may be used in the interval.

DIAGNOSIS AND TREATMENT OF COMMON DERMATOLOGIC DISEASE CATEGORIES

Tumors of Skin

Commonly encountered benign tumors of skin include seborrheic keratoses, cysts, skin tags (acrochordons), lipomas, histiocytomas, dermatofibromas, and benign nevi. Primary malignancies of skin include basal cell epitheliomas, squamous cell carcinoma, carcinoma in situ (Bowen's disease), and malignant melanomas. Actinic keratoses are classified as premalignant lesions. The major task for the primary care physician is accurate diagnosis of these lesions, because virtually all malignant ones require referral for treatment whereas usually financial resources are wasted if one refers benign lesions to a dermatologist to establish their diagnosis. In most cases an accurate diagnosis can be made by inspection.

Common Benign Tumors. Seborrheic keratoses occur most commonly on the face, neck, back, and upper chest in elderly individuals, average about 1 cm in diameter, and vary from flesh-colored to brown or black (Fig. 69–1*A*). The verrucous ("warty") surface of these lesions and their appearance of being superficially adherent to skin are recognizable features. Warts (verruca vulgaris) (see Fig. 69–1*B*) appear more papillary or raised than seborrheic keratoses and are usually not as darkly pigmented but have a verrucous surface. Skin tags are pedunculated growths, common in the neck and axilla of older persons. There may be multiple small, slightly pigmented, pedunculated lesions or larger soft, fleshy growths covered by normal skin. Cysts have a soft consistency, are movable and discrete, and are located beneath the skin surface. Synovial (ganglion) cysts, located near tendons and joints, may appear more translucent. Lipomas are softer and usually larger than cysts; typically they feel more lobulated with less distinct margins. Histiocytomas and dermatofibromas occur most commonly on the anterior shins, are firm and nodular, and usually are less than 1 cm in size. They may usually be differentiated from fibrosarcomas by their lack of continued growth and lack of invasion of subcutaneous tissue.

Basal Cell Epitheliomas (see Fig. 69–1*C*). These are the most commonly encountered malignancies of skin and almost invariably are located on sun-exposed areas. In addition to the face, torso, and extremities, examination of the ears, nasal folds, scalp, and neck is required. The earliest, most easily removable lesions are small, flesh-colored to red nodules, recognizable by their firm adherence to and outgrowth from underlying skin, their "waxy" surface appearance, and their characteristic surface telangiectasias. As they enlarge, a central ulceration often forms, typically surrounded by a raised "pearly" border. Less often, epitheliomas are brown or black, particularly in dark-skinned individuals, or appear as a scarred plaque or "fibrosing type," usually on the face.

Squamous Cell Carcinoma (see Fig. 69–1*D*). These occur particularly on sun-exposed areas of the lower lip, tongue, ears, and dorsum of the hands; they may also arise at sites of scars and actinic keratoses or form the bases of cutaneous horns. They grow more rapidly than do basal cell epitheliomas, and they sometimes metastasize. The most commonly noted morphology is that of a firm, red, asymptomatic nodule that, as it expands, develops raised, indurated margins and central ulceration on an erythematous base. A less common and more indolent type has a heaped-up, "warty" appearance that may resemble a benign verrucous lesion, although careful inspection reveals a hyperkeratotic rather than verrucous surface and firm adherence to the erythematous base. Keratoacanthomas are similar in appearance to squamous cell carcinomas and must be differentiated histologically.

Squamous cell carcinoma in situ (Bowen's disease) presents as an erythematous scaly patch, which may be difficult to differentiate form eczema or psoriasis. Its distinct irregular margins, isolated occurrence, lack of pruritus, small size, and mildly hyperkeratotic appearance should alert the clinician that a biopsy may be necessary, either at once or if a brief trial of topical corticosteroid therapy fails to produce adequate results (Fig. 69–2*B*).

Premalignant Lesions. These are actinic or senile ker-

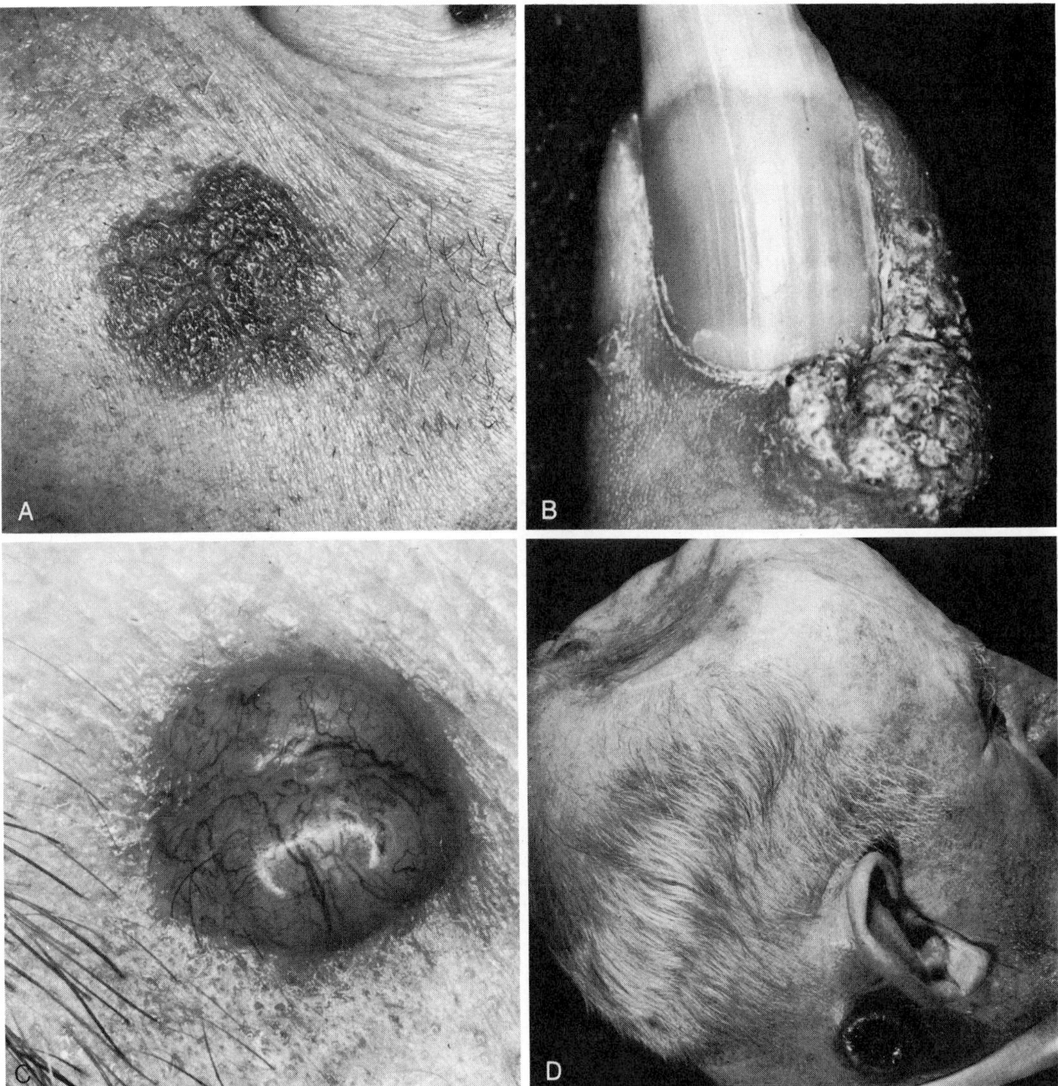

FIGURE 69–1. Typical features of seborrheic keratosis (*A*); wart (verruca vulgaris) (*B*); basal cell epithelioma (*C*); and squamous cell carcinoma (*D*). See text for descriptions.

atoses, leukoplakia, and arsenical keratoses. Sun-related actinic keratoses are persistent, raised, scaly patches or erythematous macules that have the consistency of sandpaper to the feel. The risk of developing malignancy is about 1:1000 of these lesions. Rapid growth or induration is an indication for biopsy. Leukoplakia is a white, somewhat raised plaque adherent to the mucous membranes. Arsenical keratoses occur on the palms and soles of persons with the history of prolonged arsenic ingestion.

Benign Nevi Versus Malignant Melanomas. Benign nevi may be flat or raised and may have a smooth or compound surface appearance. They are distinguishable from malignant melanomas (see Fig. 72–6) by their regular margins, uniform pigmentation ranging from tan to dark brown, and intact surface markings. Malignant melanomas occur as one of three types. The least common (~5%) is the premalignant *lentigo maligna,* an irregular, flat pigmentation generally found on the face in an elderly individual and recognizable by the flecks or fine network of black pigment mixed irregularly with the brown color of the lesion, as well as by its irregular shape. Such lesions may persist for many years before developing into invasive malignant melanomas. Lentigo maligna may be distinguished from senile lentigo, because the latter is uniformly tan or brown and shaped as a regular ellipsoid, and from freckles, because they are multiple, tan or brown in color, generally small, and confined to exposed areas of skin.

Nodular malignant melanomas, the second most common melanoma (~15%), are similar in appearance to benign blue nevi in that both are darkly pigmented, regularly shaped nodules, but nodular melanomas characteristically feature a deeper bluish hue, may be noted to be rapidly growing, and are usually irregular or ulcerated on the surface. Pyogenic granuloma is another nodular, friable, easily bleeding lesion and may require biopsy to be distinguished from amelanotic nodular melanoma.

The most common type of melanoma, *superficial spreading malignant melanoma* (70%), is more easily distinguishable from benign nevi than the nodular type, because it is usually 1 cm or more in diameter, its margins are usually quite irregular, and it often exhibits characteristic reddish, whitish, and bluish areas in addition to brown and black. These lesions are relatively flat (but slightly elevated); they may have intact surface markings in the early, curable phase.

Lentigo maligna may exist as a noninvasive lesion for 5

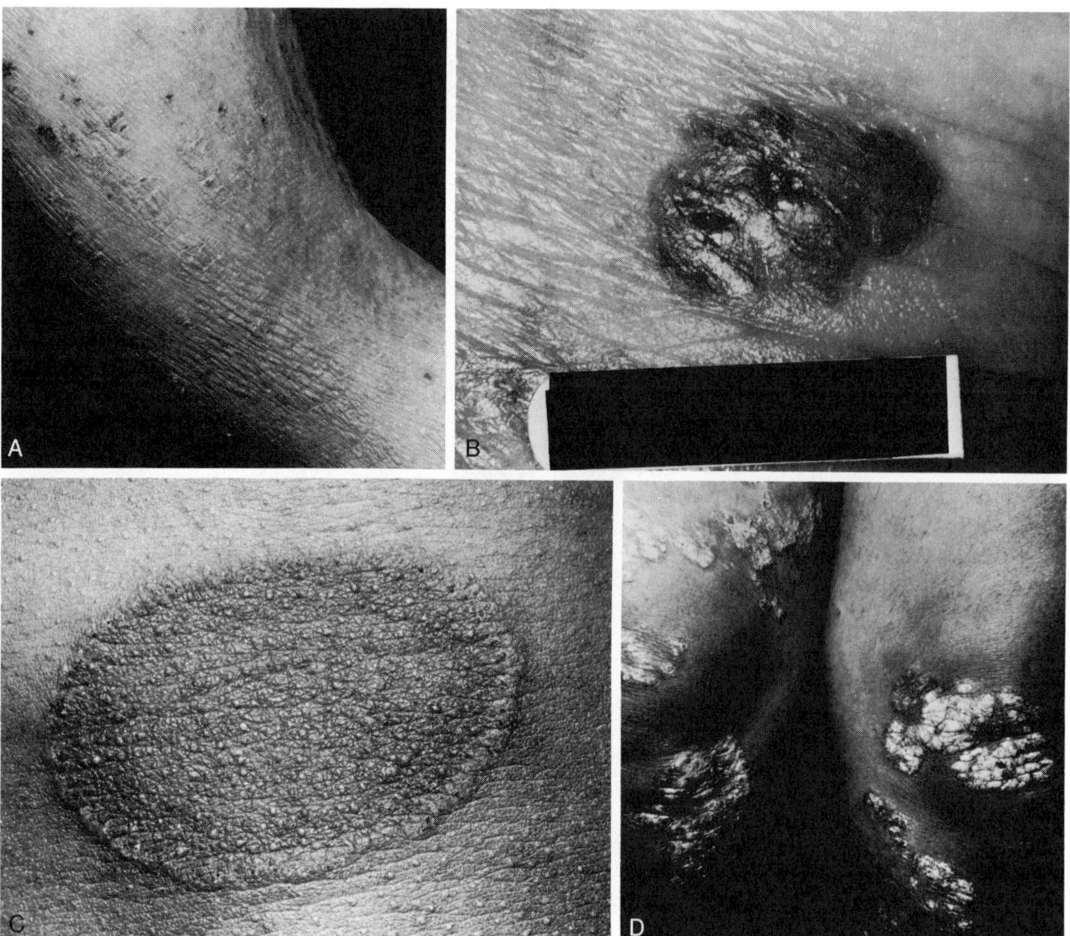

FIGURE 69–2. Typical features of chronic eczematous dermatitis with "lichenification" of skin (*A*); Bowen's disease (squamous cell carcinoma in situ) (*B*); tinea corporis ("ringworm" of smooth skin) (*C*); and psoriatic plaques (*D*). See text for descriptions.

to 50 years, whereas superficial spreading melanoma commonly remains in an early stage of invasiveness for several years. Once resected, staging is done by measuring the thickness of the primary tumor by micrometer. Lesions 0.75 mm or less in depth have an excellent prognosis for cure, whereas those 3 mm or more in thickness have a poor prognosis for 5-year survival.

Although related to sun exposure, malignant melanomas are *not* most commonly distributed on the face and dorsum of the hands but are more often found on the back in both sexes, the legs of women, and the anterior torso of men.

With the exception of congenital nevi, benign nevi are not considered to be premalignant lesions. A congenital nevus, defined as one present at birth, does have a potential for malignancy, and it is agreed that this is related to its size. It remains controversial whether to remove prophylactically small congenital nevi (<1.5 cm in diameter), but it is estimated that approximately 8% of melanomas arise in the site of a contiguous nevus. Giant hairy nevi and other congenital nevi over 1.5 cm in diameter warrant consideration of removal.

A syndrome of *familial malignant melanoma* is now recognized. Relatives of melanoma patients have a tenfold increased risk, probably via polygenic inheritance. Some in these families typically manifest numerous large *"dysplastic" nevi.* These nevi have histologic features of atypia and may be difficult to distinguish pathologically from actual malignant melanoma, except in expert hands. Dysplastic nevi are often larger (1 to 2 cm in diameter) than is common with benign nevi (usually <5mm in size), are somewhat more irregularly shaped, and may have varying shades of pigmentation. Thus, the benign "dysplastic" nevus has some features suggestive of malignant melanoma. Since affected individuals typically have large numbers of nevi, it is usual for them to be followed by a dermatologist, with removal of any lesion that appears to be enlarging or looks more atypical in size or appearance than their other nevi.

Treatment of Skin Growths

Some seborrheic keratoses and benign skin tags are pruritic or have a propensity to become irritated or infected. Such symptomatic as well as cosmetically unacceptable benign lesions may be removed by cryosurgery or excised with sharp-pointed scissors. Actinic keratoses can be treated by cryosurgery or fluorouracil cream applied twice daily to small areas for 2 to 3 weeks, with interruption of treatment if unacceptable inflammation occurs. Basal cell epitheliomas are chiefly of concern because of their locally invasive behavior. Surgical excision using an elliptical incision and leaving 3- to 4-mm borders is usually employed to remove them when small. Cryosurgery using much deeper and wider freezing than for benign lesions is often an excellent alternative. Lesions that are of unusually large size, are in difficult locations, or recur after previous therapy require special consideration and consultation. The dermatologist is often best able to proffer treatment from among excisional surgery, cryosurgery, and radiation therapy. Surgical excision is usually the treatment of choice for squamous cell carcinomas.

Suspicious pigmented lesions should be excised locally and examined histologically. If they are too large for excisional biopsy, a partial biopsy of a very suspicious area is reasonable. More extensive surgery is postponed until the malignant nature of the lesion has been confirmed. No increased risk of local recurrence, nodal metastases, or death from disease has been shown to result from dermal punch biopsy for diagnosis of malignant melanoma, but surgical excisional biopsy remains preferable as the initial approach whenever feasible. Because of the need to examine tissue histopathologically, cryosurgery or electrodesiccation is not utilized for removing nevi.

In discussing management, we should not neglect to mention the importance of using high-protection *sunscreens* and of avoiding peak hours of sunlight exposure in the long term prevention of all types of skin malignancies. Light-skinned persons, those living in warm climates, and those occupationally exposed or with a previous history of skin cancer should be warned in particular to avoid excessive exposure.

ECZEMATOUS DERMATITIS

Eczematous dermatitis is the generic term for subcategories of localized inflammatory reactions characterized by erythema with indistinct margins. In the acute phase, lesions may exhibit edema, vesiculation, oozing, and, in some cases, bullae. More chronic plaques are dry and scaly and may exhibit secondary lichenification (see Fig. 69–2*A*). Crusting may indicate superimposed bacterial infection. Pruritus is typically present. The most common subcategories of eczema are contact dermatitis; atopic eczema; stasis dermatitis; several forms of primary eczema including dyshidrosis, nummular eczema, and lichen simplex chronicus; and some types of external otitis and pruritus ani. In most cases the eczema is thought to represent abnormally intense reaction of skin to exposure to an allergen or irritant. Acute forms that are accompanied by blistering and oozing usually represent contact with an allergen, with the exception of lesions on the palms or soles.

Allergic contact dermatitis typically conforms to an area of exposure, such as exposed skin in poison ivy, earlobe in nickel earring allergy, eyelid in eye makeup allergy, or hand and forearm in soap allergy. Rubber, acrylics, metals like nickel and chromate, and topical drugs are other common dermatologic allergens. Industrial irritants produce a similar reaction on a nonallergic basis confined to the area of exposure. Even mild irritants such as polishes, bleaches, and soaps produce a reaction with repeated exposure in some people. Exposure to friction, sunlight, thermal injury, or occlusion may potentiate the irritant effect.

Atopic eczema is a more generalized, intensely pruritic form of eczema typically found in young adults with a family history of asthma, hay fever, or atopy; characteristically, it is distributed in the antecubital and popliteal fossae and on the wrists and posterior neck.

Stasis dermatitis typically develops above the medial malleolus of patients with edema secondary to chronic venous insufficiency of the lower extremities (see Chapter 12). Other forms of eczema may have a characteristic appearance and distribution. Coin-shaped, papulovesicular patches located chiefly on the extremities suggest *nummular eczema*. Eczematous dermatitis of the hands tends to develop tiny vesicles and is often referred to as *dyshidrosis*. *Eczematous external otitis* is confined to the ear canal and *pruritus ani* to the perianal region. Persistent rubbing transforms an eczematous rash into a chronically pruritic, lichenified lesion termed *lichen simplex chronicus*; this does not resolve as long as the rubbing persists. The term *neurodermatitis,* when applied to eczematous rashes in various stages of the papulovesicular and lichenified form, refers to the role of itching and resultant scratching in causing persistence of such lesions, typically located at the nape of the neck, scrotum, or perianal region. It should be noted that any dermatitis—for example, stasis dermatitis of the ankle—may be transformed into a chronic lesion by continuous scratching. The term *neurodermatitis,* however, is best avoided in favor of a morphologic term, such as *chronic eczematous dermatitis* or *lichen simplex chronicus,* since the etiology of the lesion is not strictly psychogenic.

Differential Diagnosis. The margins of a psoriatic plaque are more distinct and its surface thicker and scales more heaped-up and whiter in appearance than in eczematous dermatitis. Fungal infections of skin often have areas of central clearing with well-defined, slightly raised borders featuring small vesicles indicative of disease activity; the Swartz-Lamkins stain or KOH preparation may be necessary to confirm the fungal etiology of an inflammatory plaque. Bowen's disease (carcinoma in situ) is nonpruritic, smaller, usually a single lesion, and more persistent; it has more distinct margins and a less inflammatory appearance than do typical lesions of eczematous dermatitis (see Fig. 69–2*B*).

Management. A strenuous effort is indicated to identify the etiology by eliciting the history of exposure to an allergen or irritant. Removal from contact with such an agent is the first step in management. Use of a barrier cream and hypoallergenic makeup, or no makeup, is recommended for women allergic to cosmetics. For eczema of the hands, most physicians empirically recommend avoidance of hand- or dishwashing as much as possible, use of a mild soap (e.g., Dove), and wearing plastic or cotton-lined rubber gloves while washing dishes. Lessening edema by wrapping the legs with an Ace bandage, use of a pressure gradient (Jobst) stocking, or, if necessary, bedrest and elevation of the feet prevent or heal stasis dermatitis. Once present, eczematous dermatitis is easily worsened by repeated exposure to irritants like soap, allergens, and industrial chemicals, even in small amounts, so stringent measures to avoid reexposure are necessary, especially during the initial weeks of treatment.

Specific therapy consists, first, of measures designed to alleviate symptoms, promote healing, and prevent secondary infection and, second, of topical corticosteroid agents. Antihistamines taken at night help to relieve symptoms of itching. Acutely inflamed, oozing lesions such as acute contact or stasis dermatitis, particularly if secondarily infected, respond to wet dressings, which have a drying and débriding effect. Less severely inflamed but oozing lesions such as those typically associated with poison ivy may be covered by a shake lotion, which is soothing but has less drying effect than a wet dressing. Conversely, a topical ointment such as petrolatum may be needed to remove scales, and this will facilitate penetration of topical corticosteroids into chronic eczematous lesions, which tend to have dry, scaly, or lichenified surfaces.

A short course of an oral corticosteroid such as prednisone beginning with approximately 60 mg/day and tapered over about 15 days is indicated for very acute, extensive eruptions such as those sometimes associated with poison ivy. Less extensive eczematous lesions respond to strong topical corticosteroids such as a fluorinated steroid cream applied twice daily as a small amount massaged into the surface of the lesion; application is continued until the lesion has totally cleared. Prior treatment with topical ointments or keratolytic agents, as outlined earlier, may be necessary for thickened or scaly lesions to facilitate penetration of the topical corticosteroid into the lesion. Repeated treatments are necessary for recurrent eczema. On the face, intertriginous areas, and mucous membranes, only weak hydrocortisone preparations are used. The addition of menthol or camphor to the corticosteroid cream reduces local pruritus and thus hastens healing of chronic eczema by diminishing scratching. Over-the-counter preparations, such as Sarna lotion, containing menthol, camphor and phenol, may be applied as often as needed to relieve pruritus, in addition to the twice-daily topical corticosteroid applications.

FUNGAL DISEASES OF SKIN

Superficial fungal infections can be divided into three categories: superficial fungal infections, termed tinea; the ultrasuperficial infection of the skin called tinea versicolor; and candidal infections. For practical purposes, since treatment depends on the location of the lesion, local tinea infections may be classified according to the body area: tinea corporis (smooth skin), tinea cruris (groin), tinea pedis (feet), tinea manus (hands), tinea capitis (scalp), and so on, although they are caused by various species of fungi. Tinea versicolor (described later) generally involves the shoulders and anterior chest and requires different management. Infections with *Candida albicans* also differ in their clinical features from tinea infections, but treatment now available is effective against both types. Hence, it is more important to distinguish superficial fungal infections from other types of skin lesions than it is to identify the exact type of fungal agent involved. Tinea infections are usually single, erythematous, scaly patches or plaques with a slightly raised scaly border and some central clearing. Candidal infections are more "beefy" red in appearance, are sometimes oozing or eroded, and typically have papular, pustulovesicular, or pustular lesions along their ill-defined borders or as satellite lesions beyond their margins.

Correct diagnosis is the key to successful therapy. Since fungal infections provoke various degrees and types of eczematous reactions in the skin, clinical examination is often inadequate to ascertain with certainty whether or not fungal infection is present. If the question of fungal infection arises, a KOH preparation or Swartz-Lamkins stain of scales or vesicle roofs scraped from the lesion is extremely desirable for diagnosis. If there is no fungal infection, antifungal therapy wastes time and money. If fungal infection is present, topical corticosteroid therapy will cause the lesion to spread and will increase the extent of fungus per given area of skin. The 5 minutes devoted to the microscopic examination is worthwhile because it may prevent the patient from becoming a treatment failure requiring dermatologic referral. The KOH preparation or Swartz-Lamkin stain reveals septate branching hyphae or, in the quiescent phase of candidal infections, budding yeast forms.

Tinea Corporis. So-called "ringworm" infections of smooth skin are seen most commonly in children, who often acquire them from pets. They appear as scaly patches, generally single, with sharp, slightly scaly, rolled borders (see Fig. 69–2*C*), and central clearing if large. The distinct margins of these lesions distinguish them from eczema; absence of crusting distinguishes them from impetigo. A variety of therapeutic agents are effective, including Tinactin solution (tolnaftate), which may be applied twice daily for several weeks until the lesion has cleared, and Lotrimin (clotrimazole) or Micatin (miconazole nitrate), applied similarly.

Tinea Versicolor. These infections usually involve the chest, shoulders, and upper back. The rash consists of widespread, irregularly shaped, slightly scaly patches with either slightly increased or slightly decreased pigmentation. KOH preparation, revealing clusters of budding spores mixed with short, curved hyphae, can confirm the diagnosis if there is concern about the etiology of the rash. The typical location and chronic nature of the lesions generally distinguish tinea versicolor from secondary syphilis, pityriasis rosea, and other papulosquamous lesions of the body. Most cases are asymptomatic and, once recognized, may require no treatment. The rash can be controlled, if not permanently eradicated, by Selsun (selenium sulfide suspension, 2.5%), which may be applied with a rough washcloth for 10 minutes daily for 1 week or for 2 consecutive days/month for 6 months. In widespread lesions, Selsun may be applied to all involved areas after bathing, allowed to dry, then washed off after 8 to 24 hours. Clearing of the fungi can also be achieved following twice-daily applications for 3 weeks of 2% miconazole cream or 1% sulconazole to versicolor lesions. Ketoconazole cream and shampoo are also very effective, but more expensive. Chronic prophylaxis is desirable: the routine use of a shampoo containing selenium sulfide or zinc pyrithione and of bath soap (e.g., Fostex) containing sulfur and salicylic acid will reduce the otherwise 100% risk of recurrence.

Intertriginous Infections. Dampness and resulting maceration and irritation of skin frequently produce rashes of the body folds or intertriginous areas beneath the breasts, in the axilla, or in the groin. These may become secondarily infected. The epidermis may be eroded or denuded, particularly in warm weather, and this is greatly worsened in the groin region if the patient is incontinent. *Candida* sp. are common pathogens of the intertriginous folds with their typical "beefy" red, oozing, burning, itching, poorly marginated lesions and satellite papules and pustules. *Tinea cruris* is a more indolent, less symptomatic, generally bilateral infection, characterized by fan-shaped, well-marginated scaly patches. *Erythrasma* is a bacterial infection of the groin or axilla caused by a species of *Corynebacterium*; its lesions show a faint red-tan coloration, little or no scaling, and no elevation of margins.

Management of intertriginous infections is based on the principle of keeping the area as dry as possible. Loose-fitting boxer shorts or panties of 100% cotton are worn, or a brassiere with good support is used. Wool, nylon, or other synthetic fabric underwear is avoided. If possible, the patient should avoid hot, humid climates or areas. Greasy ointments that retain moisture are also avoided. It may be necessary for the patient to expose the involved area while lying down and use a fan or electric light bulb near the infected area for its drying effect. Diabetes and obesity should be corrected, if possible.

Specific Therapy. In the acute phase, especially if the lesions are oozing or denuded, Burow's solution compresses are employed. For more indolent or healed infections, Zeasorb or other types of powder are recommended to minimize moisture. For intertriginous rashes without secondary infection, one may employ hydrocortisone cream, but not fluorinated steroids because atrophy may develop in these areas. Prophylactically, one may use nystatin or miconazole powder liberally on top of a thin application of hydrocortisone cream. Both candidal and tineal intertriginous infections can be treated with miconazole lotion (Monistat-

Derm, 2%). Erythrasma responds to erythromycin, 250 mg taken four times daily for 5 to 7 days, or it can be treated with the topical erythromycin lotions intended for acne in a twice-daily application for 14 days.

Fungal Infections of the Feet, Hands, Scalp, and Beard Area. Acute tinea infection of the feet, manifested by blisters and vesiculopustular lesions, responds to local treatment with Tinactin powder. Unusually severe cases require the addition of systemic griseofulvin and topical Burow's solution compresses. The chronic, scaling "athlete's foot" is difficult to eradicate with local therapy, although acute flare-ups respond to Tinactin solution or miconazole lotion. Resistant cases may respond to naftafine HCl (Naftin), econazole (Spectazole), or ketoconazole (Nizoral). Scaly erythema of the hands is more often caused by contact or eczematous dermatitis than by tinea infection. Chronic tinea infection of the hands does occur, and the diagnosis may be confirmed by KOH preparation or by Swartz-Lamkins stain.

Griseofulvin may be employed in chronic infection of the hands or fingernails but is avoided for chronic infection of the feet or toenails, because toenail infections are nearly impossible to cure and chronic tinea infection of the feet has a very high recurrence rate even after prolonged therapy with griseofulvin. Even therapy for more than 9 months with orally administered ketoconazole has not been shown to permanently eradicate tinea infection involving the soles or toenails, although this therapy often works to eradicate persistent infection of the trunk, groin, hands, or fingernails that fails to respond to griseofulvin. The thickening, crumbling, and distortion of the toenails caused by chronic tinea infestation can be controlled by débridement by a podiatrist. Persistent topical antifungal therapy is recommended and occasionally results in clearing of nail infections.

Candidal infections of the hands typically involve the web spaces between the fingers or produce paronychia. The latter does not involve the nail itself and is less acute in onset and less painful than bacterial paronychia; it may be treated by frequent liberal applications of miconazole solution or clotrimazole solution. Unnecessary exposure to water should be avoided.

Tinea infections of the scalp consist of scaly patches, sometimes including an inflamed pustular reaction and loss of hairs that break off. Scalp infections occur most commonly in children and are transmissible from one child to another. They may often be recognized by the bright fluorescence of infected hairs under Wood's lamp. The inflammation may be controlled by soaking with Burow's solution for 15 minutes twice each day. Selsun (2.5% selenium sulfide) shampoos subsequently applied twice daily for 3 weeks will suppress the viability of fungal spores and may help to prevent transmission of the agent to other persons while therapy with griseofulvin is being initiated.

Griseofulvin is employed for scalp infections as well as for chronic tinea infection of the fingernails and hands. For treatment of scalp and hand infections, it may be given in a dose of 250 mg ultramicrosize three times daily with meals or milk until all clinical evidence of infection resolves, usually within 4 to 6 weeks for scalp infections, 3 months for hand infections, and up to 9 months for fingernail infections. The white blood cell count and differential of peripheral blood should be followed during oral griseofulvin therapy.

Id Reactions. Id reactions consist of vesicular or papulofollicular eruptions often involving the hands or body of a patient with a primary fungal infection located elsewhere. These reactions are thought to result from hypersensitivity to the fungal agent. They do not contain fungi but disappear when the primary site of infection is adequately treated. They can be treated with the measures employed for eczematous dermatitis.

VIRAL DISEASES OF SKIN

Viral diseases of skin are encountered commonly by both dermatologists and primary care physicians. This section discusses the diagnosis and treatment of herpes simplex and herpes zoster, and the differential diagnosis of generalized exanthems, most commonly of either viral or allergic etiology. The problem of warts (verrucae vulgares) is discussed under tumors of skin (page 876). Several other important clinical topics are discussed elsewhere: diagnosis and treatment of genital herpes infections on page 365, condylomata acuminata on page 371, molluscum contagiosum on page 371, plantar warts on page 698, and herpes infections of the eye on page 863.

Herpesvirus Infections. These skin infections, including chickenpox, herpes zoster, and herpes simplex, are characterized by the formation of a vesicle with an umbilicated surface. The initial finding in various types of herpetic infections includes a group of vesicles containing clear fluid and surrounded by erythema. Typically, the vesicles eventually rupture, leaving erosions and crust formation.

Herpes zoster represents reactivation of latent infection with chickenpox virus, is common in immunologically compromised hosts but frequently occurs in otherwise normal elderly persons, and is characterized by its confinement to a dermatomal segment. A neuritic type of pain may precede the development of skin lesions by several days. Postherpetic neuralgia is defined as neuritic pain of a dermatomal segment that persists for more than 30 days after resolution of the skin lesions. The herpetic vesicles may appear slightly cloudy; true purulence is sometimes a sign of secondary bacterial infection. Therapy with acyclovir is effective in herpes zoster but requires 800 mg orally five times per day (four times the dose for herpes simplex) for 7 to 10 days. Treatment began within the first few days will reduce the amount of pain, the severity of lesions, and the time until healing is complete.

Skin symptoms may be relieved somewhat by application of a soothing lotion (e.g., calamine lotion or alcoholic white shake lotion). Secondary infection can be treated by wet dressings (Burow's solution), followed by application of povidone-iodine ointment. The patient may need a strong analgesic during the initial several days or week of severe pain. Stool softeners should be added to avoid constipation in the elderly. A 7- to 10-day course of oral corticosteroids (e.g., prednisone, 60 mg by mouth initially, tapered over 10 days) was shown to decrease the incidence of postherpetic neuralgia in patients older than 60 years of age in one study, but it does not shorten the duration of pain or lead to more rapid resolution of the primary rash. We prescribe a limited course of prednisone in elderly persons with this infection when they are otherwise healthy, are not immunocompromised, and have no medical contraindication to corticosteroid therapy. Immunocompromised patients with zoster probably should be treated with intravenous acyclovir to avoid dissemination. Patients with zoster already showing dissemination should also be treated with intravenous acyclovir. If such patients are not known to have immunodeficiency, they should be evaluated.

Herpes simplex infections most often involve the mouth or genital area. The morphology of primary herpes simplex is somewhat similar to that of herpes zoster in that it is characterized by widespread involvement of the affected area. However, it is not confined to one dermatome. Recurrent herpes simplex of the lips usually produces only a few vesicles or erosions. Herpes simplex of the mouth must be differentiated from aphthous stomatitis, which is characterized by a single, or a few, sharply marginated erosions, somewhat larger and more painful than is typical of recurrent herpes. Herpes simplex infections require no treatment if the symptoms are mild and persist for no more than 5 to 7 days. Treatment with oral acyclovir is reasonable for severe primary herpes and for recurrent herpes that is unusually frequent or severe. Oral therapy (200 mg, five times daily for 5 days) is less toxic than intravenous therapy, is more effective than topical therapy, and is the treatment of choice if treatment is necessary. Chronic suppressive therapy is appropriate for patients with very frequent, severe recurrent herpes. In severely immunologically compromised patients, intravenous acyclovir may be preferable.

Generalized Exanthems. It is difficult to distinguish the erythematous maculopapular generalized eruption of a viral exanthem from an allergic generalized drug eruption. In the case of *viral exanthems,* lesions are more likely to be located peripherally and to involve the palms or soles, the rash is usually less pruritic, some scaling may accompany its resolution, and the rash may be morbilliform, consisting of only scattered papules. Occasional additional characteristic features of a viral illness include not only general manifestations of infection, such as fever, myalgias, headache, and cough, but also enanthem consisting of papulovesicular lesions of the soft palate, usually indicative of a coxsackievirus infection, or other particular features such as the Koplik's spots of the mouth in patients with measles or the posterior auricular lymphadenopathy of patients with rubella. If a date of exposure is known, the typical incubation period of the viral illness should coincide with onset of the rash.

In adult medicine, *drug rashes* are probably encountered much more commonly than viral exanthems. The history of onset of the rash within days to a few months after initiation of a new medication is helpful. Most commonly the rash develops within the first week of the administration of the drug, but patients occasionally develop an allergic rash after years of being on a medication. One may at times be forced to resort to a trial of discontinuing medications, either restarting them one by one or substituting structurally different but therapeutically similar compounds. Drug rashes can be accompanied by lymphadenopathy and fever (e.g., the rash of phenytoin allergy). Compared with a viral exanthem, the typical drug rash is more centrally distributed and pruritic, has a brighter red coloration, and becomes more confluent over its truncal distribution.

Virtually any drug may be associated with a rash. The most common ones are ampicillin, amoxicillin, and trimethoprim/sulfamethoxazole. Others commonly associated are allopurinol, penicillins, barbiturates, chlorpromazine, phenytoin (Dilantin), isoniazid, and the sulfonamides (including thiazides and sulfonylureas). Digoxin rarely if ever causes a rash.

Some special types of generalized rashes can be distinguished clinically from the generalized exanthems. *Toxic erythema* is a diffuse, at times rather striking, blanching erythema of the skin, usually with indistinct margins; it is typically a reaction to a bacterial toxin, as in toxic shock syndrome or scarlet fever. This type of reaction can be mimicked by allergies to some drugs, including quinidine, salicylates, and sulfonamides. *Vasculitis* of the skin may result from drug allergy or other etiologies. Vasculitis can be distinguished from the self-limited maculopapular rashes seen in most allergic reactions because it is accompanied by nonblanching palpable purpura or by ulcerations distributed predominantly over the lower extremities, or because there are other features of vasculitis, such as synovitis or glomerulonephritis. *Erythema multiforme* is a syndrome consisting of its typical rash, fever, mucous membrane lesions, and sometimes synovitis. It may reflect a drug allergy or viral infection or be of unknown etiology. The typical rash of erythema multiforme includes macular and bullous lesions in addition to papular lesions, involves the distal extremities (particularly the palms), and is especially characterized by the presence of specific iris-shaped lesions. The most severe variant of this syndrome, which involves the skin extensively with bullae and the eyes and mucous membranes with ulcerations, is termed the Stevens-Johnson syndrome. In *erythema nodosum,* crops of tender erythematous subcutaneous nodules typically develop around the ankles and lower extremities, sometimes accompanied by synovitis and fever, and slowly resolve, usually leaving a small ecchymotic area. The underlying etiology of erythema nodosum may be a drug allergy (sulfonamides, bromides, iodides, oral contraceptive pills), sarcoidosis, inflammatory bowel disease, primary tuberculosis, a variety of primary fungal infections including histoplasmosis and coccidioidomycosis, streptococcal infection, and other disorders, but frequently no specific etiology can be identified.

Treatment of generalized exanthems generally consists of rest, increased fluid intake, antihistamines, occasionally colloidal baths to relieve intense pruritus, and discontinuation of the offending agent if identified. Treatment of vasculitis is beyond the scope of this text, but small vessel systemic vasculitis (hypersensitivity angiitis) involving the skin and erythema nodosum both respond to oral corticosteroids, generally given in the latter case only when symptoms are disabling.

BACTERIAL INFECTIONS OF SKIN

Streptococci and staphylococci cause the majority of primary bacterial skin infections. Antibiotic therapy generally consists of a semisynthetic penicillin or topical antibiotics. The infections are divided into morphologic subtypes, the chief importance of which is that management differs somewhat for each type and that recognition of their characteristic features allows one to differentiate the primary skin infections from other types of lesions.

Focal infections consist of impetigo, ecthyma, folliculitis, furuncles, and carbuncles. *Impetigo,* typically a streptococcal infection most commonly involving the face in children, begins as a small vesicle that usually ruptures, leaving a superficial erosion on which forms the characteristic "honey-colored" crust. Occasionally, impetigo is manifested by bullae, which may coalesce into an exfoliative lesion. Bullous impetigo is always a staphylococcal infection. *Ecthyma* is a deeper local infection, also usually occurring in children and often involving the buttock following insect bite, trauma, scabies, eczema, or some other local lesion. It begins as a vesicle that ruptures, leaving a crust or area of exfoliation upon an indurated, erythematous base. Unlike impetigo, ecthyma may result in scarring. *Folliculitis,* usually caused by staphylococci, consists of small pustules at the bases of hair follicles, most commonly in the area of the beard or scalp. More extensive, deeper infection of a hair follicle, also usually staphylococcal in etiology, is termed a *furuncle* if only a single follicle is involved, or a *carbuncle* if several adjacent follicles with multiple sites of drainage are involved. These lesions begin as inflammatory nodules and develop purulent drainage. They occur typically on the buttocks, axillae, neck, and waist and are particularly common in obese individuals, diabetics, or debilitated persons.

Very mild impetigo is managed by gentle washcloth débridement followed by application of Burow's solution compresses and topical mupirocin (Bactroban). More severe cases of impetigo as well as most cases of ecthyma should receive oral penicillin. It is best also to use Hibiclens wash to help disinfect the entire skin surface and avoid a relapse after the 10- to 14-day antibiotic therapy. Bullous impetigo should be treated with semisynthetic penicillin on the presumption that a penicillin-resistant staphylococcal infection is the cause. Most cases of folliculitis can be eradicated by frequent washing with a chlorhexidine-containing bactericidal soap. Erythromycin, 250 mg four times daily for 10 to 14 days, is usually effective. To prevent recurrent folliculitis, the patient may be advised to use Hibiclens wash, apply bacitracin or mupiricin ointment to the anterior nares, to soak the face for 5 minutes with a hot washcloth before shaving, to use separate towels, sheets, and clothing, and either to discard razor blades or soak them in alcohol prior to using. Furuncles and carbuncles are managed with warm compresses (e.g., tap water or Burow's solution applied for 10 to 20 minutes, three to four times daily). Appearance of a necrotic white area on the surface of a large nodule is an indication for incision and drainage; smaller lesions resolve spontaneously without requiring drainage. A semisynthetic penicillin taken by mouth for 10 to 14 days is prescribed if the furuncle or carbuncle is accompanied by fever or cellulitis, if the lesion involves the face or perineal region, or if the patient is at risk from bacteremia (e.g., has an artificial joint or heart valve).

Recurrent furuncles or carbuncles represent a difficult problem in management. General measures such as changing bedding and sheets, use of clean towels, application of bacitracin or mupiricin ointment to the anterior nares, frequent bathing with a chlorhexidine-containing soap, and measures to keep intertriginous areas dry should be employed but are not always preventive. In some patients with frequent recurrent carbuncles, prophylaxis with twice-daily doses of a semisynthetic oral penicillin has prevented recurrent infection for periods of up to 6 months.

Recurrent abscesses involving apocrine sweat glands in the axillary or perineal regions are termed *hidradenitis suppurativa*. Single abscesses may be treated by orally administered antibiotics, wet compresses, and incision and drainage when necessary. Patients with frequent recurrent abscesses often respond to administration of a topical clindamycin-containing solution applied twice daily to affected areas. In extremely severe cases, plastic surgery to remove the areas of apocrine glands has been efficacious.

Cellulitis and *erysipelas* are primary spreading bacterial infections of skin. Characteristic features of cellulitis allow one to differentiate it from phlebitis and other inflammatory conditions. These include the deep violaceous hue of the lesion, its relatively sharp margins, and its degree of painfulness when compared with phlebitis, as well as lymphangitic spreading when present, accompanying lymphadenitis, fever, and leukocytosis. Any part of the body may be involved but most common is the lower extremities. Edema is a predisposing factor. Usually also there is a portal of entry—for example, an area of eczema that becomes secondarily infected or a scrape or puncture wound. In some cases no portal may be obvious, but entry can be through an area of maceration between the toes or tinea pedis. Diabetics and debilitated persons are predisposed to developing cellulitis. Streptococci and staphylococci are the most common pathogens. One should be aware, however, that enteric aerobic and anaerobic organisms may cause cellulitis in the perineum, and anaerobic organisms are typically involved when the infection develops from a diabetic foot ulcer, deep abscess, or traumatic wound. Such cases are characterized mostly by local infection with tissue necrosis and burrowing abscesses; when accompanied by spreading cellulitis and lymphangitis, streptococci or staphylococci are usually also involved.

Erysipelas, a superficial cellulitis that usually involves the face, is characterized by its very well-demarcated margin, more so than in deeper cellulitis. It usually begins as a small, erythematous plaque and rapidly spreads in the form of a painful, circumscribed infiltration.

Antibiotic therapy is indicated for both cellulitis and erysipelas. One may rely on treatment with a semisynthetic penicillin administered orally for 7 to 14 days in mild cases. More severe cases require hospitalization of the patient and treatment with intravenously administered antibiotics. As a rule, we favor hospitalization in questionable cases. Specific indications to hospitalize a patient include more than minimal involvement of the face or perineal region, a debilitated or immunosuppressed host or one with uncontrolled diabetes, or the presence of any large lesion—one with lymphangitic spreading, high fever, or rigors. Management includes elevation of the affected part, protection from trauma, and control of edema. We administer intravenous antibiotics until the patient is afebrile and the cellulitis is clearly subsiding; we then prefer to maintain oral antibiotics for at least an additional 7 to 14 days. A tetanus booster should be given if the patient has not received one within 5 years; in previously unvaccinated individuals, one must consider simultaneous administration of tetanus immunization and hyperimmune globulin.

Bacterial infections often secondarily involve lesions such as eczema or decubitus ulcers. Crusting on the surface of such a lesion, as well as purulence, is a sign of the secondary infection. When such a lesion becomes infected, in most cases therapy with a topically administered antibiotic ointment is sufficient. Occurrence of an eczematous-like rash around an area of bacterial infection, such as otitis externa, may be treated by application of Burow's soaks or compresses plus addition of a topical corticosteroid to the antibiotic solution or ointment. Infected stasis ulcers also are managed with wet compresses and antibiotic-containing ointment; systemically administered antibiotics are added if cellulitis develops. The primary cause of the ulcer must be treated, of course; in the case of stasis ulcers, this usually requires a period of bedrest with elevation of the involved extremity if the ulcer is infected. Following control of infection, recurrence of edema may be prevented by use of Ace bandages or a pressure-gradient (Jobst) stocking.

ACNE VULGARIS AND ACNE ROSACEA

Although *acne vulgaris* is most common in adolescents and young adults—and leads about 15% of adolescents to consult a physician—it may be present at any age. Physicians in internal medicine probably encounter acne rosacea at least as frequently. The diagnosis of either condition should be made from the physical examination. The comedo (plugged hair follicle–sebaceous gland resulting in a "blackhead") is characteristic of acne vulgaris. Also characteristic are "whiteheads," closed comedones produced by accumulation of material within an unruptured plugged sebaceous duct. These lesions typically are distributed most prominently on the face and neck and also involve the back and chest of some persons. Comedones are found in combination with papules and pustules, resulting from rupture of a sebaceous duct with resultant inflammatory reaction, and with cysts and scars in some cases. Rupture of plugged ducts and the consequent inflammation are related to bacterial colonization with *Propionibacterium acnes* and *Staphylococcus epidermidis*. *Acne rosacea* involves the nose, cheeks, the central third of the forehead, and chin. It consists of diffuse redness and accompanying papules and pustules without comedones. Telangiectatic venules occur frequently, and in longstanding cases patients develop hypertrophy of the nasal skin, termed rhinophyma. The diagnosis based on these features is usually straightforward in both forms of acne.

Management. Treatment of acne may be indicated to lessen emotional problems associated with having the lesions, as well as to prevent scarring. Scarring tends to occur in cystic acne, and these patients probably should be referred for treatment to a dermatologist. In fact, the problem of acne makes up a considerable proportion (27.4% in one study) of dermatologists' practice in a community.[2] Generalists may prefer to treat mild cases. Patient education is important for several reasons, not the least of which is to lessen the patient's emotional trauma from having acne. The condition results from plugging of pilosebaceous follicles, followed by bacterial colonization. There is no evidence that it is related in any systematic way to lack of cleanliness, dietary factors, or sexual activity. It cannot be prevented by washing the face, although, of course, patients with acne should employ good hygiene. Cleansing the involved areas twice daily with ordinary soap is sufficient. A well-balanced diet, reasonable amounts of rest and relaxation, avoidance of androgenic oral contraceptive steroids, and avoidance of creams and oils on the face is also recommended. Use of makeup is important for teenage girls but cosmetics should consist of nongreasy, nonmedicated compounds, preferably those labeled "noncomedogenic" or "nonacnegenic." Associated seborrheic dermatitis of the scalp may be controlled by selenium sulfide or zinc pyrithione shampoos. Clinical assessment should be sufficient to exclude an underlying endocrine disorder, such as Cushing's syndrome. Patients should understand that response to therapy is generally slow and that the disease can be controlled but is not eradicated in most cases. It reaches peak severity at ages 16 to 17 years in girls and 17 to 19 years in boys and often persists into the early 20s in both sexes. Acne may appear de novo in women in their mid-20s to mid-30s. Cystic acne may persist for several decades.

Specific treatments include topical retinoic acid, topical benzoyl peroxide, topical and oral antibiotics, and 13-*cis*-retinoic acid (isotretinoin) taken by mouth. Of these, the one that loosens keratin plugs and thus prevents and removes both open and closed comedones is topical retinoic acid, so it is useful for the noninflammatory phase of acne vulgaris. It may be applied as a cream, gel, or lotion, covering the affected area at night before retiring, in concentrations of 0.1 to 0.025%. Topical retinoic acid may produce erythema, irritation, and peeling of skin, particularly in light-skinned individuals. Sun exposure should be minimized and a No. 15 (or higher) sunscreen should be used in the morning during treatment. The dosage may be adjusted downward, as necessary, to minimize visible erythema. The 0.025% cream seems to be the best-tolerated preparation, and initial therapy should employ alternate-day applications.

Treatment of mild inflammatory acne begins with topical benzoyl peroxide. The cream or lotion is applied to affected areas once or twice daily, avoiding the eyes and mucous membranes. Information indicates that a concentration of 2.5% is as effective as 5 or 10% and is much less irritating. Like retinoic acid, benzoyl peroxide may produce a primary irritant dermatitis with redness and peeling of skin, which may be more severe in light-skinned individuals. The patient should be warned of this possible side effect but instructed to continue therapy for several weeks if the dermatitis is mild, because the reaction usually diminishes. When the reaction is severe, the dose of benzoyl peroxide may be reduced. An alternate delivery system is to use a 10% benzoyl peroxide wash twice daily instead of soap. This topical therapy generally is continued throughout the course of acne. Benzoyl peroxide is not very effective for closed comedones, which respond best to topical retinoic acid. The two preparations are most effective when used in conjunction, but the patient should apply one in the morning and the other at bedtime to avoid oxidation of the retinoic acid by the peroxide.

Antibiotics are the most effective standard treatment for severe cases characterized by inflammation. They work synergistically with topical therapy. Since they prevent new lesions but do not suppress established lesions, the patient should be cautioned not to expect immediate improvement. Tetracycline or erythromycin may be given in an initial dose of 500 mg taken orally two times daily. Once substantial clearing has occurred, the dose may be tapered gradually to the lowest effective level, at times as low as 250 mg taken every other day. Once clearing is maintained for 6 months on a low dose, trial discontinuation is recommended. The majority of cases reactivate after therapy, but additional courses can be prescribed. Side effects at these doses are few but sometimes include oral or vaginal candidal infection or nonspecific gastrointestinal upset. Tetracycline should be taken on an empty stomach and not concurrently with milk products or antacids. It must be avoided during pregnancy and in persons younger than 10 to 12 years of age. Topical 1.5% erythromycin or 1% clindamycin solutions are also effective in reducing inflammatory lesions of acne in most cases. We suggest that topical therapy be used even when oral antibiotics are given to reduce the dose of oral agents required. In addition, oral antibiotic therapy is not effective at clearing comedones.

A variety of other compounds have been tried in acne but none are of proven efficacy. As a rule, the agents just listed have replaced older types of therapy, including the use of sulfa, salicylic acid, and resorcinol.

Cystic acne lesions unresponsive to topical and oral therapy may be treated effectively by intralesional injection of 0.01 ml of a fluorinated corticosteroid compound. Lesions also can be frozen with liquid nitrogen. Patients should be warned, however, against attempting to incise and drain their own lesions. Incision of pustular lesions requires use of special instruments to avoid scarring.

The most potent agent used in treatment of acne is 13-*cis*-retinoic acid (isotretinoin, Accutane). This treatment, given orally in doses of 0.05 to 1 mg/kg/day for 15 to 20 weeks, produces improvement in most cases of both noninflammatory and inflammatory lesions. Side effects include cheilitis, common in all patients, and myalgias/arthralgias, occurring in a few patients. Others complain of anorexia, fatigue, xerosis, dryness of the nasal mucosa, and conjunctivitis. A small number of patients have persistent dry eyes (over 1 year) and a few develop vertebral periosteal thickening. The drug is a potent teratogen and is contraindicated in pregnancy. It seems prudent for a specialist with adequate experience to monitor the use of this drug. The drug reduces the size of sebaceous glands and inhibits sebum production. A single course of therapy has completely cured acne without recurrence in many cases. It has been used successfully also in a few cases of acne rosacea and hidradenitis suppurativa. The major concern with using this drug is the sometimes unpredictable increase in triglyceride levels; the increases may persist after discontinuation. For this reason, the drug should be reserved for severe cases that are unresponsive to conventional therapy. This drug is not now a first-line treatment for acne because its long-term adverse consequences are not fully known.

Management of acne rosacea includes avoidance of spicy foods, hot beverages, and alcohol, which aggravate the condition because of their vasodilating effects. Fluorinated steroids should also be avoided because they produce atrophy and worsening of telangiectasias. Exposure to sunlight should be diminished, and a sunscreen should be used. The most effective treatments are antibiotics. Tetracycline may be prescribed as for patients with acne vulgaris; it lessens the papular and pustular inflammatory lesions. Acne rosacea responds much more quickly to therapy, and the dose of tetracycline is often one half that used in acne vulgaris. Topical antibiotics are often effective, including metronidazole (MetroGel), erythromycin, and clindamycin. Almost all patients with acne rosacea require long-term maintenance therapy to remain clear of lesions.

Since the rhinophyma is a lobulated overgrowth of the sebaceous glands of the skin and does not involve the subcutaneous tissue, it is possible to excise the excess tissue, leaving a good cosmetic result when done by an experienced practitioner.

Perioral dermatitis is probably a variant of acne rosacea. Greasy cosmetics and fluorinated corticosteroids are contraindicated. Perioral dermatitis may be treated with topical metronidazole, erythromycin, or clindamycin along with 1% hydrocortisone cream. Often oral tetracycline will be necessary on a short-term (4 to 8 weeks) basis. If recurrence is seen after withdrawal of tetracycline, long-term maintenance therapy may be required.

PAPULOSQUAMOUS DISORDERS

Psoriasis, seborrheic dermatitis, and *pityriasis rosea* are the papulosquamous disorders most encountered by primary care physicians. Tinea versicolor, lichen planus, secondary syphilis, and some drug eruptions may have similar morphologic features and must be differentiated from the more common entities.

Psoriasis. Psoriasis can usually be recognized from its typical morphology—well-demarcated plaques with heaped-up whitish or silvery scales that leave punctate bleeding points when removed—and its distribution—characteristically the elbows and knees, scalp, perirectal and periumbilical regions, and nails (see Fig. 69–2*D*). The lesions are chronic and for the most part asymptomatic or only mildly pruritic. They result from an increased pool of actively proliferating keratinocytes and are not accompanied by constitutional symptoms (however, associated arthritis of several types does occur, as described in Chapter 50). Morphologically distinct forms of psoriasis are guttate psoriasis, an acute outbreak of widely distributed, small, drop-like, scaly papular lesions, often a reaction to streptococcal pharyngitis, and *pustular psoriasis,* an outbreaking of psoriatic lesions with sterile pustules, often involving the palms and soles. Nail involvement with pitting and hyperkeratotic thickening commonly accompanies psoriasis.

Seborrheic Dermatitis. This mildly pruritic, erythematous scaling lesion occurs in characteristic locations: the scalp, areas of the face around the scalp, eyebrows, nasolabial folds, behind the ears, and sometimes the axillary and pubic areas. The scales are much finer than those of psoriasis. The erythematous plaque-like rash characteristically is less well demarcated than psoriasis. It occurs most often in persons with oily skin and is often associated with acne.

Pityriasis Rosea. This self-limited, mildly pruritic eruption is most commonly seen in young adults and is possibly of viral etiology. The lesions have a characteristic distribution over the trunk. They are preceded by a "herald patch," which is usually a larger, scaly plaque. The outcropping of smaller, oval, discrete, slightly scaly plaques usually involving the trunk is then characteristic and persists for an average of 6 weeks. A scraping to rule out fungus and a serologic test to rule out secondary syphilis are recommended.

Differential Diagnosis

As a rule, the papulosquamous disorders have more well-demarcated borders than do lesions of eczematous dermatitis. They lack the central clearing and slightly rolled margins and are more widely distributed than tinea corporis. Tinea versicolor, however, usually involves the trunk more diffusely, is chronic, asymptomatic, and characterized by whitish or tan, irregularly shaped lesions. In secondary syphilis, onset of the rash is abrupt, pruritus is absent, fever is often present, and the oral and genital mucous membranes are often involved. The papulosquamous-like lesions of secondary syphilis are most prominantly distributed on the palms and soles. However, a serologic test for syphilis should be obtained in any patient with acute onset of diffuse papulosquamous lesions, even when the features are typically those of pityriasis rosea.

In lichen planus, lesions have a shiny, flat-topped, violaceous, papular appearance and are most commonly distributed along the volar surfaces of the wrists. The legs, upper chest, and back are other common sites. Occasionally lichen planus is generalized. Onset is typically abrupt, but the lesions may persist for months or years. Whitish gyrate or lacy patches of the buccal mucous membranes are a characteristic feature of many cases. The Koebner phenomenon, which occurs in psoriasis as well as in lichen planus, refers to the development of typical skin lesions along the distribution of scratches or other skin abrasions. Pruritus in lichen planus is often severe.

Drug eruptions with a pityriasis rosea-like appearance have been associated with barbiturates, antihistamines, captopril, bismuth, and gold; eruptions with a lichen planus–like appearance are described in allergy to arsenic, gold, and Atabrine. Eruptions may take various appearances and may exfoliate, but as a rule drug eruptions are more diffuse and confluent than are the papulosquamous disorders. In the final analysis, one must depend on the history of taking a pharmocologic agent and the response to a trial of discontinuing the agent to determine the approach to a patient suspected of having a drug eruption.

Management

Topical corticosteroids are mainstays in the management of all these inflammatory dermatoses. In each case, however, different approaches are taken, and there is a role for other medications designed to help alleviate symptoms or promote the effectiveness of corticosteroids. In scaly inflammatory disorders the goals are to hydrate and soften scale, remove excess scale, reduce formation of scale, reduce inflammation, and reduce itching.

Ointment will decrease water loss to the air and will hydrate scale and therefore make it softer, more flexible, and more permeable to other medications. Plain petrolatum works but is messy. Aquaphor or Eucerin is less messy (Eucerin is Aquaphor mixed 50:50 with water). Even less messy, but more expensive, is Complex 15 cream.

Keratolytic agents weaken the bond between the corneocytes of the stratum corneum. When used effectively these agents can débride scales. A salicylic acid, propylene gel (Keralyt), is very effective but will sting fissures. It is more elegant to use than petrolatum with 5 to 10% salicylic acid, which can be followed by a coat of steroid-containing ointment or cream or by coal tar or by both. Somewhat less potent but still very useful are lactic acid preparations, the strongest available being Lac-Hydrin lotion, containing 12% ammonium lactate. Urea in 15 to 20% concentration (Ultra Mide) is also effective but less potent.

Coal tar derivatives reduce the kinetics of the epidermal proliferation and thus reduce scale production. They also are photosensitizing. Estar Gel and T/Derm body oil are elegant tar preparations.

Ultraviolet radiation in the form of sunlight or mid-ultraviolet (UVB) lamps is also effective in reducing the epidermal proliferation. Severe sunburn followed by withdrawal of exposure can result in a backlash flare and should be avoided. If a sunburn occurs, one should use intensive topical steroids acutely and resume lower-dose UV therapy as soon as the skin will tolerate it. Photochemotherapy using oral psoralen plus strong long-wave UV lamps (PUVA) is much more potent, more complicated, and more risk prone but can clear the skin of about 75 or 80% of patients, who then require either maintenance treatments at reduced frequency or repeat courses to clear up subsequent relapses. In one study, the risk of skin malignancy, especially squamous cell carcinoma, was one case per 52 years of PUVA therapy after several years of follow-up and was dose related. PUVA plus UVB should be reserved for failures of topical therapy because of the risk of inducing actinic skin damage with subsequent increased risk of squamous cell carcinoma.

Topical corticosteroids are anti-inflammatory, antipruritic, and vasoconstrictive and reduce excess epidermal proliferation. The vehicle is important in providing an emollient/protective effect; ointment will work better than lotions or creams. Lotions should be reserved for hairy scalp and creams for intertriginous areas. Patients may prefer creams for daytime use but will use ointments overnight. The risk of dermal atrophy with prolonged use is negligible with 1% hydrocortisone. The more potent the steroid the higher is the risk, but the effectiveness is greater. Intertriginous areas and the face are at highest risk, but they often respond to 1% hydrocortisone. If that is not effective, 0.2% hydrocortisone valerate or 0.1% triamcinolone acetonide is a reasonable next step up the ladder. Palms and soles require the most potent agents such as Ultravate, Temovate, Diprolene, Diprosone, Halog, Florone, Lidex, and Topicort. Occlusion enhances the therapeutic efficacy of topical steroids. Ointments are partially occlusive. Plastic gloves or Saran Wrap is completely occlusive. A midpotency corticosteroid incorporated into the adhesive side of a transparent flexible plastic tape (Cordran tape) is useful for small lesions.

Chemotherapy with methotrexate should be reserved for cases unresponsive to maximum strength topical therapy, as well as to PUVA if that is appropriate. The other acceptable indication for methotrexate is severe psoriatic arthritis mutilans (see Chapter 50). Methotrexate is an antimitotic and reduces epidermal proliferation; it may be anti-inflammatory as well. Renal and hepatic function must be excellent if it is used, and alcohol consumption is a contraindication. Cirrhosis of the liver induced by the drug is the usual long-term limiting factor of methotrexate therapy.

In treating seborrheic dermatitis involving the face, fluorinated corticosteroids are contraindicated; treatment consists of application of a hydrocortisone preparation, 0.5 to 1% strength, massaged into the involved areas twice daily. For both psoriasis and seborrheic dermatitis involving the scalp, a shampoo with 2.5% selenium sulfide suspension (Selsun), 2% zinc pyrithione (Sebulon), or ketoconazole (Nizoral) daily or every other day, may be utilized for control of symptoms. Use of the shampoo to wash the face often reduces or eliminates the need to use corticosteroid treatment there. Shampooing will need to be continued indefinitely but may be tapered somewhat in frequency depending on the clinical response. The scalp may also be treated by application of a steroid lotion after shampooing.

In pityriasis rosea, there is often no pruritus. If pruritus is present, initial therapy consists of an antihistamine taken by mouth or a colloidal bath (e.g., Aveeno in 6 to 8 inches of lukewarm water) for control of itching. Dry, scaly lesions may be treated by the addition of hydrocortisone ointment to soften them, but the lesions are not steroid responsive. Severe, symptomatic cases often improve with UVB phototherapy. The rash of pityriasis rosea generally resolves spontaneously after 6 weeks and usually does not recur.

Lichen planus is difficult to treat because it responds poorly to topical corticosteroid preparations, may be severely pruritic, and may persist for up to 9 months. Management includes use of antipruritic agents like camphor, phenol, or coal tar in a lotion, fluorinated topical corticosteroids applied beneath an occlusive dressing, and the addition of a minor tranquilizer or antihistaminic agent to control itching and aid in sleep. Patients with persistent symptoms may respond to a brief course of oral corticosteroid therapy. PUVA has been effective in some patients with severe recalcitrant lichen planus.

ALOPECIA

The approach to alopecia depends on the type of hair loss. Hair loss is divided into nonscarring and scarring types, each of which has a different differential diagnosis. The other major distinction is patchy and diffuse hair loss.

Patchy Hair Loss. Alopecia areata and tinea scalp infection are the most common causes of nonscarring patchy hair loss. Alopecia areata is manifested by one or more slowly enlarging areas of hair loss, with smooth regular borders, usually involving the scalp but sometimes the beard or an eyebrow. This condition occurs most commonly in young adults but has a worse prognosis in a prepubescent child. Alopecia totalis, in which all scalp hair is lost, also has a worse prognosis. There is no scarring or scaling in the area of hair loss in alopecia areata. At the periphery of the hair loss, one can usually detect what are termed "exclamation point hairs," which represent breaking off of the hair 2 to 3 mm above the surface, giving it the appearance of an exclamation point as the top portion appears thicker than the base of the hair. Treatment of alopecia areata consists for the most part of reassurance. One may inform the patient with local hair loss due to this condition that it is generally spontaneously reversible after 6 to 12 months and rarely progresses to involve the entire scalp.

Conversely, alopecia totalis carries a poor prognosis for complete recovery and may require wearing a wig. Patients with alopecia areata may be given treatment for associated seborrhea, but there is no role for seborrhea in this or other types of hair loss. Further treatment involves use of corticosteroids, anthralin, and topical minoxidil. Corticosteroids may be applied as a lotion (Diprolene, Temovate, or Ultravate) or, in severe cases, as intralesional injections given by a dermatologist. These injections can be of some benefit, but there is a risk of localized dermal atrophy, especially if numerous repeat injections are required. Topical anthralin (Drithoscalp), to the point of causing some irritation, often stimulates regrowth. Topical minoxidil may help regrowth and prolong periods of remission.

Alopecia areata is distinguished from fungal infection of the scalp because the latter lacks the exclamation point hairs, is accompanied by scaliness, usually occurs in children, and may be recognized by fluorescence using a Wood light or by a positive KOH preparation. Other forms of nonscarring hair loss include trichotillomania, in which the patient obsessively pulls out his or her own hairs in an irregular shape or pattern, and secondary syphilis, in which hair loss is accompanied by other manifestations of the disease, including oral lesions, skin rash, fever, and a positive result on a serologic test for syphilis.

Patchy hair loss with scarring, unlike the nonscarring varieties, is rarely reversible. This may result from tinea of the scalp if secondarily infected with bacteria or from an unusually severe and inflammatory fungal infection itself. Bacterial infection of the scalp, such as a carbuncle, will leave a scar in which hair growth does not resume. Any other condition that leaves scarring of the scalp may similarly affect hair growth. In discoid lupus erythematosus, the hair loss is accompanied by scaly erythema, atrophy, and depigmentation. Other agents that affect the scalp with scarring include third-degree burns, trauma, chemical agents, herpes zoster, scalp neoplasms, and skin conditions such as lichen planus or scleroderma.

Diffuse Hair Loss. Diffuse nonscarring hair loss is most commonly androgenetic alopecia. Men are affected most frequently and most severely. This normal hereditary pattern typically involves recession of the hairline in the temporal regions, sometimes accompanied by an enlarging area of hair loss at the vertex. Women may develop a hereditary pattern of diffuse hair loss, usually beginning after 50 years of age and most prominently affecting the vertex, without progression to complete loss of hair. Temporary hair loss in both sexes may follow any condition producing high fever. On other occasions, an apparently normal woman may complain that hair is falling out profusely, even though examination reveals no areas of baldness or unusual thinning. Some women note abnormal hair loss following normal pregnancy. The explanation is that hair growth is more luxuriant during pregnancy, resulting in temporary abnormal hair loss following pregnancy as the hair returns to its usual thickness. Diffuse hair loss may also follow chemotherapy or radiotherapy, may be associated with certain diseases such as exfoliative dermatitis, systemic lupus erythematosus, or dermatomyositis, or may be associated with iron deficiency, drugs, or endocrine abnormalities, including hypothyroidism, Cushing's syndrome, and hypopituitarism. The latter are recognized by their history and by the accompanying clinical and laboratory features of these disorders. Women with diffuse hair loss should be evaluated carefully for signs of virilism on physical examination. Laboratory studies to check for iron deficiency, hyper- or hypothyroidism, and increased adrenal or ovarian androgens should be performed. Any medications taken within several months of the onset of the hair loss should be investigated to see whether or not any such medication has been associated with hair loss; anticoagulants and oral contraceptives are two common classes of medication with such an association.

In simple androgenetic alopecia in either sex, it is reasonable to use topical minoxidil (Rogaine). Responders will note fewer hairs being shed after 4 to 6 months of use. A minority of users will get significant regrowth, but most will markedly reduce further loss.

XEROSIS AND GENERALIZED PRURITUS

Xerosis, or dry skin, is a common complaint in the practice of primary care physicians as well as dermatologists. *Pruritus* of a generalized nature is usually associated with this complaint, but of course the differential diagnosis of generalized pruritus also includes medical and other conditions that are not accompanied specifically by dry skin. Xerosis itself occurs most commonly in the elderly, is usually experienced during the winter because of decreased humidity in heated houses and apartments, and usually involves the legs most prominently. Symptoms are worse at night. The shoulders, beltline, and sacrum are also frequently involved. At times, there may be no findings other than dry skin, but more severe cases often have visible dry plaques, scales, or excoriations. The preponderance of elderly patients is probably accounted for by the decreased effectiveness of the barrier function of stratum corneum that occurs with aging. Excessive bathing and use of drying soaps promote this condition. It may be referred to as senile pruritus. In the young, one must consider the possibility of an underlying internal malignancy such as Hodgkin's disease or lymphosarcoma.

Xerosis also occurs in a hereditary form. The most common type is *ichthyosis vulgaris,* inherited in the autosomal dominant pattern and manifested by the occurrence of small, polygonal, whitish scales over the arms, legs, and sometimes entire body. This condition generally worsens with aging. In ichthyosis vulgaris, the stratum corneum cells do not exfoliate as soon as normal ones, thus causing the build-up of a thickened stratum corneum layer—somewhat like a callus. This thickened layer is susceptible to dehydration and cracking. If the hyperkeratosis is thick enough on the palms and soles, fissuring may occur. Like senile and essential pruritis, the symptoms of ichthyosis vulgaris tend to diminish in the summer when the air is humid and to recur in the winter.

Generalized pruritus may occur without any primary skin lesions, sometimes secondary to other disorders.

Evaluation and Differential Diagnosis. Many patients believe that their symptoms of pruritus are caused by a dermatologic condition, and one should search for any specific manifestations of such a condition. In fact, the major task of the physician is to sort out patients whose pruritus is secondary to some skin disorder from patients whose pruritus cannot be so explained. In addition to xerosis and ichthyosis, the physician should look for the characteristic burrows of scabies; the nits associated with pediculosis; urticarial or angioedematous lesions; the typical small blisters and papular hives of the scapular areas, elbows, knees, and buttocks of dermatitis herpetiformis; and the characteristic plaques of eczematous dermatitis, lichen planus, and psoriasis. If peculiar lesions are found, a skin biopsy for diagnosis may be appropriate.

The internist is often asked to evaluate the patient for an underlying systemic illness when the complaint is generalized pruritus without primary skin lesions. The history of drug ingestion or exposure to other allergens such as pets or intestinal parasites is pertinent. An evaluation should also include testing for hypo- or hyperthyroidism, diabetes mellitus, hypercalcemia, uremia, and cholestasis. A blood count should be obtained to exclude polycythemia, iron deficiency anemia, and eosinophilia. Pruritus is also associated with the last trimester of pregnancy. The most difficult aspect of the medical work-up is deciding how far to go to exclude Hodgkin's disease, lymphoma, or other internal malignancy. One would, of course, search for lymph nodes and obtain a chest roentgenogram. If the patient were young and had unexplained ichthyosis of recent onset, if pruritus were accompanied by weight loss, fever, night sweats, or general malaise, or if the severity of the pruritus in an individual of any age were out of proportion to the finding of dry skin, then one should obtain further testing to search for underlying malignancy. Such testing might include an ultrasound examination or computed tomography of the abdomen and retroperitoneum.

Psychogenic causes of generalized pruritus are frequently considered. In our experience, such a complaint often represents exaggerated perception of pruritus by the patient who has dry skin concurrently with a psychiatric problem. The most typical example is the elderly patient with agitated depression. Psychogenic pruritus is said to be particularly severe at night, although pruritus of any cause is usually more severe at night because of the decrease in other stimuli. Only if the result of the work-up is negative for systemic causes of pruritus and if there are no dermatologic findings of the specific conditions aforementioned may one consider a psychogenic cause. If the patient's perception and concern about pruritus far exceeds what would be expected from the degree of dryness of the skin, one may be tempted to attribute the symptoms to the psyche. The diagnosis of psychogenic pruritus, however, is best made by eliciting specific features of the psychiatric disorder, such as depression, agitation, and anxiety. The diagnosis of "delusional parasitosis" can be made from the patient's bizarre description of his or her symptoms. This usually includes a rather colorful description of the perceived parasites, with bizarre overtones or accompanying delusions of internal decay, often associated with recognizable agitation or anxiety. Such patients may have schizophrenia, or, if elderly, agitated depression and senility. Once a specific psychiatric disorder of any of these types has been recognized, one may proceed with its management. If the psychiatric disorder is also accompanied by some degree of pruritus due to dry skin, this may be managed as well. However, even if a psychiatric disorder is present, one should not attribute the etiology of pruritus to it until an evaluation for other causes is negative.

Management. Environmental factors of possible significance, such as lack of humidity, exposure to fiberglass, sunburn, and excessive bathing, should be corrected or removed. Patients should also avoid coffee, alcohol, and spices since vasodilatation may worsen pruritus. Time spent in the tub or shower should be minimized. Wool clothes should not be in direct contact with the skin, and cotton clothing should be rinsed twice in order to remove all detergents. Patients with dry skin may be advised to diminish the frequency of bathing, to add a bath oil to the tub (e.g., Lubath, Domol, Nivea, Alpha Keri), or both. An emollient soap (e.g., Dove, Aveeno bar, Basis) should be used. One should also recommend use of a humidifier in the bedroom during the heating season. Patients with ichthyosis vulgaris or senile or essential dry skin should be cautioned that no cure for the condition is available, though the symptoms can be lessened. One of the most effective treatments is ammonium lactate 12% lotion (Lac-Hydrin), which tends to normalize the structure and function of the stratum corneum.

Additional treatment may include application of an emollient to the skin, such as Nivea or Eucerin skin oil or cream, Keri lotion or cream, Lubriderm lotion or cream, or white vaseline. These may be applied before bedtime. Less greasy products that are effective moisturizers are Complex 15 cream and LactiCare lotion. Menthol, 0.25%, can be added, or it may be convenient to recommend Sarna lotion (containing menthol, camphor, and phenol) for ad libitum applications. This usually controls pruritus for 15 minutes to several hours. Pramegel (menthol and pramoxine hydrochloride), a nonsensitizing topical antihistamine (also available as Prax lotion) is another useful topical antipruritic agent. Topical corticosteroids are effective antipruritic agents, but chronic use will cause dermal atrophy if preparations stronger than 1% hydrocortisone are used. For patients afflicted with insomnia caused by pruritus, one may prescribe an antihistamine with sedative properties (e.g., Benadryl) at night. Most patients with mild senile or essential pruritus, however, can be managed by altering their environment and by topical therapy, thus one may not need to resort to pharmacotherapy. If daytime antihistamine therapy is necessary, reserve Benadryl for a bedtime sedative and use instead hydroxyzine hydrochloride, 10 to 50 mg every 4 to 6 hours (the generic form is less expensive than Atarax) or chlorpheniramine maleate, 2 to 12 mg every 4 to 6 hours (now available in an inexpensive over-the-counter generic brand).

Another condition common in hot, humid climates is prickly heat resulting from maceration of the skin. Patients complain of burning or pruritus and manifest tiny vesicular papules caused by obstruction, dilatation, and rupture of sweat ducts on the neck, back, trunk, and body folds. Unlike pruritus caused by dry skin, this form of pruritus is treated by preventing maceration from too much wetness by means of a fan or air conditioner and by application of a dusting powder like Zeasorb.

URTICARIA AND ANGIOEDEMA

Urticaria, also called hives, is a local reaction characterized by nonpitting, localized plaques of edema extending into the superficial portion of the dermis. Angioedema may accompany urticaria produced by any cause and has a similar pathogenesis, but the swelling extends to subcutaneous tissue. Both urticaria and angioedema are characterized by well-demarcated, nonpitting swelling. Urticarial and angioedematous lesions are generally of rapid onset, are pruritic, develop in crops persisting for up to 72 hours, and are distributed asymmetrically. Urticarial lesions themselves range in size from small papules to giant hives, have red borders with paler central areas, and are transient, tending to fade out while new crops of lesions develop. Acute urticaria persists for less than 6 to 8 weeks; that persisting for more than 8 weeks is defined as chronic urticaria.

Etiologies. Urticaria associated with seasonal allergy or specific allergy to a drug, food, inhaled antigen, intestinal parasite, or insect bite (Hymenoptera) is IgE-mediated and usually associated with eosinophilia. The most common specific cause is food allergy, most commonly from shellfish, nuts, cheeses, strawberries, chocolate, pork, tomatoes, fresh fruits, and sometimes milk containing traces of penicillin. One must depend on obtaining a history of symptoms following exposure to the specific food to make this diagnosis, and one also depends on the history of exposure to an inhaled allergen or animal dander to identify these potential allergens as causes. If urticaria is seasonal or associated with allergic rhinitis or atopic eczema, one may also presume an allergic basis. The most commonly involved drugs are penicillin, barbiturates, codeine, and morphine, but almost any drug could be implicated as the cause of an allergic reaction. Urticaria following a viral syndrome is also common. Urticaria induced by physical agents, such as cold-induced urticaria, and those caused by trauma (dermatographism), sunburn, heat, or exercise are also IgE-mediated. Recurrent urticaria sometimes accompanied by syncope may follow exposure to cold or exercise; in these cases, an IgE-like factor has been identified in serum, and mast cells are noted to be degranulated.

Hereditary and acquired angioedema, as well as the urticarias associated with vasculitis, hepatitis, and serum sickness–like reactions, are complement mediated. In these cases, complement levels may be diminished, although the most sensitive laboratory test to identify urticaria related to vasculitis is the sedimentation rate. The urticarial lesions themselves do not differ from those associated with other etiologies. In hereditary and acquired angioedema, however, angioedema is not accompanied by urticaria, and involvement of the gastrointestinal tract, producing colic and vomiting as well as laryngeal edema, is a prominent manifestation. In these cases, the inhibitor of C1′ esterase is deficient, leading to decreased levels of C1, C4 and C2 on a chronic basis, with further decreases in levels during acute episodes. The hereditary form is transmitted by autosomal dominant inheritance, so that studies of kindreds can confirm this diagnosis. The acquired form is usually associated with an underlying lymphoproliferative disorder.

Urticaria caused by hepatitis, serum sickness, and vasculitis is probably mediated by immune complexes. In the case of vasculitis, arthralgias may accompany urticaria, and the problem is recurrent rather than being limited to a single episode. This type of vasculitis involves the arterioles, capillaries, and venules and is generally referred to as hypersensitivity or small-vessel vasculitis. The most severe form characterized by arteriolar involvement with decreased complement levels may be seen to have fragmented neutrophils surrounding the vascular lesions and is sometimes referred to as "leukocytoclastic angiitis." In these cases, small arteries may be involved, producing complications such as ulceration of the skin, peripheral neuropathy, glomerulonephritis, encephalopathy, and other lesions related to vascular ischemia. This type of small-vessel vasculitis may be idiopathic in occurrence, or it may be associated with a specific allergen, with certain recognizable disorders such as systemic lupus erythematosus, rheumatoid arthritis, and Waldenström's hypergammaglobulinemia, or with essential (mixed) cryoglobulinemia. Diagnosis of small-vessel vasculitis may be confirmed by a biopsy of the skin lesions.

Urticaria may also be produced by agents that cause mast cell degranulation directly or that alter arachidonic acid metabolism. The former is produced by opiates, curare, pilocarpine, and iodinated radiocontrast agents in some individuals. Other individuals react to aspirin, other nonsteroidal anti-inflammatory drugs, tartrazine food dye, and benzoates with urticaria or, in some cases, with perennial nonallergic rhinitis and nasal polyposis.

In many cases no specific etiology of urticaria can be identified. This is particularly the case in chronic urticaria, persisting for longer than 6 to 8 weeks. Urticaria in general is a common skin reaction, particularly of those aged 20 to 30 years. If no other etiology is identified, urticaria may be considered idiopathic, but in some cases stress and anxiety have been implicated in the absence of another etiology.

Differential Diagnosis. Angioedema may accompany urticaria of any cause, but recurrent angioedema in the absence of urticaria suggests the hereditary or acquired form of complement-mediated angioedema, as does development of laryngeal edema or prominent gastrointestinal symptoms related to angioedema. One should distinguish urticaria from erythema multiforme, a type of skin rash most prominently involving the extremities, face, and lips, and characterized by the occurrence of papules, bullae, and particularly iris-shaped macules in addition to urticaria. Whereas most forms of urticaria have no systemic manifestations, erythema multiforme is commonly associated with fever as well as arthralgias. One must distinguish urticarial lesions also from bullae and vesicles. Contact dermatitis is characterized by localized vesicular lesions at the site of contact. Whereas urticaria is characterized by nonpitting edema, vesicles and bullae contain serous fluid. Thus, bullous dermatoses should not be mistaken for urticarial reactions. Bullae may be associated with bullous impetigo, contact dermatitis, and drug eruptions. Some specific dermatologic conditions, namely pemphigus, pemphigoid, and dermatitis herpetiformis, are distinguished by the occurrence of blisters and bullae rather than the edematous "hives" of urticaria, but there may also be some erythematous edematous plaques without bullae.

Management. If a specific agent can be identified, avoidance is the first principle of management. This of course applies to urticaria induced by a drug or food or inhaled allergens. Urticaria due to cold, heat, or exercise exposure may require an alteration in lifestyle. Acute urticaria may be relieved by epinephrine 1:1000 injected subcutaneously in 0.1-ml doses, given up to a total of three to five times with a short interval between each dose. One may also inject Benadryl, 20 mg subcutaneously. Topical corticosteroids have no efficacy, but the patient with severe, acute urticaria may benefit from prednisone in an initial dose of 20 mg taken orally three times daily. Pruritus is prominent in patients with urticaria and, if severe, may be ameliorated by colloidal baths or topical camphor or menthol-containing lotions or both. The mainstays for management of urticaria are antihistamines. Cyproheptadine (Periactin) (4-mg tablets) and hydroxyzine (Atarax) (10- or 25-mg tablets) are often recommended. The dose may be titrated to achieve maximal relief of pruritus without producing oversedation. Both drugs are usually given three or four times daily, in total doses of up to 20 mg/day for cyproheptadine and 200 mg/day for hydroxyzine when given for urticaria. Benadryl also can be used in doses of 25 to 50 mg taken three to four times daily for relief of pruritus when one would also like to produce some degree of sedation. If one must avoid any sedation, try terfenadine (Seldane), 60 mg two times daily or astemizole (Hismanal) 10 mg once daily. The combination of two or more chemical classes of antihistamine simultaneously is sometimes helpful when side effects of a single agent do not permit increasing the dose. Antihistamines are effective for all types of urticaria that are IgE-mediated or idiopathic.

Urticaria that is complement-mediated requires different management. Hereditary angioedema can be treated prophylactically with attenuated androgens, which stimulate the production of C1′ esterase inhibitor in the heterozygote. Attacks can be treated with epsilon-aminocaproic acid, although use of attenuated androgens generally prevents attacks. Urticaria and other manifestations of small vessel or hypersensitivity vasculitis respond to treatment with prednisone, given for periods of several months to years in the lowest daily dosage required to suppress manifestations of the disease.

PARASITIC DISEASES OF SKIN

Scabies and *pediculosis* are the two major parasitic diseases of skin encountered in the United States. Scabies is caused by a mite (*Sarcoptes scabiei*). Pediculosis is caused by the head louse (*Pediculus humanus capitis*), the body louse (*Pediculus humanus corporis*), or the pubic louse (*Phthirus pubis*). Scabies and pediculosis share the clinical feature of intense pruritus. Whereas scabies is a generalized eruption, pediculosis is usually confined to the scalp or pubic region, and less frequently, usually in extremely unkempt individuals, the body. In most cases, the intense pruritus is accompanied by signs of excoriation. Scabies can be suspected by its distribution, usually involving the lower abdomen, back, periumbilical area, nipples, pubic region, and axillae. More extensive involvement, particularly of the wrists, web spaces between the fingers, knees, and elbows, characterizes severe cases.

The pathognomonic finding of scabies is the "burrow," which is usually a few millimeters in length and accompanied by excoriations and sometimes by vesicles or pustules or crusting from secondary bacterial infection. To find a scabetic burrow, one should search carefully for nonexcoriated lesions. The burrow is about as wide as a sewing needle and slightly irregular in direction, extending for several millimeters in length and terminating in a slightly larger portion, which has within it a gray dot, barely visible to the naked eye. This dot represents the adult female acarus. Microscopic diagnosis is made by placing a droplet of immersion oil on the skin and scraping away the overlying skin on top of the burrow until an erosion exists; the scraping is then examined under the microscope. A more thorough examination is a shave biopsy of the burrow by shaving the skin with a No. 10 or 15 scalpel blade. Place the shaved skin on a microscopic slide with a drop of potassium hydroxide or Swartz-Lamkins stain (without heating) and a coverslip. The specimen is examined under low power for the adult acarus, for egg cases, and for fecal pellets, any one of which is diagnostic.

In pediculosis, the most specific feature is the finding of tiny oval nits, attached to pubic or scalp hairs or to the seams of inner clothing in pediculosis corporis. These eggs deposited by the female lice have a translucent, shiny appearance. In severe cases, excoriations are also visible, with redness, matting of hairs, secondary bacterial infections, and lymphadenopathy. Sometimes the eyelashes are involved in pubic infections. Adult lice usually attach to skin or a hair shaft and are the color of a "freckle," but careful inspection reveals that they are raised from the skin and have legs on each side.

Differential Diagnosis. Bacterial infections are recognized by their pustular appearance. Seborrheic dermatitis exhibits white scales that could be mistaken for nits, but these are of variable size, flaky, and easily removed form the hair shafts. The patient with "senile" dry skin or itching has no burrows, complains of dryness, and is usually elderly, and the itching is worse on the legs and back as opposed to the pubic, axillary, and lower abdominal regions characteristic of parasitic diseases. Neurotic excoriations most often involve a single area of skin, but the patient with generalized pruritus of any cause may reveal excoriations over the body. In these cases, one should search carefully for burrows or nits and seek excoriations in the web spaces and other typical distributions of parasites, since scabies in particular is intensely pruritic and induces a hypersensitivity reaction after several weeks of infestation.

Dog or cat fleas also bite humans, as do bedbugs and chiggers. These lesions appear as scattered papules or as a single lesion of papular urticaria. Chigger bites are most common at the waistline, where socks and neckbands end, or in intertriginous folds. Usually, only a few scattered, papular urticarial lesions are visible.

Management. For discussion of the treatment of scabies, please consult Chapter 31, pages 367 and 375.

For pediculosis capitis, permethrin 1% rinse (NIX) is applied for 10 minutes after shampooing, then rinsed off. For pediculosis pubis, synergized pyrethrins (RID or A-200) are applied for 10 minutes, then rinsed off. Nits should be removed with a fine tooth comb. Treatment may be repeated in 1 week. Clothing and bed linens should be cleaned. This over-the-counter treatment is currently the therapy of choice, with Kwell being an alternative. Nits and lice may be removed manually from the eyelashes with forceps or the lashes treated with 0.025% physostigmine ophthalmic ointment. Retreatment is given in 7 to 10 days if necessary. It is advisable to treat simultaneously the household and sexual contacts of patients. The lice associated with pediculosis corporis are in the patient's clothing so that treatment of the body is usually unnecessary, but all clothing should be cleaned and pressed or laundered and ironed, or it may be placed in a plastic bag and sprayed with Kwell or stored for 1 month.

Bacterial infections superimposed onto parasitic lesions can be treated with antibiotic-containing ointment if mild, or with systemic antibiotics if more severe. Itching due to hypersensitivity often persists for several days to 2 weeks after treatment of scabies or pediculosis. Itching may be ameliorated by orally administered antihistamines, antipruritic lotions containing menthol or camphor, or a topical midpotency corticosteroid cream such as triamcinolone, 0.1%.

DERMATOLOGIC MANIFESTATIONS OF INTERNAL DISEASE

Vitiligo and Other Depigmented Macules. The white macules of *vitiligo* are well circumscribed, irregularly shaped, and at times surrounded by hyperpigmented margins. Such "spots" may be any size and occur on any body area, but most commonly they are found on the dorsum of the hands, the feet, and extensor surfaces; these amelanotic macules may regress but in most cases tend to enlarge slowly. The condition is familial in about one third of cases and idiopathic in most others; however, it is sometimes associated with autoimmune and endocrine disorders like adrenal insufficiency, hypothyroidism, hyperthyroidism, pernicious anemia, and diabetes mellitus. When vitiligo develops, all patients probably should be screened for thyroid function, particularly if they are older than 50 years of age, and one should search specifically for clinical features of the other disorders. No treatment of the lesions themselves is required, although patients who wish cosmetic improvement may be informed that repigmentation is reported using psoralens and ultraviolet A, whereas benzoquinone cream may induce total and permanent depigmentation in the remaining pigmented areas.

Other conditions associated with decreased skin pigmentation include congenital *tuberous sclerosis*, manifested by small oval or lance-shaped, partly hypopigmented macules of the trunk or buttocks, and *piebaldism,* manifested by circumscribed depigmented macules characteristically located on the anterior thorax and extremities, present at birth, often accompanied by a white forelock. Piebaldism usually is not accompanied by other congenital abnormalities, although rare syndromes of congenital deafness and uveitis associated with the circumscribed white macules and forelock are described. *Sarcoidosis* and *leprosy* are also associated with hypomelanotic macules, but these have some residual pigmentation, indistinct margins, and in leprosy are anesthetic. Both benign *nevi* and malignant *melanomas* may be surrounded by an area of hypopigmentation (halo). Any inflammatory skin disorder such as *eczema* or *psoriasis* may also leave an area of postinflammatory hypopigmentation after its resolution. *Tinea versicolor* is typically hypopigmented but can be recognized by its distribution on the chest and by the accompanying scaling.

Hyperpigmentation. *Excessive ACTH* due to primary Addison's disease, ACTH-producing tumors, or pituitary adenoma developing after bilateral adrenalectomy produces a generalized hyperpigmentation caused by increased melanin in skin. Pigment is most prominent over pressure points such as the knuckles, knees, and vertebrae, in the body folds, and in the palmar creases. The degree of hyperpigmentation varies; it is less intense in light-skinned individuals but is more intense after exposure to sunlight. Nonetheless, the presence of hyperpigmentation in areas not exposed to the sun is a helpful clue that the finding is due not to tanning but to the presence of this or another disorder.

Generalized brown hyperpigmentation is also a feature of *hemochromatosis, porphyria cutanea tarda, variegate porphyria, vitamin* B_{12} *deficiency, uremia, systemic sclerosis,* and *hepatic insufficiency.* The skin in hemochromatosis may be identical in appearance to that in Addison's disease, or it may have a slate gray color; a biopsy is often diagnostic. The porphyrias have accompanying distinctive skin abnormalities, including vesicles and atrophic macules in sun-exposed areas. Hypermelanosis overlying the knuckles as well as premature graying of hair sometimes accompanies vitamin B_{12} deficiency, and generalized hyperpigmentation sometimes accompanies nutritional *protein deficiency* and *sprue* as well as uremia, all of which may also be associated with a change in hair color to reddish-brown. Various shades of slate gray or brownish hyperpigmentation are also seen in *arsenic intoxication* or following treatment with some *antineoplastic drugs.* In the evaluation of all patients who appear hyperpigmented, key questions obviously include the familial and racial background of the patient and whether or not hyperpigmentation has been present since birth.

Pregnancy and *oral contraceptive pills* lead to *chloasma* or *melasma* (irregular local brown hyperpigmentation of the face, neck, and scars of the body). Hyperpigmentation locally may also follow resolution of inflammatory skin disease or radiotherapy. Local areas of hyperpigmentation include the brown and blue macules of the lips seen in *intestinal polyposis* (Peutz-Jeghers syndrome), and the *café au lait spots* (pale brown, circumscribed, oval-shaped macules of various size) associated with *neurofibromatosis* (von Recklinghausen's disease). The presence of six or more café au lait spots greater than 1.5 cm in diameter suggests neurofibromatosis; polyostotic fibrous dysplasia and pulmonary stenosis are sometimes associated with a smaller number of such spots. We emphasize that café au lait spots are also present in many normal individuals. Multiple smaller hyperpigmented macules (*lentigines*) are sometimes associated with cardiac arrhythmias, growth retardation, and deafness. Finally, multiple yellowish-red to brown macules that develop urticarial edema upon firm stroking are associated with *urticaria pigmentosa.*

Collagen Vascular Diseases. Chronic *discoid lupus erythematosus* shares some histopathologic features with *systemic lupus erythematosus* but in 80% of patients is a localized skin disorder. Both conditions are often characterized by the presence of the rash in a "butterfly" distribution on the face (bridge of the nose and malar regions). In systemic lupus erythematosus, the initial lesion is erythematous, telangiectatic, and characteristically "puffy"; subsequently, scaling may develop. Residual scarring is not common. Discoid lupus erythematosus is characterized by a red, scaly patch, somewhat similar in appearance but lacking puffiness, and with elevated borders and plugging of pilosebaceous follicles. The skin lesion of discoid lupus is chronic and typically progresses to atrophic areas of hypopigmentation, scarring, and telangiectasia. Sun exposure may exacerbate the rash in both types of lupus, but in 80% of cases discoid lupus is not accompanied by positive findings on serologic tests for antinuclear antibodies or by systemic manifestations like synovitis, polyserositis, glomerulonephritis, or encephalitis. Red, scaly patches of discoid lupus may also be located on the ears, other parts of the face, chest, upper extremities, and scalp.

Characteristic rashes are seen in other collagen vascular diseases. A puffy erythematous rash of the face and eyelids is a component of *dermatomyositis.* Early *scleroderma* is accompanied by swelling and thickening of skin, which later becomes immobile and atrophic. Localized scleroderma or *morphea* characterized by violaceous, slowly enlarging, inelastic macules or plaques has no accompanying systemic manifestations. These macules typically develop pale, depressed centers, rarely ulcerate, and may eventually lead to permanent scarring.

Photosensitivity reactions of other types should be distinguished from the rashes of collagen vascular diseases. Such reactions may represent phototoxicity or photoallergy; in these, a drug or other substance is altered by exposure to light and becomes toxic or antigenic. The reactions themselves range from urticaria to generalized papular/eczematous eruptions. Among the substances commonly encountered that produce these reactions are certain deodorants (halogenated salicylanilides), sunscreens (PABA), coal tar derivatives, griseofulvin, chlorpromazine, thiazide diuretics, tolbutamide, sulfanilamides, doxycycline, ciprofloxacin, demethylchlortetracycline (Declomycin), and psoralen. The *erythropoietic porphyrias* are associated with urticarial, vesicular, or crusting sunlight-induced reactions. All these should be distinguished from *polymorphous light eruptions,* which usually occur in the spring or early summer on initial exposure to sunlight in sensitive individuals, and consist of multiple papules and vesicles that may coalesce into an eczematous reaction on sun-exposed areas, usually the face and neck. Polymorphous light eruptions are not accompanied by systemic manifestations and are unrelated to systemic lupus erythematosus. Use of maximum protection sunscreens, with sun protection factor (SPF) of 45 or 50 is advisable, along with avoidance of sunlight by these individuals if possible. If a patient is allergic to PABA, PABA-free sunscreens (Solbar PF, Ti.Screen, Piz Buin) should be used.

Raynaud's Phenomenon. This should be distinguished from the vascular lability and cool hands and feet sometimes noted by normal young individuals, some of whom have migraine headaches. In Raynaud's phenomenon, the demarcation is sharp between normal and affected areas of the hand or finger(s), and the color changes are pronounced, marked pallor usually being followed by a phase of secondary vasodilatation in which the skin becomes deeply violaceous. Patients may develop symptoms with even brief cold exposure—for example, removing ice cubes from a refrigerator. Raynaud's phenomenon can be an isolated finding in an otherwise healthy person. It is also associated with the connective tissue diseases, including systemic lupus erythematosus, dermatomyositis, and rheumatoid arthritis; the most marked association is with progressive systemic sclerosis (scleroderma). The onset of Raynaud's phenomenon past the age of 50 years should also suggest a search for multiple myeloma or other conditions, such as essential mixed cryoglobulinenemia associated with hyperviscosity of serum. In scleroderma, Raynaud's phenomenon may precede other manifestations by many months to years or may be associated with a form of the disease (CREST syndrome) that is usually limited to Raynaud's phenomenon in association with calcinosis (subcutaneous calcific defects in the hands), telangiectasias of the hands and fingers, sclerodactyly, and motor disorder of the esophagus. Later skin changes of scleroderma involving the hands and other tissues include swelling and edema, eventually followed by thickening and tautness of skin, which becomes tightly bound to the subcutaneous tissue. Patients with CREST syndrome may develop cor pulmonale after 10 to 20 years of disease but usually do not develop renal disease.

Cutaneous Signs of Internal Malignancy. Tumors may metastasize or infiltrate skin. Biopsy usually reveals the diagnosis of direct metastases to skin and should be performed in lesions with features of metastases: firm pink to purple-colored dermal nodules. In *leukemia,* there may be multiple firm, elevated papules, pink to purple in color, often accompanied by extensive ecchymoses. In *Kaposi's sarcoma,* plaques as well as nodules, dark blue to purplish in color, accompanied by chronic swelling and thickening of the skin and located most typically on the distal extremities, are characteristic. *Mycosis fungoides* passes through three dermatologic stages, beginning with scaly, pruritic erythematous patches, progressing to well-demarcated indurated plaques, and finally developing into nodular tumors. *M. fungoides* may also occur as a generalized erythroderma in which the skin is infiltrated by lymphoma cells.

Dermal manifestations of malignancy may also represent a reaction of skin to the tumor or its products. For example, generalized erythroderma occurs in some early leukemic or lymphomatous neoplasias, but in these cases usually is thought to reflect hypersensitivity and is not accompanied by dermal infiltration. *Acanthosis nigricans* is well known as a cutaneous manifestation of internal malignancy. It appears as brown to black papules that tend to become confluent and sometimes progress to raised velvety plaques of the axillary, groin, periareolar, or umbilical regions. The association with malignancy, especially adenocarcinoma of the stomach, is strong in acanthosis nigricans of adult onset. Acanthosis nigricans, occurring at birth or before puberty, is considered to be hereditary and is not associated with malignancy. The adult onset of acanthosis may also be explained by its association with endocrinologic conditions, including Cushing's disease, acromegaly, Stein-Leventhal syndrome, and insulin-resistant diabetes. Also, the use of nicotinic acid as a cholesterol-lowering agent occasionally causes acanthosis nigricans that will resolve after discontinuation of the drug.

A variety of other skin manifestations at times have been associated with internal malignancy. The aforementioned *dermatomyositis* is thought to be associated with an internal malignancy in 8.5% of the adult-onset cases. *Migratory thrombophlebitis,* particularly involving the upper exremities or unexplained by underlying venous disease such as varicose veins, may be associated with carcinoma of the pancreas. Carcinoma of the pancreas also may be associated with unexplained development of localized *nodular fat necrosis.* Generalized *ichthyosis* or hyperkeratosis of the palms and soles with onset in adulthood and without a familial history may indicate an underlying lymphoma. The sudden development of numerous seborrheic keratoses is thought to suggest the possibility of malignancy, as may the abrupt development of multiple xanthomata involving the trunk and neck in the absence of hyperlipoproteinemia. Atypical forms of urticaria, sometimes assuming gyrate or annular patterns and unusually persistent at a single site (erythema perstans), have been associated with malignancy. The small, well-demarcated, eczematous-appearing plaques of Bowen's disease, which reveal squamous cell carcinoma in situ of the skin on biopsy, are also sometimes associated with internal malignancy of the gastrointestinal, respiratory, or genitourinary tracts, particularly if occurring on skin not exposed to sun. Finally, bullous pemphigoid with onset in the elderly and atypical dermatitis herpetiformis with onset in late middle age can indicate underlying malignancy in rare cases.

Pyoderma Gangrenosum and Other Ulcerations of Skin. These deep large ulcers, usually involving the extremities, are associated with ulcerative colitis and regional enteritis and at times are idiopathic. An atypical form of pyoderma gangrenosum has also been associated with myeloproliferative disorders, including polycythemia, myeloid metaplasia, and the myelogenous leukemias. When associated with inflammatory bowel disease, activity of the ulceration generally follows activity of the primary disease. In addition to large size, the ulcers are characterized by necrosis at the base and margins, by their overhanging margins, and by their violaceous or blue-tinged rim. Satellite bullae may occur; the initial lesion is usually a bulla, nodule, or papule that slowly enlarges and becomes necrotic. A biopsy of the edges reveals a nonspecific neutrophilic infiltrate. These ulcers are larger and less numerous than the multiple necrotic ulcerations of the lower extremities seen in hypersensitivity (small vessel) angiitis and in rheumatoid vasculitis. They are also larger than the centrally necrotic, dark-colored nodules of ecthyma gangrenosum, which is a manifestation of *Pseudomonas* sepsis. Stasis ulcers are smaller, generally 1 to 4 cm in diameter, and are recognizable by their location above the medial malleolus and associated findings of stasis hyperpigmentation, brawny edema, and eczematous dermatitis. Large purpuric areas with central necrosis may be seen in some drug allergies, including a hypersensitivity reaction to Coumadin. The multiple large areas of purpura with central necrosis seen in purpura fulminans may result from diffuse intravascular coagulation of any cause and sepsis, particularly meningococcal. These are acutely developing lesions in seriously ill patients and should not be confused with pyoderma gangrenosum and other indolent ulcerations.

Necrobiosis Lipoidica Diabeticorum. This atrophic plaque may occur in the presence or absence of diabetes mellitus. It is characteristically distributed on the anterior shins and is recognizable by the appearance of a gradually enlarging, atrophic area brownish-yellow in color, with erythematous margins and superimposed shallow ulcerations, telangiectasias, and loss of normal skin markings. If there is diagnostic uncertainty, skin biopsy is helpful. Necrobiosis lipoidica diabeticorum sometimes regresses if treated with intralesional steroid injections administered cautiously only in the active, elevated areas of disease at the periphery of the plaque. The degree of therapeutic control of the diabetes is not correlated with the skin lesion.

Granulomatous Lesions. *Sarcoidosis* may be accompanied by noncaseating granulomata of skin; these typically are small (3 to 6 mm), raised, reddish papular lesions of the face and upper body, or they may be located in scars or areas of previous injury. They are generally multiple, of variable configuration, and often result in scarring and atrophy following their resolution. They may be recognized from their typical appearance. A biopsy is diagnostic of granulomatous disease, but cultures and clinicopathologic correlation are necessary to exclude mycobacterial infection. Larger dermal plaques occur less commonly in sarcoidosis and may result in disfigurement of the nose, cheeks, and ears (lupus pernio).

Tuberculosis of skin (lupus vulgaris) is distinguished from sarcoidosis chiefly by a biopsy revealing caseation necrosis and acid-fast bacili. Lesions of lupus vulgaris may be nodular, ulcerative, or plaque-like and of any size, configuration, and location. Tuberculosis of skin is currently quite rare in the United States but may be suspected because of the persistence of the gradually enlarging lesions, which can have a central area of scarring, producing disfiguration.

Some other inflammatory lesions of skin (granuloma inguinale, chancroid, and lymphogranuloma venereum) are chiefly manifested by shallow ulcerations or erosions (and/or lymphadenopathy) and involve the genital region. They are discussed in Chapter 31. The chancre of primary syphilis is also described in Chapter 31. The lesions of tertiary syphilis (gummas) are rarely encountered nowadays; they appear as indolent ulcers of skin. Fungal infections may induce granulomatous lesions of skin. In the United States, sporotrichosis is characterized by a primary chancre with a nodular ulcerative appearance and lymphangitic spread of satellite nodules. Larger granulomatous nodules with draining sinuses are associated with rare cases of actinomycosis. The South American fungal diseases of skin are associated with large, nodular, ulcerative granulomas, which often are draining. The general principle is that any persistent unexplained nodular or ulcerative lesion of skin of significant size should be biopsied to establish the diagnosis.

REFERENCES

1. Branch WT Jr, Collins M, and Wintroub BU: Dermatologic practice: Implications for a primary care residency curriculum. J Med Educ 58:136, 1983.
2. Mendenhall RC, Ramsay DL, Girard RA, et al: A study of the practice of dermatology in the United States. Arch Dermatol 114:1456, 1978.
3. Arndt KA: Manual of Dermatologic Therapeutics, 4th ed. Boston, Little, Brown, 1989.
4. Fitzpatrick TB, et al: Dermatology in General Medicine, 4th ed. New York, McGraw-Hill, 1993.
5. Berger TG, Elias PM, and Wintroub BU: Manual of Therapy for Skin Diseases. New York, Churchill-Livingstone, 1990.
6. Flowers FP and Krusinski PA: Dermatology in Ambulatory and Emergency Medicine: A Clinical Guide with Algorithms. Chicago, Year Book Medical Publishers, 1984.
7. Moschella SL and Hurley HJ: Dermatology, 3rd ed. Philadelphia, WB Saunders, 1992.

70

Basic Assessment of Auditory Function

HOWARD H. ZUBICK, PhD
CRAIG D. BARTH, MS

The incidence of hearing loss increases as a function of age.[1] For the physician treating the adult population, an understanding of both hearing loss and assessment practice are requisite, because hearing loss is so common. When office screening is positive for hearing loss, a more detailed evaluation is warranted. Such evaluation will provide information regarding type and degree of loss, possible site of lesion, and potential and prognosis for rehabilitation when applicable.

PHYSIOLOGY

The peripheral hearing mechanism shown in Figure 70–1 is divided into three separate anatomic divisions that function interdependently. Moving in a lateral to medial fashion, these three divisions are called the outer ear, the middle ear, and the inner ear.

The peripheral hearing mechanism can also be divided into two functional divisions. The conductive or transformer mechanism, consisting of the outer and middle ears, will move relative to the amount of sound pressure at the plane of the tympanic membrane. This movement is transmitted to the inner ear via the ossicular chain. The inner ear or transducer mechanism includes the cochlea, semicircular canals, and eighth cranial nerve.

Pathology in either the outer or middle ear will reduce the conductive capability of the system. As a result, the intensity of a signal reaching the inner ear will be attenuated. Such an impairment is referred to as a conductive hearing loss.

The cochlea or end-organ of hearing is often the site of adult auditory deficits. Such deficits may occur due to the aging process, disease, or noise exposure.[2–4] Microscopic hair cells within the cochlea form the transducer and ultimate transmission points for auditory signals routed to the brain via the eighth cranial nerve. A sensory (cochlear end-organ) or neural (eighth nerve or higher) hearing loss is usually designated in combined fashion as a sensorineural hearing loss.

A hearing loss that affects the conductive mechanism (outer or middle ear) as well as the sensorineural mechanism (inner ear) is referred to as a mixed hearing loss.

SCREENING PROCEDURES

Office screening tests and examination of the outer ear and tympanic membrane are indicated whenever there is any concern regarding hearing or if there exists a history of hearing loss.

Screening for hearing loss is begun simply during the history-taking by asking about hearing. Specific inquiry regarding the ability (or inability) to understand speech is most important. In the course of simple conversation, one can quickly judge the extent to which hearing may be impaired for normal levels of speech. A predominant complaint of individuals presenting with sensorineural hearing loss is marked difficulty in understanding speech, particularly in situations in which background noise is present.[5]

QUALITATIVE TESTS

Tuning Fork Tests

Tuning fork testing, while unable to quantify the degree of hearing loss, provides a simplified method for defining the type of hearing loss (conductive, sensorineural, or mixed). The two most commonly used such tests are the Weber test and the Rinne test.

Weber Test. The shaft of the vibrating tuning fork is placed on the vertex or the midline of the frontal bone, and the patient is asked in which ear the tone is heard the loudest. The diagnostic paradigm of the Weber test is that the tone lateralizes to the ear with either the better sensorineural sensitivity or the greater conductive component.

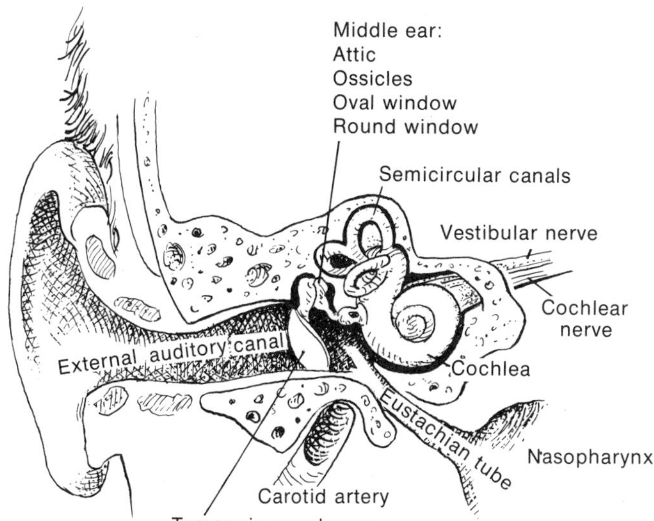

FIGURE 70–1. Clinical anatomy of the outer ear, middle ear, inner ear, and related structures.

Rinne Test. The results of the Rinne test are used to confirm or refute the findings of the Weber test. In this two-part test, the vibrating tuning fork is positioned 2 to 3 cm from the opening of the external ear canal. The patient indicates whether the air-conducted tone can be heard. Bone conduction is then assessed by repositioning the tuning fork with the stem placed against the mastoid process. The patient indicates whether the tone can be heard by bone conduction and whether it was louder by air conduction or bone conduction.

The results of the Rinne test are reported as being either positive or negative. A negative result on a Rinne test is recorded when bone conduction is reported as being louder than air conduction (BC>AC). A negative result on a Rinne test is indicative of a conductive hearing loss. Normal hearing or an unknown degree of sensorineural hearing loss is indicated when a positive result on a Rinne test is recorded (AC≥BC).

If lateralization occurs on the Weber test, masking may be required during the Rinne test to prevent contralateral participation of the nontest ear trough cross-over by bone conduction. A Barany noisebox applied to the nontest ear may be used for this purpose.

Tympanometry

Tympanometry serves as both a qualitative and quantitative objective measure of middle ear function. Varying pressure against the tympanic membrane in the sealed ear canal will result in a measurable movement of the eardrum and middle ear system relative to pressure on both sides of the drum. During tympanometry, a tone is introduced in the closed ear canal while the pressure is varied from positive to negative or negative to positive, (e.g., +200 mm H_2O to −400 mm H_2O). The tympanometer records the reflection of the tone from the drum as a function of the variation in air pressure in the sealed ear canal (Fig. 70–2). As a result, a graph depicting middle ear mobility is produced. Such a graph is called a tympanogram. A pressure peak or point of maximum compliance represents equal pressure on both sides of the tympanic membrane. The normal middle ear system displays a pressure peak in the range of +50 to −150 mm H_2O on the tympanogram. An absence of or variation in the position, or in certain cases the shape of the peak, is indicative of middle ear dysfunction. Such dysfunction is often associated with conductive hearing loss.

A normal middle ear system, regardless of the degree of

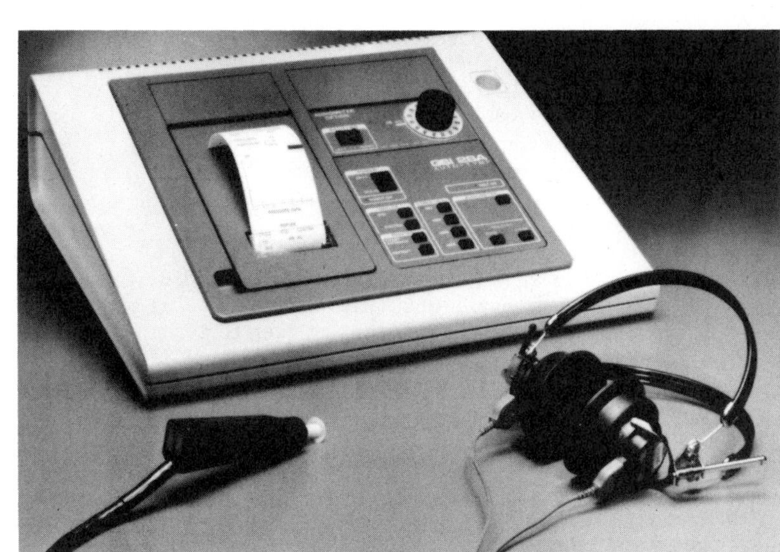

FIGURE 70–2. GSI Model 28A tympanometer. (Courtesy of Lucas Grason-Stadler, Inc.)

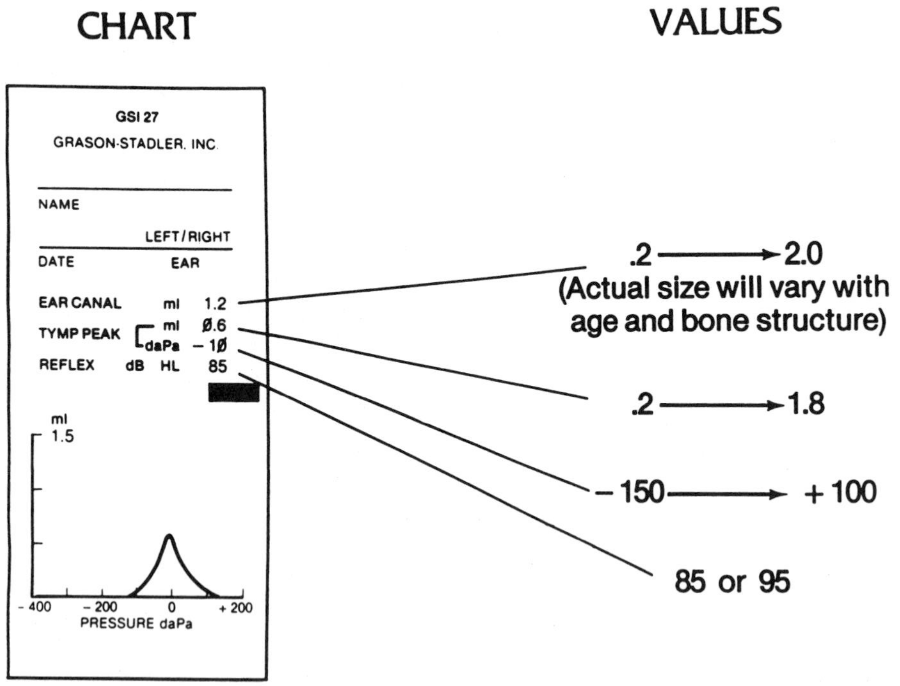

CHART
VALUES
GSI 27
GRASON-STADLER, INC.
NAME
LEFT/RIGHT
DATE
EAR
EAR CANAL ml 1.2
TYMP PEAK ml Ø.6
daPa − 1Ø
REFLEX dB HL 85
ml
1.5
− 400
− 200
0
+ 200
PRESSURE daPa
.2 → 2.0
(Actual size will vary with age and bone structure)
.2 → 1.8
− 150 → + 100
85 or 95

FIGURE 70–3. Normal tympanogram. Note the normative values to the right of the tracing. (Courtesy of Lucas Grason-Stadler, Inc.)

sensorineural hearing loss, will yield a normal tympanogram. In the elderly patient, tympanogram peak amplitude may be reduced. This reduction is likely to be caused by an overall stiffening of the tympanic membrane and ossicular chain with increasing age. The most common impairment of normal middle ear mobility is seen with a fluid-filled middle ear space (otitis media). Otoscopic determination of a retracted tympanic membrane can be correlated with negative middle ear pressure secondary to eustachian tube dysfunction and the resultant rarefied middle ear atmosphere. Representative tympanometric configurations are shown in Figures 70–3 to 70–8.

Pure Tone Audiometry

The standard pure tone audiometric evaluation should always include an assessment of both air and bone conducted threshold sensitivity. (Air conducted thresholds alone may be sufficient when hearing sensitivity is within the normal range or when performing screening measures in order to identify gross auditory deficiencies.) Hearing thresholds are determined using pure-tone stimuli at octave frequencies from 250 to 8000 Hz.

Hearing loss is reported in decibels (dB). The decibel is a measure of sound level that expresses the ratio between two sound pressures. In evaluating patients, the decibel is used to express the ratio between what is referred to as 0-dB hearing threshold level and any threshold that is greater than this 0-dB normative level.

Figure 70–9 shows a sample audiogram format that depicts hearing threshold (on the ordinate or Y-axis) as a function of frequency (on the abscissa or X-axis) in graphical form.

The audiogram is interpreted by noting the degree of hearing loss at a number of selected test frequencies critical

GSI 27
GRASON-STADLER, INC
NAME
LEFT/RIGHT
DATE
EAR
EAR CANAL ml 1.7
TYMP PEAK ml Ø.3
daPa − 3ØØ
REFLEX dB HL 1Ø5
ml
1.5
− 400
− 200
0
+ 200
PRESSURE daPa

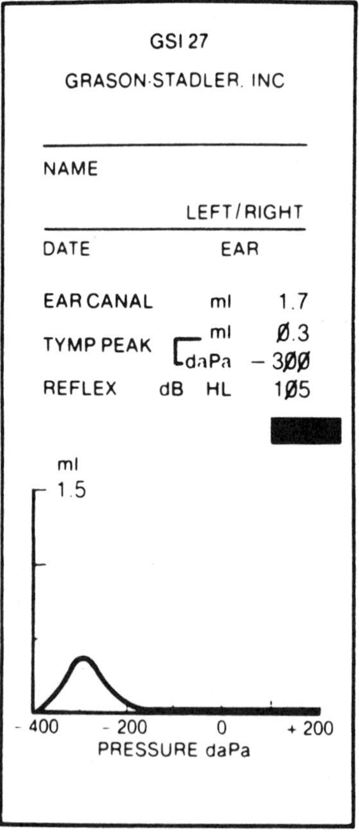

FIGURE 70–4. Abnormal tympanogram. Note the normal ear canal volume with reduced middle ear mobility and a pressure peak in the abnormal (negative) range. Possible causes of such a tympanogram include eustachian tube dysfunction or mild middle ear effusion. (Courtesy of Lucas Grason-Stadler, Inc.)

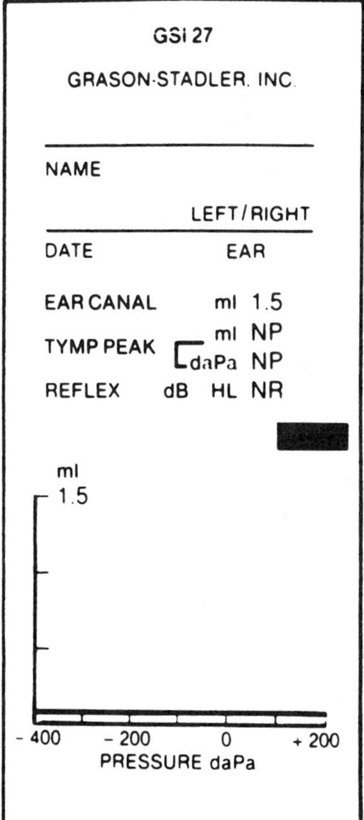

FIGURE 70–5. Abnormal tympanogram. Note the presence of normal ear canal volume with absent middle ear pressure and no middle ear mobility. The most likely cause of such a tympanogram is a fluid-filled middle ear space (otitis media). (Courtesy of Lucas Grason-Stadler, Inc.)

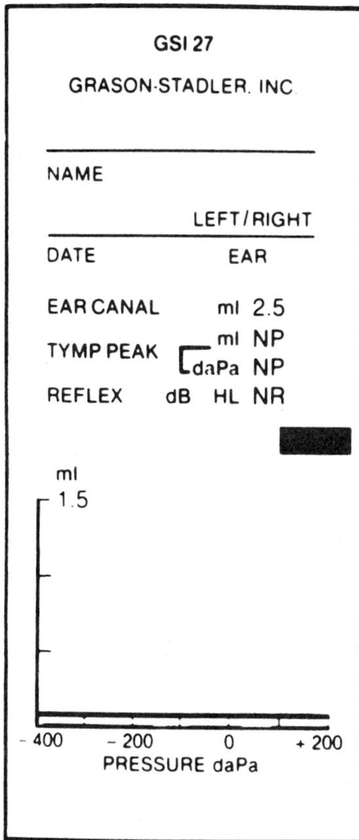

FIGURE 70–6. The abnormal tympanogram in this figure shows an abnormally large ear canal volume with no pressure peak and no mobility. The two most consistent causes of such a tympanogram are a perforated tympanic membrane and a PE tube that is patent. (Courtesy of Lucas Grason-Stadler, Inc.)

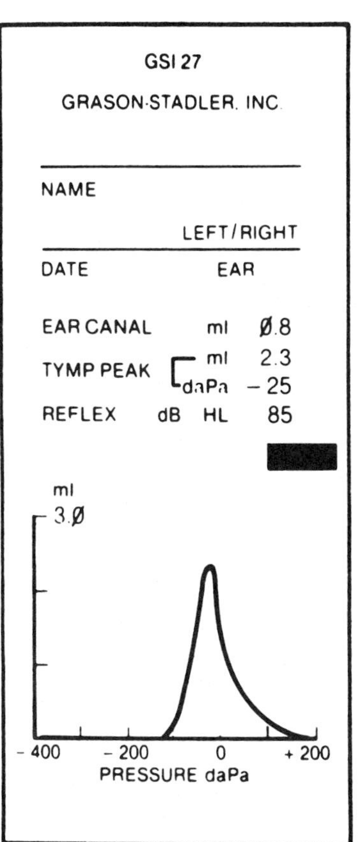

FIGURE 70–7. Abnormal tympanogram with hypermobility, normal pressure peak, and normal ear canal volume. Such a tympanogram can be caused by scar tissue on the tympanic membrane or by a monomeric (extremely thin) drum. (Courtesy of Lucas Grason-Stadler, Inc.)

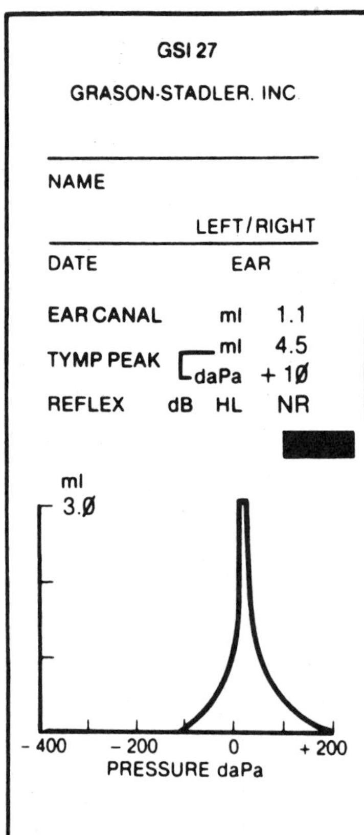

FIGURE 70–8. Tympanogram showing normal ear canal volume with a normal pressure peak. Note the extreme hypermobility that is most likely indicative of an ossicular disarticulation. (Courtesy of Lucas Grason-Stadler, Inc.)

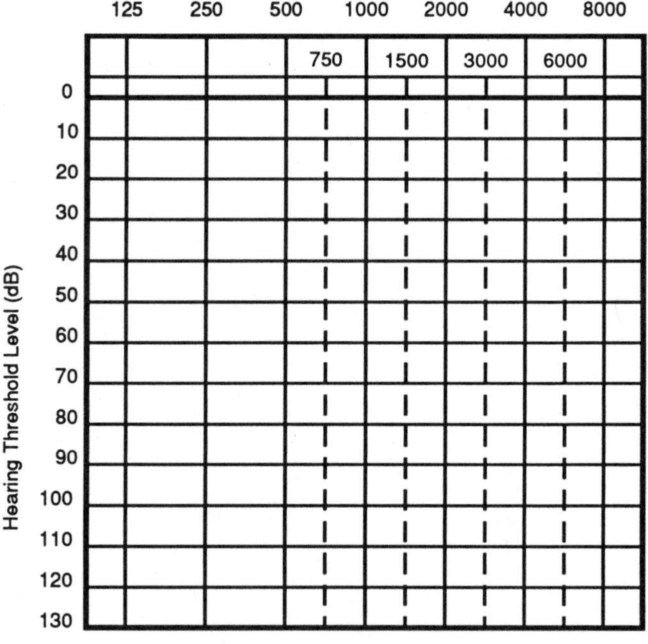

FIGURE 70–9. Sample audiogram. Hearing threshold in decibels (dB) is recorded as a function of pure tone test frequency.

SPEECH AUDIOMETRY

	SRT	DISCRIMINATION
AD	dB	%
AS	dB	%

TABLE 70–1. HEARING LOSS IN DECIBELS (dB) RELATED TO APPROXIMATE DEGREE OF IMPAIRMENT*

Hearing Loss (dB)	Degree of Impairment
0–20	Normal
20–40	Mild loss
40–70	Moderate loss
70–90	Severe loss
90–100	Profound loss

*After Goodrich A: Reference zero levels for pure tone audiometer. ASHA 1:262, 1965.

to the reception of speech. Terms relating hearing loss in decibels to degree of impairment are listed in Table 70–1. Comparison of air conduction thresholds to bone conduction thresholds provides the qualitative determination with regard to the type of loss as well as to quantitative assessment as to degree of communicative impairment. Various audiogram configurations are shown in Figures 70–10 to 70–15.

AUDIOGRAM

FREQUENCY (Hz)

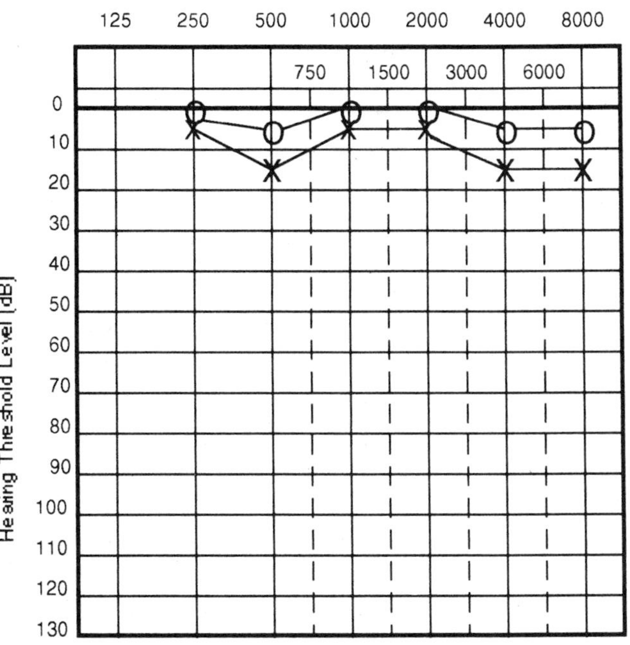

SPEECH AUDIOMETRY

	SRT	DISCRIMINATION
AD	0 dB	100 %
AS	5 dB	98 %

FIGURE 70–10. Normal hearing. Note that the speech reception thresholds for both ears are consistent with the respective pure tone averages at 500, 1000, and 2000 Hz. Speech discrimination scores are excellent, as would be expected with normal hearing.

AUDIOGRAM

FREQUENCY (Hz)

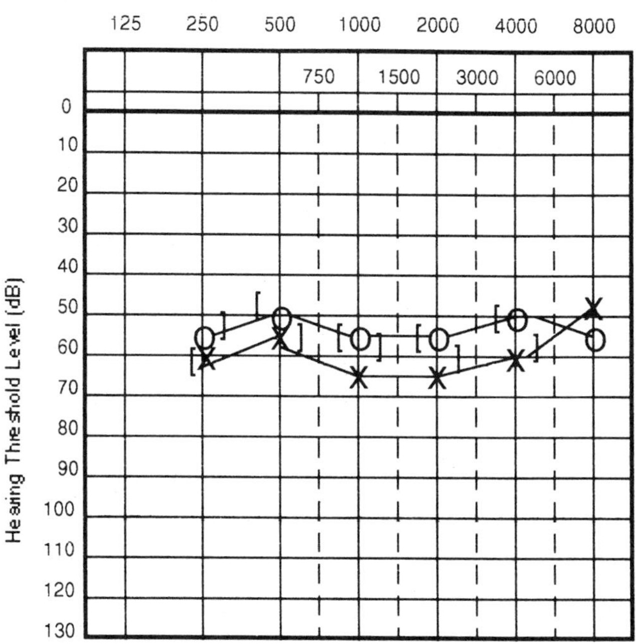

SPEECH AUDIOMETRY

	SRT	DISCRIMINATION
AD	52 dB	78 %
AS	60 dB	82 %

FIGURE 70–11. Audiogram depicting a moderate, flat, sensorineural hearing loss. SRTs are depressed relative to the degree of loss in each ear. Speech discrimination scores are also reduced.

Speech Audiometry

The patient's inability to understand normal conversational speech often precipitates the complaint and subsequent referral for hearing testing. Pure tone audiometry, although an indicator of the degree of hearing loss, does not provide a complete picture of communicative dysfunction. The effect of hearing loss on one's ability to communicate can best be evaluated by using measures of speech audiometry.

Speech audiometry consists of two essential components. The first step is to establish a threshold level for speech stimuli. This threshold level is defined as the level at which the patient can correctly repeat the stimuli on 50% of the

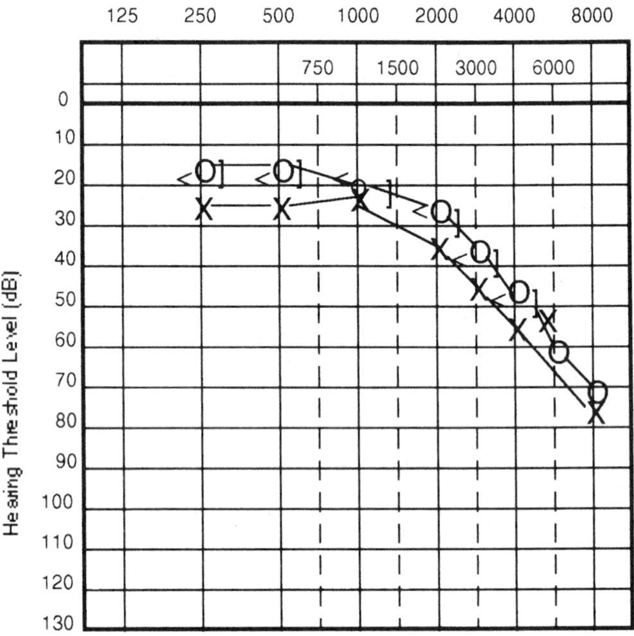

SPEECH AUDIOMETRY

	SRT	DISCRIMINATION
AD	26 dB	88 %
AS	30 dB	84 %

FIGURE 70–12. The hearing loss shown on this audiogram is a mild to moderate, sloping, high-frequency sensorineural hearing loss. The hearing loss is bilaterally symmetrical. Such a configuration is typically seen in presbycusis.

presentations. The result is called the speech reception threshold (SRT).

The SRT is obtained by presenting spondees or two-syllable words that place equal stress on each syllable. Baseball, cowboy, and hotdog are several examples of spondee words used during SRT testing. In SRT testing, the patient continues to repeat the stimulus words as they are decreased in level until threshold is reached. Generally, the SRT should be in close agreement with the pure tone average at 500, 1000, and 2000 Hz for the same ear. These frequencies are considered to be the most critical test frequencies for the reception of speech.

The SRT thus becomes an indicator of the validity of the pure tone test results as well as an indicator of basic communicative deficiency. Lack of agreement between the pure tone average and the SRT can be caused by a variety of reasons, including nonorganic hearing loss (i.e., hysteria or malingering, steeply sloping losses, tester error).

The second component is designed to evaluate the patient's speech discrimination. In discrimination testing, monosyllabic stimulus words such as chair, down, toe, and wire are presented to the test ear at a fixed suprathreshold level that remains constant throughout the test. Discrimination testing is typically done at 40-dB sensation level (SL) or level above the SRT. Due to the level at which the test is performed, any words not repeated or repeated incorrectly can not be ascribed to an inability to hear but to an inability to discriminate or understand what is heard. Speech discrimination or the ability to repeat stimulus words correctly is reported as a percentage score out of 100%. Figures 70–10 to 70–15 include examples of SRT and discrimination results.

Neurophysiology

Brain stem auditory evoked response (BAER) testing can prove useful in cases in which conventional audiometric

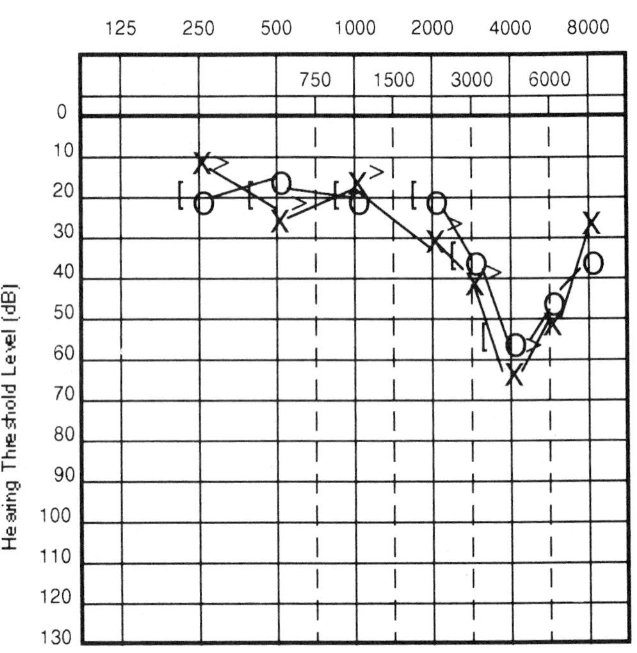

SPEECH AUDIOMETRY

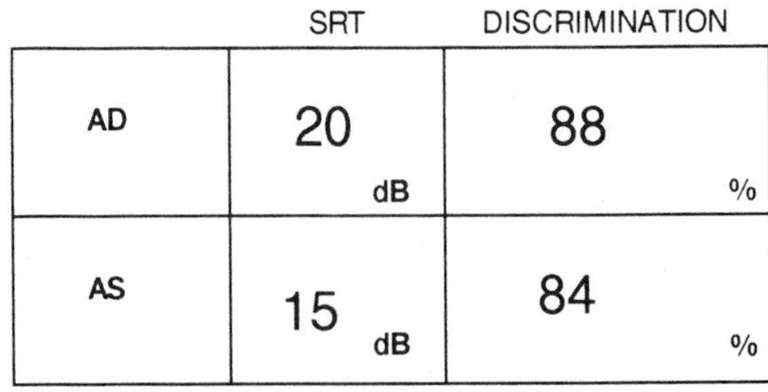

	SRT	DISCRIMINATION
AD	20 dB	88 %
AS	15 dB	84 %

FIGURE 70–13. Typical configuration of hearing loss caused by either prolonged noise exposure or sudden acoustic trauma. Note the characteristic notch between 2000 and 4000 Hz, with thresholds recovering at 6000 to 8000 Hz.

AUDIOGRAM

FREQUENCY (Hz)

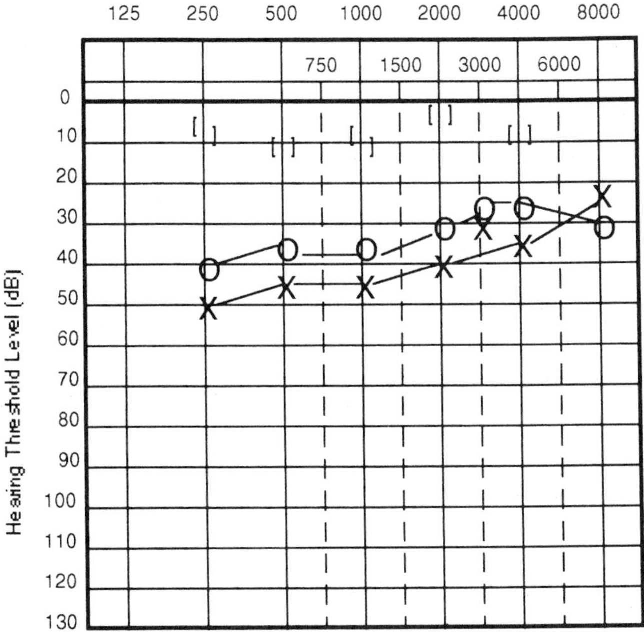

SPEECH AUDIOMETRY

	SRT	DISCRIMINATION
AD	32 dB	98 %
AS	40 dB	100 %

FIGURE 70–14. Conductive type of hearing loss. Note that speech reception thresholds are consistent with air conduction pure tone averages (500, 1000, and 2000 Hz) for each ear. Discrimination scores are typically unaffected by conductive pathologies.

evaluation has been inconclusive, such as in attempting to differentiate between a cochlear loss (e.g., Meniere's disease) and a retrocochlear loss (e.g., acoustic neuroma). BAER testing can also provide utility when in need of information from the nonparticipatory patient who either can not or will not cooperate.

BAER testing is accomplished using a basic far-field electroencephalographic (EEG) recording technique. As the patient listens to a repetitive acoustic transient sound (e.g., acoustic click or tone burst), changes in the resting EEG are monitored and recorded. The EEG information recorded via three surface electrodes placed on the scalp is analyzed with the aid of a signal averaging computer. The signal averaging computer filters, sums, averages, and amplifies the small submicrovolt changes in the resting EEG produced by the presentation of the repetitive acoustic transient delivered to the ear.

The BAER consists of from 5 to 7 peaks occurring within a 10-msec stimulus onset. The waveform is labelled with sequential Roman numerals (I to VII).[6] Wave I occurs at approximately 1.7 msec, and each subsequent wave is delayed by approximately 1 msec. Generally, BAER interpretation is based on several physical characteristics of the recorded waveform. Response interpretation may be based on evaluations of absolute peak latencies in milliseconds, interpeak latency differences in milliseconds (IPI, IWI), peak amplitudes in μV, waveform morphology, and I-V amplitude ratio. Figure 70–16 shows a sample BAER tracing with the relevant diagnostic criteria.

The BAER yields information regarding sound transmission capabilities of the auditory system as a function of time and stimulus intensity. In cases of certain types of hearing loss or degenerative neurologic disease, changes in the BAER can provide useful diagnostic information that is otherwise unattainable. Severe or profound hearing loss will likely result in the prolongation or absence of wave I

AUDIOGRAM

FREQUENCY (Hz)

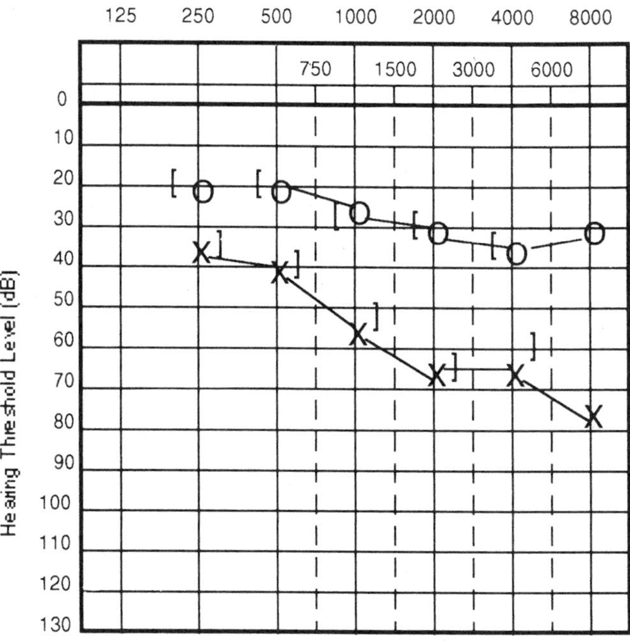

SPEECH AUDIOMETRY

	SRT	DISCRIMINATION
AD	25 dB	98 %
AS	50 dB	78 %

FIGURE 70–15. Asymmetrical hearing loss with the thresholds for the right ear better than the left. This asymmetry is also reflected in the speech reception thresholds as well as in the discrimination scores.

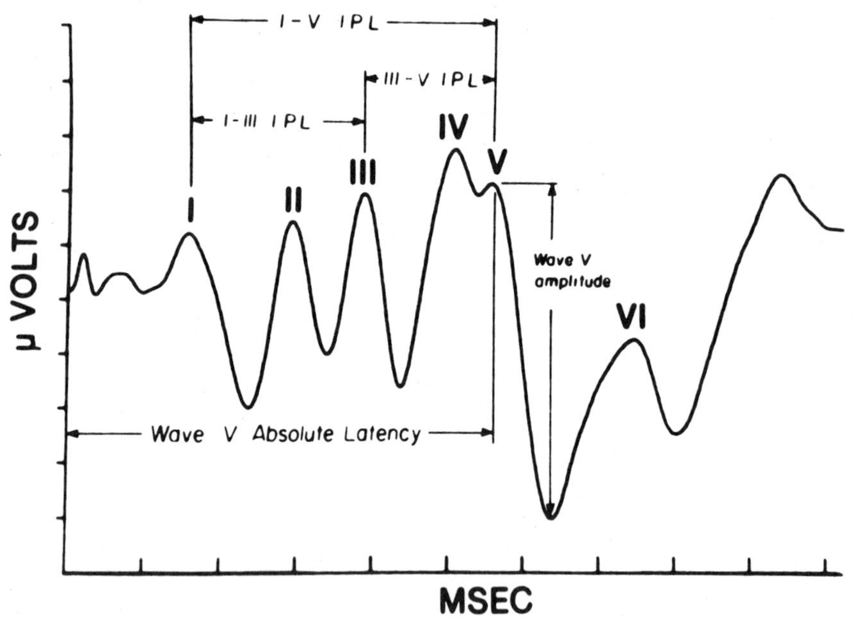

FIGURE 70–16. Normal brain stem auditory evoked response (BAER) with appropriate diagnostic landmarks. (From John T. Jacobson, *The Auditory Brain Stem Response.* Copyright © 1985 by Allyn and Bacon. Adapted by permission.)

and possibly all other later waves. Figure 70–17 represents a patient with a normally functioning right ear as evidenced by the normal BAER landmarks, whereas the left ear displays a degraded waveform and prolonged absolute and interpeak latencies. This type of response is suggestive of a retrocochlear (VIII nerve and/or brain stem) pathology. This patient, who experienced a significant high-frequency hearing loss on audiometry, which was asymmetric to the left ear, was later found on a computed tomography (CT) scan to have a left-side intracanicular acoustic neuroma that had extended into the cistern of the left cerebellopontine angle.

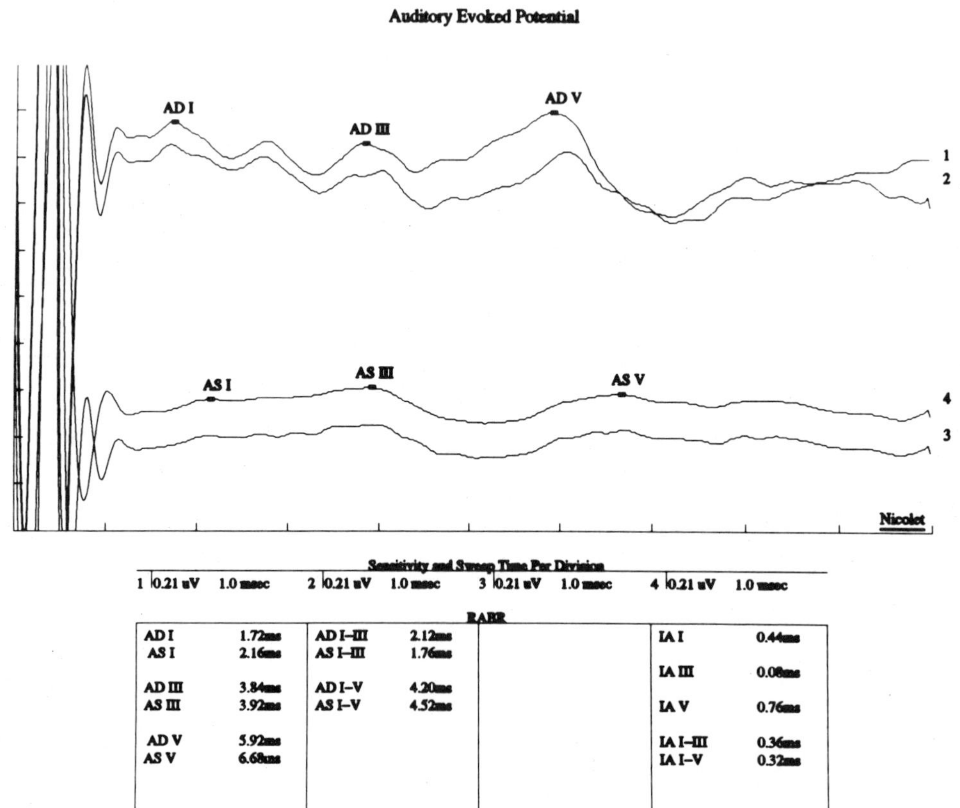

AD I	1.72ms	AD I–III	2.12ms			IA I	0.44ms
AS I	2.16ms	AS I–III	1.76ms				
						IA III	0.08ms
AD III	3.84ms	AD I–V	4.20ms				
AS III	3.92ms	AS I–V	4.52ms			IA V	0.76ms
AD V	5.92ms					IA I–III	0.36ms
AS V	6.68ms					IA I–V	0.32ms

FIGURE 70–17. Brain stem auditory evoked response (BAER) showing a normal right ear with appropriate landmarks and an abnormal left ear.

TABLE 70–2. TYPES OF HEARING LOSS AND EXPECTED OTOLOGIC AND AUDIOLOGIC FINDINGS

Conductive Loss	Abnormal otoscopic examination BC > AC Abnormal tympanograms Weber lateralizes to poorer ear Rinne negative Audiogram shows BC > AC SRT elevated Speech discrimination good-to-excellent BSAEP shows normal transmission time with delay in wave I reflecting middle ear deficit
Sensorineural Loss	Normal otoscopic examination AC ≥ BC Normal tympanograms Weber midline except in asymmetric sensorineural loss, then to better ear Rinne positive Audiogram shows AC ≥ BC Fair-to-poor speech discrimination BSAEP may show absence of waveforms, or delay in time-locked sequencing from waves I-V
Mixed Loss	Any combination of conductive and sensorineural findings

Clinical Interpretation

The interpretation of test data can be made readily by the examiner. Correlation of information from both otologic and audiologic examination provides the physician with useful diagnostic criteria in the interpretation of auditory dysfunction.[7] Table 70–2 presents previously discussed types of hearing loss with correlative findings from otologic and audiologic evaluations. Common causes of conductive and sensorineural hearing loss are presented in Table 70–3.

REHABILITATION THROUGH AMPLIFICATION

Uniform criteria for specifying when an individual requires amplification is difficult to establish. Amplification is considered when the patient has an inability to hear normal conversational speech and when this difficulty can be substantiated by audiometric testing.[8]

The United States Food and Drug Administration (FDA) has published criteria requiring a medical examination and letter of clearance from a licensed physician prior to the sale of a hearing aid.[9] Under this legislation, anyone over 18 years of age may exercise his or her right to waive the medical examination, although it is stated that this is clearly *not* in his or her best interest.

The primary physician, after determining that hearing loss is present, should plan an appropriate work-up to determine the type, degree, and possible cause of the hearing loss prior to referral for amplification. When the physician coordinates the evaluative and referral process, the entire rehabilitative program is enhanced and better serves the patient.

TABLE 70–3. COMMON CAUSES OF HEARING LOSS

Conductive Loss	Excessive cerumen Foreign objects Otitis externa or otitis media Tumors of the outer or middle ear Perforated tympanic membrane Thickened tympanic membrane Discontinuity of the ossicular chain Otosclerosis
Sensorineural Loss	Aging (presbycusis) Noise exposure (prolonged or traumatic) Drug ototoxicity Meniere's disease Vascular disorders Skull trauma Acoustic neuroma Viral illness Genetic
Mixed Loss	Any combination

Hearing Aids

Hearing aids are miniaturized amplifying devices with varying power and frequency response characteristics designed to overcome decreased auditory sensation.[10] Hearing aids may be appropriately fitted to either sensorineural, conductive, or mixed hearing loss. The popular misconception that individuals with a sensorineural loss cannot benefit from amplification should be discarded. Although there may be a select minority of patients who will not demonstrate a beneficial response to amplification, most patients can and do experience significant improvement, at least to the point that a trial fitting is warranted.

The more important components of a hearing aid include the microphone, amplifier, volume control, receiver, on-off switch, and battery for powering the electronic circuitry and components. In addition, some instruments have power-limiting or circuitry controls for altering the frequency response and gain characteristics of the instrument so that the amplifier will closely match the needs dictated by the audiogram.

The hearing aid microphone transduces the airborne sound waves into an electrical signal that is then routed to the amplifier where the intensity is then increased according to the user setting of the volume control. The amplified signal is then routed to the receiver, where it is transduced into an airborne wave. This acoustical signal is subsequently directed into the ear canal through a coupling device referred to as an earmold.

The basic audiometric evaluation allows one to assess the type and degree of hearing loss as well as how the loss is manifested in speech signal sensitivity and discrimination. The important question at this point is whether the patient requires amplification and, if so, how he or she can comfortably and effectively use it in the ear or ears selected for its use.

Prior to the recommendation for a specific hearing aid, additional information is required. Determination of the most comfortable loudness level (MCL), the level in decibels at which the patient reports being most comfortable with the listening situation, and the uncomfortable loudness level (UCL), the level in decibels at which the patient reports speech as being uncomfortably loud. The difference between the UCL and the patient's SRT is referred to as the *dynamic range,* which reflects the intensity range in decibels to which speech can be amplified without causing distress to the patient (Fig. 70–18).

Finally, the basic thesis in the amplification process is to lower the speech reception threshold or SRT to within nor-

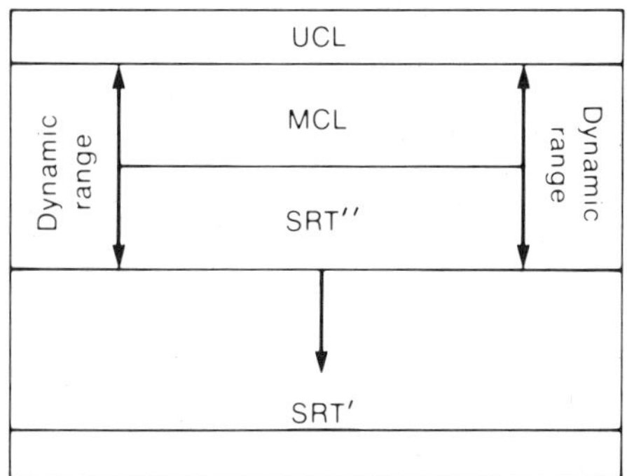

FIGURE 70–18. Hearing aid evaluation table in which SRT′ refers to the normal sensitivity range and SRT″ refers to a hearing loss in excess of 30 dB. The dynamic range is the difference between SRT″ and the uncomfortable loudness level (UCL). This represents the level to which speech can be comfortably amplified. The most comfortable loudness level (MCL) is the level in decibels within the dynamic range reported by the patient to be the most comfortable for average listening situations.

mal range, preferably below 30 dB in the better ear without causing distortion of the acoustic signal or discomfort to the patient. During the evaluative process, aided versus unaided speech testing (SRT and speech discrimination) can be utilized to determine the improvement provided with amplification. Real-ear probe microphone testing can assist in providing hearing aid frequency response and gain information in situ.

These hearing aid–related tests should be performed in a sound-controlled environment with a minimum of background noise.

Hearing aids may have similar basic internal components, but they are manufactured in differing sizes, shapes, and colors. Generally, the smaller the instrument, the better is the cosmetic appeal to the patient. It should be noted as well that the smaller the device, the less power that is made available to overcome the loss in hearing. The different types of hearing aids that are currently the most popular are:

In-the-ear (ITE): a custom-fitted instrument with miniaturized components that are placed in their own casing formed from a mold of the patient's concha and canal (Fig. 70–19)

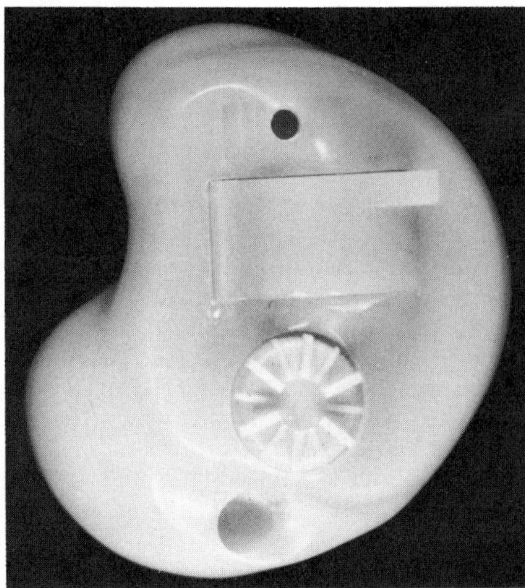

FIGURE 70–19. In-the-ear (ITE) hearing aid that fills the entire concha. (Courtesy of Argosy Electronics.)

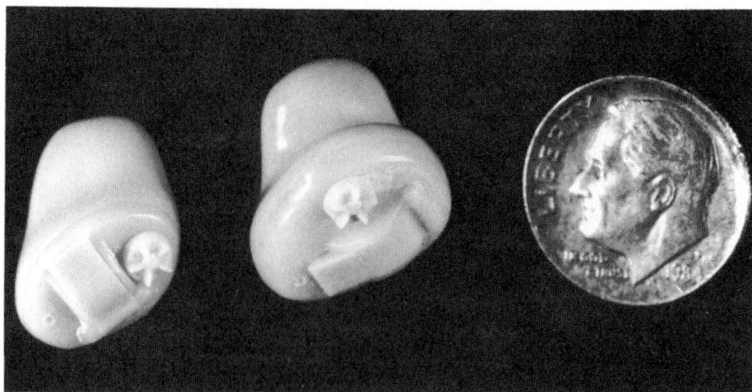

FIGURE 70–20. In-the-canal (ITC) hearing aids showing a standard size custom canal unit on the right and a custom microcanal unit on the left. (Courtesy of Argosy Electronics.)

In-the-canal (ITC): a miniature unit with all of the components housed within the canal portion of the custom mold (Fig. 70–20)

Postauricular: a premade, single-sized unit (size depending on manufacturer and model) contoured to the curvature of the auricle, resting on the helix. This type of instrument is also known as a behind-the-ear (BTE) hearing aid. The aid is coupled to the concha and canal via a custom-fitted earmold as shown in Figure 70–21.

Body type: a premade single sized unit with the microphone and amplifier housed in a case that is the size of a paging beeper, coupled to a receiver unit by a cord (Fig. 70–22). The cord is necessary to provide distance between the microphone and amplifier, which is typically worn somewhere on the chest area (usually a shirt pocket).

Table 70–4 provides a general guide to determine which type of hearing aid is most appropriate for a given patient and his or her degree and configuration of loss.

The evaluation for and the final fitting of a hearing aid is for many hearing-impaired patients only the beginning of the rehabilitative process. Individuals utilizing amplifica-

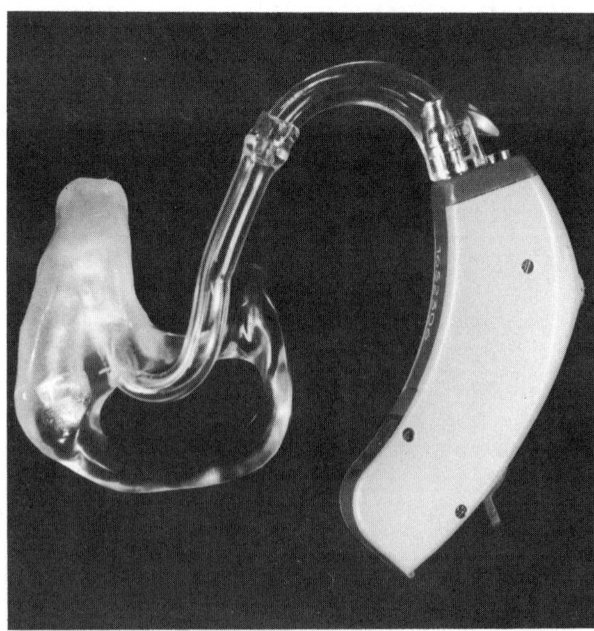

FIGURE 70–21. Behind-the-ear (BTE) instrument that is coupled to the ear by a polycarbonate earmold and connector tubing. (Courtesy of Starkey Laboratories.)

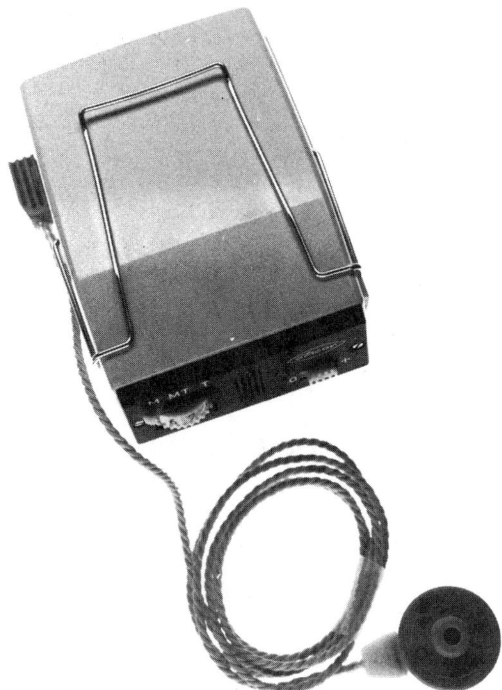

FIGURE 70–22. Body-type instrument typically worn in a shirt pocket and connected to the ear via a cord, receiver, and custom earmold (Courtesy of Oticon Corporation.)

tion often must readjust to hearing speech and environmental sounds at normal or near-normal levels once again. The interactive process between the patient and the practitioner subsequent to the final hearing aid fitting often has great impact on the ultimate success or failure for the rehabilitative efforts through the use of amplification. Counseling the patient regarding the need for realistic expectations and readjustment may be necessary. In cases of severe hearing impairment, supplemental input in the way of speech or lip-reading skills may be required in order to maximize the potential for use of residual auditory skills.

TABLE 70–4. HEARING AID FITTING GUIDE

Type of Aid	Degree of Loss	Configuration
Canal	Mild-to-moderate (25–40 dB)	Flat to gently falling
In-the-ear	Mild-to-moderate (25–60 dB)	Flat to gently falling
In-the-ear IROS*	Mild-to-moderate (20–60 dB)	High-frequency loss above 200 Hz
Postauricular	Mild-to-severe (20–90 dB)	All configurations, including low-frequency loss
Body	Severe-to-profound (70–100 dB+)	Minimal residual hearing at any frequency

*IROS = *I*psilateral *R*outing of *S*ignal, an in-ear device designed specifically for high-frequency loss.

REFERENCES

1. Metropolitan Life Insurance Company: Hearing impairment in the United States. Metropolitan Life Insurance Statistics 57:7, 1976.
2. Schuknecht H: Presbycusis. Laryngoscope 44:402, 1955.
3. Ward WD: Noise: The identification and treatment of noise induced hearing loss. Otolaryngol Clin North Am 90:89, 1969.
4. Zubick HH, Tolentino AT, and Boffa J: Hearing loss and the high speed dental handpiece. Am J Public Health 70:633, 1980.
5. Jerger J, Jerger S, and Mauldin L: Studies in impedance audiometry. III Middle ear disorders. Arch Otolaryngol 99:165, 1974.
6. Jacobson J: An Overview of the auditory brainstem response. *In* Jacobson J (ed): The Auditory Brain Stem Response. San Diego, College Hill (Allyn and Bacon), 1985.
7. Selters WA and Brackman DE: Acoustic tumor detection with brainstem electric response audiometry. Arch Otolaryngol 103:181, 1977.
8. Pestalozza G and Shore I: Clinical evaluation of presbycusis on the basis of different tests of auditory function. Laryngoscope 65:1136, 1955.
9. Federal Register: Rules of the Food and Drug Administration for the hearing aid industry. Federal Register, February 15, 1977, pp 9286–9296.
10. Teter DL: Clinical considerations of hearing aids. *In* Northern J (ed): Hearing Disorders. Boston, Little Brown, 1976.

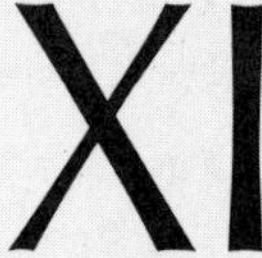

XI Screening and Preventive Medicine

71 Periodic Health Assessment of Asymptomatic Adults

WILLIAM T. BRANCH, Jr., MD
ROBERT S. LAWRENCE, MD

The effective *prevention* of disease is more efficient than the investment of time and money that characterizes *treatment* of disease. Routine examinations are still the most common reason for a physician-patient encounter,[1] and Americans have viewed the "yearly check-up" as the best way to maintain good health. In truth, although prevention is effective against infectious diseases, it is much more difficult to apply to the chronic diseases prevalent in modern industrialized nations. Nor does the finite nature of financial and human resources permit a wide-ranging battery of tests to be performed annually on all apparently healthy adults. Numerous groups of health care providers, statisticians, epidemiologists, and others, most recently the US Preventive Services Task Force, have reviewed available information and outlined recommendations for periodic health assessments.[2–5] Although data are often lacking to support all seemingly beneficial maneuvers, it has been possible to compile reasonable guidelines for the primary care practitioner.

PREVENTIVE APPROACH

"Screening" and "prevention" became catchwords in the 1960s, when many Americans began to raise questions about the appropriateness of the health care delivery system. Their concerns centered on access to, and availability of, health services for citizens at all levels of society. At the same time, it was recognized that the populations of several countries with leaner health care budgets had longer life expectancies and lower infant mortality rates.

Health care providers and policy makers promoted the development of medical technology as a means of addressing these concerns. The industry produced the instruments to facilitate batteries of diagnostic tests and helped "sell" screening to the public. By the 1970s, advocates of preventive care grew in number and included health maintenance organizations, fee-for-service providers, and special interest organizations, such as the American Cancer Society and the American Heart Association. Soon patients, consumer groups, and the public at large were requesting screening programs. To meet this higher demand and simultaneously encourage the preventive approach to health care, various mass screening efforts were initiated, ranging from blood pressure and tuberculin tests administered in mobile vans in neighborhoods and shopping areas to vast multiphasic screening centers, such as that at the Oakland site of the Kaiser Permanente Plan.[6]

Given their widespread availability, how valuable are these tests? Some argue that even though the available data do not conclusively establish their validity for disease prevention, many routine procedures are justified to serve other purposes. The visit to the doctor may be most valuable to establish a useful clinical data base if some future illness should arise, as well as to establish some degree of rapport between the patient and the provider. It follows that on the basis of this rapport a patient might be expected to report the onset of symptoms more promptly, allowing earlier treatment. With respect to the all-inclusive clinical data base, however, the limited value but sizable cost of many routinely performed tests, such as the baseline electrocardiogram[7] and routine and preadmission chest radiographs,[8,9] cast doubt on their usefulness.

SCREENING VERSUS CASE FINDING

As Sackett and Holland[10] have written, *screening* is the performance of a test or series of tests on volunteers from a general, unselected population. These tests are initiated by those administering them for the purpose of categorizing individuals into high- or low-risk groups for a given disorder. The act of screening carries with it an implicit promise of eventual beneficial outcome.

Case finding occurs when a physician tests a member of a patient population who is seeking care for a disorder. The indication for performing the test may or may not be related to the chief reason for the patient's visit, but the test has been chosen specifically to determine the presence of some problem for which the patient is considered to be at high risk because of his or her symptoms, family history, age, race, socioeconomic status, occupation, or lifestyle. Case finding, which produces a higher yield of positive findings than screening but carries no implicit guarantee of benefit, clearly justifies obtaining tests in many instances that would not be warranted for screening purposes. These may include instances such as obtaining mammography in a woman 40 to 49 years of age, in whom general screening is not recommended but whose concerns and desire to be tested, together with plausible benefit from the procedure, can justify case finding by the physician.

Ethical Questions. By suggesting that a patient undergo certain tests, the physician implies a desirable outcome. As defined by McKeown[11] over a decade ago, these implications are

1. If the disorder being sought is present, it will be found (sensitivity).
2. If the disorder is not present, it will not be suggested (specificity).
3. If the disorder is present, it can be treated.
4. Treatment will be beneficial even in terms of risk and cost.

The US Preventive Services Task Force addressed these issues by recommending screening in cases in which data from prospective trials, or convincing data from other types of studies, such as case-control studies, show benefit to the patient.[5] In some cases, in which evidence suggests but does not prove a benefit, the recommendation to perform, or not to perform, a screening test is left to the discretion of the provider.[5]

Expediency. Patient expectations have been raised by statements made in the medical and lay press regarding the benefits of preventive care. Asymptomatic persons coming to an appointment for a routine examination prefer even more tests than are are recommended by published guidelines.[12] For patients expecting such care, providers are tempted to order a battery of tests, rather than spending time explaining the limited benefit and possible disadvantages of such an approach.

Cost. If providers were to implement some of the protocols that have been promulgated for routine examinations at given intervals over a lifetime, a vast amount of health resources would be utilized. According to one estimate,[13] one of these protocols would carry with it costs equal to 5 to 10% of a total national health budget and 25% of the payments made to physicians. Such an expenditure cannot be justified unless corresponding benefit is substantiated.

Compliance. Physicians fall short of obtaining many procedures recommended by published guidelines.[14,15] Such data suggest that primary care physicians should organize systems within their practices to monitor the performance of tests that they themselves believe are necessary and should be prepared to educate their patients on the extent and purposes of screening.

With these concerns in mind, what does the practitioner hope to achieve in an optimal preventive care program? The first goal is to maintain or improve the health status of patients by decreasing morbidity, mortality, and disability rates. The second goal is to help the patient by diagnosing a disease or disorder early. The third goal is to achieve the most efficient use of time, money, personnel, and space by giving effective medical care to patients only when it is "truly needed."

In reference to the first objective, it is worth remembering that the most significant advances in improving the health status of large populations are those that have been made in the public health field. Proper sewage disposal, fluoridation of water systems, and immunization are all proven preventive measures for a wide variety of diseases.

As for the benefit to the patient of early diagnosis, Sackett[15] and others argued that in many cases of a terminal chronic disease state, early awareness merely prolongs the anxiety and depression. In some cases, an early diagnosis only seems to improve the survival of patients by prolonging the time that the disease is known to exist (i.e., the *lead time*) but does not actually alter its outcome.

RECOMMENDATIONS FOR PERIODIC HEALTH ASSESSMENT OF ASYMPTOMATIC ADULTS

Our recommendations should be applied to apparently healthy, nonpregnant, asymptomatic adults and not to those with specific complaints, previously diagnosed chronic illnesses, or known high risk of developing a particular illness. Any of the latter groups may justify more frequent visits or additional studies done for the purpose of case finding. This discussion is divided into the following sections: routine examination, tests, immunizations, counseling, the occupational and environmental history, and screening of refugees.

Routine Examination

A complete history and physical examination at the initial visit may help establish rapport with the patient as well as a data base for the future. Only a few aspects of the history and physical examination have proved to be beneficial (Table 71–1).[5] Recording of blood pressure and weight, examination of the oral cavity, testing of vision and hearing

TABLE 71–1. PERIODIC HEALTH ASSESSMENT FOR ASYMPTOMATIC NONPREGNANT ADULTS*

	Ages of Patients		
Routine Examination	*19–39 yr*	*40–64 yr*	*65 yr and over*
History	Dietary intake Physical activity Tobacco, alcohol, or drug use Sexual practices Depressive symptoms	Dietary intake Physical activity Tobacco, alcohol, or drug use Sexual practices Depressive symptoms	Functional status at home Prior symptoms of transient ischemic attack Dietary intake Physical activity Tobacco, alcohol, or drug use Depressive symptoms Abnormal bereavement Changes in cognitive function Medications that increase risk of falls
Physical Examination	Height and weight Blood pressure Tooth decay or gingivitis Signs of physical abuse	Height and weight Blood pressure Clinical breast examination (annually for women) Signs of physical abuse Malignant skin lesions Tooth decay, gingivitis, loose teeth	Height and weight Blood pressure Visual acuity Hearing and hearing aids Clinical breast examination (annually for women) Signs of physical abuse or neglect Malignant skin lesions Peripheral arterial disease Tooth decay, gingivitis, loose teeth
Laboratory/Diagnostic Procedures	Nonfasting blood cholesterol level Papanicolaou smear (every 1–3 years)	Nonfasting blood cholesterol level Papanicolaou smear (every 1–3 years) Mammogram (every 1–2 years for women beginning at age 50) Stool for occult blood (annually over age 50) Flexible sigmoidoscopy (every 10 years, beginning at age 50)	Thyroid function tests (for women) Papanicolaou smear (unless 3 previously negative) Mammogram (every 2 years until age 75–80) Stool for occult blood (annually) Flexible sigmoidoscopy (every 10 years)
Counseling	Diet and exercise: fat, cholesterol, fiber, iron (for women), calcium (for women), caloric balance, selection of exercise program Substance use: tobacco cessation, alcohol, and other drugs: limiting alcohol consumption during driving or other dangerous activities, treatment for abuse Sexual practices: sexually transmitted diseases, partner selection, condoms, anal intercourse, unintended pregnancy, and contraceptive use Injury prevention: safety belts, use of safety helmets, smoke detectors, no smoking near bedding or upholstery, violent behavior (for men), firearms (for men) Dental health: regular tooth brushing, flossing, dental visits	Diet and exercise: fat, cholesterol, complex carbohydrates, fiber, calcium (for women), caloric balance, selection of exercise program Substance use: tobacco cessation, alcohol and other drugs: limiting alcohol consumption during driving or other dangerous activities, treatment for abuse Sexual practices: sexually transmitted diseases, partner selection, condoms, anal intercourse, unintended pregnancy, and contraceptive options Injury prevention: safety belts, use of safety helmets, smoke detectors, no smoking near bedding or upholstery Dental health: regular tooth brushing, flossing, and dental visits	Diet and exercise: fat, cholesterol, complex carbohydrates, fiber, calcium (for women), caloric balance, selection of exercise program Substance abuse: tobacco cessation, alcohol and other drugs: limiting alcohol consumption during driving or other dangerous activities, treatment for abuse Injury prevention: prevention of falls, use of safety belts, smoke detectors, no smoking near bedding or upholstery, safe hot water temperature, safety helmets Dental health: regular dental visits, tooth brushing, flossing Other primary preventive measures: glaucoma testing by eye specialist
Immunizations	Tetanus-diphtheria booster (every 10 years) Measles-mumps (persons born after 1956 who are not known to be immune to measles) Rubella (women without documented immunity)	Tetanus-diphtheria booster (every 10 years)	Tetanus-diphtheria booster (every 10 years) Influenza vaccine (annually) Pneumococcal vaccine

*Adapted from US Preventive Services Task Force: Guide to Clinical Preventive Services. An Assessment of the Effectiveness of 169 Interventions. Baltimore, Williams & Wilkins, 1989.

for persons older than 65 years of age, and a breast examination for female patients should be included. Once the patient has disrobed and is being examined, however, very little additional time is needed to direct the examination toward additional maneuvers that will be of benefit in persons at special risk (Table 71–2).

The frequency of periodic health assessments following an initial examination is generally suggested to be at 2- to 5-year intervals, the longer interval for the younger age groups (16 to 60 years). Exceptions include blood pressure checks, which should be done at each visit, and breast examination and other limited aspects of the physical examination, which should be done annually. Most primary care patients will visit their doctor for some reason—for example, an episodic symptom or brief check-up—each year,[16] and these visits can provide the means for case finding during the intervals between major periodic health assessments.

Tests

Data support the obtaining of blood cholesterol periodically in all persons, plus additional tests in persons at special risk (see Table 71–2).[5]

Data from a randomized trial show a statistically significant 33% reduction in the 13-year cumulative mortality rate from colorectal carcinoma in persons aged 50 to 80 years screened annually for fecal occult blood with six rehydrated occult blood slides (two each from three consecutive stools), compared with control patients, who had very few occult blood tests done on their own.[17] Biennial occult blood testing appeared less beneficial. Rehydration resulted in 9.8% positive occult blood slide results, increasing the sensitivity but decreasing the positive predictive value of the testing. Over 13 years, 38% of the screened patients underwent colonoscopy, of whom 1.9% had cancer and 27.5%, colorectal polyps. Most of the decreased mortality could be explained by a decreased proportion of stage D cancers in the annually screened group. Data from a case-control study[18] and decision analyses[19, 20] also suggest 20 to 30% reductions in mortality from colorectal cancer by fecal occult blood testing. A case-control study of sigmoidoscopy, performed as infrequently as every 10 years, suggests a 60% reduction in mortality from colorectal cancer within reach of the sigmoidoscope.[21]

We conclude that annual screening for fecal occult blood and flexible sigmoidoscopy every 5 to 10 years will reduce mortality in persons aged 50 to 80. Rehydration of occult blood slides increases the number of colonoscopies and, hence, the cost of this approach. Further studies may reveal less costly alternatives, but until such studies are available, providers may reasonably adopt this policy. An additional possible benefit of screening is reduced mortality as patients are followed beyond 13 years if removal of polyps reduces the risk of later development of colorectal cancer.[22]

The Papanicolaou test is suggested at intervals of 2 to 3 years for sexually active women between the ages of 18 and 60 and should be performed every 3 to 5 years in women older than 60 years of age, unless they are known to have three prior negative results on Papanicolaou smears and have no postmenopausal bleeding. Mammography is recommended every 1 to 2 years for women older than 50 years of age. In women between the ages of 40 and 49, with no special risk factors for breast cancer, current data do not show benefit from routine mammography, although longer follow-up is needed to be sure that no benefit exists[23]; therefore, this recommendation is at the discretion of the patient and the provider. Despite lack of proven benefits, breast self-examination should be taught.

Some specialists recommend annual prostate-specific antigen (PSA) testing in all men aged 50 to 75 years to detect occult cancer of the prostate.[24, 25] However, the 10-year survival rate is high in men with untreated early-stage prostatic cancer.[26] Periodic PSA testing plus digital rectal examinations, followed by transrectal ultrasonography and prostate biopsies as indicated, can detect early-stage prostatic cancer but are without proven benefit. Radical prostatectomy and radiation therapy have small but not negligible mortality rates (1.5% and 0.5%, respectively) and complication rates (impotence [25%], rectal injury [1–3%], urinary incontinence [3–6%], and urethral stricture [8–18%]).[26a] No recommendation for routine screening of asymptomatic men with PSA testing seems feasible unless results of prospective trials, now under way, show net benefit in mortality.[26a] A policy of obtaining PSA levels in men at increased risk of prostatic cancer, because of race, family history, or nonspecific but suspicious symptoms or findings, could enhance potential cost-effectiveness of testing by increasing the true-positive to false-positive ratio of the PSA levels.

Immunizations

Young women should be tested serologically for rubella and should be immunized prior to pregnancy if the test result is negative. Congenital rubella now occurs most commonly in the children of unmarried inner-city teenagers; therefore, one should pay close attention to their immunization status, as well as to that of women more traditionally thought to be in the child-bearing years. A tetanus and diphtheria vaccination is recommended every 10 years. Available data support giving the measles vaccine to persons born after 1956 who are not known to be immune to measles, influenza vaccine every year, pneumococcal vaccine once to patients over the age of 65, and hepatitis B vaccine to persons at increased risk of exposure to hepatitis B.

Counseling

In view of the important role played by lifestyle and personal habits in maintaining one's health, an effective preventive care plan must include counseling by the primary care practitioner. As is widely known, issues having a significant impact on well-being include the use of alcohol and drugs, proper nutrition, exercise, smoking, contraception, safe sexual practices, prevention of osteoporosis (see later), and accident prevention, plus additional psychosocial, sexual, and family-related problems listed in Tables 71–1 and 71–2.

The recommendation by the physician for the patient to use seatbelts and a child-support for infants in automobiles may have a positive impact on accident prevention.[28] Mention of the problem of driving while intoxicated may also unearth information and lead to help for the patient, who may be concerned about a family member.

Another preventive aspect involves counseling patients who are on prescribed drugs. Oral instructions on the reasons for taking a medication, its dosage schedule, and common side effects are essential and can be supplemented by leaflets on common drugs, available from several sources.[29]

TABLE 71–2. ADDITIONAL HEALTH ASSESSMENTS FOR NONPREGNANT ADULTS IN HIGH-RISK GROUPS*

	Ages of Patients		
Routine Examination	*19–39 yr*	*40–64 yr*	*65 yr and over*
History			
Suicide risk factors	Recent divorce, unemployment, depression, alcohol or other drug abuse, serious medical illnesses, living alone, recent bereavement	Same	Same
Physical Examination			
Complete oral cavity examination	Exposure to tobacco or excessive alcohol or those with suspicion on self-examination	Same	Same
Palpation for thyroid nodules	History of upper body irradiation	Same	Same
Clinical breast examination	Family history of premenopausal breast cancer in first-degree relative		
Clinical testicular examination	Cryptorchidism, orchiopexy, or testicular atrophy		
Complete skin examination	Family or personal history of melanoma, skin cancer, or precursor lesions; increased occupational or recreational sunlight exposure		
Auscultation for carotid bruits		Hypertension, smoking, coronary artery disease, atrial fibrillation, diabetes, or history of neurologic symptoms	Same
Peripheral arterial disease		Smoking, diabetes mellitus, age over 50	
Laboratory/Diagnostic Procedures			
Fasting plasma glucose level	Marked obesity, family history, or gestational diabetes	Same	Same
VDRL†/RPR‡	Prostitution, sexual promiscuity, living in high-prevalence area, or known contact	Same	
Urinalysis	In diabetes	Same	At provider's discretion
Chlamydia testing	Women with multiple sexual partners or sexual partner with multiple contacts	Same	
Gonorrhea culture	Prostitution, sexual promiscuity, living in high-prevalence area, or known contact	Same	
Counseling and testing for HIV§	For any risk factor or known exposure	Same	
Hearing test	Noise exposure	Same	
Tuberculin skin test	Household contacts, recent immigrants, migrant workers, residents of correctional institutions or homeless shelters, immunodeficient persons	Same	Household contacts, or residents of nursing homes, homeless shelters, or institutions
Electrocardiography	Men who would endanger public safety if they experience sudden cardiac events	Men with two or more cadiac risk factors, sedentary or high-risk males planning to begin a vigorous exercise program, men who would endanger public safety	Risk factors
Mammography	Women 35 and older with family history of premenopausal breast cancer in first-degree relative	Same	
Colonoscopy	Family history of familial polyposis or cancer family syndrome	Same	Same
Bone mineral content		Perimenopausal women at increased risk for osteoporosis	
Prostate-specific antigen		Age 50 years if at risk because of black race, family history, or symptoms	Same to age 75

Table continued on opposite page

TABLE 71–2. ADDITIONAL HEALTH ASSESSMENTS FOR NONPREGNANT ADULTS IN HIGH-RISK GROUPS* *Continued*

Routine Examination	Ages of Patients: *19–39 yr*	*40–64 yr*	*65 yr and over*
Counseling			
Information on sharing and using unsterilized needles and syringes	Intravenous drug use	Same	
Back-conditioning exercises	Past history, body configuration, or activities predisposing to low back injury	Same	
Prevention of childhood injuries	Children in the home or automobile	Same	Same
Falls in the elderly	Older adults in the home	Same	
Other Primary Preventive Measures			
Discussion of hemoglobin testing	Young adults of Caribbean, Latin American, Asian, Mediterranean or African descent		
Skin protection from ultraviolet light	Increased exposure to sunlight	Same	
Discussion of aspirin therapy		Men with risk factors for myocardial infarction who lack risk factors for bleeding	Same
Discussion of estrogen replacement therapy		Perimenopausal women at risk for osteoporosis without known contraindications	Same
Immunizations			
Hepatitis B vaccine	Homosexually active men, intravenous drug use, receipt of blood products, health-related jobs with exposure to blood or blood products	Same	Same
Pneumococcal vaccine	Medical conditions that increase the risk of pneumococcal infection, including sickle cell disease, nephrotic syndrome, Hodgkin's disease, asplenia, diabetes, alcoholism	Same	
Influenza vaccine	Chronic care residency or chronic cardiopulmonary diseases, metabolic disorders, hemoglobinopathies, immunosuppression, or renal dysfunction	Same	

*Adapted from US Preventive Services Task Force: Guide to Clinical Preventive Services. An Assessment of the Effectiveness of 169 Interventions. Baltimore, Williams & Wilkins, 1989.
†VDRL = Venereal Disease Research Laboratories test.
‡RPR = rapid plasma reagin test.
§HIV = human immunodeficiency virus.

Occupational and Environmental History

The occupational and environmental history is part of the data base. Although not every patient benefits, the payoff of such a history, when it reveals clinically relevant information, is high.[30–32] Common problems are skin reactions to environmental agents, respiratory symptoms from inhaled pollutants, and orthopedic problems, especially back pain. The occupational history usually includes asking about work missed because of illness or injury, difficulty breathing on the job, changes in jobs or work assignments, exposure to loud noise or radiation, and back pain. The environmental history includes asking about hobbies or crafts, use of pesticides, exposure to chemicals, paints, sprays, or dusts, changes in residence because of health problems, or proximity of the residence to an industrial plant. When symptoms are reported, one should inquire whether they are of lesser severity when the patient is at home or on vacation, and one may inquire about ventilation systems and use of protective equipment. The physician should be familiar with occupational and environmental causes of medical problems (Table 71–3). The chemicals included in trade-name products are listed in publications such as the *Handbook of Poisoning*[33] and *Clinical Toxicology of Commercial Products.*[34]

Back pain may be prevented by educating the worker to lift by bending the knees and to carry heavy bundles clasped against the chest; nerve entrapment syndromes can be alleviated by eliminating repetitive motion at work. The physician may also help his or her patient obtain Worker's Compensation; in many states, work hastening, aggravating or contributing to a disability qualifies for compensation.[31] Regulations vary from state to state; it has been suggested that physicians, when writing a report, identify

TABLE 71–3. COMMON SYMPTOMS CAUSED BY OCCUPATIONAL AND ENVIRONMENTAL EXPOSURES*

	Agent	Potential Exposures
Immediate or Short-Term Effects		
Dermatoses (allergic or irritant)	Metals (chromium, nickel), fibrous glass, epoxy resins, cutting oils, solvents, caustic alkali, soaps	Electroplating, metal cleaning, plastics machining, leather tanning, housekeeping
Headache	Carbon monoxide, solvents	Firefighting, automobile exhaust, foundry, wood finishing, dry cleaning, painting
Acute psychoses	Lead (especially organic), mercury, carbon disulfide	Handling gasoline, seed handling, fungicide, wood preserving, viscose rayon industry
Fever, viral-like illness (polymer fume fever)	Heated fluoropolymers	Cigarette smoking plus working with polymers
Asthma or dry cough	Formaldehyde, toluene diisocyanate, animal dander	Textiles, plastics, polyurethane kits, lacquer use, animal handler
Pulmonary edema, pneumonitis	Nitrogen oxides, phosgene, halogen gases, cadmium	Welding, farming ("silo filler's disease"), chemical operations, smelting
Cardiac arrhythmias	Solvents, fluorocarbons	Metal cleaning, solvent use in painting, woodworking, or cleaning, refrigerator maintenance
Angina	Carbon monoxide (including that derived from methylene chloride)	Car repair, traffic exhaust, foundry, wood finishing, paint removal, ceramics, gas firing, indoor charcoal grill
Abdominal pain	Lead	Battery making, enameling, smelting, painting, welding, ceramics, plumbing
Hepatitis (may become a long-term effect)	Halogenated hydrocarbons, e.g., carbon tetrachloride; virus	Solvent use, lacquer use, hospital workers
Latent or Long-Term Effects		
Chronic dyspnea		
Pulmonary fibrosis	Asbestos, silica, beryllium, coal, aluminum	Mining, insulation, pipefitting, sandblasting, quarrying, metal alloy work, aircraft or electrical parts, sculpture grinding
Chronic bronchitis, emphysema	Cotton dust, cadmium, coal dust, organic solvents, cigarettes	Textile industry, battery production, soldering, mining, solvent use
Lung cancer	Asbestos, arsenic, nickel, uranium, coke-oven emissions	Insulation, pipefitting, smelting, coke ovens, shipyard work, nickel refining, uranium mining
Nasopharyngeal cancer	Wood dust, leather exposure	Woodworking, shoemaking
Bladder cancer	β-naphthylamine, benzidine dyes	Dye industry, leather, rubberworking, chemists
Peripheral neuropathy	Lead, arsenic, *n*-hexane, methyl butyl ketone, acrylamide	Battery production, plumbing, smelting, painting, shoemaking, solvent use, insecticides
Behavioral changes	Lead, carbon disulfide, solvents, mercury, manganese	Battery makers, smelting, viscose rayon industry, degreasing, repair of scientific instruments, dental amalgam workers
Extrapyramidal syndrome	Carbon disulfide, manganese	Viscose rayon industry, steel production, battery production, foundry
Aplastic anemia, leukemia	Benzene, ionizing radiation	Chemists, furniture refinishing, cleaning, degreasing, radiation workers

*From Goldman RH and Peters JM: Occupational and environmental health history. JAMA 246:2831, 1981. Copyright 1981, American Medical Association.

for themselves, their patients, and others whether they are assuming the role of advocate for the patient's claim or of adjudicator on behalf of the disability board.[35]

SCREENING OF RECENTLY ARRIVED REFUGEES

Special screening is indicated for recently arrived refugees. Those from Southeast Asia are at risk for intestinal parasites, tuberculosis, and hepatitis. In one study, more than half of recently arrived Southeast Asian refugees had intestinal parasites detected by fecal examination, most commonly *Ascaris, Trichuris,* and hookworm.[36] About 40% of the refugees had positive results on tuberculin tests, but only one had active tuberculosis identified on chest radiograph.[36] An unknown number had received bacille Calmette-Guérin vaccine. Most of the adults tested positive for antibody to hepatitis B, and 16% were hepatitis B–antigen carriers.[36] Vaccination of siblings and other family members of carriers, if antigen- and antibody-negative, is probably indicated. Other findings in refugees included dental caries, scabies, pediculosis, otitis media, and, rarely, a positive result on the Venereal Disease Research Laboratories test.[36] Persons of Hispanic background are at special risk for diabetes, cervical cancer, hypertension, tuberculosis, alcoholism, violent death, and human immunodeficiency virus infection.[37]

ADDITIONAL TESTS FOR PERSONS AT HIGH RISK

Also deserving of mention here are certain additional tests that may be administered to groups known to be at high risk for specific disorders, including the tuberculin test for inner-city and nursing home residents, thyroid testing in postmenopausal women, and tests for syphilis or gonorrhea, sickle cell anemia, thalassemia, and Tay-Sachs disease for persons at risk for these diseases. (see Table 71–2). Individuals at high risk for glaucoma include those with diabetes mellitus, arterial hypertension, or a positive family history of glaucoma, as well as the elderly. It is variously estimated that up to 5% of the population over the age of 40 years may have increased ocular tension (>20 mm Hg). On the other hand, less than 0.5% of the population older than 40 years of age has glaucoma, as manifested by loss of vision or an intraocular tension of 30 mm Hg or more.[38] And the efficacy of treatment in asymptomatic patients with borderline intraocular hypertension (20 to 30 mm Hg) is still debatable. We suggest that routine tonometric testing, usually performed with up-to-date equipment at the time of a periodic vision examination, be performed in individuals at high risk and perhaps those older than 65 years of age.

Some procedures have been excluded deliberately from these recommendations, such as the complete chemistry laboratory screening profile done by autoanalyzer and the routine chest radiograph. Extensive chemical screening (except for cholesterol) of asymptomatic individuals has not yielded information adequate to justify its performance,[39, 40] and the same can be said for routine chest radiographs.[8] Case finding may be useful on a limited basis for medical outpatient procedures, such as testing for glucose, aminotransferase, and cholesterol.[41] Bone densitometry may prove valuable in evaluating the therapy of osteoporosis but is not yet judged to be useful for screening asymptomatic women to predict future fractures.[42]

On the other hand, estrogen may prove beneficial in preventing coronary artery disease as well as osteoporosis in postmenopausal women.[43] We recommend counseling all such women on the benefits and risks of estrogen treatment in light of their risk factors and family histories. Postmenopausal women with inadequate dietary calcium intake may also be counseled to take 1000 mg/day of elemental calcium in the absence of contraindications.[44]

ACKNOWLEDGMENTS

The original contributions of H. Richard Nesson, MD, and Maria W. Willard, MPH, who were coauthors of this chapter in the first edition of this textbook, are gratefully acknowledged.

REFERENCES

1. National Ambulatory Medical Care Survey, 1977: Summary of Vital and Health Statistics Data from the National Health Survey, Series 13, No. 44. DHEW Publication No. (PHS)80–795, p 37.
2. Medical Practice Committee, American College of Physicians: Periodic health examination: A guide for designing individualized preventive health care in the asymptomatic adult. Ann Intern Med 95:729, 1981.
3. Council on Scientific Affairs: Medical evaluations of healthy persons. JAMA 249:1626, 1983.
4. Canadian Task Force on the Periodic Health Examination. Can Med Assoc J 130:1278, 1984.
5. US Preventive Services Task Force: Guide to Clinical Preventive Services: An Assessment of the Effectiveness of 169 Interventions. Baltimore, Williams & Wilkins, 1989.
6. Collen MF: Multiphasic testing as a triage to medical care. *In* Ingelfinger FJ, Ebert RV, Finland M, et al (eds): Controversy in Internal Medicine, 2nd ed. Philadelphia, WB Saunders, 1974, p 85.
7. Rubenstein LZ and Greenfield S: The baseline electrocardiogram in evaluating acute cardiac complaints. JAMA 244:2536, 1980.
8. Tape TG and Mushlin AI: The utility of routine chest radiographs. Ann Intern Med 104:663, 1986.
9. Hubbell AF, Greenfield S, Tyler JL, et al: The impact of routine admission chest x-rays on patient care. N Engl J Med 312:209, 1985.
10. Sackett DL and Holland WW: Controversy in the detection of disease. Lancet ii:357, 1975.
11. McKeown T: Validation of screening procedures. *In* Screening in Medical Care. London, Oxford University Press, 1968.
12. Woo B, Woo B, Cook EF, et al: Screening procedures in the asymptomatic adult: Comparison of physician's recommendations, patient's desires, published guidelines, and actual practice. JAMA 254:1480, 1985.
13. Spitzer WO: Epidemiological and clinical considerations. *In* Dorsey JL and Kane J (eds): Health Assessment and Preventive Care: Proceedings of the Medical Directors Conference (Medical Directors Division, Group Health Association of America), Vol 2, No 3. February 1978.
14. Romm FJ, Fletcher SW, and Hulka BS: The periodic health evaluation: Comparison of recommendations and internists' performance. South Med J 74:265, 1981.
15. Sackett DL: Can screening programs for serious diseases really improve health? Sci Forum 15:9, 1970.
16. Vital and Health Statistics: Current estimates from the Health Interview Survey, United States, 1978. Bethesda, MD, US Department of Health, Education and Welfare, National Center for Health Statistics, 1979.
17. Mandel JS, et al: Reducing mortality from colorectal cancer by screening for fecal occult blood. N Engl J Med 328:1365, 1993.
18. Selby JV, Friedman GD, Quesenberry CP, et al: Effect of fecal occult blood testing on mortality from colorectal cancer: A case-control study. Ann Intern Med 118:1, 1993.
19. Byers T and Gorsky R: Estimates of costs and effects of screening for colorectal cancer in the United States. Cancer 70:1288, 1992.
20. Wagner JL, Herdman RC, and Wadhwa S: Cost-effectiveness of colorectal cancer screening in the elderly. Ann Intern Med 115:807, 1991.
21. Selby JV, Friedman GD, Quesenberry CP, et al: A case-control study of screening sigmoidoscopy and mortality from colorectal cancer. N Engl J Med 326:653, 1992.
22. Winawer SJ, Zauber AG, Ho MN, et al: Prevention of colorectal cancer by colonoscopic polypectomy. N Engl J Med 329:1977, 1993.
23. Miller AB, Baines CJ, To T, et al: Canadian national breast screening study: 1. Breast cancer detection and death rates among women aged 40 to 49 years. Can Med Assoc J 147:1459, 1992.
24. Oesterling JE: Prostate-specific antigen: Improving its ability to diagnose early prostate cancer. JAMA 267:2236, 1992.
25. American Urological Association: American Urological Association Policy Statement. Early detection of prostate cancer and use of transrectal ultrasound. *In* American Urological Association 1992 Policy Statement Book. Baltimore, American Urological Association, 1992.
26. Johansson J-E, Adami H-O, Andersson S-O, et al: High 10-year survival rate in patients with early, untreated prostatic cancer. JAMA 267:2191, 1992.
26a. Kramer BS, Brown ML, Prorok PC, et al: Prostate cancer screening: What we know and what we need to know. Ann Intern Med 119:914, 1993.
27. Paffenbarger RS, Hyde RT, Wing AL, et al: The association of changes in physical-activity level and other lifestyle characteristics with mortality among men. N Engl J Med 328:538, 1993.
28. Attico NB, Smith RJ, Fitzpatrick MB, et al: Auto seat belts: Good prenatal, postpartum, and infant care. Am J Public Health 75:892, 1985.
29. Health and Public Policy Committee, American College of Physicians: Drug information for patients. Ann Intern Med 104:121, 1986.

30. The Occupational and Environmental Health Committee of the American Lung Association of San Diego and Imperial Counties: Taking the occupational history. Ann Intern Med 79:641, 1983.
31. Goldman RH and Peters JM: The occupational and environmental health history. JAMA 246:2831, 1981.
32. Cullen MR, Cherniack MG, and Rosenstock L: Occupational medicine (parts 1 and 2) (medical progress). N Engl J Med 322:594, 675, 1990.
33. Dreisbach RH: Handbook of Poisoning: Prevention, Diagnosis and Treatment, 10th ed. Los Altos, Lange Medical Publications, 1980.
34. Gosselin R, et al: Clinical Toxicology of Commercial Products, 4th ed. Baltimore, Williams & Wilkins, 1976.
35. Carey TS and Hadler NM: The role of the primary physician in disability determination for social security insurance and worker's compensation. Ann Intern Med 104:706, 1986.
36. Barry M, Craft J, Coleman D, et al: Clinical findings in Southeast Asian refugees. Child development and public health concerns. JAMA 249:3200, 1983.
37. U.S. Council on Scientific Affairs: Hispanic health in the United States. JAMA 265:248, 1991.
38. Frame PS and Carlson SJ: A critical review of periodic health screening using specific screening criteria. J Fam Pract 2:382, 1975.
39. Bradwell AR, Carmalt MHB, and Whitehead TP: Explaining the unexpected abnormal results of biochemic profile investigations. Lancet ii:1071, 1974.
40. Cebul RD and Beck JR: Biochemical profiles: Applications in ambulatory screening and preadmission testing of adults. Ann Intern Med 106:403, 1987.
41. Rottimann S, Dreifuss M, Clemencon D, et al: Multiple biochemical blood testing as a case-finding tool in ambulatory medical patients. Am J Med 94:141, 1993.
42. Ott S: Should women get screening bone mass measurements? Ann Intern Med 104:874, 1986.
43. Barrett-Connor E and Bush TL: Estrogen and coronary heart disease in women. JAMA 265:1861, 1991.
44. Reid IR, Ames RW, Evans MC, et al: Effect of calcium supplementation on bone loss in postmenopausal women. N Engl J Med 328:460, 1993.

72

Case Finding for Cancer

PART 1 Case Finding

I. CRAIG HENDERSON, MD
WILLIAM T. BRANCH, Jr., MD

It was pointed out in the preceding chapter that available evidence supports the use of only a limited number of screening procedures to detect asymptomatic diseases in apparently healthy adults. For detection of malignancy, such procedures include the Papanicolaou test, carried out at regular intervals to detect carcinoma of the cervix; mammographic examination to detect carcinoma of the breast beginning no later than age 50; stool examination for occult blood to detect carcinoma of the colon in individuals above ages 40 to 50 years; and sigmoidoscopic examinations at approximately 5-year intervals in persons older than 50 years of age. In other instances, the physician may seek to detect cancer by the process of *case finding* rather than screening. Some symptom may have been elicited, or the patient may be known to be at relatively high risk for the condition in question, and this often justifies a particular type of examination. In the broadest sense, one should tailor all periodic health assessments to the patient's age, sex, race, family history, and occupation.

EPIDEMIOLOGY AND IDENTIFICATION OF INDIVIDUALS AT HIGH RISK

In addition to age and sex, the major variables that determine a patient's risk of developing a malignant disease are a history of a prior cancer, family history, race, occupation, and use of alcohol and cigarettes (Table 72–1). Information collected on patients who enter primary care constitutes a data base that can be used to identify individuals for whom increased surveillance is indicated.

For most types of cancer, a history of a previous cancer in a paired organ or even in another organ system of the body may be the single highest risk factor. For example, women with a diagnosis of breast cancer are at increased risk throughout the remainder of their lifetime for developing an additional breast cancer in any remaining breast tissue, whether it is in the ipsilateral breast for patients treated with less than mastectomy or the contralateral breast. Patients who have had a diagnosis of retinoblastoma are at increased risk of developing osteogenic sarcoma either in the area irradiated as part of the treatment of the retinoblastoma or at sites distant from the primary tumor. An increased incidence of soft tissue sarcomas, brain tumors, and melanomas occur in these patients as well. Patients with a diagnosis of melanoma are more likely to develop a subsequent melanoma, and this increased risk is not entirely explained by increased sun exposure. Women diagnosed with breast cancer are at increased risk of endometrial cancer. Multiple additional examples of this type can be given, but interpretation of the recent literature is confounded by the impact of treatment. Both radiotherapy and chemotherapy may be associated with an increased risk of developing additional cancers, and it is often difficult to distinguish between the inherent risk of developing a second cancer and the effects of treatment. In any case, patients with a prior history of cancer should be monitored for the development of new cancers more carefully than the general population.

TABLE 72–1. DATA BASE TO IDENTIFY INDIVIDUALS AT INCREASED RISK OF DEVELOPING MALIGNANCY

Age and sex

Family history
- Carcinoma of the colon
- Carcinoma of the breast in first-degree relative
- Malignant melanoma
- Multiple carcinomas (uterus, stomach, lung)
- Rare familial syndromes, including von Recklinghausen's disease, medullary carcinoma of the thyroid, multiple endocrine adenomatosis, retinoblastoma, Wilms's tumor, multiple familial polyposis, Li-Fraumeni syndrome

History of prior malignancy

Race
- Fair complexioned individuals: malignant melanoma, skin cancer
- Black individuals: carcinoma of the oral cavity, esophagus, lung, stomach, pancreas, liver, prostate, and uterine cervix
- Chinese individuals from Canton, Hong Kong: nasopharyngeal carcinoma
- Japanese and Korean individuals: gastric cancer

Food and chemical ingestion
- Cigarette consumption: cancer of the oral cavity, paranasal sinuses, larynx, lung, urinary bladder, and pancreas
- Combination of alcohol and cigarette consumption: cancer of the oral cavity and esophagus
- Diet: cancer of the stomach, large bowel, endometrium, gallbladder, pancreas, breast
- Snuff dipping: cancer of the oral cavity

Occupation exposures
- Asbestos: carcinoma of the lung and malignant mesothelioma
- Polyvinyl chloride: hepatic angiocarcinoma
- Dye, rubber, and hydrocarbons: cancer of the urinary bladder
- Furniture and wood dust: cancer of the paranasal sinuses
- Petroleum: cancer of the skin and scrotum

Miscellaneous factors
- Postmenopausal conjugated estrogens: endometrial carcinoma
- Stilbestrol in utero: clear-cell cancer of the vagina
- Radiation exposure of the head or neck in childhood: thyroid cancer
- High-dose radiotherapy or chemotherapy for treatment of malignancy: leukemia
- Undescended testes: testicular cancer
- Vasectomy: prostate cancer
- Viral transmission through sexual contact or blood transmission: acquired immunodeficiency syndrome and Kaposi's sarcoma

The family history of colorectal cancer or cancer of the breast in first-degree relatives should always be sought. Familial clusters of endometrial, lung, and gastric cancer and of malignant melanomas have also been described. Other familial associations are rare but may carry high risk for the affected individual. A general question such as "Has there been a history of tumors or cancer in members of your family?" will often allow the physician to pursue this aspect in more detail. Familial associations appear in Table 72–1. In general, pedigrees associated with a high familial risk of cancer are characterized by the multifocal or bilateral development of primary tumors at a considerably younger age than for the general population.[1]

Race is an important factor in determining the risk of malignancy (see Table 72–1). Black individuals have an increased incidence (roughly twofold or greater) of carcinomas of the lung, oral cavity, esophagus, stomach, prostate, and uterine cervix. The likelihood of skin cancer and malignant melanoma is considerably greater in fair-complexioned individuals, particularly those exposed to sunlight because of climate or occupation.

Occupations associated with increased risk of cancer include shipyard, pipefitting, or insulation work leading to asbestos exposure (cancer of the lung or malignant mesothelioma); chemical work leading to polyvinyl chloride exposure (hepatic angiosarcoma); and work involving dye, rubber, or hydrocarbon exposure (cancer of the urinary bladder). Cancers of the nose and paranasal sinuses have been related to dust inhalation by wood or furniture workers.[2] Petroleum workers are at increased risk of acquiring cancer of the skin, which commonly involves the hands, head, neck, and scrotum.

The risk of developing lung cancer is closely correlated with cigarette smoking and becomes appreciable (~ 1%) after 20 pack-years; in persons who have smoked as many as three packs/day for 40 years, the aggregate risk reaches 20%.[3] Cigarettes are also associated with increased incidence of cancer of the oral cavity and paranasal sinuses, larynx, and urinary bladder. The conjunction of alcohol and tobacco use greatly increases the risk of cancer in both the oral cavity and the esophagus, whereas cigar and pipe smokers are at increased risk of oral cancer. Recognition of the carcinogenic potential of cigarettes may have contributed to the recent increased use of "smokeless" tobacco or snuff, but this, too, has been reported to increase the incidence of oral cancer by fourfold.[4] Between the 1930s and 1970s, there was a greater than 50% decrease in the mean tar content/cigarette in Britain, which may account for a 40 to 50% fall in the lung cancer mortality during the period 1960 to 1980.[5] This decrease in cancer mortality could not be accounted for by the small decrease in cigarette consumption during this period.

Exogenous hormone administration, especially the administration of conjugated estrogens, has been shown to be a risk factor for endometrial cancer when it is used to relieve postmenopausal symptoms and for clear cell carcinoma of the vagina in the offspring of patients given estrogens during pregnancy. Exogenous hormone administration is not clearly established as a risk factor for breast cancer, but nearly 60 case-control and cohort studies have been performed evaluating postmenopausal estrogen replacement therapy and oral contraceptive use.[6] The results from these individual studies are contradictory. Two meta-analyses have been performed on studies on postmenopausal estrogen replacement therapy. When all studies are considered together without regard for estrogen dose, duration of estrogen exposure, type of estrogen preparation, underlying risk of developing breast cancer, and various other confounding factors, there is a slight but statistically nonsignificant increase in risk.[7, 8] However, in one of these studies, the relative risk was determined to be 1.3 (95% confidence interval 1.2 to 1.6) among women whose estrogen use exceeded 15 years, and in this meta-analysis there also appeared to be an increased risk associated with a prior family history of breast cancer.[8] A similar meta-analysis of the case-control and cohort studies evaluating oral contraceptive use failed to demonstrate an overall risk when potential confounding factors were ignored, but the relative risk of developing a breast cancer at a young age (≤45 years old) was 1.46 among women who used oral contraceptives for durations in excess of 10 years (p = 0.001).[9] The relative risk of developing breast cancer prior to age 45 was 1.73 among women who had used oral contraceptives for more than 4 years before their first full-term pregnancy.

Radiotherapy to the head, neck, or mediastinum during childhood, especially that given in low doses for benign conditions, has been associated with thyroid malignancies in 5 to 10% of individuals up to 35 years after exposure.[3] An increased incidence of almost all types of cancer, except chronic lymphatic leukemia and possibly Hodgkin's disease and cervical cancer, has been associated with prior radiotherapy. Breast, thyroid, and bone marrow are organs considered especially sensitive to the carcinogenic effects of radiotherapy.[10] Skin cancer commonly develops in old burn or radiation scars or chronic ulcers. Radiation-induced malignancies usually occur within the radiotherapy field after a latent period of 10 to 15 years. The latent period between the administration of chemotherapy and the appearance of a second tumor is shorter, about 4 years, and almost any organ may be involved. However, secondary leukemia following chemotherapy has been reported more often than other types of malignancies.[11] The risk of developing any type of leukemia within 10 years of treatment with adjuvant melphalan for early breast cancer has been reported to be increased 11-fold.[12] A more commonly used regimen for the treatment of early breast cancer is the combination cyclophosphamide, methotrexate, and 5-fluorouracil (CMF), and the leukemogenic potential of this regimen appears to be less than that of melphalan. However, even CMF may induce as many fatal leukemias as 5/10,000 women treated.[13] Fortunately, the reduction in breast cancer mortality from the use of this therapy exceeds the risk of leukemia in most patient groups.[14] Combinations of chemotherapy and radiation are more carcinogenic than either alone, but the magnitude of this increased risk is difficult to determine. It has ranged from 5- to more than 1000-fold in various reports.[11]

Dietary factors have been estimated to contribute to more than a third of all cancer deaths.[15] These factors include overnutrition (e.g., obesity, high-fat diet), clinical or subclinical deficiencies (e.g., fibers, selenium, vitamins E and A), and the use of harmful food additives (e.g., nitrites, artificial sweeteners). The carcinogenic potential of these factors may be greatest during childhood, and it has not yet been shown that a change in habits during adult life will change cancer incidence.[6] Fortunately, dietary recommendations to reduce cancer incidence are likely to be beneficial in reducing the morbidity and mortality of other diseases as well, especially the incidence of cardiovascular diseases. These recommendations include maintenance of ideal body weight, restriction of fat intake to no more than one third of total caloric intake, and increased consumption of high-fiber foods such as fruits, vegetables, and whole-grain products.[16] Several highly publicized reports that linked coffee consumption with an increased incidence of pancreatic cancer were methodologically flawed, so this continues to be an area of controversy.

The incidence of Kaposi's sarcoma has abruptly increased in association with the epidemic of acquired immunodeficiency syndrome. Homosexuals—especially those with numerous sexual partners, heterosexuals with bisexual partners, parenteral drug users, hemophiliac patients, and patients given multiple blood transfusions are all at increased risk of developing this syndrome.[17]

In most patients, the risk of acquiring cancer depends chiefly on age and sex. In some cases, the prevalence of certain lesions may approach 1% of patients encountered, for example, cancer of the prostate in men over the age of 65 years and cancer of the breast in women over the age of 60 years. Clearly, such probabilities should be considered at the time of any office visit. Conversely, neoplasms that are most likely to occur in young adults (e.g., cancer of the testes in men and carcinoma in situ of the uterine cervix in women) differ from those most likely to occur in older persons. Figures 72–1 to 72–4 illustrate the annual incidence rates for commonly encountered malignant lesions according to age and sex.[18] The prevalence of such lesions in patients being examined for the first time or after a long hiatus generally will be two to three times the incidence rate. We recommend that clinicians familiarize themselves with these rates and include an examination of organs that are most likely to be affected at the time of each periodic health assessment.

Skin cancer is not included in Figures 72–1 to 72–4 because its incidence varies in different parts of the world and is not known exactly. In Texas and Australia, it has been reported to be the most frequently diagnosed type of malignancy and to account for more than 33% of all cancers.[19] Most squamous cell and basal cell carcinomas occur in persons older than 40 years of age, with a gradually increasing prevalence throughout aging and a moderate preponderance in men.

HISTORY AND PHYSICAL EXAMINATION

A review of systems sufficient to detect a large percentage of malignancies can be accomplished within a few minutes, often while one is examining the patient. The incremental cost of asking these questions and of performing a targeted physical examination, as outlined below, at the time of a routine patient visit has not been studied but should be cost-effective. The patient should be asked whether he or she has noticed any lumps or skin lesions that should probably be examined. Before examining the oral cavity, one might inquire whether the patient has noted any persistent ulceration or thickening. Likewise, during the breast examination the patient should be asked if she is aware of the presence of any lumps and, simultaneously, may be encouraged to perform periodic self-examinations. Other important items to investigate include a history of rectal bleeding or any change in bowel function; difficulty in urinating or redness or discoloration of the urine; and abnormal vaginal bleeding or any vaginal bleeding in a postmenopausal woman. Other complaints that

Text continued on page 921

MOST COMMON SITES OF MALIGNANCY IN AGES 30 TO 34 YEARS

WHITE WOMEN

Site	Annual Incidence per 1000 Women
Uterine cervix, carcinoma in situ	1.20*
Breast	0.25*
Uterine cervix, invasive carcinoma	0.16*
Thyroid	0.09
Malignant melanoma	0.08
Hodgkin's disease and lymphomas	0.05
Ovary	
Colorectum	0.04*
Uterus (corpus)	0.04
Lung	0.03
Brain	0.02
Leukemia	0.02
Bones, joints, and soft	0.02*
tissue	0.01*
Total incidence of invasive malignancy developing at any site	0.89
Total incidence of all malignancies	2.13

*Incidence increased in black Americans.

WHITE MEN

Site	Annual Incidence per 1000 Men
Testes	0.09
Hodgkin's disease and lymphomas	0.09
Malignant melanoma	0.07
Thyroid	0.04
Colorectum	0.03
Lung	0.03*
Brain	0.03
Leukemias	0.03
Bones, joints, and soft tissues	0.02
Buccal cavity and pharynx	0.02
Urinary bladder	0.02
Total incidence of invasive malignancy developing at any site	0.52
Total incidence of all malignancies	0.53

*Incidence increased in black Americans.

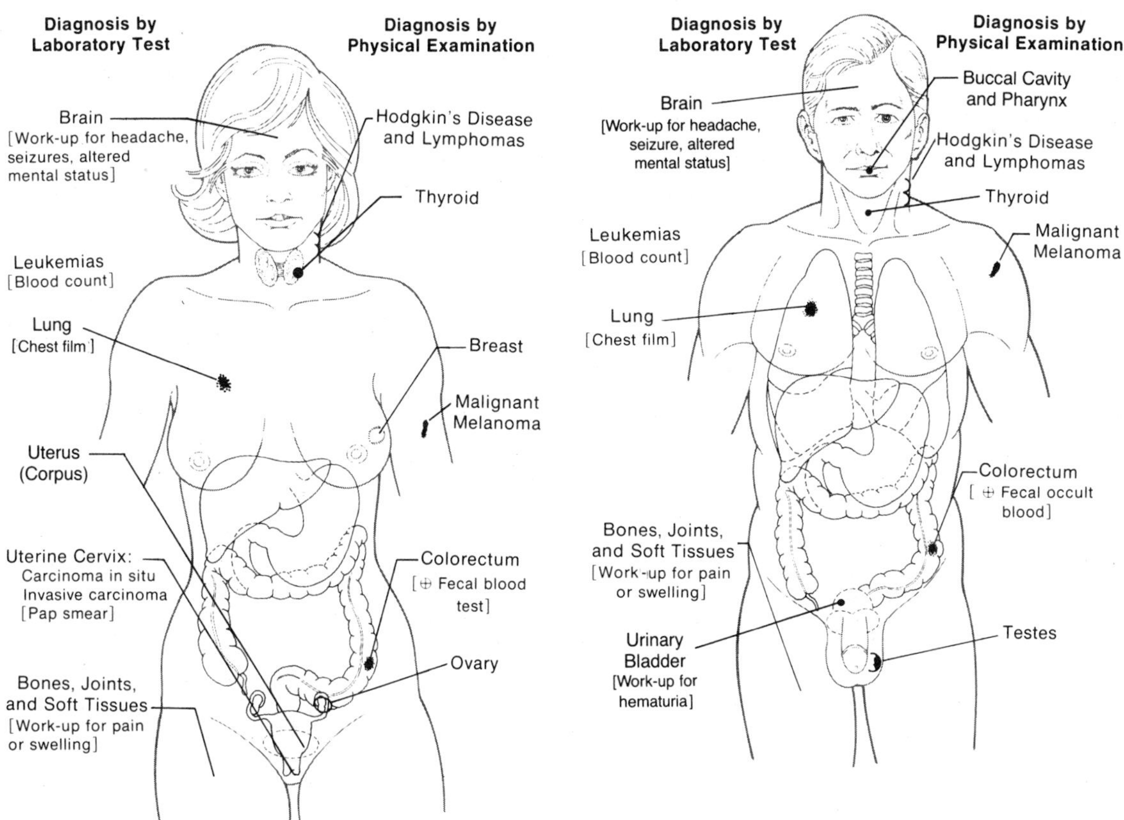

FIGURE 72–1. Data obtained from Young JL, Percy CL, et al: Surveillance Epidemiology End Results: Incidence and Mortality Data 1973–77. National Cancer Monograph 57, June 1981.

MOST COMMON SITES OF MALIGNANCY IN AGES 45 TO 49 YEARS

WHITE WOMEN

Site	Annual Incidence per 1000 Women
Breast (invasive)	1.76
Uterine cervix, carcinoma in situ	0.35*
Uterus (corpus)	0.32
Lung	0.30*
Colorectum	0.29*
Ovary	0.24
Uterine cervix, invasive carcinoma	0.18*
Breast (in situ)	0.16
Malignant melanoma	0.11
Thyroid	0.10
Hodgkin's disease and lymphomas	0.10
Total incidence of invasive malignancy developing at any site	4.01
Total incidence of all malignancies	4.63

*Incidence increased in black Americans.

WHITE MEN

Site	Annual Incidence per 1000 Men
Lung	0.58*
Colorectum	0.29
Buccal cavity and pharynx	0.16*
Urinary bladder	0.15
Hodgkin's disease and lymphomas	0.14
Malignant melanoma	0.13
Kidney	0.10
Larynx	0.10*
Brain	0.08
Pancreas	0.07*
Stomach	0.07*
Leukemias	0.07
Total incidence of invasive malignancy developing at any site	2.35
Total incidence of all malignancies	2.39

*Incidence increased in black Americans.

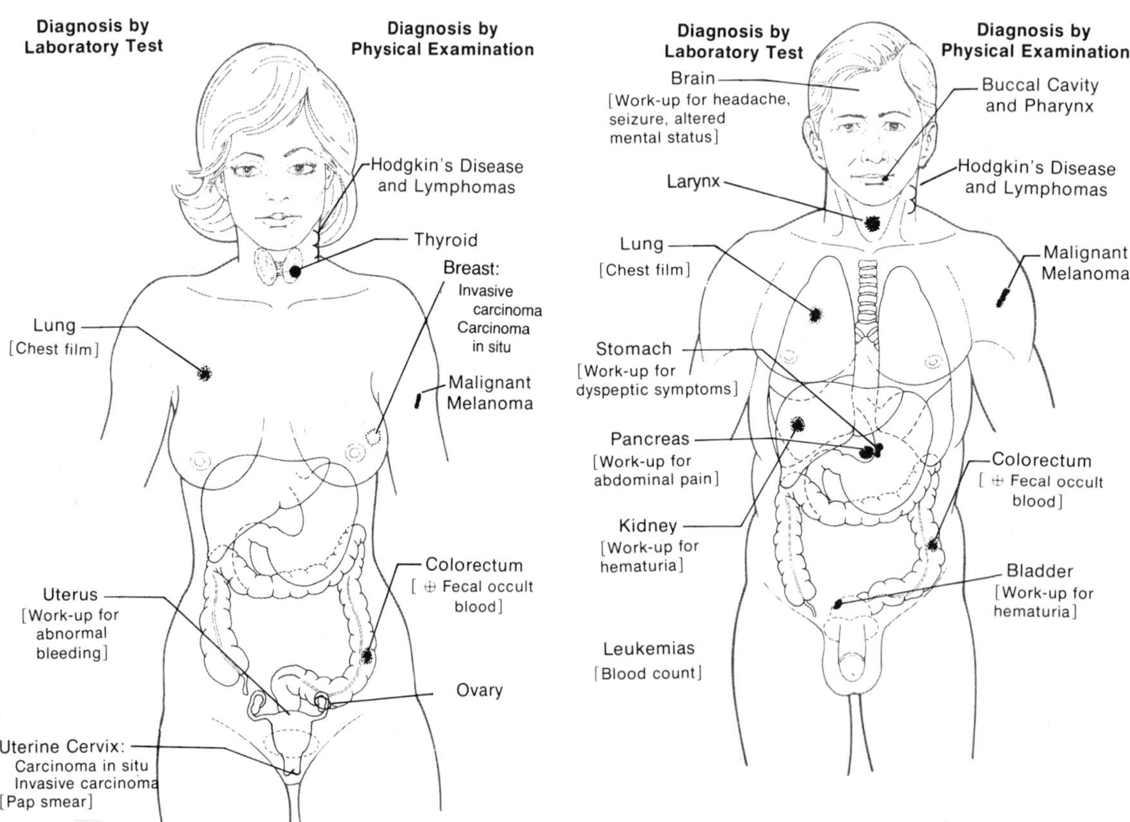

FIGURE 72–2. Data obtained from Young JL, Percy CL, et al: Surveillance Epidemiology End Results: Incidence and Mortality Data 1973–77. National Cancer Institute Monograph 57, June 1981.

MOST COMMON SITES OF MALIGNANCY IN AGES 60 TO 64 YEARS

WHITE WOMEN

Site	Annual Incidence per 1000 Women
Breast (invasive)	2.52
Uterus (corpus)	1.39
Colorectum	1.20
Lung	0.89
Ovary	0.46
Hodgkin's disease and lymphomas	0.29
Uterine cervix, invasive carcinoma	0.26*
Pancreas	0.24*
Buccal cavity and pharynx	0.23
Leukemias	0.17
Total incidence of invasive malignancy developing at any site	9.37
Total incidence of all malignancies	9.83

*Incidence increased in black Americans.

WHITE MEN

Site	Annual Incidence per 1000 Men
Lung	2.84*
Colorectum	1.65
Prostate	1.54*
Urinary bladder	0.78
Buccal cavity and pharynx	0.63*
Stomach	0.40*
Pancreas	0.37*
Hodgkin's disease and lymphomas	0.37
Larynx	0.36*
Kidney	0.30
Leukemias	0.30
Total incidence of invasive malignancy developing at any site	11.10
Total incidence of all malignancies	11.28

*Incidence increased in black Americans.

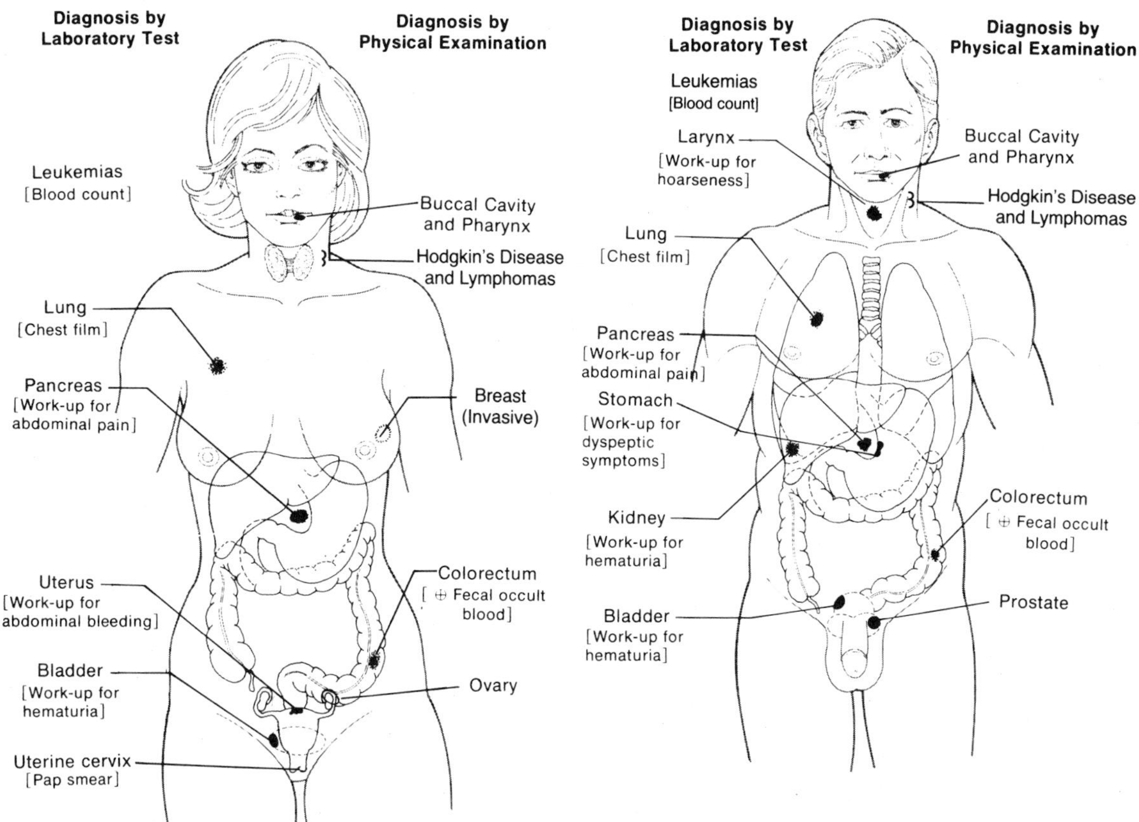

FIGURE 72–3. Data obtained from Young JL, Percy CL, et al: Surveillance Epidemiology End Results: Incidence and Mortality Data 1973–77. National Cancer Institute Monograph 57, June 1981.

MOST COMMON SITES OF MALIGNANCY IN AGES 70 TO 74 YEARS

WHITE WOMEN

Site	Annual Incidence per 1000 Women
Breast (invasive)	3.04
Colorectum	2.53
Uterus (corpus)	1.00
Lung	0.93*
Ovary	0.50
Pancreas	0.46*
Hodgkin's disease and lymphomas	0.46
Urinary bladder	0.38
Stomach	0.31*
Leukemias	0.31
Uterine cervix, invasive carcinoma	0.25*
Kidney	0.23
Buccal cavity and pharynx	0.22*
Multiple myeloma	0.20*
Brain	0.13
Total incidence of invasive malignancy developing at any site	12.44
Total incidence of all malignancies	12.83

*Incidence increased in black Americans.

WHITE MEN

Site	Annual Incidence per 1000 Men
Prostate	4.88*
Lung	4.82*
Colorectum	3.60
Urinary bladder	1.68
Buccal cavity and pharynx	0.84
Pancreas	0.74*
Stomach	0.74*
Leukemias	0.65
Hodgkin's disease and lymphomas	0.62
Kidney	0.49
Larynx	0.42*
Esophagus	0.32*
Multiple myeloma	0.28*
Brain	0.20
Malignant melanoma	0.18
Total incidence of invasive malignancy developing at any site	22.29
Total incidence of all malignancies	22.58

*Incidence increased in black Americans.

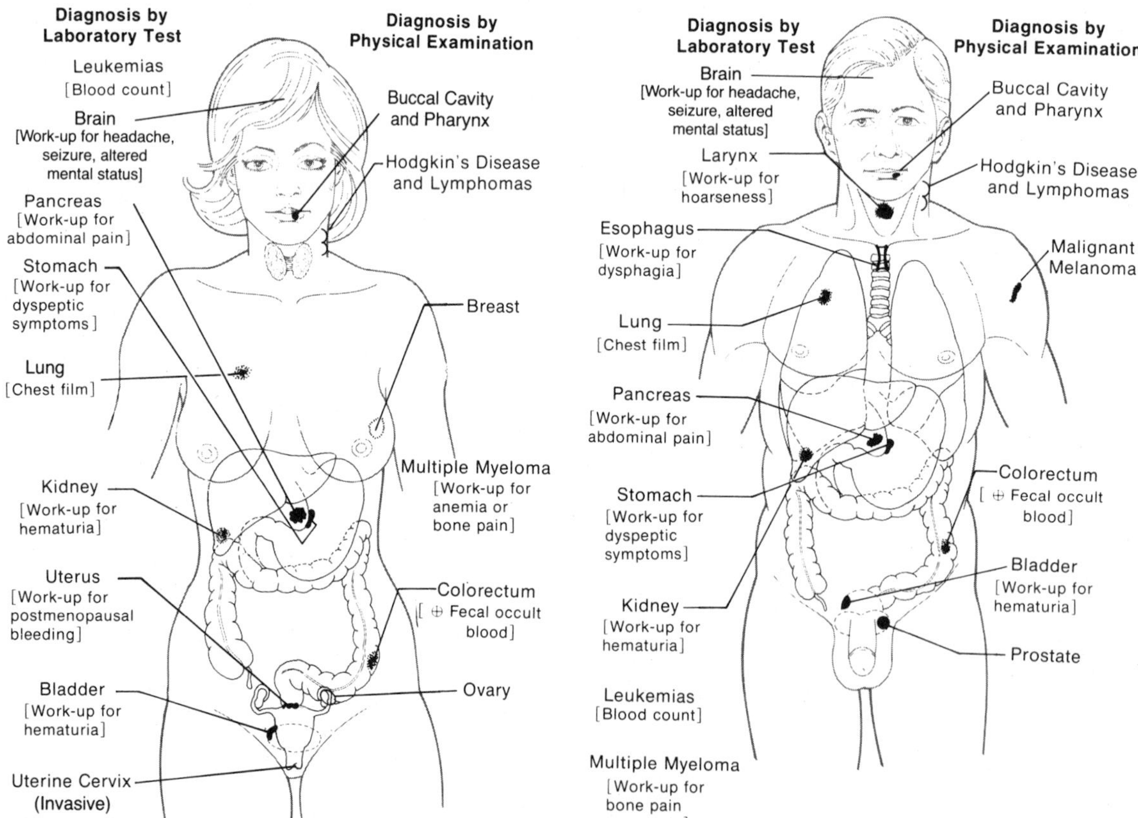

FIGURE 72–4. Data obtained from Young JL, Percy CL, et al: Surveillance Epidemiology End Results: Incidence and Mortality Data 1973–77. National Cancer Institute Monograph 57, June 1981.

require investigation include cough, hoarseness, and dysphagia; headache; unexplained fever, weight loss, or loss of appetite; and persistent, unexplained pain at any site.

Once the patient has disrobed, one should take a minute before starting to examine each organ system to observe the patient as a whole because melanomas, skin cancer involving the head and neck, and other seemingly obvious yet often overlooked abnormalities will be detected by this maneuver. Then, by spending only 3 or 4 additional minutes on the examination, one may very carefully assess the breasts, prostate, neck, testes, and other areas most likely to harbor a malignant lesion.

With calipers or a tape measure, one should carefully measure and record the precise location of all presumed or proved cancer lesions. This applies to enlarged lymph nodes, melanotic nodules, breast masses, lesions of the head and neck, hepatomegaly, abdominal masses, or lesions of the extremities. These measurements may be used as a baseline for future comparisons to assess tumor growth rate. In many instances, tumor characteristics will be distorted by subsequent biopsies or treatment, and these baseline observations by the patient's primary care physician may be the only accurate means of assigning a clinical stage to the patient. Whenever possible a primary tumor should be characterized using the TNM system. Tumor (T) size, fixation to surrounding organs, and infiltration of overlying skin should be noted. The presence of enlarged regional lymph nodes (N) and their fixation to each other or underlying structures should be recorded, along with evidence of metastases (M) distant to the site of the primary tumor and regional nodes.[20]

Skin. In Caucasians, most *skin cancers* are located on the head, neck, and upper extremities. These lesions are much less common and are more likely to involve the lower extremities in persons of darker complexions. The diagnosis should be evident from the physical examination (Fig. 72–5).

Squamous cell carcinomas often develop within premalignant actinic keratoses, which have the appearance of minimally raised erythematous patches with firmly adherent scaling and indistinct borders. Cutaneous horns sometimes contain a squamous cell carcinoma at their base. Intraepithelial squamous cell carcinoma (carcinoma in situ, Bowen's disease) appears as plaque-like, reddish, scaly papules and nodules of various sizes, which may range from a few millimeters to several centimeters in diameter and may remain unchanged for years before transforming into invasive squamous cell carcinoma. Early invasive squamous cell carcinomas appear as small, firm erythematous nodules with indistinct margins. As the lesions grow, the surface typically becomes ulcerated, with a raised, indurated border. Slowly growing lesions may fail to ulcerate and will appear as hyperkeratotic nodules. *Basal cell epitheliomas* appear as small pearly nodules with fine telangiectasias over the surface. Larger lesions typically become umbilicated; occasionally, the lesions show brown or black pigmentation or have a whitish, plaque-like, scarred appearance.

Malignant melanoma is the second or third most commonly encountered malignancy of individuals between the ages of 20 and 30 years; its absolute incidence increases in the elderly and is highest above the age of 80 years (~ 0.2/1000 persons).[18] Thus, malignant melanomas should be sought in individuals of all ages. They occur most commonly in fair-complexioned persons and on parts of the body exposed to sunlight. Although no more than 1 to 10% of melanomas in Caucasian patients are plantar melanomas, 67% of the melanomas in black Africans are reported to occur on the sole.[21] Subungual melanomas may also be rarely observed. Because they are malignancies of the melanocytes, melanomas sometimes occur by chance within a benign nevus; however, most benign nevi, including the junctional nevus, are not considered premalignant or more likely to give rise to melanomas than are melanocytes elsewhere in the epidermis.[22] Congenital nevi, certainly giant hairy nevi but also probably small congenital nevi, may be precursors of malignant melanoma.[23, 24] Recent attempts to define a "dysplastic nevus syndrome" that may also be a precursor of malignant melanoma suggest that its features are similar but more subtle than those of malignant melanoma.[25] Because these must be distinguished from more benign nevi, biopsy or removal of a nevus should be considered when the lesion is larger than average, the borders are fuzzy or irregular, the pigmentation is unusually dark, or the lesion displays two or more colors with variegated patterns. One must be able to recognize three types of malignant melanomas: the superficial spreading melanoma, the lentigo maligna, and the nodular melanoma (Fig. 72–6).

A variegated color, with shades of red, white, and blue within a brown or black lesion, and an irregular border, with an angular indentation or notch, are the most characteristic features of *superficial spreading melanomas.* The *lentigo maligna* is a flat lesion often present for many years with no apparent growth or change in appearance. Although its surface is smooth, the margins are markedly indented. It is not characterized frequently by shades of red, white, or blue, but its coloring is not uniformly brown because there are usually uneven flecks of black. These features allow one to distinguish lentigo maligna from benign lentigo senilis ("liver spots"), which have distinct round or oval margins and are uniformly pigmented. Transformation of lentigo maligna into an invasive melanoma is characterized by formation of nodular, sometimes hyperkeratotic, growth superimposed on the flat surface.

Nodular malignant melanomas are most often uniformly colored and may have regular borders closely resembling a benign blue nevus. These lesions are usually bluish-black, bluish-gray, or bluish-red in color. These shades of blue, especially if the surface or borders are irregular, should serve as an indication for biopsy, which should be done when there is the possibility of malignancy even if the lesion is more likely to be a benign nevus.

Lymphadenopathy and Soft Tissue Masses. *Hodgkin's disease* is most prevalent in individuals between 20 and 40 years of age and again becomes more prevalent in individuals above the age of 50 years. Because of the potential for cure if the involvement is local at the time of diagnosis, the neck, axillae, and inguinal regions should be palpated routinely during health assessments. Unexplained lymphadenopathy that remains more than 2 cm in diameter after a brief period of observation should be considered suspicious for malignancy. Excisional biopsy generally is recommended, unless metastatic oropharyngeal carcinoma is strongly suspected, in which case aspiration biopsy may be preferred. *Malignancies of the soft tissues* are rare but can be found at any age; firm, irregular, fixed, or enlarging soft tissue masses should be biopsied.

The Oral Cavity. Malignancies of the lip, tongue, oral cavity, pharynx, nasopharynx, and salivary glands are rarely encountered below the age of 35 years but become increasingly common (incidence of up to nearly 1.0/1000 persons) above the age of 50 years.[18] They are found most frequently in men, cigarette smokers, and blacks. Although there is little evidence that alcohol is carcinogenic in nonsmokers, there appears to be a synergistic effect between

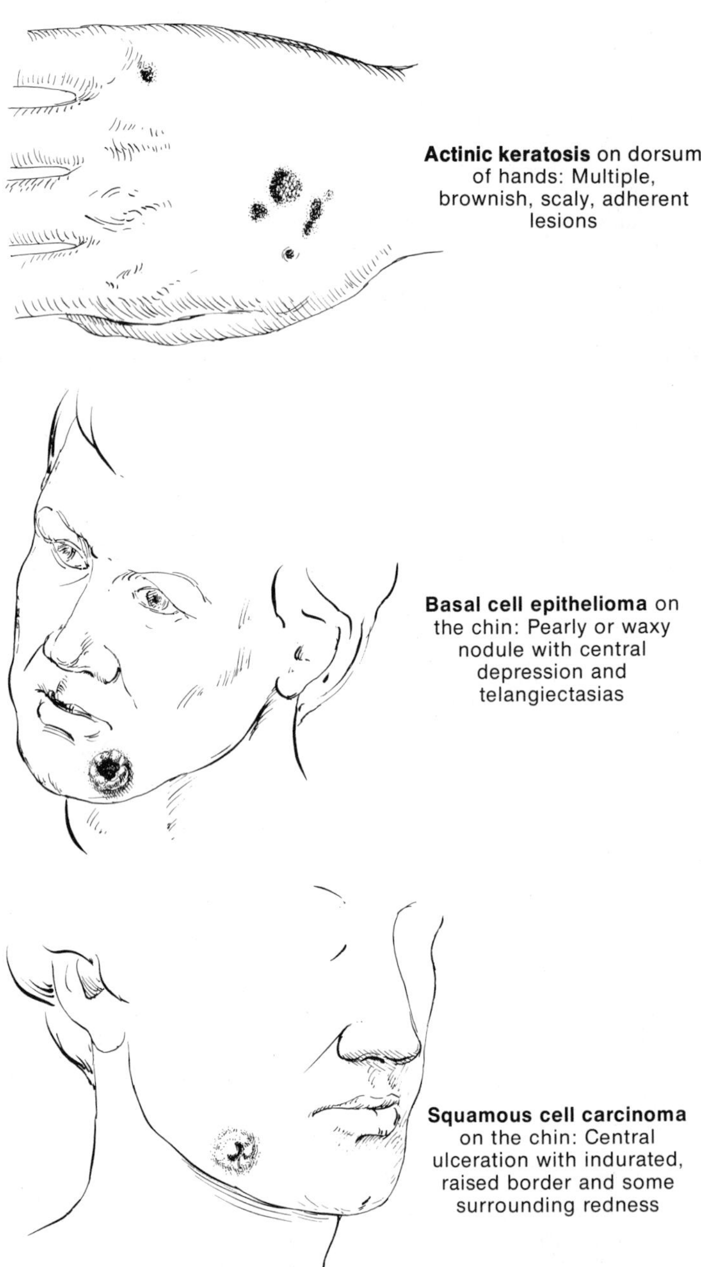

FIGURE 72–5. The most common pre-malignant and malignant lesions of the skin.

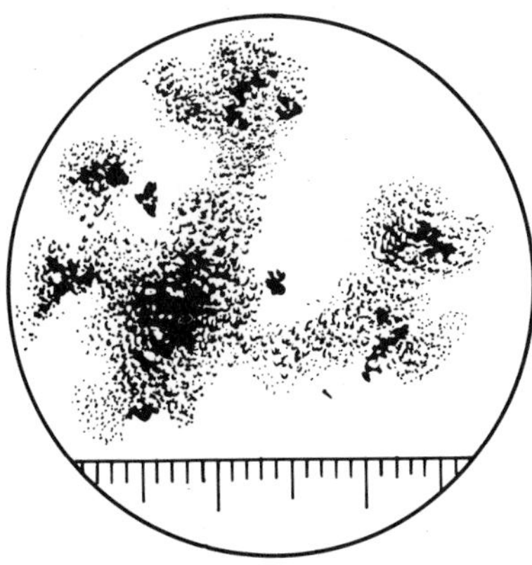

Lentigo maligna is a noninvasive flat lesion that displays a markedly indented margin and contains unevenly flecked black or reticulated areas. (This lesion has been present for many years.)

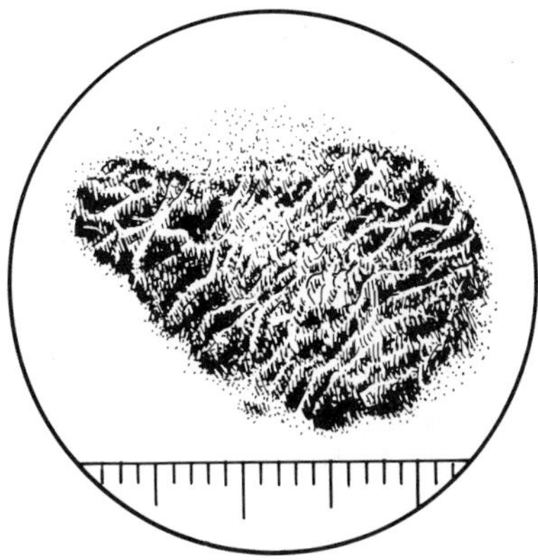

Superficial spreading melanoma displays variegated color with a light central area of bluish-white. The surface is irregularly raised.

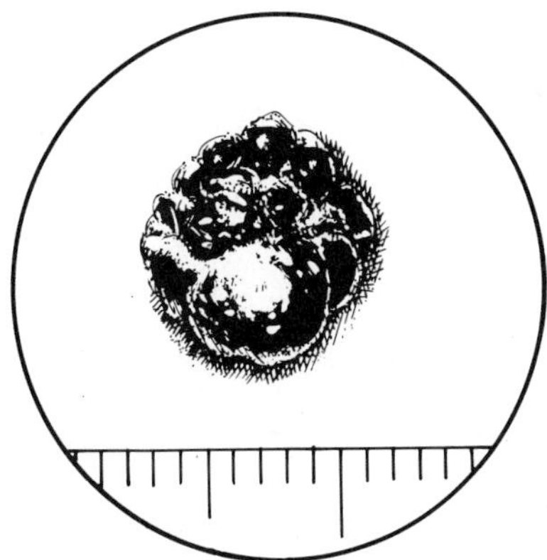

Nodular malignant melanoma is a deeply invasive lesion with an almost uniform bluish-black color. The surface is irregular, although the margins of this lesion are not notched.

FIGURE 72–6. The characteristic features of malignant melanomas.

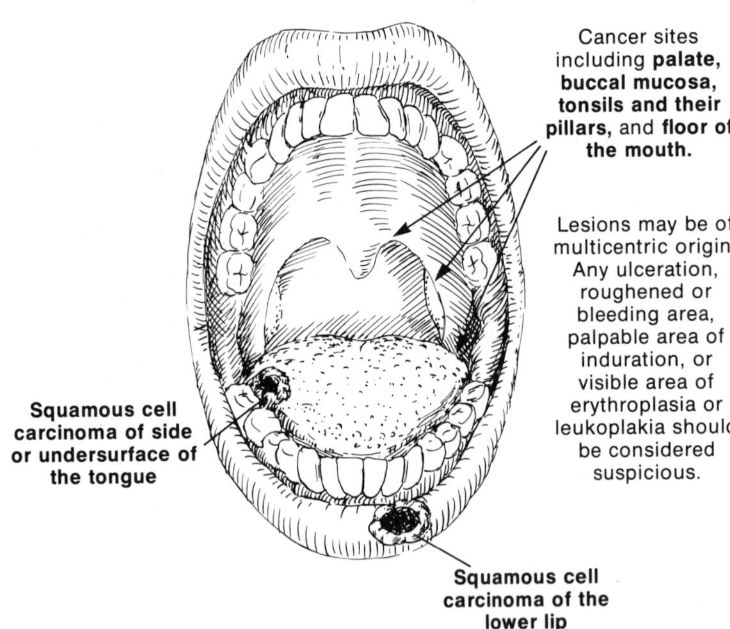

FIGURE 72–7. Most common locations of malignancies of the oral cavity.

tobacco and alcohol in the induction of oral cancers.[15] Daily consumption of 5 ounces of alcohol will increase the risk of oral cancer twofold. Daily consumption of 8 ounces will increase the risk threefold. *Tumors of the lips and oral cavity* are visible as ulcerations or roughened areas. Oral cancers are most frequently located on the undersurface of the tongue, the soft palate, and the tonsils (Fig. 72–7). They are more commonly red or pink (erythroplasia) than white (leukoplakia). Any plaquelike lesion, especially if thick or fissured, should be regarded as suspicious, as should any area of induration.

Leukoplakia is a reaction to chronic irritation and is malignant in only a minority of cases, but this can be decided only on biopsy of the lesion.

Cancer of the paranasal sinuses generally remains asymptomatic until it presents as a bloody unilateral nasal discharge or unexplained persistent rhinosinusitis. *Tumors of the nasopharynx* are often asymptomatic prior to the production of a bloody nasal discharge or development of metastatic lymph nodes in the high jugular chain.

Any painless lump of the *salivary glands,* particularly if hard, fixed, or irregular, must be regarded with suspicion, as must any solitary nodule or prominent hard nodule of the *thyroid gland.* One third of all parotid masses and two thirds of submaxillary masses are malignant (Fig. 72–8).

The Lungs. Programs designed to screen male smokers by means of chest roentgenograms yield less than 1% with cancer on the initial testing followed by 4 to 6 new cases of lung carcinoma for every 1000 persons screened each year.[26–29] None of these detection programs, however, has been shown to reduce the mortality rate from lung cancer. Although the 5-year survival of the 206 lung cancer patients diagnosed in the screened group of the Mayo Clinic study was 33%, compared with only 15% for the 160 patients in the control group, the mortality from lung cancer was nearly identical for all men randomly assigned to the screened group (3.2/1000 person-years), compared with those randomly assigned to the control group (3.0/1000 person-years). The mortality of the screened compared with the control group was similar in the Johns Hopkins study

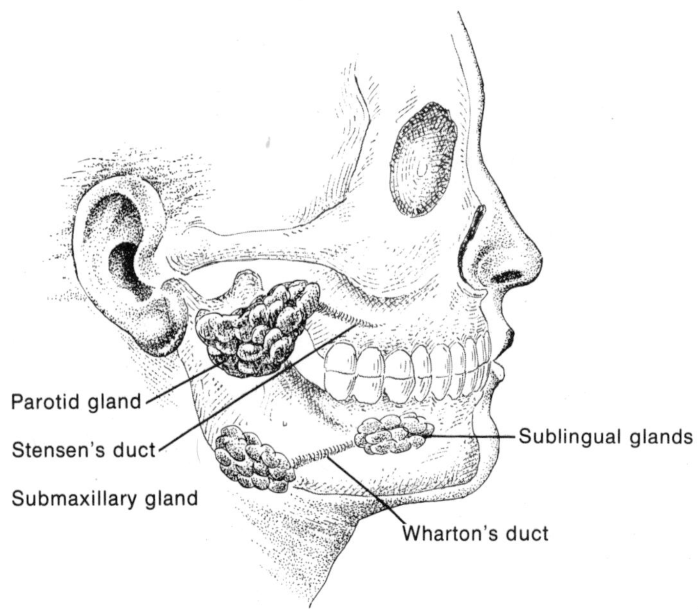

FIGURE 72–8. Location of the parotid, submandibular, and sublingual glands. Any hard, nontender nodule should be considered malignant.

(3.4 versus 3.8/1000 person-years, respectively) and the Memorial trial (2.7/1000 person-years in both groups).[27]

It is worth reviewing the natural history and clinical presentation of lung cancer to explain why screening with chest roentgenography affords no apparent reduction in mortality. Very rapidly growing small cell tumors make up 15 to 25% of tumors; at the time of their presentation with symptoms of local disease or metastases, the chest film generally reveals a hilar mass that appears to have developed abruptly. Even chest films obtained at intervals of 4 months are insufficient to detect these rapidly growing tumors prior to their clinical presentation.[27,29] Thirty per cent of lung tumors are centrally located epidermoid (squamous cell) carcinomas. Although present for months to years before becoming symptomatic, epidermoid carcinomas usually are not detectable radiographically, because of their central location, until they are locally far advanced. Even sputum cytology evaluated every 4 months did not reduce mortality in this group.[25] Thus, screening employing chest films or chest films plus sputum cytology will have no impact in about half the patients who develop lung cancer.

The remaining half of lung cancers are peripheral tumors that may be visualized radiographically as coin lesions. They may be epidermoid, large cell anaplastic, or adenocarcinoma in type. If lesions are detected when they are less than 2 cm in diameter, the 5-year survival rate of patients is reported to be 69%.[30] However, the doubling time of these tumors is thought to average 4 months.[31] For this reason, chest films, even if taken semiannually, may fail to detect a majority of peripheral carcinomas until they are larger than 2 cm.

A recent analysis of the data on the adenocarcinomas and large cell cancers of the lung diagnosed in the Memorial and Johns Hopkins studies led to the conclusion that somewhere between 10 and 19% of heavy smokers are likely to develop one of these tumor types if they live long enough.[29] The probability of detecting an early-stage or totally resectable adenocarcinoma or large-cell carcinoma on a single chest radiograph is only 0.16. Finally, the most optimistic estimate of the cure rate of this type of cancer using routine screening ranged from 5 to 18% in the two studies. For this reason, even larger screening studies for lung cancer are under consideration.[27] However, at present, it appears that screening for carcinoma of the lung remains a subject for investigation and cannot be recommended for general use in practice. This appraisal need not deter the practitioner from judicious case finding, or from adopting a vigorous approach to the patient with hemoptysis or a pulmonary nodule.

Abdomen. Any palpable, nonpulsatile mass of the abdomen is likely to be malignant; such a finding generally indicates advanced disease.

Pelvic Area. Pelvic examination and obtaining the Papanicolaou smear should begin at the initiation of sexual activity or at 18 years of age in women for the purpose of detecting carcinoma in situ of the uterine cervix (see later). Invasive carcinomas of the cervix, endometrium, and ovary become common after the age of 45 years. By age 60 to 64 years, the annual incidences of ovarian and endometrial carcinoma are 0.46 and 1.39/1000 women, respectively.[18] *Ovarian masses* may indicate malignancy in older women; they must also be regarded with suspicion in premenopausal women if they are more than 4 cm in diameter and persist beyond several menstrual cycles. Unfortunately, abdominal distention or ascites, indicative of metastases or

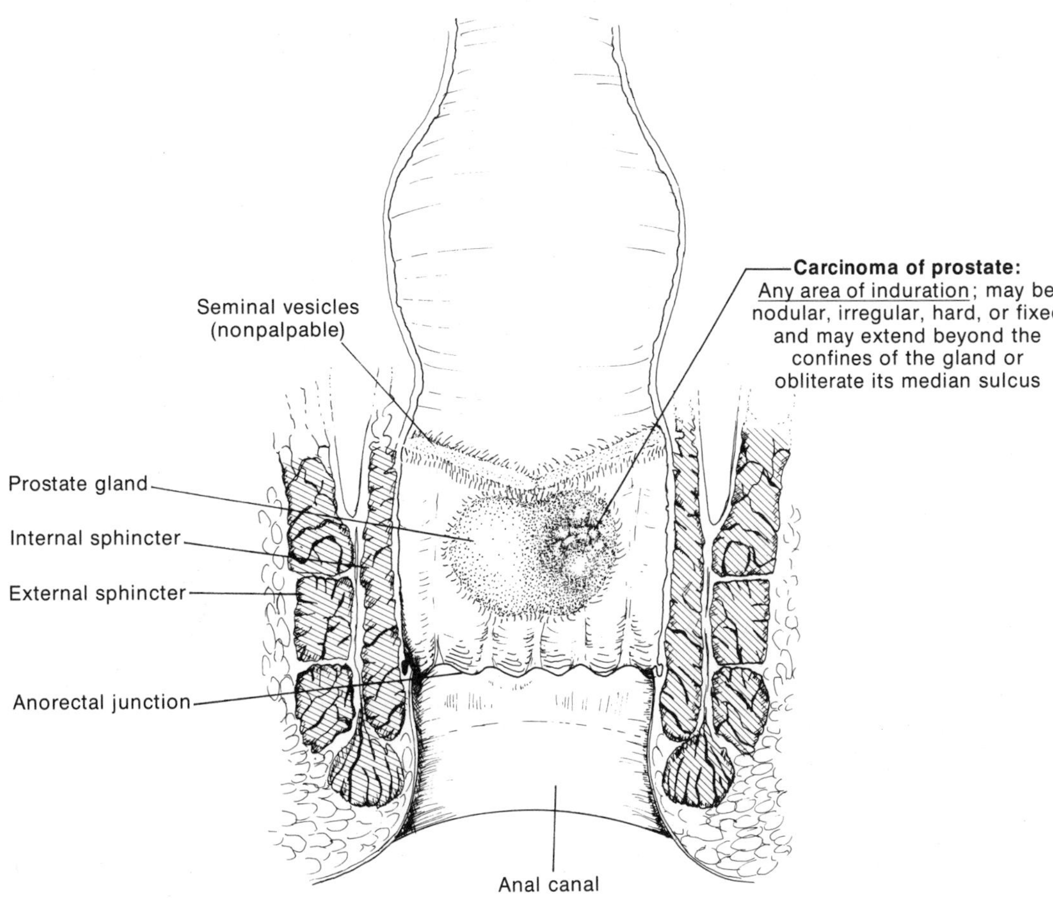

FIGURE 72–9. Carcinoma of the prostate—findings on physical examination.

local extension, is the presenting symptom in the majority of patients with ovarian carcinoma. In most cases, uterine enlargement represents fibroid tumors, and most endometrial carcinomas have a history of abnormal uterine bleeding rather than positive physical findings, whereas leiomyosarcomas are rarely encountered; however, the rapid enlargement of a *uterine mass* or its enlargement in a postmenopausal woman, as noted on physical examination, is suspicious. Biopsy of any hyperkeratotic white lesion, erosion, or nodular lesion of the vulva is indicated. Ulcerations or nodules within the vagina should be scraped and examined cytologically by the Papanicolaou technique.

Rectum and Prostate. Screening for *colorectal cancer* is discussed separately later in this chapter. *Carcinoma of the prostate* becomes common in men above the age of 50 years, and in those older than 65 years its prevalence as a clinically important lesion approaches 1%. Thus, it is particularly important during every routine health assessment in older men to spend some time palpating all aspects of the prostate gland. Palpation of the gland remains the single best screening test for detection of carcinoma, because its sensitivity (69% in one study) compares favorably with those of other methods.[32] Areas of induration or nodular irregularities possibly indicative of carcinoma (Fig. 72–9) should be biopsied.

Recently, the prostate-specific antigen (PSA) has been used as a sensitive but somewhat nonspecific test for prostate cancer. Transrectal needle biopsies may be performed when the PSA is clearly elevated (e.g., $\geqslant$ 10 ng/ml), or if slightly elevated (e.g., $\geqslant 4 < 10$ ng/ml), when transrectal ultrasonography of the prostate reveals hypoechoic areas suggesting possible malignancy.[33, 34] We do not recommend screening all men over the age of 50 years with PSA levels at this time (see Chapter 71), but it seems reasonable to screen men in the approximate age range of 50 to 74 years who are thought to be at increased risk of harboring prostate cancer, such as those with positive family histories, of black ancestry, and perhaps a history of vasectomy[34a]; equivocal or minimally suspicious findings on physical examination; recent, rapid onset of symptoms of prostatism, especially at an early age; bleeding from the prostate; or borderline elevation of a previous PSA test result. Decision analyses suggest no to modest benefit from early treatment of prostate cancer, but the results of a prospective trial now under way will be needed to determine whether survival benefits from early therapy outweigh the complications.[34b, 34c, 34d] Watchful waiting in place of treatment may be considered in men diagnosed with prostate cancer, although current evidence seems to indicate that life expectancy greater than 10 years and having a less well-differentiated tumor are factors that suggest potential benefit from treatment.

Miscellaneous. Some findings on physical examination are rarely present but may lead to the discovery of tumors. Galactorrhea, the appearance of acromegaly or Cushing's syndrome, or hyperpigmentation suggests the presence of pituitary (or adrenal) neoplasia. Ovarian and adrenal neoplasms may be manifested by virilization. Any indurated mass confined to the testes that is nontender or only mildly tender must be considered malignant. Malignant melanomas of the iris appear as dark velvety or flesh-colored tumors of the iris or angle of the anterior chamber. Brain tumors often first present with subtle changes in mental status.

PART 2 Carcinoma of the Breast

I. CRAIG HENDERSON, MD

Survival of patients with carcinoma of the breast is related most closely to the stage of the disease at the time of diagnosis. In most cases, this is determined by the size of the tumor and presence or absence of metastases to the axillary lymph nodes or of distant metastases (Table 72–2). There is a good correlation between survival and the number of lymph nodes found to be histologically involved at the time of node dissection. By convention, patients have been assigned to one of three pathologic stages. The 10-year survival of patients with no involved nodes is 65%; with one to three positive nodes, 38%; and with four or more nodes, 13%.[35]

The definitions of the breast cancer stages have changed frequently during the past 30 years, and this is often a source of confusion when physicians communicate with each other. The current staging system outlined in Table 72–2 includes both clinical and histologic criteria. Cancers that are stage I, II, or IIIA are technically operable. Patients with stage IIIB or IV may live for a decade or more after diagnosis, but there is no evidence that mastectomy or other forms of local therapy will prolong the survival of patients with these stages.[35]

Various evidence supports the concept that breast cancers represent a biologic spectrum.[35] Some tumors are inherently rapidly growing and tend to metastasize early in their course, whereas others are biologically indolent and slow to metastasize. For this reason there is a less-than-perfect correlation between prognosis and clinical-pathologic stage. A small stage I tumor thought to be "early" might be a late tumor with a very slow growth rate. A large stage III tumor might be "late" or a very aggressive, rapidly growing cancer. The intrinsic biology of a breast cancer is probably reflected more precisely in its histologic grade, thymidine-labeling index, or estrogen receptor content. For example, poorly differentiated tumors are more likely to have a high labeling index (i.e., a high percentage of cells undergoing DNA synthesis) and a low estrogen receptor content. Patients with estrogen receptor–negative tumors have a shorter interval from diagnosis to initial relapse and shorter survival.[36, 37] However, the absolute differences are

TABLE 72–2. CLINICAL-PATHOLOGIC STAGING OF CARCINOMA OF THE BREAST*

Stage Tis (in situ)

Stage I
T = Tumor less than 2 cm in diameter (may be fixed to fascia or muscle)
N = No palpable axillary nodes *or* palpable nodes not considered to contain growth. No evidence of histologic node involvement
M = No known distant metastases

Stage II
T = Tumor more than 2 cm but less than 5 cm in its greatest dimension (may be fixed to fascia or muscle)

and/or

N = Axillary nodes considered to contain growth but not fixed to one another or to surrounding structures *or* histologic node involvement of any type
M = No known distant metastases

Stage III A
T = Tumor more than 5 cm in diameter (may be fixed to fascia or muscle or cause dimpling of skin)

and/or

N = Axillary nodes, if present are fixed to one another or to other structures
M = No known distant metastases

Stage III B
T = Tumor of any size with invasion or direct involvement including ulceration or peau d'orange appearance of skin or involvement of chest wall

and/or

N = Homolateral supra- or infraclavicular node thought to contain growth

and/or

M = No known distant metastases present

Stage IV
T = Any of the above
N = Any of the above
M = Distant metastases present

*Adapted from American Joint Committee on Cancer: Manual for Staging of Cancer, 1992. Philadelphia, JB Lippincott, 1992, pp 149–194.

much greater among node-positive than node-negative patients.[38]

The mean doubling time for breast cancer is estimated to be 100 days.[39] If this is true, it would take almost 10 years to grow from a single malignant cancer cell to a size of 1 cc, a point at which most breast cancers can be relatively easily detected on physical examination. This long preclinical phase of the disease provides ample opportunity for early detection, and there is good evidence that tumors that usually metastasize late in this preclinical period can be detected prior to metastases by the use of screening mammography (discussed subsequently).

However, both the heterogeneous nature of breast cancer biology and its long preclinical lead time are sources of considerable confusion in interpreting the results of diagnostic and therapeutic trials. Comparisons of the survival or other behavior of small cohorts of patients selected at different times, from different locations, and by nonrandom methods are likely to be misleading. Patients diagnosed in screening clinics may be predominantly those with the more indolent forms of the disease and not comparable to those diagnosed because of symptoms. For this reason, all breast cancer survival data derived from nonrandom trials must be interpreted with great caution. Among patients with the best clinical-pathologic stages, some will do poorly and die of breast cancer. Among patients with the worst clinical-pathologic stages, a few will live for decades without evidence of recurrence. A breast cancer patient's prognosis should never be the sole determinant of a diagnostic or therapeutic recommendation.

EPIDEMIOLOGY AND RISK FACTORS FOR CARCINOMA OF THE BREAST

Based on a normal life expectancy, breast cancer affects approximately 10% of all women. The annual incidence among white women in the United States increases steadily with age, from 0.3 cases/1000 women 30 to 34 years of age to more than 1.9 cases/1000 women aged 50 to 54 years, and reaches 3.7 cases/1000 women at ages 70 to 74.[40] Fewer than half the lesions are confined to the breast at the time of detection, and the annual mortality rate of 27 deaths/100,000 women has remained virtually unchanged for several decades.

Although the cumulative lifetime risk of developing breast cancer is about 10%, the lifetime risk of dying of breast cancer is only about one third of this (Table 72–3).[41] This risk is spread over the interval from birth to 110 years but is greatest after the age of 65. The chance of developing breast cancer is only 2.5% and of dying of breast cancer is 0.6% between the ages of 35 and 55 years. One should be cautious about estimating the breast cancer risk for an individual patient (e.g., one with a positive family history) as simply the product of her group's relative risk and the lifetime probability of developing breast cancer.

For example, a patient in a group with a relative risk of 7.0 might be told that she has a 71% lifetime risk of developing breast cancer. In fact, no patient group has been shown to have such a high risk. In addition, it may be important to the patient to realize that her chance of dying of breast cancer is considerably less than her chance of developing breast cancer and that the chances of her dying in the next 10 to 20 years are much smaller than the calculated lifetime probability would suggest. For these reasons, it is recommended that cumulative probabilities of developing breast cancer be used cautiously, and when

TABLE 72–3. PROBABILITY OF EVENTUALLY DEVELOPING AND DYING OF BREAST CANCER—WHITE WOMEN*

Age Interval (Yr)	Risk of Developing Breast Cancer (%)	Risk of Dying of Breast Cancer (%)
Birth–110	10.20	3.60
20–30	0.04	0.00
20–40	0.49	0.09
20–110	10.34	3.05
35–45	0.88	0.14
35–55	2.53	0.56
35–110	10.27	3.56
50–60	1.95	0.33
50–70	4.67	1.04
50–110	8.96	2.75
65–75	3.17	0.43
65–85	5.48	1.01
65–110	6.53	1.53

*From Seidman H, Mushinski MH, Gelb SK, et al: Probabilities of eventually developing or dying of cancer–United States, 1985. CA Cancer J Clin *35*:36, 1985. ©American Cancer Society.

used they should be based on the data in Table 72–3 rather than on a single lifetime probability.

The factors associated with the highest risk for developing breast cancer are carcinoma in the opposite breast and a positive family history for the disease (Table 72–4). The relative risk of developing a second breast cancer subsequent to treatment of the first has been reported to be between 1.8 and 5.0. The risk is higher for women under the age of 50 years, and in several series, the cumulative risk over 10 to 20 years was 12 to 13% for this age group, compared with a cumulative incidence of 4 to 5% for women aged 50 to 70 years.[42] Simultaneous bilateral breast cancer occurs in 0.2 to 3.8% of women.

These differences in incidence seem to be related to the diligence of the search.[43] Any patient with a family history of breast cancer on the maternal or paternal side has an increased risk of breast cancer, but the greatest risk is among women who have a first-degree relative with breast cancer. The relative risk of developing breast cancer may be increased two- to threefold among women with a sister or both a mother and sister with breast cancer.[44–46] The relatives of patients whose cancers were diagnosed while they were premenopausal may be at a higher risk than the relatives of patients with postmenopausal breast cancer.[47] Relatives of patients with bilateral breast cancer have also been found to be at increased risk compared with relatives of patients with unilateral breast cancer.[47]

Patients with benign breast disease, and especially patients who have had a biopsy demonstrating benign breast disease, have been shown to be at increased risk of subsequently developing breast cancer.[48] However, no one has shown an increased risk of breast cancer in patients with "lumpy breasts," and this normal condition should not be mislabeled as "benign breast disease" or "fibrocystic disease," thus placing almost all women in a high-risk group. Recent studies suggest that most of the incurred risk attributed to benign breast disease is among the 7% of biopsied patients who have atypical hyperplasia. The relative risk of developing breast cancer in this group is 4.4 compared with 1.6 in patients with proliferative patterns but no atypia, and 0.89 in patients without a proliferative pattern at all.[49] The relative risk for patients with both atypical hyperplasia and a history of breast cancer in a first-degree relative is 8.9, and the observed incidence of breast cancer in this group was 20% over the first 15 years of follow-up. Fortunately, there appears to be attenuation of this risk with time, suggesting that patients with atypical hyperplasia need to be followed up most diligently during the first decade following this diagnosis.[50]

In situ carcinoma of the breast constituted only 1 to 2% of all breast cancers diagnosed 25 years ago, but with widespread use of screening mammography the incidence of in situ cancers has increased to 10 to 20% of breast cancers now diagnosed. At one time, the treatment of in situ cancer was identical to that for invasive breast cancer. However, long-term observation of patients treated with excisional biopsy leads to the conclusion that most of these patients will not develop an invasive breast cancer. In one series of 211 patients, the incidence of invasive breast cancer after a diagnosis of lobular carcinoma in situ was 1% per year (~ 30% over 30 years), and the incidence of subsequent invasive cancer was equally divided between the breast originally biopsied and the contralateral breast.[51]

TABLE 72–4. RISK FACTORS FOR DEVELOPING BREAST CANCER

Prior breast cancer
Invasive in the opposite breast
In situ carcinoma on biopsy
Positive family history
Sister = mother > other relatives
Benign breast disease
Atypical hyperplasia on biopsy
Hormone-related factors
Late first pregnancy
No or few pregnancies
Early menarche or late menopause

Fewer data are available on the subsequent incidence of invasive cancer in patients with in situ ductal cancer treated with excision only, but several recent reports suggest that the incidence of secondary invasive cancer after ductal carcinoma in situ may be quite similar to that for lobular carcinoma in situ.[6, 52, 53] In contrast to lobular carcinoma in situ, subsequent invasive cancers after a biopsy for ductal carcinoma in situ occur predominantly in the ipsilateral breast. Patients with carcinoma in situ must be considered at high risk for subsequent invasive cancer, but it is no longer certain that patients with this entity should be treated in the same manner as patients with invasive cancers. Increasing numbers of patients are now offered either lumpectomy (wide excision) alone or lumpectomy plus radiotherapy. The relative value of these two approaches is under evaluation in at least six independent randomized trials.

The other generally accepted risk factors for breast cancer are hormonally related.[6] The magnitude of increased risk ranges from 1.3- to 2.3-fold for factors such as having fewer than three pregnancies or more than 30 aggregate years of menstrual activity.[54] The age of a woman at the time of her first pregnancy is a more important risk factor than the number of pregnancies. Compared with nulliparous women, the relative risk of breast cancer in patients younger than age 24 years at the time of first pregnancy is 0.7, and in patients over age 35 years at the time of first pregnancy the relative risk is 1.4.[45]

Even though numerous risk factors for breast cancer can be identified, most breast cancers occur in women without attributable risk. In an American Cancer Society survey of 365,000 white women ages 30 to 84, only 21% of the premenopausal and 29% of the postmenopausal women who developed breast cancer had one or more identifiable risk factors.[55] Practically, this means that a screening program limited to women with risk factors will fail to diagnose most breast cancers.

CLINICAL FEATURES OF BREAST MALIGNANCIES

The woman with breast cancer may present with a lump in the breast, a discharge from the nipple, or skin manifestations.

Breast Lumps

The chief complaint in 80 to 90% of patients with breast carcinoma is a lump or mass in the breast, which is in many cases discovered by patients either during self-examination or, quite often, by accident; otherwise, the physician's physical examination is the most important diagnostic maneuver. Classically, *breast cancers* are firm or hard, irregular, nontender, single nodules. Often, carcinomas are not clearly delineated from, or may seem fixed to, surrounding tissues. However, of cancers detected in the Health Insurance Plan of New York (HIP) study, 61% were described initially as freely movable, 41% as regular, and 38% as soft or cystic on physical examination[56]; hence, any distinct mass or persistent area of abnormality within the breast must be considered suspicious of carcinoma.

The examination begins with the patient supine. Using three fingers, the examiner gently compresses the breast tissue, systematically palpating in concentric circles on all aspects of the breast. The axilla can be examined while the patient is supine by supporting the patient's wrist and palpating the uppermost area of the axilla; the fingers should then move downward slowly in an attempt to feel the nodes by compressing them against the chest wall.

In addition to palpation, one should carefully inspect the overlying skin and nipple areas because breast cancer often causes fibrosis or tissue retraction that results in asymmetry in the contour of the breast, inversion or flattening of a nipple, or dimpling of the skin over the breast. Lymphatic blockage can cause the skin to become thickened with enlarged pores, creating a *peau d'orange* appearance. If present, these "secondary" changes of breast carcinoma are useful in differentiating a carcinoma from other nodular lesions of benign etiology. It is particularly helpful to have the patient raise her arms over her head, press her hands against her hips, or lean forward while supported from the standing position in order to appreciate abnormalities in the breast contour, dimpling, retraction, or the peau d'orange appearance.

Several types of benign breast disease may also present as a solitary nodule. *Fibroadenomas* are very mobile, solid, firm, rubbery, well-demarcated, and nontender masses that are multiple or bilateral in 15 to 20% of instances. *Fat necrosis* within the breast or *sclerosing adenosis* from a proliferation of ductal cells produces a lump that is clinically indistinguishable from carcinoma. *Solitary large cysts* have a soft, cystic character that can often be appreciated.

The most common benign condition of the breast is a nondescript lumpiness often referred to erroneously as *fibrocystic disease,* characterized by the finding of numerous, well-delineated, mobile nodules having a firm, elastic consistency and occurring most commonly in women 35 to 60 years of age. The lesions are diffuse, most often occupy the outer upper quadrants, and may become tender during the premenstrual phase of the cycle. Another multinodular disease is *cystosarcoma phylloides,* which presents either as rapidly growing, painless nodules or, more often, as a large noninvasive mass in women of childbearing age. Whether these are benign or low-grade malignant sarcomas can be determined only after histologic examination.

Nipple Discharge

Nipple discharge is most frequently associated with various benign conditions, such as galactorrhea of endocrine or drug-induced causes, or benign organic lesions of the ductal system. *Galactorrhea* may be distinguished from local breast disease because the discharge is usually bilateral and clear or milky in appearance. The most frequent benign etiology for a nipple discharge is intraductal papilloma, which is the underlying cause of 45 to 69% of all nipple discharges and may cause either a serous or bloody discharge.[57, 58] Breast cancer is the source of only 5 to 12% of nipple discharges and may cause a serous, watery, or bloody discharge. However, in a series of 270 patients presenting with nipple discharge, all 16 patients (5.9%) in the series eventually found to have breast cancer had a hemoglobin-positive test result regardless of the gross appearance of the discharge. None of the patients whose nipple discharge was hemoglobin negative had breast cancer. However, the presence of hemoglobin in the discharge did little to increase the overall probability of breast cancer because only 7.4% of all patients with a hemoglobin-positive test result were eventually found to have breast cancer.[58]

Dermatitis

Paget's disease of the breast refers to dermatitis around the nipple associated with an invasive ductal carcinoma. Findings in Paget's disease of the breast range from itching, scaliness, and redness to nipple crusting and erosion or to gross destruction of the nipple. The condition can be distinguished from eczema or benign *seborrheic dermatitis* of the nipple because in malignant disease the findings are unilateral and fail to resolve following treatment with topical corticosteroids. Inversion or retraction of the nipple is not only a sign of Paget's disease of the breast but, of course, may also be related to an underlying carcinoma. Superficial phlebitis of the breast or *Mondor's disease* can be recognized by its characteristic distribution along the course of a vein.

Inflammatory carcinomas of the breast carry a very poor prognosis and are characterized by diffuse erythema, peau d'orange skin, and generalized breast enlargement, often without a mass. This condition could be easily mistaken for a mastitis except for the fact that mastitis is rare in patients who are not postpartum and lactating. The diagnosis of inflammatory breast cancer should be confirmed by a biopsy of both the breast and the overlying skin, where plugging of dermal lymphatics may be seen.

MAMMOGRAPHY

The diagnostic procedures currently of proven value for detecting carcinoma of the breast are mammography and xeroradiography. Although the diagnostic sensitivities of the two procedures are nearly equal, screen-film mammography is generally preferred in screening clinics because of the lower doses of radiation used. The mean dose for a two-view screen-film examination ranges between 0.066 and 0.072 rad. Xerograms more often employ doses of 0.35 to 0.45 rad.[59, 60]

Of the several other modalities that have been used or are being developed for detecting breast cancer, thermography has been found to be too insensitive and nonspecific for adoption as a screening test.[61] Breast ultrasound may be helpful in distinguishing a solid from a cystic mass in the breast, but it has limited value in screening asymptomatic women because it is unable to detect microcalcifications (see later). In addition, a proper ultrasound examination requires a dedicated unit, and this is probably an unjustifiable expense outside of centers performing large numbers of breast examinations because the same information may be obtained by needle aspiration of the mass. Breast carcinoma may be diagnosed radiographically by detecting a mass lesion, "secondary" signs of altered breast architecture, or the presence of microcalcifications.

Mass lesions have characteristics that usually allow the radiologist to distinguish benign from malignant disease. Increased density compared with surrounding tissue, irregularity or spiculation of the borders, or distortion of surrounding breast architecture suggests malignancy. Benign nodules have smooth borders and are round, lobulated, and noninvasive, although occasionally a mucin-producing papillary or medullary adenocarcinoma will have smooth borders. Fibrocystic disease has the appearance of multiple benign cysts superimposed on accentuated, dense intervening connective tissue.

If no mass is identified or if a mass appears smooth, carcinoma may be diagnosed from the presence of secondary radiographic signs. These include retraction or thickening of the skin, increased caliber of veins, or alterations of ductal architecture. Thickening of the skin identified radiographically is particularly important because it may be the only abnormality in inflammatory carcinomas.

Microcalcifications within the breast noted on mammography are often the earliest signs of carcinoma. Scattered coarse calcifications or foci with several microcalcifications are commonly associated with benign disease. However, five or more calcifications, each less than 1 mm in diameter, clustered together within 1 cc of breast tissue should be considered suspicious for breast cancer.[62] There may be one, several, or many such clusters within the breast, and biopsies must be done of each to be certain the patient does not have cancer. Even these microcalcifications will be benign in 80 to 90% of patients, but cancers diagnosed on the basis of microcalcifications alone are those with the best prognosis.[63]

Mammography is more difficult to interpret in women below the age of 50 years because of the radiodensity of the premenopausal breast tissue compared with the more radiolucent breasts of older women. Newer mammographic techniques have improved the sensitivity of mammography in younger women. In the American Cancer Society's Breast Cancer Detection Demonstration Project (BCDDP), 45.7% of the cancers diagnosed in women ages 40 to 49 years and 45.3% of the cancers diagnosed in women ages 50 to 59 years were detectable only on mammography. Ninety-two and 93.4%, respectively, of all cancers diagnosed in these two age groups were evident on mammograms.[64] Nevertheless, mammograms are still not generally recommended in very young women (less than 35 years) with very dense breasts. The incidence of false-positive and false-negative evaluations varies greatly with the equipment used and the skill of the mammographer. However, even large masses may not be apparent on radiography, and in some series, up to one third of mammograms taken in women with cancer have been reported to be falsely negative.[65] False-positive results represent a major problem as mammography is performed with increasing frequency. The ratio of nonmalignant to malignant findings on breast biopsies in the BCDDP, employing experienced mammographers, varied from 16.4 to 1 in women aged 35 to 39 years to 9.5 to 1 in those aged 40 to 44 years; 5.2 to 1 in those aged 50 to 54 years; and 2.7 to 1 in those aged 70 to 74 years.[66] Conversely, biopsies may be performed in some community hospitals on sharply defined 1-cm nodular densities with a probability of malignancy as low as 1 in 50.[67] It is important, therefore, that mammograms be interpreted cautiously and that patients be encouraged to seek a second opinion, as opposed to a breast biopsy, when findings are equivocal.

APPROACH TO THE PATIENT

The clinician faces two problems in detecting breast cancer: first, how to evaluate the patient who has positive findings or complaints; and second, how to detect breast cancer through screening techniques in asymptomatic patients.

Clinical Evaluation

In most cases, either the patient or the physician will discover a suspicious lump on physical examination. One must first decide whether the lump is indeed "suspicious." Benign lumps and cysts are usually recognizable on examination because of the flat, lobulated consistency of the underlying tissue; bilateral symmetry, increased tenderness and prominence during the premenstrual phase, and lack of skin retraction or other secondary signs of malignancy. All other palpable masses must be considered suspicious. In these cases, mammography cannot be used to exclude carcinoma because of the possibility of a false-negative result. For patients with palpable lesions, mammography is of value chiefly to exclude carcinoma in another part of the breast or in the opposite breast (present in 3 to 5% of cases[68]) prior to biopsy and to obtain a baseline study. Biopsy should never be postponed or delayed because the mammogram is negative.

It is now common practice to perform incisional or excisional biopsy of palpable masses on an outpatient basis under local anesthesia; this provides an immediate diagnosis without producing undue anxiety in women with benign lesions and affords the opportunity for those found to have malignancies to discuss the choices of therapy and prepare themselves prior to undergoing major surgery.[69] Biopsies may also be done on nonpalpable lesions evident only on mammogram under local anesthesia in the outpatient department.[70] These lesions are usually localized with needles or wires in the radiology department prior to biopsy. The biopsy specimen may be radiographed to confirm that the suspicious lesion has been removed, and a repeat mammogram should be performed after the biopsy site has healed to further confirm the complete excision of the worrisome area. It is important, particularly in cases of so-called "minimal" breast carcinoma, to have the specimens reviewed carefully by an experienced pathologist before recommending major surgery. Lesions that are totally excised should be sent for an estrogen and progesterone receptor determination because subsequent biopsies or mastectomy may provide no further cancerous tissue on which to perform these valuable tests. Lesions thought to be benign can be evaluated by frozen section before deciding that a receptor evaluation is unnecessary.

In a few instances, this approach can be modified. Cystic lesions may be aspirated with a needle. The cystic character is confirmed by obtaining clear, nonbloody fluid. If the cyst totally collapses and has not recurred after a period of observation for several months, the evaluation is completed. Recurrence of a cystic lesion following aspiration is an indication for open biopsy.

Aspiration biopsy of solid breast masses, in which a 22-gauge needle and 10-ml syringe are used to obtain a sample that is then smeared on an albumin-treated slide for examination by the Papanicolaou technique, has been reported to yield false-negative negative rates of 10 to 35%.[71] The rate of false-positive results has varied from 10 to 50% in various series,[72, 73] but this percentage appears to fall as the physician performing the aspiration has greater experience. More recently, fine-needle aspiration has been used successfully to diagnose nonpalpable breast lesions.[74] Not surprisingly, however, a substantial percentage of the aspirates of nonpalpable lesions do not contain representative material. More recently, special devices have been developed to permit both mammographic localization and guided fine-needle aspiration.[75] This system also failed to yield sufficient material for diagnosis in almost one fourth of patients. Fine-needle aspiration biopsy has a role in the diagnosis of breast cancer when used by physicians experienced in the technique. However, an incisional or excisional biopsy should always be performed in spite of a negative cytologic result if the prebiopsy clinical diagnosis was thought to be cancer, and when a lesion is almost certain to be cancerous, a fine-needle aspiration biopsy may represent a needless additional step because the cytologic evaluation may not provide the information on histologic cell type and tumor architecture necessary for the patient and physician to begin discussions on appropriate local treatment of the breast cancer.

In patients with nipple discharge or dermatitis of the nipple, mammography is more sensitive than physical examination in detecting either a subareolar mass or calcifications,[76] but only a biopsy provides definitive information. Patients whose chief complaint is scaliness, crustiness, or other findings of dermatitis around the nipple may be treated first with a short course (less than 2 weeks) of topical corticosteroids. If the nipple lesion does not clear promptly, the edge of the nipple should be biopsied and evaluated for the characteristic monolayer of Paget's cells in the epidermis on the undersurface of the nipple. Patients with hemoglobin-positive nipple discharge may have a Papanicolaou smear, prepared by expressing a small amount of the discharge at the tip of the nipple and touching a clean glass slide to the nipple. Cytologic evaluation of this smear will occasionally demonstrate cancer cells. If the smear is negative but the discharge persists, the involved duct system may be removed. This, too, is usually a simple outpatient procedure in the hands of an experienced surgeon. Identification of a benign papilloma on dissection of the duct may obviate extensive tissue removal.

Screening

Evidence suggests that tumors detected during both breast self-examination and periodic routine examinations by physicians are smaller and in earlier clinical stages than are tumors detected by accident.[77, 78] In one study, 54% of neoplasms detected by periodic physical examination were clinical stage I compared with 27% of those detected accidentally by the patient.[78]

There is considerable evidence that the addition of mammography is much more effective than physical examination alone in detecting carcinomas. Several sources of data exist on the value of routine mammography in asymptomatic women: The HIP of New York study was a randomized trial performed more than 20 years ago, but it remains a major source of data on the effect of routine screening on breast cancer mortality.[79] The BCDDP used self-selected patients and much better mammographic techniques than those used in the HIP study.[66] It is our best source of information on the sensitivity and specificity of modern mammography but is of limited use in evaluating the effectiveness of screening because no control group was included. Ongoing randomized trials in Canada and Europe may permit an assessment of the value of modern mammography in reducing breast cancer mortality.

In the HIP study, 62,000 women between the ages of 40 and 64 years were randomly assigned to receive either an annual physical examination and mammogram or a special breast evaluation only as dictated by symptoms. About the same number of cancers were diagnosed in each group. However, metastases to regional nodes at the time of diagnosis had occurred in 54% of the patients in the control group, compared with only 43% of the patients in the study group and 30% of the patients in the study group whose cancers were actually detected at a screening examination.[80] No patient had more than three screening evaluations, and these were all performed during the first 5 years of the study. The maximum reported follow-up for this study is 18 years.[79, 81] At the end of the first 5 years of follow-up, the difference in breast cancer mortality in the screened and controlled populations was 38.1%; at 10 years, this difference was 28.6% and at 18 years, 22.7%.[79] It is estimated that overall breast cancer mortality might have been decreased by 32.4% if yearly screening had continued beyond the fifth year.

Early reports from the HIP study suggested that the value of mammography in decreasing breast cancer mortality was limited to women over the age of 50 years. With longer follow-up, the differential benefit of mammography related to age at diagnosis was less evident.[81] In the HIP study, 41.5% of the cancers detected in patients aged 50 to 59 years and 19.4% of the cancers detected in patients aged 40 to 49 years were evident only on mammography and not on physical examination. In the more recent BCDDP study, 46.7% of the cancers in women aged 50 to 59 years and 45.3% of those in patients aged 40 to 49 years were detectable only on mammogram. These results have been taken as evidence that improved technology has increased the sensitivity of mammography in younger women and that any differential benefits related to age in the early studies are not likely to persist in the future.[64]

The HIP and BCDDP studies differed in another important aspect. In the HIP trial, only 7% of the cancers detected in the screened population were in situ or noninvasive. In the BCDDP study, 20% of all cancers detected were in this category.[82] It is possible that 50 to 70% of these in situ cancers would never have caused symptoms or compromised the survival of these patients (see earlier).

The observations made in the HIP trial have been reproduced in Swedish studies.[83] Communities rather than individual patients were randomly assigned, and 133,065 women over the age of 40 years were enrolled. This study design, unlike that used in the HIP study, ensures that lead time cannot account for all the apparent benefits. A single mammographic view was obtained, and screening was repeated at 2- to 3-year intervals. At the end of the tenth year, a 30% reduction in breast cancer mortality in the screened group was seen ($P = 0.0002$). As in the early reports from the HIP trial, benefits were observed only in women over the age of 50 years.

There remains the question of the extent to which exposure to radiation during mammography counterbalances the benefits of the procedure by inducing additional breast carcinomas.[84] Based on the low dose of radiation delivered using currently available technology (about 0.2 rad/exposure), the risk associated with a modern screening mammogram is now estimated to be 1 excess cancer/year/1 million women after a 10-year latency period. This risk is equal to that incurred by smoking 1.4 cigarettes, drinking 0.5 liter of wine, and traveling 10 miles by bicycle or 300 miles by car.[85]

There is little room for further debate on the general proposition that early detection with screening mammography will reduce breast cancer mortality. However, several subsidiary questions have yet to be answered.

1. *Is mammography as effective in younger women as in those over the age of 50 years?*

No one has yet shown a statistically significant survival benefit for screening women under the age of 50 years. A review of all of the published randomized and case-control studies that included women aged 40 to 49 years indicates that the effect of mammography on mortality is variable, with a 95% confidence interval surrounding the mean ranging from a 56% increase in mortality to a 33% decrease in mortality.[86] Regardless of which estimate of benefit is accepted, mammography is clearly less effective in women under the age of 50 than in those aged 50 and over. Because cancer is less common among younger women, the cost-benefit ratio for screening all women aged 40 to 49 would be higher than for screening older women even if the efficacy were identical, and for this reason many groups have recommended screening younger women at less frequent intervals, such as every 2 years. However, this may not be a reasonable recommendation if breast cancers grow more rapidly in younger women, thus shortening the interval during which a cancer without distant metastases might be detected. This possibility is suggested by an analysis of the data from the Swedish two-county trial.[87] In this study, younger women were screened once every 24 months. By the end of the second year of follow-up after an initial screening examination, the incidence of breast cancer among women aged 40 to 49 was 68% of the incidence in the unscreened control population. In contrast, the incidence among older women had reached only 29% at the end of 2 years. Analyses of this type suggest that younger women should be screened at more frequent intervals, if they are screened at all. There are no data demonstrating the value for a baseline mammogram at age 35, and for this reason the American Cancer Society has dropped this recommendation in their most recent set of guidelines.

2. *Should mammograms be repeated annually?*

No direct comparisons of different screening intervals have been made. The HIP study used a 1-year interval, the Swedish study a 2- to 3-year interval. It is possible that 80% or more of the total benefit from screening older women might be achieved by screening at 3-year intervals.

3. *Is the widespread use of screening mammography likely to lead to overtreatment?*

Frequent mammography has resulted in an increased detection of in situ lesions. These lesions may be the earliest and most curable form of breast cancer or they may designate another high-risk group, most of whom will never develop a breast cancer with malignant potential. The use of mastectomy or radiotherapy for all these patients may be overtreatment for 50 to 70% of them.

4. *Can we afford to screen all women older than the age of 40 or 50 years on an annual basis?*

If the current American Cancer Society and American College of Radiology recommendations were fully implemented, every American radiologist would need to read 8 mammograms every day.[88] In addition, frequent mammograms will also result in an increased number of biopsies and an increased frequency of complications from these procedures. The net cost of annual screening of all women aged 40 to 49 years for 10 years would be approximately $402 million (in 1984 dollars).[86] The considerable costs associated with screening make it imperative that this modality be applied appropriately in various age groups. Additional studies to refine guidelines more precisely seem justified.

Until recently, most professional societies in the United States, with the notable exception of the American College of Physicians and the U.S. Preventive Task Force, recommended baseline mammography between ages 35 and 40 years with follow-up mammography at intervals of 1 to 2 years between the ages of 40 and 49 years.[89] However, this has changed since the publication of results from a Canadian trial in which women in this age group were randomized to undergo either yearly mammography or only a baseline physical examination.[90] After a median follow-up of 7 years, no survival benefit from screening was observed. Since then, several international workshops have been held to review all of the world's data on screening younger women.[91] As a result, the American Cancer Society has discontinued recommendations for a baseline evaluation prior to age 40.[91] The U.S. National Cancer Institute has withdrawn recommendations for routine screening in women under age 50 years, and European investigators have embarked on new, larger studies for women in this younger age group. Outside of the United States, only Sweden recommends mammograms before the age of 50. All of the American organizations recommend an annual mammogram in women 50 years of age or older without an age limit for stopping. The British recommend mammograms at 3-year intervals for women aged 50 to 64 years, and the Swedish public health policy is to obtain mammograms at 2-year intervals between the ages of 55 and 74.[92] With this background of controversy, the following guidelines appear reasonable:

1. Mammography should not be used to screen women under age 40 years.
2. The use of mammography prior to the age of 50 should be a decision made jointly by each woman in consultation with her physician. Women should be informed that the benefits are likely to be small and that the optimal frequency of mammography is unknown. Further, although it is reasonable to recommend mammography at an earlier age for women in high-risk groups, there is really no evidence that mammography is more beneficial in high-risk groups than in other women.
3. Screening using combined mammography and physical examination should be made available on an annual or biennial basis to all women 50 years of age or older.

The proper approach to patients considered at high risk based on factors other than a prior invasive cancer or breast cancer in a first-degree relative is unclear. The potential list of such factors is endless, but many of the factors are associated with a very small increase in risk, whereas others, such as abnormal parenchymal patterns on mammography, are not reproducible from one study to the next. Symptoms in patients with any of these risk factors should be investigated thoroughly, but most are not an indication for more frequent mammograms. An exception to this rule may be those with biopsy-proved, atypical hyperplasia or in situ carcinoma (see earlier). Although some physicians recommend mastectomy routinely for patients in these two categories, this is a subject of intense controversy. Certainly these patients should all be considered at high risk for subsequent invasive cancer and might reasonably be followed with yearly mammograms.

Controlled studies are missing to demonstrate that prophylactic mastectomy for patients with atypical hyperplasia will reduce breast cancer mortality to a degree sufficient to justify the removal of so many breasts that will never become cancerous. Surgery is not recommended in these patients unless the patient requests this approach to decrease unacceptable levels of anxiety. Patients with lobular carcinoma in situ might reasonably be treated with bilateral mastectomies because the subsequent risk of invasive cancer is equally distributed over both breasts. Unilateral mastectomy is not recommended, but it is reasonable to follow patients with lobular carcinoma in situ as a high-risk group without further surgery of any kind.

Ductal carcinoma in situ (intraductal carcinoma) is traditionally treated with simple, unilateral mastectomy, and the increasing trend to follow these patients after excisional biopsy is very recent. Subcutaneous mastectomy is not recommended for any of these patients. This operation does not remove all the breast tissue, the goal of any surgery performed to prevent cancer. Because knowledge in this field is evolving rapidly, patients with carcinoma in situ probably should be referred for a therapeutic decision to an oncologist or oncologic surgeon with an interest in breast disease.

Recently, increased attention has been given to the possibility of preventing or substantially delaying the onset of breast cancer by the use of tamoxifen in otherwise asymptomatic women. This approach is justified in large part by the observation that the incidence of contralateral breast cancer following the treatment of one breast cancer could be reduced by 39% when adjuvant tamoxifen was given for periods of 1 to 5 years following diagnosis and initial treatment.[93] Tamoxifen is an attenuated estrogen, and it appears to have estrogenic effects on other organs of the body. Tamoxifen has been shown to reduce serum cholesterol and possibly to reduce osteoporosis as well.[94] Overall, adjuvant tamoxifen reduced the mortality from causes other than breast cancer by 12% ($p = .05$) and reduced mortality from vascular causes by 25% ($p = 0.06$).[93] These observations have provided justification for large randomized trials of tamoxifen in women at high risk for developing breast cancer, and such studies are ongoing in England and the United States. Other approaches, such as the use of retinoids, are in earlier stages of development. However, until the results of formal trials are available, none of these methods can be recommended for routine practice.

In most women below the age of 50 years, the two principal means of detection are breast self-examination and yearly examinations by physicians. Because the majority of breast tumors continue to be discovered by the patients themselves, no physician should neglect to instruct his or her patients in breast self-examination (Fig. 72–10).

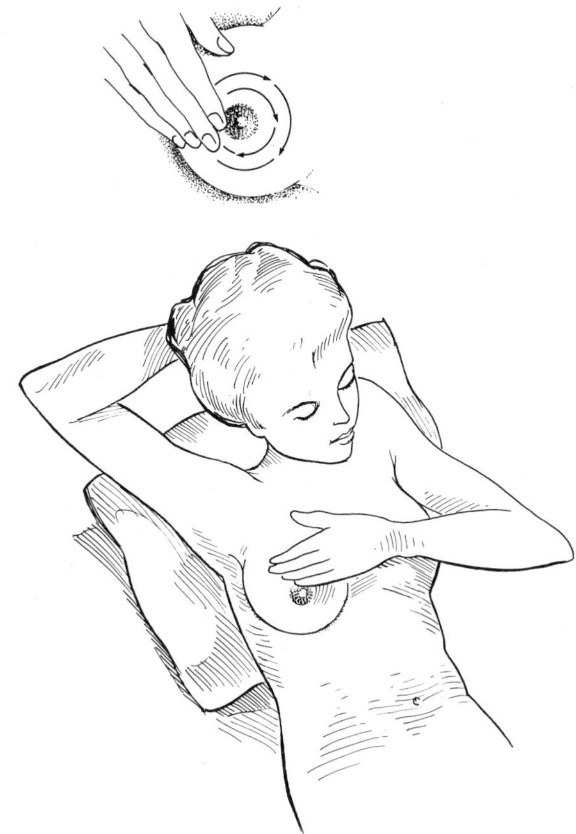

FIGURE 72–10. Breast self-examination. The patient is instructed to examine each breast with the opposite hand, either while in the bath or shower or while lying down with one hand behind the head and a small pillow beneath the shoulder. The fingers should be straight while the hand is held flat and gently pressed against the breast tissue with small circular motions, covering all areas of the breast. If a lump, dimpling, or discharge is discovered during self-examination, the patient is instructed to consult her physician for re-examination and possible diagnostic tests.

PART 3 ■ Dysplasia, Carcinoma in Situ, and Cancer of the Uterine Cervix

ELLEN E. SHEETS, MD

Although carcinoma of the uterine cervix is not a common malignancy—its incidence is about one fifth that of breast cancer—two features make screening for this lesion both useful and feasible:

1. The availability of a screening test that is inexpensive and accurate (the Papanicolaou smear for exfoliative cytologic examination)
2. Histologically identifiable premalignant changes that may antedate the development of actual cancer by many years

Indeed, the uterine cervix furnishes a model that has improved our understanding of oncogenesis in other, less accessible organs. Somewhere on the outer surface of the cervix lies the squamocolumnar junction, where endocervical columnar epithelium changes fairly abruptly into exocervical squamous epithelium, the same kind of epithelium that lines the vagina. Beginning at birth and continuing through the reproductive years, in a process of continual *squamous metaplasia,* the columnar epithelium is replaced by new squamous epithelium, and the squamocolumnar junction thus moves inward toward the internal cervical os.

Instead of normal metaplasia, an abnormal squamous epithelium, squamous intraepithelial neoplasia (so-called dysplasia), may develop in the *transformation zone* where columnar epithelium is being changed into squamous epithelium. Over many years, studies of the cervix have produced strong evidence that squamous cell carcinoma of the cervix is preceded by a progressive evolution of the lesion; low-grade cervical intraepithelial neoplasia (CIN I), otherwise known as mild dysplasia, transforms to more severe cervical intraepithelial neoplasia (CIN II/III) to carcinoma in situ (CIS), and finally to invasive cancer.[95] Thus Papanicolaou screening offers the potential for far more than just early detection of malignancy; it can be used to detect premalignant states that can be treated by simple means with the prospect of 100% cure. As shown in Figure 72–11, the premalignant lesion CIS is found in considerably younger women than is invasive cancer, and the CINs are found in still younger women. These early lesions may be detected by Papanicolaou smear or by examination of the cervix with

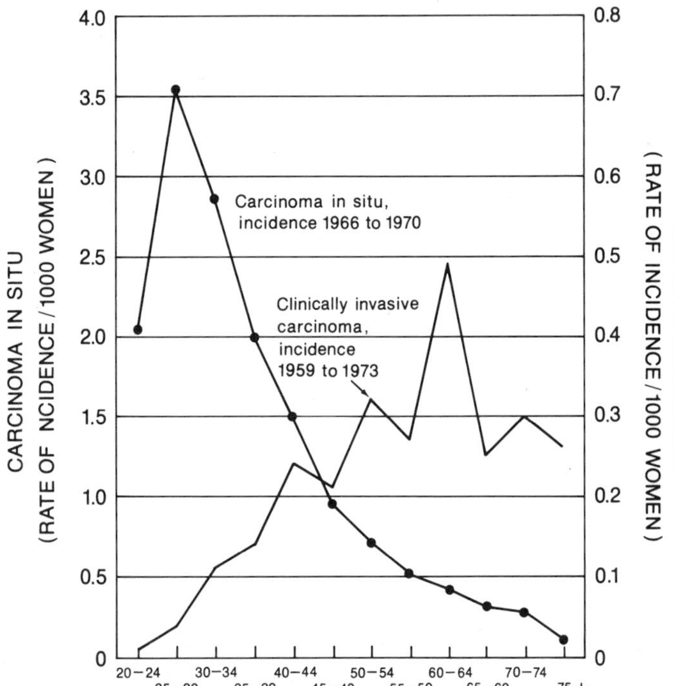

FIGURE 72–11. Age-specific rates per 1000 women for carcinoma in situ and invasive carcinoma of the uterine cervix. (Adapted from Cervical Cancer Screening Programs: The Walton Report. Can Med Assoc J 114:1003, 1976, by permission of the publisher, CMAJ.)

a low-power microscope (colposcopy). They cannot be recognized with certainty by visual inspection alone.

The reasons for a malignant rather than a normal development of the transformation zone are not yet fully understood but are strongly associated with the early onset of sexual relations (prior to age 20 years) and with multiple sexual partners.[96] Smoking and multiple sexual partners in the male partner of the patient are also risk factors. These observations, including the finding of a linkage between cervical cancer in women and penile cancer in men,[96] and of cervical cancer in second wives of men whose first wives had cervical cancer,[97] strongly suggest a sexually transmitted agent as the cause of squamous cervical cancer.[96] The role oral contraceptives play in the risk of developing premalignant or malignant changes of the cervix appears to remain in doubt.[98] Currently, the trend is toward a twofold increase in the risk of developing CIN in long-term oral contraceptive users, that is, greater than 10 years; however the vast majority of the studies contain confounding variables that have not been well controlled.[99] For many years, genital infection with type II herpes virus has been suspected as a cause, but more recently a wealth of evidence has accumulated linking infection with human papillomavirus to cervical dysplasias, CIS, and cancer.[97, 100–102] The actual virus is identified in early lesions,[102] but as the lesions become less well differentiated and closer to cancer, the intact virus is identified less often. However, sophisticated studies using DNA hybridization techniques can demonstrate the papillomavirus genome incorporated with the DNA of moderate-to-severe CIN and beyond into CIS or invasive cervical cancer.[101, 103]

Whether all CIN or CIS inevitably progress to cancer is subject to controversy, as is the rate at which this may occur. The likelihood of noting progression to a more severe lesion depends on the length of time one observes an abnormality and may be influenced by the use of cervical biopsies for initial diagnosis and follow-up. Obtaining biopsy specimens may itself be curative in some cases by removing the most abnormal areas. Regression or lack of progression occurs most frequently in CIN I, in which between 20 and 60% of lesions will regress, depending on whether biopsies are done. An increased rate of regression has been noted for patients who have undergone biopsies.[104, 105] Progression of CIN I to CIS or invasive cancer increased with the age of the patient but overall is nine times less frequent than progression of CIN III to CIS or invasive cancer.[105, 106] For CIN II/III lesions, the rate of spontaneous regression varies between 20 and 40%.[104] In cases of CIS, progression to invasive disease appears to occur in 25 to 70% of patients within a time span of about 10 years.[107]

Lack of predictability of clinical outcome has lead investigators to look for other predictors of possible progression or regression of isolated abnormalities. Initially, the type of human papillomavirus present in each lesion appeared to explain some of the controversy as to rates of progression of dysplasias to cancer. CIN I is most commonly associated with human papillomavirus types 6 and 11, whereas higher grade CIN, CIS, and invasive cancer are associated with type 16.[101, 103] Even though this association is a strong one, it essentially carries no predictive value for the individual patient as to her chance of progression to cancer.[108] Other cellular changes, such as DNA ploidy, abnormal mitoses, and chromosomal aberrations, have been studied in association with CIN in an attempt to predict clinical outcome. Although all of them have some element of predictiveness, none stands alone as the ultimate clinical test, and they vary in their expense and availability.[103, 109–112]

OBTAINING SPECIMENS FOR CERVICAL CYTOLOGIC EXAMINATION—THE PAPANICOLAOU SMEAR

The Papanicolaou test is performed as follows:

1. The cervix is exposed with a vaginal speculum lubricated only with water.
2. Two specimens are taken for cytologic examination, one from the endocervix and one from the ectocervix.
   a. Endocervical specimens are best obtained by using an endocervical brush. The tip is placed into the external os and rotated multiple times to obtain endocervical mucus and cells.
   b. Exocervical specimens are obtained by rotating a specially shaped wooden spatula (Ayre's) against the external os. Care must be taken to obtain a sample from the entire squamocolumnar junction. The clinician should locate this junction on every patient's cervix to make sure that this area is sampled with the spatula.
3. Each sample can be transferred to a glass slide individually, or both samples can be sent on the same slide. In either case, fixation should be done promptly because failure to do so may lead to cellular alterations and errors in reading. This phenomenon is described as air-drying artifact by the cytopathologist and is one of the leading causes of error in Papanicolaou smear interpretation.[113] If both specimens are sent on the same slide, the endocervical sample should be spread first with the spatula spread promptly afterwards followed by immediate fixation. The water content of the endocervical mucus provides a small protective effect to the cells contained within it, whereas the ectocervical specimen has very little moisture associated with it. Multiple studies have shown that usage of a cytobrush, as compared with a cotton-tipped moist swab, enhances the ability of the practitioner to obtain endocervical cells and to detect preinvasive disease.[114, 115]

Once the Papanicolaou smear has been properly obtained, it must be processed, examined, and interpreted appropriately. Recommendations for laboratory facilities that examine Papanicolaou smears have been recently updated by the federal government and were published in 1992 in the *Federal Register*. These recommendations include that any individual cytotechnologist must not screen more than 100 slides/day, that quality control mandates rescreening 10% of all normal Papanicolaou smear results, and that new high-grade lesions require that all previous Papanicolaou smears on that patient for an immediate 5-year period preceding the abnormal smear result be rescreened.[116]

Recently, all of the major pathology and cytology organizations and the American College of Obstetricians and Gynecologists endorsed a new reporting system for Papanicolaou smears and cervical biopsies known as the *Bethesda System*.[117] This reporting system is outlined in Table 72–5 and is compared with the descriptive Papanicolaou smear system that preceded it. The reason for the alteration in reporting was to give cytologists and pathologists more uniform guidelines to follow in reporting abnormalities.

SCREENING FOR CERVICAL NEOPLASIA

Several factors seem to be important when one considers screening for cervical cancer. The smear, as described by

TABLE 72–5. REPORTING SYSTEM (BETHESDA SYSTEM) FOR PAPANICOLAOU SMEARS AND CERVICAL BIOPSIES

Descriptive Classification	Bethesda System
No abnormal cells	No evidence of malignant cells
Atypical cells present below the level of cervical neoplasia	Atypical cells of undetermined significance, excluding infectious changes
Smear contains cells consistent with intraepithelial neoplasia; often graded as CIN† I–III, or carcinoma in situ	Squamous intraepithelial lesion, low-grade: equivalent to CIN I and changes associated with HPV*
	Squamous intraepithelial lesion, high-grade: equivalent to CIN II/III and carcinoma in situ
Smear contains cells consistent with invasive cancer	Smear consistent with invasive cancer

*HPV = human papillomavirus.
†CIN = cervical intraepithelial neoplasia.

Papanicolaou and Traut, is an easily obtained test that represents little risk to the patient, and since its introduction, overall cervical cancer mortality has decreased. Additionally, cervical cancer has been shown to be preceded by a preinvasive state that is extended to the point that virtually 100% of preinvasive disease should be detected and cured.[107, 118] Questions that remain are how often a Papanicolaou smear should be done, which age groups of patients are appropriate to screen, and at what cost should life-years be saved.

Because there are no randomized clinical trials looking at Papanicolaou smear screening intervals and reduction of mortality, large, organized, mass-screening programs and mathematical models are the most helpful tools available.[118, 119] From these data sources, several facts are clear: the initiation of mass screening, with its expected lag phase, leads to marked reduction in the incidence and mortality from cervical cancer, and the interval between Papanicolaou smears can vary by several years without affecting the apparent efficacy of screening.[107, 118–120] Data from a mass-screening program in Finland using a 5-year screening interval indicate that the incidence of invasive cervical cancer dropped over 70% in the age groups of 30 to 54 years. The corresponding mortality was reduced by 80%. It appears that the trend toward reduction of incidence and mortality has stabilized in the late 1980s, probably reflecting the ultimate effect that can be achieved with this screening program.[118] Whether decreasing the interval between screening to 3, 2, or 1 year would be more effective continues to be debated. Screening data indicate that intervals of 2, 3, 5, and 10 years retain 99%, 97%, 89%, and 69%, respectively, of the efficacy of cervical screening in reducing cervical cancer mortality.[119, 120]

No consensus currently exists regarding the duration of screening after the age of 65, although nearly half of the deaths from cervical cancer occur in women over the age of 65.[121] The approach to screening is hampered by lack of data concerning how long the transformation process takes from CIN to invasive disease in the elderly, and the understanding of the possibility of regression. Projections from the sparse data that exist, from mathematical models, and estimates made by ratios of prevalence to incidence, indicate that the conversion of CIS to invasive cancer may take as little as 1 year in women over the age of 65.[122] Further prospective studies are required to make recommendations for Papanicolaou smear screening in the elderly, although the movement is toward screen beyond the age of 65.

Cost-effectiveness of Papanicolaou smear screening depends on the endpoint of observation, but most estimates look at cost/added year of life expectancy. In 1984 dollars, annual screening starting at age 20 adds a year of life expectancy at a cost of $100,000, as compared with $700 for screening every 5 years.[120]

Interval for Screening

Despite the limitation in data that exist in regard to Papanicolaou smear screening, the American College of Obstetrics and Gynecology, in conjunction with several other major cancer organizations, issued guidelines for practitioners in 1988. They suggested that screening begin with the onset of sexual activity, or at age 18 years, whichever occurs first. After 3 consecutive normal results on yearly Papanicolaou smears and pelvic examinations, the physician may extend the interval at his or her discretion. If the patient or her sexual partner has had two or more sexual partners, they would not recommend extending the interval. These recommendations apply until age 65. Whether the College will give guidelines beyond the age of 65 is not clear.[123] In view of the controversies that exist with oral contraceptive use, yearly screening is probably indicated. Women exposed in utero to estrogens should be screened with baseline Papanicolaou smears, have careful digital examination of the vagina, and have their transformation zone mapped by colposcopy. If no abnormalities are found, then follow-up smears and vaginal examinations should be done yearly.[123]

Management of the Patient With an Abnormal Papanicolaou Smear Result

Papanicolaou smear results designated as "no abnormal cells" in the descriptive Papanicolaou smear system or as "no evidence of malignant cells" in the Bethesda System require no further evaluation. As discussed, the purpose of the Bethesda System was to clarify for cytopathologists and pathologists the various abnormalities that exist in Papanicolaou smears. The comments that follow in regard to abnormal cells seen on the smear are in accordance with the Bethesda System, and correlation to the descriptive, CIN Papanicolaou smear result will be noted where appropriate or can be compared using Table 72–5. Papanicolaou smears that are labeled "atypical cells of undetermined significance," a category that excludes any infectious process, remain controversial as to whether further evaluation is required or whether simple follow-up with a repeat Papanicolaou smear in 4 months should be done. A result that falls into any category beyond this (see Table 72–5) should be further evaluated.[117]

Patients with smears that show abnormal cells consistent with dysplasia or with malignant disease should be referred to a gynecologist who is expert in evaluating the abnormal cervix. Abnormal smears should not be repeated prior to this referral because even if a repeat specimen is interpreted as normal, the initially abnormal finding demands evaluation. Opinion concerning the ideal management of patients with abnormal results on Papanicolaou smears has evolved over the years, and there are still points of controversy; however, the basic principle is to localize and perform biopsies on areas of greatest abnormality to confirm the cytologic findings.

At present, many clinicians in the United States favor examination of the cervix with a colposcopy, a low-powered binocular lens system. The trained colposcopist can locate the lesion visually on the basis of its characteristic surface epithelium, which is determined by the underlying vascular structures.[124,125] Small biopsy specimens are taken from the abnormal areas using a special punch that provides a cuboidal tissue specimen, which can be oriented by the pathologists in the appropriate plane for sectioning. An endocervical curettage should be performed before the cervical biopsy on every patient, as long as the patient is not pregnant. For the colposcopy to be accurate, the entire squamocolumnar junction, often referred to as the transformation zone, must be visualized. If it is not visualized, which becomes increasingly more frequent as a woman approaches menopause or has had previous surgery on the cervix, then the gynecologist must decide whether further excision of the cervix is necessary for investigation of the abnormal Papanicolaou smear result. The smear is generally repeated at the time of colposcopy.

When the results of the biopsies, endocervical curettage, and repeat Papanicolaou smears are available, they should be compared to determine whether the findings on biopsy confirm the results of the smear. If the results do not agree by one degree of error or more, that is, the smear result is consistent with CIN II but the biopsy specimens are normal, then one can proceed to repeat examination with colposcopy and biopsies or move to excisional biopsy of the transformation zone (conization).[125] In patients whose repeat colposcopy still does not explain the abnormal Papanicolaou smear result, cervical conization should be performed.[126]

Recently, many gynecologists have moved to large loop excision of the transformation zone (LLETZ) for the evaluation and treatment of preinvasive disease of the cervix. Electrical excision or cauterization of the cervix has been available for many years but led to severe scarring of the cervix. Now a combination of new electrosurgical generators that combines both cutting and coagulating tissue effects and new wire loops that withstand these complex radiofrequency-blended currents has led to outpatient office usage of this technique.[127,128]

In general, preinvasive disease of the cervix can be approached by two broad categories of treatment modalities: ablation of the cervical epithelium or excision of the epithelium. The initial decision is made on the basis of the colposcopic findings. If the colposcopy is adequate, that is, if the transformation zone is seen, then ablation with cryosurgery (freezing) or laser vaporization is possible. When the colposcopy is inadequate, or when the cervical biopsies do not explain the Papanicolaou smear result, then excisional procedures such as conization by scalpel, laser, or LLETZ must be performed. In rare cases of extensive CIS or recurrent severe preinvasive disease, hysterectomy can be considered in women who do not wish further child bearing. The decision as to which method is to be used depends on the patient, her physician, and the characteristics of her preinvasive disease.[129–134] The general trend has been, however, toward removal of the transformation zone with LLETZ.[127–130] This technique has been used in lieu of cervical biopsies but does require colposcopy of the cervix to ascertain the size of the transformation zone and the nature of the cervical lesion. All methods of treatment, including hysterectomy, have a failure rate that varies from a low of 1 to 2% for hysterectomy to 10 to 15% for ablation methods. LLETZ has the least long-term data, but data thus far place the risk of recurrence at between 5 and 10%.[128,132–134] Follow-up for these procedures should be only by Papanicolaou smear on a frequent basis. Colposcopy appears to have a high false-positive rate unless it is associated with an abnormal smear result.[135]

Invasive carcinoma is treated by radical hysterectomy and pelvic lymph node dissection or by extensive radiation therapy, depending primarily on the stage of the disease, the suitability of the patient for surgery, and patient and physician preference.

PART 4 Colorectal Carcinoma

WILLIAM T. BRANCH, Jr., MD

The annual incidence of colorectal cancer in men and women is almost 1/1000 persons at the age of 50 years and continues to increase as they grow older.[135A] The prevalence of detectable cancer in a previously unscreened population is probably 3 to 4/1000 persons above the age of 45 years. Hence, asymptomatic colorectal cancer is likely to be present in several of the patients cared for by the average internist at any given time. Screening and diagnostic tests to detect colorectal cancer are now widely available and used in practice.

NATURAL HISTORY

It has been estimated that 90% of colorectal carcinomas arise from adenomatous polyps and villous adenomas.[136–138] Adenomatous polyps affect 3 to 10% of individuals over 40 years of age.[139,140] They may be classified according to their shape as pedunculated, sessile, or indeterminate, but the risk of malignancy, in general, is related to the size of the polyp.[136,140–142] Size also correlates with histology because most polyps over 2 cm in size have some villous components, and smaller polyps are mostly tubular.[140] In one study, invasive cancer was found in 1.3% of polyps that were 1.0 cm in diameter; in 9.5% of those between 1.0 and 2.0 cm; and in 46% of those greater than 2.0 cm.[141] If intramucosal in addition to invasive carcinomas are counted, the incidence of malignancy doubles for polyps at each size.[142] It is thought that the majority of intramucosal cancers will also ultimately become invasive.[142] Malignancies are rare in polyps less than 1.0 cm in diameter; at least two thirds of those less than 0.5 cm in diameter are hyperplastic rather than adenomatous polyps, in which the risk of malignancy is zero.[141, 143] Regardless of how small, if the surface of a pedunculated polyp appears irregular, or if a sessile lesion of the colon is triangular, rectangular, or odd-shaped, it is likely to be malignant.[142, 144]

Survival following detection of colorectal cancer depends on whether the malignancy has spread through the bowel wall and whether there is lymphatic involvement (Table 72–6). By the time of surgery, the tumor will have penetrated all layers of the bowel wall in 50 to 75% of patients presenting with symptoms, and about 60% have some regional lymph node metastases.[145] Recent data indicate improvements, but the 5-year survival of patients in stages B_2 and C is probably no better than 67 to 82%.[146] Of patients with negative nodes and extension limited to the muscularis (stage B_1) and of those with infiltration no deeper than the submucosa (stage A), 5-year survivals are approximately 85% and 90 to 100%, respectively.

RISK FACTORS

The high incidence of colorectal carcinoma in Western societies has been attributed to increased beef or red meat intake, a low-fiber diet,[16] dietary carcinogens, or alterations of the fecal flora. Within this population, the major known risk factors, as just noted, are age and the presence of adenomatous polyps. These are the factors of most concern for practitioners, because they affect so many patients. Risk also is about threefold greater and begins earlier in individuals with a family history of colonic carcinoma.[137] Increased risk applies also to members of families in whom carcinomas of the ovary, breast, and endometrium are clustered. Spinners, weavers, and fabric mill and asbestos workers are at higher-than-average risk.[147] Especially high risk has been associated with familial polyposis (adenomatous polyps throughout the colon and rectum), Gardner's syndrome (epidermoid cysts, osteomas of the skull and mandible, and polyps of the large and small bowel), and inflammatory bowel diseases. In familial polyposis, the occurrence of malignancy reaches 50% by age 20.[137] The eventual development of adenomatous polyps and adenocarcinomas has also been noted in a few families with multiple hyperplastic polyps.[148] In ulcerative colitis, onset of the disease before age 25 years, continuously active disease, and disease involving the entire colon are associated with the highest risk of malignancy, which remains low until the disease is of 10 years' duration but then becomes 20% per decade in those most strongly predisposed. Granulomatous colitis and ulcerative colitis involving only the rectum have much lower incidences of malignancy.[137]

TABLE 72–6. STAGING OF COLORECTAL CARCINOMA

Classification	Description	5-Year Survival (%)
A	Nodes negative; infiltration no deeper than submucosa	90–100
B_1	Nodes negative; extension into muscularis but still within bowel	85
B_2	Nodes negative; extension through entire bowel wall, including serosa if present	75–82
C_1	Nodes positive; lesion limited to bowel	45–67
C_2	Nodes positive; extension through entire bowel wall including serosa	45–67
D	Distant metastases	(survival of 6–8 months)

SCREENING

Patients in the very-high-risk groups for colorectal carcinoma will be encountered infrequently in a general medical practice. Thus, the problem for the physician will be the detection of carcinoma as early as possible in an entire population. Surveillance should begin at 40 to 50 years of age.[136] In those with positive family histories, it should begin at age 20 years. The methodologies suitable for screening are testing of stool for occult blood and flexible proctosigmoidoscopy. Serum levels of carcinoembryonic antigen are not useful for screening because they are positive infrequently in small, localized lesions, but elevated levels can be associated with cirrhosis of the liver and other conditions.[145]

Fecal Occult Blood. Current recommendations are to use impregnated guaiac slides (Hemoccult II); two specimens are collected by the patient from different parts of the stool each day for 3 days.[137, 149] Using Hemoccult is superior to testing with benzadine, which, although more sensitive, results in many false-positive reactions; or to testing with guaiac solution, which tends to deteriorate and give false-negative reactions.

Protocols for using Hemoccult II vary. Some ignore diet.[149] Others suggest a meat-free diet of high residue but low in fresh vegetable and fruit peroxidases.[137, 150] Data to ascertain dietary effects on the sensitivity and specificity of testing are not available.[149] It is judged that false-positive results can result from aspirin or iron ingestion and from exposure of stool to povidone-iodine or formalin; false negatives result from vitamin C ingestion. Slides lose sensitivity if stored at room temperature for more than 2 days and regain sensitivity if rehydrated prior to testing; however, rehydration approximately doubles the number of false-positive results and therefore is not always recommended. Equivocal results should be considered negative, but even a single minimally positive test cannot be discarded. About one fourth of the carcinomas detected in one study were positive only on the second or third test.[151] A variety of other commercially marketed tests (Fecatest, Colo-Rect, Coloscreen, Hemo-Fec) also employ guaiac, but information comparing these tests with Hemoccult II or with each other is limited.[150]

The practicality of the Hemoccult test depends on its predictive value and sensitivity when it is applied to large, asymptomatic populations. A summary of many series suggests that 2 to 6% of the results are positive.[149] Of these, about half represent false-positive reactions and half have bowel diseases, including many trivial conditions like hemorrhoids and diverticulosis, as well as adenomatous polyps and carcinomas.[137, 149, 150, 152] The predictive value of the test averages approximately 20% for benign polyps and about 5% for cancer. The high yield of cancers diagnosed in many early series was misleading, because publicity for screening undoubtedly caused individuals with symptoms or increased risk of cancer to enroll in the studies. The test also is not as sensitive as originally thought, and this is its major limitation as a screening test. Only 48 to 67% of patients with cancer and about 25% of those with adenomas have positive test results.[149, 153–155]

It is hoped that both the sensitivity and specificity of testing for fecal blood can be improved. Hemoccult is not reliably positive at fecal blood losses of less than 20 ml/day (nl 0.5 to 2.0 ml day), whereas fecal blood loss associated with colorectal cancer varies from 0 to 75 ml/day and exceeds 10 ml in fewer than 25% of daily collections. An immunochemical method positive only for human blood detects one tenth the amount detectable by the Hemoccult but is expensive, more complex to perform, and requires further validation prior to wide-scale use.[149] In a series of 150 patients proved to have colorectal carcinoma, the Hemoccult test, performed once, yielded positive results in 40% and the immunochemical method in 65% of cases.[156]

A quantitative test for fecal heme (HemoQuant) is technically more cumbersome than Hemoccult but is independent of storage and dietary factors.[149] Results of studies are conflicting on whether the sensitivity of HemoQuant (83 to 63% at 3 mg/g [~ equal to 3 ml/day of blood]) outweighs that of Hemoccult (67 to 89.5% in patients with known colon cancer in these studies).[157, 158]

Proctosigmoidoscopy. Although within the past 30 years the proportion of distal colonic carcinomas has gradually declined, 30% of bowel lesions are still thought to be within reach of the rigid sigmoidoscope.[136] An initial proctosigmoidoscopic examination done to 25 cm in a population of patients more than 50 years of age, with compression of rectal valves to identify hidden lesions, should detect 1.5 carcinomas/1000 individuals, plus adenomatous polyps in an additional 4.7 to 9.7% of patients.[159] However, on the average, proctosigmoidoscopic examinations using a rigid scope do not advance beyond 16 to 19 cm.[160]

Flexible fiberoptic sigmoidoscopes of 35- and 60-cm lengths are now available. Experienced examiners using the 60-cm scope can cover a mean of 56.4 cm of colon in 7.4 minutes.[161] The risk of perforation by experienced examiners is about 1/10,000 examinations, compared with about 1/40,000 examinations using the rigid scope.[136] Special training in endoscopy is necessary to use these instruments because inexperienced examiners, particularly when attempting to negotiate the area from the sigmoid to the descending colon, will experience higher rates of complications. A minimal proficiency with the 35-cm scope requires 6 to 10 supervised examinations, and the 60-cm scope may require considerably more.[162] Compared with the rigid sigmoidoscope, flexible sigmoidoscopy to 60 cm is estimated to increase the fraction of adenomatous polyps and carcinomas detected from approximately 30 to 50%.[136] Testing of stool for occult blood does not replace sigmoidoscopic examination in screening for carcinomas. In a large-scale prospective trial, about 25% of cancers and about 75% of polyps detected by rigid sigmoidoscopy had negative fecal blood test results.[163]

Recommendations. As a screening procedure, the fecal occult blood test has two major disadvantages: lack of high sensitivity and poor compliance. Even the well-motivated patients enrolled in clinical trials have a 30 to 50% rate of noncompliance.[149] Compliance is more difficult to achieve in the elderly, who are at highest risk for colorectal carcinoma, and the problem of noncompliance is compounded by failure of many patients with positive test results to have a complete diagnostic evaluation. Advantages are that the test is inexpensive and simple and practical to perform. The important question is whether use of the fecal occult blood test produces improved survival for patients. Uncontrolled trials established that screening for fecal blood detects a large number of asymptomatic cancers in stages A and B.[135A, 150] The apparently early stage of detected lesions, however, may represent length- and lead-time biases, so large-scale randomized trials are necessary to determine whether mortality is favorably influenced.[153–155] One well-designed trial has reported a statistically significant 33% reduction in the cumulative mortality rate for colorectal cancer in persons aged 50 to 80 years.[153a] These patients were screened annually with six rehydrated occult blood slides.[153a] Rehydration increased the sensitivity but produced more false-positive–testing slides (9.8% were positive), so that 38% of the screened patients underwent colonoscopy over 13 years. Another study has reported a 27% reduction in mortality.[155] This difference will become statistically significant if it persists,[155] and it is hoped that the benefits of screening will increase over time as colorectal polyps are detected and removed, thus preventing future development of malignancies.[154]

Flexible sigmoidoscopy, with a trained endoscopist using the 60-cm scope or a proficient primary care physician using the 35-cm scope, is preferred over rigid sigmoidoscopy for screening.[165] The chief disadvantage of sigmoidoscopy is noncompliance due to poor patient acceptance. An advantage of proctosigmoidoscopy is that it leads to no false-positive results requiring evaluation. Its advocates point out that if all adenomatous polyps of the rectosigmoid were removed during sigmoidoscopy, the subsequent development of colorectal cancer might be prevented. It is estimated that, on the average, precancerous adenomas are detectable by sigmoidoscopy for 7 to 10 years before they become invasive.[136, 166] In a report of 21,150 people who underwent a mean of 5.4 sigmoidoscopies during 6 years, with removal of polyps, the incidence of rectal cancer was 15% of that predicted based on the patients' ages.[167] A large case-control study revealed that patients dying of colorectal cancer within reach of the rigid sigmoidoscope were about one third as likely as control patients to have had rigid sigmoidoscopy in the preceding 10 years.[166] By inference, this study suggests that sigmoidoscopy with removal of polyps protects against dying from cancer occurring within reach of the scope.

A randomized trial showing that screening consisting of fecal occult blood testing reduces mortality from colorectal cancer and a case-control study whose results suggest benefit from sigmoidoscopy justify a policy of screening of asymptomatic patients.[153a, 166] A cost-effective strategy to screen persons at average risk may consist of annual fecal occult blood testing beginning between the ages of 40 and 50 years and continuing to age 80 years or older and of flexible sigmoidoscopy every 5 to 10 years beginning at the age of 50 or 55 years.[136] Assuming that a 60-cm flexible sigmoidoscopy costs about $65 (compared with $40 for a rigid sigmoidoscopy), flexible sigmoidoscopy adds less than 25% to costs and increases estimated survival by approximately 9% in this strategy.[136] However, the large number of colonoscopies performed in one randomized trial that showed decreased mortality by testing for fecal occult blood suggests that the strategy will be costly.[153a] Less costly alternatives will probably be considered. These may be based on dividing patients into those at low-risk (those with no or only small [<5mm] adenomatous polyps by age 55 or 60 years) who need no or little additional screening and into those at high-risk (those with adenomatous polyps >5mm) who may be screened periodically. Risk could be determined by performing flexible sigmoidoscopy, barium enema, or single colonoscopy; however, the last of these carries the risk of increased perforation of the colon when compared with flexible sigmoidoscopy. Until further investigations are done, the standard recommendation is to perform annual fecal occult blood testing and periodic flexible sigmoidoscopy in asymptomatic persons.

CLINICAL EVALUATION OF THE PATIENT

Diagnostic evaluations should be performed in all patients who have rectal bleeding or fecal occult blood and, because of the high prevalence of colorectal carcinomas, should also be performed in persons over the age of 40 to 50 years with suggestive symptoms or unexplained anemia. In practice, the commonest symptom of colonic carcinoma is a nonspecific change in bowel habits. Patients may describe this as a sensation of abdominal fullness or of having partial bowel movements or the inability to evacuate completely. Diarrhea, rather than constipation or obstruction, occasionally is the initial manifestation. Any such symptom, if persistent and representing a definite change in the bowel patterns of an older person, or the finding of fecal blood is sufficient to justify diagnostic evaluation. Evaluation for symptoms usually includes an air-contrast barium enema in addition to proctosigmoidoscopy. For an individual with blood in the stool, colonoscopy should be performed, followed by upper gastrointestinal and small-bowel series if bleeding persists and a source is not identified. Positive occult blood tests should not be attributed solely to diverticulosis unless other lesions have been excluded.

Diagnostic Studies, Barium Enema, and Colonoscopy

Accuracy of barium enema for cancer detection presents a problem. Single-contrast barium enemas miss about 20% of carcinomas.[168] Air-contrast studies are more costly and time consuming but provide better visualization of the rectum.[169] Their advocates state that air-contrast studies can detect polyps as small as 2 to 3 mm in diameter, or carcinomas, manifested by mucosal alterations or focal rigidity of the bowel wall, measuring 1 cm.[170] The sensitivity of high-quality air-contrast barium enemas is reported to be as high as 92.2% for detecting polyps and 93.7% for detecting carcinomas.[171] In routine practice, however, air-contrast studies may not be so sensitive. Air-contrast barium enemas identified 9 (75%) of 12 carcinomas and 24 (62.5%) of 40 adenomas in a large British trial.[135a] Barium enemas missed 33% of cancers in the large, prospective University of Minnesota trial.[172]

Colonic cleansing must be done meticulously prior to air-contrast barium enema. Otherwise the rate of false-positive findings, sometimes leading to unnecessary colonoscopic examinations, averages 17%.[173]

Colonoscopy is a sensitive but costly method for detecting mucosal lesions. It has been shown to detect 88 to 97% of colonic polyps.[141, 150, 174] Numerous reports in the literature describe colonic polyps or carcinomas detected by colonoscopy that barium enemas had failed to identify.[142, 150, 175, 176] The additional yield of carcinomas (6.5 to 13.0%) is particularly high in patients with gross rectal bleeding and those with persistent occult bleeding.[175, 176] Barium enema is sometimes performed prior to colonoscopy, to forewarn the colonoscopist of suspicious areas, anatomic variants, or unsuspected contraindications (e.g., acute inflammatory bowel disease or diverticulitis). The barium enema occasionally identifies lesions that are missed on colonoscopy, particularly lesions of the sigmoid colon, splenic and hepatic flexures, and right colon if this is not reached by the colonoscopist.[171, 177] Nevertheless, skillful colonoscopists now undertake their examinations without a preceding barium enema in otherwise healthy persons being studied because of the finding of fecal occult blood. Perforation is estimated to occur in 1/2000 colonoscopic examinations.[136]

Pedunculated polyps up to 3.4 cm in diameter can be excised during colonoscopy. Even experienced colonoscopists may find sessile polyps difficult to snare and remove completely, but often these can be extirpated by the combination of piecemeal resection by snaring and coagulation.[177, 178] Very small polyps (less than 0.5 cm), if encountered, are usually biopsied and then coagulated.[178] Larger polyps are preferably removed because the accuracy of a single colonoscopic biopsy may be as low as 79%.[142] Colonoscopists report an overall success rate of 93% in removing polyps and a complication rate of 1.5 to 2.3%.[177, 178]

APPROACH TO THE PATIENT

Because of its accuracy for detecting colonic lesions, colonoscopy should be performed in all patients with gross rectal bleeding or positive test results for fecal occult blood. If another explanation accounts for the bleeding, such as hemorrhoids or aspirin ingestion, and if the fecal occult blood test results reverts to negative on repeated testing, it may be reasonable to rely on proctosigmoidoscopy plus a technically excellent air-contrast barium enema. Hemorrhoids, however, are commonly present in elderly persons and should not be assumed to be the source of bleeding without careful assessment.

When identified, it is generally recommended that polypoid lesions greater than 1.0 cm in diameter be excised during colonoscopy. The colonoscopist should search the entire colon for lesions in addition to any already identified on barium enema. Lesions with the radiographic features of carcinoma invading the intestinal wall require partial colectomy.[142, 177, 178] Colonoscopic excision of a polyp found to have intramucosal carcinoma or invasive carcinoma that has not yet reached the stalk may be adequate therapy; however, if the malignancy is poorly differentiated, has invaded the stalk, or is in a broad-based polyp, colectomy is generally recommended.[142]

Polypectomy can sometimes be deferred in small lesions (less than 1 cm in diameter) if the barium enema is repeated in 1 year.[141] Using serial barium enemas, Marshak and colleagues followed 480 small, perfectly rounded polyps on long pedicles and reported only three malignant transformations after 4 to 8 years.[144] One may also elect to follow-up some slightly larger (1.0- to 1.5-cm), benign-appearing polyps radiographically in very elderly patients or those whose life expectancies are limited by medical illness. In most cases, however, it seems preferable to remove polyps rather than to subject the patient to a lifetime of annual endoscopic or barium enema examinations.

Following excision of benign polyps, it is recommended that endoscopy be repeated in 3 years.[179] Data suggest that this strategy detects important colonic lesions (polyps >1 cm in diameter or with high-grade dysplasia or invasive cancer) as effectively as a stragegy that consists of performing first follow-up colonoscopy 1 year after removal of a benign adenoma.[179] Patients found to have colorectal cancer require more frequent surveillance to detect synchronous lesions that may have been missed as well as suture line recurrences and metachronous lesions. Colonoscopy in these patients should be done at 3 months, if not completed at the time of diagnosis, and again at 1 year and at 3 years after the diagnosis.[150]

ACKNOWLEDGMENTS

The contributions to this chapter of Arthur J. Siegel, MD, and Gordon Vineyard, MD, in the first edition of this text are gratefully acknowledged.

REFERENCES

1. Fraumeni JF Jr, Hoover RN, Devesa SS, and Kinlen LJ: Epidemiology of cancer. *In* DeVita VT Jr, Hellman SH, and Rosenberg SA (eds): Cancer Principles and Practice of Oncology, 3rd ed. Philadelphia, Lippincott, 1989, pp 196–227.
2. Roush GC, Meigs JW, Kelly J, et al: Sinonasal cancer and occupation: A case-control study. Am J Epidemiol 111:183, 1980.
3. Costanza ME, Li FP, Green HL, and Patterson WB: Cancer prevention and detection: Strategies for practice. *In* Cancer, A Manual for Practitioners. Boston, American Cancer Society, Massachusetts Division, 1986, pp 14–35.
4. Winn DM, Blot WJ, Shy CM, et al: Snuff dipping and oral cancer among women in the southern United States. N Engl J Med 304:745, 1981.
5. Peto RAD: Keynote address: The control of lung cancer. *In* Lung Cancer: Causes and Prevention. Geneva, Verlag Chemie International, 1984, pp 1–19.
6. Henderson IC: What can a woman do about her risk of dying of breast cancer? Curr Probl Cancer 14:165, 1990.
7. Dupont WD and Page DL: Menopausal estrogen replacement therapy and breast cancer. Arch Intern Med 151:67, 1991.
8. Steinberg KK, et al: A meta-analysis of the effect of estrogen replacement therapy on the risk of breast cancer. J Am Med Assoc 265:1985, 1991.
9. Romieu I, Berlin JA, and Colditz G: Oral contraceptives and breast cancer: Review and meta-analysis. Cancer 66:2253, 1990.
10. Boice JD: Cancer following medical irradiation. Cancer 47:1081, 1981.
11. Penn I: Second neoplasms following radiotherapy or chemotherapy for cancer. Am J Clin Oncol 5:83, 1982.
12. Fisher B, Rockette H, Fisher ER, et al: Leukemia in breast cancer patients following adjuvant chemotherapy or postoperative radiation: The NSABP experience. J Clin Oncol 3:1640, 1985.
13. Curtis RE, John MA, Boice JD, et al: Risk of leukemia after chemotherapy and radiation treatment for breast cancer. N Engl J Med 326:1745, 1992.
14. Henderson IC: Breast cancer therapy—The price of success. N Engl J Med 326:1774, 1992.
15. Doll R and Peto R: The Causes of Cancer. New York, Oxford University Press, 1981.
16. Newell GR: Nutrition and diet. Cancer 51:2420, 1983.
17. Blattner WA, Biggar RJ, Weiss SH, et al: Epidemiology of human T-lymphotropic virus type III and the risk of the acquired immunodeficiency syndrome. Ann Intern Med 103:665, 1985.
18. Young JL, Percy CL, et al: Surveillance Epidemiology End Results: Incidence and Mortality Data 1973–77. National Cancer Institute Monograph 57, June 1981.
19. Stoll HL Jr: Squamous cell carcinoma. *In* Fitzpatrick TB, Arndt KA, Clark WH, et al (eds): Dermatology in General Medicine. New York, McGraw-Hill, 1971, p 407.
20. American Joint Committee on Cancer: Manual for Staging of Cancer. Philadelphia, JB Lippincott, 1983.
21. Feibleman CE, Stoll H, and Maize JC: Melanomas of the palm, sole, and nailbed: A clinicopathologic study. Cancer 46:2492, 1980.
22. Clark WH Jr and Mihm MC Jr: Moles and malignant melanoma. *In* Fitzpatrick TB, Arndt KA, Clark WH, et al (eds): Dermatology in General Medicine. New York, McGraw-Hill, 1971, p 491.
23. Alper J, Holmes LB, and Mihm MC: Birth marks with serious medical significance: Nevocellular nevi, sebaceous nevi, and multiple café au lait spots. J Pediatr 95:696, 1979.
24. Rhodes AR, Sober AJ, Mihm MC, et al: Possible risk factors for cutaneous malignant melanoma. Clin Res 28:252A, 1980.
25. Clark WH, Reimer RR, Green MH, et al: Origin of malignant familial melanoma from heritable melanocytic lesions. Arch Dermatol 114:731, 1978.
26. Brett GZ: Earlier diagnosis and survival in lung cancer. Br J Med 4:260, 1969.
27. Fontana RS, Sanderson DR, Woolner LB, et al: Screening for lung cancer. A critique of the Mayo Lung Project. Cancer 67:1155, 1991.
28. Tockman MS: Survival and mortality from lung cancer in a screened population: The Johns Hopkins study. Chest 89(Suppl):324, 1986.
29. Flehinger BJ, Kimmel M, and Melamed MR: Natural history of adenocarcinoma-large cell carcinoma of the lung: Conclusions from screening program in New York and Baltimore. J Natl Cancer Inst 80:337, 1988.
30. Jackman RJ, Good CA, Clagett OT, et al: Survival rates in peripheral bronchogenic carcinomas up to four centimeters in diameter presenting as solitary pulmonary nodules. J Thorac Cardiovasc Surg 57:1, 1969.
31. Weiss W: Peripheral measurable bronchogenic carcinoma: Growth rate and period of risk after therapy. Am Rev Respir Dis 103:198, 1971.
32. Guinan P, Bush I, Ray V, et al: The accuracy of the rectal examination in the diagnosis of prostate carcinoma. N Engl J Med 303:499, 1980.
33. Cooner WH, Mosley BR, Rutherford CL, et al: Prostate cancer detection in a clinical urological practice by ultrasonography, digital rectal examination and prostate specific antigen. J Urol 143:1146, 1990.
34. Catalona WJ, Smith DS, Ratliff TL, et al: Measurement of prostate-specific antigen in serum as a screening test for prostate cancer. N Engl J Med 324:1156, 1991.

34a. Giovannucci E, Ascherio A, Rimm EB, et al: A prospective cohort study of vasectomy and prostate cancer in US men. JAMA 269:873, 1993.

34b. Fleming C, Wasson JH, Albertsen PC: A decision analysis of alternative treatment strategies for clinically localized prostate cancer. JAMA 269:2650, 1993.

34c. Kramer BS, Brown ML, Prorok PC: Prostate cancer screening: What we know and what we need to know. Ann Intern Med 119:914, 1993.

34d. Chodak GW, Thisted RA, Gerber GS, et al: Results of conservative management of clinically localized prostate cancer. N Engl J Med 330:242, 1994.

35. Henderson IC and Canellos GP: Cancer of the breast. I. The past decade. N Engl J Med 302:17, 1980.
36. Henderson IC: Prognostic factors. *In* Harris JR, Hellman S, Henderson IC, and Kinne DW (Eds): Breast Diseases. Philadelphia, JB Lippincott, 1991, pp 332–346.
37. McGuire WL and Clark GM: Prognostic factors and treatment decisions in axillary node-negative breast cancer. N Engl J Med 326:1756, 1992.
38. Fisher B, Redmond C, Fisher ER, and Caplan R: Relative worth of estrogen or progesterone receptor and pathologic characteristics of differentiation as indicators of prognosis in node negative breast cancer patients: Findings from national surgical adjuvant breast and bowel project protocol B-06. J Clin Oncol 6:1076, 1988.
39. Gullino PM: Natural history of breast cancer. Cancer 39:2697, 1977.
40. Krieger N: Rising incidence of breast cancer. J Natl Cancer Inst 80:2, 1988.
41. Seidman H, Mushinski MH, Gelb SK, et al: Probabilities of eventually developing or dying of cancer—United States, 1985. CA Cancer J Clin 35:36, 1985.
42. Adami HO, Bergstrom R, and Hansen J: Age at first primary as a determinant of the incidence of bilateral breast cancer: Cumulative and relative risks in a population-based case-control study. Cancer 55:643, 1985.
43. Leis HP Jr: Managing the remaining breast. Cancer 46:1026, 1980.
44. Adami H, Hansen J, Jung B, et al: Characteristics of familial breast cancer in Sweden. Cancer 48:1688, 1981.
45. Lipnick R, Speizer FE, Bain C, et al: A case-control study of risk indicators among women with premenopausal and early postmenopausal breast cancer. Cancer 53:1020, 1984.
46. Ottman R, King MC, Pike MC, and Henderson BE: Practical guide for estimating risk for familial breast cancer. Lancet ii:556, 1983.
47. Anderson DE and Badzioch MD: Risk of familial breast cancer. Cancer 56:383, 1985.
48. Love SM, Gelman RS, and Silen W: Fibrocystic "disease" of the breast—a nondisease? N Engl J Med 307:1010, 1982.

49. Dupont WD and Page DL: Risk factors for breast cancer in women with proliferative breast disease. N Engl J Med 312:146, 1985.
50. Dupont WD and Page DL: Relative risk of breast cancer varies with time since diagnosis of atypical hyperplasia. Hum Pathol 20:723, 1989.
51. Haagensen C, Lane N, Lattes R, et al: Lobular neoplasia (so-called lobular carcinoma in situ) of the breast. Cancer 42:737, 1978.
52. Lagios MD, Margolin FR, and Westdahl PR: Mammographically detected duct carcinoma in situ: Frequency of local recurrence following tylectomy and prognostic effect of nuclear grade on local recurrence. Cancer 63:618, 1989.
53. Schnitt SJ, Silen W, Sadowsky NL, et al: Ductal carcinoma in situ (intraductal carcinoma) of the breast. N Engl J Med 318:898, 1988.
54. Henderson BE: Endogenous and exogenous endocrine factors. Hematol Oncol Clin North Am 577, 1989.
55. Seidman H, Stellman SD, and Mushinski MH: A different perspective on breast cancer risk factors: Some implications of the nonattributable risk. CA Cancer J Clin 32:301, 1982.
56. Venet L, Strax P, Venet W, et al: Adequacies and inadequacies of breast examinations by physicians in mass screening. Cancer 28:1546, 1971.
57. Haagensen CD: Diseases of the Breast. Philadelphia, WB Saunders, 1971.
58. Chaudary MA, Millis RR, Davies GC, et al: Nipple discharge. Ann Surg 196:651, 1982.
59. Dodd GD: Mammography: State of the art. Cancer 53:652, 1984.
60. Moskowitz M: Mammography in medical practice. A rational approach. JAMA 240:1898, 1978.
61. Moskowitz M, Milbrath J, Gartside P, et al: Lack of efficacy of thermography as a screening tool for minimal and stage I breast cancer. N Engl J Med 295:249, 1976.
62. Egan RL, McSweeney MB, and Sewell CW: Intramammary calcifications without an associated mass in benign and malignant diseases. Radiology 137:1, 1980.
63. Moskowitz M: The predictive value of certain mammographic signs in screening for breast cancer. Cancer 51:1007, 1983.
64. Smart CR and Beahrs OH: Breast cancer screening results as viewed by the clinician. Cancer 43:851, 1979.
65. Egan RL: Breast biopsy priority: Cancer versus benign preoperative masses. Cancer 35:612, 1975.
66. Baker LH: Breast Cancer Detection Demonstration Project: Five-year summary report. CA Cancer J Clin 32:194, 1982.
67. Hall FM: Screening mammography—potential problems on the horizon (sounding board). N Engl J Med 314:53, 1986.
68. Edeiken S: Mammography in the symptomatic woman. Cancer 63:1412, 1989.
69. Walker GM, Foster RS, McKegney CP, et al: Breast biopsies: Comparison of outpatient and inpatient experience. Arch Surg 113:942, 1978.
70. Hall FM and Frank HA: Progress in radiology: Preoperative localization of nonpalpable breast lesions. Am J Radiol 132:101, 1979.
71. Kline TS and Neal HS: Needle aspiration biopsy: Critical appraisal, eight years and 3,267 specimens later. JAMA 239:36, 1978.
72. Barrows GH, Anderson TJ, Lamb JL, and Dixon JM: Fine-needle aspiration of breast cancer. Cancer 58:1493, 1986.
73. Bell DA, Hajdu SI, Urban JA, and Gaston JP: Role of aspiration cytology in the diagnosis and management of mammary lesions in office practice. Cancer 51:1182, 1983.
74. Helvie MA, Baker DE, Adler DD, et al: Radiographically guided fine-needle aspiration of nonpalpable breast lesions. Radiology 174:657, 1990.
75. Dent DM, Kirkpatrick AE, McGoogan E, et al: Stereotaxic localisation and aspiration cytology of impalpable breast lesions. Clin Radiol 40:380, 1989.
76. Osteen RT: Paget Disease and the Nipple in Breast Disease, 2nd ed. Harris JR, Hellman S, Henderson IC, and Kinne DW (eds). Philadelphia, JB Lippincott, 1991, pp 797–804.
77. Huguley CM and Brown RL: The value of breast self-examination. Cancer 47:989, 1981.
78. Greenwald P, Nasca PC, Lawrence CE, et al: Effect of breast self-examination and routine physician examinations on breast-cancer mortality. N Engl J Med 299:271, 1978.
79. Shapiro S: Determining the efficacy of breast cancer screening. Cancer 63:1873, 1989.
80. Shapiro S: Evidence on screening for breast cancer from a randomized trial. Cancer 39:2772, 1977.
81. Shapiro S: Report on the International Workshop on Information Systems in Breast Cancer Detection. Cancer (Suppl):2645, 1989.
82. Seidman H, Gelb SK, Silverberg E, et al: Survival experience in The Breast Cancer Detection Demonstration Project. CA Cancer J Clin 37:258, 1987.
83. Nystrom L, Rutqvist L, Wall S, et al: Breast cancer screening with mammography: Overview of Swedish randomized trials. Lancet 341:973, 1993.
84. Bailar JC: Screening for early breast cancer. Pros and cons. Cancer 39:2783, 1977.
85. Kopans DB, Meyer JE, and Sadowsky N: Medical progress: Breast imaging. N Engl J Med 310:960, 1984.
86. Eddy DM, Hasselblad V, McGivney W, and Hendee W: The value of mammography screening in women under age 50 years. J Am Med Assoc 259:1512, 1988.
87. Tabar L, Faberberg G, Day NE, and Holmberg L: What is the optimum interval between mammographic screening examinations? An analysis based on the latest results of the Swedish Two-County Breast Cancer Screening Trial. Br J Cancer 55:547, 1987.
88. Hall FM: Screening mammography—potential problems on the horizon. N Engl J Med 314:53, 1986.
89. Stomper PC and Gelman RS: Mammography in symptomatic and asymptomatic patients. Hematol Oncol Clin North Am 611, 1989.
90. Miller AB, Baines CJ, TO Twall C: Canadian National Breast Screening Study: 1. Breast cancer detection and death rates among women aged 40–49 years. Can Med Assoc J 147:1459–1476, 1992.
91. Fletcher S, Black W, Harris R, et al: Report of the International Workshop on Screening for Breast Cancer. J Natl Cancer Inst 85:1644–1656, 1993.
92. Dodd GD: American Cancer Society Guidelines on Screening for Breast Cancer: An overview. CA Cancer J Clin 42:177–180, 1992.
93. Early Breast Cancer Trialists' Collaborative Group: Systemic treatment of early breast cancer by hormonal, cytotoxic, or immune therapy: 151 randomised trials involving 32,000 recurrences and 25,000 deaths among 77,000 women. Lancet 339:1, 71, 1992.
94. Love RR: Tamoxifen therapy in primary breast cancer: Biology, efficacy, and side effects. J Clin Oncol 7:803, 1989.
95. Richart RM and Barron BA: A follow-up study of patients with cervical dysplasia. Am J Obstet Gynecol 105:386, 1969.
96. Devesa SS: Descriptive epidemiology of cancer of the uterine cervix. Obstet Gynecol 63:605, 1984.
97. Levine RU, Crum CP, Herman E, et al: Cervical papillomavirus infection and intraepithelial neoplasia: A study of male sexual partners. Am J Obstet Gynecol 64:16, 1984.
98. Brinton LA: Oral contraceptives and cervical neoplasia. Contraception 43:581, 1991.
99. Jones CJ, Brinton LA, Hamman RF, et al: Risk factors for in situ cervical cancer: Results from a case-control study. Cancer Res 50:3657, 1990.
100. Meisels A and Morin C: Human papilloma virus and cancer of the uterine cervix. Gynecol Oncol 12:S111, 1981.
101. Durst M, Gissman L, Ekenberg H, et al: A papillomavirus DNA from a cervical carcinoma and its prevalence in cancer biopsy samples from different geographic regions. Proc Natl Acad Sci U S A 80:3812, 1983.
102. Reid R, Stanhope CR, Herschman BR, et al: Genital warts and cervical cancer IV. A colposcopic index for differentiating subclinical papilloma virus infection from cervical intraepithelial neoplasia. Am J Obstet Gynecol 149:815, 1984.
103. Crum CP, Ikenberg H, Richart RM, et al: Human papilloma virus type 16 and early cervical neoplasia. N Engl J Med 310:880, 1984.
104. Kataja V, Syrjanson KI, Mantyjarvi R, et al: Prospective follow-up of cervical HPV infections: Life table analysis of histopathological, cytological and colposcopic data. Eur J Epidemiol 5:1, 1989.

105. van Oortmardsen GJ and Habbema JD: Epidemiological evidence for age-dependent regression of preinvasive cervical cancer. Br J Cancer 64:559, 1991.
106. Jordan SW, Smith NL, and Dike LS: The significance of cervical cytologic dysplasia. Acta Cytol 25:237, 1981.
107. Eddy DM: Appropriateness of cervical cancer screening. Gynecol Oncol 12:S168, 1981.
108. de Villiers EM, Wagner D, Scheider A, et al: Human papillomavirus DNA in women without and with cytological abnormalities: Results of a 5-year follow-up study. Gynecol Oncol 44:33, 1992.
109. Fu YS, Cheng L, Huang I, et al: DNA ploidy analysis of cervical condyloma and intraepithelial neoplasia in specimens obtained by punch biopsy. Anal Quant Cytol Histol 11:187, 1989.
110. Chatelain R, Schunck T, Schindler EM, et al: Diagnosis of prospective malignancy in koilocytic dysplasias of the cervix with DNA cytometry. J Reprod Med 34:505, 1989.
111. Kashyap V, Das DK, and Luthra UK: Microphotometric nuclear DNA analysis in cervical dysplasia of the uterine cervix: Its relation to the progression to malignancy and regression to normalcy. Neoplasm 37:497, 1990.
112. Murty VV, Mitra AB, Das BC, et al: Chromosomal phenotypes in patients with precancerous lesions of the uterine cervix progressed to cancer during follow-up. Oncology 45:384, 1988.
113. Gay JD, Donaldson LD, and Goellner JR: False-negative results in cervical cytologic studies. Acta Cytol 29:1043, 1985.
114. Kristensen GB, Holund B, and Grinsted P: Efficacy of the cytobrush versus the cotton swab in the collection of endocervical cells. Acta Cytol 33:849, 1989.
115. Selvaggi SM: Spatula/cytobrush vs spatula/cotton swab detection of cervical condylomatous lesions. J Reprod Med 34:629, 1989.
116. Specific list for categorization of laboratory test systems, assays and examinations by complexity. Federal Register 57:7245, 1992.
117. National Cancer Institute: The 1988 Bethesda System for reporting cervical/vaginal cytological diagnoses: National Cancer Institute Workshop. JAMA 262:931, 1989.
118. Louhivuori MA: Effect of a mass screening program on the risk of cervical cancer. Cancer Detect Prev 15:471, 1991.
119. Eddy DM: The frequency of cervical cancer screening: Comparison of a mathematical model with empirical data. Cancer 60:1117, 1987.
120. Eddy DM: Screening for cancer in adults. The value of preventive medicine. Ciba Found Symp 110:88, 1985.
121. US Department of Health and Human Services, Public Health Service, National Center for Health Statistics: Vital Statistics of the United States. Washington, DC, US Government Printing Office, 2, PHS-88–1102, 1984.
122. Mandelblatt J, Schechter C, Fahs M, et al: Clinical implications of screening for cervical cancer under Medicare: The natural history of cervical cancer in the elderly: What do we know? What do we need to know? Am J Obstet Gynecol 164:644, 1991.
123. American College of Obstetricians and Gynecologists: Report of the task force on routine cancer screening. ACOG Committee Opinion 68, April 1989.
124. Kolstad P and Stofl A: Atlas of Colposcopy. Baltimore, University Park Press, 1972.
125. McCord ML, Stovall TG, Summitt RL Jr, et al: Discrepancy of cervical cytology and colposcopic biopsy: Is cervical conization necessary? Obstet Gynecol 77:715, 1991.
126. Ramirez EJ, Hernandez E, and Miyazana K: Cervical conization findings in women with dysplastic cervical cytology and normal colposcopy. J Reprod Med 35:359, 1990.
127. Wright TC Jr, Gagnon S, Richart RM, et al: Treatment of cervical intraepithelial neoplasia using the loop electrosurgical excision procedure. Obstet Gynecol 79:173, 1992.
128. Whiteley PF and Olah KS: Treatment of cervical intraepithelial neoplasia: Experience with the low-voltage diathermy loop. Am J Obstet Gynecol 162:1272, 1990.
129. Chappatte OA, Byrne DL, Raju KS, et al: Histological differences between colposcopic-directed biopsy and loop excision of the transformation zone (LETZ). A cause for concern. Gynecol Oncol 43:46, 1991.
130. Wright TC Jr, Richart RM, Fenenczy A, et al: Comparison of specimens removed by CO_2 laser conization and the loop electrosurgical excision procedure. Obstet Gynecol 79:147, 1992.
131. Turner MJ, Rasmussen MJ, Flannelly GM, et al: Outpatient loop diathermy conization as an alternative to inpatient knife conization of the cervix. J Reprod Med 37:314, 1992.
132. Benedlet JL, Miller DM, and Nickerson KG: Results of conservative management of cervical intraepithelial neoplasia. Obstet Gynecol 79:105, 1992.
133. Hellberg D and Nilsson S: 20-year experience of follow-up of the abnormal smear with colposcopy and histology and treatment by conization or cryosurgery. Gynecol Oncol 38:166, 1990.
134. Ferenczy A: Comparison of cryo- and carbon dioxide laser therapy for cervical intraepithelial neoplasia. Obstet Gynecol 66:793, 1985.
135. Lopes A, Mor-Yoset S, Pearson S, et al: Is routine colposcopic assessment necessary following laser ablation of cervical intraepithelial neoplasia? Br J Obstet Gynaecol 97:175, 1990.
135a. Hardcastle JD, Farrands PA, Balfour TW, et al: Controlled trial of faecal occult blood testing in the detection of colorectal cancer. Lancet ii:1, 1983.
136. Eddy DM: Cost-effectiveness of colorectal cancer screening. *In* Levin B and Riddell RH (eds): Frontiers in Gastrointestinal Cancer. New York, Elsevier, 1984.
137. Winawer SJ, Sherlock P, Schottenfeld D, et al: Screening for colon cancer. Gastroenterology 70:783, 1976.
138. Sherlock P, Lipkin M, and Winawer SJ: Predisposing factors in colon carcinoma. Adv Intern Med 20:121, 1975.
139. Colon adenomas—To burn or not to burn. Selected summaries. Gastroenterology 71:1101, 1977.
140. Morson BC: Evolution of cancer of the colon and rectum. Cancer 34:845, 1974.
141. Panish JF: State of the art. Management of patients with polypoid lesions of the colon—Current concepts and controversies. Am J Gastroenterol 71:315, 1979.
142. Garbrielsson N, Granqvist S, Ohlsen H, et al: Malignancy of colonic polyps. Diagnosis and management. Acta Radiol 19:479, 1978.
143. Granqvist S, Gabrielsson N, and Sundelin P: Diminutive colonic polyps—Clinical significance and management. Endoscopy 11:36, 1979.
144. Marshak RH, Lindner AE, and Maklanski D: Adenomatous polyps of the colon—A rational approach. JAMA 235:2856, 1976.
145. Kaufman SD, Deckers PJ, and Gunderson LL: Cancer of the colon and rectum. *In* Cancer, A Manual for Practitioners. Boston, American Cancer Society, Massachusetts Division, 1978, p 184.
146. Enker WE, Laffer UT, and Block GE: Enhanced survival of patients with colon and rectal cancer is based on wide anatomic resection. Ann Surg 190:350, 1979.
147. Vezzoni P, Clemente C, and Gennari L: Adenocarcinoma of the large intestine. Tumori 63:565, 1977.
148. Beacham CH, Shields HM, and Raffensperger EC: Juvenile and adenomatous gastrointestinal polyposis. Am J Dig Dis 23:1137, 1977.
149. Simon JB: Occult blood screening for colorectal carcinoma: A critical review. Gastroenterology 88:820, 1985.
150. Sherlock P, Lipkins M, and Winawer SJ: The prevention of colon cancer. Am J Med 68:917, 1980.
151. Greegor DA: Occult blood testing for detection of asymptomatic colon cancer. Cancer 28:131, 1971.
152. Winawer S, Ginther M, Weston E, et al: Impact of modifications in fecal occult blood test on screening program of colorectal neoplasia. Gastroenterology 74:1151, 1978.
153. Allison JE, Feldman R, and Tekawa IS: Hemoccult screening in detecting colorectal neoplasia: Sensitivity, specificity and predictive value. Ann Intern Med 112:328, 1990.
153a. Mandel JS, Bond JH, Church TR, et al: Reducing mortality from colorectal cancer by screening for fecal occult blood. N Engl J Med 328:1365, 1993.
154. Hardcastle JD, Thomas W, Chamberlain J, et al: Randomised, controlled trial of faecal occult blood screening for colorectal cancer. Results for first 107,349 subjects. Lancet i:1160, 1989.

155. Kronborg O, Fenger C, Olsen J, et al: Repeated screening for colorectal cancer with fecal occult blood test: A prospective randomized study at Funen, Denmark. Scand J Gastroenterol 24:599, 1989.
156. Songster CL, Barrows GH, and Jarrett DD: Immunochemical detection of fecal occult blood—The fecal smear punch-disc test: A new noninvasive screening test for colorectal cancer. Cancer 45:1099, 1980.
157. Ahlquist DA, McGill DB, Schwartz S, et al: Fecal blood levels in health and disease. N Engl J Med 312:1422, 1985.
158. St John DJB, Young GP, McHutchinson JG, et al: Comparison of the specificity and sensitivity of Hemoccult and HemoQuant in screening for colorectal neoplasia. Ann Intern Med 117:376, 1992.
159. Winawer SJ, Melamed M, and Sherlock P: The potential of endoscopy, biopsy and cytology in the diagnosis and management of patients with cancer. Clin Gastroenterol 5:575, 1976.
160. Nivatvongs S and Fyrd DS: How far does the proctosigmoidoscope reach? A prospective study of 1000 patients. N Engl J Med 303:380, 1980.
161. Lipshutz GR, Katon RM, McCool MF, et al: Flexible sigmoidoscopy as a screening procedure for neoplasia of the colon. Surg Gynecol Obstet 148:19, 1979.
162. Zucker GM, Madura MJ, Chmiel JS, et al: The advantages of the 30-cm flexible sigmoidoscope over the 60-cm flexible sigmoidoscope. Gastrointest Endosc 30:59, 1984.
163. Winawer SJ: Detection and diagnosis of colorectal cancer. Cancer 51:2519, 1983.
164. Nivatvongs S, Gilbertson VA, Goldberg SM, et al: Distribution of large bowel cancers detected by occult blood test in asymptomatic patients. Dis Colon Rectum 25:420, 1982.
165. Winawer S, Schottenfeld D, and Sherlock P: Screening for colorectal cancer: The issues. Gastroenterology 88:841, 1985.
166. Selby JV, Friedman GD, Quesenberry CP, et al: A case-control study of screening sigmoidoscopy and mortality from colorectal cancer. N Engl J Med 326:653, 1992.
167. Gilbertsen VA and Nelms JM: The prevention of invasive cancer of the rectum. Cancer 41:1137, 1978.
168. Miller RE: Detection of colon carcinoma in the barium enema. JAMA 231:1195, 1974.
169. Johnson CD, Carlson HC, Taylor WF, et al: Barium enemas of carcinoma of the colon: Sensitivity of double- and single-contrast studies. AJR 140:1143, 1983.
170. Dodd BD and Goldstein HM: Newer radiological techniques in the diagnosis of gastrointestinal cancer. Clin Gastroenterol 5:597, 1976.
171. Ott DJ, Gelfand DW, and Ramquist NA: Cause of error in gastrointestinal radiology. VI. Barium enema examination. Gastrointest Radiol 5:99, 1980.
172. Gilbertson VA, McHugh RB, Schuman L, et al: The earlier detection of colorectal cancers. A preliminary report of the results of the occult blood study. Cancer 45:2899, 1980.
173. Knutson CO, Williams HC, and Max MH: Detection of intracolonic lesions by barium contrast enema. The importance of adequate bowel preparation for diagnostic accuracy. JAMA 242:2206, 1979.
174. Leinicke JL, Dodds WJ, Hagar WJ, et al: A comparison of colonoscopy and roentgenography for detecting polypoid lesions of the colon. Gastrointest Radiol 2:125, 1977.
175. Hunt R: Rectal bleeding. Clin Gastroenterol 7:719, 1978.
176. Tedesco FJ, Waye JD, Raskin JB, et al: Colonoscopic evaluation of rectal bleeding. A study of 304 patients. Ann Intern Med 89:907, 1978.
177. Schwesingl WH, Levine BA, and Ramos R: Complications of colonoscopy. Surg Gynecol Obstet 148:270, 1979.
178. Bess MA and Spencer RJ: Colonoscopic polypectomies. Mayo Clin Proc 54:32, 1979.
179. Winawer SJ, Zauber AG, O'Brien MJ, et al: Randomized comparison of surveillance intervals after colonoscopic removal of newly diagnosed adenomatous polyps. N Engl J Med 328:901, 1993.

73

Immunization for Adults

WILLIAM C. TAYLOR, MD
SUSAN M. LETT, MD, MPH

CLINICAL OVERVIEW

In the United States, deaths from vaccine-preventable diseases occur primarily in adults. Approximately 50,000 to 70,000 adults die each year from pneumococcal, influenza, and hepatitis B infections (in comparison, only about 1000 children die from these infections). There are several reasons for the poor record of adult immunization compared with that for children. Even clinicians who are knowledgeable and committed to effective immunization do not ensure the appropriate and complete immunization of their patients. Thus, ongoing education about the efficacy and safety of vaccines is imperative for both physicians and patients. The paradigm for clinical primary prevention is epitomized by immunization: after providing the patient with sufficient information about the benefits and risks of an intervention, and after the patient has consented, the clinician offers the patient an intervention that has been proved to increase the likelihood that the patient will remain free of a disease. Although this process may describe most clinical primary prevention, proof of effectiveness is more clearly established for immunizations than for virtually all other clinical interventions.

The National Coalition for Adult Immunization has developed its *Standards for Adult Immunization Practice* to help improve immunization levels among adults. Development of and improvement in the *systems* that involve immunization are essential. Major improvements in office practice could decrease missed opportunities for immunization. A patient's immunization status should be evaluated at his or her every encounter with the health-care system. Physicians should follow only valid contraindications when deferring immunization. Providers should develop recall and reminder systems. Computerization of office systems can facilitate this process for the patients already being served by a health-care system. Providing patients with a copy of their immunization records is also important. Health policy development and enforcement, in both the public and private sector, are essential components of the systems needed to improve adult immunization. Appropriate immunizations should be required for all staff, patients, and students in a variety of health, educational, and other occupational settings.

Other factors contribute to the underimmunization of adults. Among them may be the concerns that many patients have had about the safety and efficacy of vaccines and that physicians have had about liability. The National Childhood Vaccine Injury Act (NCVIA) of 1986 (which also applies to adults) was passed to address these issues. It requires that patients be provided with sufficient information about the benefits and risks of vaccination versus disease before their consent is obtained. It also requires the complete recording of patients' immunization data in the medical record and the reporting of adverse events and explains how to file a claim with the federal "no fault" National Vaccine Injury Compensation Program. Although the act has placed additional legal obligations on the physician in terms of obtaining informed consent, recordkeeping, and reporting, it has ensured that patients make informed choices prior to immunization. In addition, it has been extremely successful in reducing physician and vaccine manufacturer liability in the case of vaccination-related injuries.

SOURCES OF INFORMATION

The US Centers for Disease Control provides frequent updates of current recommendations in its periodical *Morbidity and Mortality Weekly Reports;* included are the recommendations from the Advisory Committee on Immunization Practices (ACIP). The Centers for Disease Control also provides information via telephone at 404-639-8209. For information about the National Vaccine Injury Compensation Program and filing claims, call 1-800-338-2382.

GENERAL PRINCIPLES

Immunization is the protection against disease or sequelae through administration of either antibodies (passive immunization) or an agent that stimulates an immune response (active immunization). Active immunity may be stimulated by a vaccine, a suspension of live or inactivated microorganisms or of some component of a microorganism, or a toxoid, a modified toxin from a microorganism. Passive immunity may be provided with immune globulin (IG) derived from pooled human plasma, containing various antibodies depending on the population that served as the

TABLE 73–1. COMMONLY USED INVALID CONTRAINDICATIONS TO VACCINES

Invalid Contraindication	Comments
A minor reaction to a previous dose	All vaccines can be given
A mild illness with low fever, a mild diarrheal illness, or both, in an otherwise healthy individual	All vaccines can be given
Current antimicrobial therapy or convalescent phase of an illness	All vaccines can be given
Recent exposure to an infectious disease	All vaccines can be given
Pregnancy	Pregnant women can receive all vaccines except MMR. Household contacts of pregnant women can receive all vaccines.
Breast feeding	Mothers who breast feed can be vaccinated. Children being breast-fed should be vaccinated.
Allergies to penicillin	No vaccines in the United States contain penicillin
Allergies to antibiotics	Only significant allergies: anaphylaxis to neomycin (e.g., MMR, IPV) or streptomycin (e.g., IPV).
Allergies to duck meat or feathers	No vaccines in the United States contain duck antigens
A family history of allergies or seizures, or of an adverse event, unrelated to immunosuppression, after vaccination	No contraindication

source; with specific IGs, obtained from donors with high levels of antibodies to specific antigens; or with antitoxins, solutions of antibodies obtained from animals with high levels of a particular antibody to a particular toxin.

Although most immunizations can be performed simultaneously, several exceptions should be noted. Some vaccines for international travelers should not be given simultaneously; combinations that are best avoided include cholera vaccine with either typhoid fever or yellow fever vaccine.

Immunizations with some live vaccines, if not performed on the same day, should be separated by a 1-month interval (e.g., measles-mumps-rubella [MMR] and yellow fever vaccines, and single-antigen MMR vaccines that are not given in the MMR combination). However, these restrictions do not apply to MMR vaccine (or its single-antigen components) and oral polio vaccine (OPV).

Blood and other antibody-containing blood products (e.g., immune globulin [IG] preparations) may interfere with the ability of some live vaccines to induce immunity. Interference has been best documented for measles vaccine, but also for rubella vaccine. Guidelines under development by the Centers for Disease Control suggest that physicians wait, if possible, for 3 to 11 months before giving measles vaccine to persons who have received immune globulin and other blood products.* The effect of IG preparations on the response to mumps and varicella vaccine is unknown. However, commercial immune globulin preparations contain antibodies to these viruses.

IG preparations should be given at least 2 weeks after administration of MMR vaccine or its individual components. MMR vaccine or its components should not be given after administration of an IG preparation before the intervals recommended below. If administration occurs within any of these intervals, the vaccination should be repeated unless serologic testing indicates that specific antibodies have been produced. However, the postpartum vaccination of rubella-suspectible women with rubella or MMR vaccine should not be delayed because of the receipt of Rho(D) IG or any other blood product during the last trimester of pregnancy or at delivery. These women should be vaccinated immediately after delivery and tested at least 3 months later to ensure that rubella (and, if necessary, measles) immunity was established. If simultaneous administration of IG preparations with MMR or its components is necessary, the MMR vaccine should be administered at a site remote from that chosen for the IG preparations. In addition, serologic testing for immunity or reimmunization should be done at the appropriate interval.

OPV and yellow fever vaccines may be given at any time, in combination with or after administration of IG products. Although published data are not yet available, it is thought that administration of IG should not interfere with the immune response to concurrently administered oral typhoid vaccine (Ty21a).

Preferred route and site of administration, as well as dose, are best determined from manufacturers' package inserts; in the United States, the content of these inserts is regulated by the US Food and Drug Administration. The deltoid area is usually preferred for most intramuscular and subcutaneous immunizations; hepatitis B vaccine and rabies vaccine must be given in the deltoid muscle in adults. Administration in the gluteus has been associated with vaccine failure. An exception should be made for administration of large volumes, which are best injected in the buttocks; the upper, outer quadrant should be used to avoid damage to the sciatic nerve.

Anaphylactic reactions to vaccine components (including reactions to eggs for vaccines such as influenza, measles, mumps, and yellow fever vaccines that are grown in eggs or chick embryo tissue culture) are almost always an absolute contraindication to vaccine administration. In addition, oral polio vaccine should not be given to persons who might expose immunocompromised patients (either through household contact or occupation).

In general, misconceptions about vaccine contraindications frequently impede appropriate immunization (Table 73–1). A clinician's task is to provide factual information to dispel concerns that are unfounded. Persons with mild upper respiratory or gastrointestinal illnesses with temperatures of less than 38°C can be immunized safely.

Accurate notation in the medical record of all immunizations, including the date of administration, agent administered, dose, site, manufacturer and lot number, when the next dose is due and providing the patient with an immunization record, constitutes good medical practice. The name, address, title, and signature of the health care provider administering the vaccine are required by the NCVIA.

*Suggested waiting periods are 3 months after administration of tetanus, hepatitis A, or hepatitis B IG or a transfusion with reconstituted red blood cells; 4 months after administering rabies IG; 5 months after administering varicella or measles IG; 6 months after administering packed red blood cells, whole blood, or measles IG to immunocompromised patients; 7 months after administering plasma/platelet products; 8 months after administering replacement of humoral immune deficiencies or treatment of idiopathic thrombocytopenic purpura (ITP) with 400 mg/kg of IG intravenously; 10 months after treatment of ITP with 1000 mg/kg IG intravenously; and 11 months after administering 2 g/kg IG intravenously for Kawasaki's disease.

NATIONAL CHILDHOOD VACCINE INJURY ACT OF 1986

As described earlier, the NCVIA was developed to ensure that patients are adequately informed about immunizations, to decrease litigation associated with vaccine-related injuries, and to protect the supply of vaccines. Despite its name, its legal requirements apply to the immunization of both adults and children.

Since April 15, 1992, physicians in the United States have been required to provide certain information about vaccines to their patients, including benefits and risks. They are also required to document immunizations in their patients' permanent medical records, as described earlier, and to report the occurrence of adverse events related to the administration of vaccines and toxoids covered by the NCVIA (as listed in Table 73–2). Vaccines and toxoids may be added to the table by the Secretary of Health and Human Services.

Vaccine Information Materials (VIMs) have been prepared by the U.S. Public Health Service (USPHS) for those vaccines and toxoids covered by the NCVIA. They contain a description of the benefits of the vaccine, a description of the risks associated with the disease, information about who should and who should not receive a vaccine, a description of the adverse events, the reporting mechanism for adverse events, and information for filing claims with the National Vaccine Injury Compensation Program. For vaccines and toxoids not covered by NCVIA, the USPHS has prepared *Important Information Statements* (IISs), which are designed to provide pertinent information to patients.

All physicians administering vaccines and toxoids covered by the NCVIA must use VIMs prepared by the USPHS, regardless of whether these agents were purchased through federal contracts or purchased privately. Physicians using vaccines and toxoids not covered by the NCVIA, but purchased through federal contracts, must use IISs. Those administering agents not covered by the act, but purchased privately, may develop alternative materials.

PATIENT CHARACTERISTICS

Healthy Adults (Table 73–3)

Tetanus and Diphtheria. All healthy adults should be immunized against tetanus and diphtheria with combined tetanus and diphtheria toxoid every 10 years. If a three-dose primary series has not been given, adults should receive two doses at least 4 weeks apart, followed by a third dose at least 6 months later.

Measles, Mumps, and Rubella. Persons born before 1957 are likely to have been infected with both measles and mumps virus and can therefore usually be considered to be

Text continued on page 952

TABLE 73–2. ON THE BASIS OF THE NATIONAL CHILDHOOD VACCINE INJURY ACT OF 1986, THE VACCINES AND TOXOIDS, ADVERSE EVENTS, AND INTERVALS FROM VACCINATION TO ONSET OF ADVERSE EVENT REQUIRED FOR REPORTING OR COMPENSATION IN THE UNITED STATES*

		Interval from Vaccination to Onset of Event	
Vaccine/toxoid	**Adverse Event**	*For Reporting*	*For Compensation*
DTP,† P,‡	Anaphylaxis or anaphylactic shock	24 hours	24 hours
DTP/Poliovirus combined	Encephalopathy (or encephalitis)¶	7 days	3 days
	Shock-collapse or hypotonic-hyporesponsive collapse§	7 days	3 days
	Residual seizure disorder§§	§§	3 days
Measles, Mumps, and Rubella; DT‖, Td‡‡, T**	Anaphylaxis or anaphylactic shock	24 hours	24 hours
	Encephalopathy (or encephalitis)¶	15 days (for measles, mumps, and rubella vaccines); 7 days (for DT, Td, and T)	15 days (for measles, mumps, and rubella vaccine); 3 days (for DT, Td, and T)
	Residual seizure disorder§§		15 days (for measles, mumps, or rubella vaccine); 3 days for DT, Td, or T)
OPV††	Paralytic poliomyelitis in a nonimmunodeficient recipient	30 days	30 days
	in an immunodeficient recipient	6 months	6 months
	in a vaccine-associated community case	No limit	Not applicable
Inactivated polio vaccine	Anaphylaxis or anaphylactic shock	24 hours	24 hours
All vaccines	Any acute complication or sequela (including death) of above events	No limit	Not applicable
	Events described as contraindications to additional doses of vaccine (see manufacturer's package insert)	(See package insert)	

*From Immunization Practices Advisory Committee: Recommendations of the Immunization Practices Advisory Committee. Update on adult immunizations. MMWR 40:1–94, 1991.

†DTP = diphtheria and tetanus toxoids and pertussis vaccine, adsorbed (pediatric).

‡P = pertussis vaccine.

¶*Encephalopathy* means any significant acquired abnormality of, injury to, or impairment of function of the brain. Among the frequent manifestations of encephalopathy are focal and diffuse neurologic signs, increased intracranial pressure, or changes lasting at least 6 hours in level of consciousness, with or without convulsions. The neurologic signs and symptoms of encephalopathy may be temporary with complete recovery or may result in various degrees of permanent impairment. Signs and symptoms such as high-pitched and unusual screaming, persistent inconsolable crying, and bulging fontanel are compatible with an encephalopathy, but in and of themselves are not conclusive evidence of encephalopathy. Encephalopathy usually can be documented by slow wave activity on an electroencephalogram.

§*Shock-collapse* or *hypotonic-hyporesponsive collapse* may include signs or symptoms such as decrease or loss of muscle tone, paralysis (partial or complete), hemiplegia, hemiparesis, loss of color or turning pale white or blue, unresponsiveness to environmental stimuli, depression of or loss of consciousness, prolonged sleeping with difficulty being aroused, or cardiovascular or respiratory arrest.

‖DT = diphtheria and tetanus toxoids, absorbed.

**T = tetanus toxoid, adsorbed.

††OPV = oral poliovirus vaccine, live, trivalent.

‡‡Td = tetanus diphtheria toxoids, adsorbed (adult).

§§*Residual seizure disorder* may have occurred if no other seizure or convulsion unaccompanied by fever or accompanied by a fever of <102° F occurred before the first seizure or convulsion after the administration of the vaccine involved, and if, in the case of measles-, mumps-, or rubella-containing vaccines, the first seizure or convulsion occurred within 15 days after vaccination, or, in the case of any other vaccine, the first seizure or convulsion occurred within 3 days after vaccination, and, if two or more seizures or convulsions unaccompanied by fever or accompanied by a fever of <102° F occurred within 1 year after vaccination. The terms *seizure* and *convulsion* include grand mal, petit mal, absence, myoclonic, tonic-clonic, and focal motor seizures and signs.

TABLE 73–3. IMMUNOBIOLOGICS AND SCHEDULES FOR ADULTS (≥18 YEARS OF AGE) IN THE UNITED STATES*

Immunobiologic Generic Name	Primary Schedule and Booster(s)	Indications	Major Precautions and Contraindications	Special Considerations
Toxoids				
Tetanus/diphtheria toxoid, adsorbed (for adult use) (Td)	Two doses intramuscularly (IM) 4 weeks apart; third dose 6–12 months after second dose. Booster every 10 years.	All adults.	Except in the first trimester, pregnancy is not a contraindication. History of a neurologic reaction or immediate hypersensitivity reaction following a previous dose. History of severe local (Arthus-type) reaction following previous dose. Such individuals should not be given further routine or emergency doses of Td for 10 years.	Tetanus prophylaxis in wound management. (See below)
Live-Virus Vaccines				
Measles vaccine, live	One dose subcutaneously (SC); second dose at least 1 month later, at entry into college or post-high school education, beginning medical facility employment, or before traveling. Susceptible travelers should receive one dose.	All adults born after 1956 without documentation of live vaccine on or after first birthday, physician-diagnosed measles, or laboratory evidence of immunity; persons born before 1957 are generally considered immune.	Pregnancy; immunocompromised persons; history of anaphylactic reactions following egg ingestion or receipt of neomycin.	MMR† is the vaccine of choice if recipients are likely to be susceptible to rubella and/or mumps as well as to measles. Persons vaccinated between 1963 and 1967 with a killed measles vaccine alone, killed vaccine followed by live vaccine, or with a vaccine of unknown type should be revaccinated with live measles virus vaccine.
Mumps vaccine, live	One dose SC; no booster.	All adults believed to be susceptible can be vaccinated. Adults born before 1957 can be considered immune.	Pregnancy; immunocompromised persons; history of anaphylactic reaction following egg ingestion.	MMR is the vaccine of choice if recipients are likely to be susceptible to measles and rubella as well as to mumps.
Rubella vaccine, live	One dose SC; no booster.	Indicated for adults, both male and female, lacking documentation of live vaccine on or after first birthday or laboratory evidence of immunity, particularly young adults who congregate in places such as hospitals, colleges, or military, and susceptible travelers.	Pregnancy; immunocompromised persons; history of anaphylactic reaction following receipt of neomycin.	Women pregnant when vaccinated or who become pregnant within 3 months of vaccination should be counseled on the theoretical risks to the fetus. The risk of rubella vaccine–associated malformations in these women is so small as to be negligible. MMR is the vaccine of choice if recipients are likely to be susceptible to measles or mumps as well as to rubella.
Smallpox vaccine (vaccinia virus)	THERE ARE NO INDICATIONS FOR THE USE OF SMALLPOX VACCINE IN THE GENERAL CIVILIAN POPULATION.			Laboratory workers working with orthopoxviruses or health-care workers involved in clinical trials of vaccinia-recombinant vaccines.
Yellow fever attenuated virus, live (17D strain)	One dose SC 10 days to 10 years before travel; booster every 10 years.	Selected persons traveling or living in areas where yellow fever infection exists.	It is prudent on theoretical grounds to avoid vaccinating a pregnant woman unless she must travel where the risk of yellow fever is high. Immunocompromised persons; history of hypersensitivity to egg ingestion.	Some countries require a valid International Certificate of Vaccination showing receipt of vaccine. If the only reason to vaccinate a pregnant woman is an international requirement, efforts should be made to obtain a waiver letter.

Live-Virus and Inactivated-Virus Vaccines				
Polio vaccines: Enhanced potency inactivated poliovirus vaccine (eIPV) Oral poliovirus vaccine, live (OPV)	eIPV preferred for primary vaccination; two doses SC 4 weeks apart; a third dose 6–12 months after second; for adults with a completed primary series and for whom a booster is indicated, either OPV or eIPV can be administered. If immediate protection is needed, OPV is recommended.	Persons traveling to areas where wild poliovirus is epidemic or endemic. Certain health-care personnel. Incompletely vaccinated adults, especially in households of children to be immunized with OPV.	It is prudent on theoretical grounds to avoid vaccinating pregnant women. However, if immediate protection against poliomyelitis is needed, OPV is recommended. OPV should not be given to immunocompromised individuals or to persons with known or possibly immunocompromised family members. eIPV is recommended in such situations.	Although a protective immune response to eIPV in the immunocompromised person cannot be assured, the vaccine is safe, and some protection may result from its administration.
Inactivated-Virus Vaccines				
Hepatitis B (HB) inactivated-virus vaccine	Two doses IM 4 weeks apart; third dose 5 months after second; booster doses not necessary within 7 years of primary series.	Adults at increased risk of occupational, environmental, social, or family exposure.	Pregnancy should *not* be considered a vaccine contraindication if the woman is otherwise eligible. Because the vaccine contains only noninfectious HBsAg particles, the risk should be negligible.	Prevaccination serologic screening for susceptibility before vaccination may or may not be cost effective depending on costs of vaccination and testing and on the prevalence of immune persons in the group.
Influenza vaccine (inactivated whole-virus and split-virus vaccine)	Annual vaccination with current vaccine. Either whole- or split-virus vaccine may be used.	Adults with high-risk conditions, residents of nursing homes or other chronic-care facilities, medical-care personnel, or healthy persons ≥65 years.	History of anaphylactic hypersensitivity to egg ingestion.	No evidence exists of maternal or fetal risk when vaccine is administered in high-risk pregnancy. However, it is reasonable to wait until the second or third trimester, if possible, before vaccination.
Human diploid cell rabies vaccine (HDCV) (inactivated, whole-virion); rabies vaccine, adsorbed (RVA)	Pre-exposure prophylaxis: two doses 1 week apart; third dose 3 weeks after second. If exposure continues, booster doses every 2 years, or an antibody titer determined and a booster dose administered if titer is inadequate (<5). Postexposure prophylaxis: All postexposure treatment should begin with soap and water. 1) Persons who have a) previously received postexposure prophylaxis with HDCV, b) received recommended IM pre-exposure series of HDCV, c) received recommended ID† pre-exposure series of HDCV in the United States, or d) have a previously documented rabies antibody titer considered adequate: two doses of HDCV, 1.0 ml IM, one each on days 0 and 3. 2) Persons not previously immunized as above: HRIG 20 IU/kg body weight, half infiltrated at bite site if possible; remainder IM in a separate syringe and at a different anatomic site than the vaccine; and five doses of HDCV, 1.0 ml IM one each on days 0, 3, 7, 14, 28.	Veterinarians, animal handlers, certain laboratory workers, and persons living in or visiting countries for >1 month where rabies is a constant threat.	If there is substantial risk of exposure to rabies, pre-exposure vaccination may be indicated during pregnancy. Corticosteroids and immunosuppressive agents can interfere with the development of active immunity; history of anaphylactic or type III hypersensitivity reaction to previous dose of HDCV.	Complete pre-exposure prophylaxis does not eliminate the need for additional therapy with rabies vaccine after a rabies exposure. The decision for postexposure use of HDCV depends on the species of biting animal, the circumstances of biting incident, and the type of exposure (e.g., bite, saliva contamination of wound). The type of and schedule for postexposure prophylaxis depends on the person's previous rabies vaccination status, or the result of a previous or current serologic test for rabies antibody. For postexposure prophylaxis, HDCV should always be administered IM, *not* ID.

Table continued on following page

TABLE 73–3. IMMUNOBIOLOGICS AND SCHEDULES FOR ADULTS (≥18 YEARS OF AGE) IN THE UNITED STATES* *Continued*

Immunobiologic Generic Name	Primary Schedule and Booster(s)	Indications	Major Precautions and Contraindications	Special Considerations
Inactivated Bacteria Vaccines				
Cholera vaccine	Two 0.5 ml doses SC or IM or two 0.2-ml doses ID 1 week to 1 month apart; booster doses (0.5 ml IM or 0.2 ml ID) every 6 months.	Travelers to countries requiring evidence of cholera vaccination for entry.	No specific information on vaccine safety during pregnancy. Use in pregnancy should reflect actual increased risk. Persons who have had severe local or systemic reactions to a previous dose.	One dose sometimes satisfies International Health Regulations. Vaccination should not be considered an alternative to continued careful selection of foods and water.
Haemophilus influenzae type b conjugated vaccine (HbCV)	One dose (0.5 ml) IM	Severely immunocompromised individuals, post–solid organ transplant on chronic suppressive therapy, asplenia. It should be considered in those with HIV infection.	No specific information on vaccine safety during pregnancy.	No efficacy data available for adults; not indicated for adult contacts of children with invasive disease.
Meningococcal polysaccharide vaccine (tetravalent A, C, W135, and Y)	One dose in volume and by route specified by manufacturer; need for boosters unknown.	Travelers visiting areas of a country that are recognized as having epidemic meningococcal disease.	Pregnancy unless there is substantial risk of infection.	
Plague vaccine	Three IM doses; first dose 1.0 ml; second dose 0.2 ml 1 month later; third dose 0.2 ml 5 months after second; booster doses (0.2 ml) at 1- to 2-year intervals if exposure continues.	Selected travelers to countries reporting cases, or in which avoidance of rodents, rabbits and fleas is impossible; all laboratory and field personnel working with *Yersinia pestis*.	Pregnancy, unless there is substantial and unavoidable risk of exposure; persons with known hypersensitivity to any of the vaccine constituents, or who have had severe local or systemic reactions to a previous dose.	Prophylactic antibiotics may be recommended for definite exposure whether or not the exposed person has been vaccinated.
Pneumococcal polysaccharide vaccine (23 valent)	One dose (0.5 ml) IM or SC; revaccination recommended for those at highest risk ≥6 years after the first dose.	Adults who are at increased risk of pneumococcal disease and its complications because of underlying health conditions; older adults, especially those ≥65 years of age who are healthy.	The safety of vaccine for pregnant women has not been evaluated; it should not be given during pregnancy unless the risk of infection is high.	
Inactivated Bacteria and Live-Bacteria Vaccines				
Typhoid vaccine, SC and oral	Two 0.5-ml doses SC 4 or more weeks apart, booster 0.5 ml SC or 0.1 ml ID every 3 years if exposure continues. Four oral doses on alternate days; revaccination with the entire four-dose series every 5 years.	Travelers to areas where there is a recognized risk of exposure to typhoid.	Severe local or systemic reaction to a previous dose. Acetone-killed and dried vaccines should not be administered ID.	Vaccination should not be considered an alternative to continued careful selection of foods and water.
Live-Bacteria Vaccine				
Bacille Calmette-Guérin vaccine (BCG)	One dose ID or percutaneously. (See package label.)	For children only, who have prolonged close contact with untreated or ineffectively treated active tuberculosis patients, or resistant organisms. Children belonging to groups with high rates of new infection.	Pregnancy, unless there is unavoidable exposure to infective tuberculosis; immunocompromised patients.	In the United States, tuberculosis-control efforts are directed toward early identification and treatment of cases, and preventive therapy with isoniazid.

Immune Globulins¶				
Immune globulin (IG)	Hepatitis A prophylaxis: *Pre-exposure:* one IM dose of 0.02 ml/kg for anticipated risk of 2–3 months; IM dose of 0.06 ml/kg for anticipated risk of 5 months; repeat appropriate dose at above intervals if exposure continues.	Nonimmune persons traveling to developing countries.		For travelers, IG is not an alternative to continued careful selection of foods and water. Frequent travelers should be tested for hepatitis A antibody. IG is not indicated for persons with antibody to hepatitis A.
	Postexposure: one IM dose of 0.02 ml/kg administered within 2 weeks of exposure.	Household and sexual contacts of persons with hepatitis A; staff, attendees, and parents of diapered attendees in daycare center outbreaks.		
	Measles prophylaxis (immunocompetent): 0.25 ml/kg IM (maximum 15 ml) administered within 6 days after exposure. Measles prophylaxis (immunocompromised) 0.5 ml/kg [maximum 15 ml] administered within 6 days of exposure)	Exposed susceptible contacts of measles cases.	IG should *not* be used to control measles.	Recipients of IG for measles prophylaxis should receive live measles vaccine 3 months later.
Hepatitis B immune globulin (HBIG)	0.06 ml/kg IM as soon as possible after exposure (with HB vaccine started at a different site); a second dose of HBIG should be administered 1 month later (percutaneous/mucous-membrane exposure) or 3 months later (sexual exposure) if the HB vaccine series has not been started.	Following percutaneous or mucous-membrane exposure to blood known to be HBsAg‖ positive (within 7 days); following sexual exposure to a person with acute HBV or an HBV carrier (within 14 days).		
Tetanus immune globulin (TIG)	250 U IM.	Part of management of nonclean, nonminor wound in a person with unknown tetanus toxoid status, with less than two previous doses or with two previous doses and a wound more than 24 hours old.		
Rabies immune globulin, human (HRIG)	20 IU/kg, up to half infiltrated around wound; remainder IM, in a syringe and at a different anatomic site than the vaccine.	Part of management of rabies exposure in persons lacking a history of recommended pre-exposure or postexposure prophylaxis with HDCV.		Although preferable to administer with the first dose of vaccine, can be administered up to the eighth day after the first dose of vaccine.
Varicella-zoster immune globulin (VZIG)	Persons <50 kg: 125 U/10 kg IM; persons >50 kg: 625 U.	Immunocompromised patients known or likely to be susceptible with close and prolonged exposure.		

*From Immunization Practices Advisory Committee: Recommendations of the Immunization Practices Advisory Committee. Update on adult immunizations. MMWR 40:1–94, 1991.

†MMR = measles = mumps = rubella vaccine.

‡ID = intradermal.

§HIV = human immunodeficiency virus.

‖HB_sAg = hepatitis B surface antigen.

¶After administration of antibody-containing products and blood, administration of measles, mumps, rubella and varicella vaccines should be deferred for the appropriate intervals.

immune to both. Nonimmune, healthy, nonpregnant adults born after 1956, who are not otherwise at increased risk (see later) and who do not have documentation of at least one dose of live measles vaccine given on or after his or her first birthday or serologic proof of immunity should be vaccinated. Measles vaccine is recommended to be administered as combined MMR vaccine. As discussed later, those at increased risk require two doses of live measles vaccine, given at least 1 month apart, with the first dose being administered on or after the individual's first birthday. Persons who received killed measles vaccine in the period from 1963 to 1967 need to receive at least one dose of live vaccine.

Measles is the only disease for which prophylactic immunization of susceptible individuals shortly after exposure can prevent infection. Therefore, all susceptible individuals should be vaccinated within 72 hours of exposure; immunization during this time period is most likely to be protective.

Mumps vaccine (also recommended to be administered as MMR) should be given to healthy, nonpregnant adults born after 1956 unless they demonstrate serologic evidence of immunity or have had mumps vaccination on or after the first birthday. Rubella vaccine (also recommended to be administered as MMR vaccine) is indicated for all adults without evidence of immunity based on serologic evidence or on documentation of immunization occurring on or after the first birthday. Rubella vaccination is particularly important for nonpregnant women of childbearing age to protect against congenital rubella syndrome. Some authorities recommend vaccination of nonpregnant women of childbearing age without serologic testing.

MMR should not be given to persons who (1) are pregnant, (2) are immunocompromised (exception: those with human immunodeficiency virus [HIV] infection), or (3) have a history of anaphylaxis to eggs or neomycin. If an individual has received any blood or other antibody-containing blood products within the last 11 months, MMR vaccine administration should be deferred according to the guidelines mentioned in the General Principles section of this chapter.

Many clinicians have concerns about the inadvertent administration of MMR vaccine to a pregnant woman. The risks of exposing live viral vaccine to the fetus are theoretical and have not been substantiated for any vaccine, even that for rubella. No cases of congenital rubella syndrome (CRS) have been reported to be associated with administration of rubella vaccine within 3 months pre- or postconception. Before vaccinating women of childbearing age, providers should inform them about the theoretical risks and advise them against becoming pregnant for 3 months.

Influenza. Although yearly influenza vaccination of adults not in a special occupational group or high-risk situation (see later) is considered routine only among the elderly (e.g., those above the age of 64), it is reasonable to offer influenza vaccine to all healthy, nonpregnant persons interested in receiving it to reduce their risk of illness from influenza. Pregnant women at high risk should also be vaccinated.

Pneumococcal Infection. Healthy persons over the age of 65 should be offered immunization against pneumococcal disease with the current 23-valent vaccine. Revaccination of healthy persons is not generally recommended, but revaccination of certain high-risk groups should be considered.

Other Immunizations. Healthy adults may be candidates for other immunizations based on special occupations or high-risk situations (see later).

Pregnant Women

Immunization is best avoided during the first trimester of pregnancy. Live vaccines should generally be avoided during all of pregnancy except where the benefit clearly outweighs the risk (e.g., yellow fever vaccine before travel to areas where risk of disease is substantial, or oral polio vaccine for immediate protection of previously unvaccinated women in situations in which risk of exposure is high). Tetanus and diphtheria toxoid is indicated for pregnant women who are not already appropriately immunized; the risk of neonatal tetanus is thereby reduced. IG is indicated for pregnant women exposed to hepatitis A or measles unless there is serologic evidence of immunity. If given after exposure to rubella, IG will *not* prevent infection or viremia. It does *not* guarantee protection against fetal infection. The only circumstance in which IG might be useful is for unimmunized women exposed to rubella who choose not to abort. Varicella IG (VZIG) is indicated for nonimmune pregnant women exposed to varicella. VZIG reduces the chance that pregnant women will experience complications of varicella. It is not known whether the fetus will be protected against malformations. Pregnancy is not a contraindication to immunization against hepatitis B for persons exposed or at high risk (see later). Influenza and pneumococcal vaccines can also be given to pregnant women at high risk (see later).

Persons with Compromised Immunity[9]

Alcoholism. Pneumococcal and influenza vaccines are indicated for patients with alcoholism and alcoholic liver disease.

Asplenia. Persons with functional asplenia (e.g., persons with sickle cell disease) or who have had their spleens removed surgically should receive pneumococcal vaccine every 6 years. *Haemophilus influenzae* type b conjugate (Hib) vaccine and meningococcal vaccine are also recommended for persons without a functioning spleen.

Long-Term Immunosuppressive Therapy. Because of a fear that vaccination, especially with tetanus toxoid, may trigger a nonspecific immune response (leading to organ rejection or exacerbation of autoimmune disease) in patients on immunosuppressive therapy, primary immunizations should, if possible, be given before immunosuppressive therapy is begun. There is no evidence of this phenomenon with influenza, Hib, pneumococcal, or hepatitis B vaccine. Influenza, Hib and pneumococcal vaccines are recommended for all chronically immunosuppressed patients. Transplant recipients should be revaccinated against pneumococcal disease every 6 years. Hepatitis B vaccine is recommended as well when indicated, including in patients with renal disease, as noted above.

Human Immunodeficiency Virus Infection. Pneumococcal vaccine as well as annual influenza vaccine have been recommended for persons infected with HIV. Hib vaccine should be considered. Tetanus-diphtheria immunity should be maintained in the same manner as for persons not infected with HIV.

Malignancy. Patients whose immunity is compromised because of malignancy should be immunized against influenza, Hib, and pneumococcal diseases; the degree of immune compromise must be determined on an individual basis. Immunizations should be given before cycles of radiation or chemotherapy. Pneumococcal vaccine should be given before scheduled splenectomy. Patients with severe immune compromise, such as persons with hematologic malignancies, should not receive live-virus preparations.

Renal Failure. Immunizations are best administered early in the course of renal disease, when immune function is likely to be better. Yearly influenza vaccine may be supplemented by amantadine prophylaxis during periods of high risk of exposure to influenza A. Pneumococcal vaccine is indicated, with revaccination every 6 years for those with nephrotic syndrome. Hepatitis B vaccine is ideally given early in the course of disease to patients likely to need dialysis or transplantation.

Immune Globulin Use in Persons with Compromised Immunity.[9] When immunocompromised individuals have been exposed to varicella, they must be carefully and individually evaluated. An immunocompromised patient who is believed to be susceptible and who has had significant exposure to varicella should receive varicella zoster IG within 96 hours of exposure. Similarly, IG is indicated for immunocompromised individuals after they have been exposed to measles. Exposed symptomatic HIV-infected individuals and severely immunocompromised individuals should receive IG irrespective of previous immunization status. Some authorities recommend that tetanus IG (TIG) be given to HIV-infected individuals who sustain a significant wound exposure, regardless of immunization status.

Other High-Risk Medical Conditions

In addition to persons with the conditions noted above, persons with conditions that increase the likelihood of serious adverse consequences from lower respiratory tract infection should have influenza vaccine. These conditions include (1) acquired or congenital heart diseases that alter circulatory dynamics, (2) any condition that produces compromised pulmonary function, (3) diabetes mellitus and other metabolic diseases that predispose to more severe infections, and (4) chronic hemoglobinopathies, including sickle cell disease.

Similarly, high-risk conditions in addition to those mentioned in previous sections for which pneumococcal vaccine is recommended include (1) congestive heart failure, (2) chronic pulmonary disease, and (3) diabetes mellitus.

Occupational Groups

Workers in certain jobs should be considered candidates for immunizations in addition to those advocated for the general population. Such immunizations serve either to protect the worker from infection to which the occupation puts the worker at higher risk or to reduce the likelihood that the worker will transmit infections to others. As mentioned earlier, an ethical dilemma may be perceived in the latter situation, when the person receiving the immunization (and its attendant risk) is not the person who will receive the primary benefit from the immunization. In this situation, meticulous attention to fully informed consent is particularly germane.

Health-Care Workers. Immunization against hepatitis B is recommended for health-care workers who are exposed to blood or blood products. Immunization against influenza is also strongly recommended. Documented immunity to rubella is recommended for those who might otherwise transmit rubella to pregnant patients or fellow workers. Measles immunity is also strongly advised. Persons born after 1956 without documentation of two doses of live measles vaccine and one dose of mumps vaccine (or serologic evidence of immunity to both) should be vaccinated. However, a large proportion of the measles cases among health-care workers have occurred in those born before 1957. Therefore, it is recommended that health-care facilities consider requiring at least one dose of measles vaccine for older health-care workers at risk of exposure. Immunity to poliomyelitis is recommended for health-care workers who might be exposed to patients excreting polioviruses; the inactivated virus preparation should be used for adults unless immediate protection is required.

Providers of Essential Community Services. Such essential workers as police, firefighters, and teachers may be considered candidates for annual immunization against influenza. Emergency medical personnel who have exposure to blood should also receive immunization against hepatitis B.

Child-Care Workers. Persons working in child care centers should have immunity against mumps, measles, and rubella. In the absence of immunity, MMR should be given unless contraindicated. For nonpregnant adults without immunity against poliomyelitis, enhanced-potency inactivated polio vaccine is recommended in nonurgent situations unless there is a history of anaphylactic reactions to neomycin, which appears in trace amounts in the vaccine. Vaccination of child care workers against influenza is reasonable annually. Also recommended is the administration of IG to child care workers if an outbreak of hepatitis A occurs. Vaccination of child care workers against *H. influenzae* type b is not recommended because adults do not usually acquire this organism from children, nor do they usually transmit it to children.

Laboratory Workers. Except for those working in specialized laboratories where exposure may occur to anthrax, plague, rabies, smallpox, or tularemia, the only additional vaccination recommended for most laboratory workers who handle blood or blood products is hepatitis B vaccine.

Workers Exposed to Animals. For workers at risk, protection against rabies through routine immunization is recommended. Similarly recommended is protection against plague for workers exposed to animals in areas (such as the southwestern United States) where plague is endemic. For those with frequent exposure to animal products potentially infected with anthrax, an anthrax vaccine is available.

High-Risk Living Situations or Behaviors

College Students. Unless immunity is confirmed by serologic evidence, measles vaccination (usually MMR) is recommended for college students born after 1956, even those who have already received one dose of measles vaccine. Mumps vaccination (also usually MMR) should be given to college students born after 1956 unless there is a history of adequate mumps immunization or serologic evidence of immunity. For rubella, vaccination (again, usually MMR) is indicated for all college students unless there is serologic evidence of immunity or a documented history of adequate immunization. In the absence of previous immunization against rubella, vaccination has been recommended without serologic testing. MMR should not be given to persons who (1) are pregnant, (2) may become pregnant within 3 months, (3) are immunocompromised (exception: those with HIV infection), or (4) have a history of anaphylaxis to eggs or neomycin. If an individual has received blood or other antibody-containing blood products within the last 11 months, administration of MMR vaccine should be deferred according to the guidelines mentioned in the General Principles section of this chapter.

Institutionalized Persons with Developmental Disabilities. Because of a high prevalence of infection with hepatitis B among institutionalized persons with developmental disabilities, it is reasonable to screen for previous hepatitis B infection and immunize those without documented immunity.

International Travelers. Immunization requirements for international travelers are discussed in detail in Chapter 74.

Nursing Home Residents. Residents of nursing homes should receive yearly immunization against influenza. Pneumococcal vaccine is also recommended. Like their non-institutionalized counterparts, their tetanus-diphtheria immunization status should also be up-to-date.

Persons with Unprotected Exposure to Multiple Sex Partners. Persons with unprotected exposure to multiple sex partners should be informed about the associated health risks, including the increased risk of acquiring hepatitis B. For those who continue the behavior, it is reasonable to screen for previous hepatitis B infection and immunize those without documented immunity.

Prison Inmates. In addition to receiving routine immunizations, inmates of prisons should be considered for hepatitis B vaccine. Before vaccination, screening for hepatitis B immunity is appropriate.

Users of Illicit Intravenous Drugs. In addition to tetanus and other routine immunizations, users of illicit intravenous drugs who share needles are at increased risk for hepatitis B. It is appropriate to screen persons who engage in such behavior for immunity to hepatitis B, and to vaccinate those found not to be immune.

Accidental Exposures or Bites

Immunizations for accidental exposures and bites are beyond the scope of this chapter. For more information on topics such as tetanus prophylaxis for wound management; management after exposure to hepatitis A, hepatitis B, meningococcal infections, and tuberculosis; and management after bites by animals, snakes, and spiders, see text citations in the references.[1–8]

NEW VACCINES IN DEVELOPMENT FOR USE IN ADULTS

A live attenuated varicella vaccine and two killed-virus hepatitis A vaccines are nearing licensure. When available, varicella vaccine will be targeted for nonimmune adults working in the health-care profession, teachers, day-care personnel, and others working with children. Adults who will be targeted for hepatitis A vaccine will include international travelers, staff of day-care and other custodial centers, food handlers, military personnel, and populations with high levels of endemic infection (e.g., Native Americans).

Pertussis is an important cause of persistent cough illness in adults. Studies of adults with prolonged cough have identified pertussis in up to 25% of cases. Vaccine-induced immunity wanes and is absent 12 years after the last dose is given at school entry. By the time most individuals reach adolescence and adulthood, they are susceptible. Adults have a primary role in the current epidemiology of pertussis. They serve as major reservoirs of infection for infants and children who may develop severe disease.

Routine immunization of adults with pertussis vaccine is currently not recommended because of the frequency of adverse reactions after immunization of older individuals with whole-cell preparations. Purification of pertussis antigens has led to the licensure of acellular pertussis vaccine for use in children. One recent study demonstrated acellular pertussis vaccine to be both safe and to induce a significant antibody response in adults.[10] Acellular pertussis vaccine could potentially be formulated with diphtheria and tetanus toxoid to create a TdaP booster. If acellular vaccines are licensed for use in adolescents and adults, they will contribute to decreased morbidity in persons of all age groups, including infants and children.

REFERENCES

1. CDC: Recommendations of the Immunization Practices Advisory Committee (ACIP). Update on adult immunizations. MMWR 40(RR-12):1–94, 1991.
2. CDC: Recommendations of the Immunization Practices Advisory Committee (ACIP). General recommendations on immunization. MMWR 38:205–227, 1989. (New recommendations due in 1994).
3. Control of Communicable Diseases in Man. American Public Health Association.
4. Centers for Disease Control: Health Information for International Travel. Atlanta, Georgia: Department of Health and Human Services, Public Health Service, 1989, HHS publication no. (CDC) 89-8280.
5. Centers for Disease Control: National Childhood Vaccine Injury Act: Reporting requirements for permanent vaccination records and for reporting selected events after vaccination. MMWR 37:197–200, 1988.
6. World Health Organization: Vaccination Certificate Requirements and Health Advice for International Travel. Geneva, World Health Organization, 1988.
7. American College of Physicians Task Force on Adult Immunization and Infectious Disease Society of America: Guide for Adult Immunization, 2nd ed. Philadelphia, American College of Physicians, 1990.
8. Adult immunizations. *In* Guide to Clinical Preventive Services: Report of the US Preventive Services Task Force. Baltimore, Williams & Wilkins, 1989, pp 363–368.
9. CDC: Recommendations of the Advisory Committee (ACIP): Use of Vaccines and Immune Globulins in Persons with Altered Immunocompetence. MMWR 42(RR-4):1–18, 1993.
10. Edwards KM, Decker MD, Graham Mezzatesta J, et al: Adult immunization with acellular pertussis vaccine. JAMA 269:53–56, 1993.

74

Health Advice for Travelers

ROBERT P. SMITH, Jr., MD, MPH

The rapid expansion of international travel to remote areas of the world exposes millions of Americans to unfamiliar health hazards. Although the risk of serious illness is small, proper medical preparation for international travel is too often neglected by both prospective tourists and their physicians. More than one half of North American travelers to malarious areas use inadequate malaria prophylaxis.[1] Fortunately, up-to-date resources for physicians are now readily available. Health Information for International Travel, the comprehensive sourcebook on immunization requirements and malaria prophylaxis from the Centers for Disease Control (CDC), is updated annually.[2] State health departments also offer advice on medical preparation for travel, as do specialized traveler's clinics in some urban areas. Physicians with office computers can benefit from new software with continuously updated recommendations.

Travel to industrialized areas of the world, such as Canada, Western Europe, or Australia and New Zealand, seldom requires special precautions, thus this chapter focuses on issues pertinent to travel in the developing areas of the world. The degree of preparation necessary for travel in the tropics varies with the type of travel and itinerary. For example, tourists to Caribbean resorts rarely require immunizations or malaria prophylaxis, but a health worker on assignment to rural Haiti may benefit from a polio booster, typhoid and hepatitis B vaccine, immune globulin, and an antimalaria regimen. The risk of travel-associated illness increases with the duration of the trip, the amount of rural travel, and the adoption of local village lifestyles.

Although serious illness is a rare occurrence among tropical travelers, at least one third of tourists to tropical areas experience a minor illness that may result in discomfort, worry, and a blighted itinerary.[3, 4] Respiratory infections and gastrointestinal (constipation and diarrhea) and skin ailments account for the majority of traveler's illnesses. Peace Corps statistics reveal that automobiles are the greatest threat to North Americans living in the tropics, due to treacherous roads in poor repair, faulty vehicles, and lax enforcement of rules of the road.[5] Life-threatening infectious disease is quite rare, but malaria,[6] typhoid fever (1 to 5 per 10^5 travelers),[7] hepatitis A, and bacterial and amebic dysentery[8] continue to cause significant morbidity.

PRETRIP EVALUATION

Physicians should encourage a pretrip office visit by their patients to review current medical problems, to ensure an adequate supply of essential medications, and to counsel patients regarding necessary immunizations and malaria prophylaxis. This visit should be planned at least 6 weeks before departure to tropical areas to allow adequate time for scheduling vaccinations.

Physicians should tailor advice to persons with chronic disease to the individual's health status and the demands of the planned trip. Insulin-dependent diabetic patients may need to modify their insulin regimen, taking into account changes in time zones and daily activities. The American Diabetes Association provides a pamphlet with specific suggestions.[9] Patients with diabetes or cardiopulmonary disease or who are on certain medications are more susceptible to heat illness (Table 74–1).[10] However, with judicious planning, these need not be reasons to avoid travel to hot climates.

Jet travel poses a small risk to patients with severe cardiopulmonary disease because cabin pressures in high-altitude aircraft are similar to those at 5000 to 8000 feet of altitude.[11] Supplemental oxygen may be prudent for these patients. They should also be warned to avoid small, unpressurized aircraft.

Patients with achlorhydria or who are taking cimetidine or antacids are more susceptible to enteric infections and

TABLE 74–1. DRUGS THAT CAN PREDISPOSE TO HEAT STROKE

Anticholinergic drugs: atropine, scopolamine, benztropine mesylate
Phenothiazine
Tricyclic antidepressants
Monoamine oxidase inhibitors
Diuretics

TABLE 74–2. INFORMATION FOR TRAVELERS TO THE TROPICS

1. Avoid all untreated water, including ice.
   Safe water: Boiled 10 minutes or treated with one of the following:
   Iodine tablets (1 per quart, allow 30 minutes)
   2% Tincture of iodine (5 drops/qt, allow 30 minutes)
   Probably safe: Sealed bottled water
2. Carbonated soft drinks, beer, coffee, tea, undiluted fruit juice, and pasteurized milk are safe to drink.
3. Avoid fresh leafy vegetables or raw vegetables unless known to be carefully washed in treated water. Only eat fruits you can peel or slice yourself.
4. Avoid undercooked or "buffet style" meats, fish, shellfish. Eat well-cooked food served hot.
5. Avoid dairy products in rural areas (milk, ice cream, soft cheese) unless known to be pasteurized.
6. Use a diethyltoluamide-containing insect repellent when mosquitoes are active.
7. Swim with care. Inquire about undertow at ocean beaches and *Bilharzia* (schistosomiasis) in freshwater lakes and streams.
8. Avoid over-the-counter drugs unless you know what they are. Avoid drug injections for minor illness.
9. Remember to take your malaria pills as prescribed.
10. Check your health insurance policy to ensure coverage abroad.

should carefully follow the usual precautions regarding food and water. Immunosuppressed patients cannot receive some live viral vaccines and are obviously at greater risk from infections.

Most travelers to the tropics benefit from a review of commonsense precautions regarding food, water, and climate (Table 74–2). A small medical kit is often appropriate if extensive travel is planned, given the difficulty in obtaining familiar medications in certain countries (Table 74–3). A handout summarizing the treatment of travelers' diarrhea (see Tables 74–6 and 74–7) is also appropriate.

More thorough preparations for prolonged travel (e.g., Peace Corps volunteers, foreign aid workers) should include careful physical and dental examinations and contingency plans for medical assistance abroad. The International Association for Medical Assistance for Travelers (IAMAT, 350 5th Avenue, Suite 5620, New York, NY 10001) offers names of English-speaking physicians throughout the world and other information on the reliability of medical facilities abroad.

Immunizations

Immunizations against infectious diseases are sometimes *required* for entry into foreign countries (i.e., cholera, yellow fever), and these requirements are listed annually in Health Information for International Travel.[2]

Other immunizations, although not required, are *recommended* on the basis of risk of exposure. There is little argument over the benefit of an overdue tetanus-diphtheria booster, but the value of typhoid, polio, cholera, and yellow fever vaccines varies with the proposed itinerary. All too often, appropriate immunizations are neglected because they are not a requirement for international travel. Table 74–4 summarizes the array of immunizations available for protection of the tropical traveler.

Timing of immunizations is important. Immune globulin should not be given prior to live attenuated vaccines because it may interfere with an effective immune response. However, adequate immunity to yellow fever and oral polio vaccine is obtained when given simultaneously with immune globulin. If possible, immune globulin should be given no sooner than 14 days after live vaccines.

TABLE 74–3. TRAVELER'S MEDICAL KIT

Prescription Items
Antimalarial
Antibiotic—trimethoprim-sulfamethoxazole (160 mg/800 mg) or ciprofloxacin (500 mg tablets) for empiric treatment of severe diarrhea or urinary tract infection; erythromycin (250-mg tablets) for severe respiratory or soft tissue infections
Antihistamine—diphenhydramine (Benadryl) for systemic allergy (e.g., urticaria); can also be used as a soporific
Antimotion sickness—meclizine (Antivert, 25 mg) or transdermal scopolamine for prevention of motion sickness
Antinausea remedy—prochlorperazine (Compazine, 25-mg rectal suppositories) for severe nausea, vomiting
Antispasmodic—loperamide (Imodium) for treatment of diarrhea, abdominal cramps with turista; should not be used for dysentery
For rapid ascent to high altitude—acetazolamide (Diamox), 250 mg tid 2 days prior to ascent and for 2–3 days after arrival at high altitude

Nonprescription Items
Aspirin or acetaminophen (Tylenol)—for treatment of minor arthralgias, febrile illness
Antibiotic ointment (Bacitracin, Neosporin)—for use in cuts and abrasions
Bismuth subsalicylate (Pepto-Bismol), 8 oz liquid in bottle—for treatment of turista
Decongestant (pseudoephedrine preparation)—with a cold, a nasal spray decongestant may be helpful prior to air travel
0.5% Hydrocortisone skin cream (Cort-Aid)—for sunburn, insect bites, contact dermatitis
Sunscreen (5% PABA as ingredient) and sunblocker (No. 15 rating)
Iodine water purification tablets (Potable Aqua, Globaline, Coughlan's)
Insect repellent (containing diethyltoluamide)
Glucose-electrolyte powder—powdered mix for replacement of fluid losses
Povidone-iodine liquid (Betadine)—for cleansing dirty cuts
Antifungal foot powder (Tinactin, Desitin)
Thermometer in plastic case
Moleskin
Band-Aids, sterile gauze and adhesive tape, Ace bandage, and scissors

If immunizations are given at separate sites, up to three live vaccines or a live vaccine and a killed vaccine can be administered on the same day. Yellow fever vaccine can be obtained only at a limited number of officially designated

TABLE 74–4. IMMUNIZATIONS FOR THE TRAVELER

Routine
These vaccinations should be up-to-date for all travelers:
Diphtheria-tetanus (booster every 10 years)
Measles*
Mumps*
Rubella*
Poliomyelitis*
Sometimes required for international travel
Cholera (valid for 6 months)
Yellow fever* (valid for 10 years)
Often recommended for tropical travel to rural areas
Typhoid
Immune globulin for hepatitis A prophylaxis (renew every 3–6 months, depending on dose)
Vaccines for special circumstances
Rabies (HDCV—booster every 2 years)
Meningococcal
Plague
Hepatitis B
Japanese B encephalitis
Discontinued or unavailable
Smallpox, typhus

*Live attenuated viral vaccine.
HDCV = human diploid-cell rabies vaccine.

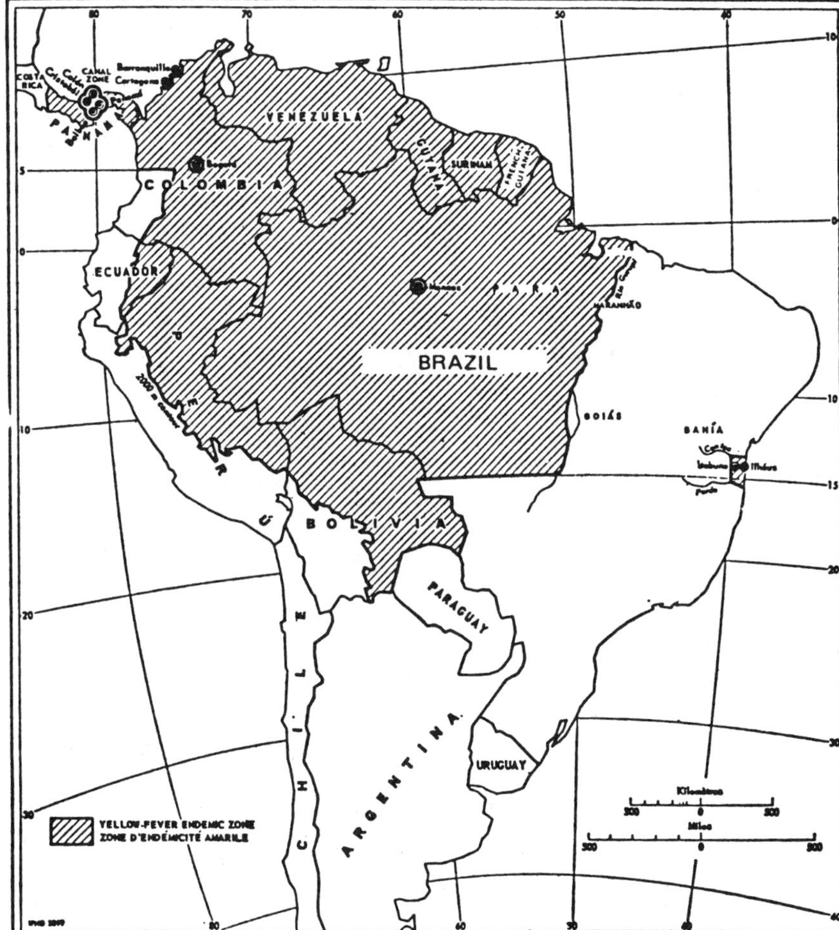

FIGURE 74–1. Yellow fever endemic zones in the Americas. (From Centers for Disease Control: Health information for international travel. MMWR (Suppl), 1991, p 127.)

centers, thus health providers should direct their patients to these sites well in advance of departure.

Live attenuated viral vaccines are generally contraindicated in pregnant or immunosuppressed patients, although polio and yellow fever immunizations are sometimes recommended for susceptible pregnant women with unavoidable high risk of exposure. Oral polio and typhoid vaccines should not be given to immunosuppressed patients or family members of these patients. Killed vaccines such as cholera should also be avoided in pregnancy, given the frequent occurrence of febrile reactions to these vaccines.

Routine Vaccinations

Travelers should bring up-to-date their routine vaccinations (e.g., diphtheria-tetanus) prior to departure. Individuals in a susceptible age group (birthdate after 1957) and without a history of a measles booster should receive one prior to travel. If there is no history of rubella or mumps immunity, a combined measles-mumps-rubella vaccine is recommended.

Most American adults have received complete immunizations to polio with either the inactivated or oral live vaccines. However, decreased immunity in adults is not unusual. As polio is endemic (and epidemic) in most of the developing world, a polio booster is recommended for tropical travel, particularly if the trip includes close contact with local populations. Because of the remote risk of vaccine-acquired polio, the inactivated (eIPV) vaccine is preferable in previously unvaccinated or partially vaccinated adults.[12] Individuals with immunologic deficiency should also receive the inactivated vaccine.

Vaccines Sometimes Required

Yellow Fever. Although seldom required for entry, yellow fever vaccine is recommended for all travelers to the endemic zones in South America, Africa, and Trinidad (Figs. 74–1 and 74–2), with the possible exception of brief travel restricted to large urban areas. Yellow fever vaccine is an effective, safe, attenuated live viral vaccine that confers immunity for at least 10 years. The highest-risk areas are the lowland rain forests in continental South America and Panama and the forest-savannah interface in equatorial Africa.[13] The CDC provides weekly updates on areas of reported yellow fever, but substantial underreporting is likely.

Cholera. The killed vaccine for cholera is not very effective and is usually advised only to satisfy immigration authorities, for whom a single dose or a medical letter of exemption will suffice. Although no longer a WHO-required vaccination for entry to another country from the United States, it is sometimes required when travelers travel between cholera-endemic countries. Travelers are at very low risk of contracting cholera (1 per 500,000) unless given to indiscreet dietary habits in the midst of an epidemic.[14, 15] Complete cholera immunization (two doses in the primary series) is reasonable for American health care workers in a cholera-endemic area and for persons with gastric achlorhydria who are at higher risk of cholera infection.

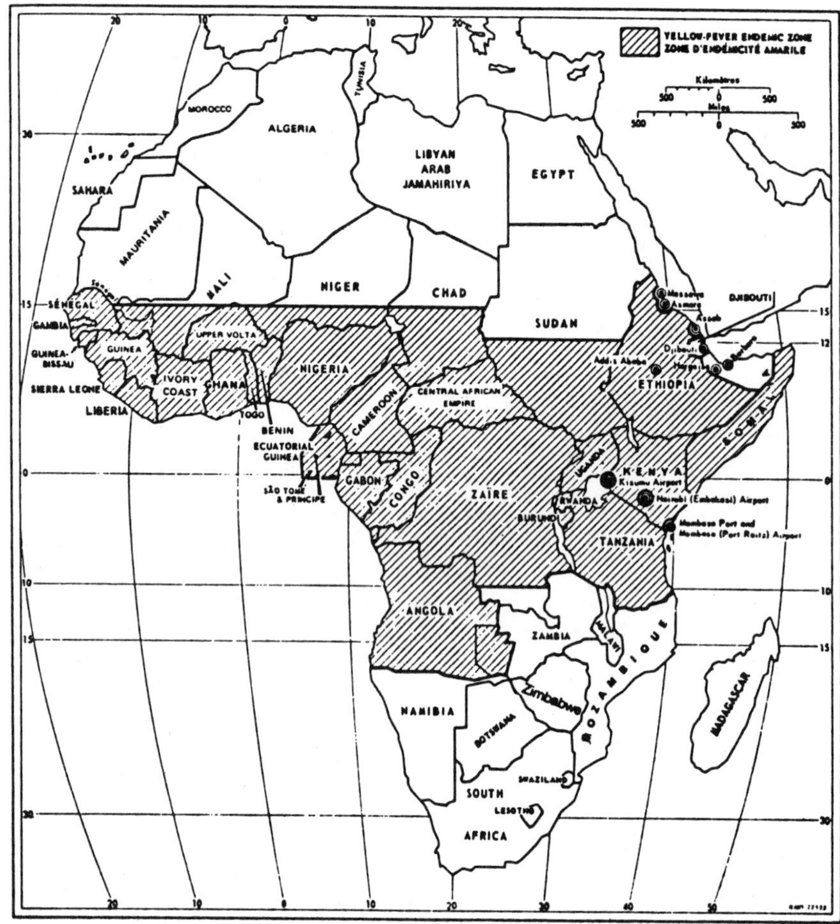

FIGURE 74–2. Yellow fever endemic zones in Africa. (From Centers for Disease Control: Health information for international travel. MMWR (Suppl), 1991, p 126.)

Vaccines Often Recommended for Tropical Travel

Typhoid. The greatest risk of typhoid occurs among American travelers to India, Peru, Pakistan, and Chile, but all travelers to areas off the usual tourist routes in the developing world are at risk of typhoid exposure through contaminated food and water, thus vaccination is recommended.[16] Risks are highest in children, the elderly, and those with close contact with local populations. A live-attenuated oral typhoid vaccine (Ty21a) has largely replaced the parenteral killed vaccine. It is equally effective, and, unlike the killed vaccine, well tolerated.[16] The oral vaccine is contraindicated for immunosuppressed persons. It should not be given concurrently with antibiotics or an antimalarial regimen.

Passive Immunization Against Hepatitis A. Immune globulin provides passive protection against hepatitis A for 3 to 6 months, depending on the dose administered. Hepatitis A is prevalent in most tropical and developing areas of the world, as well as the Mediterranean littoral. The risk of acquisition of hepatitis A by unimmunized travelers to remote areas in the tropics is high, thus use of immune globulin is strongly advised.[8, 17] Prophylaxis may be omitted by short-term travelers to western-style hotels and resorts. Gamma globulin is free of the risk of human immunodeficiency virus (HIV) and other infectious disease transmission.[3, 18] The immune globulin injection must be repeated every 6 months for continuous protection. Travelers with extensive experience in developing countries may choose to check their immune status to hepatitis A. If serology is positive, immune globulin prophylaxis is unnecessary. An inactivated hepatitis A vaccine that has been shown to be safe and effective is licensed in Europe and is due to be released in the United States soon.

Vaccines for Special Circumstances

Rabies. Rabies is prevalent in domestic and wild animals in Africa, Latin America, and the Indian subcontinent. Peace Corps volunteers, anthropologists, biologists, and others planning prolonged residence in an endemic area should consider pretrip immunization with three doses of human diploid-cell rabies vaccine (HDCV). Although postexposure immunization is still required in the event of a bite, the pretrip vaccination provides some protection to the person who is unable to get immediate medical attention and eliminates the need for rabies immune globulin, which is seldom available in the tropics. Immunization, given either intradermally or intramuscularly, requires a booster dose every 2 years. The HDCV vaccine, although expensive, is well tolerated and more effective than its predecessor, the duck embryo vaccine. However, rare systemic allergic reactions (1 per 1000 vaccinations) have been reported following booster doses of HDCV. The concurrent use of chloroquine at the time of rabies vaccination may blunt the antibody response to the vaccine. Therefore, rabies immunization should be completed prior to chloroquine use if possible.[19]

Meningococcal. Sub-Saharan Africa experiences annual (dry season) meningococcal epidemics. Visitors planning prolonged residence or involvement in health care in these countries may benefit from pretrip vaccination with

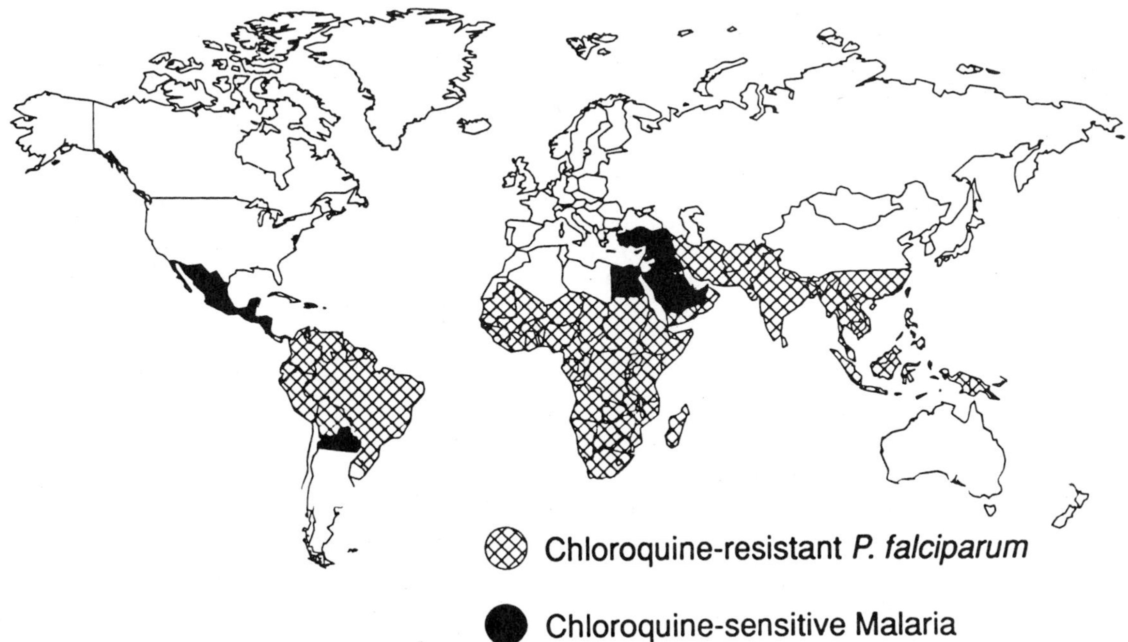

FIGURE 74–3. Distribution of malaria and chloroquine-resistant *Plasmodium falciparum,* 1992. (From Centers for Disease Control: Health information for international travel, 1991. No. HHS (CDC) 91-8280. Washington, DC, US Department of Health and Human Services, Public Health Service, 1992.)

quadrivalent meningococcal vaccine. Because of meningococcal outbreaks in India and Nepal, travelers to these areas (especially trekkers) should also consider vaccination.

Plague. Plague vaccine is rarely indicated for travelers, with the exception of those anticipating long-term residence in mountainous areas of rural Africa, Asia, or South America, and particularly if the traveler may be in contact with wild rodents and their fleas.

Hepatitis B. Hepatitis B prevalence is many times higher in South Africa, Africa, and Asia than it is in the United States. Therefore, all health-care workers on assignment in these areas should be vaccinated against this virus, and, because venereal transmission is possible, hepatitis B vaccine may be advisable in nonimmune visitors anticipating immersion in local daily life. Travelers to the Far East occasionally inquire about protection against Japanese B encephalitis, an arboviral disease endemic to much of Asia, Nepal, and the Western Pacific.

Japanese B Encephalitis

Travelers to the Far East may benefit from vaccination against Japanese B encephalitis, an arboviral disease endemic to much of Asia, Nepal, and the Western Pacific. Risk of Japanese B encephalitis is very low for short-term travelers and for those who visit only urban areas.

Discontinued or Unavailable Vaccines

Smallpox vaccine is contraindicated for travelers because of global eradication of the disease (last case, 1977) and the risk of vaccine-related illness. It is no longer required for entry into any country.

Reports of typhus acquired during travel are so rare that vaccine is no longer produced in the United States or Canada.

Malaria Prophylaxis

Travel-acquired malaria has increased markedly among Americans during the past decade, largely owing to a resurgence of malaria in the developing world and to increased travel to these areas by unprotected tourists (Fig. 74–3). The CDC's *Health Information for International Travel* provides extensive up-to-date information on the risk of malaria by locale and time of year. All travelers to malarious areas, even for a brief trip, should take antimalarial medication (Table 74–5).

Although chloroquine has been the cornerstone of malaria chemoprophylaxis, the continued spread of chloroquine-resistant strains of *Plasmodium falciparum* has limited its usefulness in most malarious countries. Chloroquine is still effective against *P. falciparum* in Central America north of the Panama Canal, the Dominican Republic, and Haiti. It can also be used in malarious countries without *P. falciparum* (e.g., Egypt, Iraq, and Turkey). Chloroquine is taken weekly for 1 to 2 weeks prior to entry into the malarious zone and is continued during the stay and for 4 weeks after departure. Side effects (e.g., rash, nausea, telogen effluvium) are rare. Retinopathy does not occur with the doses used for prophylaxis, unless the drug is continued for more than 5 years.[20, 21]

Most malarious areas of the world are now host to strains of chloroquine-resistant *P. falciparum* malaria (see Fig. 74–3). Travelers at risk for malaria exposure in these countries are generally advised to use mefloquine for prophylaxis. Like chloroquine, mefloquine is taken weekly and is continued for 4 weeks after departure from the malarious zone. Use of mefloquine is not recommended for travelers who are pregnant, on β-blockers, or with a history of seizures or psychiatric disorders. Doxycycline (100 mg/day orally) is an alternative drug for chemoprophylaxis in chloroquine-resistant areas. If neither mefloquine nor doxycycline can be used, travelers to these areas may take chloroquine along with a treatment dose (three tablets) of pyrimethamine-sulfadoxine (Fansidar). The treatment dose of pyrimethamine-sulfadoxine should be used only for the empiric treatment of severe febrile illness in the absence of immediate access to medical care. Pyrimethamine-sulfadoxine has been associated with a significant risk (1:11,000 to 1:25,000 users) of fatal cutaneous reactions and should not be used for malaria prophylaxis.[23]

Individuals with intense exposure to malaria during a prolonged stay should consider the addition of primaquine (15-mg base per day for 14 days) at the end of their period of exposure. Primaquine eradicates latent malaria parasites in the liver that are merely suppressed by chloroquine. Primaquine candidates should be screened for glucose-6-phosphate dehydrogenase (G6PD) deficiency prior to its use. Terminal prophylaxis with primaquine is not necessary for short-term visitors to the tropics.

In addition to chemoprophylaxis, travelers to malarious areas should use diethyltoluamide insect repellents when out at dawn or dusk and a mosquito net if sleeping in an unscreened dwelling. As none of these measures is 100% effective, all travelers to malarious areas should be reminded to report to their physician any febrile illness occurring within a few months of their return.

Resistant patterns of malarial parasites are in constant evolution, as underscored by reports of mefloquine-resistant strains of malaria from Southeast Asia.[22] Physicians should check the CDC's *Health Information for Travelers* for current recommendations or call the CDC Malaria Hotline at (404) 332–4555.

PRECAUTIONS WHILE TRAVELING

Many tropical travelers are unaware of simple precautions. Physicians should briefly review these "rules of the road" with their patients at the pretrip office visit or provide them with a handout (see Table 74–2) or a more detailed pamphlet such as *Health Hints for the Tropics.*[24]

Water. Tapwater (including ice) is often contaminated with enteric organisms in the developing world despite frequent testimonials to its safety by local authorities. It is best to avoid drinking water entirely unless it is properly purified by 10 minutes of boiling or by chemical treatments. Iodine tablets (Potable Aqua, Globaline) are more effective than chlorine (Halazone) tablets against protozoan cysts. Bottled water, if carbonated and sealed, is generally safe, as are carbonated soft drinks, beer, and undiluted fruit drinks.

Food. Although exotic cuisine is one of the delights of travel, the wise tourist will limit intake of certain foods. Raw fruits and vegetables often harbor enteric parasites because of the widespread use of nightsoil and the frequent use of untreated water to "freshen" them. Therefore, fresh salads must be passed by and fruits chosen only when they can be peeled by the traveler (i.e., bananas, oranges, mangoes) or washed in treated water. Undercooked meats are a source of toxoplasmosis, trichinosis, and tapeworm and should be avoided. Raw shellfish is responsible for several possible enteric infections, including hepatitis A and Norwalk virus. Even dairy products may be unsafe in rural areas where milk is not pasteurized and may lead to infections such as *Campylobacter* enteritis, brucellosis, or tuberculosis. Breads and canned foods are safe. In general, travelers should choose well-cooked foods served hot and ignore "buffet style" cold luncheons.

Climate. Physiologic adaptation to a hot climate requires at least 2 weeks of acclimatization. Underestimation of the effects of heat, the need for adaptation, and the rapidity of insensible fluid loss during exercise in a hot, dry environment may lead to heat exhaustion or heat cramps. Tourists should plan a gradual approach to physical activity, keep well hydrated, and salt their foods generously. Actual heat stroke is extremely rare among tourists, but the risk may be enhanced by certain medications (see Table 74–1).

The effects of intense sunlight are also often underestimated. Fair-skinned individuals should use high potency (No. 15) benzophenone sunscreens (and lip balms), hats, and protective clothing to ensure a gradual tan. Sunscreens should be applied 0.5 to 1 hour prior to sun exposure and reapplied after swimming or sweating.

Altitude. Acute mountain sickness is common among travelers arriving at elevations above 10,000 feet. It may occur as low as 8000 feet. Symptoms include headache, dyspnea on exertion, dizziness, nausea, and insomnia. These symptoms usually subside after 2 to 3 days at high altitude. Double-blind trials have demonstrated the effectiveness of acetazolamide (Diamox), 250 mg tid in preventing acute mountain sickness when given 2 days prior to arrival at high altitude and continued for 2 to 3 days after arrival.[25] It is not known yet whether acetazolamide can prevent the more serious complications of altitude illness (pulmonary and cerebral edema) that rarely afflict hikers and skiers at very high elevations, usually above 12,000 feet.

Traffic. Automobiles and their drivers are the greatest health hazard for the tropical traveler. Cars and drivers should be selected with care, seat belts worn, and night driving discouraged.

Swimming. Undertow is a potential hazard on ocean beaches with good surf but no swimmers. Schistosomiasis is endemic in many freshwater ponds and streams in the tropics, thus swimming or bathing sites should be chosen

TABLE 74–5. MALARIA CHEMOPROPHYLAXIS

Indication	Drug	Dose
All malarious areas, except those with chloroquine-resistant strains of *Plasmodium falciparum*	Chloroquine phosphate	Adult: 500 mg po weekly (300-mg base) Child: 8.3 mg/kg/wk (not to exceed 500 mg total dose/wk)
Areas with chloroquine-resistant *P. falciparum*	Mefloquine	Adult: 250 mg po weekly (228-mg base) Child: See manufacturer's recommendation based on weight
Terminal prophylaxis for individuals at heavy risk of malaria exposure	Primaquine phosphate (rule out G6PD deficiency first)	Adult: 26.3 mg (15 mg base)/day for 14 days during last 2 weeks of chloroquine prophylaxis Child: 0.5 mg/kg/day for 14 days (not to exceed 26.3 mg [15 mg base]/day)

G6PD = glucose-6-phosphate dehydrogenase.

with care. Stagnant or slow-flowing streams near village washing and wading areas are particularly dangerous.

Insects. In addition to causing malaria, mosquitoes serve as vectors of a variety of viral and parasitic diseases. Use of a diethyltoluamide-containing insect repellent is helpful. Light-colored, long-sleeved shirts and blouses and trousers and slacks should be worn at dawn and dusk when most mosquito species are active. A mosquito net is a good idea if the traveler is sleeping in an unscreened dwelling.

Animal Bites. Peace Corps statistics record a tenfold increased incidence of animal bites in their volunteers over the rate expected in North America. Given the prevalence of rabies, contact with domestic animals should be limited to family pets and avoided completely if an animal appears ill. Animal bites should be washed carefully with soap and water, and rabies prophylaxis should be obtained as soon as possible.

Medication. Potentially dangerous drugs such as chloramphenicol are sold over-the-counter in many developing countries. Travelers should not take medication blindly or at the suggestion of local pharmacists. They should also avoid injected drugs for mild illnesses, since the use of unsterile needles is frequent.

Prevention and Treatment of Travelers' Diarrhea

The bane of travelers from temperate zones to the tropics, travelers' diarrhea afflicts 30 to 50% of North Americans visiting the developing world. Enterotoxigenic *Escherichia coli* are the major cause of travelers' diarrhea, although other enteric pathogens such as *Campylobacter, Shigella,* vibrios, and rotavirus may be important as well.[26]

"Turista" often begins during the first week of tropical travel and lasts 3 to 4 days. Abdominal cramps, nausea, and 3 to 15 watery bowel movements per day are typical. Dehydration is the major complication.

Although salad eaters and those adventurous enough to purchase meals from street vendors are at greatest risk, even fastidious individuals who follow the usual food and water precautions are susceptible.[27, 28] Numerous regimens designed to avoid turista persist in travel folklore, but there are only two proven preventive approaches (Table 74–6). The first, requiring doses of bismuth subsalicylate (Pepto-Bismol) qid is cumbersome.[29, 30] The second, the use of prophylactic antibiotics such as doxycycline, trimethoprim-sulfamethoxazole (TM/SZ) or oral quinolones, put travelers at risk of drug side effects (doxycycline:photosensitivity, vaginitis, candidiasis; TM/SZ:rash) and could potentiate infection by more troublesome organisms such as salmonella.[31–33] Prophylactic use of antibiotics should be limited to travelers planning short stays for whom 1 or 2 days of diarrhea would pose a major problem and to other travelers with underlying illness that might be exacerbated by turista.

TABLE 74–6. TRAVELERS' DIARRHEA

Prevention
Bismuth subsalicylate (Pepto-Bismol), 60 ml qid or 2 tablets (262 mg) qid
Trimethoprim/sulfamethoxazole, 160 mg TM/800 mg SZ (one tablet qd)
Doxycycline, 100 mg/day
Norfloxacin, 400 mg/day
Ciprofloxacin, 500 mg/day

Treatment
1. Fluid replacement (avoid dairy products)
2. Bismuth subsalicylate, 30 ml (1 oz) every 0.5 hr for a total of 8 doses (240 ml); may repeat on day 2 OR
   Trimethoprim/sulfamethoxazole, 1 double-strength tablet bid for 3–5 days OR
   Trimethoprim, 200 mg bid for 3–5 days (for sulfa-allergic patient) OR
   Ciprofloxacin, 500 mg bid for 3–5 days

3.* Loperamide, 4 mg; then 1 capsule (2 mg) after each loose movement, up to 8 capsules within 24 hours
   Diphenoxylate HCl (with atropine sulfate—Lomotil); do not exceed 2 tablets qid

*For symptom relief only; do not use in dysentery.

TABLE 74–7. FORMULA FOR TREATMENT OF DIARRHEAL DISEASE*

Prepare 2 separate glasses of the following:

Glass Number 1	
Orange, apple, or other fruit juice (rich in potassium)	8 oz
Honey or corn syrup (contains glucose necessary for absorption of essential salts)	$\frac{1}{2}$ tsp
Salt, table (contains sodium and chloride)	1 pinch
Glass Number 2	
Water (carbonated or boiled)	8 oz
Soda, baking (contains sodium bicarbonate)	$\frac{1}{4}$ tsp

Drink alternately from each glass until thirst is quenched. Supplement as desired with carbonated beverages, water, or tea made with boiled or carbonated water. Avoid solid foods and milk until recovery occurs. It is important that infants continue breast-feeding and receive plain water while receiving these solutions.

*From Centers for Disease Control: Health Information for International Travel, 1983. U.S. Department of Health and Human Services, Public Health Services, Aug., 1983.

A preferable alternative for most travelers is to treat turista at its onset. Mild symptoms may be treated with either bismuth subsalicylate or loperamide alone, while more severe symptoms respond to TM/SZ or ciprofloxacin.[34–38] This usually limits illness to 1 to 1.5 days' duration. A combination regimen of loperamide and an oral antibiotic is the most effective treatment for turista.[38] Maintaining adequate fluid intake is crucial; travelers should carry with them a recipe for replacement of fluid losses, such as that advocated by the CDC or electrolyte packets that can be reconstituted (Table 74–7). Bowel antiperistalsis agents help control symptoms but may exacerbate incipient dysentery and should not be used if patients have bloody diarrhea or a high fever. Kaopectate is of no benefit. Iodohydroxy-chloroquine (Enterovioform), an over-the-counter remedy in many countries, should be avoided because it is ineffective and causes subacute myelo-optic neuropathy.

Turista may recur repeatedly during long stays in the tropics, but travelers with persistent or recurrent diarrhea should be checked for other enteric pathogens.

High fever and bloody diarrhea or tenesmus (the dysentery syndrome) are not typical of turista and require immediate medical attention. True dysentery is fortunately uncommon among tourists to the tropics.

THE RETURNING TRAVELER (Table 74–8)

The asymptomatic traveler returning from a tour in the tropics seldom harbors latent infection.[39] Routine studies are usually unnecessary, with the possible exception of a PPD test and perhaps a complete blood count with differential and liver function tests. The symptomatic returnee, however, warrants thorough investigation.

Physicians should carefully review details of the itiner-

TABLE 74–8. DIAGNOSTIC STUDIES IN TROPICAL TRAVELERS

Asymptomatic Returnee	
Short-term	None
Long-term (over 1 month)	
Low-risk trip	None
High-risk trip*	CBC with differential Liver function tests PPD (Stool O and P optional)
Febrile Traveler	CBC with differential Liver function tests, chest film Urinalysis + culture Thick and thin smears for malaria × 3 (if returning from malarious area) Blood cultures × 2–3 *If negative, consider:* Stool cultures × 3 Stool O and P × 3 PPD *Brucella* agglutinins Liver ultrasound Schistosomiasis serology for individuals with risk by history
Traveler with Diarrhea	CBC with differential Liver function tests Fecal smear for leukocytes Stool cultures × 3 Stool O and P × 3 (Blood cultures, malaria smears if febrile)
Traveler with Eosinophilia	
Asymptomatic	Consider drug allergy Stool O and P × 3
Symptomatic	Stool O and P × 3 *If negative, consider:* Enterotest of duodenal aspirate Schistosomiasis serology if at risk Urine examination for *S. haematobium* ova if at risk Filariasis serology and blood smear examination if at risk

*Rural travel, health-care workers, biologists, anthropologists, and so on.
CBC = complete blood count; PPD = purified protein derivative.

ary to assess the risk of exotic illness. For example, a businessman returning from a stay in a western-style hotel in a major city in the tropics is very unlikely to acquire endemic disease. But a student hiking through rural areas runs a significant risk of exposure to local diseases. Physicians should inquire about diet (e.g., rare meats, shellfish, raw milk), contact with local populations, swimming, exposure to insects, and the type of dwellings visited. A careful review of any medications taken abroad is important. An estimate of the possible incubation period of the illness helps to limit the differential diagnosis (Table 74–9).

Fever. Any febrile illness occurring within 6 months of return must be taken seriously, particularly if the patient has been in a malarious area. Falciparum malaria is life threatening and has protean manifestations. It often presents as a "flu-like" illness without a characteristic fever pattern.[41] Although falciparum malaria appears within a few months of return, vivax and ovale malaria may remain latent for up to 3 years. Physicians should carefully examine both thick and thin blood smears for malaria in all travelers with persistent or recurrent fever. If the results of initial smears are negative but clinical suspicion remains high, empiric antimalarial therapy may be justified while considering other possibilities. Malaria serology can be obtained for confirmation.

Typhoid and paratyphoid fevers are also important considerations in the febrile traveler. There is frequently no history of gastrointestinal distress and few clues on physical examination. Blood, stool, and urine cultures should be obtained. Rarely, bone marrow culture is necessary to confirm the diagnosis.

Liver function tests are important in all febrile travelers to rule out viral hepatitis. Amebic liver abscess may present solely with fever and no antecedent diarrhea. Right upper quadrant tenderness is common but not universal. An ultrasound study of the liver usually reveals the defect, and amebic serology is positive despite the frequent occurrence of negative results on stool examinations.

Further work-up of the febrile traveler should be guided by a careful history, physical examination, and review of the itinerary and of likely differential diagnoses.[42] Other important considerations include brucellosis, tuberculosis, rickettsial diseases, arboviruses, and endemic parasitic disease like filariasis, schistosomiasis, and leishmaniasis.

Because of the remote risk of viral hemorrhagic fever (Lassa, Ebola, Marburg) in the febrile returnee from rural west or central Africa (particularly if the results of malaria smears are negative), early infectious disease consultation is advisable.[43]

Diarrhea. Travelers' diarrhea rarely lasts for more than a week unless complicated by lactose intolerance. The returning traveler with persistent diarrhea must be investigated for treatable enteric bacteria and parasites. *Campylobacter* enteritis is a particularly common bacterial cause of persistent or relapsing diarrhea. Other important considerations include salmonella, Shigella and noncholera vibrios. *Giardia* is the most commonly encountered intestinal parasite, with *Entamoeba histolytica* and helminths occurring relatively infrequently. If the traveler used antibiotics during the trip, pseudomembranous enterocolitis should also be considered.

A stool smear for polymorphonuclear leukocytes is usually positive in invasive bacterial diarrhea. Three stool cultures, including media for *Campylobacter,* should be obtained, along with a careful examination for ova and parasites. Antacids, laxatives, antibiotics, and barium studies interfere with stool examination for parasites, thus stool collections should be delayed several days to 1 week if these

TABLE 74–9. INCUBATION PERIODS OF TRAVELERS' INFECTIONS

Short (1–7 Days)	*Rare*
Travelers' diarrhea	Yellow fever
*Campylobacter**	Leptospirosis
Shigella	Relapsing fever*
Salmonella enteritis*	
Dengue	
Ciguatera poisoning*	
Intermediate (7–27 Days)	*Rare*
Malaria*	Typhus
Typhoid, paratyphoid*	Q fever*
Hepatitis A	Trypanosomiasis*
Amebiasis*	Viral hemorrhagic fever
Giardiasis*	Schistosomiasis
Brucellosis*	(Katayama fever)*
	Poliomyelitis
Long (>27 Days)	*Rare*
Malaria*	Leishmaniasis*
Hepatitis B*	Schistosomiasis*
	Tuberculosis*
	Filariasis*
	Rabies

*Prolonged or relapsing course possible.

substances have been used. Inexperienced technicians may mistake *Entamoeba coli,* a nonpathogen, or leukocytes for *E. histolytica.*[44] Other nonpathogenic amebae, such as *Endolimax nana,* are not treated, although they may indicate a higher likelihood of concurrent *E. histolytica* infection. Travelers infected with *Balantidium coli* or *Dientamoeba fragilis* are usually treated with tetracyclines. *Blastocystis hominis* is frequently identified in stool samples from travelers with diarrhea, but its possible role as a pathogen is uncertain, and treatment is not generally recommended.

If the results of stool cultures and ova and parasite examinations are negative but symptoms persist, an empiric trial of metronidazole or quinacrine for presumed giardiasis is reasonable.

Chronic diarrhea without an obvious infectious cause requires a logical approach to its long differential diagnosis, as outlined in Chapter 27. Physicians should keep in mind the possibility of tropical sprue, particularly in travelers who have lived in Southeast Asia or the Caribbean.[45] These individuals develop a malabsorption syndrome with weight loss, steatorrhea, and often a sore tongue. Blunting of intestinal microvilli is seen on small bowel biopsy. Tropical sprue usually responds to a combination of tetracycline and vitamin B_{12} and folate supplements.

Rash. Many diseases cause fever and rash, including arboviruses (i.e., dengue), rickettsia, relapsing fever, rubella, rubeola, leptospirosis, syphilis, typhoid, filariasis, and acute schistosomiasis. However, physicians should always remember the more likely possibility of drug allergy caused by antibiotics or by the traveler's antimalarial regimen.

Boils acquired during tropical travel are usually due to *Staphylococcus.* However, myiasis is possible, particularly if the boil forms an ulcerated crater or movement is perceived within the lesion. Application of petroleum jelly over the ulceration often results in emerging of the offending larva.

Chronic indolent skin lesions require expert evaluation, with consideration of atypical mycobacteria, leprosy, fungi, cutaneous diphtheria, tropical ulcer, leishmaniasis, and yaws. A biopsy is usually needed to make a specific diagnosis.

Eosinophilia. Asymptomatic individuals with eosinophilia most likely have light helminth infestion caused by *Strongyloides, Ascaris, Trichuris,* or hookworm. Rarely, filariasis, trichinosis, schistosomiasis, or clonorchiasis may be the cause of unexplained eosinophilia. Protozoan (*Giardia, E. histolytica*) infections do not typically produce eosinophilia. Stool collections for ova and parasite examinations to yield a specific diagnosis are a reasonable first step, but additional studies may be required, depending on the traveler's risk of exposure to different parasites.

Eosinophilia in the presence of fever often indicates drug allergy, but filariasis and schistosomiasis are concerns in the traveler returning from an endemic area.

REFERENCES

1. Lobel HO, Campbell CC, Pappaionou M, et al: Use of prophylaxis for malaria by American travelers to Africa and Haiti. JAMA 257:2626, 1987.
2. Centers for Disease Control: Health information for international travel 1991. MMWR (Suppl), 1992.
3. Kendrick MA: Study of illness among Americans returning from international travel. J Infect Dis 126:694, 1972.
4. Peltola H, Kyronseppa H, Holsa P, et al: Trips to the South—a health hazard. Scand J Infect Dis 15:375, 1983.
5. Gangarosa EJ, Kendrick MA, Loewenstein MS, et al: Global travel and travelers' health. Aviat Space Environ Med 51:265, 1980.
6. Centers for Disease Control: Malaria Surveillance Annual Summary, 1977. Atlanta, US Public Health Service, Centers for Disease Control, 1977.
7. Steffen R: Typhoid vaccine, for whom? (Letter) Lancet ii:615, 1982.
8. Steffen R, Rickenbach M, Wilhelm U, et al: Health problems after travel to developing countries. J Infect Dis 156:84, 1987.
9. American Diabetes Association: Vacationing with Diabetes. New York, American Diabetes Association.
10. Kilbourne EM, Choc K, Jones TS, et al: Risk factors for heat stroke. JAMA 247:3332, 1982.
11. Gong H: Advising patients with pulmonary diseases on air travel (Editorial). Ann Intern Med 111:549, 1989.
12. Mann JM, Bernier RH, and Hinman AR: Poliomyelitis vaccination for the international traveler. Am Fam Physician 26:135, 1982.
13. Centers for Disease Control: Yellow fever vaccine. Ann Intern Med 100:540, 1984.
14. Snyder J and Blake PA: Is cholera a problem for U.S. travelers? JAMA 247:2268, 1982.
15. Morger H, Steffen R, and Schar M: Epidemiology of cholera in travelers, and conclusions for vaccine recommendations. BMJ 286:184, 1983.
16. Woodruff BA, Pavia AT, and Blake PA: A new look at typhoid vaccination: Information for the practicing physician. JAMA 265:756, 1991.
17. Christenson B: Epidemiological aspects of acute viral hepatitis A in Swedish travelers to endemic areas. Scand J Infect Dis 17:5, 1985.
18. Centers for Disease Control: Safety of therapeutic immune globulin preparations with respect to transmission of HTLV-III/LAV infection. MMWR 35:231, 1986.
19. Pappaioanou M, Fishbein D, Orresen D, et al: Antibody response to pre-exposure human diploid-cell rabies vaccine given concurrently with chloroquine. N Engl J Med 314:280, 1986.
20. Appleton B, Wolfe MS, and Mishtowt GI: Chloroquine as a malaria suppressive: Absence of visual effects. Milit Med 225, 1973.
21. Editorial: Malaria prophylaxis for long-term visitors. BMJ 287:1454, 1983.
22. Lobel HO, Bernard KW, Williams SL, et al: Effectiveness and tolerance of long-term malaria prophylaxis with mefloquine. JAMA 265:361, 1991.
23. Miller KD, Lobel HO, Satriale RF, et al: Severe cutaneous reactions among American travelers using pyrimethamine-sulfadoxine (Fansidar) for malaria prophylaxis. Am J Trop Med Hyg 35(3):451, 1986.
24. Health Hints for the Tropics. 8th ed. Supplement to Tropical Medicine and Hygiene News. Wheaton, MD, American Society of Tropical Medicine and Hygiene, 1980.
25. Larson EB, Roach RC, Schoene RB, et al: Acute mountain sickness and acetazolamide: Clinical efficacy and effect on ventilation. JAMA 248:328, 1982.
26. Merson MH, Morris GK, Sack DA, et al: Travelers' diarrhea in Mexico. N Engl J Med 294:1299, 1976.
27. Tjoa WS, DuPont HL, Sullivan P, et al: Location of food consumption and travelers' diarrhea. Am J Epidemiol 106:61, 1977.
28. Steffen R, van der Linde F, Gyr K, et al: Epidemiology of diarrhea in travelers. JAMA 249:1176, 1983.
29. DuPont HL, Sullivan P, Evans DG, et al: Prevention of travelers' diarrhea (emporiatric enteritis): Prophylactic administration of subsalicylate bismuth. JAMA 243:237, 1980.
30. DuPont HC, Ericsson CD, Johnson PC, et al: Prevention of travelers' diarrhea by the tablet formulation of bismuth subsalicylate. JAMA 257:1347, 1987.
31. Sack DA, Kaminsky DC, Sack RB, et al: Prophylactic doxycycline for travelers' diarrhea. N Engl J Med 298:758, 1978.
32. DuPont HL, Galindo E, Evans DG, et al: Prevention of travelers' diarrhea with trimethoprim/sulfamethoxazole and trimethoprim alone. Gastroenterology 84:75, 1983.
33. Scott DA, Haberberger RL, Thornton SA, et al: Norfloxacin for the prophylaxis of travelers' diarrhea in US military personnel. Am J Trop Med Hyg 42:160, 1990.

34. Graham Dy, Estes MK, and Gentry LO: Double-blind comparison of bismuth subsalicylate and placebo in the prevention and treatment of enterotoxigenic *E. coli*–induced diarrhea in volunteers. Gastroenterology 85:1017, 1983.
35. Johnson PC, Ericsson CD, DuPont HL, et al: Comparison of loperamide with bismuth subsalicylate for the treatment of acute travelers' diarrhea. JAMA 255:757, 1986.
36. DuPont L, Reves RR, Galindo E, et al: Treatment of travelers' diarrhea with trimethoprim/sulfamethoxazole and with trimethoprim alone. N Engl J Med 307:841, 1982.
37. Ericsson CD, DuPont HL, Mathewson JJ, et al: Treatment of travelers' diarrhea with sulfamethoxazole and trimethoprim and loperamide. JAMA 263:257, 1990.
38. Ericsson CD, Johnson PC, DuPont HL, et al: Ciprofloxacin or trimethoprim-sulfamethoxazole as initial therapy for travelers' diarrhea: A placebo-controlled trial. Ann Intern Med 106:216, 1987.
38a. DuPont HL and Ericsson CD: Prevention and treatment of traveler's diarrhea. N Engl J Med 328:1821–1827, 1993.
39. Effersoe P: Check-ups after tours of duty to the tropics. Scand J Infect Dis 9:137, 1979.
40. Brown K and Phillips SM: Tropical diseases of importance to the traveler. Annu Rev Intern Med 59, 1984.
41. Kean H and Reilly PC Jr: Malaria—the mime: Recent lessons from a group of civilian travelers. Am J Med 61:159, 1976.
42. Wolfe MS: Management of the returnee from exotic places. J Occup Med 21:691, 1979.
43. Zweighaft RM, Fraser DW, and Hattwick MA: Lassa fever: Response to an imported case. N Engl J Med 297:803, 1977.
44. Krogstad DJ, Spencer HC Jr, and Healy GR: Amebiasis. N Engl J Med 298:262, 1978.
45. Klipstein FA and Falaiye JM: Tropical sprue in expatriates from the tropics living in the continental U.S. Medicine 43:475, 1969.

75

Antibiotic Prophylaxis for Transient Bacteremias

J. BARCLAY ADAMS, MD, PhD

Transient bacteremias are a common occurrence in some dental and medical procedures and pose a risk of initiating a serious infection. This risk can be diminished in some cases by the prophylactic use of antibiotics. This chapter offers recommendations for such use applicable to situations that might occur in an office practice of general medicine. The topics discussed include procedures that might be done in the office (e.g., sigmoidoscopy or minor superficial surgery) and questions that might arise in the course of consultation for colleagues in dentistry or radiology. Procedures of medical subspecialty practice (e.g., colonoscopy or cystoscopy) and issues in more invasive surgical practice or in obstetrical practice are excluded.

A decision to recommend prophylactic use of antibiotics when a transient bacteremia may occur is a compound of judgments of the risk of potential infection, the risk and the cost of antibiotic treatment, and the likelihood of benefit of prophylaxis. In many circumstances the small amount of data available allows some latitude in judgments. Reasonable and thoughtful individuals differ in their recommendations.

CONDITIONS AT RISK

Abnormalities of the anatomy in the circulatory system and implanted foreign bodies are potential sites for the establishment of infection. The risks may be modulated by systemic factors that compromise host defenses.

In the circulatory system turbulent flow or endothelial damage can set up a matrix of fibrin and platelets to which bacteria can adhere to establish an infection. Such fibrin matrices occur in the heart with damaged or abnormal valves and put them at risk for the development of bacterial endocarditis.[1, 2] Valves with fixed murmurs clearly fall into this category of risk. Mitral valve prolapse, the most common valvular variant,[3] is emerging as the most common seat of endocarditis.[4]

Because of its prevalence mitral valve prolapse warrants special consideration. The diagnosis of mitral valve prolapse encompasses a spectrum of conditions. The prolapse can be manifest on physical examination as an isolated systolic click, a click with an intermittent murmur, or a click with a fixed murmur. Mitral valve prolapse, myxomatous degeneration, and regurgitant flow can be manifest as ultrasonographic findings. The interpretation of ultrasonographs depends on the criteria selected for definition of mitral prolapse. The findings of color Doppler studies of mitral regurgitation can be discordant with auscultatory findings, although there is a strong trend associating the general severity of regurgitation as assessed by auscultation versus color Doppler.[5] Some patients with mitral valve prolapse are at increased risk of endocarditis, but it is not known where in the spectrum of mitral valve prolapse lies the threshold of significant risk.[6]

Other valvular lesions carry the risk of endocarditis. Among them are aortic stenosis or insufficiency, mitral stenosis or insufficiency, and disease of the tricuspid or pulmonic valves.[2] Hypertrophic obstructive cardiomyopathy is associated with endocarditis.[7] Prior bacterial endocarditis carries an increased risk of a new infection, although a substantial fraction of cases can be attributed to illicit use of intravenous drugs.[8] An increased frequency of bacterial endocarditis has been reported in small studies of patients with systemic lupus erythematosus.[9] It is not known whether this may be caused by Libman-Sacks lesions, which can be difficult to detect, or to other compromise of host defenses. Prosthetic valves, both mechanical and bioprosthetic, carry a high risk of endocarditis.[10]

Of the many species of bacteria residing in the mouth and bowel, strikingly few establish endocarditis with significant frequency. This selection may be on the basis of the adhesive qualities of the bacterial coating. The bacterial endocarditis from bacteremias from oral sources are dominantly species of viridans streptococci. The dominant bacteria establishing endocarditis from the gut and genitourinary sources are species of group D streptococci and much less frequently gram-negative bacilli. From skin, *Staphylococcus epidermidis* and *S. aureus* are the most frequent causes of endocarditis.[1, 2]

Nonvalvular heart lesions with flow from a high-pressure chamber to a low-pressure chamber entail a risk of endocarditis. These lesions are ventricular septal defect, patent ductus arteriosus, and coarctation of the aorta. Surgically constructed arteriopulmonary shunts are at high risk. Atrial septal defects, atherosclerotic plaques, coronary artery disease, repaired cardiac lesions with closure of defects, and coronary artery bypass grafts have very low risk of endocarditis.[2] Cardiac pacemaker infections at times remote from implantation are rare and are not thought to be caused by bacteremias from medical procedures.[10] Atheromatous plaques and arterial aneurysms are at very low risk for infection. Without prosthetic materials, healed vascular surgery including arteriovenous shunts do not carry a risk of infection. With prosthetic materials vascular grafts more than 1 year after implantation appear to carry a very small risk of infection, with the possible exception of arteriovenous shunts.[11–13] The bacteria of prosthetic arteriovenous shunt infections are usually those of the skin. Interestingly, vena cava filters have not been reported to have a significant risk of infection via hematogenous seeding.[14]

Remote postoperative infection at fixed orthopedic hardware, such as screws or plates, is very rare and thought not to arise from transient bacteremia. Infection attributable to bacteremia from dental or medical procedures late after the implantation of prosthetic joints occurs seldom if ever, but the consequences of prosthetic joint infection are serious. There is controversy with regard to the estimation of the importance of this risk.[15, 16]

An established breast implant is rarely the site of infection, and those that occur are usually caused by *S. aureus*.[17] Bacteremic infection at the site of genitourinary prostheses has been observed.[18] Cerebrospinal fluid shunts have not been reported to be infected by hematogenous sources.[19] Viridans streptococcal bacteremia has been observed as a cause of peritonitis in patients with continuous ambulatory peritoneal dialysis catheters.[20] Several bacterial species have been reported as causing infections with peritoneovenous shunts, but it is not known whether transient bacteremias due to procedures were causal.[21] Hematogenous spread to an intraocular lens implant has not been reported.[22]

The risk of infection in any situation can be modulated by systemic factors that compromise host defense mechanisms. Acquired immunodeficiency syndrome (AIDS) greatly increases the risk of infections. A high rate of bacterial endocarditis has been noted in this population, although much of the excess may be caused by illicit intravenous drug administration.[23] The patient who has had a splenectomy is at risk of overwhelming sepsis. It would be reasonable to take this into account when performing manipulations that would result in transient bacteremias, although there have been no reports of such events.[24] Substantial renal insufficiency, liver failure, poorly controlled diabetes, treatment with corticosteroids, immune suppression for transplantation, and some courses of chemotherapy all can impede host response to infection.[25, 26] Increased risk of endocarditis in patients with inflammatory bowel disease has been observed.[27] It is not known whether this is due to increased exposure to bacteremia or to some compromise of immune response.

SOURCES OF BACTEREMIA

The sites of natural carriage of bacteria are the nares, the mouth, the lower bowel, the vagina, and the skin. When the integrity of the epithelial surfaces of these sites is violated, bacteria may gain entry to the blood stream. It has been demonstrated that normal activities such as chewing, tooth brushing, and defecation give rise to transient bacteremias.[28] The low incidence of development of hematogenous infection suggests that bacterial doses below a minimal threshold must usually be clinically insignificant.

Since the gingival crevice is populated with a large variety of bacteria, dental procedures that cause gingival bleeding,[25] including professional cleaning and scaling, and endodentistry, cause detectable bacteremias.[29] Dental procedures confined to the crown of the tooth and anesthetic injections through uninfected gingiva do not appear to give rise to significant bacteremias.[30] Dental extraction always gives rise to a bacteremia that can be of high grade if coming from an abscess.

The importance of bacteremias induced by manipulation of the lower intestinal tract is disputed. Fecal flora have been reported in the blood stream after digital rectal examination and after a barium enema.[31] There is evidence implicating sigmoidoscopy in some cases of endocarditis.[32] Bacteremia may be more frequent and of higher grade after a biopsy is done or when the bowel is distended.[31]

Urinary catheterization can cause bacteremia. However,

even for a colonized bladder, transient catheterization does not appear to carry significant risk.[33]

Bacteremias are caused by manipulation or drainage of infected skin lesions and are thought to be the source of bacteria for some endocarditis and some vascular shunt infections.

PROPHYLAXIS

For patients at risk for the establishment of infection through transient bacteremias, primary prophylaxis consists of minimizing local infections that may be the source of seeding of the blood stream. Good dental and gingival hygiene should be maintained. Prompt attention should be given to skin lesions to prevent the establishment of a local infection.

Topical antibiotics can reduce the burden of bacteremia in dental procedures.[30] The application of chlorhexidine to the gingiva is recommended in oral surgery.[34]

Recommendations for the use of systemic antibiotics to prevent the establishment of infection by a transient bacteremia are based largely on anecdotal evidence and on the use of experimental animal models of uncertain relevance to human disease.[35–38] The most studied infection is bacterial endocarditis. It has been estimated that the chance that an at-risk patient without antibiotic prophylaxis develops endocarditis is as low as one in 115,000 episodes of bacteremia.[39] The low frequency of infections makes prospective controlled trials of prophylaxis in a patient population not practicable. Fewer than 20% of cases of bacterial endocarditis can be attributed to bacteremias caused by procedures.[2, 40] Recommended regimens are not always successful in the prevention of endocarditis.[41] The reduction in the total number of cases of bacterial endocarditis by universal practice of the recommended prophylaxis would be modest. Nonetheless, three case-control studies have assembled some evidence on the efficacy of antibiotic prophylaxis in the reduction of risk in bacterial endocarditis. Two studies have been restricted to native cardiac lesions. One study that suggests 91% efficacy must be assessed with some caution, because the study is based on only eight cases.[42] A much larger study estimated the efficacy at 49%, but this result was not statistically significant.[40] The third study focused on prosthetic valves and found clear evidence for the benefits of prophylaxis.[43] Arguments can be advanced that even at relatively low levels of efficacy, prophylaxis is worthwhile.[44]

In the selection of antibiotics it is not possible to cover all potential pathogens, and attention is focused only on those that are most often found to cause disease. Eradication of an established infection requires bactericidal antibiotics. However, prevention of the establishment of an infection can be accomplished by bacteriostatic antibiotics and those that merely alter bacterial adhesiveness.[25, 38] Bacteremias arising from medical and dental manipulations are naturally cleared by the body in only a few minutes. The experimental animal models indicate that sustaining serum antibiotic levels for a few hours is sufficient to prevent the development of a fixed infection.

A recommendation for antibiotic prophylaxis must weigh the risk of infection against the risk of an adverse reaction to the antibiotic program. Antibiotics can cause minor or serious allergic reactions. Even brief prophylactic programs have caused pseudomembranous colitis.[45, 46] Gentamicin can cause renal failure. The use of antibiotics can select for resistant bacterial strains in the patient's flora. The risk of infection from bacteremia is so low that the risks of adverse reactions to antibiotics can be comparable in magnitude.[47, 48] To be effective, a program must also be accepted by both the patient and the practitioner as tolerable in convenience and cost.

High serum levels of erythromycin provide good protection in animal models against the common infective agents of mouth flora, principally the viridans streptococci, in bacteremias,[49] although the human levels are not bactericidal.[50] Erythromycin has also a very low frequency of allergic reactions. Two doses are needed for adequate duration of serum levels. Unfortunately, the doses needed for prophylaxis frequently cause gastrointestinal distress. The frequency of this reaction is lower with the esters, erythromycin ethylsuccinate and erythromycin stearate. The newer macrolides now available, clarithromycin and azithromycin, offer a spectrum of antibiotic coverage similar to erythromycin and have the advantage of less gastrointestinal upset.[51] There is no reason to suppose that these medications are less effective than is erythromycin in the prevention of the development of an established infection after transient bacteremia; however, trials of their use in this way in animal models have not yet been carried out. Until such trials are reported, clarithromycin 1 g po 1 hour before the procedure might be an acceptable last alternative if the standard regimens are intolerable or completely impractical.

The penicillins provide good antibiotic coverage for transient bacteremias of mouth flora that are likely to establish infections. Ampicillin and amoxicillin have a broader spectrum of activity than has penicillin, and these drugs offer some benefit in prophylaxis against bowel and urinary tract flora. Amoxicillin is the most reliably absorbed of the penicillins, making it the oral penicillin of choice. Ampicillin is recommended for parenteral use. Both amoxicillin and ampicillin must be given in two separate doses. Some patients find the recommended 3-g dose of amoxicillin difficult to take. An attractive alternative of 1 g of amoxicillin plus 1 g of probenecid has been advanced.[52] This one-dose program gives an adequate duration of satisfactory serum levels.

Clindamycin is a reasonable choice for patients who are intolerant of erythromycin and who are allergic to the penicillins. The risk of pseudomembranous colitis following its use in a single dose appears to be very small.[53]

For patients at especially high risk, gentamicin can be added to therapy with amoxicillin or ampicillin for improved coverage of mouth flora. This drug must be given parenterally, but it need be given only once. The use of gentamicin always entails the risk of renal failure. Doses must be limited for smaller patients.

Coverage of gastrointestinal and genitourinary flora must prevent the establishment of infection by enterococci. In low-risk situations, amoxicillin or ampicillin may provide adequate therapy, but in moderate- or high-risk situations because of the relative resistance of some of these bacteria to penicillins, an aminoglycoside (e.g., gentamicin) should be added.

For patients who are allergic to penicillin and who are at high risk, vancomycin can be used alone for oral flora and vancomycin plus gentamicin can be used for gastrointestinal and genitourinary flora. However, vancomycin must be given intravenously and is expensive. Therapy with teicoplanin may offer an alternative to vancomycin and may have fewer side effects.[53]

RECOMMENDATIONS

A set of recommendations for specific use of antibiotics in specific conditions is set forth in Tables 75–1 to 75–5.

TABLE 75–1. RELATIVE RISK OF ANATOMIC CONDITIONS

Conditions with high risk of infection
Prosthetic cardiac valves and valve xenografts
Surgically constructed arterial pulmonary shunts
Heart valves with history of prior endocarditis
Conditions with moderate risk of infection
Heart valves with murmur
Hypertrophic stenotic cardiomyopathy with murmur
Unrepaired ventricular septal defect
Arteriovenous shunts with prosthetic material
Prosthetic vascular grafts during first year after implantation
Urogenital implants
Systemic lupus erythematosus
Peritoneovenous shunts
Peritoneal dialysis catheter
Prosthetic joints that have been reoperated
Conditions with low risk of infection
Prosthetic joints
Cardiac pacemakers
Cerebrospinal fluid drainage shunts
Conditions with negligible risk of infection
Mitral prolapse without murmur
Repaired ventricular or atrial septal defect
Autologous vein grafting, both coronary and peripheral
Prosthetic vascular grafts more than 1 year after implantation
Breast implants
Fixed orthopedic hardware
Intraocular lens implants
Vena cava filters
Arterial aneurysms
Atherosclerotic plaques

These are generally consonant with current recommendations of committees.[31, 34, 53–55] Controversy surrounds several points. Some favor more vigorous prophylaxis for prosthetic joints.[56] The available systemic studies would seem to support the recommendations made here.[57] Some advocate more vigorous prophylaxis for cardiac pacemakers.[58] Practices with sigmoidoscopy vary.[31] Some favor prophylaxis for all detected lesions of mitral valve prolapse. The recommendations here for prophylaxis of mitral valve prolapse with only a murmur are based on an estimate of the risk and benefit of prophylaxis.[6] As a matter of practicality, they do not require that every patient suspected of mitral valve prolapse have echocardiography. Table 75–1 offers a rough scale for the potential of various conditions for the establishment of an infection. Table 75–2 is a rough guide to the levels of bacteremia expected in various procedures. Table 75–3 contains doses, routes, and schedules for the antibiotics recommended for adult patients. Table 75–4 gives recommendations for the selection of a regimen for oral flora from Table 75–3 using the risk of infection and the level of bacteremia given in Tables 75–1 and 75–2. Table 75–5 does the same for gastrointestinal and genitourinary flora.

TABLE 75–2. LEVELS OF SOURCES OF BACTEREMIA

Sources of high levels of bacteremia
Extraction of tooth from abscess
Periodontal surgery on highly infected gingiva
Incision of abscess
Sources of moderate levels of bacteremia
Professional dental cleaning
Scaling of teeth
Periodontal surgery
Endodentistry
Sigmoidoscopy with inflammatory bowel disease or biopsy
Sources of low levels of bacteremia
Sigmoidoscopy without inflammatory bowel disease
Barium enema
Catheterization of the infected bladder
Sources of negligible levels of bacteremia
Dental procedures restricted to the crown of the tooth
Tooth brushing by patient
Rectal examination
Routine pelvic examination
Catheterization of sterile bladder

TABLE 75–3. ANTIBIOTIC REGIMENS FOR PROPHYLAXIS FOR ADULTS

Erythromycin
Erythromycin ethylsuccinate 800 mg po 2 hours before and 400 mg po 6 hours after the procedure *or* erythromycin stearate 1 g po 2 hours before and 500 mg po 6 hours after the procedure
Amoxicillin
Amoxicillin 3 g po 1 hour before and 1.5 g po 6 hours after the procedure *or* amoxicillin 1 g po plus probenecid 1 g po 1 hour before the procedure
Clindamycin oral
Clindamycin 300 mg po 1 hour before and 150 mg po 6 hours after the procedure
Clindamycin parenteral
Clindamycin 300 mg in 50 ml IV over 10 minutes 30 minutes before and 150 mg in 50 ml IV over 10 minutes 6 hours after the procedure
Ampicillin
Ampicillin 2 g IV or IM 30 minutes before and 1 g IV or IM 6 hours after the procedure
Gentamicin
Gentamicin 1.5 mg/kg not to exceed 80 mg IV or IM 30 minutes before and same dose 6 hours after the procedure
Vancomycin
Vancomycin 1 g IV over 1 hour starting 1 hour before the procedure
Dicloxacillin
Dicloxacillin 1 g po 1 hour before and 500 mg 6 hours after procedure

IM = intramuscularly; IV = intravenously; po = by mouth.

For conditions with low, moderate, or high risk for infection for which incision of a skin abscess is planned, a minimal program of prophylaxis would be one of the regimens from Table 75–3—dicloxacillin, erythromycin, or oral clindamycin. For an abscess that is likely to contain staphylococci, breast prostheses should be considered at low (not negligible) risk. Usually the appropriate treatment of a skin abscess would itself require a more prolonged course of antibiotic therapy.

The absence of a fully satisfactory oral program for some situations can pose a practical problem. In office practice the use of vancomycin intravenously or even gentamicin intramuscularly can be daunting. A routine periodontal

TABLE 75–4. RECOMMENDED ANTIBIOTIC REGIMENS FOR ORAL FLORA

	High-Level Bacteremia	Low- or Moderate-Level Bacteremia
High risk of infection	Ampicillin plus gentamicin or vancomycin alone	Amoxicillin or erythromycin or clindamycin oral
Medium risk of infection	Erythromycin or amoxicillin or clindamycin oral	Erythromycin
Low risk of infection	Erythromycin	None

TABLE 75–5. RECOMMENDED ANTIBIOTIC REGIMENS FOR GASTROINTESTINAL OR GENITOURINARY FLORA

	High-Level Bacteremia	Low- or Moderate-Level Bacteremia
High risk of infection	Ampicillin plus gentamicin or vancomycin plus gentamicin	Amoxicillin
Medium risk of infection	Amoxicillin	None
Low risk of infection	Amoxicillin	None

surgery or a urinary tract evaluation for the patient who is intolerant of penicillin or erythromycin may require coordination with a hospital day surgery or outpatient service or expensive intravenous administration at the patient's home. A difficult decision that involves balancing cost and convenience versus risks is required.

Doses of penicillin that are appropriate for prophylaxis of rheumatic fever are inadequate prophylaxis for transient bacteremias. If a patient is on chronic penicillin treatment for any reason, it should be presumed that the flora are resistant to penicillin, and one of the alternative regimens should be used. Because of the rapid emergence of antibiotic resistance in flora, procedures needing antibiotic prophylaxis should be spaced by more than 1 week whenever possible.

The estimation of risk listed in Table 75–1 might be increased by one rank if there is a concurrent systemic condition that might impede normal host defense mechanisms. The most important of these are listed in Table 75–6. In the case of advanced AIDS, the risk may be so great that prophylactic antibiotics may be required even if there is no anatomic abnormality at unusual risk of infection.

The estimation of the level of bacteremia in Table 75–2 might be increased by one rank for manipulations in fields that have an unusually heavy bacterial population or that cause exceptional loss of integrity of the mucosal surface.

If anticipatory prophylaxis has not been given in a situation in which it might be appropriate, there is some reason to believe that giving a course of antibiotics up to 48 hours after the procedure could diminish the risk of infection.[59]

As with decisions on the use of postmenopausal estrogen replacement, in some cases it might be appropriate to invite the patient to participate in the decision regarding the use of prophylactic antibiotics. The risks, potential benefits, and uncertainties associated with different potential courses of action could be frankly discussed with the patient. If desired by the patient, the practitioner could offer a recommendation, but the patient could make a choice in keeping with his or her own values.

An active practitioner will at times be required to deal with circumstances that are not covered by any guidelines. It is hoped that the recommendations in this chapter can be of some help in the necessary exercise of sound clinical judgment.

TABLE 75–6. SYSTEMIC CONDITIONS INCREASING RISK OF INFECTION

Diabetes mellitus in poor control
Renal insufficiency of substantial degree
Hepatic insufficiency
Steroids used orally or parenterally
Chemotherapy affecting the immune system
Acquired immunodeficiency syndrome
Splenectomized patient
Rheumatoid arthritis for prosthetic joints

REFERENCES

1. Weinstein L: Infective endocarditis. *In* Braunwald E (ed): Heart Disease, 3rd ed. Philadelphia, WB Saunders, 1988, pp 1093–1134.
2. Durack DT: Infective and noninfective endocarditis. *In* Hurst JW, Schlant RC, Rackley CE, et al (eds): The Heart, Arteries, and Veins, 7th ed. New York, McGraw-Hill, 1990, pp 1230–1255.
3. Levy D and Savage D: Prevalence and clinical features of mitral valve prolapse. Am Heart J 113(5):1281, 1987.
4. McKinsey DS, Ratts TE, and Bisno AL: Underlying cardiac lesions in adults with infective endocarditis: The changing spectrum. Am J Med 82(4):681, 1987.
5. Rahko PS: Prevalence of regurgitant murmurs in patients with valvular regurgitation detected by Doppler echocardiography. Ann Intern Med 111(6):466, 1989.
6. MacMahon SW, Roberts JK, Kramer-Fox R, et al: Mitral valve prolapse and infective endocarditis. Am Heart J 113(5):1291, 1987.
7. Alessandri N, Pannarale G, del Monte F, et al: Hypertropic obstructive cardiomyopathy and infective endocarditis: A report of seven cases and a review of the literature. Eur Heart J 11(11):1041, 1990.
8. Baddour LM: Twelve-year review of recurrent native-valve infective endocarditis: A disease of the modern antibiotic era. Rev Infect Dis 10(6):1163, 1988.
9. Luce EB, Montgomery MT, and Redding SW: The prevalence of cardiac valvular pathosis in patients with systemic lupus erythematosus. Oral Surg Oral Med Oral Pathol 70(5):590, 1990.
10. Heimberger TS and Duma RJ: Infections of prosthetic heart valves and cardiac pacemakers. Infect Dis Clin North Am 3(2):221, 1989.
11. Karchmer AW and Bisno AL: Infections of prosthetic heart valves and vascular grafts. *In* Bisno AL and Waldvogel FA (eds): Infections Associated with Indwelling Medical Devices. Washington, DC, American Society for Microbiology, 1989, pp 129–159.
12. Zibari GB, Rohr MS, Landreneau MD, et al: Complications from permanent hemodialysis vascular access. Surgery 104(4):681, 1988.
13. Freischlag JA and Moore WS: Infection in prosthetic vascular grafts. *In* Rutherford RB (ed): Vascular Surgery, 3rd ed. Philadelphia, WB Saunders, 1989, pp 510–521.
14. Greenfield LJ: Deep vein thrombosis: Prevention and management. *In* Wilson SE, Veith FJ, Hobson RW, and Williams RA (eds): Vascular Surgery: Principles and Practice. New York, McGraw Hill, 1987, pp 722–735.
15. Brause BD: Infected orthopedic prostheses. *In* Bisno AL and Waldvogel FA (eds): Infections Associated with Indwelling Medical Devices. Washington, DC, American Society for Microbiology, 1989, pp 111–127.
16. Field EA and Martin MV: Prophylactic antibiotics for patients with artificial joints undergoing oral and dental surgery: Necessary or not? Br J Oral Maxillofac Surg 29(5):341, 1991.
17. Freedman AM and Jackson IT: Infections in breast implants. Infect Dis Clin North Am 3(2):275, 1989.
18. Blum MD: Infections of genitourinary prostheses. Infect Dis Clin North Am 3(2):259, 1989.
19. Venes JL: Infections of CSF shunt and intracranial pressure monitoring devices. Infect Dis Clin North Am 3(2):289, 1989.
20. Vas SI: Infections of continuous ambulatory peritoneal dialysis catheters. Infect Dis Clin North Am 3(2):301, 1989.
21. Conn HO: Complications of peritoneovenous shunts. ASAIO Trans 35(2):176, 1989.
22. Carlson AN, Tetz MR, and Apple DJ: Infectious complications of modern cataract surgery and intraocular lens implantation. Infect Dis Clin North Am 3(2):339, 1989.
23. Daar ES and Meyer RD: Medical management of AIDS pa-

tients: Bacterial and fungal infections. Med Clin North Am 76(1):173, 1992.
24. Terezhalmy GT and Hall EH: The asplenic patient: A consideration for antimicrobial prophylaxis. Oral Surg Oral Med Oral Pathol 57(1):114, 1984.
25. Barco CT: Prevention of infective endocarditis: A review of the medical and dental literature. J Periodontol 62(8):510, 1991.
26. Heimdahl A and Nord CE: Antimicrobial prophylaxis in oral surgery. Scand J Infect Dis 70(Suppl):91, 1990.
27. Kreuzpaintner G, Horstkotte D, Heyll A, et al: Increased risk of bacterial endocarditis in inflammatory bowel disease. Am J Med 92(4):391, 1992.
28. Everett ED and Hirschmann JV: Transient bacteremia and endocarditis prophylaxis: A review. Medicine 56(1):61, 1977.
29. Heimdahl A, Hall G, Hedberg M, et al: Detection and quantitation by lysis-filtration of bacteremia after different oral surgical procedures. J Clin Microbiol 28(10):2205, 1990.
30. Bender IB, Naidorf IJ, and Garvey GJ: Bacterial endocarditis: A consideration for physician and dentist. J Am Dent Assoc 109(3):415, 1984.
31. Rosen L, Abel ME, Gordon PH, et al: Practice parameters for antibiotic prophylaxis—supporting documentation: The Standards Task Force. American Society of Colon and Rectal Surgeons. Dis Colon Rectum 35(3):278, 1992.
32. Norfleet RG: Infectious endocarditis after fiberoptic sigmoidoscopy: With a literature review. J Clin Gastroenterol 13(4):448, 1991.
33. Colachis SC: Prevention of bacterial endocarditis. JAMA 265(13):1686, 1991.
34. Dajani AS, Bisno AL, Chung KJ, et al: Prevention of bacterial endocarditis: Recommendations of the American Heart Association. JAMA 264(22):2919, 1990.
35. Glauser MP and Francioli P: Relevance of animal models to the prophylaxis of infective endocarditis. J Antimicrob Chemother 20(Suppl)A:87, 1987.
36. Baddour LM, Christensen GD, Lowrance JH, and Simpson WA: Pathogenesis of experimental endocarditis. Rev Infect Dis 11(3):452, 1989.
37. Ricci MA, Mehran RJ, Petsikas D, et al: Species differences in the infectibility of vascular grafts. J Invest Surg 4(1):45, 1991.
38. Durack DT: Prophylaxis of infective endocarditis. *In* Mandell GL, Douglas RG, and Bennett JE (eds): Principles and Practice of Infectious Diseases, 3rd ed. New York, Churchill Livingstone, 1990, pp 716–721.
39. Pogrell MA and Welsby PD: The dentist and prevention of infective endocarditis. Br Dent J 139:12, 1975.
40. van der Meer JT, van Wijk W, Thompson J, et al: Efficacy of antibiotic prophylaxis for prevention of native-valve endocarditis. Lancet 339(8786):135, 1992.
41. van der Bijl P and Maresky LS: Failures of endocarditis prophylaxis: Selective review of the literature and a case report. Ann Dent 50(1):5, 1991.
42. Imperiale TF and Horwitz RI: Does prophylaxis prevent post-dental infective endocarditis? A controlled evaluation of protective efficacy. Am J Med 88(2):131, 1990.
43. Horstkotte D, Friedrichs W, Pippert H, et al: Benefits of endocarditis prevention in patients with prosthetic heart valves (Ger). Z Kardiol 75(1):8, 1986.
44. Gould I and Buckingham JK: Antibiotic prophylaxis and endocarditis. Lancet 339(8795):738, 1992.
45. Manzione NC: Pseudomembranous colitis associated with endocarditis prophylaxis for endoscopy. Gastrointest Endosc 37(4):501, 1991.
46. Freiman JP, Graham DJ, and Green L: Pseudomembranous colitis associated with single-dose cephalosporin prophylaxis. JAMA 262(7):902, 1989.
47. Bor DH and Himmelstein DU: Endocarditis prophylaxis for patients with mitral valve prolapse: A quantitative analysis. Am J Med 76(4):711, 1984.
48. Jacobson JJ, Schweitzer SO, and Kowalski CJ: Chemoprophylaxis of prosthetic joint patients during dental treatment: A decision-utility analysis. Oral Surg Oral Med Oral Pathol 72(2):167, 1991.
49. Kaye D: Prophylaxis for infective endocarditis: An update. Ann Intern Med 104(3):419, 1986.
50. Cannell H, Kerawala C, Sefton AM, et al: Failure of two macrolide antibiotics to prevent post-extraction bacteremia. Br Dent J 171(6):170, 1991.
51. Neu HC: New macrolide antibiotics: Azithromycin and clarithromycin. Ann Intern Med 116(6):517, 1992.
52. Paulsen O, Hoglund P, and Schalen C: Pharmacokinetic comparison of two models of endocarditis prophylaxis with amoxicillin. Scand J Infect Dis 21(6):669, 1989.
53. Simmons NA, Ball AP, Cawson RA, et al: Antibiotic prophylaxis and infective endocarditis. Lancet 339(8804):1292, 1992.
54. Antibiotic prophylaxis of infective endocarditis: Recommendations from the Endocarditis Working Party of the British Society of Antimicrobial Chemotherapy. Lancet 335(8681):88, 1990.
55. Infection control during gastrointestinal endoscopy: Guidelines for clinical application. Gastrointest Endosc 34(Suppl 3):37S, 1988.
56. Grant A and Hoddinott C: Joint replacement, dental surgery, and antibiotic prophylaxis. BMJ 304(6832):959, 1992.
57. Thyne GM and Ferguson JW: Antibiotic prophylaxis during dental treatment in patients with prosthetic joints. J Bone Joint Surg Br 73(2):191, 1991.
58. Vlay SC: Prevention of bacterial endocarditis in patients with permanent pacemakers and automatic internal cadioverter defibrillators (Editorial). Am Heart J 120(6):1490, 1990.
59. Pogrel A: Antibiotics: Better late than never? Br Dent J 170(7):249, 1991.

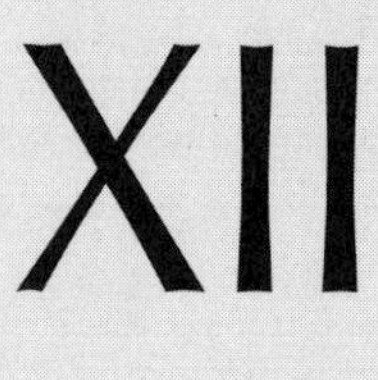

Social-Psychiatric Problems

76

The Medical Interview and Related Skills

MACK LIPKIN, Jr., MD

IMPORTANCE OF THE MEDICAL INTERVIEW

The interview is the major medium of medical care.[1–4] In most settings, the most time spent by physicians and patients together is in the interview. The interview delimits the problems considered by the physician. It determines whether the full range of problems present will be detected.[5] The interview determines the accuracy and completeness of historical data. It creates expectations for the physician and patient about what is necessary.[6] These strongly influence the diagnostic approaches and therapeutic solutions that the physician will consider or that the patient will accept in a given case.[7] The interview determines whether or not the patient and physician will understand each other and whether the physician's orders such as prescriptions, self-care, lifestyle changes, or diagnostic tests will be followed.[8] The satisfaction of patients with their care is determined by the interview together with the perceived skill and appropriate behavior of the provider.[9, 10] Likewise, the satisfaction of the physician is influenced by the interview. With skilled use of science, self, and suggestion, each practitioner through the interview has the opportunity to maximize help to the patient. The interview is the most used clinical tool. An average practitioner may expect to do about 160,000 interviews in a 40-year professional life time.

Even though both common sense and empiric study confirm that the interview is central to effective and satisfying medical care, few physicians calibrate, sharpen, or maintain this basic medical tool. Why this is so is not known. Perhaps because it is so important it is very sensitive. Like many human basics—parenting, teaching, sex—it is seldom taught or studied, even by those who do it often.[12, 13]

Similarly, although there is new interest in research and teaching about the interview, it remains relatively understudied.[14] It is also little taught and then often by amateurs or persons who bring to the teaching only limited experience with *medical* patients seen in the "real world" at a realistic pace. Most physicians leave training having never been observed interviewing. It is an area filled with arbitrary dogmatism and folk belief.

This chapter is intended to aid the physician's work with patients. It begins with the structure and function of the initial interview. It describes elements of effective technique appropriate for each interview phase. The chapter then discusses specific common and important situations in which basic interview technique must be varied to maximize effectiveness or prevent serious error. Briefly, methods of working on one's interview techniques are discussed, since reading about interviewing has the same limited value as reading about skiing, flying, or tennis. To do these well, one must learn how, practice, keep practicing, and reinforce and refine approaches over time.

The territory covered in the subject of "interviewing" is vast. Maps for it are preliminary. Each interview, however, has structure, and certain functions are completed during each interview. Effectiveness includes performing each function well and integrating all structural elements skillfully.

While it is possible to outline the structure of an interview, the structural elements do not necessarily occur sequentially. Effective interviewing uses a flexible approach that responds to each situation and patient, and to what problems the patient and situation present.

Skilled interviewers pursue multiple goals simultaneously. One may receive, process, and elicit from the patient data concerning a fact, an appearance, an affect, and mentation, all at the same time. Similarly, one can initiate a caring relationship from the first moment of contact, assess the patient's personal and cognitive styles, develop hypotheses about the patient's priority problems, and begin care. The elements and functions are separated and ordered here for purposes of presentation, recognizing that the elements blend in skillful interviews.

The importance of the interview is different but complementary for the physician and patient, as shown in Table 76–1. The items shown, sometimes summarized as the physician-patient relationship, are factors important to each participant. Each affects the outcome of the interview. These are matters too important to leave to chance or token learning. Fortunately, effective and satisfying interviewing can be taught and amply rewards the time spent.[15]

TABLE 76–1. IMPORTANCE OF THE MEDICAL INTERVIEW

Physician's Perspective	Patient's Perspective
Major medium of care	Major medium of care
Major time spent on interview	Major time spent on interview
Defines problem	Defines helping
Defines specific problems	Creates feeling of being understood
Provides context for understanding problems	Provides context for adapting to illness and understanding care
Establishes contract	Ensures goals are met
Medium of patient education	Learning how to care for self
Promotes compliance	Therapeutic alliance
Professional satisfaction	Health needs met: personally supported
Interpersonal satisfaction	Personal satisfaction
Builds practice	Social needs facilitated
Facilitates healing	Comforts and cures

FUNCTIONS OF THE INTERVIEW

The functions of the interview may be accomplished in any phase of an interview and facilitate the achievement of the goals of the patient and physician. Bird and Cohen-Cole have described a model to focus on three principal functions: information gathering, emotion handling, and behavior management, shown in Table 76–2.[16–18]

These three functions and several other important ones, including active listening, listening at multiple levels, letting the patient do the work, establishing rapport, and eliciting sensitive and personal relevant information, are elaborated in the following discussions of the structural elements of the interview, shown in Table 76–3.

STRUCTURAL ELEMENTS OF THE INTERVIEW

Optimizing the Environment

The physical conditions of the interview are significant. They may present barriers to communication. They reflect the physician's regard for the patient's comfort, and they offer learning about the patient through the patient's manipulation of the environment (Table 76–4). Finally, the physical setting offers the first opportunity to treat through suggestion.

The physical setting is a positive statement of the context that the physician chooses to provide for his or her work with patients. The physical setting allows the physician to express nonverbally what he or she regards as important. Thus, the physician can maximize privacy even if he or she works in a rigid or impoverished setting by drawing the curtains or by moving the patient to where no one else can hear. The physician can eliminate distractions by turning off the television or radio, by drawing the curtain, by turning off the telephone and beeper, and by indicating to the staff that during an interview, he or she should be disturbed only for urgent problems. "Do not disturb" can be a rule, on a sign or in a code such as a light. The physician can eliminate physical barriers (e.g., the bed rail, the desk, the examining table) between himself or herself and the patient. This puts the physician and the patient at the same level, which enhances the opportunity for good eye contact, a full view of each other, and touching. The arrangement of chairs can be a message about relative status or about caring. If there is no choice but to have a high and a low seating arrangement, maximizing the patient's choice by entering after the patient and letting the patient choose where to sit provides useful insight concerning issues of power and authority. Finally, active manipulation of an environment to make it suit both the physician and the patient suggests that the physician will have an active, effective approach to problems.[19]

Although knowledge about the effects of spatial arrangements and decor on mood and receptivity is considerable, none is specific to the physician's office. It is clear, however, that the choices that the physician makes or does not make add up to a statement. The patient is most likely to be comfortable and satisfied if the setting is congruent with the other features that the physician expresses about himself or herself. Patients have cultural- and social class–determined expectations about the physician's office. A pa-

TABLE 76–2. THREE-FUNCTION MODEL OF THE MEDICAL INTERVIEW*

	Objective	Skills
I. Information gathering	Accurate data Efficient collection	Open-ended questions Open to closed cone Avoid leading or multiple questions Facilitate Direct Summarize and check
II. Emotion management	Patient satisfaction Relief of distress Detection and management of psychiatric illness Physician satisfaction Improved physical outcomes Therapeutic alliance	Empathy (name the emotion) Reassurance (show understanding) Support/create a partnership Show respect
III. Behavior management	Lifestyle change Increase coping	Educate Motivate

*From Bird J, Cohen-Cole SA, and Mance R: The three-function model of the medical interview. (In preparation)

tient is most likely to be comfortable with what he or she expects. Thus, decor should be appropriate to the expectations of the practice population. Most patients expect a mix of science and art, of the personal and professional.

Opening

Observation of the patient is the first learning opportunity for the physician in the interview. It is desirable to observe the patient actively prior to any conversation. By observing the patient leaving the waiting area and coming into the office or examining room or by walking the patient into the room, a host of impressions and hypotheses are generated in the alert, focused observer. In particular, general well-being, gait, coloring, grooming, social class, style, and affect can be noted—not conclusively, but in a flow of impressions that raises questions to be answered by further data. Some physicians worry that no useful data can be garnered through observation prior to any conversation. A test of this is to see how rich impressions are in a crowd, preferably a public crowd with some heterogeneity. In seconds most persons have a host of impressions, such as liking or disliking, attraction or aversion, class and race, and potential for interaction. All persons have initial impressions. To the extent that one can focus and be aware of initial impressions, one can better control their effect and can use them as sources of very useful hypotheses.

TABLE 76–3. STRUCTURAL ELEMENTS OF THE INTERVIEW

Optimizing the physical environment
The opening
Observation
Preparing self to listen
The greeting
Introduction and conveying interest
Surveying problems, developing hypotheses
Organizing the flow of the interview
Developing the life context of the patient and illness
Management of personal and sensitive information
Active listening
Letting the patient do the work
Listening at multiple levels
Negotiating and contracting
Completing coverage with closed questions
Developing a therapeutic alliance
Closing

Each interview starts with an opening. This is the most useful period for the efficient collection of data. Every effort should be made to be prepared, through a state of passive alertness, to receive data about the patient at the onset of the initiation of contact. Microanalysis of taped interviews shows the importance of this phase. Beckman and Frankel have shown that in only 23% of cases is the patient able to complete an opening statement without interruption.[5] Interruptions occur, after the first expressed concern, at an average of 18 seconds into the interview! Since patients often begin by testing the waters and reserve sensitive or feared subjects until they feel safe and able to talk comfortably with the interviewer, the effects of such interruptions are important. Burack and Carpenter have suggested that 76% of somatic and only 6% of psychosocial complaints are identified by the physician.[20] The chief, that is, first, complaint is not necessarily the most important from either the patient's or physician's perspective. Interruptions, such as "Tell me more about that," often are made with the best of intentions, to focus on the first problem or to show interest. Nevertheless they interfere with the patient's ability to state problems.

The Greeting

The richest data of the interview derive from the opening; it is critical, therefore, that the physician has his or her mind and senses keenly attuned and is not to be distracted by the effort of creating the greeting. The greeting, therefore, should be prepared and tuned through thoughtful practice.

The contents of the greeting are important. The patient must quickly learn that the physician is interested in communicating and that he or she does not wish to be anony-

TABLE 76–4. ENVIRONMENTAL FEATURES OF THE INTERVIEW

Provide privacy
Eliminate distractions (television, radio)
Take active steps to avoid interruptions (telephone, staff, beeper)
Lower physical barriers (bed rail, height differentials)
Arrange seating equality or offer choice
Be conscious of what the decor communicates and be responsible for it
Model active problem-solving

mous. The first step is that the physician should state his or her name clearly. Next the physician should define the role or reason for the interaction, if it is in doubt—for example, as in a consultation. Finally, the physician should check that his or her notions of the patient's name and its pronunciation are correct.

There is debate presently about the value of using a stereotyped opening in interviewing. By always using the same opening, the physician can be reasonably sure that the variations in response derive mainly from the patient and not from himself or herself. The disadvantage is loss of appropriateness. Probably the best thing to do is to use a stereotyped opening long enough to provide a vivid and active sense of the common variations and then to become flexible and intuitive. If the greeting is chosen intuitively, the physician should note his or her own response in order to provide data about how he or she is responding to the patient.

Novice interviewers often begin with a social rather than professional greeting. Greetings such as "How are you?" or "Glad to meet you" require an awkward shift to data collection. It is best to be clearly professional from the outset, such as "How are you feeling today?"

Introduction and Conveying Interest

Having made mutual greetings, the introductory phase of the interview begins. Conveying interest from the start opens the patient up. A person is much better able to talk about difficult matters if he or she is relaxed in the setting and physically comfortable. The many concerns that patients have make them appropriately anxious—"Will I be believed, will you listen to all that is on my mind, will you help, in which domains, and will it hurt?" If the patient is also physically uncomfortable, this distracts significantly. The physician's attention to the patient's physical discomfort frees the patient to participate in the work ahead and shows explicitly that the physician is prepared to be helpful. It also conditions the patient to being helped, thus facilitating therapeutic efforts. At this point in an interview, however, it is premature to do very much other than arrange the chair, be sure the patient's posture is comfortable, and attend to the patient's immediate discomforts such as a full bladder or severe pain.

In addition to greeting the patient warmly and with clarity, making the patient comfortable, and showing interest in his or her immediate physical comfort, the physician's nonverbal messages should be consciously controlled. Virtually all studies of doctor-patient interactions show the importance and impact of nonverbal behavior on the opening.[21] Whether the physician is interested or not is communicated most clearly through posture, eye contact, and verbal tone. Carkhuff and associates have studied the postures most conducive to effective interaction and communication.[22] By experimentally varying your postures and noting both your feelings and the reactions of others, one can easily determine which postures lead to comfort and which to discomfort. Spiegel and Machotka have identified major measurable categories of body language.[23] Direction of gaze relates reliably to issues of dominance and superiority, as does turning of the head, but not of the body. Physical distance increases subordination. Arm positions strongly affect dominance relationships. These authors conclude that looking directly at the other person while not bowing the head is the most friendly and intimate position of gaze. Sitting with legs open (i.e., not crossed at knee or ankle), facing the patient directly, with arms open and palms exposed is the most facilitative posture. Frequent but not constant eye contact facilitates. Constant eye contact is experienced as aggressive or erotic. No eye contact is experienced as haughty, submissive, or both.

Calibrating the Interview

As with any other scientific instrument, the physician's interviewing tool must be "calibrated" each time it is used in new circumstances. That is, the physician must consciously attempt to understand fully how his or her techniques are working or not working in each encounter with each patient. It is essential to ascertain what the patient is able to communicate, what the barriers to communication are, and to be able to overcome these barriers.

The first step is to recognize barriers to communication. Some important ones are noted in Table 76–5.[24]

Surveying Problems ("What Else?") and Developing Hypotheses

Surveying problems consists of asking the patient to name the problems that he or she wishes the physician to deal with or know about. If the patient has made an opening statement without interruption, he or she will on average have cited three problems on a first visit.[5] Patients often forget or suppress matters that they had intended to bring up. Hence, after the opening statement, it is helpful to summarize what has been heard and then ask "What else?" after hearing each problem described, until the patient runs out of problems to discuss. In a few minutes, this familiarizes the physician and the patient with the full menu of problems and thus permits sensible priority setting and contracting between them.

There are five reasons to survey problems. First, patients often reserve presenting difficult or embarrassing problems, hoping the physician will be distracted by the initial problem and overlook the other problems. Second, surveying the full set of problems lets the physician and the patient pick priority issues without creating a feeling of helplessness because other more important problems are not addressed. Third, the variety of problems and their presentation gives extremely helpful information about the patient. For example, it shows whether a patient is hypochondriac ("My teeth itch and my nose, let me tell you about all the awful . . ."), obsessive ("I just happen to have a list here, doctor"), or has a health belief model different from your own.[25] Fourth, it serves to remind the patient of important issues forgotten or suppressed. Finally, it allows the physician to communicate to the patient his or her wishes con-

TABLE 76–5. BARRIERS TO COMMUNICATION*

Physical environment: bed rails, discordant eye level, and so on
Patient barriers
- Physical attributes: e.g., pain, sensory lack, deafness, blindness, delirium, intoxication
- Psychological and behavioral barriers:
  - Beliefs, attitudes, personal values, emotions, behaviors such as personality styles (if not noted), mental disorders, coping style, and cultural conditioning

Physician barriers
- Physical barriers
- Psychological and behavioral barriers: beliefs, attitudes and values, behaviors

*From The Working Group on Curriculum: Faculty Development Course on Teaching of the Medical Interview. Brown University, 1983.

cerning sharing of responsibility in the interview and in care.[26]

Studies of physician behavior, pioneered by Elstein and colleagues,[7] suggest that practicing physicians do not follow decision-making strategies like those modeled in the clinical-pathologic conferences of the Massachusetts General Hospital by starting with a full case presentation and ending in a closely reasoned differential diagnosis. Rather, they rapidly develop one to six hypotheses about the nature of the principal problem based on key cues or on patterns, and devote the rest of the interview to ruling these in or out. Inexperienced physicians ask questions more systematically (i.e., unrelated to patterns or cues) and experienced physicians ask fewer, more cogent questions resulting in more rapid diagnosis. Effective clinicians tolerate ambiguity as long as necessary and avoid premature closure. As well, they continue to use open-minded thinking, which generates many and varied hypotheses. Testing of hypotheses involves assessment of the probability that the hypothesized entity is present, an assessment of its potential seriousness, an assessment of the value of treatment in such cases, and some subjective sense of how interesting the entity is.[27] Some clinicians tend to use models and classifications learned as house officers.[28] A survey of problems creates the security that an adequate range of problems is under discussion.

Organizing the Flow of the Interview

During the course of the interview, the interviewer needs to achieve a series of goals. These include understanding the priority problem(s) and developing hypotheses about it and generating a way to pursue it diagnostically and therapeutically. Included also is understanding the patient as a person with respect to personality style, coping, strengths and weaknesses, family and social setting, and health belief systems. Goals also include developing trust, caring, and a way of working with the patient based on mutual interests.

To accomplish these multiple ends, the interviewer needs a system to be able to give full attention to and to be able to think about the dense flood of information present in every patient encounter. The best method is to organize the interview around a narrative so that the patient can do the work of telling his or her story of illness while the interviewer can receive, store, and ponder the information being provided. If the physician has to be thinking constantly about the next question or thinking while the patient is talking, he or she will significantly diminish his or her capacity to listen, remember, and analyze.

A useful way to organize the patient's story of illness is to suggest that the patient go back to the beginning of the illness ("When did you last feel completely well?") or of the episode ("What happened as things changed this time?"). Ask the patient to tell the story in sequence. Allowing this to happen creates a *narrative thread.*

Once the narrative thread is established, the physician can suggest digressions and have a smooth way to get back on track. For example, if the patient is talking about when he last felt well, the physician can digress to find out about the life setting. Questions such as "Where were you then?" or "What was happening in your life then?" can rapidly enrich the physician's information about the life context."Who was at home then?" gives information about who the patient has close to him or her. After hearing enough, the physician can easily bring the patient back to the narrative thread by asking "So what happened next?" The narrative thread permits the physician to control the flow in a natural way that every patient understands instinctively since everyone knows how stories are organized. Furthermore, psychosocial issues can be introduced without diverging from the context of the interview, and the physician can return to the main topic whenever he or she has heard enough.

In organizing the flow, the quality of information provided is important. The physician interviews to obtain succinct, accurate, and detailed information. It is not reasonable to expect lay persons to understand this or to know intuitively what content, level of detail, or quality of detail to provide. As well, many patients have had encounters with physicians who discouraged detail or did not want to know much about the illness, the treatments, or the patient as a person attempting to adapt to illness. To get appropriate information, one has to *train* the patient to provide it. This is done efficiently by taking the first several occasions after the opening statement to show the patient what is needed. An interruption coupled with an explanation is effective: interrupting to ask, "Can you remember precisely when that was?," "Can you tell me exactly what you were feeling?" will quickly condition the patient to provide the level of information required.

Forms of Questions. One of the most powerful discreet skills in interviewing is the ability to control the *form* of questions to elicit the desired *form* of response. In surveying problems and in initiating discussion of an area, the use of an open-ended form of question is critical. Practitioners who use more *open-ended questions* elicit more information from their patients than those who do not use them.[29] Open-ended questions introduce an area of inquiry without biasing or shaping the content of the response. The power of open-ended questions cannot be overemphasized. "Tell me more about that" or "How was that for you?" allows the patient to tell the story without bias and without limits as to the aspects of the problem under discussion. Therefore, the patient can pick what is important from his or her perspective, can introduce elements the interviewer would never think of, and thus provide much richer information more efficiently. The usual fear of open-ended questions is precisely related to their power. Some interviewers believe that they must maintain control for the sake of efficiency. They fear that an open-ended question will lead the patient to ramble or provide more information than is desired. Therefore, they stick to closed questions and lead the patient. This invariably narrows the inquiry, which *does not* improve diagnosis, for the interviewer then must think of all possibilities rather than allowing the patient to stimulate a broader range of diagnostic questions. The opportunity is lost to learn enough about patients to know how to work with and help them maximally. Interviews using exclusively closed-ended questions almost always produce major distortions or omissions about the case.

Developing the Life Context of the Patient and Illness (Table 76–6)

Efficiently developing the personal background of the patient frustrates many internist and general practitioner interviewers. Although most physicians wish to have better-quality information about the patient as a person, some believe that they do not have the time to elicit the data or they feel frustrated in their attempts to "get the patient to open up." One reason for these difficulties is that many patients have been trained, through their experience in the health-care system, to believe that physicians do not want

TABLE 76–6. DEVELOPING THE LIFE CONTEXT

- Prepare the patient
  - Greet personally
  - Set patient at ease
  - Negotiate seriously and respectfully
- Establish the narrative
- Reinforce psychosocial discussion
  - Echo or inquire about the first personal issue mentioned
  - Rather than reassure, listen with interest
- Do not allow psychosocial inquiry to overwhelm the other priority tasks

to hear personal information. For this reason alone, the steps already described make a major difference in the development of a relationship and in obtaining needed psychosocial information (properly greeting and introducing oneself to the patient, setting the patient at ease and seeing to physical and psychological comfort, surveying problems with interest, and developing a narrative thread).

To explore the life context (see Table 76–6), a major useful technique is to use the *initial* psychosocial comment of the patient to express interest in such information. Thus, the first time the patient mentions a family member, a job, parents, or whatever, inquire about the person or event mentioned. This can be done simply by echoing (after "I hurt so bad my husband had to . . ." the physician then says ". . . your husband?"). Or the physician can be explicit and say something like "Tell me more about your husband." This demonstrates to the patient that material other than physical symptoms is of interest. If the narrative thread is in place, the physician can hear as much as he or she wishes about the husband and then pick up the thread. Few patients fail to respond to this technique. For those few who question or resist a particular line of inquiry, the physician can state straightforwardly that he or she needs to know something of the life setting in which the illness developed in order to be most helpful. Most patients understand the importance of their life as the context of the development of their illness and the setting for their ongoing care, and many appreciate the interest shown.[30, 31]

Management of Sensitive and Personal Aspects of the Illness and the Person. Eliciting sensitive and personal information is central to the performance of effective and complete care. Yet it is taxing to both the physician and patient.[32] Often both the physician and patient collude to avoid dealing with delicate or painful topics. They raise realistic objections: the personal information will not be kept private, raising painful subjects will lead to discomfort without benefit, and it is unfair to deal with painful material in a patient already sick and therefore troubled. The only way to allay such doubts or objections is to be certain that they are not true. Thus, preparation for privacy and talking about the need may be in order. Preparation for privacy begins with the physical setting of the interview—it must be out of earshot of others and safeguarded against interruption. Records must be confidential, or private records must be kept separately. Alternatively, one can learn to write in a code or Aesopian language that allows remembrance of key information. Remember, however, that all medical records can be made public under certain legal circumstances, such as cases involving controlled substances or felonies.

The fact that painful personal material taxes the sick person is often true—but it is also often helpful or necessary. Certainly, if the physician feels unable to help deal with distressing reactions to illness or personal problems in a patient's life, he or she is right not to get involved in it. Is he or she therefore neglectful as a doctor? This depends on one's view of the role of a physician. Psychological issues are central to care for several reasons. They contribute to disease etiology[33]; they often determine the timing and extent of health care–seeking behavior[34–36]; they usually account for denial, which contributes to morbidity or death in some cases; and they can contribute positively to compliance or negatively to failure to adhere to a treatment regimen.[8, 37] In some patients, the occasion of illness can induce growth and increased maturity and well-being. No other health professionals have the leverage of physicians for potential help. In many instances, only a physician is capable of sorting through the complex biopsychosocial influences in patients' disease and their adjustment to it. If the goal of the physician is to comfort always and cure occasionally, then not to gather the full range of necessary and relevant information is deficient. In addition, difficult and delicate information may be needed to accomplish even the limited goals of biotechnical care if it reveals such items as susceptibilities due to family illness, exposure to stigmatized infections, failure to take medication, or the like. As well, a physician needs personal, sensitive, and intimate knowledge of the patient's life to fashion appropriate care approaches and conditions. Medical students sometimes rationalize that patients should not be subjected to invasive inquiry in order to avoid their own discomfort. Yet patients welcome such discussion more often than not. Well done, it is almost always comforting and sometimes growth-inducing for the patient to discuss difficult feelings and issues with a primary care physician. It promotes a feeling of being understood and not isolated. It may help by showing the patient that what had felt scary, unique, or shameful is common, normal, and manageable. Some of the healing impact of primary care physicians derives from the simple communication of understanding, positive regard, and caring.[38]

Often, however, the patient and physician must overcome prior conditioning that personal and sensitive information is not welcomed or considered relevant by doctors.[39, 40] The technique of eliciting and managing sensitive and personal information derives from simple principles. Essentially, patients respond to empathy, interest, and understanding.[41, 42] The most effective way to begin demonstrating to the patient that personal feelings and experience are important in the process of care is to take the first opportunity to inquire about them. After doing this several times, the patient will realize that the physician wants to know and understand more than a narrow account of disease. The inquiry can be direct, "How did that feel for you?" or indirect, "It sounds like you were really angry." This is described as "naming the feeling." Understanding may be stated, "I can understand that you felt sad," or demonstrated, "Anyone would feel that way under the circumstances." Empty reassurance is unhelpful. But providing supportive information is reassuring and further shows the patient that the physician understands him or her. Finally, nonverbal and verbal communication of the physician's positive regard for the patient helps the patient to accept. This is accomplished verbally by direct statements of regard, "I admire how well you are coping," or "It takes a strong person to face these feelings of weakness and helplessness."

The fear that inquiry into personal issues will swamp one in uncontrollable digressions about irrelevant life experience is usually unjustified. Once it is established between the physician and patient that personal events are relevant and of interest, the patient can outline their extent and the physician can indicate further interest or a desire to go on, or perhaps to come back to the issue later. In fact, one *does not* want to get too deeply involved in hidden and important issues until one knows enough about the patient to know how to react, how to be helpful, and how the patient is coping. Thus, it is best early on to inquire mainly about who is in the family or home, what the life context is, and the like. This shows how the patient deals with self, feelings, and relationships. Extensive probing can come later when the physician knows how to be direct but unhurtful. Several investigators argue that the process of care is more efficient if sensitive psychosocial issues are raised and discussed when relevant.[4, 43] If one spends more time initially to get an accurate picture of the person, the real problems, the life context, and coping, this saves time later owing to efficient working together with less patient testing of the physician, less ineffective prescribing and unfocused test ordering, and the healing benefit of a supportive relationship.[44]

On Active Listening. The preceding sections have discussed initial aspects of an interview shaped to maximize effectiveness. However, shaping the environment and the initial interaction with the patient are necessary but not sufficient steps to effective interviewing. Equally important are methods to control, in effect, the internal environment so that the physician is maximally able to listen. One approaches every interview with expectations and goals that one wants to meet. The physician may have some prejudices (prejudgments) about what this patient presents and may have other pressures, such as keeping to schedule, things at home, and work waiting. If the physician is a ward resident, added to these pressures is the panel of waiting patients with quantities of "scut" work. Students and interns have the pressures of uncertain competence and of being watched and evaluated. Taken together, such concerns create loud noise in your "seven receptive channels." Miller has shown that the average person can process seven plus or minus two bits of information simultaneously.[45] If channels are closed or occupied due to fatigue, appetites such as hunger, or distractions like the beeper, intercom, and telephone, few bits are left for the patient.

In contrast, if the physician is able temporarily to put everything else aside, both internally and externally, several goals can be better met. The physician can observe multiple entities simultaneously. He or she will be able to tune into the verbal content and the nonverbal communications and to develop rich hypotheses and keep track of them. As well, the physician will convey to the patient that he or she is listening attentively. This is invariably appreciated and leads to cooperation.

There are a number of ways to prepare oneself to interview. First, take care of outstanding business so that interruptions during the interview are minimized. Second, the physician should meet personal needs in advance: physical comfort, emptying one's bladder, grooming, eating, and so on. Third, he or she should have a clear mind and should approach the interview in an alert, relaxed, and helpful manner. How to accomplish this depends on the physician's own characteristic methods of achieving temporary focus. Successful ways to achieve readiness to listen have in common the suggestion to oneself that what is about to happen is completely new and fresh, that it (like an athletic or intellectual event) requires total attention, and that one is at peace or calm. Some imagine themselves about to do some other favorite activity—ski down a mountain, dive in, serve in tennis. Some use self-hypnosis to achieve attentiveness. Some view themselves helping this new patient in a comprehensive, subtle, and satisfying way.[46]

Regardless of the technique used, the key is to prepare consciously to listen physically, psychologically, and institutionally. When done routinely, the ability to listen actively grows rapidly. It is useful for the physician to have a fixed routine to ensure that this is accomplished at every patient visit. The physician should decide on a routine way to prepare. A sensible place to do so is at the threshold of the room in which the patient is waiting.

Having attained attentiveness, one functions most effectively if able to maintain active listening. This is enhanced by an upright and relaxed posture, letting the patient do the work, consciously rejecting distracting external stimuli, and refocusing internal thoughts and feelings as information about one's response to the patient.

Letting the Patient Do the Work. When possible, organize the interview so as to be free to think and feel about what is being said without the distraction of preparing the next question. One method is to establish a narrative thread. This allows the patient to tell the story of the illness with minimal interruptions. A second strategy involves having a well-practiced repertoire of efficient interventions—"minimal encouragers"—that guide the patient to greater clarity or relevance without effort on the physician's part. These include echoing, nodding, and specific guiding comments and gestures. Echoing consists of repeating a phrase or word just used by the patient to show interest in that aspect of the subject and to encourage elaboration thereon. Some excellent interviewers seldom speak but are like orchestra conductors using their heads and hands. They use gestures to mean "come on" or "stop," they nod when the going is appropriate and desired, and turn away, gaze down, or gently shake their heads "no" when they do not want to hear more. These nonverbal mannerisms are extremely effective when used preconsciously (i.e., in a reflexive way accessible to awareness). Some excellent interviewers have no idea that they do this. A good way to know what you do is to videotape yourself interviewing and review the tape with the sound turned off. Most physicians are surprised to see the amount and variety of things they express nonverbally.[23, 47–50]

Listening at Multiple Levels. Listening at multiple levels refers to listening for the direct meaning of the patient's words and for as much other information as can be inferred. This involves noting and correctly interpreting subtleties of syntax, changes in tense, correlations of content and affective expression or meaningful changes of subject, "phrases" of body language, meaningful metaphors, missing information, and so on.[46, 48] Details of learning to accomplish nonliteral information-gathering from the interview are beyond the complexity feasible here. But to illustrate: a change in voice or a change from "I" to "you" in a patient's story of the illness may indicate the patient's need for distance from the events being described—hence, you as a practitioner may be able to help the patient deal with or work through a difficulty in handling feelings in this area. If it involves the work-up or treatment, a syntax change may point to resistance to therapies. Similarly, a change in tense may indicate a wish to put an event behind, to have the chance to do it over, or to do it better this time. Such data are more heuristic for hypothesis generation, than definitive.

Negotiating and Contracting

Both the physician and patient enter each interview with implicit and explicit goals and expectations. For the physician, these include goals such as diagnosing acutely; treating cleverly; getting paid; generating referrals; feeling satisfied, competent, and important; and getting to know the patient as a person. For the patient, these include getting all problems addressed and relieved; not being hurt; not being embarrassed, shamed, or humiliated[51]; trusting or liking the doctor; saving money; getting healthier; or growing as a person.

Physician and patient pairs differ in expectations and in their degree of mutuality or conflict. An important source of conflict concerning expectations has to do with differing models of care and healing. Parsons first clearly delineated the modal model of care in Western medicine as a dyadic relationship involving reciprocal roles with the physician in a dominant or paternalistic position.[52] Szasz and Hollender expanded this view by describing a spectrum of possible relationships, ranging from the entirely physician-dominated (e.g., caring for a comatose patient) to an entirely patient-dominated situation in which the physician does exactly what the patient wishes.[53]

Lazare and associates[54] and Quill[26] have focused on the processes of reaching agreement rather than on the initial positions of either party.[26, 54] They conceptualize the interview as a dyadic encounter in which implicit and explicit goals and expectations are negotiated mutually. Without such negotiations, neither side feels satisfied and each side will probably engage in disruptive steps to meet preferred goals and expectations. For example, a physician may believe that intravenous (IV) lines are essential for treatment of endocarditis in a drug addict, but the patient may feel that the IV line threatens already precarious autonomy. Negotiation through clarification of needs makes it possible for the physician to help the patient meet autonomy needs in different ways that enable the patient to accept the limits created by IV therapy. For example, the physician can give the addict control over diet, mobility, smoking, and so on.

Lazare has created a taxonomy of conflicts and suggested approaches to clinical negotiation. In brief, he describes conflicts about the definition of the problem, conflicts over goals for and conditions of treatment, and conflicts about the relationship between the physician and patient. Conflict may be explicit or implicit, displaced or direct, and conscious or unconscious.[55] Some conflicts need not be addressed, if unimportant. But major conflicts will eventually become important. It is wise to deal with them early on in the relationship.

Fisher and Ury of the Harvard Negotiating Project have written a useful description of techniques of "getting to yes."[56] They show that it is more effective to find mutual interests than to bargain over positions. For example, both the physician and patient may agree that relief of pain is important and thus avoid a struggle over pain medication hazards. Lazare emphasizes the value of creating a warm atmosphere based on communication of caring and trust. By acknowledging the importance of a patient's position (to the patient), it is possible to separate the person from the problem. Having a variety of options available to use permits one to make concessions and still meet goals. Clarity about the nature of the conflict is critical.

Table 76–7 describes the basic negotiation techniques described by Lazare and by Fisher and Ury.

TABLE 76–7. NEGOTIATING TECHNIQUES

Create a suitable atmosphere
Trust, respect, caring
Establish expertise
Use empathy, understanding, and positive regard
Clarify the conflict
Be clear about the problem
Don't bargain over positions
Make your intentions explicit
Be objective *and* subjective (i.e., separate facts from values and feelings)
General negotiating strategies
Expand the clinician's definition of the problem (e.g., include values and feelings)
Relate likely outcomes to the patient's goals
Educate, separate the people from problem
Focus on areas of agreement
Specific negotiating strategies
Make concessions initially
Provide samples of plans (e.g., treatment)
Share control
Confront and clarify resistance
Invent options or alternatives
Have alternatives available
Know your bottom line
Walk around or exaggerate the resistance (i.e., some problems can be eliminated by reframing them in a way that eliminates the conflict. Others melt when the problem is shown to be absurd through exaggeration)

Using Closed-Ended Questions to Complete Coverage of Problems

Having heard the patient's story in his or her own words a practitioner will have generated multiple hypotheses. The patient will have given data to support or reject some but not all of the hypotheses. The physician may wish additional information on specific points, such as those covered in a review of systems. At this point one weaves a "safety net" under the open-ended, exploratory phase of the interview by systematically covering points not settled during the patient's free-form story of illness. One can now check for internal consistency by reviewing portions of the story. One can reassess the patient's mental status, if needed, by asking the patient to recall some items introduced earlier (e.g., the physician's name, the receptionist's name), by asking the patient to do simple arithmetic derived from the story (you had ulcer surgery in 1958, how old were you then?), by asking the patient to interpret some aspect of the story (this is like interpreting proverbs), or by other informal and nonthreatening means.

In this phase of an interview, it is appropriate to use closed-ended questions in closed cones of questioning. A closed cone is a set of questions that pursues a specific algorithm to an endpoint. Closed-ended questions require short and specific answers. They encourage specificity rather than elaboration as do open-ended questions. Closed-ended questions have forms like "Did you smoke?" "Is there heart disease in your family?" "What medications do you take?" With closed-ended questions one is sure of the meaning of the answers. They permit one to test hypotheses directly. Their disadvantage is that they cover only explicitly mentioned material. Because several closed-ended questions produce negative answers, medical interviewers may falsely assume that all such questions would elicit negative answers. This can lead to premature closure and a resulting false assumption that the answers to questions *not asked* are negative. In general, it is most powerful to use open-ended questions in developing hypotheses and closed-ended ones in testing them.

Developing a Therapeutic Alliance

Although the term "compliance" is widely used,[37] the phrase "therapeutic alliance" has definite advantages because it suggests mutually negotiated work involving both the patient and physician. The therapeutic alliance is especially critical in primary care since the ambulatory patient controls and is responsible for the taking of tests and medications.

Some of the techniques for developing the therapeutic alliance have been already covered, such as setting the patient at ease; using empathy, understanding and positive regard; negotiating and contracting; and elaborating the life context of the story of illness. DeMatteo and others argue that the central determinant in compliance is interviewing, which can create an attitude of willingness to help oneself.[8] In the health belief model of Rosenstock,[57] "compliance" is determined by the patient's view of the seriousness of the problem; that is, a person's likeliness to act according to the health belief model is proportional to the perceived cost of acting compared with the perceived cost of not acting. Both the patient's sense of cooperation and the seriousness of the illness are surely factors; hence, it is useful to discuss the therapeutic alliance directly with a patient and to review with the patient his or her reactions to what has been found and what is planned.

It is useful to survey for *barriers to compliance*.[24] These include a health explanatory model different from the practitioner's (e.g., the hot-cold model of Puerto Ricans and the *ut siong* of the Chinese); they include negative feelings or misunderstandings about the nature of the problem, such as fear of the side effects or knowing someone who did poorly with the suggested remedy; or fundamental personality or psychological barriers such as inability to relinquish control, denial of the problem, or displacement of anger about the problem to the provider or care system.[58, 59] Failure to detect and deal with such problems leads to frustrating ineffectiveness.

Some practitioners and lay persons believe that patient education is central to effective compliance. This is certainly true of understanding *how* to comply. It is less true of understanding *why* the physician is proposing a diagnostic or therapeutic plan. The value of education concerning the whys of the care depends on the model of healing held by the patient. Patient education is essential for consumer-oriented middle class American patients. However, laborious or defensive justification of the regimen may be counterproductive for those patients who have strong needs to see the physician as powerful, magical, or omnipotent. For such patients, education may not be necessary and may undermine their coping with their illness.[60] When patient education is sensitive, includes what patients need to know, is what they are able to absorb, and is what they expect (e.g., patients in New York expect a good doctor to criticize their smoking whether or not they intend to quit), it will be useful.[61]

Closing the Interview

Ending the interview is often rushed over in order to get on to the next patient or activity. Effective closing matters. The physician can check to ascertain the patient's understanding of what was found and what is planned. This is the most effective time to reinforce learning and the therapeutic alliance. It is the time to reinforce return arrangements and to review the status of the contract between the physician and patient. The physician can reinforce caring for the patient through focused attention and care with these details. Finally, it is the best time to clarify what the patient can do if care is needed before the next scheduled visit (Table 76–8).

TABLE 76–8. CLOSING THE INTERVIEW

Review and confirm the contract
Involve the patient actively
Review the main points: start with most important, repeat the main points
Demonstrate interest and caring
Reinforce return arrangements
Clarify and review arrangements for interim contact

In reviewing the contract, the return arrangements, and the interim arrangements, the patient should be allowed and encouraged to be as active as possible; that is, the patient should be asked what the main purposes of the visit were and if they were covered. The patient should be asked what his or her understanding is of what has been found, accomplished, and planned. Then, if further actions are needed—going for tests, taking drugs, or changing lifestyle—the patient should be asked to describe them in detail. Making the patient active increases the probability of learning, it communicates and reinforces the patient's responsibility, and it reveals and then eliminates misunderstandings.

Making clear what to do if care is needed between visits is especially useful. It communicates to patients that the physican has a professional concern for detail and is willing to assume continuing care for them. If these arrangements are not clarified, anxious or dependent patients may test the physician's caring by calling in order to check whether or not he or she is committed to their care. If one does not have a fail-safe on-call arrangement (and who does?), it is also a sensible strategy in selected cases to give the patient one's home telephone number. Paradoxically, this leads to fewer calls, to more secure relations with patients, and occasionally to saving a life.

RETURN VISITS

Return visits differ from initial visits in several important respects. Although there is no longer a need to introduce oneself, it is useful to survey problems anew because a new set of needs has arisen. The physician needs to learn of changes between visits, to review prior patient learning, to check on the effect and execution of diagnostic and therapeutic interventions, and to strengthen and deepen the relationship initiated in the prior visit. The patient will have reacted to the prior visit and may have important feelings, facts, or thoughts to discuss.

Despite these differences, many requirements of first and return visits are the same. It is valuable, again, to observe the patient before initiation of talking: after doing this several times, one's ability to note changes in each patient increases. It is important to greet the patient properly. It is useful to set the patient at ease and to ensure the patient's and one's own physical comfort prior to beginning. It helps to be ready to listen actively. The contract should be reviewed and, if necessary, renegotiated.

The common habit of reviewing the chart at the outset of return visits conveys a sense of disorganization and last-minute preparation. Furthermore, if one is absorbed in reading the patient's chart, one is not observing the patient and renewing the relationship. It is better to review past notes and the problem list and locate necessary laboratory and other data prior to the patient's arrival.

New issues regarding the therapeutic alliance arise in return visits. The patient will have had an opportunity to try what was agreed upon and will have reactions to the prior visit. It is useful, therefore, to review specific aspects of the prior visit: whether the items agreed upon were done; if so, how the patient reacted to them; if not, why not; and any new problems. In particular, without cueing the patient, ask "What medications are you taking?" and for each, "How are you taking it, in what dose, at what time?" Go over the patient's modifications of the regimen and try to accept as many as are safe. Also, there usually have been problems left unexplored during the initial visit because of time pressure. If the physician remembers to deal with them later, this strongly conveys a sense of thoroughness and concern to the patient (Table 76–9).

TERMINATION

Termination refers to ending the physician-patient relationship because the physician or the patient leaves or because the patient's care passes to another. Occasionally, termination is due to incompatibility or dissatisfaction. For whatever reason, it arouses a complex of feelings both the patient *and the physician* experience on occasions of loss. Thus, the best predictor of a patient's responses to termination is the reaction to prior losses. Often, the patient feels grief, sadness, or rejection. Somatization or return of initial complaints may occur.

One way to deal with physicians' feelings of loss is through mastery of effective management of the termination. This includes letting the patient know you are leaving as soon as possible but not more than 5 or 6 months ahead. The reasons for leaving may be discussed, but the patient should not be subjected to a long apologia. It is best to introduce the subject early in the visit to allow the patient time to react. If necessary, extra time should be scheduled to discuss leaving. The patient *should not* be told on the last visit. It is helpful to allow the patient time to plan future care and to convey choice and mastery to the patient in this planning. Residency programs and group practices should plan for termination.

Despite such plans, termination can be difficult. Patients who somatize, are hypochondriac, are very dependent, or are sick and have complications suffer personally and are probably at increased risk at times of physician loss. Even with extra time, one can expect some to do badly regardless of the physician's efforts. It sometimes seems as if the patient has reverted to the point at which his or her treatment began. If this occurs, reassurance that recovery will be quick with the new physician can be given realistically, provided the follow-up plan is appropriate.[62]

ADAPTING THE INTERVIEW TO THE PATIENT AND THE SITUATION

The effectiveness of interviews depends on the ability of each participant to adapt to the needs and style of the other. Although some patients handle their physician masterfully, in general the physician is expected to do most of the adapting. The more one is able to recognize and accommodate to a patient's needs for specific forms of communication, the more varied a group of patients one can interview effectively. In practice, both the physician and the patient exhibit selection. Inflexible physicians tend to have homogeneous practices. Flexible physicians tend to have more varied and complex practices.

TABLE 76–9. RETURN VISIT

Resurvey problems
Review contract
Review execution of plans
Diagnostics
Therapeutics
Survey for changes in problems
Complications
Progression
Resolution
Cover problems not dealt with previously

Some physicians question whether it is sensible or honest to adapt one's style to the patient's. This depends on one's goals. Clearly, it is sensible and helpful to alter one's approach if the patient cannot work with the physician's usual style. Judgment enters in knowing when such adaptation is called for and whether it is preferable (or possible) to make the necessary change or to refer. This depends on the physician's range of styles and on the availability of alternative practitioners who can do what you cannot. In many communities, certain physicians are recognizably better at handling certain sorts of patients and thus have frequent referrals or are sought by their "type" of patient.

Variations in the physical environment require adaptation to compensate for less-than-ideal conditions. At the bedside, this most notably includes lack of privacy. When loss of privacy is uncorrectable, the interviewer should not attempt to discuss matters that would compromise the patient by disclosure to room- or wardmates. The same consideration applies to a lesser extent when the privacy of the records is at issue or is a concern to the patient.

Important physical variations in the patient that alter interviewing are too numerous to include in detail. Deaf patients are similar to patients who speak a foreign language except that it is possible to communicate with literate deaf patients by writing. Writing everything out, however, is time consuming and frustrating. For many deaf or foreign language–speaking patients, use of an interpreter is desirable. The main problem then is that the interpreter interferes by "interpreting" *meaning* in addition to content. All who use interpreters have had the experience of asking a short question only to hear its interpretation go on at length or, conversely, to have the patient go on at length only to get a terse summary! If the interpreter is a family member, care must be taken not to compromise your relationship through breaching the privacy needs of the patient. Finally, frequently one finds the patient relating only to the interpreter, through eye contact and affective or cultural bonding. This can be corrected by having the interpreter sit behind the patient. Thus, both patient and interpreter have eye contact with you rather than with each other.

Blind patients present less of a linguistic problem but some diminution of exchange occurs because of loss of visual nonverbal material. Touch and increased attention to tone compensate to some extent.

Physical symptoms can greatly interfere with an interview. Patients who are *short of breath* should be helped by asking questions that allow short answers. Using written questionnaires also may help, as may a nod code. If used, a nod code should be made explicit and be monitored for accuracy from time to time. Patients in *pain* may be expected to be inattentive, irritable, and anxious, with resultant increase in inaccuracy and in brief or noncooperative answers. Again, this should be handled with conscious adaptation—treating the pain if this will not interfere with diagnosis; keeping one's inquiry brief and relevant to the present problem; saving the exhaustive, exhausting aspects of "completeness," such as questions related to not immediately relevant past history or prevention and health maintenance, for a later time when the patient feels better.

Goffman brilliantly describes patients with a problem they perceive as stigmatizing.[63] "Stigma" is any deviation from the ideal felt by a patient to be perceptible to the person with whom the patient is interacting—although it usually applies to socially stigmatized patients such as homosexuals or alcoholics or to patients with obvious physical stigmata such as deafness, mutilation, blindness, or colostomy stomas. As Goffman puts it, these patients may have "spoiled identities," resulting in a series of maneuvers to gain acceptance, to develop social support and a peer group, and to avoid discredit or bias against themselves or members of their stigmatized class. To do this, they strictly limit those to whom they reveal their problem by controlling information about themselves and the problem. They go to places that "cover" the problem, where they can pass as normal—thus, deaf persons go to noisy places, blind people to dark places, male homosexuals to the armed services or all-male gyms. They reframe their stigma as a good, leading to handicap "chauvinism" and the creation of in-groups. The in-group has privileged access to intimate information and often creates a special language with key words to show in-group membership. Physicians can utilize this process by showing that they understand the in-group, which then lets them in as "honorary members." This is accomplished by asking about the phenomena if one is not familiar with them ("I am not familiar with what it is like to have a colostomy—can you tell me what it is like for you"); or by indicating familiarity if genuine ("My patients who have AIDS often have problems such as whom to tell, how to deal with the feelings about having caused this oneself in some sense, and so forth. How has it been for you?").

Certain variations in mental status or the developmental stage of the patient require adaptation of interview technique. More time must be spent on relating to and putting pediatric patients at ease. Respect for autonomy combined with reassurance about confidentiality is helpful for adolescents.[64] Identifying barriers to communication such as deafness or senility is needed in aged patients.[65] For children, adolescents, and impaired elderly patients, questions need to be structured, simple, very clear, free of specialized vocabulary or jargon, and limited to one item of inquiry at a time. Slowing one's normal pace of speech helps these patients. Simplifying does not mean shortening if in shortening questions one becomes more abstract and therefore harder to comprehend. Suppression of the physician's frustration helps, because many of these patients get worse when feeling inadequate or censured for their incapacity. Elderly patients need increased focus on functions and their social situations. They usually have multiple problems. They may not remember well, thus they need extra help in checking on medication usage.

Delirious patients require prompt diagnosis and several distinct interview strategies. Diagnosis depends on a high index of suspicion. Delirium is defined as a syndrome of rapid onset (of a few hours to days) with impairment of consciousness, disorientation, decreased memory, and disruption of speech, perception, or motor function. It ranges from the patient who is obviously confused, hallucinatory, restless, worried, and paranoid to the person with a subtle confusion and disturbance of memory and thought detectable only through formal mental-status testing. Delirium is present in 10% of hospitalized patients and in close to one half of geriatric hospitalized patients. It should *always* be considered in ill patients older than 60 years of age, in patients with primary cranial involvement, and in older patients with secondary compromise of cerebral blood flow or metabolism. Delirium is often terrifying to an elderly patient who suddenly becomes confused, forgetful, and incapable of self-care. The interviewer should not push the patient to the point of painful awareness of memory loss or confusion. One should keep to essentials and be slow, clear, and simple. After the mental status is assessed, physicians should offer orientation frequently—saying who they are, where the patient is, what the place and is, and what is happening. Since most delirium is reversible, this fact may be pointed out to the patient, who can be assured that the new incapacity is temporary. The staff and family should be instructed to treat the patient the same way: clearly, simply, and with frequent orientating comments. Staff should reinforce effective function and should be kept as constant as possible. Sedatives and hypnotics should be discontinued or used only when absolutely necessary.[66]

INTERVIEW TECHNIQUE AS A FUNCTION OF THE PATIENT'S PERSONALITY

Adapting to the "personality style" of the patient requires acute observation and skill. Various empiric schemata exist for description of personality and temperament.[67] A literature also exists based on clinical experience, which describes "problem," "hateful," or "difficult" patients.[68–71] Personality style refers to a constellation of behaviors that characterize the thought, interaction, and feeling demonstrated by the person or group. It includes the cognitive style: the conscious ways the person experiences and describes the world and ideas. It characterizes how the person usually relates to others. As well, each style may include features of such disparate things as grooming, sense of truth, handwriting, and speech content of metaphors, qualifiers, and so on.[72]

One of the most useful clinical classifications is Shapiro's group of hysterical, obsessive, impulsive, and paranoid "neurotic" styles.[73] These recognizable paradigms of behavior have explicit implications for management. Along with the borderline, narcissistic, and dependent paradigms of behavior, these are patient types one must recognize *early* in an interview to avoid predictable problems.[74–76] These states are *dimensions* rather than exclusive types. A person may exhibit elements of more than one personality style: many excellent artists, for example, have elements both of hysterical and obsessive styles. Borderlines mix styles and can be hysterical, paranoid, and impulsive in rapid succession. No judgments or values are implicit: these are descriptive and predictive categories. Finally, men and women are equally well described as "hysterical," a useful term when used descriptively rather than pejoratively, although often the term "histrionic" is now substituted.[77,78]

Hysterical Patient

The hysterical patient's personality style is characterized by a dominant concern to *feel* strongly. Hysterics relate so as to maintain strong feelings regardless of their effect. Because their attention in an event is on feeling, they tend to be vague in factual description and to be inconsistent or contradictory about details. Because they are trying to be pleasing or to elicit strong feelings, hysterics are easily led in an interview. Often, they relate to others effectively. They rapidly sense what the interviewer wants to hear and provide it "in spades." If the interviewer wants to learn that the patient has a diagnosis in their specialty, for example, the hysteric obliges with "correct" answers to the closed-ended or leading questions posed to them. Because the hysterics are hyperacute in sensing what the physician is looking for, it is essential in dealing with them to **use open-ended questions** that do not indicate a preferred answer or subject matter. Instead of asking "Did you then have chest pain?", which will produce the answer "Yes," ask "What happened next?"

Recognition of hysterics, with whom one should be especially careful to remain open-ended, is straightforward. Hysterics are often instantly engaging. They may engage personal, sexual, or clinical interest. Such patients often are flamboyant—in appearance, in relating style, or in their description of illness. They exaggerate extremely (the worst pain, the most wonderful doctor absolutely). Since they focus on the interpersonal aspect of events, they can accurately describe how they felt but are vague, circumstantial, or even contradictory about facts, such as when something occurred or what drugs they took. Some, but not all, show inappropriate affect—they describe pain with a smile, depression with fondness. One way to understand them is to recognize that they desire unconsciously to merge with other persons and then find this intolerable because of the loss of self that results. Thus, their rapidly formed, falsely close relationships with others often end with abrupt withdrawal. They are incautious initially and then defend, by means of distance, by leaving, or by disrupting the relationship. It is hard for a physician to recognize that the wonderful rapport developed with a fascinating patient was itself the reason why the patient dropped out of care. Hence, these patients often produce feelings of disappointment, rejection, and anger.

In the long term, hysterics are helped (or as they might put it, saved) if the physician recognizes their personality style. Their cognitive style leads them to give false or misleading information, thus they are at risk for unnecessary work-up and therapy. Due to their difficulty with genuine intimacy, they often drop out of care with risk to themselves. Finally, hysterics frequently somatize; that is, they experience psychological difficulties or conflicts as physical sensations. This also puts them at risk for harm from pursuit of diagnostic possibilities mimicked by their somatization. Finally, blatant or acting-out hysterics are often dismissed with resultant omission of necessary care.[73]

Obsessive-Compulsive Patient

Obsessive persons are familiar to all medical personnel. In mild obsessives, one is merely aware of especially tuned orderliness. This extends to pattern of speech: precise; to dress: neat; to command of information: detailed. Such patients often appeal because they are so good. When decompensated, obsessives use magic and irrational methods to keep the chaos and helplessness of everyday life under control. They get upset at any deviation from their expectations; they make lists; they perseverate about details; and they fret about or blow up over simple decisions that require normal arbitrariness. Such patients may experience hypochondriasis when they are losing their sense of self-mastery. As Shapiro notes, they exhibit machine-like rigidity and actively seek out bases for uncertainty by worrying over every detail.[73] They couple this with fixation of attention on the minor and manageable, shutting out the rest. If focused on recombinant DNA, this may be productive. If focused on wasteful behaviors such as compulsive cleaning, it isolates. At times, obsessive-compulsives demonstrate ritualistic behavior coupled with a distorted sense of reality.

There are several reasons to recognize the obsessive-compulsive patient. First, if the patient is decompensating, the associated behaviors may lead to care-seeking through hypochondriasis, or they may produce dangerous indecisiveness, resulting in a failure to follow through on care. Simply refocusing the fixated patient on healthy areas in which they do have mastery will lead to restoration of well-being. Second, such patients do poorly with too much uncertainty or ambiguity. Thus, one should alter questioning toward simple, clear, and closed questions. Similarly, providing simple clear directions helps these patients, whereas elaborate directions overwhelm them. Third, it is easy to get into a struggle with obsessive patients who need to go into exquisite detail just when the physician's time is short. Such struggles can be reframed by structuring questions so as to give the patient control. Assign their obsessiveness to them by asking them, for example, to go home and make a list of the things they must check on to bring to the next visit. This will free the physician of the burden of wrestling with the patient about the problem's definition.

Paranoid Patient

Paranoid personalities differ from paranoid schizophrenics in that their problems are lifelong and merely neurotic. But they do also span a spectrum of severity from the mild to the near-psychotic. They show a cognitive style characterized by *suspicious thinking* that in some cases is absurd, in others insightful or shrewd. For instance, they will wonder why the physician is asking what he or she is asking and omitting what he or she is not asking. They question the physician's confidentiality. Such persons are especially rigid. This derives from their preoccupation that reality should confirm their suspicions—hence they also ignore facts that might allay their fears. Because their concerns feel urgent, they are intense in search of confirmation. Whereas hysterics blur facts and obsessives list them, paranoids heighten the importance of minor facts and continually isolate for focus those facts that confirm their fears. This leads to variable but critical distortions of reality. Paranoids confirm their inner fears and fantasies through projection. The paranoid sees events clearly, then interprets them idiosyncratically. Paranoids show problems with autonomy and also often seem excessively arrogant or submissive. Taken altogether, paranoids are similar to obsessives but are more primitive and engaged.[73]

The implications of the paranoid style for the physician are several. First, whereas the problem with an obsessive is to get past nit-picking details and clarifications, the paranoid may quickly get into struggles over control or autonomy and may become suspicious of or threatened by the physician's personality or by the threats implicit in the illness or the cure. Thus, the paranoid may withhold information, may use rejection to manage threatening aspects of the findings, and may attack the physician's style or technical skill. The basic method of dealing with this is to avoid struggles over "irrational" fears and to create a sense of safety for the patient. This is done by noting and supporting (e.g., explicitly praising) the patient's heightened command of facts and the patient's insistence on autonomy and self-control. Giving the patient control over many aspects of the process (you tell me, please make lists, please see what you can discover, feel free to get an independent opinion) heighten autonomy and the sense of safety.

Dependent Patient

The dependent patient is one of the most difficult for some physicians, the favored type for others. These patients enter into a relationship with the physician similar to that of an infant with a mother, sucking at the physician for support and input. They call often and expect the physician to have a fascination with their every belch and bowel movement. They rage at and otherwise punish the physician who does not provide the desired support. Some such patients respond to behavior-shaping. If one ignores their oral clinging and rewards their independent behavior with attention and praise, some dependents can grow in the doctor-patient interaction to be interdependent. Others, who never respond, need firm and clear limits. When the physician specifies when and how often he or she will respond, these patients learn that they must control their neediness and that their escalating demands will be met with pleasant refusal to interact. This helps them, and it saves the physician effort and stress. It is useful in such cases, however, for the physician to ask whether he or she has inadvertently fed into the situation by reinforcing dependent or clinging behavior. If so, the physician must not reinforce the dependent behavior by responding to it with intermittent support in the future. The hardest reinforcement schedule to extinguish is that of intermittent positive reinforcement.[69, 76]

Narcissistic Patient

Narcissistic patients act and feel as if *only they matter*. They demand the best service, describe their place in life grandiosely, seem arrogant or superior, and describe their value and strengths at unbearable length, suffering interruption or humor poorly. They require the care of the most important physician or exaggerate the importance of whoever is caring for them. They are riddled with thinly compensated anxiety about their own inadequacy and danger. They usually respond promptly to recognition of their importance, to explanation of how well they are being safeguarded, and to explanations as to how their own actions can make them into even more superior patients.

Impulsive Patients

The impulsive personality is characteristic of persons with many psychiatric labels, including sociopaths, psychopaths, addicts, alcoholics, and others. These persons combine lack of intentional action with sudden acts based on whim. They display poor judgment in emphasizing only those predictable aspects of their actions that are temporarily pleasing to them. They focus on short-term gain at the expense of long-term well-being. They say things like "I just did it" or "I just had to do it." In some cases, they feel remorse or guilt combined with a sense that outside agents are responsible—"He made me do it" or "It just happened to me." Often, the impulses of such persons are flamboyant, very gratifying, or self-destructive. Usually, impulsive persons can plan short-term activities very effectively. The effect of their dissociation from (or absence of) intentionality and dominance by impulse is a career marked by sudden ups and downs and by erratic involvements in both cognitive and affective domains.

Practically, the paradigm has three implications for working with impulsive characters. First, it is important to recognize and expect that their impulsive character will lead to disruptions and unsatisfactory aspects of their work with the physician. This alerts one not to make matters worse by taking their characteristic behavior personally or by rejecting the patient through anger. Second, it is sometimes useful to explicitly discuss erraticism and impulsivity with the patient and to suggest the possibility of choice! A few will benefit thereby. Finally, physicians often introduce unrealistic demands and use the subsequent failure as a basis for dismissing the impulsive patient from concern or from care. It is useful to be clear with oneself when this is happening and to set up challenges for impulsive patients only about important issues.[73]

Borderline Patient

Borderline patients are often confused with many of the aforementioned types because they show many of the same characteristics. These persons have extremely disturbed psychological development. They exhibit little sense of self. They often describe themselves as emotionally tumultuous while also feeling empty. They feel unable to distinguish themselves from those with whom they are relating, leading to frequent disruptions of relations and parallel needs for emotional intensity periodically defended against by distance. They are often hostile, expecting to be hurt. They are impulsive and frequently abuse substances or themselves. They somatize. They often have psychotic ideation and micropsychoses. They exhibit histories of polypsychiatry, polypharmaceuticals, and polysurgery. They are often demanding and threatening in medical situations, which leads to overly intense searches for obscure diagnoses and to iatrogenic harm due to needless drugs, procedures, or surgery.[75, 79]

Recognition of borderlines is rewarding for a physician since one can then defend oneself and the patient from harmful relationships. One should proceed slowly with the work-up while gradually developing the relationship. With them, one must independently confirm data about prior medical care. One should remove illness as a reason for visits by planning visits on a fixed schedule. One should avoid marginally indicated or addicting medications. One must remain supportive and be as flexible as possible given the intensity of the demands such patients present. Borderlines are often hypochondriac. They also sometimes create factitious illnesses,[80] thus careful documentation and inclusion of other health-care personnel in these cases are useful protections for the physician and patient. As with hysterics, the interviewing of borderlines can be a roller coaster of emotion and conflict. It is wise never to suggest symptoms to them, to remain as open-ended in questioning as possible, and to control one's affect so as to remain positive, supportive, and firm.

INTERVIEWING MORE THAN ONE PERSON AT A TIME

It is sometimes desirable, necessary, or unavoidable to interview more than one person at a time, such as when a patient is not competent, when the bond between the patient and someone else (e.g., a parent or a child) is very strong, or when there is need to include someone else for reasons of patient education or compliance. Sometimes diagnostic consideration or sometimes the creation of a good care plan requires interviewing a family. Most often, the additional person is the spouse, parent or child, or close friend. Sometimes, however, it may be a guardian, a social service representative, a police guard, or another member of the health-care team.

The role of the additional party to an interview determines the interview technique to some extent. When the additional person is related to the patient, the more one can initially allow the patient and relative to interact the more one can learn. By allowing the others to set the tone, determine agenda, or take initiative, the physician can learn the interactional pattern; learn who is dominant and how they relate, show affection, handle communications between themselves, solve problems and prepare themselves to deal with outsiders such as the physician. Carefully follow the basic format but include each party and give each person initial attention, empathy, understanding, and positive regard. If the family is present, respect and attention given to each member initially can be invaluable in creating a working relationship between the health-care team and the patient and family. The family or significant others can play a crucial role in developing a strong therapeutic alliance, especially in accomplishing lifestyle changes and in home care. Correspondingly, the family can be a major source of disruption of therapeutic plans and agreements unless adequately consulted and convinced. They can present alternative explanatory models or raise rational or irrational folk beliefs that change the patient's perception of the problem. Thus, especially in situations requiring considerable cross-cultural accommodation, it is useful to see the spouse or family in order for them to obtain appreciation of and support for the physician's orientation and person. Additionally, the family may be needed to confirm controversial data or to complete information.

A dilemma in seeing family members is that some of what the physician and the patient have discussed may involve confidences that exclude the family. Similarly, family members may want to disclose information that they do not want the patient to hear. There is no general approach to such situations; they involve individual judgments based on as full information as possible. However, it is best to discuss confidentiality before seeing others so as not to become triangulated among members of power struggles or disputes. Seeing the patient and others together can be followed by asking the patient to go to the examining room to prepare. Then one can see each party alone gracefully.

Those close to a very sick patient will have adaptational needs of their own. They are subject to the full range of mental mechanisms used by persons under stress. It is often most helpful to begin by dealing with or at least acknowledging their needs, by asking something like "How has this been for you?" This demonstrates caring and softens displacement toward the physician. Clarification of the person's own agenda and one's own role creates a basis for effective interaction and makes an ally of the family member.

DYING PATIENTS

Epicurus wrote, "So death, the most terrifying of ills, is nothing to us, since so long as we exist, death is not with us: but when death comes, then we do not exist. It does not then concern either the living or the dead, since for the former it is not, and the latter are no more."[81] Nevertheless, the study, knowledge, and management of the events of dying now has its own journal (*The Journal of Thanatology*), institutions (hospices), and bureaucracies. The determinants of the behavior of dying patients include most especially their premoribund personality and experience—particularly their prior history of grieving or giving up. Cultural issues and rituals about dying are paramount in importance. They are present in every culture, including those found in the United States.[82]

In addition to the illness, which may be dominant in the patient's adjustment, dying patients face a predictable group of problems: fear of the unknown, loss of those things to which they are presently attached, and loss of their future or potential.[83] Kubler-Ross has identified a series of stages through which the dying patient is alleged to pass.[84] In my experience, these events may occur but not necessarily in the order given by Kubler-Ross. Dying patients do experience elements of anger, denial, depression, bargaining, and acceptance, but the physician must determine which applies. A dying patient, for example, may be angry about the diagnosis, denying loss of family, bargaining about the future, and accepting of the loss of potential. Thus, the approach to the dying patient must be reassessed frequently and be sensitive to change and development.

The clinician dealing with a dying patient must decide which aspects of the patient's situation are presently of priority and must ascertain how the patient is coping in that domain at the time of intervention or discussion. Negotiation is key: these patients have their own priorities that must be identified and respected while realizing they also will change. Dying patients do need help in their coping. Avoidance by the health-care team of the pain of dying deprives the patient of needed help toward acceptance. This does not imply that the zeal of some to force patients to cope with death when such is not their wish is correct. Rather, one should open the door to discussion and let the patient enter when ready. Using open-ended questions to allow the patients to say what is on their minds, surveying problems, and picking priorities together is effective with dying patients. They should be allowed to bring up issues related to their dying or adjustment to it and to have an opportunity to discuss them with their primary physician or someone else. It is very helpful simply to allow the patient to discuss fears, pain, and other feelings. This discharges some and leads to clarification of others. It shows the patient that he or she is not alone. However, if the patient steadfastly signals denial or distaste for the subject, it is not the physician's business to impose the thanatologic imperative on them: that they must deal with their problems or be judged deficient. While it is difficult to do, it often helps dying patients to speak plainly to them of one's own sense of loss, sadness, and helplessness. It helps to allow them to make clear choices, subject to later confirmation, concerning the extent of intensive care they desire, where they would like to experience their dying, and whether or not they wish the family to have a role in decision-making about them.[85]

It is often a great comfort to the family to have explicit discussion of what to expect and how the dying will (concretely) look to them. Family members need support through their loss and need help to accept the horrors of deterioration and of intensive care. Framing what is being done as "care" rather than as "giving up" can transform the experience from a nightmare to a final act of love, caring, and courage. Ethical dilemmas arise when the family's wishes conflict with the patient's wishes.

Improving Interviewing Skills and Knowledge

The skills and knowledge described in this chapter may be new to many physicians, even those who are nevertheless excellent interviewers. They are neither necessary nor sufficient to be an effective interviewer. The knowledge, skills, and attitudes found in a core curriculum concerning the medical interview are discussed in detail elsewhere.[1]

Practitioners interested in improving their formal knowledge or their practical skill in interviewing have many options. Initially, it helps to define one's needs either alone or through use of an authoritative consultant. Feedback about interviews can take a variety of forms. One can ask patients for feedback, recognizing that unless the relationship is exceptionally trusting and honest the answers may be skewed in the direction the patient feels the physician wants. Second, one can record the interviews using audio- or videotaping. Audiotaping omits the nonverbal visual content of the interview and therefore is less distracting, allowing one to focus on the verbal tone, content, and process. Videotape has the advantage of capturing nonverbal visual material but can be distracting in the taping and in the review. Material thus obtained can be reviewed by oneself, with one or more colleagues or with an expert. If review is done, it is sometimes done by pre-establishing criteria of excellence such as items mentioned in this chapter or elsewhere.[1] As well, it is sometimes done using "process recall." In this technique, pioneered by Kagan,[86] one stops the interview at moments of important affect, interaction, or content. One then attempts to recall what gave rise to the thought or feeling and to figure out ways to do it better or to enhance one's sensitivity in such situations.

The affective dimensions of interviewing are difficult to work on alone, both because they are subtle and because often the problems result from one's own defenses. Group experiences are available through the American Academy on Physician and Patient[88] for work on the human dimensions of medical practice and interviewing. They can change the feeling of a person's practice from one of burden to one of exhilaration.[89] It is frequently observed that students enter medical school idealistically and hopefully and relating effectively with their peers and colleagues. The same students often change and may adopt an authoritarian style, exhibit decreased interpersonal skills, and ultimately experience decreased satisfaction in their work. To a large extent, this is a function of their inadequate understanding and mastery of the human dimensions of practice. These dimensions should be worked on by all those not fully satisfied with their practice to increase satisfaction and to reduce risk of ineffectiveness, early burnout, and psychological withdrawal from practice.

Having developed satisfying and effective interviewing and interpersonal skills in medical interviewing, through self-directed initiatives or formal course or other work, ongoing maintenance and enhancement of skill and sensitivity are undertaken by some. Balint groups are groups of practitioners meeting with an expert to discuss cases that are particularly difficult, meaningful, or instructive. Such groups meet weekly to monthly for several hours and discuss technical, interpersonal, or personal aspects of management.[30] In my group work, patients are sometimes interviewed in weekly conferences. This permits the members to get feedback about their interviewing as well as help with difficult cases. It benefits the patient, who gets practical input from the group. Interviewing is a complex skill requiring integration of knowledge, skill, and affective dimensions into a preconscious behavioral repertoire. Thus, some feel it to be most effectively worked on in intensive, focused courses. Week-long courses now available through the American Academy on Physician and Patient permit focused and undistracted learning of interviewing.[87]

CONCLUSION

This chapter attempts to synthesize data and experience about interviewing. Interviewing is critical both to data collection and to development of a satisfying and effective physician-patient relationship. The chapter provides a practical framework for understanding and improving the structure and function of interviews and an approach to adaptation of the interview style as needed to accommodate differing patient styles. Interviewing can be improved through focused learning and repeated practice. If this is done, greater satisfaction, improved medical skill, and improved therapeutic alliances result. Interviewing is the core clinical skill. Therefore, your interviewing skills deserve lifelong maintenance and growth.

REFERENCES

1. Lipkin M Jr, Quill T, and Napodano RJ: The medical interview: A core curriculum for residencies in internal medicine. Ann Intern Med 100:277, 1984.
2. Hampton JR, Harrison MJG, Mitchell JRH, et al: Relative contributions of history-taking, physical examination, and laboratory investigation to diagnosis and management of medical outpatients. BMJ 2:486, 1975.
3. Reiser DE, Schroder AK, and Schmock CL (eds): Patient Interviewing: The Human Dimension. Baltimore, Williams & Wilkins, 1980, pp 1–239.
4. Greco RS and Pittenger RA: One Man's Practice: Effects of Developing Insight on Doctor-Patient Transactions. London, Tavistock, 1966, pp 1–124.
5. Beckman HB and Frankel RM: The effect of physician behavior on the collection of data. Ann Intern Med 101:693, 1984.
6. Starfield B, Steinwachs D, Morris I, et al: Patient-doctor agreement about problems: Influence on outcome of care. JAMA 242:344, 1979.
7. Elstein AS: Psychological research on diagnostic reasoning. *In* Lipkin M, Putnam SM, and Lazare A (eds): The Medical Interview. New York, Springer-Verlag, 1994.
8. DeMatteo MR and DiNicola PD: Achieving Patient Compliance. New York, Pergamon Press, 1982.
9. Roter DL: Patient participation in the patient-provider interaction: The effects of patient question-asking on the quality of interaction, satisfaction and compliance. Health Educ Monogr 5:281, 1977.
10. Stiles WB and Putnam SM: Coding categories for investigating medical interviews: A meta classification. *In* Lipkin M, Putnam SM, and Lazare A (eds): The Medical Interview. New York, Springer-Verlag, 1994.
11. Lipkin M, et al.: Performing the interview. *In* Lipkin M, Putnam SM, and Lazare A (eds): The Medical Interview. New York, Springer-Verlag, 1994.
12. Platt FW and McMath JC: Clinical hypocompetence: The interview. Ann Intern Med 91:898, 1979.
13. Duffy DL, Hammerman D, and Cohen MA: Communication skills of house officers: A study in a medical clinic. Ann Intern Med 93:354, 1980.
14. Wasserman RC and Inui TS: Systematic analysis of clinician-patient interaction: A critique of recent approaches with suggestions for future research. Med Care 21:279, 1983.
15. Cohen-Cole SA: Training others in liaison psychiatry: Literature review and methodologic proposals. Gen Hosp Psychiatry 2:282, 1980.
16. Cohen-Cole SA. The Medical Interview: The Three-Function Approach. St. Louis, CV Mosby, 1991.
17. Cohen-Cole SA: The Medical Interview: The Three-Function Approach. St. Louis, CV Mosby, 1991.
18. Lazare A and Putnam SM: The three functions of the medical interview. *In* Lipkin M, Putnam SM, and Lazare A (eds): The Medical Interview. New York, Springer-Verlag, 1994.
19. Erickson MH, Rossi EL, and Rossi S: Hypnotic Realities: The

Induction of Clinical Hypnosis and Forms of Indirect Suggestion. New York, Halsted Press of John Wiley & Sons, 1976.
20. Burack RS and Carpenter RR: The predictive value of the presenting complaint. J Fam Prac 16:749, 1983.
21. Hall JA: Affective and nonverbal aspects of the medical visit. *In* Lipkin M, Putnam SM, and Lazare A (eds): The Medical Interview. New York, Springer-Verlag, 1994.
22. Carkhuff R: Art of Helping. Amherst, MA, Human Resources Development Press, 1972.
23. Spiegel JP and Machotka P: Messages of the Body. New York, Free Press, 1974.
24. Quill TE: Barriers to effective communication. *In* Lipkin M, Putnam SM, and Lazare A (eds): The Medical Interview. New York, Springer-Verlag, 1994.
25. Kleinman A, Eisenberg J, and Good B: Culture, illness and care. Ann Intern Med 88:251, 1978.
26. Quill TE: Partnerships in patient care: A contractual approach. Ann Intern Med 98:228, 1983.
27. Weinstein MC and Fineberg HV: Clinical Decision Analysis. Philadelphia, WB Saunders, 1980.
28. Charap MH, Levin RI, and Weinglass J: Physician choices in the management of angina pectoris. Am J Med 79:461, 1985.
29. Roter D and Hall JA: Physicians' interviewing styles and medical information obtained from patients. J Gen Intern Med 2:325, 1987.
30. Balint M: The Doctor, His Patient, and the Illness. London, Pitman, 1957.
31. MacKinnon RA and Michels R: Psychiatric Interview in Clinical Practice. Philadelphia, WB Saunders, 1971.
32. Bird B: Talking with Patients. Philadelphia, JB Lippincott, 1973.
33. Weiner H: Psychobiology of Human Disease. New York, Elsevier, 1957.
34. Mechanic D: Medical Sociology: A Selective View. New York, Free Press, 1968.
35. White K, Williams TF, and Greenberg B: Ecology of medical care. N Engl J Med 265:885, 1961.
36. Mechanic D: Social-psychologic factors affecting the presentation of bodily complaints. N Engl J Med 206:1132, 1972.
37. Haynes RB, Taylor DW, and Sackett DL: Compliance in Health Care. Baltimore, Johns Hopkins University Press, 1979.
38. Rogers C: Characteristics of a helping relationship. *In* Rogers C: On Becoming a Person. Boston, Houghton Mifflin, 1961.
39. Korsch BM, Gazzi EK, and Frances V: Gaps in doctor-patient communication: Doctor-patient interaction and patient satisfaction. Pediatrics 92:855, 1968.
40. Frances V, Korsch BM, and Morris MJ: Gaps in doctor-patient communication: Patient response to medical advice. N Engl J Med 280:535, 1969.
41. Rogers C: On Becoming a Person. Boston, Houghton Mifflin, 1961.
42. Hall JA, Roter DL, and Rand CS: Communication of affect between patient and physician. J Health Soc Behav 22:18, 1981.
43. Lipkin M: Care of Patients. New York, Oxford University Press, 1974.
44. Cassel J: The contribution of the social environment to host resistance. Am J Epidemiol 104:107, 1976.
45. Miller GA: The magical number seven plus or minus: Some limits on our capacity for processing information. Psychol Rev 63:81, 1956.
46. Lankton SR and Lankton CH: The Answer Within: A Clinical Framework of Eriksonian Hypnotherapy, Part 3. New York, Brunner-Mazel, 1983.
47. Darwin C: Expression of the Emotions in Man and Animals. Chicago, University of Chicago Press, 1965.
48. Feldman SS: Mannerisms of Speech and Gestures in Everyday Life. New York, International University Press, 1959.
49. Goffman E: Relations in Public. New York, Harper Colophon, 1977.
50. Hall ET: The Silent Language. New York, Doubleday, 1973.
51. Lazare A: Shame, humiliation, and stigma in the medical encounter. *In* Lipkin M, Putnam SM, and Lazare A (eds): The Medical Interview. New York, Springer-Verlag, 1994.
52. Parsons T: Illness and the role of the physician: A sociological perspective. Am J Orthopsychiatry 21:452, 1951.
53. Szasz TS and Hollender MH: A contribution to the philosophy of medicine: The basic models of the doctor-patient relationship. Arch Intern Med 97:585, 1956.
54. Lazare A, Eisenthal S, and Frank A: Clinician-patient relations II: Conflict and negotiation. *In* Lazare A: Outpatient Psychiatry: Diagnosis and Treatment, 2nd ed. Baltimore, Williams & Wilkins, 1989, pp 137–152.
55. Lazare A: Personal communication, 1984.
56. Fisher R and Ury W: Getting to Yes: Negotiating Agreement Without Giving In. Boston, Houghton Mifflin, 1981.
57. Rosenstock IM: The health belief model and preventive health behavior. Health Educ Monogr 2:354, 1974.
58. Kleinman A: Patients and Healers in the Context of Culture. Berkeley, University of California Press, 1979.
59. Harwood A: Mainland Puerto Ricans. *In* Harwood A: Ethnicity and Medical Care. Cambridge, Harvard University Press, 1981, pp 397–481.
60. Beecher HK: Placebos and placebo reactions. *In* Beecher HK: Measurement of Subjective Response. New York, Oxford, 1959, pp 65–72.
61. Bruner JS: Toward a Theory of Instruction, Cambridge, Harvard, 1966.
62. Lichstein P: Terminating the patient-clinician relationship. *In* Lipkin M, Putnam SM, Lazare A (eds): The Medical Interview. New York, Springer-Verlag, 1994.
63. Goffman E: Stigma: Notes on the Management of Spoiled Identity. Englewood Cliffs, NJ, Prentice-Hall, 1963.
64. Esman AH: The Psychology of Adolescence. New York, International University Press, 1975.
65. Strain J, Putnam SM, Goldberg R: The mental status examination. *In* Lipkin M, Putnam SM, Lazare A (eds): The Medical Interview. New York, Springer-Verlag, 1994.
66. Lipowski ZJ: Delirium: Acute Brain Failure in Man. Springfield, IL, Charles C Thomas, 1980.
67. Thomas A and Chess S: Dynamics of Psychological Development. New York, Brunner-Mazel, 1980, pp 216–232.
68. Drossman DA: The problem patient: Evaluation and care of medical patients with psychosocial disturbances. Ann Intern Med 88:366, 1978.
69. Lipp MR: Respectful Treatment: The Human Side of Medical Care. New York, Harper & Row, 1977.
70. Groves JE: Taking care of the hateful patient. N Engl J Med 298:883, 1978.
71. Putnam SM, Lipkin M, Lazare A, et al: Personality styles. *In* Lipkin M, Putnam SM, Lazare A (eds): The Medical Interview. New York, Springer-Verlag, 1994.
72. Corsini RJ: Current Personality Theories. Itasca, IL, FE Peacock, 1977.
73. Shapiro D: Neurotic Styles. New York, Basic Books, 1965.
74. Koenigsberg HW, Kernberg OF, and Schonen J: Diagnosing borderline conditions in an outpatient setting. Arch Gen Psychiatr 40:49, 1983.
75. Kernberg OF: Severe Personality Disorders: Psychotherapeutic Strategies. New Haven, CT, Yale University Press, 1984.
76. Kahana RJ and Bibring GL: Personality type in medical management. *In* Zinberg NE (ed): Psychiatry and Medical Practice in a General Hospital. New York, International University Press, 1964.
77. Lazare A: The hysterical character in psychoanalytic theory: Evolution and confusion. Arch Gen Psychiatr 25:131, 1971.
78. Lazare A, Klerman GL, and Armor D: Oral, obsessive and hysterical personality patterns: replications of factor analysis in an independent sample. J Psychiatr Res 7:275, 1970.
79. Kernberg OF: Neurosis, psychosis and the borderline states. *In* Kaplan HI and Sadock BJ (eds): Comprehensive Textbook of Psychiatry, 4th ed. Baltimore, Williams & Wilkins, 1984, pp 621–630.
80. Ford CV: The Somatizing Disorders. New York, Elsevier, 1983, pp 135–154.
81. Epicurus: Letter to Menoeceus (Translated by C Bailey). *In* Enright DJ (ed): Oxford Book of Death. New York, Oxford University Press, 1983, p 8.
82. Sudnow D: Passing On: The Social Organization of Dying. Englewood Cliffs, NJ, Prentice-Hall, 1967.
83. Parkes CM: Bereavement: Studies of Grief in Adult Life. New York, International University Press, 1972.
84. Kubler-Ross E: On Death and Dying. New York, Macmillan, 1969.

85. Quill TE: Death and Dignity. New York, WW Norton, 1993.
86. Kagan N: Counseling psychology, interpersonal skills and health care. *In* Stone GC, Cohen F, and Adler NE: Health Psychology. San Francisco, Jossey-Bass, 1980, pp 465–485.
87. Clark WD: SREPCIM's first course in medical interviewing. SREPCIM Newsletter 5:60, 1983.
88. American Academy on Physician and Patient, 3000 Chestnut Ave., Baltimore, MD, 21211.

77

Management of Depression

MALCOLM P. ROGERS, MD

Regardless of the framework in which depressions are differentially defined, understood, and treated, all medical practitioners can agree that they are commonly encountered in clinical practice. One epidemiologic survey in the United States has found the lifetime prevalence of any affective disorder to be 7.8%, with a female: male ratio of 2:1.[1] Many, if not most, of these patients will have been examined initially by a physician who does not specialize in psychiatry. Many patients will discuss it with their physician only if he or she seems interested and willing to deal with such matters. Some types of depression may develop in the context of a medical illness for which a physician is already treating the patient. On the other hand, depression may appear, instead, in a disguised manner as a multitude of somatic complaints and may range in severity from temporary and generally adaptive grief reactions to protracted, disabling, and sometimes life-threatening major depressions.

Suicides occur more commonly in men and are generally the product of a depressive illness. They occur at the rate of approximately 31,000 per year, making this the third most common cause of death for persons between the ages of 15 and 34 years; for all ages, suicide ranks eighth as a cause of death.[2] Suicide attempts are approximately 10 times as frequent. The level of disability in depression exceeds that found in most common chronic medical disorders.[3]

Statistics alone, however, cannot capture the enormity of the personal suffering of those who experience depression and of the people who are closest to them. The loss of productive work, the painful effects of disturbed interpersonal relationships, and the wasted human potential are incalculable.

Despite the shortcomings in our understanding of different types of depression, current treatment is generally effective. Primary care practitioners have important contributions to make in the early recognition of abnormal depressive states, in the provision of direct treatment, and in skillful referral.

Evaluation

Although at times the patient's primary complaint is depression, sometimes its manifestations are subtle and are recognized only when looked for. Numerous studies have confirmed that primary care physicians have large numbers of patients coming for office visits for psychiatric problems. According to one study, they accounted for 14% of the visits, making psychiatric problems the fourth most common reason for going to see the physician.[4] It is also evident from many studies that one third to two thirds of such psychiatric complaints are improperly diagnosed—in part because the symptoms are disguised or "masked." One study revealed that 20 to 30% of patients do not report their emotional or behavioral problems to their primary care physicians.[5] They are much more likely to describe their distress in somatic terms. Other studies have clearly documented a pattern of increasing visits and laboratory testing around the time of the developing psychiatric disorder.

In an effort to identify depression in primary care patients, several studies have employed depression self-rating scales, such as the Zung Self-Rating Scale or Beck Depression Inventory. Figures ranging from a 12 to 17% incidence of moderate-to-severe depression have emerged, along with evidence that pharmacologic intervention has a beneficial effect.[6, 7] In a retrospective analysis of depression in one physician's family practice, 60% of patients initially had a somatic complaint or no complaint, whereas 40% had fatigue, nervousness, or depression. Somatic complaints ranged widely but leading the list were musculoskeletal pain, pulmonary infection, desire for "health maintenance or blood pressure check," irregular menses, headaches, and dizziness.[8] Thus the primary care physician should be especially attuned to the wide spectrum of presentations of "masked" depression.

How can the primary care physician facilitate the diagnosis of depression? To begin with, by providing a conducive atmosphere, by listening, by exploring subtle cues, and by asking a few open-ended questions, such as "How are things in general?" or "How are your spirits?" Such relatively simple and innocent questions are often revealing and give patients permission to discuss psychosocial issues.

Much of the information communicated in an interview is nonverbal. The tone and timing of what the patient says, the way the patient looks, and the feelings that are evoked within the physician are often much more revealing than the actual words spoken. Various affective states are contagious; for example, the physician may feel somewhat depressed after talking with a depressed patient. Intuition and self-awareness, therefore, are important in the recognition of the more subtle manifestations of depression.

The physician's capacity to listen to and accept without avoidance strong depressive affects is in itself very important. If a physician can calmly inquire into the reason for the sudden tears rather than abruptly changing the subject, the psychological meaning of a depressive state may be quickly clarified. The evaluation process is also the beginning of a therapeutic intervention.

Finally, one approaches the experience of the interview as a particular moment in time in the patient's life. One must assess when the patient was last his or her "normal self," when and what changed that, and if or how much the current presentation differs from that of the baseline. The interview itself must be considered as a process within the overall course of the patient's life. How significant is it for the patient to acknowledge depressive symptoms, why now, and what impact is that likely to have on the depression? One is dealing with a dynamic, evolving process, and it is often helpful to see the patient at least for a second visit before launching into any longer-term treatment for a major depression.

Differential Diagnosis

The differential diagnosis of mood disorders is briefly summarized in Table 77–1. As a first priority, one searches for the most serious and at times, life-threatening depressions, termed *major depressive episodes*. These depressions generally require specific somatic therapies, such as antidepressant medication or electroconvulsive therapy.

MOOD DISORDERS

Major Depression

The present nomenclature for mood disorders as contained in the *Diagnostic and Statistical Manual of Mental Disorders*,[9] or DSM III-R as it is more commonly known, is still evolving. (DSM IV is due for publication in the near future.) Older adjectives such as *endogenous* or *involutional* depression may be more familiar and in some cases (e.g., *psychotic* depression) continue to be used to describe subtypes of major depression. All of these terms identify a severe pattern of depression, which is not simply a symptom or a reaction to a loss but represents a complex psychophysiologic state that sometimes occurs spontaneously. It implies a total body reaction that lasts from weeks to months and includes somatic symptoms, such as insomnia, anorexia, constipation and psychomotor retardation (the observation of slowness of physical movement), or psychomotor agitation (increased physical activity marked by anxiety, pacing, and hand-wringing).

The term psychotic depression applies to the most extreme cases (~10%) in which the physiologic symptoms are present, but the patient suffers as well from a distortion of reality (e.g., hallucinations or delusions) that is most often affectively congruent (e.g., self-deprecatory voices, delusions of having sinned or being bad).

A major depressive episode is defined by at least a sustained 2-week period of depressed mood or loss of interest or pleasure and at least four of the following symptoms (which are not attributable to a medical disorder): significant weight loss or gain; insomnia (especially early morning awakening) or hypersomnia; psychomotor agitation or retardation; fatigue; feelings or worthlessness or excessive guilt; diminished concentration or indecisiveness; and suicidal ideation.

It is important to note that such a constellation of symp-

TABLE 77–1. DIFFERENTIAL DIAGNOSIS OF DEPRESSION

Major Depressive Disorders	
Major depression (unipolar disorder): Single or recurrent episode	Present >2 weeks: Persistent dysphoric mood and global loss of interest; altered appetite, sleep, and psychomotor state; fatigue, feelings of worthlessness, and diminished concentration and libido; and suicidal ideation
Bipolar disorder (manic-depressive illness)	Presence of manic episode
Other Depressive Conditions	
Uncomplicated bereavement (grief reaction)	Reaction to death of loved one; differs from major depression in lacking marked functional impairment, feelings of worthlessness, or psychomotor retardation
Adjustment disorder w/depressed mood	Maladaptive reaction to stress with tearfulness and depressed mood
Dysthymic disorder (characterologic depression or depressive neurosis)	Prolonged depressed mood or loss of interest (>2 years) but less severe than major depression
Cyclothymic disorder	Chronic (>2 years) mood swings but less severe than bipolar disorder
Organic affective syndrome	Disturbance in mood due to specific organic factor, such as reserpine intake or hypothyroidism
Depressions secondary to other psychiatric illness	Secondary to wide range of other disorders, personality disorders, anxiety disorders, schizophrenia, and so on

toms has usually been present for weeks to months and not simply for several days. There is often a diurnal variation, such that the symptoms are more pronounced in the morning and improve somewhat during the day. There may or may not be an obvious triggering stress, such as a loss. In any event, the depressive episode generally has an intractable quality, as though the patient were caught in a web of circular and self-generating despair. The withdrawal from friends, family, and often work only intensifies the sufferer's sense of worthlessness. Very often one has the feeling that the patient is so self-absorbed in the process that he or she is unreachable through talking or reasoning. The disturbance in concentration is sometimes so severe that it simulates dementia (the "pseudodementia of depression"). Most such syndromes remit spontaneously in 6 months or so, provided that suicide does not intervene. The social and economic consequences, however, may be more difficult to reverse.

A summary of the important characteristics of major affective disorders that distinguish them from less severe or more transient depressive reactions (to be described further on) might include the following: there persists a sense of personal worthlessness, a lack of hope for the future, and a disruption of normal diurnal cycles, accompanied by sleep and appetite disturbances and loss of sexual interest.

If possible, seeing the patient during a second visit several days later will help to clarify the relative intractability of such a syndrome. A previous history of a major clinical depression of the same sort, or previous episode of mania, can help to establish the presence of a major affective disturbance. A positive family history for depression or alcoholism may lend support to the diagnosis. This diagnosis leads one to prescribe antidepressant medication in most cases and electroconvulsive therapy (ECT) in some cases.

Manic-Depressive Illness, Bipolar Disorder

The presence of a manic episode at some time in the past or as a recurrent mental state points to a diagnosis of bipolar affective disturbance or manic-depressive disease. Compared with other types of affective disturbance, it is uncommon (estimated to be 0.4 to 1.2% of the adult population) and is equally distributed between men and women.[10]

Mania is characterized by a marked increase in energy, an escalating rush of activity and speech, flight of ideas, grandiosity, irritability, and most significantly a serious impairment in judgment, such that this rush of energy and activity has frequently very destructive effects. Flight of ideas refers to a sequential series of sentences or phrases, the content of which relates to the preceding and following idea but taken as a whole is nonsensical. Such episodes frequently involve unchecked and wasteful expenditures of money on wild and unworkable schemes. Since the patients are often feeling euphoric, the complaints about their behavior are usually made by family members struggling to contain the inappropriate and extravagant actions of the patient. Prolonged sleeplessness is frequently present.

On encountering such patients, the examining physician may feel exhausted or amused. The patient's rate of speech is usually markedly increased, sometimes with clang associations (words juxtaposed because of rhyme), puns, and rapid switching of topics. Episodes of mania may alternate with episodes of major depression, between which there are usually periods of normal functioning.

A previous history of manic or hypomanic episodes and a family history of affective disease or alcoholism may assist in making the diagnosis. In acute stages, especially when delusions are present, it may be difficult to distinguish bipolar disease from schizophrenia (see Chapter 82). But, as with the unipolar disorders, an accurate diagnosis implies the use of very specific chemotherapeutic agents, namely mood stabilizers like lithium carbonate. In acute situations, the use of antipsychotic medications may also be needed. These are discussed in more detail later.

BEREAVEMENT AND ADJUSTMENT REACTIONS

At the other end of the spectrum are the nonpathologic "depressive" reactions, such as grief reactions or other transient situational reactions with depressive content. By and large these represent adaptive responses to the inevitable losses that occur in life—for example, the loss of a loved one or the sudden loss of health. They may range from the normal, brief depressive reactions and inevitable minor ups and downs of life to the more serious grief reactions triggered by major, sometimes catastrophic, losses. Maladaptive excessive reactions to stress are currently defined as adjustment disorders with depressed mood. Absence of a family or personal history of past depressions and rapid resolution of these reactions helps to distinguish them from major depression.

Individuals confronted with the loss of some important person or object to which they have been strongly attached undergo a mourning process that is characterized by intense sadness, preoccupation with the lost object, and often somatic symptoms, which may be symbolically connected with the loss or may represent psychophysiologic responses. Unlike the case in major pathologic depressions, in uncomplicated bereavement the loss of self-esteem and feelings of worthlessness do not play a central part. The grief appears in direct response to the loss, both in its timing and its proportion to the magnitude of the loss. Although the grief reaction to the death of a spouse, for example, may have a relatively long course, in the range of 3 months to 1 year, it does not generally interfere for long with basic functioning in other interpersonal relationships or in work. Clinical experience indicates that the mourning process is instrumental in allowing the bereaved individual gradually to accept the loss and to begin to substitute other attachments and love objects.

In some instances, of course, what begins as a normal grief reaction may develop into a pathologic depression. Various studies have indicated that such major life changes make an individual more vulnerable both to serious psychiatric illness and to physical illness. Strongly felt ambivalence toward the lost object may complicate the mourning process. In general, the more diverse the patient's other interests and attachments and the greater the source of social support, the more uncomplicated the adjustment will be.

DYSTHYMIC AND CYCLOTHYMIC DISORDERS

Between the extremes of major affective disturbances and normal depressive or grief reactions exist other types of depressions that are commonly encountered in clinical practice. This category, here referred to as dysthymic and cyclothymic disorders, includes patients whose depressions are not as severe as the major affective disorders but constitute psychopathologic states.

The term *dysthymic disorder* replaced the earlier term depressive neurosis and represents a shift from a psychodynamic to a more descriptive classification. In the older nomenclature, persistent mood disturbance was seen as a type of personality disorder. Now this middle ground of less severe but persistent mood disorders and their interrelationship to major affective disorders is being re-examined. For an adult, a chronic low-grade depressed mood and diminished interest of 2 years' duration is required for diagnosis of dysthymic disorder; the changes may be persistent or intermittent, with intervening normal moods not lasting more than a few months. When the mood disturbances involve alternating hypomanic episodes (not reaching the severity of mania), the term *cyclothymic disorder* is used.

Results from the National Institute of Mental Health (NIMH) Epidemiologic Catchment Area (ECA) project indicate that about 4% of the adult population meets the criteria for dysthymic disorder. Klerman has postulated that there may be at least two different pathways to the development of this disorder. His 1978 naturalistic follow-up study indicated that 85% of depressed patients are symptom-free at 1 year.[11] That leaves a significant number of patients who do not fully recover—for some, the result of inadequate treatment; but for others, the result of resistance to even the most comprehensive treatment. Keller and colleagues have demonstrated a higher vulnerability to relapse in the immediate postrecovery period of major depressive episodes. About 20% of patients who had a relapse remained chronically depressed as in dysthymic disorder.[12] These same investigators have coined the term *double depression*; that is, the development of acute major depressive episodes superimposed on chronic unresolved dysthymic depression without intercurrent periods of normal mood.[13]

The other major route to dysthymic disorder involves the insidious onset of depressive features in adolescence and young adulthood. Chronically impaired self-esteem often creates interpersonal difficulties and social isolation, although such patients may be able to function relatively well in their jobs. As they progress into their 30s and 40s, episodes of double depression begin to occur. Whether such chronic interpersonal difficulties are best viewed as underlying personality disturbances or as a "forme fruste" of affective disorder is unclear at present. Akiskal conceptualized the personality traits commonly seen in dysthymic patients—chronic pessimism, low self-confidence, self-critical attitudes, passivity, and interpersonal dependency—as sequelae of the initiating affective disorder in adolescence.

Akiskal has proposed a third pathway leading to dysthymia that occurs secondary to chronic medical diseases (particularly neurologic or rheumatologic diseases of early onset) or in some cases leading to chronic nonaffective psychiatric disorders.[14] He and others have recommended a trial of antidepressant medication, intended to identify and benefit those dysthymic disorders that represent primary affective disorders.[15] Psychotherapy is almost always indicated for dysthymia, which is discussed further in the section on treatment.

ORGANIC AFFECTIVE SYNDROMES

These depressions clinically mimic the major affective disorders and dysthymia but are different in that they are caused by an underlying organic factor, such as the onset of a serious medical illness or the institution of a pharmacologic agent. For these reasons, of course, it is important to consider carefully the timing of the patient's depression in relation to any new medications or changes in the dose of medications and to evaluate the patient's overall medical health for occult diseases. Illnesses like hypothyroidism, occult malignancies, anemia, primary neurologic diseases, and a host of other somatic processes may resemble psychogenic depression. An accurate diagnosis depends primarily on careful review of systems and, when necessary, a workup for a medical disorder.

Medications that may produce depression include antihypertensive medications (e.g., reserpine, α-methyldopa, and propranolol), steroids, anti-inflammatory agents, and many others. Depression may result from digitalis toxicity or sometimes from inappropriate use of minor tranquilizers like diazepam. Such biologic stresses may act in synergism with psychological susceptibility to depressive reactions.

Premenstrual Syndrome

Premenstrual depression, or late luteal phase dysphoric disorder, as proposed in DSM III-R, has been difficult to characterize. It has been found to correlate highly with a previous history of a depressive syndrome (57% of women with unipolar depression and 90% of women with a secondary depression).[16] Although different affective subtypes may occur within the broad spectrum of premenstrual syndrome, including the predominance of hostility, anxiety, or depression, the most common symptoms in unselected women (63%) as well as in women with active major depression (51%) are depression, hypersomnia, increased appetite, and paradoxically, either increased or decreased levels of energy.[17] A careful menstrual history, therefore, may provide supporting evidence for a depressive diagnosis in female outpatients.

DEPRESSIONS SECONDARY TO OTHER PSYCHIATRIC ILLNESS

Depressions sometimes occur in response to other psychiatric disturbances and are usually classified separately. The aftermath of an acute psychotic episode, especially schizophrenia, may be characterized by a prolonged period of depression that is often referred to as postpsychotic depression. Other psychiatric disturbances, such as obsessive-compulsive or panic disorders, are also frequently accompanied by clinical depression. In such instances, the treatment of the primary psychiatric disorder should prevail.

ETIOLOGY OF DEPRESSION

Although the purpose of this chapter is to provide a practical outline for the approach to the diagnosis and treatment of depression for the primary care physician, it nevertheless seems appropriate to devote some attention to the various explanations for the various depressive states. Numerous psychological and biologic models have attempted to explain the causative mechanisms in depression. None seems sufficient to explain fully the various manifestations of depression. In any given clinical situation, one or more of the explanations may seem particularly applicable. These theories provide conceptual frameworks that, in clinical situations, help the physician to organize and make sense of the clinical history. Although both psychological and biologic models exist, the two are not mutually exclusive; both are more or less relevant in any given clinical situation.

Psychological Models

The concept of loss is central to many of the psychological explanations. One should always look for a sense of loss or disappointment coinciding with the onset of of the depressive syndrome. The loss may include not only the loss of a loved one but also the loss of a body function or an expectation.

The failure to live up to one's ego ideal is a common feature of both the major affective disturbances and especially dysthymia. Within this conceptual framework, one looks for the ideal, whether explicit or implicit, that was disappointed. To be loved, to see oneself as good and loving, and to achieve a level of recognition commensurate with one's ambitions are some of the more common ideals represented. A criticism from another, a rejection in a relationship, an inability to pursue a particular goal, an awareness of negative emotions that may conflict with one's ego ideal may all trigger a depressive reaction of varying degrees. It is helpful to consider the expectation in the context of what seems realistic, and the working out of a possible discrepancy between these two may constitute an important path in a subsequent psychotherapeutic approach. Guilt over such failures and the related self-hatred are important psychodynamic aspects of this process. Although such self-hatred (aggression turned inward toward the self) has been emphasized in earlier writings on the subject, more recent investigations have demonstrated that this factor by no means excludes the possibility of overt, outward hostility.

Another model of depression, developed by Beck in particular, emphasizes the cognitive distortion in depressive mood states.[18] The hopelessness and helplessness so commonly described in depression are thought to reflect a peculiar "cognitive" triad: a negative concept of self, a negative interpretation of one's experiences, and a negative view of the future. Although these cognitive processes are commonly encountered in depressive states, in some cases they may reflect ingrained personality traits and in other instances may merely be part of the temporary depressive state. Keeping this framework in mind, the physician should remain aware that the negative events described by the patient may reflect the patient's perception much more than the external reality. Being aware of such assumptions and distortions on the part of the patient and pointing them out when appropriate may be an important part of the psychotherapeutic process.

The concept of learned helplessness developed by Seligman and Groves has also been fruitful.[19] They have developed experimental animal models in which the early experience of helplessness in avoiding noxious stimuli is repeated in later life, despite new available options. The paradigm suggests that helplessness and an inability to cope can become fixed, learned patterns of response. Clinical histories often reveal that an accumulation of negative experiences in early life may leave an individual helpless to deal with adversity later. The absence of positive models to emulate further reinforces a negative self-image.

Another animal model of depression is derived from early observations of the effect of attachment and separation on child development. In work carried out primarily by Harlow and associates, separating a rhesus monkey infant from its mother replicates a sequential behavioral response of protest, withdrawal, and apparent despair similar to clinical depression.[20] The timing of the separation is an important variable. The earlier the separation occurs during infancy, the more traumatic the experience appears to be. The experimental work at least provides an analogy for the frequent clinical finding of early losses and separations in the life of patients who later develop affective disorders. In many of these situations, the loss, which may have been either the actual death of a parent or, even more traumatic, the lack of care and acceptance of affection given to a child or abuse by one or both parents, may predispose toward the development of depressions. In evaluating a patient's current symptoms and history, one looks for disturbances of self-esteem that might have been derived from such earlier experiences.

One may also view depressions from the point of view of social interaction and support. The assumption of a helpless posture by the depressed patient generally elicits more support or some intervention from family and friends. There is some evidence that lack of adequate social support initially may enhance an individual's vulnerability for developing depressions following life stresses.

Conceptualizing depressive states as reverberating vicious cycles may also be useful. Feeling depressed and less worthy, patients generally become more withdrawn and reduce their level of activities. They tend thus to deprive themselves of the usual sources that help to sustain their self-esteem. In addition, they may increase behaviors—for example, overeating and procrastination—that tend only to confirm their negative self-concept. Thinking, then, in terms of the behaviors involved and of the rewards or punishments that might continue to shape them is another valuable dimension along which to consider a patient's history.

Biologic Models

It has long been noted that both depression and manic depression have some familial pattern. Many early studies indicated that for parents, siblings, and children of manic-depressive index cases, the incidence of manic depression was in the range of 10%. Twin studies have also tended to support some genetic predisposition to depression. Higher morbidity risks have been found in relatives of bipolar patients than in relatives of patients with major depression. A major obstacle to clarifying the genetics has been the heterogeneous nature of mood disorders.

Although at present the precise role of genetic factors in affective disturbances is far from settled, from a practical standpoint a physician evaluating a patient with depression should look closely for the presence of affective disturbances in parents, children, and other near relatives.[21]

Over the last 2 decades, considerable attention has also been paid to the biochemistry of depression.[22] The so-called "biogenic amine hypothesis" was based primarily on the dual observations that reserpine, which was known to deplete biogenic amine storage, could precipitate depression in some patients and that the effective antidepressant medications, both the tricyclic antidepressants and the monoamine oxidase (MAO) inhibitors, had the biochemical effect of increasing the effective availability of various biogenic amine substances at the postsynaptic membrane. It also postulated that the reverse was true in mania. That hypothesis proved to be a catalyst for much of the subsequent research, although the results of many studies have been inconsistent with the hypothesis.[23] Abnormalities in other neurotransmitters such as serotonin, dopamine, and acetylcholine have been postulated in affective disorders, perhaps in combination with norepinephrine.

Biologic Markers

Although no adequate biochemical model for depression currently exists, various biologic alterations or markers have been identified. They have begun to provide helpful research tools for the identification of subtypes of affective disorders. The principal biologic markers that have been investigated widely are the dexamethasone suppression test (DST), the thyroid-stimulating hormone (TSH) response to thyrotropin-releasing hormone (TRH),[24] delayed rapid eye movement (REM) sleep latency,[25] and urinary methoxyhyroxyphenyglycol (MHPG), a metabolite of norepinephrine.[26]

Overall, the expectation that such markers would be used in clinical practice, to aid in diagnosis or identify subtypes most likely to respond to particular antidepressant medications, has not been met. Nevertheless they remain as important pieces of the puzzle and potential probes in developing a better understanding of the underlying biology of major depression.

THERAPY

Psychotherapeutic Approaches

Any consideration of treatments begins with attention to the psychotherapeutic alliance. Trust, confidence, and rapport are crucial to the success of any intervention, whether it be psychotherapeutic or somatic, such as antidepressant therapy or ECT. Attentive and empathic listening is likely to strengthen this alliance. A feeling of being understood offers significant relief in itself. When there is genuine understanding and empathy, patients perceive it. By the same token, they are quick to recognize its absence. Honest reassurance based on a true understanding of the problem tends to work well. The physician need not understand everything about the problem, but he or she must be aware of the patient's perception of it. Considerable pressure may be exerted for the physician to supply immediate reassurance for the patient's fears, but it is best to temporize, at least until one has explored what fears may exist. Premature reassurance may widen the gap between the patient and the physician.

One may justifiably express optimism about the patient's recovery from depression, emphasizing the self-limited nature of most depressions and the proven benefits of both antidepressants and ECT in accelerating the process. Such a positive approach is most appropriate in the major affective disturbances and in organic affective states. It may help to acknowledge that the patient's sense of hopelessness and futility about treatment may make it impossible for the patient to share that optimism. In doing so, it is important not to minimize the real despair that the patient may be feeling, but it can be pointed out that such hopelessness is generally part of the illness itself.

The initial interview and often much of the subsequent psychotherapy are aimed at clarifying the losses or other sources of the depression and at defining the parameters of the depressive response. Obviously such clarification is important from a diagnostic point of view in guiding subsequent treatment, but, in addition, it helps the patient to begin taking a more objective view of what is happening and begin making the depression more comprehensible.

One pursues the patient's affects wherever they may lead. It is important not to avoid them and not to make assumptions about what lies behind them. For instance, if a patient begins to become tearful, one should inquire into the thoughts that are causing the sadness. Sometimes the patient may not even know. By tracing the sequence of associations leading to the affects, the central issues tend to emerge in clearer form. Affects do not lie. One is much more likely to become confused or lost in a morass of intellectualizations. In a useful simplification, the late Elvin Semrad characterized the psychotherapeutic process as a sequence of helping the patient to acknowledge, bear, and put into perspective painful affects.[27]

Guilt is a frequently encountered affect in depression, often underlying a need for self-punishment and suffering. Clarification and acknowledgment of its source generally lessen its impact. Recent losses have a way of reactivating reactions to prior loss. Unfulfilled wishes and expectations, juxtaposed upon aging and lost opportunities, are common depressive themes.

Another aspect of the psychotherapeutic approach is to help mobilize a patient to initiate behavioral changes that would clearly bring relief. Very often the decisions and behaviors that can begin to undo the depression are obvious both to the physician and to the patient. For example, it may be clear that a certain destructive relationship must end or that some other difficult task cannot be avoided if improvement is to occur. The problem is often in taking the initial step and in passing the first hurdle. This is not a matter of the physician's telling a confused patient what to do (i.e., imposing his or her own solution to the problem). It is, rather, a process of encouraging and supporting a direction that the patient has come to view as necessary. The taking of an initial positive action often tends to generate its own energy. Distorted, negative perceptions of the self, the outside world, and the future are frequently at the core of a depressive posture. Challenging and correcting those distortions, and the self-defeating behaviors that accompany them, lie at the heart of the cognitive therapy approach pioneered by Beck.[28]

At times the patient's depression may arise from the psychopathology of an interpersonal relationship. A patient may be blaming himself or herself for the difficulties in a relationship, sometimes suspecting that the problem lies more in the other person but lacking the self-confidence or self-assertiveness to confront it. An independent validation of these perceptions may enable the patient to deal more effectively with the other person.

Controlled studies have demonstrated the efficacy of interpersonal psychotherapy (IPT), which focuses on educating the patient about the nature of depression and the particular interpersonal issues related to it, whether grief, role disputes, role transitions, or interpersonal deficits.[29] IPT has been shown not only to improve social functioning but also to prevent recurrences.[30]

The psychotherapeutic relationship between the physician and the patient offers special assistance in both being more objective than most other relationships and being free from exploitation. Ideally, the patient can be assured that the physician operates together with him in his best interest. That kind of therapeutic alliance generally allows for an evaluation of the therapeutic interaction itself. The therapeutic interaction can be viewed as a microcosmic example of the patient's general patterns of interrelationships. The kinds of intense and inappropriate attitudes and feelings that the patient directs towards the physician, based primarily on prior relationships, is referred to as *transference*. Similarly, the physician's response to the patient is referred to as *countertransference.* The relationship provides in some respects, an active, almost laboratory-like situation in which the exploration of interpersonal relationships may occur. At times, referral to group psychotherapy may enhance the patient's awareness of his or her impact on others.

Many of these psychotherapeutic techniques are, of course, complicated and for proper psychotherapy require the experience of a skilled psychotherapist. Yet most of these elements are also present in somewhat modified form in most physician-patient relationships, and it would be a mistake to underestimate the importance of the psychotherapeutic aspects of this relationship. We will return to the subject of the referral process later.

Approaches to Specific Mood Disorders

In uncomplicated *bereavement,* one can assure patients of their normality and of the importance of going through the process. Inevitably, considerable remembering is involved and also sharing of the remembrances with other people. Anniversaries accentuate these reactions. The eventual redirection of energy and attachments should be encouraged. At times, basically normal grief reactions may be complicated by guilt or ambivalent feelings toward the lost person or object. Attention to the details about funeral arrangements, burial plot locations, or personal effects that remind the bereaved of the loss may help in assessing the affective status of the bereaved. Generally in these situations the physician's pointing out the normality of the process and its characteristic features and perhaps sharing the patient's grief on an occasion or two will be sufficient. The physician can reassure the patient that he or she is available if further help is required.

The approach for the patient with major depression or bipolar disorder, as mentioned previously, is often to take a strong and positive stance with regard to the effectiveness of treatment. Generally a somatic therapy is indicated, and the patient will need to be educated about such treatments (see discussion of somatic treatments later). It is frequently impossible to carry on detailed conversations with patients in psychotic or near-psychotic states of depression, in which thinking may be so distorted as to defy a reasoning approach. Much of the psychotherapeutic effort is in encouraging and facilitating the patient's taking the necessary somatic treatment. In general, the decision about more formal psychotherapy, as one would suggest with a dysthymic disorder, for example, must await the course of somatic therapy. At that point, the potential benefits of psychotherapy can be reassessed.

With the manic or hypomanic patient, one of the physician's first efforts is to slow him or her down both in speech and in action. It is particularly important to try to contain destructive behaviors, such as reckless spending and socially embarrassing displays of erratic behavior. Family members, who often have the most to lose, usually must play an important role in this kind of containment. As with major depression, the value of continuing psychotherapy is often best assessed after the initial crisis is brought under control.

In the more chronic but less severe depressions (dysthymic and cyclothymic disorders), guidelines are somewhat less clear. Antidepressant and other psychotropic medications may have a role. For patients in whom the depressed state seems more deeply ingrained as part of the character, gentle confrontation (by providing evidence of the patient's own contributions to his or her troubles and cognitive distortions) may become the primary means of effecting change. Joint meetings with family and sometimes group psychotherapy may assist in the confrontation process, since it is often those around such a patient who feel most of the distress. At times one must accept that little change will be likely. A long-term supportive relationship, in which the physician acknowledges helplessness to change the situation in combination with expressions of admiration for the patient's capacity to carry on so well despite suffering, may yield best results.

In contrast, some dysthymic patients are likely to blame themselves and experience considerable guilt, anxiety, inhibitions, and other symptoms more typical of a neurosis. These patients are most apt to benefit from formal, skilled psychotherapy. Clarification and the development of insight to unconscious repetitive patterns of behavior and therapeutic use of transference are some of the classic psychotherapeutic approaches that work best. The motivation for change and self-understanding is highest in these patients, and the principles of psychodynamics are most applicable.

In the organic affective syndromes, one attempts to distinguish as much as possible the symptoms that are organic in nature from those that basically represent psychologic responses to illness. Are the fatigue and loss of interest experienced by a person with lupus, for example, part of the illness itself or simply reactions to the disability resulting from the medical illness? This differentiation requires detailed discussions of the onset of the depressive reaction in relation to the timing of physical symptoms. At times one's approach with these patients is similar to that of the patient with a grief reaction but with particular attention to the exact loss created by the organic disease. Does the illness mean loss of income, loss of respect, loss of valued activities, or loss of body image, sexual functioning, appetite, and so on?

Naturally, with drug-induced depressions the physician must discontinue the drug when possible and also be prepared to add additional somatic therapies if the former is not sufficient. Many of these patients have an underlying predisposition toward depression, and the role of psychotherapy, as with the major affective disturbances, can be reassessed following the somatic management.

SOMATIC APPROACHES

Pharmacotherapy with antidepressants, mood stabilizers, or ECT are useful primarily in the management of the major affective disturbances. In general, the physician should evaluate the patient on more than one occasion before using any somatic treatment for depression in order to clarify the severity and constancy of the depressive symptoms. Before the initiation of treatment the patient's own perceptions and reactions to medication or ECT need to be explored as well. More will be said on this subject in connection with each of these specific treatments.

Antidepressants

There are three major categories of antidepressant medications: the tricyclics, the newer generation agents, and the MAO inhibitors. The efficacy of all of the antidepressants in the treatment of major depression is similar—in the range of 70%. However, for any given patient, for reasons not yet well understood, one antidepressant may turn out to be more efficacious than another. Usually, the initial

TABLE 77–2. ANTIDEPRESSANTS AND USUAL DOSAGE RANGES

Tricyclics	
Imipramine (Tofranil, Imavate, Presamine)	75–300 mg/day
Amitriptyline (Elavil, Amitril, Endep)	75–300 mg/day
Doxepin (Sinequan, Adapin)	75–300 mg/day
Desipramine (Norpramin, Pertofrane)	75–200 mg/day
Nortriptyline (Aventyl, Pamelor)	50–100 mg/day
Protriptyline (Vivactil)	15–60 mg/day
Chlomipramine (Anafranil)	75–300 mg/day
Trimipramine (Surmontil)	75–300 mg/day
New Generation of Antidepressants	
Amoxapine (Asendin)	100–400 mg/day
Trazodone (Desyrel)	50–600 mg/day
Maprotiline (Ludiomil)	50–300 mg/day
Fluoxetine (Prozac)	20–40 mg/day
Sertraline (Zoloft)	50–100 mg/day
Paroxetine (Paxil)	20–40 mg/day
Bupropion (Wellbutrin)	150–300 mg/day

choices are made on the basis of side effect profiles. Many psychiatrists now begin with the newer agents such as bupropion, fluoxetine, sertraline, or paroxetine because of their relatively lower incidence of bothersome side effects.

Tricyclics. The tricyclic antidepressants have been in use for more than 30 years. The tertiary amines, imipramine, amitriptyline, and doxepin are converted to their demethylated secondary amine metabolites, desipramine, nortriptyline, and protriptyline, respectively, which retain pharmacologic activity and are used clinically as separate entities (Table 77–2).

Pharmacologic Actions. The principal pharmacologic action of these agents is the blockade of the "amine pump," which actively transports released amine neurotransmitters across the cell membrane of the presynaptic nerve from the synaptic cleft. This activity in the central nervous system may account for the antidepressant effect. Variance in the relative blockade of serotonin compared with norepinephrine among different agents provides at least a theoretical basis for variability of clinical response among patients.[29] Attention has also focused on variations in the binding of antidepressants to receptor sites. These differences are closely correlated with patterns of side effects (Table 77–3): muscarinic receptor blockade with dry mouth, blurred vision, and other anticholinergic side effects; histamine (H_1) receptor blockade with sedation; α_1-adrenergic receptor blockade with postural hypotension; and α_2-adrenergic receptor blockade with blockage of the antihypertensive effects of clonidine, α-methyldopa, and guanethidine. These receptor effects may also be relevant to the mechanism of the antidepressant effect.

Sedation and anticholinergic manifestations account for the majority of side effects of tricyclic antidepressants. The most common anticholinergic side effects are dry mouth, blurred vision, constipation, and urinary retention. Other side effects include sweating, tremors, and weight gain. With the exception of urinary retention, these side effects are usually tolerated by the patient and are not indications to stop treatment. Major side effects that may lead to discontinuation of a drug include (1) orthostatic hypotension; (2) acute closure in narrow-angle glaucoma; (3) acute urinary retention in prostatic hypertrophy; and (4) completion of partial heart block.

In certain circumstances the side effects of a tricyclic agent can be used advantageously: in agitated depressions, sedation is desirable; doxepin, a highly sedating antidepressant, might be a logical choice in this circumstance. In retarded depressions, the stimulation of imipramine is an advantage.

Anticholinergic side effects that are bothersome in young patients can produce medically urgent problems in the elderly: (1) a dry mouth prevents retention of dentures, causing decreased food intake; (2) constipation leads to fecal impaction; (3) benign prostatic hypertrophy leads to acute urinary retention; and (4) mild cognitive deficits may progress to disorientation and memory impairment or to a florid delirium with assaultive behavior and visual hallucinations. These side effects are potentiated by over-the-counter drugs that contain antihistamines or sedatives, which may be taken without the physician's knowledge. In addition, drugs are metabolized more slowly in the elderly. Thus, starting doses are lower and increases more gradual. In patients with a particular vulnerability to anticholinergic side effects, desipramine or nortriptyline would be the tricyclic of choice.

In a medically ill population, multiple drug regimens are common. Drug interactions should be noted. Depressed hypertensive patients treated with guanethidine, clonidine, or

TABLE 77–3. POTENCY OF ANTIDEPRESSANTS IN BLOCKING RECEPTORS*

	Antihistamine (Sedation)	Anti-α-Adrenergic (Orthostatic Hypotension)	Anticholinergic (e.g., Dry Mouth, Constipation)	Serotonin S_2 (Ejaculatory Problems)
Tricyclics				
Amitriptyline	+ + +	+ + + +	+ + + +	+
Desipramine	+	+ +	+	+
Doxepin	+ + + +	+ + + +	+ + +	+
Imipramine	+ +	+ + +	+ + +	+
Nortriptyline	+ +	+ + +	+ +	+
Trimipramine	+ + + +	+ + + +	+ + +	+
Protriptyline	+ +	+ +	+ + + +	+
Newer Antidepressants				
Amoxapine	+ +	+ + +	+	+ + + +
Maprotiline	+ + +	+ + +	+	
Trazodone	+	+ + + +		
Bupropion				
Fluoxetine	+		+	+
Sertraline	+		+	+
Paroxetine	+		+	+

*From Richelson E: Synaptic pharmacology of antidepressants: An update. McLean Hosp J 13:67–88, 1988.

α-methyldopa should receive doxepin or one of the newer antidepressants like fluoxetine, which do not block the antihypertensive effects of these drugs.

Dosage and Timing. The typical starting dose is between 50 and 75 mg. The dosage is then increased gradually to approximately 150 mg/day, depending on the drug (see Table 77–2). Frequently, the initial dose is given at bedtime to take advantage of the sedative side effects. Patients at risk for suicide should not be given large quantities of tricyclics (generally not more than a 1-week supply); total doses equivalent to 2.5 g of imipramine (which would be only 50 pills at a strength of 50 mg) may be fatal if taken in an overdose.

Patient Education. All patients should be told that there is approximately a 2-week delay from the time of establishing the therapeutic dosage to the time when the full antidepressant effect can be noted. Sometimes the lag time may be 1 month. It is also important to forewarn patients of the most common side effects, particularly dry mouth and orthostatic hypotension; the latter can be minimized by having the patient get up gradually from a lying position. It is also helpful to discuss the patient's view of medications in general. Some patients may strongly resist medications for fear of giving in and losing control, fear of addiction, or fear of side effects. When possible, it is helpful to wait until the patient agrees to the need to take the medication. Although predicting success may help to maximize the placebo effect of these compounds, it may also be useful to point out their limitations—namely, their inability to solve complex social and situational problems, even though the patient's mood, sleep, appetite, and other endogenous symptoms may improve. In dealing with the frequent fear that patients may no longer be solving problems on their own if they resort to medication, it is well to point out that the medication functions in many respects simply as an aid to patients, who alone must still solve most of the problems. The frequency with which patients are unable to tolerate these medications is generally underestimated, and it takes a great deal of encouragement and support to carry the patient through an adequate clinical trial.

Maintenance. After a positive response has been obtained, the question arises as to whether or not to continue the medication on a maintenance schedule. In general, if the patient has experienced depression for the first time, it is reasonable at around 9 months to taper the doses of the drug gradually over a period of a few months and discontinue it if no relapse occurs. In patients with a history of prior attacks, it may be reasonable to continue the medication on a maintenance schedule, probably at full dosage as judged from the most recent studies. The evidence from three separate studies comparing relapse rate in placebo versus maintenance tricyclic-treated groups is that maintenance therapy reduces the relapse rate by about one half.[32]

Use of Drug Combinations. When hallucinations and delusions are a prominent aspect of a depression, an antipsychotic agent such as a phenothiazine or butyrophenone is used in combination with an antidepressant agent. In a patient with bipolar disorder on an antidepressant, lithium is used as an adjunct for prophylaxis. If hypomania occurs despite lithium prophylaxis, the antidepressant is stopped and a neuroleptic agent is substituted. A reversible neurotoxicity with symptoms similar to those of the malignant neuroleptic syndrome has been described. A review of the literature, however, concluded that the benefits of the combined neuroleptic and lithium treatment outweighed the risks of this syndrome. The symptoms are most likely to occur within 2 weeks of treatment.[33]

Newer Generation Agents

Over the past decade a number of new antidepressant agents have been introduced. Despite the initial claims for increased efficacy and shortened onset of action, in general they do not appear to be more efficacious than the older generation of antidepressants. On the other hand, they clearly have different pharmacologic actions and very different side effect profiles. Some of their advantages and disadvantages are still being identified.

Specific Serotonin (5 HT) Reuptake Inhibitors (SSRIs). The introduction of fluoxetine (Prozac) in the United States in 1987 has dramatically changed the choice of antidepressant medications. The distinct advantages of this class of antidepressants are the relative lack of anticholinergic side effects, the absence of weight gain, and the lack of cardiovascular toxicity (see Table 77–3). The principal side effects have been nausea, overstimulation or insomnia, and ejaculatory disturbances (primarily delay). The ejaculatory disturbances are secondary to blockade of 5 HT_2 receptors, while the clinical antidepressant effect is apparently derived from their potent effects in blocking the uptake of 5 HT into the presynaptic neuron.

A small percentage of patients appear to lose weight. For these reasons fluoxetine rapidly became the most frequently prescribed antidepressant drug and was touted in the popular media as a "breakthrough drug for depression."[35] Then a report was published about six patients on fluoxetine, previously nonsuicidal, who developed intense suicidal preoccupation after 2 to 7 weeks of treatment.[36] The report received a disproportionate amount of attention, due mainly to a campaign against the drug launched by the Citizens Commission on Human Rights, a Church of Scientology group. In July 1991, after reviewing the available scientific data, the United States Food and Drug Administration (FDA) rejected a petition from this group seeking the removal of the drug from the market. However, the distorted negative publicity with wide exposure on talk shows across the United States often necessitates some explanation and reassurance to patients as to the relative safety of this medication.

A second agent of this type, sertraline (Zoloft), was released in 1992 and a third agent, paroxetine (Paxil), was released early in 1993. Both appear to date to have an efficacy and side effect profile very similar to fluoxetine, but without the associated controversy.

Another distinct advantage of the SSRIs is that the therapeutic dosage is frequently the same as the starting, minimal dosage, for fluoxetine 20 mg, for sertraline 50 mg, and for paroxetine 20 mg. Occasionally the dosage is doubled or tripled if there is no improvement after the usual lag time, which is 2 to 4 weeks. Because of their stimulatory effects, the entire dosage of the medication is generally taken in the morning.

Aside from their use in depression, the SSRIs have also been shown to be beneficial in the treatment of anxiety disorders—specifically, obsessive-compulsive disorder and panic disorder. This is useful to remember, because many patients with affective disorders also have concomitant anxiety disorders.

Bupropion. Bupropion (Wellbutrin) was introduced in 1989 and represents a structurally distinct compound, interestingly without reuptake blockade effects on either serotonin or norepinephrine, and the most specific blocking effect on dopamine uptake. Its efficacy in the treatment of major depression is comparable with the tricyclics.[37] Like the SSRIs, it has minimal anticholinergic and antihistaminic properties and no known cardiovascular toxicity and is not associated with weight gain. Its stimulating effect is generally less pronounced than the SSRIs.

Concern about seizures arose in the early trials of bupropion, largely in relation to larger dosages (450 mg/day or >150 mg/single dose) and in patients who were also bulimic. Careful subsequent studies have shown a rate of new seizures at approximately 0.4%, which is not much different from all the other antidepressant drugs that are known to lower the seizure threshold slightly. As a practical matter, bupropion is contraindicated in patients with bulimia or anorexia nervosa and those with a past history of seizures or factors that might predispose them to seizures (e.g., alcohol or substance abuse). The usual starting dosage is 75 mg three times a day, with a maximal dosage 450 mg/day given in dosages no larger than 150 mg three times a day.

Amoxapine. Amoxapine (Asendin) is a derivative of the antipsychotic drug loxapine. Its mechanism of action is through reuptake blockade of norepinephrine primarily and serotonin secondarily. It is as effective an antidepressant as imipramine and amitriptyline, and many of its side effects are similar, primarily sedation and anticholinergic symptoms.[38] Rare side effects associated with overdosage reported in the literature include treatment-resistant seizures,[39, 40] acute renal failure,[39] and permanent neurologic sequelae.[40]

An unusual property of amoxapine and its minor metabolite 7-hydroxyamoxapine is dopamine receptor-blocking activity,[38] a property associated with the therapeutic effects of antipsychotic drugs. Plasma neuroleptic levels in patients on moderate doses of amoxapine are equivalent to levels of patients on antipsychotic drugs.[41] Despite these levels, the incidence of neuroleptic side effects such as akathisia, dystonia, or parkinsonism is low. There are, however, case reports of galactorrhea probably secondary to hyperprolactinemia, as well as tardive dyskinesia.

Because of its unique antipsychotic properties, amoxapine may be a particularly good choice for the treatment of psychotic depressions.

Tetracyclics. Maprotiline (Ludiomil) is the first available tetracyclic compound. A potent norepinephrine reuptake inhibitor, its clinical efficacy and incidence of side effects, including cardiotoxicity, are similar to those of traditional tricyclic antidepressants.[42, 43] Case reports of seizures, both at therapeutic doses as well as following overdose, have led to speculation that maprotiline is more likely to lower the seizure threshold. Maprotiline offers no clear advantage over traditional antidepressants.

Triazolopyridine Derivatives. Trazodone (Desyrel) has emerged as a chemically and pharmacologically distinct addition. Its mode of action is primarily as a serotonin reuptake inhibitor; its overall antidepressant effect is equal to that of traditional antidepressants.[44] It has the advantage of low (relative to the tricyclics) anticholinergic toxicity,[45] but the disadvantage of orthostatic hypotension and ventricular irritability. Finally priapism requiring surgical intervention has been reported.[46] For these reasons, it has largely been supplanted by the newer SSRI drugs.

Monoamine Oxidase Inhibitors. The antidepressant effect of MAO inhibitors was first observed in tuberculous patients treated with iproniazid in the 1950s.[47] Clinical trials with MAO inhibitors for the treatment of depression were discontinued because of the high incidence of hypertensive crises with resultant cerebrovascular accidents. When the tyramine (or "cheese") effect was delineated in Europe, MAO inhibitors were reintroduced into the United States in the 1970s and are presently experiencing a renaissance in the pharmacopoeia of psychiatry.

The most commonly used MAO inhibitors today are tranylcypromine (Parnate), an analog of amphetamine, and phenelzine (Nardil), a hydrazine derivative with low hepatotoxicity. They are presently indicated for the treatment of tricyclic-resistant depression; major depressions characterized by dysphoria, hypersomnia, and hyperphagia; agoraphobia; and generalized anxiety with and without panic attacks. They have been used in the treatment of bulimia and obsessive-compulsive disorder. They are least effective in the treatment of major depression with classic symptoms of anorexia, insomnia, and anhedonia.

The most common side effect is orthostatic hypotension. Insomnia can be problematic. Dose-related anorgasmy and inhibited ejaculation and impotence have been reported.[48] The most severe and yet least frequent side effect is hypertensive crisis precipitated by ingestion of tyramine-containing foodstuffs (e.g., cheese, Chianti wine, pickled herring) or sympathomimetic agents (e.g., pressor agents and over-the-counter stimulants or sinus preparations). It is manifested by hypertension, throbbing headache, photophobia, stiff neck, and palpitations. If the hypertension persists, intravenous phentolamine (Regitine) should be used.

Other serious drug interactions include that with meperidine (Demerol), which can be fatal in combination with MAO inhibitors by producing hypotension or hypertension, hyperpyrexia, and coma. Oral hypoglycemics are potentiated by MAO inhibitors, and dosages may need to be reduced. Tricyclic antidepressants were at one time considered an absolute contraindication; in recent years, however, the combination has been shown to be a potent treatment for previously unresponsive depressions.

Cardiac Side Effects of Antidepressants. A frequent concern regarding the use of antidepressant medications in patients with major affective disturbances is cardiotoxicity: specifically, orthostatic hypotension, tachycardia (an anticholinergic effect), and cardiac arrhythmia, including ventricular irritability, conduction delays, and, rarely, even torsades de pointes (due to quinidine-like effects). Patients with pre-existing conduction defects or history of a recent myocardial infarction are not good candidates for tricyclic agents, or MAO inhibitors.

Among the newer agents, bupropion, fluoxetine, sertraline, and paroxetine are least likely to be associated with cardiac arrhythmias and represent the best choices for patients with conduction defects or ventricular irritability.

Refractory Patients. Patients who fail to respond (~30%) after 3 to 4 weeks at a full therapeutic dosage (150 mg of a tricyclic or an equivalent dosage for the new agents) should have a serum level of the antidepressant measured. If the level is low or in the low to mid-therapeutic range, their daily dosage should be increased to a tricyclic equivalent of 250 to 300 mg/day, provided that they are able to tolerate the side effects. There may be marked individual variations in patients' dosage requirements to obtain a therapeutic level or a clinical response. The serum level of nortriptyline has been the most frequently studied antidepressant correlating plasma concentration to clinical response. There is a U-shaped relationship between these two variables, creating a "therapeutic window." Thus, patients with levels below 40 to 50 ng/ml show little response to the drug, and with levels exceeding 140 to 170 ng/ml the therapeutic effect declines. The threshold level of clinical response to amitriptyline, imipramine, or desipramine is different from that of nortriptyline. It is generally from 95 to 120 ng/ml, and thereafter clinical efficacy appears to increase in a linear fashion rather than showing a U-shaped distribution. The determination of serum levels of tricyclics still remains a rather specialized laboratory procedure, although it is becoming more widely available.

After confirming that the patient has been compliant with antidepressant therapy, and, indeed, continues to fit the diagnostic criteria for major depressive episode, a failure to respond would suggest that a different antidepressant drug be given, generally one with a different pharmacologic profile (Table 77–4). If there is no response to an adequate trial of a second or even a third drug, various drug combinations should be considered. The usual first choice would be the addition of lithium carbonate, which has been shown to augment the antidepressant effects of other antidepressants.[49] Probably the preferred next step is a combination of a tricyclic antidepressant (TCA), such as desipramine, and fluoxetine.[50] Other combinations are sometimes tried, and the option of ECT should be strongly considered for patients not responding to a trial of antidepressants. Beyond the first step of ensuring an adequate trial of an antidepressant, the primary care physician should refer the treatment-resistant patient with depression to a psychiatrist.

Lithium Carbonate. In 1949, while investigating lithium urate in the treatment of nephrotoxicity in patients with gout, J. F. Kade made the serendipitous observation that lithium produced a quieting effect. From that initial observation, lithium has become well established since the 1960s in the treatment of acute mania and especially for prophylaxis of recurrent bipolar affective disorders. Lithium is an ion that exists naturally as a salt and has similar chemical properties to sodium, both in size and in charge. It is used as a lithium carbonate preparation.

It is best established for prophylaxis of recurrent manic episodes.[51] It also appears to reduce recurrent depressive episodes in bipolar illness, although the evidence for this is less well accepted. Maintenance lithium treatment in bipolar illness can be expected to decrease both the amplitude and the frequency of the moods swings. Most investigators have reported about a 70% efficacy. Some patients continue to have moderate mood swings that are attenuated by lithium.

In acute manic episodes, antipsychotic preparations, such as haloperidol and chlorpromazine, bring about a more rapid control of the disorder. Although lithium is more specifically antimanic than the neuroleptics, this effect is not exerted before approximately 5 to 14 days. Consequently, lithium is generally used in combination with a neuroleptic in treating acute manic attacks.

The relative contraindications for the use of lithium include significant cardiac disease, renal disease, organic brain damage, restriction of dietary salt intake, hypothyroidism, pregnancy, and breast-feeding. Salt-depleting measures, including thiazide diuretics, excessive heat and sweating, severe vomiting, or diarrhea, may diminish renal excretion of lithium and tend to elevate serum levels.

Lithium-induced hypothyroidism occurs in 5 to 20% of all patients treated and is more likely to appear in women. Classic symptoms of hypothyroidism accompany the biochemical change that may lead to myxedema if undetected.

TABLE 77–4. TREATMENT-RESISTANT DEPRESSION

1. Give adequate trial and sufficient dosage for sufficient time.
2. Check compliance with serum level.
3. Check diagnostic accuracy.
4. Switch to a different type of antidepressant.
5. Add lithium carbonate.
6. Try a combination of a tricyclic antidepressant and fluoxetine.
7. Use electroconvulsive therapy.

Determination of baseline thyroid functions prior to institution of lithium, followed by annual checks or checks when clinically indicated, allows proper treatment with thyroid preparations. Nephrogenic diabetes insipidus is manifested by polyuria and polydipsia and may respond to a decrease in lithium dosage or to the addition of a thiazide diuretic (the latter requires frequent evaluations of lithium and potassium levels). Changes in renal pathology, such as focal glomerular sclerosis and interstitial fibrosis, may occur in patients with acute lithium intoxication and in those with nephrogenic diabetes insipidus.[52, 53] Approximately one in seven patients may develop pathologic changes correlating with length of treatment and the presence of polyuria. A few of these patients have associated elevated creatinines or decreased creatinine clearances, but frank renal failure in lithium treatment is rare.[52] Cardiovascular malformations, particularly Ebstein's anomaly, occur at a much greater rate in the children of women on lithium during pregnancy[54]; therefore, lithium should be discontinued in women planning pregnancy. Other side effects include elevated blood glucose levels and elevated white blood cell counts.

Dosage and Administration. The initial dosage of lithium carbonate is generally 300 mg three times a day. It reaches a steady state in 5 to 6 days. Blood samples should be drawn approximately 12 hours after the last intake of lithium. Initially, lithium levels should be checked twice a week, with decreasing frequency as the level stabilizes. The therapeutic range is between 0.8 and 1.4 mEq/l, with the total medication dosage of 600 to 1200 mg/day given in two divided doses.

Side Effects. The toxic levels are close to the therapeutic levels, and side effects are common. At levels of 1.0 to 1.5 mEq/l, the acute side effects are generally mild. The most common are anorexia, gastric discomfort, diarrhea, vomiting, thirst, polyuria, and tremor. The more serious side effects usually occur at levels greater than 1.5 mEq/l and include muscle fasciculation, twitching, confusion, and ataxia, progressing in severe toxicity to somnolence and sometimes seizures.

Alternatives to Lithium. When lithium is either ineffective or not tolerated because of side effects, several anticonvulsant medications have been used as alternatives. Spurred on by observations of the psychiatric sequelae of temporal lobe epilepsy, various investigators have begun to explore the use of carbamazepine (Tegretol) and valproate (Depakene, Depakote) in bipolar disorder. Sometimes carbamazepine is used in combination with lithium or with a neuroleptic. It may be particularly helpful in the control of "rapid-cycling" bipolar patients, who have four or more affective episodes per year. Valproate may also have a role in stabilizing "rapid-cyclers" and appears to be useful in treating acute mania as well as being preventative in maintenance therapy.[55]

Electroconvulsive Therapy (ECT). ECT is an empirically derived treatment procedure developed in the late 1930s by two Italian physicians, Bini and Cerletti. Much resistance to its use remains, but in selected cases its judicious administration offers the most rapid and effective antidepressant therapy. Almost all comparative studies have found ECT to be more efficacious (~70 to 90% response) than is tricyclic antidepressant therapy (50 to 70%).[56] ECT is the treatment of choice in major depression when the patient is suicidal and the need for the most rapid recovery is mandatory. The only other indication for ECT is an extremely agitated psychotic state in a patient suffering from either mania or catatonic schizophrenia.

The major contraindication is increased intracranial pressure caused by any space-occupying lesion in the brain. A relative contraindication is a recent myocardial infarction, since arrhythmias may occur during the induced seizure. With adequate oxygenation, however, the risk of arrhythmia is less than that in tricyclic therapy.

Since the early days of its use, which have given rise to its distorted representation as a brutal torture, the use of ECT has been modified in several ways. First, general anesthesia is used. Prior to the induction of an ECT seizure, the patient is anesthetized with a short-acting barbiturate, such as sodium methohexital (Brevital). An anesthetist or anesthesiologist administers the anesthetic. Prior to treatment, the patient is given atropine to block the vagal-stimulating effects of ECT. After anesthesia, a muscle relaxant, such as succinylcholine, is given to block the seizure so that only minimal clonic movements of the fingers and toes will be apparent. Prior to the administration of ECT, the patient is preoxygenated with 95 to 100% oxygen. The treatments are frequently given unilaterally—that is, with one electrode being placed in the midforehead and the other one in the temporal region of the nondominant hemisphere. This placement tends to reduce the temporary memory loss of a few hours' duration that follows the treatment but may not be as effective as conventional, bilateral treatment.

The number of treatments varies, although depressive reactions usually respond in 6 to 12 treatments. Some patients, particularly elderly individuals, may respond to as few as three treatments. In some instances, ECT may be given safely as an outpatient procedure.

ECT may be preferred over antidepressant chemotherapy in patients with pre-existing cardiovascular disease (excluding recent myocardial infarctions) or breast-feeding mothers with severe postpartum depression. High-risk medical patients can be given ECT in a closely monitored medical setting, and many people believe that when so used ECT is safer than prolonged tricyclic therapy.

Side Effects. Memory loss and confusion are now the most common side effects of ECT. The memory loss is characterized by short-term decrease in the ability to acquire new information as well as some amnesia for recent events. Memory loss does not usually appear until the fourth treatment and is proportional to the number of treatments received. Most lost memory returns within 3 to 6 weeks. Confusion with disorientation and impairment of social functioning may appear as an acute organic brain syndrome following ECT. Unilateral placement, although not as rapidly effective as bilateral ECT (with electrodes placed at each temple), does tend to decrease the amount of memory loss and confusion.

Hospitalization. The need to hospitalize a patient with severe affective disturbances arises in several situations, the most frequent of which is a high potential of suicide. A high energy state, agitation, psychosis, profound hopelessness, and the presence of specific suicidal thoughts—for example, thoughts of jumping from a particular building—all indicate a high suicidal potential. A patient in this state of mind should not be left alone. The degree of care and supervision that can be provided by family and friends will in part determine the need for hospitalization. Patients who are strongly opposed to hospitalization but who represent a clear and immediate danger with regard to suicide may need involuntary hospitalization.

One is more likely to defer hospitalization when the patient is continuing to function in an adequate fashion, either at home or at work. As long as these demands are not perceived as overwhelming, they may continue to provide an important source of self-esteem. However, when a patient reaches the point of damaging his or her reputation, risking loss of employment and family by gross errors of judgment, hospitalization is warranted.

PROGNOSIS

Certainly the prognosis depends on the type of depression. In the major affective disorders, either unipolar or bipolar, one would expect the acute episode to resolve within 6 months to 1 year. Treatment rapidly accelerates the recovery. In both illnesses, there is a relatively high likelihood of recurrence, probably on the order of 50%. If recurrences develop, prophylactic maintenance therapy with either lithium or an antidepressant is indicated.

For dysthymia, the potential for recurrence and chronicity is by definition high. Lasting remission depends to some extent on the resolution of the underlying conflicts, when they can be identified, and in some cases antidepressant drug therapy. Similarly, the alteration of characterologic patterns, although difficult, holds out the greatest hope for the characterologic depressions.

Although much has been made of the prophylactic benefits of lithium or antidepressant treatments, it should be kept in mind that psychotherapy, either by altering intrapsychic functioning or by altering a patient's interpersonal environment, may produce some basic lasting changes that protect against recurrence in the long term. Indeed, in a study of 150 neurotically depressed patients (now diagnosed as dysthymic disorder), who were treated with tricyclic agents and psychotherapy, alone and in combination, for 8 months, both modalities seemed to play a unique role.[57] Although the combination offered no significant diminution in relapse rate during the 8-month interval compared with drug treatment alone, psychotherapy did improve social adjustment, as measured by improvement in the marital situation and in personal relationships with friends and family.

Above all, one should remember that most depressions are self-limited and highly responsive to treatment. There are ample grounds for feeling and communicating optimism about the resolution of depression.

ACKNOWLEDGMENTS

I am grateful for Ms. Chris Henry's assistance in the preparation of this chapter, for the thoughtful review of Dr. Michael Mufson, and for the helpful contributions made in the previous edition by Dr. Patricia Maguire.

REFERENCES

1. Weissman MM, Bruce ML, Leaf PJ, et al: Affective disorders. *In* Robins LN and Regier DA (eds): Psychiatric Disorders in America: The Epidemiologic Catchment Area Study. New York, The Free Press, 1991.
2. Silverberg E, Boring CC, and Squires TC: Cancer statistics, 1990. CA Cancer J Clin 40:9, 1990.
3. Wells KB, Stewart A, Hays RD, et al: The functioning and well-being of depressed patients: Results from the medical outcomes study. JAMA 262:914, 1989.
4. Widmer RB and Cadoret RJ: Depression: The great imitator in family practice. J Fam Pract 17:485, 1983.
5. Good MJD, Good BJ, and Clear PD: Do patient attitudes influence physician recognition of psychosocial problems in primary care? J Fam Pract 25:53, 1987.

6. Wright JH, Bell RA, and Kuhn CC: Depression in family practice patients. South Med J 73:1031, 1980.
7. Nielson AC and Williams TA: Depression in ambulatory medical patients. Arch Gen Psychiatry 37:999, 1980.
8. Justin RG: Incidence of depression in one family physician's practice. J Fam Pract 3:438, 1976.
9. Diagnostic and Statistical Manual of Mental Disorders, 3rd ed. Washington, DC, American Psychiatric Association, 1987.
10. Goodwin F and Jamison K: Manic Depressive Illness. Oxford, Oxford University Press, 1990.
11. Klerman GL: Long-term treatment of affective disorders. *In* Lipton MA (ed): Psychopharmacology: A Generation of Progress. New York, Raven Press, 1978, pp 1303–1331.
12. Keller MB, Klerman GL, Lavori PN, et al: Treatment received by depressed patients. JAMA 248:1848, 1982.
13. Keller MB and Shapiro RW: "Double depression": Superimposition of acute depressive episodes on chronic depressive disorders. Am J Psychiatry 139:438, 1982.
14. Akiskal HS: Characterologic manifestations of affective disorders: Toward a new conceptualization. Integr Psychiatry 2:83, 1984.
15. Akiskal HS: Dysthymic disorder: Psychopathology of proposed chronic depressive subtypes. Am J Psychiatry 140:1, 1983.
16. Kashiwazi T, McClure JN, and Wetzel R: Premenstrual affective syndrome and affective disorder. Dis Nerv System 37:116, 1976.
17. Halbreich U, Endicott J, and Nee J: Premenstrual depressive changes—value of differentiation. Arch Gen Psychiatry 40:535, 1983.
18. Beck A: Depression: Clinical, Experimental, and Theoretical Aspects. New York, Harper & Row, 1967.
19. Seligman M and Groves D: Nontransient learned helplessness. Psychonom Sci 19:191, 1979.
20. Young L, Suomi S, Harlow H, et al: Early stress and later response to separation in rhesus monkeys. Am J Psychiatry 130:400, 1973.
21. Rainer JD: Genetics and psychiatry. *In* Kaplan HI and Sadock BJ (eds): Comprehensive Textbook of Psychiatry, IV. Baltimore, Williams & Wilkins, 1985, pp 25–42.
22. Gold PN, Goodwin FK, and Chrousos GP: Relation to the neurobiology of stress: Clinical and biochemical manifestations of depression (2 Parts). N Engl J Med 319:348, 1988.
23. Chiong BN: The evidence against the catecholamine hypothesis. Psychiatr Opin 16:10, 1979.
24. Loosen PT and Prange AJ Jr: Serum thyrotropin response to thyrotropin-releasing hormone in psychiatric patients: A review. Am J Psychiatry 139:405, 1982.
25. Gillin JC: Sleep studies in affective illness: Diagnostic, therapeutic and pathophysiological implications. Psychiatr Ann 13:367, 1983.
26. Schildkraut JJ, Orsulak PJ, Schatzberg AF, et al: Towards biochemical classification of depressive disorders. 1: Differences in urinary excretion of MHPG and other catecholamine metabolites in clinically defined subtypes of depressions. Arch Gen Psychiatry 135:1427, 1978.
27. Semrad EV: Teaching psychotherapy of psychotic patients; Supervision of beginning residents. *In* Van Buskirk D (ed): The Clinical Approach. New York, Grune & Stratton, 1969.
28. Beck AT, Rush AJ, Shaw BF, and Emery G: Cognitive Therapy of Depression. New York, Guilford, 1979.
29. Klerman GL, Weissman MM, Rounsaville BJ, and Cevron ES: Interpersonal Therapy for Depression. New York, Basic Books, 1984.
30. Frank E, Kupfer DJ, Wagner EF, et al: Efficacy of interpersonal psychotherapy as a maintenance treatment of recurrent depression: Contributing factors. Arch Gen Psychiatry 48:1053, 1991.
31. Richelson E: Are receptor studies useful for clinical practice? J Clin Psychiatry 44:4, 1983.
32. Frank E and Kupfer DJ: Maintenance treatment of recurrent unipolar depression: Pharmacology and psychotherapy. *In* Kemali D and Racagni G (eds): Chronic Treatments in Neuropsychiatry. New York, Raven Press, 1985.
33. Prakesh R, Kilwala S, and Ban TA: Neurotoxicity with combined administration of lithium and a neuroleptic. Compr Psychiatry 23:567, 1982.
34. Richelson E: Synaptic pharmacology of antidepressants: An update. Mclean Hosp J 13:67, 1988.
35. Newsweek Magazine. March 26, 1990, pp 38–41.
36. Teicher MH, Glod C, and Cole JO: Emergence of intense suicidal preoccupation during fluoxetine treatment. Am J Psychiatry 147:207, 1990.
37. Settle EC: Bupropion: A novel antidepressant—update 1989. Int Drug Ther Newslett 24:29, 1989.
38. Lydiard RB and Gelenberg AJ: Amoxapine—an antidepressant with some neuroleptic properties? A review of its chemistry, animal pharmacology and toxicity, human pharmacology and clincial efficacy. Pharmacotherapy 1:163, 1981.
39. Pumariega AJ, Miller B, and Rivers-Bulkeley N: Acute renal failure secondary to amoxapine overdosage. JAMA 248:3141, 1982.
40. Goldberg MJ and Spector R: Amoxapine overdosage: Report of two patients with severe neurologic damage. Ann Intern Med 96:463, 1982.
41. Gohen BM, Harris PQ, Alterman RI, et al: Amoxapine: Neuroleptic as well as antidepressant? Am J Psychiatry 139:1165, 1982.
42. Robinson DS: Adverse reactions, toxicities, and drug interactions of new antidepressants: Anticholinergic, sedative, and other side effects. Psychopharmacol Bull 20:280, 1984.
43. Glassman AM: The newer antidepressant drugs and their cardiovascular effects. Psychopharmacol Bull 20:272, 1984.
44. Ayd FJ Jr and Settle EC Jr: Trazodone: A novel broad-spectrum antidepressant. Mod Probl Pharmopsychiatry 18:49, 1982.
45. Gershon S and Newton R: Lack of anticholinergic side effects with a new antidepressant trazodone. J Clin Psychiatry 41:100, 1980.
46. Priapism with trazodone. Med Lett 26:35, 1983.
47. Bloch RG, Doneief AS, Buchberg AS, et al: Clinical effects of isoniazid and iproniazid in the treatment of pulmonary TB. Ann Intern Med 40:881, 1954.
48. MAO inhibitors for depression. Med Lett 22:58, 1980.
49. Zusky PM, Biederman J, Rosenbaum JF, et al: Adjunct low-dose lithium carbonate in treatment-resistant depression: A placebo-controlled study and review. J Clin Psychopharmacol 8:120, 1988.
50. Nelson JC, Mazure CM, Bowers MB, and Jatlow PI: A preliminary, open study of the combination of fluoxetine and desipramine or rapid treatment of major depression. Arch Gen Psychiatry 48:303, 1991.
51. Davis JM: Overview: Maintenance therapy in psychiatry. II: Affective disorders. Am J Psychiatry 133:1, 1976.
52. DePaulo JR Jr, Correr EI, and Sapir DG: Renal toxicity of lithium and its implications. Johns Hopkins Med J 149:15, 1981.
53. Hestbach J, Hansen HE, Amdensen A, et al: Chronic renal lesions following long-term treatment with lithium. Kidney Int 12:205, 1977.
54. Weistein MR and Goldfield MD: Cardiovascular malformations with lithium use in pregnancy. Am J Psychiatry 132:529, 1975.
55. McElroy SL and Pope HC Jr (eds): Use of Anticonvulsants in Psychiatry: Recent Advances. Clinton, NJ, Oxford Health Care, 1988.
56. Crowe RR: Current concepts: Electroconvulsive therapy—a current perspective. N Engl J Med 311:163, 1984.
57. Klerman GL, DiMascio A, Weissman M, et al: Treatment of depression by drugs and psychotherapy. Am J Psychiatry 131:186, 1974.

78

Anxiety Disorders

SARAH L. MINDEN, MD
ALISON FIFE, MD

Anxiety, or nervousness, is a universal feeling. It is also one of the complaints most frequently made by patients to their physicians. Recent estimates suggest that 15% of patients seen in general practice and 76% of patients seen in an outpatient family practice suffer from anxiety.[1] Current and lifetime prevalence rates for various forms of anxiety have been reported for various communities (Table 78–1), further demonstrating how common these disorders are.[2–5] Indeed in 1991, the anxiolytic alprazolam (Xanax) was the third most frequently prescribed drug in the United States.[6]

As a set of symptoms, anxiety may be an appropriate response to a stressful situation or may reflect an underlying medical or psychiatric illness. It is simultaneously a subjective state, characterized by a vague uneasiness or specific fears or intolerable panic, and a physical state marked by shortness of breath, palpitations, chest discomfort, paresthesias, dizziness, nausea, headache, and tremulousness. What confuses the diagnostician is that these same symptoms may equally suggest a panic attack, an episode of hyperventilation, a myocardial infarction, or a pulmonary embolus. Since each of these disorders has a specific treatment of its own, the psychiatric no less than the medical, accurate diagnosis is essential. Even though the medical presentation may be confusing, a detailed medical and psychosocial history, a thorough physical assessment with relevant laboratory work, and a careful mental status examination will in most cases point to the correct diagnosis.

78–1. PREVALENCE RATES FOR ANXIETY DISORDERS

	Prevalence Rate (%)	
Disorder	*1 Month to 1 Year*	*Lifetime*
All anxiety disorders	7.3[3, 4]	14.6[3, 5]
Panic disorder	0.4–1.2[2]	1.6
Obsessive-compulsive disorder	1.3–2.0[2–4]	2.5[3, 5]
Phobia	6.2[3, 4]	12.5[3, 5]
Agoraphobia	2.5–6.3[2, 3]	12.6[3]
Social phobia	1.3[3]	2.8[3]
Simple phobia	5.1[3]	10.0[3]
Generalized anxiety disorder	2.3–6.4[2, 3]	—
Post-traumatic stress disorder	—	1.0[3]

ASSESSMENT

History

Patients describe their anxiety symptoms in different ways. One person may say that he or she has a lump in his or her throat, that his or her ears are ringing, or that he or she is short of breath whereas another may speak in more psychological terms of tension, worry, or stress. These differences simply reflect different individuals' ways of thinking about themselves and their discomforts and not that one person has a medical illness and that the other has a psychiatric disorder. The clinician needs to know precisely when the symptoms began and how they progressed. What brings on the anxiety and what relieves it? Is the anxiety acute or chronic, a new symptom, or a habitual way of experiencing life? Is there a family history of similar symptoms? How has the patient's life been affected? Was there a precipitating event, or do the symptoms seem to be independent of external circumstances? It is important to keep an open mind: attributing causality too readily to a temporally related stressful situation may obscure the signs of a physical illness underlying the anxiety symptoms. Still, there are some events that typically make people anxious: loss of a loved one through death, divorce, or relocation; threatened loss as in a serious medical illness; change, as in a new job or marriage; problems in relationships at home or at work; developmental states and transitions such as adolescence and retirement.

When evaluating a patient's symptoms, we want to know what kind of person he or she is. Is the patient someone who usually manages well but is now overwhelmed for some reason, or has he or she chronically been unable to deal with life's difficulties? Is the person usually self-sufficient and confident or dependent and easily frustrated? What can we learn of his or her capacity for pleasure, for productive work, and for achieving satisfying relationships? Does this person stoically minimize pain or exaggerate the slightest discomfort? Is the person openly frightened or denying any worries, and are these responses appropriate to the situation? What supports exist in terms of family and friends, or has the person alienated potential help?

Approach to the Anxious Patient

The key to gathering a complete and accurate history is attentive, patient, and respectful listening. Many anxious people complain at length about symptoms that are vague, idiosyncratic, and at odds with our usual notions of anatomy and physiology. The more frightened a patient is by the symptoms, the more insistent he or she will be. The dramatic tone that the person gives to the account in the hope of engaging interest in the problems may have the unintended consequence of alienating the listener. When a patient feels that the symptoms are discounted as "all in the head," as trivial in comparison with the next person's complaints, or as irksome and boring to the physician, there can only be contention, disappointment, and frustration on both sides. Such patients tend to become increasingly urgent in their demands for attention, and physicians are bound to feel increasingly helpless and angry. The patient may feel misunderstood and neglected; the physician may feel abused and deceived. The patient may leave to find help elsewhere or may be unwittingly (or even intentionally) driven away. Alternatively, a chronically tense and hostile relationship may evolve. A genuine sense of working together to solve the patient's problems can be fostered by the physician's empathy and respect.

Examination

Physical examination of the anxious patient may reveal signs of autonomic arousal: tachycardia, mild systolic hypertension, rapid respirations, sweating, cold and clammy hands, coarse tremor, tense facial expression, easy startle, and restlessness. It may also reveal an underlying disease state producing these symptoms. The mental status examination is crucial for distinguishing functional from organic causes of anxiety and for differentiating among various psychiatric disorders. Disorientation and deficits in attention, memory, and other cognitive functions should prompt a thorough investigation for organic disease. Diagnostic features of psychiatric disorders associated with anxiety are described later.

Formulation

The data gathered through the history and examination can be formulated in the following general ways. (1) The anxiety is "normal," an understandable and typical response to a common human experience and is not indicative of physical or mental illness. (2) The nervousness is the presenting symptom of a specific medical illness such as hyperthyroidism. (3) The anxiety is the major symptom of a specific psychiatric illness such as generalized anxiety disorder or panic disorder, or one of many symptoms that comprise a psychiatric syndrome such as post-traumatic stress disorder or obsessive-compulsive disorder. (4) The nervousness is real and painful, but the diagnosis remains unclear and continuing observation is required.

CURRENT THEORIES OF ANXIETY

The cause of anxiety is unknown. Although biologic and psychological theories are often set in contrast to one another, a comprehensive approach to a patient's difficulties usually reflects both perspectives and makes use of pharmacologic as well as psychological interventions. Research in both areas allows for optimism, but methodologic problems and contradictory results abound. Under such circumstances a broad conceptual framework is perhaps most useful: When human beings believe that they are in danger, the body prepares for fight or flight. The cortex activates skeletal muscle through pyramidal and extrapyramidal pathways. The limbic system stimulates the hypothalamus to activate the sympathetic nervous system to release pituitary hormones that circulate to peripheral endocrine glands, causing them to release their hormones (thyroxine, cortisol, epinephrine, and norepinephrine). As a result, there is an end-organ increase in heart rate, blood pressure, and respiratory rate, causing the person to experience palpitations, dyspnea, circumoral numbness, and tingling fingertips. Selective vasoconstriction may lead to lightheadedness and fainting. Virtually the same symptoms will result whether the process begins with the brain perceiving a threat or with dysfunction in the endocrine system (e.g., excess thyroxine). If the stress is ongoing or if for some reason the system cannot return to normal, a state of chronic arousal results. There may be alterations in various neurotransmitter systems and, as some believe, lasting end-organ change or damage, resulting in various gastrointestinal disorders, cardiovascular disease, autoimmune disease, or cancer. Researchers in recent decades have illuminated many of the neuroanatomic, neurochemical, and endocrinologic processes that underlie the autonomic hyperactivity associated with anxiety. Comprehensive reviews of these many areas can be found in several references.[7–10]

Although symptoms of anxiety can be induced in the laboratory, subjective experience of the event is colored by expectations, attitudes, and beliefs,[11] indicating that more than biology is involved in feeling nervous. Sigmund Freud, for example, thought of anxiety as signaling that a person's wishes to gratify instinctual desires (e.g., love and hate) were in conflict with equally strong wishes to win the approval of others. He argued that imagined disapproval produces anxiety and compels the person to find an acceptable compromise. Aggressive impulses, for example, may be sublimated effectively into sporting activities, practical jokes, and so forth. In the neuroses, however, fears of retaliation or disapproval are exaggerated and a set of defenses are erected to nullify the anxiety and contain the unacceptable desires. The person may forget the wishes (repression), claim opposite impulses (reaction formation), or try to justify them (rationalization). Excessive use of these defenses and others does not, in the end, effectively contain the anxiety, and instead leads to painful and self-defeating personality traits and symptoms.[12, 13] Through psychotherapy, patients may gain insight into maladaptive behaviors and underlying conflicts and find more effective ways of resolving them.

Behaviorists and learning theorists argue that a phobia may develop when a traumatic event or other painful stimulus is contemporaneously paired with a neutral event so that the individual comes to experience the nontraumatic phenomenon with the same kind of anxiety as if it were the traumatic event. Researchers have found support for the corollary, namely, that anxiety and related increases in blood pressure and heart rate can be modulated by pairing anxiety-inducing experiences with calming or neutral events (e.g., biofeedback, systematic desensitization, and other cognitive behavioral therapies).[14, 15]

DIFFERENTIAL DIAGNOSIS

Anxiety or, generically, nervousness, is a symptom. Diagnosis of the underlying psychiatric or medical disorder determines management and treatment.

"Normal" Anxiety

Nervousness is not likely to be pathologic when it is associated with a specific situation that would make anyone anxious, when it is not too intense, and when it is of limited duration. We expect someone to be nervous when hospitalized, facing surgery, or experiencing a major loss or life change. Although the somatic sensations of fear and anxiety may be identical, with anxiety there is no real danger and there is a tendency to wonder why there is such alarm. "Normal" anxiety has social and cultural determinants and can be a positive force toward learning new skills and achieving goals. Mastery of anxiety enhances self-esteem and confidence.

Psychological Disorders Presenting with Anxiety

Generalized Anxiety Disorder. A person with generalized anxiety disorder is tense and distracted, worried without reason, hypervigilant, and easily startled. He or she is often acutely aware of each heart beat and is alarmed by its seemingly rapid or irregular rhythm. The person may be irritable and urgently plead for relief. He or she is shaky, fidgets, and paces and feels "on edge" or "about to explode." One is fatigued, yet has trouble falling asleep and may awaken frequently; another may have a constant headache, a band of pressure around the head, or a throbbing behind the eyes; still another may feel unable to take a full breath or complain of a lump in the throat, butterflies in the stomach, sweating, a dry mouth, constipation or diarrhea, or urinary frequency. A person may have difficulty concentrating, working, socializing, or having fun. The physical examination and laboratory evaluation reveal only a sinus tachycardia, rapid, shallow respirations, slightly elevated systolic blood pressure, and a fine tremor with cool, clammy extremities. Many patients attempt to treat their symptoms with drugs or alcohol or become addicted to minor tranquilizers offered indiscriminately by physicians.

Generalized anxiety disorder begins in early adulthood and is twice as common in women. It affects more than 2% of the general population but is much more common in medical settings. The cause is unknown. In some cases there is a precipitating event such as a loss, trauma, or conflict with another person. In other cases, it is a chronic state that ebbs and flows over many years without apparent reason. Generalized anxiety may be part of the clinical picture of major depression, panic disorder, obsessive-compulsive disorder, social phobia, and agoraphobia. It is often the most apparent symptom of alcoholism in patients who deny the extent of their addiction.[16] Treatment usually involves a combination of psychotherapy and pharmacotherapy. For some, relaxation therapy is very useful (details of all treatments are discussed later). Prognosis depends on the duration of symptoms, the existence of an identifiable precipitating stressor, the patient's basic personality features, and the quality of interpersonal relationships.

Several references provide comprehensive reviews of diagnostic and therapeutic issues in anxiety disorders.[8–10, 17–20]

Panic Disorder. The patient with panic disorder describes a sudden, overwhelming feeling of terror that comes "like a bolt out of the blue." It is accompanied by hyperventilation, numbness, and tingling in the fingers and around the mouth. During an attack, which usually lasts for only a few minutes, the patient is dizzy, lightheaded, trembling, and weak-kneed and sometimes has blurred vision and perceptual distortions and may faint. There may also be a cold sweat, pounding palpitations, and chest pain that is sharp and stabbing or mimics angina. Some patients imagine that they will "drop dead of a heart attack," "pass out," "go crazy," or "lose control." Many are ashamed to be seen in this helpless, frightened state, and their fears make it difficult to leave home or to be where help is not readily available (e.g., tunnels, bridges, crowded stores). Expecting an attack at any moment, a secondary anticipatory anxiety develops, indistinguishable from generalized anxiety disorder. In the extreme case, one finds a severely incapacitated person, homebound, needing constant companionship, unable to work, socialize, or travel. A careful search for the initial symptoms of panic is important because specific remedies are available.

It has been estimated that 2 million Americans suffer from this disorder.[21] Panic attacks typically start in the third decade and may occur several times a week for many months. These episodes may come and go over the years or evolve into a chronic agoraphobic state (see the next section). There is often a family history of either panic attacks or agoraphobia, and there may be an association with mitral valve prolapse.[22]

Phobic Disorder. A phobia is an unreasonable fear and avoidance of an object, situation, or activity. The phobic individual knows that his or her fear is irrational but cannot control the panic. Agoraphobia refers to a fear of public spaces (e.g., elevators, crowds, airplanes), places from which there is no escape and no hiding from view. Although agoraphobia typically begins in young adults (usually women), these patients may not seek treatment for some years. The onset often, but not invariably, follows a stressful event, and the course is a fluctuating one with exacerbations and partial remissions. Generally, patients give a history of panic attacks, but they may have been forgotten or minimized; rarely, none may have occurred.[23]

An intense fear of looking foolish while eating, speaking, or appearing in public is considered a social phobia, while a simple phobia refers to fearful avoidance of particular objects or situations such as heights, the dark, or animals. The severity of the phobia can be measured by how assiduously the person avoids the situation and by the degree to which usual activities are altered or given up. Phobias are common, affecting more than 6% of the general population (see Table 78–1), and can be quite disabling, particularly when complicated by depression and substance abuse and by vocational and social impairment.[23] Phobias are generally chronic conditions in adults, but children and adolescents, who are especially susceptible to simple and social phobias, often outgrow them. Social phobias may arise under specific circumstances, for example, in response to disfigurement from surgery or an accident or to visible signs of a medical condition.[24] Current treatments include psychotherapy, medication, and behavior therapy.

Post-traumatic Stress Disorder. Following an exceptionally stressful event that is, according to DSM III-R, outside the range of usual human experience,[25] a person may experience a typical cluster of symptoms: emotional deadening, recurrent nightmares and intrusive memories, inability to experience pleasure, feelings of estrangement from others, and symptoms typical of generalized anxiety or panic attacks or both. There may be difficulty sleeping, concentrating, and remembering, loss of appetite, irritability, and depression. A survivor of a group tragedy may feel intense guilt. Situations and people reminiscent of the original event tend to be avoided because they intensify the symptoms and may provoke irrational or even violent behavior; there may be amnesia for all or part of the traumatic event. Precipitants are typically events of undisputed stress—war, rape, incest, torture, serious accidents, and natural catastrophes—that are experienced with an understandable fear of annihilation, profound helplessness, and loss of control.[26, 27] It is this set of feelings that is continually re-experienced by the victim. The diagnosis of post-traumatic stress disorder would not typically be made with stressors such as divorce, death of a loved one, or serious illness, although some individuals may be especially sensitive to relatively common stresses.[28]

The symptoms may immediately follow the event, remit in time, become chronic, or not emerge for an extended period. The resultant disability depends on a combination of the nature and severity of the stressor, the personality and coping skills of the victim, and the availability of emotional support during and following the crisis. Avoiding intimacy, emotional blunting, and loss of interest can threaten relationships, work, and leisure activities. Anxiety and depression can lead to alcohol and drug abuse, chronic maladjustment, or suicide attempts.

Obsessive-Compulsive and Somatoform Disorders. Psychoanalytic theory, as we have seen, argues that when anxiety can neither be faced nor contained by the defenses, other symptoms develop: phobias, obsessions, compulsions, and various somatic preoccupations.[29] An alternative theory, based on the effectiveness of serotonin reuptake blockers such as clomipramine in controlling obsessive-compulsive symptoms, suggests that the disorder results from dysregulation of the serotonergic neurotransmitter system.[30] In either case, obsessions are recurrent, persistent, unwanted thoughts or impulses that include images of violence, ruminations of self-doubt, and fears of contamination. Compulsions are ritualistic behaviors such as excessive hand washing, counting, and checking. People may know that their intrusive thoughts or compelling rituals are irrational but feel unable to control them. They experience mounting tension if they try to resist them and are relieved only when they give in to them.

In conversion disorder, the intolerable anxiety that arises from an unacceptable wish (e.g., to strike someone) may be "converted" into a physical symptom that prevents the action but also symbolically conveys it (e.g., an arm raised in anger, but "paralyzed"). Similarly, patients with somatization disorder may deny feeling anxious but instead present a great number of physical complaints for which no organic cause can be found. The hypochondriacal patient does experience considerable anxiety, but it is always about physical symptoms, which are unrealistically feared as signs of a serious illness. In exploring the histories of these kinds of patients, one is often struck by experiences that in someone else would produce anxiety or depression. During the course of a successful psychotherapy, these feelings in fact do come to the fore. The somatoform disorders can coexist with organic disease, and, in up to one third of patients, physical illness may eventually emerge.[31]

Depression. Depression and anxiety coexist in many patients.[32] There is some evidence that the same neurotransmitters are involved, since tricyclic antidepressants and monoamine oxidase inhibitors (MAOIs) are known to be effective in both syndromes. In some cases, either the depression or the anxiety will be more prominent, but in others, it may be difficult to determine which is the primary disorder. Some have argued for a diagnostic category of mixed anxiety-depression (which will be included in ICD-10)[33] and note that a single pharmacologic agent is often appropriate for treating both types of symptoms.

Physical Disorders Presenting with Anxiety

Many physical disorders present with symptoms of nervousness. As we have seen, these autonomic experiences are the end of a common neural and endocrine pathway: The same sensations may result from either a hyperactive thyroid gland or the as-yet-unknown sources of psychologic anxiety. In diagnosing the anxiety disorders, special care must be taken to ensure that there is not a concurrent medical condition producing the symptoms. In most cases a thorough review of systems, a careful physical examination, and relevant laboratory tests will clarify the situation. Nevertheless, underlying medical disorders are often overlooked when psychiatric symptoms are prominent.[34–36] Some diseases are notoriously difficult to diagnose (e.g. multiple sclerosis and systemic lupus erythematosus) and require prolonged observation before they can be comfortably excluded. Furthermore, our prejudices and biases may interfere with good clinical judgment when so-called "typical" patients appear. For example, the young woman who has recently been divorced and is overwhelmed with caring for several children may too quickly be dismissed as anxious without a thorough evaluation of her thyroid function.

Endocrine Disorders. Patients with hyperthyroidism, like patients with generalized anxiety disorder, complain of nervousness, distractibility, irritability, and fatigue. They may also describe palpitations, dyspnea, and sweating, but their hands tend to be warm and moist, whereas those of the patient with anxiety are cold and clammy. Both kinds of patients may have increased appetites, but the anxious patient will likely gain weight whereas the hyperthyroid patient will not. The tremor in anxiety is coarser and more irregular, and anxious patients are generally not heat intolerant, do not sweat excessively, and should not have dyspnea on exertion. In hyperthyroidism the fatigue coexists with a kind of inner "driven" or "turned-on" feeling and is present on waking in the morning. For many patients with mild or early hyperthyroidism these distinctions can be difficult to make, and the possibility of thyroid disease must be kept in mind—especially when a patient's personal style is to explain physical events in psychological terms.

Hypoglycemia may also produce symptoms that are indistinguishable from those of anxiety. Once a "fashionable" explanation for nervousness and fatigue in nondiabetic patients, the diagnosis of hypoglycemia should be based on strict criteria (symptoms occurring simultaneously with low blood sugar levels 2 hours after a carbohydrate-rich meal). Both endogenous and exogenous excess of corticosteroids can produce emotional lability, anxiety, depression, poor concentration, confusion, and psychosis,[37, 38] as can hypoparathyroidism. Pheochromocytoma may cause symptoms that are identical to those of a panic attack, but paroxysmal hypertension and an association of the panic with physical exertion, headache, profuse diaphoresis, and abdominal pressure may point to the correct diagnosis. The paroxysmal events associated with pheochromocytoma tend to be less frequent and less intense than panic attacks, and there is not the same fear of dying or going crazy or phobic avoidance.[39] In addition, the presence of neurofibromatosis, hemangioblastoma, and thyroid cancer, as well as hypertension provoked by smoking, anesthesia, guanethidine, or ganglionic blocking agents suggests pheochromocytoma.[40]

Premenstrual syndrome (late luteal phase dysphoric disorder) is characterized by mood changes, nervousness, irritability, and tearfulness in the week or two before the menstrual period. It is not known how prevalent these symptoms are nor how they relate to the affective disorders. Similar symptoms may occur during menopause. Whether a woman considers these symptoms reason to seek medical attention depends on their severity and her personality, sociocultural background, and current life circumstances.

Neurologic Disorders. A number of neurologic disorders have prominent behavioral symptoms. A temporal lobe seizure may cause fear or a sense of unreality (depersonalization or derealization) along with other simple or complex emotional, perceptual, and behavioral phenomena. The presence of hallucinations (especially olfactory and gustatory), forced thoughts, dreamy states, staring spells, and recurrent stereotypic behaviors should raise the possibility of this diagnosis. Temporal lobe epileptics may experience emotions more intensely than do other people and tend to have temper outbursts, labile mood states, severe depression, and anxiety.[41] Because temporal lobe epilepsy may also be associated with characteristic personality traits, distinguishing it from functional psychiatric disorders is difficult. However, because medication is effective in controlling the episodic phenomena, although not the personality changes, the clinician should routinely inquire about unusual experiences. These may be difficult for the patient to describe and typically last for a few seconds up to 1 minute. Useful diagnostic data like postictal clouding of consciousness or an abnormal electroencephalogram (EEG) (even with nasopharyngeal leads) may be absent.

Delirium from any cause (e.g., alcohol or drug intoxication and withdrawal, brain tumor, viral encephalitis, or central nervous system [CNS] vasculitis) can present anxiety-like symptoms. However, other evidence of diffuse brain dysfunction (e.g., disorientation, inattention, impaired memory, disorganized thinking, perceptual disturbances that worsen at night, and diffuse slowing on EEG) will be present. These symptoms themselves, as well as any diagnostic and treatment procedures that the patient might undergo, may induce considerable anxiety in an already confused individual.

Transient ischemic attacks involving the vertebrobasilar system may mimic panic attacks because they can cause dizziness, visual disturbances, strange physical sensations, and confused behavior.

Cardiopulmonary Disorders. Hyperdynamic β-adrenergic circulatory state is a diagnostic label that has been applied to recurrent attacks of palpitations, chest discomfort, dyspnea, and a preoccupation with cardiac function; it remains unclear whether this is simply another form of panic disorder with prominent cardiovascular symptoms. Although spells of paroxysmal atrial tachycardia (PAT) occur episodically and are frightening, like panic attacks, they tend to end more abruptly and to produce heart rates above 140 beats/min. PAT, but not panic attack, can be ended by carotid sinus massage.[42]

Patients with mitral valve prolapse may experience symptoms typical of panic disorder. Indeed, several studies have found that groups of patients with panic attacks have a higher incidence of mitral valve prolapse than has the general population.[22] It is unknown whether one causes the other or whether both disorders result from some single underlying, possibly genetic, abnormality.

Hyperventilation can create the somatic symptoms of acute panic but, unlike true panic disorder, symptoms can be reproduced by rapid breathing for a few minutes and readily stopped by rebreathing carbon dioxide. Patients with hyperventilation may put more emphasis on symptoms such as lightheadedness, blurred vision, and tingling around the mouth and fingers. There may also be carpopedal spasm.

Symptoms Without Signs. Patients who have vague and atypical symptoms for which no organic cause can be found or who have prominent psychological difficulties are often diagnosed as hypochondriacal or "hysterical" and referred for psychiatric treatment. Although there may be evidence to support a psychiatric diagnosis, follow-up studies have found bona fide organic disease in 10 to 30% of such patients.[43] Disorders such as multiple sclerosis, myasthenia gravis, Huntington's disease, Wilson's disease, combined systems disease, systemic lupus erythematosus, and acute intermittent porphyria are notoriously difficult to diagnose in the early stages. When patients are told, or interpret their physicians as saying, "It's all in your head," they understandably feel misunderstood, angry, and hurt. Demoralized by persistent symptoms, they become pessimistic about ever receiving help and fear the progression of a serious illness while "no one is watching." The stage is then set for a difficult doctor-patient relationship even after a diagnosis is established. It is unwise to perform endless tests for unexplained subjective symptoms, but it is important to convey to the patient that his or her complaints are taken seriously. Reassurance and ongoing concern should be supported by regularly scheduled times for re-evaluation and frank discussion of positive and negative findings.

Medications and Drugs of Abuse. A great number of medications and drugs of abuse produce the characteristic symptoms of anxiety, either as a predictable side effect (e.g., terbutaline) or as an idiosyncratic reaction in susceptible individuals (e.g., corticosteroids).[37, 38] The Boston Collaborative Drug-Related Programs found that of 9000 patients with 90,000 drug exposures, more than 200 experienced moderately severe symptoms, such as agitation, bizarre and unusual feelings, depersonalization, anxiety, depression, fatigue, nervousness, malaise, and nightmares. The two agents most likely to produce psychiatric disturbances were prednisone (of which one sixth of the reactions that occurred were psychiatric in nature) and isoniazid (of which nearly one third of reactions were neuropsychiatric).[44] Whereas fewer than 1% of patients taking less than 40 mg/day of prednisone will have psychiatric symptoms, 18% developed them at doses of over 80 mg/day.[38]

Perhaps the drug that is most responsible for nervousness, irritability, and "the jitters" is caffeine. Twenty to 30% of Americans consume more than the intoxicating daily dose of 500 mg in coffee, tea, colas, cocoa, and over-the-counter medications. Only "five cups of coffee, two headache tablets, and a cola drink" total 700 mg.[45] An intoxicated patient may experience palpitations and, on withdrawal, lethargy, emotional lability, headache, and distractibility. The diagnosis depends on the resolution of symptoms with cessation of the drug. Similar reactions can occur with aminophylline, theophylline, and the stimulants amphetamine, phencyclidine, and cocaine. Hallucinogens like lysergic acid diethylamide (LSD), mescaline, and cannabis may produce anxiety reactions depending on the individual's personality and the circumstances under which the drugs are consumed.

Withdrawal from alcohol, barbiturates, benzodiazepines, and opiates typically involves an initial period of nervousness, irritability, tremulousness, insomnia, and malaise. Each agent has, in addition, typical signs of withdrawal, and a unique course. Patients who have been hospitalized for medical or surgical problems and who suddenly develop evidence of autonomic hyperactivity are most likely withdrawing from some substance on which they are physiologically dependent.

The list of drugs that have been known to produce nervousness is long: lidocaine and propranolol; ethosuximide and primidone; salicylates and other nonsteroidal anti-inflammatory agents; epinephrine and isoproterenol; atropine, trihexyphenidyl, benztropine mesylate, and scopolamine (often found in over-the-counter medications); thyroid preparations; estrogens; antihistamines; and levodopa.[46]

TREATMENT

General Approach

Once a diagnosis has been made, a treatment plan ought to be tailored to each individual patient, depending on diagnosis, age, medical status, personality, and life circumstances. Attention should be paid also to a patient's reliability and potential for abusing medication. There are two goals of any treatment: relief of symptoms and resolution of underlying causes.

Effective management of anxiety is multidimensional. It depends to a great extent on a positive therapeutic relationship between the patient and the clinician. Medication may be indicated for specific disorders, and meditation, relaxation, and biofeedback may be useful for responsive individuals who will learn and practice these techniques.

The major dilemma facing the primary care physician is when to treat a patient and when to refer him or her to a psychiatrist. This depends to some degree on the physician's interest, personality style, type of practice, and time availability. Treating emotional disorders can be rewarding for those who like working with these kinds of patients and frustrating and painful for those who do not. Treatment is most successful when there is enough time to get to know the patient well and to listen and explore his or her feelings in an unhurried way. This may involve as little as 30 minutes every month or as much as 1 hour every week. As in all psychotherapeutic arrangements, there should be an initial discussion about the goals of treatment, the frequency and duration of meetings, fees, how missed appointments will be handled, and how the physician may be reached in an emergency. Firm yet supportive limits may be set on unreasonable demands for extra time, inappropriate emergency calls, and unusual requests that suggest a desire for greater intimacy.

Treatment by the primary care physician is appropriate in many cases of mild to moderately severe anxiety or anxiety clearly related to a stressful situation (e.g., divorce). When the patient is psychotic or suicidal, incapacitated by symptoms, or disrupting the lives of others, he or she should be referred to a psychiatrist. Somatoform disorders are sometimes treated more successfully by the internist, because of the low rate of follow-up on psychiatric referrals, the tendency of these patients to deny any psychological distress, and the need for periodic medical re-evaluation.

When the primary care physician elects to treat the patient, alternatives should be discussed: The patient ultimately is the one to choose. It is important to formulate an explicit treatment plan, and reviewing the case with a psychiatrist may be helpful. Consultation can be repeated whenever there are difficulties or prior to ending treatment. Peer supervision is standard practice among psychiatrists, especially when working with difficult patients.

A patient is referred to a psychiatrist when help is needed to establish a diagnosis and treatment plan or when the primary physician wants the psychiatrist to assume the care of the patient. The way that a referral is handled will often determine the outcome. One patient may experience a psychiatric referral as a covert message that he or she is "crazy"; another may feel rejected; still another may worry that a serious disease will be missed. Such concerns can be diminished by addressing them directly. Generally, the referral should be suggested only after a thorough evaluation has been completed. Since so much depends on the understanding between the patient and the primary physician, taking time to establish a strong relationship is more important than quick relief. In this context, a promise of continued availability will be taken as genuine.

It also helps to explain in detail to the patient what to expect from the referral. The patient should be told the specific symptoms and diagnostic considerations that have prompted the referral and the reasons behind seeking the specialized services of a psychiatrist. The patient should know in advance that the initial meeting usually lasts an hour and that, in addition to inquiring about the current symptoms, the psychiatrist will probably ask about family, work, and other life circumstances, both past and present. The psychiatrist may want to see the patient for a second time or offer ongoing treatment. The patient should be told that information pertinent to his or her care will be provided to the primary physician but that whatever else is shared with the psychiatrist will be kept confidential.

Psychiatric consultations are most effective when the referring physician talks with the psychiatrist beforehand to clarify the reasons for the referral (e.g., consultation versus treatment) and to pass on important information about the patient. Given the structure of most psychiatric practices—fixed hourly sessions, many of which may already be assigned to patients in ongoing treatment—it is helpful to know whether the psychiatrist has time available to treat the patient, if that is what is desired. If treatment is not possible, the primary physician and psychiatrist can decide whether the patient should be seen for an evaluation and referred to someone else who can provide the necessary treatment.

When psychiatric help is unavailable in a particular community or when the patient refuses the referral, the primary physician may have to treat the patient despite a preference or judgment not to do so. Talking over the case with a psychiatrist may be especially important under these circumstances.

SPECIFIC TREATMENTS

Psychotherapy

Psychotherapy offers an opportunity for a patient to express thoughts and feelings freely to another person who implicitly promises nonjudgmental attention. Most psychotherapies are based on the notion that symptoms reflect underlying wishes, fears, or conflicts.[47, 48] An insight-oriented or psychodynamic psychotherapist helps the patient to uncover these unconscious feelings and understand their origins and how they have led to the present difficulties. This task requires a specially trained clinician and commitment of the patient to long-term psychotherapy. The goal of such treatment is greater self-awareness and change in long-standing, undesirable patterns of behavior and personality traits.

When a patient is interested, instead, in symptom relief and return to a usual level of functioning, briefer therapy is possible. Supportive psychotherapy is more directive than insight-oriented therapy: The therapist may point out maladaptive behaviors and suggest ways to amend them or may recommend changes in life circumstances that might improve the situation. Such therapy also may make explicit the connections between symptoms and inner feelings and wishes, although in a less complete way than does dynamic psychotherapy. There tends to be more direct guidance, reassurance, support, and lower expectations for major change. For example, a young woman's anxiety improved when she was able to talk about her anger at her husband's drinking and her fears of being abandoned. She could then see that her symptoms occurred whenever he was late from work. This type of supportive psychotherapy can be practiced effectively by the primary care physician as well as by the specialist.

Behavioral Therapy

Based on the theory that anxiety is a learned set of responses to a particular set of circumstances, behavioral therapists believe that new, anxiety-free reactions can be acquired instead (desensitization).[49, 50] Patients may be taught meditation, deep muscle relaxation, self-hypnosis, and undergo systematic desensitization. Alternatively, they may be exposed to an anxiety-provoking stimulus in flooding or immersion techniques or taught to stop obsessional thoughts. There is evidence for a decrease in the level of autonomic arousal with certain relaxation techniques. These procedures have proved effective for some patients with panic disorder, phobias, and obsessive-compulsive disorders (see further on).

Pharmacotherapy

In this section we describe the kinds of medications that are available for treating anxiety (Table 78–2); later, we present the standard treatments for specific disorders and discuss some of the management issues involved. Since this is a brief overview, clinicians are advised to consult authoritative texts regarding doses, drug interactions, and adverse effects before prescribing medication. This is especially important with medically ill and elderly patients. See the references for reviews of all aspects of pharmacotherapy for anxiety disorders.[9, 10, 17, 18, 19, 51, 52]

While no one ought to be deprived of medication that may relieve painful anxiety, indiscriminate use should be discouraged. Despite the safety of the benzodiazepines, the most effective anxiolytics available, they can induce psychological and physiologic dependence and thus create their own problems. Medication for anxiety is most appropriate when symptoms interfere with a patient's capacity to function and when the anxiety is the result of a specific stressful situation or event. There is no reason to "treat" the usual tensions of everyday life.

Although there are many effective pharmacologic agents for anxiety, all treat only the symptoms and do not alter the underlying disorder. It is important that both the clinician and the patient recognize that to achieve more substantial resolution of the anxiety disorder, psychotherapy or behavioral therapy is required. In most cases, some degree of change in the patient and his or her life situation is necessary.

The way that medication is offered sets the stage for discontinuing it and minimizing the risk of dependency. When the patient and the physician collaborate in helping the patient tolerate an acute stress and regain more effective functioning, medication becomes only one of a number of aids in that process. From the beginning it should be clear that the medication will only be taken for a limited time with a clearly marked end point. The patient should be familiar with the type of medication, anticipated positive and negative effects, and the dose and schedule of administration.

All patients have feelings about medications. Some people view pills magically, as a tangible representation of the physician's caring. Withholding medication, then, can be seen as a cruel and threatening deprivation. With such transformations it is clear that medication received from a highly valued physician, even if no longer necessary, is at best reluctantly given up. Considerable conflict can develop when the physician does not believe that a patient should be taking a medication that the patient strongly desires. Other patients tend to see their anxiety as their "fault," not as a medical disorder, but as a sign of weakness or failure. These patients need help understanding that their symptoms may be caused by biochemical dysregulation and that medication is an appropriate and effective treatment. They generally require reassurance that they will not become addicted and "permission" to obtain symptomatic relief. Still others expect instant and complete relief; they become discouraged and stop their medication unless they are told in advance, and reminded, that recovery can be a fairly prolonged process that often requires not only a variety of interventions but also great patience.

Attention to patients' feelings about medication prior to initiating treatment often resolves concerns that otherwise emerge during treatment, typically as an inability to tolerate side effects or as an exaggerated response to such effects. By understanding the patient's worries, the clinician can anticipate problems and provide extra support.

Benzodiazepines. These are the most commonly used drugs for anxiety; they are effective and safe when taken as prescribed. Typical side effects include sedation, ataxia, and impaired intellectual functioning, but these are dose related, occur early in treatment, and generally resolve. Until patients have become acclimatized to the drug, they should not drive or operate machinery. All other CNS depressants, such as alcohol, over-the-counter sleeping pills, cold remedies, and antihistamines, should be avoided. Although benzodiazepines decrease blood pressure, cardiac output, and respiration, clinically these effects are rarely important. These drugs ought to be avoided in pregnancy. Drug interactions are minimal, compared with barbiturates, because the benzodiazepines have little effect on hepatic microsomal enzymes. Diazepam, however, may increase levels of phenytoin and digoxin, whereas disulfiram, β-blockers, and cimetidine increase levels of the long-acting benzodiazepines.[52]

The various benzodiazepines offer similar anti-anxiety effectiveness, and differ primarily in terms of their half-

TABLE 78–2. MEDICATIONS USED TO TREAT ANXIETY DISORDERS*[1]

Medication	Usual Dose	Major Side Effects and Limitations	Uses and Advantages
Long-Acting Benzodiazepines		***All Benzodiazepines***	***All Benzodiazepines***
Diazepam (Valium)	2–10 mg bid–qid	Possible CNS depression, sedation, confusion, ataxia, fatigue, dizziness, headache, dysarthria, anterograde amnesia; loss of efficacy with prolonged use (4 months for anxiolytics and 2 to 4 weeks for hypnotics); dependence, tolerance, and withdrawal syndromes[3]; potentiate alcohol effects; reversible dementia in elderly and patients with renal disease.	Generalized anxiety disorder
Chlordiazepoxide (Librium)	5–10 mg tid–qid	Advise caution when driving or operating machinery. Taper slowly to avoid withdrawal syndrome. Watch for abuse. Avoid in pregnant and nursing women. Be alert to drug interactions and adjust doses accordingly.	***Some Benzodiazepines***
Clorazepate (Azene, Tranxene)	15–30 mg/24 hr	***Long-Acting Benzodiazepines***	Insomnia
Prazepam (Centrax)	30–60 mg/24 hr	Accumulation with frequent dosing, especially in elderly and patients debilitated with renal or hepatic disease; use lower doses and infrequent dosing.	Seizure disorders
Flurazepam[2] (Dalmane)	15–30 mg hs		Muscle spasticity
Clonazepam (Klonopin)	0.5 mg bid–tid		Alcohol withdrawal
Halazepam (Paxipam)	20–40 mg tid–qid		Panic disorder
			Mixed anxiety and depression
Short-Acting Benzodiazepines		***Short-Acting Benzodiazepines***	
Oxazepam (Serax)	10–15 mg tid–qid	Early withdrawal syndrome[3] (18 hours to 3 days) after taking the drug for 1 week to 4 months	
Lorazepam (Atrivan)	1 mg bid–tid		
Temazepam[2] (Restoril)	15–30 mg hs		
Triazolam[2] (Halcion)	0.125–0.5 mg hs		
Alprazolam (Xanax)	0.25–0.5 mg tid (3–8 mg/24 hr for panic disorder)		
Azaspirones			
Buspirone (Buspar)	5–20 mg tid	Slow onset of action (1–4 weeks); less effective in patients previously treated with a benzodiazepine; dizziness, insomnia, stimulation, nausea, headache, drowsiness, tinnitus, fatigue, GI symptoms, nervousness. Advise caution when driving or operating machinery. Do not administer concurrently or within 2 weeks of a monoamine oxidase inhibitor. Avoid in pregnant and nursing women. Consider potential drug interactions.	Generalized anxiety disorder. Less sedation, less interaction with alcohol, less psychomotor impairment and longer clinical efficacy than benzodiazepines; nonaddictive; no abuse potential; tolerated well by elderly; usually no withdrawal symptoms
Antihistamines			
Hydroxyzine (Vistaril, Atarax)	50–100 mg qid	Anticholinergic effects;[4] sedation, dizziness, poor coordination; potentiate effects of alcohol. Advise caution when driving or operating machinery. Use cautiously in patients with prostatic hypertrophy, narrow-angle glaucoma, stenosing peptic ulcer, and bladder neck obstruction. Avoid in pregnant and nursing women and in patients taking other CNS depressants.	Generalized anxiety disorder
Diphenhydramine (Benadryl)	25–50 mg tid–qid		
β-Blockers			
Propranolol (Inderal)	Performance anxiety: 10–20 mg 1 hr before event. Social phobia: 20–40 mg bid–tid	Bradycardia, lightheadedness, ataxia, dizziness, hearing loss, hypnogogic hallucinations, drowsiness, irritability, confusion, insomnia, depression, fatigue, weakness, GI symptoms. Use cautiously in patients with asthma, cardiac disease, and diabetes. Avoid in pregnant and nursing women. Consider possible drug interactions.	Performance anxiety. Social phobia

TABLE 78–2. MEDICATIONS USED TO TREAT ANXIETY DISORDERS*[1] *Continued*

Medication	Usual Dose	Major Side Effects and Limitations	Uses and Advantages
Tricyclic Antidepressants (Tertiary Amines)[6]		***All Tricyclics***	***All Tricyclics***
Imipramine (Tofranil) Amitriptyline (Elavil, Endep) Doxepin (Sinequan, Adapin)	50–300 mg/24 hr 50–300 mg/24 hr 50–300 mg/24 hr	Moderate to high anticholinergic effects[4]; sedating; moderate cardiac effects[5]; exacerbate alcohol effects; withdrawal symptoms (anxiety, flu-like syndrome); potentially lethal in overdose; may lower seizure threshold or precipitate mania. Increase and decrease slowly in small increments. Avoid use with monoamine oxidase inhibitors. Advise caution when driving or operating heavy machinery. Avoid in pregnant or nursing women. Consider drug interactions.	Panic disorder Phobias Depression with anxiety
Tricyclic Antidepressants (Secondary Amines)[6]			***Secondary Amines***
Nortriptyline (Aventyl, Pamelor)	75–150 mg/24 hr		Fewer anticholinergic effects[4]; fewer cardiac effects[5]
Desipramine (Norpramine, Pertofrane)	150–300 mg/24 hr	May cause allergic reaction	
Other Antidepressants			
Amoxapin (Asendin)	200–400 mg/24 hr	Low to moderate anticholinergic effects[4]; risk of tardive dyskinesia; extrapyramidal reactions in 1% of patients.	Depression with anxiety
Trazadone (Desyrel)	150–400 mg/24 hr	Sedation, lightheadedness, malaise, weakness, fatigue, headache, insomnia, priapism; GI effects. Advise caution when driving or operating machinery.	Depression with anxiety Few anticholinergic effects[4] Few cardiac effects[5]
Monoamine Oxidase Inhibitors[6]			
Phenelzine (Nardil) Isocarboxazid (Marplan) Tranylcypromine (Parnate)	30–90 mg/24 hr 10–30 mg/24 hr 30–60 mg/24 hr	Risk of hypertensive crisis with tyramine-containing foods and certain medications; moderate to high cardiac effects[5]; insomnia, weight gain, anorgasmia, headache, dizziness, lethargy; anticholinergic effects[4]; may precipitate hypomania. Increase and decrease slowly in small increments. Advise carefully regarding medication and dietary restrictions and signs of impending hypertensive crisis. Do not use in pregnant and nursing women. Consider drug interactions, especially TCAs, CNS depressants, narcotics, and sympathomimetic and catecholamine-releasing agents.	Panic disorder Agoraphobia Social phobia
Selective Serotonin Reuptake Inhibitors[6]			
Clomipramine (Anafranil)	150–250 mg/24 hr	Similar side effects to TCAs. Do not administer within 14 days of a monoamine oxidase inhibitor or postmyocardial infarction; may precipitate seizures; may induce hypomania; possible liver injury; weight gain; impotence and ejaculatory failure in men. Advise caution when driving or operating machinery.	Obsessive-compulsive disorder
Fluoxetine (Prozac)	10–20 mg/24 hr	Stimulation, insomnia, anorexia, headache, GI symptoms, weight loss; may precipitate seizures and hypomania. Advise caution when driving or operating machinery. Do not use within 5 weeks of a monoamine oxidase inhibitor. Consider drug interactions.	

GI = gastrointestinal; CNS = central nervous system; TCA = tricyclic antidepressant.

*From Guze B, Richeimer S, and Szuba M: The Psychiatric Drug Handbook. St. Louis, Mosby–Year Book, 1992; Derogatis LR and Wise TN: Anxiety and Depressive Disorders in the Medical Patient. Washington, DC, American Psychiatric Association Press, 1989; Roy-Byrne PP and Wingerson D: Pharmacotherapy of anxiety disorders. *In* Tasman A and Riba MB: American Psychiatric Press Review of Psychiatry, Vol 11. Washington, DC, American Psychiatric Press, 1992, pp 260–284.

1. Only the major side effects associated with these medications are listed in this table. The dose ranges represent typical minimum doses and recommended maximum doses for maintenance therapy. Readers should consult specialized pharmacologic sources for complete information and select appropriate doses and dosing schedules for individual patients.
2. These drugs are marketed as hypnotics.
3. Benzodiazepine withdrawal syndrome: anxiety, insomnia, gastrointestinal disturbance, restlessness, tremor, ataxia, and possible seizures.
4. Anticholinergic effects: dry mouth, constipation, blurred vision, urinary retention, impotence, tachycardia, difficulty initiating urination. Use caution with patients with benign prostatic hypertrophy or at risk for urinary retention or angle-closure glaucoma.
5. Cardiac effects: postural hypotension, depression of the myocardium, prolonged conduction times, inverted or flattened T valves, tachycardia, bradycardia, palpitations, ventricular extrasystoles. Use caution with patients with bundle-branch block or atrioventricular block.
6. Only antidepressants that are used for anxiety disorders or symptoms are listed.

lives (see Table 78–2). Those with longer half-lives, like diazepam and chlordiazepoxide, undergo oxidative metabolism through a number of intermediate steps, producing long-acting metabolites. These drugs continue to accumulate for four to five times the half-life so that a steady state may not be achieved for 1 to 2 weeks. The effect of a given dose is not fully apparent until the steady state is reached; hence, increasing the dose before this may result in excessive blood levels. On the other hand, once the steady state exists, a long half-life permits a single daily dose and a "natural" gradual tapering when the drug is discontinued.[1]

The shorter-acting benzodiazepines are metabolized more quickly and do not have active metabolites. Their duration of action is shorter, and multiple daily doses are required. A steady state is achieved within several days so that effects of a given dose can be determined more quickly. Withdrawal reactions, however, may be more pronounced (see later).

These pharmacokinetic factors are most important in patients with liver disease and in the elderly in whom alterations in drug distribution, metabolism, and excretion lead to decreased clearance and higher plasma concentrations. At 20 years of age, the half-life of diazepam is about 20 hours; by 80 years of age it has increased to 90 hours. The shorter-acting drugs like oxazepam do not increase their half-lives with a patient's age and are, therefore, more appropriate for the elderly.[1] In addition, among elderly patients adverse CNS effects are both more likely and more dangerous.

Other than these considerations, the choice of a benzodiazepine depends on clinician familiarity, previous effectiveness for a particular patient, and the half-life of the drug. Because patients develop a physiologic dependence on benzodiazepines, withdrawal states occur and have been reported in 10 to 15% of patients following abrupt discontinuation.[1] Symptoms range from sleeplessness, headaches, anorexia, and tremulousness to hypotension, hyperthermia, neuromuscular irritability, and seizures. The reactions have been observed not only in patients who had taken high doses of diazepam and chlordiazepoxide for 6 weeks but also in patients on standard doses for longer periods. Whereas anxiety symptoms reappear after 1 to 3 weeks, withdrawal symptoms typically begin as early as 3 days after discontinuing the short-acting preparations and 4 to 10 days after stopping drugs with longer half-lives.[1] Milder withdrawal symptoms may persist for a number of months. Thus, to avoid dependence, benzodiazepines should be used for as short a time as possible and should always be discontinued by gradual tapering.

Perhaps the greatest drawback of the benzodiazepines is the psychological dependence that can develop. Even though there is evidence that these drugs may not retain their effectiveness after 6 months, some patients cannot do without them. If symptoms develop after gradually discontinuing the drug, talking with the patient about his or her worries and determining whether new stresses exist will help to differentiate physiologic withdrawal from the return of the original symptoms or from anxieties related to breaking the dependency. Occasional patients, however, do well only with long-term use of these medications.[53]

Benzodiazepines are best prescribed for a limited time (e.g., 2 to 3 weeks), during which a small initial dose is gradually increased until symptoms abate or side effects become troublesome, and then slowly discontinued. While the risks of dependency are made clear, the patient should also be assured that if symptoms return, another short course can be tried. Medication should be prescribed in small amounts without refills. Despite reasonable concern about the numbers of anxiolytics prescribed, most people do not abuse these medications. Indeed, there is equal risk in being too sparing in their use and prolonging needless suffering.[1]

Azaspirones. Buspirone (Buspar), a nonbenzodiazepine anxiolytic, produces virtually no sedation, cognitive effects, psychomotor retardation, or addiction and can be as effective as the benzodiazepines. Buspirone is indicated in the treatment of generalized anxiety disorder but not of panic attacks or alcohol withdrawal; it may have some role in treating patients with depressive, phobic, and obsessive-compulsive symptoms alongside generalized anxiety.[51] Buspirone does not produce muscle relaxation and is not an anticonvulsant. It is well absorbed after an oral dose, metabolized by the liver, and eliminated by the kidneys, and it reaches peak plasma levels within 60 to 90 minutes. The half-life ranges from 2 to 11 hours, and there are no active metabolites. Unlike the benzodiazepines, buspirone affects the serotonergic system and possibly other neurotransmitter systems. The response time for buspirone is much longer than that of the benzodiazepines—2 to 4 weeks—and thus may be less desirable for acutely anxious patients.

Patients who previously used benzodiazepines have been observed to have less of a clinical response to buspirone. Side effects include dizziness, nausea, insomnia, headache, upper respiratory tract complaints, restlessness, and agitation.[51]

Barbiturates and Meprobamate. With benzodiazepines and azaspirones available, there is no reason for using barbiturates or meprobamate. There is little margin of safety between therapeutic and lethal doses of these drugs. Their addiction potential is high, and withdrawal reactions can be severe. As respiratory depressants, the barbiturates can cause fatal overdoses and are dangerous in patients with pulmonary disorders. Other drugs that should no longer be used for similar reasons are ethchlorvynol, glutethimide, and methaqualone.

Antihistamines and β-Blockers. Sedating antihistamines like hydroxyzine (Vistaril, Atarax) and diphenylhydramine (Benadryl) have been prescribed for patients who abuse other anti-anxiety drugs because they have unpleasant side effects that make them less desirable. These drugs lose their effectiveness over time, produce excessive sedation and paradoxical excitement, lower the seizure threshold, and have troublesome anticholinergic effects. Propranolol (Inderal) has been used for similar reasons, that is, to avoid the dependency that develops with benzodiazepines. It blocks the peripheral sympathetic nervous system symptoms of anxiety, such as palpitations and tremors, but has uncertain effects on the mental aspects.[51] The Food and Drug Administration has not approved propranolol for use with anxiety, and side effects of slowed heart rate, lightheadedness, and dizziness, as well as fatigue, depression, and poor concentration, may be problematic.[52] With other agents now available, there is little reason to use antihistamines and β-blockers for anxiety.[51]

Antidepressant and Antipsychotic Medications. Antidepressants are the drugs of choice for panic disorder (see later). Neuroleptics are indicated for anxiety of psychotic proportions and are not appropriate for treating generalized anxiety or panic attacks. Because of their long-term effects (tardive dyskinesia), they should not be used for nonpsychotic anxiety.

TREATMENT APPROACHES FOR SPECIFIC DISORDERS

"Normal Anxiety" and Physical Disorders Presenting with Anxiety. The patient whose anxiety is to be expected, given a particular situation such as the stress of a developmental stage, loss of a loved one, or change in life circumstances, generally is helped by clarifying the nature of the stress and by offering the reassurance that most people in this situation would also be anxious. Emphasizing that the anxiety will be short lived and encouraging the patient to find ways to minimize it (e.g., seeking out friends, physical exercise, taking a break) are helpful. In many cases this can be a growth experience.

The patient who has a medical illness that presented with anxiety needs to hear that mental symptoms are as much a part of certain disorders as physical ones and that they ought not to be considered shameful. It is good practice to explore emotional reactions to illness with a patient, because all of us experience some degree of anxiety when we are unwell, or when we are forced to give up, even temporarily, our usual adult independent activities. Validation of such feelings not only reflects a respectful and satisfying physician-patient relationship, but it also prepares the basis for an uneventful recovery even in complicated psychosocial situations.

Generalized Anxiety Disorder and Post-traumatic Stress Syndrome. In addition to manifest anxiety, generalized anxiety disorder may involve a chronic pattern of poor coping requiring personality and environmental changes that can be achieved only through nonpharmacologic means; that is, through psychotherapy. For some patients, however, a short course of benzodiazepines may calm their anxiety and allow them to make better use of psychotherapy. When the risk of dependence presents a problem and when rapid relief of symptoms is not important, buspirone may be indicated. A poor response to these medications should raise the possibility of other diagnoses, particularly depression or alcoholism. Relapse rates are high in generalized anxiety disorder, so that typically patients are treated for a number of months, withdrawn to a drug-free state, and retreated for a limited time when symptoms return. With the assurance that treatment will be available when needed, most patients are willing to taper and discontinue medication when both their symptoms and the precipitating crisis have resolved.

Benzodiazepines are helpful for acute post-traumatic anxiety, but less for chronic symptoms, especially when substance abuse is present. Ultimately, however, recovery depends on developing, through psychotherapy, a genuine sense of mastery over the residual effects of the trauma. When the patient is depressed, heterocyclic antidepressants are the treatment of choice.

Panic Attacks, Agoraphobia, and Social Phobia. For patients with panic attacks with or without agoraphobia, the heterocyclic antidepressants, some benzodiazepines (clonazepam [Klonopin], alprazolam [Xanax]), and the MAOIs (phenelzine [Nardil]) are the drugs of choice. Unlike the treatment of generalized anxiety disorder in which medication is given to provide symptomatic relief within a relatively brief time period because of appropriate concern about dependence, treatment of panic disorder depends on nonaddictive medications (except for alprazolam) that are used for more prolonged intervals.

Imipramine and desipramine have been used most extensively. Nortriptyline and fluoxetine may also be effective, but other antidepressants have not been evaluated thoroughly for this disorder. Full antidepressant doses are required, as are therapeutic blood levels, and a treatment effect may not be apparent for 8 to 12 weeks.[51] Patients should be informed of side effects such as postural hypotension, sedation, palpitations, dry mouth, urinary retention, impaired sexual function, and constipation. Patients should also be told that the drug must be given a trial of up to 12 weeks before an effect may be noticed. Therapy should be continued for 6 to 12 months and the medication then tapered and stopped. If the attacks return, the patient should be reassessed.

Because of the need to assiduously avoid foods and beverages containing tyramine as well as sympathomimetic medications and narcotics lest a hypertensive crisis be precipitated, MAOIs should be tried only after there has been a clear treatment failure with a heterocyclic drug (Table 78–3). It is important to ensure that the latter drugs were prescribed at adequate doses for a long enough time and that the diagnosis is correct.

The physician must carefully review with the patient which foods and medications should be avoided and provide a written summary (see Table 78–3). Patients should be told to go immediately to the emergency room if they develop a severe headache, flushing, or palpitations. These drugs must only be given to patients who will reliably adhere to dietary restrictions. In addition, several weeks should elapse between taking tricyclic or other antidepressants and the MAOIs, because of reports of a syndrome with delirium, seizures, hyperpyrexia, and rarely death.

TABLE 78–3. DIETARY AND PHARMACOLOGIC RESTRICTIONS FOR PATIENTS TAKING MAOIs*

Foods and Drinks

All cheeses (fresh cottage and cream cheese are safe)
Pizza, fondue, salad dressings, sour cream, and Italian dishes containing cheeses
Aged or fermented meats or fish, including aged corned beef, salami, sausage, pepperoni, summer sausage, pickled herring
Liver of any type or liverwurst
Broad bean pods, English or Chinese
Extracts of meat or yeast (yeast in baked products [bread] are safe)
Any spoiled food, including bananas, pineapples, avocados (fresh fruits are safe)
Beer, ale, red wine, sherry, vermouth, cognac (other alcoholic drinks, including gin, vodka, and whiskey, are safe in moderation)

Medications

Nasal decongestants, sinus medications, and cold medications, including Dristan, Contac, etc.
Asthma inhalants (pure steroid asthma inhalants are safe)
Allergy and hay fever medications
All narcotics, including Demerol (codeine is safe)
Amphetamines, including diet pills
Sympathomimetic medications of any type, including epinephrine, isoproterenol, methoxamine, levarterenol, norepinephrine, methylphenidate, phenylpropanolamine, ephedrine, cyclopatamine, pseudoephedrine, tyramine, Vetaraminol, and phenylephrine
Any local anesthetic containing epinephrine (local anesthetics without epinephrine are safe)
Levodopa (dopamine) for parkinsonism
Antihistamines
Antidepressants, including tricyclics and serotonin reuptake inhibitors
Note: Diabetics may find the need for decreased insulin dosage, and hypertensive patients may require less antihypertensive medication while on MAOIs

To Be Consumed in Small Amounts, Only If Fresh, and Only by Patients Who Do Not Have Symptoms Following Their Consumption:

Chocolate, anchovies, caviar, coffee, colas, figs, raisins, dates, sauerkraut, mushrooms, beets, rhubarb, curry powder, junket, Worcestershire sauce, soy sauce, licorice, snails, yogurt

Not to be taken for 2 days before starting and for 2 weeks after stopping MAOIs (within 6 weeks of stopping Prozac [fluoxetine]). However, several weeks should elapse before starting MAOI therapy after stopping therapy with another type of antidepressant.

*Adapted from Sheehan DV: Monoamine oxidase inhibitors and alprazolam in the treatment of panic disorder and agoraphobia. Psychiatr Clin North Am 8:49, 1985.

Other side effects are similar to those of the tricyclics. MAOIs are contraindicated in patients with liver and kidney disease, pheochromocytoma, cardiovascular disease, and hypertension as well as in disorders like asthma and chronic bronchitis in which pressor agents may be required.[54] It is unwise to use these drugs in patients older than 60 years of age. Because of the risks involved with these medications, many primary physicians prefer to refer patients who may need them to psychiatrists.

The benzodiazepines, alprazolam and clonazepam, are safer and more rapid in their antipanic effects than the MAOIs; thus, they are often used for patients with disabling panic. Treatment begins with small doses (e.g., 0.25 mg of alprazolam three times daily), which may be increased in small increments every few days to a therapeutic level (e.g., up to 4 to 6 mg of alprazolam per 24 hr). Treatment is continued for 6 to 12 months, then tapered by 0.5 mg or less every week. It may be difficult to distinguish between transient withdrawal effects and return of the panic attacks; the former will resolve in a few weeks if the patient can be supported through this uncomfortable period.[51] Since relapse rates are high, patients should be assured that medication will be available when needed. An antidepressant can be started after the panic is under control, allowing the benzodiazepine to be discontinued after only a brief period. As it is with other anxiety disorders, psychotherapy is important for dealing with the secondary anticipatory anxiety.

Social phobia has been treated effectively with phenelzine. Propranolol can eliminate the discomforting symptoms associated with public speaking and other forms of performance anxiety without the adverse cognitive effects of the benzodiazepines.[51]

Obsessive-Compulsive Disorder and Somatoform Disorders. The serotonin reuptake blockers, clomipramine and fluoxetine, have been reported to be effective for perhaps one third of patients with obsessive-compulsive symptoms, although there appears to be no effect on social functioning. Clomipramine is strongly anticholinergic and sedating and can interfere with sexual functioning, whereas fluoxetine can be excessively stimulating and cause gastrointestinal symptoms, insomnia, and headache. It may take 8 to 16 weeks to see an effect with these drugs.[51] Behavioral therapy, particularly relaxation-assisted systematic desensitization and response prevention, has also had some positive results.

The somatoform disorders are best treated with psychotherapy, although it is often difficult to convince patients that a psychological treatment will be of value for their somatic symptoms (see Chapter 81). During the course of treatment, more obvious symptoms of anxiety or depression often emerge. When they do, the appropriate medication may be instituted. In such cases, however, there are two risks: The patient may lose interest in understanding the psychological basis of the symptoms and may have a recrudescence of somatic concern around expected drug side effects. It often helps to make these possibilities explicit. The clinician can distinguish the specific psychological symptoms (e.g., depression, anxiety) that are being targeted now for treatment from the original somatic complaints and also help the patient to recognize his or her proclivity to worry about unfamiliar physical sensations.

REFERENCES

1. Ballenger JC: Psychopharmacology of the anxiety disorders. Psychiatr Clin North Am 7:757, 1984.
2. Weissman MM and Merikangas KR: The epidemiology of anxiety and panic disorders: An update. J Clin Psychiatry 47(Suppl): 11, 1986
3. Schatzberg AF: Overview of anxiety disorders: Prevalence, biology, course, and treatment. J Clin Psychiatry 52(Suppl 7):5–9, 1991.
4. Myers JK, Weissman MM, Tischler GL, et al: Six-month prevalence of psychiatric disorders in three communities. Arch Gen Psychiatry 41:959, 1984.
5. Robins LN, Helzer JE, Weissman MM, et al: Lifetime prevalence of specific psychiatric disorders in three sites. Arch Gen Psychiatry 41:949, 1984.
6. What are pharmacists dispensing most often? Pharmacy Times, April 1991.
7. Winokur G and Coryell W (eds): Biologic systems: Their relationship to anxiety. Psychiatr Clin North Am II:287, 1988.
8. Papp L, Coplan J, Gorman JM, et al (eds): Neurobiology of anxiety. *In* American Psychiatric Press Review of Psychiatry, Vol 11. Washington, DC, American Psychiatric Press, 1992, pp 307–322.
9. Curtis GC, Thyer BA, and Rainey JM (eds): Symposium on anxiety disorders. Psychiatr Clin North Am 8:1, 1985.
10. Derogatis LR and Wise TN: Anxiety and Depressive Disorders in the Medical Patient. Washington, DC, American Psychiatric Press, 1989.
11. Jefferson JW: Biologic systems and their relationship to anxiety. Psychiatr Clin North Am 11:463, 1988.
12. Freud S: Inhibitions, symptoms and anxiety. *In* Standard Edition of the Complete Psychological Works of Sigmund Freud, Vol 20. London, Hogarth Press, 1962, pp 77–175.
13. Freud A: The Ego and the Mechanisms of Defense. New York, International Universities Press, 1966.
14. Marks I: Behavioral therapy for anxiety disorders. Psychiatr Clin North Am 8:25, 1985.
15. Brown TA, Hertz RM, and Barlow DH: New developments in cognitive-behavioral treatment of anxiety disorders. *In* Tasman A and Riba MB (eds): American Psychiatric Press Review of Psychiatry, Vol 11. Washington, DC, American Psychiatric Press, 1992, pp 285–306.
16. Kushner MG, Sher KJ, and Beitman BD: The relation between alcohol problems and the anxiety disorders. Am J Psychiatry 147:685, 1990.
17. Update on anxiety and panic disorders. J Clin Psychiatry 47(Suppl):1–39, 1986.
18. Roy-Bryne PP (ed): Panic disorder. Psychiatr Ann 18:447, 1988.
19. Sussman N (ed): Anxiety disorder. Psychiatr Ann 18:134, 1988.
20. American Psychiatric Association: Diagnostic and Statistical Manual of Mental Disorders, 3rd ed. Washington, DC, American Psychiatric Association, 1987.
21. Sheehan DV: Current concepts in psychiatry: Panic attacks and phobias. N Engl J Med 307:156, 1982.
22. Crowe RR: Mitral valve prolapse and panic disorder. Psychiatr Clin North Am 8:63, 1985.
23. Liebowitz MR: Diagnostic issues in anxiety disorders. *In* Tasman A and Riba MB: American Psychiatric Press Review of Psychiatry, Vol 11. Washington, DC, American Psychiatric Press, 1992, pp 247–259.
24. Stein MB, Heuser IJ, Juncos JL, and Uhde TW: Anxiety disorders in patients with Parkinson's disease. Am J Psychiatry 147:217, 1990.
25. Horowitz MJ, Wilner N, Kaltreider N, et al: Signs and symptoms of posttraumatic stress disorder. Arch Gen Psychiatry 37:85, 1980.
26. Friedman MJ: Post-Vietnam syndrome: Recognition and management. Psychosomatics 22:931, 1981.
27. Burgess AW and Holstrum L: The rape trauma syndrome. Am J Psychiatry 131:981, 1974.
28. Kaltreider NB, Wallace A, and Horowitz MJ: A field study of the stress response syndrome: Young women after hysterectomy. JAMA 242:1499, 1979.
29. Nemiah JC: Somatoform disorders. *In* Kaplan HI, Freedman AM, and Sadock BJ (eds): Comprehensive Textbook of Psychiatry, 3rd ed. Baltimore, Williams & Wilkins, 1980, pp 1525–1544.
30. Zohar J and Insel TR: Diagnosis and treatment of obsessive compulsive disorder. Psychiatr Ann 18:168, 1988.

31. Hall RCW: Anxiety. *In* Hall RCW (ed): Psychiatric Presentations of Medical Illness: Somatopsychic Disorders. New York, SP Medical & Scientific Books, 1980, pp 13–35.
32. Breir A, Charney DS, and Heninger GR: The diagnostic validity of anxiety disorders and their relationship to depressive illness. Am J Psychiatr 142:787, 1985.
33. Fogelson DL, Bystritsky A, and Sussman N: Interrelationships between major depression and the anxiety disorders: Clinical relevance. Psychiatr Ann 18:158, 1988.
34. Koranyi EK: Morbidity and rate of undiagnosed physical illness in a psychiatric clinic population. Arch Gen Psychiatry 36:414, 1979.
35. Hall RCW, Gardner ER, Popkin MK, et al: Unrecognized physical illness prompting psychiatric admission: A prospective study. Am J Psychiatry 138:629, 1981.
36. Hall RCW, Popkin MK, Devaul RA, et al: Physical illness presenting as psychiatric disease. Arch Gen Psychiatry 35:1315, 1978.
37. Ling MHM, Perry PJ, and Tsuang MT: Side effects of corticosteroid therapy: Psychiatric aspects. Arch Gen Psychiatry 38:471, 1981.
38. Boston Collaborative Drug Surveillance: Acute adverse reactions to prednisone in relation to dosage. Clin Pharmacol Ther 13:694, 1972.
39. Starkman MN, Zelnick TC, Nesse RM, et al: Anxiety in patients with pheochromocytoma. Arch Intern Med 145:248, 1985.
40. Holland OB: Pheochromocytoma. *In* Isselbacher KJ, Adams RD, Braunwald E, et al (eds): Principles of Internal Medicine. New York, McGraw-Hill, 1980, pp 1736–1741.
41. Benson DF and Blumer D: Psychiatric Aspects of Neurologic Disease. New York, Grune & Stratton, 1975, pp 151–198.
42. Raj AB and Sheehan DV: Medical evaluation of the anxious patient. Psychiatr Ann 18:176, 1988.
43. Lazare A: Hysteria. *In* Hackett TP and Cassem NH (eds): Massachusetts General Hospital Handbook of General Hospital Psychiatry. St. Louis, CV Mosby, 1978, pp 117–140.
44. Boston Collaborative Drug Related Programs: Psychiatric side effects of non-psychiatric drugs. Semin Psychiatry 3:406, 1971.
45. Greden JF: Caffeine and tobacco dependence. *In* Kaplan HI, Freedman AM, and Sadock BJ (eds): Comprehensive Textbook of Psychiatry, 3rd ed. Baltimore, Williams & Wilkins, 1980, pp 1645–1651.
46. Hall RCW, Stickney SK, and Gardner ER: Behavioral toxicity of non-psychiatric drugs. *In* Hall RCW (ed): Psychiatric Presentations of Medical Illness: Somatopsychic Disorders. New York, SP Medical & Scientific Books, 1980, pp 337–406.
47. Karasu TB: Psychotherapy of the medically ill. Am J Psychiatry 136:1, 1979.
48. Karasu TB (ed): The Psychiatric Therapies. Washington, DC, American Psychiatric Association, 1984.
49. Brown TA, Herz RM, and Barlow DH: New developments in cognitive-behavioral treatment of anxiety disorders. *In* Tasman A and Ribam B (eds): American Psychiatric Press Review of Psychiatry, Vol 11. Washington, DC, American Psychiatric Press, 1992, pp 285–306.
50. Marks I: Behavioral psychotherapy for anxiety disorders. Psychiatr Clin North Am 8:25, 1985.
51. Roy-Byrne PP and Wingerson D: Pharmacotherapy of anxiety disorders. *In* Tasman A and Riba MB (eds): American Psychiatric Press Review of Psychiatry, Vol 11. Washington, DC, American Psychiatric Press, 1992, pp 260–284.
52. Geenberg AJ: Anxiety. *In* Bassuk EL, Schonover SC, and Greenberg AJ: The Practitioner's Guide to Psychoactive Drugs. New York, Plenum Medical Book Company, 1983, pp 167–201.
53. Greenblatt DJ, Shader RI, and Abernethy DR: Current status of benzodiazepines. N Engl J Med 309:410, 1983.
54. Schoonover SC: Depression. *In* Bassuk EL, Schoonover SC, and Gelenberg AJ: The Practitioner's Guide to Psychoactive Drugs. New York, Plenum Medical Book Company, 1983, pp 19–77.

79

The Difficult Doctor-Patient Encounter

DON R. LIPSITT, MD

Patients whose behavior evokes feelings of vexation, frustration, and even hate in the caregiver are commonly referred to as "difficult." Encounters with these patients mobilize in physicians not the curiosity and gratification of other diagnostic challenges to the physician's skills, but rather the tendency to add to a colorful lexicography of assorted names, labels, and epithets applied to these medical provocateurs. Words like "gomer," "turkey," "crock," "demander," "clinger," "help-rejecting complainer," and "borderline" are a reflection of the distress experienced by physicians and a testimony to the failure of medical education to bring enlightenment to physicians about the interpersonal, behavioral, and psychological nuances of doctor-patient interactions.

New emphasis on primary care medicine has enhanced physician awareness of the importance of the doctor-patient relationship. Much of medical education has heretofore focused on the episodic, the symptomatic, and the acute, with little opportunity for the student of medicine to synthesize data from the integrated physical, psychological, and social dimensions of the patient's reality. Because most patients who are ultimately at risk of being labeled difficult are first encountered and often followed up by primary care physicians, it will serve the well-being of both if the nature of these patients and their help-seeking behavior can be better understood by those most likely to provide medical care for them.

This chapter describes how dysfunctional doctor-patient relations evolve with the difficult patient; will attempt a classification consistent with present psychiatric nosology; and will offer suggestions for understanding treatment and management.

PATIENTS WHO ARE DIFFICULT

A fairly extensive literature alludes to the varieties of difficult or problem patients seen in medical practice.[1, 2] Generally, they have been seen by physicians over long periods of time, to whom they offer multiple complaints and exhibit refractoriness to a wide variety of therapeutic efforts.[3] Ultimately, the physician's interest flags, and he or she may, in desperation, recommend more and more radical treatments or refer to other physicians. Mounting experiences of "failure" engender disappointment, frustration, anger, guilt, a decrement in the physician's self-esteem, and even hate[4]—feelings that are, in all likelihood, also experienced by the patient through a process that may remain entirely at a nonverbal level. Usually at this point in the process, the physician experiences the patient as difficult or as a problem. As in the case of a beleaguered parent with an intractable child, there is often a reciprocal failure in both parties to identify expectations, to communicate meaningfully, and to negotiate an acceptable common goal.

Few systematic studies have shed light on the characteristics and personality factors that contribute to a difficult doctor-patient relationship. Available literature is largely anecdotal and impressionistic and focuses almost exclusively on the patient side of the doctor-patient equation. Collective experience and published reports suggest that the so-called difficult patient is one who generates in the physician reactions that are based more on "illness behavior"[5] than on the medical complexity of the case. Such patients almost certainly uniformly threaten the physician's sense of control, not only over the relationship itself but also, and especially, over the physician's own emotions.

In medical education, the tendency to devalue affect as a potentially therapeutic tool may further diminish the physician's capacity to empathize with patients who manifest certain personality traits; in some circumstances, a conscious withholding of empathy guards against the physician's unconscious fear of becoming too much like the disliked patient.

In some cases, negative feelings toward certain types of patients (e.g., alcoholic, suicidal, epileptic, or obese patients) arise from unconscious early experiences in the physician. The unconscious elements of unresolved personal conflict give rise to *transference* in patients and *countertransference* in physicians, both at the risk of complicating or even nullifying a successful doctor-patient encounter. An example would be the immediate dislike each could feel for the other without having had even a few minutes to experience one another.

The effort required to maintain emotional distance from patients who create discomfort is sometimes seen as contributing to the stress experienced by physicians in medical practice.[6] Certainly, patients who mobilize feelings of helplessness and ineptness in their physicians are high on the "difficult" list. A certain amount of helplessness and dependence in the *patient* is experienced as desirable because these evoke the physician's natural tendency to be nurturant, protective, directive, and controlling, behaviors that amplify self-esteem by bolstering the physician's self-image as competent, responsible, knowledgeable, and caring. But when dependency and helplessness in the patient exceed a delicate threshold, they arouse similar feelings in physicians; when the physician depends on a "good" outcome in the patient for his or her own professional gratification, he or she is often distressed by his or her awareness of helplessness to diminish the patient's complaints. Studies have shown that any dimension of the doctor-patient relationship that contributes to a lack of control by the physician generates professional dissatisfaction even more than does the lack of a personal relationship.[7]

Consistent with the impression that problems with affect are at the very core of difficult doctor-patient encounters is the similarity of the profile of the so-called difficult patient to descriptions of psychiatric patients, even when no bona fide psychiatric diagnosis is warranted.[8, 9] Patients who consult their physicians with complaints for which no physical basis is found are often, but certainly not always, too quickly regarded as hypochondriacs, somatizers, or "worried well,"[10, 11] even before sufficient historical links are explored between physical complaint and transient social and personal circumstances contributing to bodily stress. Disparate illness belief models, expectations, and divergent attributions of patients and physicians easily lead to misperception, misdiagnosis, and untherapeutic behavior. A recent study showed that physicians underestimated patients' discomfort or pain and levels of anxiety 25% of the time.[12] In urgent care settings, underestimation was even more frequent for discomfort, pain, anxiety, and activity limitation, suggesting that increased time pressure reduces opportunity to understand (diagnose) the patient. Underestimation correlated strongly with levels of patient dissatisfaction, another factor contributing to dysfunctional doctor-patient encounters.

Studies like this call attention not only to time and empathic response as important ingredients of the effective patient-physician relationship but also to the doctor's vital role as a kind of "interpreter," one who must translate the language of the patient into a comprehensible model of illness not always concordant with the well-learned "medical model." The level of ability to do this will pivot around cultural and ethnic factors,[13] deep-seated values and biases, and the physician's privately (sometimes unconsciously) held definitions of what constitutes a "good physician" and a "good patient." The ability of the physician to help the patient "organize the illness" (à la Balint[14]) will depend in large measure on his or her skill as an "interpreter." To the extent that the physician fails at this kind of interpretation and organization, thwarted efforts at diagnosis and treatment commonly lead to perceptions of the patient as deviant, odd, or difficult. In such a setting, negotiation for care becomes problematic, and at times, impossible.

"Easy" Versus "Difficult" Patients

Medical sociologists have thoroughly described the "sick role" and its relevance to the illness behavior of individuals who seek medical care.[15] "Good" patients follow a relatively ritualistic pattern in their search for care and treatment. Most individuals (they do not become patients until seen by a physician) first identify a reason for consulting a physician; it may be a perceived change in a pre-existing illness, an observed change, or worrisome sensations. Most commonly, the presentation is in terms of pain or bodily sensations. Our culture teaches (and thus our physicians learn) that the "preferred" mode of complaining is physical. It is thus usually both the patient's and the physician's selected pathway to diagnosis and treatment. To the extent that both patient and physician are thinking along similar lines, the physician's "decision-tree" approach to diagnosis may lead to the kind of evaluation the patient expected. If the evaluation leads to suspicion of and confirmation of, say, a diseased gallbladder, the deserved patienthood status with its "sick role" rights and obligations is conferred on the patient. Both patient and physician are "pleased"; successful medical or surgical treatment brings even further gratification to both participants. The expectations, treatment, and outcome have been met satisfactorily in this medical encounter. The patient was a good historian, played by the rules defining the sick role, and established a concordant relationship with the physician. They had similar expectations, understood each other, spoke the same language. This was a "good" patient, an "easy" patient.

Consider the patient for whom physical evaluation results in a diagnosis of "no disease." This may be sufficient reassurance for some; for others, there is puzzlement, disbelief, or even intensified concern. The physician's heightened efforts to reassure are met with augmented concern in the patient. Medical explanation does not suffice; the patient feels sick, the doctor says "not sick." Conferring of "sick role" privileges is denied; the patient begins to feel fraudulent, reprimanded, accused, misunderstood, and resentful. The physician feels irritated, burdened, baffled, and impatient. A dysfunctional relationship emerges from a sense that the patient wants ("demands," "clings," "is entitled") more than the physician is able ("inept") or willing ("uncaring") to give. The patient feels guilty for "wasting the doctor's time," and the physician feels victimized, exploited, manipulated,[16] rejected, and angry. Expectations, treatment, and outcome have not been satisfactorily met in this encounter. The patient was a "poor historian," did not play by the rules, and established a discordant relationship that was not therapeutic and was perhaps antitherapeutic. Doctor and patient had disparate expectations, did not understand each other, and did not speak the same language. This was a "bad" patient, a "difficult" patient. But in the nature of such encounters, it is usually the patient and not the physician who is labeled.

The labeling process often precludes further meaningful diagnostic exploration. Energy is spent on maintaining distance (often effectively achieved through the label itself) rather than on investigating what went wrong on both sides of the doctor-patient relationship. Connectedness between patient and physician is both a complicating and an enabling factor in a caring and health-promoting relationship. The patient seeks connectedness to the physician to rectify a perceived disruption to an ordered life (whether social, emotional, or physical). The physician seeks connectedness through empathy, while maintaining sufficient separateness to be objective and not to encourage unrealistic expectations (professional stance).

Both need to feel gratified without mobilizing sexual, aggressive, or other confounding feelings; failure in this process encourages such behaviors as seductiveness, hostility, dependency, and garrulousness. The physician must be nurturant without expecting nurturance in return. The line between social intimacy and a therapeutic medical alliance can indeed be very thin; it is prone to easy violation. Part of the physician's very difficult task is to learn ways to promote connectedness through an alliance that permits dependency without compromising separateness. Patients who are regarded as difficult are those who strain the boundaries of this task. Indeed, both patient and physician must at times be reminded of the limits of propriety in professional medical encounters.

Some Examples

Clearly, some patients are prone to test the delicate balance of concordant relationships more readily than others. Likewise, it should not be overlooked that some physicians have trouble in this area as well; the physician who prematurely closes off the patient's meaningful history-giving is one example.

Patients whose behavior is most floridly deviant are generally not those who are regarded as belonging to the category of "difficult patients." The drug abuser, the malingerer, the seductive patient, the threateningly hostile individual, or the clearly psychotic patient does not openly challenge the traditional doctor-patient relationship as much as does the covertly angry, the personality-disordered, the hypochondriacal, the factitious, or the somatizing patient. Whereas the former patients may be annoying to the physician, they do not evoke early empathic doctoring patterns that are later thwarted, nor do they introduce the degree of diagnostic uncertainty and affective response that the latter patients do.

Somatoform Disorders

For the primary care physician, perhaps the largest number of difficult patients will emerge from those having somatoform disorders. According to Katon and others, "somatization is the single most common medical problem facing primary care providers, accounting for between a third and a half of primary care contacts."[17] These writers have also shown that the greatest proportion of somatization phenomena is accounted for by cultural idioms of distress, social uses and misuses of the sick role, and family styles of communication and coping. The problem, therefore, of "interpreting" or "translating" the patient's complaints is much more complex than merely defining a sign or a symptom. For the physician to fail at this translation is to under-identify a condition that requires not further expensive evaluation but supportive cognitive approaches that will help maintain the patient at an optimal functioning level.

Somatization is the process by which psychologic events are converted to physiologic and somatic responses. It is believed to represent an immature bodily response to stressful circumstances (internal or external) that catalyze a regression (especially in the adult) to physical behavior more common to the young child. The process may be triggered by emotional conflict, interpersonal difficulties, or socioenvironmental distress. The symptoms, themselves without physical basis, may have various meanings and secondary elaborations: they camouflage the "real" stress by focusing attention on the physical complaint; they influence (usually unconsciously) the nature of the impaired relationship; they maintain connectedness to others when abandonment seems imminent; they call attention to important losses by identifying with others with similar symptoms; they atone for unconscious shame and guilt for personal transgressions; they represent manifestations of masked depression, anxiety, or panic disorder.[18] Fixation on the physical complaint, usually including pain, assumes such intensity for some that it becomes a way of life.[19] For these patients, it serves the purpose of relating to others, communicating, seeking love and attention, and manipulating their world.

An example is Mrs. B, a 38-year-old married woman with two children, who complained of unremitting midabdominal pain for 2.5 years, since the anniversary of a spontaneous abortion of a third pregnancy. She recounts an extensive history of visits to "highly reputable" doctors, innumerable endoscopic studies, and treatment with many medications with either no relief or worsening of her distress. She angrily describes the failure of doctors to "find what is wrong" and is concerned that perhaps a tumor has been missed. She recounts stories of acquaintances who have had medical mishaps following misdiagnoses. Occasional physicians, she says, have promised she would be well with treatment only to ultimately dismiss her completely ("they throw up their hands") or to suggest that she see a psychiatrist ("how could I have this pain if it was psychosomatic?"). She complains that "doctors always leave me," although on one occasion she proudly proclaims that *she* made a change on her own because her doctor was "an asshole."

Her personal history is replete with disappointments and a sense of deprivation, although she grew up in a well-to-do, privileged, and educated family. She married a professional man and gave up opportunities to pursue further education and a possible career for the "pleasures of motherhood." She had diligently raised two boys, now in their teens, and had eagerly tried to become pregnant "before I reached mid-life." A late pregnancy terminated abruptly in the loss of a female fetus. She described her loss as "mildly disappointing," although she began to be preoccupied with multiple physical symptoms, none of which were identified as "anything serious" by her physician. As her multiplicity of symptoms was replaced by a more focused abdominal pain, she pursued medical treatment with great intensity, seeking out "the most prestigious physicians."

The fixity of her physical symptom and its failure to respond to various treatments induced or was caused by a depression that further intensified her belief that she was suffering a serious physical disease. Her involvement with her physical distress took on a life of its own and consumed all her waking hours. She agreed to a psychiatric consultation for the depression secondary to her unremitting pain, but only with assurance that she could return to her primary care physician. Her physician, in consultation with the psychiatrist, then agreed to see her regularly (i.e., not to "throw up his hands"), to manage her conservatively, to limit the extent of further physical work-up, and to explore, over time, through continuous history-taking, the patient's disappointment over loss of the coveted third child, which aggravated a whole series of prior disappointments in her life. Availability (with proper limit-setting), constancy, and continuity eventually yielded a diminution of symptom intensity, a lifting of depression, and a decrease in reliance on questionably useful medications in this patient with a somatoform disorder (hypochondriasis).

Such patients profoundly vex physicians by their persistence, their entrenched behavior, and their refractoriness to therapeutic endeavors.[20] Although the symptom complaints are physical, the severity of the disorder warrants its inclusion in the psychiatric diagnostic nomenclature as one of the somatoform disorders.[21]

Somatoform disorders include somatization disorder, conversion disorder, psychogenic pain disorder, and hypochondriasis. In each of these conditions, the somatic preoccupation can achieve the intensity of delusional belief, resistant to reassurance or "psychologic explanation." The common remark by physicians to these patients that "there is nothing wrong" is perceived as a hostile accusation of craziness, sure proof to the patient of misunderstanding (speaking different languages). Hasty offers of psychiatric referral are usually rejected because of the negative (to the patient) implications as well as the threat of further abandonment, a feeling state that may have been, in fact, a contributing precipitant to the disorder.

Physicians who attempt to "cure" such patients through customary medical ministrations are certain to experience the dysfunctional relationship just described. These patients perceive the physician as a helper who, with an armamentarium of drugs, procedures, and tests, will compensate the patient for collective past and present deprivations. Overzealous efforts to meet this expectation imply the correctness of the patients' perceptions, causing intensification of efforts to obtain what is felt to be the patients' due.

The Elderly

Long lives are likely to be accompanied by all varieties of illness, both chronic and acute. Failing memories may generate inadequate histories. Milder physical complaints are prone to be minimized or dismissed by the physician but exaggerated by the patient, sometimes even before symptoms are thoroughly assessed. Buffeted emotionally by multiple losses and social stresses, elderly people frequently live alone and lose the social contacts and stimulation of activity that keeps them connected to their world. They begin to experience increased alienation, and their interests are directed more toward the functioning of their bodies rather than events in their environment.

Mrs. M, an alert 84-year-old widow of 5 years, moved from a home shared with her husband until his death from repeated strokes to a small apartment removed from her usual friends. Until her husband's death, she had been athletically inclined, bowling and playing golf regularly—"good ways to keep my mind off my troubles." Always considered vigorous, energetic, and stoic, she pursued her athletic interests with her friends until increasingly painful osteoarthritis made her "give it all up." She continued to drive her own car for some time, but eventually this too had to be forfeited, and her two grown children made arrangements for her to have a homemaker as well as a social worker who visited her in her apartment. She had formed a relationship with a kindly and highly regarded family doctor in her community who saw her in regular but infrequent visits and provided conservative palliative management while acknowledging her strength and independence.

At a time that both her physician and her social worker went on vacation, she began to experience pain in the rectum, back, and abdomen. Annoyed by her daughter's inference that "you've always been strong, mother, it's all psychosomatic," she complained of increasing pain, began staying in bed, and was ultimately admitted to the hospital complaining of faintness, headaches, and difficulty in walking. Thorough medical and neurologic evaluation (including computed tomographic scan and lumbar puncture) failed to establish a physical diagnosis. In the hospital, she was observed to cry fitfully, although clandestinely. With nursing staff, she talked about the difficulties of being "cooped up" in a small apartment, her anger at her son for intimations of nursing home placement, her previous enjoyment of physical activity, and fond memories of her husband. When the reports of negative study results were given to her, she said "I guess my daughter was right, it *is* all psychosomatic." Although she stayed in bed much of the time in the hospital and requested pain medications for her recent symptoms and her chronic arthritis, she gradually ambulated with the assistance of a walker. She brightened noticeably at news of her social worker's return and a planned visit to the patient in the hospital. She was markedly improved and ready for discharge on the day before the scheduled return of her physician from vacation.

Such patients are sometimes erroneously labeled malingerers or hypochondriacs, or sometimes worse. This patient was able to escape such appellations because she was unusually intelligent, alert, and communicative, thus likable. Nonetheless, she demonstrates the very real (and unconscious) inter-relatedness of uncomplicated bereavement and sadness with somatic illness (somatization) occasioned by a concatenation of factors: isolation from friends and physical activity, loss of supports of physician and social worker, reawakening of sadness over husband's death, and intimations by son and daughter that she was "crazy," no longer independent, and ready for "total dependent care." Her experienced family physician probably understood her personality and her past history and provided the connectedness she needed with a revered successful man (a surrogate for her deceased successful husband). No psychiatric diagnosis was necessary, although she manifested elements of psychogenic pain disorder and uncomplicated bereavement (from DSM-IV diagnostic criteria). Psychiatric consultation alone, which formulated and discussed with her the "causes" of her pain, constituted adequate "psychiatric" treatment.

Personality Styles and Disorders

Another group of patients likely to be cast as "difficult" are those whose personality traits and behavior patterns may be exaggerated in stressful situations. Whereas some individuals may have characteristically disordered personalities, others function well under normal circumstances but may appear to be psychopathologic when difficulty arises in coping with illness, relationships, or work. Kahana and Bibring have described how normal personality types, under anxiety-producing circumstances, may complicate medical management and the doctor-patient relationship.[22] It behooves the physician to recognize and "diagnose" normal personality styles to account for, but not overreact emotionally to, the behaviors and attitudes of individuals whose illness is cloaked in the exaggerated mantle of their personality types.

The seven basic categories of personality types are (1) the dependent, overdemanding personality; (2) the orderly, controlled personality; (3) the dramatizing, emotionally involved, captivating personality; (4) the long-suffering, self-sacrificing patient; (5) the guarded, querulous patient; (6) the patient with the feeling of superiority; and (7) the patient who seems uninvolved or aloof. Recognizing some of the predictable ways in which each type responds to illness enables the physician to better understand the meaning of illness to each, the characteristic efforts to cope, and the maladaptive responses to the stress of illness. Medical care can then be formulated and planned in ways that can have optimal benefit through helping the patient to adapt to illness and comply with the therapeutic regimens.

An example of the type of patient with a feeling of superiority is Mr. C, a 30-year-old male advertising executive admitted to the hospital for a flare-up of his ulcerative colitis the day after he was told his job was terminated. His physician initially found him pleasant and cooperative as he went through the admission evaluation and the beginning of fairly standard treatment. Although he was assured that he was responding well to the medical regimen, he was experienced by his hospital physician and the nursing staff as being "difficult, demanding, and cocky." What had originally been described as "charm" and a "likable personality" was now perceived as manipulative, controlling, and trouble-making behavior, which was found to obstruct treatment by house staff and nurses alike.

As the patient's interpersonal struggles escalated and he repeatedly asked to review his chart, a psychiatric consultation was requested to assist with a treatment plan. He accepted the psychiatrist reluctantly but quickly assumed a receptive and deferential demeanor. He talked freely with the psychiatrist, describing his life of a "playboy," supported by his wealthy parents. He traced an early history through stories of great achievement, aplomb, and autonomy, at the same time extolling his uncommon ability to endure personal abstinence and control. He spoke of others—both his colleagues and his former doctors—in demeaning terms, while strongly praising his absent internist, a highly regarded professor much the patient's senior but addressed by his first name by the patient. He was hypercritical of nurses who "ordered" him around and of house officers who "are wet behind the ears." In describing his ordinal position in his family, he said he was "top banana."

The psychiatrist expressed to the patient his admiration for the patient's knowledge of his disease, as well as his capacity for having useful ideas about what he needed in order to get better, but he did not allow himself to engage in the patient's efforts to devalue, diminish, or criticize his caretakers. Rather he explained that staff who had known him for only a short time needed all the help they could get from him to assist them in applying their expertise. The patient shook hands respectfully with the psychiatrist and thanked him for the opportunity "to tell my story—I'm always ready to talk to anybody who's willing to hear me talk about myself."

To the nursing and medical staff, the psychiatrist described the patient as having a narcissistic personality characterized by the following: a fondness for holding forth about himself, an aura of superiority bordering on grandiosity, a need to diminish others and to set some staff members against others by exploitative and manipulative behavior, relationships alternating between the polarities of overidealization and devaluation, and a sense of entitlement that, if unmet, led to anger and demandingness. Many of these characteristics disguised a deep-seated sense of shame or low self-esteem, especially in response to the stress of his serious physical disease.

An understanding of the aforementioned qualities made it possible for staff to maintain their professional stance, to give the patient control of his care where appropriate, but to set limits and guidelines when necessary. Staff were able to avoid the pitfall of taking criticism personally and were able to see it as an ingredient of the patient's character structure. They could also appreciate that the intensified dependency occasioned by the patient's flare-up and the absence of his regular doctor contributed to his anxiety, irritability, and need to overemphasize his autonomy. The remainder of his hospital stay proceeded without further difficulty when a treatment plan was worked out "collaboratively" with the patient.

One study notes that patients who ask to read their hospital charts are often those identified as having personality disorders giving rise to conflict-ridden relationships in the hospital setting.[23, 24] Although personality disorders are more likely to surface under the stress of hospitalization, they will often emerge in the ambulatory treatment of patients over time. The use of proper diagnostic descriptors will help the physician avoid punitive labeling and maintain a therapeutic relationship with the patient.

Adherence to standard diagnostic nomenclature (DSM-IV) will help the physician avoid negative countertransference reactions that lead to dysfunctional doctor-patient relationships. The pathologic forms of normal personality styles are described as paranoid personality disorder, schizoid personality disorder, schizotypal personality disorder, histrionic personality disorder, narcissistic personality disorder, antisocial personality disorder, borderline personality disorder, avoidant personality disorder, dependent personality disorder, compulsive personality disorder, passive-aggressive personality disorder, and atypical, mixed, or other personality disorder.

Although each category of disorder has special characteristics that can disrupt an effective working alliance between doctor and patient, special attention has been drawn to the borderline personality[25] because of marked unpredictability, instability of mood, severe identity disturbance that may easily lead to suicidal impulses, and a propensity for sudden displays of unanticipated anger. The usual appearance of social adaptability, intelligence, and productivity often cloak deep-seated character problems, often leaving the physician unsuspecting of extreme reactions to illness.[26–28]

Factitious Illness and Malingering

Other patients who generate strong negative feelings among physicians are those who deceive intentionally. However, because such patients have only episodic contacts with physicians, they do not form lasting relationships and are therefore not commonly included in the rubric of "difficult patients." They include patients described in psychiatric nomenclature (DSM-IV) as having factitious disorders and being malingerers; they are not so much interested in any treatment as they are in seeking either to "enjoy" the status of "patient" or obtaining a medical diagnosis for personal gain of one sort or another. The usual response of physicians to these patients, when they are detected, is anger and rejection. Psychotherapeutic treatment is seldom sought, accepted, or responded to. Nonetheless, psychiatric referral is indicated.

Masked Anxiety and Depression

Finally, patients with anxiety disorders and various depressive syndromes so often present only with somatic complaints that the basic illness is often missed.[29, 30] Persistent failure to make the global diagnosis while attempting to treat individual physical complaints may in time frustrate both physician and patient to the point at which the relationship becomes dysfunctional, and a label of "difficult" may bring diagnostic assessment to premature closure. Because such large numbers of patients with mental health problems are seen first and sometimes exclusively by their primary care physician, accuracy of diagnosis of the anxiety disorders and depressive syndromes masked by somatic complaints is especially critical (see Chapters 77, 78, and 81).

PRINCIPLES OF MANAGEMENT

"Difficult" patients can be experienced as less "troublesome" and even *gratifying* by the primary care physician who will take the time to cultivate a few fundamental techniques to facilitate relationships with these individuals.

Understanding the Meaning of Symptoms. Traditional medical education and training, as well as realities of time and money, condition the physician to seek rapid understanding, diagnosis, treatment, and closure of a patient's complaint. However, the presenting complaint is frequently not the problem. Failure to recognize this will often lead to misdiagnosis, prolonged and sometimes unnecessary evaluations, and even major errors in decision-making. Some patients with a specific physical complaint may often need less reassurance that they "don't have anything" than they need understanding that the complaint may have been triggered by serious etiologic factors, such as grief, anxiety, depression, and phobia. Premature "physical" reassurance may foreclose the patient's opportunity to be understood and treated properly. Palliative treatment with medications (rather than listening) may intensify emotional states like hopelessness, disappointment, isolation, hostility, and helplessness, which (unknowingly to the patient) may have precipitated the presenting symptom. It may even be discovered that some patients temporarily must retain their symptoms pending sufficient opportunity to develop a trusting context in which it finally becomes "safe" to relinquish symptomatology. Acceptable diagnostic classification (e.g., DSM-IV) is always preferable to vague labeling.

Physician's Awareness of Personal Feelings. Negative (and sometimes even excessively positive) feelings and attitudes in the physician toward a patient (both conscious and unconscious) can short-circuit the evaluative process and lead to misdiagnosis and inadequate treatment. When the physician can recognize that the caretaker's own experience of feelings of helplessness, anger, depression, loss of control, sexual stimulation, frustration, or anxiety often implies coexistence of similar affects in the patient, these affects can be respected as legitimate data of the doctor-patient relationship. As such, they can contribute to the understanding and proper treatment of the whole patient rather than acting as impediments to a working relationship.

Need for Therapeutic Restraint. A tendency to hastily dispose of the troublesome patient sometimes contributes to overzealous treatment of a patient's presenting complaints. Prescription of the latest "miracle drugs" with abundant verbal reassurance is often responded to with intensification rather than diminution of symptoms. Attempts to translate somatic presentations into psychologic formulations are often similarly too emphatic and premature. Many patients bring their complaints to their primary physician not only because they do not understand their origin but also because they are not "psychologically ready" to accept a different interpretation of their problem than the one they are temporarily "comfortable" with. The natural process of thorough history-taking, adequate physical examination, proper (but not excessive) laboratory studies, and sufficient listening time, perhaps over a span of several visits, builds the relational framework until a patient is readied for clarification, interpretation, and perhaps referral (although explication of a psychological basis for symptoms need not always be coupled with psychiatric referral). Patients who are especially resistant to psychiatric referral can be discussed with a psychiatrist consultant and managed by the primary physician over time.

Limit-Setting. All physicians wish to be regarded by their patients as kind, compassionate, and gentle. For some, this wish interferes with the need to set therapeutic limits or to communicate clearly to the patient. Defining realistic limits helps both patient and physician dispel mounting frustration and anger by containing expectations and ministrations within the real confines of time and resources available. The physician who cannot comfortably, and gently, tell the patient that he or she has "run out of time today" may find himself or herself trying to nudge the patient out of the consulting room by hastily scribbling a prescription or by engaging in seemingly interminable hand-on-doorknob discussions. The physician whose compassionate demeanor encourages patients to call "at all hours" may find it difficult to nonpunitively say to a patient, after assessing the nonurgency of the call, "I know you have a lot to talk about, but it is not possible for me to give you the kind of attention right now (e.g., at a meeting, about to leave the hospital, in the middle of dinner, or too late at night) that is needed to listen carefully to what you have to say; please call my secretary and make another appointment so we can talk unhurriedly"—an approach that offers the patient something (another appointment) at the same time as setting the limit. Likewise, in sitting with a garrulous patient, it is far more effective (and honest) to openly (rather than clandestinely) look at one's watch and call an end to the visit rather than let tensions mount and bodies squirm. Familiarizing oneself with techniques of limit-setting can help enormously to reduce the number of unnecessary prescriptions and feelings of stress and guilt that sometimes are generated by daily medical practice.

The Matter of Referring. Most physicians pride themselves on being able to make expeditious and appropriate referrals. But patients who are not "psychologically minded" will find it difficult to comprehend the reason for psychiatric consultation and may experience referral as rejection rather than empathic helpfulness. The time and delicacy with which a referral is handled may make the difference between a therapeutic and nontherapeutic experience. Some patients are more receptive to referral for consultation when they are reassured that the relationship with their primary physician will continue. If the primary doctor-patient relationship is a strong one, the patient will usually comply with the physician's recommendation. In those occasional instances, however, when a patient balks or refuses consultation or referral outright, the physician may exercise one of several options: (1) continue to see the patient in regular visits, each time further clarifying the meaning and purpose of the referral; (2) ask the advice of a psychiatrist colleague—before referring the patient—about techniques of referral or maintenance of the patient; or (3) keep the patient in treatment but ask a psychiatrist to provide on-site consultation in the physician's office, an approach that sometimes dispels the patient's fears of abandonment or stereotypes of psychiatric intervention.

"Supporting" and "Getting to Know" the Patient. Support is more than comfort and maintenance; when properly used, it is a therapeutic intervention. The sensitivity and character of the physician's relationship to the patient can improve or impede the patient's ability to give a good history, raise or quell anxiety, affect what the patient "hears" of what the doctor says, and change a "compliant" patient into one who is "noncompliant." A supportive physician conveys interest in and a sense of worth and purpose to the patient, creating a setting in which the patient's telling of his or her "story" is the beginning of treatment as well as diagnosis. Patients' symptoms often arise in the throes of loneliness, frustration, depression, stress, and hopelessness. The disconnectedness from others that arises in this context is often restored through the interested, empathic figure of the physician. The supportive physician not only recognizes and accepts the patient's transient need for dependence but also promotes health by finding the patient's strengths and autonomy. A supportive relationship does not imply endless availability or sympathy; even a few minutes of focused empathic caring can bring significant help to the symptomatic patient. For the physician, getting to know the patient may transform him or her, over time, from a "difficult patient" or a "somatizer" into a person with some likeable attributes and strengths (as well as weaknesses), and provide rewarding as well as challenging aspects of care. Ignoring these precepts can result in iatrogenic illness.

CONCLUSIONS

When an individual experiences distress, he or she tries to make sense of it. An upsetting event is interpreted in the light of past experience, present circumstances, and one's general fund of knowledge; if part of a familiar world, the event is readily adapted to or dismissed, but if not in the context of one's known reality, it may be perceived as "disease." This perturbation engenders a sense of disequilibrium, discomfort, and disconnectedness from meaningful others, catalyzing help seeking from relatives, friends, or professionals. Distress perceived as coming from the body generally propels the individual to seek help from a physician.

To the extent that patient and physician address the same problem, a concordant relationship ensues and "healing" takes place; a discordant relationship results from misunderstanding and miscommunication. The failure to interpret the "true" nature of the complaint sows the seeds of dysfunctional relationships and creates "difficult patients" who are "help rejecting." The behavior that first brought the patient appropriately to the doctor may now be seen as clinging dependency that is demanding and manipulative, characteristics that evoke negative responses in the physician.

The doctor's function is ideally to "make the patient whole again." If successful, he or she will restore the patient's connectedness to his or her world, by healing the deviance and disruption that is the patient's symptomatic disease. For some particularly traumatized, deprived, or support-deficient individuals, the physician may need to provide a lifelong adaptive bridge to the patient's world of continuing and threatening stress. These are the patients for whom the continuity of visits—even if irregular and at wide intervals—can make the difference between adaptation and decompensation, whether in the physical, psychologic, or social realms. Primary care physicians who can accept this task experience a challenging and gratifying role in comprehensive health care and promotion.

REFERENCES

1. Wright AL and Morgan WJ: On the creation of "problem" patients. Soc Sci Med 30:951, 1990.
2. Cohen J: Diagnosis and management of problem patients in general practice (Editorial). J R Coll Gen Pract [Occas Pap] 37:295, 1987.
3. Kaplan C, Lipkin M Jr, and Gordon GH: Somatization in primary care: Patients with unexplained and vexing medical complaints. J Gen Intern Med 3:177, 1988.
4. Groves JE: Taking care of the hateful patient. N Engl J Med 298:883, 1978.
5. Pilowsky I: The diagnosis of abnormal illness behavior. Aust N Z J Psychiatry 5:136, 1971.
6. McCue J: The effects of stress on physicians and their medical practice. N Engl J Med 306:458, 1981.
7. Ort RS, Ford AB, and Liske RE: The doctor-patient relationship as described by physicians and medical students. J Health Hum Behav 5:25, 1964.
8. Geertsma RH, MacAndrew C, and Stoller RJ: Medical student orientations toward the emotionally ill. Arch Neurol Psychiatry 81:377, 1959.
9. Goodwin JM, Goodwin JS, and Kellner R: Psychiatric symptoms in disliked medical patients. JAMA 241:1117, 1979.
10. Lipsitt DR: Who are the "worried well"? (Editorial). Gen Hosp Psychiatry 4:93, 1982.
11. Barsky A: Patients who amplify bodily sensations. Ann Intern Med 91:63, 1979.
12. Wartman SA, Morlock LL, Malitz FE, et al: Impact of divergent evaluations by physicians and patients of patients' complaints. Public Health Rep 98:141, 1983.
13. Mechanic D: Social and psychological factors affecting the presentation of complaints. N Engl J Med 286:1132, 1972.
14. Balint M: The Doctor, His Patient and the Illness. New York, International Universities Press, 1957.
15. Parsons T: The Social System. New York, The Free Press, 1951.
16. Mackenzie TB, Rosenberg SD, Bergen BJ, et al: The manipulative patient: An interactional approach. Psychiatry 41:264, 1978.
17. Katon W, Kleinman A, and Rosen G: Depression and somatization: A review. Parts I and II. Am J Med 72:127, 1982.
18. Katon W (ed): Panic disorder, somatization, medical utilization, and treatment. Am J Med 92:15, 1992.
19. Ford CV: The Somatizing Disorders: Illness as a Way of Life. New York, Elsevier, 1983.
20. Lipsitt DR: Medical and psychological characteristics of "crocks." Int J Psychiatry Med 1:15, 1970.
21. Diagnostic and Statistical Manual of Mental Disorders (Fourth edition) DSM-IV. American Psychiatric Association, Washington, DC, 1994.
22. Kahana RJ and Bibring GL: Personality types in medical management. *In* Zinberg NE (ed): Psychiatry and Medical Practice in a General Hospital. New York, International Universities Press, 1964.
23. Altman JH, Reich P, Kelly MJ, et al: Patients who read their hospital charts. N Engl J Med 302:169, 1980.
24. Lipsitt DR: The patient and the record (Editorial). N Engl J Med 302:167, 1980.
25. Reiser DE and Levenson H: Abuses of the borderline diagnosis: A clinical problem with teaching opportunities. Am J Psychiatry 141:1528, 1984.
26. Stoudemire A and Thompson TL II: The borderline personality in the medical setting. Ann Intern Med 96:76, 1982.
27. Groves JE: Management of the borderline patient on a medical or surgical ward: The psychiatric consultant's role. Int J Psychiatry Med 6:337, 1975.
28. Groves JE: Borderline personality disorder. N Engl J Med 305:259, 1981.
29. Kroenke K: Symptoms in medical patients: An untended field. Am J Med 92:35, 1992.
30. Linn LS and Yager J: Recognition of depression and anxiety by primary physicians. Psychosomatics 25:593, 1984.

80

Chronic Pain Syndrome: Integrating the Medical and Psychiatric Evaluation and Treatment

MICHAEL J. MUFSON, MD

OVERVIEW OF THE PROBLEM

The treatment of the patient with chronic pain poses challenging and complex problems for physicians in a wide variety of specialties. Such patients in their search for relief often establish strained relationships with physicians that can be characterized by mutual suspicion and antagonism, resulting in a breakdown of the therapeutic alliance. The patient may then be extruded from care or referred to a psychiatrist or other specialists for management. This can result in a cycle of referrals in which the patient continues to hope for a "cure" while the physician, unable to tolerate the demands of the patient, refers the patient anew.

The report of the Institute of Medicine's Committee on Pain, Disability, and Chronic Illness Behavior underscores the problems in treating this group of patients: "On the basis of the available evidence, the Committee believes that health care providers are not adequately trained to manage patients with pain. Primary care providers should (1) appreciate the complexity of chronic pain associated with illness behavior and psychosocial and cultural influences on pain; (2) be aware of commonly overlooked physical and psychiatric disorders that may account for the pain or contribute to it; (3) be able to make appropriate referrals of chronic pain patients to practitioners in other disciplines; (4) understand the impact of health care providers on the course of chronic pain problems and disability."[1]

The focus of this chapter is on describing the diagnostic heterogeneity of this group of patients and on presenting the difficulties in attempting to define a prototypical "pain patient." A review of these complex patients shows that they fall into many different medical and psychiatric diagnostic categories and often elude a simple diagnosis. Acknowledging the heterogeneity of these patients, a systematic approach to their medical and psychiatric evaluation and management is provided in the hope of presenting clinicians with a useful framework from which they can better understand and manage patients with chronic pain.

BACKGROUND

The neurobiologic components of pain are complex, and the reader is referred to the detailed examinations of Yaksh, Campbell, and Basbaum for a comprehensive review of the peripheral and central substrates of pain.[2–4] As the clinician works with patients suffering from chronic pain, however, it becomes clear that it is impossible to simply reduce pain to its neuroanatomic and biologic substrates or, at the other extreme, to reduce it solely to a psychological phenomenon.

Cassel examines pain in its true context—that of the person who is suffering.[5] He writes that "suffering is ultimately a personal matter" and that this is true for pain as well. He rejects the dualism of mind versus body, pointing out the central role of the "person" in human illness and suffering. Cassel describes how suffering occurs when the person experiences a state of severe distress associated with events threatening the person's intactness. He points out that suffering can occur in relation to a variety of aspects of the person's identity, including social role, group identification, sense of self as an individual, or the relation of the self to a transcendent source of meaning. Finally, Cassel persuasively argues how suffering can occur when *physicians* do not validate a patient's pain and how people in pain report suffering when they "feel out of control, when the pain is overwhelming, when the source of the pain is unknown, when the meaning of pain is dire, or when the pain is chronic."[5]

Loesser provides another useful framework for conceptualizing chronic pain in a model that he calls the "layers of pain." He identifies four concepts that any model of pain must take into account: (1) nociception, (2) pain, (3) suffering, and (4) pain behavior.

He defines nociception as the detection of potentially tissue-damaging events by specialized nerve endings connected to the A-delta and C fiber afferents. Nociception leads to pain, which he defines as the "perceived noxious input to the nervous system." Loesser emphasizes that pain can exist without nociception, as seen in central pain states such as tic douloureux, postherpetic neuralgia, causalgia, and phantom limb pain. Pain is ultimately the *private experience* of the individual and usually leads to suffering. The private experience reflects the person's past social, cultural, and psychological experience.[6]

Suffering, according to Loesser, is the negative affective response that pain has generated in higher nervous centers. Suffering is the emotional component of pain and is also influenced by the individual's prior experience, expectations, and social interactions. Pain behavior, on the other hand, represents all forms of behavior generated by the individual that reflect the presence of pain and how the individual interacts with the world. This includes the patient's behavior in relation to physicians and family members and to all forms of help-seeking behavior. Loesser emphasizes the need to evaluate what combination of the four factors is playing a role in the genesis of the patient's pain and to then direct therapies at those specific factors.[6]

Engel postulated that there are "pain-prone patients" in whom pain is related to feelings of aggression, guilt, loss, and depression. Engel emphasized that pain cannot be understood only in the neuroanatomic realm and underscored the importance of psychological factors in chronic pain. He postulated that painful states would emerge when pain-prone individuals felt the need to suffer, faced a potential loss, or had guilt feelings because of aggressive impulses. He related these psychological aspects of pain to early experience with punitive and abusive parents.[7]

Blumer updated this concept in his description of the "pain-prone disorder," or the "dysthymic pain disorder." He postulated that these patients characteristically have continuous pain and somatic preoccupations, denial of conflicts, and idealization of self and family relations. The premorbid traits in these patients include masochistic relationships, intolerance of success, "courting" of failures, and what he terms "ergomania," that is, relentless activity and overachievement. He also emphasized a family history of alcoholism, chronic pain, crippled relatives, and unipolar depression, and he viewed these patients as anhedonic and dysthymic.[8–10] Blumer sees the pain-prone disorder as a variant of major depressive disorder, in which pain is an expression of muted depression, and recommends antidepressants as the treatment of choice.[9] Although there may be a subgroup of patients who fall into this category, few studies have validated Blumer's concept. The coexistence of chronic pain and depressive disorder is a complex one and is focused on later in this chapter.

DSM III-R addresses chronic pain under the category of somatoform pain disorder. The diagnosis is based on the presence of preoccupation with pain in the absence of "adequate" physical findings to account for the pain or its intensity, or if an extensive diagnostic evaluation does not reveal organic pathology. In some cases psychological factors are considered etiologic, such as when there is a clear temporal relationship between a psychological conflict and initiation or exacerbation of pain.[11] The diagnosis of somatoform pain disorder, however, does not address the multiple "layers" of pain in a meaningful fashion, ignores the role of suffering, and gives little guidance to the clinician regarding how to evaluate the involvement of psychological factors that may be complexly and subtly woven into the fabric of the chronic pain syndrome.

Other approaches used to explain chronic pain include learning theory, which emphasizes learning and conditioning factors as influences on pain behavior,[12] and social modeling theory, which focuses on the "sick role" and pain behavior as related to modeled instruction and the response of the social environment to the patient's expression of pain.[13]

In summary, the pathophysiology of chronic pain is still unclear, and the assessment of a patient with chronic pain remains a difficult task with a variety of theoretical approaches.[14, 15] As Bouckoms points out, "chronic pain rarely has either a clear etiology for its continuation or a specific anatomic deficit."[16]

CHARACTERISTICS OF PATIENTS WITH CHRONIC PAIN

Various approaches have been taken in attempts to define the characteristics of patients with chronic pain. Given the heterogeneity of these patients, it is not surprising that these attempts are filled with contradictory findings.

Pilowsky and Spence, for example, examined patients who were convinced that their pain was caused by physical disease despite a lack of physical findings substantiating their complaints. These patients showed little phobic concern about their pain, though they were convinced it was organically based; they were preoccupied with symptoms and rejected the idea that their pain was related to psychological factors.[17]

Some investigators have used the Minnesota Multiphasic Personality Inventory (MMPI) to elucidate characteristics of patients with chronic pain, emphasizing elevations in the hypochondriasis and hysteria scales. Given that MMPI scales were designed for patients without physical illness and the fact that chronic pain may lead to elevations in these scales over time due to somatic dysfunction, these characteristics have not been uniformly helpful in diagnosing this group of patients. As summarized by Romano, Turner, and Moore, although some studies "suggest relationships between MMPI scales and outcome after back surgery, highly accurate predictions regarding a particular patient's response to surgery cannot be made reliably, and considerable caution is needed in clinical decision-making in individual cases."[18]

Blumer and Heilbroner's assertion that chronic pain is a variant of depressive disease is highly controversial.[9] Whereas Blumer and Heilbroner argue that more than 90% of people who have pain disorders suffer from a depressive illness, Pilowsky and associates found that only 10% of patients in a pain clinic had depressive illness, and Reich found that only 29% of 43 patients with chronic pain had a depressive disorder by DSM III criteria.[19, 20] Katon found that 32% of 37 patients with chronic pain had a major depressive disorder when assessed with the National Institute of Mental Health (NIMH) Diagnostic Interview Schedule.[21] His study showed that 59.5% of the patients had one first-degree relative with chronic pain; 29.7% had a family member with affective illness; and 37.8% had a family member with alcohol abuse.

The diagnosis of major depression in patients with chronic pain is complicated by the fact that it is often difficult to distinguish primary major affective symptomatology from symptoms arising as an adjustment reaction to the pain state or from an organic illness underlying the pain. Indeed, the task of diagnosing major depressive illness based on simple diagnostic criteria remains controversial.[22, 23] The prevalence of depressive symptoms in the general population (13 to 20%) and lifetime rates of major depressive disorder (2.9 to 12.6%) must be considered when attributing depression to the pain syndrome alone.[24]

France and associates, using the dexamethasone suppression test (DST) to differentiate depressive disorder from chronic pain, found that their patients' abnormal cortisol responses related to the presence of symptoms and signs of major depression and not to chronic pain per se. They argue against the notion of chronic pain as a variant of depressive disorder.[25]

Finally, the impact of the chronic pain syndrome on a person's mood must be evaluated. There is little research into the relationship between antecedent chronic pain and the subsequent emergence of a depressive disorder secondary to the ongoing psychosocial impact of a chronic pain syndrome.

Despite the lack of consistency in characterizing patients with chronic pain, from a clinical standpoint there are often certain features that the physician must consider when treating these patients. Recognizing these clinical features will help the clinician to understand the patient's plight, thus facilitating the development of a therapeutic relationship.

The patient has often been evaluated by a wide variety of specialists. These specialists may include the internist, surgeon, orthopedist, neurosurgeon, neurologist, anesthesiologist, and other subspecialist depending on the location of the pain. Several consequences result from having *multiple consultations.* The patient may hear a variety of opinions and feel at a loss to know which one to accept. Furthermore, the patient may see so many specialists that his or her care becomes unfocused, and he or she no longer knows which physician, if any, is taking responsibility for managing his or her care. Finally, there is often little communication among the specialists, leading to the potential for misinterpretation of the information that the patient presents to each new physician. For the characterologically disturbed patient, this is an ideal setting for *splitting* to emerge, when one physician is portrayed as the benevolent good physician and the other physicians are experienced as "bad."

Some patients may be involved in *litigation* concerning an injury related to the onset of their pain. Although this can be a complicating factor in the evaluation, there are no conclusive studies showing that compensation issues perpetuate pain symptoms. Some studies even demonstrate the persistence of symptoms despite settlements of claims.[26, 27] All too often, patients do not receive thorough evaluations because a lawsuit is pending. Whereas Guck and associates reported financial compensation to be associated with successful outcome of nonsurgical treatment of chronic pain,[28] Dworkin found employment history more predictive of long-term outcome than compensation or litigation.[29] Dworkin argues that there has been too much emphasis on the relationship between litigation and treatment outcome. Suffice it to say that this issue must be assessed as part of the total evaluation but in and of itself should not exclude a full work-up or the initiation of appropriate treatment.

As the consultation continues, the patient with chronic pain may receive *narcotics* and become dependent on them for pain relief, beginning the escalating cycle of increasing demand for higher doses due to narcotic tolerance and decreasing relief. The patient may seek out narcotic prescriptions from several physicians and often becomes dependent on the physicians as well as the narcotic. If a physician abruptly terminates the narcotic prescription, the patient may feel abandoned and enraged. Narcotics are often prescribed by the physician as an attempt to "do something" to relieve the patient's pain. Both the physician and the patient find this more satisfactory than "tolerating" the pain until the evaluation is complete.

As the patient feels more frustrated with an unending search for a solution to the pain syndrome, he or she may become increasingly angry at physicians. The physicians, on the other hand, may become easily frustrated and less tolerant towards the patient, who by now is both more dependent and demanding. This creates a stalemate, which usually ends with the patient seeking care elsewhere or being referred for yet another consultation by the specialist who feels at a loss to offer the patient anything further.

The patient by this juncture is often determined to find an understanding ear. He or she has often been told that "It's all in your head" and may become preoccupied with proving this "accusation" false. Such patients are in a tug of war with their physicians. They are angry at not being cured, alienated from the medical care system, and feel helpless with nowhere to turn. The remainder of this chapter describes an organized approach to the evaluation and multidisciplinary management of the patient by medical and psychiatric colleagues that can benefit both the patient and his or her referring physician and help to avoid a therapeutic impasse.

INITIAL CONSULTATION: ESCAPING THE IMPASSE

It is often apparent from the beginning of the consultation that the referring physician has become frustrated in working with the patient who is in chronic pain and, as such, may have limited his or her investigation of a medical problem underlying the pain syndrome. This frustration is often reflected in the phrasing of the questions that arise in the internist's mind.

Questions commonly asked in this context include:

Is the pain psychosomatic?
Is the pain "functional"?
Is the patient "neurotic or crazy"?
Is the pain "out of proportion" to the findings?
Is the patient a "malingerer"?

These questions most often are a reflection of the fact that there is no simple explanation for the patient's pain, and the physician is experiencing helplessness and a loss of control as the patient's demands for pain relief and a cure escalate. Often at this point a review of the medical evaluation can help to break the impasse and alleviate the patient's anxiety.

MEDICAL CONSULTATION

Reviewing the Medical Evaluation

The medical consultant must first establish an open working relationship with the patient and primary care physician or other referring specialist. The nature of the relationship between the patient and the referring physician may be explored as well as what the patient has been told by his or her primary care physician. This avoids splitting the treatment. As illustrated in Table 80–1, there are a wide variety of medical syndromes associated with chronic pain—some are common, but some are rare. The patient may have an as yet undiagnosed malignancy, early multiple sclerosis, or causalgia. This necessitates caution in invoking a psychiatric diagnosis or implicating emotional factors in the etiology of the pain syndrome. The medical

TABLE 80–1. MEDICAL DIAGNOSES ASSOCIATED WITH CHRONIC PAIN SYNDROMES*

Head and Neck
Headache syndromes
Cervical disc disease
Cervical spondylitis
Neuralgias (e.g., trigeminal, postherpetic)
Lesions of the ear, nose, oral cavity (e.g., infection, tumor)
Sinusitis
Suboccipital and cervical musculoskeletal disorders
TMJ syndrome
"Phantom tooth pain"
Myofascial pain
Atypical facial pain

Shoulder, Arm, and Hand
Vascular disease of limb
Post-traumatic syndromes
Causalgia
Cervical disc disease
Brachial plexus lesions
Collagen disease of limb
Vasodilating diseases

Chest
Referred from abdomen or gastrointestinal tract
Postherpetic neuralgia
Postoperative sternal pain
Muscle pain
Angina pectoris
Inflammation

Joint and Connective Tissue Pain
Arthropathies
Spondyloarthropathies

Abdominal
Neurologic origin
Visceral origin
Endometriosis
Postsurgical pain
Adhesions
Syndrome of generalized disease

Neuropathies
Diabetic
Postherpetic
Trigeminal

Female Genitalia: Uterus, Ovaries, Adnexa
Ovarian cyst
Endometriosis
Dysmenorrhea
Uterine retroversion
Pelvic malignancy
Pelvic inflammatory disease
Ectopic pregnancy
Idiopathic pelvic pain

Male Genitalia
Prostate disease
Urethral disease
Epididymitis
Torsion of the testicle
Tumors
Trauma
Hydrocele
Varicocele
Priapism
Inflammation (e.g., condylomas, herpes)

Leg, Foot, Hip, and Thigh
Neuropathy
Sciatic pain
Post-traumatic syndromes
Causalgia
Phantom limb pain
Musculoskeletal syndromes

Low Back Pain
Lumbosacral disc disease
Arachnoiditis
Post-traumatic pain syndrome
Spinal stenosis
Myofascial pain syndrome
Osteoporosis
Paget's spondylitis
Ankylosing spondylitis
Osteoarthritis
Axial-skeletal joint dysfunction

Rectum and Perineum
Inflammation
Tumor

*Adapted from Merskey H: Classification of chronic pain, descriptions of chronic pain syndromes, and definitions of pain terms. Pain 3(Suppl):S13–S24, 1986.

evaluation must be reviewed comprehensively, exploring with the patient's physicians their working diagnoses and ensuring that all relevant medical causes for the pain have been investigated. Once this has been accomplished, a psychiatric consultation can explore if a major psychiatric disorder or emotional conflict underlies or perpetuates the pain syndrome (see Table 80–1).

Psychiatric Consultation

Once the medical reevaluation has been completed, the psychiatric consultant should reformulate the questions commonly asked by the referring physician and specify questions that provide a more useful psychological framework from which to operate. Rather than relying on such antiquated concepts as "functional versus organic," the psychiatric assessment should focus on the following issues:

Is the pain syndrome a presenting feature of, or associated with, a major psychiatric disorder? Is there a comorbid psychiatric and medical disorder?

Is the pain syndrome associated with psychological factors in the patient's life including unrecognized emotional conflicts, psychodynamic issues, or family conflict? Is the pain associated with more symbolic aspects of the symptoms including loss, punishment, suffering, or identification?

This allows the psychiatrist to move away from the ambiguous terms like "psychosomatic," "supratentorial," and "functional," which have little clinical meaning and contribute little to understanding the nature of the pain syndrome.

CHRONIC PAIN IN THE CONTEXT OF MAJOR PSYCHIATRIC DISORDERS

Chronic pain syndromes may be associated with a wide variety of major psychiatric disorders. Table 80–2 provides a list of psychiatric disorders in which chronic pain can present as a major symptom.[20, 21] It is important to emphasize that not all patients referred for psychiatric evaluation will have a major psychiatric disorder. Katon found that 13.5% of his patients had no psychiatric diagnosis. One of the main tasks of the psychiatric consultant is to delineate which patient group needs further evaluation medically or psychiatrically and which patients have no evidence of psychiatric disorder.

Katon also describes how certain patients have either major depressive episodes or alcohol abuse that precede the onset of the pain syndrome. He envisions the pain syndrome as an expression of the patient's psychiatric illness. For example, the patient with major depressive illness may selectively focus on the somatic components of the depressive syndrome (e.g., headache, back pain) and minimize the depressive elements. The chronic pain syndrome may then ensue with reinforcers from the social system (e.g., disability payments, changes in the family system, opiate treatment) that perpetuate the pain syndrome.[21]

Our clinical experience supports Katon's theory that a subgroup of patients with major affective disorder report that they have difficulty recalling which came first, "the depression or the pain syndrome." If the depression resolves with antidepressants and the pain syndrome remits, the patient can then recall how the pain complaint emerged from the mood disorder. Often, however, patients are not able to make this distinction as clearly as the clinician would hope, especially when the pain becomes influenced by social reinforcers. It remains clear, however, that major

TABLE 80–2. PSYCHIATRIC DISORDERS ASSOCIATED WITH CHRONIC PAIN AS A PRESENTING FEATURE

1. Adjustment reaction
2. Major depressive disorder
3. Schizophrenia
4. Paranoid disorder
5. Somatoform pain disorder
6. Somatization disorder
7. Hypochondriasis
8. Anxiety disorder
9. Drug dependence
10. Personality disorder
11. Malingering
12. Münchausen's syndrome/factitious disorders

depressive disorder must be ruled out in patients suffering from chronic pain.

Individuals with *psychotic disorders* can present pain as a reflection of a delusional idea involving body parts or express pain as part of a personalized psychotic belief (e.g., evil forces inside the body causing pain; a body organ malfunctioning resulting in a painful perception). Such syndromes are well documented in Kraeplin's early descriptions of patients with schizophrenia. He describes patients with morbid tactile sensations including heat, pain, and burning that receive a "very strange interpretation." The patient is terribly tormented, notices that "every part of his body is misused"; he feels "internal stirrings"; his "body is twisted . . . his testicles burst . . . God pierces his foot with a wire . . . Very commonly these sensations are associated with electricity . . ."[30] Patients with depression, psychosis, and pain syndromes carry an increased risk for suicide. The primary care physician and the psychiatrist must be alert to this potential throughout the evaluation process and recognize acute suicidality as an emergency when it arises.

Patients with *paranoid disorders* often complain of pain to their internist, while not discussing their delusional beliefs. When they present to the psychiatrist, their bizarre ideation surrounding the pain syndrome or delusions involving the pain (often genital pain) emerge.

In the *somatoform pain disorder,* the patient often gives the history of a psychological stress temporally related to the onset of the pain, for example, a man with the onset of chest pain following death of his child who was undergoing open heart surgery, or the patient who becomes preoccupied with chest pain after recovering from a myocardial infarction. In these situations this diagnosis can only be entertained after a complete medical work-up. Psychogenic pain syndromes are the exception, not the rule.

Chronic pain syndromes can also be seen in patients with *hypochondriasis.* Barsky and Klerman in a detailed review emphasized the need to understand hypochondriasis from a variety of conceptual frameworks. Hypochondriasis is seen as a disorder characterized by physical symptoms disproportionate to demonstrable organic disease; a fear of disease and a conviction that one is sick; a preoccupation with one's body; and the persistent and unsatisfactory pursuit of medical care.[31, 32] Hypochondriasis can exist with or without a pre-existing psychiatric illness. Psychotic patients, as described earlier, can present with hypochondriacal delusions. Their beliefs exist in the context of a psychotic or paranoid disorder, whereas the purely hypochondriacal patient is not psychotic.

Barsky elaborates the need to understand the psychodynamics of the patient with hypochondriasis in terms of the unconscious gratification that bodily symptoms can hold. Hypochondriasis can also be a manifestation of a perceptual or cognitive disorder or may be a reflection of a learned social behavior. He argues that a more concise term for such patients would be "amplifying somatic style," a term allowing for the presence or absence of concomitant medical disease, psychiatric disorder, or intrapsychic conflict.[32] This framework is very useful in approaching patients with chronic pain who have no major psychiatric disorder. Barsky emphasizes the need to assess the influence of psychological factors including childhood experiences, modeling of a sick family member, the meaning of the symptom to the patient, and psychologically significant precipitants including losses and important life events on the patient.[32]

It is well known that patients can present to primary care physicians and cardiologists with chest pain as a manifestation of *panic-anxiety disorder.* In Fishbain's review, 62.5% of chronic patients in their study had anxiety disorders ranging from panic disorder and generalized anxiety disorder to obsessive-compulsive disorder and post-traumatic stress disorder.[35]

Somatization disorder is another complex psychiatric syndrome in which chronic pain can present. In his review of this disorder, Lipowski emphasizes the syndrome as one in which the patient experiences and communicates somatic distress and symptoms in the absence of pathologic findings.[33] He points out how these patients respond to stress in a somatic rather than psychological mode and neither recognize nor understand the relationship between their distress and psychological factors in their lives. Of import is his conclusion, as well, that the cornerstone of treatment is *comprehensive medical, psychiatric, and psychosocial evaluation with unambiguous discussion of the medical and psychiatric assessment.*

Patients with a history of *alcohol and drug abuse* not infrequently present to physicians with the complaint of chronic pain in an attempt to procure narcotic analgesics or minor tranquilizers. This type of patient is often difficult to evaluate in terms of delineating the true etiology of the pain, especially if the person is presenting with pain in an attempt to obtain drugs.

Payne presents a rational approach for evaluating pain in the drug abuser. He rightly emphasizes the need for recognizing tolerance and physical dependence, being alert to "drug-abuse behaviors" including drug hoarding, unauthorized dose escalations, prescription forging, obtaining multiple and simultaneous prescriptions, and excessive negotiations and struggles around drug doses.[34] Such patients need referral to either drug and alcohol programs or inpatient pain units or detoxification units.

Patients with a wide variety of *personality disorders* including histrionic, dependent, schizotypal, borderline, passive-aggressive, narcissistic, compulsive, and paranoid can present with chronic pain.[20, 35] Little is written about patients with narcissistic vulnerabilities and borderline disorders who present to physicians complaining of chronic pain. These patients, when under stress, can present to emergency rooms and primary care physicians complaining of a wide variety of pain syndromes that fluctuate with the level of their internal emotional distress. They often describe the pain as tearing their bodies apart and experience this as intolerable. The pain reflects a somatic expression of their disorganized internal emotional state and is often not recognized during the initial evaluation in the generalist's office.

Patients with Münchausen's syndrome can also present with complaints of pains in an attempt to engage the physician in a comprehensive evaluation. As Spiro points out, Münchausen's syndrome can be seen in association with a variety of psychological disorders, including personality disorders and psychosis, or exist independently as a primary disorder. Associated findings are illnesses requiring extensive treatment early in life, employment in the medical world, and family members in the medical field. This should be distinguished from malingering, in which there is a conscious attempt for secondary gain (e.g., financial reward, avoiding work, evading prosecution) through the complaint of painful symptoms.

PSYCHOLOGICAL FACTORS ASSOCIATED WITH CHRONIC PAIN SYNDROME

Some 20 to 50% of patients evaluated by the psychiatrist are not diagnosed as suffering from a major psychiatric disorder. The clinician must thus also investigate the patient's emotional life as it relates to the pain syndrome. This includes an examination of unconscious conflicts and the meaning of the pain to the individual, including the religious and symbolic meanings of the pain. The evaluation must also include an assessment of couples and family dynamics and the role that the pain plays in the context of the patient's involvement in the medical care system. Finally, the psychiatrist must piece together the complexities of the patient's life history and the role of pain in that life history.

Table 80–3 lists the variety of psychological factors found to serve as important emotional factors sustaining chronic pain syndromes.

A comprehensive psychological history must include the life circumstances related to the onset of the pain, the history of pain syndromes in other family members, losses in the patient's life and early developmental history as it relates to illness, and prior episodes of pain. It is also necessary to evaluate the functioning of the family and marital unit. The spouse can often be a valuable observer of pain behavior or, on the other hand, be a person supporting the pathologic behavior.

The psychiatrist also needs to attend to the patient's relationship with the physicians or hospital (institution) to evaluate displacement of emotional conflict (e.g., anger) into the medical arena in the form of a pain syndrome.

Patients should be assessed for a history of physical or sexual abuse, especially in women with pelvic pain.[36–38] Finally, the clinician needs to assess whether ongoing litigation is playing a role in sustaining the pain syndrome. Delineating such psychological factors can be a complicated process, and often patients deny such conflicts or refuse to talk about them to the internist, exclusively focusing on the pain. In such patients a psychiatric consultation can be very useful in providing a context that allows the patient to explore such conflicts. This consultation may by necessity be extended and often leads to therapy so that the patient has time to examine such issues in some depth.

In summary, the role of the psychiatrist is to define if there is a major psychiatric disorder present in the patient, to evaluate if there are psychological factors associated with the pain syndrome, and to evaluate if these problems exist comorbidly with a pain syndrome secondary to a medical disorder or exist independently and are etiologic to the pain syndrome.

After such an evaluation is completed, recommendations can be made regarding treatment. This can range from psychotropic medication to psychotherapy, couples therapy, family therapy, or inpatient hospitalization.

TABLE 80–3. PSYCHOLOGICAL FACTORS IN CHRONIC PAIN SYNDROMES

1. Symbolic identification
2. Unresolved grief
3. Marital discord
4. Family discord
5. Sexual conflict
6. Anger at physicians/medical institutions
7. Pain as a reflection of suffering
8. Physical abuse
9. Incest
10. Litigation

MEDICAL MANAGEMENT OF CHRONIC PAIN (Table 80–4)

Pharmacologic Approach to Chronic Pain

Non-narcotic analgesics form the foundation of the pharmacologic treatment of chronic pain. These drugs include aspirin, acetaminophen, and new nonsteroidal anti-inflammatory drugs (NSAIDs) (e.g., etodolac, fenoprofen, ibuprofen, ketorolac, naproxen).[39] Aspirin and acetaminophen can be used concurrently with NSAIDs to increase analgesia, but there is little evidence that two NSAIDs used conjointly provided increased pain relief. Anticonvulsants (e.g., carbamazepine, clonazepam, phenytoin) also have been used to treat pain in neuralgic syndromes. This includes trigeminal neuralgia, postherpetic neuralgia, glossopharyngeal neuralgia, and diabetic neuropathy. Baclofen is also used as an adjunctive treatment, and both baclofen and anticonvulsants can be used in additive fashion with antidepressants.[39–45] Phenothiazines also have been added to drug regimens but carry excessive risk of sedation and extrapyramidal side effects.

The primary problem seen in the use of these medications is undermedication and inappropriate administration. Analgesics should be administered at fixed time intervals that reflect the pharmokinetics of the chosen medication; dosages should be increased to appropriate levels before being considered ineffective.

The psychiatrist may also be involved in the use of antidepressants. The psychiatrist can help to evaluate whether these medications should be used in antidepressant doses or in subtherapeutic doses that may have analgesic effect. Furthermore, the psychiatrist can help to monitor blood levels of antidepressants that can provide an important guide in treatment.

Approximately 50 to 60% of patients with chronic pain benefit from adjunctive analgesic effects of antidepressants. The benefit can be in some cases due to treatment of major depressive disorder, when it is present or may be an independent analgesic effect. The mechanism of the latter effect remains unknown but may be related to their effect on biogenic amine systems and their augmentation of endogenous pain inhibitory mechanisms. Their efficacy has been demonstrated most clearly in deafferentation pain but appears to be also useful in arthritic disorders and low back pain.[39]

If non-narcotic analgesics fail, opiates can be considered

TABLE 80–4. MEDICAL MANAGEMENT OF CHRONIC PAIN

Pharmacologic Treatments
- Non-narcotic analgesics
- Narcotic analgesics
- Adjuvants
  - Antidepressants
  - Anticonvulsants
  - Phenothiazines
  - Narcotic analgesics

Pathway Modulation
- Transepidermal nerve stimulation
- Acupuncture

Physical Medicine
- Physical therapy
- Heat, cold, hydrotherapy

Anesthesia
- Local and regional blocks
- Ganglion blocks
- Epidural anesthesia

in a case-by-case basis. Opiates are now considered a potential treatment option in managing chronic pain. Carefully screened patients without a history of substance abuse or psychiatric disorder can often benefit from narcotics, even in pain syndromes that are not caused by malignancy. The narcotics should be dispensed by a single practitioner under strict guidelines as outlined by Portenoy.[46]

Pathway Modulation

In addition to medication, the primary care practitioner must be familiar with the many other alternatives to medication, such as transcutaneous nerve stimulation (the application of controlled low-voltage electrical pulses to the nervous system by passing electrical current through the skin). These devices are contraindicated in patients with cardiac pacemakers.

"Hyperstimulation analgesia" may also explain the use of acupuncture as an adjunctive treatment in chronic pain syndromes. The use of this treatment remains controversial but is often requested by patients.[47, 48] They should receive an open discussion about the current state of knowledge on this modality to help them in their decision.

Physical Medicine

Physical remedies include heat and cold applications that theoretically relieve pain through effects on peripheral nerve endings. Heat should be used conservatively in cases with anesthesia or in cases with a hemorrhagic diathesis. Cold treatments are contraindicated in patients with cold hypersensitivity and in cases of patients with cold agglutinins and cryoglobulins.

Physical therapy has become a mainstay of the treatment of chronic pain. Rehabilitation necessitates a dynamic relationship between the primary care physician, the physical therapist, and the patient. The goal is to increase function, relieve pain, and prevent disuse atrophy, contractures, and psychological regression. An ongoing program of physical therapy forms the backbone of patients with low back pain and recovery from post-traumatic pain syndromes.

Anesthesia

So-called "therapeutic blocks" include the contributions of anesthesiologists to the pain treatment regimen. Anesthesiologists can recommend whether local or regional blocks, ganglion blocks, or epidural anesthesia will be useful in each particular case.

Behavioral Techniques

Behavioral techniques are extremely useful in helping a patient to manage chronic pain. These techniques encourage active participation from the patient and can provide the patient with a sense of control over the pain. The mainstays of these treatments are hypnosis and progressive muscle relaxation. These services can be provided by psychiatric consultants or by behavioral therapists experienced in treating chronic pain.

Difficult-to-Manage Patient with Chronic Pain—Inpatient Pain Units

Certain patients, often with characterologic disturbances, present difficulties that go beyond the traditional physician-patient relationship. This may include the demand for frequent visits, drug-seeking behavior, demands that the physician "cure" the patient, or refusal to be an active participant in the treatment program, whereas the patient takes on a passive, resigned role awaiting the doctor's treatment that will make the pain vanish.

Often due to the sense of urgency that patients with chronic pain present with, physicians feel obligated to "do something" in response. This may include prescribing analgesics, seeking referrals, or sending the patient to a psychiatrist. Often discussing the goals and realistic expectations of treatment is the most productive first step in long-term management and an alternative to "doing something" with medication or invasive procedures.

In certain cases, patients are refractory to both conventional medical and psychiatric treatment. In these instances, the physician should seriously consider a referral to an inpatient pain service. These programs provide a multidisciplinary approach in a structured setting. Such a referral removes the primary care physicians from the battle with the patient and attempts to remobilize the patient in the rehabilitation process.

If the patient refuses this referral, a psychiatric referral can help to address the behavioral and psychological aspects of the patient's pain syndrome, also with the hope of engaging him or her in treatment.

Establishing Goals of Treatment

Long-term management begins by the primary care-taking physician presenting the patient with explicit and specific goals of the evaluation and treatment. This includes communicating to the patient the understanding that it is unlikely that the chronic pain will disappear, that the patient will have to learn how to cope with the pain, and that the treatment will necessitate a multidisciplinary approach often involving physical therapy or rehabilitation medicine, behavioral techniques, medication, and, when necessary, psychiatric intervention.

Early on in the development of the treatment plan, the physician should explore the patient's feelings with regard to mistrust and anger that may have developed in the context of the patient's encounters with the medical system. Furthermore, the physician must emphasize that the patient cannot play a passive role in treatment but will be expected to actively participate in a broad-based rehabilitation program.

Working Closely With Colleagues

Due to the complexity of treatment in patients with chronic pain, many physicians are often involved in providing care. This creates a ripe setting for patient misunderstanding on the one hand and the potential for "splitting" the "good doctor" versus the "bad doctor" on the other hand.

To avoid misunderstanding or distortion by the patient and to avoid making comparisons, the doctors must keep open lines of communication with each other and define specific expectations of the patient. The patient must understand the cause of the pain as the physician formulates the etiology, and the physician must use language the patient understands. If the etiology is unclear or unknown, the patient must be told. If the cause appears to be related to a psychiatric disorder, the patient must be referred to a psychiatrist. All too often the primary care physician supports the patient's denial that psychiatric problems may be part of the pain syndrome.

If pain medications or narcotics are prescribed, only one physician should be in charge of dispensing the medication. Patients should be told in no uncertain terms that receiving drugs from more than one physician at a time is counterproductive. Also, if the patient has become drug dependent, a referral to a psychiatrist or drug treatment program is mandatory.

Once the patient is engaged in treatment, he or she can begin a multidisciplinary program. This most often involves physical therapy and behavioral techniques including hypnosis, biofeedback, or relaxation techniques. The combination of such techniques should be tailored to the patient's pain syndrome and personality style. Special attention should be paid to *pain behavior,* focusing on how the patient can change this maladaptive behavior and still receive the treatment that he or she needs. Pain behavior that alienates the physicians and family should be addressed openly.

It is important to note that certain patients with chronic pain refuse treatment as prescribed. This occurs most often in character disorders and in drug-seeking patients. Physicians must be able to set limits in such cases and not allow the patient to dictate the terms of treatment. Physicians should not feel compelled to prescribe narcotics or to cure the patient. Rather they too must recognize that treatment of patients with chronic pain demands patience and most of all a clear, deliberate plan of treatment.

Most often a multidisciplinary approach as outlined above can create a productive treatment plan that benefits the patient and also allows the physician to continue in a relationship with the patient that addresses the multiple layers of the chronic pain syndrome.

REFERENCES

1. Institute of Medicine: Pain and Disability: Clinical, Behavioral and Public Policy Perspectives. Washington, DC, National Academy Press, 1987, p 11.
2. Campbell J, Raja SN, Cohen DC, et al: Peripheral neural mechanisms of nociception. *In* Wall P and Melzack R (eds): Textbook of Pain. New York, Churchill Livingstone, 1989, pp 22–45.
3. Yaksh TL and Aimone LD: The central pharmacology of pain transmission. *In* Wall P and Melzack R (eds): Textbook of Pain. New York, Churchill Livingstone, 1989, pp 181–205.
4. Basbaum AI and Fields H: Endogenous pain control mechanisms: Review and hypothesis. Ann Neurol 4:451–462, 1978.
5. Cassel E: The nature of suffering and the goals of medicine. N Engl J Med 306:639–645, 1982.
6. Loesser J and Fordyce WE: Chronic pain. *In* Carr JL and Dengerink HA (eds): Behavioral Science in the Practice of Medicine. New York, Elsevier, 1983, pp 331–345.
7. Engel G: Psychogenic pain and the pain prone patient. Am J Med 26:899–918, 1959.
8. Blumer D: Chronic Pain As a Psychobiologic Phenomenon: The Pain Prone Disorder in Psychiatric Aspects of Neurologic Disease, Vol 11. New York, Grune & Stratton, 1982, pp 79–84.
9. Blumer D and Heilbroner M: Dysthymic pain disorder: The treatment of chronic pain as a variant of depression. *In* Tollison CD (ed): Handbook of Chronic Pain Management. Baltimore, Williams & Wilkins, 1989, pp 197–209.
10. Blumer D and Heilbroner M: Antidepressant treatment for chronic pain. Psychiatr Ann 14:796–800, 1984.
11. American Psychiatric Association: DSM III-R. Washington, DC, American Psychiatric Association, 1987, pp 264–267.
12. Fordyce W: Learning Processes in Pain in the Psychology of Pain. New York, Raven Press, 1986, pp 49–65.
13. Craig KD: Modeling and social learning factors in chronic pain. *In* Bonica JJ, Lindblom V, and Iggo A (eds): Advances in Pain Research and Therapy, Vol 5. New York, Raven Press, 1983, pp 813–826.
14. Wall PP and Melzack R (eds): Textbook of Pain. New York, Churchill Livingstone, 1989.
15. Holden AV and Winslow N (eds): Neurobiology of Pain. Manchester, University Press, 1983.
16. Bouckoms A: Recent developments in the classification of pain. Psychosomatics 26(8):637–645, 1985.
17. Pilowsky I and Spence ND: Pain and illness behavior: A comparative study. J Psychosom Res 20:131–134, 1976.
18. Romano J, Turner J, and Moore J: Psychological evaluation. *In* Tollison C (ed): Handbook of Chronic Pain Management. Baltimore, Williams & Wilkins, 1989, pp 38–51.
19. Pilowsky I, Chapman CR, and Bonica JJ: Pain, depression and illness behavior in a pain clinic population. Pain 4:183–192, 1977.
20. Reich J: Psychiatric diagnosis of chronic pain patients. Am J Psychiatry 140:1495–1498, 1983.
21. Katon WK: Chronic pain: Lifetime psychiatric diagnoses and family history. Am J Psychiatry 142:1156–1160, 1985.
22. Davidson J, Turnbull C, Strickland RN, et al: Comparative diagnostic criteria for melancholia and endogenous depression. Arch Gen Psychiatry 41:506–511, 1984.
23. Zimmermal M, Coryell W, Pfohl B, et al: The validity of four definitions of endogenous depression. Arch Gen Psychiatry 43:234–244, 1986.
24. Smith A and Weissman M: Epidemiology. *In* Paykel ES (ed): Handbook of Affective Disorders. New York, Guilford Press, 1992, pp 111–129.
25. France R, Krishnan KR, Trainor M, et al: Differentiation of depression from chronic pain with dexamethasone suppression test and DSM. Am J Psychiatry 141:577–581, 1984.
26. Mendelson G: Not cured by a verdict: Effect of legal settlement on compensation claimants. Med J Aust 2:132–141, 1982.
27. Merskey H: Psychiatry and the cervical sprain syndrome. Canad Med Assoc J 130:119–121, 1984.
28. Guck TP, Meilman PW, Skulety FM, et al: Prediction of long-term outcome of multidisciplinary pain treatment. Arch Phys Med Rehab 67:293–296, 1986.
29. Dworkin RH, Handlin DS, Richlin DM, et al: Unraveling the effects of compensation, litigation and employment on treatment response in chronic pain. Pain 23:49–59, 1985.
30. Kraeplin E: Dementia, Praecox, and Paraphrenia. New York, Krieger, 1971.
31. Barsky AJ and Klerman GL: Overview: Hypochondriasis, bodily complaints and somatic styles. Am J Psychiatry 140(3):273–283, 1983.
32. Barsky A: Parents who amplify bodily sensations. Ann Intern Med 91:6370–6375, 1979.
33. Lipowski ZJ: Somatization: The concept and its clinical application. Am J Psychiatry 145:1358–1368, 1988.
34. Payne R: Pain in the drug abuser. *In* Foley K and Payne R (eds): Current Therapy of Pain. Toronto, BC Decker, 1988, pp 46–54.
35. Fishbain D, Goldberg M, Meaghen B, et al: Male and female chronic pain patients categorized by DSM-III psychiatric diagnostic criteria. Pain 26:181–197, 1986.
36. Nadelson C, Notman M, and Ellis E: Psychosomatic aspects of obstetrics and gynecology. Psychosomatics 24:871–884, 1983.
37. Grass RJ and Doerr H: Borderline syndromes and incest in chronic pelvic pain patients. Int J Psychiatry Med 10:74–96, 1980.
38. Walker E, Katon W, Harrop-Griffiths J, et al: Relationship of chronic pelvic pain to psychiatric diagnoses and childhood sexual abuse. Am J Psychiatry 145:1, 75–80, 1988.
39. Abramowicz M (ed): Drugs for Pain. Med Lett 35(887):1–6, 1993.
40. Maciewicz R, Bouckoms A, and Martin L: Drug therapy of neuropathic pain. Clin J Pain 1:39–49, 1985.
41. Atkinson J: Psychopharmacologic agents in the treatment of

pain syndromes. *In* Tollison C (ed): Handbook of Chronic Pain Management. Baltimore, Williams & Williams, 1989, pp 69–103.
42. Rogers M and Mufson M: Using antidepressants in rheumatoid arthritis. J Musculoskel Med 7(1):38–56, 1991.
43. Portenoy R: Pain polyneuropathy. *In* Pain: Mechanisms and syndromes. Neurol Clin 7(2):265–288, 1989.
44. Fromm G: Trigeminal neuralgia and related disorders. *In* Pain: Mechanisms and syndromes. Neurol Clin 7(2):305–319, 1989.
45. Max M, Lynch S, Muir J, et al: Effects of desipramine, amitriptyline, and fluoxene on pain in diabetic neuropathy. N Engl J Med 326(19):1250–1256, 1992.
46. Portenoy R: Chronic opioid therapy in non-malignant pain. J Pain Symptom Man 15(1):S46–S62, 1990.
47. North M: Neural stimulation techniques. *In* Tollinson C (ed): Handbook of Chronic Pain Management. Baltimore, Williams & Wilkins, 1989, pp 136–146.
48. Meyerson B: Electrostimulation procedures: Effects, presumed rationales, and possible mechanisms. *In* Bonica J (ed): Advances in Pain Research and Therapy. New York, Raven Press, 1983, pp 495–534.

81

Somatization in Primary Care

CRAIG B. KAPLAN, MD, MA
MACK LIPKIN, Jr., MD

Most physicians recall vexing patients who suffer from persistent physical complaints that remain unexplained despite every diagnostic and therapeutic effort. These patients are common in both primary care and specialty medical practices. They use much medical care, are frequently subjected to repeated diagnostic tests and invasive procedures, and often frustrate and anger their physicians.

Most are individuals who express psychological illness or social distress as somatic body sensations. They seem unable to acknowledge or complain directly about this distress, experiencing it as physical symptoms instead. Although we do not presently understand their disease processes (in the biomedical sense of disturbed cellular or organ function), these patients suffer greatly as a result of this process. This chapter describes for the clinician the differential diagnosis and etiology of somatization, as well as its detection and management.

Barsky and Klerman define somatization as ". . . the expression of emotional discomfort and psychosocial stress in the physical language of bodily symptoms."[1] Smith defines it as "an alternative way (somatic) to express psychiatric disease or psychological stress when a patient is unable to use the emotional route of expression."[2] The thread common to these definitions and others is the patient's experience of sensory body complaints when psychological or social problems are present and when there is no presently measurable pathophysiologic disturbance sufficient to explain the symptoms. When physical illness is present, symptoms are out of proportion to what might be expected based on objective findings. We label such body complaints as being somatized. We stress that we use the term "somatization" to indicate a general process rather than a specific diagnostic category or disorder. Patients with many different psychological diagnoses (to be described later) somatize. Rather than expressing these disorders directly (e.g., altered mood, anxiety), they express them as physical symptoms. "Somatization" describes this process.

SIGNIFICANCE

Cross-cultural studies of somatization suggest that it is probably a universal human phenomenon that occurs in many, if not all, cultures.[3–5] Data from the United States and Great Britain suggest that somatizing patients are an important problem for primary care physicians. Katon and coworkers concluded that 25 to 75% of visits to primary care physicians were primarily due to psychosocial stress manifested by somatic complaints.[6] In a busy Birmingham, Alabama practice, Burnum found that, of 909 patients seen in 3 months, 98 had major psychiatric problems and 65 combined them with physical disease.[7] Collyer, a family physician, estimated that 28% of his patient contacts involved emotional illness and that these contacts took up 48% of his time.[8] He found that 3.6% of families accounted for 32% of his time in practice. Almost all of these families included two patients or more who had depression and vague complaints. Cummings and VandenBos state that as many as 60% of primary care patients recurrently present with somatic symptoms that express psychosocial distress.[9] In their review of studies of mental disorder in health maintenance organizations, they concluded that "the failure to provide mental health service (had) the potential of bankrupting the health care financing system due to overutilization of primary care physicians by somatizing patients." One study done in a large northwest health maintenance organization demonstrated that 51% of patients who were "high" utilizers (top 10%) were identified as having a mental health disorder by their physicians or by meeting criteria for mental health disorder on standardized tests.[10]

The importance of somatization has also been emphasized by two major epidemiologic studies. The Epidemiologic Catchment Area (ECA) study,[11] using a probability sample in five well-defined population groups, found that, of patients with any of 13 common mental disorders, 58% had seen their general medical practitioner in the prior 6 months. Compared with patients without mental disorder, these patients had a twice-increased probability of using medical care.

Although not all patients identified in these studies as having emotional or mental disorders somatize, many of them do. Regier and associates and Schurman and colleagues used data from the National Ambulatory Medical Care Survey to demonstrate that approximately 70% of patients with primary or secondary diagnoses of emotional disorders gave a somatic complaint as the reason for their visits to physicians.[12, 13] Among the most common complaints were constitutional symptoms, headache, dizziness, abdominal or extremity pain, and requests for check-ups. Internists, family practitioners, and general practitioners each carry about 25% of these patients.[12]

DIFFERENTIAL DIAGNOSIS

Most individuals experience minor pains or sensory disturbances in the course of daily activity. Such disturbances become symptoms when they are labeled as abnormal and lead the individual to seek medical care. Psychiatric disorders or significant psychosocial stress may increase the likelihood that an individual will label physiologic sensations as abnormal. Alternatively, stress and psychiatric disorders can produce new symptoms directly. When this process occurs as a result of transient stress that temporarily overwhelms the individual's usual means of coping, we refer to it as transient or acute somatization. In contrast, chronic somatization is a long-lasting process that usually occurs in the context of specific psychiatric disorders.

Transient, Acute Somatization

Probably the most common form of somatization seen in primary care settings, this process occurs when individuals face sudden stressful situations that overwhelm their usual means of coping. During such times, these individuals may experience disturbing body sensations and interpret them as abnormal. Rarely is there a history of prolonged symptoms, and health care seeking is not usually a dominant aspect of their lives. Such individuals do not commonly have diagnosable psychiatric illnesses and usually accept stress as a cause of their symptoms.

Chronic Somatization

Chronic somatization is found in association with the disorders listed in Table 81–1. Studies in varied populations suggest that somatization is most frequently associated with depression, anxiety reactions, and somatoform disorders.[6, 14–16] These disorders are discussed in detail elsewhere in this text. Here we discuss their relevance to somatization.

Depression

Depression is one of the most common disorders underlying somatization in primary care.[17–19] Depressed patients often present to primary care physicians without the symptoms of depressed affect or mood, presenting instead with classic somatic or "vegetative" complaints (e.g., insomnia, fatigue, weight loss, inability to concentrate), nonspecific cardiopulmonary and gastrointestinal symptoms, or localized pain. Sometimes termed "masked depression," these patients may lack the ability to label and report emotions (alexithymia) or be unable to reveal feelings using usual words or language.[20] They may also use coping mechanisms to selectively deny or minimize the feelings associated with depression. Goldberg and Bridges have shown in England that depressed patients who present with somatic symptoms are recognized as depressed less often than are patients who present with mood symptoms.[21, 22] Other studies have shown that increased physical symptoms are often a prelude to depressive episodes.[23] This presentation may account for the consistently low rates of recognition for depression reported in primary care settings (although index of suspicion, recording habits, and training deficits also contribute).

Somatized symptoms associated with depression may respond to appropriate antidepressant therapy. Lesse described favorable responses to antidepressant medication in his neuropsychiatric practice; however, Rickels demonstrated that depressed patients in a general practice responded differently to medication than did those in a psychiatric clinic.[24, 25] Depressed patients with diurnal variations in mood, sleep disturbances, severe anorexia, psychomotor changes, and guilty rumination may be more likely to respond to medication than may those with unexplained or atypical somatic complaints.[26] Patients seen in a psychiatric practice as opposed to a medical practice may respond in a similar manner. However, many clinicians

TABLE 81–1. SETTINGS IN WHICH CHRONIC SOMATIZATION IS FOUND

Depression	Factitious disorders and malingering
Anxiety/panic disorder	Psychophysiologic disorders
Somatoform disorders	Character or personality disorders
Hypochondriasis	Psychoses
Conversion	Transient emotional stress
Somatization disorder	
Psychogenic pain	

attempt a course of tricyclic antidepressants with somatizing, depressed patients.

Anxiety Disorders

Among mental disorders, anxiety disorders are second only to substance abuse in prevalence. Panic disorder is particularly common, occurring in up to 1 to 5% in the general population, with prevalences of 6 to 10% in a primary care setting and 10 to 14% in one cardiology clinic.[27] Patients who have panic attacks may focus selectively on one or more physical symptoms and deny their anxious feelings. Katon studied 55 patients with panic disorder referred from a primary care service.[27] Presenting somatic complaints were epigastric pain (28%), tachycardia (25%), chest pain (22%), dizziness or vertigo (18%), shortness of breath (13%), headache (11%), and syncope (9%). The symptoms were paroxysmal and were not necessarily associated with certain environmental stimuli or situations. Like depression, panic disorder is often unrecognized by physicians. In one study, 70% of patients had visited more than ten physicians before they were diagnosed and treated.[28] Treatment of panic attacks with benzodiazepines or tricyclic antidepressants decreases the frequency and severity of attacks in most cases.

Somatoform Disorders

For these patients, somatization is a chronic, long-lived process but is not associated with a specific psychiatric disorder such as depression or panic disorder. These patients are classified by the *Diagnostic and Statistical Manual of Mental Disorders* (DSM III-R) as having a somatoform disorder.[29] Somatoform disorders are defined as "symptoms suggesting a physical disorder for which there are no demonstrable organic findings or known physiologic mechanisms, and for which there is positive evidence, or a strong presumption, that the symptoms are linked to psychological factors or conflicts." There are four major somatoform disorders: (1) somatization disorder, (2) conversion disorder, (3) hypochondriasis, and (4) psychogenic pain. The clinical features of these disorders may overlap considerably with each other.

Somatization Disorder. Patients with strictly defined somatization disorder have histories of multiple physical symptoms of several years' duration, beginning before 30 years of age. For each symptom, patients must have taken medications, been seen by physicians, or altered their life patterns. DSM III-R criteria require that there be at least 13 of a list of 37 possible symptoms in seven areas: neurologic, gastrointestinal, female genital tract, psychosexual, cardiopulmonary, regional pain, and "sickly all their lives."[29] Somatization disorder has been studied extensively under older names of hysteria or Briquet's syndrome, and the diagnosis has high stability and validity over time. Most patients are female, with an estimated prevalence of approximately 1% in psychiatric practice, although the prevalence may be as high as 5% in primary care settings.[30] Patients with somatization disorder often have emotional as well as somatic disturbances and may have chaotic relationships with others. Smith and associates studied patients referred from primary care practices and found that their per capita personal health care expenditure was approximately nine times that of an age-matched control group.[31] Physician expenditures for these patients were 14 times that for the control group (most of this increase was related to inpatient charges). A single psychiatric consultation with recommendations to the primary provider decreased the cost of caring for this group of patients, primarily by decreasing inpatient charges, without detrimental effects on their functional status.[32]

Conversion Disorder. Patients with conversion disorder have an alteration in physical functioning or symptoms suggesting a physical disorder, but without a pathophysiologic explanation. Historically, they presented with losses or alterations in sensory or voluntary motor function, such as blindness, paralysis, or anesthesia. Currently they present with symptoms such as chest and abdominal pain. Psychological factors are frequently prominent and important, as evidenced by a close temporal relationship of symptom onset with psychological stress or by observation that the symptoms either unconsciously resolve a conflict (primary gain) or enable the patient to avoid some noxious activity and obtain support from the environment (secondary gain). Accurate diagnosis of conversion disorder can be difficult to make. In one study, 20 to 50% of patients initially given this diagnosis eventually developed recognizable diseases (e.g., multiple sclerosis) that explained their symptoms.[33]

Hypochondriasis. Hypochondriacs interpret normal sensations as evidence of illness or "overreact" to minor abnormal sensations (e.g., abdominal cramps, minor muscular aches).[1] Instead of ignoring transient physical sensations, hypochondriacal patients become fearful and convinced that they have a serious illness. These fears and beliefs persist despite medical reassurance and impair social and occupational function. Hypochondriacal patients become preoccupied with their bodies and may be measurably more skilled than other people at detecting body sensations.[34] They often feel abandoned and can be hostile toward others, including physicians. The illness may be a presenting feature of anxiety and depression, and it is important to search for these conditions.[35] The epidemiology and treatment of hypochondriasis in the primary care setting are not well studied. Factors associated with better prognosis include acute onset, short duration, young age, high socioeconomic status, and no organic disease or doctor-shopping.

Psychogenic Pain. The final major somatoform disorder is psychogenic pain. In this condition, severe and prolonged pain is the prominent disturbance. The pain is inconsistent with or out of proportion to the physical findings, and there may be evidence of a temporal relationship of symptoms to psychological stress. For some shamed or guilty patients, pain may serve as unconscious punishment.[34] The diagnosis of psychogenic pain overlaps with that of chronic pain syndrome, which is defined as more than 6 months of pain in one or more body sites that significantly interferes with life activities. Although chronic pain syndrome is not a DSM III-R diagnosis, it is a common form of somatization in the United States today and is most often diagnosed in pain clinics and by psychologists. Chronic pain has many features of depression, including similar findings on psychological testing and response to antidepressant treatment. In a study of patients in the chronic pain program at the University of Washington, 57% satisfied DSM III criteria for major depression; 35% met criteria for psychogenic pain.[19]

The diagnostic categorization of the somatoform disorders is confusing. Definitions overlap: many patients have features of more than one category, whereas others may not meet criteria for any one specific disorder. Although it is probably valuable to recognize and separately classify chronically somatizing patients who are neither depressed nor anxious as having a somatoform disorder, further characterization does not predict therapy or outcome.

Other Disorders Associated With Somatization

Other disorders associated with somatization include factitious disorders and malingering, psychoses, and personality disorders. Unlike the somatoform disorders, in which underlying processes are unconscious, factitious disorders and malingering are the conscious production of a simulated or actual somatic illness. Patients with factitious disorders have no apparent goals, except those of receiving medical care and preserving secondary gain, whereas malingerers seek specific goals such as winning lawsuits or obtaining disability payments. Psychotic patients may have somatic delusions that present as bizarre complaints ("I have fire shooting up my spine and out my ears." "My insides are rotting out.").

Personality disorders frequently coexist with other psychological disorders in somatizing patients and, when present, may affect prognosis adversely.[14, 15, 36, 37] Many patients have histrionic personality disorders or traits. Patients with borderline or narcissistic personality disorders may relate to others in pathologic ways through their somatic complaints. Patients with dependent traits may benefit from symptoms as they facilitate more access to and closer association with physicians upon whom they can depend. Recognizing personality disorders or their traits may allow physicians to reduce conflict, formulate limit setting strategies, and frame diagnostic or therapeutic plans in more acceptable ways.[38–40]

Many studies of somatizing patients report a small subset of patients who have "no defined" psychiatric disorder. Not all patients who seem to be somatizing have a strictly defined psychiatric disorder. One possibility is that these patients do indeed suffer from milder forms of depression, anxiety, or somatization disorder, but that they fail to meet the relatively strict psychiatric criteria for these disorders. Recent literature has termed these patients "subsyndromal," and it appears that they have illness severity and health care utilization intermediate between patients without psychiatric disorders and those who meet strict psychiatric criteria.[41]

MECHANISMS OF SOMATIZATION

Somatization may be understood from four different perspectives: neurobiologic, psychodynamic, behavioral, and sociocultural. While we present them as distinct from one another, we stress that they are ways of understanding a patient's somatizing behavior and that no single perspective is "right" or "correct" for all patients. One perspective may satisfactorily facilitate understanding of some patients, whereas multiple perspectives may be necessary for others.

Neurobiologic Perspective

Neurobiologic theories of somatization have been reviewed by Miller,[42] who emphasizes two concepts. The first—corticofugal inhibition—conceptualizes somatization as a process of abnormal central nervous system regulation of incoming sensory information. Afferent sensory pathways are subject to central inhibition by corticofugal neurons in order to regulate the amount of incoming sensory information. Abnormalities in corticofugal inhibition may occur, causing either over- or underinhibition of sensory input.

The second means of conceptualizing somatization from the neurobiologic perspective is based on the observation that the two sides of the human brain are not symmetric in their functions. For most individuals, the right hemisphere is considerably less involved with language than the left hemisphere but may be more involved in processing emotions. Patients with deficient communication between hemispheres may be unable to express emotions verbally since such verbal expression requires communication of emotions from right to left hemispheres. Therefore, such patients would be unable to express emotions directly, expressing them instead as physical complaints.

Psychodynamic Perspective

From the psychodynamic perspective, reviewed by Rodin,[43] physical sensations occur as expressions of underlying conflict. Somatization is, therefore, viewed as a defense mechanism that resolves conflicting emotions. Some psychodynamic theories view somatizing patients as manifesting a latent need for nurturance and support, which they obtain from the medical and paramedical community. Other theories speculate that somatizing patients are unable to clearly separate physical from psychological experiences and that this inability might be related to unempathic parents who encouraged them (not always consciously) as children to respond to feelings in somatic terms rather than by direct verbalization.

Behavioral Perspective

Patient behaviors are reinforced by the environment in which they occur. Balint observed that patients "negotiated" the form of their illness with their physicians.[44] Patients presented to their physicians with several interpretations of the illness, some emotional ("I'm sad.") and some somatic ("My chest hurts."). The physician then reinforced the physical symptoms ("Tell me about your chest pain.") and ignored the emotional content. This served to reinforce the patient's somatic complaints and diminished the perceived importance of feelings. Physician responses "shaped" patient behavior and the ultimate form of the illness.

Katon and coworkers conceptualized an "illness maintenance system" as the constellation of environmental reinforcers that maintains abnormal illness behavior in any given patient.[6] This system consists of beneficial (from the patient's psychological perspective) changes in family structure, disability payments, or medical care that result from the patient's medical complaints and consequently reinforce them. To correct abnormal illness behavior, these illness maintenance systems must be identified and altered.

In this context, understanding the family dynamics of somatizing patients (both current and family of origin) may be particularly rewarding, because families often function as illness maintenance systems. By responding to illness behavior with more attention in the form of frequent visits, telephone calls, or release from family responsibilities, family members can unwittingly become important reinforcers. Additionally, in families with significant interpersonal conflict, illness in a family member often enables the family to avoid open conflict and its associated stress. Illness behavior may therefore persist because of the role it plays in reducing open conflict and maintaining family harmony.

Sociocultural Perspective

Members of each culture learn from each other "correct" behaviors for dealing with emotions and feelings. For some cultures, direct expression of emotions is permissible; for others, it is not and is highly stigmatized. When a culture does not allow direct communication of emotional content, one means available to express emotions is through physical symptoms. Although not directly labeled as emotional in origin, these physical complaints are recognized as such by others in the culture and responded to appropriately. Somatization in effect serves to notify others of emotional stress or mental illness in ways that are acceptable and not stigmatizing. Since different cultures have different "rules" for the expression of emotions, somatizing behavior varies from one culture to another. Members of one cultural group (particularly one that accepts more direct routes of emotional expression) may therefore not correctly interpret somatizing behavior in members of another culture that stigmatizes emotional behavior. Whatever the cultural origin of physicians, their training makes them members of a biotechnical medical subculture and may make it difficult for them to correctly interpret somatizing behavior in their patients. Misunderstanding the indirect communication conveyed by somatized behaviors, physicians take patients' physical complaints literally. Nations and associates described this phenomenon in a rural Appalachian health care clinic.[45]

Neurobiologic, psychodynamic, behavioral, and sociocultural perspectives may represent explanations for somatization from different levels of the biopsychosocial hierarchy. Just as heart failure can be understood from different perspectives (biochemical, cellular, organ, and others) so can somatization. As with heart failure, no one perspective is exclusive of the others. Each leads to improved understanding and therapy. Some may be more useful for a given patient than others. A view of somatization that integrates these different perspectives is necessary for fully understanding and treating these patients. Somatization is truly a biopsychosocial phenomenon in which neurobiologic, psychodynamic, behavioral, and sociocultural systems interact to produce symptoms, perceptions, and behavior. In order to help somatizing patients, physicians need to appreciate all of these interactions and use a multisystem approach to diagnosis and therapy.

DIAGNOSIS

Recognizing somatization can be difficult and frustrating, although there are certain clues that may indicate that symptoms arise from underlying psychosocial distress. We stress that diagnosing somatization is not merely a process of "ruling out" other organic causes. Rather, it is a *positive* process, achieved by maintaining a high index of suspicion, carefully listening to symptoms, attending to certain diagnostic clues, and learning about the patient's cultural and personal beliefs.

Remember that psychiatric disorders associated with somatization have high prevalences in primary care settings. They are, therefore, much more common than the rare diseases such as pheochromocytoma, heavy metal intoxication, and porphyria that are often investigated repeatedly in this population. This warrants a high index of suspicion for psychological illness when patients present with lengthy histories of undiagnosed or unsuccessfully treated complaints. Listen for and inquire early in the diagnostic process about psychological information concerning the patient's mood, sources of stress (personal, family, occupational), and prior history of psychological problems. Gathering psychological data as you gather biological data will identify psychological distress earlier. More important, it avoids conveying the impression to the patient that you are turning to a psychological line of inquiry as a last resort. Most somatizing patients are very alert to such a change in diagnostic strategy, because it often indicates that the physician has concluded that this is "all in their head" and that they need to see a psychiatrist. They therefore experience the psychological line of inquiry as prelude to a rejection and may become angry or strongly resistant.

Throughout the information-gathering process, the physician should be alert to clues to somatization. Lipkin suggested 11 positive criteria useful for the diagnosis of "psychogenic" symptoms (Table 81–2).[46] The presence of several of these criteria increases the likelihood that somatization exists. Another clue to somatization is the "disease syndrome-illness behavior discrepancy" described by Pilowsky.[47] When told by physicians that they are healthy or given a relatively benign explanation for their complaints, these patients react with persistent complaints and demands, in contrast to most patients, who react with relief or resignation to the physician's explanations. Detecting this behavioral discrepancy may help to identify patients who are somatizing.

Formal assessment techniques have also been used for detecting somatization and related emotional disorders in the medical setting. Some tests for depression have been used extensively in medical patients. These brief, self-administered tests can be completed by patients in the office and are easy to score. However, they are more sensitive than specific; a normal score virtually rules out significant depression, but an abnormal score does not confirm it. Patients with abnormal scores should be investigated more fully. For somatizing patients, the Somatization, Anxiety, and Depression subscales of the Minnesota Multiphasic Personality Inventory may be helpful. We emphasize strongly that, although these tests may provide adjunctive information to the clinician, they should not take the place

TABLE 81–2. POSITIVE CRITERIA FOR DIAGNOSIS OF PSYCHOGENIC SYMPTOMS

1. The patient has features of the hysterical personality style—dramatic, shallow affect, vague, contradictory or inconsistent, quickly relating emotionally (positively or negatively), distractable, suggestible, unrealistic.
2. The illness begins in a psychologically meaningful setting.
3. The illness or symptom has an idiosyncratic (symbolic) meaning for the patient.
4. The description of the symptom is vague, inconsistent, or bizarre.
5. The symptoms have persisted despite allegedly specific medical therapy.
6. A great deal of medical attention is given to the patient but with limited curing (many physicians or many visits).
7. The patient denies the psychological role of the symptoms (a normal person would consider the psychological possibility).
8. There is associated psychiatric illness—depression, schizophrenia, schizoaffective disorder, addiction, other disorders.
9. Polysurgery has occurred (usually to organs such as the appendix or gallbladder, or for adhesions or trapped nerves).
10. Alexithymia is present.
11. The symptom functions to communicate for the patient to the physician (or significant others) about psychological conflicts or pains.

(From Lipkin M Jr: Psychiatry and medicine. *In* Kaplan H and Sadock B (eds): Comprehensive Textbook of Psychiatry. Baltimore, Williams & Wilkins, 1987. © Williams & Wilkins, 1987.)

of the sensitive, thorough interview process that we have outlined.

MANAGEMENT

In general, the most important aspect of management in any setting is the development of an empathic, trusting, caring physician-patient relationship. Establishing the therapeutic relationship is critical to both diagnosis and treatment. Its constancy and dependability should be emphasized repeatedly to the patient. Over time, the relationship can be used to promote healthy growth and development. Expression of feelings and emotions can be encouraged and, through physician demonstrations of acceptance, respect, and positive regard, patients can grow toward greater self-esteem.

This is not to say that relationships with somatizing patients are easy to establish, however. These patients can be very frustrating; physicians often find themselves feeling angry, hopeless, or helpless. While these feelings can be barriers to the development of a therapeutic relationship,[48, 49] they may be diagnostically valuable.[49, 50] Recognizing anger or frustration with a patient, especially early in the relationship, may indicate the presence of a personality disorder or other psychological illness.

Several core attitudes help the authors to deal with these emotions. Remember that these patients are reacting in the best and (without help) only way available to them. In addition, they challenge both our diagnostic and therapeutic skills in a way that more routine patients do not. Finally, they are fascinating, giving us important insight into the relationship between the mind and the body.

Acute, Transient Somatization

Somatization in patients undergoing acute situational stress is often transient and has a good prognosis. These patients do not have long histories of somatization and are often willing to consider or accept psychological or psychophysiologic explanations for their symptoms. Often it is necessary only to tell them that the experience of stress as physical symptoms is a common and normal phenomenon. Reassure them that you have thoroughly considered their symptoms and suggest that periodic follow-up is needed without further extensive investigation. When stress is severe or likely to be prolonged, these patients will often readily accept referral to mental health providers for stress management or therapy.

Chronic Somatization

Chronically somatizing patients require a more complex management strategy. Because these patients consider their symptoms to be physical problems, they strongly resist psychological explanations and usually refuse psychiatric referral. Even when successfully referred, few respond to insight-oriented psychotherapy.

Primary care providers can treat these patients, however. Effective management strategies in the primary care setting can reduce costs and improve patient and physician satisfaction with care. Specific management suggestions are outlined below (Table 81–3).

TABLE 81–3. CHRONIC SOMATIZATION: MANAGEMENT STRATEGY

1. Find mutually acceptable language/labels for symptoms.
2. Talk specifically about appropriate goals.
3. Don't dispute the reality of the complaint.
4. Respectfully evaluate symptoms.
5. Schedule follow-up regularly, independently of symptom status.
6. Use medications only when indicated.
7. Refer when appropriate and emphasize that referral is not dismissal.

Find and use mutually acceptable language to explain the symptoms to the patient, avoiding the use of psychological labels (e.g., depression, anxiety, stress). Explanations that attempt to relate the symptom to anxiety or depression frequently prove fruitless: patients have usually heard them before and quickly anticipate rejection. In fact, many patients actually believe the opposite explanation ("I feel depressed because of my symptoms."). It is much more helpful to base daily interaction on the somatic complaint. Descriptive physiologic explanations such as "You have abnormally tense muscles in your abdomen (or chest)" tend to be more acceptable to patients and to their families. In time, as trust and acceptance within the relationship builds, patients themselves may initiate exploration of the relationship between their psychosocial issues and symptoms, in turn accepting psychological labels. We emphasize, however, that this may take months or years and is rarely possible during the first several visits.

Establish appropriate goals for yourself and negotiate goals explicitly with the patient. This seldom involves a *cure*: It is almost never possible in the short term and promising it dooms the physician and the patient to disappointment. Rather than cure or complete resolution of symptoms, it is better to set less global, more realistic goals. For the physician, realistic goals might be decreasing the numbers of urgent telephone calls and unscheduled or emergency visits, decreasing doctor-shopping, and avoiding unnecessary hospitalizations or invasive procedures. For the patient, positive, realistic goals might include acceptance by the physician, improved coping with symptoms, increased feelings of control of themselves or their symptoms, or improved social or occupational functioning.

Don't dispute the reality or severity of physical complaints. Remember that their symptoms are very real to these patients. If the physician suggests that the patient's symptoms are not as severe as he or she states, this may convince the patient that he or she (and his or her complaints) is not being taken seriously. Patients are helped by feeling that physicians truly believe them when they say that they are suffering. Explicit acknowledgment of the suffering ("I can see how much you've suffered with all of these symptoms") early in the relationship will promote a sense of trust and acceptance. Paying close attention to and fully clarifying patients' illness stories, and demonstrating understanding of underlying beliefs and expectations for care will also convince them that they are being taken seriously.

Each symptom should be respectfully evaluated using the interview, physical examination, and judicious use of diagnostic tests. It is important to do a careful physical examination, no matter how unusual the symptoms, because patients often judge how seriously you take them by whether or not you actually examine them. Not all complaints merit diagnostic tests and, when necessary, tests should be used in a conservative, step-wise fashion. Attempt to negotiate diagnostic tests, particularly if patients indicate that they think they are necessary. It may help to ask the patient to agree, in return for ordering some diagnostic tests, to accept the conservative management strategy outlined here if test results are negative.

Schedule follow-up visits at regular intervals (every 2 to 4 weeks) so that they are not contingent on the presence of symptoms. Basing frequency of visits on the number or severity of symptoms merely reinforces and maintains them. Follow-up appointments scheduled regularly regardless of symptom severity stress the importance of the relationship, de-emphasizing symptoms. Unless suggested by the patient, attempting to lengthen times between appointments may actually lead to worsening symptoms.

Once you and the patient commit to regular follow-up appointments, it is appropriate to set limits on telephone calls and "drop-in" visits. Rules for these behaviors should be set early in the relationship. One rule is that patients consider the practitioner the primary care physician and agree not to doctor-shop or to see other practitioners without mutual discussion. Another is that the patient will reserve all except emergency complaints for regularly scheduled sessions. If the patient calls in between scheduled visits, the discussion should be limited to assessing that there is no objective emergency or psychological crisis requiring immediate action. If not, further discussion should be gently deferred until the next scheduled appointment. Surprisingly, patients almost always accept such arrangements once they realize that the relationship is not dependent on the continued presence of physical symptoms and complaints.

Medications should be avoided in most instances. If used, they should be prescribed to treat defined disorders such as depression or reduce (not remove) specific target symptoms. Patients should be told of these conditions for prescribing at the onset of drug treatment, and a specific time should be set, after which the medications will be discontinued if benefit is not observed or is lost. Some associated conditions should be treated, however. Major depression should be treated since antidepressants have proven efficacy. Severe somatizers often deserve an empiric trial of tricyclic antidepressants because of the frequency of concomitant masked depression. Anxiolytics may help if used specifically for anxiety or panic disorder. Treatment with narcotics, hypnotics, or sedatives is ineffective, and patients may easily become dependent on them.

These patients are hard for primary care providers to refer to mental health providers since they resist the psychological labelling required to justify referral. Even when successfully referred, those with somatoform disorders do not respond well to insight-oriented therapy offered within mental health settings. Frequently they end up back in medical settings for chronic management. A consultation model, in which patients are asked to see mental health providers for one or several visits in order to help the primary care provider, is often better accepted. When possible, such consultation can help by confirming the presence of a psychological disorder or identifying difficult personality styles or disorders. Helpful suggestions for discussing referral with patients have been offered by Bursztajn and Barsky.[51] Perhaps better than referral or consultation is care conjointly provided by primary care and psychiatric personnel (as well as by other ancillary services) in multidisciplinary clinics.

Disability is an important issue. Many patients are involved in disability proceedings when first seen or soon become involved in them. We attempt to estimate the degree of the patient's psychological rather than physical disability. Immediate coping needs often dictate a brief respite from circumstances causing psychological stress, but we emphasize that such respites should be limited and coupled with positive expectations about future functional recovery. Long-term or permanent disability probably harms most patients, thus we avoid such outcomes.

A final major barrier to a successful relationship is the emotional reaction of the physician to the patient. As pointed out earlier, physicians often have strong reactions to somatizing patients, ranging from despair to outright anger. We find that many of these occur as a result of frustration with one's inability to achieve cure or resolution of symptoms. Abandoning such unrealistic goals in favor of more limited goals of reducing destructive behaviors and improving coping improves negative emotional reactions. Openly discussing these emotional responses with other care providers will also help practitioners to understand and cope with them.

This management strategy requires multiple visits scheduled regularly over months to years. For both the physician and the patient, the process can seem slow and frustrating. At these times, it is important to emphasize to the patient that cure is unlikely and that, if cure were possible or likely, someone long ago would have identified a curable process. Listening empathically to the patient's frustration or anger without responding defensively will further reinforce your trustworthiness. For the physician it helps to remember that these are *chronic* illnesses that undergo exacerbations and remissions, and one should keep in mind the appropriate and realistic therapeutic goals described earlier. Even if patients do not accept referral to mental health care providers or achieve sudden insight into the psychological basis of symptoms, they can and do improve with the management strategy that we have outlined.

SUMMARY

Somatizing patients experience or express emotional discomfort and psychosocial distress as physical symptoms. Somatization occurs in a broad spectrum of illnesses, in association with a wide variety of mental disorders, including depression, anxiety, and the somatoform disorders. Because these illnesses frequently present in primary care settings, primary care providers must detect and treat them. The diagnosis is based on positive criteria. Care rests on conservative medical management and evaluation; a physician-patient relationship based on acceptance, caring, and trust; reinforcement of positive behaviors and elimination of destructive ones; and the gradual use of the relationship to promote a healthy attitude in the patient.

REFERENCES

1. Barsky AJ and Klerman GL: Overview: Hypochondriasis, bodily complaints, and somatic styles. Am J Psychiatry 140:273–283, 1983.
2. Smith RC: A clinical approach to the somatizing patient. J Fam Pract 21:294–301, 1985.
3. Kirmayer LJ: Culture, affect, and somatization, Part I. Transcultural Psychiatr Res Rev 21:159–188, 1984.
4. Kirmayer LJ: Culture, affect, and somatization, Part II. Transcultural Psychiatr Res Rev 21:237–262, 1984.
5. Kleinman A: The Illness Narratives: Suffering, Healing, and the Human Condition. New York, Basic, 1988.
6. Katon W, Ries RK, and Kleinman A: The prevalence of somatization in primary care. Compr Psychiatry 25:208–215, 1984.
7. Burnum JF: Is writing a list of symptoms a sign of an emotional disorders? N Engl J Med 313:690–691, 1985.
8. Collyer JA: Psychosomatic illness in a solo family practice. Psychosomatics 20:762–767, 1979.
9. Cummings NA and VandenBos GR: The twenty years Kaiser-Permanente experience with psychotherapy and medical utili-

zation: Implications for national health policy and national health insurance. Health Policy Q 1:159–175, 1981.
10. Katon W, Von Korff M, Lin E, et al: Distressed high utilizers of medical care: DSM-III-R diagnoses and treatment needs. Gen Hosp Psychiatry 12:1–8, 1990.
11. Regier DA, Myers JK, Kramer M, et al: The NIMH epidemiologic catchment area program. Arch Gen Psychiatry 41:934–941, 1984.
12. Regier DA, Goldberg ID, and Taube CA: The de facto U.S. mental health services system. Arch Gen Psychiatry 35:685–693, 1978.
13. Schurman RA, Kramer PD, and Mitchell JB: The hidden mental health network. Arch Gen Psychiatry 253:89–94, 1985.
14. Katon W, Ries RK, and Kleinman A: A prospective DSM-III study of 100 consecutive somatization patients. Compr Psychiatry 25:305–314, 1984.
15. Slavney PR, Teitelbaum ML, and Chase GA: Referral for medically unexplained somatic complaints: The role of histrionic traits. Psychosomatics 26:103–109, 1985.
16. Ford CV and Folks DG: Conversion disorders: An overview. Psychosomatics 26:371–383, 1985.
17. Katon W, Kleinman A, and Rosen G: Depression and somatization: A review, Part I. Am J Med 72:127–135, 1982.
18. Katon W, Kleinman A, and Rosen G: Depression and somatization: A review, Part II. Am J Med 72:241–247, 1982.
19. Katon W: Depression: Relationship to somatization and chronic medical illness. J Clin Psychiatry 45:4–11, 1984.
20. Lesser IM: Alexithymia. N Engl J Med 312:690–692, 1985.
21. Goldberg DP and Bridges K: Somatic presentations of psychiatric illness in primary care settings. J Psychosom Res 32:137–144, 1988.
22. Bridges KW and Goldberg DP: Somatic presentation of DSM-III psychiatric disorders in primary care. J Psychosom Res 29:563–569, 1985.
23. Widmer RB and Cadoret RJ: Depression in primary care: Changes in pattern of patient visits and complaints during a developing depression. J Fam Pract 7:293–302, 1978.
24. Lesse S: Behavioral problems masking severe depression. Am J Psychother 33:41–53, 1979.
25. Rickels K, Jenkins BW, Zamostein B, et al: Pharmacotherapy in neurotic depression: Differential population responses. J Nerv Ment Dis 145:475–485, 1968.
26. Bielski RJ and Freidel RO: Prediction of tricyclic antidepressant response: A critical review. Arch Gen Psychiatry 33:1479–1489, 1976.
27. Katon W: Panic disorder and somatization. Am J Med 77:101–106, 1984.
28. Sheehan DV, Ballenger J, and Jacobsen G: Treatment of endogenous anxiety with phobic, hysterical, and hypochondriacal symptoms. Arch Gen Psychiatry 37:51–59, 1980.
29. American Psychiatric Association: Diagnostic and Statistical Manual of Mental Disorders, 3rd rev ed. Washington, DC, American Psychiatric Association, 1987.
30. deGruy F, Columbia L, and Dickinson L: Somatization disorder in a family practice. J Fam Pract 25:45–51, 1987.
31. Smith GR, Monson RA, and Ray DC: Patients with multiple unexplained symptoms: Their characteristics, functional health, and health care utilization. Arch Intern Med 146:69–72, 1986.
32. Smith GR, Monson RA, and Ray DC: Psychiatric consultation in somatization disorder. N Engl J Med 314:1407–1413, 1986.
33. Lazare A: Conversion symptoms. N Engl J Med 305:745–748, 1981.
34. Engel GL: "Psychogenic" pain and the pain-prone patient. Am J Med 26:899–918, 1959.
35. Barsky AJ: Patients who amplify bodily sensations. Ann Intern Med 91:63–70, 1979.
36. Slavney PR and Teitelbaum ML: Patients with medically unexplained symptoms: DSM-III diagnoses and demographic characteristics. Gen Hosp Psychiatry 7:21–25, 1985.
37. Folks DG and Ford CV: Psychiatric disorders in geriatric medical/surgical patients. I: Report of 195 consecutive consultations. South Med J 78:239–402, 1985.
38. Leigh H and Reiser MF: The patient's personality. *In* Leigh H and Reiser MF (eds): The Patient: Biological, Psychological, and Social Dimensions of Medical Practice. New York, Plenum, 1980, pp 253–269.
39. Reich J: Personality disorders. Primary Care 14:725–736, 1987.
40. Tollefson GD: Personality disorders. Am Fam Physician 27:215–223, 1983.
41. Escobar JI, Golding JM, Hough RL, et al: Somatization in the community: Relationship to disability and use of services. Am J Public Health 77:837–840, 1987.
42. Miller L: Neuropsychological concepts of somatoform disorders. Int J Psychiatry Med 14:31–46, 1984.
43. Rodin G: Somatization and the self: Psychotherapeutic issues. Am J Psychother 38:257–263, 1984.
44. Balint M: The Doctor, the Patient, and the Illness. New York, International Universities Press, 1972.
45. Nations MK, Camino LA, and Walker FB: "Hidden" popular illnesses in primary care: Residents' recognition and clinical implications. Cult Med Psychiatry 9:223–240, 1985.
46. Lipkin M Jr: Psychiatry and medicine. *In* Kaplan H and Sadock B (eds): Comprehensive Textbook of Psychiatry. Baltimore, Williams & Wilkins, 1987.
47. Pilowsky I: A general classification of abnormal illness behaviors. Br J Med Psychol 51:131–137, 1978.
48. Gorlin R and Zucker HD: Physicians' reactions to patients: A key to teaching humanistic medicine. N Engl J Med 308:1059–1063, 1983.
49. Zinn WM: Doctors have feelings too. JAMA 259:3296–3298, 1988.
50. Levinson W: Frustrating patients: Using our feelings as diagnostic clues. J Gen Intern Med 6:259–260, 1991.
51. Bursztajn H and Barsky AJ: Facilitating patient acceptance of psychiatric referral. Arch Intern Med 145:73–75, 1985.

82

Psychotic Disorders

MICHAEL J. MUFSON, MD

Psychotic disorders constitute a wide range of states characterized by the presence of symptoms that interfere with an individual's reality testing. The impairment in reality testing is most often severe and interferes with the person's abilities to think, function at work, and organize goal-directed behavior.

Psychotic symptoms include delusions, hallucinations, thought disorder (e.g., loose associations; personalized, illogical, and incoherent thinking), and disturbances in modulation of affect and grossly disorganized behavior. It is important to note that psychosis may occur in a wide variety of neurologic, medical, and toxic states as well as in psychiatric disorders (e.g., schizophrenia and bipolar illness).

This chapter focuses on the diagnosis and treatment of these disorders, emphasizing the differential diagnosis of acute and chronic psychotic states and the need to differentiate psychoses seen in the psychiatric disorders from those seen in medical and neurologic illnesses.

ACUTE PSYCHOSIS

Acute psychotic states can be seen in both psychiatric and medical conditions. The most important characteristic of the acute psychotic state is the *abrupt* onset. The clinical picture includes the psychotic symptoms noted earlier, and the clinician's task is to determine whether the psychotic symptoms are part of an acute organic brain syndrome, secondary to an acute psychiatric process, or an exacerbation of a chronic recurrent psychotic process such as schizophrenia.

The causes of acute psychosis associated with medical, toxic, and neurologic conditions are listed in Table 82–1. Perhaps the most common source of acute psychosis is the confusional state. The distinguishing features of the confusional state are reviewed in Chapter 57. The important hallmarks are an impairment of consciousness, an increased or decreased psychomotor state, a disruption of thinking, an impairment in attention and memory, and perceptual disturbances. Emotional changes are frequent and range from depression to euphoria, anxiety, and irritability. The importance of recognizing that a psychosis is secondary to an acute medical or neurologic disorder, of course, is that treatment of the underlying cause produces resolution of the syndrome. Obtaining a complete clinical history is often the most important step in establishing the etiology. This is especially true in drug abuse, acute exacerbation of a chronic psychosis, alcohol-related states, and acute neurologic emergencies.

ORGANIC BRAIN SYNDROMES

The organic brain syndromes can be grouped into several categories: (1) delirium; (2) dementia; and (3) drug intoxication and withdrawal.

Delirium

Delirium, or acute confusional state, refers to an acute clouding of consciousness. Delirium is characterized by confusion; fluctuations in the level of consciousness including lucid intervals of variable duration; disorganized thinking; reduced ability to maintain attention to external stimuli; and impaired ability to shift attention to new stimuli. The confusional state includes disorientation and memory impairment and may be accompanied by psychotic symptoms including paranoid delusions and visual and auditory hallucinations. Vivid dreams and nightmares may occur and merge with hallucinations.[1,2]

The most common medical problems that present with acute confusion and behavioral disorders with psychotic symptoms are hypoglycemia, toxic-metabolic encephalopathies, delirium tremens due to alcohol withdrawal, drug withdrawal, and toxic psychoses induced by drugs. Meningitis, intracranial hemorrhage, hypertensive encephalopathy, and other disorders listed in Table 82–1 must also be considered.

One should suspect an underlying medical or neurologic basis to the psychotic state if the onset is quite abrupt, if the patient is older than 40 years of age and has no prior history of psychotic episodes, if the patient has a history of alcoholism or drug abuse, or if the patient is receiving medication that can provoke a confusional state. The acute schizophrenic psychoses, on the other hand, generally have their onset over a period of weeks to months. Abnormal

TABLE 82–1. CAUSES OF ORGANIC PSYCHOSES

Medical and Surgical Conditions Associated with Delirium and Psychotic Symptoms	Neurologic Diseases Associated with Cognitive Impairment and Psychotic Symptoms
Septicemia	Temporal lobe seizures
Pneumonia	Presenile and senile dementias
Hypoglycemia	Wernicke's encephalopathy and Kosakoff's syndrome (thiamine deficiency)
Encephalitis, meningitis, brain abscess, carcinomatosis	Vitamin B_{12} deficiency (pernicious anemia)
Drug or alcohol withdrawal (delirium tremens); barbiturate withdrawal	Hydrocephalus: normal pressure
Encephalopathy	Brain neoplasms
Hypo- or hyperthyroidism	Wilson's disease
Adrenal dysfunction	Niemann-Pick disease
Uremia/renal failure	Huntington's chorea
Hepatic encephalopathy	Subdural hematoma
Electrolyte disturbances	Head trauma (traumatic delirium)
CNS involvement by systemic lupus erythematosus, AIDS, syphilis	Subarachnoid hemorrhage
Acute intermittent porphyria	Infarcts
Postcardiac arrest state and cardiac failure	CNS infections (eg., HIV)
Hypoxia/respiratory failure	
Toxic States Associated with Delirium	**Genetic Disorders**
Antiparkinsonian agents (e.g., amantadine, carbidopa, L-dopa)	Klinefelter's syndrome
Amphetamines, cocaine, PCP	Turner's syndrome
Antibiotics (acyclovir, amphotericin B)	Porphyria
Corticosteroids	Metachromatic leukodystrophy
Lithium toxicity	Phenylketonuria
Anticonvulsants (e.g., phenobarbital, phenytoin, valproate)	Wilson's disease
Bromocriptine	**Abstinence Syndromes**
Cimetidine	Alcohol
Isoniazid, chloroquine	Barbiturates
Antidepressants (especially amitriptyline)	Sedatives (e.g., methaqualone)
MAO inhibitors	Benzodiazepines
Anticholinergics (e.g., antihistamines, benztropine)	
Cardiac agents (e.g., propranolol, clonidine, digitalis, lidocaine, quinidine, procainamide)	
Bromism	
Disulfiram	
Indomethacin	
Pentazocine	
Opiates	
Phenothiazines (especially thioridazine)	

AIDS = acquired immunodeficiency syndrome; CNS = central nervous system; PCP = phencyclidine hydrochloride.

vital signs, tremulousness, and other signs and symptoms of drug abuse/withdrawal are helpful in establishing a diagnosis (Table 82–2).

Whenever an organic illness causing behavioral disturbances is a possibility, it is essential that the patient be thoroughly examined. If necessary, one may administer haloperidol (2 to 5 mg, given intramuscularly or intravenously) to control the patient's behavior and permit examination without causing excessive sedation.[3] Failure to examine the patient with a behavioral disorder because the patient is uncooperative is not a defense against negligence if the patient has been brought for examination. Since hypoglycemia and thiamine deficiency are readily reversible causes of behavioral disturbances, all delirious or comatose patients should receive intravenous glucose and thiamine at the time of presentation.

Dementia and Beclouded Dementia

The essential feature of dementia is impairment of short- or long-term memory associated with impairment in intellectual functioning. In dementia there are often associated personality changes, and this disorder develops insidiously, often without confusion in the early stages, and in most cases is irreversible. The most common causes include Alzheimer's disease and multi-infarct dementia. Treatable disorders that may present with this picture include subdural hematomas, normal-pressure hydrocephalus, cerebral neoplasm, Parkinson's disease, vitamin B_{12} deficiency, and hypothyroidism.

Such patients may show changes in personality, including increased irritability, hostility, depression, or euphoria and emotional lability and can become frankly paranoid with delusional thinking.[4, 5] As the disease progresses, the patient also manifests a lack of sociability and becomes unable to care for himself or herself. The onset of the illness late in life, as well as concomitant memory loss and disorientation, should suggest that dementia rather than schizophrenia is the underlying problem. The medical evaluation should be directed to determine if a potentially reversible cause of dementia is present (see Chapter 57).

Demented patients may also develop acute confusion superimposed on the senile dementia, "beclouded dementia," and this can present as an acute psychosis. This state is often precipitated by drugs (e.g., minor tranquilizers, L-dopa, lidocaine, ritalin) or acute illness. The psychosis resolves over time with removal of the offending drug or with resolution of the acute illness.

Drug Intoxication and Withdrawal

The essential features of intoxication are abnormal behavior and a substance-specific syndrome caused by a recent ingestion of a psychoactive substance. Similarly, in

TABLE 82–2. SYMPTOMS AND SIGNS OF DRUG OVERDOSE OR WITHDRAWAL*†

Drug	Acute Intoxication and Overdose	Withdrawal Syndrome
Hallucinogens LSD,[1] psilocybin; mescaline; PCP,[2] STP,[3] MDMA,[4] bromo-DMA[5]	*Pupils* dilated (normal or small with PCP); *BP* elevated; *heart rate* increased; *tendon reflexes* hyperactive; *temperature elevated;* face flushed; euphoria; anxiety or panic; paranoid thought disorder; sensorium often clear; affect inappropriate; illusions; time and visual distortions; visual hallucinations; depersonalization; with PCP cyclic coma or extreme hyperactivity, drooling, blank stare, mutism, amnesia, analgesia, nystagmus (sometimes vertical), gait ataxia, muscle rigidity, impulsive, often violent behavior	None
CNS Stimulants Amphetamines; cocaine; methylphenidate; phenmetrazine; phenylpropanolamine; most antiobesity drugs	*Pupils* dilated and reactive; *respiration* shallow; *BP* elevated; *heart rate* increased *tendon reflexes* hyperactive; *temperature* elevated; cardiac arrhythmias; dry mouth; sweating; tremors; sensorium hyperacute or confused; paranoid ideation; hallucinations; impulsivity; hyperactivity; stereotype; convulsions; coma	Muscular aches; abdominal pain; chills, tremors; voracious hunger; anxiety; prolonged sleep; lack of energy; profound psychological depression; sometimes suicidal; exhaustion
Cannabis Group Marijuana; hashish; THC[6]; hash oil	*Pupils* dilated and reactive; *respiration* shallow; *BP* decreased on standing; *heart rate* increased; increased appetite; euphoria, anxiety; sensorium often clear; dreamy, fantasy state; time-space distortions; hallucinations rare; tachycardia, ataxia, and pallor in children	Nonspecific symptoms including anorexia nausea, insomnia, restlestness, irritability, anxiety
Opioids Heroin; morphine; codeine; meperidine; methadone; hydromorphone; opium; pentazocine; propoxyphene	*Pupils* constricted (may be dilated with meperidine or extreme hypoxia); *respiration* depressed; *BP* decreased; *temperature* decreased; *reflexes* diminished; stupor or coma; pulmonary edema; constipation; convulsions with propoxyphene or meperidine	*Pupils* dilated; *pulse* rapid; gooseflesh; abdominal cramps; muscle jerks; "flu" syndrome; vomiting, diarrhea; tremulousness; yawning; anxiety
CNS Sedatives Barbiturates; chlordiazepoxide; diazepam; flurazepam; glutethimide; meprobamate; methaqualone; others	*Pupils* in mid-position and fixed (but dilated with glutethimide or in severe poisoning); *BP* decreased; *respiration* depressed; *tendon reflexes* depressed; drowsiness or coma; nystagmus; confusion; ataxia, slurred speech; delirium; convulsions or hyperirritability with methaqualone overdosage; serious poisoning rare with benzodiazepines alone	Tremulousness; insomnia sweating; fever; clonic blink reflex; anxiety cardiovascular collapse; agitation; delirium; hallucinations; disorientation; convulsions
Anticholinergics Atropine, belladonna; henbane; scopolamine; trihexyphenidyl; benztropine mesylate; procyclidine; propantheline bromide	*Pupils* dilated and fixed; *heart rate* increased; *temperature* elevated; decreased bowel sounds; drowsiness or coma; flushed, dry skin and mucous membranes; sensorium clouded; amnesia; disorientation, visual hallucinations; body image alterations; confusions	Gastrointestinal and musculoskeletal symptoms

*From Acute drug abuse reactions. Med Lett 27:77, 1985.
†Mixed intoxications produce complex combinations of signs and symptoms.
[1]Lysergic acid diethylamide.
[2]Phencyclidine.
[3]2,5-Dimethoxy-4-methylamphetamine.
[4]3,4-Methylenedioxymethamphetamine.
[5]DMA 4-bromo-2,5-dimethoxyamphetamine.
[6]Delta-9-tetrahydrocannabinol.
BP = blood pressure.

withdrawal there is the development of specific signs and symptoms following cessation or reduction of a substance that the person has been using regularly.[6] The physician should thus be familiar with the specific signs and symptoms of drug intoxication and withdrawal (see Table 82–2). For example, in the case of psychosis induced by hallucinogens, amphetamines, phencyclidine hydrochloride (PCP), or cocaine, one must often rely on the acute onset of symptoms and the history of drug abuse obtained from the patient's family. The diagnosis can be confirmed by obtaining a toxic screen and by observing the course of the illness, which will subside spontaneously while the patient is kept under observation. Drug-induced psychosis usually resolves within 48 to 72 hours. If the psychotic process continues beyond that period, one must raise the question of whether the drug abuse has precipitated a latent psychotic process such as yet undiagnosed schizophrenia.[7]

PSYCHOTIC SYNDROMES ASSOCIATED WITH SEIZURE DISORDERS

Psychotic symptoms related to epilepsy and temporal lobe epilepsy bear special mention. Psychosis occurs in approximately 7% of patients suffering from epilepsy. The prevalence of epilepsy in patients with psychosis is about 2%, approximately three to seven times the prevalence in the adult population. Of note is that psychosis is found four to twelve times more frequently in the patients with temporal lobe epilepsy. Most of these cases are brief psychotic episodes, but in some cases persistent psychotic states emerge. These psychotic states present independently of the seizure state and are not associated with confusion or seizure activity. They are often referred to as epileptic psychosis and should be distinguished from the brief psychotic episodes.[8, 9]

Patients with complex partial seizures may be mistakenly diagnosed as having schizophrenia, either because manifestations of the psychomotor seizures mimic the hallucinations and the psychotic behavior of schizophrenia or because some patients with psychomotor epilepsy develop chronic psychosis. Paranoid psychoses during interictal periods can be present in more than one third of patients with psychomotor epilepsy.[8]

Quite commonly, the symptoms of complex partial seizures include a primary visual aura that may mimic a visual hallucination. The patient's behavior during the seizure can appear bizarre, also suggesting the possibility of a psychosis. Other manifestations of partial seizures can be transient, and the patient may describe a visual hallucination or repetitive vision occurring several times during the day. This can be mistaken for symptoms of psychosis. During the seizure the patient may exhibit quasipurposeful, complex automatisms. These automatisms may be interrupted by lip smacking, eye blinking, or staring, and speech is arrested. The patient is often amnestic for the episode, but sometimes partial recall is found regarding the ictal event. The event itself may be followed by postictal states that usually consist of sound sleep but sometimes are characterized by fatigue, depression, or elation. A nondiagnostic electroencephalogram, even if performed when the patient has been deprived of sleep or with nasopharyngeal leads, does not exclude the diagnosis of complex partial seizures, and a trial of anticonvulsant therapy may be necessary.

In an acute episode, however, a differential diagnosis in certain individuals may be difficult to make, with the epileptic psychosis manifesting religious and paranoid delusions. A trial of antipsychotic agents in the acute phase may be indicated. They may be used in conjunction with anticonvulsant agents such as carbamazepine (Tegretol). After acute symptoms are controlled, the neuroleptic may be withdrawn gradually, while observing the patient closely for a recrudescence of symptoms. Since reports indicate that high or rapidly increasing doses of neuroleptics can precipitate seizures, they must be used judiciously and in conjunction with the anticonvulsant.

ACUTE PSYCHOSIS: THE FORMAL PSYCHIATRIC DISORDERS

Brief Reactive Psychoses and Schizophreniform Disorders

A wide variety of psychiatric disorders can present with psychotic symptoms (Table 82–3). Brief reactive psychoses can occur following a wide variety of psychosocial stressors (e.g., loss of loved one, combat trauma). The clinical picture includes emotional turmoil and at least one psychotic symptom (e.g., incoherence, delusions, hallucinations, disorganized behavior). The symptoms last between a few hours and 2 weeks, followed by a return to the premorbid level of functioning. Associated symptoms may include a feeling of confusion and complaints of disorientation and memory lapses, making the distinction from a toxic state or dissociative state difficult. Behavioral changes may include bizarre posturing, screaming, or muteness. Suicidal or aggressive behavior may also be present.

TABLE 82–3. PSYCHIATRIC SYNDROMES ASSOCIATED WITH PSYCHOTIC SYMPTOMS

1. Brief reactive psychosis
2. Schizophreniform reactions
3. Schizophrenia; acute or chronic
4. Paranoid delusional disorders
5. Schizoaffective disorder
6. Schizophrenia in association with mental retardation
7. Manic depressive illness
8. Delusional depression
9. Somatic delusional disorders

Schizophreniform reactions differ in that they do not necessarily follow a major stress and have a longer duration. In contrast to schizophrenia, there is a tendency toward more acute onset and resolution, more likelihood of recovery and return to premorbid functioning, and a lower frequency of family history suggesting first-degree relatives with schizophrenia.[10, 11] The clinical features may be identical to those of schizophrenia, but the duration is less than 6 months.

Management of Acute Psychotic Reactions

The management of the acute psychosis secondary to organic brain syndromes consists of defining and treating the underlying cause. It is important to note that confusional states may continue for days beyond the resolution of metabolic imbalances or the removal of the offending medication. This is true especially in the elderly.

In the toxic psychoses, one generally expects a resolution within 72 hours after the patient is drug free. If the psychotic state continues for more than 1 week, the clinician must suspect the existence of a more chronic psychotic state that has been exacerbated by use of drugs. In delirium with acute psychotic symptoms, patients often need interpersonal support and respond best to the familiar faces of family or friends. For the delirious patient, haloperidol (0.5 to 2 mg orally) often helps to resolve the psychotic symptoms. In the intensive care unit setting intravenous haloperidol may be used judiciously.[3]

In drug-induced psychosis, as seen in toxic states from cocaine, amphetamine, or PCP, patients are best managed with reassurance. In extreme cases of agitation in which self-mutilation is feared, restraints may be necessary. Phenothiazines should be avoided in drug-induced psychosis because they may increase agitation as the patient attempts to combat the sedating and dysphoric effects of the antipsychotic agent. Minor tranquilizers are the drugs of choice if sedation is necessary, although they too can cause dysphoric reactions.

For schizophreniform disorders and brief reactive psychoses, antipsychotic medication can help to resolve the acute psychotic symptoms. These patients need ongoing psychotherapy to help address the psychosocial stresses associated with the acute state and to help the patient understand and integrate what is a most frightening experience. Referral to a psychiatrist is indicated.

CHRONIC AND RECURRENT PSYCHOSES

Schizophrenia

Schizophrenia is a heterogeneous group of disorders manifested by the presence of psychotic features during the active phase of the illness and by characteristic symptoms involving multiple psychological processes during the course of the illness (Table 82–4). Schizophrenia develops at some time in the lifetime of 1% of the population and is a rather common cause of psychosis in patients seen by the

TABLE 82–4. DIAGNOSTIC CRITERIA FOR A SCHIZOPHRENIC DISORDER*

A. At least one of the following during a phase of illness:
   Thought Disorder
   1. Bizarre delusions (content is patently absurd and has no possible basis in fact), such as delusions of being controlled, thought broadcasting, thought insertion, or thought withdrawal
   2. Somatic, grandiose, religious, nihilistic, or other delusions without persecutory or jealous content
   3. Delusions of persecutory or jealous content is accompanied by hallucinations
   4. Incoherence, marked loosening of associations, markedly personalized or illogical thinking, poverty of content of speech
   Perceptual Disorder
   5. Auditory hallucinations in which either a voice keeps up a running commentary on the individual's behavior or thoughts or two or more voices converse with each other
   6. Auditory hallucinations on several occasions with content of more than one or two words, having no apparent relation to depression or elation
   Disorder of Affect
   7. Thought disorder associated with blunted, flat, or inappropriate affect
   Disorder of Social or Motor Behavior
   8. Thought disorder associated with catatonic or grossly disorganized behavior; isolation, detachment, failure to form interpersonal relationships
B. Deterioration from a previous level of functioning in areas such as work, social relations, and self-care
C. Duration: Continuous signs of the illness for at least 6 months at some time during the person's life, with some signs of the illness at present. The 6-month period must include an active phase during which there were symptoms from A, with or without a prodromal or residual phase, as defined below.
   Prodromal phase: A clear deterioration in functioning before the active phase of the illness not due to disturbance in mood or to a substance abuse disorder and involving two of the symptoms noted below
   Residual phase: Persistence, following the active phase of the illness, of two of the symptoms below
   Prodromal or residual symptoms
   1. Social isolation or withdrawal
   2. Marked deterioration in role functioning as a wage earner, student, or homemaker
   3. Peculiar behavior (e.g., collecting garbage, talking to self in public)
   4. Marked impairment in personal hygiene
   5. Blunted, flat, or inappropriate affect
   6. Digressive, vague, overelaborate, circumstantial, or metaphonic speech
   7. Odd, bizarre, magical thinking (e.g., clairvoyance, telepathy, overvalued ideas, ideas of reference)
   8. Unusual perceptual experience (e.g., recurrent illusions, sensory presence of force, or person not actually present)
D. Onset of prodromal or active phase before 45 years of age
E. Not due to organic mental disorder, medical illness, or mental retardation

*Adapted from American Psychiatric Association Diagnostic and Standard Manual of Mental Disorders, Third Edition, Revised. Washington, DC, American Psychiatric Association, 1987.

internist. Despite ongoing intensive research into this disorder, the etiology remains unknown. The genetic diathesis toward schizophrenia is inherited, and its expression often, although not exclusively, occurs in the context of psychosocial stress.[11–13]

Patients with this illness have a variable prognosis, and it is often difficult to predict future social functioning after the first episode of psychosis. Quite often there is a deterioration from the previous level of functioning that involves impairment in such areas of life as work, social relationships, and self-care. Other individuals, however, appear to function at nearly normal levels, whereas some are totally incapacitated.

The differential diagnosis is broad (see Tables 82–1, 82–2, and 82–3) and includes organic mental disorders (e.g., delirium, dementia, intoxication, withdrawal), drug-induced psychoses (especially amphetamine, PCP, cocaine), paranoid disorders, affective disorders (specifically acute manic psychosis or delusional depression), neurologic disorders (temporal lobe epilepsy), multiple sclerosis, Huntington's disease, Wilson's disease (especially in adolescents), endocrinopathies, and mental retardation associated with genetic disorders (e.g., Klinefelter's syndrome, Turner's syndrome, metachromatic leukodystrophy). As such, the initial psychotic episode necessitates a comprehensive medical, neurologic, and endocrinologic evaluation to rule out disorders that can mimic schizophrenia.

The role of the generalist in dealing with psychotic patients may extend beyond the initial period of diagnosis. At the very least, the physician will serve as a point of entry into the medical system. It is necessary to know when to refer patients to a psychiatrist and when they must be hospitalized. This is especially important given the *increased risk of impulsive suicides* in schizophrenic patients.

A considerable number of chronic schizophrenics may also choose to seek regular care from the general physician. Many of these patients are reluctant to be followed by a psychiatrist, and in some cases they may be able to function well while being managed by a generalist. This requires that the physician be familiar with the principles of psychotherapy and pharmacotherapy for psychotic patients and be familiar also with the utilization of community resources (e.g., day hospitals, groups, structured work settings) necessary for treatment and the prevention of social isolation.

Diagnosing Schizophrenia

The diagnosis of schizophrenia is not based on any single feature of the illness but should be made when the patient's symptoms fit into a consistent pattern. No single feature in itself is diagnostic of this disorder. Even a patient with hallucinations should not be considered to have schizophrenia unless there is other evidence of the illness. The diagnosis is made by assessing the acute episode and by placing it in the historical context of the patient's psychological life history.

The psychosis of schizophrenia is marked by prodromal, active, and residual phases. The *prodrome* of psychosis is characterized by social withdrawal, impairment in functioning, peculiar behavior, decreased self-care, disturbances in communication, and the beginning of bizarre or personalized ideation. Parents or relatives can often identify a gradual change in personality. The length of the prodrome is variable but suggests poor prognosis when it has taken an insidious, downhill course over years.

The *active* phase of psychotic symptoms is manifested by delusions, hallucinations, florid thought disorder, and grossly disorganized behavior. The specific psychotic symptoms are noted in Table 82–4. The onset of the active phase is often associated with a psychosocial stressor such as marriage, graduation, leaving home, initial sexual encounters, new jobs, or the death of a parent. The use of amphetamines or other stimulants or hallucinogens can exacerbate an underlying psychosis in the prodromal phase.

The *residual* phase is similar to the prodromal phase but is most commonly characterized by affective flattening, impairment in role functioning, and persistent delusions or hallucinations accompanied by less intense affect. The distortion in thinking in chronic schizophrenia is characterized by highly personal and idiosyncratic thinking. Language assumes personalized meanings and, in the extreme case, can become incoherent. Patients typically display ideas of reference in which highly personalized meanings are ascribed to daily events. Delusions may be present wherein the person believes that he or she is being persecuted, controlled by outside forces, or involved in a religious scheme. Body sensations may be misinterpreted in a bizarre fashion, and patients with psychosis can complain to their physician about unusual pain syndromes or feelings of falling apart or decaying inside. Perceptual disorders consist of hallucinations, most often auditory but in some cases visual, tactile, or olfactory. The latter should raise the question of temporal lobe dysfunction, and the presence of visual hallucinations should raise the question of toxic or drug-induced psychosis or drug withdrawal, although visual hallucinations can be seen in the schizophrenic episode itself.[14]

The schizophrenic patient also exhibits an affective disturbance with typical features. Most characteristic is an inappropriate affect such as laughing when talking about sad events or an unmodulated affect with unexplained periods of laughing, crying, or anxiety. The patient may over time exhibit "flattening" of affect, with a paucity of facial expressions, few or no spontaneous movements, and a failure to respond either with sadness or happiness as would be expected during a conversation. This syndrome may be difficult to distinguish from the parkinsonian side effect of neuroleptics. Such persons often avoid eye contact with the examiner, and their speech has a monotonous quality. Although psychomotor retardation and sad affect can be seen in depression, the schizophrenic patient often does not spontaneously report the depressive themes of hopelessness or worthlessness seen in depressed patients; rather, he or she responds not at all or inappropriately to the situation and is preoccupied with internal stimuli or delusional beliefs. In postpsychotic depression, however, the distinguishing features of major depressive disorder versus psychosis are less clear, and a psychiatric evaluation may be indicated to help in the diagnosis and treatment (i.e., to determine the potential value of antidepressants).[15]

Differential Diagnosis and Types of Schizophrenia

Schizophrenia is often divided into subtypes, depending on the prominent features manifested. These types are currently classified as disorganized (what used to be called hebephrenic), catatonic, paranoid, and residual. The types are a reflection of clinical symptoms over time, and often in one individual the symptoms may change from one acute episode to the next. The prognostic and treatment implications of the types are not well defined.

Catatonia. The features of the clinical picture of catatonia include catalepsy, waxy flexibility, negativism, mutism, and bizarre postures and mannerisms.[13, 16] It is important to note that during catatonic excitement, the patient may harm himself or herself or attempt to harm others. Such patients require close supervision until the condition is controlled.

Catatonia may be seen in a *wide variety of organic states* and is not pathognomonic of schizophrenia. The differential diagnosis includes psychiatric disorders (e.g., schizophrenia, manic-depressive illness, conversion reactions, and dissociative states), neurologic disorders (including basal ganglia disorders, frontal lobe tumors, diffuse brain trauma, encephalitis), metabolic disorders, and toxic drug states, particularly those induced by PCP and neuroleptics (e.g., neuroleptic malignant syndrome).[16]

Paranoid Disorders. It is also important to distinguish schizophrenia from the *paranoid* disorders. These disorders usually occur in mid or late adult life and are characterized by persistent delusions of persecution or delusional jealousy in the absence of schizophrenic symptoms (i.e., thought disorder or bizarre delusions). Some classify these disorders as either simple delusional disorder (paranoid disorder without hallucinations) or as hallucinatory delusional disorder (paranoid disorder with hallucinations).[17, 18] The individuals can function at work and in daily living activities without impairment. Their social and marital functioning, on the other hand, can be severely impaired.

Their family histories appear to indicate that these are distinct syndromes independent of schizophrenia. Their social histories reveal isolation; these individuals are chronically suspicious and may refuse to seek medical help. They ignore serious medical problems and may be brought to the physicians by relatives or social agencies. It is often difficult to enlist their help in caring for their illnesses, especially in terms of taking medication or consenting to procedures. This can raise complex medicolegal questions centering on refusal of treatment and the need for guardianship. The response of such patients to neuroleptics is variable. The delusions often remain chronic and unremitting, despite treatment with antipsychotic agents.

It is also important to note that the paranoid syndrome may be seen in other psychiatric disorders, including paranoid schizophrenia, mania, delusional depression, and the paranoid personality style.

Numerous medical and neurologic conditions can also present with symptoms of paranoid ideation or delusions. These include temporal lobe epilepsy, multiple sclerosis, Huntington's chorea, Alzheimer's disease, hepatic encephalopathy, central nervous system tumor, chronic subdural hematomas, confusional states, uremia, systemic lupus erythematosus, hypothyroidism, and vitamin B_{12} deficiency. Treatment with steroids may also induce this picture.[19]

Paranoia is often seen in alcohol intoxication or withdrawal or as a chronic alcohol-related disorder associated with auditory hallucinations.[20, 21] Drug abuse, especially with amphetamines and cocaine, must also be excluded in cases of paranoia occurring in individuals without a past history of paranoid disorder.

Some patients with paranoia have fixed somatic delusions, which are often referred to as "hypochondriacal delusions." These patients express beliefs that they emit a foul odor or have infestations in their skin or that they have internal parasites. They can complain of bizarre pain syndromes, or they may believe that their body is deformed. Such individuals can consult multiple internists in an attempt to gain an explanation for the symptoms. Antipsychotic medication may be beneficial.

A last entity worth mentioning is paranoid illness of the elderly. This refers to paranoid symptoms or delusions that are expressed in the absence of intellectual deterioration (dementia) or confusional states or major depressive disorder. Some refer to this disorder as late paraphrenia.[22] It is especially prominent among individuals living alone and among those with sensory deficits. This disorder also responds variably to antipsychotic agents but in some cases the response may be dramatic and allow the individual to continue to live at home.

Schizoaffective Disorders. The term schizoaffective disorder has been used in a variety of ways since its inception in 1940 by Kasanin. There remains a debate as to its meaning and validity.[23, 24] Currently this diagnosis is favored when the clinical picture manifests a full-blown affective syndrome with mood-incongruent psychotic features. The picture often resembles that of schizophrenia but is associated with marked lability of affect. Antipsychotic agents may treat the former but not the latter. The unmodulated affect may continue to make the individual appear psychotic, and often this lability resolves with lithium treatment. The patient treated with lithium appears calmer and less psychotic and returns to a higher level of function. The diagnosis can be difficult to make and necessitates a psychiatric evaluation.

"Propf 's Schizophrenia." In another group of patients, the psychosis appears to coexist with mental retardation or minimal brain damage.[25] The British refer to Propf's schizophrenia as psychosis grafted on mental retardation.[15] Psychosis in this group can be very difficult to manage and often leads to severe personality disorganization. Long-term inpatient care is frequently necessary, and the use of neuroleptics is complicated by an increased incidence of severe side effects and increased risk of tardive dyskinesia.

Affective Disorders. Both bipolar and unipolar affective disorders may present with psychotic symptoms.

Manic-Depressive Disorders. The hallmark of manic-depressive disease is a period of persistently elevated or irritable mood alternating with depressive episodes.

During the manic phase of manic-depressive illness, patients may experience delusions and hallucinations that are either paranoid or grandiose in nature. Their thoughts may be incoherent due to flight of ideas and pressured speech. The individual is distractible and easily drawn to unimportant stimuli in the environment. Symptoms of mania can include increased energy and libido with promiscuity, diminished need for sleep, talkativeness, and psychomotor agitation. The patient can be irritable and express full-blown paranoid delusions and ideas of reference.[26] This behavior closely resembles that of acute paranoid schizophrenia.

Mixed affective states with features of both mania and depression are not uncommon. This is often referred to as dysphoric mania.

Establishing the correct diagnosis depends not only on a careful assessment of the clinical features at the time of presentation but also on consideration of the patient's premorbid personality, family history, response to previous treatment (e.g., lithium), and recurrence of episodes during longitudinal follow-up.

Most patients with manic-depressive illness also have a family history that is positive for bipolar or unipolar affective disorders in first-degree relatives.[26]

Treatment with lithium is effective in manic psychosis but not in true schizophrenia. In the acute manic psychosis, however, a neuroleptic will be needed to help sedate the patient, especially in light of the fact that it will take 7 to 10 days for the lithium to exert its antimanic action. In patients who do not tolerate lithium or who are refractory to it, carbamazepine and valproic acid are now considered acceptable alternatives or adjuncts. Both require medical monitoring of side effects (e.g., by complete blood counts, liver function tests).[26–28]

Delusional Depressive Disorders. Delusional depressions can also be difficult to distinguish from schizophrenia in the acute stage. The content, however, of delusional thoughts in delusionally depressed individuals is different from that found in schizophrenics. Delusions of the depressed patient reflect self-degradation, gloominess, and hopelessness. Individuals believe that they are being persecuted because they have sinned.[29] Of importance to the general physician is that patients may express to their internist the belief that they are severely ill or consumed with cancer. Somatic and hypochondriacal delusions are common in delusional depression but resolve with treatment of the depression. Hallucinations are less common but can involve voices berating the individual for worthlessness or sinfulness. Delusionally depressed patients represent a suicide risk and must be treated promptly. The initial treatment includes both neuroleptic and tricyclic agents.[29] The neuroleptic can help to prevent a tricyclic-induced exacerbation of the psychotic thinking and may help to resolve the delusions. Improvement can be expected in a 2- to 4-week period in most cases. In severe cases with acute suicidal ideation, electroconvulsive therapy may be indicated.

Management of Schizophrenia

Once the diagnosis of schizophrenia is made (i.e., other psychiatric, medical, and neurologic disorders are ruled out), the physician must turn his or her attention to management.

Management of schizophrenia should be designed to enable the patient to function as normally as possible and to prevent exacerbations of the psychosis. The latter is a particularly important goal because an exacerbation can be extremely disruptive to the social arrangements laboriously constructed by a patient and his or her family after recovery from the acute psychosis.

Individuals experience psychotic episodes as a disintegration of self that is both frightening and emotionally painful. Despite outward denial, the individual fears a recurrence and often needs the help of a physician to gain the support necessary for moving forward in life activities. The involvement of community and family support, in addition to a psychotherapeutic relationship, ensures compliance with medication and helps the patient to address the numerous social and psychological problems that he or she will encounter: job stresses, depression, loss of self-esteem. It is important for the patient in remission to maintain the optimal level of functioning that he or she can attain.

Psychotherapy. Psychotherapy and pharmacotherapy are considered to be of complementary value in the treatment of schizophrenia. There is evidence that social adjustment is improved by psychotherapy,[30] although psychotherapy cannot substitute for the independent beneficial effects of drug therapy.

The initial stages of therapy with a schizophrenic focus on building a trusting alliance with the patient. Following an acute psychotic episode, such patients may feel the need to deny their problem and may fear ongoing therapy, which is a reminder that they are ill. Such patients may mistrust the therapist and balk at being on neuroleptics given their sedative effects. Finally, patients fear talking with a psychiatrist or physician because during such conversations they re-experience the pain and suffering associated with the ego disorganization. The psychotic state is a frightening period for patients, and they may feel that talking about it may cause another episode, whereas avoiding the subject makes them feel safer.

In the context of this mistrust and fear, it may be difficult to engage the patient in treatment. The physician needs to be available and make clear that he or she is there to help the individual get better. This can be demonstrated by initially allowing the patient to choose what to talk about and by re-emphasizing the fact that the therapeutic venture is designed to help the patient avoid another psychotic episode. Medication should be seen as helping achieve this goal and should be maintained at antipsychotic doses. Pa-

TABLE 82–5. ANTIPSYCHOTIC AGENTS

Generic Name	Trade Name	Class	Antipsychotic Dosage Range*	Prominent Adverse Effects
Low-Potency Agents				
Chlorpromazine	Thorazine	Phenothiazine	400–1200 mg	Sedation
Thioridazine	Mellaril	Phenothiazine	200–800 mg	EPS, akathisia, anticholinergic effects, photosensitivity, drowsiness, postural hypotension, moderate sedation
Intermediate-Potency Agents				
Thiothixene	Navane	Thioxanthene	20–40 mg	EPS, akathisia, anticholinergic effects, galactorrhea, rash, less sedation than Thorazine
Perphenazine	Trilafon	Phenothiazine	32–64 mg	
High-Potency Agents				
Haloperidol	Haldol	Butyrophenone	10–30 mg	EPS, dystonia, blood dyscrasias, low sedation, photosensitivity
Trifluoperazine	Stelazine	Phenothiazine	15–40 mg	
Fluphenazine	Prolixin	Phenothiazine	5–15 mg	
New Antipsychotics				
Clozapine	Clozaril	Dibenzodiazepine	250–500 mg (range of 25–900 mg)	1–2% evidence agranulocytosis or leukopenia; *weekly* monitoring of hematologic status required; 3–5% seizure incidence; sedation, diarrhea; weight gain; hypotension; fever; tachycardia

EPS = extrapyramidal side effects.
*Per 24 hr (maintenance dose).

tients often attempt to negotiate lower doses, and noncompliance is not uncommon.

As the relationship is established, the therapy can address real life issues. Therapy focuses on reality testing and limit setting in a supportive fashion. To be successful, the therapeutic alliance must be achieved. Before a patient can respond to goals and limits and realize that these are in his or her best interests, the patient must trust the physician.

The physician must be aware of the transference that develops in such therapeutic relationships and that this may be reflected in the patient's behavior (e.g., hostility, overdependence, child-like behavior, testing the physician's tolerance). Through trust and negotiating the transference, the patient can learn to experience the outside world in a less anxiety-provoking fashion.

The physician should listen sympathetically and empathetically to the patient's thoughts and ideas; he or she may choose to avoid commenting on the validity of delusional thinking but should never agree with or enter into the patient's delusions. Ultimately, it is hoped that the patient can be taught to distinguish personalized ideas and delusions from external reality. The goals for the patient should be realistic—keeping regular appointments, seeing a therapist, and understanding the psychological origin of some of his or her behaviors is all that is possible for many chronic schizophrenics. Others can return to work and live independently or in a structured setting away from home.

Early intervention at times of stress, particularly if this involves the loss of someone close to the patient, may prevent decompensation. After a period of psychosis or depression, as the patient struggles to regain a more normal level of social functioning, emphasis should be placed at first on providing support rather than on investigating the origin of the psychosis. Following this period of regaining equilibrium, which usually lasts for 9 to 10 months, the physician may attempt to impart an understanding of the factors that led to the psychotic episode and perhaps teach the patient better methods of coping with stress.

Many psychotic episodes are precipitated by stressful circumstances, but patients often hide or deny these problems. Many months of therapy may pass before they can be discussed. Depressive phases, which often follow psychotic episodes, may require a major effort to keep the patient from becoming discouraged and dropping out of therapy.

Ultimately, it is hoped that the patient may learn to understand and cope better with his or her limitations, but it must be emphasized that the risk of suicide is substantial, particularly during the early stages of illness, in intelligent, young schizophrenics, who are struggling with severe losses caused by the psychotic break. Throughout the course of schizophrenia, the patient will be vulnerable to stress. The physician must be a source of support and hope for the future, despite setbacks or periods of hopelessness.

Pharmacotherapy. The use of neuroleptic agents now allows many schizophrenic patients to function in the community following brief hospitalizations. A variety of compounds, including phenothiazines, piperazines, and butyrophenones (e.g., haloperidol) are available to the clinician (Table 82–5). The basic antipsychotic effects of these drugs appear to be identical, so that the choice of an agent depends on its potential for adverse effects.[31, 32]

If a patient has responded to a particular agent, however, it is generally recommended that the agent be used in the future to treat recurrent episodes.

A response to antipsychotics occurs over a period of months for delusions and hallucinations whereas other symptoms, such as idiosyncratic thinking and personalized ideation, subside even more slowly. Following the acute psychotic episodes, dosages may need to be reduced if sedation is a problem; otherwise, dosages should be kept in the therapeutic range and should not be decreased until the prospect of a drug holiday is considered. This usually occurs approximately 1 year after the acute episode at a period in which stress is minimal and family support is available in case of a relapse. In practice, the clinician should become familiar with several drugs in order to take advantage of minimizing side effects in individual patients.

Low-potency drugs like chlorpromazine (Thorazine) and thioridazine (Mellaril) have more sedative and anticholinergic properties but fewer extrapyramidal side effects than do the high-potency agents. Compared with high-potency agents, the low-potency drugs are also more likely to produce postural hypotension and may have arrhythmogenic properties. Agents that are less sedating, such as perphenazine (Trilafon), are useful in adolescent patients in terms of compliance.

For elderly persons who are more vulnerable to anticholinergic effects and for persons subject to cardiac arrhythmias, the high-potency drugs like haloperidol (Haldol) and trifluoperazine (Stelazine) are preferred. Haloperidol, given intramuscularly, may also be preferred in some emergency situations when it is important to control the patient's behavior without causing sedation. Drugs of intermediate potency like acetophenazine (Tindal) and thiothixene (Navane) have fewer extrapyramidal side effects but are more strongly anticholinergic that are the high-potency agents.

Clozapine is a new antipsychotic drug recommended for use in treatment-resistant schizophrenics. Its virtues include improvement in positive symptoms (e.g., delusions, hallucinations) and negative symptoms (e.g., social withdrawal, emotional blunting) of psychosis in formerly refractory patients with negligible extrapyramidal side effects. Its major drawback is the risk of agranulocytosis (incidence of 1.3%), necessitating weekly white cell counts. Its side effects, which are often problematic, include sedation and fatigue, sialorrhea, weight gain, hypotension, nausea and vomiting, tachycardia, and fever. There is also a risk for seizure activity and sinus tachycardia.[33, 34]

Adverse Effects. The anticholinergic, sedative, hypotensive, and cardiotoxic effects chiefly ascribed to low-potency agents have been mentioned. All phenothiazine and related compounds may cause liver toxicity, usually manifested by reversible cholestatic jaundice, and may cause reversible but often severe granulocytopenia. The incidence of agranulocytosis is reported to be fewer than 1 in 10,000 patients treated with antipsychotic medication. (As mentioned above, clozapine causes leukopenia more commonly [1.3%].) The incidence of cholestatic jaundice is thought to be less than 2% and is becoming increasingly rare in modern preparations of the drugs.[32]

The extrapyramidal side effects of antipsychotic drugs are closely related to their basic antipsychotic effect. The extrapyramidal effects may be classified as acute dystonic reactions, akathisia, drug-induced parkinsonism, and tardive dyskinesia. Estimates of the incidence of these reactions vary, ranging from 2.2 to 95% of patients treated with neuroleptics.[35] Patients should be forewarned about these possible effects so that they do not become excessively frightened if they do occur.

Acute dystonic reactions consist of the abrupt onset of muscle spasms that generally involve the head and neck. Typically, the masseter muscles may be so tightly contracted that the mouth cannot be opened. Spasm of the external ocular muscles may cause painful persistent upward gaze associated with torticollis. The trunk may be affected, more commonly in children, and shoulder shrugging, tortipelvis, opisthotonos, and scoliosis may occur. Bizarre writhing movements of the limbs may be seen as well.[35] Such reactions usually occur within 48 hours of starting medications and are dose related. They can be relieved by the parenteral administration of antiparkinsonian or antihistaminic drugs.

It is important to recognize akathisia because it may be mistaken for increased psychotic agitation. This condition has been described as an uncontrollable restlessness, particularly manifested by fidgeting, pacing, and restless legs.[35] In the more severe form (tasikinesia), the patient is only comfortable when in motion. The patients may tap their feet or appear fidgety and constantly shift their legs. This may result in difficulty in sleeping because of an inability to lie still and fall asleep. It may not respond to antiparkinsonian drugs and may require a reduction in the dosage of medication or a change to a different agent (e.g., from high-potency to intermediate-potency agent).

Drug-induced parkinsonism is clinically indistinguishable from idiopathic parkinsonism. Symptoms are related to use of high doses, particularly of high-potency agents, but may also reflect individual predisposition, since the syndrome is more often encountered in older patients. The symptoms of drug-induced parkinsonism include rigidity, mask-like facies, stooped posture, and a festinating gait identical to that seen in idiopathic parkinsonism; tremor at rest is less characteristic of the drug-induced syndrome. Levodopa is not effective for drug-induced parkinsonism, but patients can be treated with benztropine (Cogentin), 1 mg twice daily or trihexyphenidyl (Artane), 2 to 4 mg twice daily, continued for several months, or by reducing the dose of the phenothiazine or switching to an agent with fewer extrapyramidal effects. It is generally not recommended that antiparkinsonian drugs be given prophylactically to patients receiving antipsychotic medications, because the former agents may be subject to abuse by psychotic patients or may produce toxic brain syndromes.

Tardive dyskinesia rarely occurs in patients treated with neuroleptics for less than several months. Its prevalence varies greatly from one study to another, with conservative estimates being 15 to 20% and rising to 70% in high-risk populations (e.g., in the elderly). The relationship between tardive dyskinesia and drug exposure remains uncertain. There are no data to clarify if one drug or class of drugs correlates with increased risk. The syndrome consists of repetitive, stereotyped involuntary movements of the mouth, lips, and tongue, sometimes accompanied by choreiform movements of the limbs and trunk. Sucking and smacking movements, puffing of the cheeks, and protrusion of the tongue are characteristic of the full-blown syndrome. Earlier signs of tardive dyskinesia include subtle vermiform movements of the surface of the tongue and floor or the mouth. Rarely, the hands and fingers move in a repetitive pattern.[36]

The symptoms of this condition can become more pronounced as the dose of an antipsychotic medication is lowered, in what is referred to as a "withdrawal dyskinesia."

To date there is no known definitive treatment for tardive dyskinesia. No drugs have been found to be either safe or effective over time in the treatment of this disorder. The effort is focused on prevention through prudent use of the antipsychotic medications. Periodic evaluation for movement disorders enables prompt diagnosis and early discontinuation of the antipsychotic agent. A wide variety of agents (including dopamine depleters; reserpine; γ-aminobutyric acid agonists; baclofen; diazepam; clonazepam; anticholinergics; lithium; and propranolol) have been used to treat tardive dyskinesias. All have been associated with anecdotal successes, but none has produced definitive treatment.[36]

Antipsychotic agents may also produce symptoms of sluggishness and weakness. An akinetic state closely resembling depression has been described that may respond to antiparkinsonian agents such as trihexyphenidyl.[37]

Other side effects of neuroleptic agents include pigmentary retinopathy in patients receiving more than 800 mg/day of thioridazine. This agent also causes inhibition of ejaculation, which can be a troubling side effect and result in noncompliance. It is worth noting that the various side effects caused by neuroleptics are often poorly tolerated by the psychotic individual, who may discontinue medication without informing the physician. Noncompliance should always be suspected in a patient who becomes psychotic while supposedly under treatment with neuroleptics.

Patients are also susceptible to heat pyrexia, especially in the summer. Patients present temperatures over 39.4° C (103° F) and must be treated as a medical emergency. Transient nausea, diarrhea, restlessness, and insomnia have been reported to occur 1 to 2 weeks after withdrawal from neuroleptic agents.[38]

In addition to hyperpyrexia, patients on neuroleptics can develop the neuroleptic malignant syndrome (NMS).[39] Men are more frequently affected than women, and younger patients (80% younger than 40 years old) are more susceptible than are older patients. It appears most often within 2 weeks of starting treatment with neuroleptics or during increasing dosage but can occur months into treatment on a stable dosage. This is a potentially lethal disorder that is characterized by hyperthermia, diverse extrapyramidal reactions, altered consciousness, and autonomic instability.[40,41]

The alterations in consciousness can range from alertness to stupor or coma, and the neurologic manifestations range from generalized rigidity to dyskinesias. The muscle rigidity can lead to rhabdomyolysis and subsequent myoglobinuria and acute renal failure. Autonomic dysfunction includes profuse diaphoresis, tachycardia, and fluctuating blood pressure. Laboratory abnormalities include elevated creatine phosphokinase (>15,000) and blood urea nitrogen; leukocytosis; and abnormal liver functions. Neuroleptic malignant syndrome must be differentiated from catatonia caused by a variety of etiologies, such as neurologic problems (encephalitis) and metabolic disorders (e.g., hyperparathyroidism). It must also be distinguished from central hyperthermia, heat stroke (which may develop in patients on neuroleptics), and malignant hyperthermia. Treatment rests on the discontinuation of the neuroleptic agent and supportive medical treatment of the hyperthermia and associated coagulopathy, aspiration pneumonia, anemia, cardiovascular collapse, and acute renal failure.[40,41]

The muscle relaxant dantrolene has been used successfully to treat this syndrome. This drug, which interferes with the release of calcium from the sarcoplasmic reticulum, produces muscle relaxation and has provided dramatic relief of the symptoms of NMS. It also has central effects on γ-aminobutyric acid metabolism. In addition, a number of reports describe beneficial results with bromocriptine (in combination with dantrolene) and amantadine.[40] Benzodiazepines are also helpful in relieving symptoms of NMS, often at high doses (100 mg/day po). Patients reportedly respond within hours of treatment; however, due to the long elimination half-life of neuroleptics, treatment to relieve the NMS must be ongoing for several days.

Long-Term Management. Several aspects of the long-term care of schizophrenic patients are frequently dealt with by generalists. Schizophrenic patients under the care of the state are often lacking in good medical care. When seen for medical evaluation, they are often suffering from physical disorders that are yet undiagnosed; this should lead the primary care physician to a careful evaluation of such patients—the psychotic state should not be the sole area of concern. The generalist may be managing the use of the antipsychotic medication. Compliance can be a problem in the suspicious schizophrenic or the patient with somatic delusions. The drug can be presented to the patient as a medicine used for controlling the symptoms of an illness (in this case delusions and hallucinations), because many patients will accept medications only in the context of this medical model. For the severely psychotic and noncompliant individual, weekly intermuscular injections of fluphenazine are an alternative method of treatment.

Evidence that maintenance therapy with antipsychotic medications prevents a relapse in the years after the acute onset of schizophrenia was shown consistently in numerous studies.[42] In several studies, about 85% of patients on drug therapy could be maintained at home, compared with about 45% of those on placebo.[43] Thus, maintenance therapy would be prescribed for almost all patients with chronic schizophrenia if there were not the potential for the development of irreversible tardive dyskinesia. Because of this possibility, the advantages and disadvantages of maintenance therapy should be weighed carefully in every patient. The impact of neuroleptics on social adjustment over the long term is less clear than their impact on preventing acute decompensations.[42,43]

Prognosis in schizophrenia appears to relate to the patient's ability to hold a job, maintain social relations, and avoid rehospitalization.

Early manifestations of tardive dyskinesia should be sought in all patients receiving neuroleptic agents, particularly at times of dosage reductions. Patients themselves are usually unaware of manifestations of the dyskinesia, which are more noticeable to the physician or to the patient's family.[44] If dyskinesias appear, an effort should be made to discontinue the drug gradually if possible. When psychotic relapse and dyskinesia occur simultaneously, low-potency agents, which have milder extrapyramidal side effects, may be tried.

Hospitalization. Symptoms of schizophrenia in themselves do not constitute an indication for hospitalization. Hospitalization, however, may serve to remove the acutely psychotic patient from conflicts in the family and provide a structured environment in which the patient can feel safe. The decompensated schizophrenic often experiences hospitalization as a relief, and most physicians hospitalize schizophrenic patients for a first psychotic episode. Hospitalization is imperative for patients judged to be a threat to themselves or to others. The duration of hospitalization depends on the patient's response to therapy and may range from a few weeks to several months or longer.

Supportive Treatment. The psychotic state is frightening for the patient and family alike. It heralds, in the case of schizophrenia, the beginning of a lifelong illness that necessitates ongoing treatment and contacts with medical and psychiatric personnel. During this period, hopes for the future that an adolescent and the family once shared are often shattered; both patients and families often need to deny the severity of the illness and thus do not plan appropriately.

The approach to treatment must include establishing a trusting relationship with both the family and the patient, emphasizing the realities of the problems to be faced and yet not taking away all hope of a return to a modest level of functioning. In the past families have often suffered from the guilt of feeling that they "produced" the psychotic child. They need support and education about the current understanding of schizophrenia, its etiology, and its prognosis. The emphasis should be on ensuring ongoing treatment for the patient and on providing support for the family. Once an alliance is established, deeper-rooted psychological issues may emerge that will necessitate the involvement of a psychiatrist or a family therapist.

A key role for the primary physician is that of a consistent figure who has known the family and who can provide support throughout the frequently arduous treatment. The physician can be the most important figure in helping the family to accept the tragic reality of chronic psychosis and in facilitating a transition into the psychiatric system when necessary.

REFERENCES

1. Lipowski ZJ: Delirium, clouding of consciousness and confusion. J Nerv Ment Dis 145:227, 1967.
2. Strub R and Black F: Acute Confusional States in Neurobehavioral Disorders: A Clinical Approach. Philadelphia, FA Davis, 1988, pp 107–139.
3. Adams F: Emergency intravenous sedation of the delirious, medically ill patient. J Clin Psychiatry 49(Suppl):12, 1988.
4. Katzman R: Alzheimer's disease. N Engl J Med 314:22–27, 1986.
5. Wragg R and Jeste D: Overview of depression and psychosis in Alzheimer's disease. Am J Psychiatry 146(5):577, 1989.
6. Diagnostic and Statistical Manual of Mental Disorders, 3rd ed, Revised. Washington, DC, American Psychiatric Association, 1987, pp 165–172.
7. Bowers M: Psychoses precipitated by psychomimetic drugs. Arch Gen Psychiatry 34:832, 1977.
8. McKenna PJ, Kane JM, and Parrish K: Psychotic syndromes in epilepsy. Am J Psychiatry 142:895, 1985.
9. Blumer D: Temporal lobe epilepsy and its psychiatric significance. *In* Benson DF and Blumer D (eds): Psychiatric Aspects of Neurologic Disease. New York, Grune & Stratton, 1975, pp 171–198.
10. Day M and Semrad EV: Schizophrenic reactions. *In* Nicholi AM (ed): The Harvard Guide to Modern Psychiatry. Cambridge, MA, Belknap Press of Harvard University, 1978, pp 199–242.
11. Gottesman I: Schizophrenia Genesis. New York, WH Freeman, 1991.
12. Bebbington P and McGuffin P: Schizophrenia: The Major Issues. London, Heinemann Professional Publishing, 1988.
13. Hamilton M (ed): Fish's Schizophrenia, 3rd ed. Bristol, John Wright & Sons, Ltd., 1984.
14. Goodwin D, Alderson P, and Rosenthal R: Clinical significance of hallucinations in psychiatric disorders. Arch Gen Psychiatry 24:76, 1971.
15. Plasky P: Antidepressant usage in schizophrenia. Bullentin 17(4):649, 1991.
16. Gelenberg A: The catatonic syndrome. Lancet 1:1339, 1976.
17. Kendler K: The nosologic validity of paranoia. Arch Gen Psychiatry 37:699, 1980.
18. Kendler K: Paranoid psychosis, delusional disorders and schizophrenia. Arch Gen Psychiatry 38:547, 1981.
19. Manschreck T and Petin M: The paranoid syndrome. Lancet 2:251, 1978.
20. Cutting J: A reappraisal of alcoholic psychoses. Psychol Med 8:285, 1978.
21. Victor M and Hope J: The phenomenon of auditory hallucinations in chronic alcoholism. J Nerv Mental Dis 126:451, 1958.
22. Post F: Persistent Persecutory States of the Elderly. London, Oxford University Press, 1966.
23. Procci W: Schizoaffective psychosis: Fact or fiction? Arch Gen Psychiatry 33:1167, 1976.
24. Samson JA, Simpson JC, Tsuang MT: Outcome studies of schizoaffective disorders. Schizophr Bull 114:543, 1988.
25. Bellak L: Schizophrenic syndrome related to minimal brain dysfunction. Schizophr Bull 15:480, 1979.
26. Goodwin F and Jamison K: Manic Depressive Illness. New York, Oxford, 1990.
27. Ballenger J: The use of anticonvulsants in manic depressive illness. J Clin Psychol 49 (Suppl 11):21, 1988.
28. Fawcett J: Valproate use in acute mania and bipolar disorder. J Clin Psychiatry 50 (Suppl 3):10, 1989.
29. Nelson JC and Bowers MD. Delusional unipolar depression. Arch Gen Psychiatry 35:1321–1381, 1978.
30. Gunderson J, Frank AF, Katz HM: Effects of psychotherapy in schizophrenia. II: Comparative outcome of two forms of treatment. Schizophr Bull 10:564, 1984.
31. Schulz S and Pato C: Pharmacologic treatment of schizophrenia. Psychiatr Ann 19(10):536, 1989.
32. Levinson D and Simpson G: Serious nonextrapyramidal adverse effects of neuroleptics: Sudden death, agranulocytosis, and hepatotoxicity. *In* Meltzer H (ed): Psychopharmacology: The Third Generation of Progress. New York, Raven Press 1987, pp 1431–1436.
33. Kane J, Honigfeld G, Singer J: Clozapine for the treatment-resistant schizophrenic. Arch Gen Psychiatry 45:789, 1988.
34. Baldesssarini R and Frankenburg F: Clozapine. N Engl J Med 234:746, 1991.
35. Sovner R and DiMascio A: Extrapyramidal syndromes and other neurological side effects of psychotropic drugs. *In* Lipton MA, DiMascio A, and Killiam KF (eds): Psychopharmacology: A Generation of Progress. New York, Raven Press, 1978, pp 1021–1032.
36. Casey D: Tardive dyskinesia. *In* Meltzer H (ed): Psychopharmacology: The Third Generation of Progress. New York, Raven Press, 1987, pp 1411–1419.
37. Van Patten T: Akinetic depression in schizophrenia. Arch Gen Psychiatry 35:1101, 1978.
38. Gardos G, Cole JO, and Tarsy D: Withdrawal syndromes associated with antipsychotic drugs. Am J Psychiatry 135:1321, 1978.
39. Levenson JL: Neurologic malignant syndrome. Am J Psychiatry 142:1137, 1985.
40. Kaufman C and Wyatt R: Neuroleptic malignant syndrome. *In* Meltzer H (ed): Psychopharmacology: The Third Generation of Progress. New York, Raven Press, 1987, pp 1421–1430.
41. Geizer B and Baxter L: Neuroleptic malignant syndrome. N Engl J Med 313(3):16306, 1985.
42. Kane J and Lieberman J: Maintenance pharmacotherapy in schizophrenia. *In* Meltzer H (ed): Psychopharmacology: The Third Generation of Progress. New York, Raven Press, 1987, pp 1103–1109.
43. Quitkin F, Rifkin A, Kane J, et al: Long-acting oral versus injectable antipsychotic drugs in schizophrenics: One-year double-blind comparison in multiple-episode schizophrenics. Arch Gen Psychiatry 35:889, 1978.
44. Alexopoulos GS: Lack of complaints in schizophrenics with tardive dyskinesia. J Nerv Ment Dis 167:125, 1979.

83

Substance Abuse and Addiction in Primary Care Medicine

HENRIETTA N. BARNES, MD
JUDYANN BIGBY, MD

The primary care physician encounters the disease of addiction every day. Its faces are varied: the truck driver who drinks 8 cups of coffee a day and smokes 2 packs of cigarettes; the lawyer who needs daily alprazolam to calm her nerves when arguing a court case; the teacher with a past history of intravenous drug use who tests positive for the human immunodeficiency virus (HIV); and the young hypertensive construction worker who drinks a six-pack with his friends after work. Both the patients' characteristics and the pharmacology of the drug affect the clinical presentation of addiction, but the underlying illness is the same: the repeated use of a psychoactive substance over time despite adverse consequences.

The primary care physician must be equally skilled at recognizing a patient's problem with addiction early and providing appropriate intervention and at managing a patient with recurrent relapses or progressive disease. This chapter will describe the disease of addiction and the primary physician's role, with particular emphasis on detection and management in the office setting.

THE DISEASE OF ADDICTION

Clinical experience teaches us that patients addicted to one psychoactive substance frequently have problems with other psychoactive substances. Patients with severe addictions will routinely substitute one drug for another if their drug of choice is unavailable. Traditionally, smoking cigarettes, using intravenous opiate, and alcoholism have been considered separate disorders. A more useful paradigm describes these problems as different manifestations of a single disorder, addiction. In addiction, the compulsive, repetitive use of a psychoactive substance, whether episodic or daily, becomes a central activity in the person's life in spite of his or her knowledge of negative effects. The conflict between the person's perceived need for a drug and his or her awareness of the adverse effects of drug use results in denial of the seriousness of these adverse consequences.

But what evidence is there that these illnesses are more accurately described as one disorder? About 10% of adult Americans who use alcohol develop problems with it.[1] Similarly, only about 10% of servicemen who had used intravenous opiates while in Southeast Asia during the Vietnam War continued to have problems with intravenous drug abuse on return to the United States.[2] Similar figures are suggested for the percentage of people who try cocaine and become addicted. We know from twin and adoption studies and recent work on brain wave patterns that there is a hereditary component in the development of alcoholism.[3] Together, these data suggest that one of every 10 Americans has a genetic or familial predisposition for developing an addiction to a psychoactive substance.

A patient susceptible to addiction must be informed about environmental risk factors. A family history of alcohol abuse, reflecting both environmental and genetic factors, increases threefold a person's risk of developing drinking problems.[4] The patterns of drug use in one's family or social circle influence the likelihood of developing problems. Vaillant noted that families from Mediterranean backgrounds in which lower-proof alcoholic beverages (wine) were used as a beverage with meals had lower rates of alcohol problems than families with English or Scandinavian backgrounds, where higher-proof spirits are more common and drinking is usually done in taverns or bars.[4] Occupations with common characteristics, such as availability of alcohol, lack of immediate supervision, and high stress, are associated with higher rates of drinking problems.[5] Whether these occupations cause drinking problems or whether people with a propensity for drinking problems gravitate toward them is unknown. Certainly, the intersection of a genetic susceptibility to addiction with social availability and acceptance of drug use presents a very risky crossroad for affected patients.

The natural history of addiction covers a spectrum of nonuse, use, misuse, abuse, and dependence. Alcohol and drug use is learned behavior that starts with initial experimentation. The vast majority of users finds a level of use that maximizes the mood-altering pleasures of a drug with minimal negative consequences. People in this category may experience episodes of misuse, which range from minor (embarrassing behavior while intoxicated) to severe (fatal automobile crash) consequences. Women who consume more than 12 drinks per week (15 drinks for men) are at increased risk of problems due to drinking. A small percentage of users have continued problems due to drug use and are unable to control their drug use consistently. An even smaller number develop severe, recurrent problems, including physiologic dependence on the drug.[6]

Although some people with addiction follow the course best described by Jellinek of continued downward progression to death or recovery,[7] patterns of substance abuse and dependence are usually much more variable. Addiction is like other chronic medical problems: a person may have exacerbations or relapses as well as periods of remission. Most people who use psychoactive substances will move in and out of different categories of use many times.

Several factors influence the presentation of addiction. The pharmacology of the drug is perhaps the most salient, but the route of administration and the legal status of the drug play important roles. For example, can a stable pattern of snorting cocaine two or three times a year be described as "nonproblematic" use, or does its illegality ipso facto make this activity misuse or abuse? The answers to these questions depend not only on medical knowledge of substance abuse but also on the social and cultural mores of both patient and physician.

The major classes of drugs of abuse are stimulants, sedatives, and hallucinogens. The most significant public health burden results from the stimulant nicotine (discussed in Chapter 9), followed by the sedative ethyl alcohol, alone or in combination with other drugs. The other sedatives (opiates and sedative hypnotics), stimulants (cocaine and amphetamines), and the hallucinogens account for a small fraction of problems related to drugs in the general population, although the high prevalence of intravenous drug use in inner cities has had devastating effects. The pharmacology of each drug dictates the pattern of abuse and dependence.

The stimulants cause an increase in energy, heart rate, and blood pressure mediated through the dopaminergic system. The usual routes of administration for cocaine—smoking, intravenous injection, and nasal insufflation—provide rapid onset of action. A relatively short half-life of 2 to 3 hours allows for an intense, short-lived effect, followed by a "crash," manifested by dysphoria and craving for the drug. Cocaine users susceptible to addiction tend to develop a typical pattern of abuse: binges during which the drug is administered every few hours until the supply is gone or the user is too emotionally depleted to continue. Within 18 to 24 months, cocaine abusers have either stopped using the drug through treatment or substitution of another drug or have suffered devastating medical or economic consequences.

Sedatives, including ethyl alcohol, opiates and sedative-hypnotics, cause an initial increase in activity due to release of inhibitions, followed by sedation, decreasing levels of consciousness, and in high doses, respiratory depression, coma, and death. In contrast to stimulants, sedative drug abuse presents a more indolent course. Alcohol abuse usually develops after several years of heavy drinking. Drinkers and their families can persist in dysfunctional states of alcohol abuse for years. Although alcohol is toxic to virtually every organ system, there is enormous variability in a drinker's susceptibility to alcohol-related medical problems. Heroin addicts in England who have access to sterile needles and a medicinal supply of heroin or opiate addicts in methadone programs in the United States have maintained stable patterns of opiate dependence for years. The majority of medical complications in intravenous opiate use result from the use of nonsterile needles and an illegal, unpredictable supply of drug.

The hallucinogens form a class of drugs that produce states of altered perception, such as heightened meaning of trivial sensations or loss of the sense of boundary between self and the environment. Many of these drugs have either stimulant or depressant effects at other doses than those used for hallucinogenic effect. Included in this group are lysergic acid diethylamide (LSD), mescaline, and 5-methoxy 3,4-methylenedioxyamphetamine (MMDA). Phencyclidine piperidine (PCP), an arylcyclohexylamine, is a related compound with both central nervous system stimulant and sedative effects in addition to hallucinogenic properties. Easy to synthesize, PCP is frequently used to cut other street drugs, such as heroin or cocaine.

PREVALENCE OF ADDICTION AND THE PRIMARY CARE PHYSICIAN'S ROLE

Substance abuse and addiction are highly prevalent in the community and in all medical care settings. An estimated 20 million Americans suffer from alcoholism, and 76 million, representing 43% of all Americans, have been exposed to alcoholism in the family.[1,8] Illicit drug use declined from 12% of the population 12 years and older in 1985 to 7% of the population in 1988. Cocaine use has declined except among those who use it on a regular basis. Among the 8 million who use cocaine, 10% use it at least once/week. Heroin use has recently increased, especially among young men.[9]

Alcohol use alone is associated with 70% of drownings, 25% of fires, 50% of traffic fatalities, 50% or more of homicides, 30% of suicides, and 67% of sexual assaults. An estimated 20 to 50% of inpatient hospital admissions are related to alcohol abuse or alcoholism, and 15 to 25% of patients in the ambulatory care setting suffer from alcoholism. Alcoholism and related disorders cost the United States over $427 billion dollars in health care expenditures and even more in lost productivity and antisocial behavior.[1] Alcohol use has been linked to excessive deaths due to cancer, cardiovascular disease, and unintentional injuries. Opioid and cocaine use have been indirectly related to homicide, either due to criminal activity to support a habit or to activity related to drug trafficking.[10] HIV infection among heterosexuals is commonly related to sexual contact with a partner who uses intravenous drugs.

Primary care physicians are uniquely placed to educate patients about the use of psychoactive drugs and the prevention of substance abuse problems. Knowledgeable physicians may successfully screen for substance abuse using standardized screening tools, such as the CAGE questionnaire (Table 83–1), asking about adverse consequences of substance use, and following up on behavioral, symptomatic, and physical signs of substance use, abuse, and addiction. Research on treatment for substance abuse has

TABLE 83–1. CAGE QUESTIONNAIRE

1. Have you ever tried to *CUT DOWN* on your drinking?
   Why? Was it difficult? How did you do it? Why did you start drinking again?
2. Have you ever been *ANNOYED* about criticism of your drinking?
   Who criticized you? Why was your drinking criticized? What was your response? Did you try to stop drinking or cut down?
3. Have you ever felt *GUILTY* about your drinking?
   What caused the guilt? How do you act when you are drinking? Do you always remember what you have done when you have been drinking? Have you ever resolved not to drink as a consequence of your behavior while drinking?
4. Have you ever had a morning *EYE OPENER*?
   Do you have the shakes in the morning? Do you ever wake up in the middle of the night and need a drink to go back to sleep? Do you start drinking in the morning to make it through the day?

demonstrated that treatment is effective. Walsh and colleagues demonstrated that inpatient treatment was effective in achieving improved job performance and decreasing alcohol and drug use among workers who were heavy drinkers.[11] In another study, heavy drinkers were randomly assigned to regular counseling about their drinking and monitoring of liver function tests, or to no counseling. The workers who were counseled cut down on their drinking and had fewer hospital admissions and lower mortality.[12] Other studies have demonstrated that treatment is effective in decreasing drug use, criminal behavior, and unemployment.[13, 14]

Given the risk for, and the prevalence of, substance abuse and addiction and the efficacy of screening and treatment, the primary care physician should assume an active role in the management of substance abuse by identifying patients at risk and those in the early stages of the disorder, making effective interventions, and recommending referrals for treatment.

Clinical Presentations

The primary care physician should assume that every patient uses some psychoactive drug, most likely caffeine, nicotine, or ethyl alcohol. The challenge is to determine what drugs a patient uses, whether their use poses any problems for the patient, and, if so, how severe those problems are. Understanding where a patient's drug use falls on the spectrum of use-misuse-abuse-dependence is crucial in planning appropriate intervention. Because of the fluidity of an individual's drug use, several assessments over time may be necessary for accurate diagnosis. Furthermore, the psychological denial of patients with significant problems of addiction may hamper the collection of accurate data.

Four Diagnostic Criteria. The primary care physician must assess the patient's drug use in four areas:

1. Loss of control over substance use
2. Adverse consequences secondary to use
3. Evidence of physiologic addiction (tolerance or withdrawal symptoms)
4. Quantity of use

Exploration of possible consequences of drug use is most important. Because early problems with drug use are primarily behavioral, the personal, social and family histories may provide the most data: loneliness, alienation, marital discord, children with behavioral problems, or leisure activities that revolve around the use of a drug. Problems with work performance or frequent job change usually indicate a severe problem with addiction, because many people suffering from an addiction, especially those in highly skilled occupations, continue to perform adequately on the job despite severe problems elsewhere in their lives. Health effects may be quite nonspecific: anxiety, irritability, insomnia, abdominal pain, or sexual dysfunction. Manifestations of loss of control over drug use include repeated attempts to limit drug use or continued use despite acknowledgment of adverse effects. The phenomenon of tolerance—the need for increasing amounts of the drug to achieve the desired effect, or conversely, the apparent lack of effect despite high doses of the drug—and subsequent withdrawal symptoms are most notable with the sedative drugs. Symptoms of mild alcohol or sedative withdrawal include difficulty sleeping, gastric distress, and anxiety. Opiate withdrawal may present as a flulike illness with rhinorrhea, chilliness, piloerection, and abdominal pain. Patients dependent on stimulants are less likely to visit the doctor because of symptoms of acute withdrawal—extreme dysphoria and exhaustion—but may present with fatigue, apathy, and weight loss. Knowing the quantity of drug used is most helpful in anticipating the severity of withdrawal symptoms on discontinuing the drug.

Screening for substance abuse answers the question "Do I need to assess this patient further for problems of addiction?" Although an experienced clinician may rely primarily on cues from the patient's history or affect to answer this question, formal screening instruments provide an efficient and accurate approach. The CAGE questionnaire (see Table 83–1), developed for alcohol abuse and adapted for drug use, consists of four questions that cover the first three parameters described earlier.[15] A positive answer to any two of the four questions has a sensitivity or specificity of about 75% in outpatient medical populations.[16] An affirmative answer to the question "Have you ever had a drinking problem?" and answering "within the last 24 hours" to the question "When was your last drink?" had a similar sensitivity and specificity when used to screen new patients presenting to an ambulatory medical clinic.[17] Because addiction is initially a behavioral disorder, laboratory tests are not useful in screening for substance abuse in the office setting.[18]

A positive result on the screening test, affective clues such as defensiveness or anxiety, or data suggestive of addiction from the medical history require confirmation with a detailed substance abuse history exploring the four areas outlined earlier. A trial of controlled drinking or abstinence may add useful data about the patient's ability to control his or her drug use. In early stages of substance abuse, the physical examination is either normal or yields nonspecific data, such as weight loss (stimulant abuse) or unexplained hypertension (alcohol use or withdrawal). Signs of chronic liver disease secondary to alcohol abuse or recurrent skin infections from intravenous drug use document the severity of the addiction but represent such late-stage disease that they should not be part of a case-finding strategy. Similarly, laboratory test results such as elevated liver transaminases and elevated mean corpuscular volume may be indicators of only late-stage problems with addiction. The number and constellation of signs and symptoms rather than any single indicator provides the most accurate picture of the patient's position on the spectrum of substance use-abuse-dependence.[4] If there is disagreement between the primary care physician and the patient about the diagnosis, a consultation with a substance abuse specialist for a diagnostic evaluation may be helpful.

Office Interventions

Having confirmed a problem of substance abuse, the primary care physician must discuss his or her concerns with the patient and recommend appropriate treatment. This process includes presenting the diagnosis to the patient, establishing treatment goals, and negotiating a therapeutic plan.

Effective techniques for discussing the diagnosis include

Using *specific* data from the history and physical examination to support the diagnosis. "Mrs. Jones, your fatigue and lack of energy, as well as your constipation, and the trouble you mentioned with your teenage daughter lead me to think that your real difficulty is not your chronic back pain, but a problem with your use of Percocet."

Providing support and hope. "I can understand that this must seem like a very difficult problem, but it's one that I can help you with."

Educating the patient. "Many people don't realize that medications like Percocet are not that helpful for chronic pain because as your body gets used to it, you must take higher and higher doses to achieve the same amount of pain relief."

The goals of treatment are to reverse the adverse consequences of alcohol and drug use by decreasing or discontinuing use. For people with occasional episodes of misuse, education about risks (e.g., driving after drinking) or recommendations to limit the amount of drug use may be appropriate. However, because most people with more severe forms of addiction have problems controlling the amount of drug use, total abstinence is the recommended goal. For those suffering from a severe, progressive course of addiction, a decrease in the frequency and duration of relapses may prove to be a more realistic goal.

In the primary care setting, the majority of patients with problems need only a brief intervention: a discussion of the physician's concerns about the patient's use of alcohol or drugs, followed by a recommendation to limit or discontinue drug use. This brief intervention, coupled with educational materials and follow-up, appears to be as effective as more intensive treatment for patients with minimal-to-moderate alcohol problems.[6] Other patients, who have more severe addiction problems or who have not responded positively to a brief intervention, require a referral to specialized treatment services, to self-help groups, such as Alcoholics Anonymous (AA), or both. Occasionally, a trial of controlled drinking or enlisting the help of a family member may provide the encouragement needed for a patient to accept treatment. However, the physician should be aware that family members may have their own agendas or may be participating in the patient's denial of an addiction problem.

Pharmacologic agents may be useful in preventing relapse if their use is part of a comprehensive treatment program. The most commonly used agents are those that block symptoms of withdrawal or craving (clonidine for opiate dependence, desipramine in cocaine addiction) or alter the desired effect of a drug (disulfiram for ethyl alcohol, naltrexone for narcotics).

The primary care physician plays a significant role in the ongoing care of patients with addictions regardless of whether they have received specialized treatment. In early recovery, the physician should monitor the patient for signs of relapse (decline in attendance at treatment or self-help groups, continued or increasing anxiety and irritability, resumption of social behaviors associated with alcohol or drug use) and work actively with the patient on relapse prevention. Because most patients relapse several times before achieving stable abstinence, the physician can help the patient anticipate possible relapse and frame the experience as a learning opportunity rather than as an excuse to return to drug use. Despite appropriate attempts at intervention, some patients continue to drink or use drugs in a harmful way, even while seeing their primary care physician for other illnesses. The physician should continue to document their problems with substance abuse and remind these patients that treatment is available if and when they are ready to address their addiction. Reassessment of drug and alcohol use should become part of the periodic health examination for all patients with a history of addiction (Fig. 83–1).

Making Referrals and Options for Treatment

Once the patient and the physician have decided that there is a problem and agree to formulate a treatment plan, the physician can help the patient choose appropriate therapy depending on the patient's medical and social situation and the availability of resources in the community. The physician should be familiar with different resources from patient education programs to inpatient treatment.

Before making a referral for treatment, the physician and the patient should discuss the goals for treatment. Abstinence may be one goal. Other, more immediate goals should also be discussed, including efforts to prevent the loss of a job, to respond to threats of divorce or dissolution of a relationship, to prevent further legal problems, or to maintain or prevent further deterioration of health. The physician should consider the patient's individual circumstances, such as the need for child care, insurance status, sociocultural and ethnic background, and previous treatment.

Outpatient treatment, including day treatment, workplace–based counseling through an employee assistance program, and group, individual, and family counseling, is available in most communities. It is less restrictive than inpatient treatment and allows patients to try to continue to fulfill work and family obligations. It is less expensive than inpatient treatment, but because some high-risk individuals may fail outpatient treatment and then require inpatient treatment, the difference in costs may be minimal.[11] Outpatient treatment generally works best for individuals who have intact social situations, including supportive family, no previous recent treatment failure, no major medical consequences of substance abuse, and no history of major withdrawal.

Inpatient treatment, consisting of detoxification if necessary, individual and group counseling, intensive education, and skill building, is generally available, but access to inpatient treatment may depend solely on insurance status. Most departments of health at the state or municipal level provide up-to-date information on treatment resources. Inpatient admission should be considered for patients with poor social supports, an impending catastrophe (e.g., divorce or loss of job), a major medical problem, a history of major withdrawal, and recent failure to improve with outpatient treatment. Inpatient therapy is also appropriate for individuals with significant denial and lack of insight.

There are several ways to improve the effectiveness of a referral. The physician should emphasize that specialized treatment for substance abuse is necessary, just as it may

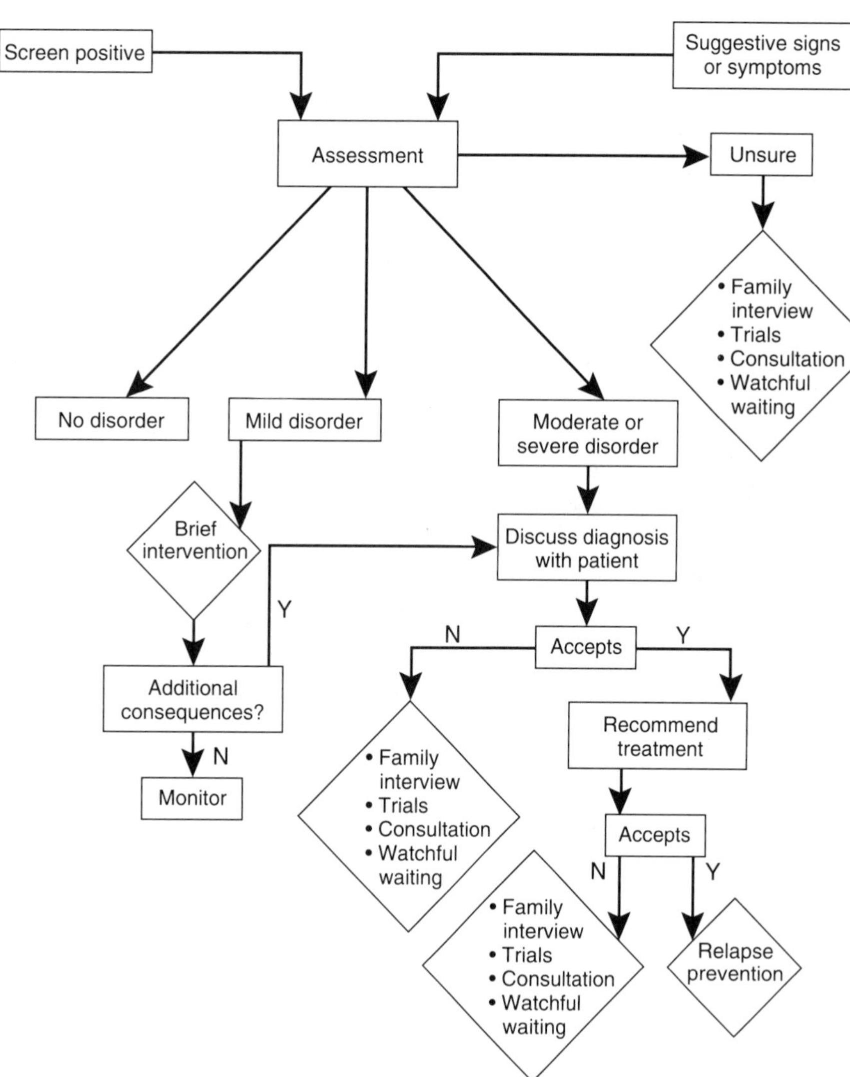

FIGURE 83–1. Diagnosis and treatment of addiction in the office setting. (From Brown RL: Identification and office management of alcohol and drug disorders. *In* Fleming MF and Barry KL (eds): Addictive Disorders. St. Louis, MO, Mosby–Year Book, 1992.)

be for any other serious medical problem, and that treatment is effective. Once a patient accepts the need for treatment, the physician should contact a substance abuse treatment program while the patient is still in the office. If the patient can be seen immediately the referral will be more effective.[14] Physicians should refer patients to specific individuals or programs with expertise in treating substance abuse. Not all social workers, psychologists, or psychiatrists are experienced in substance abuse treatment. It is important to involve the family in the treatment and the referral. The physician should explain to the patient exactly what treatment he or she will receive and how it will help him or her to stop drinking or using drugs. It helps if the physician is knowledgeable about the treatment program and can answer questions about treatment.

Self-help programs, such as AA, Cocaine Anonymous, and Narcotics Anonymous, are useful adjuncts to treatment but are also helpful even if the patient will not accept any other treatment. These programs provide individuals with the opportunity to learn about substance abuse and demonstrate that substance abusers can get better. The only requirement for membership is a desire to stop drinking or using other substances. Each autonomous AA group sponsors a weekly meeting whose character reflects the ethnic and socioeconomic makeup of the surrounding community or a particular common interest, such as gender or sexual preference. Because of the diversity of AA meetings, patients should be encouraged to attend several different meetings to find the most compatible one or ones. At these meetings, AA members share their experiences with alcohol and drugs and their recovery. No one is required to speak, and anonymity is maintained by using only first names.

The appeal of self-help programs is the warm and supportive fellowship in the groups. The program may use a set of 12 steps or principles to help individuals accept the role of drugs in their lives and develop new skills to deal with the common stresses of life without drinking or using drugs. Some members follow the steps explicitly; others use them as general precepts for healthful living. Simple, easy-to-remember phrases are used to help individuals identify how to stay sober ("One day at a time," "90 meetings in 90 days," "Keep coming back"), and to describe an impending slip ("Stinking thinking"). Physicians can refer patients to AA or other self-help meetings by calling the number listed in the local telephone book and describing to the intake person the type of meeting that may be right for the patient. Often, the central office will volunteer to have someone take the patient to a meeting. Family members can be referred to Al-Anon, a parallel program for individuals whose lives are affected by another person's use of alcohol or drugs.

TABLE 83–2. PRIMARY CARE OF THE PATIENT WITH SUBSTANCE USE DISORDERS

1. Screen and counsel for all conditions as appropriate for age and gender.
2. Counsel about increased risk for accidents or unintentional injuries.
3. Counsel and screen for sexual and physical abuse.
4. Counsel and screen for sexually transmitted disease.
5. Discuss prevention of human immunodeficiency virus transmission.
6. Screen intravenous drug users for hepatitis B and tuberculosis.

If the patient refuses treatment, the physician should continue to provide primary care for the patient, emphasizing substance abuse as a major problem.

Management of Medical Problems

The physician who provides primary care to patients who are substance abusers must know when and how to prescribe psychoactive and potentially addictive medications to these patients, who frequently have medical problems due to drug abuse. This section reviews specific issues related to the primary care of the patient who is a substance abuser or addict, the outpatient management of alcohol and opiate withdrawal, and prescription of psychoactive and addictive medications.

Primary Care of Patients with Substance Abuse Disorders

The primary care physician should provide routine screening and counseling about preventable conditions to patients with substance abuse disorders just as he or she provides these services to any other patient. However, there are some special issues to consider in the primary care of substance abusers (Table 83–2). Moderate-to-heavy alcohol use and alcoholism are associated with increased mortality,[19] primarily because of increased deaths from cirrhosis, cerebrovascular disease, and accidents. The physician should educate the patient about these consequences and how use of excess alcohol may compound other risks for cardiovascular disease, such as smoking or family history.

The physician can also reinforce the danger of driving under the influence of alcohol or drugs and the relationship between alcohol and drug use and accidents, unintentional injuries, and acts of violence.[10] Frequently, this discussion provides an opportunity to identify women who are at risk for physical and sexual abuse, either because of their own drinking or drug use or that of their partners.[20]

Physicians should also understand that individuals who abuse or are addicted to alcohol or other drugs may be at increased risk for sexually transmitted diseases, including HIV, because intoxication may lead to increased and unprotected sexual activity. Although HIV infection is most clearly linked with intravenous drug use, chronic alcohol use suppresses the immune system[21] and may increase the risk of infection with exposure to HIV. The physician can play an important role in counseling patients about the relationship between HIV and substance use and suggest testing for HIV when it is appropriate. The physician should also discuss protection against HIV transmission, including safe sexual practices and avoidance of injection of drugs and needle sharing. Condoms have been found to be protective against transmission of gonorrhea, herpes, and chlamydia and can be recommended for protection against transmission of HIV.[22]

Patients who are known to use drugs intravenously are at increased risk for hepatitis B infection and tuberculosis. Patients should be screened appropriately for these organisms. The hepatitis B vaccine should be offered to individuals who are not infected or immune.

Treatment of Withdrawal and Detoxification

Moderate-to-severe withdrawal from alcohol or other sedatives may pose a life-threatening risk, whereas withdrawal from opiates or stimulants, although uncomfortable, is seldom associated with significant morbidity. Although severe alcohol withdrawal should be treated in an environment where the patient is observed closely, mild alcohol withdrawal is a common presenting condition in the outpatient or office setting and often can be managed on an outpatient basis.

Symptoms of alcohol withdrawal occur after physiologic dependence to alcohol has developed. Because tolerance to the chronic use of alcohol causes compensatory changes in the central nervous system, an abrupt withdrawal or decrease in alcohol consumption may result in a withdrawal syndrome. Although the severity of symptoms of alcohol withdrawal is dependent on the dose and duration of alcohol consumption, the course of alcohol withdrawal is not predictable.

Withdrawal usually begins 4 to 8 hours after a decrease in consumption. Typically, the first signs of withdrawal are tremulousness, anxiety, insomnia, irritability, nausea, and vomiting. Tachycardia, tremor, mild hypertension, and nystagmus are physical signs of early alcohol withdrawal. In addition, the patient may be easily startled, diaphoretic, and hyper-reflexive. Hallucinations may develop 24 hours after decreased alcohol consumption. They are usually auditory hallucinations, but visual hallucinations may also occur. Alcohol withdrawal seizures usually occur 12 to 48 hours after the last drink but may occur as late as 10 days later, especially if the patient is also dependent on benzodiazepines. Delirium tremens usually occurs 3 to 4 days after the last drink but may occur as late as 14 days. Patients with delirium tremens or impending delirium tremens have a high morbidity, particularly if other illnesses, such as pneumonia, trauma, or pancreatitis are present. Prompt hospitalization and intensive monitoring have reduced mortality significantly.[23]

Some patients with withdrawal can be managed in the outpatient setting (Table 83–3). If a patient has only mild signs of withdrawal, no mental status changes, has no history of alcohol withdrawal seizures or delirium tremens,

TABLE 83–3. SEVERITY OF ALCOHOL WITHDRAWAL

	Symptoms	Treatment
Mild	Nausea, tremor, tachycardia, anxiety	Education, support with or without outpatient detoxification*
Moderate	Same as mild plus hypertension, paroxysmal sweats, agitation, flushing	Outpatient detoxification*
Severe	Same as moderate plus hallucinations, clouding of sensorium, vomiting, thought disturbance, fever, delirium	Inpatient detoxification

*If the patient has intact social supports, no history of major withdrawal, and no major medical problems. Also consider drinking frequency, daily consumption, and duration of heavy drinking.

comes from a stable social environment, and has access to close follow-up, his or her addiction problem can be managed in the outpatient setting. Patients with a history of drinking around the clock, consuming a fifth or more of alcohol a day, and drinking for a prolonged period of time are at high risk for severe withdrawal. Patients with comorbid diseases, such as hypertension, coronary artery disease, or diabetes, whose conditions might be exacerbated by alcohol withdrawal, should not be managed in the outpatient setting.

Although patients with signs of mild withdrawal can often be managed without medication, pharmacologic treatment with benzodiazepines is more common. Diazepam is appropriate because its half-life is similar to the half-life of alcohol. Physicians can prescribe diazepam, 10 to 15 mg 4 times a day, for the first day and have the patient return the following day. If the patient is stable, the physician can decrease the dose by one third or one half on each subsequent day over 3 to 4 days, when the patient should no longer require medication. The physician should educate reliable family members about the signs and symptoms of withdrawal that warrant immediate medical attention. Patients should also be treated for possible thiamine and folate deficiency by prescribing thiamine, 100 mg daily for 3 days, and folate, 1 mg daily.

Opiate withdrawal begins 6 to 12 hours after the last dose of narcotic, depending on the half-life of the drug. The signs of mild withdrawal include lacrimation, rhinorrhea, diaphoresis, yawning, restlessness, and insomnia. Other signs, including mydriasis, piloerection, fasciculations, and abdominal pain, are common as withdrawal progresses. Tachycardia, hypertension, tachypnea, fever, nausea and vomiting, and diarrhea indicate severe withdrawal.

Although in principle a narcotic could be used to treat opiate withdrawal, the potential for abuse outweighs the benefits. Methadone cannot be prescribed legally for an outpatient with signs of opiate withdrawal. A single dose of 0.2 mg of clonidine can be given to block the α-adrenergic effects of opiate withdrawal. If there is no significant hypotension, clonidine, 0.1 mg by mouth every 4 to 6 hours, can be used in conjunction with a clonidine patch. The dose can be tapered over 10 days.[24]

The profound depression of cocaine withdrawal often responds to antidepressants. However these patients frequently need more supervision and support than is available in an office setting. Patients withdrawing from cocaine should be referred to specialized treatment programs.

Prescribing Psychoactive and Potentially Addictive Drugs

Addicted patients may have other psychiatric or medical conditions that require treatment with a psychoactive drug, for example, narcotics for an acute pain syndrome. Physicians should apply the same general principles for prescribing drugs to patients with substance abuse as they apply to other patients. First, physicians should be aware of the abuse potential of any drug prescribed, including knowing the potential mood-altering qualities of the drugs and understanding that the prescribed pills will possibly be sold on the street. The physician should document in the patient's chart the rationale for prescribing the drug (including a specific diagnosis), the intended duration of treatment, the number of pills prescribed, and the number of refills. The physician should also document the patient's understanding of this information.

When writing prescriptions for controlled substances, the physician should spell out the number of pills prescribed and give no refills. Keeping prescription pads in secure places and not using pads with preprinted Drug Enforcement Agency numbers can prevent illegal use.

Substance abuse patients frequently request drugs for treatment of pain, insomnia, anxiety, or depression. Specific requests should be fully evaluated and prescriptions written only when medically indicated. Anxiety, sleeplessness, and depression are common transient symptoms during recovery and in general do not require prescription medications. These symptoms usually resolve in 6 to 12 months. The physician should offer alternative, nonpharmacologic or nonaddicting medications to treat these symptoms.

CONCLUSIONS

Substance abuse and addiction are common problems facing the primary care physician. The consequences of alcohol, opiate, sedative hypnotic, and stimulant abuse are varied but can be identified through appropriate screening. Office interventions and effective referrals are helpful in getting patients to abstain from harmful substances. The primary care physician can play an important role in educating patients about the risks for, and consequences of, substance abuse and addiction.

BIBLIOGRAPHY

Barnes HN, Aronson MD, and Delbanco TL (eds): Alcoholism. A Guide for the Primary Care Physician. New York, Springer-Verlag, 1987.

Fleming MF and Barry KL: Addictive Disorders. St. Louis, Mosby–Year Book, 1992.

Kinney J: Clinical Manual of Substance Abuse. St. Louis, Mosby–Year Book, 1991.

REFERENCES

1. National Institute on Alcohol Abuse and Alcoholism: Seventh Special Report to the U.S. Congress on alcohol and health. Washington, D.C., Public Health Service 1990, DHHS Publication No. (ADM) 90-1656.
2. Newman RG: The need to redefine "addiction." N Engl J Med 308:1096–1098, 1983.
3. Galanter M (ed): Recent Developments in Alcoholism, Vol 9. New York, Plenum Press, 1991.
4. Vaillant GE: The Natural History of Alcoholism: Causes, Patterns and Paths to Recovery. Cambridge, Harvard University Press, 1983.
5. Plant ML: Drinking Careers. London, Tavistock, 1979.
6. Institute of Medicine: Broadening the Base of Treatment for Alcohol Problems. Washington, D.C.: National Academy Press, 1990.
7. Jellinek EM: Phases of alcohol addiction. Q J Stud Alcohol 13:673–684, 1952.
8. Schoenborn CA: Exposure to alcoholism in the family: United States, 1988. Advance data from vital and health statistics; No. 205. Hyattsville, MD: National Center for Health Statistics, 1991.
9. National Institute on Drug Abuse: Drug Abuse and Drug Abuse Research. The Third Triennial Report to Congress. Rockville, MD. US Department of Health and Human Services 1991, DHHS Publication No. (ADM) 91-1704.
10. Tardiff K: Patterns and major determinants of homicide in the United States. Hosp Community Pract 36:632–639, 1985.
11. Walsh DC, Hingson RW, Merrigan DM, et al: A randomized trial of treatment options for alcohol-abusing workers. N Engl J Med 325:775–782, 1991.

12. Kristenson H, Ohlin H, Hulten-Nosslin RB, et al: Identification and intervention of heavy drinking in middle-aged men: Results and follow-up of 24–60 months of a long-term study with randomized controls. Alcohol Clin Exp Res 7:203–209, 1983.
13. McLellan AT, Laborsky L, O'Brien CP, et al: Is treatment for substance abuse effective? JAMA 247:1423–1428, 1982.
14. Goldberg HI, Mullen M, Ries RK, et al: Alcohol counseling in a general medical clinic. A randomized control trial of strategies to improve referral and show rates. Med Care 29:JS49–JS56, 1991.
15. Mayfield D, McLeod G, and Hall P: The CAGE questionnaire. Validation of a new alcoholism screening instrument. Am J Psychiatry 131:1121–1123, 1974.
16. Ewing JA: Detecting alcoholism: The CAGE questionnaire. JAMA 252:1905–1907, 1984.
17. Cyr MG and Wartman SA: The effectiveness of routine screening questions in the detection of alcoholism. JAMA 259:51–54, 1988.
18. Bush B, Shaw S, Cleary P, et al: Screening for alcohol abuse using the CAGE questionnaire. Am J Med 82:231–235, 1987.
19. Klatsky AL, Friedman GD, and Siegelaub AB: Alcohol and mortality. A ten-year Kaiser-Permanente experience. Ann Intern Med 95:139–145, 1981.
20. Rath GD, Jarratt LG, and Leonardson G: Rates of domestic violence against adult women by men partners. J Am Board Fam Pract 2:227–233, 1989.
21. Bagsra O: Effects of alcohol ingestion on in vitro susceptibility of peripheral blood mononuclear cells to infection with HIV and selected T-cell function. Alcoholism 13:636–643, 1989.
22. Stone KM, Grimes DA, and Magder LS: Primary prevention of sexually transmitted diseases. A primer for clinicians. JAMA 255:1763–1766, 1986.
23. Naranjo CA and Sellers M: Clinical assessment and pharmacotherapy of the alcohol withdrawal syndrome. *In* Galanter M (ed): Recent Advances in Alcoholism, Vol 4. New York and London, Plenum Press, 1986, pp 265–282.
24. Gold MS, Pottash AC, Sveny DR, and Kleber HD: Opiate withdrawal using clonidine. JAMA 243:343–346, 1980.

84

Disorders of Eating

WILLIAM T. BRANCH, Jr., MD
JANE SILLMAN, MD

OBESITY

Obesity is not a single disease, and thus no single etiologic factor can be isolated in obese patients. In a society placing a strong positive value on thinness, all obese patients experience psychological and social strains as well as biologic alterations. Evaluation and treatment of an obese patient should integrate a thorough understanding of the biologic etiologies and risks of obesity as well as its social and psychological consequences (Table 84–1).

Definition

Obesity refers to an excessive amount of adipose tissue. *Overweight* refers to a body weight in excess of a standard such as an average or desirable weight but does not indicate whether the excess is due to fat, muscle, bone, or fluid. There are different ways to measure obesity. Relative weight is the measure used by the insurance industry and in many epidemiologic studies, including the Framingham study. It is the weight of a person divided by the "desirable" weight for a person of medium frame. The desirable weights most often used are those published by the Metropolitan Life Insurance Company, which are the weights associated with the lowest mortality at any given height (Tables 84–2 and 84–3).[1] Body weights greater than 20% above desirable are defined as obese and are associated with increased health risks.

The body mass index (BMI), also referred to as the Quetelet Index, is currently used more often than the life insurance tables by researchers. The BMI is determined by dividing a person's weight in kilograms by his or her height in meters squared.[2] A BMI of greater than 27 kg/m^2 is

TABLE 84–1. BIOLOGIC, PSYCHOLOGICAL, AND SOCIAL FACTORS KNOWN TO INFLUENCE PREVALENCE, RISK, ETIOLOGY AND TREATMENT OF OBESITY*

Factor	Prevalence	Health Risk	Etiology	Treatment
Biologic	Genetic Age Physical activity Body structure	Coronary artery disease Hypertension Diabetes mellitus Pulmonary function Osteoarthritis Obstetric complications Cholecystitis Hirsutism	Genetic Ventromedial nucleus of hypothalamus Hypothyroidism Cushing's syndrome Male hypogonadism Number of fat cells, set point for weight Drugs: phenothiazines, tricyclics	Diet: 1400 cal/day, men : 1200 cal/day, women Drugs Surgery: gastric bypass, or gastroplasty
Psychological	Anxiety Depression Stress	Body image Minnesota Multiphasic Personality Inventory Self-blame or guilt Self-consciousness Self-disgust	Learning hunger Developmental obesity Reactive obesity Eating response to external clues Decreased tendency to exercise Defense against depression, anxiety, or loneliness	Motivation Educate patient to count calories Diet attractive and palatable Set realistic goals Doctor-patient relationship Work with patient's distorted body image
Social	Sex Race Economic status Educational level Availability of food Cost of food Physician activity habits Advertising	Reduced social mobility Education Employment Earning capacity Negative attitudes Family Physicians and nutritionists	Eating behavior Sedentary activity Marital discord Unique position in family Unsolvable life situations	Family support Exercise program Eating habits Cost of food Fad diets

*Developed by Ralph B. Freidin, MD

defined as overweight or obesity by many authorities and corresponds to a relative weight 20% above desirable. Though the BMI is actually a measure of overweight, it has been shown to correlate well with body fat.[3]

In practice, triceps skinfold thickness determined with a skin caliper correlates best with more sophisticated research methods of measuring total body *fat.* Measurements can be compared with charts indicating minimum skinfold thickness indicative of obesity according to the patient's age, sex, and ethnicity.

The "pinch test" is a simple method for estimating the amount of subcutaneous fat during routine office examination. By picking up a skinfold in the midtriceps area, below the scapulae, lower part of the chest wall, buttocks, or thigh, one can arrive at a fair assessment of whether the patient has normal (<0.5 inch) or excessive (>1 inch) subcutaneous fat stores. In men, the greater omentum can store large amounts of fat, and the expanding waistline may be the only clue. However, when the patient's weight is 10 or 20% above desirable level for estimated body frame, the clinical diagnosis rarely is in doubt.

The distribution of body fat has clinical importance. There are two main patterns of fat distribution. In truncal, or "male"-pattern obesity, fat is concentrated in the abdominal region. This pattern is associated with an increased risk of coronary artery disease, diabetes, hypertension, hyperlipidemia, stroke, and death.[4–6] In gluteal, or "female"-pattern obesity, fat is concentrated in the hips and thighs. This pattern is not an independent risk factor. These two patterns are quantitated by determining the waist-to-hip ratio. Patients with truncal obesity have an elevated waist-to-hip ratio.

TABLE 84–2. DESIRABLE WEIGHT (APPROXIMATE) OF WOMEN ACCORDING TO HEIGHT AND BODY FRAME

Height		Frame		
Ft	*In*	*Small*	*Medium*	*Large*
4	8	92–98	96–107	104–119
4	9	94–101	98–110	106–122
4	10	96–104	101–113	109–125
4	11	99–107	104–116	112–128
5	0	102–110	107–119	115–131
5	1	105–113	110–122	118–134
5	2	108–116	113–126	121–138
5	3	111–119	116–130	125–142
5	4	114–123	120–135	129–146
5	5	118–127	124–139	133–150
5	6	122–131	128–143	137–154
5	7	126–135	132–147	141–158
5	8	130–140	136–154	145–163
5	9	134–144	140–155	149–168
5	10	138–148	144–159	153–173

TABLE 84–3. DESIRABLE WEIGHT (APPROXIMATE) OF MEN ACCORDING TO HEIGHT AND BODY FRAME

Height		Frame		
Ft	*In*	*Small*	*Medium*	*Large*
5	1	112–120	118–129	126–141
5	2	115–123	121–133	129–144
5	3	118–126	124–136	132–148
5	4	121–129	127–139	135–152
5	5	124–133	130–143	138–156
5	6	128–137	134–147	142–161
5	7	132–141	138–152	147–166
5	8	136–145	142–156	151–170
5	9	140–150	146–160	155–174
5	10	144–154	150–165	159–179
5	11	148–158	154–170	164–184
6	0	152–162	158–175	168–189
6	1	156–167	162–180	173–194
6	2	160–171	167–185	178–199
6	3	164–175	172–190	182–204

TABLE 84–4. PREVALENCE OF OBESITY IN AMERICA BY AGE, SEX AND RACE*

Age	Men: *Black* (%)	Men: *White* (%)	Women: *Black* (%)	Women: *White* (%)
21	8.3	15.1	18.1	16.6
30	12.0	21.0	36.4	25.9
40	16.4	23.1	46.1	26.5
50	13.2	23.9	52.7	41.9
60	19.1	18.6	46.7	37.8
70	8.8	14.8	32.6	30.9
80	10.0	13.7	28.1	26.7

*Adapted from the Ten-State Nutrition Survey 1968–1970. US Department of Health, Education, and Welfare Pub. No. (HSM) 72–8131, pp iii–85.

TABLE 84–5. INFLUENCE OF OVERWEIGHT ON LIFE EXPECTANCY FOR MEN AND WOMEN*†

$$\frac{\textbf{Observed Deaths Among Overweight}}{\textbf{Expected Deaths of Those of Normal Weight}} \times 100$$

Age at Initial Examination	*Men*	*Women*
20–29	180	134
30–39	169	152
40–49	152	150
50–64	131	138
All ages	150	147

*Adapted from Armstrong DM, et al: Obesity and its relation to health and disease. JAMA, 147:1007, 1951. Copyright 1951, American Medical Association.
†Data from Metropolitan Life Insurance Company on applicants given higher premium owing to their weight but without other medical impairments or past medical history, followed up from 1925–1950.

Prevalence

In the United States Public Health Service Ten-State Nutrition Survey (Table 84–4), between 11 and 39% of white male adolescents and between 9 and 19% of white female adolescents were designated obese. The figures for black male adolescents were slightly less than for their white counterparts. Between 5 and 25% of adult men were obese, compared with a prevalence of 10 to 55% of adult women. In all age-matched groups, more black than white adult women were obese. The opposite was found for adult men.

Regardless of ethnic background, men of lower socioeconomic status have a lower prevalence of obesity. The opposite is true for women, in whom the prevalence is 30% among women of low socioeconomic status, compared with 4% among women of high socioeconomic status.[7]

Acculturation with American society also seems to influence the prevalence of obesity. Women who are recent immigrants tend to have more obesity (24%) than do fourth-generation women (15%) of the same ethnic background and same socioeconomic status.[8] These differences are not so marked for men. Marriage is associated with obesity in men but not in women.[9]

OBESITY AS A HEALTH RISK FACTOR

Obesity is a risk factor for one's physical, social, and emotional well-being. It may reduce life expectancy, aggravate the progression of other diseases, or modify one's social and economic status.

Actuarial studies (Table 84–5 and Fig. 84–1) usually show a progressive increase of excessive mortality with overweight. This effect is greater for men than women and more marked for younger than older patients.

Obesity is unequivocally related to hypertension, hypercholesterolemia, non–insulin-dependent diabetes mellitus, and excess occurrence of certain cancers.[1] In other medical problems, such as chronic obstructive pulmonary disease and osteoarthritis of the knees, hips, or spine, obesity contributes to disability. In morbid obesity (two or three times or 100 lb [45 kg] above desirable weight) and the pickwickian syndrome, obesity entails a clear-cut threat to life.[1]

Some studies show a direct association, particularly among young men, between being moderately overweight (excess body weight of 20%) and the risk of developing coronary disease.[10–13] Other studies fail to demonstrate that obesity makes a significant contribution to future coronary artery disease at all[14] or when other risk factors, such as age, sex, blood pressure, smoking, and serum cholesterol level, are controlled.[15, 16] However, recently the Nurses' Health Study demonstrated a strong association between obesity and risk of coronary heart disease in women. After controlling for hypertension, diabetes, and elevated cholesterol level, obesity itself was still associated with a modest increase in coronary risk.[17]

The cohort of men followed up longitudinally in the Framingham study experienced minimum mortality at relative weights of 100 to 109% and considerably higher mortality at weights 120% above desirable.[13] Smokers experience much higher mortality at all weights,[18] although underweight smokers experience higher mortality than persons of average weight.[8, 13]

Weight reduction is recommended for individuals with excessive weight of 20% or more above desirable. Weight loss is strongly recommended in persons with potentially reversible adverse health factors related to obesity, such as diabetes mellitus or a family or gestational history of dia-

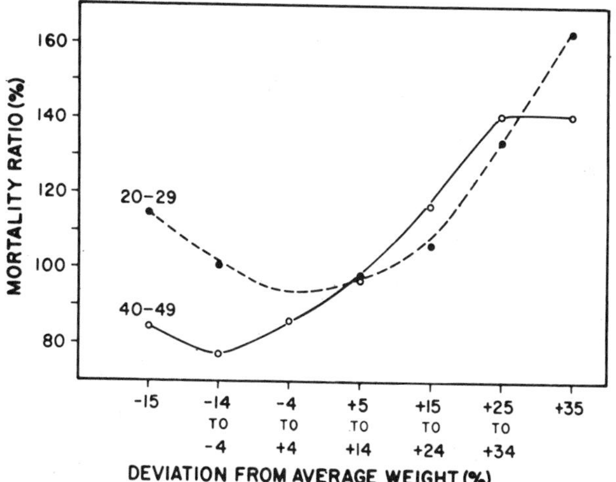

FIGURE 84–1. Effects of body weight on death rate. The death rate for deviations from the mean body weight has been plotted for persons aged 20 to 29 years and 40 to 49 years. The 100% figure on the ordinate represents the number of deaths per 100,000 insured subjects of all weights in each age group. The deviations from this 100% figure represent greater or lesser numbers of deaths in the subgroups of the population, whose deviations in body weight are plotted on the abscissa. (Reproduced with permission, from Bray GA, et al: Obesity: A serious symptom. Ann Intern Med 77:779, 1972.)

betes, hyperlipidemia, hypertension, or coronary heart disease.

In addition to physical risks, being obese has social and psychological consequences. Although these forms of morbidity are not uniformly present, they certainly cause unhappiness in many patients and may stimulate their seeking care sooner than might the risks to their physical health. In modern American society, slimness is the ideal of health and beauty. Much of the social stigma associated with obesity arises from the prejudice that unlike individuals with other chronic conditions, obese patients are responsible for their own plight. Fat people may internalize social condemnation and develop feelings of personal inferiority. Those with a poor sense of inner security, adolescents in particular, are especially vulnerable.[19]

These personal feelings and this social stigma may interfere with the development of normal social or sexual relations. This may limit social mobility and dating opportunities and also hinder educational and employment opportunities. For example, although obesity and intelligence are not correlated, obese adolescents appear to have less chance of acceptance to the college of their choice than nonobese peers.[20]

ETIOLOGIC CONSIDERATIONS

In evaluating an obese patient, it is important to recognize that excessive deposition of adipose tissue reflects an imbalance of caloric* consumption over metabolic expenditure. This usually results from a multiplicity of factors interacting simultaneously within the patient.

Genetic Factors

There is evidence that genetic factors contribute to differences in body weight. In one study, the BMI of adopted children was found to be similar to the BMIs of their biologic parents, but not to the BMIs of their adoptive parents.[21] In a study of twins, Bouchard and coworkers overfed 12 pairs of monozygotic twins for several months. Weight gain among the whole group ranged from 4.3 to 13.3 kg, but the variance within monozygotic pairs was much smaller, suggesting that the genotype determined the amount of weight gain.[22]

Diet

Overeating is the usual cause of obesity but has been hard to study because obese subjects have been noted to under-report their caloric intake more than lean subjects.[23, 24] Reliable ways to measure intake are needed because metabolic ward studies do not reflect normal living situations.

Composition of the diet is also a factor. Animal experiments have shown that rodents given a high-fat or high-sucrose diet eat more than needed for weight maintenance and gain weight.[25, 26] Epidemiologic evidence suggests that fat intake, especially saturated fat, is associated with weight gain in middle-aged women.[27]

Energy Expenditure

The main components of energy expenditure are the basal metabolic rate, the thermic effect of food, and physical activity. Of these three, decreases in physical activity are most important in causing obesity.

The basal metabolic rate is the energy used by someone resting in bed in the morning in a fasting state. In most sedentary adults, the basal metabolic rate accounts for 50 to 70% of their daily energy expenditure.[28] Obesity is associated with a high "absolute" metabolic rate. However, at any given body size, an individual can have a high, normal, or low "relative" metabolic rate.[28] Studies in Pima Indians have shown that a low relative metabolic rate was a modest risk factor for weight gain.[29]

The thermic effect of food refers to the increase in the basal metabolic rate in response to food and accounts for about 10% of daily energy expenditure. There have been many studies of the thermic effect of food in obese individuals, with 60% reporting a slight decrease and 40% showing no difference. It appears unlikely that a decreased thermic effect contributes significantly to the development of obesity.[29]

Physical activity represents 20 to 40% of daily energy expenditure and is an important factor in the development of obesity. Epidemiologically, the highest frequency of overweight men is found in groups with sedentary occupations. The development of the double-labeled water technique[30] has provided researchers with a way to measure the effect of physical activity on energy expenditure. Studies of Pima Indians by using this technique have demonstrated an inverse relationship between physical activity and obesity.[29]

Drugs

Some commonly prescribed drugs that can cause weight gain are glucocorticoids, phenothiazines, and tricyclic antidepressants, especially amitryptyline. The antihistamine cyproheptadine leads to weight gain by stimulating an increase in food intake. The weight gain reported with estrogen treatment is largely due to fluid retention. However, progestins, including medroxyprogesterone, may increase weight.[25]

Psychological Factors

Not all or even the majority of obese persons suffer psychological disturbances.[31] Being obese may compensate for a stressful and frustrating life. In others, however, obesity is associated with, and directly related to, severe personality and developmental disturbances. Despite the diversity and individual nuances of the psychological factors to which obese patients are prone, only two psychological disturbances seem related directly to obesity and overeating: hunger awareness and disturbance of body image. In assessing the origins of an individual's weight problem, a primary care physician should evaluate these areas as they pertain to the development of the patient's obesity.

Some obese persons, particularly those who gained weight as a child or adolescent, may have a basic disturbance in the way they sense hunger. Their eating habits may reflect external signals (i.e., sight, availability of food, and apparent passage of time) rather than the internal cues of hunger pangs that control the appetites of nonobese people.[32] These obese persons and some others, such as those with bulimia, seem to have trouble distinguishing between hunger and other states of bodily need or emotional arousal.[33] Eating thus can become a pseudosolution for the personality problems of these patients.

Hunger is not an innate response but rather is acquired

*The term *calorie* in this chapter means kilocalorie.

during early emotional development.[34] During this early period of personal development, some mothers may not feel good about themselves and thus feel incapable of giving anything except what is easily accessible—food. Sensations and emotions become confused, and possibly eating becomes a method of allaying anxiety for the child.

Obesity occurring in adulthood is sometimes a reaction to a significant psychological trauma,[35] frequently, a loss of a loved one through separation or death. In these patients, overeating becomes a method of warding off feelings of loneliness, depression, or anxiety. This coping mechanism leads to the possibility that in some obese patients, dieting may uncover depression.

A distorted body image is another behavioral disturbance to which obese patients are subject. Patients particularly prone to develop a disturbed body image are those whose obesity begins during childhood or adolescence, those who have associated emotional disturbances, and those whose family and peers give a strongly negative evaluation to obesity. Body image disturbances tend not to be part of the clinical picture of obesity starting during adulthood in an otherwise emotionally stable person.[36]

Some obese patients view their own bodies as loathsome and may feel that others regard their bodies with contempt. For others, whose obesity began in childhood, excessive fat tissue may be an attempt to gain strength and guard themselves from a hostile external environment. Such patients may dissociate the size of their body from the quantity of food they eat. Snacks eaten when no one is looking may not count as food.

Bulimia (discussed later) develops in a subset of patients who use food to relieve dysphoric feelings and may have distorted body images. Distorted perceptions of the body frequently persist after weight reduction,[37] although they sometimes gradually change with long-term psychotherapy.[38]

DISEASES ASSOCIATED WITH OBESITY

Laurence-Moon-Biedl syndrome is a recessively inherited disease characterized by mental retardation, retinitis pigmentosa, hypogonadism, obesity, and polydactyly. von Gierke's disease is a glycogen storage disease appearing in infancy with hepatomegaly, skeletal retardation with osteoporosis, ketonuria, and hypoglycemia. Obesity may develop as the patient grows older.

Obesity developing rapidly following head injury, encephalitis, or neurosurgery may be due to hypothalamic dysfunction. Similarly, hypothalamic tumors may be associated with obesity. However, in over 2300 cases of craniopharyngiomas and other lesions of the hypothalamus, the incidence of obesity was only 12%, which is identical to that of the general population. There are very few well-documented cases in which the hypothalamic lesion is the probable cause of obesity. Although high levels of insulin can be demonstrated in these patients, there is little else to distinguish them from patients with essential obesity except the history of rapid onset of weight gain in the absence of life crises, but frequently associated with headaches, visual disturbances, and impaired reproductive function (amenorrhea in women and decreased libido in men).[39]

The frequency of pure endocrine disorders causing obesity as seen in primary care practice is unknown, but they are uncommon. About 60% of patients with hypothyroidism have a modest weight gain, which results from accumulation of myxedematous fluid as well as adipose tissue. Cushing's disease may cause a moderate weight gain distributed in the face, thorax, and abdomen while sparing the buttocks and extremities. In women, obesity, hirsutism, and infertility suggest the Stein-Leventhal syndrome. About half of men with hypogonadism—Klinefelter's syndrome being the most frequent cause—will be modestly overweight with some increase in adipose tissue as well as a reduced muscle mass.

Life Events

Stopping cigarette smoking is usually associated with increased hunger and food intake and moderate weight gain. Other events that often lead to the development of obesity are pregnancy, decrease in physical activity due to job change, and surgery.[25]

MANAGEMENT

Patient Selection

It is important to evaluate the suitability of the patient for weight reduction and his or her motivation to lose. Obesity alone is not an absolute indication for treatment. Despite the risk to the patient's physical well-being from being overweight, obesity may act as a defense against underlying psychological problems—in particular, depression and distorted body image. Weight loss may uncover these psychological problems, with which the patient has more trouble coping than his or her obesity. Distortion of body image is frequent in patients whose obesity began in childhood. Depression is a significant problem for both juvenile and adult onset of obesity. As such, it is important not to disturb the delicate balance that each patient has established unless, and until, the patient is ready to do so. The "ideal" weight for some patients may be 20, 30, or even 50 pounds "overweight." In such a patient, it would be better to help the patient accept his or her obesity than to cause a sense of guilt, anxiety, and worthlessness about not being able to limit caloric consumption.

The stimulus for most patients to become interested in losing weight is cosmetic, precipitated by social circumstances, such as dating, marriage, or employment. Prevention of physical illness is an uncommon motivation to lose weight. If treatment is initiated or suggested before the patient develops a strong motivation, the weight-reducing program will be ineffective, and the doctor-patient relationship may also be compromised.

Benefits of Losing Weight

There are no clear data that losing weight has an effect on mortality. However, modest weight loss in the range of 15 to 20 lb has been shown to have benefits. Patients with non–insulin-dependent diabetes mellitus who lose modest amounts of weight have improved diabetic control, and some may be able to stop oral agents.[2] Weight loss in hypertensive patients leads to decreases in blood pressure and in the doses and need for antihypertensive treatment.[40] Hyperlipidemia also improves with weight loss.[2, 40] Weight loss in the range of 10 to 15 lb over a 10-year period has been shown to decrease the risk of symptomatic knee osteoarthritis in women.[41] The prevalence and severity of sleep apnea is reduced by weight loss. Other documented benefits are reduced work absenteeism and greater social interaction.[2]

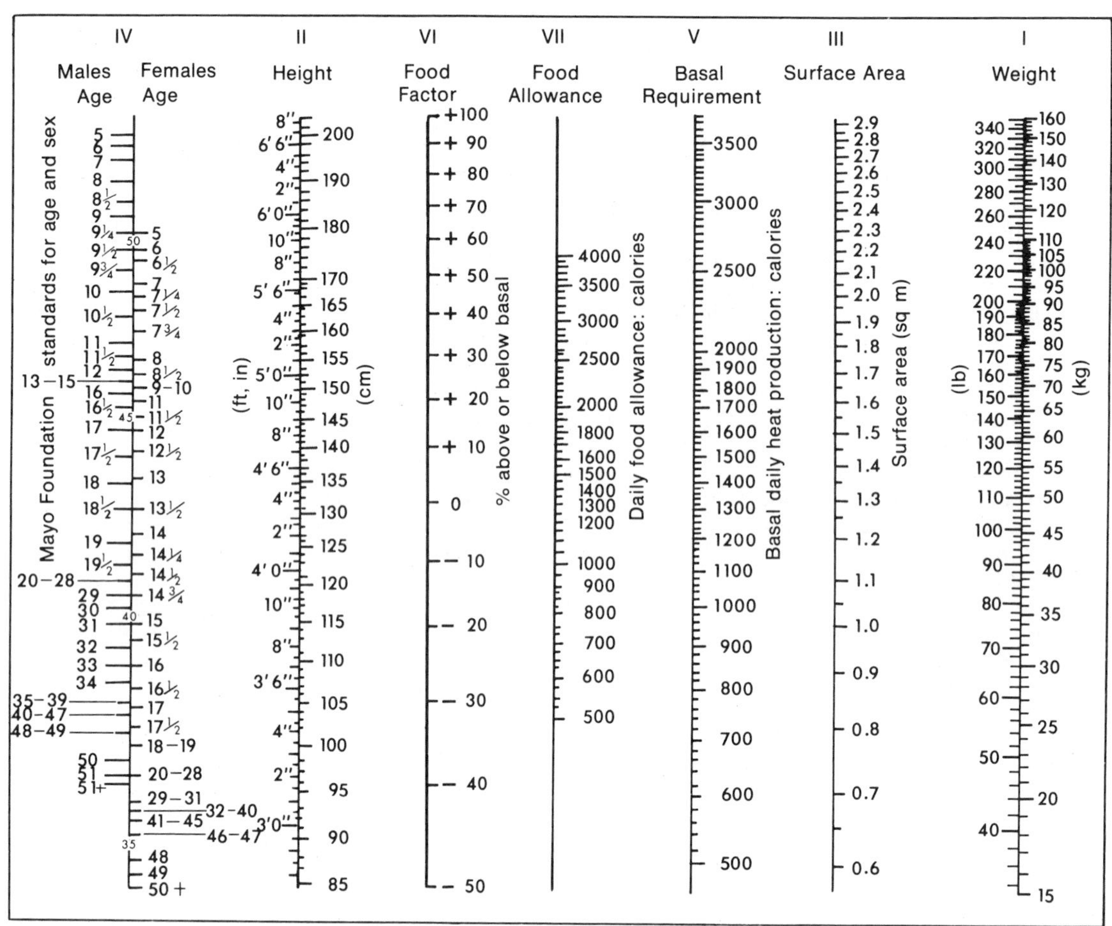

FIGURE 84–2. The Food Nomogram.

1. Locate patient's actual weight on Scale I by means of a pin.
2. Place the edge of a ruler against the pin and swing the other end of the ruler to the patient's height on Scale II.
3. Transfer the pin to the point where the ruler crosses Scale III.
4. Holding the ruler against the pin on Scale III, swing the left-hand end of the ruler to patient's age and sex on Scale IV. (Use the age at last birthday.)
5. Transfer the pin to where the ruler now crosses Scale V, which gives the basal calories for 24 hours and represents the calories of food required when fasting and resting in bed (basal calories).
6. To these basal calories add an allowance for activity. From Table 84–6 estimate the patient's percentage of calories above the basal and locate this point on Scale VI. (Since activity varies in different occupations, estimates of the per cent increase to be added for activity can be found in this figure. As most people who are obese are homemakers or are engaged in a sedentary occupation, a 50% increase for activity is the figure most often added to the basal calories.) With the ruler, connect this point with the point located previously on Scale V, and where that line now crosses Scale VII, you will find the amount of food calories that are expended by the patient daily.

Possible Adverse Effects of Weight Cycling

Several studies have evaluated the effects of weight cycling, where people repeatedly lose and regain weight. In the Framingham study, men and women with highly variable body weights had an increased risk of heart disease and death from heart disease.[42] Weight cycling may result in faster regaining of weight[2] and in a greater increase in the percentage of body fat.

Approach to Treatment

A long-term commitment to diet modification and lifestyle change is necessary for effective weight control. The most helpful approach is one that combines diet, increased exercise, and behavior modification. Patients need to set realistic goals for weight loss that relate to their health status.[43]

Dietary Treatment

Control of caloric consumption is essential to any management plan for obesity. Patients who were obese at some time in the past must have consumed more calories than they metabolized. The patient's present caloric consumption may be only maintaining excessive weight gained in the past. Patients able to reduce caloric consumption below their metabolic needs will succeed in losing weight (see Fig. 84–2).

In general, anywhere from 10 to 60% of patients undergoing diet therapy are able to lose 20 or more pounds while in treatment.[44] The long-term results of dietary programs are less successful. It appears that between 10 and 20% of patients who initially lose weight will maintain or increase their weight loss with the passage of time. The remaining patients will return to their initial weight or become even heavier.[45–48] Thus the physician should encourage gradual,

TABLE 84–6. PER CENT INCREASE TO BE ADDED TO BASAL CALORIES TO OBTAIN DAILY CALORIC EXPENDITURE

20%: for people confined to house, bed, a room, chair, or a wheelchair, as following a fracture of the leg, a crippling type of arthritis, a stroke or paralysis, heart disease, and in early convalescence from an illness.

30%: for people with moderately restricted activity but who are up and about. This generally includes people in late convalescence not confined to the house but permitted to sit on the lawn, take short motor trips or short walks, or be a sports spectator. This group also includes most retired elderly people who voluntarily or on doctor's recommendations restrict physical activity to the minimum sufficient to prevent boredom.

40%: for people with slightly restricted activity. The largest group here are housewives who do not do their own housework or engage in outside work.

50%: for people in the following light or home occupations: the white-collar occupations, machinery operators, housewives who do their own work, domestic servants, chauffeurs, and similar workers.

60%: for people who are moderately heavy workers such as manual laborers, farmers, truck drivers, and expressmen. This also applies to most adolescents who are obese.

70 TO 100%: for people who are engaged in heavy work, e.g., stevedores, lumberjacks, and steelworkers.

steady weight loss, followed by the long-term adoption of an isocaloric diet.

Many kinds of weight-reducing diets can be used by a motivated patient. A simple diet requiring few directions and incorporating some (but not all) of present eating habits is probably best. Negotiation over what should be limited or given up usually enhances the therapeutic relationship with the patient and assists him or her to stay on the diet.

The diet should satisfy all nutrient needs except kilocalories. There are two levels of caloric restriction in common use: low-calorie diets and very-low-calorie diets. Low-calorie diets provide 1000 to 1500 calories/day and are the appropriate treatment for moderately obese patients. Referral to a nutritionist can be extremely helpful in designing a low-calorie diet that is acceptable to a patient. Most commercial diet programs offer low-calorie diets.

For an adult woman, daily intake of about 1000 to 1200 calories and for an adult man, 1200 to 1400 calories is appropriate (Table 84–6). The diet should be palatable (Table 84–7), and liberal use of low-calorie, high-residue vegetables, such as raw celery, carrots, or cauliflower, may enhance compliance by providing a sense of satiety. The patient should be able to follow the diet at home and away from home without a sense of being different. The diet should minimize hunger between meals and should retain the patient's eating habits. With slight caloric modification, it should become the patient's permanent pattern of eating.

In addition to caloric restriction, interest has focused on the composition of the diet. Currently, low-fat, increased complex carbohydrate diets are favored because they induce weight loss in addition to lowering cholesterol.[45, 49, 52, 53] Restriction of alcohol and refined sugar is also appropriate, as they both provide energy but no nutrients. Low carbohydrate diets induce a mild ketosis leading to decreased appetite and induce the additional utilization of about 100 caolories/day but are not shown to increase weight loss[50] and are not recommended because they increase cholesterol and lead to volume depletion.[51] So-called fantasy diets, which may claim effectiveness owing to special "enzymatic" or other effects, are of unproven value and usually are not well evaluated for hazard.[45, 54]

Very-low-calorie diets are diets in the 800-calorie range. They are appropriate only for high-risk and morbidly obese patients. These diets, usually in the form of high-protein liquid formulas, should be used only with the supervision of a physician. Some carbohydrate is used to prevent electrolyte imbalance, or the diet is supplemented by 3 to 5 g of sodium chloride, 3 g of potassium (40 mEq), 1.5 to 2 liters of noncaloric fluid, and a multivitamin capsule each day.[55] Limited use of these diets is reputedly not associated with cardiac arrhythmias or myocardial wasting if supplements and high-nutrient proteins are employed and careful medical follow-up is provided.[55] A flavored powder (Cambridge Plan) available over-the-counter contains 300 calories: 30 g of protein, 45 g of carbohydrate, and 100% of the recommended daily allowance of vitamins and minerals. Sudden death was reported with use of liquid protein diets without adequate mineral and fluid supplements[56, 57]; the more adequately supplemented over-the-counter preparations available today may still be hazardous without careful medical supervision.[57]

Although rapid weight loss is achieved by using very-low-calorie, high-nutrient protein diets, the resultant rapid weight loss is often followed by a rapid regaining of weight.[55] It is not clear that incorporation of a behavioral modification program along with these diets solves this problem.

Doctor-Patient Relationship

The inconsistent results of the same diet administered by different physicians and nutritionists suggest that the skills and attitudes of the caregivers are as important as the particulars of the diet.[44] A physician's behavior can influence the management of obese patients in several ways. For example, the degree to which a physician is either too accepting or too critical of the patient's inability to meet his or her goals may strongly influence motivation to remain in treatment. Through understanding obesity within the psychological and social context of a patient's lifestyle, and the present and past stresses with which he or she is coping, a physician can offer empathetic listening that gives the patient the personal security to pursue weight loss.

If the physician is prescribing the diet, it is important to demonstrate a commitment to helping the patient by offering return appointments. This is particularly true during the first 6 or 8 weeks for patients who need support or listening, as well as a sense of being in control of their treatment.

The physician's attitude and behavior can also be a negative influence.[58, 59] In one study of patients cared for in a medical outpatient department, there was only a one in four chance that a patient who was more than 20% overweight encountered a physician who would both recognize the patient's weight problem and propose a program for managing it. Physicians not only tended to underestimate the personal strengths of these patients but also associated negative characteristics, such as weakness and unattractiveness, with obese patients.[60] From these studies, one can understand why feelings of shame, self-denigration, and embarrassment that occur during the medical encounter are a common reason given by patients for terminating weight-reducing programs.[61] It is important for physicians and others who treat obesity to understand their own feelings about obese people and recognize how these attitudes may add to already-present difficulties and frustrations.

TABLE 84–7. TIPS FOR COOKING WITH FEWER CALORIES*

- By cooking with low fat, the number of calories in food can be halved. Gravy, fried foods, and rich sauces are avoided.
- Main meals:
  - Fish baked in foil with sliced tomatoes, onions, salt, pepper, and oregano; or with lemon or lime juice; or with white wine or sherry, mushrooms, and seasonings.
  - Chicken without skin or wings baked in white wine, with fresh or water-packed mushrooms, sliced onion rings, and parsley; or in orange juice and sprinkled with ginger; or in tomato juice with sliced onions and pepper.
  - Flank steak, bottom or top round, cooked on a rack to let fat drip, with barbecue sauce on top.
  - Spaghetti with meatballs that have been broiled on a rack until fully cooked, in onions and garlic simmered in water plus tomatoes and seasonings.
- Soups—refrigerate stock overnight to remove hardened fat.
- Gravy substitute—damp water-packed or fresh mushrooms steamed in top of a double boiler with minced onion, garlic, parsley, salt, and pepper.
- Vegetables:
  - Green beans with basil, oregano or curry; or mixed with mushrooms or celery.
  - Spinach with vinegar.
  - Broccoli with garlic salt and lemon juice.
  - Tomatoes simmered with minced onion, parsley, oregano, and bay leaf.
- Desserts:
  - Baked cored apple sprinkled with cinnamon and filled with diet black cherry soda.
  - Stewed sliced pear simmered in diet black cherry soda.
  - Banana flambé, with orange juice, sprinkled with cinnamon, baked or broiled.
  - Apple brown betty: sprinkle 1/4 inch of raisin bran in bottom of pie pan, add sliced apples, sprinkle with cinnamon, cover with foil and bake.

*Adapted from Massachusetts General Hospital Department of Dietetics: Low Calorie Cooking Tips.

Exercise

Exercise alone causes limited weight loss, usually in the range of 4 to 7 lb. It has the additional beneficial effects of increasing high-density lipoprotein levels and increasing lean body mass and, if continued for a long time, helping patients maintain weight loss. Patients should be encouraged to incorporate increased exercise into their daily life.

Behavioral Modification

The keystone of all management plans that are aimed at permanent weight loss is a permanent change in eating habits. There is no painless method to control one's eating behavior. Long-term weight loss always means long-term caloric restriction. To assist in overcoming the difficulties of changing eating habits and to combat the patient's frustrations, techniques of behavioral change have been applied to the treatment of obesity. Although not adequately validated in clinical studies, it appears that a multifaceted approach to reprogramming the environment (making inappropriate eating more difficult while facilitating appropriate eating and stimulating social or personal reinforcement of constructive eating habits) addresses the biologic, psychological, and social aspects of obesity and thus is likely to succeed. These programs of behavioral modification are successful in the short run.[62, 63] There are few reports on long-term follow-up. In one Swedish study, 104 of 107 severely obese patients were evaluated 4 years after a behavior modification program combined with nutrition counseling, exercise, and jaw wiring. Thirty-three had left the program, eight had gained weight, 17 had lost 0 to 5 kg, and 49 had lost from 5 kg to more than 20 kg.[64]

Most behavioral programs employ a combination of the following components: (1) a period of self-monitoring and recording of body weight, food intake, and the feelings or environmental factors associated with eating; (2) goal setting; (3) nutritional, exercise, and health counseling; (4) tangible operant consequences (reward and punishment); (5) aversion therapy; (6) social reinforcement in the form of therapist, group, or family support; (7) covert conditioning and cognitive reconstructive strategies; (8) self-presented consequences; and (9) stimulus-control procedures.[62] The relative mix of these ideas is best determined by the individual needs of the patient. In general, behavior-oriented treatment of an obese patient probably should incorporate ideas that focus on personal control as well as those that stress environmental control. Personal control (e.g., helping the patient identify uncomfortable feelings such as anxiety or depression, or other factors, such as alcohol consumption, and deal with them without eating) may predominate in the treatment of patients whose primary need is to feel differently about problematic situations that previously led to excessive eating. On the other hand, the person who habitually consumes ice cream while watching television in bed might do better with a program stressing environmental control (e.g., use small plates and cocktail forks, and agree to prohibit eating in bed or while watching television).

Hospital-based and community clinics as well as commercial groups and *Weight Watchers International* offer programs employing behavioral modification for obesity, in addition to supportive group sessions. The latter may be helpful, although drop-out rates from some expensive proprietary clinics are reported to be as high as 70% after 3 months.[45] Overeaters Anonymous, modeled after Alcoholics Anonymous, offers group support and 12-step programs and is free. Many patients who remain involved with Overeaters Anonymous have been able to manage their eating and maintain weight loss.

Drugs

In research programs, treatment with investigational drugs has been effective in producing weight loss. Short-term use of drugs and some caloric restriction has caused weight loss similar to that achieved with very-low-calorie diets.

In a long-term trial, patients with severe obesity were treated with both fenfluramine and phentermine in small doses in addition to diet and behavior modification for up to 3.5 years. Patients maintained weight loss while on drug treatment but regained weight when the drug was changed to placebo. Patients on fenfluramine and phentermine had better control of hunger, increased satiety, and better adherence to diet (Table 84–8).[65]

Both fenfluramine and phentermine are sympathomimetic amines related chemically to the amphetamines, drugs that have been extensively abused and can cause dependence. Although dependence and abuse are possible, neither was observed in the long-term trial in which the drugs were dispensed in low doses under carefully monitored conditions. Both drugs suppress appetite. Fenfluramine is thought to work by increasing brain serotonin, whereas phentermine increases levels of dopamine and norepinephrine. Side effects of both drugs are dry mouth

TABLE 84–8. DRUGS USED IN THE TREATMENT OF OBESITY

Drug	Dose	Side Effects	Contraindication
Fenfluramine (Pondimin)	Initial dose, 20 mg tid with meals Maximum dose, 40 mg tid with meals	Dry mouth Diarrhea or constipation Rebound depression Sedation	History of significant depression Drug abuse
Phentermine (Ionamin)	15 mg q AM; maximum dose, 30 mg q AM	Dry mouth Diarrhea or constipation CNS* stimulation Insomnia	Drug abuse Symptomatic CAD† Moderate-to-severe HT‡
Combined treatment	Fenfluramine, 60-mg delayed release, and phentermine, 15 mg in the morning		

*CNS = central nervous system.
†CAD = coronary artery disease.
‡HT = hypertension.

and gastrointestinal disturbances, and both diarrhea and constipation. Their central nervous system effects differ. Fenfluramine can cause sedation and depression, which may occur after stopping the drug, whereas phentermine is more likely to cause nervousness and difficulty sleeping.

Drug therapy should be considered only in the treatment of high-risk or morbidly obese patients and should always be used as only one component of a broader management plan that includes dietary treatment, increased physical activity, and behavior modification.

Surgical Procedures

Surgery is considered for patients with morbid obesity who fail to respond to dietary therapy. Gastric bypass with gastrojejunostomy and gastroplasty employing vertical banding of the stomach are currently used to reduce the volume of the stomach and control eating.[45, 66, 67] Considerable weight loss is often achieved but is not inevitable because patients can continue to consume liquids and snacks on a regular basis and thereby overcome the effect of the surgery. Adverse effects include an approximately 0.3 to 0.5% operative mortality, occasional persistent nausea and vomiting, and vitamin deficiencies.[45, 68] Gastric procedures have largely replaced intestinal bypass surgery because the latter is associated with long-term complications including synovitis, calcium oxalate renal calculi, hepatic fibrosis, and intestinal pseudo-obstruction.

In England, jaw wiring by using dental splints of the type used to treat fractured jaws has been used to provide an obstacle to eating.[69] This noninvasive procedure has been acceptable to patients. Their appearance and speech have not been significantly affected, and they remain able to drink but not eat. Significant weight loss is often, but not always, achieved because patients can overdrink. Surgery and jaw wiring should be considered only in the management of morbidly obese patients.

GENERAL APPROACH TO MANAGING PATIENTS WHO OVEREAT

Considering the broad origins of obesity and the many biologic, psychological, and social risks of being obese, it is not surprising that no single treatment emerges as the most successful method of weight reduction.

The following steps are offered as a general approach.

Evaluate the Patient's Motivation. If the patient has been overweight for years, it is important to know why he or she wants to lose weight *now*. What is at stake: job, college application, boyfriend, girlfriend, or spouse? The precipitating forces behind the patient's request may be sufficient to convince the physician of the patient's intentions. In other cases, the causes are less clear. Although an individual may be intellectually committed to losing weight, it is important to see how willing he or she is to be actively involved before undertaking an elaborate program. This determination can be made by asking the patient to keep a record of weight each morning at the same time for 2 weeks while on a simple diet. If a patient is unable to complete this simple task of being aware of, and responsible for, his or her weight, it is likely that treatment not only will be unsuccessful but also may create a struggle with the physician that compromises the effective treatment of other illnesses.

If a patient's motivation is poor, one should reconsider the appropriateness of selecting the patient for weight reduction therapy.

Determine the Age of and Factors Related to the Onset of Obesity. Is this juvenile-onset obesity *(developmental)*, or is it obesity that began in adulthood *(reactive)?* If it is the former, how did the patient learn to respond to hunger as a child? If the latter, can an important loss or event in the patient's life be identified that precipitated the excessive caloric intake?

These data are important in estimating the likelihood of weight loss, as well as in assessing the degree to which a patient is prepared to deal with psychological issues in a broad approach to eating behavior. Patients who have been obese since childhood are less successful in weight reduction than are those who developed obesity in adulthood.[70] Likewise, treating a young adult whose obesity began following the death of his father may have minimal long-term success unless the patient's feelings about his father are addressed as part of the program. One should be especially careful when dealing with adolescents, who should be encouraged to feel good about their bodies, and to employ only moderate, common-sense measures for long-term weight control. If psychological issues associated with obesity appear too threatening to a patient and the physician judges that they will lead to psychological regression, then the suitability of the patient for weight reduction therapy ought to be reassessed.

Determine the Previous History of Weight Loss. Has there been a previous history of successful weight loss? When did it occur, and what led up to it? How long did it last, and what were the issues surrounding the patient's loss of motivation and regaining of weight? Aside from assessing whether a patient is better prepared to handle stresses than before, the primary care physician should be prepared to help patients respond to stress that develops during the course of treatment.

Obtain a Detailed History of Patient's Daily Diet and Eating Patterns. The physician may wish to obtain the history directly, or to refer the patient to a nutritionist for assistance. When asking an obese patient what he or she eats, one should realize that these patients may not count snacks eaten when no one is looking. Another suggestion is to find out which foods the patient enjoys most, so that one does not inadvertently deny items that are especially satisfying. Dieting should not be punishment.

Find out when in the day the patient first begins to eat. How much is consumed between meals? Does he or she eat on arriving home from work, before dinner, or after dinner? Where in the house does eating occur—bedroom, closet, bathroom, or kitchen?

The patient's success in modifying and controlling behavior should be emphasized more than the pounds lost. Do not emphasize "going on a diet" because it implies "going off a diet" in the future. Focus on the development of new eating habits. Have the patient separate eating from other activities, limit times and places of eating, avoid buying high-calorie foods, reduce the portions of food and put leftovers away before they are eaten, eat slowly, and put utensils down between bites.

Unrestricted nutritional exchange strategies avoid eliminating particularly gratifying foods and lead to establishing more reasonable long-term habits.

A therapeutic diet should be nutritionally balanced and should not cause excessive hunger. Three meals/day, particularly a morning meal, are more effective than one or two meals a day in controlling appetite.

Estimate Caloric Intake Needed to Achieve Established Goal. This goal should be mutually set by patient and physician, both in the amount of weight and rate at which it is to be lost. A nutritionist can be helpful in creating the actual diet. In general, a low-calorie diet of 1200 calories/day for a man or 1000 calories/day for a woman will result in a 500-calorie negative balance/day. Weight loss will proceed at 1 to 2 lb/week. Realistic goal setting increases the patient's changes of success and, thus, of achieving a more positive self-evaluation.

Give the Patient Increasing Responsibility for Diet Control and Weight Reduction. Knowing what the daily and weekly goals are and being motivated to weigh himself or herself every day, the patient can assume increasing responsibility for the outcome of treatment. As the patient becomes increasingly responsible for the outcome, the physician or nutritionist can take on a less directive and more supportive role. Scheduling frequent visits (i.e., every week or every 2 weeks), particularly at the outset, is an important way to support the patient. The price of unrealistic expectations is defeat and shame. One should never make a patient feel guilty. A way to be supportive is to inform the person that all patients have difficulty losing weight and that everyone occasionally goes off the diet. This is particularly important around holidays, when patients may either enjoy the foods that everyone else is eating and feel guilty or do not and feel angry. Long-term change in eating habits, not episodic weight loss, is the ultimate goal.

On the other hand, the physician should not accept persistent inability to lose weight. If this occurs, re-explore the patient's motivation.

Prescribe Physical Activities. Five calories are expended per minute of walking. If a patient has a stable diet, addition of 30 minutes of walking per day will yield a weight loss of about 15 lb over a year.

Carefully Observe the Patient's Emotional Status. There have been multiple reports of emotional problems, particularly depression, and even severe psychosis occurring when patients are being treated for obesity. This is more frequent in patients whose obesity began in childhood or in those undergoing radical caloric restriction.[36]

Work on Developing Family and Social Supports. Changing the patient's eating habits is difficult to achieve without adequate social support. Initially, the support will come from the physician, but ultimately, one must strive to make the patient's family or friends a source of self-reward. The eating behavior of the patient's friends or family also needs to be addressed. Meetings with family may be helpful in some cases.

Terminate Treatment Appropriately. Too abrupt a withdrawal from the physician or nutritionist can have a rebound effect that returns the patient to previous eating patterns.[71]

BULIMIA AND ANOREXIA NERVOSA

Serious eating disorders—bulimia and anorexia nervosa—are now recognized to be increasingly prevalent. Because these disorders affect entire families and require medical as well as psychiatric expertise, internists and family physicians are often involved in their management. Bulimia is a disorder of binge-eating followed by "purging." Diagnostic criteria listed in the *Diagnostic and Statistical Manual of Mental Disorders* (DSM-III-R) include (1) recurrent episodes of binge eating (rapid consumption of a large amount of food in discrete periods of time); (2) a feeling of lack of control over eating behavior during the eating binges; (3) the person regularly engages in self-induced vomiting, use of laxatives or diuretics, strict dieting or fasting, or vigorous exercise to prevent weight gain; (4) a minimum average of two binge-eating episodes/week for at least 3 months; and (5) persistent overconcern with body shape and weight. Additional features may be present, including the following: highly caloric foods are consumed during the binge; binging occurs secretly or inconspicuously; it is terminated by sleep, vomiting, or complete satiety; and alternating binges and fasts produce frequent weight fluctuations of 10 pounds or more.[72]

The criteria for diagnosis of anorexia nervosa, as abstracted from DSM-III-R, include (1) refusal to maintain body weight over a minimum normal weight for age and height, that is, weight loss leading to maintenance of body weight 15% below that expected, or failure to make expected weight gain during a period of growth, leading to body weight 15% below that expected; (2) intense fear of gaining weight or becoming fat, even though underweight; (3) disturbance in the way in which one's body weight, size, or shape is experienced, that is, the person claims to "feel fat," even when emaciated or believes that one area of the body is "too fat" even when obviously underweight; and (4) in females, absence of at least three consecutive menstrual cycles when otherwise expected to occur (primary or secondary amenorrhea). (A woman may be considered to have amenorrhea if her periods occur only following hormone, e.g., estrogen, administration.)[72] Other features usually present in anorexia nervosa include onset before 25 years of age, unusual hoarding or handling of food, presence of lanugo hair and bradycardia, periods of overactivity, and sometimes, episodes of bulimia or self-induced vomiting.[73]

Prevalence and Features of the Patients

Although bulimia is not always easily separable from dieting and overeating (two thirds of college women binge eat at least once/year), surveys report bulimia meeting DSM-III-R criteria in 3.8% of women seen at a college mental health center[74] and in up to 10.3% of suburban shoppers, of whom 4.7% practiced bulimia at the time of the survey.[75] Anorexia nervosa is estimated to occur in as many as 1 in 200 white female adolescents in the United States. It is much less common in African-American women.[76] Both disorders are 10 to 20 times more common in women than in men, and 40% of severely bulimic women have a history of anorexia.[77] Eighty per cent of anorectic women develop their symptoms within 7 years of menarche.[78] They are typically described as "model children," responsive to their parents' needs, and growing up in a tightly enmeshed family, who may have difficulty experiencing their own feelings and "differentiating their desires and feelings from those of their parents."[78] Bulimic patients tend to be more socially outgoing. Unlike the "thin" anorectic patient, they often appear physically healthy. Although they are also reported to be "high achievers," depression, alcohol or drug abuse, kleptomania, and sexual promiscuity in women or homosexuality in men are relatively common.[78] Bulimia begins during a period of severe dietary restriction in most patients.[31] Two answers to screening questions are correlated with bulimia: a "no" response to "Are you satisfied with your eating patterns?" and a "yes" response to "Do you ever eat in secret?"[79]

Psychological Factors

Bulimia usually develops within a milieu of preoccupation with weight, distorted body image, and perhaps depression, anxiety, or other dysphoric feelings relieved by food intake. The child given food rather than emotional comfort from its mother is one model for bulimia and anorexia. The family addressing problems around the dinner table is another frequent association. Other features of bulimic girls include feelings of inadequacy and passivity, looking to men for confirmation of their worth, gaining positive feedback from losing weight, and lacking assertiveness or a sense of self-worth.[77, 80]

Binges are typically preceded first by difficulty controlling the impulse and then by a heightened sense of anticipation, sometimes leading to a shopping spree. The binge itself occurs in secret. Some patients report eating continuously without even being aware of what they are eating. The food is usually highly caloric "junk food." Purging occurs by self-induced vomiting, by diuretic abuse, and/or by surreptitious use of laxatives, which some patients erroneously believe prevents absorption of the food. Patients are typically depressed after binging. Ritualistic exercise, such as excessive jogging or cycling, is common in patients with bulimia nervosa.

Bulimics are divided into several groups.[77, 78] Models, jockeys, dancers, prize fighters, wrestlers, and even socialites may control weight semirationally with purging but in general do not engage in binges. Mild or transient bulimia is common in college women. Intractable bulimia associated with multiple episodes of binging and purging, often in a single day, occurs less commonly. Some older women have lifelong, stable bulimia, which often occurs at the end of a busy day and is incorporated into a stable pattern of behavior.[77]

Anorectic patients have a much more distorted body image. Unlike bulimic patients, who are aware of their preoccupation and tend to maintain normal body weight, anorectics have an obsession with thinness that amounts to a delusion. They often develop the illness or are noted to have symptoms at a younger age than do bulimics and generally are more introverted and perfectionistic. Some (about 15%) purge. Others control weight by obsessive exercise. Some anorectics are preoccupied with bizarre foods or may prepare elaborate meals for others. Their pursuit of weight loss is relentless. Not only are they unaware of hunger but they also deny fatigue, and they often seem unaware of anger, depression, anxiety, and other emotions.[78] They tend to maintain an immaculate appearance. Psychologically, controlling their eating may work to defend the ego against a feared loss of control, or against being subsumed by others.

Physiologic Consequences

Binge eating produces gastric dilatation and may induce pancreatitis. Self-induced vomiting may produce gastric or esophageal rupture or a Mallory-Weiss tear, gastroesophageal reflux, erosion by gastric acid of dental enamel, hoarseness, and dehydration. Surreptitious laxative abuse can lead to hypokalemia, hypocalcemia, and aperistalsis of the colon and may cause the physician to plan an elaborate evaluation for chronic diarrhea. Osmotic-type diarrhea, a positive stool phenolphthalein test result, and melanosis coli may be noted with laxative abuse. Diuretic and laxative abuse at times produce sufficient dehydration and electrolyte imbalance to cause renal damage.[81] Multiple doses of ipecac to induce vomiting may cause cardiomyopathy.[82] Sudden death may result from electrolyte imbalance.[83]

The many physiologic effects of anorexia nervosa are chiefly consequences of the malnutrition and are probably not causally related to the syndrome.[78] Included are dry, scaly skin, a sallow, carotenemic color, lanugo hair, low blood pressure, and bradycardia. A body fat content of 17% is required for gonadotropin cycling at menarche; once lost because of decreased weight, a fat content of about 22% may be needed to restore menses.[78] The amenorrhea of anorectic women is characterized by a lack of withdrawal bleeding after receiving progesterone, by low serum follicle-stimulating and luteinizing hormone levels, and by lack of the bursts of luteinizing hormone secretion seen in normal women in response to luteinizing hormone–releasing factor throughout the day.[78] They have normal levels of free thyroxine (T_4) and thyroid-stimulating hormone, but low triiodothyronine (T_3) and increased reverse T_3 levels, suggesting poor peripheral conversion of T_4 to T_3. They may have an abnormal dexamethasone suppression test result but maintain normal secretion and diurnal cycling of adrenocorticotropic hormone. Human growth hormone may be elevated, but the anabolic effects of growth hormone, mediated by somatomedin, which is produced in the liver and other tissues, are lacking. These hormonal effects appear at least in part to represent an adaptation to the malnourished state.[78] Vasopressin secretion can be partially impaired. Myocardial wasting with decreased left ventricular wall thickness occurs as a consequence of malnutrition. Arrhythmias, Q-T interval prolongation, and conduction defects of the heart are probably related to acid-base and electrolyte imbalance.[83] Other effects include mild anemia and leukopenia, constipation, decreased serum cholesterol and albumin levels, and elevated serum carotene level.

Medical Management

The diagnoses of bulimia and anorexia nervosa are made from the patient history. Emaciation to the extent produced by anorexia is rarely caused by a medical problem that remains occult. Among the diagnostic tests that can be considered to rule out other medical illness are blood counts, sedimentation rate, serum electrolytes, amylase, total protein and albumin, renal and liver function tests, serum carotene (usually decreased in malabsorption, increased in anorexia), T_4 and T_3 determinations, sigmoidoscopy, stool examination for blood, fat, and parasites, a lateral film of the skull, and gastrointestinal radiographs, including small-bowel follow-through.[78] One may also obtain plasma cortisol levels. Severity of the malnutrition is evaluated by baseline weight, height and triceps skinfold measurements, albumin and serum transferrin levels, and skin testing for *Candida* antigen.[78]

The physician should be aware of, and monitor the patient for, the complications of bulimia and anorexia listed earlier (Table 84–9). Usually, serum electrolytes and the electrocardiogram are followed in repetitively bulimic and in anorectic patients. Indications for hospitalization include severe hypokalemia despite oral potassium replacement therapy, arrhythmias, onset of lethargy or listlessness in the previously active anorectic patient, depression and associated risk of suicide, and weight loss that is severe, rapidly progressive, or falls below the agreed-on minimal weight.

Nutritional management of anorexia has undergone changes in recent decades.[76] A nihilistic approach was replaced in the late 1960s by use of tube feeding and intravenous hyperalimentation. Complications and the lack of long-term changes in patients' behavior after such treatment led to the current approach of intervention for severe weight loss, with outpatient medical, psychiatric, and sometimes pharmacologic and/or behavioral therapy for most patients.

Outpatient nutritional supplements designed to increase caloric intake to 250 to 500 calories above daily energy requirements are recommended for patients with moderate malnutrition.[78] It is suggested that physicians and patients agree on a minimum weight, below which the patient will be hospitalized. This avoids arguments, excuses, or blame laying on the patient when the need arises to hospitalize. In general, a more than 40% loss from normal body weight or a 25 to 30% weight loss in fewer than 3 months warrants hospitalization.[76, 78] The goal is a weight gain of 1 to 2 kg/week by oral supplements or tube feeding.[78] Peripheral or central intravenous hyperalimentation, gradually increasing caloric delivery from one half to full daily requirements over 3 days, maintained until body weight reaches 80% of normal, is recommended for patients refusing to eat, vomiting, or otherwise unable to tolerate oral feeding.[78] Thiamine is administered prior to feeding, and electrolytes, blood sugar, calcium, phosphate, and magnesium levels are closely monitored.

Tricyclic antidepressants, fluoxetine, and trazodone have successfully diminished binging in bulimic patients.[84] The agents are less clearly beneficial in patients with anorexia nervosa, although prior anorexia nervosa does not preclude a positive response in bulimia. Bupropion is avoided because it has been linked to a higher rate of seizures in bulimic patients, and monoamine oxidase inhibitors are contraindicated because of the likelihood of dietary indiscretion in these patients. Full antidepressant doses are employed in patients on pharmacotherapy, and blood levels may be helpful to monitor compliance and the possible effect of purging on drug absorption.

Psychiatric and Behavioral Therapy

The physician's support during follow-up may help the patient attain a sense of autonomy and may encourage family involvement in the treatment program.[78] It is recommended that the physician strive to be absolutely honest, objective, and dependable in dealing with these pa-

TABLE 84–9. COMPLICATIONS OF BULIMIA AND ANOREXIA NERVOSA*

	Behavioral Components				
Organ System	*Intentional Malnourishment*	*Binge-Eating*	*Self-Induced Vomiting*	*Cathartic Abuse*	*Diuretic Abuse*
Endocrine/metabolic	Amenorrhea, infertility, hypothyroidism (rare)	—	—	Hypocalcemia	—
Cardiovascular/pulmonary	Heart failure	Heart failure, refeeding edema	Aspiration pneumonitis	Myocarditis (from ipecac abuse), hypokalemic cardiomyopathy	—
Renal/electrolyte	Reduced glomerular filtration rate, tubular dysfunction	—	Metabolic alkalosis, hypokalemia	Hypokalemia, kaliopenic nephropathy	Hypokalemia, hyponatremia
Hematologic	Anemia, leukopenia, thrombocytopenia	—	—	—	—
Alimentary tract	Constipation, hemorrhoid exacerbation	Gastric dilatation or rupture, pancreatitis	Oral cavity trauma, tooth enamel erosion, esophagitis, Mallory-Weiss syndrome, esophageal rupture, parotid enlargement	Hypokalemic ileus, melanosis coli, cathartic colon	—
Neurologic/psychiatric	Depression, hypothermia, lack of REM† sleep	Electroencephalographic abnormalities	—	—	—

*Reproduced with permission, from Harris RT: Bulimarexia and related serious eating disorders with medical complications. Ann Intern Med 99:800, 1983.
†REM = rapid eye movement.

tients, who will sensitively detect evasiveness, inconsistency, or judgmental attitudes from the physician.[78] The physician is the liaison between the patient and other health-care providers. He or she should work closely with the psychiatrist. If it becomes necessary to hospitalize, brief admission to a medical facility followed by transfer to a psychiatric facility is often advantageous.

Group therapy is recommended for college students with mild bulimia. Intractable bulimia in college students usually requires intensive psychotherapy and careful medical follow-up. Some of the patients require hospitalization. Stable bulimia in older women responds poorly to intervention, but psychotherapy should be considered.[77, 78]

Whereas classic psychoanalysis is not often successful, insight-oriented psychotherapy and family therapy are effective in some anorectic patients.[78] Bruch makes the point that the patient is not amenable to psychotherapy until the worst malnutrition is corrected.[85] The goal of lasting recovery requires changes in the patient's image of himself or herself and possibly in family dynamics. Bruch begins therapy by giving the patient a simple explanation: preoccupation with weight loss is a "cover-up" for the patient's doubts about self-worth. He or she is then told that a great deal is known about the problem and that therapy is for the patient's—not the parents'—benefit. Psychotherapy addresses the patient's basic mistrust; his or her tendency to hide this under a "facade of pleasing cooperation"; and the family's interactions that interfered with normal development, including the patient's overinvolvement with his or her parents' aspirations and his or her tight enmeshment with the family. If successful, the psychotherapy should lead to discovery of the "validity and worthwhileness of the patient's core personality."[85]

Behavioral therapy is often employed for anorexia with the proviso that too many external manipulations may hamper the patient's developing rational self-control.[78, 85] For severely malnourished anorectics, a sequence of hospitalization, bed confinement, supervised eating, behavioral therapy, psychotherapy, and family therapy, and possibly pharmacotherapy is as good as or better than any other approach.[78, 86] Outcomes are fairly good in treated patients, with one half to three fourths achieving greater than 75% of normal weight and menstruating, though less than one third of patients attained normal eating habits.[78] The mean mortality rate in several series was 6%. Inanition, severe electrolyte disturbances, suicide, and aspiration caused the majority of deaths.[78]

ACKNOWLEDGMENT

The contributions of Ralph B. Freidin, M.D., who wrote the original version of this chapter in the first edition, on which this version is based, are gratefully acknowledged.

REFERENCES

1. Consensus Development Panel on the Health Implications of Obesity: Health implications of obesity. National Institutes of Health Consensus Development Conference Statement. Ann Intern Med 103:1073, 1985.
2. NIH Technology Assessment Conference Panel: Methods for voluntary weight loss and control. Ann Intern Med 116:942, 1992.
3. Keys A, et al: Indices of relative weight and obesity. J Chron Dis 25:329, 1972.
4. Larsson B, Svardsudd K, Welin L, et al: Abdominal adipose tissue distribution, obesity, and risk of cardiovascular disease and death: 13 year follow up of participants in the study of men born in 1913. BMJ 288:1401, 1984.
5. Kissebah A, Vydelingum N, Murray R, et al: Relation of body fat distribution to metabolic complications of obesity. J Clin Endocrinol Metab 54:254, 1982.
6. Krotkiewski M, Bjorntorp P, Sjostrom L, et al: Impact of obesity on metabolism in men and women. J Clin Invest 72:1150, 1983.
7. Moore ME, Stunkard A, Srole L: Obesity, social class and mental illness. JAMA 181:962, 1962.
8. Goldblatt PB, Moore ME, Stunkard A: Social factors in obesity. JAMA 192:1039, 1965.
9. Sobal J, Rauschenbach B, Frongillo E: Marital status, fatness and obesity. Soc Sci Med 35:915, 1992.
10. Stamler J, Berkson DM, Lindberg H, et al: Coronary risk factors. Med Clin North Am 50:229, 1966.
11. Chapman JM, Coulson JH, Clark VA, et al: The differential effect of serum cholesterol, blood pressure and weight on incidence of myocardial infarction and angina pectoris. J Chron Dis 23:631, 1971.
12. Hubert H: Obesity as an independent risk factor for cardiovascular disease: A 26-year followup of the participants in the Framingham Heart Study. Circulation 67:968, 1983.
13. Garrison RJ and Castelli WP: Weight and thirty-year mortality of men in the Framingham Study. Ann Intern Med 103:1006, 1985.
14. Barrett-Connor E: Obesity, atherosclerosis and coronary heart disease. Ann Intern Med 103:1010, 1985.
15. Kannel WB, et al: Relation of body weight to development of coronary artery disease. Circulation 35:734, 1967.
16. Keys A, Colditz G, Stampfer M, et al: Coronary heart disease: Overweight and obesity as risk factors. Ann Intern Med 77:15, 1972.
17. Manson J, Colditz G, Stampfer M, et al: A prospective study of obesity and risk of coronary heart disease in women. N Engl J Med 322:882, 1990.
18. Lew E and Garfinkel L: Variations in mortality by weight among 750,000 men and women. J Chron Dis 32:563, 1979.
19. Maddox GL, et al: Overweight as social deviance and disability. J Health Soc Behav 9:287, 1968.
20. Canning H and Mayer J: Obesity: Its possible effect on college acceptance. N Engl J Med 275:1172, 1966.
21. Stunkard A, Sorensen T, Hanis C, et al: An adoption study of human obesity. N Engl J Med 314:193, 1986.
22. Bouchard C, Tremblay A, Després J, et al: The response to long-term overfeeding in identical twins. N Engl J Med 322:1477, 1990.
23. Bandini L, Schoeller D, Cyr H, et al: Validity of reported energy intake in obese and nonobese adolescents. Am J Clin Nutr 52:421, 1990.
24. Lichtman S, Pisarska K, Berman E, et al: Discrepancy between self-reported and actual caloric intake and exercise in obese subjects. N Engl J Med 327:1893, 1992.
25. Bray G: Classification and evaluation of the obesities. Med Clin North Am 73:161, 1989.
26. Kanarek R and Hirsch E: Dietary-induced overeating in experimental animals. Fed Proc 36:154, 1977.
27. Romieu I, Willett W, Stampfer M, et al: Energy intake and other determinants of relative weight. Am J Clin Nutr 47:406, 1988.
28. Ravussin E and Swinburn B: Pathophysiology of obesity. Lancet 340:404, 1992.
29. Ravussin E, Lillioja S, Knowler W, et al: Reduced rate of energy expenditure as a risk factor for body-weight gain. N Engl J Med 318:467, 1988.
30. Schoeller D and Fjeld C: Human energy metabolism: What have we learned from the doubly labeled water method? Annu Rev Nutr 11:355, 1991.
31. Wadden TA and Stunkard AJ: Social and psychological consequences of obesity. Ann Intern Med 103:1062, 1985.
32. Schachter S: Obesity and eating. Science 161:751, 1968.
33. Stunkard A: The relationship of gastric motility and hunger. A summary of the evidence. Psychosom Med 33:123, 1971.
34. Bruch H: Instinct and interpersonal experience. Comp Psychiat 11:495, 1970.
35. Stunkard AJ and Rush J: Dieting and depression reexamined. Ann Intern Med 81:526, 1974.

36. Louderback L: Fat Power: Whatever You Weigh is Right. New York, Hawthorne Books, 1970, pp 47–52.
37. Glucksman ML, et al: The response of obese patients to weight reduction. II. A quantitative evaluation of behavior. Psychosom Med 30:359, 1968.
38. Stunkard AJ and Mendelsen M: Obesity and the body image: I. Characteristics of disturbances in the body image of some obese patients. Am J Psychiatry 123:1296, 1967.
39. Bray GA and Gallagher TF: Manifestations of hypothalamic obesity in man: A comprehensive investigation of eight patients and a review of the literature. Medicine 54:301, 1975.
40. Puddey I, Parker M, Beilin L, et al: Effects of alcohol and caloric restrictions on blood pressure and serum lipids in overweight men. Hypertension 20:533, 1992.
41. Felson D, Zhang Y, Anthony J, et al: Weight loss reduces the risk for symptomatic knee osteoarthritis in women. Ann Intern Med 116:535, 1992.
42. Lissner L, Odell P, D'Agostino R, et al: Variability of body weight and health outcomes in the Framingham population. N Engl J Med 324:1839, 1991.
43. Garrow J: Treatment of obesity. Lancet 340:409, 1992.
44. Feinstein AR: The treatment of obesity: An analysis of methods, results, and factors which influence success. J Chron Dis 11:349, 1960.
45. Elliot DL, Goldberg L, and Girard DE: Obesity: Pathophysiology and practical management. J Gen Intern Med 2(3):188, 1987.
46. Fellows HH: Studies of relatively normal obese individuals during and after weight reduction. Am J Med Sci 181:301, 1931.
47. Bray GA: The myth of diet on management of obesity. Am J Clin Nutr 23:1141, 1970.
48. Sohar E and Sneh E: Follow-up of obese patients: 14 years after successful reducing diet. Am J Clin Nutr 20:845, 1973.
49. Kendall A, Levitsky D, Strupp B, et al: Weight loss on a low-fat diet: Consequence of the imprecision of the control of food intake in humans. Am J Clin Nutr 53:1124, 1991.
50. Werner SC: Comparison between weight reduction on a high-calorie, high-fat diet and on an isocaloric regimen high in carbohydrate. N Engl J Med 252:661, 1955.
51. Council on Foods and Nutrition: A critique of low-carbohydrate ketogenic reduction regimes. A review of Dr. Atkins' Diet Revolution. JAMA 224:1415, 1973.
52. Weinsier RL, Johnston MH, Doleys DM, et al: Dietary management of obesity: Evaluation of the time-energy displacement diet in terms of its efficacy and nutritional adequacy for long-term weight control. Br J Nutr 47:367, 1982.
53. Weinsier RL, Bacon JA, and Birch R: Time-calorie displacement diet for weight control: A prospective evaluation of its adequacy for maintaining normal nutritional status. Int J Obes 7:539, 1983.
54. Mirkin GB and Shore RN: The Beverly Hills diet. JAMA 246:2235, 1981.
55. Wadden TA, Stunkard AJ, and Brownell KD: Very low calorie diets: Their efficacy, safety, and future. Ann Intern Med 99:675, 1983.
56. Felig P: Four questions about protein diets. N Engl J Med 298:1025, 1978.
57. Lantigna RA, Amtruda JM, Biddle TL, et al: Cardiac arrhythmias associated with a liquid protein diet for the treatment of obesity. N Engl J Med 303:735, 1980.
58. Maddox GL and Liederman V: Obesity as a social disability with medical implications. J Med Educ 44:214, 1969.
59. Maiman LA, et al: Attitudes toward obesity and the obese among professionals. J Am Diet Assoc 74:331, 1979.
60. Maddox GL, et al: Overweight as a problem of medical management in a public outpatient clinic. Am J Med Sci 252:394, 1966.
61. Stunkard A and Reader J: The management of obesity. NY State J Med 58:78, 1958.
62. Mahoney MJ: *In* Enelow AJ and Henderson JB (eds): The Behavioral Treatment of Obesity in Applying Behavioral Science to Cardiovascular Risk. Proceedings of a Conference. Seattle, 1974. American Heart Association, 1975, pp 121–131.
63. Stunkard AJ: New therapies for eating disorders: Behavioral modification of obesity and anorexia nervosa. Arch Gen Psychiatry 26:39, 1972.
64. Bjorvell H and Rossner S: Long term treatment of severe obesity: Four year follow up of results of combined behavioural modification programme. BMJ 291:379, 1985.
65. Weintraub M, Sundaresan P, Schuster B, et al: Long-term weight control: The National Heart, Lung, and Blood Institute funded multimodal intervention study. Clin Pharmacol Ther 51:581, 1992.
66. Carey LC, Martin EWJ, and Mojzisik C: The surgical treatment of morbid obesity. Curr Probl Surg 21:7, 1984.
67. Gastric operations for obesity. Med Lett 26:113, 1984.
68. Freeman JP and Burchett H: Failure rate with gastric partitioning for morbid obesity. Am J Surg 145:113, 1983.
69. Garrow J: Dental splinting in the treatment of hyperphagic obesity. Proc Nutr Soc 33:29A, 1974.
70. Bruch H: Eating Disorders, Obesity, Anorexia Nervosa, and the Person Within. Philadelphia, WB Saunders, 1976.
71. Freidin RB and Lazerson AM: Terminating the physician-patient relationship in primary care. JAMA 24:819, 1979.
72. American Psychiatric Association: Diagnostic and Statistical Manual of Mental Disorders, 3rd ed, revised (DSM-III-R). Washington, D.C., American Psychiatric Association, 1987, pp 65–69.
73. Feighner JP, Robins E, Guze SB, et al: Diagnostic criteria for use in psychiatric research. Arch Gen Psychiatry 26:57, 1972.
74. Stangler R and Printz A: DSM-III: Psychiatric diagnosis in a university population. Am J Psychiatry 137:937, 1980.
75. Pope HG Jr, Hudson JI, and Yurgelun-Todd D: Anorexia nervosa and bulimia among three hundred suburban women shoppers. Am J Psychiatry 141:2, 1984.
76. Schwabb AD, Lippe BM, Chang RJ, et al: Anorexia nervosa (UCLA Conference). Ann Intern Med 94:371, 1981.
77. Lowenkopf EL: Bulimia: Concept and therapy. Comp Psychiatry 24:546, 1983.
78. Balaa M and Drossman DA: Eating disorders. Dis Mon 31:1, 1985.
79. Freund KM, Graham SM, Lesky LG, et al: Detection of bulimia in a primary care setting. J Gen Intern Med 8:236, 1993.
80. Bosking-Lodahl M: Cinderella's step sisters: A feminist perspective on anorexia nervosa and bulimia. Signs (Winter):342, 1976.
81. Harris RT: Bulimarexia and related serious eating disorders with medical complications. Ann Intern Med 99:800, 1983.
82. Palmer EP and Guay AT: Reversible myopathy secondary to abuse of ipecac in patients with major eating disorders. N Engl J Med 313:1457, 1985.
83. Isner JM, Roberts WC, Heymsfield SB, et al: Anorexia nervosa and sudden death. Ann Intern Med 102:49, 1985.
84. Arana GW and Hyman SE: Handbook of Psychiatric Drug Therapy, 2nd ed, Boston, Little, Brown, 1991, p 48.
85. Bruch H: Anorexia nervosa: Therapy and theory. Am J Psychiatry 139:12, 1982.
86. Agras WS and Kraemer HC: The treatment of anorexia nervosa: Do different treatments have different outcomes? *In* Stunkard AJ and Sellar E (eds): Eating and Its Disorders. New York, Raven Press, 1984.

85

Sexual Problems

MARTYN A. VICKERS, Jr., MD
LILI A. GOTTRIED, MD

Patients with sexual problems may have overt complaints and express a clear request for guidance and help. More frequently, however, conflicts over sexuality are expressed as or along with depression, anxiety, alcoholism, or other behavioral problems. Although the frequency of sexual problems encountered is in part a function of the physician's comfort and ease in dealing with these topics, some experts estimate that in half of married couples an area of sexual incompatibility may manifest itself in somatic symptoms or as general emotional unrest. In one survey it was found that the incidence of sexual problems reported by patients increased from 7.9 to 14% when the physician routinely asked about sexual symptoms in a general review of symptoms.[1]

Awareness of the effects of major illness or surgery on sexual functioning, whether physiologic or psychological, is crucial. In cases of minor illness, such as that of an adolescent with venereal disease, the patient may benefit from an opportunity to express fears about sequelae or from discussion that may lift some of the taboos and perceived shame surrounding this condition. A young woman who has had a recent abortion may be puzzled by her lack of sexual interest. The change in body image of a woman following mastectomy or hysterectomy often causes sexual inhibitions and can be overcome with a sensitive exploration of the patient's or couple's perceptions. Patients who have had myocardial infarction need a clear discussion of the sexual implications of their illness. All patients nowadays require counseling about safe sexual practices.

Openness about sexual expression and increasing expectations have generated recognition of a variety of specific sexual dysfunctions. These demand additional expertise from physicians. The opportunity to offer help with sexual problems has increased in the past few years, with newly expanded knowledge of the physiology of sexual response and methods of treatment. The scope of sexuality in practice is defined to a great extent by the physician's interest, attitudes, and receptivity to such problems. Patients are sensitive to discomfort or bias on the part of their physicians, which will hamper open communication. Some physicians feel uneasy or incompetent in dealing with sexual problems. The physician must explore the boundaries of his or her personal and ethical positions on sexuality. Inhibitions or discomfort with homosexuality or sexual deviance should be taken into account. The seductive potential of a detailed discussion of sexual practices may be disturbing to both the patient and the physician. It is desirable and important for the practitioner to establish a level of involvement with sexual issues at which he or she is comfortable and to have appropriate sources for referral beyond that point.

OBTAINING A SEXUAL HISTORY

The physician must project ease with sexual topics to neutralize the threatening aspects of revealing sexual concerns. Ideally, this history is pursued as nonjudgmentally as would be a history involving the respiratory or cardiovascular systems.

A working knowledge of normal sexual physiology underlies a meaningful history and accurate problem identification. The physician's goal is to deal constructively with overt complaints in a nonthreatening fashion or to allow underlying concerns to surface more freely. Questions on sexual function are naturally appended to a gynecologic or urogenital review of systems. Initial questions can be directed toward the perceived adequacy rather than the frequency of sexual intercourse with the spouse or partner. This establishes an atmosphere of openness that invites patients to raise specific sexual concerns. The goal of the primary physician is to communicate that sexuality is part of health and a legitimate sphere for discussion. Initial interviewing, however, should refrain from voyeuristic probing into details about sexual activity, which might make patients anxious or defensive.

Once a sexual problem is identified, the next goal is to obtain a more specific history. This information includes details about the onset and progression of the problem, its chronicity, and the patient's perceptions of its cause. Issues of communication between the patient and partner, attempted remedial measures, and overall expectations are relevant. A complaint of impotence, for example, requires information on when the symptoms first arose and under what circumstances, the frequency of recurrence, and what feelings have occurred in the partner. Relationship to organic illness, drugs, and alcohol may be critical. Communication requires use of common but appropriate words for sexual parts and activities rather than the vernacular. Slang and joking, even when used by patients, are inappropriate; yet a common understanding of terms must take into account the patient's background and educational level.

NORMAL VERSUS DISORDERED SEXUALITY

Disorders of sexual function can be classified by the level of the sexual response at which they arise. A working knowledge of the physiologic substrate of sexual behavior, as defined through the studies of Masters and Johnson,[2] is basic to such understanding. Men and women share the same neurophysiologic capacities, and the sexual experience passes through similar stages; an initial excitement phase, the arousal plateau, orgasm, and resolution. Dysfunction may arise in either sex at any of these levels. Interference with initial excitement, for example, is appreciated as loss of libido in men and frigidity in women. Dysfunctions after arousal, such as impotence, may involve the early or late excitement phase. Orgasmic dysfunctions include ejaculatory disturbances in men and anorgasmia in women.

Capacity for the normal sexual response extends beyond biologic and neurophysiologic capacities into the interpersonal dimension of psychosexual functioning. This has been characterized by Levine (see later).

Both partners are willing to make love. Each is able to relax. Nonsexual concerns disappear from awareness. A special alteration of consciousness supervenes marked by exclusive attention to one's own and one's partner's pleasurable sensation. The concern for the partner's sensations inconspicuously results in the formation of a feedback system whereby clues from the skin, breathing, posture, and utterances are used somewhat automatically to direct what happens next. The pleasure and excitement of each partner is infectious and augments the pleasure and excitement of the other. The rights of each partner to give and receive sexual pleasure are fully acceptable to both. Sex is completed with a high degree of personal pleasure and also with a sense of having shared a meaningful experience.[3]

Categorization of sexual dysfunctions as organic versus functional or psychogenic is based on the biologic model; a fuller appreciation of the sexual experience suggests a more complex pathogenesis. Sexual dysfunction may arise from ignorance or misinformation, be a symptom of poor communication or deterioration of a relationship, or arise from organic causes or psychiatric illness. The assessment of a specific case requires consideration on all these levels.

Impotence may serve as an example of how these various factors influence a specific dysfunction. In some cases, the symptom may arise from misinformation or misunderstanding over experiences or expectations. Frequent male concerns relate to penile size (erect or nonerect), potential for repetitive orgasm, or satisfaction of a partner. Similar concerns over body image and feelings of sexual inadequacy may arise in women over breast size. In such cases, reassurance about normal anatomy and explanations of sexual capacities for receiving and delivering pleasurable sexual experience may dispel such anxiety over performance.

Masturbation is a frequent source of guilt in men and women that interferes with sexual function and creates anxiety over presumed self-destructive effects. Reassurance about the normal spectrum of masturbatory behavior and its role in sexual experience can often dispel such feelings. Dysfunction may sometimes arise from a lack of knowledge about sexual anatomy or the relationship of working parts. Sympathetic counseling can lead to prompt resolution in these cases.

Differing sexual expectations between partners can lead to deterioration in the relationship. Conversely, conflicts in nonsexual areas can be manifest as sexual incompatibility. Although one partner may experience the dysfunction, successful therapy demands that both partners participate in therapy.[2] Counseling for couples may be the necessary intervention. Discussing the specifics of these issues with the couple in the office is the important first step in accurate diagnosis of sexual dysfunction. When a principally sexual problem is identified, or when disordered sexual function is found to be the major causative issue, specific treatment or referral is appropriate. To sort out these issues, the physician should be conversant with the major areas of sexual dysfunction. Although analogous problems can arise in men and women, separate consideration at this level is helpful.

SPECIFIC SEXUAL DYSFUNCTIONS IN MEN

Impotence

Impotence is defined as either primary (a lifelong absence of erection sufficient to accomplish coitus) or secondary (preceded at some time by adequate function). Primary impotence is rare. Organic causes include hypogonadism, penile arterial hypoplasia, penile venous dysfunction, or congenital neural abnormalities. Primary impotence is more frequently psychogenic in nature. Masters and Johnson report a variety of situations that may result in deep-seated psychological conflicts, such as severe sexual repression, disturbed mother-son relationship, and traumatic sexual experience.[2] Such conflicts may require formal psychiatric intervention. The history enables the primary physician to distinguish these cases from transient dysfunction or worries over sexual performance.

Secondary impotence is an acquired loss of erectile capacity sufficient to accomplish coitus. Occasional erectile failure may be universal in men, so that the diagnosis implies a frequency of failure at least in 25% of attempts at coitus. Secondary impotence is much more prevalent than primary impotence. Martin reported prevalence rates of impotence of 8% in men younger than 40 years of age up to 30% in men older than 60 years of age.[3]

In the past, a clear distinction was made between organic and psychogenic impotence. However, questions have been raised about the concept of purely psychogenic impotence. Subtle or undetected physical problems may exist in patients who develop impotence under conditions of psychological stress. Because of the psychological reactions to full or partial loss of potency, a vicious cycle can be created wherein psychological feedback further inhibits erectile capacity because of secondary depression and anxiety.

Physiology

Male sexual response is divided into four parts: (1) erection, (2) emission, (3) ejaculation, and (4) orgasm. Each portion has a separate neurologic mechanism. Frequently, patients may have impairment in one of these mechanisms

TABLE 85–1. CLASSIFICATION OF PHYSICAL (ORGANIC) CAUSES OF SECONDARY IMPOTENCE

Endocrine
Hypergonadotropic hypogonadism (primary testicular failure)
Hypogonadotropic hypogonadism secondary to pituitary or hypothalamic disease
Diabetes mellitus
Acromegaly
Adrenal neoplasms (with or without Cushing's syndrome)
Hyperprolactinemic states (pituitary adenomas)
Chromophobe adenoma
Hypothyroidism
Hyperthyroidism

Urologic
Peyronie's disease
Prostatitis
Phimosis
Priapism

Neurologic
Autonomic peripheral neuropathy (including diabetic neuropathy)
Degenerative disease (amyotrophic lateral sclerosis)
Spinal cord tumors or transection
Multiple sclerosis
Tabes dorsalis

Vascular
Athero-obstructive aortoiliac disease
Aneurysm
Arteritis

Chronic Medical Illnesses of Other Types That Often Are Associated with Impotence:

Cardiorespiratory
Cardiomyopathy
Coronary insufficiency
Pulmonary insufficiency (emphysema)

Hematologic
Hodgkin's disease
Leukemia, acute and chronic
Severe chronic sickle cell anemia

Infectious
Genital tuberculosis

Organ System Failure
Cirrhosis
Chronic renal failure
Toxicologic agents (lead, herbicides)

Surgical
Aortoiliac surgery
Radical pelvic surgery (cystectomy)
Postprostatectomy, suprapubic and transurethral (sometimes), perineal (frequently)
Pelvic irradiation

while the others remain intact. The ability to have an erection requires intact neural, vascular, hormonal, and psychological functioning. Erection is predominantly parasympathetic via the reflex arcs and occurs at S2, S3, and S4. Recent attention has been focused on the determination of the final neurotransmitter. Seminal emission is a manifestation of sympathetic activity of the thoracolumbar sympathetic trunk (T12–L3).[4] Orgasm is a psychic integration of all the various events. Finally, detumescence is caused by the release of epinephrine.

Evaluation and Treatment of Primary Impotence

Although primary impotence is rarely organic, an organic cause must be excluded prior to institution of definitive therapy. Office testing of the S2–S4 nerve roots (vibratory perception, bulbocavernous reflex), serum testosterone assay, and penile sleep monitoring are essential. If these studies are normal, referral to a urologist for pharmacologic penile injections or to a sex therapist for behaviorally based treatment is appropriate.[5] We are presently studying whether success rates can be improved by combining injection therapy with sex therapy.

If, on the other hand, the sleep studies suggest organic erectile dysfunction, a formal evaluation of the penile arterial and venous systems should be performed using duplex ultrasonography, pelvic arteriography, and dynamic pharmacocavernosometry.

Evaluation of Secondary Impotence

Organic cause may play a role in many cases of secondary impotence. Of cases of secondary impotence, 20 to 52% are primarily due to well-defined physical disorders.[6] Diabetes is a frequent cause of erectile failure, related to its adverse neurologic or vascular effects. Approximately one half of all diabetic men eventually suffer problems of impotence. Criteria for differentiating organic causes from functional causes of secondary impotence are elusive. Performance anxiety may frequently exacerbate a decrease in function related to underlying neurologic or vascular disease. Our current understanding of impotence suggests that the preferred strategy is to search first for an organic component with attention to psychogenic influences rather than to separate all impotence into either organic or psychogenic.[7]

Specific features in the history, nevertheless, may be helpful in distinguishing predominantly organic from psychogenic causes of impotence. Organic impotence most commonly arises in the setting of manifest chronic illness, such as vascular insufficiency or diabetes mellitus. The onset is usually insidious but is relentlessly progressive over a period of months or years. Organic causes may at first leave libido relatively intact. Such impotence is relatively complete once established, in contrast to that of psychogenic causes, which may be under great influence from life events and are more likely to begin abruptly after a crisis or interpersonal conflict. Organic impotence usually extends to all partners and occurs in all settings. The history of occasional erections and sporadic successful intercourse, however, does not rule out organic impotence, especially if related to endocrinologic dysfunction.[8] Sustained penile rigidity on awakening or during masturbation suggests psychogenic dysfunction.[9]

Differential Diagnosis

A partial list of medical conditions that may contribute to the organic type of impotence appears in Table 85–1. Drugs affecting the neurologic or vascular system can create a blockade in the neurophysiologic pathways responsible for erection (parasympathetic) and ejaculation (sympathetic) (Table 85–2.) Virtually any chronic illness may have

TABLE 85–2. DRUGS IMPAIRING SEXUAL RESPONSE

Alcohol
Benzodiazepines
Chlordiazepoxide (Librium)
Diazepam (Valium)
Oxazepam (Serax)
Chlorazepate (Tranxene)
Antidepressants, monoamine oxidase inhibitor type
Antidepressants, tricyclic type
Antischizophrenic agent (major tranquilizers)
Phenothiazines
Butyrophenones
Thioxanthenes
Antihypertensive drugs
Clonidine (Catapres)
Guanethidine (Ismelin)
Rauwolfia-reserpine
α-Methyldopa (Aldomet)
Propranolol (Inderal and other β-blockers)
Thiazides

an indirect negative impact on sexual response or performance.[10] It must be remembered, however, that the psychological reaction of patients to illness plays a strong role in the dynamics of these problems. Changes in self-image or sense of basic competence may be directly related to illness after, for example, a myocardial infarction. Anxiety about the risks of intercourse may be neutralized by counseling and, when appropriate, by graded submaximal exercise testing to establish the safety of coitus in the cardiac patient.[11] Determining the cause of organic impotence is more difficult when the problem arises in a previously healthy person or in someone with chronic but asymptomatic illness. In such patients, organic impotence is most often related to drugs or alcohol; autonomic peripheral neuropathy, frequently accompanying diabetes mellitus; endocrinologic dysfunction; or vascular insufficiency.[12]

Several investigators have reported on the frequency and causes of impotence in medical outpatients. Slag and associates reported a 34% prevalence of impotence among 1180 men followed at a Veterans Administration outpatient clinic: 25% of cases related to side effects of medications; 14% were psychogenic; 7% were neurologic; 6% were urologic; 10% were primary hypogonadism; 9% were secondary hypogonadism; 5% were hypothyroidism; 1% were hyperthyroidism; 4% were hyperprolactinemia; and 19% were miscellaneous or unknown.[13] In the past 3 years, fewer than 2% of patients evaluated for erectile dysfunction at the Men's Diagnostic and Treatment Center at the Brigham and Women's Hospital have had the physical stigmata or biochemical evidence of hypogonadism, hyperprolactinemia, or thyroid imbalance. Arterial insufficiency was suggested as a factor in more than half of 178 men with organic impotence.[14] Penile venous incompetence has been demonstrated in more than 60% of men with erectile dysfunction who failed to respond to intracavernosal smooth muscle relaxants.[15]

The important influence of drugs further complicates the evaluation of erectile dysfunction in chronic illness. A wide variety of prescribed drugs may impair the sexual response, as shown in Table 85–2. Almost all antihypertensive drugs have been implicated as causing erectile dysfunction.[16] Centrally acting drugs, like α-methyldopa, clonidine and reserpine, and peripheral blockers (e.g., guanethidine and propanalol) can unmask or intensify the symptoms of impotence. Seldom, however, does change of antihypertensive medications result in improvement of erectile dysfunction.

Alcohol, sedative-hypnotics, psychotropic drugs, and narcotics are other classes of drugs that interfere with sexual function. The physician must consider these drugs as compounding causes. When the underlying illness is identified (e.g., diabetes mellitus), it is important to emphasize that organic and psychogenic factors may coexist. Guidance, reassurance, and specific counseling may allow for improved function.

Hypogonadotropic hypogonadism, producing decreased levels of serum testosterone, follicle-stimulating hormones, and luteinizing hormones (LH), can result from diseases of the pituitary or hypothalamus. These can sometimes be differentiated by testing the pituitary reserve, determined by measuring the LH response to luteinizing hormone–releasing hormone (LHRH). Others patients have primary testicular failure (hypergonadotropic hypogonadism) with a low testosterone and elevated gonadotropin levels. An excess of prolactin is another cause of erectile dysfunction. Specific treatment to reduce prolactin levels by appropriate surgery or with medication, such as bromocriptine mesylate, is required. Hyperprolactinemia is commonly accompanied by low testosterone levels that may require correction with intramuscular (IM) testosterone. Correction of clearly low levels may be of benefit; however, treatment of borderline low serum testosterone with IM testosterone rarely corrects erectile dysfunction and has the attendant risk of stimulating growth of an occult prostatic cancer. In general, testosterone treatment in patients with low levels of this hormone enhances sexual interest and the frequency of sex acts, and it may have less effect on erectile function.

Vasculogenic impotence has assumed new importance for several reasons, the most important of which is the attribution of impotence to arteriosclerosis of the internal pudendal and penile arteries. Penile ultrasonography can identify arteriogenic impotence, and surgical treatment with revascularization is available. The possibility of a vascular lesion of the penis, with or without concomitant peripheral vascular disease, should always be considered.

Assessment

Although a urologist may ultimately be called on to perform special diagnostic tests, the primary physician usually makes the first inquiry about the patient's disorder. The general physician must decide to what extent patients with a complaint of impotence require an evaluation for organic disease.

It is important to set aside adequate time for a careful history and physical examination. The onset and progression of the problem and the current level of functioning of the patient are carefully documented. A detailed sexual history, particularly concerning the presence or absence of nocturnal erections, other types of sexual dysfunction, dysfunction with different sexual partners, possible psychogenic factors, present and past illnesses, medications, drinking behavior, and family history of diabetes are all important. A history of sudden onset of the impotence, of its selective occurrence, or of nonsexual erections present in the morning on awakening, during masturbation, or during fantasizing is useful in suggesting a psychological origin. A progressive organic disorder is suggested by a sequence of deterioration that consists initially of decreased rigidity and frequency of erection and progresses through problems with inability to maintain an erection, achieving an erection only under very stimulating sexual circumstances, and decreased frequency of nonsexual erections leading eventually to a total loss of erectile ability. Identification of systemic diseases that may be associated with dysfunction is important, as is identification of prior surgical procedures or medications that might affect potency.

The initial physical examination should be directed toward identifying vascular, neurologic, hormonal, or other factors that could be associated with the inability to maintain an erection. A vascular etiology may be suggested by absent peripheral pulses, femoral bruits, or trophic skin changes. More commonly, however, penile arterial insufficiency exists in the presence of normal peripheral pulses. Doppler studies and penile/brachial indices may indicate diminished penile blood flow. Duplex ultrasonography of the penis with Doppler after intracavernosal injection of papaverine is required for confirmation of penile arterial patency.[17] Penile corporovenous dysfunction is assessed with dynamic pharmacocavernosometry.[18]

The initial neurologic examination should include testing of perianal sensation (S1–S5), strength of small muscles in the feet (S1–S2), and sphincter tone (S2–S4). Anal and bulbocavernosus reflexes (i.e., contraction of the anal sphincter on stroking with a tongue blade; contraction of the scrotum on squeezing the penile bulb) should be evaluated to exclude peripheral sacral neurologic disease. Internal pudendal sensory neural function is assessed by vibratory testing using a tuning fork or biothesiometer, which is gently applied to the lateral aspects of the penis and the glans penis. Direct evaluation of the cavernosal motor supply requires sophisticated electromyogram (EMG) analysis. Indirect evidence of its integrity comes from changes of penile circumference and rigidity during sleep, as detected by the nocturnal penile tumescence (NPT) monitor.

Identification of normal secondary sexual characteristics, gynecomastia, and testicular size are important. Small, soft testes or evidence of incomplete virilization suggests hypogonadism. Gynecomastia suggests hyperprolactinemia. The lower genitourinary tract should be examined, with particular attention to penile abnormalities (i.e., penile curvature or scar).

Laboratory studies should include a multichannel serum analysis and measurement of fasting or 2-hour postprandial blood sugar. A testosterone level may be considered if the patient has remained unable to have an erection under all conditions for more than 3 months. Levels of follicle-stimulating hormone, LH, and prolactin are obtained to clarify the cause of a low serum testosterone.

When there remains a significant doubt as to whether the erectile dysfunction is on a primary organic or psychogenic basis, NPT may be very helpful. Totally absent penile tumescence and rigidity during rapid eye movement (REM) sleep is suggestive of organic impotence.[19–21] Likewise, normal tumescence and rigidity (the presence of at least one episode of penile rigidity equalling or exceeding 550 g and lasting 5 minutes, during two consecutive study nights) implies psychogenic impotence.[22]

Management

The extent of the diagnostic evaluation and therapy recommended by the physician should depend on the patient's motivation and on the extent to which psychogenic or organic factors, or both, are causal. Some individuals with psychogenic impotence are depressed. These patients often have a low level of libido. Reassuring the patient that he has normal erectile capacity may be all that is required. Behavioral therapy, beginning with nongenital sensate focusing, is designed to treat the larger number of individuals in whom performance-related anxiety is a major contributor to impotence. In this approach, the patient and his partner perform exercises, initially without the demand to achieve an erection, and progress, after anxiety abates, to each new step until intercourse is performed. Published reports of these modifications and others of the Masters and Johnson method either contain no group of untreated patients with whom to compare the outcomes or were poorly controlled for confounding variables such as the patient's age, motivation, and availability of a cooperative partner. Nevertheless, at least one third of individuals seeking out and undergoing this therapy reported that it had been successful.[1] Success is more likely when the patient's libido is active and the marital or sexual relationship is stable. Yohimbine has yet to be proved effective in psychogenic or organic impotence through a complete double-blinded cross-over study.

Medical and Surgical Therapy

Correction of endocrinologic abnormalities, hypogonadism, or hyperprolactinemia will frequently result in remission of erectile dysfunction. Revascularization of the penis, in patients with obstruction within the pudendal arterial system, has had success rates of 30 to 40% in highly selected patients (young patients with a history of a straddle injury).[23] Neurologic erectile dysfunction has been widely and successfully treated with pharmacologic agents (e.g., papaverine, phentolamine, and PGE_1). Patients with corporovenous dysfunction have been treated with ligation and excision of the incompetent penile veins. Long-term follow-up of these patients is not yet available. Success rates of 40 to 50% have been experienced at 2-year follow-ups.[24] Other therapeutic options for this group of patients includes a penile prosthesis or a vacuum constriction device. The latter is relatively inexpensive and is well received by patients with a stable sexual relationship.

More than 80% of all patients with organic erectile dysfunction are suitable candidates for the Pharmacologic Erection Program (PEP), utilizing papaverine, phentolamine, PGE_1, or any combination of these three drugs. The program begins with in-office pharmacologic testing. The first step is to determine the dosage of intracavernosally injected vasoactive substance that will induce 15 to 30 minutes of penile rigidity sufficient for vaginal penetration. The patient is then instructed on the technique of sterile corporal injection. He is taught to apply a rubber band about the base of his penis, cleanse its lateral aspect with an alcohol wipe, steady the penis in a horizontal position, insert a 27-gauge needle at a 90-degree angle into the left or right corpus cavernosum and slowly inject a vasoactive substance. On occasion, the patient may be unable to perform the injection due to lack of manual dexterity, tremors, obesity, or needle phobia. In these situations, the sexual partner can be taught to perform the injection.

At his next visit, the patient performs a self-injection with supervision. He is then provided the following: (1) one ampule containing 10 ml of a vasoactive drug or a drug combination, 10 27-gauge ½″ needles and 10 1-ml syringes; (2) printed illustrations of the injection technique; (3) the office telephone number to call if he has questions about PEP; (4) an emergency telephone number to call if the office is closed; and (5) a printed form to be signed that contains a detailed description of the attendant risks of the PEP program. Priapism and fibrosis are the major side effects of using papavarine, phentolamine, or PGE_1, which are vasodilators and not specifically contraindicated, if used cautiously, in patients with underlying stable vascular or coronary artery disease.

Each patient is informed of the importance of seeking emergency medical treatment if his drug-induced erection lasts for more than 4 hours. If he adheres to the drug dosage, determined by in-office testing, and injects only once each 48-hour period, it is extremely unlikely that he will experience priapism. In fact, in the past 3 years, spanning several thousand at-home injections, we have needed to see and treat only one patient on one occasion for drug-induced priapism.

The second global option for this group of patients is a penile prosthesis. A variety of prostheses are available that are semirigid and inflatable. Improvements in design of the prosthesis and the surgical technique in implantation has resulted in these devices being functionally and cosmetically acceptable. The vacuum constriction device is another option that is available for patients with organic disease independent of its primary etiology.

Premature Ejaculation

Premature ejaculation is a common dysfunction that can often be treated effectively by the primary care or family physician. The sexually normal male has voluntary control over his ejaculatory reflex, which allows him to thrust while he is at a high level of arousal, until he chooses to "let go" and ejaculate.[25] As with impotence, performance anxiety is often a secondary stress contributing to premature ejaculation. Counseling with the patient and partner and instruction in behavioral modification techniques or sensate focus exercises are often effective as initial therapy. Start/stop ejaculator control exercises or squeeze techniques are described in several sources.[1, 25] These involve controlled stimulation by the partner to enable the man to recognize levels of sensations that precede the threshold of ejaculation. Start/stop exercises can establish such awareness and lead to improved control in 90% of cases. The squeeze technique described by Masters and Johnson is similarly effective in the treatment of this problem. When results are poor after such approaches, masturbation at some time prior to intercourse may help to control prematurity. This condition may require a referral for sexual counseling.

Ejaculatory failure, or the inability of the erect penis to ejaculate, is a rare disorder, involving less than 0.5% of men, but becomes more common with advancing years. When the condition is encountered, organic causes in the genitourinary system as well as drugs should be considered. Behavior modification or sexual therapy approaches may be successful in the absence of urologically defined abnormalities.

Retrograde ejaculation, or expulsion of semen into the bladder rather than through the external urethral meatus, is most frequently caused by damage of the sympathetic nerves during retroperitoneal surgery or by damage to the internal urethral sphincter during transurethral surgery. In the former case, sympathomimetics (imipramine or ephedrine) given 30 minutes before intercourse, may tighten the bladder neck sufficiently to prevent a retrograde ejaculation. In the latter situation, pharmacologic manipulation is seldom beneficial. The risk and probability of developing retrograde ejaculation should be discussed with the patient prior to the transurethral procedure.

SPECIFIC SEXUAL DYSFUNCTIONS IN WOMEN

In women, as in men, impairment of sexual response may occur at the excitement or orgasmic phase and is primary or secondary.[26] Problems with excitement, analogous to impotence in men, are defined as frigidity or general unresponsiveness. They involve the inability to attain or maintain the characteristic lubrication and swelling of the genitalia and are characterized as primary if there has never been a sexual response in any setting. This can occur despite the desire to engage in sexual activity, but there is usually a lack of erotic feeling. There is some evidence that an important cause of decreased sexual interest may be due to suppression of ovulation, as by oral contraceptives.[27] Orgastic dysfunction is a specific inhibition of the orgastic component of the sexual response, despite intact desire and an erotic response. There is frequently confusion about the old argument of vaginal or coital orgasm versus clitoral orgasm, which are known now to be identical physiologically and to involve a subjective response. Orgastic dysfunction is primary if the woman has never experienced an orgasm, either during a sexual encounter or through masturbation.

As in men, primary orgastic dysfunction in women can arise from serious, deep-seated fears involving close interpersonal relationships. These patients commonly need referral for psychotherapy. More often, however, lack of education about orgasm, guilt about sexual abandon, or fear of working openly with the partner on satisfying techniques is the problem. Whether manifested as frigidity or as orgastic blockade, secondary dysfunctions are partner-specific, not present during masturbation, or new in onset. They often have to do with conflict within the relationship; guilt, as during an illicit affair; or anxiety and depression not specifically related to the sexual act. As mentioned earlier, losses of self-esteem, through illness, through change in body image after surgery or with aging, or through job loss or dissatisfaction, can upset the delicate mechanisms necessary for the complete sexual response. The approach to these problems is analogous to that in men. In addition, clitoral stimulation by the patient or her partner is sometimes employed as a technique to facilitate orgasm.

A third dysfunction, after frigidity and anorgasmia, is specific to women. This is vaginismus, which is the involuntary spastic contraction of the outer one third of the vagina, so that the introitus is literally closed to any object. This is thought to represent a phobic avoidance of penetration, and although it can be associated with other phase dysfunctions, it is sometimes found alone, with intact desire, arousal, and orgasmic phases. Vaginismus is often a complaint that is made or recognized at the time of a pelvic examination. Treatment, involving sequential dilatation in a relaxed setting by the patient and eventually with her partner, has an excellent outcome, approaching 90% success in the motivated person.

A final female dysfunction is dyspareunia, which involves pain during coitus. Although it may be simply a matter of inadequate lubrication, dyspareunia often signals the need for a diligent search for significant pelvic disease. Chronic pelvic infections, endometriosis, chemical or atrophic vaginitis, or a variety of structural gynecologic disorders may be considered as the basis of dysfunction.

ACKNOWLEDGMENT

We wish to acknowledge the contributions of Arthur J Siegel, MD, and Jerome Richie, MD, who co-wrote this chapter in the first and second editions.

REFERENCES

1. Masters WH and Johnson VE: Human Sexual Inadequacy. Boston, Little, Brown, 1970.
2. Masters WH and Johnson VE: The Human Sexual Response. Boston, Little, Brown, 1970.
3. Martin CE: Marital and sexual factors in relation to age, disease, and longevity. *In* Wirt RD, Winokur G, and Roff M (eds): Life History Research in Psychopathology, Vol 4. Minneapolis, University of Minnesota Press, 1975.
4. Kuntz A: The Autonomic Nervous System, 4th ed. Philadelphia, Lea & Febiger, 1965.
5. Vickers M, DeNobrega A, Dluhy R: Diagnosis and treatment of psychogenic erectile dysfunction in a urological setting. J Urol 149:1258–1261, 1993.
6. Jonas U, Thou W, and Stief G: Erectile Dysfunction. New York, Springer-Verlag, 1991.
7. Bohlan JG: Sleep reaction monitoring in the evaluation of male erectile failure. Urol Clin North Am 8:119, 1981.
8. Spark RE, White RA, and Connolly BB: Impotence is not always psychogenic. JAMA 243:750, 1980.
9. Seagraves K, Segraves R, and Schoenberg H: Use of sexual history to differentiate organic from psychogenic impotence. Arch Sex Behav 16(2):125, 1987.
10. Weiss HD: The physiology of human penile erection. Ann Intern Med 76:793, 1972.
11. Hellerstein H and Friedman EJ: Sexual activity and the postcoronary patient. Arch Intern Med 125:125, 1970.
12. Barry JM and Hodges CV: Impotence: A diagnostic approach. J Urol 119:575, 1978.
13. Slag M, Morley JE, Elson MK, et al: Impotence in medical clinic outpatients. JAMA 249:1736, 1983.
14. Virag R, Bouilly P, and Frydman D: Is impotence an arterial disorder? A study of arterial risk factors in 440 impotent men. Lancet 1:181, 1985.
15. Rajfer J, Rosciszewski A, and Mehringer M: Prevalence of corporeal venous leakage in impotent men. J Urol 140:69, 1988.
16. Kaplan HS: The New Sex Therapy. New York, Brunner Maxel, 1974.

16a. Mulligan T, Schmitt B: Testosterone for erectile failure. J Gen Intern Med 8:517, 1993.

17. Benson C and Vickers M: Sexual impotence caused by vascular disease: Diagnosis with duplex sonography. AJR Am J Roentgenol 153:11499, 1989.
18. Vickers M, Benson C, Dluhy R, and Ball R: The current cavernosometric criteria for corporovenous dysfunction are too strict. J Urol 147:614, 1992.
19. Van Arsdalen KN and Wein AJ: A critical review of diagnostic tests used in the evaluation of the impotent male. World J Urol 1:218, 1983.
20. Hosking J, Bennet T, Hampton JR, et al: Diabetic impotence: Studies of nocturnal erection during REM sleep. BMJ 2:1394, 1979.
21. Wasserman MD, Pollak CP, Spielman AJ, et al: The differential diagnosis of impotence. The measurement of nocturnal penile tumescence. JAMA 243:2038, 1980.
22. Karacan I, Salis P, Thorby J, and Williams R: The autogenicity of nocturnal penile tumescense. Waking and Sleeping 1:27, 1976.
23. Zorgniotti AW: Diagnosis and Management of Impotence. Philadelphia, BC Decker, 1991.
24. Knoll LD, Furlow WL, Benson RC: Penile venous surgery for the management of cavernosal venous leakage. Int J Impotence Res 2:21–27, 1990.
25. Kaplan HS: How to overcome premature ejaculation. New York, Brunner/Mazel, 1989.
26. Levine SB: Marital sexual dysfunction: Female dysfunctions. Ann Intern Med 86:558, 1977.
27. Adams DB, Gold AR, and Burt AD: Rise in female-initiated sexual activity at ovulation and its suppression by oral contraceptives. N Engl J Med 299:1145, 1978.

86

Sleep Disorders

QUENTIN REGESTEIN, MD

Obligatory but enigmatic, sleep derives from the circadian rhythms found in all living creatures and from the ecologic niche of human beings, who must depend on vision but see relatively poorly at night. The disorders of sleep include insomnia, hypersomnia, or pathologic conditions precipitated or aggravated by sleep. Significant insomnia afflicts about 15% of adults, according to epidemiologic surveys; sleep apnea appears to be quite common, especially in older age groups, whereas the parasomnias appear particularly during childhood. Medical conditions commonly affect sleep because of their disturbing symptoms, or because of side effects from their treatments. In turn, disordered sleep may alter and worsen various disease problems, and therefore most physicians will see patients who have sleep disorders.

Normal sleep means quiet recumbency, lessened responsiveness, and arousability. Polygraph measurements divide it into distinct stages. As these stages progress from light to deep, the electroencephalographic background rhythm progressively slows in frequency: stage I, "light sleep" or "drowsy," shows breaking up of the alpha (8 to 13 Hz) rhythm and appearance of the theta (3 to 7 Hz) rhythm; stage II, "medium sleep," shows predominance of theta activity; and stages III and IV, "deep" or "slow-wave sleep," respectively, show at least 20% and at least 50% delta (1 to 3 Hz) rhythms. Hallmark patterns additionally mark the stages: stage I has slow eye movements; stage II has "K complexes" (an evoked potential–like sharp positive wave followed by a negative wave) and "spindles" (brief 12 to 14 Hz patterns). Rapid eye movement (REM) sleep, "dreaming," or "paradoxic" sleep has an electroencephalogram (EEG) like that of stage I but bursts of eye movements and quiescent electromyographic muscle activity.

The different stages are associated with different clinical problems. Deep sleep entails the least cortical activation. Therefore, enuresis, night terrors, and sleepwalking occur in deep sleep because these unremembered automatisms escape cortical suppression. REM sleep manifests autonomic arousal and therefore may precipitate episodes of nocturnal angina, cardiac arrhythmias, or peptic ulcer distress.

From infancy through senescence, sleep gradually becomes less solid. The older person takes longer to fall asleep, has less deep sleep, and has more intervening wakeful periods. When this natural decline develops sufficiently to reinforce some chronic disruptor of sleep, insomnia may supervene with apparent spontaneity.

A person's total sleep time varies more between nights than between weeks. Although adults may average 7 to 8 hours of nightly sleep, twin studies suggest that total sleep time is a constitutional trait. It varies widely from the few per cent of individuals who need fewer than 4 hours to those less fortunate few saddled with more than 9 hours of sleep per night.

INSOMNIA

Fifteen to twenty-five per cent of Americans admit various degrees of insomnia in epidemiologic surveys, and about 10% use sleeping pills.[1] These figures much increase in older age groups.

Physicians often neglect to specifically diagnosis insomnia or else rapidly jump to a diagnosis without considering the alternatives. A nonspecific prescription for hypnotic drugs often ensues. The underestimation by the insomniac of polygraphically recorded sleep time further confuses clinical concepts of insomnia. Defining insomnia as any complaint of insufficient sleep provides clinical guidance. Although insomnia is frequently attributed to noise or other environmental disturbance, most people living near airports and railroads sleep well. Insomnia is serenely ascribed to psychopathology, despite the uninterrupted sleep observed in many individuals with severe thought or personality disorders. A systematic diagnostic investigation is therefore preferred over casual and obvious explanations for insomnia, especially in recurrent cases. Such an investigation should be done after obvious interferences with sleep have been removed, such as irregular sleep schedules, drugs that affect the nervous system, disturbing activity near bedtime, or disruptive disease symptoms.

Transient Insomnia After Bereavement. Unexpected loss provokes insomnia, especially among those with higher arousal tendencies or additional provocations for insomnia, such as caffeine. Sleep may return quickly in adaptable persons, but less so in the ill or rigid. Psychological regression may induce sleep-disrupting habits, such as irregular arising times or over-reliance on sedatives. After a year, apparent reaction to devastating loss implies psychopathology, as do sleepless reactions to the vicissitudes of life, such as examinations, tax season, or job deadlines. Reminders of losses, such as an anniversary or a retrial, may reprecipitate transient insomnia.

Primary Insomnia. Primary insomnia often begins in the fourth decade with a prolonged sleep onset time. Such patients may suffer a plethora of forced thoughts on retiring. Thereafter, they may drop into lighter sleep early in the night and progress to deeper sleep as the night wears on, the reverse of normal patterns. Sleep returns rapidly after any brief night awakenings. The patient awakens in the morning from relatively deep sleep and may remain sleepy for a half hour or more. The sleep onset difficulty may disappear on trips away from home. Afflicted individuals tend to be alert, introspective, cautious, scrupulous people who frequently anticipate or ruminate. "To me nothing is trivial," said one. Some are prone to anxiety and depression when distressed, simmer down slowly after excitement, and are aroused for hours after an argument or squash game in the evening.

Psychiatric Problems. Prior to any investigations, insomnia is often attributed to insufficient coping with life's challenges. In fact, major character or thought disorders do not necessarily interfere with sleep, and anxious people who practice sleep hygiene may sleep well. A patient's self-diagnosed neurosis may motivate fruitless referral for psychotherapy to relieve insomnia before any sleep hygiene is attempted. Failure to adhere to sleep-promoting regimens better justifies such referral.

Endogenous depression is the most frequently unrecognized psychiatric cause of insomnia. Unexplained early wakening may progress to fitful sleep for the entire night. The individual may deny depressed or sad feelings or crying spells but have other depressive symptoms, such as lessened enjoyment; sardonic attitudes; appetite or weight loss; unexplained diarrhea or constipation; intolerance of repetitive stimuli, such as lights, noises, television, traffic, or commotion; temperamental outbursts; increased pains; accentuated suspicion; worry about occult disease; or energy decline. After negative physical examination and screening tests results, bedtime sedatives may prove but transiently effective and the patient, increasingly desperate.

The increased arousal caused by many psychiatric disorders will be manifest day and night. Therefore, disorders involving anxiety, phobia, affective changes, and paranoid states often cause insomnia, in contradistinction to problems associated with decreased arousal, such as psychopathy, mental subnormality, or schizophrenias marked predominantly by apathy and affective blunting.

Drugs. The commonest drugs disrupting sleep are caffeine, alcohol, and nicotine. Caffeine has a 12- to 20-hour duration of action[2] and lightens polygraphically recorded sleep of laboratory volunteers. Often, patients will be unaware of the volumes of cola drinks they consume daily. Those who consume the equivalent of 6 or more cups of coffee are likely to use sedatives as well and be groggier in the morning.[3] Alcohol is the commonest hypnotic drug but lightens sleep and increases body temperature and body movements later in the night.[4] Chronic alcoholics have more broken sleep that persists months[5] after quitting using alcohol. Nicotine has direct stimulant effects, as indicated not only by its appetite-suppressing and addictive properties but also by the deeper sleep of those who quit smoking.[6] Heavy smokers frequently awaken to smoke one or two cigarettes. Their nightly withdrawal state is indicated by the high importance they attach to the morning's first cigarette. The chronic lung disease developed through smoking may lessen breathing during sleep and thus cause wake periods. Individuals addicted to nasal decongestants may suffer sleep disruption.

Prescription drugs that disrupt sleep include β-blockers, β-agonists, xanthines, methyldopa, levodopa, methysergide, antibronchospastics, and antiarrhythmics. These agents presumably disrupt sleep through their actions on the neurotransmitters regulating sleep. β-Blockers may exert central nervous system effects for several weeks after they are discontinued.[7] Exogenous hormones, including steroids or thyroid hormone, and antiarrhythmic drugs may also disrupt sleep. Diuretics may induce the restless legs syndrome, presumably through electrolyte imbalance or diminished peripheral circulation. Sedatives taken during the day or at bedtime may worsen sleep by habituation and withdrawal states or through cortical disinhibition in some patients. Stimulating antidepressants may lessen sleep, especially among elderly patients.

Movement Disorders. Although parkinsonian tremor and the stereotypies of neurodegenerative conditions may disappear during sleep, some motor movements occur or worsen during this time. Sudden leg or whole body jerks commonly occur as an individual falls asleep and do not occur thereafter. Other movements, like teeth grinding, twitches, talking, sitting up, or even walking may occur without disturbing sleep. Common movement problems disrupting sleep are the restless legs syndrome[8] and nocturnal myoclonus.

Restless legs syndrome involves an agitated feeling deep in the legs, with twitches and small leg movements when the legs are at rest. An irresistible need to walk around continually compels the patient to leave bed before falling asleep. Mild pain or crampiness may be present, and paresthesias may begin peripherally and rise as far as the abdomen. Inexplicably, the symptoms sometimes disappear as soon as the patient stands up, only to recur again at rest.

This symptom complex stems from conditions that impair lower motor neuron or peripheral nerve function, such as peripheral vascular disease, electrolyte imbalances often involving the use of diuretics, diabetes mellitus, avitaminoses, intervertebral disk disease, paraneoplastic syndromes, and neurogenic amyotrophies. Neuroleptic akathisia, muscle cramps, or anxious restlessness may also be involved.

Nocturnal myoclonus, or "periodic movements," involves discrete twitches, usually in the legs, that occur every 20 to 30 seconds for lengthy periods during the night. These may cause lightened sleep or wakefulness but may occur without change of sleep stage. If such movements are undetected or unremembered, the patient may have daytime sleepiness rather than insomnia. The affected person's bed partner may detect these movements and should be interviewed. Myoclonic jerks may rarely be provoked by stimulant or antidepressant medication but remain otherwise unexplained.

Insomnia in Old Age

Insomnia complaints increase with age; 25 to 45% of those over 70 years of age complain of significant insomnia. Although one hears that old people "need" less sleep, most of them obtain average amounts with the help of naps. However, sleep becomes lighter and more interrupted with age. Average sleep of healthy individuals over 50 years old is reportedly 24 minutes less than that of similar subjects aged 30 to 49 years.[9] Sleep is preserved in old people who retain intact cerebral functioning, as evidenced by tests of intelligence and cerebral blood flow. Biologic timing systems,[10] which adjust bodily circadian rhythms to support the internal economy and control of the body, depend primarily on the external light-dark schedule after about age 45 years, thus amplifying the effects of any sleep scheduling irregularities.

Against this background of more fragile sleep, some elderly have difficulties that further worsen sleep. Some of them remain in bed too long in a fruitless search for more sleep. Their greater morbidity entails more sleep-disrupting symptoms, such as joint pain irritated by movement, reflux esophagitis aggravated by lying down, or nocturnal angina. They also use disproportionately large amounts of sedatives, which are excreted more slowly and which may further impair the cerebral functions that support sound sleep. Although dementia impairs sleep, agitation often remits when psychotropic drugs are discontinued.[11] Age also causes a higher incidence of snoring, sleep apnea, and nocturnal myoclonus.

Treatments

A careful routine of sleep hygiene should be instituted in all cases of insomnia not easily remedied by the removal of obvious irritants. Maintaining a daily sleep chart of rising times, naps, retiring times, and sleep quality will provide baseline measurements against which treatments may be judged (Fig. 86–1). Rising at a regular clock time fosters a regular circadian rhythm[10] and should be done 7 days a week; a regular bedtime will help ensure a regular rising time. Ideally, all drugs that affect the nervous system should be gradually discontinued. Although caffeine and alcohol tend to be readily discontinued by those with significant insomnia, careful individualized behavioral techniques, use of nicotine chewing gum, or skin patches, and an optimistic long-term approach are usually needed to encourage withdrawal from nicotine. Prolonged in-bed times, often maintained by unemployed insomniacs, should be avoided in favor of a regular amount of total daily in-bed time, according to the individual's estimated preinsomnia baseline. One should avoid irregular naps, large suppers, and evening disturbances. Periodic and systematic review of sleep charts, the patient's practices, adherence to clinic suggestions, and progress should be undertaken until optimal habits are induced or the insomnia is controlled by the patient. The restriction of total in-bed times to the patient's estimated sleep time, with 15-minute increments prescribed until sleep occupies at least 90% of in-bed time, can be adjusted by daily telephone reports.

Treatment of hyperarousal insomnia aims to lower arousal level at bedtime. Scrupulous sleep hygiene, relaxing, predictable evening routines, restriction of annoying and arousing activities to an earlier time, and progressive muscle relaxation exercises or meditation techniques all help. These are practiced in a supine position with legs uncrossed and arms at the side in an undisturbed place outside the bedroom once or twice a day until they are well mastered and induce a feeling of relaxation. Thereafter, they are done on nights that risk little insomnia, such as

A

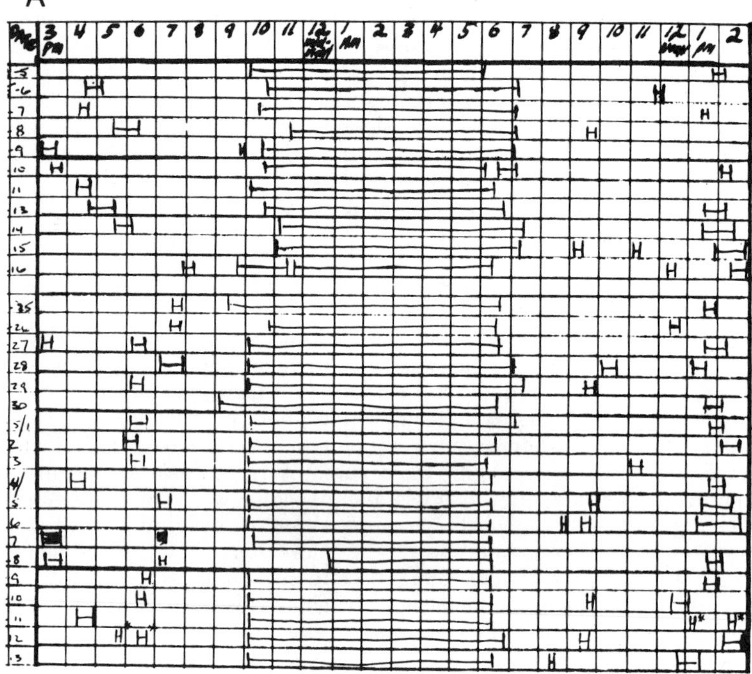

B

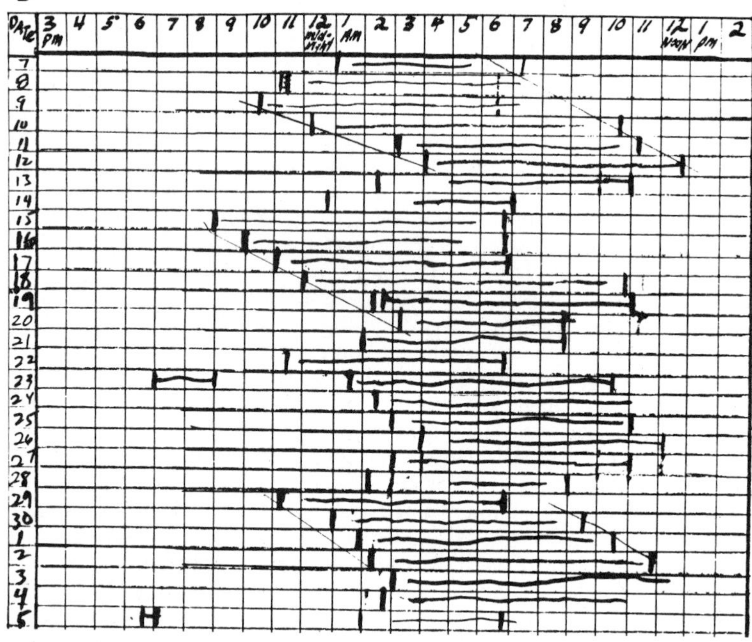

FIGURE 86–1. Sleep charts. The amount and solidness of sleep and regularity of bedtimes and arising times and of naps are shown. Events such as use of alcohol or medication or occurrence of parasomnias (qv) can also be indicated, and clinical progress is monitored. *A,* Chart A was made by a 43-year-old man with idiopathic hypersomnia. It shows a pattern of solid sleep and multiple naps. Timing of possible stimulant use is suggested by clusters of naps around 9.00 AM, 1.30 PM, and 4.30 to 6.30 PM. *B,* Chart B records the sleep schedule of a 34-year-old graduate student with delayed sleep phase syndrome. Obligatory morning meetings, progressive bedtime delays, and exhaustion (as indicated by sudden early bedtime and naps) result in repeated sleep delay patterns that last for approximately 1 week.

weekends and vacations. After several weeks, they are then applied every bedtime.

Clinical dilemmas may ensue as the hyperaroused individual resents sacrificing habits like occasional alcohol or late sleeping. Discussions of the imposed choices may resolve such problems.

Bedtime sedatives may be highly effective in such patients and risk little habituation because these thoughtful individuals wish to reserve them for particularly problematic nights. Their availability in the medicine chest may lessen fearfulness, thus promoting sleep.

The treatment of endogenous depression usually requires an adequate trial of antidepressant medication. In diagnostically unclear cases, sleep charts should be gathered for at least 2 weeks before medication is taken. Thereafter, good rapport and the education of the patient about these complex drugs are mandatory. This requires explanation of the lag period prior to therapeutic action and the probable side effects of such drugs. Sedating tricyclic antidepressants, such as doxepin or trazodone, may be taken at bedtime in doses that gradually increase to the point of causing mild dry mouth. Patients who are insistent, agitated, severely distressed, uncooperative, or unable to work merit psychiatric consultation.

When drug-induced insomnia is diagnosed, withdrawal of the offending drug provides a decisive diagnostic test as well as an effective treatment. When continued administration of the drug is required, a balance must be struck between the relief of insomnia and of other problems.

When antihypertensive β-blockers are incriminated, the

patient may be switched to peripherally acting agents, such as angiotensin-converting enzyme inhibitors or calcium-channel blockers. Clinical dilemmas may arise when adrenergic drugs are required by an asthmatic insomniac. Optimizing drug regimens by use of minimal doses, shorter-acting medications later in the day, or greater reliance on inhaled steroids may lessen sleep disruption.

To obtain interpretable diagnostic test results, hypnotics must be withdrawn, tapered over weeks or months to prevent worsening insomnia. Some patients who sleep poorly on fixed doses of bedtime sedatives may have only drug withdrawal insomnia, which can be remedied by exquisitely gradual withdrawal. This may require randomly mixing capsules containing slightly less medication in with the month's drug supply and use of small decrements, for example, one eighth of a capsule or crushed tablet powder. Some patients reduce medication doses to a minimum below which insomnia repeatedly reappears. Further diagnostic re-evaluation is then warranted.

Restless leg syndrome may be relieved by treatment of the primary condition, a bedtime hot bath, vitamin E, bedtime clonazepam or other benzodiazepines, carbamazepine, baclofen, propoxyphene, codeine, or L-dopa.

Use of Sedatives

About 3 to 4% of American adults use prescribed sleeping pills, mostly less than once a week. About one third of users take them daily for 2 months or less, but a quarter of them take such drugs even more often.[1] Research literature offers little guidance on use of sedatives, however. The arbitrary division of central nervous system depressant drugs into sedatives, hypnotics, and minor tranquilizers derives from marketing rather than pharmacologic considerations and excludes many agents from insomnia studies. A small minority of hypnotic drug studies are of adequate design.[12] Studies of next-day hangover, for instance, use mostly young volunteers[13] rather than the older insomnia patients more likely to use such medications. Nevertheless, 80% of those using prescription hypnotics felt they were helped "quite a bit/a lot,"[1] demand for them remains high, and experience plus common sense can still guide prescribing practice.

A careful routine of sleep hygiene will help hypnotics work and prevent sedatives from masking remediable problems.

A working concept is needed about how sedatives might improve or worsen the patient's sleep. Drugs are most likely to relieve insomnia caused by transient problems, hyperarousal, and relapsing anxiety; are least likely to help in affective or neurodegenerative disorders; and are unlikely to be worthy expedients against the ravages of polypharmacy. They may distort the polygraphic architecture of sleep for weeks after they are discontinued.[14]

Intermittent rather than regular use of hypnotics prevents drug tolerance and may lessen withdrawal reactions. Frequently, drug-induced sleep three nights a week provides sufficient relief for the grateful patient who carefully prevents over-reliance on sedatives. For some patients, the security of sleeping pills in the medicine chest permits falling asleep.

Physician and patient should discuss how long sedatives will be prescribed before a gradual withdrawal regimen is instituted. When withdrawal proves arduous, the pace of drug withdrawal should be readjusted to approximately a one eighth reduction of daily dose per week, using a proportion of powder from capsules or crushed pills. Decremental steps can be extended to once monthly as needed.

Alcohol and Related Drugs. Alcohol remains the most used hypnotic drug,[15] but it can either disturb or increase sleep. In practice, response to alcohol varies widely, and a glass of wine with dinner may benefit some.[16] Encrusted with a plethora of physiologic responses and personal attitudes, individual responses to humankind's oldest sedative become less predictable. It is metabolized at about 10 to 20 mg%/hour, roughly equivalent to one drink/hour, and should produce no hangover from moderate intake.

Chloral hydrate, the oldest prescription hypnotic, along with chloral betane and triclofos sodium, is metabolized into trichloroethanol. Trichloroethanol peaks in concentration 20 to 60 minutes after ingestion, acts rapidly, and is excreted by the liver with a half-life of about 8 hours. It induces hepatic enzymes and may speed the metabolism of dicumarol or warfarin. Chloral hydrate also comes in syrup form and costs about an eighth as much as triazolam, temazepam, or flurazepam.

Barbiturates. Habituation is common with barbiturates, partly because of their hepatic enzyme induction. Concomitantly administered anticoagulants, antidepressants, tetracycline, digitoxin, and corticosteroids, therefore, may require dosage adjustments.[15] Habituation, individual sensitivity, and differences in proportion of body fat rather than the individual barbiturate determine the appearance of any hangover. Barbiturate habituation may be remedied by exquisitely gradual withdrawal.

The usefulness of barbiturates in seizure disorders and other states of central nervous system electrical excitability and their effectiveness in some cases of insomnia explain the continued use of these agents. Although chronic use of barbiturates in usual doses, for example, 100 mg of pentobarbital, may cause lessened deep sleep and increased nocturnal wakeful episodes, lower doses, for example, 50 mg of pentobarbital, may relieve insomnia.

Benzodiazepines. These agents largely replaced older sedatives because of their wider safety margins. One patient took 2000 mg of diazepam, increased his plasma diazepam to 100 times the usual therapeutic concentration, and retained normal vital signs.[17] However, shorter-acting benzodiazepines in overdose may be fatal.[18]

These drugs are often classified by the rate of elimination for them or their active metabolites (see also Chapter 78). Age, proportion of fat, available binding proteins, and elimination half-life affect drug clearance, whereas central nervous system sensitivity, use of nicotine and other drugs, and sex all affect drug responsiveness. Volume of distribution for diazepam has a fivefold range among the elderly, and total drug clearance commonly has an even wider range. Thus, generalizations depend on research averages, which summarize a wide range of individual drug responses, making prediction for the individual patient difficult. Generally considered long-acting drugs are chlorazepate, diazepam, flurazepam, ketazolam, halazepam, prazepam, and quazepam. Intermediate are alprazolam, clonazepam, chlordiazepoxide, estazolam, flunitrazepam, loprazolam, lorazepam, nitrazepam, oxazepam, and temazepam. Short-acting drugs are adinazolam, brotizolam, midazolam, triazolam, as are the similar nonbenzodiazepines zolpidem and zopiclone.

Patients may prefer agents that act quickly. Each agent increases sleep quality compared with placebo, although the more rapidly excreted agents may increase wakefulness later in the night. As one might expect, evidences of pharmacologic action persist longer with the more slowly eliminated compounds. Next-day ease of sleep onset, mood, and anxiety reduction all may be greater with longer-acting medications, although subjective sleepiness may be the same and test performance may be the same compared with those of shorter-acting agents. The total dose may determine next-day status more than elimination half-life.[13] Chronic administration of shorter-acting agents may induce anxiety, hostility, or nocturnal wakefulness and amnesia, possibly because of sedative withdrawal or inverse agonist effects.[18A] Rebound insomnia may be greater after withdrawal from short-acting agents. Even difficulties on withdrawal from longer-acting agents may be seen, especially lessened sleep, and therefore withdrawal should be gradual, for example, decrease of daily dose by one eighth each week for 8 weeks.

In choosing among benzodiazepines, those with a rapid onset but a long enough half-life to prevent continual withdrawal problems, such as diazepam, might be considered first. When anxiety is present, longer-acting drugs may be considered. When depression is present, some patients respond well to alprazolam, others to diazepam. Should next-day hangover be present, intermediate- or shorter-acting drugs should be considered. Drugs should be taken perhaps 45 to 60 minutes prior to bedtime if they have a slow onset of action. Chlordiazepoxide is more water soluble, less rapidly absorbed, and possibly for this reason, less preferred by patients. The absorption of chlorazepate is also less certain. Shorter-acting agents have more amnestic properties.

Other Agents. Methyprylon has achieved favorable ratings in several studies compared with other older hypnotics.[15] It has a rapid onset of action.

Over-the-Counter Agents. Patients will often inquire about these drugs, which are used twice as much as prescription hypnotics, usually with low frequency.[15] Methapyrilene, possibly the most frequently used hypnotic after alcohol, owes its continued presence to a legal grandfather clause. It is mild and anticholinergic and causes excitatory effects in overdose. Diphenhydramine blocks central histamine H receptors, causing sleepiness. Never systematically assessed as a hypnotic agent for insomnia patients, it has weaker central actions in vitro than the sedating antidepressants. It may induce drowsiness rather than deeper sleep; its popularity may derive from its mildness. Reportedly aspirin, on intermittent use, relieves insomnia, especially later night awakening.[19] A warm milk drink also improves sleep compared with placebo treatment.[20]

Further Choices Among Sedatives

Features of a particular insomnia patient may favor use of a specific agent. When liver disease is present, oxazepam excretion is not slowed; other water-soluble, renally excreted drugs such as phenobarbital or chlordiazepoxide may be of use. The more lipid-soluble, shorter-acting benzodiazepines are transformed to inactive metabolites by the liver and may therefore be of value when renal impairments are present. Carefully noted responses of an observant patient provide a tailor-made bioassay by which dosage regimens in such situations may be judged. The use of stomach antacids or achlorhydria delays the absorption of chlordiazepoxide. The well-motivated alcoholic patient may get a psychologic boost by substituting one 500-mg chloral hydrate dose for each ounce of alcohol previously used for hypnotic purposes. Use of this cross-tolerant drug may thus facilitate alcohol withdrawal. For the depressed patient, alprazolam or diazepam may be considered, but a sedating antidepressant may be more effective. The epileptic patient may remedy insomnia by taking most of the dose of phenobarbital or clonazepam at bedtime. When sedatives are prescribed for drug abusers, those with slow onset, for example, temazepam or phenobarbital, may be of value. Should a liquid dosage form be desired, chloral hydrate syrup is available.

Insomnia in Other Medical Conditions

Insomnia commonly derives from itch, pain, or dyspnea. Itch may emerge when the lights go out at bedtime as internal sensations replace distracting visual information. The recumbent position may worsen pain from reflux esophagitis. The autonomic arousal of REM sleep may precipitate pains of peptic ulcer or nocturnal angina. Prolapsed mitral valve syndrome incurs a high incidence of disordered sleep, possibly from increased catecholamine sensitivity.[21] Arthritis of large joints or intervertebral disk disease may be aggravated by body movements during sleep.

Treatment of primary symptoms, for example, by analgesics, such as for pain or itch, antihistamines, or antacids, should be optimized before nighttime sedation is used. Timed-release aspirin or long-acting nonsteroidal anti-inflammatory agents for arthritis pain, tetranitrate tablets or transdermal nitroglycerin for nocturnal angina, and antacids or ranitidine at bedtime exemplify attempts to suppress symptoms in favor of restful sleep. Symptom-suppression regimens may be systematically fashioned by gradual adjustment of dosages according to several nights' average results as documented on a sleep chart that records drug dosages, bedtimes, sleep periods, symptomatic episodes, and arising times (see Fig. 86–1).

Although disease symptoms can cause or aggravate insomnia, the reverse is also true—that sleeplessness itself worsens certain symptoms. Experimenters have observed a worsening of "fibrositis syndrome" after deep-sleep deprivation.[22] Pre-existing problems, such as cardiac arrhythmias, epileptic states, and psychologic difficulties, may be much worsened by insomnia.

Insomnia may also be a common result of many disorders.[23] Chronic uremia from any cause as well as the scheduling and other effects of dialysis often cause insomnia. Liver failure with portacaval shunting may increase ammonia levels or blood aromatic amnio acids and thus cause severe insomnia through central nervous system effects. The toxemia of chronic liver or kidney failure also impairs daytime arousal. Chronic dementia may induce reversion to frequent periods of daytime sleep and nighttime wakefulness. Epilepsy, especially temporal lobe epilepsy or temporal lobe dysfunction, may involve severe, unrelenting insomnia, occasionally with increased hypnic jerks, auditory or visual hallucinations at sleep onset, frequent wakenings throughout the night, or nightmares. Cushing's syndrome, exogenous steroids, or Addison's disease all may cause severe insomnia. Hyperthyroidism may provoke insomnia in some patients. Normal hormonal changes, such as those found premenstrually, may worsen sleep. Menopausal women manifest double the premenopausal incidence of insomnia complaints and may experience fitful sleep that is remedied in some cases by replacement estrogens, even in elderly women. Although women in early pregnancy may sleep more, late pregnancy commonly disrupts sleep through motor movements of the unborn child, nocturia, or finding a comfortable recumbent position.

The chronic insomnia caused by chronic disease may elicit pessimism about its remediability; treatment is often conceived of as bedtime sedatives alone. However, when the primary disease lowers daytime arousal, such medications may further impair next-day behavioral function through slow drug elimination or increased sensitivity to sedation and thus blunt the amplitude of the sleep-wake cycle. In fact, vigorous sleep hygiene prevents aggravating the existing problem by insomniac habits, such as late morning sleeping or caffeine use, and provides a background against which the intermittent use of bedtime sedatives can help. Steroids may provoke a latent mood disorder, and the resulting insomnia may require psychotropic drugs. Treating the insomnia of hyperthyroidism requires suppression of the primary condition.

HYPERSOMNIA

Excessive daytime sleepiness previously excited too little clinical concern because it seemed benign and inconvenient rather than incapacitating. Many individuals manage to push themselves through somnolent lives. Others rely on daily routines that keep them busy and mobile. They may never seek help for their somnolence until family members insist. Embarrassing naps at work or a traffic accident may precipitate consultation. Somnolent people develop low standards for subjective wakefulness and may feel no difficulty except in retrospect after successful treatment. This can make them incautious in situations demanding alertness and too satisfied with partial relief.

Certain monotonous situations elicit sleepiness, such as protracted meetings, television watching, and turnpike driving. Even when sleep inappropriately supervenes, casual explanations rather than systematic investigation may result. Sleepy patients have often been sent away with normal thyroid function and glucose tolerance test results and reassurance, but the medical and popular literature has recently sensitized physicians and patients to the potential seriousness of excessive sleepiness.

Objective tests permit the quantification of sleepiness by a simple daily log, kept for 1 week, in which the patient, at predetermined times, chooses a phrase or checks a 100-mm line to designate the degree of wakefulness. The resulting score is a valid measurement of sleepiness. Continuous performance tests involve scored tasks requiring sustained attention. Sorting a deck of cards by suit (normal range is 30 to 45 seconds) or an electric toy task, compared with the patient's average performance, may be done twice or more daily at predetermined times. For some, measurements of physical endurance, for example, number of push-ups or weight lifts, correlate with sleepiness, and therefore can be used to judge treatment response.

The Multiple Sleep Latency Test measures sleepiness by polygraphically monitoring the interval between lying down on a comfortable bed and falling asleep.[24] Five 20-minute trials are done every 2 hours beginning at 10 AM. A maximum of 10 minutes' sleep is allowed. The average sleep latency for narcoleptic individuals is less than 5 minutes, for other sleepy individuals 7 to 9 minutes, for young normal individuals 8 to 12 minutes, and for elderly individuals, about 14 minutes.[25]

Sleep Apnea Syndrome[26–28]

Sleep apnea is most commonly due to partial upper airway obstruction to airflow. Slight encroachments on the radius of the airway, as from nasal blockage, bogginess of pharyngeal mucosa, enlarged uvula, fat deposits, or a large tongue base, may induce increased inspiratory efforts. The resulting negative pressure partially collapses the pharyngeal airway and thus decreases pulmonary ventilation. Acromegaly, enlarged tonsils, jaw retrusion, or neck masses may also initiate this process. Use of sedatives, alcohol, or β-blockers aggravates sleep apnea, presumably through relaxation of pharyngeal structures. As arterial oxygen saturation falls, pulmonary hypertension develops, with occasional right-sided heart failure. Increased right ventricular afterload may induce leftward intraventricular septum shift and thus lower cardiac output. Purely "central" sleep apnea, in which little or no respiratory effort is made during periods of airflow stoppage, occurs less commonly than obstructive apnea and is usually related to primary neurologic disease or to chronic hypercapnia with carbon dioxide receptor hyposensitivity. Chronic obstructive lung disease with hypercapnia sometimes provokes sleep apnea. In chronically hypoxic individuals who operate on the sharply descending segment of the oxyhemoglobin dissociation curve, a decline in arterial PO_2 during sleep apnea may produce a large loss in blood oxygen saturation. At some critical blood oxygen level, which decreases with age, the patient will awaken for multiple, brief, unremembered episodes during which he or she draws a breath. Cardiac arrhythmias are commonly found, usually a bradycardia-tachycardia sequence concomitant with hypoxic episodes and the subsequent resumption of breathing. Almost any arrhythmia, however, including high-grade ventricular ectopy, may occur.

Clinically, obstructive apnea presents most often in middle-aged men with upper body obesity who snore loudly. Sleepiness, declining work performance, morning headaches, or psychological changes may be the chief complaint of the patient, who characteristically fails to remember the apneic spells. The patient's wife, concerned about loud snoring or respiratory pauses during sleep, may insist on the consultation. Physical examination, in addition to obesity, reveals moderate hypertension in about half of cases.[28a] Young and thin snorers often have upper airway structural compromise, for example, jaw retrusion or nasal blockage. Floppy eyelid syndrome[29] and depression[30] may also be associated with sleep apnea.

Milder variants of sleep apnea occur commonly in asymptomatic individuals. In one series of randomly selected adults, 13% of the men showed oxygen saturation drops to between 68 and 72%.[31] Those who snore but have no other symptoms have a disproportionately high incidence of hypertension, and many are found to have sleep apnea.

Management of sleep apnea depends on the severity of the problem. Cardiac monitoring in these individuals characteristically reveals a wide variation of nocturnal heart rate that may suggest this disorder. Sleep studies will confirm the diagnosis in symptomatic individuals. A polygraphic recording of night sleep quantifies the number of apnea periods (diagnosis usually requires that there be $\geq$ 35 episodes/7 hours), the grade of any arrhythmia, the degree of oxygen desaturation (via earlobe oximetry), and the amount of sleep disturbance. Cephalometry may reveal an undersized mandible pushing the tongue back into a compromised pharynx. When no major health risk exists, such as severe sleepiness while driving or high-grade cardiac arrhythmias, conservative measures like weight reduction and avoidance of sedatives may constitute decisive therapy. Mechanical aids to prevent the patient from sleeping on the back or flexing the neck rarely help but can be accomplished with a harness or a ball-containing sock pinned to the back of the pajama shirt and a Thomas neck collar. Medroxyprogesterone, a respiratory stimulant, 60 to 120 mg/day, alleviates sleep apnea in some pickwickian patients, as can protriptyline, an antidepressant. Low-flow oxygen carries the risk of prolonging the apneic spells but reportedly helps some patients with central sleep apnea and hypercapnia.[32] Surgical alteration of the upper airway for obstructive sleep apnea may involve reduction of the uvula, removing a small rim of palate, resection of redundant pharyngeal folds, tonsillectomy, osteotomy and advancement of the mandible, or midline section of the hyoid bone. Continuous positive-pressure airway insufflation by closely fitting facemask can relieve obstructive sleep apnea. This requires much cooperation, has a long-term compliance of about 70%, but avoids medications and surgery. Gradual increase of pressure after bedtime ("ramp" function) and lower pressure during exhalation ("BiPAP") may increase patient tolerance. For patients with dangerous arrhythmias, heart failure, unrelieved severe somnolence, severe blood oxygen desaturation during sleep, massive obesity, inability to cooperate, or otherwise untreatable obstructive sleep apnea, tracheostomy must be considered. Relief is swift and progressive; difficulties with a thick neck, periostomal infection, and tracheomalacia may occur; and a rigorous routine for ambulatory tracheostomy maintenance must be developed.[33]

Idiopathic Hypersomnia[33a, 33b]

This unrelenting tendency toward drowsiness frequently involves a familial tendency, often develops during adolescence or after a severe viral illness, and often remains undiagnosed for decades. Even during childhood, when subjective sleepiness is absent, some patients prefer low-energy behaviors, for example, avoiding sports. Sleep is of rapid onset, uninterrupted, and prolonged. On awakening, about half of patients suffer "sleep drunkenness," an impairment of alertness, initiative, and mood for an hour or more.

A daytime nap or even two may be obligatory (see Fig. 86–1). Despite requirements of work, school, or the military, the patient cannot tolerate shortened sleep. One or two alcoholic drinks may put him or her to sleep, but he or she increasingly relies on caffeine, which may worsen morning incapacitation. Patients may episodically manifest depression along with irritability and fatigability.

Physical examination occasionally reveals a systolic blood pressure of 115 mm Hg or less and a resting heart rate in the low 60s.

Among diagnostic tests, subjective rating scales show scores for extreme sleepiness, often at consistent times of day. The EEG frequently shows mild, nonspecific changes, such as symmetric bursts of theta activity, with the patient falling asleep. Laboratory night sleep is usually normal and prolonged if the patient is allowed to sleep in the morning; multiple sleep latency and continuous performance tests show impairments.

Idiopathic hypersomnia differs from sedative use, toxicities, and the effects of chronic stimulants or their withdrawal in its persistence in the prolonged drug-free state. Hypersomniac depressions are episodic. Neurologic and endocrinologic problems cause fatigue more than sleep or else show specific features, as do sleep apnea and narcolepsy. Uremic or hepatic encephalopathies cause somnolence and broken rather than uninterrupted sleep. Chronic fatigue syndrome has a shorter course and shows problems more with energy than with sleep.

Idiopathic hypersomnia patients show a wide range of treatment responsiveness. Many derive no benefit from drugs and live with rigorous sleep hygiene and scheduled naps. Caffeine, amphetamines, pemoline, stimulating antidepressants, or methysergide has proved valuable to some. Stimulants taken prior to bedtime may lessen morning sleep drunkenness. Amphetamines should be used at preset times to maintain rather than restore wakefulness and require a weekly drug holiday.

Irremediable idiopathic hypersomnia impairs every aspect of behavioral functioning and causes work disability.[34] Physician support should focus on the details of habits and activities related to sleep to progressively optimize the patient's individual situation.

NARCOLEPSY[35–38]

Narcolepsy often appears during the second or third decades of life but becomes diagnosed years later. It can run in families and is associated with specific blood antigens. The classic symptoms include irresistible sleep attacks, cataplexy, sleep paralysis, and hypnogogic hallucinations, but mindless automatic behavior, disrupted nocturnal sleep, depression, and much-impaired concentration all may be present, chronically interfering with the patient's work and social life.

Sleep attacks without other classic symptoms happen in about a third of patients and may supervene in monotonous situations or in the midst of such activities as swimming or skiing. They tend to be 5 to 10 minutes in duration, temporarily refresh the patient, but occur daily, often two or three times.

Cataplexy is a brief bilateral paresis occurring suddenly, with emotion, such as laughter, anger, or surprise happening in over half of patients. A weakening in knees or arms is more common than falling down. Consciousness is preserved. Falling may be slow; cataplexy causes fewer accidents than sleep attacks.

Sleep paralysis is a sudden awakening with inability to move or speak. The attack lasts less than a minute, may involve anxiety, and happens in about a quarter of patients.

Hypnagogic hallucinations occur in the transition between wake and sleep and may involve misapprehensions of common noises such as a child's crying or a doorbell, music, or voices. Visual hallucinations may be vivid or dreamlike, for example, a face appears. Occasionally a feeling, for example, of a person in the room, may be present. The frequency and intensity of these vary widely and affect about a quarter of patients.

Narcolepsy severity varies from an occasional nap to alertness deficits that interfere with school or work performance or cause accidents.[38]

Objective tests reveal severe somnolence. The Multiple Sleep Latency Test yields an average sleep latency of less than 5 minutes and REM sleep in two of the five naps. Early REM onset may be observed in other conditions, such as depression; withdrawal from stimulants, antidepressants, or sedatives; abnormal sleep-wake schedule; use of catecholamine-blocking drugs; or recent surgery or trauma. Absence of haplotypes DR-2 or DQW1 virtually rules out narcolepsy.

Narcolepsy differs from idiopathic hypersomnia in its brief naps and lack of prolonged, uninterrupted night sleep. The undrugged narcoleptic finds his or her best time shortly after awakening, unlike the sleep-drunken hypersomniac. Frequent cataplexy is pathognomonic of narcolepsy. Sleep apnea of adult onset, unlike narcolepsy, usually begins in thickset middle-aged men who snore. Some narcoleptics have coexisting sleep apnea. Unremembered insomnia from nocturnal myoclonus causes sleepiness unrelieved by a brief nap and usually begins in older age groups. Depression with lethargy is accompanied by mood disturbance, indecisiveness, self-reproach, anhedonia, agitation, somatic concerns, and appetite and bowel disturbance; it remits episodically.

Narcolepsy management requires daily documentation of the sleep-wake schedule, including naps and sleep hygiene. Some patients with mild narcolepsy will prefer to manage their condition by prescheduled naps alone.

Stimulants will be needed for most patients. They should be used on arising at morning and prior to predictable slump periods. Drug attempts to induce evening wakefulness usually impair nocturnal sleep. A weekly drug holiday assures continued therapeutic action and causes little inconvenience when the stimulant dosage remains moderate. Pemoline stimulates for 8 to 10 hours; 18.75-mg tablets can be taken on arising and around noon, depending on when sleepiness appears, to a total of about 6 tablets daily. Methylphenidate and dextroamphetamine have a 2- to 5-hour duration of action and must be used accordingly, up to 60 mg daily; use of slow-release tablets complicates assessment of drug action. Some patients prefer caffeine to other stimulants. Constant preparation, quantity, and dosage times permit judging and optimizing its therapeutic effects. Stimulant antidepressants relieve most cataplexy and may lessen sleepiness.

Fostering a stable regimen in more difficult cases requires regular office visits for review of sleep charts, optimization of treatment regimens, and fostering adjustment to a chronic disease.

DISORDERS OF BODILY TIMING

The external light-dark cycle drives bodily clocks, which in turn control circadian rhythms, that is, predictable daily oscillations in substances and functions, such as electrolytes, enzymes, hormones, body temperature, mitosis rates, neuronal firing rates, and sleep scores on behavioral tests.[39] Artificial light and jet travel can produce rapid shifts in external light-dark cycles that are too abrupt for the immediate resynchronization of bodily rhythms. When external and internal cycles are thus incongruent, bodily timing of sleep and wake is temporarily inappropriate to the new circumstances and sleep may occur at "wrong" clock times. Regular sleep-wake scheduling in the setting of a regular light-dark cycle, therefore, prevents a sleep-disrupting divergence of external and internal rhythms. Sleep-wake rhythms should generally be shifted slowly to permit gradual readjustment of underlying timing systems.

Irregular Schedules. Erratic wake times are usually found in the sleep deprived, who compensate by sleeping late on weekends, or in the unemployed or others who lack regular morning obligations. The vagaries of social, family, work, or school obligations may lessen the regularity of bedtimes. Insomnia patients are often surprised when a daily sleep log contradicts their impression that they arise and retire at regular times. A 2- or 3-week log of arising times and bedtimes should be kept. Irregular arising times can be summarized as a range from earliest to latest, but an occasional transgression of a steady schedule must be distinguished from wandering, irregular sleep timing.

Jet Lag. The abrupt relocation to a different time zone leaves the individual with a disparity between internal and environmental circadian rhythms. Travel westward, in the direction of the setting sun, conforms more with the tendency of internal timing systems toward delayed sleep times and wake times, whereas travel eastward clashes with this tendency and requires longer adjustment periods until bodily rhythms, for example, temperatures and sleep-wake cycles, resynchronize.

Delayed Sleep Phase Syndrome. Some people sleep well only after late bedtimes,[40, 41] require a rising time late in the morning, and protest the tyranny of morning work schedules. They may settle into occupations that permit late rising or continually attempt earlier arising, often with the fruitless help of multiple alarm clocks or calls from friends. Many such patients are "night people" who are maximally productive at normal bedtimes. The tendency of the bodily timing systems toward delayed sleep and arising times is accentuated in these individuals. This syndrome sometimes induces depression and antidepressant drug treatment failure. When time of arising reverts to normal earlier clock times, coexisting depression often disappears.

Night Workers. Some who work at night, especially those with changing work schedules, suffer inadequate sleep. There are many night workers,[42] and most of them simply cope with their sleep problems. Youth and a relatively low sleep requirement help some adjust to such schedules.

Treatment

Insomnia caused by timing disorders may be remedied by gradual refashioning of the patient's sleep-wake schedule. For problems due to irregular scheduling, the insomnia patient picks a regular clock time to arise that he or she rigidly observes. Thereafter, a desirable retiring time usually becomes evident. In the absence of other problems, the sleep-wake cycle will gradually conform with the schedule.[43] The sudden disruption of sleep-wake patterns can be lessened by a gradual shift, for example, retiring and arising 10 minutes earlier every day for 3 weeks prior to a trip eastward through 6 time zones. This will induce a schedule over 3 hours earlier, which constitutes half the change required. One fully adjusts to westward trips in approximately 1 day for every time zone crossed.

The treatment of the delayed sleep-phase syndrome first demands inducing regular, if inconveniently late, sleep schedules. Thereafter, three treatments are possible. First, gradually advancing bedtimes, for example, 10 minutes earlier every second night, slowly against the physiologic tendency to delay. Alternatively, 2- to 3-hour delay of bedtimes each day, rigidly maintaining the desired arising time once reached. Thirdly, bright light exposure, for example, by reading for an hour with two unshaded fluorescent or two high-watt bulbs positioned in the visual field between the eyes and the text, is done on the second half of the patient's night (most effective) or on arising (more convenient).

PARASOMNIAS[44]

Parasomnias are untoward behaviors that occur during sleep. The transitional state between sleep and wakefulness may evoke unusual behaviors. Hypnic jerks are sudden, brief, isolated whole body or limb jerks that occur as an individual is falling asleep and are frequently found in normal individuals.

Sleepwalking occurs mostly in childhood but occasionally lasts into adulthood. A family history and a history of sleep-talking are frequently found. Episodes supervene during deep sleep[45] and therefore usually early in the night. Sleep-walking involves slow, poorly coordinated movements, little responsiveness to stimuli, and amnesia for the event. The patient who lives alone may find evidence of pseudopurposful behaviors, such as a dish retrieved from the cupboard, the following morning. Although rare, dangerous events occur, such as falling downstairs, starting an automobile, or walking into the street. Episodes may vary in frequency from once or twice a year to several times monthly. There are no specific EEG findings in this automatism. More circumscribed and repetitive movements during sleep involve the jaw (bruxism), which can cause atypical facets on teeth, the head (jactatio capitis), or the extremities (myoclonus).[46] These must be differentiated from more integrated motor patterns found in states of partial arousal, in which confused activities, for example, putting dishes in the clothes dryer, or impulsive or even aggressive acts, such as hitting the bed partner, may occur. Aggressive or defensive behavior may occur during REM sleep in older persons, possibly from degeneration of REM-sleep motor inhibitory centers.[47]

Night terrors also occur during deep sleep and are attacks of sudden screaming, sweating, great elevation of heart rate, and sometimes sleepwalking. The patient is confused, inconsolable, and amnestic for the event.

Nightmares are much more common than night terrors, occur during REM sleep, and are therefore found after the first few hours of the night. They involve a bad dream, for example, of mutilation, death, horrid monsters, or being attacked. Often, the patient awakens with aroused emotions and memory of the dream but little autonomic arousal, compared with that occurring with night terrors. Conditions that increase REM, such as use of central catecholamine–depleting drugs; withdrawal from stimulants, sedatives, anticonvulsants, or antidepressants; and severe depression or major psychologic trauma, such as rape or combat, all may induce "REM pressure" and therefore, nightmares. More rarely, chronic nightmares without such provocations may occur, beginning sometimes with distressing experiences and express psychopathology.[48]

Bedwetting, or enuresis, is found in 1 to 3% of adults. Causes include anomalies of the urethra, cystitis, diabetes, and neuronal immaturity or degeneration. Episodes occur mostly during deep sleep.

Treatment

The suppression of parasomnias aims to increase neocortical function, which inhibits them, and decrease factors that may initiate the expression of autonomous motor patterns, such as fever, use of stimulants, or psychologic disquiet. Most parasomnias do not occur every night, and therefore a careful record of sleep schedule, time of parasomnia occurrence, and presence of other relevant factors, such as use of alcohol or strenuous exercise during the preceding day, may reveal aggravating influences.

Sleepwalking may provoke much anxiety. Initially, a piece of twine fixed to the bed, tied around one ankle and long enough to permit free movements in bed may both lessen the patient's fear of sleepwalking and prevent departure from the room. Discontinuation of caffeine, nicotine, and other chronically used central nervous system–acting drugs is mandatory. Individual patients differ in the drugs that may suppress their sleepwalking; some are helped by sedatives, such as diazepam or alcohol, others by antidepressants or anticonvulsants. Drug use is often reserved for periods of high risk or trips away from home.

Bruxism is treated by a mouth guard or splint to protect teeth. Repetitive head movements or banging is not well treated save by removing hard sources of head bruising.

Night terrors may partially respond to sleep hygiene. Empiric trials of diazepam, antidepressants, or anticonvulsants may be warranted, but psychotherapy may relieve the terrors.

When no specific etiology for nightmares is found, antidepressants, especially monoamine oxidase inhibitors, may suppress them, for example, phenelzine, 15 to 30 mg at bedtime, or tranylcypromine, 10 to 20 mg at bedtime. Such drugs taken during the day gradually diminish the symptom. Nightmares due to psychologic trauma are often temporary and treated with psychotherapy.

Bedwetting of no specific origin in adults may be treated with bladder training. Increasing intervals between urinary urge and micturition are instituted, for example, 20 minutes each time for a week, then 40, 60, and 90 minutes thereafter. This, subsequently increasing diurnal fluid intake and evening fluid restriction raises the threshold against the urinary reflex at night. Insomnia due to nocturia may also be thus treated. When mental subnormality precludes such treatment, imipramine suppresses bedwetting; desmopressin may abolish it.

REFERENCES

1. Balter MB and Baner ML: Patterns of prescribing and use of hypnotic drugs in the United States. *In* Clift AD (ed): Sleep Disturbance and Hypnotic Drug Dependence. Amsterdam, Excerpta Medica, 1975, pp 261–293.
2. Hollingworth HL: The influence of caffeine on mental and motor efficiency. Arch Psychol (Frankf) 20:1, 1912.
3. Goldstein A, Kaizer S, and Whitley O: Quantitative and qualitative difference associated with habituation to coffee. Clin Pharmacol Ther 10:489, 1969.
4. Mullin FJ, Kleitman N, and Cooperman NR: Studies on the physiology of sleep. X. The effect of alcohol and caffeine on motility and body temperature during sleep. Am J Physiol 106:478, 1933.
5. Pikorny AD: Sleep disturbances, alcohol and alcoholism: A review. *In* Williams RL and Karacan I (eds): Sleep Disorders: Diagnosis and Treatment. New York, John Wiley & Sons, 1978, pp 233–260.
6. Soldatos CR, Kales JD, Scharf MB, et al: Cigarette smoking associated with sleep difficulty. Science 207:551, 1980.
7. Helson L and Dugne L: Acute brain syndrome after propranolol. Lancet i:98, 1978.
8. Ekbom KA: Restless legs syndrome. Neurology 10:868, 1960.
9. Bixler EO, Kales A, Jacoby JA, et al: Nocturnal sleep and wakefulness: Effects of age and sex in normal sleepers. Int J Neurosci 23:33, 1984.
10. Moore-Ede MC, Sulzman FM, and Fuller CA: The Clocks That Time Us. Cambridge, MA, Harvard University Press, 1982.
11. Learoyd BM: Psychotropic drugs and the elderly patient. Med J Aust 1:1131, 1972.
12. Williams RL and Karacan I: Pharmacology of Sleep. New York, John Wiley & Sons, 1976, p 142.
13. Johnson LC and Chernik DA: Sedative-hypnotics and human performance. Psychopharmacology 76:101, 1982.
14. Oswald I and Priest RG: Five weeks to escape the sleeping pill habit. BMJ 2:1093, 1965.
15. Mendelson WB: The Use and Misuse of Sleeping Pills. New York, Plenum Press, 1980.
16. Mishara BL and Kastenbaum R: Wine in the treatment of long-term geriatric patients in mental institutions. J Am Geriatr Soc 22:88, 1974.
17. Greenblatt DJ, Woo E, Allen MD, et al: Rapid recovery from massive diazepam overdose. JAMA 240:1872, 1978.
18. Lheureux P, Debailleul G, DeWitte O, et al: Zolpidem intoxication mimicking narcotic overdose. Hum Exp Toxicol 9:105, 1990.
18a. Adam K and Oswald I: Can a rapidly-eliminated hypnotic cause daytime anxiety? Pharmacopsychiatry 22:115, 1989.
19. Hauri PJ and Silhertarb PM: Effects of aspirin on the sleep of insomniacs. Curr Ther Res 28:867, 1980.

20. Southwell PR, Evons CR, and Hunt JN: Effect of a hot milk drink on movements during sleep. BMJ 2:429, 1972.
21. Clark RW, Bondoulas H, Schaal SF, et al: Adrenergic hyperactivity and cardiac abnormality in primary disorders of sleep. Neurology 30:113, 1980.
22. Moldofsky H and Scarisbrick D: Induction of neurasthenic musculoskeletal pain syndrome by selective sleep stage deprivation. Psychosom Med 38:35, 1976.
23. Regestein QR: Sleep disorders. *In* Stoudemire A and Fogel BS (eds): Principles of Medical Psychiatry, 2nd ed. Oxford, New York, 1992.
24. Richardson GS, Corskadon MA, Flagg W, et al: Excessive daytime sleepiness in man: Multiple sleep latency measurement in narcoleptic and control subjects. Electroencephalogr Clin Neurophysiol 45:621, 1978.
25. Carskadon MA, Van den Hoed J, and Dement W: Sleep and daytime disturbances in the aged. J Geriatr Psychiatry 13:135, 1980.
26. Strohl KP, Cherniak NS, and Gothe B: Physiologic basis of therapy for sleep apnea. Am Rev Respir Dis 134:791, 1986.
27. Kryger MH, Roth T, and Dement WC: Principles and Practice of Sleep Medicine. Philadelphia, WB Saunders, 1989.
28. Kuna ST and Sant-Ambrogio G: Pathophysiology of upper airway closure during sleep. JAMA 266:1384, 1991.
28a. Guilleminault C: Natural history, cardiac impact and long-term follow-up of sleep apnea syndrome. *In* Guilleminault C, Lugaresi E (eds): Sleep/Wake Disorders. New York, Raven Press, 1983, pp 107–125.
29. Woog JJ: Obstructive sleep apnea and the floppy eyelid syndrome. Am J Ophthalmol 3:314, 1990.
30. Millman RP, Foyel BS, McNamara ME, et al: Depression as a manifestation of sleep apnea: Reversal with nasal continuous positive airway pressure. J Clin Psychiatry 50:348, 1989.
31. Block AJ, Boysen PG, Wynne JW, et al: Sleep apnea, hypoxia and oxygen desaturation in normal subjects. N Engl J Med 300:513, 1979.
32. Martin RJ, Sanders MH, Gray BA, et al: Acute and long-term ventilatory effects of hyperoxia in the adult sleep apnea syndrome. Am Rev Respir Dis 125:175, 1982.
33. Dye JP: Living with a tracheostomy for sleep apnea. N Engl J Med 308:1167, 1983.
33a. Roth B: Narcolepsy and Hypersomnia. Basel, Karger, 1980, pp 207–227.
33b. Guilleminault C: Idiopathic central nervous system hypersomnia. *In* Kryger MH, Roth T, and Dement WC. Principles and Practice of Sleep Medicine. Philadelphia, WB Saunders, 1989, pp 347–350.
34. Broughton R, Nevsimalova S, and Roth B: The socio-economic effects of idiopathic hypersomnia: Comparisons with controls and with compound narcoleptics. *In* Popovicin L, et al (eds): Sleep. Basel, S. Karger, 1980, pp 229–233.
35. Yoss RE and Daly DD: Narcolepsy. Med Clin North Am 44:953, 1960.
36. Regestein QR, Reich P, and Mufson MJ: Narcolepsy: An initial clinical approach. J Clin Psychiatry 44:166, 1983.
37. Guilleminault HC: Narcolepsy syndrome. *In* Kryger MH, Roth T, and Dement WC: Principles and Practice of Sleep Medicine. Philadelphia, WB Saunders, 1989, pp 338–345.
38. Aldrich MS: Automobile accidents in patients with sleep disorders. Sleep 12:487, 1989.
39. Wever R: The circadian multi-oscillator system of man. Int J Chronobiol 3:19, 1975.
40. Weitzman ED, Czeisler CA, Zimmerman JC, et al: Chronobiological disorders: Analytic and therapeutic techniques. *In* Guilleminault C (ed): Sleeping and Waking Disorders: Indications and Techniques. Menlo Park, CA, Addison-Wesley, 1982, pp 297–329.
41. Czeisler CA, Richardson GS, Coleman RM, et al: Chronotherapy: Resetting the circadian clocks of patients with delayed sleep phase insomnia. Sleep 4:1, 1981.
42. Czeisler CA, Moore-Ede MC, and Coleman RM: Rotating shift work schedules that disrupt sleep are improved by applying circadian principles. Science 217:460, 1982.
43. Webb WB and Agnew HW: Regularity in the control of the free-running sleep-wakefulness rhythm. Aerospace Med 45:701, 1974.
44. Thorpy MJ and Glovinsky PB: Parasomnias. Psychiatr Clin North Am 10:623, 1987.
45. Broughton RJ: Sleep disorders: Disorders of arousal? Science 159:1070, 1968.
46. Gastant H, Batini C, Broughton R, et al: Electroencephalographic study of non-epileptic episodic phenomena during sleep. *In* Fischgold H (ed): Sommeil de Nuit. Paris, Masson, 1965, pp 215–236.
47. Mahowald M and Schenck CH: REM sleep behavior disorder. *In* Kryger M, Roth T, and Dement WC: Principles and Practice of Sleep Medicine. Philadelphia, WB Saunders, 1989, pp 389–401.
48. Kales A, Soldatos CR, Caldwell AB, et al: Nightmares: Clinical characteristics and personality patterns. Am J Psychiatry 137:1197, 1980.

Index

Note: Page numbers in *italics* indicate illustrations; those followed by t refer to tables.

ISBN 0-7216-4338-8